S0-AHC-951

Drug Information Handbook for Dentistry

3rd Edition | **1997-98**

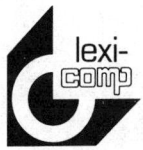
lexi-comp

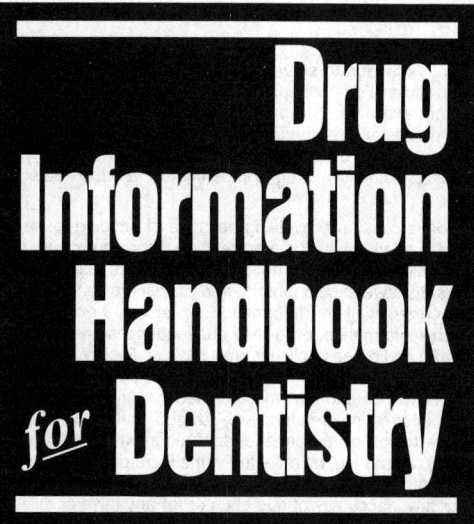

Drug Information Handbook for Dentistry

3rd Edition ▮▮ *1997-98*

Richard L. Wynn, BSPharm, PhD
Professor of Pharmacology
Baltimore College of Dental Surgery
Dental School
University of Maryland at Baltimore
Baltimore, Maryland

Timothy F. Meiller, DDS, PhD
Professor
Oral Medicine and Diagnostic Sciences
Baltimore College of Dental Surgery
Professor of Oncology
Greenebaum Cancer Center
University of Maryland at Baltimore
Baltimore, Maryland

Harold L. Crossley, DDS, PhD
Associate Professor of Pharmacology
Dental School
University of Maryland at Baltimore
Baltimore, Maryland

LEXI-COMP INC
Hudson (Cleveland)

NOTICE

This handbook is intended to serve the user as a handy reference and not as a complete drug information resource. It does not include information on every therapeutic agent available. The publication covers a combination of commonly used drugs in dentistry and medicine and is specifically designed to present important aspects of drug data in a more concise format than is typically found in medical literature, exhaustive drug compendia, or product material supplied by manufacturers.

Drug information is constantly evolving because of ongoing research and clinical experience and is often subject to interpretation. While great care has been taken to ensure the accuracy of the information presented, the reader is advised that the authors, editors, reviewers, contributors, and publishers cannot be responsible for the continued currency of the information or for any errors, omissions, or the application of this information, or for any consequences arising therefrom. Therefore, the author(s) and/or the publisher shall have no liability to any person or entity with regard to claims, loss, or damage caused, or alleged to be caused, directly or indirectly, by the use of information contained herein. Because of the dynamic nature of drug information, readers are advised that decisions regarding drug therapy must be based on the independent judgment of the clinician, changing information about a drug (eg, as reflected in the literature and manufacturer's most current product information), and changing medical practices. The editors are not responsible for any inaccuracy of quotation or for any false or misleading implication that may arise due to the text or formulas as used or due to the quotation of revisions no longer official.

The editors, authors, and contributors have written this book in their private capacities. No official support or endorsement by any federal or state agency or pharmaceutical company is intended or inferred.

The publishers have made every effort to trace the copyright holders for borrowed material. If they have inadvertently overlooked any, they will be pleased to make the necessary arrangements at the first opportunity.

If you have any suggestions or questions regarding any information presented in this handbook, please contact our drug information pharmacist at

1-800-837-LEXI (5394)

This manual was produced using the FormuLex™ Program — A complete publishing service of Lexi-Comp Inc.

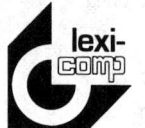

Lexi-Comp Inc
1100 Terex Road
Hudson, Ohio 44236
(216) 650-6506

ISBN 0-916589-55-2

TABLE OF CONTENTS

About the Authors 3
Editorial Advisory Panel 4
Preface to the Third Edition 6
Acknowledgments 7
Use of the Drug Information Handbook for Dentistry 8
FDA Pregnancy Categories 10

Drug Monographs 11

Oral Medicine Topics

Part I. Dental Management and Therapeutic Considerations in Medically Compromised Patients
Cardiovascular Diseases 912
Respiratory Diseases 924
Endocrine Disorders 927
Rheumatoid Arthritis, Osteoarthritis,
and Joint Prostheses 930
Nonviral Infectious Diseases 932
Systemic Viral Diseases 934

Part II.

Dental Management and Therapeutic Considerations in Patients With Specific Oral Conditions
Oral Pain 940
Oral Bacterial Infections 945
Oral Fungal Infections 948
Oral Viral Infections 951
Oral Nonviral Soft Tissue Ulcerations or Erosions 955
Dentin Hypersensitivity; High Caries Index; Xerostomia 959
Temporomandibular Dysfunction (TMD) 963

Other Oral Medicine Topics
Patients Requiring Sedation 965
Patients Undergoing Cancer Therapy 967
Chemical Dependency and Dental Practice 971
Animal and Human Bites Guidelines 976
Systemic Considerations Related to Natural Products for
Weight Loss 979
Dental Office Emergencies 984
Suggested Readings 991

Appendix
Abbreviations and Measurements
Common Symbols & Abbreviations 1004
Apothecary/Metric Conversions 1006
Pounds-Kilograms Conversion 1007
Temperature Conversion 1007
Body Surface Area of Adults and Children 1008
Average Weights and Surface Areas 1009
Calcium Channel Blockers & Gingival Hyperplasia
Calcium Channel Blockers & Gingival Hyperplasia 1010
Cancer Chemotherapy
Cancer Chemotherapy Regimens - Adults 1011
Comparative Drug Charts
Corticosteroid Equivalencies Comparison 1017
Corticosteroids, Topical Comparison 1018
Narcotic Agonist Charts 1019
Nonsteroidal Anti-Inflammatory Agents, Comparative
Dosages, and Pharmacokinetics 1021

TABLE OF CONTENTS

Dental Drug Interactions

Dental Drug Interactions: Update on Drug Combinations
Requiring Special Considerations 1022

Infectious Disease Information

Occupational Exposure to Bloodborne Pathogens
(Universal Precautions) 1030
Antimicrobial Activity Against Selected Organisms 1034
Antimicrobial Prophylaxis in Surgical Patients 1042
Organisms Isolated in Head & Neck Infections 1044
Predominant Cultivable Microorganisms of the Oral
Cavity 1045

Laboratory Values

Reference Values for Adults 1046

Over-The-Counter Dental Products

Artificial Saliva Products............................... 1050
Dentifrice Products 1051
Denture Adhesive Products 1060
Denture Cleanser Products 1062
Mouth Pain, Cold Sore, Canker Sore Products............. 1063
Oral Rinse Products 1067

Sugar-Free Liquid Pharmaceuticals

Sugar-Free Liquid Pharmaceuticals Listing 1070

Miscellaneous

Allergic Skin Reactions to Drugs 1076
Common Oral-Facial Infections and
Antibiotics for Treatment........................... 1077
Controlled Substances 1078
Drugs Associated With Adverse Hematologic Effects 1079
Herbal Medicines 1081
Poison Information Centers 1086
Prescription Writing 1100
Safe Writing Practices 1103
Top 200 Prescribed Drugs 1104
Vasoconstrictor Interactions With Antidepressants 1108
What's New 1109

Therapeutic Category Index 1111

Alphabetical Index 1147

ABOUT THE AUTHORS

Richard L. Wynn, BSPharm, PhD

Richard L. Wynn, PhD, is Professor of Pharmacology at the Baltimore College of Dental Surgery, Dental School, University of Maryland at Baltimore. Dr Wynn has served as a dental educator, researcher, and teacher of dental pharmacology and dental hygiene pharmacology for his entire professional career. He holds a BS (pharmacy; registered pharmacist, Maryland), an MS (physiology) and a PhD (pharmacology) from the University of Maryland. Dr Wynn chaired the Department of Pharmacology at the University of Maryland Dental School from 1980 to 1995. Previously, he chaired the Department of Oral Biology at the University of Kentucky College of Dentistry. He has to his credit over 160 publications including original research articles, textbooks, textbook chapters, monographs, and articles in continuing education journals. He has given over 300 continuing education seminars to dental professionals in the U.S., Canada, and Europe. Dr Wynn has been a consultant to drug industry for 16 years. His research laboratories have contributed to the development of new analgesics and anesthetics. He is a consultant to the U.S. Pharmacopeia, Dental Drugs and Products section, a consultant to the Academy of General Dentistry, and a former consultant to the Council on Dental Education, Commission on Accreditation. He is a featured columnist and his drug review articles, entitled *Pharmacology Today*, appear in each issue of General Dentistry, a journal published by the Academy. He is currently funded by drug industry and government agencies for research on the emetogenic nature of pain, mechanisms of postoperative nausea, and animal models of acupuncture. One of his primary interests continues to be keeping dental professionals informed on all aspects of drug use in dental practice.

Timothy F. Meiller, DDS, PhD

Dr Meiller is Professor of Oral Medicine and Diagnostic Sciences at the Baltimore College of Dental Surgery and Professor of Oncology in the Program of Oncology at the Greenebaum Cancer Center, University of Maryland at Baltimore.

Dr Meiller teaches Oral Medicine at the Dental School and serves as an attending faculty at the Greenebaum Cancer Center. He is a Diplomate of the American Board of Oral Medicine. He is a graduate of Johns Hopkins University and the University of Maryland Dental and Graduate Schools, holding a DDS and a PhD in Immunology/Virology. He maintains an active general dental practice and is a consultant to the National Institutes of Health. He is currently engaged in ongoing investigations into cellular immune dysfunction in oral diseases associated with AIDS and in other medically compromised patients.

Harold L. Crossley, DDS, PhD

Dr Crossley is an Associate Professor of Pharmacology at the Baltimore College of Dental Surgery, Dental School, University of Maryland at Baltimore. A native of Rhode Island, Hal received a Bachelor of Science degree in Pharmacy from the University of Rhode Island in 1964. He later was awarded the Master of Science (1970) and Doctorate degrees (1972) in the area of Pharmacology. The University of Maryland Dental School in Baltimore awarded Dr Crossley the DDS degree in 1980. He is the Director of Conjoint Sciences and Preclinical Studies at the School of Dentistry and maintains an intramural part-time private dental practice. Dr Crossley has co-authored a number of articles dealing with law enforcement on both a local and federal level. This liaison with law enforcement agencies keeps him well-acquainted with the "drug culture". He has been appointed to the Governor's Commission on Prescription Drug Abuse and the Maryland State Dental Association's Well-Being Committee.

Drawing on this unique background, Dr Crossley has become nationally and internationally recognized as an expert on street drugs and chemical dependency as well as the clinical pharmacology of dental drugs.

EDITORIAL ADVISORY PANEL

4

PREFACE TO THE THIRD EDITION

The authors of the *Drug Information Handbook for Dentistry*, wish to congratulate and thank the practitioners and students that have made the previous editions a great success. We have sincerely endeavored to consistently respond to constructive comments and suggestions of the readership and as a result have incorporated new ideas into this third edition.

The philosophy and soul of the text remain the same. Complete cross-referencing of generic, brand names, medical conditions, oral conditions, therapeutic indications, and prescribing guidelines allow the practitioner or staff members to access needed information quickly and succinctly. This third edition is reformatted to allow all of the drug monographs to appear alphabetically now numbering over 1300 detailed monographs. The complete alphabetical index at the back of the text assists in inquiries where the reader may be unsure of accurate drug names. This index adds key Oral Medicine and Appendix headings to help the reader to access other topics in the text, regardless of where the inquiry begins.

The text remains an excellent companion to a complete oral medicine and medical reference library. It compliments a sound foundation in oral and systemic disease, focusing on therapeutic considerations, dental office management and prescribing guidelines. The active general practitioner, specialist, dental hygienist, and advanced students of dentistry and dental hygiene will be better prepared for patient evaluation and treatment with this third edition as an ideal drug reference database.

Timothy F. Meiller

Richard L. Wynn

Harold L. Crossley

ACKNOWLEDGMENTS

This handbook exists in its present form as a result of the concerted efforts of many individuals, including Jack D. Bolinski, DDS, and Brad F. Bolinski who recognized the need for a comprehensive dental and medical drug compendium; the publisher and president of Lexi-Comp Inc, Robert D. Kerscher; Lynn D. Coppinger, managing editor; John E. Janosik, PharmD; Leonard L. Lance, RPh, and David C. Marcus, systems analyst.

Other members of the Lexi-Comp staff include Diane Harbart, MT (ASCP), medical editor; Barbara F. Kerscher, production manager; Jeanne Wilson, Beth Daulbaugh, Leslie Ruggles, and Julie Katzen, project managers; Alexandra Hart, composition specialist; Jacqueline L. Mizer, Tracey J. Reinecke, and Jennifer Harbart, production assistants; Brian B. Vossler, Jerry M. Reeves, and Marc L. Long, sales managers; Jay L. Katzen, product manager; Kenneth J. Hughes, manager, authoring systems; Kristin M. Thompson, Matthew C. Kerscher, Tina L. Collins, Mary M. Murphy, and Eddie W. Norman, sales and marketing representatives; Edmund A. Harbart, vice-president, custom publishing division; Jack L. Stones, vice-president, reference publishing division; Dennis P. Smithers and Sean Conrad, system analysts; and Thury L. O'Connor, vice-president of technology.

In addition, the authors wish to thank their families, friends, and colleagues who supported them in their efforts to complete this handbook.

USE OF THE DRUG INFORMATION HANDBOOK FOR DENTISTRY

The *Drug Information Handbook for Dentistry, 3rd Edition* is organized into six sections: Introductory text, drug monographs, oral medicine topics, appendix, therapeutic category index, and alphabetical index

INTRODUCTORY TEXT

The first section is a compilation of information pertinent to the use of this handbook.

ALPHABETICAL LISTING OF DRUG MONOGRAPHS

The drug information section of the handbook, in which over 1300 drugs are listed alphabetically, incorporates drugs commonly prescribed in dentistry as well as medications that dental patients may currently be taking. Extensive cross-referencing is provided by brand names and synonyms.

Each monograph is consistent in its format and may include all or some of the following fields:

Generic Name	U.S. Adopted Name
Pronunciation Guide	Phonetic listing of generic name
Related Information	Cross-reference to other pertinent drug information found elsewhere in the book
Brand Names	Common trade names
Canadian/Mexican Brand Names	Trade names found in Canada and Mexico if different from the U.S.; complete listing is located in the Alphabetical Index
Therapeutic Category	Unique systematic classification of medications
Synonyms	Other names or accepted abbreviations of the drug in the U.S., Canada, and Mexico
Use	Information pertaining to appropriate dental and medical indications of the drug
Restrictions	DEA classification for federally scheduled controlled substances and their associated prescribing limits
Usual Dosage	The amount of the drug to be typically given or taken during therapy
Mechanism of Action	How the drug works in the body to elicit a response
Local Anesthetic/Vasoconstrictor Precautions	Specific information to prevent potential drug interactions related to anesthesia
Effects on Dental Treatment	How drug therapy affects the dental treatment/ diagnosis with suggested management approaches
Other Adverse Effects	Side effects grouped by percentage of incidence with oral manifestations reported
Contraindications	Information pertaining to inappropriate use of the drug
Warnings/Precautions	Cautions and hazardous conditions related to use of the drug
Drug Interactions	A list of agents that when combined may affect the therapy
Drug Uptake	Information includes onset and duration of effect, absorption, time to peak serum concentration, and serum half-life
Pregnancy Risk Factor	Five categories established by the FDA to indicate the potential of a systemically absorbed drug for causing birth defects
Breast-feeding Considerations	Information pertaining to drug administration while breast-feeding
Dosage Forms	Information with regard to form, strength, and availability of the drug
Dietary Considerations	Information regarding effect of food with drug
Generic Available	Indicated by a "yes" or "no"
Comments	Additional pertinent information

8

(continued)

Selected Readings | Sources and literature where the user may find additional information

ORAL MEDICINE TOPICS

The third section contains text on Oral Medicine topics and is divided into two major parts.

In each of the two major parts, the systemic condition or the oral disease state is described briefly, followed by the pharmacologic considerations, with which the dentist must be familiar. Selected readings have been listed for further inquiry.

Part I: **Dental Management and Therapeutic Considerations in Medically Compromised Patients** focuses on common medical conditions and their associated drug therapies with which the dentist must be familiar. Patient profiles with commonly associated drug regimens are described.

Part II: **Dental Management and Therapeutic Considerations in Patients With Specific Oral Conditions and Other Oral Medicine Topics** focus on therapies the dentist may choose to prescribe for patients suffering from oral disease or are in need of special care. Some overlap between these sections has resulted from systemic conditions that have oral manifestations and vice-versa. Cross-references to the descriptions and the monographs for individual drugs described elsewhere in this handbook allow for easy retrieval of information. Example prescriptions of selected drug therapies for each condition are presented so that the clinician can evaluate alternate approaches to treatment. Seldom is there a single drug of choice.

Those drug prescriptions listed represent prototype drugs and popular prescriptions and are examples only. The therapeutic index is available for cross-referencing if alternatives or additional drugs are sought.

APPENDIX

The Appendix section offers a compilation of tables, guidelines, and conversion information which can often be helpful when considering patient care. This section is broken down into various sections for ease of use. The Appendix also includes descriptions of most over-the-counter drugs and oral care products. There are also presentations of drug interactions and drugs under development.

THERAPEUTIC CATEGORY INDEX

The Therapeutic Category Index provides a useful listing by an easy-to-use therapeutic classification system.

ALPHABETICAL INDEX

The Alphabetical Index provides a quick reference for generic, American/Canadian/Mexican brand names, and major headings from the chapters. From this index, the reader can cross-reference to the drug monographs and to Oral Medicine topics.

FDA PREGNANCY CATEGORIES

Throughout this book there is a field labeled Pregnancy Risk Factor (PRF) and the letter A, B, C, D, or X immediately following which signifies a category. The FDA has established these five categories to indicate the potential of a systemically absorbed drug for causing birth defects. The key differentiation among the categories rests upon the reliability of documentation and the risk:benefit ratio. Pregnancy Category X is particularly notable in that if any data exists that may implicate a drug as a teratogen and the risk:benefit ratio is clearly negative, the drug is contraindicated during pregnancy.

These categories are summarized as follows:

A   Controlled studies in pregnant women fail to demonstrate a risk to the fetus in the first trimester with no evidence of risk in later trimesters. The possibility of fetal harm appears remote.

B   Either animal-reproduction studies have not demonstrated a fetal risk but there are no controlled studies in pregnant women, or animal-reproduction studies have shown an adverse effect (other than a decrease in fertility) that was not confirmed in controlled studies in women in the first trimester and there is no evidence of a risk in later trimesters.

C   Either studies in animals have revealed adverse effects on the fetus (teratogenic or embryocidal effects or other) and there are no controlled studies in women, or studies in women and animals are not available. Drugs should be given only if the potential benefits justify the potential risk to the fetus.

D   There is positive evidence of human fetal risk, but the benefits from use in pregnant women may be acceptable despite the risk (eg, if the drug is needed in a life-threatening situation or for a serious disease for which safer drugs cannot be used or are ineffective).

X   Studies in animals or human beings have demonstrated fetal abnormalities or there is evidence of fetal risk based on human experience, or both, and the risk of the use of the drug in pregnant women clearly outweighs any possible benefit. The drug is contraindicated in women who are or may become pregnant.

ALPHABETICAL LISTING OF DRUGS

A-200™ Pyrinate [OTC] *see* Pyrethrins *on page 753*
A and D™ Ointment [OTC] *see* Vitamin A and Vitamin D *on page 899*
Abbokinase® *see* Urokinase *on page 886*

Abciximab (ab sik′ si mab)
Brand Names ReoPro™
Therapeutic Category Platelet Aggregation Inhibitor
Synonyms C7E3; 7E3
Use Adjunct to percutaneous transluminal coronary angioplasty or atherectomy (PTCA) for the prevention of acute cardiac ischemic complications in patients at high risk for abrupt closure of the treated coronary vessel
Usual Dosage I.V.: 0.25 mg/kg bolus followed by an infusion of 10 mcg/minute for 12 hours
Local Anesthetic/Vasoconstrictor Precautions No information available to require special precautions
Effects on Dental Treatment No effects or complications reported
Pregnancy Risk Factor C

Abelcet™ Injection *see* Amphotericin B Lipid Complex *on page 61*
ABLC *see* Amphotericin B Lipid Complex *on page 61*

Acarbose (ay′ car bose)
Related Information
Endocrine Disorders & Pregnancy *on page 927*
Brand Names Precose®
Therapeutic Category Alpha-Glucosidase Inhibitor; Hypoglycemic Agent, Oral
Use Treatment of noninsulin-dependent diabetes mellitus (NIDDM); as monotherapy or in combination with a sulfonylurea when diet plus acarbose or a sulfonylurea does not result in adequate glycemic control
Usual Dosage Oral:
　Adults: Dosage must be individualized on the basis of effectiveness and tolerance while not exceeding the maximum recommended dose of 100 mg 3 times/day
　　Initial dose: 25 mg 3 times/day with the first bite of each main meal
　　Maintenance dose: Should be adjusted at 4- to 8-week intervals based on 1-hour postprandial glucose levels and tolerance. Dosage may be increased from 25 mg 3 times/day to 50 mg 3 times/day. Some patients may benefit from increasing the dose to 100 mg 3 times/day. Maintenance dose ranges: 50-100 mg 3 times/day.
　　Maximum dose:
　　　≤60 kg: 50 mg 3 times/day
　　　>60 kg: 100 mg 3 times/day
　　Patients receiving sulfonylureas: Acarbose given in combination with a sulfonylurea will cause a further lowering of blood glucose and may increase the hypoglycemic potential of the sulfonylurea. If hypoglycemia occurs, appropriate adjustments in the dosage of these agents should be made.
　　Elderly: Mean steady-state AUC and maximum concentrations of acarbose were 1.5 times higher in elderly compared to young volunteers; however, these differences were not statistically significant
　　Dosing adjustment in renal impairment: Cl_{cr} <25 mL/minute: Peak plasma concentrations were 5 times higher and AUCs were 6 times larger than in volunteers with normal renal function; however, long term clinical trials in diabetic patients with significant renal dysfunction have not been conducted and treatment of these patients with acarbose is not recommended
Local Anesthetic/Vasoconstrictor Precautions No information available to require special precautions
Effects on Dental Treatment No effects or complications reported
Drug Uptake
　Absorption: <2% absorbed as active drug

Accolate® *see* Zafirlukast *on page 905*
Accupril® *see* Quinapril Hydrochloride *on page 756*
Accutane® *see* Isotretinoin *on page 475*

Acebutolol Hydrochloride (a se byoo′ toe lole hye droe klor′ ide)
Brand Names Sectral®
Canadian/Mexican Brand Names Monitan® (Canada); Rhotral® (Canada)
Therapeutic Category Antiarrhythmic Agent, Class II; Antiarrhythmic Agent (Supraventricular & Ventricular); Beta-Adrenergic Blocker, Cardioselective
Use Treatment of hypertension, ventricular arrhythmias, angina

Usual Dosage Oral:

Adults: 400-800 mg/day in 2 divided doses; maximum: 1200 mg/day

Elderly: Initial: 200-400 mg/day; dose reduction due to age related decrease in Cl_{cr} will be necessary; do not exceed 800 mg/day

Mechanism of Action Competitively blocks beta$_1$-adrenergic receptors with little or no effect on beta$_2$-receptors except at high doses; exhibits membrane stabilizing and intrinsic sympathomimetic activity

Local Anesthetic/Vasoconstrictor Precautions No information available to require special precautions

Effects on Dental Treatment Non-cardioselective beta-blockers (ie, propranolol, nadolol) enhance the pressor response to epinephrine, resulting in hypertension and bradycardia. This has not been reported for acebutolol, a cardioselective beta-blocker. Therefore, local anesthetic with vasoconstrictor can be safely used in patients medicated with acebutolol. Many nonsteroidal anti-inflammatory drugs such as ibuprofen and indomethacin can reduce the hypotensive effect of beta-blockers after 3 or more weeks of therapy with the NSAID. Short-term NSAID use (ie, 3 days) requires no special precautions in patients taking beta-blockers.

Other Adverse Effects

>10%: Fatigue

1% to 10%:

Cardiovascular: Chest pain, edema, bradycardia, hypotension

Central nervous system: Headache, dizziness, insomnia, depression, abnormal dreams

Dermatologic: Rash

Gastrointestinal: Constipation, diarrhea, dyspepsia, nausea, flatulence

Genitourinary: Micturition (frequency)

Neuromuscular & skeletal: Arthralgia, myalgia

Ocular: Abnormal vision

Respiratory: Dyspnea, rhinitis, cough

<1%:

Cardiovascular: Ventricular arrhythmias, heart block, heart failure

Central nervous system: Cold extremities

Gastrointestinal: Dry mouth, anorexia

Genitourinary: Impotence, urinary retention

Miscellaneous: Facial swelling

Drug Interactions

Decreased effect of beta-blockers:

Barbiturates (increased liver metabolism of beta-blockers to result in lower serum levels)

NSAIDs (attenuate the hypotensive therapeutic effects of beta-blockers)

Rifampin (increased liver metabolism of beta-blockers to result in lower serum levels)

Increased effects of beta-blockers:

Calcium channel blockers (increase serum levels of beta-blockers by unknown mechanism to enhance hypotension)

Beta-blockers increase the effects of:

Epinephrine (vasoconstrictor; initial hypertensive episode followed by bradycardia) only from non-cardioselective type beta-blockers

Phenylephrine (Neosynephrine®; enhanced pressor response)

Theophylline (inhibit theophylline metabolism causing increase in serum concentrations)

Drug Uptake

Absorption: Oral: Well absorbed (40%)

Serum half-life: 6-7 hours average

Time to peak: 2-4 hours

Pregnancy Risk Factor B

Selected Readings

Foster CA and Aston SJ, "Propranolol-Epinephrine Interaction: A Potential Disaster," *Plast Reconstr Surg*, 1983, 72(1):74-8.

Wong DG, Spence JD, Lamki L, et al, "Effect of Nonsteroidal Anti-Inflammatory Drugs on Control of Hypertension of Beta-Blockers and Diuretics," *Lancet*, 1986, 1(8488):997-1001.

Wynn RL, "Dental Nonsteroidal Anti-Inflammatory Drugs and Prostaglandin-Based Drug Interactions, Part Two," *Gen Dent*, 1992, 40(2):104, 106, 108.

Wynn RL, "Epinephrine Interactions With Beta-Blockers," *Gen Dent*, 1994, 42(1):16, 18.

Aceon® *see* Perindopril Erbumine *on page 676*

Acephen® [OTC] *see* Acetaminophen *on next page*

Aceta® [OTC] *see* Acetaminophen *on next page*

Acetaminofen (Mexico) *see* Acetaminophen *on next page*

Acetaminophen (a seet a min' oh fen)

Related Information

Oral Pain *on page 940*

Brand Names Acephen® [OTC]; Aceta® [OTC]; Anacin-3® [OTC]; Apacet® [OTC]; Banesin® [OTC]; Dapa® [OTC]; Datril® [OTC]; Dorcol® [OTC]; Feverall™ [OTC]; Genapap® [OTC]; Halenol® [OTC]; Neopap® [OTC]; Panadol® [OTC]; Tempra® [OTC]; Tylenol® [OTC]; Valadol® [OTC]

Canadian/Mexican Brand Names Atasol® (Canada); Pediatrix® (Canada); 222 AF® (Canada); Tantaphen® (Canada); Algitrin® (Mexico); Analphen® (Mexico); Febrin® (Mexico); Minofen® (Mexico); Neodol® (Mexico); Sinedol® (Mexico); Sinedol® 500 (Mexico); Temperal® (Mexico); Cilag® (Mexico); Winasorb® (Mexico); Tylex® 750 (Mexico)

Therapeutic Category Analgesic, Non-narcotic; Antipyretic

Synonyms Acetaminofen (Mexico); Paracetamol (Mexico)

Use

Dental: Treatment of postoperative pain

Medical: Treatment of pain and fever; does not have anti-inflammatory effects

Usual Dosage Oral:

Children <12 years: 10-15 mg/kg/dose every 4-6 hours as needed; do not exceed 5 doses (2.6 g) in 24 hours

Adults: 325-650 mg (1-2 tablets) every 4-6 hours or 1000 mg 3-4 times/day; do not exceed 4 g/day

Mechanism of Action Inhibits the synthesis of prostaglandins in the CNS and peripherally blocks pain impulse generation; produces antipyresis by inhibition of hypothalamic heat-regulating center

Local Anesthetic/Vasoconstrictor Precautions No information available to require special precautions

Effects on Dental Treatment No effects or complications reported

Other Adverse Effects No data reported

Oral manifestations: No data reported

Contraindications Patients with known Glucose-6-phosphate dehydrogenase (G-6-PD) deficiency; hypersensitivity to acetaminophen

Warnings/Precautions May cause severe hepatic toxicity on overdose; use with caution in patients with alcoholic liver disease; chronic daily dosing in adults of 5-8 g of acetaminophen over several weeks or 3-4 g/day of acetaminophen for 1 year have resulted in liver damage

Drug Interactions Rifampin can interact to reduce the analgesic effectiveness of acetaminophen; barbiturates, carbamazepine, hydantoins, sulfinpyrazone can increase the hepatotoxic potential of acetaminophen; chronic ethanol abuse increases risk for acetaminophen hepatotoxicity

Drug Uptake

Onset: 1-3 hours

Time to peak serum concentration: 0.5-2 hours

Duration: 3-4 hours

Serum half-life: 1-4 hours

Pregnancy Risk Factor B

Breast-feeding Considerations May be taken while breast-feeding

Dosage Forms

Caplet: 160 mg, 325 mg, 500 mg

Drops: 48 mg/mL (15 mL); 60 mg/0.6 mL (15 mL)

Elixir: 120 mg/5 mL, 160 mg/5 mL, 167 mg/5 mL, 325 mg/5 mL

Liquid, oral: 160 mg/5 mL, 500 mg/15 mL

Solution: 100 mg/mL (15 mL); 120 mg/2.5 mL

Suppository, rectal: 120 mg, 125 mg, 300 mg, 325 mg, 650 mg

Tablet: 325 mg, 500 mg, 650 mg

Tablet, chewable: 80 mg, 160 mg

Dietary Considerations May be taken with food

Generic Available Yes

Comments Doses of acetaminophen >5 g/day for several weeks can produce severe, often fatal liver damage. Hepatotoxicity caused by acetaminophen is potentiated by chronic alcohol consumption. It has been reported that a combination of two quarts of whiskey a day with 8-10 acetaminophen tablets daily resulted in severe liver toxicity. People who consume alcohol at the same time that they use acetaminophen, even in therapeutic doses, are at risk of developing hepatotoxicity.

Selected Readings

Barker JD Jr, de Carle DJ, and Anuras S, "Chronic Excessive Acetaminophen Use in Liver Damage," *Ann Intern Med*, 1977, 87(3):299-301.

Dionne RA, Campbell RA, Cooper SA, et al, "Suppression of Postoperative Pain by Preoperative Administration of Ibuprofen in Comparison to Placebo, Acetaminophen, and Acetaminophen Plus Codeine," *J Clin Pharmacol*, 1983, 23(1):37-43.

Licht H, Seeff LB, and Zimmerman HJ, "Apparent Potentiation of Acetaminophen Hepatotoxicity by Alcohol," *Ann Intern Med*, 1980, 92(4):511.

Acetaminophen and Codeine (a seet a min′ oh fen & koe′ deen)

Brand Names Capital® and Codeine; Phenaphen® With Codeine; Tylenol® With Codeine

Canadian/Mexican Brand Names Lenoltec® With Codeine (Canada); Novo-Gesic-C8® (Canada); Novo-Gesic-C15® (Canada); Novo-Gesic-C30® (Canada); Tylex® CD (Mexico)

Therapeutic Category Analgesic, Narcotic

Use
Dental: Treatment of postoperative pain
Medical: Relief of pain

Usual Dosage
Children: Not recommended in pediatric dental patients
Adults: Based on codeine (30-60 mg/dose) every 4-6 hours; 1-2 tablets every 4 hours to a maximum of 12 tablets/24 hours

Mechanism of Action
Acetaminophen: Inhibits the synthesis of prostaglandins in the CNS and peripherally blocks pain impulse generation; produces antipyresis by inhibition of hypothalamic heat-regulating center
Codeine: Binds to opiate receptors (mu and kappa subtypes) in the CNS causing inhibition of ascending pain pathways, altering the perception of and response to pain

Local Anesthetic/Vasoconstrictor Precautions No information available to require special precautions

Effects on Dental Treatment No effects or complications reported

Other Adverse Effects
>10%:
Central nervous system: Lightheadedness, dizziness, sedation
Gastrointestinal: Nausea, vomiting
1% to 10%: Gastrointestinal: Constipation

Oral manifestations: <1%: Dry mouth

Contraindications Patients with known G-6-PD deficiency; hypersensitivity to acetaminophen; hypersensitivity to codeine

Warnings/Precautions Use with caution in patients with hypersensitivity reactions to other phenanthrene derivative opioid agonists (morphine, hydrocodone, hydromorphone, levorphanol, oxycodone, oxymorphone); respiratory diseases including asthma, emphysema, COPD, or severe liver or renal insufficiency; some preparations contain sulfites which may cause allergic reactions; may be habit-forming

Enhanced analgesia has been seen in elderly patients on therapeutic doses of narcotics; duration of action may be increased in the elderly; the elderly may be particularly susceptible to the CNS depressant and constipating effects of narcotics

Drug Interactions
With codeine component: Increased toxicity of CNS depressants, phenothiazines, tricyclic antidepressants, guanabenz, MAO inhibitors (may also lead to a decrease in blood pressure)
With acetaminophen component: Refer to Acetaminophen monograph

Drug Uptake
Acetaminophen:
Onset: 1-3 hours
Time to peak serum concentration: 0.5-2 hours
Duration: 3-4 hours
Serum half-life: 1-4 hours
Codeine:
Onset (analgesia): Oral: 30-45 minutes
Time to peak serum concentration: 1-2 hours
Duration: 4-6 hours
Serum half-life: 2.5-3.5 hours

Pregnancy Risk Factor C

Breast-feeding Considerations Both acetaminophen and codeine may be taken while breast-feeding

Dosage Forms
Capsule:
#2: Acetaminophen 325 mg and codeine phosphate 15 mg (C-III)
#3: Acetaminophen 325 mg and codeine phosphate 30 mg (C-III)
#4: Acetaminophen 325 mg and codeine phosphate 60 mg (C-III)
(Continued)

Acetaminophen and Codeine *(Continued)*

Elixir: Acetaminophen 120 mg and codeine phosphate 12 mg per 5 mL with alcohol 7% (C-V)

Suspension, oral, alcohol free: Acetaminophen 120 mg and codeine phosphate 12 mg per 5 mL (C-V)

Tablet: Acetaminophen 500 mg and codeine phosphate 30 mg (C-III); acetaminophen 650 mg and codeine phosphate 30 mg (C-III)

Tablet:

#1: Acetaminophen 300 mg and codeine phosphate 7.5 mg (C-III)

#2: Acetaminophen 300 mg and codeine phosphate 15 mg (C-III)

#3: Acetaminophen 300 mg and codeine phosphate 30 mg (C-III)

#4: Acetaminophen 300 mg and codeine phosphate 60 mg (C-III)

Dietary Considerations May be taken with food

Generic Available Yes

Comments Codeine products, as with other narcotic analgesics, are recommended only for acute dosing (ie, 3 days or less). The most common adverse effect you will see in your dental patients from codeine is nausea, followed by sedation and constipation. Codeine has narcotic addiction liability, especially when given long term. Because of the acetaminophen component, this product should be used with caution in patients with alcoholic liver disease.

Selected Readings

Dionne RA, "New Approaches to Preventing and Treating Postoperative Pain," *J Am Dent Assoc*, 1992, 123(6):26-34.

Dionne RA, Campbell RA, Cooper SA, et al, "Suppression of Postoperative Pain by Preoperative Administration of Ibuprofen in Comparison to Placebo, Acetaminophen, and Acetaminophen Plus Codeine," *J Clin Pharmacol*, 1983, 23(1):37-43.

Forbes JA, Butterworth GA, Burchfield WH, et al, "Evaluation of Ketorolac, Aspirin, and an Acetaminophen-Codeine Combination in Postoperative Oral Surgery Pain," *Pharmacotherapy*, 1990, 10(6 Pt 2):77S-93S.

Gobetti JP, "Controlling Dental Pain," *J Am Dent Assoc*, 1992, 123(6):47-52.

Acetaminophen and Dextromethorphan

(a seet a min' oh fen & dex troe meth or' fan)

Brand Names Bayer® Select® Chest Cold Caplets [OTC]; Drixoral® Cough & Sore Throat Liquid Caps [OTC]

Therapeutic Category Analgesic, Non-narcotic; Antipyretic; Antitussive

Use Treatment of mild to moderate pain and fever; symptomatic relief of coughs caused by minor viral upper respiratory tract infections or inhaled irritants; most effective for a chronic nonproductive cough

Local Anesthetic/Vasoconstrictor Precautions No information available to require special precautions

Effects on Dental Treatment No effects or complications reported

Selected Readings

Barker JD Jr, de Carle DJ, and Anuras S, "Chronic Excessive Acetaminophen Use in Liver Damage," *Ann Intern Med*, 1977, 87(3):299-301.

Dionne RA, Campbell RA, Cooper SA, et al, "Suppression of Postoperative Pain by Preoperative Administration of Ibuprofen in Comparison to Placebo, Acetaminophen, and Acetaminophen Plus Codeine," *J Clin Pharmacol*, 1983, 23(1):37-43.

Licht H, Seeff LB, and Zimmerman HJ, "Apparent Potentiation of Acetaminophen Hepatotoxicity by Alcohol," *Ann Intern Med*, 1980, 92(4):511.

Acetaminophen and Diphenhydramine

(a seet a min' oh fen & dye fen hye' dra meen)

Brand Names Arthritis Foundation® Nighttime [OTC]; Excedrin® P.M. [OTC]; Midol® PM [OTC]

Therapeutic Category Analgesic, Non-narcotic

Use Relief of mild to moderate pain; sinus headache

Local Anesthetic/Vasoconstrictor Precautions No information available to require special precautions

Effects on Dental Treatment 1% to 10%: Dry mouth

Selected Readings

Barker JD Jr, de Carle DJ, and Anuras S, "Chronic Excessive Acetaminophen Use in Liver Damage," *Ann Intern Med*, 1977, 87(3):299-301.

Dionne RA, Campbell RA, Cooper SA, et al, "Suppression of Postoperative Pain by Preoperative Administration of Ibuprofen in Comparison to Placebo, Acetaminophen, and Acetaminophen Plus Codeine," *J Clin Pharmacol*, 1983, 23(1):37-43.

Licht H, Seeff LB, and Zimmerman HJ, "Apparent Potentiation of Acetaminophen Hepatotoxicity by Alcohol," *Ann Intern Med*, 1980, 92(4):511.

Acetaminophen and Isometheptene Mucate

(a seet a min' oh fen & eye soe me thep' teen myoo' kate)

Brand Names Midrin®

Therapeutic Category Analgesic, Non-narcotic; Antimigraine Agent

Use Relief of migraine and tension headache

Local Anesthetic/Vasoconstrictor Precautions No information available to require special precautions

Effects on Dental Treatment No effects or complications reported

Comments Should not exceed 5 g in 12 hours; may cause drowsiness; avoid alcohol and other CNS depressants

Selected Readings
Barker JD Jr, de Carle DJ, and Anuras S, "Chronic Excessive Acetaminophen Use in Liver Damage," *Ann Intern Med*, 1977, 87(3):299-301.
Dionne RA, Campbell RA, Cooper SA, et al, "Suppression of Postoperative Pain by Preoperative Administration of Ibuprofen in Comparison to Placebo, Acetaminophen, and Acetaminophen Plus Codeine," *J Clin Pharmacol*, 1983, 23(1):37-43.
Licht H, Seeff LB, and Zimmerman HJ, "Apparent Potentiation of Acetaminophen Hepatotoxicity by Alcohol," *Ann Intern Med*, 1980, 92(4):511.

Acetaminophen and Phenyltoloxamine

(a seet a min' oh fen & fen il to lox' a meen)

Brand Names Percogesic® [OTC]

Therapeutic Category Analgesic, Non-narcotic

Use Relief of mild to moderate pain

Local Anesthetic/Vasoconstrictor Precautions No information available to require special precautions

Effects on Dental Treatment No effects or complications reported

Selected Readings
Barker JD Jr, de Carle DJ, and Anuras S, "Chronic Excessive Acetaminophen Use in Liver Damage," *Ann Intern Med*, 1977, 87(3):299-301.
Dionne RA, Campbell RA, Cooper SA, et al, "Suppression of Postoperative Pain by Preoperative Administration of Ibuprofen in Comparison to Placebo, Acetaminophen, and Acetaminophen Plus Codeine," *J Clin Pharmacol*, 1983, 23(1):37-43.
Licht H, Seeff LB, and Zimmerman HJ, "Apparent Potentiation of Acetaminophen Hepatotoxicity by Alcohol," *Ann Intern Med*, 1980, 92(4):511.

Acetaminophen, Aspirin, and Caffeine

(a seet a min' oh fen, as' pir in, & kaf' een)

Brand Names Excedrin®, Extra Strength [OTC]; Gelpirin® [OTC]; Goody's® Headache Powders

Therapeutic Category Analgesic, Non-narcotic

Use Relief of mild to moderate pain

Local Anesthetic/Vasoconstrictor Precautions No information available to require special precautions

Effects on Dental Treatment No effects or complications reported

Other Adverse Effects See individual agents

Selected Readings
Barker JD Jr, de Carle DJ, and Anuras S, "Chronic Excessive Acetaminophen Use in Liver Damage," *Ann Intern Med*, 1977, 87(3):299-301.
Desjardins PJ, Cooper SA, Gallegos TL, et al, "The Relative Analgesic Efficacy of Propiram Fumarate, Codeine Aspirin, and Placebo in Post-Impaction Dental Pain," *J Clin Pharmacol*, 1984, 24(1):35-42.
Dionne RA, Campbell RA, Cooper SA, et al, "Suppression of Postoperative Pain by Preoperative Administration of Ibuprofen in Comparison to Placebo, Acetaminophen, and Acetaminophen Plus Codeine," *J Clin Pharmacol*, 1983, 23(1):37-43.
Forbes JA, Butterworth GA, Burchfield WH, et al, "Evaluation of Ketorolac, Aspirin, and an Acetaminophen-Codeine Combination in Postoperative Oral Surgery Pain," *Pharmacotherapy*, 1990, 10(6 Pt 2):77S-93S.
Forbes JA, Keller CK, Smith JW, et al, "Analgesic Effect of Naproxen Sodium, Codeine, a Naproxen-Codeine Combination and Aspirin on the Postoperative Pain of Oral Surgery," *Pharmacotherapy*, 1986, 6(5):211-8.
Licht H, Seeff LB, and Zimmerman HJ, "Apparent Potentiation of Acetaminophen Hepatotoxicity by Alcohol," *Ann Intern Med*, 1980, 92(4):511.

Acetaminophen, Chlorpheniramine, and Pseudoephedrine

(a seet a min' oh fen, klor fen ir' a meen, & soo doe e fed' rin)

Brand Names Alka-Seltzer® Plus Cold Liqui-Gels Capsules [OTC]; Aspirin-Free Bayer® Select® Allergy Sinus Caplets [OTC]; Co-Hist® [OTC]; Sinutab® Tablets [OTC]

Therapeutic Category Analgesic, Non-narcotic; Antihistamine/Decongestant Combination

Use Temporary relief of sinus symptoms

Local Anesthetic/Vasoconstrictor Precautions Use with caution since pseudoephedrine is a sympathomimetic amine which could interact with epinephrine to cause a pressor response

Effects on Dental Treatment
Chlorpheniramine: Prolonged use will cause significant xerostomia
Pseudoephedrine: Up to 10% of patients could experience tachycardia, palpitations, and dry mouth; use vasoconstrictor with caution

(Continued)

Acetaminophen, Chlorpheniramine, and Pseudoephedrine *(Continued)*

Other Adverse Effects See individual agents

Selected Readings

Barker JD Jr, de Carle DJ, and Anuras S, "Chronic Excessive Acetaminophen Use in Liver Damage," *Ann Intern Med*, 1977, 87(3):299-301.

Dionne RA, Campbell RA, Cooper SA, et al, "Suppression of Postoperative Pain by Preoperative Administration of Ibuprofen in Comparison to Placebo, Acetaminophen, and Acetaminophen Plus Codeine," *J Clin Pharmacol*, 1983, 23(1):37-43.

Licht H, Seeff LB, and Zimmerman HJ, "Apparent Potentiation of Acetaminophen Hepatotoxicity by Alcohol," *Ann Intern Med*, 1980, 92(4):511.

Acetasol® HC Otic *see* Acetic Acid, Propanediol Diacetate, and Hydrocortisone *on next page*

Acetazolamide (a set a zole' a mide)

Brand Names AK-Zol®; Diamox®; Diamox® Sequels®

Canadian/Mexican Brand Names Acetazolam® (Canada); Apo-Acetazolamide® (Canada); Novo-Zolamide® (Canada)

Therapeutic Category Anticonvulsant, Miscellaneous; Antiglaucoma Agent; Carbonic Anhydrase Inhibitor; Diuretic, Carbonic Anhydrase Inhibitor

Use Lowers intraocular pressure to treat glaucoma, also as a diuretic, adjunct treatment of refractory seizures and acute altitude sickness; centrencephalic epilepsies (sustained release not recommended for anticonvulsant)

Usual Dosage Note: I.M. administration is not recommended because of pain secondary to the alkaline pH

Children:

Glaucoma:

Oral: 8-30 mg/kg/day or 300-900 mg/m^2/day divided every 8 hours

I.M., I.V.: 20-40 mg/kg/24 hours divided every 6 hours, not to exceed 1 g/day

Edema: Oral, I.M., I.V.: 5 mg/kg or 150 mg/m^2 once every day

Epilepsy: Oral: 8-30 mg/kg/day in 1-4 divided doses, not to exceed 1 g/day; sustained release capsule is not recommended for treatment of epilepsy

Adults:

Glaucoma:

Chronic simple (open-angle): Oral: 250 mg 1-4 times/day or 500 mg sustained release capsule twice daily

Secondary, acute (closed-angle): I.M., I.V.: 250-500 mg, may repeat in 2-4 hours to a maximum of 1 g/day

Edema: Oral, I.M., I.V.: 250-375 mg once daily

Epilepsy: Oral: 8-30 mg/kg/day in 1-4 divided doses, not to exceed 1 g/day; **sustained release capsule is not recommended for treatment of epilepsy**

Altitude sickness: Oral: 250 mg every 8-12 hours (or 500 mg extended release capsules every 12-24 hours). Therapy should begin 24-48 hours before and continue during ascent and for at least 48 hours after arrival at the high altitude.

Urine alkalinization: Oral: 5 mg/kg/dose repeated 2-3 times over 24 hours

Elderly: Oral: Initial: 250 mg twice daily; use lowest effective dose

Mechanism of Action Reversible inhibition of the enzyme carbonic anhydrase resulting in reduction of hydrogen ion secretion at renal tubule and an increased renal excretion of sodium, potassium, bicarbonate, and water to decrease production of aqueous humor; also inhibits carbonic anhydrase in central nervous system to retard abnormal and excessive discharge from CNS neurons

Local Anesthetic/Vasoconstrictor Precautions No information available to require special precautions

Effects on Dental Treatment No effects or complications reported

Other Adverse Effects

>10%:

Gastrointestinal: Anorexia, diarrhea, malaise, metallic taste

Genitourinary: Increased urination

Neuromuscular & skeletal: Muscular weakness

<1%:

Central nervous system: Fever, fatigue, mental depression, drowsiness

Dermatologic: Rash

Endocrine & metabolic: Hyperchloremic metabolic acidosis, hypokalemia

Gastrointestinal: GI irritation, dryness of mouth

Genitourinary: Dysuria, renal calculi

Hematologic: Bone marrow suppression, blood dyscrasias, elevation of blood glucose

Neuromuscular & skeletal: Paresthesia

Ocular: Myopia

Miscellaneous: Black stools

Drug Interactions Acetazolamide increases lithium excretion and alters excretion of other drugs by alkalinization of urine (such as amphetamines, quinidine, procainamide, methenamine, phenobarbital, salicylates)

Drug Uptake
Onset of action:
Extended release capsule: 2 hours
I.V.: 2 minutes
Peak effect:
Extended release capsule: 3-6 hours
Tablet: 1-4 hours
I.V.: 15 minutes
Duration:
Extended release capsule: 18-24 hours
Tablet: 8-12 hours
I.V.: 4-5 hours
Serum half-life: 2.4-5.8 hours

Pregnancy Risk Factor C

Acetic Acid and Aluminum Acetate Otic see Aluminum Acetate and Acetic Acid on page 39

Acetic Acid, Propanediol Diacetate, and Hydrocortisone

(a see′ tik as′ id, pro pa′ neh dye′ ole dye as′ e tate, & hye droe kor′ ti sone)

Brand Names Acetasol® HC Otic; VōSol® HC Otic

Therapeutic Category Otic Agent, Anti-infective

Use Treatment of superficial infections of the external auditory canal caused by organisms susceptible to the action of the antimicrobial, complicated by swelling

Local Anesthetic/Vasoconstrictor Precautions No information available to require special precautions

Effects on Dental Treatment No effects or complications reported

Other Adverse Effects Transient burning or stinging may be noticed occasionally when the solution is first instilled into the acutely inflamed ear

Acetohexamide (a set oh hex′ a mide)

Related Information
Endocrine Disorders & Pregnancy on page 927

Brand Names Dymelor®

Therapeutic Category Antidiabetic Agent; Hypoglycemic Agent, Oral; Sulfonylurea Agent

Use Adjunct to diet for the management of mild to moderately severe, stable, noninsulin-dependent (type II) diabetes mellitus

Usual Dosage Adults: Oral (elderly patients may be more sensitive and should be started at a lower dosage initially): 250 mg to 1.5 g/day in 1-2 divided doses; doses >1.5 g/day are not recommended; if dose is ≤1 g, administer as a single daily dose

Mechanism of Action Believed to cause hypoglycemia by stimulating insulin release from the pancreatic beta cells; reduces glucose output from the liver (decreases gluconeogenesis); insulin sensitivity is increased at peripheral target sites (alters receptor sensitivity/receptor density); potentiates effects of ADH; may produce mild diuresis and significant uricosuric activity

Local Anesthetic/Vasoconstrictor Precautions No information available to require special precautions

Effects on Dental Treatment Use salicylates with caution in patients taking acetohexamide because of potential increased hypoglycemia. Phenylbutazone is the only NSAID reported to significantly increase hypoglycemic effects of acetohexamide. NSAIDs such as ibuprofen, naproxen and others may be safely used. Acetohexamide-dependent diabetics (noninsulin-dependent, type II) should be appointed for dental treatment in mornings to minimize chance of stress-induced hypoglycemia.

Other Adverse Effects
>10%:
Central nervous system: Headache, dizziness
(Continued)

Acetohexamide *(Continued)*

Gastrointestinal: Constipation, diarrhea, heartburn, anorexia, epigastric fullness

1% to 10%: Dermatologic: Rash, hives, photosensitivity

<1%:

Endocrine & metabolic: Hypoglycemia

Hematologic: Aplastic anemia, hemolytic anemia, bone marrow depression, thrombocytopenia, agranulocytosis

Drug Interactions

Monitor patient closely; large number of drugs interact with sulfonylureas

Decreased effect: Decreased hypoglycemic effect when coadministered with cholestyramine, diazoxide, hydantoins, rifampin, thiazides, loop or thiazide diuretics, and phenylbutazone

Increased effect: Increased hypoglycemia when coadministered with salicylates or beta-adrenergic blockers; MAO inhibitors; oral anticoagulants, NSAIDs, sulfonamides, phenylbutazone, insulin, clofibrate, fenfluramine, fluconazole, gemfibrozil, H_2 antagonists, methyldopa, tricyclic antidepressants

Drug Uptake

Onset of effect: 1 hour

Peak hypoglycemic effects: 8-10 hours

Duration: 12-24 hours, prolonged with renal impairment

Serum half-life:

Parent compound: 0.8-2.4 hours

Metabolite: 5-6 hours

Pregnancy Risk Factor D

Acetohydroxamic Acid *(a see' toe hye drox am ik as' id)*

Brand Names Lithostat®

Therapeutic Category Urinary Tract Product

Synonyms AHA

Use Adjunctive therapy in chronic urea-splitting urinary infection

Local Anesthetic/Vasoconstrictor Precautions No information available to require special precautions

Effects on Dental Treatment No effects or complications reported

Acetophenazine Maleate *(a set oh fen' a zeen mal' ee ate)*

Brand Names Tindal®

Therapeutic Category Antipsychotic Agent

Use Management of manifestations of psychotic disorders

Usual Dosage Adults: Oral: 20 mg 3 times/day up to 60-120 mg/day

Hospitalized schizophrenic patients may require doses as high as 400-600 mg/day

Not dialyzable (0% to 5%)

Mechanism of Action Antagonizes the effects of dopamine in the basal ganglia and limbic areas of the forebrain; this activity appears responsible for the antipsychotic efficacy, as well as the production of extrapyramidal symptoms; increases the secretion of prolactin and has a marked suppressive effect on the chemoreceptor trigger zone; also produces peripheral blockade of cholinergic neurons

Local Anesthetic/Vasoconstrictor Precautions No information available to require special precautions

Effects on Dental Treatment Orthostatic hypotension and nasal congestion possible in dental patients. Since the drug is a dopamine antagonist, extrapyramidal symptoms of the TMJ is a possibility; increased motor activity of head, face, and neck may occur. This drug is also an anticholinergic causing xerostomia.

Other Adverse Effects

>10%:

Cardiovascular: Hypotension, orthostatic hypotension

Central nervous system: Pseudoparkinsonism, akathisia, dystonias, tardive dyskinesia (persistent), dizziness

Gastrointestinal: Constipation

Ocular: Pigmentary retinopathy

Respiratory: Nasal congestion

Miscellaneous: Decreased sweating

1% to 10%:

Dermatologic: Increased sensitivity to sun, skin rash

Endocrine & metabolic: Changes in menstrual cycle, ejaculatory disturbances, changes in libido, pain in breasts

    Gastrointestinal: Weight gain, nausea, vomiting, stomach pain
    Genitourinary: Difficulty in urination
    Neuromuscular & skeletal: Trembling of fingers
<1%:
    Central nervous system: Neuroleptic malignant syndrome (NMS)
    Dermatologic: Discoloration of skin (blue-gray)
    Endocrine & metabolic: Galactorrhea
    Genitourinary: Priapism
    Hematologic: Agranulocytosis, leukopenia
    Hepatic: Cholestatic jaundice, hepatotoxicity
    Ocular: Cornea and lens changes, pigmentary retinopathy
    Miscellaneous: Impairment of temperature regulation, lowering of seizures
      threshold
Drug Interactions No data reported
Drug Uptake
  Duration: ~24 hours, permitting daily dosing
  Absorption: Tissue saturation, particularly in high lipid tissues such as the
    central nervous system
  Serum half-life: Range: 20-40 hours
Pregnancy Risk Factor C

Acetylcholine Chloride (a se teel koe′ leen klor′ ide)
Brand Names Miochol®
Therapeutic Category Cholinergic Agent, Ophthalmic; Ophthalmic Agent,
  Miotic
Use Produces complete miosis in cataract surgery, keratoplasty, iridectomy and
  other anterior segment surgery where rapid miosis is required
Usual Dosage Adults: Intraocular: 0.5-2 mL of 1% injection (5-20 mg) instilled
  into anterior chamber before or after securing one or more sutures
Mechanism of Action Causes contraction of the sphincter muscles of the iris,
  resulting in miosis and contraction of the ciliary muscle, leading to accommo-
  dation spasm
Local Anesthetic/Vasoconstrictor Precautions None
Effects on Dental Treatment Ophthalmic use of acetylcholine has no effect
  on dental treatment
Other Adverse Effects <1%:
  Cardiovascular: Bradycardia, hypotension, flushing
  Central nervous system: Headache
  Ocular: Altered distance vision, decreased night vision, transient lenticular
    opacities
  Respiratory: Breathing difficulty
  Miscellaneous: Sweating
Drug Interactions No data reported
Drug Uptake
  Onset of miosis: Occurs promptly
  Duration: ~10 minutes
Pregnancy Risk Factor C

Acetylcysteine (a se teel sis′ teen)
Brand Names Mucomyst®; Mucosil™
Therapeutic Category Antidote, Acetaminophen; Mucolytic Agent
Use Adjunctive mucolytic therapy in patients with abnormal or viscid mucous
  secretions in acute and chronic bronchopulmonary diseases; pulmonary
  complications of surgery and cystic fibrosis; diagnostic bronchial studies; anti-
  dote for acute acetaminophen toxicity
Usual Dosage
  Acetaminophen poisoning: Children and Adults: Oral: 140 mg/kg; followed by
    17 doses of 70 mg/kg every 4 hours; repeat dose if emesis occurs within 1
    hour of administration; therapy should continue until all doses are adminis-
    tered even though the acetaminophen plasma level has dropped below the
    toxic range

  Inhalation: Acetylcysteine 10% and 20% solution (Mucomyst) (dilute 20%
    solution with sodium chloride or sterile water for inhalation); 10% solution
    may be used undiluted
    Children: 3-5 mL of 20% solution or 6-10 mL of 10% solution until nebulized
      given 3-4 times/day
    Adolescents: 5-10 mL of 10% to 20% solution until nebulized given 3-4
      times/day
    Note: Patients should receive an aerosolized bronchodilator 10-15 minutes
      prior to acetylcysteine
(Continued)

21

Acetylcysteine *(Continued)*

Meconium ileus equivalent: Children and Adults: 100-300 mL of 4% to 10% solution by irrigation or orally

Mechanism of Action Exerts mucolytic action through its free sulfhydryl group which opens up the disulfide bonds in the mucoproteins thus lowering mucous viscosity. The exact mechanism of action in acetaminophen toxicity is unknown; thought to act by providing substrate for conjugation with the toxic metabolite.

Local Anesthetic/Vasoconstrictor Precautions No information available to require special precautions

Effects on Dental Treatment No effects or complications reported

Other Adverse Effects
>10%:
  Gastrointestinal: Vomiting
  Miscellaneous: Unpleasant odor during administration
1% to 10%:
  Gastrointestinal: Stomatitis, nausea
  Hematologic: Hemoptysis
  Local: Irritation
  Respiratory: Bronchospasm
  Miscellaneous: Rhinorrhea, drowsiness, clamminess, chills
<1%: Dermatologic: Skin rash

Drug Interactions No data reported

Drug Uptake
Oral:
  Peak plasma levels: 1-2 hours
Onset of action: Inhalation: Mucus liquefaction occurs maximally within 5-10 minutes
Duration: Can persist for >1 hour
Serum half-life:
  Reduced acetylcysteine: 2 hours
  Total acetylcysteine: 5.5 hours

Pregnancy Risk Factor B

Aches-N-Pain® [OTC] *see* Ibuprofen *on page 447*

Achromycin® *see* Tetracycline *on page 829*

Achromycin® V *see* Tetracycline *on page 829*

Aciclovir (Mexico) *see* Acyclovir *on next page*

Acidulated Phosphate Fluoride *see* Fluoride *on page 374*

A-Cillin® *see* Amoxicillin Trihydrate *on page 58*

Aclovate® *see* Alclometasone Dipropionate *on page 28*

Acrivastine and Pseudoephedrine

(ak' ri vas teen & soo doe e fed' rin)

Brand Names Semprex-D®

Therapeutic Category Antihistamine/Decongestant Combination

Use Temporary relief of nasal congestion, decongest sinus openings, running nose, itching of nose or throat, and itchy, watery eyes due to hay fever or other upper respiratory allergies

Usual Dosage Adults: 1 capsule 3-4 times/day
  Dosing comments in renal impairment: Do not use

Mechanism of Action Acrivastine is an analogue of triprolidine and it is considered to be relatively less sedating than traditional antihistamines; believed to involve competitive blockade of H_1-receptor sites resulting in the inability of histamine to combine with its receptor sites and exert its usual effects on target cells

Pseudoephedrine: Directly stimulates alpha-adrenergic receptors of respiratory mucosa causing vasoconstriction; directly stimulates beta-adrenergic receptors causing bronchial relaxation, increased heart rate and contractility

Local Anesthetic/Vasoconstrictor Precautions Use with caution since pseudoephedrine is a sympathomimetic amine which could interact with epinephrine to cause a pressor response

Effects on Dental Treatment Up to 10% of patients could experience tachycardia, palpitations, and dry mouth; use vasoconstrictor with caution

Other Adverse Effects
>10%: Central nervous system: Drowsiness, headache
1% to 10%:
  Cardiovascular: Tachycardia, palpitations
  Central nervous system: Nervousness, dizziness, insomnia, vertigo, lightheadedness, fatigue, weakness

Gastrointestinal: Nausea, vomiting, dry mouth, diarrhea
Genitourinary: Difficult urination
Respiratory: Pharyngitis, cough increase
Miscellaneous: Diaphoresis
<1%:
Endocrine & metabolic: Dysmenorrhea
Gastrointestinal: Dyspepsia
Drug Interactions Increased toxicity with MAO inhibitors (hypertensive crisis) sympathomimetics, CNS depressants, alcohol (sedation)
Pregnancy Risk Factor B

ACT *see* Dactinomycin *on page 248*

ACT® **[OTC]** *see* Fluoride *on page 374*

Actagen® **[OTC]** *see* Triprolidine and Pseudoephedrine *on page 878*

Actagen-C® *see* Triprolidine, Pseudoephedrine, and Codeine *on page 879*

ACTH® *see* Corticotropin *on page 233*

Acthar® *see* Corticotropin *on page 233*

Actidose-Aqua® **[OTC]** *see* Charcoal *on page 179*

Actidose® **With Sorbitol [OTC]** *see* Charcoal *on page 179*

Actifed® **[OTC]** *see* Triprolidine and Pseudoephedrine *on page 878*

Actifed® **With Codeine** *see* Triprolidine, Pseudoephedrine, and Codeine *on page 879*

Actigall™ *see* Ursodiol *on page 887*

Actimmune® *see* Interferon Gamma-1B *on page 465*

Actinex® *see* Masoprocol *on page 526*

Actinomycin D *see* Dactinomycin *on page 248*

Actisite® *see* Tetracycline Periodontal Fibers *on page 830*

Activase® *see* Alteplase *on page 37*

Acutrim® Precision Release® **[OTC]** *see* Phenylpropanolamine Hydrochloride *on page 687*

Acyclovir (ay sye' kloe veer)
Related Information
Oral Viral Infections *on page 951*
Systemic Viral Diseases *on page 934*
Brand Names Zovirax®
Canadian/Mexican Brand Names Avirax® (Canada); Acifur® (Mexico)
Therapeutic Category Antiviral Agent, Oral; Antiviral Agent, Parenteral; Antiviral Agent, Topical
Synonyms Aciclovir (Mexico)
Use
Dental: Treatment of initial and prophylaxis of recurrent mucosal and cutaneous herpes simplex (HSV-1 and HSV-2) infections
Medical: In medicine, herpes simplex encephalitis, herpes zoster, genital herpes infection, varicella-zoster infections in healthy, nonpregnant persons >13 years of age, children <12 months of age who have a chronic skin or lung disorder or are receiving long-term aspirin therapy, and immunocompromised patients; for herpes zoster, acyclovir should be started within 72 hours of the appearance of the rash to be effective; acyclovir will not prevent postherpetic neuralgias
Usual Dosage
Dosing weight should be based on the smaller of lean body weight or total body weight
Adult determination of lean body weight (LBW) in kg:
LBW males: 50 kg + (2.3 kg x inches >5 feet)
LBW females: 45 kg + (2.3 kg x inches >5 feet)
Treatment of herpes simplex virus infections: I.V.
Children and Adults:
Mucocutaneous HSV infection 750 mg/m²/day divided every 8 hours or 5 mg/kg/dose every 8 hours for 5-10 days
HSV encephalitis: 1500 mg/m²/day divided every 8 hours for 5-10 days
I.V.: 5 mg/kg/dose every 8 hours for 5-10 days
Treatment of herpes simplex virus infections: Adults:
Oral: Treatment: 200 mg every 4 hours while awake (5 times/day)
Topical: ¹/₂" ribbon of ointment for a 4" square surface area every 3 hours (6 times/day)
Treatment of varicella-zoster virus (chickenpox) infections:
Oral:
Adults: 600-800 mg/dose every 4 hours while awake (5 times/day) for 7-10 days or 1000 mg every 6 hours for 5 days

(Continued)

Acyclovir *(Continued)*

Children: 10-20 mg/kg/dose (up to 800 mg) 4 times/day for 5 days; begin treatment within the first 24 hours of rash onset

I.V.: Children and Adults: 1500 mg/m^2/day divided every 8 hours or 10 mg/kg/dose every 8 hours for 7 days

Treatment of herpes zoster infections:

Oral:

Adults (immunocompromised): 800 mg every 4 hours (5 times/day) for 7-10 days

Children (immunocompromised): 250-600 mg/m^2/dose 4-5 times/day for 7-10 days

I.V.: Children and Adults (immunocompromised): 7.5 mg/kg/dose every 8 hours

Prophylaxis in immunocompromised patients:

Varicella zoster or herpes zoster in HIV-positive patients: Adults: Oral: 400 mg every 4 hours (5 times/day) for 7-10 days

Bone marrow transplant recipients: Children and Adults: I.V.:

Autologous patients who are HSV seropositive: 150 mg/m^2/dose (5 mg/kg) every 12 hours; with clinical symptoms of herpes simplex: 150 mg/m^2/dose every 8 hours

Autologous patients who are CMV seropositive: 500 mg/m^2/dose (10 mg/kg) every 8 hours; for clinically symptomatic CMV infection, consider replacing acyclovir with ganciclovir

Prophylaxis of herpes simplex virus infections: Adults: 200 mg 3-4 times/day or 400 mg twice daily

Mechanism of Action Inhibits DNA synthesis and viral replication by competing with deoxyguanosine triphosphate for viral DNA polymerase and incorporation into viral DNA

Local Anesthetic/Vasoconstrictor Precautions No information available to require special precautions

Effects on Dental Treatment No effects or complications reported

Other Adverse Effects

Systemic: 1% to 10%:

Central nervous system: Lethargy, dizziness, seizures, confusion, agitation, coma, headache

Dermatologic: Rash

Gastrointestinal: Nausea, vomiting

Neuromuscular & skeletal: Tremor

Renal: Elevated creatinine

Oral manifestations: No data reported

Contraindications Hypersensitivity to acyclovir

Warnings/Precautions

Systemic: Use with caution in patients with pre-existing renal disease or in those receiving other nephrotoxic drugs concurrently; use with caution in patients with underlying neurologic abnormalities, serious hepatic or electrolyte abnormalities, or substantial hypoxia

Topical: No data reported

Drug Interactions Systemic: Increased CNS side effects with zidovudine and probenecid

Drug Uptake

Absorption: Oral: 15% to 30%

Time to peak serum concentration:

Oral: 1.5-2 hours

I.V.: Within 1 hour

Serum half-life:

Adults: 3.3 hours

Children 1-12 years: 2-3 hours

Influence of food: Does not appear to affect absorption

Pregnancy Risk Factor C

Breast-feeding Considerations May be taken while breast-feeding

Dosage Forms

Capsule: 200 mg

Injection: 500 mg (10 mL); 1000 mg (20 mL)

Ointment, topical: 5% [50 mg/g] (3 g, 15 g)

Suspension, oral (banana flavor): 40 mg/mL

Tablet: 800 mg

Dietary Considerations May be taken with food

Generic Available No

Adagen™ *see* Pegademase Bovine *on page 662*

Adalat® *see* Nifedipine *on page 619*
Adalat® CC *see* Nifedipine *on page 619*

Adapalene (a dap′ a leen)
Brand Names Differin®
Therapeutic Category Acne Products
Use Topical treatment of acne vulgaris
Usual Dosage Topical: Adults: Apply once daily, before retiring, in a thin film to affected areas after washing
Mechanism of Action Retinoids act through one of the known high affinity binding proteins for retinoic acid. The activity of adapalene in the epidermis appears to be mediated mainly by its specific binding to b and g nuclear retinoic acid receptors (RARs). This binding profile differs from tretinoin, which binds to a, b and g RARs. Furthermore, unlike tretinoin, adapalene does not bind to cellular retinoic acid binding proteins (CRABPs) or to nuclear retinoid X receptors. The relevance to therapeutic efficacy of these differences between retinoids is not yet fully understood. However, future research will probably result in other novel retinoids, each with distinct advantages for treating particular diseases based upon receptor-specific targeting.
Local Anesthetic/Vasoconstrictor Precautions No information available to require special precautions
Effects on Dental Treatment No effects or complications reported
Generic Available No

Adapin® *see* Doxepin Hydrochloride *on page 298*
Adeflor® *see* Vitamins, Multiple *on page 901*
Adenocard® *see* Adenosine *on this page*
Adenoscan® *see* Adenosine *on this page*

Adenosine (a den′ oh seen)
Brand Names Adenocard®; Adenoscan®
Therapeutic Category Antiarrhythmic Agent (Supraventricular); Antiarrhythmic Agent, Miscellaneous
Synonyms 9-Beta-D-ribofuranosyladenine
Use Treatment of paroxysmal supraventricular tachycardia (PSVT)
Usual Dosage Rapid I.V. push (over 1-2 seconds) via peripheral line:
Children: Pediatric advanced life support (PALS): Treatment of SVT: 0.1 mg/kg; if not effective, give 0.2 mg/kg
Alternatively: Initial dose: 0.05 mg/kg; if not effective within 2 minutes, increase dose by 0.05 mg/kg increments every 2 minutes to a maximum dose of 0.25 mg/kg or until termination of PSVT; medium dose required: 0.15 mg/kg
Maximum single dose: 12 mg

Adults: 6 mg; if not effective within 1-2 minutes, 12 mg may be given; may repeat 12 mg bolus if needed
Maximum single dose: 12 mg

Note: Patients who are receiving concomitant theophylline therapy may be less likely to respond to adenosine therapy
Note: Higher doses may be needed for administration via peripheral versus central vein
Mechanism of Action Slows conduction time through the A-V node, interrupting the re-entry pathways through the A-V node, restoring normal sinus rhythm
Local Anesthetic/Vasoconstrictor Precautions No information available to require special precautions
Effects on Dental Treatment No effects or complications reported
Other Adverse Effects
>10%:
Cardiovascular: Flushing of face, arrhythmias, palpitations
Respiratory: Shortness of breath, dyspnea
1% to 10%:
Cardiovascular: Chest pain
Central nervous system: Dizziness, numbness or tingling in arms
Gastrointestinal: Nausea
Respiratory: Cough
<1%:
Cardiovascular: Hypotension, hypoventilation
Central nervous system: Lightheadedness, headache, dizziness, apprehension
Dermatologic: Burning sensation
(Continued)

Adenosine *(Continued)*

Gastrointestinal: Nausea, metallic taste
Neuromuscular & skeletal: Heaviness in arms, neck and back pain
Ocular: Blurred vision
Miscellaneous: Sweating, tightness in throat, pressure in head, groin, and chest

Drug Uptake

Duration: Very brief
Serum half-life: <10 seconds, thus adverse effects are usually rapidly self-limiting

Pregnancy Risk Factor C

Comments Short action an advantage; not effective in atrial flutter, atrial fibrillation, or ventricular tachycardia

Adipex-P® *see* Phentermine Hydrochloride *on page 683*

Adlone® *see* Methylprednisolone *on page 569*

ADR *see* Doxorubicin Hydrochloride *on page 299*

Adrenalin® *see* Epinephrine (Dental) *on page 313*

Adriamycin® PFS *see* Doxorubicin Hydrochloride *on page 299*

Adriamycin® RDF *see* Doxorubicin Hydrochloride *on page 299*

Adrucil® Injection *see* Fluorouracil *on page 376*

Adsorbocarpine® *see* Pilocarpine *on page 691*

Adsorbotear® Ophthalmic Solution [OTC] *see* Artificial Tears *on page 75*

Advil® [OTC] *see* Ibuprofen *on page 447*

Advil® Cold & Sinus Caplets [OTC] *see* Pseudoephedrine and Ibuprofen *on page 750*

Aeroaid® [OTC] *see* Thimerosal *on page 838*

AeroBid® *see* Flunisolide *on page 372*

AeroBid-M® *see* Flunisolide *on page 372*

Aerolate® *see* Theophylline/Aminophylline *on page 832*

Aerolate III® *see* Theophylline/Aminophylline *on page 832*

Aerolate JR® *see* Theophylline/Aminophylline *on page 832*

Aerolate SR® S *see* Theophylline/Aminophylline *on page 832*

Aerosporin® *see* Polymyxin B Sulfate *on page 704*

AeroZoin® [OTC] *see* Benzoin *on page 104*

Afrin® Nasal Solution [OTC] *see* Oxymetazoline Hydrochloride *on page 649*

Afrinol® [OTC] *see* Pseudoephedrine *on page 749*

Aftate® [OTC] *see* Tolnaftate *on page 855*

AgNO₃ *see* Silver Nitrate *on page 787*

AHA *see* Acetohydroxamic Acid *on page 20*

AHF *see* Antihemophilic Factor (Human) *on page 68*

Akarpine® *see* Pilocarpine *on page 691*

AKBeta® *see* Levobunolol Hydrochloride *on page 493*

AK-Chlor® *see* Chloramphenicol *on page 182*

AK-Con® *see* Naphazoline Hydrochloride *on page 605*

AK-Dilate® Ophthalmic Solution *see* Phenylephrine Hydrochloride *on page 685*

AK-Homatropine® Ophthalmic *see* Homatropine Hydrobromide *on page 426*

Akineton® *see* Biperiden *on page 113*

AK-Nefrin® Ophthalmic Solution *see* Phenylephrine Hydrochloride *on page 685*

Akne-Mycin® Topical *see* Erythromycin, Topical *on page 324*

AK-Neo-Dex® Ophthalmic *see* Neomycin and Dexamethasone *on page 609*

AK-Pentolate® *see* Cyclopentolate Hydrochloride *on page 240*

AK-Poly-Bac® *see* Bacitracin and Polymyxin B *on page 94*

AK-Pred® *see* Prednisolone *on page 718*

AK-Spore® *see* Bacitracin, Neomycin, and Polymyxin B *on page 94*

AK-Spore H.C.® Ophthalmic Ointment *see* Bacitracin, Neomycin, Polymyxin B, and Hydrocortisone *on page 95*

AK-Spore H.C.® Ophthalmic Suspension *see* Neomycin, Polymyxin B, and Hydrocortisone *on page 610*

AK-Spore H.C.® Otic *see* Neomycin, Polymyxin B, and Hydrocortisone *on page 610*

AK-Spore® Ophthalmic Solution *see* Neomycin, Polymyxin B, and Gramicidin *on page 610*

AK-Sulf® *see* Sodium Sulfacetamide *on page 793*

AK-Taine® *see* Proparacaine Hydrochloride *on page 737*

AK-Tracin® *see* Bacitracin *on page 93*

AK-Trol® *see* Neomycin, Polymyxin B, and Dexamethasone *on page 610*

Akwa Tears® **Solution [OTC]** *see* Artificial Tears *on page 75*

AK-Zol® *see* Acetazolamide *on page 18*

Ala-Quin® **Topical** *see* Clioquinol and Hydrocortisone *on page 216*

Alazide® *see* Hydrochlorothiazide and Spironolactone *on page 431*

Albalon-A® **Ophthalmic** *see* Naphazoline and Antazoline *on page 604*

Albalon® **Liquifilm**® *see* Naphazoline Hydrochloride *on page 605*

Albendazole (al ben' da zole)

Brand Names Albenza®

Therapeutic Category Anthelmintic

Use Treatment of parenchymal neurocysticercosis and cystic hydatid disease of the liver, lung, and peritoneum; albendazole may also be useful in the treatment of ascariasis, trichuriasis, enterobiasis, hook worm, strongyloidiasis, giardiasis, and microsporidiosis in AIDS

Usual Dosage Oral:

Children ≤2 years:

Neurocysticercosis: 15 mg/kg for 8 days; repeat as necessary

Hook worm, pin worm, round worm: 200 mg as a single dose may be repeated in 3 weeks

Strongyloidiasis and tape worm: 200 mg/day for 3 days, may repeat in 3 weeks

Children >2 years and Adults:

Hydatid disease: 800-1200 mg/day in divided doses for 28 days followed by a 2-week drug-free period, then repeated for a duration of therapy ranging from 1-12 months determined by the size, number, and location of cysts

Neurocysticercosis: 15 mg/kg for 8-30 days and repeat the cycle as necessary

Round worm, pin worm, hook worm: 400 mg as a single dose; treatment may be repeated in 3 weeks

Giardiasis: Strongyloidiasis and tape worm: 400 mg/day for 3 days; treatment may be repeated in 3 weeks (giardiasis is a single course)

Mechanism of Action Albendazole appears to cause selective degeneration of cytoplasmic microtubules in intestinal and tegmental cells of intestinal helminths, and larvae; glycogen is depleted, glucose uptake and cholinesterase secretion are impaired, and desecratory substances accumulate intracellularly. ATP production decreases causing energy depletion, immobilization, and worm death.

Local Anesthetic/Vasoconstrictor Precautions No information available to require special precautions

Effects on Dental Treatment No effects or complications reported

Other Adverse Effects (Percentages of occurrence were not available for all adverse effects at the time of this writing)

Central nervous system: Dizziness, headache, fever

Dermatologic: Alopecia, rash, pruritus

Gastrointestinal: Abdominal pain, anorexia, constipation, diarrhea, dry mouth, epigastric pain, nausea, vomiting

Hematologic: Eosinophilia, neutropenia

Hepatic: Increased LFTs, jaundice

Warnings/Precautions Corticosteroids should be administered 1-2 days before albendazole therapy in patients with neurocysticercosis to minimize inflammatory reactions

Drug Interactions Carbamazepine may accelerate albendazole metabolism; dexamethasone increases plasma levels of albendazole metabolites

Drug Uptake

Absorption: Oral absorption is poor (<5%); may increase up to 4.5 times when administered with a fatty meal; albendazole itself is essentially undetectable in plasma; albendazole sulfoxide is probably the active agent

Serum half-life: ~8.5 hours

Pregnancy Risk Factor X

Generic Available No

Selected Readings

Liu LX and Weller PF, "Antiparasitic Drugs," *N Engl J Med*, 1996, 334:1178-84.

Albenza® *see* Albendazole *on this page*

Albuterol (al byoo' ter ole)

Related Information

Respiratory Diseases *on page 924*

(Continued)

Albuterol *(Continued)*

Brand Names Proventil®; Ventolin®; Volmax®

Canadian/Mexican Brand Names Apo-Salvent® (Canada); Novo-Salmol® (Canada); Sabulin® (Canada); Volmax® (Canada); Salbulin® (Mexico); Salbutalan® (Mexico)

Therapeutic Category Adrenergic Agonist Agent; Antiasthmatic; Beta-2-Adrenergic Agonist Agent; Bronchodilator

Synonyms Salbutamol (Mexico)

Use Bronchodilator in reversible airway obstruction due to asthma or COPD

Usual Dosage

Oral:

Children:

2-6 years: 0.1-0.2 mg/kg/dose 3 times/day; maximum dose not to exceed 12 mg/day (divided doses)

6-12 years: 2 mg/dose 3-4 times/day; maximum dose not to exceed 24 mg/day (divided doses)

Children >12 years and Adults: 2-4 mg/dose 3-4 times/day; maximum dose not to exceed 32 mg/day (divided doses)

Elderly: 2 mg 3-4 times/day; maximum: 8 mg 4 times/day

Inhalation MDI: 90 mcg/spray:

Children <12 years: 1-2 inhalations 4 times/day using a tube spacer

Children ≥12 years and Adults: 1-2 inhalations every 4-6 hours; maximum: 12 inhalations/day

Exercise-induced bronchospasm: 2 inhalations 15 minutes before exercising

Inhalation: Nebulization: 2.5 mg = 0.5 mL of the 0.5% inhalation solution to be diluted in 1-2.5 mL of NS **or** 0.01-0.05 mL/kg of 0.5% solution every 4-6 hours; intensive care patients may require more frequent administration; minimum dose: 0.1 mL; maximum dose: 1 mL diluted in 1-2 mL normal saline

<5 years: 1.25-2.5 mg every 4-6 hours as needed

>5 years: 2.5-5 mg every 4-6 hours as needed

Hemodialysis effects: Not removed by hemodialysis

Mechanism of Action Relaxes bronchial smooth muscle by action on beta$_2$-adrenergic receptors with little effect on heart rate

Local Anesthetic/Vasoconstrictor Precautions No information available to require special precautions

Effects on Dental Treatment No effects or complications reported

Other Adverse Effects

>10%:

Cardiovascular: Tachycardia, palpitations, pounding heartbeat

Gastrointestinal: GI upset, nausea

1% to 10%:

Cardiovascular: Flushing of face, hypertension or hypotension

Central nervous system: Nervousness, CNS stimulation, hyperactivity, insomnia, dizziness, lightheadedness, drowsiness, headache, weakness

Gastrointestinal: Dry mouth, heartburn, vomiting, unusual taste

Genitourinary: Difficult urination

Neuromuscular & skeletal: Muscle cramping, tremor

Respiratory: Coughing

Miscellaneous: Increased sweating

<1%:

Neuromuscular & skeletal: Chest pain

Respiratory: Paradoxical bronchospasm

Miscellaneous: Loss of appetite, unusual paleness

Drug Interactions Increased toxicity: Cardiovascular effects are potentiated in patients also receiving MAO inhibitors, tricyclic antidepressants, sympathomimetic agents (eg, amphetamine, dopamine, dobutamine), inhaled anesthetics (eg, enflurane)

Drug Uptake

Time to peak: 2-3 hours

Duration of action: 4-6 hours

Serum half-life: 2.7-5 hours

Pregnancy Risk Factor C

Alcaine® *see* Proparacaine Hydrochloride *on page 737*

Alclometasona (Mexico) *see* Alclometasone Dipropionate *on this page*

Alclometasone Dipropionate

(al kloe met' a sone dye pro' pee oh nate)

Brand Names Aclovate®

Canadian/Mexican Brand Names Logoderm® (Mexico)

Therapeutic Category Corticosteroid, Topical (Low Potency)

Synonyms Alclometasona (Mexico)

Use Treats inflammation of corticosteroid-responsive dermatosis (low potency topical corticosteroid)

Usual Dosage Topical: Apply a thin film to the affected area 2-3 times/day

Mechanism of Action Stimulates the synthesis of enzymes needed to decrease inflammation, suppress mitotic activity, and cause vasoconstriction

Local Anesthetic/Vasoconstrictor Precautions No information available to require special precautions

Effects on Dental Treatment No effects or complications reported

Other Adverse Effects

1% to 10%: Topical: Itching, burning, erythema, dryness, irritation, papular rashes

<1%: Topical: Hypertrichosis, acneiform eruptions, hypopigmentation, perioral dermatitis, maceration of skin, skin atrophy, striae, miliaria

Drug Interactions No data reported

Pregnancy Risk Factor C

Alconefrin® Nasal Solution [OTC] see Phenylephrine Hydrochloride on page 685

Aldactazide® see Hydrochlorothiazide and Spironolactone on page 431

Aldactone® see Spironolactone on page 798

Aldesleukin (al des loo' kin)

Brand Names Proleukin®

Therapeutic Category Antineoplastic Agent, Miscellaneous; Biological Response Modulator

Synonyms IL-2; Interleukin-2

Use Primarily investigated in tumors known to have a response to immunotherapy, such as melanoma and renal cell carcinoma; has been used in conjunction with LAK cells, TIL cells, IL-1, and interferon

Usual Dosage All orders should be written in million International units (million IU) (refer to individual protocols)

Adults: Metastatic renal cell carcinoma:

Treatment consists of two 5-day treatment cycles separated by a rest period. 600,000 units/kg (0.037 mg/kg)/dose administered every 8 hours by a 15-minute I.V. infusion for a total of 14 doses; following 9 days of rest, the schedule is repeated for another 14 doses, for a maximum of 28 doses per course.

Investigational regimen: I.V. continuous infusion: 4.5 million units/m²/day in 250-1000 mL of D_5W for 5 days

Dose modification: Hold or interrupt a dose rather than reducing dose; refer to protocol

Retreatment: Patients should be evaluated for response ~4 weeks after completion of a course of therapy and again immediately prior to the scheduled start of the next treatment course. Additional courses of treatment may be given to patients only if there is some tumor shrinkage following the last course and retreatment is not contraindicated. Each treatment course should be separated by a rest period of at least 7 weeks from the date of hospital discharge. Tumors have continued to regress up to 12 months following the initiation of therapy.

Mechanism of Action IL-2 promotes proliferation, differentiation, and recruitment of T and B cells, natural killer (NK) cells, and thymocytes; IL-2 also causes cytolytic activity in a subset of lymphocytes and subsequent interactions between the immune system and malignant cells; IL-2 can stimulate lymphokine-activated killer (LAK) cells and tumor-infiltrating lymphocytes (TIL) cells. LAK cells (which are derived from lymphocytes from a patient and incubated in IL-2) have the ability to lyse cells which are resistant to NK cells; TIL cells (which are derived from cancerous tissue from a patient and incubated in IL-2) have been shown to be 50% more effective than LAK cells.

Local Anesthetic/Vasoconstrictor Precautions No information available to require special precautions

Effects on Dental Treatment No effects or complications reported

Other Adverse Effects

>10%:

Cardiovascular: Hypotension, dizziness, sensory dysfunction, sinus tachycardia, arrhythmias, pulmonary congestion

Dermatological: Pruritus, erythema, rash, dry skin, exfoliative dermatitis

Gastrointestinal: Nausea, vomiting, fever, chills, pain, fatigue, weakness, malaise, edema, weight gain, diarrhea, stomatitis, anorexia, GI bleeding

(Continued)

Aldesleukin *(Continued)*

Hematological: Anemia, thrombocytopenia, leukopenia, coagulation disorders; elevated bilirubin, BUN, serum creatinine, transaminase, and alkaline phosphatase; hypomagnesemia, acidosis, hypocalcemia, hypophosphatemia

Neurological: Mental status changes

Pulmonary: Dyspnea, pulmonary edema, jaundice

Renal: Oliguria, anuria, proteinuria

1% to 10%:

Cardiovascular: Bradycardia, premature ventricular contractions (PVCs), myocardial ischemia, myocardial infarction, cardiac arrest, syncope

Central nervous system: Sensory disorders

Dermatologic: Purpura

Endocrine & metabolic: Hypokalemia, hypoproteinemia, hyponatremia, alkalosis, hypocholesterolemia

Gastrointestinal: Dyspepsia, constipation, weight loss

Hepatic: Ascites

Hematologic: Leukocytosis, eosinophilia

Local: Injection site reactions

Neuromuscular & skeletal: Arthralgia, myalgia

Renal: Hematuria, renal impairment

Respiratory: Respiratory failure, tachypnea, wheezing

<1%:

Cardiovascular: Congestive heart failure

Central nervous system: Coma, seizures

Dermatologic: Alopecia

Endocrine & metabolic: Hypothyroidism, hypercalcemia

Gastrointestinal: Pancreatitis

Genitourinary: Urinary frequency

Neuromuscular & skeletal: Arthritis, muscle spasm

Miscellaneous: Allergic reactions

Drug Uptake

Absorption: Oral: Not absorbed

Serum half-life:

Initial: 6-13 minutes

Terminal: 20-120 minutes

Pregnancy Risk Factor C

Comments 22 million units = 1.3 mg

1 Cetus Unit = 6 International Units

1.1 mg = 18×10^6 International Units (or 3×10^6 Cetus Units)

1 Roche Unit (Teceleukin) = 3 International Units

Aldoclor® *see* Chlorothiazide and Methyldopa *on page 188*

Aldomet® *see* Methyldopa *on page 566*

Aldoril® *see* Methyldopa and Hydrochlorothiazide *on page 567*

Alendronate Sodium (a len′ droe nate sow′ dee um)

Brand Names Fosamax®

Therapeutic Category Biphosphonate Derivative

Use Symptomatic treatment of Paget's disease and heterotopic ossification due to spinal cord injury or after total hip replacement, hypercalcemia associated with malignancy

Usual Dosage Oral:

Adults: Patients with osteoporosis or Paget's disease should receive supplemental calcium and vitamin D if dietary intake is inadequate

Osteoporosis in postmenopausal women: 10 mg once daily. Safety of treatment for >4 years has not been studied (extension studies are ongoing).

Paget's disease of bone: 40 mg once daily for 6 months

Retreatment: Relapses during the 12 months following therapy occurred in 9% of patients who responded to treatment. Specific retreatment data are not available. Retreatment with alendronate may be considered, following a 6-month post-treatment evaluation period, in patients who have relapsed based on increases in serum alkaline phosphatase, which should be measured periodically. Retreatment may also be considered in those who failed to normalize their serum alkaline phosphatase.

Elderly: No dosage adjustment is necessary

Local Anesthetic/Vasoconstrictor Precautions No information available to require special precautions

Effects on Dental Treatment No effects or complications reported

Other Adverse Effects 1% to 10%:
Gastrointestinal: Abdominal pain, GI disturbances
Neuromuscular & skeletal: Musculoskeletal pain
Drug Uptake
Absorption: Poor from the GI tract; pharmacokinetic studies are lacking

Alersule Forte® *see* Chlorpheniramine, Phenylephrine, and Methscopolamine *on page 193*

Aleve® (Naproxen Sodium) (OTC) *see* Naproxen *on page 606*

Alfenta® *see* Alfentanil Hydrochloride *on this page*

Alfentanil Hydrochloride (al fen' ta nil hye droe klor' ide)
Related Information
Narcotic Agonist Charts *on page 1019*
Brand Names Alfenta®
Canadian/Mexican Brand Names Alfenta® (Canada); Rapifen® (Mexico)
Therapeutic Category Analgesic, Narcotic; General Anesthetic, Intravenous
Use Analgesic adjunct given by continuous infusion or in incremental doses in maintenance of anesthesia with barbiturate or nitrous oxide (NO_2) or a primary anesthetic agent for the induction of anesthesia in patients undergoing general surgery in which endotracheal intubation and mechanical ventilation are required
Usual Dosage Doses should be titrated to appropriate effects; wide range of doses is dependent upon desired degree of analgesia/anesthesia

Children <12 years: Dose not established
Adults: Dose should be based on ideal body weight; see table.

Alfentanil

Indication	Approximate Duration of Anesthesia (min)	Induction Period (Initial Dose) (mcg/kg)	Maintenance Period (Increments/ Infusion)	Total Dose (mcg/kg)	Effects
Incremental injection	≤30	8-20	3-5 mcg/kg or 0.5-1 mcg/kg/ min	8-40	Spontaneously breathing or assisted ventilation when required.
	30-60	20-50	5-15 mcg/kg	Up to 75	Assisted or controlled ventilation required. Attenuation of response to laryngoscopy and intubation.
Continuous infusion	>45	50-75	0.5-3.0 mcg/kg/ min average infusion rate 1-1.5 mcg/kg/min	Dependent on duration of procedure	Assisted or controlled ventilation required. Some attenuation of response to intubation and incision, with intraoperative stability.
Anesthetic induction	>45	130-245	0.5-1.5 mcg/kg/ min or general anesthetic	Dependent on duration of procedure	Assisted or controlled ventilation required. Administer slowly (over three minutes). Concentration of inhalation agents reduced by 30%-50% for initial hour.

Mechanism of Action Binds to opiate receptors (mu and kappa subtypes) in the CNS causing inhibition of ascending pain pathways, altering the perception of and response to pain; produces generalized CNS depression
Local Anesthetic/Vasoconstrictor Precautions No information available to require special precautions
Effects on Dental Treatment Erythromycin inhibits the liver metabolism of alfentanil resulting in increased sedation and prolonged respiratory depression
Other Adverse Effects
Hematologic: Antidiuretic hormone release
Ocular: Miosis
>10%:
Cardiovascular: Bradycardia, peripheral vasodilation
Central nervous system: Drowsiness, sedation, increased intracranial pressure
Gastrointestinal: Nausea, vomiting, constipation
(Continued)

31

Alfentanil Hydrochloride (Continued)

1% to 10%:
  Cardiovascular: Cardiac arrhythmias, orthostatic hypotension
  Central nervous system: Confusion, CNS depression
  Ocular: Blurred vision
<1%:
  Central nervous system: Convulsions, mental depression, paradoxical CNS
    excitation or delirium, dizziness, dysesthesia
  Dermatologic: Skin rash, hives, itching
  Respiratory: Respiratory depression, bronchospasm, laryngospasm
  Miscellaneous: Physical and psychological dependence with prolonged use,
    cold, clammy skin, biliary or urinary tract spasm

Drug Interactions Increased toxicity: CNS depressants (eg, benzodiazepines,
barbiturates, phenothiazines, tricyclic antidepressants), erythromycin, reserpine, beta-blockers

Drug Uptake
  Serum half-life: Adults: 83-97 minutes

Pregnancy Risk Factor C

Selected Readings
  Bartkowski RR, Goldberg ME, Larijani GE, et al, "Inhibition of Alfentanil Metabolism by
    Erythromycin," *Clin Pharmacol Ther*, 1989, 46(1):99-102.
  Bartkowski RR and McDonnell TE, "Prolonged Alfentanil Effect Following Erythromycin
    Administration," *Anesthesiology*, 1990, 73(3):566-8.

Alferon® N *see* Interferon Alfa-N3 *on page 463*

Alglucerase (al gloo′ ser ase)

Brand Names Ceredase® Injection

Therapeutic Category Enzyme, Glucocerebrosidase

Synonyms Glucocerebrosidase

Use Long-term enzyme replacement in patients with confirmed Type I
Gaucher's disease who exhibit one or more of the following conditions:
Moderate to severe anemia; thrombocytopenia and bleeding tendencies; bone
disease; hepatomegaly or splenomegaly

Usual Dosage Usually administered as a 20-60 units/kg I.V. infusion given with
a frequency ranging from 3 times/week to once every 2 weeks

Mechanism of Action Glucocerebrosidase is an enzyme prepared from
human placental tissue. Gaucher's disease is an inherited metabolic disorder
caused by the defective activity of beta-glucosidase and the resultant accumulation of glucosyl ceramide laden macrophages in the liver, bone, and spleen;
acts by replacing the missing enzyme associated with Gaucher's disease.

Local Anesthetic/Vasoconstrictor Precautions No information available to
require special precautions

Effects on Dental Treatment No effects or complications reported

Other Adverse Effects These reactions do not normally require discontinua-
tion of therapy
>10%: Local: Discomfort, burning, and swelling at the site of injection
<1%:
  Central nervous system: Fever, chills
  Gastrointestinal: Abdominal discomfort, nausea, vomiting

Pregnancy Risk Factor C

Comments Injection should be diluted in 0.9% sodium chloride injection to a
final volume ≤100 mL.

Alkaban-AQ® *see* Vinblastine Sulfate *on page 895*

Alka-Mints® [OTC] *see* Calcium Carbonate *on page 140*

Alka-Seltzer® Plus Cold Liqui-Gels Capsules [OTC] *see* Acetaminophen, Chlorpheniramine, and Pseudoephedrine *on page 17*

Alkeran® *see* Melphalan *on page 536*

Allbee® With C [OTC] *see* Vitamin B Complex With Vitamin C *on page 900*

Allbee® With C *see* Vitamins, Multiple *on page 901*

Allegra® *see* Fexofenadine Hydrochloride *on page 361*

Aller-Chlor® [OTC] *see* Chlorpheniramine Maleate *on page 191*

Allerest® 12 Hour Capsule [OTC] *see* Chlorpheniramine and Phenylpropanolamine *on page 190*

Allerest® 12 Hour Nasal Solution [OTC] *see* Oxymetazoline Hydrochloride *on
page 649*

Allerest® Eye Drops [OTC] *see* Naphazoline Hydrochloride *on page 605*

Allerest® Maximum Strength [OTC] *see* Chlorpheniramine and Pseudoephedrine
on page 191

Allerfrin® [OTC] *see* Triprolidine and Pseudoephedrine *on page 878*

Allerfrin® w/Codeine *see* Triprolidine, Pseudoephedrine, and Codeine *on page 879*

Allergan® Ear Drops *see* Antipyrine and Benzocaine *on page 70*

Allergic Skin Reactions to Drugs *see page 1076*

AllerMax® [OTC] *see* Diphenhydramine Hydrochloride *on page 288*

Allerphed® [OTC] *see* Triprolidine and Pseudoephedrine *on page 878*

Allopurinol (al oh pure' i nole)

Brand Names Zyloprim®

Canadian/Mexican Brand Names Apo-Allopurinol® (Canada); Novo-purol® (Canada); Purinol® (Canada); Atisuril® (Mexico); Unizuric® 300 (Mexico)

Therapeutic Category Uric Acid Lowering Agent; Uricosuric Agent

Synonyms Alopurinol (Mexico)

Use Prevention of attacks of gouty arthritis and nephropathy; also used to treat secondary hyperuricemia which may occur during treatment of tumors or leukemia; prevent recurrent calcium oxalate calculi

Usual Dosage Oral:

Children ≤10 years: 10 mg/kg/day in 2-3 divided doses **or** 200-300 mg/m^2/day in 2-4 divided doses, maximum: 800 mg/24 hours

Alternative:

<6 years: 150 mg/day in 3 divided doses

6-10 years: 300 mg/day in 2-3 divided doses

Children >10 years and Adults: Daily doses >300 mg should be administered in divided doses

Myeloproliferative neoplastic disorders: 600-800 mg/day in 2-3 divided doses for prevention of acute uric acid nephropathy for 2-3 days starting 1-2 days before chemotherapy

Gout:

Mild: 200-300 mg/day

Severe: 400-600 mg/day

Dosing adjustment in renal impairment: Must be adjusted due to accumulation of allopurinol and metabolites; removed by hemodialysis. See table.

Adult Maintenance Doses of Allopurinol*

Creatinine Clearance (mL/min)	Maintenance Dose of Allopurinol (mg)
140	400 qd
120	350 qd
100	300 qd
80	250 qd
60	200 qd
40	150 qd
20	100 qd
10	100 q2d
0	100 q3d

*This table is based on a standard maintenance dose of 300 mg of allopurinol per day for a patient with a creatinine clearance of 100 mL/min.

Hemodialysis: Administer dose posthemodialysis or administer 50% supplemental dose

Mechanism of Action Allopurinol inhibits xanthine oxidase, the enzyme responsible for the conversion of hypoxanthine to xanthine to uric acid. Allopurinol is metabolized to oxypurinol which is also an inhibitor of xanthine oxidase; allopurinol acts on purine catabolism, reducing the production of uric acid without disrupting the biosynthesis of vital purines.

Local Anesthetic/Vasoconstrictor Precautions No information available to require special precautions

Effects on Dental Treatment No effects or complications reported

Other Adverse Effects

>10%: Dermatologic: Skin rash (usually maculopapular), exfoliative, urticarial or purpuric lesions

1% to 10%:

Central nervous system: Drowsiness, chills, fever

Dermatologic: Alopecia

Gastrointestinal: Nausea, vomiting, diarrhea, abdominal pain, gastritis, dyspepsia

(Continued)

33

Allopurinol *(Continued)*

Hepatic: Increased alkaline phosphatase, AST, and ALT, hepatomegaly, hyperbilirubinemia, and jaundice; hepatic necrosis has been reported

<1%:

Central nervous system: Headache, somnolence, neuritis

Dermatologic: Toxic epidermal necrolysis and Stevens-Johnson syndrome have been reported

Hematologic: Bone marrow depression has been reported in patients receiving allopurinol with other myelosuppressive agents

Idiosyncratic: Reaction characterized by fever, chills, eosinophilia, arthralgia, nausea, and vomiting, leukopenia, leukocytosis

Local: Thrombophlebitis

Neuromuscular & skeletal: Peripheral neuropathy, paresthesia

Ocular: Cataracts

Renal: Renal impairment

Miscellaneous: Epistaxis, vasculitis

Drug Interactions

Decreased effect with alcohol

Increased toxicity:

Allopurinol prolongs half-life of oral anticoagulants

Allopurinol increases serum half-life of theophylline

Allopurinol may compete for excretion in renal tubule with chlorpropamide and increase chlorpropamide's serum half-life

Allopurinol inhibits metabolism of azathioprine and mercaptopurine

Thiazide diuretics enhance toxicity of allopurinol

Use with ampicillin may increase the incidence of skin rash

Urinary acidification with large amounts of vitamin C may increase kidney stone formation

Drug Uptake

Decreases in serum uric acid occur in 1-2 days with nadir achieved in 1-2 weeks

Absorption:

Oral: ~80% of dose absorbed from GI tract; peak plasma concentrations are seen 30-120 minutes after administration

Rectal: Poor and erratic

Serum half-life:

Normal renal function:

Parent drug: 1-3 hours

Oxypurinol: 18-30 hours

Pregnancy Risk Factor C

Alomide® see Lodoxamide Tromethamine *on page 509*

Alophen Pills® [OTC] see Phenolphthalein *on page 682*

Alopurinol (Mexico) see Allopurinol *on previous page*

Alpha₁-PI see Alpha₁-Proteinase Inhibitor, Human *on this page*

Alpha₁-Proteinase Inhibitor, Human

(al fa won pro' tee in ase in hi' bi tor, hyu' min)

Brand Names Prolastin® Injection

Therapeutic Category Antitrypsin Deficiency Agent

Synonyms Alpha₁-PI

Use Congenital alpha₁-antitrypsin deficiency

Usual Dosage Adults: I.V.: 60 mg/kg once weekly (at a rate ≥0.08 mL/kg/minute)

Mechanism of Action Human alpha₁-proteinase inhibitor is prepared from the pooled human plasma of normal donors and is intended for use in the therapy of congenital alpha₁-antitrypsin deficiency. Alpha₁-antitrypsin (AAT) is the principal protease inhibitor in the serum and exists as a single polypeptide glycoprotein. Production of AAT occurs in the liver hepatocyte and secretion occurs at a rate to maintain serum concentrations of 150-200 mg/dL. The major physiologic role of the antiprotease is that of combining with proteolytic enzymes to render them inactive. Several proteases can be inactivated by AAT including trypsin, chymotrypsin, coagulation factor XI, plasmin, thrombin, and neutrophil elastase.

Local Anesthetic/Vasoconstrictor Precautions No information available to require special precautions

Effects on Dental Treatment No effects or complications reported

Other Adverse Effects <1%:

Central nervous system: Dizziness, lightheadedness, fever <102°F (delayed up to 12 hours after treatment)

Hematologic: Leukocytosis

Drug Uptake Serum half-life, elimination (parent compound): 4.5-5.2 days
Pregnancy Risk Factor C
Comments Sodium content of 1 L after reconstitution: 100-210 mEq

Alphagan® *see* Brimonidine Tartrate *on page 121*
Alphamin® *see* Hydroxocobalamin *on page 439*
Alphamul® **[OTC]** *see* Castor Oil *on page 161*
AlphaNine® *see* Factor IX Complex (Human) *on page 350*
Alphatrex® *see* Betamethasone *on page 109*
Alpidine® *see* Apraclonidine Hydrochloride *on page 72*

Alprazolam (al pray′ zoe lam)

Related Information
  Patients Requiring Sedation *on page 965*
  Temporomandibular Dysfunction (TMD) *on page 963*
Brand Names Xanax®
Canadian/Mexican Brand Names Apo-Alpraz® (Canada); Novo-Aloprazol® (Canada); Nu-Alprax® (Canada); Tafil® (Mexico)
Therapeutic Category Antianxiety Agent; Benzodiazepine; Tranquilizer, Minor
Use Treatment of anxiety; adjunct in the treatment of depression; management of panic attacks
Usual Dosage Oral:
  Children <18 years: Safety and dose have not been established
  Adults: 0.25-0.5 mg 2-3 times/day, titrate dose upward; maximum: 4 mg/day
Mechanism of Action Binds at stereospecific receptors at several sites within the central nervous system, including the limbic system, reticular formation; effects may be mediated through GABA
Local Anesthetic/Vasoconstrictor Precautions No information available to require special precautions
Effects on Dental Treatment Significant dry mouth will occur in over 10% of patients; normal salivary flow occurs with cessation of drug therapy
Other Adverse Effects
  >10%:
    Cardiovascular: Tachycardia, chest pain
    Central nervous system: Drowsiness, fatigue, impaired coordination, light-headedness, memory impairment, insomnia, anxiety, depression, headache
    Dermatologic: Rash
    Endocrine & metabolic: Decreased libido
    Gastrointestinal: Dry mouth, constipation, decreased salivation, constipation, nausea, vomiting, diarrhea, increased or decreased appetite
    Neuromuscular & skeletal: Dysarthria
    Ocular: Blurred vision
    Miscellaneous: Sweating
  1% to 10%:
    Cardiovascular: Syncope, hypotension
    Central nervous system: Confusion, nervousness, dizziness, akathisia
    Dermatologic: Dermatitis
    Gastrointestinal: Weight gain or loss
    Neuromuscular & skeletal: Rigidity, tremor, muscle cramps
    Otic: Tinnitus
    Respiratory: Nasal congestion, hyperventilation
    Miscellaneous: Increased salivation
Drug Interactions Alprazolam will produce an additive CNS depressant effect when co-administered with other psychotropic medications, anticonvulsants and antihistamines; the blood level of alprazolam can be increased by cimetidine (Tagamet®) and by oral contraceptives; the clinical significance of this effect is unclear; fluvoxamine (Floxyfral) can increase alprazolam plasma concentrations resulting in increased psychomotor impairment
Drug Uptake
  Serum half-life: 12-15 hours
  Time to peak serum concentration: Within 1-2 hours
Pregnancy Risk Factor D
Dosage Forms Tablet: 0.25 mg, 0.5 mg, 1 mg, 2 mg
Dietary Considerations May be taken with food or water to avoid upset
Generic Available No

Alprostadil (al pross′ ta dil)

Brand Names Caverject® Injection; Prostin VR Pediatric® Injection
Therapeutic Category Prostaglandin
  (Continued)

Alprostadil *(Continued)*

Synonyms PGE$_1$; Prostaglandin E$_1$

Use Temporary maintenance of patency of ductus arteriosus in neonates with ductal-dependent congenital heart disease until surgery can be performed. These defects include cyanotic (eg, pulmonary atresia, pulmonary stenosis, tricuspid atresia, Fallot's tetralogy, transposition of the great vessels) and acyanotic (eg, interruption of aortic arch, coarctation of aorta, hypoplastic left ventricle) heart disease.

Investigationally used for the treatment of pulmonary hypertension in infants and children with congenital heart defects with left-to-right shunts

Usual Dosage

Patent ductus arteriosus (Prostin VR Pediatric®):

I.V. continuous infusion into a large vein, or alternatively through an umbilical artery catheter placed at the ductal opening: 0.05-0.1 mcg/kg/minute with therapeutic response, rate is reduced to lowest effective dosage; with unsatisfactory response, rate is increased gradually; maintenance: 0.01-0.4 mcg/kg/minute

PGE$_1$ is usually given at an infusion rate of 0.1 mcg/kg/minute, but it is often possible to reduce the dosage to $^1/_2$ or even $^1/_{10}$ without losing the therapeutic effect. The mixing schedule is shown in the table.

Add 1 Ampul (500 mcg) to:	Concentration (mcg/mL)	Infusion Rate	
		mL/min/kg Needed to Infuse 0.1 mcg/kg/min	mL/kg/24 h
250 mL	2	0.05	72
100 mL	5	0.02	28.8
50 mL	10	0.01	14.4
25 mL	20	0.005	7.2

Therapeutic response is indicated by increased pH in those with acidosis or by an increase in oxygenation (pO$_2$) usually evident within 30 minutes

Erectile dysfunction (Caverject®):

Vasculogenic, psychogenic, or mixed etiology: Individualize dose by careful titration; usual dose: 2.5-60 mcg (doses >60 mcg are not recommended); initiate dosage titration at 2.5 mcg, increasing by 2.5 mcg to a dose of 5 mcg and then in increments of 5-10 mcg depending on the erectile response until the dose produces an erection suitable for intercourse, not lasting >1 hour; if there is absolutely no response to initial 2.5 mcg dose, the second dose may increased to 7.5 mcg, followed by increments of 5-10 mcg

Neurogenic etiology (eg, spinal cord injury): Initiate dosage titration at 1.25 mcg, increasing to a doses of 2.5 mcg and then 5 mcg; increase further in increments 5 mcg until the dose is reached that produces an erection suitable for intercourse, not lasting >1 hour

Note: Patient must stay in the physician's office until complete detumescence occurs; if there is no response, then the next higher dose may be given within 1 hour; if there is still no response, a 1-day interval before giving the next dose is recommended; increasing the dose or concentration in the treatment of impotence results in increasing pain and discomfort

Mechanism of Action Causes vasodilation by means of direct effect on vascular and ductus arteriosus smooth muscle

Local Anesthetic/Vasoconstrictor Precautions No information available to require special precautions

Effects on Dental Treatment No effects or complications reported

Other Adverse Effects

>10%:

Cardiovascular: Flushing

Central nervous system: Fever

Genitourinary: Penile pain

Respiratory: Apnea

1% to 10%:

Cardiovascular: Bradycardia, hypotension, hypertension, tachycardia, cardiac arrest, edema

Central nervous system: Seizures, headache, dizziness

Endocrine & metabolic: Hypokalemia

Gastrointestinal: Diarrhea

Genitourinary: Prolonged erection, penile fibrosis, penis disorder, penile rash, penile edema

Hematologic: Disseminated intravascular coagulation

Local: Injection site hematoma, injection site ecchymosis

Neuromuscular & skeletal: Back pain

Respiratory: Upper respiratory infection, flu syndrome, sinusitis, nasal congestion, cough

Miscellaneous: Sepsis, localized pain in structures other than the injection site

<1%:

Cardiovascular: Cerebral bleeding, congestive heart failure, second degree heart block, shock, supraventricular tachycardia, ventricular fibrillation, hyperemia

Central nervous system: Hyperirritability, hypothermia, jitteriness, lethargy

Endocrine & metabolic: Hypoglycemia, hyperkalemia

Gastrointestinal: Gastric regurgitation

Genitourinary: Anuria, balanitis, urethral bleeding, penile numbness, yeast infection, penile pruritus and erythema, abnormal ejaculation

Hematologic: Anemia, bleeding, thrombocytopenia

Hepatic: Hyperbilirubinemia

Neuromuscular & skeletal: Hyperextension of neck, stiffness

Renal: Hematuria

Respiratory: Bradypnea, bronchial wheezing

Miscellaneous: Peritonitis

Drug Uptake

Serum half-life: 5-10 minutes

Pregnancy Risk Factor X

Comments Therapeutic response is indicated by an increase in systemic blood pressure and pH in those with restricted systemic blood flow and acidosis, or by an increase in oxygenation (pO$_2$) in those with restricted pulmonary blood flow; response usually evident within 30 minutes. Alprostadil has also been used investigationally for the treatment of pulmonary hypertension in infants and children with congenital heart defects with left-to-right shunts. Alprostadil was administered via continuous infusion into the right pulmonary artery.

AL-R® [OTC] *see* Chlorpheniramine Maleate *on page 191*

Altace™ *see* Ramipril *on page 762*

Alteplase (al' te place)

Brand Names Activase®

Canadian/Mexican Brand Names Lysatec-rt-PA® (Canada)

Therapeutic Category Thrombolytic Agent

Use Management of acute myocardial infarction for the lysis of thrombi in coronary arteries; management of acute massive pulmonary embolism (PE) in adults; to improve neurologic recovery and decrease disability in adults following acute ischemic stroke, and most common type of stroke, caused by blood clots that block blood flow, treatment must start within 3 hours of the start of the stroke and only after bleeding in the brain has been ruled out by a cranial computerized tomography (CT) scan

Usual Dosage

Coronary artery thrombi: I.V.: Front loading dose: Total dose is 100 mg over 1.5 hours (for patients who weigh <65 kg, use 1.25 mg/kg/total dose). Add this dose to a 100 mL bag of 0.9% sodium chloride for a total volume of 200 mL. Infuse 15 mg (30 mL) over 1-2 minutes; infuse 50 mg (100 mL) over 30 minutes. Begin heparin 5000-10,000 unit bolus followed by continuous infusion of 1000 units/hour. Infuse 35 mg/hour (70 mL) for next 2 hours.

Acute pulmonary embolism: 100 mg over 2 hours

Mechanism of Action Initiates local fibrinolysis by binding to fibrin in a thrombus (clot) and converts entrapped plasminogen to plasmin

Local Anesthetic/Vasoconstrictor Precautions No information available to require special precautions

Effects on Dental Treatment No effects or complications reported

Other Adverse Effects

1% to 10%:

Cardiovascular: Hypotension

Central nervous system: Fever

Dermatologic: Ecchymosis

Gastrointestinal: GI hemorrhage, nausea, vomiting

Genitourinary: GU hemorrhage

<1%:

Hematologic: Retroperitoneal hemorrhage, gingival hemorrhage, intracranial hemorrhage rapid lysis of coronary artery thrombi by thrombolytic agents

(Continued)

ALPHABETICAL LISTING OF DRUGS

Alteplase (Continued)

    may be associated with reperfusion-related atrial and/or ventricular arrhythmias

    Miscellaneous: Epistaxis

Drug Interactions Increased effect: Anticoagulants, aspirin, ticlopidine, dipyridamole, and heparin are at least additive

Pregnancy Risk Factor C

ALternaGEL® [OTC] see Aluminum Hydroxide *on next page*

Altretamine (al tret' a meen)

Brand Names Hexalen®

Therapeutic Category Antineoplastic Agent, Alkylating Agent

Use Palliative treatment of persistent or recurrent ovarian cancer following first-line therapy with a cisplatin- or alkylating agent-based combination

Usual Dosage Oral (refer to protocol):

  Adults: 4-12 mg/kg/day in 3-4 divided doses for 21-90 days

    Alternatively: 240-320 mg/m²/day in 3-4 divided doses for 21 days, repeated every 6 weeks

    Alternatively: 260 mg/m²/day for 14-21 days of a 28-day cycle in 4 divided doses

  Temporarily discontinue (for ≥14 days) & subsequently restart at 200 mg/m²/day if any of the following occurs:

    if GI intolerance unresponsive to symptom measures

    WBC <2000/mm³

    granulocyte count <1000/mm³

    platelet count <75,000/mm³

    progressive neurotoxicity

Mechanism of Action Although altretamine clinical antitumor spectrum resembles that of alkylating agents, the drug has demonstrated activity in alkylator-resistant patients; probably requires hepatic microsomal mixed-function oxidase enzyme activation to become cytotoxic. The drug selectively inhibits the incorporation of radioactive thymidine and uridine into DNA and RNA, inhibiting DNA and RNA synthesis; metabolized to reactive intermediates which covalently bind to microsomal proteins and DNA. These reactive intermediates can spontaneously degrade to demethylated melamines and formaldehyde which are also cytotoxic.

Local Anesthetic/Vasoconstrictor Precautions No information available to require special precautions

Effects on Dental Treatment No effects or complications reported

Other Adverse Effects

  >10%:

    Central nervous system: Peripheral sensory neuropathy, neurotoxicity

    Gastrointestinal: Nausea, vomiting

    Hematologic: Anemia, thrombocytopenia, leukopenia

  1% to 10%:

    Central nervous system: Seizures

    Gastrointestinal: Anorexia, diarrhea, stomach cramps

    Hepatic: Increased alkaline phosphatase

  <1%:

    Central nervous system: Dizziness, depression

    Dermatologic: Rash, alopecia

    Hematologic: Myelosuppression

    Hepatic: Hepatotoxicity

    Neuromuscular & skeletal: Tremor

Drug Interactions

  Decreased effect: Phenobarbital may increase metabolism of altretamine

  Increased toxicity: May cause severe orthostatic hypotension when administered with MAO inhibitors; cimetidine may decrease metabolism of altretamine

Drug Uptake

  Absorption: Oral: Well absorbed (75% to 89%)

  Serum half-life: 13 hours

  Peak plasma levels: 0.5-3 hours after dose

Pregnancy Risk Factor D

Alu-Cap® [OTC] see Aluminum Hydroxide *on next page*

Aludrox® [OTC] see Aluminum Hydroxide and Magnesium Hydroxide *on page 40*

Aluminio, Hidroxido De (Mexico) see Aluminum Hydroxide *on next page*

38

Aluminum Acetate and Acetic Acid
(a loo' mi num as' e tate & a see' tik as' id)
Brand Names Otic Domeboro®
Therapeutic Category Otic Agent, Anti-infective
Synonyms Acetic Acid and Aluminum Acetate Otic; Burow's Otic
Use Treatment of superficial infections of the external auditory canal
Local Anesthetic/Vasoconstrictor Precautions No information available to require special precautions
Effects on Dental Treatment No effects or complications reported
Other Adverse Effects 1% to 10%: Irritation

Aluminum Carbonate (a loo' mi num kar' bun ate)
Brand Names Basaljel® [OTC]
Therapeutic Category Antacid
Use Hyperacidity; hyperphosphatemia
Local Anesthetic/Vasoconstrictor Precautions No information available to require special precautions
Effects on Dental Treatment Aluminum carbonate prevents gastrointestinal absorption of tetracycline by forming a large ionized chelated molecule with the tetracyclines in the stomach. Aluminum carbonate prevents GI absorption of ketoconazole and itraconazole by increasing the pH in the GI tract. Any of these drugs should be administered at least 1 hour before aluminum carbonate.
Other Adverse Effects
>10%: Gastrointestinal: Constipation, chalky taste, stomach cramps, fecal impaction
1% to 10%: Gastrointestinal: Nausea, vomiting, discoloration of feces (white speckles)
<1%: Endocrine & metabolic: Hypophosphatemia, hypomagnesemia

Aluminum Chloride (a loo' mi num klor' ide)
Brand Names Gingi-Aid® Gingival Retraction Cord; Gingi-Aid® Solution; Hemodent® Gingival Retraction Cord
Therapeutic Category Astringent
Use
Dental: Hemostatic; gingival retraction
Medical: Hemostatic
Mechanism of Action Precipitates tissue and blood proteins causing a mechanical obstruction to hemorrhage from injured blood vessels
Local Anesthetic/Vasoconstrictor Precautions No information available to require special precautions
Effects on Dental Treatment No effects or complications reported
Other Adverse Effects No data reported

Oral manifestations: No data reported
Contraindications No data reported
Warnings/Precautions Since large amounts of astringents may cause tissue irritation and possible damage, only small amounts should be applied
Drug Interactions No data reported
Breast-feeding Considerations May be taken while breast-feeding
Dosage Forms
Retraction cord impregnated with aqueous solution of aluminum chloride containing 1.0 mg or 2.0 mg/inch in lengths of 72 inches
Retraction cord impregnated with an aqueous 10% solution of aluminum chloride and dried, containing 0.9 mg/inch or 1.8 mg/inch in lengths of 84 inches
Aqueous solution, 10 g aluminum chloride/100 mL water packaged in 15 and 30 mL bottles
Dietary Considerations No data reported

Aluminum Hydroxide (a loo' mi num hye drok' side)
Brand Names ALternaGEL® [OTC]; Alu-Cap® [OTC]; Alu-Tab® [OTC]; Amphojel® [OTC]; Dialume® [OTC]; Nephrox Suspension [OTC]
Therapeutic Category Antacid; Antidote, Hyperphosphatemia
Synonyms Aluminio, Hidroxido De (Mexico)
Use Treatment of hyperacidity; hyperphosphatemia
Usual Dosage Oral:
Peptic ulcer disease:
Children: 5-15 mL/dose every 3-6 hours or 1 and 3 hours after meals and at bedtime
(Continued)

Aluminum Hydroxide *(Continued)*

    Adults: 15-45 mL every 3-6 hours or 1 and 3 hours after meals and at bedtime

  Prophylaxis against gastrointestinal bleeding:
    Children: 5-15 mL/dose every 1-2 hours
    Adults: 30-60 mL/dose every hour
    Titrate to maintain the gastric pH >5

  Hyperphosphatemia:
    Children: 50-150 mg/kg/24 hours in divided doses every 4-6 hours, titrate dosage to maintain serum phosphorus within normal range
    Adults: 500-1800 mg, 3-6 times/day, between meals and at bedtime

  Antacid: Adults: 30 mL 1 and 3 hours postprandial and at bedtime

Mechanism of Action Neutralizes hydrochloride in stomach to form Al (Cl)$_3$ salt + H$_2$O]

Local Anesthetic/Vasoconstrictor Precautions No information available to require special precautions

Effects on Dental Treatment Aluminum OH prevents gastrointestinal absorption of tetracycline by forming a large ionized chelated molecule with the tetracyclines in the stomach. Aluminum OH prevents GI absorption of ketoconazole and itraconazole by increasing the pH in the GI tract. Any of these drugs should be administered at least 1 hour before Al(OH)$_3$.

Other Adverse Effects
  >10%: Gastrointestinal: Constipation, chalky taste, stomach cramps, fecal impaction
  1% to 10%: Gastrointestinal: Nausea, vomiting, discoloration of feces (white speckles)
  <1%: Endocrine & metabolic: Hypophosphatemia, hypomagnesemia

Drug Interactions Decreased effect: Tetracyclines, digoxin, indomethacin, or iron salts, isoniazid, allopurinol, benzodiazepines, corticosteroids, penicillamine, phenothiazines, ranitidine, ketoconazole, itraconazole

Pregnancy Risk Factor C

Aluminum Hydroxide and Magnesium Carbonate

  (a loo' mi num hye drok' side & mag nee' zhum kar' bun nate)

Brand Names Gaviscon® Liquid [OTC]

Therapeutic Category Antacid

Use Temporary relief of symptoms associated with gastric acidity

Local Anesthetic/Vasoconstrictor Precautions No information available to require special precautions

Effects on Dental Treatment Aluminum hydroxide prevents gastrointestinal absorption of tetracycline by forming a large ionized chelated molecule with the tetracyclines in the stomach. Aluminum hydroxide prevents GI absorption of ketoconazole and itraconazole by increasing the pH in the GI tract. Any of these drugs should be administered at least 1 hour before aluminum hydroxide.

Other Adverse Effects 1% to 10%:
  Endocrine & metabolic: Hypermagnesemia, aluminum intoxication (prolonged use and concomitant renal failure), osteomalacia, hypophosphatemia
  Gastrointestinal: Constipation, diarrhea

Comments Sodium content per 5 mL Gaviscon® liquid: 0.6 mEq

Aluminum Hydroxide and Magnesium Hydroxide

  (a loo' mi num hye drok' side & mag nee' zhum hye drok' side)

Brand Names Aludrox® [OTC]; Maalox® [OTC]; Maalox® Therapeutic Concentrate [OTC]

Therapeutic Category Antacid

Synonyms Magnesium Hydroxide and Aluminum Hydroxide

Use Antacid, hyperphosphatemia in renal failure

Local Anesthetic/Vasoconstrictor Precautions No information available to require special precautions

Effects on Dental Treatment Aluminum hydroxide prevents gastrointestinal absorption of tetracycline by forming a large ionized chelated molecule with the tetracyclines in the stomach. Aluminum hydroxide prevents GI absorption of ketoconazole and itraconazole by increasing the pH in the GI tract. Any of these drugs should be administered at least 1 hour before aluminum hydroxide.

Other Adverse Effects
  >10%: Gastrointestinal: Constipation, chalky taste, stomach cramps, fecal impaction

1% to 10%: Gastrointestinal: Nausea, vomiting, discoloration of feces (white speckles)

<1%: Endocrine & metabolic: Hypophosphatemia, hypomagnesemia

Comments Sodium content of 5 mL (Maalox®): 1.3 mg (0.06 mEq)

Aluminum Hydroxide and Magnesium Trisilicate

(a loo' mi num hye drok' side & mag nee' zhum trye sil' i kate)

Brand Names Gaviscon®-2 Tablet [OTC]; Gaviscon® Tablet [OTC]

Therapeutic Category Antacid

Use Temporary relief of hyperacidity

Local Anesthetic/Vasoconstrictor Precautions No information available to require special precautions

Effects on Dental Treatment Aluminum hydroxide prevents gastrointestinal absorption of tetracycline by forming a large ionized chelated molecule with the tetracyclines in the stomach. Aluminum hydroxide prevents GI absorption of ketoconazole and itraconazole by increasing the pH in the GI tract. Any of these drugs should be administered at least 1 hour before aluminum hydroxide.

Comments Sodium content per tablet:

Gaviscon®: 0.8 mEq

Gaviscon®-2: 1.6 mEq

Aluminum Hydroxide, Magnesium Hydroxide, and Simethicone

(a loo' mi num hye drok' side, mag nee' zhum hye drok' side, & sye meth' i kone)

Brand Names Di-Gel® [OTC]; Gas-Ban DS® [OTC]; Gelusil® [OTC]; Maalox® Plus [OTC]; Magalox Plus® [OTC]; Mylanta®-II [OTC]; Mylanta® [OTC]

Therapeutic Category Antacid; Antiflatulent

Use Temporary relief of hyperacidity associated with gas; may also be used for indications associated with other antacids

Local Anesthetic/Vasoconstrictor Precautions No information available to require special precautions

Effects on Dental Treatment Aluminum hydroxide prevents gastrointestinal absorption of tetracycline by forming a large ionized chelated molecule with the tetracyclines in the stomach. Aluminum hydroxide prevents GI absorption of ketoconazole and itraconazole by increasing the pH in the GI tract. Any of these drugs should be administered at least 1 hour before aluminum hydroxide.

Other Adverse Effects

>10%: Gastrointestinal: Chalky taste, stomach cramps, constipation, decreased bowel motility, fecal impaction, hemorrhoids

1% to 10%: Gastrointestinal: Nausea, vomiting, discoloration of feces (white speckles)

<1%: Endocrine & metabolic: Hypophosphatemia, hypomagnesemia

Miscellaneous: Dehydration or fluid restriction

Comments Sodium content of 5 mL:

Maalox® Plus: 1.3 mg (0.06 mEq)

Mylanta®: 0.7 mg (0.03 mEq)

Mylanta®-II: 1.14 mg (0.05 mEq)

Aluminum Sulfate and Calcium Acetate

(a loo' mi num sul' fate & kal' see um as' e tate)

Brand Names Bluboro® [OTC]; Boropak® [OTC]; Domeboro® Topical [OTC]; Pedi-Boro® [OTC]

Therapeutic Category Topical Skin Product

Use Astringent wet dressing for relief of inflammatory conditions of the skin and to reduce weeping that may occur in dermatitis

Local Anesthetic/Vasoconstrictor Precautions No information available to require special precautions

Effects on Dental Treatment No effects or complications reported

Alupent® *see* Metaproterenol Sulfate *on page 550*

Alu-Tab® [OTC] *see* Aluminum Hydroxide *on page 39*

Amantadina, Clorhidrato De (Mexico) *see* Amantadine Hydrochloride *on this page*

Amantadine Hydrochloride (a man' ta deen hye droe klor' ide)

Related Information

Respiratory Diseases *on page 924*

Systemic Viral Diseases *on page 934*

(Continued)

Amantadine Hydrochloride *(Continued)*

Brand Names Symadine®; Symmetrel®

Canadian/Mexican Brand Names Endantadine® (Canada); PMS-Amantadine® (Canada)

Therapeutic Category Anti-Parkinson's Agent; Antiviral Agent, Oral

Synonyms Amantadina, Clorhidrato De (Mexico)

Use Symptomatic and adjunct treatment of parkinsonism; prophylaxis and treatment of influenza A viral infection; treatment of drug-induced extrapyramidal symptoms

Usual Dosage

Children:

1-9 years: (<45 kg): 5-9 mg/kg/day in 1-2 divided doses to a maximum of 150 mg/day

10-12 years: 100–200 mg/day in 1-2 divided doses

Prophylaxis: Administer for 10-21 days following exposure if the vaccine is concurrently given or for 90 days following exposure if the vaccine is unavailable or contraindicated and re-exposure is possible

Adults:

Parkinson's disease: 100 mg twice daily

Influenza A viral infection: 200 mg/day in 1-2 divided doses

Prophylaxis: Minimum 10-day course of therapy following exposure if the vaccine is concurrently give or for 90 following exposure if the vaccine is unavailable or contraindicated and re-exposure is possible

Elderly patients should take the drug in 2 daily doses rather than a single dose to avoid adverse neurologic reactions

Mechanism of Action As an antiviral, blocks the uncoating of influenza A virus preventing penetration of virus into host; antiparkinsonian activity may be due to its blocking the reuptake of dopamine into presynaptic neurons and causing direct stimulation of postsynaptic receptors

Local Anesthetic/Vasoconstrictor Precautions No information available to require special precautions

Effects on Dental Treatment Prolonged use of amantadine may cause significant xerostomia

Other Adverse Effects

1% to 10%:

Cardiovascular: Orthostatic hypotension, peripheral edema

Central nervous system: Insomnia, depression, anxiety, irritability, dizziness, hallucinations, ataxia, headache, somnolence, nervousness, dream abnormality, agitation, fatigue

Dermatologic: Livedo reticularis

Gastrointestinal: Nausea, anorexia, constipation, diarrhea, dry mouth

Respiratory: Dry nose

<1%:

Cardiovascular: Congestive heart failure, hypertension

Central nervous system: Psychosis, weakness, slurred speech, euphoria, confusion, amnesia, instances of convulsions

Dermatologic: Skin rash, eczematoid dermatitis

Endocrine & metabolic: Decreased libido

Gastrointestinal: Vomiting

Genitourinary: Urinary retention

Hematologic: Leukopenia, neutropenia

Neuromuscular & skeletal: Hyperkinesis

Ocular: Visual disturbances, oculogyric episodes

Respiratory: Dyspnea

Drug Interactions Anticholinergic drugs may potentiate CNS side effects of amantadine; these include trihexyphenidyl (Artane®) and benztropine (Cogentin®)

Drug Uptake

Onset of antidyskinetic action: Within 48 hours

Absorption: Well absorbed from GI tract

Serum half-life:

Normal renal function: 2-7 hours

End stage renal disease: 7-10 days

Time to peak: 1-4 hours

Pregnancy Risk Factor C

Amaphen® *see* Butalbital Compound *on page 133*

Amaryl® *see* Glimepiride *on page 398*

Ambenonium Chloride (am be noe' nee um klor' ide)

Brand Names Mytelase® Caplets®

Therapeutic Category Cholinergic Agent

Use Treatment of myasthenia gravis

Local Anesthetic/Vasoconstrictor Precautions No information available to require special precautions

Effects on Dental Treatment Increased salivation

Other Adverse Effects

>10%:

Gastrointestinal: Diarrhea, nausea, stomach cramps

Miscellaneous: Increased sweating and mouth watering

1% to 10%:

Genitourinary: Urge to urinate

Ocular: Small pupils, lacrimation

Respiratory: Increased bronchial secretions

<1%:

Cardiovascular: Bradycardia, A-V block

Central nervous system: Seizures, headache, dysphoria, drowsiness

Local: Thrombophlebitis

Neuromuscular & skeletal: Muscle spasms, weakness

Ocular: Miosis, diplopia

Respiratory: Laryngospasm, respiratory paralysis

Miscellaneous: Hypersensitivity, hyper-reactive cholinergic responses

Ambenyl® Cough Syrup see Bromodiphenhydramine and Codeine on page 122

Ambien™ see Zolpidem Tartrate on page 909

Amcill® see Ampicillin on page 62

Amcinonida (Mexico) see Amcinonide on this page

Amcinonide (am sin' oh nide)

Related Information

Corticosteroids, Topical Comparison on page 1018

Brand Names Cyclocort®

Canadian/Mexican Brand Names Visderm® (Mexico)

Therapeutic Category Corticosteroid, Topical (Medium/High Potency)

Synonyms Amcinonida (Mexico)

Use Relief of the inflammatory and pruritic manifestations of corticosteroid-responsive dermatoses (high potency corticosteroid)

Usual Dosage Adults: Topical: Apply in a thin film 2-3 times/day

Mechanism of Action Stimulates the synthesis of enzymes needed to decrease inflammation, suppress mitotic activity, and cause vasoconstriction

Local Anesthetic/Vasoconstrictor Precautions No information available to require special precautions

Effects on Dental Treatment No effects or complications reported

Other Adverse Effects

1% to 10%: Topical: Itching, maceration of skin, skin atrophy, burning, erythema, dryness, irritation, papular rashes

<1%: Topical: Hypertrichosis, acneiform eruptions, hypopigmentation, perioral dermatitis, striae, miliaria

Drug Interactions No data reported

Drug Uptake

Absorption: Adequate through intact skin; increases with skin inflammation or occlusion

Pregnancy Risk Factor C

Amcort® see Triamcinolone on page 862

Amen® see Medroxyprogesterone Acetate on page 533

Amesec® [OTC] see Aminophylline, Amobarbital, and Ephedrine on page 47

A-Methapred® see Methylprednisolone on page 569

Amfepramone (Canada) see Diethylpropion Hydrochloride on page 276

Amgenal® Cough Syrup see Bromodiphenhydramine and Codeine on page 122

Amicar® see Aminocaproic Acid on page 46

Amikacina, Sulfato De (Mexico) see Amikacin Sulfate on next page

Amikacin Sulfate (am i kay' sin sul' fate)

Brand Names Amikin®

Canadian/Mexican Brand Names Amikin® (Canada); Amikin® (Mexico); Amikafur® (Mexico); Amikayect® (Mexico); Biclin® (Mexico); Gamikal® (Mexico); Yectamid® (Mexico)

Therapeutic Category Antibiotic, Aminoglycoside

Synonyms Amikacina, Sulfato De (Mexico)

Use Treatment of documented gram-negative enteric infection resistant to gentamicin and tobramycin (bone infections, respiratory tract infections, endocarditis, and septicemia); documented infection of mycobacterial organisms susceptible to amikacin including *Pseudomonas, Proteus, Serratia,* and gram-positive *Staphylococcus*

Usual Dosage Individualization is critical because of the low therapeutic index

Use of ideal body weight (IBW) for determining the mg/kg/dose appears to be more accurate than dosing on the basis of total body weight (TBW)

In morbid obesity, dosage requirement may best be estimated using a dosing weight of IBW + 0.4 (TBW - IBW)

Initial and periodic peak and trough plasma drug levels should be determined, particularly in critically ill patients with serious infections or in disease states known to significantly alter aminoglycoside pharmacokinetics (eg, cystic fibrosis, burns, or major surgery)

Once daily dosing: Higher peak serum drug concentration to MIC ratios, demonstrated aminoglycoside postantibiotic effect, decreased renal cortex drug uptake, and improved cost-time efficiency are supportive reasons for the use of once daily dosing regimens for aminoglycosides. Current research indicates these regimens to be as effective for nonlife-threatening infections, with no higher incidence of nephrotoxicity, than those requiring multiple daily doses. Doses are determined by calculating the entire day's dose via usual multiple dose calculation techniques and administering this quantity as a single dose. Doses are then adjusted to maintain mean serum concentrations above the MIC(s) of the causative organism(s). (Example: 14-35 mg/kg as a single dose/24 hours; peak (maximum) serum concentration may approximate 40-55 mcg/mL and trough (minimum) serum concentration <3 mcg/L). Further research is needed for universal recommendation in all patient populations and gram-negative disease; exceptions may include those with known high clearance (eg, children, patients with cystic fibrosis or burns who may require shorter dosage intervals) and patients with renal function impairment for whom longer than conventional dosage intervals are usually required.

Children and Adults: I.M., I.V.: 5-7.5 mg/kg/dose every 8 hours

Mechanism of Action Inhibits protein synthesis in susceptible bacteria by binding to ribosomal subunits

Local Anesthetic/Vasoconstrictor Precautions No information available to require special precautions

Effects on Dental Treatment No effects or complications reported

Other Adverse Effects

1% to 10%:

Central nervous system: Neurotoxicity

Otic: Ototoxicity (auditory), ototoxicity (vestibular)

Renal: Nephrotoxicity

<1%:

Cardiovascular: Hypotension

Central nervous system: Headache, drowsiness, weakness

Dermatologic: Rash

Gastrointestinal: Nausea, vomiting

Hematologic: Eosinophilia

Neuromuscular & skeletal: Paresthesia, tremor, arthralgia

Respiratory: Difficulty in breathing

Miscellaneous: Drug fever

Drug Interactions

Increased toxicity of aminoglycoside: Indomethacin I.V., amphotericin, loop diuretics, vancomycin, enflurane, methoxyflurane, cephalosporins

Increased toxicity of depolarizing and nondepolarizing neuromuscular blocking agents and polypeptide antibiotics with administration of aminoglycosides

Drug Uptake

Absorption: I.M.: May be delayed in the bedridden patient

Serum half-life (dependent on renal function):

Adults:

Normal renal function: 1.4-2.3 hours

Anuria: End stage renal disease: 28-86 hours
Time to peak serum concentration:
I.M.: Within 45-120 minutes
I.V.: Within 30 minutes following 30-minute infusion
Pregnancy Risk Factor C

Amikin® see Amikacin Sulfate *on previous page*
Amilorida Clorhidrato De (Mexico) see Amiloride Hydrochloride *on this page*

Amiloride and Hydrochlorothiazide
(a mil′ oh ride & hye droe klor oh thye′ a zide)
Brand Names Moduretic®
Therapeutic Category Diuretic, Combination
Synonyms Hydrochlorothiazide and Amiloride
Use Antikaliuretic diuretic, antihypertensive
Local Anesthetic/Vasoconstrictor Precautions No information available to require special precautions
Effects on Dental Treatment No effects or complications reported
Other Adverse Effects See individual agents

Amiloride Hydrochloride (a mil′ oh ride hye droe klor′ ide)
Brand Names Midamor®
Therapeutic Category Diuretic, Potassium Sparing
Synonyms Amilorida Clorhidrato De (Mexico)
Use Counteracts potassium loss induced by other diuretics in the treatment of hypertension or edematous conditions including CHF, hepatic cirrhosis, and hypoaldosteronism; usually used in conjunction with more potent diuretics such as thiazides or loop diuretics; investigational solution for cystic fibrosis
Usual Dosage Oral:
Children: Although safety and efficacy have not been established by the FDA in children, a dosage of 0.625 mg/kg/day has been used in children weighing 6-20 kg
Adults: 5-10 mg/day (up to 20 mg)
Elderly: Initial: 5 mg once daily or every other day
Mechanism of Action Interferes with potassium/sodium exchange (active transport) in the distal tubule, cortical collecting tubule and collecting duct by inhibiting sodium, potassium-ATPase; decreases calcium excretion; increases magnesium loss
Local Anesthetic/Vasoconstrictor Precautions No information available to require special precautions
Effects on Dental Treatment No effects or complications reported
Other Adverse Effects
1% to 10%:
Central nervous system: Headache, weakness, fatigability, dizziness
Endocrine & metabolic: Hyperkalemia, hyperchloremic metabolic acidosis, dehydration, hyponatremia, gynecomastia
Gastrointestinal: Nausea, diarrhea, vomiting, abdominal pain, gas pain, appetite changes, constipation
Genitourinary: Impotence
Neuromuscular & skeletal: Muscle cramps
Respiratory: Cough, dyspnea
<1%:
Cardiovascular: Angina pectoris, orthostatic hypotension, arrhythmias, palpitations, chest pain
Central nervous system: Vertigo, nervousness, insomnia, depression
Dermatologic: Skin rash or dryness, pruritus, alopecia
Gastrointestinal: GI bleeding, thirst, heartburn, flatulence, dyspepsia
Genitourinary: Decreased libido, urinary frequency, bladder spasms
Hepatic: Jaundice
Neuromuscular & skeletal: Joint pain, tremor, neck/shoulder pain, back pain
Ocular: Increased intraocular pressure
Renal: Polyuria, dysuria
Respiratory: Shortness of breath
Drug Interactions Increased risk of amiloride-associated hyperkalemia: Triamterene, spironolactone, angiotensin-converting enzyme (ACE) inhibitors, potassium preparations, indomethacin
Drug Uptake
Absorption: Oral: ~15% to 25%
Onset: 2 hours
Duration: 24 hours
(Continued)

45

Amiloride Hydrochloride *(Continued)*

Serum half-life:
Peak serum concentration: 6-10 hours
Pregnancy Risk Factor B

2-Amino-6-Mercaptopurine *see* Thioguanine *on page 838*

Aminocaproic Acid *(a mee noe ka proe′ ik as′ id)*
Brand Names Amicar®
Therapeutic Category Hemostatic Agent
Synonyms Aminocaproico, Acido (Mexico)
Use Treatment of excessive bleeding from fibrinolysis
Usual Dosage In the management of acute bleeding syndromes, oral dosage regimens are the same as the I.V. dosage regimens in adults and children

Chronic bleeding: Oral, I.V.: 5-30 g/day in divided doses at 3- to 6-hour intervals

Acute bleeding syndrome:
Children: Oral, I.V.: 100 mg/kg or 3 g/m² during the first hour, followed by continuous infusion at the rate of 33.3 mg/kg/hour or 1 g/m²/hour; total dosage should not exceed 18 g/m²/24 hours
Traumatic hyphema: Oral: 100 mg/kg/dose every 6-8 hours
Adults:
Oral: For elevated fibrinolytic activity, give 5 g during first hour, followed by 1-1.25 g/hour for approximately 8 hours or until bleeding stops
I.V.: Give 4-5 g in 250 mL of diluent during first hour followed by continuous infusion at the rate of 1-1.25 g/hour in 50 mL of diluent, continue for 8 hours or until bleeding stops
Maximum daily dose: Oral, I.V.: 30 g
Mechanism of Action Competitively inhibits activation of plasminogen to plasmin, also, a lesser antiplasmin effect
Local Anesthetic/Vasoconstrictor Precautions No information available to require special precautions
Effects on Dental Treatment No effects or complications reported
Other Adverse Effects
1% to 10%:
Cardiovascular: Hypotension, bradycardia, arrhythmia
Central nervous system: Dizziness, headache, tinnitus, malaise, weakness, fatigue
Dermatologic: Rash
Gastrointestinal: GI irritation, nausea, cramps, diarrhea
Hematologic: Decreased platelet function, elevated serum enzymes
Neuromuscular & skeletal: Myopathy
Respiratory: Nasal congestion
<1%:
Central nervous system: Convulsions
Genitourinary: Ejaculation problems
Neuromuscular & skeletal: Rhabdomyolysis
Renal: Renal failure
Drug Interactions No data reported
Drug Uptake Serum half-life: 1-2 hours
Pregnancy Risk Factor C

Aminocaproico, Acido (Mexico) *see* Aminocaproic Acid *on this page*
Amino-Cerv™ Vaginal Cream *see* Urea *on page 884*

Aminoglutethimide *(a mee noe gloo teth′ i mide)*
Brand Names Cytadren®
Therapeutic Category Antiadrenal Agent; Antineoplastic Agent, Adjuvant
Use Suppression of adrenal function in selected patients with Cushing's syndrome; also used successfully in postmenopausal patients with advanced breast carcinoma and in patients with metastatic prostate carcinoma as salvage (third-line hormonal agent)
Usual Dosage Adults: Oral: 250 mg every 6 hours may be increased at 1- to 2-week intervals to a total of 2 g/day; give in divided doses, 2-3 times/day to reduce incidence of nausea and vomiting
Mechanism of Action Blocks the enzymatic conversion of cholesterol to delta-5-pregnenolone, thereby reducing the synthesis of adrenal glucocorticoids, mineralocorticoids, estrogens, aldosterone, and androgens
Local Anesthetic/Vasoconstrictor Precautions No information available to require special precautions

Effects on Dental Treatment Over 10% of patients likely to experience nausea; approximately 10% may experience orthostatic hypotension

Other Adverse Effects Most adverse effects will diminish in incidence and severity after the first 2-6 weeks

>10%:
  Central nervous system: Headache, dizziness, drowsiness, and lethargy are frequent at the start of therapy, clumsiness
  Dermatologic: Systemic lupus erythematosus, skin rash
  Gastrointestinal: Nausea, vomiting, anorexia
  Hepatic: Cholestatic jaundice
  Neuromuscular & skeletal: Myalgia
  Renal: Nephrotoxicity
  Respiratory: Pulmonary alveolar damage
1% to 10%:
  Cardiovascular: Hypotension and tachycardia, orthostatic hypotension
  Central nervous system: Headache
  Endocrine & metabolic: Hirsutism in females, adrenocortical insufficiency
  Hematologic: Rare cases of neutropenia, leukopenia, thrombocytopenia, pancytopenia, and agranulocytosis have been reported
  Neuromuscular & skeletal: Muscle pain
<1%: Endocrine & metabolic: Adrenal suppression, lipid abnormalities (hypercholesterolemia), hyperkalemia, hypothyroidism, goiter

Drug Interactions Aminoglutethimide enhances elimination of dexamethasone resulting in reduction of steroid response; increased clearance of digitoxin after 3-8 weeks of aminoglutethimide therapy resulting in decreased effect of digitoxin; aminoglutethimide increases the metabolism of theophylline; decrease in anticoagulant response to warfarin

Drug Uptake
  Onset of action (adrenal suppression): 3-5 days
  Serum half-life: 7-15 hours; shorter following multiple administrations than following single doses (induces hepatic enzymes increasing its own metabolism)

Pregnancy Risk Factor D

Amino-Opti-E® [OTC] *see* Vitamin E *on page 900*

Aminophyllin™ *see* Theophylline/Aminophylline *on page 832*

Aminophylline, Amobarbital, and Ephedrine
(am in off′ i lin, am oh bar′ bi tal, & e fed′ rin)
Brand Names Amesec® [OTC]
Therapeutic Category Antiasthmatic; Bronchodilator
Use Symptomatic relief of asthma
Local Anesthetic/Vasoconstrictor Precautions Use vasoconstrictors with caution since ephedrine may enhance cardiostimulation and vasopressor effects of sympathomimetics
Effects on Dental Treatment Do not prescribe any erythromycin product to patients taking theophylline products. Erythromycin will delay the normal metabolic inactivation of theophyllines leading to increased blood levels; this has resulted in nausea, vomiting and CNS restlessness
Other Adverse Effects See individual agents

Aminosalicilico, Acido *see* Aminosalicylate Sodium *on this page*

Aminosalicylate Sodium (a mee′ noe sa lis′ i late sow′ dee um)
Brand Names Sodium P.A.S.
Canadian/Mexican Brand Names Tubasal® (Canada); Salofalk® (Mexico)
Therapeutic Category Antitubercular Agent; Nonsteroidal Anti-inflammatory Agent (NSAID), Oral
Synonyms Aminosalicilico, Acido
Use Treatment of tuberculosis with combination drugs
Usual Dosage Oral:
  Children: 150-300 mg/kg/day in 3-4 equally divided doses
  Adults: 150 mg/kg/day in 2-3 equally divided doses (usually 12-14 g/day)
Mechanism of Action Aminosalicylic acid (PAS) is a highly specific bacteriostatic agent active against *M. tuberculosis*. Most strains of *M. tuberculosis* are sensitive to a concentration of 1 µg/mL; structurally related to para-aminobenzoic acid (PABA) and its mechanism of action is thought to be similar to the sulfonamides, a competitive antagonism with PABA; disrupts plate biosynthesis in sensitive organisms
Local Anesthetic/Vasoconstrictor Precautions No information available to require special precautions
(Continued)

Aminosalicylate Sodium *(Continued)*

Effects on Dental Treatment No effects or complications reported

Other Adverse Effects

1% to 10%: Gastrointestinal: Nausea, vomiting, diarrhea, abdominal pain

<1%:

Cardiovascular: Vasculitis

Central nervous system: Fever

Dermatologic: Skin eruptions

Endocrine & metabolic: Goiter with or without myxedema

Hematologic: Leukopenia, agranulocytosis, thrombocytopenia, hemolytic anemia

Hepatic: Jaundice, hepatitis

Drug Interactions A small reduction in digoxin (Lanoxin®) plasma levels may result from coadministration with aminosalicylate sodium; probenecid increases the serum concentration of aminosalicylate sodium

Drug Uptake

Absorption: Readily absorbed >90%

Pregnancy Risk Factor C

Amiodarona, Clorhidrato De (Mexico) *see* Amiodarone Hydrochloride *on this page*

Amiodarone Hydrochloride (a mee' oh da rone hye droe klor' ide)

Related Information

Cardiovascular Diseases *on page 912*

Brand Names Cordarone®

Canadian/Mexican Brand Names Braxan® (Mexico); Cardiorona® (Mexico)

Therapeutic Category Antiarrhythmic Agent, Class III; Antiarrhythmic Agent (Supraventricular & Ventricular)

Synonyms Amiodarona, Clorhidrato De (Mexico)

Use Management of resistant, life-threatening ventricular arrhythmias or supraventricular arrhythmias unresponsive to conventional therapy with less toxic agents

Usual Dosage Oral:

Children (calculate doses for children <1 year on body surface area):

Loading dose: 10-15 mg/kg/day or 600-800 mg/1.73 m^2/day for 4-14 days or until adequate control of arrhythmia or prominent adverse effects occur (this loading dose may be given in 1-2 divided doses/day); dosage should then be reduced to 5 mg/kg/day or 200-400 mg/1.73 m^2/day given once daily for several weeks; if arrhythmia does not recur, reduce to lowest effective dosage possible; usual daily minimal dose: 2.5 mg/kg/day; maintenance doses may be given for 5 of 7 days/week

Adults: Ventricular arrhythmias: 800-1600 mg/day in 1-2 doses for 1-3 weeks, then 600-800 mg/day in 1-2 doses for 1 month; maintenance: 400 mg/day; lower doses are recommended for supraventricular arrhythmias

Mechanism of Action Class III antiarrhythmic agent which inhibits adrenergic stimulation, prolongs the action potential and refractory period in myocardial tissue; decreases A-V conduction and sinus node function

Local Anesthetic/Vasoconstrictor Precautions No information available to require special precautions

Effects on Dental Treatment This drug is indicated only for life-threatening arrhythmias; dental treatment would not be a consideration during these emergencies

Other Adverse Effects With large dosages (≥400 mg/day), adverse reactions occur in ~75% patients and require discontinuance in 5% to 20%

>10%:

Central nervous system: Ataxia, fatigue, malaise, dizziness, headache, insomnia, nightmares

Dermatologic: Photosensitivity

Gastrointestinal: Nausea, vomiting

Neuromuscular & skeletal: Tremor, paresthesias, muscle weakness

Respiratory: Pulmonary fibrosis (cough, fever, dyspnea, malaise), interstitial pneumonitis

Miscellaneous: Alveolitis

1% to 10%:

Cardiovascular: Congestive heart failure, cardiac arrhythmias (atropine-resistant bradycardia, heart block, sinus arrest, paroxysmal ventricular tachycardia), myocardial depression, flushing, edema, coagulation abnormalities

Endocrine & metabolic: Hypothyroidism or hyperthyroidism (less common), decreased libido

Gastrointestinal: Constipation, anorexia, abdominal pain

Hepatic: Abnormal liver function tests

Ocular: Visual disturbances

Miscellaneous: Abnormal taste and smell, abnormal salivation

<1%:

Cardiovascular: Hypotension, vasculitis

Central nervous system: Pseudotumor cerebri

Dermatologic: Skin rash, alopecia, slate blue discoloration of skin, photosensitivity

Endocrine & metabolic: Hyperglycemia, hypertriglyceridemia

Genitourinary: Epididymitis

Hematologic: Thrombocytopenia

Hepatic: Cirrhosis, severe hepatic toxicity (potentially fatal hepatitis)

Ocular: Optic neuritis, corneal microdeposits, photophobia

Drug Interactions Cytochrome P-450 3A enzyme inhibitor

Amiodarone appears to interfere with the hepatic metabolism of several drugs resulting in significantly increased plasma concentrations; see table.

Amiodarone Common Drug Interactions

Drug	Interaction
Anticoagulants, oral	The effects of the anticoagulant is increased due to inhibition of its metabolism
β-adrenergic receptor antagonists	β-blocker effects are enhanced by amiodarone's inhibition of the β-blocker's hepatic metabolism
Calcium channel antagonists	Additive effects of both drugs resulting in a reduction in cardiac sinus conduction, atrioventricular nodal conduction and myocardial contractility
Digoxin	Digoxin concentrations may be increased with resultant increases in activity and potential for toxicity
Flecainide	Flecainide plasma concentrations are increased
Phenytoin	Phenytoin serum concentrations are increased due to reduction in phenytoin metabolism, with possible symptoms of phenytoin toxicity
Procainamide	Procainamide serum concentrations may be increased
Quinidine	Quinidine serum concentrations may be increased and can potentially cause fatal cardiac dysrhythmias

Drug Uptake

Onset of effect: 3 days to 3 weeks after starting therapy

Peak effect: 1 week to 5 months

Duration of effect after discontinuation of therapy: 7-50 days

Note: Mean onset of effect and duration after discontinuation may be shorter in children versus adults

Serum half-life: Oral chronic therapy: 40-55 days (range: 26-107 days); shortened in children versus adults

Pregnancy Risk Factor C

Ami-Tex LA® *see* Guaifenesin and Phenylpropanolamine *on page 409*

Amitone® **[OTC]** *see* Calcium Carbonate *on page 140*

Amitriptilina Clorhidrato De (Mexico) *see* Amitriptyline Hydrochloride *on page 51*

Amitriptyline and Chlordiazepoxide

(a mee trip′ ti leen & klor dye az e pox′ ide)

Brand Names Limbitrol®

Therapeutic Category Antidepressant, Tricyclic; Antipsychotic Agent

Synonyms Chlordiazepoxide and Amitriptyline

Use Treatment of moderate to severe anxiety and/or agitation and depression
(Continued)

Amitriptyline and Chlordiazepoxide *(Continued)*

Local Anesthetic/Vasoconstrictor Precautions Use with caution; epinephrine, norepinephrine and levonordefrin have been shown to have an increased pressor response in combination with TCAs

Effects on Dental Treatment

Amitriptyline: The most anticholinergic and sedating of the antidepressants; pronounced effects on the cardiovascular system; long-term treatment with TCAs such as amitriptyline increases the risk of caries by reducing salivation and salivary buffer capacity. In a study by Rundergren, et al, pathological alterations were observed in the oral mucosa of 72% of 58 patients; 55% had new carious lesions after taking TCAs for a median of 5½ years. Current research is investigating the use of the salivary stimulant pilocarpine (Salagen®) to overcome the xerostomia from amitriptyline.

Chlordiazepoxide: Over 10% of patients will experience dry mouth which disappears with cessation of drug therapy

Other Adverse Effects See individual agents

Selected Readings

Boakes AJ, Laurence DR, Teoh PC, et al, "Interactions Between Sympathomimetic Amines and Antidepressant Agents in Man," *Br Med J*, 1973, 1(849):311-5.

Jastak JT and Yagiela JA, "Vasoconstrictors and Local Anesthesia: A Review and Rationale for Use," *J Am Dent Assoc*, 1983, 107(4):623-30.

Larochelle P, Hamet P, and Enjalbert M, "Responses to Tyramine and Norepinephrine After Imipramine and Trazodone," *Clin Pharmacol Ther*, 1979, 26(1):24-30.

Mitchell JR, "Guanethidine and Related Agents. III Antagonism by Drugs Which Inhibit the Norepinephrine Pump in Man," *J Clin Invest*, 1970, 49(8):1596-604.

Rundegren J, van Dijken J, Mörnstad H, et al, "Oral Conditions in Patients Receiving Long-Term Treatment With Cyclic Antidepressant Drugs," *Swed Dent J*, 1985, 9(2):55-64.

Svedmyr N, "The Influence of a Tricyclic Antidepressive Agent (Protriptyline) on Some of the Circulatory Effects of Noradrenaline and Adrenalin in Man," *Life Sci*, 1968, 7(1):77-84.

Amitriptyline and Perphenazine

(a mee trip′ ti leen & per fen′ a zeen)

Brand Names Etrafon®; Triavil®

Therapeutic Category Antidepressant, Tricyclic; Phenothiazine Derivative

Synonyms Perphenazine and Amitriptyline

Use Treatment of patients with moderate to severe anxiety and depression

Local Anesthetic/Vasoconstrictor Precautions

Amitriptyline: Use with caution; epinephrine, norepinephrine and levonordefrin have been shown to have an increased pressor response in combination with TCAs

Perphenazine: No information available to require special precautions

Effects on Dental Treatment

Amitriptyline: The most anticholinergic and sedating of the antidepressants; pronounced effects on the cardiovascular system; long-term treatment with TCAs such as amitriptyline increases the risk of caries by reducing salivation and salivary buffer capacity. In a study by Rundergren, et al, pathological alterations were observed in the oral mucosa of 72% of 58 patients; 55% had new carious lesions after taking TCAs for a median of 5½ years. Current research is investigating the use of the salivary stimulant pilocarpine (Salagen®) to overcome the xerostomia from amitriptyline.

Perphenazine: Significant hypotension may occur, especially when the drug is administered parenterally; orthostatic hypotension is due to alpha-receptor blockade, the elderly are at greater risk for orthostatic hypotension

Tardive dyskinesia: Prevalence rate may be 40% in elderly; development of the syndrome and the irreversible nature are proportional to duration and total cumulative dose over time

Extrapyramidal reactions are more common in elderly with up to 50% developing these reactions after 60 years of age; drug-induced **Parkinson's syndrome** occurs often; **Akathisia** is the most common extrapyramidal reaction in elderly

Increased confusion, memory loss, psychotic behavior, and agitation frequently occur as a consequence of anticholinergic effects

Antipsychotic associated sedation in nonpsychotic patients is extremely unpleasant due to feelings of depersonalization, derealization, and dysphoria

Other Adverse Effects

>10%:

Central nervous system: Dizziness, drowsiness, headache

Gastrointestinal: Dry mouth, constipation, increased appetite, nausea, unpleasant taste, weight gain

Neuromuscular & skeletal: Weakness

1% to 10%:
  Cardiovascular: Arrhythmias, hypotension
  Central nervous system: Confusion, delirium, hallucinations, nervousness, restlessness, Parkinsonian syndrome, insomnia
  Endocrine & metabolic: Sexual function impairment
  Gastrointestinal: Diarrhea, heartburn
  Genitourinary: Difficult urination
  Neuromuscular & skeletal: Fine muscle tremors
  Ocular: Blurred vision, eye pain
  Miscellaneous: Excessive sweating
<1%:
  Central nervous system: Anxiety, seizures
  Dermatologic: Alopecia
  Endocrine & metabolic: Breast enlargement, galactorrhea, SIADH
  Genitourinary: Testicular swelling
  Hematologic: Agranulocytosis, leukopenia, eosinophilia
  Hepatic: Cholestatic jaundice, increased liver enzymes
  Ocular: Increased intraocular pressure, photosensitivity
  Otic: Tinnitus
  Miscellaneous: Trouble with gums, decreased lower esophageal sphincter tone may cause GE reflux, allergic reactions

Selected Readings

Boakes AJ, Laurence DR, Teoh PC, et al, "Interactions Between Sympathomimetic Amines and Antidepressant Agents in Man," *Br Med J*, 1973, 1(849):311-5.

Jastak JT and Yagiela JA, "Vasoconstrictors and Local Anesthesia: A Review and Rationale for Use," *J Am Dent Assoc*, 1983, 107(4):623-30.

Larochelle P, Hamet P, and Enjalbert M, "Responses to Tyramine and Norepinephrine After Imipramine and Trazodone," *Clin Pharmacol Ther*, 1979, 26(1):24-30.

Mitchell JR, "Guanethidine and Related Agents. III Antagonism by Drugs Which Inhibit the Norepinephrine Pump in Man," *J Clin Invest*, 1970, 49(8):1596-604.

Rundegren J, van Dijken J, Mörnstad H, et al, "Oral Conditions in Patients Receiving Long-Term Treatment With Cyclic Antidepressant Drugs," *Swed Dent J*, 1985, 9(2):55-64.

Svedmyr N, "The Influence of a Tricyclic Antidepressive Agent (Protriptyline) on Some of the Circulatory Effects of Noradrenaline and Adrenalin in Man," *Life Sci*, 1968, 7(1):77-84.

Amitriptyline Hydrochloride (a mee trip' ti leen hye droe klor' ide)

Brand Names Elavil®; Endep®; Enovil®

Canadian/Mexican Brand Names Apo-Amitriptyline® (Canada); Levate® (Canada); Novo-Tryptin® (Canada); Anapsique® (Mexico); Tryptanol® (Mexico)

Therapeutic Category Antidepressant, Tricyclic

Synonyms Amitriptilina Clorhidrato De (Mexico)

Use Treatment of various forms of depression, often in conjunction with psychotherapy; analgesic for certain chronic and neuropathic pain, prophylaxis against migraine headaches

Usual Dosage

Children: Pain management: Oral: Initial: 0.1 mg/kg at bedtime, may advance as tolerated over 2-3 weeks to 0.5-2 mg/day at bedtime

Adolescents: Oral: Initial: 25-50 mg/day; may give in divided doses; increase gradually to 100 mg/day in divided doses

Adults:
  Oral: 30-100 mg/day single dose at bedtime or in divided doses; dose may be gradually increased up to 300 mg/day; once symptoms are controlled, decrease gradually to lowest effective dose
  I.M.: 20-30 mg 4 times/day

Mechanism of Action Increases the synaptic concentration of serotonin and/or norepinephrine in the central nervous system by inhibition of their reuptake at the presynaptic neuronal membrane

Local Anesthetic/Vasoconstrictor Precautions Use with caution; epinephrine, norepinephrine and levonordefrin have been shown to have an increased pressor response in combination with TCAs

Effects on Dental Treatment The most anticholinergic and sedating of the antidepressants; pronounced effects on the cardiovascular system; long-term treatment with TCAs such as amitriptyline increases the risk of caries by reducing salivation and salivary buffer capacity. In a study by Rundergren, et al, pathological alterations were observed in the oral mucosa of 72% of 58 patients; 55% had new carious lesions after taking TCAs for a median of 5½ years. Current research is investigating the use of the salivary stimulant pilocarpine (Salagen®) to overcome the xerostomia from amitriptyline.

Other Adverse Effects Anticholinergic effects may be pronounced; moderate to marked sedation can occur (tolerance to these effects usually occurs)

>10%:
  Central nervous system: Dizziness, drowsiness, headache
(Continued)

Amitriptyline Hydrochloride (Continued)

Gastrointestinal: Dry mouth, constipation, increased appetite, nausea, weakness, unpleasant taste, weight gain

1% to 10%:

Cardiovascular: Hypotension, postural hypotension, arrhythmias, tachycardia, sudden death

Central nervous system: Nervousness, restlessness, parkinsonian syndrome, insomnia, sedation, weakness, fatigue, anxiety, impaired cognitive function, seizures have occurred occasionally, extrapyramidal symptoms are possible

Gastrointestinal: Diarrhea, heartburn, constipation

Genitourinary: Sexual function impairment, urinary retention

Neuromuscular & skeletal: Tremor

Ocular: Eye pain, blurred vision

Miscellaneous: Excessive sweating

<1%:

Central nervous system: Anxiety, seizures

Dermatologic: Alopecia, photosensitivity

Endocrine & metabolic: Breast enlargement, galactorrhea, rarely SIADH

Genitourinary: Testicular swelling

Hematologic: Leukopenia, eosinophilia, rarely agranulocytosis

Hepatic: Cholestatic jaundice, increased liver enzymes

Ocular: Increased intraocular pressure

Otic: Tinnitus

Miscellaneous: Trouble with gums, decreased lower esophageal sphincter tone may cause GE reflux; allergic reactions

Drug Interactions

Decreased effect: Phenobarbital may increase the metabolism of amitriptyline; amitriptyline blocks the uptake of guanethidine and thus prevents the hypotensive effect of guanethidine

Increased toxicity: Clonidine has caused hypertensive crisis; amitriptyline may be additive with or may potentiate the action of other CNS depressants such as sedatives or hypnotics; with MAO inhibitors, hyperpyrexia, hypertension, tachycardia, confusion, seizures, and **deaths have been reported**; amitriptyline may increase the prothrombin time in patients stabilized on warfarin; amitriptyline potentiates the pressor and cardiac effects of sympathomimetic agents such as isoproterenol, epinephrine, etc; cimetidine and methylphenidate may decrease the metabolism of amitriptyline

Additive anticholinergic effects seen with other anticholinergic agents

Drug Uptake

Onset of action: 7-21 days

Serum half-life: Adults: 9-25 hours (15-hour average)

Time to peak serum concentration: Within 4 hours

Pregnancy Risk Factor D

Selected Readings

Boakes AJ, Laurence DR, Teoh PC, et al, "Interactions Between Sympathomimetic Amines and Antidepressant Agents in Man," Br Med J, 1973, 1(849):311-5.

Jastak JT and Yagiela JA, "Vasoconstrictors and Local Anesthesia: A Review and Rationale for Use," J Am Dent Assoc, 1983, 107(4):623-30.

Larochelle P, Hamet P, and Enjalbert M, "Responses to Tyramine and Norepinephrine After Imipramine and Trazodone," Clin Pharmacol Ther, 1979, 26(1):24-30.

Mitchell JR, "Guanethidine and Related Agents. III Antagonism by Drugs Which Inhibit the Norepinephrine Pump in Man," J Clin Invest, 1970, 49(8):1596-604.

Rundegren J, van Dijken J, Mörnstad H, et al, "Oral Conditions in Patients Receiving Long-Term Treatment With Cyclic Antidepressant Drugs," Swed Dent J, 1985, 9(2):55-64.

Svedmyr N, "The Influence of a Tricyclic Antidepressive Agent (Protriptyline) on Some of the Circulatory Effects of Noradrenaline and Adrenalin® in Man," Life Sci, 1968, 7(1):77-84.

Amlexanox (am lex' an ox)

Related Information

Oral Nonviral Soft Tissue Ulcerations or Erosions on page 955

Brand Names Aphthasol®

Therapeutic Category Anti-inflammatory, Locally Applied

Use For treating signs a symptoms of canker sores (minor aphthous ulcers)

Usual Dosage Administer directly on ulcers 4 times/day following oral hygiene, after meals, and before going to bed

Local Anesthetic/Vasoconstrictor Precautions No information available to require special precautions

Effects on Dental Treatment No effects or complications reported

Other Adverse Effects

Local: Stinging or burning at the administration site

Oral manifestations: No data reported

Contraindications Known hypersensitivity to any of its components

Dosage Forms Paste: 5%

Generic Available No

Comments Treatment of canker sores with amlexanox showed a 76% median reduction in ulcer size compared to a 40% reduction with placebo. Greer, et al, reported an overall mean reduction in ulcer size of 1.82 mm^2 for patients treated with 5% amlexanox versus an average reduction of 0.52 mm^2 for the control group.

Selected Readings Greer RO, Lindenmuth JE, Juarez T, et al, "A Double-Blind Study of Topically Applied 5% Amlexanox in the Treatment of Aphthous Ulcers," *J Oral Maxillofacial Surg*, 1993, 51:243-8.

Amlodipina, Besilato De (Mexico) *see* Amlodipine *on this page*

Amlodipine (am loe' di peen)

Related Information

Calcium Channel Blockers & Gingival Hyperplasia *on page 1010*
Cardiovascular Diseases *on page 912*

Brand Names Norvasc®

Canadian/Mexican Brand Names Norvas® (Mexico)

Therapeutic Category Antianginal Agent; Calcium Channel Blocker

Synonyms Amlodipina, Besilato De (Mexico)

Use Treatment of hypertension and angina

Usual Dosage Adults: Oral: Initial dose: 2.5-5 mg once daily; usual dose: 5-10 mg once daily; maximum dose: 10 mg once daily

Hemodialysis effects: Hemodialysis and peritoneal dialysis does not enhance elimination; supplemental dose is not necessary

Dosage adjustment in hepatic impairment: 2.5 mg once daily

Mechanism of Action Inhibits calcium ion from entering the "slow channels" or select voltage-sensitive areas of vascular smooth muscle and myocardium during depolarization, producing a relaxation of coronary vascular smooth muscle and coronary vasodilation; increases myocardial oxygen delivery in patients with vasospastic angina

Local Anesthetic/Vasoconstrictor Precautions No information available to require special precautions

Effects on Dental Treatment Other drugs of this class can cause gingival hyperplasia (ie, nifedipine) but there have been no reports for amlodipine

Other Adverse Effects

>10%: Cardiovascular: Peripheral edema

1% to 10%:

Cardiovascular: Edema, flushing, palpitations
Central nervous system: Headache, fatigue, dizziness, somnolence
Dermatologic: Dermatitis, rash
Endocrine & metabolic: Sexual difficulties
Gastrointestinal: Nausea, abdominal pain
Respiratory: Shortness of breath
Neuromuscular & skeletal: Muscle cramps

<1%:

Cardiovascular: Hypotension, bradycardia, arrhythmias, abnormal EKG, ventricular extrasystoles
Dermatologic: Alopecia, petechiae
Gastrointestinal: Weight gain, anorexia
Neuromuscular & skeletal: Joint stiffness
Respiratory: Nasal congestion, cough
Miscellaneous: Sweating, epistaxis

Drug Interactions No data reported

Drug Uptake

Onset of action: 30-50 minutes
Peak effect: 6-12 hours
Duration: 24 hours
Absorption: Oral: Well absorbed
Serum half-life: 30-50 hours

Pregnancy Risk Factor C

Selected Readings

Wynn RL, "An Update on Calcium Channel Blocker-Induced Gingival Hyperplasia," *Gen Dent*, 1995, 43:218-22.

Wynn RL, "Calcium Channel Blockers and Gingival Hyperplasia," *Gen Dent*, 1991, 39(4):240-3.

Amlodipine and Benazepril (am loe' di peen & ben ay' ze pril)

Brand Names Lotrel™

Therapeutic Category Angiotensin-Converting Enzyme (ACE) Inhibitors; Calcium Channel Blocker

Use Treatment of hypertension

Local Anesthetic/Vasoconstrictor Precautions No information available to require special precautions

Effects on Dental Treatment Other drugs of this class can cause gingival hyperplasia (ie, nifedipine) but there have been no reports for amlodipine

Selected Readings

Wynn RL, "An Update on Calcium Channel Blocker-Induced Gingival Hyperplasia," *Gen Dent*, 1995, 43:218-22.

Wynn RL, "Calcium Channel Blockers and Gingival Hyperplasia," *Gen Dent*, 1991, 39(4):240-3.

Ammonia Spirit, Aromatic (a moe' nee ah spear' it, air oh mat' ik)

Brand Names Aromatic Ammonia Aspirols®

Therapeutic Category Respiratory Stimulant

Use Respiratory and circulatory stimulant, treatment of fainting

Usual Dosage Used as "smelling salts" to treat or prevent fainting

Local Anesthetic/Vasoconstrictor Precautions No information available to require special precautions

Effects on Dental Treatment No effects or complications reported

Other Adverse Effects 1% to 10%:

Gastrointestinal: Nausea, vomiting

Respiratory: Irritation to nasal mucosa, coughing

Oral manifestations: No data reported

Contraindications Hypersensitivity to ammonia or any component

Drug Interactions No data reported

Pregnancy Risk Factor C

Breast-feeding Considerations No data reported

Dosage Forms

Inhalant, crushable glass perles: 0.33 mL, 0.4 mL

Solution: 30 mL, 60 mL, 120 mL

Dietary Considerations No data reported

Generic Available Yes

Ammonium Chloride (a moe' nee um klor' ide)

Therapeutic Category Metabolic Alkalosis Agent; Urinary Acidifying Agent

Use Diuretic or systemic and urinary acidifying agent; treatment of hypochloremic states

Usual Dosage Metabolic alkalosis: The following equations represent different methods of correction utilizing either the serum HCO_3^-, the serum chloride, or the base excess

Mechanism of Action Increases acidity by increasing free hydrogen ion concentration

Local Anesthetic/Vasoconstrictor Precautions No information available to require special precautions

Effects on Dental Treatment No effects or complications reported

Other Adverse Effects 1% to 10%:

Cardiovascular: Bradycardia

Central nervous system: Mental confusion, coma, headache

Dermatologic: Rash

Endocrine & metabolic: Metabolic acidosis secondary to hyperchloremia

Gastrointestinal: Gastric irritation, nausea, vomiting

Local: Pain at site of injection

Respiratory: Hyperventilation

Drug Uptake

Absorption: Rapid from GI tract, complete within 3-6 hours

Pregnancy Risk Factor C

Ammonium Lactate *see* Lactic Acid With Ammonium Hydroxide *on page 487*

Amobarbital (am oh bar' bi tal)

Brand Names Amytal®

Canadian/Mexican Brand Names Amobarbital® (Canada)

Therapeutic Category Barbiturate; Hypnotic; Sedative

Use

Oral: Hypnotic in short-term treatment of insomnia, to reduce anxiety and provide sedation preoperatively

I.M., I.V.: Control status epilepticus or acute seizure episodes. Also used in catatonic, negativistic, or manic reactions and in "Amytal® Interviewing" for narcoanalysis

Usual Dosage
Children: Oral:
Sedation: 6 mg/kg/day divided every 6-8 hours
Insomnia: 2 mg/kg or 70 mg/m²/day in 4 equally divided doses
Hypnotic: 2-3 mg/kg

Adults:
Insomnia: Oral: 65-200 mg at bedtime
Sedation: Oral: 30-50 mg 2-3 times/day
Preanesthetic: Oral: 200 mg 1-2 hours before surgery
Hypnotic:
Oral: 65-200 mg at bedtime
I.M., I.V.: 65-500 mg, should not exceed 500 mg I.M. or 1000 mg I.V.

Mechanism of Action Interferes with transmission of impulses from the thalamus to the cortex of the brain resulting in an imbalance in central inhibitory and facilitatory mechanisms

Local Anesthetic/Vasoconstrictor Precautions No information available to require special precautions

Effects on Dental Treatment No effects or complications reported

Other Adverse Effects
>10%:
Central nervous system: Dizziness, lightheadedness, "hangover" effect, drowsiness, CNS depression, fever
Local: Pain at injection site
1% to 10%:
Central nervous system: Confusion, mental depression, unusual excitement, nervousness, faint feeling, headache, insomnia, nightmares
Gastrointestinal: Nausea, vomiting, constipation
<1%:
Cardiovascular: Hypotension
Central nervous system: Hallucinations
Dermatologic: Skin rash, exfoliative dermatitis urticaria, Stevens-Johnson syndrome
Hematologic: Agranulocytosis, megaloblastic anemia, thrombocytopenia
Local: Thrombophlebitis
Respiratory: Respiratory depression, apnea, laryngospasm

Drug Interactions
Barbiturates can induce hepatic microsomal enzymes resulting in increased metabolism and, therefore, decreased effects of anticoagulants, corticosteroids, doxycycline
Increased toxicity when combined with other CNS depressants or antidepressants, respiratory and CNS depression may be additive

Drug Uptake
Onset of action:
I.V.: Within 5 minutes
Oral: Within 1 hour
Serum half-life, biphasic:
Initial: 40 minutes
Terminal: 20 hours

Pregnancy Risk Factor D

Amobarbital and Secobarbital
(am oh bar' bi tal & see koe bar' bi tal)

Brand Names Tuinal®
Therapeutic Category Barbiturate; Hypnotic
Synonyms Secobarbital and Amobarbital
Use Short-term treatment of insomnia
Local Anesthetic/Vasoconstrictor Precautions No information available to require special precautions
Effects on Dental Treatment No effects or complications reported
Other Adverse Effects
>10%:
Central nervous system: Dizziness, lightheadedness, drowsiness, "hangover" effect
Local: Pain at injection site
1% to 10%:
Central nervous system: Confusion, mental depression, unusual excitement, nervousness, faint feeling, headache, insomnia, nightmares

(Continued)

Amobarbital and Secobarbital *(Continued)*

Gastrointestinal: Constipation, nausea, vomiting
<1%:
Central nervous system: Hallucinations
Cardiovascular: Hypotension
Dermatologic: Skin rash, exfoliative dermatitis, Stevens-Johnson syndrome
Hematologic: Agranulocytosis, megaloblastic anemia, thrombocytopenia
Local: Thrombophlebitis
Respiratory: Respiratory depression

Amonidrin® [OTC] *see Guaifenesin on page 407*
Amoxapina (Mexico) *see Amoxapine on this page*

Amoxapine (a mox' a peen)

Brand Names Asendin®
Canadian/Mexican Brand Names Demolox® (Mexico)
Therapeutic Category Antidepressant, Tricyclic
Synonyms Amoxapina (Mexico)
Use Treatment of neurotic and endogenous depression and mixed symptoms of anxiety and depression
Usual Dosage Once symptoms are controlled, decrease gradually to lowest effective dose. Maintenance dose is usually given at bedtime to reduce daytime sedation. Oral:

Children: Not established in children <16 years of age
Adolescents: Initial: 25-50 mg/day; increase gradually to 100 mg/day; may give as divided doses or as a single dose at bedtime
Adults: Initial: 25 mg 2-3 times/day, if tolerated, dosage may be increased to 100 mg 2-3 times/day; may be given in a single bedtime dose when dosage <300 mg/day
Elderly: Initial: 25 mg at bedtime increased by 25 mg weekly for outpatients and every 3 days for inpatients if tolerated; usual dose: 50-150 mg/day, but doses up to 300 mg may be necessary

Maximum daily dose:
Inpatient: 600 mg
Outpatient: 400 mg

Mechanism of Action Reduces the reuptake of serotonin and norepinephrine and blocks the response of dopamine receptors to dopamine
Local Anesthetic/Vasoconstrictor Precautions Use with caution; epinephrine, norepinephrine and levonordefrin have been shown to have an increased pressor response in combination with TCAs
Effects on Dental Treatment Long-term treatment with TCAs such as amoxapine increases the risk of caries by reducing salivation and salivary buffer capacity
Other Adverse Effects
>10%:
Central nervous system: Dizziness, drowsiness, headache, weakness
Gastrointestinal: Dry mouth, constipation, increased appetite, nausea, unpleasant taste, weight gain
1% to 10%:
Cardiovascular: Arrhythmias, hypotension
Central nervous system: Confusion, delirium, hallucinations, nervousness, restlessness, parkinsonian syndrome, insomnia, tardive dyskinesia
Gastrointestinal: Diarrhea, heartburn
Genitourinary: Difficult urination, sexual function impairment
Neuromuscular & skeletal: Fine muscle tremors
Ocular: Blurred vision, eye pain
Miscellaneous: Excessive sweating
<1%:
Central nervous system: Anxiety, seizures, neuroleptic malignant syndrome
Dermatologic: Photosensitivity, alopecia
Endocrine & metabolic: Breast enlargement, galactorrhea, SIADH
Genitourinary: Testicular swelling
Hematologic: Agranulocytosis, leukopenia, eosinophilia
Hepatic: Cholestatic jaundice, increased liver enzymes
Ocular: Increased intraocular pressure
Otic: Tinnitus
Miscellaneous: Trouble with gums, decreased lower esophageal sphincter tone may cause GE reflux, allergic reactions
Drug Interactions
Decreased effect of clonidine, guanethidine

Increased effect of CNS depressants, sympathomimetics, anticholinergic agents

Increased toxicity of MAO inhibitors (hyperpyrexia, tachycardia, hypertension, seizures and death may occur); similar interactions as with other tricyclics may occur

Drug Uptake

Onset of antidepressant effect: Usually occurs after 1-2 weeks

Absorption: Oral: Rapidly and well absorbed

Serum half-life:

Parent drug: 11-16 hours

Active metabolite (8-hydroxy): Adults: 30 hours

Time to peak serum concentration: Within 1-2 hours

Pregnancy Risk Factor C

Selected Readings

Boakes AJ, Laurence DR, Teoh PC, et al, "Interactions Between Sympathomimetic Amines and Antidepressant Agents in Man," *Br Med J*, 1973, 1(849):311-5.

Jastak JT and Yagiela JA, "Vasoconstrictors and Local Anesthesia: A Review and Rationale for Use," *J Am Dent Assoc*, 1983, 107:623-30.

Larochelle P, Hamet P, and Enjalbert M, "Responses to Tyramine and Norepinephrine After Imipramine and Trazodone," *Clin Pharmacol Ther*, 1979, 26(1):24-30.

Mitchell JR, "Guanethidine and Related Agents. III Antagonism by Drugs Which Inhibit the Norepinephrine Pump in Man," *J Clin Invest*, 1970, 49(8):1596-604.

Rundegren J, van Dijken J, Mörnstad H, et al, "Oral Conditions in Patients Receiving Long-Term Treatment With Cyclic Antidepressant Drugs," *Swed Dent J*, 1985, 9(2):55-64.

Svedmyr N, "The Influence of a Tricyclic Antidepressive Agent (Protriptyline) on Some of the Circulatory Effects of Noradrenaline and Adrenaline® in Man," *Life Sci*, 1968, 7(1):77-84.

Amoxicillin and Clavulanic Acid

(a mox i sil' in & klav yoo lan' ick as' id)

Related Information

Animal and Human Bites Guidelines *on page 976*

Dentin Hypersensitivity; High Caries Index; Xerostomia *on page 959*

Oral Bacterial Infections *on page 945*

Brand Names Augmentin®

Canadian/Mexican Brand Names Clavulin® (Canada); Clavulin® (Mexico)

Therapeutic Category Antibiotic, Penicillin

Use

Dental: Treatment of orofacial infections when beta-lactamase-producing staphylococci and beta-lactamase-producing *Bacteroides* are present

Medical: Treatment of otitis media, sinusitis, and infections caused by susceptible organisms involving the lower respiratory tract, skin and skin structure, and urinary tract; spectrum same as amoxicillin with additional coverage of beta-lactamase producing *B. catarrhalis*, *H. influenzae*, *N. gonorrhoeae*, and *S. aureus* (not MRSA). The expanded coverage of this combination makes it a useful alternative when penicillinase-producing bacteria are present and patients cannot tolerate alternative treatments.

Usual Dosage Oral:

Children <40 kg: 20-40 mg (amoxicillin)/kg/day in divided doses every 8 hours

Children >40 kg and Adults: 250-500 mg every 8 hours or 875 mg every 12 hours for at least 7 days; maximum dose: 2 g/day

Mechanism of Action Interferes with bacterial cell wall synthesis during active multiplication, causing cell wall death and resultant bactericidal activity against susceptible bacteria. Clavulanic acid binds and inhibits beta-lactamases that inactivate amoxicillin resulting in an antibiotic combination having an expanded spectrum of activity.

Local Anesthetic/Vasoconstrictor Precautions No information available to require special precautions

Effects on Dental Treatment Prolonged use of penicillins may lead to development of oral candidiasis

Other Adverse Effects <1%:

Dermatologic: Rash, urticaria

Gastrointestinal: Nausea, vomiting, diarrhea

Genitourinary: Vaginitis

Oral manifestations: No data reported

Contraindications Known hypersensitivity to amoxicillin, clavulanic acid, or penicillin

Warnings/Precautions In patients with renal impairment, doses and/or frequency of administration should be modified in response to the degree of renal impairment; high percentage of patients with infectious mononucleosis have developed rash during therapy; a low incidence of cross-allergy with cephalosporins exists; incidence of diarrhea is higher than with amoxicillin alone

(Continued)

Amoxicillin and Clavulanic Acid *(Continued)*

Drug Interactions Efficacy of oral contraceptives may be reduced; probenecid may cause increased amoxicillin levels; amoxicillin may increase the effect of anticoagulants

Drug Uptake Amoxicillin pharmacokinetics are not affected by clavulanic acid
Onset: Rapid and nearly complete
Time to peak serum concentration:
Capsule: 2 hours
Suspension: 1 hour
Serum half-life:
Adults with normal renal function: ~1 hour for both agents
Children: 1-2 hours
Influence of food: No effect

Pregnancy Risk Factor B

Breast-feeding Considerations
Amoxicillin: May be taken while breast-feeding
Clavulanic acid: No data reported

Dosage Forms
Suspension, oral:
125 (banana flavor): Amoxicillin trihydrate 125 mg and clavulanic acid 31.25 mg per 5 mL (75 mL, 150 mL)
200: Amoxicillin 200 mg and clavulanic acid 28.5 mg per 5 mL (50 mL, 75 mL, 100 mL)
250 (orange flavor): Amoxicillin trihydrate 250 mg and clavulanic acid 62.5 mg per 5 mL (75 mL, 150 mL)
400: Amoxicillin 400 mg and clavulanic acid 57 mg per 5 mL (50 mL, 75 mL, 100 mL)
Tablet:
250: Amoxicillin trihydrate 250 mg and clavulanic acid 125 mg
500: Amoxicillin trihydrate 500 mg and clavulanic acid 125 mg
875: Amoxicillin trihydrate 875 mg and clavulanic acid 125 mg
Tablet, chewable:
125: Amoxicillin trihydrate 125 mg and clavulanic acid 31.25 mg
250: Amoxicillin trihydrate 250 mg and clavulanic acid 62.5 mg

Dietary Considerations May be taken with meals or on an empty stomach; may mix with milk, formula, or juice

Generic Available No

Comments In maxillary sinus, anterior nasal cavity, and deep neck infections, beta-lactamase-producing staphylococci and beta-lactamase-producing *Bacteroides* usually are present. In these situations, antibiotics that resist the beta-lactamase enzyme are indicated. Amoxicillin and clavulanic acid is administered orally for moderate infections. Ampicillin sodium and sulbactam sodium (Unasyn®) is administered parenterally for more severe infections.

Selected Readings
Wynn RL and Bergman SA, "Antibiotics and Their Use in the Treatment of Orofacial Infections," *Gen Dent*, 1994, 42(Pt 1):398-402 and 42(Pt 2):498-502.

Amoxicillin Trihydrate *(a mox i sil′ in trye hye′ drate)*

Related Information
Animal and Human Bites Guidelines *on page 976*
Cardiovascular Diseases *on page 912*
Dentin Hypersensitivity; High Caries Index; Xerostomia *on page 959*
Oral Bacterial Infections *on page 945*

Brand Names A-Cillin®; Amoxil®; Larotid®; Polymox®; Trimox®; Utimox®; Wymox®

Canadian/Mexican Brand Names Apo-Amoxi® (Canada); Novamoxin® (Canada); Nu-Amoxi® (Canada); Pro-Amox® (Canada); Acimox® (Mexico); Amoxifur® (Mexico); Amoxisol® (Mexico); Amoxivet® (Mexico); Gimalxina® (Mexico); Grunicina® (Mexico); Hidramox® (Mexico)

Therapeutic Category Antibiotic, Penicillin

Use
Dental: Antibiotic for standard prophylactic regimen for dental patients who are at risk
Medical: Treatment of sinusitis, otitis media, and infections caused by susceptible organisms involving the respiratory tract, skin, and urinary tract

Usual Dosage Oral:
Children:
<15 kg: 750 mg
15-30 kg: 1500 mg
>30 kg: 3000 mg (full adult dose)

Follow-up dose should be half the initial dose; total pediatric dose should not exceed total adult dose

Adults: Prevention of subacute bacterial endocarditis: 3 g 1 hour before procedure, then 1.5 g 6 hours after initial dose

Mechanism of Action Interferes with bacterial cell wall synthesis during active multiplication, causing cell wall death and resultant bactericidal activity against susceptible bacteria

Local Anesthetic/Vasoconstrictor Precautions No information available to require special precautions

Effects on Dental Treatment Prolonged use of penicillins may lead to development of oral candidiasis

Other Adverse Effects 1% to 10%:

Central nervous system: Seizures, fever

Dermatologic: Rash (especially patients with mononucleosis)

Gastrointestinal: Diarrhea

Miscellaneous: Superinfection

Oral manifestations: No data reported

Contraindications Hypersensitivity to amoxicillin, penicillin, or any component

Warnings/Precautions In patients with renal impairment, doses and/or frequency of administration should be modified in response to the degree of renal impairment; a high percentage of patients with infectious mononucleosis have developed rash during therapy with amoxicillin; a low incidence of cross-allergy with other beta-lactams and cephalosporins exists

Drug Interactions Efficacy of oral contraceptives may be reduced with amoxicillin; disulfiram, probenecid may cause increased amoxicillin levels; allopurinol may increase the potential for amoxicillin rash

Drug Uptake

Onset: Oral: Rapid and nearly complete

Time to peak serum concentration: 2 hours (capsule) and 1 hour (suspension)

Serum half-life:

Adults with normal renal function: 0.7-1.4 hours

Children: 1-2 hours

Influence of food: No effect

Pregnancy Risk Factor B

Breast-feeding Considerations May be taken while breast-feeding

Dosage Forms

Capsule: 250 mg, 500 mg

Drops, pediatric: 50 mg/mL (15 mL, 30 mL)

Suspension, oral: 125 mg/5 mL (5 mL unit dose, 80 mL, 100 mL, 150 mL, 200 mL); 250 mg/5 mL (5 mL unit dose, 80 mL, 100 mL, 150 mL, 200 mL)

Tablet, chewable: 125 mg, 250 mg

Dietary Considerations Peak concentrations may be delayed with food; may be taken with food; may be mixed with formula, milk, or juice

Generic Available Yes

Selected Readings

Council on Dental Therapeutics, American Heart Association, "Preventing Bacterial Endocarditis," *J Am Dent Assoc*, 1991, 122(2):87-92.

Dajani AS, Bisno AL, Chung KJ, et al, "Prevention of Bacterial Endocarditis. Recommendations by the American Heart Association," *JAMA*, 1990, 264(22):2919-22.

Wynn RL, "Amoxicillin Update," *Gen Dent*, 1991, 39(5):322,4,6.

Amoxil® *see* Amoxicillin Trihydrate *on previous page*

Amphetamine Sulfate (am fet' a meen sul' fate)

Therapeutic Category Amphetamine; Central Nervous System Stimulant, Amphetamine

Use Treatment of narcolepsy; exogenous obesity; abnormal behavioral syndrome in children (minimal brain dysfunction); attention deficit hyperactive disorder (ADHD)

Usual Dosage Oral:

Narcolepsy:

Children:

6-12 years: 5 mg/day, increase by 5 mg at weekly intervals

>12 years: 10 mg/day, increase by 10 mg at weekly intervals

Adults: 5-60 mg/day in 2-3 divided doses

Attention deficit disorder: Children:

3-5 years: 2.5 mg/day, increase by 2.5 mg at weekly intervals

>6 years: 5 mg/day, increase by 5 mg at weekly intervals not to exceed 40 mg/day

(Continued)

Amphetamine Sulfate (Continued)

Short-term adjunct to exogenous obesity: Children >12 years and Adults: 10 mg or 15 mg long-acting capsule daily, up to 30 mg/day; or 5-30 mg/day in divided doses (immediate release tablets only)

Mechanism of Action The amphetamines are noncatechol sympathomimetic amines with pharmacologic actions similar to ephedrine. They require breakdown by monoamine oxidase for inactivation; produce central nervous system and respiratory stimulation, a pressor response, mydriasis, bronchodilation, and contraction of the urinary sphincter; thought to have a direct effect on both alpha- and beta-receptor sites in the peripheral system, as well as release stores of norepinephrine in adrenergic nerve terminals. The central nervous system action is thought to occur in the cerebral cortex and reticular-activating system. The anorexigenic effect is probably secondary to the CNS-stimulating effect; the site of action is probably the hypothalamic feeding center

Local Anesthetic/Vasoconstrictor Precautions Use vasoconstriction with caution in patients taking amphetamine sulfate. Amphetamines enhance the sympathomimetic response of epinephrine and norepinephrine leading to potential hypertension and cardiotoxicity.

Effects on Dental Treatment No effects or complications reported

Other Adverse Effects

>10%:

Cardiovascular: Irregular heartbeat

Central nervous system: False feeling of well being, nervousness, restlessness, insomnia

1% to 10%:

Cardiovascular: Hypertension

Central nervous system: Mood or mental changes, dizziness, lightheadedness, headache

Endocrine & metabolic: Changes in libido

Gastrointestinal: Diarrhea, nausea, vomiting, stomach cramps, constipation, anorexia, weight loss dry mouth

Ocular: Blurred vision

Miscellaneous: Increased sweating

<1%:

Cardiovascular: Chest pain

Central nervous system: CNS stimulation (severe), Tourette's syndrome, hyperthermia, seizures, paranoia

Dermatologic: Skin rash, hives

Miscellaneous: Tolerance and withdrawal with prolonged use

Drug Interactions Increased toxicity of MAO inhibitors (hyperpyrexia, hypertension, arrhythmias, seizures, cerebral hemorrhage, and death has occurred)

Pregnancy Risk Factor C

Amphojel® [OTC] see Aluminum Hydroxide on page 39

Amphotericin B (am foe ter' i sin bee)

Related Information

Oral Fungal Infections on page 948

Brand Names Fungizone®

Therapeutic Category Antifungal Agent, Oral Nonabsorbed; Antifungal Agent, Systemic; Antifungal Agent, Topical

Use Treatment of severe systemic infections and meningitis caused by susceptible fungi such as Candida species, Histoplasma capsulatum, Cryptococcus neoformans, Aspergillus species, Blastomyces dermatitidis, Torulopsis glabrata, and Coccidioides immitis; fungal peritonitis; irrigant for bladder fungal infections; topically for cutaneous and mucocutaneous candidal infections; orally for the treatment of oral candidiasis caused by susceptible strains of Candida albicans

Usual Dosage

I.V.:

Children:

Test dose (not required): I.V.: 0.1 mg/kg/dose to a maximum of 1 mg; infuse over 30-60 minutes

Initial therapeutic dose: 0.25 mg/kg gradually increased, usually in 0.25 mg/kg increments on each subsequent day, until the desired daily dose is reached

Maintenance dose: 0.25-1 mg/kg/day given once daily; infuse over 2-6 hours. Once therapy has been established, amphotericin B can be administered on an every other day basis at 1-1.5 mg/kg/dose; cumulative dose: 1.5-2 g over 6-10 week

Adults:

Test dose (not required).: 1 mg infused over 20-30 minutes

Initial dose: 0.25 mg/kg administered over 2-6 hours, gradually increased on subsequent days to the desired level by 0.25 mg/kg increments per day; in critically ill patients, may initiate with 1-1.5 mg/kg/day with close observation

Maintenance dose: 0.25-1 mg/kg/day or 1.5 mg/kg over 4-6 hours every other day; do not exceed 1.5 mg/kg/day; cumulative dose: 1-4 g over 4-10 weeks

Duration of therapy varies with nature of infection: Histoplasmosis, *Cryptococcus*, or blastomycosis may be treated with total dose of 2-4 g

I.T.:

Children.: 25-100 mcg every 48-72 hours; increase to 500 mcg as tolerated

Adults: 25-300 mcg every 48-72 hours; increase to 500 mcg to 1 mg as tolerated

Oral: 1 mL (100 mg) 4 times/day

Topical: Apply to affected areas 2-4 times/day for 1-4 weeks of therapy depending on nature and severity of infection

Mechanism of Action Binds to ergosterol altering cell membrane permeability in susceptible fungi and causing leakage of cell components with subsequent cell death

Local Anesthetic/Vasoconstrictor Precautions No information available to require special precautions

Effects on Dental Treatment No effects or complications reported

Other Adverse Effects

>10%:

Central nervous system: Fever, chills, headache, malaise, generalized pain

Endocrine & metabolic: Hypokalemia, hypomagnesemia

Gastrointestinal: Anorexia

Hematologic: Anemia

Renal: Nephrotoxicity

1% to 10%:

Cardiovascular: Hypotension, hypertension, flushing

Central nervous system: Delirium, arachnoiditis, pain along lumbar nerves

Gastrointestinal: Nausea, vomiting

Genitourinary: Urinary retention

Hematologic: Leukocytosis, bone marrow depression

Local: Thrombophlebitis

Neuromuscular & skeletal: Paresthesia (especially with I.T. therapy)

Renal: Renal tubular acidosis, renal failure

<1%:

Cardiovascular: Cardiac arrest

Central nervous system: Convulsions

Dermatologic: Maculopapular rash

Genitourinary: Anuria

Hematologic: Coagulation defects, thrombocytopenia, agranulocytosis, leukopenia

Hepatic: Acute liver failure

Ocular: Vision changes

Otic: Hearing loss

Respiratory: Dyspnea

Drug Interactions Increased toxicity: Cyclosporine and aminoglycosides (nephrotoxicity), corticosteroids (hypokalemia)

Drug Uptake

Serum half-life, biphasic:

Initial: 15-48 hours

Terminal: 15 days

Time to peak: Within 1 hour following a 4- to 6-hour dose

Pregnancy Risk Factor B

Dosage Forms Suspension, oral: 100 mg/mL (24 mL with dropper)

Amphotericin B Lipid Complex

(am foe ter' i sin bee lip' id kom' pleks)

Brand Names Abelcet™ Injection

Therapeutic Category Antifungal Agent, Systemic

Synonyms ABLC

Use Treatment of aspergillosis in patients who are refractory to or intolerant of conventional amphotericin B therapy. This indication is based on results obtained primarily from emergency use studies for the treatment of aspergillosis; orphan drug status for cryptococcal meningitis

(Continued)

Amphotericin B Lipid Complex *(Continued)*

Usual Dosage

Children and Adults: I.V.: 2.5-5 mg/kg/day as a single infusion **Note:** Significantly higher dose of ABLC are tolerated; it appears that attaining higher doses with ABLC produce more rapid fungicidal activity *in vivo* than standard amphotericin B preparations

Dosing adjustment in renal impairment: None necessary; effects of renal impairment are not currently known

Hemodialysis: No supplemental dosage necessary

Peritoneal dialysis effects: No supplemental dosage necessary

Continuous arterio-venous or veno-venous hemofiltration (CAVH/CAVHD): No supplemental dosage necessary

Local Anesthetic/Vasoconstrictor Precautions No information available to require special precautions

Effects on Dental Treatment No effects or complications reported

Other Adverse Effects

>10%:

Metabolic: Increased serum creatinine

Miscellaneous: Chills, fever, multiple organ failure

1% to 10%:

Cardiovascular: Hypotension, cardiac arrest

Central nervous system: Headache

Dermatologic: Rash

Gastrointestinal: Nausea, vomiting, diarrhea, gastrointestinal hemorrhage

Metabolic: Bilirubinemia, hypokalemia, acidosis

Respiratory: Respiratory failure, dyspnea, pneumonia

Urogenital: Renal failure

Miscellaneous: Pain, abdominal pain

Warnings/Precautions Anaphylaxis has been reported with amphotericin B desoxycholate and other amphotericin B-containing drugs. Facilities for cardiopulmonary resuscitation should be available during administration due to the possibility of anaphylactic reaction. If severe respiratory distress occurs, the infusion should be immediately discontinued and the patient should not receive further infusions. During the initial dosing, the drug should be administered intravenously and under close clinical observation by medically trained personnel. Acute reactions (including fever and chills) may occur 1-2 hours after starting an intravenous infusion. These reactions are usually more common with the first few doses and generally diminish with subsequent doses.

Dosage Forms Injection: 5 mg (20 mL)

Ampicillin *(am pi sil' in)*

Related Information

Cardiovascular Diseases *on page 912*

Dental Drug Interactions: Update on Drug Combinations Requiring Special Considerations *on page 1022*

Brand Names Amcill®; Amplin®; Omnipen®; Penamp®; Polycillin®; Principen®; Totacillin®

Canadian/Mexican Brand Names Ampicin® [Sodium] (Canada); Apo-Ampi® [Trihydrate] (Canada); Jaa Amp® [Trihydrate] (Canada); Nu-Ampi® [Trihydrate] (Canada); Pro-Ampi® [Trihydrate] (Canada); Taro-Ampicillin® [Trihydrate] (Canada); Anglopen® (Mexico); Binotal® (Mexico); Dibacilina® (Mexico); Flamicina® (Mexico); Lampicin® (Mexico); Marovilina® (Mexico); Pentrexyl® (Mexico); Sinaplin® (Mexico)

Therapeutic Category Antibiotic, Penicillin

Use

Dental: Alternate antibiotic for the prevention of bacterial endocarditis in patients undergoing dental procedures. It is used in those patients unable to take oral medications; it is also used in those patients considered high risk and not candidates for the standard regimen of prevention of bacterial endocarditis.

Medical: Treatment of susceptible bacterial infections (nonbeta-lactamase-producing organisms); susceptible bacterial infections caused by streptococci, pneumococci, nonpenicillinase-producing staphylococci, *Listeria*, meningococci; some strains of *H. influenzae*, *Salmonella*, *Shigella*, *E. coli*, *Enterobacter*, and *Klebsiella*

Usual Dosage

Children: Initial: 50 mg/kg, the follow-up dose is half the initial dose

Adults:

Prevention of bacterial endocarditis in patients unable to take oral medications: I.M., I.V.: 2 g 30 minutes before procedure, then 1 g I.M. or I.V. or oral administration of amoxicillin 1.5 g 6 hours after initial dose

In patients considered high risk and not candidates for standard regimen: I.M., I.V.: 2 g ampicillin plus gentamicin 1.5 mg/kg (not to exceed 80 mg) 30 minutes before procedure, followed by amoxicillin 1.5 g orally 6 hours after initial dose; alternatively, the parenteral regimen may be repeated 8 hours after initial dose

Mechanism of Action Interferes with bacterial cell wall synthesis during active multiplication, causing cell wall death and resultant bactericidal activity against susceptible bacteria

Local Anesthetic/Vasoconstrictor Precautions No information available to require special precautions

Effects on Dental Treatment Prolonged use of penicillins may lead to development of oral candidiasis

Other Adverse Effects

>10%:

Dermatologic: Rash (appearance of a rash should be carefully evaluated to differentiate a nonallergic ampicillin rash from a hypersensitivity reaction; incidence is higher in patients with viral infections, *Salmonella* infections, lymphocytic leukemia, or patients that have hyperuricemia)

Gastrointestinal: Diarrhea, vomiting

1% to 10%: Gastrointestinal: Severe abdominal cramps and/or pain

Oral manifestations: >10%: Oral candidiasis after chronic dosing

Contraindications Known hypersensitivity to ampicillin or other penicillins

Warnings/Precautions Dosage adjustment may be necessary in patients with renal impairment; a low incidence of cross-allergy with other beta-lactams exists; high percentage of patients with infectious mononucleosis have developed rash during therapy with ampicillin. Appearance of a rash should be carefully evaluated to differentiate a nonallergic ampicillin rash from a hypersensitivity reaction. Ampicillin rash occurs in 5% to 10% of children receiving ampicillin and is a generalized dull red, maculopapular rash, generally appearing 3-14 days after the start of therapy. It normally begins on the trunk and spreads over most of the body. It may be most intense at pressure areas, elbows, and knees.

Drug Interactions Efficacy of oral contraceptives may be reduced with ampicillin; probenecid may cause increased penicillin levels; ampicillin may increase the effect of anticoagulants; allopurinol may increase the potential for amoxicillin (ampicillin) rash

Drug Uptake

Absorption: Oral: 50%

Time to peak serum concentration: Oral: Within 1-2 hours

Serum half-life: Adults and Children: 1-1.8 hours

Pregnancy Risk Factor B

Breast-feeding Considerations Excreted into breast milk in small amounts like amoxicillin which is compatible with breast-feeding

Dosage Forms

Capsule, as anhydrous: 250 mg, 500 mg

Capsule, as trihydrate: 250 mg, 500 mg

Drops, pediatric, as trihydrate: 100 mg/mL (20 mL)

Injection, as sodium: 125 mg, 250 mg, 500 mg, 1 g, 2 g, 10 g

Suspension, oral, as trihydrate: 100 mg/mL (20 mL); 125 mg/5 mL (5 mL unit dose, 100 mL, 150 mL, 200 mL); 250 mg/5 mL (5 mL unit dose, 80 mL, 100 mL, 150 mL, 200 mL); 500 mg/5 mL (5 mL unit dose, 100 mL)

Dietary Considerations Should be taken on an empty stomach; food decreases rate and extent of absorption

Generic Available Yes

Selected Readings

Council on Dental Therapeutics, American Heart Association, "Preventing Bacterial Endocarditis," *J Am Dent Assoc*, 1991, 122(2):87-92.

Dajani AS, Bisno AL, Chung KJ, et al, "Prevention of Bacterial Endocarditis. Recommendations by the American Heart Association," *JAMA*, 1990, 264(22):2919-22.

Ampicillin and Probenecid (am pi sil' in & proe ben' e sid)

Brand Names Polycillin-PRB®; Proampacin®

Therapeutic Category Antibiotic, Penicillin

Use Uncomplicated infections caused by susceptible strains of *Neisseria gonorrhoeae* in adults

Local Anesthetic/Vasoconstrictor Precautions No information available to require special precautions

(Continued)

Ampicillin and Probenecid *(Continued)*

Effects on Dental Treatment >10% oral candidiasis after chronic dosing
Other Adverse Effects
>10%:
  Central nervous system: Headache
  Dermatologic: Rash
  Gastrointestinal: Anorexia, nausea, vomiting, diarrhea, oral candidiasis
  Neuromuscular & skeletal: Gouty arthritis (acute)
1% to 10%:
  Cardiovascular: Flushing of face
  Central nervous system: Dizziness
  Dermatologic: Skin rash, itching
  Gastrointestinal: Sore gums, severe abdominal or stomach cramps and pain
  Genitourinary: Painful urination
  Renal: Renal calculi
<1%:
  Central nervous system: Seizures
  Hematologic: Leukopenia, hemolytic anemia, aplastic anemia
  Hepatic: Hepatic necrosis
  Renal: Urate nephropathy, nephrotic syndrome
  Miscellaneous: Anaphylaxis, penicillin encephalopathy, lymphocytic leukemia
Drug Interactions Avoid concomitant use with ketorolac since its half-life is increased two-fold and levels and toxicity are significantly increased by probenecid; allopurinol theoretically has an additional potential for ampicillin rash
Pregnancy Risk Factor B

Ampicillin Sodium and Sulbactam Sodium
(am pi sil' in so' dee um & sul' bak tam so' dee um)
Related Information
  Dental Drug Interactions: Update on Drug Combinations Requiring Special Considerations *on page 1022*
Brand Names Unasyn®
Canadian/Mexican Brand Names Unasyna® (Mexico); Unasyna® Oral (Mexico)
Therapeutic Category Antibiotic, Penicillin
Use
  Dental: Parenteral beta-lactamase-resistant antibiotic combination to treat more severe orofacial infections where beta-lactamase-producing staphylococci and beta-lactamase-producing *Bacteroides* are present
  Medical: Treatment of susceptible bacterial infections involved with skin and skin structure, intra-abdominal infections, gynecological infections; spectrum is that of ampicillin plus organisms producing beta-lactamases such as *S. aureus*, *H. influenzae*, *E. coli*, *Klebsiella*, *Acinetobacter*, *Enterobacter*, and anaerobes
Usual Dosage Unasyn® (ampicillin/sulbactam) is a combination product. Each 3 g vial contains 2 g of ampicillin and 1 g of sulbactam. Sulbactam has very little antibacterial activity by itself, but effectively extends the spectrum of ampicillin to include beta-lactamase producing strains that are resistant to ampicillin alone. Therefore, dosage recommendations for Unasyn® are based on the ampicillin component.

  I.M., I.V.:
    Children: 100-200 mg ampicillin/kg/day divided every 6 hours; maximum dose: 8 g ampicillin/day
    Adults: 1-2 g ampicillin every 6-8 hours; maximum dose: 8 g ampicillin/day
Mechanism of Action Interferes with bacterial cell wall synthesis during active multiplication, causing cell wall death and resultant bactericidal activity against susceptible bacteria; addition of sulbactam, a beta-lactamase inhibitor, to ampicillin extends the spectrum of ampicillin to include beta-lactamase producing organisms
Local Anesthetic/Vasoconstrictor Precautions No information available to require special precautions
Effects on Dental Treatment Prolonged use of penicillins may lead to development of oral candidiasis
Other Adverse Effects
  >10%: Local: Pain at injection site (I.M.)
  1% to 10%:
    Dermatologic: Rash
    Gastrointestinal: Diarrhea

Local: Pain at injection site (I.V.)

Oral manifestations: <1%: Candidiasis, hairy tongue

Contraindications Hypersensitivity to ampicillin, sulbactam or any component, or penicillins

Warnings/Precautions Dosage adjustment may be necessary in patients with renal impairment; a low incidence of cross-allergy with other beta-lactams exists; high percentage of patients with infectious mononucleosis have developed rash during therapy with ampicillin. Appearance of a rash should be carefully evaluated to differentiate a nonallergic ampicillin rash from a hypersensitivity reaction. Ampicillin rash occurs in 5% to 10% of children receiving ampicillin and is a generalized dull red, maculopapular rash, generally appearing 3-14 days after the start of therapy. It normally begins on the trunk and spreads over most of the body. It may be most intense at pressure areas, elbows, and knees.

Drug Interactions Efficacy of oral contraceptives may be reduced with ampicillin and sulbactam; probenecid results in increased amoxicillin levels; allopurinol may increase the potential for amoxicillin/ampicillin rash

Drug Uptake
Absorption: Oral: 50%
Time to peak serum concentration: Ampicillin: 1-2 hours
Duration: Ampicillin: 6 hours
Serum half-life:
Ampicillin: 1-1.8 hours
Sulbactam: 1-1.3 hours

Pregnancy Risk Factor B

Breast-feeding Considerations
Ampicillin: Excreted into breast milk in small amounts like amoxicillin which is compatible with breast-feeding
Sulbactam sodium: No data reported

Dosage Forms Powder for injection: 1.5 g [ampicillin sodium 1 g and sulbactam sodium 0.5 g]; 3 g [ampicillin sodium 2 g and sulbactam sodium 1 g]

Dietary Considerations No data reported

Generic Available No

Comments In maxillary sinus, anterior nasal cavity, and deep neck infections, beta-lactamase-producing staphylococci and beta-lactamase-producing *Bacteroides* usually are present. In these situations, antibiotics that resist the beta-lactamase enzyme should be administered. Amoxicillin and clavulanic acid is administered orally for moderate infections. Ampicillin sodium and sulbactam sodium (Unasyn®) is administered parenterally for more severe infections.

Selected Readings
Wynn RL and Bergman SA, "Antibiotics and Their Use in the Treatment of Orofacial Infections," *Gen Dent*, 1994, 42(Pt 1):398-402 and 42(Pt 2):498-502.

Amplin® *see* Ampicillin *on page 62*

Amrinona, Lactato De (Mexico) *see* Amrinone Lactate *on this page*

Amrinone Lactate (am′ ri none lak′ tate)

Brand Names Inocor®

Therapeutic Category Adrenergic Agonist Agent

Synonyms Amrinona, Lactato De (Mexico)

Use Treatment of low cardiac output states (sepsis, congestive heart failure); adjunctive therapy of pulmonary hypertension; normally prescribed for patients who have not responded well to therapy with digitalis, diuretics, and vasodilators

Usual Dosage Dosage is based on clinical response
Note: Dose should not exceed 10 mg/kg/24 hours

Children and Adults: 0.75 mg/kg I.V. bolus over 2-3 minutes followed by maintenance infusion of 5-10 mcg/kg/minute; I.V. bolus may need to be repeated in 30 minutes

Mechanism of Action Inhibits myocardial cyclic adenosine monophosphate (cAMP) phosphodiesterase activity and increases cellular levels of cAMP resulting in a positive inotropic effect and increased cardiac output; also possesses systemic and pulmonary vasodilator effects resulting in pre- and afterload reduction; slightly increases atrioventricular conduction

Local Anesthetic/Vasoconstrictor Precautions No information available to require special precautions

Effects on Dental Treatment No effects or complications reported

(Continued)

Amrinone Lactate *(Continued)*

Other Adverse Effects
1% to 10%:
    Cardiovascular: Arrhythmias, hypotension (may be infusion rate-related), ventricular and supraventricular arrhythmias
    Gastrointestinal: Nausea
    Hematologic: Thrombocytopenia (may be dose-related)
<1%:
    Cardiovascular: Chest pain
    Central nervous system: Fever
    Gastrointestinal: Vomiting, abdominal pain, anorexia
    Hepatic: Hepatotoxicity
    Local: Pain or burning at injection site

Drug Interactions No data reported

Drug Uptake
Onset of action: I.V.: Within 2-5 minutes
Peak effect: Within 10 minutes
Duration: Dose dependent (~30 minutes low dose, ~2 hours higher doses)
Serum half-life:
    Adults, normal volunteers: 3.6 hours
    Adults with CHF: 5.8 hours

Pregnancy Risk Factor C

Amvisc® *see* Sodium Hyaluronate *on page 791*

Amyl Nitrite *(am′ il nye′ trite)*

Therapeutic Category Vasodilator, Coronary

Use Coronary vasodilator in angina pectoris; adjunct in treatment of cyanide poisoning; used to produce changes in the intensity of heart murmurs

Usual Dosage Adults: 1-6 inhalations from one capsule are usually sufficient to produce the desired effect

Local Anesthetic/Vasoconstrictor Precautions No information available to require special precautions

Effects on Dental Treatment No effects or complications reported

Other Adverse Effects
1% to 10%:
    Cardiovascular: Postural hypotension, cutaneous flushing of head, neck, and clavicular area
    Central nervous system: Headache
<1%:
    Dermatologic: Skin rash
    Hematologic: Hemolytic anemia

Drug Interactions Increased toxicity: Alcohol

Drug Uptake
Onset of action: Angina relieved within 30 seconds
Duration: 3-15 minutes

Pregnancy Risk Factor C

Amytal® *see* Amobarbital *on page 54*

Anacin® [OTC] *see* Aspirin *on page 78*

Anacin-3® [OTC] *see* Acetaminophen *on page 14*

Anadrol® *see* Oxymetholone *on page 650*

Anafranil® *see* Clomipramine Hydrochloride *on page 219*

Ana-Kit® *see* Insect Sting Kit *on page 459*

Anamine® Syrup [OTC] *see* Chlorpheniramine and Pseudoephedrine *on page 191*

Anaplex® Liquid [OTC] *see* Chlorpheniramine and Pseudoephedrine *on page 191*

Anaprox® (Naproxen Sodium) *see* Naproxen *on page 606*

Anaspaz® *see* Hyoscyamine Sulfate *on page 445*

Anatuss® [OTC] *see* Guaifenesin, Phenylpropanolamine, and Dextromethorphan *on page 410*

Anbesol® Maximum Strength [OTC] *see* Benzocaine *on page 102*

Ancef® *see* Cefazolin Sodium *on page 164*

Ancobon® *see* Flucytosine *on page 368*

Andro® *see* Testosterone *on page 825*

Andro-Cyp® *see* Testosterone *on page 825*

Andro®/Fem Injection *see* Estradiol and Testosterone *on page 326*

Android® *see* Methyltestosterone *on page 570*

Andro-L.A.® *see* Testosterone *on page 825*

Androlone® *see* Nandrolone *on page 604*
Androlone®**-D** *see* Nandrolone *on page 604*
Andronate® *see* Testosterone *on page 825*
Andropository® *see* Testosterone *on page 825*
Andryl® *see* Testosterone *on page 825*
Anergan® *see* Promethazine Hydrochloride *on page 733*
Anexsia® **5/500** *see* Hydrocodone and Acetaminophen *on page 431*
Anexsia® **7.5/650** *see* Hydrocodone and Acetaminophen *on page 431*
Anexsia® **10/660** *see* Hydrocodone and Acetaminophen *on page 431*
Animal and Human Bites Guidelines *see page 976*

Anisotropine Methylbromide
(an iss oh troe' peen meth' il broe' mide)
Brand Names Valpin® 50
Canadian/Mexican Brand Names Miradon® (Canada)
Therapeutic Category Anticholinergic Agent; Antispasmodic Agent, Gastro-intestinal
Use Adjunctive treatment of peptic ulcer
Usual Dosage Adults: Oral: 50 mg 3 times/day
Mechanism of Action Blocks the action of acetylcholine at parasympathetic sites in smooth muscle, secretory glands, and the CNS; increases cardiac output, dries secretions, antagonizes histamine and serotonin
Local Anesthetic/Vasoconstrictor Precautions No information available to require special precautions
Effects on Dental Treatment Dry mouth and orthostatic hypotension possible
Other Adverse Effects
>10%:
  Cardiovascular: Palpitations
  Gastrointestinal: Constipation
  Miscellaneous: Decreased sweating, dry mouth, nose, throat, or skin
1% to 10%: Decreased flow of breast milk, decreased salivary secretion
<1%:
  Cardiovascular: Orthostatic hypotension
  Central nervous system: Confusion, drowsiness, headache, loss of memory, weakness, tiredness
  Dermatologic: Skin rash
  Gastrointestinal: Bloated feeling, nausea, vomiting
  Genitourinary: Decreased urination
  Ocular: Increased intraocular pain, blurred vision, increased sensitivity to light
Drug Interactions No data reported
Drug Uptake
Absorption: Poor (~10%) from GI tract
Pregnancy Risk Factor C

Anistreplase (a niss' tre place)
Related Information
Cardiovascular Diseases *on page 912*
Brand Names Eminase®
Therapeutic Category Thrombolytic Agent
Use Management of acute myocardial infarction (AMI) in adults; lysis of thrombi obstructing coronary arteries, reduction of infarct size; and reduction of mortality associated with AMI
Usual Dosage Adults: I.V.: 30 units injected over 2-5 minutes as soon as possible after onset of symptoms
Mechanism of Action Activates the conversion of plasminogen to plasmin by forming a complex exposing plasminogen-activating site and cleavage of a peptide bond that converts plasminogen to plasmin; plasmin being capable of thrombolysis, by degrading fibrin, fibrinogen and other procoagulant proteins into soluble fragments, effective both outside and within the formed thrombus/embolus
Local Anesthetic/Vasoconstrictor Precautions No information available to require special precautions
Effects on Dental Treatment No effects or complications reported
Other Adverse Effects
>10%:
  Cardiovascular: Arrhythmias, hypotension, perfusion arrhythmias
  Hematologic: Bleeding or oozing from cuts
1% to 10%: Anaphylactic reaction
(Continued)

Anistreplase *(Continued)*

<1%:
  Central nervous system: Headache, chills
  Dermatologic: Rash
  Gastrointestinal: Nausea, vomiting
  Hematologic: Anemia, eye hemorrhage
  Respiratory: Bronchospasm
  Miscellaneous: Epistaxis, sweating
Drug Interactions Increased efficacy and bleeding potential: Anticoagulants (heparin, warfarin), antiplatelet agents (aspirin)
Drug Uptake
  Duration: Fibrinolytic effect persists for 4-6 hours following administration
  Serum half-life: 70-120 minutes
Pregnancy Risk Factor C

Anodynos-DHC® [5/500] *see* Hydrocodone and Acetaminophen *on page 431*

Anoquan® *see* Butalbital Compound *on page 133*

Ansaid® *see* Flurbiprofen Sodium *on page 381*

Antabuse® *see* Disulfiram *on page 293*

Antazoline-V® Ophthalmic *see* Naphazoline and Antazoline *on page 604*

Anthra-Derm® *see* Anthralin *on this page*

Anthralin (an' thra lin)

Brand Names Anthra-Derm®; Drithocreme®; Drithocreme® HP 1%; Dritho-Scalp®; Lasan™; Lasan HP-1™
Canadian/Mexican Brand Names Anthraforte® (Canada); Anthranol® (Canada); Anthrascalp® (Canada); Anthranol® (Mexico)
Therapeutic Category Antipsoriatic Agent, Topical; Keratolytic Agent
Synonyms Antralina (Mexico)
Use Treatment of psoriasis (quiescent or chronic psoriasis)
Usual Dosage Adults: Topical: Generally, apply once a day or as directed. The irritant potential of anthralin is directly related to the strength being used and each patient's individual tolerance. Always commence treatment for at least one week using the lowest strength possible.

  Skin application: Apply sparingly only to psoriatic lesions and rub gently and carefully into the skin until absorbed. Avoid applying an excessive quantity which may cause unnecessary soiling and staining of the clothing or bed linen.

  Scalp application: Comb hair to remove scalar debris and, after suitably parting, rub cream well into the lesions, taking care to prevent the cream from spreading onto the forehead

  Remove by washing or showering; optimal period of contact will vary according to the strength used and the patient's response to treatment. Continue treatment until the skin is entirely clear (ie, when there is nothing to feel with the fingers and the texture is normal)
Mechanism of Action Reduction of the mitotic rate and proliferation of epidermal cells in psoriasis by inhibiting synthesis of nucleic protein from inhibition of DNA synthesis to affected areas
Local Anesthetic/Vasoconstrictor Precautions No information available to require special precautions
Effects on Dental Treatment No effects or complications reported
Other Adverse Effects
  1% to 10%: Topical: Transient primary irritation of uninvolved skin; temporary discoloration of hair and fingernails, may stain skin, hair, or fabrics
  <1%: Topical: Skin rash, excessive irritation
Drug Interactions Increased toxicity: Long-term use of topical corticosteroids may destabilize psoriasis, and withdrawal may also give rise to a "rebound" phenomenon, allow an interval of at least 1 week between the discontinuance of topical corticosteroids and the commencement of therapy
Pregnancy Risk Factor C

AntibiOtic® Otic *see* Neomycin, Polymyxin B, and Hydrocortisone *on page 610*

Antihemophilic Factor (Human)

(an tee hee moe fil' ik fak' tor, hyu' min)
Brand Names Hemofil® M; Humate-P®; Kōate®-HP; Kōate®-HS; KoGENate®; Monoclate-P®; Profilate® OSD
Therapeutic Category Antihemophilic Agent; Blood Product Derivative
Synonyms AHF; Factor VIII

Use Management of hemophilia A in patients whom a deficiency in factor VIII has been demonstrated

Usual Dosage I.V.: Individualize dosage based on coagulation studies performed prior to and during treatment at regular intervals. One AHF unit is the activity present in 1 mL of normal pooled human plasma; dosage should be adjusted to actual vial size currently stocked in the pharmacy.

Hospitalized patients: 20-50 units/kg/dose; may be higher for special circumstances. Dose can be given every 12-24 hours and more frequently in special circumstances.

Formula to approximate percentage increase in plasma antihemophilic factor:

Units required = desired level increase (desired level - actual level) x plasma volume (mL)

Total blood volume (mL blood/kg) = 70 mL/kg (adults); 80 mL/kg (children)

Plasma volume = total blood volume (mL) x [1 - Hct (in decimals)]

Example: For a 70 kg adult with a Hct = 40% : plasma volume = [70 kg x 70 mL/kg] x [1 - 0.4] = 2940 mL

To calculate number of units of factor VIII needed to increase level to desired range (highly individualized and dependent on patient's condition):

Number of units = desired level increase [desired level - actual level] x plasma volume (in mL)

Example: For a 100% level in the above patient who has an actual level of 20% the number of units needed = [1 (for a 100% level) - 0.2] x 2940 mL = 2352 units

Mechanism of Action Protein (factor VIII) in normal plasma which is necessary for clot formation and maintenance of hemostasis; activates factor X in conjunction with activated factor IX; activated factor X converts prothrombin to thrombin, which converts fibrinogen to fibrin and with factor XIII forms a stable clot

Local Anesthetic/Vasoconstrictor Precautions No information available to require special precautions

Effects on Dental Treatment No effects or complications reported

Other Adverse Effects <1%:

Cardiovascular: Flushing, tachycardia

Central nervous system: Headache

Gastrointestinal: Nausea, vomiting

Neuromuscular & skeletal: Paresthesia

Sensitivity reactions: Allergic vasomotor reactions, tightness in neck or chest

Drug Uptake

Serum half-life, biphasic: 4-24 hours with a mean of 12 hours (biphasic: 12 hours is usually used for dosing interval estimates)

Pregnancy Risk Factor C

Antihemophilic Factor (Porcine)

(an tee hee moe fil' ik fak' ter, por' seen)

Brand Names Hyate®:C

Therapeutic Category Antihemophilic Agent

Use Treatment of congenital hemophiliacs with antibodies to human factor VIII:C and also for previously nonhemophiliac patients with spontaneously acquired inhibitors to human factor VIII:C; patients with inhibitors who are bleeding or who are to undergo surgery

Usual Dosage Clinical response should be used to assess efficacy rather than relying upon a particular laboratory value for recovery of factor VIII:C.

Initial dose:

Antibody level to human factor VIII:C <50 Bethesda units/mL: 100-150 porcine units/kg (body weight) is recommended

Antibody level to human factor VIII:C >50 Bethesda units/mL: Activity of the antibody to porcine factor VIII:C should be determined; **an antiporcine antibody level** >20 Bethesda units/mL indicates that the patient is unlikely to benefit from treatment; for lower titers, a dose of 100-150 porcine units/kg is recommended

If a patient has previously been treated with Hyate®:C, this may provide a guide to his likely response and, therefore, assist in estimation of the preliminary dose

Subsequent doses: Following administration of the initial dose, if the recovery of factor VIII:C in the patient's plasma is not sufficient, a further higher dose should be administered; if recovery after the second dose is still insufficient, a third and higher dose may prove effective

(Continued)

Antihemophilic Factor (Porcine) *(Continued)*

Mechanism of Action Factor VIII:C is the coagulation portion of the factor VIII complex in plasma. Factor VIII:C acts as a cofactor for factor IX to activate factor X in the intrinsic pathway of blood coagulation.

Local Anesthetic/Vasoconstrictor Precautions No information available to require special precautions

Effects on Dental Treatment No effects or complications reported

Other Adverse Effects 1% to 10%:
Central nervous system: Fever, headache, chills
Dermatologic: Skin rashes
Gastrointestinal: Nausea, vomiting

Pregnancy Risk Factor C

Comments Sodium ion concentration is not more than 200 mmol/L; the assayed amount of activity is stated on the label, but may vary depending on the type of assay and hemophilic substrate plasma used

Antihemophilic Factor (Recombinant)
(an tee hee moe fil' ik fak' tor, ree kom' be nant)

Brand Names Bioclate®; Hexlixate®; Recombinate®

Therapeutic Category Antihemophilic Agent

Synonyms Factor VIII Recombinant

Use Management of hemophilia A in patients whom a deficiency in factor VIII has been demonstrated

Local Anesthetic/Vasoconstrictor Precautions No information available to require special precautions

Effects on Dental Treatment No effects or complications reported

Other Adverse Effects <1%:
Cardiovascular: Flushing, tachycardia
Central nervous system: Headache
Gastrointestinal: Nausea, vomiting
Neuromuscular & skeletal: Paresthesia, tightness in neck or chest
Miscellaneous: Allergic vasomotor reactions

Anti-Inhibitor Coagulant Complex
(an tee-in hi' bi tor coe ag' yoo lant kom' pleks)

Brand Names Autoplex® T; Feiba VH Immuno®

Therapeutic Category Hemophilic Agent

Use Patients with factor VIII inhibitors who are to undergo surgery or those who are bleeding

Usual Dosage Dosage range: 25-100 factor VIII correctional units per kg depending on the severity of hemorrhage

Local Anesthetic/Vasoconstrictor Precautions No information available to require special precautions

Effects on Dental Treatment No effects or complications reported

Other Adverse Effects <1%:
Cardiovascular: Hypotension, flushing
Central nervous system: Fever, headache, chills
Dermatologic: Rash, urticaria
Hematologic: Disseminated intravascular coagulation
Miscellaneous: Anaphylaxis, indications of protein sensitivity

Pregnancy Risk Factor C

Antilirium® see Physostigmine on page 690

Antimicrobial Prophylaxis in Surgical Patients see page 1042

Antiminth® [OTC] see Pyrantel Pamoate on page 751

Antipyrine and Benzocaine (an tee pye' reen & ben' zoe kane)

Brand Names Allergan® Ear Drops; Auralgan®; Auroto®; Otocalm® Ear

Therapeutic Category Otic Agent, Analgesic; Otic Agent, Cerumenolytic

Synonyms Benzocaine and Antipyrine

Use Temporary relief of pain and reduction of swelling associated with acute congestive and serous otitis media, swimmer's ear, otitis externa; facilitates ear wax removal

Local Anesthetic/Vasoconstrictor Precautions Information available to require special precautions

Effects on Dental Treatment No effects or complications reported

Other Adverse Effects <1%:
Dermatologic: Edema, burning, stinging, tenderness
Miscellaneous: Hypersensitivity reactions

Antirabies Serum, Equine Origin
(an tee ray′ beez seer′ um, ee′ kwine or′ eh gin)
Therapeutic Category Serum
Synonyms ARS
Use Rabies prophylaxis
Local Anesthetic/Vasoconstrictor Precautions No information available to require special precautions
Effects on Dental Treatment No effects or complications reported
Other Adverse Effects 1% to 10%:
Dermatologic: Urticaria
Local: Pain
Miscellaneous: Serum sickness
Comments Because of a significantly lower incidence of adverse reactions, Rabies Immune Globulin, Human is preferred over Antirabies Serum Equine

Antispas® see Dicyclomine Hydrochloride on page 273

Antithrombin III (an tee throm′ bin three)
Brand Names ATnativ®; Thrombate III™
Therapeutic Category Blood Product Derivative
Synonyms ATIII; Heparin Cofactor I
Use Agent for hereditary antithrombin III deficiency
Usual Dosage After first dose of antithrombin III, level should increase to 120% of normal; thereafter maintain at levels >80%. Generally, achieved by administration of maintenance doses once every 24 hours; initially and until patient is stabilized, measure antithrombin III level at least twice daily, thereafter once daily and always immediately before next infusion. 1 unit = quantity of antithrombin III in 1 mL of normal pooled human plasma; administration of 1 unit/1 kg raises AT-III level by 1% to 2%; assume plasma volume of 40 mL/kg

Initial dosage (units) = [desired AT-III level % - baseline AT-III level %] x body weight (kg) divided by 1%/units/kg, eg, if a 70 kg adult patient had a baseline AT-III level of 57%, the initial dose would be (120% - 57%) x 70/1%/units/kg = 4,410 units

Measure antithrombin III preceding and 30 minutes after dose to calculate *in vivo* recovery rate; maintain level within normal range for 2-8 days depending on type of surgery or procedure

Mechanism of Action Antithrombin III is the primary physiologic inhibitor of *in vivo* coagulation. It is an alpha$_2$-globulin. Its principal actions are the inactivation of thrombin, plasmin, and other active serine proteases of coagulation, including factors IXa, Xa, XIa, XIIa, and VIIa. The inactivation of proteases is a major step in the normal clotting process. The strong activation of clotting enzymes at the site of every bleeding injury facilitates fibrin formation and maintains normal hemostasis. Thrombosis in the circulation would be caused by active serine proteases if they were not inhibited by antithrombin III after the localized clotting process. Patients with congenital deficiency are in a prethrombotic state, even if asymptomatic, as evidenced by elevated plasma levels of prothrombin activation fragment, which are normalized following infusions of antithrombin III concentrate.
Local Anesthetic/Vasoconstrictor Precautions No information available to require special precautions
Effects on Dental Treatment No effects or complications reported
Other Adverse Effects <1%:
Central nervous system: Dizziness, lightheadedness, fever
Cardiovascular: Chest tightness, chest pain, vasodilatory effects, edema
Dermatologic: Hives, hematoma formation
Endocrine & metabolic: Fluid overload
Gastrointestinal: Nausea, foul taste in mouth, cramps, bowel fullness
Ocular: Film over eye
Renal: Diuretic effects
Respiratory: Shortness of breath
Pregnancy Risk Factor C

Antithymocyte Globulin (Equine) see Lymphocyte Immune Globulin, Anti-thymocyte Globulin (Equine) on page 518

Antithymocyte Immunoglobulin see Lymphocyte Immune Globulin, Anti-thymocyte Globulin (Equine) on page 518

Anti-Tuss® **Expectorant [OTC]** see Guaifenesin on page 407

Antivert® see Meclizine Hydrochloride on page 530

Antralina (Mexico) see Anthralin on page 68

Antrizine® see Meclizine Hydrochloride on page 530

Anturane® *see* Sulfinpyrazone *on page 811*

Anxanil® *see* Hydroxyzine *on page 443*

Apacet® [OTC] *see* Acetaminophen *on page 14*

Apatate® [OTC] *see* Vitamin B Complex *on page 899*

Aphrodyne™ *see* Yohimbine Hydrochloride *on page 905*

Aphthasol® *see* Amlexanox *on page 52*

A.P.L.® *see* Chorionic Gonadotropin *on page 203*

Aplisol® *see* Tuberculin Purified Protein Derivative *on page 882*

Aplonidine *see* Apraclonidine Hydrochloride *on this page*

Apraclonidine Hydrochloride
(a pra kloe' ni deen hye droe klor' ide)

Brand Names Alpidine®; Iopidine®

Therapeutic Category Alpha-2-Adrenergic Agonist Agent, Ophthalmic

Synonyms Aplonidine; p-Aminoclonidine

Use Prevention and treatment of postsurgical intraocular pressure elevation

Usual Dosage Adults: Ophthalmic: Instill 1 drop in operative eye 1 hour prior to laser surgery, second drop in eye upon completion of procedure

Mechanism of Action Apraclonidine is a potent alpha-adrenergic agent similar to clonidine; relatively selective for alpha$_2$-receptors but does retain some binding to alpha$_1$-receptors; appears to result in reduction of aqueous humor formation; its penetration through the blood-brain barrier is more polar than clonidine which reduces its penetration through the blood-brain barrier and suggests that its pharmacological profile is characterized by peripheral rather than central effects.

Local Anesthetic/Vasoconstrictor Precautions No information available to require special precautions

Effects on Dental Treatment No effects or complications reported

Other Adverse Effects

1% to 10%:

Central nervous system: Lethargy

Gastrointestinal: Dry mouth

Ocular: Upper lid elevation, conjunctival blanching, mydriasis, burning and itching eyes, discomfort, conjunctival microhemorrhage, blurred vision

Respiratory: Dry nose

<1%:

Sensitivity reactions: Allergic response

Miscellaneous: Some systemic effects have also been reported including GI, CNS, and cardiovascular symptoms (arrhythmias)

Drug Uptake

Onset of action: 1 hour

Maximum IOP: 3-5 hours

Pregnancy Risk Factor C

Apresazide® *see* Hydralazine and Hydrochlorothiazide *on page 428*

Apresoline® *see* Hydralazine Hydrochloride *on page 428*

Aprodine® [OTC] *see* Triprolidine and Pseudoephedrine *on page 878*

Aprodine® w/C *see* Triprolidine, Pseudoephedrine, and Codeine *on page 879*

Aprotinin (a proe tye' nin)

Brand Names Trasylol®

Therapeutic Category Hemostatic Agent

Use Reduction or prevention of blood loss in patients undergoing coronary artery bypass surgery when a high index of suspicion of excessive bleeding potential exists; this includes open heart reoperation, pre-existing coagulopathy, operations on the great vessels, and patients whose religious beliefs prohibit blood transfusions

Usual Dosage

Test dose: **All** patients should receive a 1 mL I.V. test dose at least 10 minutes prior to the loading dose to assess the potential for allergic reactions

Regimen A (standard dose):

2 million units (280 mg) loading dose I.V. over 20-30 minutes

2 million units (280 mg) into pump prime volume

500,000 units/hour (70 mg/hour) I.V. during operation

Regimen B (low dose):

1 million units (140 mg) loading dose I.V. over 20-30 minutes

1 million units (140 mg) into pump prime volume

250,000 units/hour (35 mg/hour) I.V. during operation

Mechanism of Action Serine protease inhibitor; inhibits plasmin, kallikrein, and platelet activation producing antifibrinolytic effects; a weak inhibitor of plasma pseudocholinesterase. It also inhibits the contact phase activation of coagulation and preserves adhesive platelet glycoproteins making them resistant to damage from increased circulating plasmin or mechanical injury occurring during bypass

Local Anesthetic/Vasoconstrictor Precautions No information available to require special precautions

Effects on Dental Treatment No effects or complications reported

Other Adverse Effects Increase in postoperative renal dysfunction compared to placebo; anaphylactic reactions have been reported in <0.5% of cases; such reactions are more likely to occur with repeated administration

Drug Uptake
Serum half-life: 150 minutes

Pregnancy Risk Factor C

Aquacare® **[OTC]** *see* Urea *on page 884*

Aquachloral® **Supprettes**® *see* Chloral Hydrate *on page 180*

AquaMEPHYTON® *see* Phytonadione *on page 690*

Aquaphyllin® *see* Theophylline/Aminophylline *on page 832*

AquaSite® **Ophthalmic Solution [OTC]** *see* Artificial Tears *on page 75*

Aquasol A® **[OTC]** *see* Vitamin A *on page 898*

Aquasol E® **[OTC]** *see* Vitamin E *on page 900*

Aquatag® *see* Benzthiazide *on page 105*

AquaTar® **[OTC]** *see* Coal Tar *on page 225*

Aquatensen® *see* Methyclothiazide *on page 565*

Aralen® **Phosphate** *see* Chloroquine Phosphate *on page 187*

Aralen® **Phosphate With Primaquine Phosphate** *see* Chloroquine and Primaquine *on page 186*

Aredia™ *see* Pamidronate Disodium *on page 655*

Arfonad® *see* Trimethaphan Camsylate *on page 873*

Argesic®**-SA** *see* Salsalate *on page 779*

Arginine Hydrochloride (ar′ ji neen hye droe klor′ ide)
Brand Names R-Gene®
Therapeutic Category Metabolic Alkalosis Agent
Use Pituitary function test (growth hormone); management of severe, uncompensated, metabolic alkalosis (pH ≥7.55) **after** optimizing therapy with sodium, potassium, or ammonium chloride supplements
Usual Dosage I.V.:
Growth hormone (pituitary function) reserve test:
Children: 500 mg (5 mL) kg/dose administered over 30 minutes
Adults: 30 g (300 mL) administered over 30 minutes
Metabolic alkalosis: Children and Adults: Usual dose: 10 g/hour
Acid required (mEq) =
[1] 0.2 (L/kg) x wt (kg) x [103 - serum chloride] (mEq/L) **or**
[2] 0.3 (L/kg) x wt (kg) x base excess (mEq/L) **or**
[3] 0.5 (L/kg) x wt (kg) x [serum HCO_3 - 24] (mEq/L)
Give ½ to ⅔ of calculated dose and re-evaluate

Note: Arginine hydrochloride should never be used as an alternative to chloride supplementation but used in the patient who is unresponsive to sodium chloride or potassium chloride supplementation

Mechanism of Action
Stimulates pituitary release of growth hormone and prolactin through origins in the hypothalamus; patients with impaired pituitary function have lower or no increase in plasma concentrations of growth hormone after administration of arginine. Arginine hydrochloride has been used for severe metabolic alkalosis due to its high chloride content.
Arginine hydrochloride has been used investigationally to treat metabolic alkalosis. Arginine contains 475 mEq of hydrogen ions and 475 mEq of chloride ions/L. Arginine is metabolized by the liver to produce hydrogen ions. It may be used in patients with relative hepatic insufficiency because arginine combines with ammonia in the body to produce urea.

Local Anesthetic/Vasoconstrictor Precautions No information available to require special precautions

Effects on Dental Treatment No effects or complications reported

Other Adverse Effects
1% to 10%: Rapid I.V. infusion may produce flushing, local irritation, nausea & vomiting

(Continued)

Arginine Hydrochloride *(Continued)*

    Central nervous system: Headache
    Neuromuscular & skeletal: Numbness
<1%:
    Endocrine & metabolic: Hyperglycemia, hyperkalemia, increased serum gastrin concentration, hyperchloremia
    Gastrointestinal: Abdominal pain, bloating

Drug Uptake
  Absorption: Oral: Well absorbed
  Time to peak serum concentration: Within 2 hours

Pregnancy Risk Factor C

Argyrol® S.S. 20% *see* Silver Protein, Mild *on page 787*

Aristocort® Forte *see* Triamcinolone *on page 862*

Aristocort® Intralesional Suspension *see* Triamcinolone *on page 862*

Aristocort® Tablet *see* Triamcinolone *on page 862*

Aristospan® *see* Triamcinolone *on page 862*

Arlidin® *see* Nylidrin Hydrochloride *on page 631*

Arm-a-Med® Isoetharine *see* Isoetharine *on page 470*

Arm-a-Med® Isoproterenol *see* Isoproterenol *on page 472*

Arm-a-Med® Metaproterenol *see* Metaproterenol Sulfate *on page 550*

A.R.M.® Caplet [OTC] *see* Chlorpheniramine and Phenylpropanolamine *on page 190*

Armour® Thyroid *see* Thyroid *on page 844*

Aromatic Ammonia Aspirols® *see* Ammonia Spirit, Aromatic *on page 54*

Arrestin® *see* Trimethobenzamide Hydrochloride *on page 873*

ARS *see* Antirabies Serum, Equine Origin *on page 71*

Artane® *see* Trihexyphenidyl Hydrochloride *on page 871*

Artha-G® *see* Salsalate *on page 779*

Arthritis Foundation® Nighttime [OTC] *see* Acetaminophen and Diphenhydramine *on page 16*

Arthropan® [OTC] *see* Choline Salicylate *on page 202*

Articaine Hydrochloride with Epinephrine

Canadian/Mexican Brand Names Ultracaine DS® (Canada); Ultracaine DS Forte® (Canada)

Therapeutic Category Local Anesthetic, Injectable

Use Anesthesia for infiltration and nerve block anesthesia in clinical dentistry

Usual Dosage Adults:
Ultracaine DS® Forte:
  Infiltration:
    Volume: 0.5-2.5 mL
    Total dose: 20-100 mg
  Nerve block:
    Volume: 0.5-3.4 mL
    Total dose: 20-136 mg
  Oral surgery:
    Volume: 1-5.1 mL
    Total dose: 40-204 mg

Ultracaine DS®:
  Infiltration:
    Volume: 0.5-2.5 mL
    Total dose: 20-100 mg
  Nerve block:
    Volume: 0.5-3.4 mL
    Total dose: 20-136 mg
  Oral surgery:
    Volume: 1-5.1 mL
    Total dose: 40-204 mg
Maximum dose: 7 mg/kg

To date, Ultracaine® has not been administered to children <4 years of age, nor in doses >5 mg/kg in children between the ages of 4 and 12

Mechanism of Action Blocks nerve conduction by interfering with the permeability of the nerve axonal membrane to sodium ions; this results in the loss of the generation of the nerve axon potential

Local Anesthetic/Vasoconstrictor Precautions No information available to require special precautions

Effects on Dental Treatment No effects or complications reported

Other Adverse Effects

Cardiovascular: Myocardial depression, arrhythmias, tachycardia, bradycardia, blood pressure changes

Central nervous system: Excitation, depression, nervousness, dizziness, headache, drowsiness, unconsciousness, convulsions, chills

Dermal: Allergic reactions include cutaneous lesions, urticaria, edema, itching, reddening of skin

Gastrointestinal: Vomiting, allergic reactions include nausea and diarrhea

Local: Reactions at the site of injection, swelling, burning, ischemia, tissue necrosis

Neuromuscular & skeletal: Tremors

Ocular: Visual disturbances, blurred vision, blindness, double vision, pupillary constriction

Otic: Tinnitus

Respiratory: Allergic reactions include wheezing, acute asthmatic attacks

Oral manifestations: No data reported

Contraindications Known hypersensitivity to any of its components and/or local anesthetics of the amide group; in the presence of inflammation and/or sepsis near the injection site; in patients with severe shock, any degree of heart block, paroxysmal tachycardia, known arrhythmia with rapid heart rate, narrow-angle glaucoma, cholinesterase deficiency, existing neurologic disease, severe hypertension; when articaine with epinephrine is used, the caution required of any vasopressor drug should be followed

Warnings/Precautions Articaine should be used cautiously in persons with known drug allergies or sensitivities, or suspected sensitivity to the amide-type local anesthetics. Avoid excessive premedications with sedatives, tranquilizers, and antiemetic agents. Inject slowly with frequent aspirations and if blood is aspirated, relocate needle. Articaine should be used with extreme caution in patients having a history of thyrotoxicosis or diabetes. Due to the sulfite component of the articaine preparation, hypersensitivity reactions may occur occasionally in patients with bronchial asthma.

Drug Interactions Solutions containing epinephrine should be used with caution, if at all, in patients taking MAO inhibitors or tricyclic antidepressants because severe prolonged hypertension may result

Breast-feeding Considerations Articaine is unlikely to be transferred to mother's milk since it is rapidly metabolized and eliminated

Dosage Forms Injection:

Ultracaine DS®: Articaine hydrochloride with epinephrine [1:200,000] and sodium metabisulfite [0.5 mg/mL] and an antioxidant and water for injection (1.7 mL [50s])

Ultracaine DS Forte®: Articaine hydrochloride 4% with epinephrine [1:100,000] and sodium metabisulfite [0.5 mg/mL] and an antioxidant and water for injection (1.7 mL) [50s]

Articulose-50® see Prednisolone on page 718
Artificial Saliva Products see page 1050

Artificial Tears (ar ti fish' il tears)

Brand Names Adsorbotear® Ophthalmic Solution [OTC]; Akwa Tears® Solution [OTC]; AquaSite® Ophthalmic Solution [OTC]; Bion® Tears Solution [OTC]; Comfort® Tears Solution [OTC]; Dakrina® Ophthalmic Solution [OTC]; Dry Eye® Therapy Solution [OTC]; Dry Eyes® Solution [OTC]; Dwelle® Ophthalmic Solution [OTC]; Eye-Lube-A® Solution [OTC]; HypoTears PF Solution [OTC]; HypoTears Solution [OTC]; Isopto® Plain Solution [OTC]; Isopto® Tears Solution [OTC]; Just Tears® Solution [OTC]; Lacril® Ophthalmic Solution [OTC]; Liquifilm® Tears Solution [OTC]; Liquifilm® Forte Solution [OTC]; LubriTears® Solution [OTC]; Moisture® Ophthalmic Drops [OTC]; Murine® Solution [OTC]; Murocel® Ophthalmic Solution [OTC]; Nature's Tears® Solution [OTC]; Nu-Tears® Solution [OTC]; Nu-Tears® II Solution [OTC]; OcuCoat® Ophthalmic Solution [OTC]; OcuCoat® PF Ophthalmic Solution [OTC]; Puralube® Tears Solution [OTC]; Refresh® Ophthalmic Solution [OTC]; Refresh® Plus Ophthalmic Solution [OTC]; Tear Drop® Solution [OTC]; TearGard® Ophthalmic Solution [OTC]; Teargen® Ophthalmic Solution [OTC]; Tearisol® Solution [OTC]; Tears Naturale® Free Solution [OTC]; Tears Naturale® II Solution [OTC]; Tears Naturale® Solution [OTC]; Tears Plus® Solution [OTC]; Tears Renewed® Solution [OTC]; Ultra Tears® Solution [OTC]; Viva-Drops® Solution [OTC]

Therapeutic Category Ophthalmic Agent, Miscellaneous
Synonyms Hydroxyethylcellulose; Polyvinyl Alcohol
Use Ophthalmic lubricant; for relief of dry eyes and eye irritation
(Continued)

Artificial Tears *(Continued)*

Local Anesthetic/Vasoconstrictor Precautions No information available to require special precautions

Effects on Dental Treatment No effects or complications reported

Other Adverse Effects 1% to 10%: Ocular: May cause mild stinging or temporary blurred vision

A.S.A. [OTC] *see Aspirin on page 78*

Asacol® *see Mesalamine on page 546*

Ascorbic Acid (a skor´ bik as´ id)

Brand Names Ascorbicap® [OTC]; Cecon® [OTC]; Cee-1000® T.D. [OTC]; Cetane® [OTC]; Cevalin®; Ce-Vi-Sol® [OTC]; Cevita® [OTC]; C-Span® [OTC]; Flavorcee® [OTC]; Vita-C® [OTC]

Canadian/Mexican Brand Names Apo-C® (Canada); Ascorbic® 500 (Canada); Redoxon® (Canada); Revitalose® C-1000® (Canada); Ce-Vi-Sol® (Mexico); Redoxon® Forte (Mexico)

Therapeutic Category Urinary Acidifying Agent; Vitamin, Water Soluble

Synonyms Ascorbico, Acido (Mexico); Cevitamic Acid (Canada)

Use Prevention and treatment of scurvy and to acidify the urine

Investigational use: In large doses to decrease the severity of "colds"; dietary supplementation

Usual Dosage Oral, I.M., I.V., S.C.:

Recommended daily allowance (RDA):
<6 months: 30 mg
6 months to 1 year: 35 mg
1-3 years: 40 mg
4-10 years: 45 mg
11-14 years: 50 mg
>14 years and Adults: 60 mg

Children:
Scurvy: 100-300 mg/day in divided doses for at least 2 weeks
Urinary acidification: 500 mg every 6-8 hours
Dietary supplement: 35-100 mg/day

Adults:
Scurvy: 100-250 mg 1-2 times/day for at least 2 weeks
Urinary acidification: 4-12 g/day in 3-4 divided doses
Prevention and treatment of colds: 1-3 g/day
Dietary supplement: 50-200 mg/day

Mechanism of Action Not fully understood; necessary for collagen formation and tissue repair; involved in some oxidation-reduction reactions as well as other metabolic pathways, such as synthesis of carnitine, steroids, and catecholamines and conversion of folic acid to folinic acid

Local Anesthetic/Vasoconstrictor Precautions No information available to require special precautions

Effects on Dental Treatment No effects or complications reported

Other Adverse Effects

1% to 10%: Renal: Hyperoxaluria
<1%:
Cardiovascular: Flushing
Central nervous system: Faintness, dizziness, headache, fatigue, flank pain
Gastrointestinal: Nausea, vomiting, heartburn, diarrhea

Contraindications Large doses during pregnancy

Warnings/Precautions Diabetics and patients prone to recurrent renal calculi (eg, dialysis patients) should not take excessive doses for extended periods of time

Drug Interactions

Decreased effect:
Aspirin decreases ascorbate levels, increases aspirin
Fluphenazine decreases fluphenazine levels
Warfarin decreases effect
Increased effect: Iron enhances absorption; oral contraceptives increase contraceptive effect

Drug Uptake

Absorption: Oral: Readily absorbed; an active process and is thought to be dose-dependent

Pregnancy Risk Factor A (C if used in doses above RDA recommendation)

Breast-feeding Considerations Compatible

Dosage Forms

Capsule, timed release: 500 mg

Crystals: 4 g/teaspoonful (1000 g)
Drops: 100 mg/mL (50 mL)
Injection: 250 mg/mL (2 mL, 30 mL); 500 mg/mL (1 mL, 2 mL, 50 mL)
Liquid: 35 mg/0.6 mL (50 mL)
Powder: 4 g/teaspoonful (1000 g)
Syrup: 500 mg/5 mL (5 mL, 10 mL, 120 mL, 480 mL)
Tablet: 25 mg, 50 mg, 100 mg, 250 mg, 500 mg, 1000 mg
Tablet:
  Chewable: 100 mg, 250 mg, 500 mg
  Timed release: 500 mg, 1500 mg, 1 g
Generic Available Yes

Ascorbic Acid and Ferrous Sulfate *see* Ferrous Sulfate and Ascorbic Acid *on page 361*

Ascorbicap® [OTC] *see* Ascorbic Acid *on previous page*

Ascorbico, Acido (Mexico) *see* Ascorbic Acid *on previous page*

Ascriptin® [OTC] *see* Aspirin *on next page*

Asendin® *see* Amoxapine *on page 56*

Asmalix® *see* Theophylline/Aminophylline *on page 832*

Asparaginase (a spare' a ji nase)
Brand Names Elspar®
Canadian/Mexican Brand Names Leunase® (Mexico)
Therapeutic Category Antineoplastic Agent, Miscellaneous
Synonyms L-asparaginase
Use Treatment of acute lymphocytic leukemia, lymphoma; used for induction therapy
Usual Dosage Refer to individual protocols; dose must be individualized based upon clinical response and tolerance of the patient

I.M. administration is **preferred** over I.V. administration; I.M. administration may decrease the risk of anaphylaxis

Asparaginase is available from 2 different microbiological sources: One is from *Escherichia coli* and the other is from *Erwinia carotovora*. The *Erwinia* is restricted to patients who have sustained anaphylaxis to the *E. coli* preparation.

I.M., I.V.: 6000 units/m^2 every other day for 3-4 weeks or daily doses of 1000-20,000 units/m^2 for 10-20 days; other induction regimens have been utilized

Desensitization should be performed before administering the first dose of asparaginase to patients who developed a positive reaction to the intradermal skin test or who are being retreated. One schedule begins with a total of 1 unit given I.V. and doubles the dose every 10 minutes until the total amount given in the planned dose for that day.

Asparaginase Desensitization

Injection No.	Elspar Dose (IU)	Accumulated Total Dose
1	1	1
2	2	3
3	4	7
4	8	15
5	16	31
6	32	63
7	64	127
8	128	255
9	256	511
10	512	1,023
11	1,024	2,047
12	2,048	4,095
13	4,096	8,191
14	8,192	16,383
15	16,384	32,767
16	32,768	65,535
17	65,536	131,071
18	131,072	262,143

(Continued)

Asparaginase *(Continued)*

For example, if a patient was to receive a total dose of 4000 units, he/she would receive injections 1 through 12 during the desensitization

Mechanism of Action Some malignant cells (ie, lymphoblastic leukemia cells and those of lymphocyte derivation) must acquire the amino acid asparagine from surrounding fluid such as blood, whereas normal cells can synthesize their own asparagine. asparaginase is an enzyme that deaminates asparagine to aspartic acid and ammonia in the plasma and extracellular fluid and therefore deprives tumor cells of the amino acid for protein synthesis.

There are two purified preparations of the enzyme, one from *Escherichia coli* and one from *Erwinia carotovora*. These two preparations vary slightly in the gene sequencing and have slight differences in enzyme characteristics. Both are highly specific for asparagine and have less than 10% activity for the D-isomer. The preparation from *E. coli* has had the most use in clinical and research practice.

Local Anesthetic/Vasoconstrictor Precautions No information available to require special precautions

Effects on Dental Treatment No effects or complications reported

Other Adverse Effects

>10%:

Gastrointestinal: Pancreatitis occurs in <15% of patients but may progress to severe hemorrhagic pancreatitis

Miscellaneous: Hypersensitivity and anaphylactic reactions occur in ~10% to 40% of patients and can be fatal. This reaction is more common in patients receiving asparaginase alone or by I.V. administration. Hypersensitivity appears rarely with the first dose and more commonly after the second or third treatment. Hypersensitivity may be treated with antihistamines and/or steroids. If an anaphylactic reaction occurs, a change in treatment to the *Erwinia* preparation may be made, since this preparation does not share antigenic cross-reactivity with the *E. coli* preparation. Note that allergic reactions to the *Erwinia* preparation may also occur and ultimately develop in 5% to 20% of patients.

1% to 10%:

Endocrine & metabolic: Hyperuricemia

Gastrointestinal: Mouth sores

<1%:

Central nervous system: Disorientation, drowsiness, seizures, and coma which may be due to elevated NH_4 levels, hyperthermia, fever, malaise

Endocrine & metabolic: Transient diabetes mellitus

Gastrointestinal: Weight loss

Hematologic: Inhibition of protein synthesis will cause a decrease in production of albumin, insulin (resulting in hyperglycemia), serum lipoprotein, antithrombin III, and clotting factors II, V, VII, VIII, IX, and X. The loss of the later two proteins may result in either thrombotic or hemorrhagic events. These protein losses occur in 100% of patients. Leg vein thrombosis.

Hepatic: Increases in serum bilirubin, ST, alkaline phosphatase, and possible decrease in mobilization of lipids

Miscellaneous: Hypersensitivity reactions include hypotension, rash, pruritus, urticaria, laryngeal spasm, chills

Renal: Azotemia

Respiratory: Coughing

Drug Uptake

Absorption: Not absorbed from GI tract, therefore, requires parenteral administration; I.M. administration produces peak blood levels 50% lower than those from I.V. administration (I.M. may be less immunogenic)

Serum half-life: 8-30 hours

Pregnancy Risk Factor C

Comments Myelosuppressive effects:

WBC: Mild

Platelets: Mild

Onset (days): 7

Nadir (days): 14

Recovery (days): 21

Aspergum® [OTC] *see* Aspirin *on this page*

Aspirin (as' pir in)

Related Information

Cardiovascular Diseases *on page 912*

Dental Drug Interactions: Update on Drug Combinations Requiring Special Considerations *on page 1022*

ALPHABETICAL LISTING OF DRUGS

Oral Pain *on page 940*
Rheumatoid Arthritis, Osteoarthritis, and Joint Prostheses *on page 930*

Brand Names Anacin® [OTC]; A.S.A. [OTC]; Ascriptin® [OTC]; Aspergum® [OTC]; Bayer® Aspirin [OTC]; Bufferin® [OTC]; Easprin®; Ecotrin® [OTC]; Empirin® [OTC]; Measurin® [OTC]; Synalgos® [OTC]; ZORprin®

Canadian/Mexican Brand Names ASA® (Canada); Apo-ASA® (Canada); Asaphen® (Canada); Entrophen® (Canada); Novasen® (Canada)

Therapeutic Category Analgesic, Non-narcotic; Anti-inflammatory Agent; Antiplatelet Agent; Antipyretic

Use
Dental: Treatment of postoperative pain
Medical: Treatment of pain and fever; may be used as prophylaxis of myocardial infarction and transient ischemic episodes; management of rheumatoid arthritis, rheumatic fever, osteoarthritis, and gout (high dose)

Usual Dosage Analgesic: Oral:
Children: 10-15 mg/kg/dose every 4-6 hours, up to a total of 60-80 mg/kg/24 hours
Adults: 325-650 mg (1-2 tablets) every 4-6 hours, up to 4 g/day

Mechanism of Action Inhibits prostaglandin synthesis by decreasing the activity of the enzyme, cyclo-oxygenase, which results in decreased formation of prostaglandin precursors, acts on the hypothalamic heat-regulating center to reduce fever, blocks thromboxane synthetase action which prevents formation of the platelet-aggregating substance thromboxane A_2

Local Anesthetic/Vasoconstrictor Precautions No information available to require special precautions

Effects on Dental Treatment Use with caution in patients with platelet and bleeding disorders, renal dysfunction, erosive gastritis, or peptic ulcer disease, previous nonreaction does not guarantee future safe taking of medication; do not use aspirin in children <16 years of age for chickenpox or flu symptoms due to the association with Reye's syndrome

Avoid aspirin if possible, for 1 week prior to surgery because of the possibility of postoperative bleeding; use with caution in impaired hepatic function

Elderly are a high-risk population for adverse effects from nonsteroidal anti-inflammatory agents. As much as 60% of elderly with GI complications to NSAIDs can develop peptic ulceration and/or hemorrhage asymptomatically. Also, concomitant disease and drug use contribute to the risk for GI adverse effects. Use lowest effective dose for shortest period possible. Consider renal function decline with age. Use with caution in patients with history of asthma

Other Adverse Effects
>10%: Gastrointestinal: Nausea, vomiting, dyspepsia, epigastric discomfort, heartburn, stomach pains
1% to 10%: Gastrointestinal: Ulceration

Oral manifestations: No data reported

Contraindications Bleeding disorders (factor VII or IX deficiencies), hypersensitivity to salicylates or other NSAIDs, tartrazine dye and asthma

Warnings/Precautions Use with caution in patients with platelet and bleeding disorders, renal dysfunction, erosive gastritis, or peptic ulcer disease, previous nonreaction does not guarantee future safe taking of medication; do not use aspirin in children <16 years of age for chickenpox or flu symptoms due to the association with Reye's syndrome

Avoid aspirin if possible, for 1 week prior to surgery because of the possibility of postoperative bleeding; use with caution in impaired hepatic function

Elderly are a high-risk population for adverse effects from nonsteroidal anti-inflammatory agents. As much as 60% of elderly with GI complications to NSAIDs can develop peptic ulceration and/or hemorrhage asymptomatically. Also, concomitant disease and drug use contribute to the risk for GI adverse effects. Use lowest effective dose for shortest period possible. Consider renal function decline with age. Use with caution in patients with history of asthma

Drug Interactions Concomitant use of aspirin may result in possible decreased serum concentration of NSAIDs; aspirin may antagonize effects of probenecid; aspirin may increase methotrexate serum levels. Aspirin may displace valproic acid from binding sites which can result in toxicity; warfarin and aspirin result in increased bleeding; NSAIDs and aspirin result in increased GI adverse effects.

Drug Uptake
Absorption: Rapid
Time to peak serum concentration: ~1-2 hours
Serum half-life:
Parent drug: 15-20 minutes
(Continued)

79

Aspirin *(Continued)*

Salicylates (dose-dependent): From 3 hours at lower doses (300-600 mg), to 5-6 hours (after 1 g) to 10 hours with higher doses

Influence of food: Decreases rate but not extent of absorption (oral)

Pregnancy Risk Factor C (D if full-dose aspirin in 3rd trimester)

Breast-feeding Considerations Use cautiously due to potential adverse effects in nursing infants

Dosage Forms

Suppository, rectal: 120 mg, 200 mg, 300 mg, 600 mg

Tablet: 325 mg, 500 mg

Tablet:

Buffered: 325 mg with magnesium-aluminum hydroxide 150 mg

Chewable, children's: 81 mg

Controlled release: 800 mg

Enteric coated: 165 mg, 325 mg, 500 mg, 650 mg, 975 mg

Gum: 227.5 mg (16s, 40s)

Timed release: 800 mg

With caffeine: 400 mg with 32 mg caffeine

Dietary Considerations Should be taken with water, food, or milk to decrease GI effects

Generic Available Yes

Comments Anti-inflammatory actions of aspirin are not seen clinically at doses <3500 mg/day. Patients taking one aspirin tablet daily as an antithrombotic and who require dental surgery should be given special consideration in consultation with the physician before removal of the aspirin relative to prevention of postoperative bleeding.

Selected Readings

Desjardins PJ, Cooper SA, Gallegos TL, et al, "The Relative Analgesic Efficacy of Propiram Fumarate, Codeine Aspirin, and Placebo in Post-Impaction Dental Pain," *J Clin Pharmacol*, 1984, 24(1):35-42.

Forbes JA, Butterworth GA, Burchfield WH, et al, "Evaluation of Ketorolac, Aspirin, and an Acetaminophen-Codeine Combination in Postoperative Oral Surgery Pain," *Pharmacotherapy*, 1990, 10(6 Pt 2):77S-93S.

Forbes JA, Keller CK, Smith JW, et al, "Analgesic Effect of Naproxen Sodium, Codeine, a Naproxen-Codeine Combination and Aspirin on the Postoperative Pain of Oral Surgery," *Pharmacotherapy*, 1986, 6(5):211-8.

Aspirin and Codeine (as' pir in & koe' deen)

Related Information

Dental Drug Interactions: Update on Drug Combinations Requiring Special Considerations *on page 1022*

Oral Pain *on page 940*

Brand Names Empirin® With Codeine

Canadian/Mexican Brand Names Coryphen® Codeine (Canada)

Therapeutic Category Analgesic, Narcotic

Use

Dental: Treatment of postoperative pain

Medical: Relief of pain

Usual Dosage Oral:

Children: Not recommended in pediatric dental patients

Adults: 1-2 tablets every 4-6 hours as needed for pain; maximum: 12 tablets over 24 hours

Mechanism of Action Aspirin inhibits prostaglandin synthesis, acts on the hypothalamus heat-regulating center to reduce fever, blocks prostaglandin synthetase action which prevents formation of the platelet-aggregating substance thromboxane A_2; codeine binds to opiate receptors (mu and kappa subtypes) in the CNS causing inhibition of ascending pain pathways, altering the perception of and response to pain

Local Anesthetic/Vasoconstrictor Precautions No information available to require special precautions

Effects on Dental Treatment Use with caution in patients with platelet and bleeding disorders, renal dysfunction, erosive gastritis, or peptic ulcer disease, previous nonreaction does not guarantee future safe taking of medication; do not use aspirin in children <16 years of age for chickenpox or flu symptoms due to the association with Reye's syndrome

Avoid aspirin if possible, for 1 week prior to surgery because of the possibility of postoperative bleeding; use with caution in impaired hepatic function

Elderly are a high-risk population for adverse effects from nonsteroidal anti-inflammatory agents. As much as 60% of elderly with GI complications to NSAIDs can develop peptic ulceration and/or hemorrhage asymptomatically. Also, concomitant disease and drug use contribute to the risk for GI adverse effects. Use lowest effective dose for shortest period possible. Consider renal function decline with age. Use with caution in patients with history of asthma

Other Adverse Effects
>10%:
  Central nervous system: Lightheadedness, dizziness, sedation, depression
  Gastrointestinal: Nausea, heartburn, stomach pains, dyspepsia, epigastric discomfort, vomiting
1% to 10%: Gastrointestinal: Ulceration, constipation

  Oral manifestations: <1%: Dry mouth
Contraindications Hypersensitivity to aspirin or codeine
Warnings/Precautions Use with caution in patients with impaired renal function, erosive gastritis, or peptic ulcer disease

Enhanced analgesia has been seen in elderly patients on therapeutic doses of narcotics; duration of action may be increased in the elderly; the elderly may be particularly susceptible to the CNS depressant and constipating effects of narcotics

Drug Interactions
Aspirin: Concomitant use of aspirin may result in possible decreased serum concentration of NSAIDs; aspirin may antagonize effects of probenecid; aspirin may increase methotrexate serum levels. Aspirin may displace valproic acid from binding sites which can result in toxicity; warfarin and aspirin result in increased bleeding; NSAIDs and aspirin result in increased GI adverse effects.
Codeine: Increased toxicity when given with CNS depressants, phenothiazines, tricyclic antidepressants (TCAs), other narcotic analgesics, MAO inhibitors

Drug Uptake
Aspirin:
  Absorption: Rapid
  Time to peak serum concentration: ~1-2 hours
  Serum half-life:
  Parent drug: 15-20 minutes
  Salicylates (dose-dependent): From 3 hours at lower doses (300-600 mg), to 5-6 hours (after 1 g) to 10 hours with higher doses
  Influence of food: Decreases rate but not extent of absorption (oral)
Codeine:
  Onset of effect: 0.5-1 hour
  Time to peak serum concentration: 1-1.5 hours
  Duration of effect: 4-6 hours
  Serum half-life: 2.5-3.5 hours

Pregnancy Risk Factor C
Breast-feeding Considerations
Aspirin: Cautious use due to potential adverse effects in nursing infants
Codeine: Codeine not contraindicated with breast-feeding
Dosage Forms Tablet:
#2: Aspirin 325 mg and codeine phosphate 15 mg
#3: Aspirin 325 mg and codeine phosphate 30 mg
#4: Aspirin 325 mg and codeine phosphate 60 mg
Dietary Considerations May be taken with food or milk to minimize GI distress
Generic Available Yes
Comments Codeine products, as with other narcotic analgesics, are recommended only for limited acute dosing (ie, 3 days or less). The most common adverse effect you will see in your dental patients from codeine is nausea, followed by sedation and constipation. Codeine has narcotic addiction liability, especially when given long term. The aspirin component has anticoagulant effects and can affect bleeding times.
Selected Readings
Dionne RA, "New Approaches to Preventing and Treating Postoperative Pain," *J Am Dent Assoc*, 1992, 123(6):26-34.
Gobetti JP, "Controlling Dental Pain," *J Am Dent Assoc*, 1992, 123(6):47-52.

Aspirin and Meprobamate (as′ pir in & me proe ba′ mate)
Brand Names Equagesic®
Therapeutic Category Skeletal Muscle Relaxant, Long Acting
Synonyms Meprobamate and Aspirin
Use Adjunct to treatment of skeletal muscular disease in patients exhibiting tension and/or anxiety
Local Anesthetic/Vasoconstrictor Precautions No information available to require special precautions
(Continued)

Aspirin and Meprobamate *(Continued)*

Effects on Dental Treatment Use with caution in patients with platelet and bleeding disorders, renal dysfunction, erosive gastritis, or peptic ulcer disease, previous nonreaction does not guarantee future safe taking of medication; do not use aspirin in children <16 years of age for chickenpox or flu symptoms due to the association with Reye's syndrome

Avoid aspirin if possible, for 1 week prior to surgery because of the possibility of postoperative bleeding; use with caution in impaired hepatic function

Elderly are a high-risk population for adverse effects from nonsteroidal anti-inflammatory agents. As much as 60% of elderly with GI complications to NSAIDs can develop peptic ulceration and/or hemorrhage asymptomatically. Also, concomitant disease and drug use contribute to the risk for GI adverse effects. Use lowest effective dose for shortest period possible. Consider renal function decline with age. Use with caution in patients with history of asthma

Other Adverse Effects See individual agents

Comments Abrupt discontinuation after sustained use (generally >10 days) may cause withdrawal symptoms

Selected Readings
Desjardins PJ, Cooper SA, Gallegos TL, et al, "The Relative Analgesic Efficacy of Propiram Fumarate, Codeine Aspirin, and Placebo in Post-Impaction Dental Pain," *J Clin Pharmacol*, 1984, 24(1):35-42.

Forbes JA, Butterworth GA, Burchfield WH, et al, "Evaluation of Ketorolac, Aspirin, and an Acetaminophen-Codeine Combination in Postoperative Oral Surgery Pain," *Pharmacotherapy*, 1990, 10(6 Pt 2):77S-93S.

Forbes JA, Keller CK, Smith JW, et al, "Analgesic Effect of Naproxen Sodium, Codeine, a Naproxen-Codeine Combination and Aspirin on the Postoperative Pain of Oral Surgery," *Pharmacotherapy*, 1986, 6(5):211-8.

Aspirin-Free Bayer® Select® Allergy Sinus Caplets [OTC] *see* Acetaminophen, Chlorpheniramine, and Pseudoephedrine *on page 17*

Astemizole *(a stem' mi zole)*

Brand Names Hismanal®

Canadian/Mexican Brand Names Adistan® (Mexico); Antagon-1® (Mexico); Astemina® (Mexico)

Therapeutic Category Antihistamine

Use Perennial and seasonal allergic rhinitis and other allergic symptoms including urticaria

Usual Dosage Oral:
Children:
<6 years: 0.2 mg/kg/day
6-12 years: 5 mg/day
Children >12 years and Adults: 10-30 mg/day; give 30 mg on first day, 20 mg on second day, then 10 mg/day in a single dose

Mechanism of Action Competes with histamine for H_1-receptor sites on effector cells in the gastrointestinal tract, blood vessels, and respiratory tract; binds to lung receptors significantly greater than it binds to cerebellar receptors, resulting in a reduced sedative potential

Local Anesthetic/Vasoconstrictor Precautions No information available to require special precautions

Effects on Dental Treatment Up to 10% of patients taking astemizole may have significant dry mouth which will disappear with cessation of drug therapy; no erythromycin products or antifungals (ketoconazole, itraconazole) should be given since cardiotoxicities could occur (See respective monographs in Dental Drug Monographs section)

Other Adverse Effects
1% to 10%:
Central nervous system: Drowsiness, headache, fatigue, nervousness, dizziness
Gastrointestinal: Appetite increase, weight increase, nausea, diarrhea, abdominal pain, dry mouth
Neuromuscular & skeletal: Arthralgia
Respiratory: Pharyngitis
<1%:
Cardiovascular: Palpitations, edema
Central nervous system: Depression
Dermatologic: Angioedema, photosensitivity, rash
Hepatic: Hepatitis
Neuromuscular & skeletal: Myalgia, paresthesia
Respiratory: Bronchospasm
Miscellaneous: Thickening of mucous, epistaxis

Drug Interactions Increased toxicity: CNS depressants (sedation), triazole antifungals (torsade de pointes and other cardiotoxicities have been reported), macrolide antibiotics (cardiotoxicity)

Drug Uptake Long-acting, with steady-state plasma levels seen within 4-8 weeks following initiation of chronic therapy

Serum half-life: 20 hours

Time to peak serum concentration: Oral: Long-acting, with steady-state plasma levels of parent compound and metabolites seen within 4-8 weeks following initiation of chronic therapy; peak plasma levels appear in 1-4 hours following administration

Pregnancy Risk Factor C

Dosage Forms Tablet: 10 mg

Dietary Considerations Should be taken on an empty stomach

Generic Available No

AsthmaNefrin® see Epinephrine, Racemic on page 314

Astramorph™ PF Injection see Morphine Sulfate on page 590

Atarax® see Hydroxyzine on page 443

Atenolol (a ten′ oh lole)

Related Information

Cardiovascular Diseases on page 912

Brand Names Tenormin®

Canadian/Mexican Brand Names Apo-Atenol® (Canada); Novo-Atenol® (Canada); Nu-Atenol® (Canada); Taro-Atenol® (Canada)

Therapeutic Category Antianginal Agent; Beta-Adrenergic Blocker, Cardio-selective

Use Treatment of hypertension, alone or in combination with other agents; management of angina pectoris, postmyocardial infarction patients

Unlabeled use: Acute alcohol withdrawal, supraventricular and ventricular arrhythmias, and migraine headache prophylaxis

Usual Dosage

Oral:

Children: 1-2 mg/kg/dose given daily

Adults:

Hypertension: 50 mg once daily, may increase to 100 mg/day; doses >100 mg are unlikely to produce any further benefit

Angina pectoris: 50 mg once daily, may increase to 100 mg/day; some patients may require 200 mg/day

Postmyocardial infarction: Follow I.V. dose with 100 mg/day or 50 mg twice daily for 6-9 days postmyocardial infarction

I.V.: Postmyocardial infarction: Early treatment: 5 mg slow I.V. over 5 minutes; may repeat in 10 minutes; if both doses are tolerated, may start oral atenolol 50 mg every 12 hours or 100 mg/day for 6-9 days postmyocardial infarction

Mechanism of Action Competitively blocks response to beta-adrenergic stimulation, selectively blocks beta$_1$-receptors with little or no effect on beta$_2$-receptors except at high doses

Local Anesthetic/Vasoconstrictor Precautions No information available to require special precautions

Effects on Dental Treatment Non-cardioselective beta-blockers (ie, propranolol, nadolol) enhance the pressor response to epinephrine, resulting in hypertension and bradycardia. This has not been reported for atenolol, a cardioselective beta-blocker. Therefore local anesthetic with vasoconstrictor can be safely used in patients medicated with atenolol. Many nonsteroidal anti-inflammatory drugs such as ibuprofen and indometacin can reduce the hypotensive effect of beta-blockers after 3 or more weeks of therapy with the NSAID. Short-term NSAID use (ie, 3 days) requires no special precautions in patients taking beta-blockers.

Other Adverse Effects

1% to 10%:

Cardiovascular: Persistent bradycardia, hypotension, chest pain, edema, heart failure, second or third degree A-V block, Raynaud's phenomena

Central nervous system: Dizziness, fatigue, insomnia, lethargy, confusion, mental impairment, depression, headache, nightmares

Gastrointestinal: Constipation, diarrhea, nausea

Genitourinary: Impotence

<1%:

Respiratory: Dyspnea (especially with large doses), wheezing

Miscellaneous: Cold extremities

(Continued)

Atenolol *(Continued)*

Drug Interactions

Decreased effect of beta-blockers:

Barbiturates (increased liver metabolism of beta-blockers to result in lower serum levels)

NSAIDs (attenuate the hypotensive therapeutic effects of beta-blockers)

Rifampin (increased liver metabolism of beta-blockers to result in lower serum levels)

Increased effects of beta-blockers:

Calcium channel blockers (increase serum levels by unknown mechanism to enhance hypotension)

Beta-blockers increase the effects of:

Epinephrine (vasoconstrictor; initial hypotensive episode followed by bradycardia) only from non-cardioselective type beta-blockers

Phenylephrine (Neosynephrine®; enhanced pressor response)

Theophylline (inhibit theophylline metabolism causing increase in serum concentrations)

Drug Uptake

Absorption: Incomplete from GI tract

Serum half-life, beta:

Adults:

Normal renal function: 6-9 hours, longer in those with renal impairment

End stage renal disease: 15-35 hours

Time to peak: Oral: Within 2-4 hours

Pregnancy Risk Factor C

Selected Readings

Foster CA and Aston SJ, "Propranolol-Epinephrine Interaction: A Potential Disaster," *Plast Reconstr Surg*, 1983, 72(1):74-8.

Wong DG, Spence JD, Lamki L, et al, "Effect of Non-Steroidal Anti-Inflammatory Drugs on Control of Hypertension of Beta-Blockers and Diuretics," *Lancet*, 1986, 1(8488):997-1001.

Wynn RL, "Dental Nonsteroidal Anti-Inflammatory Drugs and Prostaglandin-Based Drug Interactions-Part Two," *Gen Dent*, 1992, 40(2):104, 106, 108.

Wynn RL, "Epinephrine Interactions With Beta-Blockers," *Gen Dent*, 1994, 42(1):16, 18.

Atenolol and Chlorthalidone *(a ten' oh lole & klor thal' i done)*

Brand Names Tenoretic®

Therapeutic Category Antihypertensive Agent, Combination

Use Treatment of hypertension with a cardioselective beta-blocker and a diuretic

Local Anesthetic/Vasoconstrictor Precautions No information available to require special precautions

Effects on Dental Treatment Non-cardioselective beta-blockers (ie, propranolol, nadolol) enhance the pressor response to epinephrine, resulting in hypertension and bradycardia. This has not been reported for atenolol, a cardioselective beta-blocker. Therefore local anesthetic with vasoconstrictor can be safely used in patients medicated with atenolol. Many nonsteroidal anti-inflammatory drugs such as ibuprofen and indometacin can reduce the hypotensive effect of beta-blockers after 3 or more weeks of therapy with the NSAID. Short-term NSAID use (ie, 3 days) requires no special precautions in patients taking beta-blockers.

Other Adverse Effects See individual agents

Comments May contain povidone as inactive ingredient

Selected Readings

Foster CA and Aston SJ, "Propranolol-Epinephrine Interaction: A Potential Disaster," *Plast Reconstr Surg*, 1983, 72(1):74-8.

Wong DG, Spence JD, Lamki L, et al, "Effect of Non-Steroidal Anti-Inflammatory Drugs on Control of Hypertension of Beta-Blockers and Diuretics," *Lancet*, 1986, 1(8488):997-1001.

Wynn RL, "Dental Nonsteroidal Anti-Inflammatory Drugs and Prostaglandin-Based Drug Interactions-Part Two," *Gen Dent*, 1992, 40(2):104, 106, 108.

Wynn RL, "Epinephrine Interactions With Beta-Blockers," *Gen Dent*, 1994, 42(1):16, 18.

ATG *see* Lymphocyte Immune Globulin, Anti-thymocyte Globulin (Equine) *on page 518*

Atgam® *see* Lymphocyte Immune Globulin, Anti-thymocyte Globulin (Equine) *on page 518*

ATIII *see* Antithrombin III *on page 71*

Ativan® *see* Lorazepam *on page 513*

ATnativ® *see* Antithrombin III *on page 71*

Atovaquone *(a toe' va kwone)*

Related Information

Systemic Viral Diseases *on page 934*

Brand Names Mepron™
Therapeutic Category Antiprotozoal
Use Acute oral treatment of mild to moderate *Pneumocystis carinii* pneumonia (PCP) in patients who are intolerant to co-trimoxazole
Usual Dosage Adults: Oral: 750 mg 2 times/day with food for 21 days
Mechanism of Action Mechanism has not been fully elucidated; may inhibit electron transport in mitochondria inhibiting metabolic enzymes
Local Anesthetic/Vasoconstrictor Precautions No information available to require special precautions
Effects on Dental Treatment No effects or complications reported
Other Adverse Effects
>10%:
Central nervous system: Headache, fever, insomnia, anxiety
Dermatologic: Rash
Gastrointestinal: Nausea, diarrhea, vomiting
Respiratory: Cough
1% to 10%:
Central nervous system: Asthenia, dizziness
Dermatologic: Pruritus
Endocrine & metabolic: Hypoglycemia, hyponatremia
Gastrointestinal: Abdominal pain, constipation, anorexia, dyspepsia
Hematologic: Anemia, neutropenia, leukopenia
Renal: Elevated creatinine and BUN
Respiratory: Cough
Miscellaneous: Elevated amylase and liver enzymes, oral *Monilia*
Drug Interactions No data reported
Drug Uptake
Absorption: Decreased significantly in single doses >750 mg; increased three-fold when administered with a high-fat meal
Serum half-life: 2.9 days
Pregnancy Risk Factor C

Atozine® *see* Hydroxyzine *on page 443*
Atrofen™ *see* Baclofen *on page 95*
Atromid-S® *see* Clofibrate *on page 217*

Atropine Sulfate (a' troe peen sul' fate)
Related Information
Cardiovascular Diseases *on page 912*
Brand Names Sal-Tropine®
Canadian/Mexican Brand Names Tropyn® Z (Mexico)
Therapeutic Category Anticholinergic Agent; Anticholinergic Agent, Ophthalmic; Antidote, Organophosphate Poisoning; Antispasmodic Agent, Gastrointestinal; Bronchodilator; Ophthalmic Agent, Mydriatic
Use
Dental: Preoperative medication to inhibit salivation and secretions;
Medical: Treatment of sinus bradycardia; management of peptic ulcer; treat exercise-induced bronchospasm; antidote for organophosphate pesticide poisoning; produce mydriasis and cycloplegia for examination of the retina and optic disc and accurate measurement of refractive errors; uveitis
Usual Dosage
Children:
Oral: These doses may be exceeded in certain cases
7-16 lbs: 0.1 mg
17-24 lbs: 0.15 mg
24-40 lbs: 0.2 mg
40-65 lbs: 0.3 mg
65-90 lbs: 0.4 mg
>90 lbs: 0.4 mg
Preanesthetic: I.M., I.V., S.C.:
<5 kg: 0.02 mg/kg/dose 30-60 minutes preop then every 4-6 hours as needed
>5 kg: 0.01-0.02 mg/kg/dose to a maximum 0.4 mg 30-60 minutes preop; minimum dose: 0.1 mg
Adults:
Oral: Usual: 0.4 mg 1 hour prior to dental appointment
Preanesthetic: I.M., I.V., S.C.: 0.4-0.6 mg 30-60 minutes preop and repeat every 4-6 hours as needed
Mechanism of Action Blocks the action of acetylcholine at parasympathetic sites in smooth muscle, secretory glands, and the CNS; increases cardiac output, dries secretions, antagonizes histamine and serotonin
(Continued)

Atropine Sulfate *(Continued)*

Local Anesthetic/Vasoconstrictor Precautions No information available to require special precautions
Effects on Dental Treatment Xerostomia
Other Adverse Effects
>10%:
Dermatologic: Dry skin
Gastrointestinal: Constipation, dry mouth and throat
Local: Irritation at injection site
Respiratory: Dry nose
Miscellaneous: Decreased sweating
1% to 10%:
Endocrine & metabolic: Decreased flow of breast milk
Gastrointestinal: Difficulty in swallowing
Ophthalmic: Increased sensitivity to light

Oral manifestations: Dry mouth
Contraindications Hypersensitivity to atropine sulfate or any component; angle-closure glaucoma; tachycardia; thyrotoxicosis; obstructive disease of the GI tract; obstructive uropathy
Warnings/Precautions Use with caution in children with spastic paralysis; use with caution in elderly patients. Low doses cause a paradoxical decrease in heart rates. Some commercial products contain sodium metabisulfite, which can cause allergic-type reactions. May accumulate with multiple inhalational administration, particularly in the elderly. Heat prostration may occur in hot weather. Use with caution in patients with autonomic neuropathy, prostatic hypertrophy, hyperthyroidism, congestive heart failure, cardiac arrhythmias, chronic lung disease, biliary tract disease
Drug Interactions Decreased effect of phenothiazines, levodopa, cisapride, methacholine, haloperidol; increased anticholinergic effects of amantadine, phenothiazines, TCAs, meperidine, antihistamines, quinidine, MAO inhibitors
Drug Uptake
Absorption: Well absorbed from all dosage forms
Serum half-life: 2-3 hours
Pregnancy Risk Factor C
Breast-feeding Considerations May be taken while breast-feeding
Dosage Forms
Injection: 0.05 mg/mL (5 mL); 0.1 mg/mL (5 mL, 10 mL); 0.3 mg/mL (1 mL, 30 mL); 0.4 mg/mL (1 mL, 20 mL, 30 mL); 0.5 mg/mL (1 mL, 5 mL, 30 mL); 0.8 mg/mL (0.5 mL, 1 mL); 1 mg/mL (1 mL, 10 mL)
Tablet: 0.4 mg
Tablet, soluble: 0.4 mg, 0.6 mg
Dietary Considerations No data reported
Generic Available Yes

Atrovent® *see* Ipratropium Bromide *on page 467*
A/T/S® Topical *see* Erythromycin, Topical *on page 324*

Attapulgite *(at a pull' gite)*
Related Information
Oral Nonviral Soft Tissue Ulcerations or Erosions *on page 955*
Brand Names Children's Kaopectate® [OTC]; Diasorb® [OTC]; Kaopectate® Advanced Formula [OTC]; Kaopectate® Maximum Strength Caplets; Rheaban® [OTC]
Therapeutic Category Antidiarrheal
Use Symptomatic treatment of diarrhea
Usual Dosage Oral:
Children:
<3 years: Not recommended
3-6 years: 750 mg/dose up to 2250 mg/24 hours
6-12 years: 1200-1500 mg/dose up to 4500 mg/24 hours

Adults: 1200-1500 mg after each loose bowel movement or every 2 hours; 15-30 mL up to 8 times/day, up to 9000 mg/24 hours
Mechanism of Action Controls diarrhea because of its absorbent action
Local Anesthetic/Vasoconstrictor Precautions No information available to require special precautions
Effects on Dental Treatment Do not give oral drugs concomitantly with Kaopectate® due to decreased GI absorption
Other Adverse Effects The powder, if chronically inhaled, can cause pneumoconiosis, since it contains large amounts of silica
1% to 10%: Constipation (dose related)

<1%: Fecal impaction

Drug Interactions Decreased GI absorption of orally administered clindamycin, tetracyclines, penicillamine, digoxin

Drug Uptake Absorption: Not absorbed from GI tract

Pregnancy Risk Factor B

Attenuvax® *see* Measles Virus Vaccine, Live *on page 529*

Augmentin® *see* Amoxicillin and Clavulanic Acid *on page 57*

Auralate® *see* Gold Sodium Thiomalate *on page 404*

Auralgan® *see* Antipyrine and Benzocaine *on page 70*

Auranofin (au rane' oh fin)
Related Information
Rheumatoid Arthritis, Osteoarthritis, and Joint Prostheses *on page 930*
Brand Names Ridaura®
Therapeutic Category Gold Compound
Use Management of active stage of classic or definite rheumatoid arthritis in patients that do not respond to or tolerate other agents; psoriatic arthritis; adjunctive or alternative therapy for pemphigus
Usual Dosage Oral:
Children: Initial: 0.1 mg/kg/day divided daily; usual maintenance: 0.15 mg/kg/day in 1-2 divided doses; maximum: 0.2 mg/kg/day in 1-2 divided doses

Adults: 6 mg/day in 1-2 divided doses; after 3 months may be increased to 9 mg/day in 3 divided doses; if still no response after 3 months at 9 mg/day, discontinue drug
Mechanism of Action The exact mechanism of action of gold is unknown; gold is taken up by macrophages which results in inhibition of phagocytosis and lysosomal membrane stabilization; other actions observed are decreased serum rheumatoid factor and alterations in immunoglobulins. Additionally, complement activation is decreased, prostaglandin synthesis is inhibited, and lysosomal enzyme activity is decreased.
Local Anesthetic/Vasoconstrictor Precautions No information available to require special precautions
Effects on Dental Treatment No effects or complications reported
Other Adverse Effects
>10%:
Dermatologic: Itching, skin rash
Gastrointestinal: Stomatitis
Ocular: Conjunctivitis
Renal: Proteinuria
1% to 10%:
Dermatologic: Hives, alopecia
Gastrointestinal: Glossitis
Hematologic: Eosinophilia, leukopenia, thrombocytopenia
Renal: Hematuria
<1%:
Dermatologic: Angioedema
Gastrointestinal: Ulcerative enterocolitis, GI hemorrhage, gingivitis, metallic taste
Hematologic: Agranulocytosis, anemia, aplastic anemia
Hepatic: Hepatotoxicity
Neuromuscular & skeletal: Peripheral neuropathy
Respiratory: Interstitial pneumonitis
Miscellaneous: Difficulty in swallowing
Drug Interactions Increased toxicity: Penicillamine, antimalarials, hydroxychloroquine, cytotoxic agents, immunosuppressants
Pregnancy Risk Factor C

Aureomycin® *see* Chlortetracyline Hydrochloride *on page 199*

Auro® Ear Drops [OTC] *see* Carbamide Peroxide *on page 152*

Aurothioglucose (aur oh thye oh gloo' kose)
Related Information
Rheumatoid Arthritis, Osteoarthritis, and Joint Prostheses *on page 930*
Brand Names Solganal®
Therapeutic Category Gold Compound
Use Adjunctive treatment in adult and juvenile active rheumatoid arthritis; alternative or adjunct in treatment of pemphigus; psoriatic patients who do not respond to NSAIDs
Usual Dosage I.M.: Doses should initially be given at weekly intervals
(Continued)

Aurothioglucose *(Continued)*

Children 6-12 years: Initial: 0.25 mg/kg/dose first week; increment at 0.25 mg/kg/dose increasing with each weekly dose; maintenance: 0.75-1 mg/kg/dose weekly not to exceed 25 mg/dose to a total of 20 doses, then every 2-4 weeks

Adults: 10 mg first week; 25 mg second and third week; then 50 mg/week until 800 mg to 1 g cumulative dose has been given; if improvement occurs without adverse reactions, give 25-50 mg every 2-3 weeks, then every 3-4 weeks

Mechanism of Action Unknown, may decrease prostaglandin synthesis or may alter cellular mechanisms by inhibiting sulfhydryl systems

Local Anesthetic/Vasoconstrictor Precautions No information available to require special precautions

Effects on Dental Treatment No effects or complications reported

Other Adverse Effects

>10%:
  Dermatologic: Itching, skin rash, exfoliative dermatitis, reddened skin
  Gastrointestinal: Gingivitis, glossitis, metallic taste, stomatitis

1% to 10%: Renal: Proteinuria

<1%:
  Central nervous system: Encephalitis, EKG abnormalities, fever
  Dermatologic: Alopecia
  Gastrointestinal: Ulcerative enterocolitis
  Genitourinary: Vaginitis
  Hematologic: Agranulocytosis, aplastic anemia, eosinophilia, leukopenia, thrombocytopenia
  Hepatic: Hepatotoxicity
  Respiratory: Pharyngitis, bronchitis, pulmonary fibrosis, interstitial pneumonitis
  Neuromuscular & skeletal: Peripheral neuropathy
  Ocular: Conjunctivitis, corneal ulcers, iritis
  Renal: Glomerulitis, hematuria, nephrotic syndrome
  Miscellaneous: Anaphylactic shock, allergic reaction (severe)

Drug Interactions Increased toxicity: Penicillamine, antimalarials, hydroxychloroquine, cytotoxic agents, immunosuppressants

Drug Uptake

Absorption: I.M.: Erratic and slow
Serum half-life: 3-27 days (half-life dependent upon single or multiple dosing)
Time to peak serum concentration: Within 4-6 hours

Pregnancy Risk Factor C

Auroto® *see* Antipyrine and Benzocaine *on page 70*

Autoplex® T *see* Anti-Inhibitor Coagulant Complex *on page 70*

AVC™ Cream *see* Sulfanilamide *on page 810*

AVC™ Suppository *see* Sulfanilamide *on page 810*

Aveeno® Cleansing Bar [OTC] *see* Sulfur and Salicylic Acid *on page 813*

Aventyl® Hydrochloride *see* Nortriptyline Hydrochloride *on page 629*

Avitene® *see* Microfibrillar Collagen Hemostat *on page 579*

Avlosulfon® *see* Dapsone *on page 251*

Axid® *see* Nizatidine *on page 626*

Axotal® *see* Butalbital Compound *on page 133*

Aygestin® *see* Norethindrone *on page 627*

Azacitidine *(ay za sye' ti deen)*

Brand Names Mylosar®

Therapeutic Category Antineoplastic Agent, Miscellaneous

Synonyms AZA-CR; 5-Azacytidine; 5-AZC; Ladakamycin; NSC-102816

Use Refractory acute lymphocytic and myelogenous leukemia

Local Anesthetic/Vasoconstrictor Precautions No information available to require special precautions

Effects on Dental Treatment No effects or complications reported

Other Adverse Effects 1% to 10%:
  Cardiovascular: Hypotension with rapid infusion
  Central nervous system: Fever
  Dermatologic: Rash
  Gastrointestinal: Nausea, vomiting, diarrhea,
  Hematologic: Myelosuppression (granulocyte nadir is 14-17 days)
  Hepatic: Hepatotoxicity

Neuromuscular & skeletal: Neuropathies (dose dependent) and neurologic toxicity

AZA-CR *see* Azacitidine *on previous page*
Azactam® *see* Aztreonam *on page 91*
5-Azacytidine *see* Azacitidine *on previous page*
Azatadina, Maleato De (Mexico) *see* Azatadine Maleate *on this page*

Azatadine and Pseudoephedrine
(a za' ta deen & soo doe e fed' rin)
Brand Names Trinalin®
Therapeutic Category Antihistamine/Decongestant Combination
Synonyms Pseudoephedrine and Azatadine
Use Perennial and seasonal allergic rhinitis and other allergic symptoms including urticaria
Local Anesthetic/Vasoconstrictor Precautions
Azatadine: No information available to require special precautions
Pseudoephedrine: Use with caution since pseudoephedrine is a sympathomimetic amine which could interact with epinephrine to cause a pressor response
Effects on Dental Treatment
Azatadine: This drug has atropine-like effects and the patient may experience drowsiness, dry mouth, nose and throat
Pseudoephedrine: Up to 10% of patients could experience tachycardia, palpitations, and dry mouth; use vasoconstrictor with caution
Other Adverse Effects See individual agents

Azatadine Maleate (a za' ta deen mal' ee ate)
Brand Names Optimine®
Canadian/Mexican Brand Names Idulamine® (Mexico)
Therapeutic Category Antihistamine
Synonyms Azatadina, Maleato De (Mexico)
Use Treatment of perennial and seasonal allergic rhinitis and chronic urticaria
Usual Dosage Children >12 years and Adults: Oral: 1-2 mg twice daily
Mechanism of Action Azatadine is a piperidine-derivative antihistamine; has both anticholinergic and antiserotonin activity; has been demonstrated to inhibit mediator release from human mast cells *in vitro*; mechanism of this action is suggested to prevent calcium entry into the mast cell through voltage-dependent calcium channels
Local Anesthetic/Vasoconstrictor Precautions No information available to require special precautions
Effects on Dental Treatment This drug has atropine-like effects and the patient may experience drowsiness, dry mouth, nose and throat
Other Adverse Effects
>10%:
Central nervous system: Slight to moderate drowsiness
Respiratory: Thickening of bronchial secretions
1% to 10%:
Central nervous system: Headache, fatigue, nervousness, dizziness
Gastrointestinal: Appetite increase, weight increase nausea, diarrhea, abdominal pain, dry mouth
Neuromuscular & skeletal: Arthralgia
Respiratory: Pharyngitis
<1%:
Cardiovascular: Palpitations, edema
Central nervous system: Depression
Dermatologic: Angioedema, photosensitivity, rash
Hepatic: Hepatitis
Neuromuscular & skeletal: Myalgia, paresthesia
Respiratory: Bronchospasm
Miscellaneous: Epistaxis
Drug Interactions Increased effect/toxicity: Procarbazine, CNS depressants, tricyclic antidepressants, alcohol
Drug Uptake
Absorption: Oral: Rapid and extensive
Serum half-life: ~8.7 hours
Pregnancy Risk Factor B

Azathioprine (ay za thye' oh preen)
Brand Names Imuran®
Canadian/Mexican Brand Names Azatrilem® (Mexico)
(Continued)

Azathioprine *(Continued)*

Therapeutic Category Immunosuppressant Agent

Synonyms Azatioprina (Mexico)

Use Adjunct with other agents in prevention of rejection of solid organ transplants; also used in severe active rheumatoid arthritis unresponsive to other agents; **azathioprine is an imidazolyl derivative of 6-mercaptopurine**

Usual Dosage I.V. dose is equivalent to oral dose

Children and Adults: Renal transplantation: Oral, I.V.: 2-5 mg/kg/day to start, then 1-3 mg/kg/day maintenance

Adults: Rheumatoid arthritis: Oral: 1 mg/kg/day for 6-8 weeks; increase by 0.5 mg/kg every 4 weeks until response or up to 2.5 mg/kg/day

Mechanism of Action Antagonizes purine metabolism and may inhibit synthesis of DNA, RNA, and proteins; may also interfere with cellular metabolism and inhibit mitosis

Local Anesthetic/Vasoconstrictor Precautions No information available to require special precautions

Effects on Dental Treatment No effects or complications reported

Other Adverse Effects Dose reduction or temporary withdrawal allows reversal

>10%:

Central nervous system: Fever, chills

Gastrointestinal: Nausea, vomiting, anorexia, diarrhea

Hematologic: Thrombocytopenia, leukopenia, secondary infection, anemia

1% to 10%:

Dermatologic: Skin rash

Hematologic: Pancytopenia

Hepatic: Hepatotoxicity

<1%:

Cardiovascular: Hypotension

Dermatologic: Alopecia, rash, maculopapular rash, Aphthous stomatitis

Neuromuscular & skeletal: Arthralgias, which include myalgias, rigors

Ocular: Retinopathy

Respiratory: Dyspnea

Miscellaneous: Rare hypersensitivity reactions

Drug Interactions Increased toxicity: Allopurinol (reduce azathioprine dose to $1/3$ to $1/4$ of normal dose). The use of angiotensin-converting enzyme inhibitors to control hypertension in patients on azathioprine has been reported to induce severe leukopenia.

Drug Uptake

Serum half-life:

Parent drug: 12 minutes

6-mercaptopurine: 0.7-3 hours

End stage renal disease: Slightly prolonged

Pregnancy Risk Factor D

Azatioprina (Mexico) *see* Azathioprine *on previous page*

5-AZC *see* Azacitidine *on page 88*

Azdone® *see* Hydrocodone and Aspirin *on page 433*

Azelaic Acid *(a zeh lay' ik as' id)*

Brand Names Azelex®

Therapeutic Category Topical Skin Product, Acne

Use Treatment of mild to moderate acne vulgaris

Usual Dosage Adults: Topical: After skin is thoroughly washed and patted dry, gently but thoroughly massage a thin film of azelaic acid cream into the affected areas twice daily, in the morning and evening. The duration of use can vary and depends on the severity of the acne. In the majority of patients with inflammatory lesions, improvement of the condition occurs within 4 weeks.

Local Anesthetic/Vasoconstrictor Precautions No information available to require special precautions

Effects on Dental Treatment No effects or complications reported

Drug Uptake

Absorption: ~3% to 5% penetrates the stratum corneum; up to 10% is found in the epidermis and dermis; 4% is systemically absorbed

Serum half-life: Healthy subjects: 12 hours after topical dosing

Azelex® *see* Azelaic Acid *on this page*

Azithromycin *(az ith roe mye' sin)*

Brand Names Zithromax™

Therapeutic Category Antibiotic, Macrolide

Synonyms Z-PAKS™

Use

Dental: Alternate antibiotic in the treatment of common orofacial infections caused by aerobic gram-positive cocci and susceptible anaerobes

Medical: Treatment against most respiratory pathogens (eg, *S. pyogenes*, *S. pneumoniae*, *S. agalactiae*, viridans *Streptococcus*, *M. catarrhalis*, *C. trachomatis*, *Legionella* sp, *Mycoplasma pneumoniae*, *S. aureus*)

Usual Dosage Oral:

Children: Safe use has not been established

Adults: 250 mg twice daily first day then 250 mg/day for 4 days

Mechanism of Action Inhibits RNA-dependent protein synthesis at the chain elongation step; binds to the 50S ribosomal subunit resulting in blockage of transpeptidation

Local Anesthetic/Vasoconstrictor Precautions No information available to require special precautions

Effects on Dental Treatment No effects or complications reported

Other Adverse Effects

1% to 10%: Gastrointestinal: Diarrhea, nausea, abdominal pain, cramping, vomiting

Oral manifestations: No data reported

Contraindications Hepatic impairment, known hypersensitivity to azithromycin, other macrolide antibiotics, or any Zithromax™ components; use with pimozide

Warnings/Precautions Use with caution in patients with hepatic dysfunction; hepatic impairment with or without jaundice has occurred chiefly in older children and adults; it may be accompanied by malaise, nausea, vomiting, abdominal colic, and fever; discontinue use if these occur; may mask or delay symptoms of incubating gonorrhea or syphilis, so appropriate culture and susceptibility tests should be performed prior to initiating azithromycin; pseudomembranous colitis has been reported with use of macrolide antibiotics

Drug Interactions Aluminum- and magnesium-containing antacids decrease serum levels of azithromycin by 24% but not total absorption; azithromycin increases serum levels of alfentanil, anticoagulants, astemizole, terfenadine, loratadine, bromocriptine, carbamazepine, cyclosporine, digoxin, disopyramide, theophylline, and triazolam

Drug Uptake

Absorption: Rapid from the GI tract

Time to peak serum concentration: 2.3-4 hours

Serum half-life, terminal: 68 hours

Influence of food: Decreases rate and extent of absorption

Pregnancy Risk Factor C

Breast-feeding Considerations No data reported

Dosage Forms

Capsule, as dihydrate: 250 mg

Capsule (Z-PAKS™): 6 capsules/box

Suspension, oral (single-dose packets): 1 g

Dietary Considerations Should be taken at least 1 hour prior to or 2 hours after a meal; should not be taken with food

Generic Available No

Selected Readings

"Pimozide (Orap) Contraindicated With Clarithromycin (Biaxin) and Other Macrolide Antibiotics," *FDA Medical Bulletin*, October 1996, 3.

Azmacort™ *see* Triamcinolone *on page 862*

Azo Gantanol® *see* Sulfamethoxazole and Phenazopyridine *on page 809*

Azo Gantrisin® *see* Sulfisoxazole and Phenazopyridine *on page 812*

Azo-Standard® *see* Phenazopyridine Hydrochloride *on page 679*

Aztreonam (az' tree oh nam)

Brand Names Azactam®

Therapeutic Category Antibiotic, Miscellaneous

Use Treatment of patients with documented aerobic gram-negative bacillary infection in which beta-lactam therapy is contraindicated (eg, penicillin or cephalosporin allergy); used for urinary tract infections, lower respiratory tract infections, septicemia, skin/skin structure infections, intra-abdominal infections, and gynecological infections; as part of a multiple-drug regimen for the empirical treatment of neutropenic fever in persons with a history of beta-lactam allergy or with known multidrug-resistant organisms

Usual Dosage

Children >1 month: I.M., I.V.: 90-120 mg/kg/day divided every 6-8 hours

(Continued)

Aztreonam *(Continued)*

Cystic fibrosis: 50 mg/kg/dose every 6-8 hours (ie, up to 200 mg/kg/day); maximum: 6-8 g/day

Adults:

Urinary tract infection: I.M., I.V.: 500 mg to 1 g every 8-12 hours

Moderately severe systemic infections: 1 g I.V. or I.M. or 2 g I.V. every 8-12 hours

Severe systemic or life-threatening infections (especially caused by *Pseudomonas aeruginosa*): I.V.: 2 g every 6-8 hours; maximum: 8 g/day

Mechanism of Action Monobactam which is active only against gram-negative bacilli (unlikely cross-allergenicity with other beta-lactams); inhibits bacterial cell wall synthesis during active multiplication, causing cell wall destruction

Local Anesthetic/Vasoconstrictor Precautions No information available to require special precautions

Effects on Dental Treatment No effects or complications reported

Other Adverse Effects

1% to 10%:

Dermatologic: Rash vomiting

Gastrointestinal: Diarrhea, nausea

Local: Thrombophlebitis, pain at injection site

<1%:

Cardiovascular: Hypotension

Central nervous system: Seizures, confusion, headache, vertigo, insomnia, dizziness, numb tongue, weakness, fever

Endocrine & metabolic: Breast tenderness

Gastrointestinal: Pseudomembranous colitis

Genitourinary: Vaginitis

Hepatic: Hepatitis, jaundice, elevation of liver enzymes

Hematologic: Thrombocytopenia, eosinophilia, leukopenia, neutropenia

Neuromuscular & skeletal: Muscular aches

Ocular: Diplopia

Otic: Tinnitus

Respiratory: Sneezing

Miscellaneous: Anaphylaxis, aphthous ulcer, altered taste, halitosis

Drug Interactions No data reported

Drug Uptake

Absorption: I.M.: Well absorbed; I.M. and I.V. doses produce comparable serum concentrations

Serum half-life:

Normal renal function: 1.7-2.9 hours

End stage renal disease: 6-8 hours

Time to peak: Within 60 minutes (I.M., I.V. push) and 90 minutes (I.V. infusion)

Pregnancy Risk Factor B

Azulfidine® *see* Sulfasalazine *on page 810*

Azulfidine® EN-tabs® *see* Sulfasalazine *on page 810*

Babee® Teething [OTC] *see* Benzocaine *on page 102*

BAC *see* Benzalkonium Chloride *on page 102*

B-A-C® *see* Butalbital Compound *on page 133*

Bacampicillin Hydrochloride (ba kam pi sil' in hye droe klor' ide)

Brand Names Spectrobid®

Therapeutic Category Antibiotic, Penicillin

Synonyms Carampicillin Hydrochloride

Use Treatment of susceptible bacterial infections involving the urinary tract, skin structure, upper and lower respiratory tract; activity is identical to that of ampicillin

Local Anesthetic/Vasoconstrictor Precautions No information available to require special precautions

Effects on Dental Treatment No effects or complications reported

Other Adverse Effects

1% to 10%: Gastrointestinal: Gastric upset, diarrhea, nausea

<1%:

Dermatologic: Rash

Gastrointestinal: Pseudomembranous colitis

Hematologic: Agranulocytosis

Hepatic: Mild elevation in AST

Miscellaneous: Hypersensitivity reactions

Comments Each mg of bacampicillin is equivalent to ampicillin 700 mcg

Bacid® [OTC] *see* Lactobacillus acidophilus and Lactobacillus bulgaricus *on page 488*

Baciguent® [OTC] *see* Bacitracin *on this page*

Baci-IM® *see* Bacitracin *on this page*

Bacillus Calmette-Guérin (BCG) Live

(ba sil′ us kal met′ gwair en′ (bee see jee) live)

Brand Names TheraCys™; TICE® BCG

Therapeutic Category Biological Response Modulator; Vaccine, Live Bacteria

Synonyms BCG

Use BCG vaccine is no longer recommended for adults at high risk for tuberculosis in the United States. BCG vaccination may be considered for infants and children who are skin test-negative to 5 tuberculin units of tuberculin and who cannot be given isoniazid preventive therapy but have close contact with untreated or ineffectively treated active tuberculosis patients or who belong to groups which other control measures have not been successful.

In the United States, tuberculosis control efforts are directed toward early identification, treatment of cases, and preventive therapy with isoniazid.

Usual Dosage Children >1 month and Adults:

Immunization against tuberculosis: 0.2-0.3 mL percutaneous; initial lesion usually appears after 10-14 days consisting of small red papule at injection site and reaches maximum diameter of 3 mm in 4-6 weeks; conduct postvaccinal tuberculin test in 2-3 months; if test is negative, repeat vaccination

Immunotherapy for bladder cancer: TICE® BCG vaccine 6 x 10⁸ viable organisms in 50 mL NS (preservative free) instilled into bladder and retained for 2 hours weekly for 6 weeks

Mechanism of Action BCG live is an attenuated strain of Bacillus Calmette-Guérin used as a biological response modifier; BCG live, when used intravesicular for treatment of bladder carcinoma *in situ*, is thought to cause a local, chronic inflammatory response involving macrophage and leukocyte infiltration of the bladder. By a mechanism not fully understood, this local inflammatory response leads to destruction of superficial tumor cells of the urothelium. Evidence of systemic immune response is also commonly seen, manifested by a positive PPD tuberculin skin test reaction, however, its relationship to clinical efficacy is not well-established. BCG is active immunotherapy which stimulates the host's immune mechanism to reject the tumor.

Local Anesthetic/Vasoconstrictor Precautions No information available to require special precautions

Effects on Dental Treatment No effects or complications reported

Other Adverse Effects

1% to 10%:

Genitourinary: Bladder infection, dysuria, urinary frequency, prostatitis

Miscellaneous: Flu-like syndrome

<1%:

Dermatologic: Skin ulceration, abscesses

Renal: Hematuria

Miscellaneous: Rarely anaphylactic shock in infants, lymphadenitis, tuberculosis in immunosuppressed patients

Pregnancy Risk Factor C

Comments

Live, attenuated vaccine

Live culture preparation of bacillus Calmette-Guérin (BCG) strain of *Mycobacterium bovis* and is a substrain of Pasteur Institute strain designed for use as active immunizing agent against tuberculosis

Bacitracin (bass i tray′ sin)

Brand Names AK-Tracin®; Baciguent® [OTC]; Baci-IM®

Canadian/Mexican Brand Names Bacitin® (Canada)

Therapeutic Category Antibiotic, Ophthalmic; Antibiotic, Topical; Antibiotic, Miscellaneous

Use Treatment of susceptible bacterial infections (staphylococcal pneumonia and empyema); due to toxicity risks, systemic and irrigant uses of bacitracin should be limited to situations where less toxic alternatives would not be effective; oral administration has been successful in antibiotic-associated colitis

Usual Dosage Do not administer I.V.:

Children: I.M.: 800-1200 units/kg/day divided every 8 hours

Adults: Antibiotic-associated colitis: Oral: 25,000 units 4 times/day for 7-10 days

(Continued)

93

Baclofen (Continued)

Effects on Dental Treatment No effects or complications reported

Other Adverse Effects

>10%: Central nervous system: Drowsiness, vertigo, dizziness, psychiatric disturbances, insomnia, slurred speech, weakness, ataxia, hypotonia

1% to 10%:
Cardiovascular: Hypotension
Central nervous system: Fatigue, confusion, headache, insomnia
Dermatologic: Rash
Gastrointestinal: Nausea, constipation
Genitourinary: Urinary frequency

<1%:
Cardiovascular: Palpitations, chest pain, syncope
Central nervous system: Euphoria, excitement, depression, hallucinations
Gastrointestinal: Dry mouth, anorexia, taste disorder, abdominal pain, vomiting, diarrhea
Genitourinary: Enuresis, urinary retention, dysuria, impotence, inability to ejaculate, nocturia
Neuromuscular & skeletal: Paresthesia
Renal: Hematuria
Respiratory: Dyspnea

Drug Interactions

Decreased effect of baclofen has been caused by lithium
Increased effect of baclofen has been caused by opiate analgesics, benzodiazepines, hypertensive agents
Increased toxicity: CNS depressants and alcohol (sedation), tricyclic antidepressants (short-term memory loss), guanabenz (sedation), MAO inhibitors (decreased blood pressure, CNS, and respiratory effects)

Drug Uptake

Onset of action: Muscle relaxation effect requires 3-4 days
Absorption: Oral: Rapid; absorption from GI tract is thought to be dose dependent
Serum half-life: 3.5 hours
Time to peak serum concentration: Oral: Within 2-3 hours

Pregnancy Risk Factor C

Dosage Forms

Injection, intrathecal: 0.5 mg/mL, 2 mg/mL
Tablet: 10 mg, 20 mg

Generic Available No

Bacticort® Otic see Neomycin, Polymyxin B, and Hydrocortisone on page 610

Bactocill® see Oxacillin Sodium on page 641

Bactrim™ see Trimethoprim and Sulfamethoxazole on page 874

Bactrim™ DS see Trimethoprim and Sulfamethoxazole on page 874

Bactroban® see Mupirocin on page 593

Baker's P&S Topical [OTC] see Phenol on page 682

Balanced Salt Solution (bal' anced salt soe loo' shun)

Brand Names BSS® Ophthalmic

Therapeutic Category Ophthalmic Agent, Miscellaneous

Use Intraocular irrigating solution; also used to soothe and cleanse the eye in conjunction with hard contact lenses

Local Anesthetic/Vasoconstrictor Precautions No information available to require special precautions

Effects on Dental Treatment No effects or complications reported

BAL in Oil® see Dimercaprol on page 287

Balnetar® [OTC] see Coal Tar, Lanolin, and Mineral Oil on page 226

Bancap® see Butalbital Compound on page 133

Bancap HC® [5/500] see Hydrocodone and Acetaminophen on page 431

Banesin® [OTC] see Acetaminophen on page 14

Banophen® [OTC] see Diphenhydramine Hydrochloride on page 288

Banthine® see Methantheline Bromide on page 554

Barbidonna® see Hyoscyamine, Atropine, Scopolamine, and Phenobarbital on page 444

Barbita® see Phenobarbital on page 680

Barc™ [OTC] see Pyrethrins on page 753

Baridium® see Phenazopyridine Hydrochloride on page 679

Barophen® see Hyoscyamine, Atropine, Scopolamine, and Phenobarbital on page 444

Basaljel® [OTC] *see* Aluminum Carbonate *on page 39*

Base Ointment *see* Zinc Oxide *on page 908*

Bayer® Aspirin [OTC] *see* Aspirin *on page 78*

Bayer® Select® Chest Cold Caplets [OTC] *see* Acetaminophen and Dextromethorphan *on page 16*

BCG *see* Bacillus Calmette-Guérin (BCG) Live *on page 93*

BCNU *see* Carmustine *on page 157*

B-D Glucose® [OTC] *see* Glucose *on page 400*

Because® [OTC] *see* Nonoxynol 9 *on page 627*

Beclometasona (Mexico) *see* Beclomethasone Dipropionate *on this page*

Beclomethasone Dipropionate
(be kloe meth′ a sone dye pro′ pee oh nate)

Related Information
Respiratory Diseases *on page 924*

Brand Names
Beclovent®; Beconase®; Beconase AQ®; Vancenase®; Vancenase® AQ; Vanceril®

Canadian/Mexican Brand Names
Beclodisk® (Canada); Becloforte® (Canada); Propaderm® (Canada); Aerobec® (Mexico); Beconase® Aqua (Mexico); Becotide® 100 (Mexico); Becotide® 250 (Mexico); Becotide® Aerosol (Mexico)

Therapeutic Category
Anti-inflammatory Agent; Corticosteroid, Inhalant

Synonyms
Beclometasona (Mexico)

Use
Oral inhalation: Treatment of bronchial asthma in patients who require chronic administration of corticosteroids

Nasal aerosol: Symptomatic treatment of seasonal or perennial rhinitis and nasal polyposis

Usual Dosage
Nasal inhalation and oral inhalation dosage forms are not to be used interchangeably

Nasal:
  Children 6-12 years: 1 spray in each nostril 3 times/day
  Adults: 1 spray in each nostril 2-4 times/day

Oral inhalation:
  Children 6-12 years: 1-2 inhalations 3-4 times/day; alternatively 2-4 inhalations twice daily; do not exceed 10 inhalations/day
  Adults: 2 inhalations 3-4 times/day; alternatively 2-4 inhalations twice daily; do not exceed 20 inhalations/day; patients with severe asthma should be started on 12-16 inhalations/day (divided 3-4 times/day) and dose should be adjusted downward according to the patient's response

Mechanism of Action
Controls the rate of protein synthesis, depresses the migration of polymorphonuclear leukocytes, fibroblasts, reverses capillary permeability, and lysosomal stabilization at the cellular level to prevent or control inflammation

Local Anesthetic/Vasoconstrictor Precautions
No information available to require special precautions

Effects on Dental Treatment
Localized infections with *Candida albicans* or *Aspergillus niger* have occurred frequently in the mouth and pharynx with repetitive use of oral inhaler of beclomethasone. Positive cultures for oral *Candida* may be present in up to 75% of patients. These infections may require treatment with appropriate antifungal therapy or discontinuance of treatment with beclomethasone inhaler.

Other Adverse Effects
>10%:
  Local: Growth of *Candida* in the mouth, irritation and burning of the nasal mucosa
  Respiratory: Cough, hoarseness

1% to 10%:
  Gastrointestinal: Dry mouth
  Local: Epistaxis, nasal ulceration

<1%:
  Central nervous system: Headache
  Dermatologic: Skin rash
  Respiratory: Bronchospasm, rhinorrhea, nasal stuffiness, sneezing, nasal septal perforations
  Miscellaneous: Difficulty in swallowing

Drug Interactions
No data reported

Drug Uptake
Therapeutic effect: Within 1-4 weeks of use

(Continued)

Beclomethasone Dipropionate *(Continued)*

Inhalation:
  Absorption: Readily absorbed; quickly hydrolyzed by pulmonary esterases prior to absorption
  Absorption: 90%
  Serum half-life:
    Initial: 3 hours
    Terminal: 15 hours

Pregnancy Risk Factor C

Beclovent® *see* Beclomethasone Dipropionate *on previous page*

Beconase® *see* Beclomethasone Dipropionate *on previous page*

Beconase AQ® *see* Beclomethasone Dipropionate *on previous page*

Becotin® Pulvules® *see* Vitamins, Multiple *on page 901*

Beepen-VK® *see* Penicillin V Potassium *on page 668*

Beesix® *see* Pyridoxine Hydrochloride *on page 753*

Beldin® [OTC] *see* Diphenhydramine Hydrochloride *on page 288*

Belix® [OTC] *see* Diphenhydramine Hydrochloride *on page 288*

Belladonna (bel a don' a)

Therapeutic Category Anticholinergic Agent; Antispasmodic Agent, Gastrointestinal

Use Decrease gastrointestinal activity in functional bowel disorders and to delay gastric emptying as well as decrease gastric secretion

Local Anesthetic/Vasoconstrictor Precautions No information available to require special precautions

Effects on Dental Treatment >10%: Dry mouth

Other Adverse Effects
>10%:
  Gastrointestinal: Constipation
  Miscellaneous: Decreased sweating; dry mouth, nose, throat, or skin
1% to 10%:
  Endocrine & metabolic: Decreased flow of breast milk, difficulty in swallowing
  Ocular: Increased sensitivity to light
<1%:
  Cardiovascular: Ventricular fibrillation, tachycardia, palpitations, ataxia, orthostatic hypotension
  Central nervous system: Confusion, drowsiness, headache, loss of memory, tiredness
  Dermatologic: Skin rash
  Gastrointestinal: Bloated feeling
  Genitourinary: Difficult urination, nausea, vomiting
  Neuromuscular & skeletal: Weakness
  Ocular: Increased intraocular pain, blurred vision

Belladonna and Opium (bel a don' a & oh' pee um)

Brand Names B&O Supprettes®

Canadian/Mexican Brand Names PMS-Opium & Beladonna (Canada)

Therapeutic Category Analgesic, Narcotic

Use Relief of moderate to severe pain associated with rectal or bladder tenesmus that may occur in postoperative states and neoplastic situations; pain associated with ureteral spasms not responsive to non-narcotic analgesics and to space intervals between injections of opiates

Usual Dosage Adults: Rectal: 1 suppository 1-2 times/day, up to 4 doses/day

Mechanism of Action Anticholinergic alkaloids act primarily by competitive inhibition of the muscarinic actions of acetylcholine on structures innervated by postganglionic cholinergic neurons and on smooth muscle; resulting effects include antisecretory activity on exocrine glands and intestinal mucosa and smooth muscle relaxation. Contains many narcotic alkaloids including morphine; its mechanism for gastric motility inhibition is primarily due to this morphine content; it results in a decrease in digestive secretions, an increase in GI muscle tone, and therefore a reduction in GI propulsion.

Local Anesthetic/Vasoconstrictor Precautions No information available to require special precautions

Effects on Dental Treatment This drug has atropine-like effects and the patient may experience drowsiness, dry mouth, nose and throat

Other Adverse Effects
>10%:
  Gastrointestinal: Constipation, dry mouth
  Miscellaneous: Decreased sweating; dry nose, throat, or skin

1% to 10%: Decreased flow of breast milk, difficulty in swallowing, increased sensitivity to light

<1%:

Cardiovascular: Orthostatic hypotension, ventricular fibrillation, tachycardia, palpitations

Central nervous system: Confusion, drowsiness, headache, loss of memory, weakness, tiredness, ataxia, CNS depression

Dermatologic: Skin rash

Endocrine & metabolic: Antidiuretic hormone release

Gastrointestinal: Bloated feeling, nausea, vomiting, constipation

Genitourinary: Difficult urination, urinary retention

Ocular: Increased intraocular pain, blurred vision

Respiratory: Respiratory depression

Miscellaneous: Biliary or urinary tract spasm, histamine release, physical and psychological dependence, sweating

Drug Interactions Increased effect/toxicity: CNS depressants, tricyclic antidepressants

Drug Uptake

Onset of action:

Belladonna: 1-2 hours

Opium: Within 30 minutes

Pregnancy Risk Factor C

Belladonna, Phenobarbital, and Ergotamine Tartrate

(bel a don' a, fee noe bar' bi tal, & er got' a meen tar' trate)

Brand Names Bellergal-S®; Bel-Phen-Ergot S®; Phenerbel-S®

Therapeutic Category Ergot Alkaloid and Derivative

Use Management and treatment of menopausal disorders, gastrointestinal disorders and recurrent throbbing headache

Local Anesthetic/Vasoconstrictor Precautions No information available to require special precautions

Effects on Dental Treatment >10%: Dry mouth

Other Adverse Effects

>10%:

Cardiovascular: Peripheral vascular effects (numbness and tingling of fingers and toes)

Central nervous system: Drowsiness, dizziness

Gastrointestinal: Constipation, diarrhea, nausea, vomiting

Local: Irritation at injection site, localized edema

Miscellaneous: Decreased sweating; dry mouth, nose, throat, or skin

1% to 10%:

Cardiovascular: Precordial distress and pain, transient tachycardia or bradycardia

Endocrine & metabolic: Decreased flow of breast milk

Gastrointestinal: Difficulty in swallowing

Ocular: Increased sensitivity to light

Neuromuscular & skeletal: Muscle pains in the extremities, weakness in the legs

<1%:

Cardiovascular: Orthostatic hypotension, ventricular fibrillation, tachycardia, palpitation, ataxia

Central nervous system: Confusion, drowsiness, headache, loss of memory, tiredness

Dermatologic: Skin rash

Gastrointestinal: Bloated feeling, nausea, vomiting

Genitourinary: Difficult urination

Neuromuscular & skeletal: Weakness

Ocular: Increased intraocular pain, blurred vision

Bellergal-S® see Belladonna, Phenobarbital, and Ergotamine Tartrate on this page

Bel-Phen-Ergot S® see Belladonna, Phenobarbital, and Ergotamine Tartrate on this page

Bemote® see Dicyclomine Hydrochloride on page 273

Benadryl® [OTC] see Diphenhydramine Hydrochloride on page 288

Benazepril Clorhidrato De (Mexico) see Benazepril Hydrochloride on this page

Benazepril Hydrochloride (ben ay' ze pril hye droe klor' ide)

Related Information

Cardiovascular Diseases on page 912

Brand Names Lotensin®

(Continued)

Benazepril Hydrochloride *(Continued)*

Therapeutic Category Angiotensin-Converting Enzyme (ACE) Inhibitors

Synonyms Benazepril Clorhidrato De (Mexico)

Use Treatment of hypertension, either alone or in combination with other antihypertensive agents

Usual Dosage Adults: Oral: 20-40 mg/day as a single dose or 2 divided doses; maximum daily dose: 80 mg

Mechanism of Action Competitive inhibition of angiotensin I being converted to angiotensin II, a potent vasoconstrictor, through the angiotensin I-converting enzyme (ACE) activity, with resultant lower levels of angiotensin II which causes an increase in plasma renin activity and a reduction in aldosterone secretion

Local Anesthetic/Vasoconstrictor Precautions No information available to require special precautions

Effects on Dental Treatment No effects or complications reported

Other Adverse Effects

1% to 10%:
Central nervous system: Headache, dizziness, fatigue, somnolence, postural dizziness
Gastrointestinal: Nausea
Respiratory: Transient cough

<1%:
Cardiovascular: Hypotension, tachycardia
Central nervous system: Anxiety, insomnia, nervousness, asthenia
Dermatologic: Rash, photosensitivity, angioedema
Endocrine & metabolic: Hyperkalemia
Gastrointestinal: Constipation, gastritis, vomiting, melena
Genitourinary: Impotence, urinary tract infection
Neuromuscular & skeletal: Hypertonia, paresthesia, arthralgia, arthritis, myalgia
Respiratory: Asthma, bronchitis, dyspnea, sinusitis
Miscellaneous: Sweating

Drug Interactions See table.

Drug-Drug Interactions With ACEIs

Precipitant Drug	Drug (Category) and Effect	Description
Antacids	ACE Inhibitors: decreased	Decreased bioavailability of ACEIs. May be more likely with captopril. Separate administration times by 1-2 hours.
NSAIDs (indomethacin)	ACEIs: decreased	Reduced hypotensive effects of ACEIs. More prominent in low renin or volume dependent hypertensive patients.
Phenothiazines	ACEIs: increased	Pharmacologic effects of ACEIs may be increased.
ACEIs	Allopurinol: increased	Higher risk of hypersensitivity reaction possible when given concurrently. Three case reports of Stevens-Johnson syndrome with captopril.
ACEIs	Digoxin: increased	Increased plasma digoxin levels.
ACEIs	Lithium: increased	Increased serum lithium levels and symptoms of toxicity may occur.
ACEIs	Potassium preps/ potassium sparing diuretics increased	Coadministration may result in elevated potassium levels.

Drug Uptake

Reduction in plasma angiotensin-converting enzyme activity: Oral:
Peak effect: 1-2 hours after administration of 2-20 mg dose
Duration of action: >90% inhibition for 24 hours has been observed after 5-20 mg dose
Reduction in blood pressure:
Peak effect after single oral dose: 2-6 hours
Maximum response With continuous therapy: 2 weeks
Absorption: Rapid (37% of each oral dose); food does not alter significantly; metabolite (benazeprilat) itself unsuitable for oral administration due to poor absorption
Serum half-life:
Parent drug: 0.6 hour

Metabolite elimination: 22 hours (from 24 hours after dosing onward)
Metabolite: 1.5-2 hours after fasting or 2-4 hours after a meal
Time to peak: 1-1.5 hours (unchanged parent drug)
Pregnancy Risk Factor D

Bendroflumethiazide (ben droe floo meth eye' a zide)
Related Information
Cardiovascular Diseases *on page 912*
Brand Names Naturetin®
Therapeutic Category Diuretic, Thiazide Type
Synonyms Bendroflumetiacida (Mexico)
Use Management of mild to moderate hypertension; treatment of edema associated with congestive heart failure, pregnancy, or nephrotic syndrome
Mechanism of Action Like other thiazide diuretics, it inhibits sodium, chloride, and water reabsorption in the renal distal tubules, thereby producing diuresis with a resultant reduction in plasma volume; hypothetically may reduce peripheral resistance through increased prostacyclin synthesis
Local Anesthetic/Vasoconstrictor Precautions No information available to require special precautions
Effects on Dental Treatment No effects or complications reported
Other Adverse Effects
1% to 10%:
Cardiovascular: Orthostatic hypotension
Endocrine & metabolic: Hyponatremia, hypokalemia
Gastrointestinal: Anorexia, upset stomach, diarrhea
<1%:
Central nervous system: Drowsiness
Endocrine & metabolic: Hyperuricemia
Gastrointestinal: Nausea, vomiting
Genitourinary: Uremia
Hematologic: Aplastic anemia, hemolytic anemia, leukopenia, agranulocytosis, thrombocytopenia
Hepatic: Hepatitis, hepatic function impairment
Neuromuscular & skeletal: Paresthesia
Renal: Polyuria
Miscellaneous: Allergic reactions
Drug Interactions
Thiazides tend to elevate blood glucose in diabetics and thus may antagonize the hypoglycemic effect of antidiabetic drugs.
GI tract absorption of thiazides are impaired by cholestyramine (Questran®) and colestipol (Colestid®).
Thiazides increase plasma lithium concentrations; lithium toxicity may occur
Pregnancy Risk Factor D
Selected Readings
Hunninghake DB, King S and LaCroix K, "The Effect of Cholestyramine and Colestipol on the Absorption of Hydrochlorothiazide," *Int J Clin Pharmacol Ther Toxicol*, 1982, 20(4):151-4.
Hurtig HI, and Dyson WL, "Lithium Toxicity Enhanced by Diuresis," *N Engl J Med*, 1974, 290(13):748-9.
Petersen V, Hvidt S, Thomsen K, et al, "Effect of Prolonged Thiazide Treatment on Renal Lithium Clearance," *Br Med J*, 1974, 2(924):143.

Bendroflumetiacida (Mexico) *see* Bendroflumethiazide *on this page*
Benemid® *see* Probenecid *on page 724*
Benoquin® *see* Monobenzone *on page 589*
Benoxyl® *see* Benzoyl Peroxide *on page 104*

Bentiromide (ben teer' oh mide)
Brand Names Chymex®
Therapeutic Category Diagnostic Agent, Pancreatic Exocrine Insufficiency
Synonyms BTPABA
Use Screening test for pancreatic exocrine insufficiency
Usual Dosage Oral:
Children 6-12 years: 14 mg/kg (maximum dose: 500 mg) followed with 8 oz of water immediately and 2 hours postdosing and an additional 16 oz of water during hours 2-6 postdosing
Children >12 years and Adults: Administer following an overnight fast and morning void, single 500 mg dose and follow with 8 oz of water immediately and 2 hours postdosing and an additional 16 oz of water during hours 2-6 postdosing
Mechanism of Action Cleaved by the pancreatic enzyme chymotrypsin causing a release of para-aminobenzoic acid (PABA), percentage of PABA
(Continued)

Bentiromide *(Continued)*

metabolites recovered in urine reflects enzymatic activity of chymotrypsin providing a way of determining pancreatic function

Local Anesthetic/Vasoconstrictor Precautions No information available to require special precautions

Effects on Dental Treatment No effects or complications reported

Other Adverse Effects

1% to 10%:
Central nervous system: Headache
Gastrointestinal: Diarrhea

<1%:
Central nervous system: Drowsiness
Gastrointestinal: Flatulence, nausea, vomiting, heartburn
Hepatic: Elevations in liver function tests
Neuromuscular & skeletal: Weakness

Drug Uptake

Time to peak serum concentration: Oral: Within 2-3 hours

Pregnancy Risk Factor B

Bentyl® Hydrochloride *see* Dicyclomine Hydrochloride *on page 273*

Benylin® Cough Syrup [OTC] *see* Diphenhydramine Hydrochloride *on page 288*

Benylin® DM [OTC] *see* Dextromethorphan *on page 266*

Benylin® Expectorant [OTC] *see* Guaifenesin and Dextromethorphan *on page 408*

Benza® [OTC] *see* Benzalkonium Chloride *on this page*

Benzac AC Wash® *see* Benzoyl Peroxide *on page 104*

Benzac W Wash® *see* Benzoyl Peroxide *on page 104*

Benzalkonium Chloride *(benz al koe' nee um klor' ide)*

Brand Names Benza® [OTC]; Zephiran® [OTC]

Therapeutic Category Antibacterial, Topical

Synonyms BAC

Use Surface antiseptic and germicidal preservative

Local Anesthetic/Vasoconstrictor Precautions No information available to require special precautions

Effects on Dental Treatment No effects or complications reported

Other Adverse Effects 1% to 10%: Hypersensitivity

Benzamycin® *see* Erythromycin and Benzoyl Peroxide *on page 323*

Benzedrex® [OTC] *see* Propylhexedrine *on page 745*

Benzmethyzin *see* Procarbazine Hydrochloride *on page 727*

Benzocaine *(ben' zoe kane)*

Related Information

Mouth Pain, Cold Sore, Canker Sore Products *on page 1063*

Brand Names Anbesol® Maximum Strength [OTC]; Babee® Teething [OTC]; Benzocol® [OTC]; Benzodent® [OTC]; Hurricaine® [OTC]; Maximum Strength Anbesol® [OTC]; Maximum Strength Orajel® [OTC]; Numzitdent® [OTC]; Numzit Teething® [OTC]; Orabase®-B [OTC]; Orabase®-O [OTC]; Orajel® Brace-Aid Oral Anesthetic [OTC]; Orajel® Maximum Strength [OTC]; Orajel® Mouth-Aid [OTC]; Orasept® [OTC]; Orasol® [OTC]; Oratect® [OTC]; Spec-T® [OTC]; Vicks Children's Chloraseptic® [OTC]; Vicks Chloraseptic® Sore Throat [OTC]; ZilaDent® [OTC]

Canadian/Mexican Brand Names Graneodin-B® (Mexico)

Therapeutic Category Local Anesthetic, Topical

Use

Dental: Ester-type local anesthetic for temporary relief of pain associated with toothache, minor sore throat pain and canker sore

Medical: Local anesthetic (ester derivative); temporary relief of pain associated with pruritic dermatosis, pruritus, minor burns, acute congestive and serious otitis media, swimmer's ear, otitis externa, hemorrhoids, rectal fissures, anesthetic lubricant for passage of catheters and endoscopic tubes

Usual Dosage Children and Adults:

Mucous membranes: Dosage varies depending on area to be anesthetized and vascularity of tissues

Oral mouth/throat preparations: Do not administer for >2 days or in children <2 years of age, unless directed by a physician; refer to specific package labeling

Mechanism of Action Local anesthetics bind selectively to the intracellular surface of sodium channels to block influx of sodium into the axon. As a result, depolarization necessary for action potential propagation and subsequent nerve function is prevented. The block at the sodium channel is reversible. When drug diffuses away from the axon, sodium channel function is restored and nerve propagation returns.

Local Anesthetic/Vasoconstrictor Precautions No information available to require special precautions

Effects on Dental Treatment No effects or complications reported

Other Adverse Effects 1% to 10%:
Dermatologic: Angioedema, contact dermatitis
Local: Burning, stinging

Oral manifestations: No data reported

Contraindications Known hypersensitivity to benzocaine, other ester-type local anesthetics, or other components in the formulation; ophthalmic use

Warnings/Precautions Not intended for use when infections are present

Drug Interactions May antagonize actions of sulfonamides

Drug Uptake
Absorption: Topical: Poorly absorbed after administration to intact skin, but well absorbed from mucous membranes and traumatized skin
Onset: ~1 minute
Duration: 15-20 minutes

Pregnancy Risk Factor C

Breast-feeding Considerations No data reported

Dosage Forms
Mouth/throat preparations:
Cream: 5% (10 g)
Gel: 6.3% (7.5 g); 7.5% (7.2 g, 9.45 g, 14.1 g); 10% (6 g, 9.45 g, 10 g, 15 g); 15% (10.5 g); 20% (9.45 g, 14.1 g)
Liquid: (3.7 mL); 5% (8.8 mL); 6.3% (9 mL, 22 mL, 14.79 mL); 10% (13 mL); 20% (13.3 mL)
Lotion: 0.2% (15 mL); 2.5% (15 mL)
Lozenges: 5 mg, 6 mg, 10 mg, 15 mg
Ointment: 20% (5 g, 15 g)
Topical for mucous membranes:
Gel: 6% (7.5 g); 20% (2.5 g, 3.75 g, 7.5 g, 30 g)
Liquid: 20% (3.75 mL, 9 mL, 13.3 mL, 30 mL)

Dietary Considerations No data reported

Generic Available Yes

Benzocaine and Antipyrine *see* Antipyrine and Benzocaine *on page 70*

Benzocaine and Cetylpyridinium Chloride *see* Cetylpyridinium Chloride and Benzocaine *on page 179*

Benzocaine, Butyl Aminobenzoate, Tetracaine, and Benzalkonium Chloride

(ben' zoe kane, byoo' til a meen oh benz' oh ate, tet' ra kane, & benz al koe' nee um klor' ide)

Brand Names Cetacaine®

Therapeutic Category Local Anesthetic, Topical

Synonyms Tetracaine Hydrochloride, Benzocaine Butyl Aminobenzoate and Benzalkonium Chloride

Use Topical anesthetic to control pain or gagging

Local Anesthetic/Vasoconstrictor Precautions No information available to require special precautions

Effects on Dental Treatment No effects or complications reported

Other Adverse Effects Dose related and may result from high plasma levels
1% to 10%: Contact dermatitis, burning, stinging, angioedema
<1%: Methemoglobinemia in infants, tenderness, urticaria, edema, urethritis

Comments This is the only topical anesthetic which comes in an easy to spray bottle, however, sensitization may result from any one of the ingredients

Benzocaine, Gelatin, Pectin, and Sodium Carboxymethylcellulose

(ben' zoe kane, jel' a tin, pek' tin, & sow' dee um kar box ee meth il sel' yoo lose)

Brand Names Orabase® With Benzocaine [OTC]

Therapeutic Category Local Anesthetic, Topical

Use Topical anesthetic and emollient for oral lesions
(Continued)

Benzocaine, Gelatin, Pectin, and Sodium Carboxymethylcellulose *(Continued)*

Local Anesthetic/Vasoconstrictor Precautions No information available to require special precautions

Effects on Dental Treatment No effects or complications reported

Other Adverse Effects Dose related and may result from high plasma levels
1% to 10%: Contact dermatitis, burning, stinging, angioedema
<1%: Methemoglobinemia in infants, tenderness, urticaria, edema, urethritis

Benzocol® [OTC] *see Benzocaine on page 102*

Benzodent® [OTC] *see Benzocaine on page 102*

Benzoic Acid and Salicylic Acid

(ben zoe' ik as' id & sal i sil' ik as' id)

Brand Names Whitfield's Ointment [OTC]

Therapeutic Category Antifungal Agent, Topical

Synonyms Salicylic Acid and Benzoic Acid

Use Treatment of athlete's foot and ringworm of the scalp

Local Anesthetic/Vasoconstrictor Precautions No information available to require special precautions

Effects on Dental Treatment No effects or complications reported

Benzoin (ben' zoin)

Brand Names AeroZoin® [OTC]; TinBen® [OTC]; TinCoBen® [OTC]

Therapeutic Category Pharmaceutical Aid; Protectant, Topical

Synonyms Gum Benjamin

Use Protective application for irritations of the skin; sometimes used in boiling water as steam inhalants for their expectorant and soothing action

Local Anesthetic/Vasoconstrictor Precautions No information available to require special precautions

Effects on Dental Treatment No effects or complications reported

Benzonatate (ben zoe' na tate)

Related Information
Patients Undergoing Cancer Therapy *on page 967*

Brand Names Tessalon® Perles

Canadian/Mexican Brand Names Beknol® (Mexico); Pebegal® (Mexico); Tesalon® (Mexico)

Therapeutic Category Antitussive; Local Anesthetic, Oral

Synonyms Benzonatato (Mexico)

Use Symptomatic relief of nonproductive cough

Usual Dosage Children >10 years and Adults: Oral: 100 mg 3 times/day or every 4 hours up to 600 mg/day

Mechanism of Action Tetracaine congener with antitussive properties; suppresses cough by topical anesthetic action on the respiratory stretch receptors

Local Anesthetic/Vasoconstrictor Precautions No information available to require special precautions

Effects on Dental Treatment No effects or complications reported

Other Adverse Effects 1% to 10%:
Central nervous system: Sedation, headache, dizziness
Dermatologic: Skin rash
Gastrointestinal: GI upset
Neuromuscular & skeletal: Numbness in chest
Ocular: Burning sensation in eyes
Respiratory: Nasal congestion

Drug Interactions No data reported

Drug Uptake
Onset of action: Therapeutic: Within 15-20 minutes
Duration: 3-8 hours

Pregnancy Risk Factor C

Benzonatato (Mexico) *see Benzonatate on this page*

Benzoyl Peroxide (ben' zoe il peer ox' ide)

Brand Names Benoxyl®; Benzac AC Wash®; Benzac W Wash®; Benzoyl Peroxide®; BlemErase® [OTC]; Clearasil® [OTC]; Dermoxyl® [OTC]; Desquam-E®; Desquam-X®; Dryox® [OTC]; Fostex® BPO [OTC]; Loroxide® [OTC]; Neutrogena® [OTC]; Oxy-5® [OTC]; Oxy-10® [OTC]; PanOxyl® [OTC]; PanOxyl®-AQ; Perfectoderm® [OTC]; Persa-Gel®; Vanoxide® [OTC]

Canadian/Mexican Brand Names Acetoxyl® (Canada); Acnomel® B.P.5 (Canada); H₂Oxyl® (Canada); Oxyderm® (Canada); Solugel® (Canada)

Therapeutic Category Acne Products; Topical Skin Product

Use Adjunctive treatment of mild to moderate acne vulgaris and acne rosacea

Usual Dosage Children and Adults:

  Cleansers: Wash once or twice daily; control amount of drying or peeling by modifying dose frequency or concentration

  Topical: Apply sparingly once daily; gradually increase to 2-3 times/day if needed. If excessive dryness or peeling occurs, reduce dose frequency or concentration; if excessive stinging or burning occurs, remove with mild soap and water; resume use the next day.

Mechanism of Action Releases free-radical oxygen which oxidizes bacterial proteins in the sebaceous follicles decreasing the number of anaerobic bacteria and decreasing irritating-type free fatty acids

Local Anesthetic/Vasoconstrictor Precautions No information available to require special precautions

Effects on Dental Treatment No effects or complications reported

Other Adverse Effects 1% to 10%: Dermatologic: Irritation, contact dermatitis, dryness, erythema, peeling, stinging

Drug Interactions Increased toxicity: Benzoyl peroxide potentiates adverse reactions seen with tretinoin

Drug Uptake

  Absorption: ~5% through the skin; gels are more penetrating than creams

Pregnancy Risk Factor C

Benzoyl Peroxide® *see* Benzoyl Peroxide *on previous page*

Benzoyl Peroxide and Hydrocortisone

(ben′ zoe il peer ox′ ide & hye droe kor′ ti sone)

Brand Names Vanoxide-HC®

Therapeutic Category Acne Products; Corticosteroid, Topical (Low Potency); Topical Skin Product

Use Treatment of acne vulgaris and oily skin

Local Anesthetic/Vasoconstrictor Precautions No information available to require special precautions

Effects on Dental Treatment No effects or complications reported

Other Adverse Effects See individual agents

Benzphetamine Hydrochloride

(benz fet′ a meen hye droe klor′ ide)

Brand Names Didrex®

Therapeutic Category Anorexiant

Use Short-term adjunct in exogenous obesity

Local Anesthetic/Vasoconstrictor Precautions Use with caution since amphetamines have actions similar to epinephrine and norepinephrine

Effects on Dental Treatment No effects or complications reported

Other Adverse Effects

  >10%:

  Cardiovascular: Irregular heartbeat

  Central nervous system: False feeling of well being, nervousness, restlessness, insomnia

  1% to 10%:

  Cardiovascular: Hypertension

  Central nervous system: Mood or mental changes, dizziness, lightheadedness, headache

  Endocrine & metabolic: Changes in libido

  Gastrointestinal: Diarrhea, nausea, vomiting, stomach cramps, constipation, anorexia, weight loss dry mouth

  Ocular: Blurred vision

  Miscellaneous: Increased sweating

  <1%:

  Cardiovascular: Chest pain

  Central nervous system: CNS stimulation (severe), Tourette's syndrome, hyperthermia, seizures, paranoia, tolerance and withdrawal with prolonged use

  Dermatologic: Skin rash, hives

Benzthiazide (benz thye′ a zide)

Related Information

  Cardiovascular Diseases *on page 912*

Brand Names Aquatag®; Exna®; Hydrex®; Marazide®; Proaqua®

(Continued)

Benzthiazide *(Continued)*

Therapeutic Category Diuretic, Thiazide Type

Use Management of mild to moderate hypertension; treatment of edema in congestive heart failure and nephrotic syndrome

Usual Dosage Oral:
Children: 1-4 mg/kg/day in 3 divided doses
Adults: 50-200 mg/day

Mechanism of Action Like other thiazide diuretics, it inhibits sodium, chloride, and water reabsorption in the renal distal tubules, thereby producing diuresis with a resultant reduction in plasma volume; hypothetically may reduce peripheral resistance through increased prostacyclin synthesis

Local Anesthetic/Vasoconstrictor Precautions No information available to require special precautions

Effects on Dental Treatment No effects or complications reported

Other Adverse Effects
1% to 10%:
Cardiovascular: Orthostatic hypotension
Endocrine & metabolic: Hyponatremia, hypokalemia
Gastrointestinal: Anorexia, upset stomach, diarrhea
<1%:
Central nervous system: Drowsiness
Endocrine & metabolic: Hyperuricemia
Gastrointestinal: Nausea, vomiting
Genitourinary: Uremia
Hematologic: Aplastic anemia, hemolytic anemia, leukopenia, agranulocytosis, thrombocytopenia
Hepatic: Hepatitis, hepatic function impairment
Neuromuscular & skeletal: Paresthesia
Renal: Polyuria
Miscellaneous: Allergic reactions

Drug Interactions
Thiazides tend to elevate blood glucose in diabetics and thus may antagonize the hypoglycemic effect of antidiabetic drugs.
GI tract absorption of thiazides are impaired by cholestyramine (Questran®) and colestipol (Colestid®).
Thiazides increase plasma lithium concentrations; lithium toxicity may occur.

Drug Uptake
Onset of action: Within 2 hours
Duration: 12 hours

Pregnancy Risk Factor D

Selected Readings
Hunninghake DB, King S and LaCroix K, "The Effect of Cholestyramine and Colestipol on the Absorption of Hydrochlorothiazide," *Int J Clin Pharmacol Ther Toxicol*, 1982, 20(4):151-4.
Hurtig HI, and Dyson WL, "Lithium Toxicity Enhanced by Diuresis," *N Engl J Med*, 1974, 290(13):748-9.
Petersen V, Hvidt S, Thomsen K, et al, "Effect of Prolonged Thiazide Treatment on Renal Lithium Clearance," *Br Med J*, 1974, 2(924):143.

Benztropine Mesylate *(benz' troe peen mes' i late)*

Brand Names Cogentin®

Canadian/Mexican Brand Names PMS-Benztropine® (Canada)

Therapeutic Category Anticholinergic Agent; Anti-Parkinson's Agent

Use Adjunctive treatment of Parkinson's disease; also used in treatment of drug-induced extrapyramidal effects (except tardive dyskinesia) and acute dystonic reactions

Usual Dosage Use in children <3 years of age should be reserved for life-threatening emergencies
Drug-induced extrapyramidal reaction: Oral, I.M., I.V.:
Children >3 years: 0.02-0.05 mg/kg/dose 1-2 times/day
Adults: 1-4 mg/dose 1-2 times/day

Acute dystonia: Adults: I.M., I.V.: 1-2 mg
Parkinsonism: Oral:
Adults: 0.5-6 mg/day in 1-2 divided doses; if one dose is greater, give at bedtime; titrate dose in 0.5 mg increments at 5- to 6-day intervals
Elderly: Initial: 0.5 mg once or twice daily; increase by 0.5 mg as needed at 5-6 days; maximum: 6 mg/day

Mechanism of Action Thought to partially block striatal cholinergic receptors to help balance cholinergic and dopaminergic activity

Local Anesthetic/Vasoconstrictor Precautions No information available to require special precautions

Effects on Dental Treatment Dry mouth, nose and throat very prevalent in patients taking this drug

Other Adverse Effects

>10%:

Gastrointestinal: Constipation, dry mouth

Miscellaneous: Decreased sweating; dry nose, throat, or skin

1% to 10%: Decreased flow of breast milk, difficulty in swallowing, increased sensitivity to light

<1%:

Cardiovascular: Coma, tachycardia, orthostatic hypotension, ventricular fibrillation, palpitations, ataxia

Central nervous system: Drowsiness, nervousness, hallucinations; the elderly may be at increased risk for confusion and hallucinations, headache, loss of memory, weakness, tiredness

Dermatologic: Skin rash

Gastrointestinal: Nausea, vomiting, bloated feeling

Genitourinary: Difficult urination

Ocular: Blurred vision, mydriasis, increased intraocular pain

Drug Interactions

Decreased effect: May increase gastric degradation of levodopa and decrease the amount of levodopa absorbed by delaying gastric emptying - the opposite may be true for digoxin

Increased toxicity: Central anticholinergic syndrome can occur when administered with narcotic analgesics, phenothiazines and other antipsychotics, tricyclic antidepressants, quinidine and some other antiarrhythmics, and antihistamines

Drug Uptake

Onset of action:

Oral: Within 1 hour

Parenteral: Within 15 minutes

Duration of action: 6-48 hours (wide range)

Pregnancy Risk Factor C

Benzylpenicilloyl-polylysine (ben' zil pen i sil' oil pol i lie' seen)

Brand Names Pre-Pen®

Therapeutic Category Diagnostic Agent, Penicillin Allergy Skin Test

Use Adjunct in assessing the risk of administering penicillin (penicillin or benzylpenicillin) in adults with a history of clinical penicillin hypersensitivity

Usual Dosage PPL is administered by a scratch technique or by intradermal injection. For initial testing, PPL should always be applied via the scratch technique. **Do not give intradermally to patients who have positive reactions to a scratch test.** PPL test alone does not identify those patients who react to a minor antigenic determinant and does not appear to predict reliably the occurrence of late reactions.

Scratch test: Use scratch technique with a 20-gauge needle to make 3-5 mm nonbleeding scratch on epidermis, apply a small drop of solution to scratch, rub in gently with applicator or toothpick. A positive reaction consists of a pale wheal surrounding the scratch site which develops within 10 minutes and ranges from 5-15 mm or more in diameter.

Intradermal test: Use intradermal test with a tuberculin syringe with a 26- to 30-gauge short bevel needle; a dose of 0.01-0.02 mL is injected intradermally. A control of 0.9% sodium chloride should be injected at least 1.5" from the PPL test site. Most skin responses to the intradermal test will develop within 5-15 minutes.

Interpretation:

(-) Negative: No reaction

(±) Ambiguous: Wheal only slightly larger than original bleb with or without erythematous flare and larger than control site

(+) Positive: Itching and marked increase in size of original bleb
Control site should be reactionless

Mechanism of Action Elicits IgE antibodies which produce type I accelerate urticarial reactions to penicillins

Local Anesthetic/Vasoconstrictor Precautions No information available to require special precautions

Effects on Dental Treatment No effects or complications reported

Other Adverse Effects

1% to 10%: Local: Intense local inflammatory response at skin test site

<1%:

Local: Pruritus, erythema, wheal, urticaria, edema

Sensitivity reactions: Systemic allergic reactions occur rarely

(Continued)

107

Benzylpenicilloyl-polylysine *(Continued)*

Drug Interactions Decreased effect: Corticosteroids and other immunosuppressive agents may inhibit the immune response to the skin test

Pregnancy Risk Factor C

Bepridil Hydrochloride *(be' pri dil hye droe klor' ide)*

Related Information

Calcium Channel Blockers & Gingival Hyperplasia *on page 1010*
Cardiovascular Diseases *on page 912*

Brand Names Vascor®

Canadian/Mexican Brand Names Bapadin® (Canada)

Therapeutic Category Antianginal Agent; Calcium Channel Blocker

Use Treatment of chronic stable angina; due to side effect profile, reserve for patients who have been intolerant of other antianginal therapy; bepridil may be used alone or in combination with nitrates or beta-blockers

Usual Dosage Adults: Oral: Initial: 200 mg/day, then adjust dose at 10-day intervals until optimal response is achieved; maximum daily dose: 400 mg

Mechanism of Action Bepridil, a type 4 calcium antagonist, possesses characteristics of the traditional calcium antagonist, inhibiting calcium ion from entering the "slow channels" or select voltage-sensitive areas of vascular smooth muscle and myocardium during depolarization and producing a relaxation of coronary vascular smooth muscle and coronary vasodilation. However, bepridil may also inhibit fast sodium channels (inward) which may account for some of its side effects (eg, arrhythmias); a direct bradycardia effect of bepridil has been postulated via direct action on the S-A node.

Local Anesthetic/Vasoconstrictor Precautions No information available to require special precautions

Effects on Dental Treatment Other drugs of this class can cause gingival hyperplasia (ie, nifedipine) but there have been no reports for bepridil

Other Adverse Effects

>10%:
  Central nervous system: Dizziness, asthenia, headache
  Gastrointestinal: Nausea, dyspepsia, abdominal pain, GI distress
1% to 10%:
  Cardiovascular: Bradycardia, palpitations
  Central nervous system: Nervousness
  Gastrointestinal: Diarrhea, anorexia, dry mouth
  Miscellaneous: Flu syndrome
<1%:
  Cardiovascular: Ventricular premature contractions, hypertension, torsade de pointes, edema, syncope, prolonged Q-T intervals
  Central nervous system: Fever, psychotic behavior, akathisia
  Dermatologic: Rash
  Genitourinary: Sexual difficulties
  Hematologic: Agranulocytosis
  Neuromuscular & skeletal: Tremor, myalgia, arthritis
  Ocular: Blurred vision
  Respiratory: Nasal congestion, cough, pharyngitis
  Miscellaneous: Sweating, taste change

Drug Interactions Bepridil increases digoxin serum concentrations by over 30% and enhances the cardiac effects of digoxin

Drug Uptake

Onset of action: 1 hour
Absorption: Oral: 100%
Serum half-life: 24 hours
Time to peak: 2-3 hours

Pregnancy Risk Factor C

Beractant *(ber akt' ant)*

Brand Names Survanta®

Therapeutic Category Lung Surfactant

Use Prevention and treatment of respiratory distress syndrome (RDS) in premature infants

Prophylactic therapy: Body weight <1250 g in infants at risk for developing or with evidence of surfactant deficiency
Rescue therapy: Treatment of infants with RDS confirmed by x-ray and requiring mechanical ventilation (administer as soon as possible - within 8 hours of age)

Usual Dosage

Prophylactic treatment: Give 100 mg phospholipids (4 mL/kg) intratracheally as soon as possible; as many as 4 doses may be administered during the first 48 hours of life, no more frequently than 6 hours apart. The need for additional doses is determined by evidence of continuing respiratory distress; if the infant is still intubated and requiring at least 30% inspired oxygen to maintain a PAO_2 ≤80 torr.

Rescue treatment: Administer 100 mg phospholipids (4 mL/kg) as soon as the diagnosis of RDS is made

Mechanism of Action Replaces deficient or ineffective endogenous lung surfactant in neonates with respiratory distress syndrome (RDS) or in neonates at risk of developing RDS. Surfactant prevents the alveoli from collapsing during expiration by lowering surface tension between air and alveolar surfaces.

Local Anesthetic/Vasoconstrictor Precautions No information available to require special precautions

Effects on Dental Treatment No effects or complications reported

Other Adverse Effects During the dosing procedure:

Cardiovascular: Transient bradycardia, vasoconstriction, hypotension, hypertension, pallor

Respiratory: Oxygen desaturation, endotracheal tube blockage, hypocarbia, hypercarbia, apnea, pulmonary air leaks, pulmonary interstitial emphysema

Miscellaneous: Increased probability of post-treatment nosocomial sepsis

Drug Interactions No data reported

Berocca® see Vitamin B Complex With Vitamin C and Folic Acid on page 900

Berubigen® see Cyanocobalamin on page 237

Beta-2® see Isoetharine on page 470

Beta-Carotene (bay' tah kare' oh teen)

Brand Names Max-Caro® [OTC]; Provatene® [OTC]; Solatene®

Therapeutic Category Vitamin, Fat Soluble

Use Reduces severity of photosensitivity reactions in patients with erythropoietic protoporphyria (EPP)

Usual Dosage Oral:

Children <14 years: 30-150 mg/day

Adults: 30-300 mg/day

Mechanism of Action The exact mechanism of action in erythropoietic protoporphyria has not as yet been elucidated; although patient must become carotenemic before effects are observed, there appears to be more than a simple internal light screen responsible for the drug's action. A protective effect was achieved when beta-carotene was added to blood samples. The concentrations of solutions used were similar to those achieved in treated patients. Topically applied beta-carotene is considerably less effective than systemic therapy.

Local Anesthetic/Vasoconstrictor Precautions No information available to require special precautions

Effects on Dental Treatment No effects or complications reported

Other Adverse Effects

>10%: Dermatologic: Carotenodermia (yellowing of palms, hands, or soles of feet, and to a lesser extent the face)

<1%:

Central nervous system: Dizziness

Dermatologic: Ecchymoses

Gastrointestinal: Diarrhea

Neuromuscular & skeletal: Arthralgia

Drug Interactions Fulfills vitamin A requirements, do not prescribe additional vitamin A

Pregnancy Risk Factor C

Betachron E-R® see Propranolol Hydrochloride on page 743

Betadine® [OTC] see Povidone-Iodine on page 713

9-Beta-D-ribofuranosyladenine see Adenosine on page 25

Betagan® see Levobunolol Hydrochloride on page 493

Betalin®S see Thiamine Hydrochloride on page 837

Betamethasone (bay ta meth' a sone)

Related Information

Corticosteroid Equivalencies Comparison on page 1017

Corticosteroids, Topical Comparison on page 1018

Respiratory Diseases on page 924

(Continued)

Betamethasone *(Continued)*

Brand Names Alphatrex®; Betatrex®; Beta-Val®; Celestone®; Cel-U-Jec®; Diprolene®; Diprolene® AF; Diprosone®; Maxivate®; Selestoject®; Teladar®; Urticort®; Valisone®

Canadian/Mexican Brand Names Selestoject® [Sodium Phosphate] (Canada); Betnesol® [Disodium Phosphate] (Canada); Diprolene® Glycol [Dipropionate] (Canada); Occlucort® (Canada); Rhoprolene® (Canada); Rhoprosone® (Canada); Taro-Sone® (Canada); Topilene® (Canada); Topisone® (Canada)

Therapeutic Category Anti-inflammatory Agent; Corticosteroid, Systemic; Corticosteroid, Topical (Medium/High Potency)

Use

Dental: Treatment of a variety of oral diseases of allergic, inflammatory or autoimmune origin

Medical: Inflammatory dermatoses such as seborrheic or atopic dermatitis, neurodermatitis, anogenital pruritus, psoriasis, inflammatory phase of xerosis

Usual Dosage

Children:

Oral: 0.0175-0.25 mg/kg/day divided every 6-8 hours **or** 0.5-7.5 mg/m²/day divided every 6-8 hours

I.M.: 0.0175-0.125 mg base/kg/day divided every 6-12 hours **or** 0.5-7.5 mg base/m²/day divided every 6-12 hours

Adults:

Oral: 0.6-7.2 mg/day in 2-4 doses

I.M., I.V.: Betamethasone sodium phosphate: 0.6-9 mg/day divided every 12-24 hours

Mechanism of Action Controls the rate of protein synthesis, depresses the migration of polymorphonuclear leukocytes, fibroblasts, reverses capillary permeability, and lysosomal stabilization at the cellular level to prevent or control inflammation

Local Anesthetic/Vasoconstrictor Precautions No information available to require special precautions

Effects on Dental Treatment No effects or complications reported

Other Adverse Effects >10%:

Central nervous system: Insomnia

Gastrointestinal: Increased appetite, indigestion

Oral manifestations: No data reported

Contraindications Systemic fungal infections; hypersensitivity to betamethasone or any component

Warnings/Precautions Use with caution in patients with hypothyroidism, cirrhosis, ulcerative colitis; do not use occlusive dressings on weeping or exudative lesions and general caution with occlusive dressings should be observed; discontinue if skin irritation or contact dermatitis should occur; do not use in patients with decreased skin circulation.

Drug Interactions Decreased effect of any systemic corticosteroid by barbiturates, phenytoin, rifampin

Drug Uptake

Absorption: Oral: Rapid

Time to peak serum concentration: I.V.: Within 10-36 minutes

Serum half-life: Oral: 6.5 hours

Pregnancy Risk Factor C

Breast-feeding Considerations No data reported

Dosage Forms

Base (Celestone®), Oral:

Syrup: 0.6 mg/5 mL (118 mL)

Tablet: 0.6 mg

Injection: Sodium phosphate salt (Celestone® Phosphate, Cel-U-®, Selestoject®): 4 mg betamethasone phosphate/mL (equivalent to 3 mg betamethasone/mL) (5 mL)

Injection, suspension: Sodium phosphate and acetate salt (Celestone® Soluspan®): 6 mg/mL (3 mg of betamethasone sodium phosphate and 3 mg of betamethasone acetate per mL) (5 mL)

Dietary Considerations May be taken with food to decrease GI distress

Generic Available Yes

Betamethasone and Clotrimazole
(bay ta meth' a sone & kloe trim' a zole)

Brand Names Lotrisone®

Therapeutic Category Antifungal Agent, Topical; Corticosteroid, Topical (Medium/High Potency)

Use Topical treatment of various dermal fungal infections

Local Anesthetic/Vasoconstrictor Precautions No information available to require special precautions

Effects on Dental Treatment No effects or complications reported

Other Adverse Effects See individual agents

Betapace® see Sotalol Hydrochloride on page 796

Betapen®-VK see Penicillin V Potassium on page 668

Betaseron® see Interferon Beta-1b on page 464

Betatrex® see Betamethasone on page 109

Beta-Val® see Betamethasone on page 109

Betaxolol Hydrochloride (be tax' oh lol hye droe klor' ide)

Related Information
Cardiovascular Diseases on page 912

Brand Names Betoptic®; Betoptic® S; Kerlone®

Therapeutic Category Antiglaucoma Agent; Beta-Adrenergic Blocker, Cardioselective; Beta-Adrenergic Blocker, Ophthalmic

Use Treatment of chronic open-angle glaucoma and ocular hypertension; management of hypertension

Usual Dosage Adults:
Ophthalmic: Instill 1 drop twice daily
Oral: 10 mg/day; may increase dose to 20 mg/day after 7-14 days if desired response is not achieved; initial dose in elderly patients: 5 mg/day

Mechanism of Action Competitively blocks beta$_1$-receptors, with little or no effect on beta$_2$-receptors; ophthalmic reduces intraocular pressure by reducing the production of aqueous humor

Local Anesthetic/Vasoconstrictor Precautions No information available to require special precautions

Effects on Dental Treatment Non-cardioselective beta-blockers (ie, propranolol, nadolol) enhance the pressor response to epinephrine, resulting in hypertension and bradycardia. This has not been reported for betaxolol, a cardioselective beta-blocker. Therefore local anesthetic with vasoconstrictor can be safely used in patients medicated with betaxolol. Many nonsteroidal anti-inflammatory drugs such as ibuprofen and indomethacin can reduce the hypotensive effect of beta-blockers after 3 or more weeks of therapy with the NSAID. Short-term NSAID use (ie, 3 days) requires no special precautions in patients taking beta-blockers.

Other Adverse Effects
1% to 10%:
Cardiovascular: Bradycardia, palpitations, edema, congestive heart failure
Central nervous system: Dizziness, fatigue, lethargy, headache
Dermatologic: Erythema, itching
Ocular: Mild ocular stinging and discomfort, tearing, photophobia, decreased corneal sensitivity, keratitis
Miscellaneous: Cold extremities
<1%:
Cardiovascular: Chest pain
Central nervous system: Nervousness, depression, hallucinations
Hematologic: Thrombocytopenia

Drug Interactions
Decreased effects of beta-blockers:
Barbiturates (increased liver metabolism of beta-blockers to result in lower serum levels)
NSAIDs (attenuate the hypotensive therapeutic effects of beta-blockers)
Rifampin (increased liver metabolism of beta-blockers to result in lower serum levels)
Increased effects of beta-blockers:
Calcium channel blockers (increase serum levels by unknown mechanism to enhance hypotension)
Beta-blockers increase the effects of:
Epinephrine (vasoconstrictor; initial hypertensive episode followed by bradycardia)
Phenylephrine (Neosynephrine®; enhanced pressor response)
(Continued)

Betaxolol Hydrochloride *(Continued)*

Theophylline (inhibit theophylline metabolism causing increase in serum concentrations)

Drug Uptake
Onset of action: 1-1.5 hours
Duration: ≥12 hours
Absorption: Systemically absorbed
Serum half-life: 12-22 hours
Time to peak: Within 2 hours

Pregnancy Risk Factor C

Selected Readings
Foster CA and Aston SJ, "Propranolol-Epinephrine Interaction: A Potential Disaster," *Plast Reconstr Surg*, 1983, 72(1):74-8.
Wong DG, Spence JD, Lamki L, et al, "Effect of Nonsteroidal Anti-Inflammatory Drugs on Control of Hypertension of Beta-Blockers and Diuretics," *Lancet*, 1986, 1(8488):997-1001.
Wynn RL, "Dental Nonsteroidal Anti-Inflammatory Drugs and Prostaglandin-Based Drug Interactions, Part Two," *Gen Dent*, 1992, 40(2):104, 106, 108.
Wynn RL, "Epinephrine Interactions With Beta-Blockers," *Gen Dent*, 1994, 42(1):16, 18.

Bethanechol Chloride (be than' e kole klor' ide)

Brand Names Duvoid®; Myotonachol™; Urabeth®; Urecholine®
Canadian/Mexican Brand Names PMS-Bethanechol® Chloride (Canada)
Therapeutic Category Cholinergic Agent
Use Nonobstructive urinary retention and retention due to neurogenic bladder; treatment and prevention of bladder dysfunction caused by phenothiazines; diagnosis of flaccid or atonic neurogenic bladder; gastroesophageal reflux

Usual Dosage
Children:
Oral:
Abdominal distention or urinary retention: 0.6 mg/kg/day divided 3-4 times/day
Gastroesophageal reflux: 0.1-0.2 mg/kg/dose given 30 minutes to 1 hour before each meal to a maximum of 4 times/day
S.C.: 0.15-0.2 mg/kg/day divided 3-4 times/day

Adults:
Oral: 10-50 mg 2-4 times/day
S.C.: 2.5-5 mg 3-4 times/day, up to 7.5-10 mg every 4 hours for neurogenic bladder

Mechanism of Action Stimulates cholinergic receptors in the smooth muscle of the urinary bladder and gastrointestinal tract resulting in increased peristalsis, increased GI and pancreatic secretions, bladder muscle contraction, and increased ureteral peristaltic waves

Local Anesthetic/Vasoconstrictor Precautions No information available to require special precautions

Effects on Dental Treatment This is a cholinergic agent similar to pilocarpine and expect to see salivation and sweating in patients

Other Adverse Effects
Oral: <1%:
Cardiovascular: Hypotension, cardiac arrest, flushed skin
Gastrointestinal: Abdominal cramps, diarrhea, nausea, vomiting
Respiratory: Bronchial constriction
Miscellaneous: Sweating, salivation, vasomotor response
Subcutaneous: 1% to 10%:
Cardiovascular: Hypotension, cardiac arrest, flushed skin
Gastrointestinal: Abdominal cramps, diarrhea, nausea, vomiting
Respiratory: Bronchial constriction
Miscellaneous: Sweating, salivation, vasomotor response

Drug Interactions
Decreased effect: Procainamide, quinidine
Increased toxicity: Bethanechol and ganglionic blockers cause critical fall in blood pressure; cholinergic drugs or anticholinesterase agents

Drug Uptake
Onset of action:
Oral: 30-90 minutes
S.C.: 5-15 minutes
Duration of action:
Oral: Up to 6 hours
S.C.: 2 hours
Absorption: Oral: Variable

Pregnancy Risk Factor C

Betimol® Ophthalmic *see* Timolol Maleate *on page 847*

Betoptic® *see* Betaxolol Hydrochloride *on page 111*

Betoptic® S *see* Betaxolol Hydrochloride *on page 111*

Bexophene® *see* Propoxyphene and Aspirin *on page 742*

Biamine® *see* Thiamine Hydrochloride *on page 837*

Biavax® II *see* Rubella and Mumps Vaccines, Combined *on page 775*

Biaxin™ Filmtabs® *see* Clarithromycin *on page 212*

Bicalutamide (bye ka loo' ta mide)
Brand Names Casodex®

Therapeutic Category Androgen; Antineoplastic Agent, Hormone

Use Combination therapy with a luteinizing hormone-releasing hormone (LHRH) analog for the treatment of advanced prostate cancer

Usual Dosage Adults: Oral: 1 tablet once daily (morning or evening), with or without food. It is recommended that bicalutamide be taken at the same time each day; start treatment with bicalutamide at the same time as treatment with an LHRH analog.

Local Anesthetic/Vasoconstrictor Precautions No information available to require special precautions

Effects on Dental Treatment No effects or complications reported

Drug Uptake
Absorption: Rapid and complete
Serum half-life: Active enantiomer is 5.8 days

Bicillin® C-R 900/300 Injection *see* Penicillin G Benzathine and Procaine Combined *on page 665*

Bicillin® C-R Injection *see* Penicillin G Benzathine and Procaine Combined *on page 665*

Bicillin® L-A *see* Penicillin G Benzathine, Parenteral *on page 665*

BiCNU® *see* Carmustine *on page 157*

Biltricide® *see* Praziquantel *on page 716*

Biocal® [OTC] *see* Calcium Carbonate *on page 140*

Bioclate® *see* Antihemophilic Factor (Recombinant) *on page 70*

Bion® Tears Solution [OTC] *see* Artificial Tears *on page 75*

Biperiden (bye per' i den)
Brand Names Akineton®

Therapeutic Category Anti-Parkinson's Agent

Use Treatment of all forms of Parkinsonism including drug induced type (extrapyramidal symptoms)

Local Anesthetic/Vasoconstrictor Precautions No information available to require special precautions

Effects on Dental Treatment Dry mouth, nose and throat very prevalent in patients taking this drug

Other Adverse Effects
>10%:
Gastrointestinal: Constipation
Miscellaneous: Decreased sweating; dry mouth, nose, throat, or skin
1% to 10%:
Endocrine & metabolic: Decreased flow of breast milk
Gastrointestinal: Difficulty in swallowing
Ocular: Increased sensitivity to light
<1%:
Cardiovascular: Orthostatic hypotension, ventricular fibrillation, tachycardia, palpitations, ataxia
Central nervous system: Confusion, drowsiness, headache, loss of memory, tiredness
Dermatologic: Skin rash
Gastrointestinal: Bloated feeling, nausea, vomiting
Genitourinary: Difficult urination
Neuromuscular & skeletal: Weakness
Ocular: Increased intraocular pain, blurred vision

Bisac-Evac® [OTC] *see* Bisacodyl *on this page*

Bisacodilo (Mexico) *see* Bisacodyl *on this page*

Bisacodyl (bis a koe' dil)
Brand Names Bisac-Evac® [OTC]; Bisacodyl Uniserts®; Bisco-Lax® [OTC]; Carter's Little Pills® [OTC]; Clysodrast®; Dacodyl® [OTC]; Deficol® [OTC]; Dulcolax® [OTC]; Fleet® Laxative [OTC]; Theralax® [OTC]
(Continued)

Bisacodyl *(Continued)*

Canadian/Mexican Brand Names Apo-Bisacodyl® (Canada); PMS-Bisacodyl® (Canada); Dulcolan® (Mexico)

Therapeutic Category Laxative, Stimulant

Synonyms Bisacodilo (Mexico)

Use Treatment of constipation; colonic evacuation prior to procedures or examination

Usual Dosage

Children:

Oral: >6 years: 5-10 mg (0.3 mg/kg) at bedtime or before breakfast

Rectal suppository:

<2 years: 5 mg as a single dose

>2 years: 10 mg

Adults:

Oral: 5-15 mg as single dose (up to 30 mg when complete evacuation of bowel is required)

Rectal suppository: 10 mg as single dose

Tannex:

Enema: 2.5 g in 1000 mL warm water

Barium enema: 2.5-5 g in 1000 mL barium suspension

Do not give >10 g within 72-hour period

Mechanism of Action Stimulates peristalsis by directly irritating the smooth muscle of the intestine, possibly the colonic intramural plexus; alters water and electrolyte secretion producing net intestinal fluid accumulation and laxation

Local Anesthetic/Vasoconstrictor Precautions No information available to require special precautions

Effects on Dental Treatment No effects or complications reported

Other Adverse Effects <1%:

Central nervous system: Vertigo

Endocrine & metabolic: Electrolyte and fluid imbalance (metabolic acidosis or alkalosis, hypocalcemia)

Gastrointestinal: Mild abdominal cramps, nausea, vomiting, rectal burning

Drug Interactions Decreased effect: Milk, antacids; decreased effect of warfarin

Drug Uptake

Onset of action:

Oral: 6-10 hours

Rectal: 0.25-1 hour

Absorption: Oral, rectal: <5% absorbed systemically

Pregnancy Risk Factor C

Bisacodyl Uniserts® *see Bisacodyl on previous page*

Bisco-Lax® [OTC] *see Bisacodyl on previous page*

Bismatrol® (subsalicylate) [OTC] *see Bismuth on this page*

Bismuth *(biz' muth)*

Brand Names Bismatrol® (subsalicylate) [OTC]; Devrom® (subgallate) [OTC]; Pepto-Bismol® (subsalicylate) [OTC]; Pink Bismuth® (subsalicylate) [OTC]

Therapeutic Category Antidiarrheal

Synonyms Bismuth Subgallate; Bismuth Subsalicylate

Use Symptomatic treatment of mild, nonspecific diarrhea; indigestion, nausea, control of traveler's diarrhea (enterotoxigenic *Escherichia coli*); as an adjunct in the treatment of *Helicobacter pylori*-associated peptic ulcer disease

Usual Dosage Oral:

Nonspecific diarrhea: Subsalicylate:

Children: Up to 8 doses/24 hours:

3-6 years: $1/3$ tablet or 5 mL every 30 minutes to 1 hour as needed

6-9 years: $2/3$ tablet or 10 mL every 30 minutes to 1 hour as needed

9-12 years: 1 tablet or 15 mL every 30 minutes to 1 hour as needed

Adults: 2 tablets or 30 mL every 30 minutes to 1 hour as needed up to 8 doses/24 hours

Prevention of traveler's diarrhea: 2.1 g/day or 2 tablets 4 times/day before meals and at bedtime

Subgallate: 1-2 tablets 3 times/day with meals

Mechanism of Action Bismuth subsalicylate exhibits both antisecretory and antimicrobial action. This agent may provide some anti-inflammatory action as well. The salicylate moiety provides antisecretory effect and the bismuth exhibits antimicrobial directly against bacterial and viral gastrointestinal pathogens. Bismuth has some antacid properties.

Local Anesthetic/Vasoconstrictor Precautions No information available to require special precautions

Effects on Dental Treatment No effects or complications reported

Other Adverse Effects

>10%: Discoloration of the tongue (darkening), grayish black stools

<1%:

Central nervous system: Anxiety, confusion, slurred speech, headache, mental depression, weakness

Gastrointestinal: Impaction may occur in infants and debilitated patients

Neuromuscular & skeletal: Muscle spasms

Otic: Loss of hearing, buzzing in ears

Drug Interactions

Decreased effect: Tetracyclines and uricosurics

Increased toxicity: Aspirin, warfarin, hypoglycemics

Drug Uptake

Absorption: Minimally absorbed across the GI tract while the salt (eg, salicylate) may be readily absorbed

Pregnancy Risk Factor C (D in third trimester)

Bismuth Subgallate *see* Bismuth *on previous page*

Bismuth Subsalicylate *see* Bismuth *on previous page*

Bisoprolol and Hydrochlorothiazide

(bis oh' proe lol & hye droe klor oh thye' a zide)

Brand Names Ziac™

Therapeutic Category Antihypertensive Agent, Combination; Beta-Adrenergic Blocker; Diuretic, Thiazide Type

Use Treatment of hypertension

Local Anesthetic/Vasoconstrictor Precautions No information available to require special precautions

Effects on Dental Treatment Non-cardioselective beta-blockers (ie, propranolol, nadolol) enhance the pressor response to epinephrine, resulting in hypertension and bradycardia. This has not been reported for bisoprolol, a cardioselective beta-blocker. Therefore local anesthetic with vasoconstrictor can be safely used in patients medicated with bisoprolol. Many nonsteroidal anti-inflammatory drugs such as ibuprofen and indomethacin can reduce the hypotensive effect of beta-blockers after 3 or more weeks of therapy with the NSAID. Short-term NSAID use (ie, 3 days) requires no special precautions in patients taking beta-blockers.

Other Adverse Effects

>10%: Central nervous system: Fatigue

1% to 10%:

Cardiovascular: Chest pain, edema, bradycardia, hypotension

Central nervous system: Headache, dizziness, depression, abnormal dreams

Dermatologic: Rash

Endocrine & metabolic: Hypokalemia, fluid and electrolyte imbalances (hypocalcemia, hypomagnesemia, hyponatremia), hyperglycemia

Gastrointestinal: Constipation, diarrhea, dyspepsia, nausea, dyspnea, insomnia, flatulence

Genitourinary: Micturition (frequency)

Hematologic: Rarely blood dyscrasias

Neuromuscular & skeletal: Arthralgia, myalgia

Ocular: Abnormal vision, photosensitivity

Renal: Prerenal azotemia

Respiratory: Rhinitis, cough

Bisoprolol Fumarate (bis oh' proe lol fyoo' ma rate)

Related Information

Cardiovascular Diseases *on page 912*

Brand Names Zebeta®

Therapeutic Category Antianginal Agent; Beta-Adrenergic Blocker, Cardioselective

Use Treatment of hypertension, alone or in combination with other agents

Unlabeled use: Angina pectoris, supraventricular arrhythmias, PVCs

Usual Dosage Oral:

Adults: 5 mg once daily, may be increased to 10 mg, and then up to 20 mg once daily, if necessary

Elderly: Initial dose: 2.5 mg/day; may be increased by 2.5-5 mg/day; maximum recommended dose: 20 mg/day

(Continued)

Bisoprolol Fumarate *(Continued)*

Mechanism of Action Selective inhibitor of beta$_1$-adrenergic receptors; competitively blocks beta$_1$-receptors, with little or no effect on beta$_2$-receptors at doses <10 mg

Local Anesthetic/Vasoconstrictor Precautions No information available to require special precautions

Effects on Dental Treatment Non-cardioselective beta-blockers (ie, propranolol, nadolol) enhance the pressor response to epinephrine, resulting in hypertension and bradycardia. This has not been reported for bisoprolol, a cardioselective beta-blocker. Therefore local anesthetic with vasoconstrictor can be safely used in patients medicated with bisoprolol. Many nonsteroidal anti-inflammatory drugs such as ibuprofen and indomethacin can reduce the hypotensive effect of beta-blockers after 3 or more weeks of therapy with the NSAID. Short-term NSAID use (ie, 3 days) requires no special precautions in patients taking beta-blockers.

Other Adverse Effects
>10%: Central nervous system: Fatigue, lethargy
1% to 10%:
Cardiovascular: Hypotension, chest pain, heart failure, Raynaud's phenomena, heart block, edema, bradycardia
Central nervous system: Headache, dizziness, insomnia, confusion, depression, abnormal dreams
Dermatologic: Rash
Gastrointestinal: Constipation, diarrhea, dyspepsia, nausea, flatulence, anorexia
Genitourinary: Micturition (frequency), impotence, urinary retention
Neuromuscular & skeletal: Arthralgia, myalgia
Ocular: Abnormal vision
Respiratory: Dyspnea, rhinitis, cough

Drug Interactions
Decreased effects of beta-blockers:
Barbiturates (increased liver metabolism of beta-blockers to result in lower serum levels)
NSAIDs (attenuate the hypotensive therapeutic effects of beta-blockers)
Rifampin (increased liver metabolism of beta-blockers to result in lower serum levels)
Increased effects of beta-blockers:
Calcium channel blockers (increase serum levels by unknown mechanism to enhance hypotension)
Beta-blockers increase the effects of:
Epinephrine (vasoconstrictor; initial hypertensive episode followed by bradycardia)
Phenylephrine (Neosynephrine®; enhanced pressor response)
Theophylline (inhibit theophylline metabolism causing increase in serum concentrations)

Drug Uptake
Absorption: Rapid and almost complete from GI tract
Serum half-life: 9-12 hours
Time to peak: 1.7-3 hours

Pregnancy Risk Factor C

Selected Readings
Foster CA and Aston SJ, "Propranolol-Epinephrine Interaction: A Potential Disaster," *Plast Reconstr Surg*, 1983, 72(1):74-8.
Wong DG, Spence JD, Lamki L, et al, "Effect of Nonsteroidal Anti-Inflammatory Drugs on Control of Hypertension of Beta-Blockers and Diuretics," *Lancet*, 1986, 1(8488):997-1001.
Wynn RL, "Dental Nonsteroidal Anti-Inflammatory Drugs and Prostaglandin-Based Drug Interactions, Part Two," *Gen Dent*, 1992, 40(2):104, 106, 108.
Wynn RL, "Epinephrine Interactions With Beta-Blockers," *Gen Dent*, 1994, 42(1):16, 18.

Bistropamide *see* Tropicamide *on page 881*

Bitolterol Mesylate *(bye tole′ ter ole mes′ i late)*

Related Information
Respiratory Diseases *on page 924*

Brand Names Tornalate®

Therapeutic Category Antiasthmatic; Beta-2-Adrenergic Agonist Agent; Bronchodilator

Use Prevention and treatment of bronchial asthma and bronchospasm

Usual Dosage Children >12 years and Adults:
Bronchospasm: 2 inhalations at an interval of at least 1-3 minutes, followed by a third inhalation if needed

Prevention of bronchospasm: 2 inhalations every 8 hours; do not exceed 3 inhalations every 6 hours or 2 inhalations every 4 hours

Mechanism of Action Selectively stimulates beta$_2$-adrenergic receptors in the lungs producing bronchial smooth muscle relaxation; minor beta$_1$ activity

Local Anesthetic/Vasoconstrictor Precautions No information available to require special precautions

Effects on Dental Treatment No effects or complications reported

Other Adverse Effects

>10%: Neuromuscular & skeletal: Trembling

1% to 10%:

Cardiovascular: Flushing of face, hypertension, pounding heartbeat

Central nervous system: Dizziness, lightheadedness, nervousness

Gastrointestinal: Dry mouth, nausea, unpleasant taste

Respiratory: Bronchial irritation, coughing

<1%:

Cardiovascular: Chest pain, arrhythmias, tachycardia

Central nervous system: Insomnia

Respiratory: Paradoxical bronchospasm

Drug Interactions Increased toxicity: Cardiovascular effects are potentiated in patients also receiving MAO inhibitors, tricyclic antidepressants, sympathomimetic agents (eg, amphetamine, dopamine, dobutamine), inhaled anesthetics (eg, enflurane)

Drug Uptake

Duration: 4-8 hours

Serum half-life: 3 hours

Time to peak serum concentration (colterol): Inhalation: Within 1 hour

Pregnancy Risk Factor C

Black Draught® [OTC] *see* Senna *on page 785*

Blanex® *see* Chlorzoxazone *on page 200*

BlemErase® [OTC] *see* Benzoyl Peroxide *on page 104*

Blenoxane® *see* Bleomycin Sulfate *on this page*

Bleomycin Sulfate (blee oh mye' sin sul' fate)

Brand Names Blenoxane®

Canadian/Mexican Brand Names Bleolem (Mexico)

Therapeutic Category Antineoplastic Agent, Antibiotic

Synonyms BLM; NIM

Use Palliative treatment of squamous cell carcinoma, testicular carcinoma, germ cell tumors, and the following lymphomas: Hodgkin's, lymphosarcoma and reticulum cell sarcoma; sclerosing agent to control malignant effusions

Usual Dosage Refer to individual protocols; 1 unit = 1 mg

May be administered I.M., I.V., S.C., or intra-cavitary

Children and Adults:

Test dose for lymphoma patients: I.M., I.V., S.C.: 1-5 units of bleomycin before the first dose; monitor vital signs every 15 minutes; wait a minimum of 1 hour before administering remainder of dose

Single agent therapy:

I.M./I.V./S.C.: Squamous cell carcinoma, lymphosarcoma, reticulum cell sarcoma, testicular carcinoma: 0.25-0.5 units/kg (10-20 units/m^2) 1-2 times/week

Continuous intravenous infusion: 15 units/m^2 over 24 hours daily for 4 days

Combination agent therapy:

I.M./I.V.: 3-4 units/m^2

I.V.: ABVD: 10 units/m^2 on days 1 and 15

Maximum cumulative lifetime dose: 400 units

Mechanism of Action Inhibits synthesis of DNA; binds to DNA leading to single- and double-strand breaks; isolated from *Streptomyces verticillus*

Local Anesthetic/Vasoconstrictor Precautions No information available to require special precautions

Effects on Dental Treatment No effects or complications reported

Other Adverse Effects

>10%:

Cardiovascular: Raynaud's phenomenon

Central nervous system: Fever, chills

Dermatologic: Pruritic erythema

Gastrointestinal: **Emetic potential: Moderately low (10% to 30%);** stomatitis, nausea, vomiting, anorexia, weight loss

Integument: Approximately 50% of patients will develop erythema, induration, hyperkeratosis, and peeling of the skin. Hyperpigmentation, alopecia,

(Continued)

117

Bleomycin Sulfate *(Continued)*

nailbed changes may occur; this appears to be dose-related and is reversible after cessation of therapy.

Local: Pain at tumor site, phlebitis

Miscellaneous: Mild febrile reaction, mucocutaneous toxicity, patients may become febrile after intracavitary administration

1% to 10%:

Idiosyncratic: Similar to anaphylaxis and occurs in 1% of lymphoma patients; may include hypotension, confusion, fever, chills, and wheezing. May be immediate or delayed for several hours; symptomatic treatment includes volume expansion, pressor agents, antihistamines, and steroids.

<1%:

Cardiovascular: Myocardial infarction, cerebrovascular accident

Dermatologic: Skin thickening

Hepatic: Hepatotoxicity

Renal: Renal toxicity

Respiratory: Tachypnea, rales; dose-related when total dose is >400 units or with single doses >30 units. Pathogenesis is poorly understood, but may be related to damage of pulmonary, vascular, or connective tissue. Manifested as an acute or chronic interstitial pneumonitis with interstitial fibrosis, hypoxia, and death. Symptoms include cough, dyspnea, and bilateral pulmonary infiltrates noted on CXR. It is controversial whether steroids improve symptoms of bleomycin pulmonary toxicity.

Drug Uptake

Absorption: I.M. and intrapleural administration produces serum concentrations of 30% of I.V. administration; intraperitoneal and S.C. routes produce serum concentrations equal to those of I.V.

Serum half-life (biphasic): Dependent upon renal function:

Normal renal function:

Initial: 1.3 hours

Terminal: 9 hours

End stage renal disease:

Initial: 2 hours

Terminal: 30 hours

Time to peak serum concentration: I.M.: Within 30 minutes

Pregnancy Risk Factor D

Bleph®-10 *see* Sodium Sulfacetamide *on page 793*

Blephamide® *see* Sodium Sulfacetamide and Prednisolone Acetate *on page 794*

BLM *see* Bleomycin Sulfate *on previous page*

Blocadren® Oral *see* Timolol Maleate *on page 847*

Bluboro® [OTC] *see* Aluminum Sulfate and Calcium Acetate *on page 41*

Blue® [OTC] *see* Pyrethrins *on page 753*

Bonine® [OTC] *see* Meclizine Hydrochloride *on page 530*

Boric Acid *(bor' ik as' id)*

Brand Names Borofax® Topical [OTC]; Dri-Ear® Otic [OTC]; Swim-Ear® Otic [OTC]

Therapeutic Category Pharmaceutical Aid

Use

Ophthalmic: Mild antiseptic used for inflamed eyelids

Otic: Prophylaxis of swimmer's ear

Topical ointment: Temporary relief of chapped, chafed, or dry skin, diaper rash, abrasions, minor burns, sunburn, insect bites, and other skin irritations

Local Anesthetic/Vasoconstrictor Precautions No information available to require special precautions

Effects on Dental Treatment No effects or complications reported

Comments Not a corrosive substance

Borofax® Topical [OTC] *see* Boric Acid *on this page*

Boropak® [OTC] *see* Aluminum Sulfate and Calcium Acetate *on page 41*

B&O Supprettes® *see* Belladonna and Opium *on page 98*

Botox® *see* Botulinum Toxin Type A *on this page*

Botulinum Toxin Type A *(bot' yoo lin num tok' sin type aye)*

Brand Names Botox®

Therapeutic Category Ophthalmic Agent, Toxin

Use

Treatment of strabismus and blepharospasm associated with dystonia (including benign essential blepharospasm or VII nerve disorders in patients ≥12 years of age)

Unlabeled uses: Treatment of hemifacial spasms, spasmodic torticollis (ie, cervical dystonia, clonic twisting of the head), oromandibular dystonia, spasmodic dysphonia (laryngeal dystonia) and other dystonias (ie, writer's cramp, focal task-specific dystonias)

Orphan drug: Treatment of dynamic muscle contracture in pediatric cerebral palsy patients

Usual Dosage

Strabismus: 1.25-5 units (0.05-0.15 mL) injected into any one muscle

Subsequent doses for residual/recurrent strabismus: Re-examine patients 7-14 days after each injection to assess the effect of that dose. Subsequent doses for patients experiencing incomplete paralysis of the target may be increased up to two fold the previously administered dose. Maximum recommended dose as a single injection for any one muscle is 25 units.

Blepharospasm: 1.25-2.5 units (0.05-0.10 mL) injected into the orbicularis oculi muscle

Subsequent doses: Each treatment lasts approximately 3 months. At repeat treatment sessions, the dose may be increased up to twofold if the response from the initial treatment is considered insufficient (usually defined as an effect that does not last >2 months). There appears to be little benefit obtainable from injecting >5 units per site. Some tolerance may be found if treatments are given any more frequently than every 3 months. The cumulative dose should not exceed 200 units in a 30-day period

Mechanism of Action Botulinum A toxin is a neurotoxin produced by *Clostridium botulinum*, spore-forming anaerobic bacillus, which appears to affect only the presynaptic membrane of the neuromuscular junction in humans, where it prevents calcium-dependent release of acetylcholine and produces a state of denervation. Muscle inactivation persists until new fibrils grow from the nerve and form junction plates on new areas of the muscle-cell walls. The antagonist muscle shortens simultaneously ("contracture"), taking up the slack created by agonist paralysis; following several weeks of paralysis, alignment of the eye is measurably changed, despite return of innervation to the injected muscle.

Local Anesthetic/Vasoconstrictor Precautions No information available to require special precautions

Effects on Dental Treatment No effects or complications reported

Other Adverse Effects

>10%: Ocular: Dry eyes, lagophthalmos, ptosis, photophobia, vertical deviation

1% to 10%:
Dermatologic: Diffuse skin rash
Ocular: Swelling of eyelid, blepharospasm

<1%: Ocular: Ectropion, keratitis, diplopia, entropion

Drug Interactions Increased effect: Botulinum toxin may be potentiated by aminoglycosides

Drug Uptake

Strabismus:
Onset of action: 1-2 days after injection
Duration of paralysis: 2-6 weeks

Blepharospasm:
Onset: 3 days after injection
Peak: 1-2 weeks
Duration of paralysis: 3 months

Pregnancy Risk Factor C

BQ® Tablet [OTC] *see* Chlorpheniramine, Phenylpropanolamine, and Acetaminophen *on page 194*

Breonesin® [OTC] *see* Guaifenesin *on page 407*

Brethaire® *see* Terbutaline Sulfate *on page 822*

Brethine® *see* Terbutaline Sulfate *on page 822*

Bretylium Tosylate (bre til' ee um toe' si late)

Related Information

Cardiovascular Diseases *on page 912*

Brand Names Bretylol®

Canadian/Mexican Brand Names Bretylate® (Canada)

(Continued)

Bretylium Tosylate *(Continued)*

Therapeutic Category Antiarrhythmic Agent, Class III; Antiarrhythmic Agent (Supraventricular & Ventricular)

Use Treatment of ventricular tachycardia and fibrillation; used in the treatment of other serious ventricular arrhythmias resistant to lidocaine

Usual Dosage (**Note**: Patients should undergo defibrillation/cardioversion before and after bretylium doses as necessary)

Children:
I.M.: 2-5 mg/kg as a single dose
I.V.: Initial: 5 mg/kg, then attempt electrical defibrillation; repeat with 10 mg/kg if ventricular fibrillation persists at 15-minute intervals to maximum total of 30 mg/kg
Maintenance dose: I.M., I.V.: 5 mg/kg every 6-8 hours

Adults:
Immediate life-threatening ventricular arrhythmias, ventricular fibrillation, unstable ventricular tachycardia: Initial dose: I.V.: 5 mg/kg (undiluted) over 1 minute; if arrhythmia persists, give 10 mg/kg (undiluted) over 1 minute and repeat as necessary (usually at 15- to 30-minute intervals) up to a total dose of 30-35 mg/kg
Other life-threatening ventricular arrhythmias:
Initial dose: I.M., I.V.: 5-10 mg/kg, may repeat every 1-2 hours if arrhythmia persist; give I.V. dose (diluted) over 8-10 minutes
Maintenance dose: I.M.: 5-10 mg/kg every 6-8 hours; I.V. (diluted): 5-10 mg/kg every 6 hours; I.V. infusion (diluted): 1-2 mg/minute (little experience with doses >40 mg/kg/day)
2 g/250 mL D_5W (infusion pump should be used for I.V. infusion administration)
Rate of I.V. infusion: 1-4 mg/minute
1 mg/minute = 7 mL/hour
2 mg/minute = 15 mL/hour
3 mg/minute = 22 mL/hour
4 mg/minute = 30 mL/hour

Mechanism of Action Class II antiarrhythmic; after an initial release of norepinephrine at the peripheral adrenergic nerve terminals, inhibits further release by postganglionic nerve endings in response to sympathetic nerve stimulation

Local Anesthetic/Vasoconstrictor Precautions No information available to require special precautions

Effects on Dental Treatment No effects or complications reported

Other Adverse Effects
>10%: Cardiovascular: Hypotension (both postural and supine)
1% to 10%: Gastrointestinal: Nausea, vomiting
<1%:
Cardiovascular: Transient initial hypertension, increase in PVCs, bradycardia, angina, flushing, syncope
Central nervous system: Vertigo, confusion, hyperthermia
Dermatologic: Rash
Gastrointestinal: Diarrhea, abdominal pain
Neuromuscular & skeletal: Muscle atrophy and necrosis with repeated I.M. injections at same site
Ocular: Conjunctivitis
Renal: Renal impairment
Respiratory: Respiratory depression, nasal congestion
Miscellaneous: Hiccups

Drug Interactions
Increased toxicity: Other antiarrhythmic agents
Additive toxicity or effect by bretylium, pressor catecholamines, digitalis

Drug Uptake
Onset of antiarrhythmic effect:
I.M.: May require 2 hours
I.V.: Within 6-20 minutes
Peak effect: 6-9 hours
Duration: 6-24 hours
Serum half-life: 7-11 hours; average: 4-17 hours

Pregnancy Risk Factor C

Bretylol® *see* Bretylium Tosylate *on previous page*

Brevicon® *see* Ethinyl Estradiol and Norethindrone *on page 339*

Brevital® Sodium *see* Methohexital Sodium *on page 559*

Bricanyl® *see* Terbutaline Sulfate *on page 822*

Brimonidine Tartrate (bri moe' ni deen tar' trate)

Brand Names Alphagan®

Therapeutic Category Alpha-2-Adrenergic Agonist Agent, Ophthalmic

Use Lowering of intraocular pressure in patients with open-angle glaucoma or ocular hypertension

Usual Dosage Ophthalmic: Adults: One drop in affected eye(s) three times daily (approximately every 8 hours)

Local Anesthetic/Vasoconstrictor Precautions No information available to require special precautions

Effects on Dental Treatment No effects or complications reported

Drug Interactions MAO inhibitors may cause an exaggerated adrenergic response if taken concurrently or within 21 days of discontinuing MAO inhibitor

Brofed® Elixir [OTC] *see* Brompheniramine and Pseudoephedrine *on page 123*

Bromaline® Elixir [OTC] *see* Brompheniramine and Phenylpropanolamine *on page 123*

Bromanate® DC *see* Brompheniramine, Phenylpropanolamine, and Codeine *on page 125*

Bromanate® Elixir [OTC] *see* Brompheniramine and Phenylpropanolamine *on page 123*

Bromanyl® Cough Syrup *see* Bromodiphenhydramine and Codeine *on next page*

Bromarest® [OTC] *see* Brompheniramine Maleate *on page 124*

Bromatapp® [OTC] *see* Brompheniramine and Phenylpropanolamine *on page 123*

Brombay® [OTC] *see* Brompheniramine Maleate *on page 124*

Bromfed® Syrup [OTC] *see* Brompheniramine and Pseudoephedrine *on page 123*

Bromfed® Tablet [OTC] *see* Brompheniramine and Pseudoephedrine *on page 123*

Bromocriptina (Mexico) *see* Bromocriptine Mesylate *on this page*

Bromocriptine Mesylate (broe moe krip' teen mes' i late)

Brand Names Parlodel®

Canadian/Mexican Brand Names Apo® Bromocriptine (Canada); Cryocriptina® (Mexico); Serocryptin® (Mexico)

Therapeutic Category Anti-Parkinson's Agent; Ergot Alkaloid and Derivative

Synonyms Bromocriptina (Mexico)

Use Usually used with levodopa or levodopa/carbidopa to treat Parkinson's disease - treatment of parkinsonism in patients unresponsive or allergic to levodopa

Prolactin-secreting pituitary adenomas, acromegaly, amenorrhea/galactorrhea secondary to hyperprolactinemia in the absence of primary tumor

The indication for prevention of postpartum lactation has been withdrawn voluntarily by Sandoz Pharmaceuticals Corporation

Usual Dosage Adults: Oral:

Parkinsonism: 1.25 mg 2 times/day, increased by 2.5 mg/day in 2- to 4-week intervals (usual dose range is 30-90 mg/day in 3 divided doses), though elderly patients can usually be managed on lower doses

Hyperprolactinemia: 2.5 mg 2-3 times/day

Acromegaly: Initial: 1.25-2.5 mg increasing as necessary every 3-7 days; usual dose: 20-30 mg/day

Mechanism of Action Semisynthetic ergot alkaloid derivative with dopaminergic properties; inhibits prolactin secretion and can improve symptoms of Parkinson's disease by directly stimulating dopamine receptors in the corpus stratum

Local Anesthetic/Vasoconstrictor Precautions No information available to require special precautions

Effects on Dental Treatment No effects or complications reported

Other Adverse Effects Incidence of adverse effects is high, especially at beginning of treatment and with dosages >20 mg/day

1% to 10%:

Cardiovascular: Hypotension

Central nervous system: Mental depression, stuffy nose, confusion, hallucinations

Gastrointestinal: Nausea, constipation, anorexia

Miscellaneous: Raynaud's phenomenon, leg cramps

<1%:

Cardiovascular: Hypertension, myocardial infarction, syncope

(Continued)

Bromocriptine Mesylate *(Continued)*

Central nervous system: Dizziness, drowsiness, fatigue, insomnia, headache, seizures

Gastrointestinal: Vomiting, abdominal cramps

Drug Interactions

Decreased effect: Amitriptyline, butyrophenones, imipramine, methyldopa, phenothiazines, reserpine, may decrease bromocriptine's efficacy at reducing prolactin

Increased toxicity: Ergot alkaloids (increased cardiovascular toxicity)

Drug Uptake

Serum half-life (biphasic):

Initial: 6-8 hours

Terminal: 50 hours

Time to peak serum concentration: Oral: Within 1-2 hours

Pregnancy Risk Factor C (See Contraindications)

Bromodiphenhydramine and Codeine

(brome oh dye fen hye' dra meen & koe' deen)

Brand Names Ambenyl® Cough Syrup; Amgenal® Cough Syrup; Bromanyl® Cough Syrup; Bromotuss® w/Codeine Cough Syrup

Therapeutic Category Antihistamine; Cough Preparation

Synonyms Codeine and Bromodiphenhydramine

Use Relief of upper respiratory symptoms and cough associated with allergies or common cold

Local Anesthetic/Vasoconstrictor Precautions No information available to require special precautions

Effects on Dental Treatment

Bromodiphenhydramine: 1% to 10%: Dry mouth

Codeine: <1%: Dry mouth

Bromofeniramina Maleato De (Mexico) *see* Brompheniramine Maleate *on page 124*

Bromotuss® w/Codeine Cough Syrup *see* Bromodiphenhydramine and Codeine *on this page*

Bromphen® [OTC] *see* Brompheniramine Maleate *on page 124*

Bromphen® DC w/Codeine *see* Brompheniramine, Phenylpropanolamine, and Codeine *on page 125*

Brompheniramine and Phenylephrine

(brome fen ir' a meen & fen il ef' rin)

Brand Names Dimetane® Decongestant Elixir [OTC]

Therapeutic Category Antihistamine/Decongestant Combination

Use Temporary relief of symptoms of seasonal and perennial allergic rhinitis, and vasomotor rhinitis, including nasal obstruction

Local Anesthetic/Vasoconstrictor Precautions

Brompheniramine: No information available to require special precautions

Phenylephrine: Use with caution since phenylephrine is a sympathomimetic amine which could interact with epinephrine to cause a pressor response

Effects on Dental Treatment

Brompheniramine: Prolonged use may decrease salivary flow

Phenylephrine: Up to 10% of patients could experience tachycardia, palpitations, and dry mouth; use vasoconstrictor with caution

Other Adverse Effects

>10%:

Cardiovascular: Tachycardia

Central nervous system: Slight to moderate drowsiness, nervousness, transient stimulation, insomnia

Respiratory: Thickening of bronchial secretions

1% to 10%:

Central nervous system: Headache, fatigue, nervousness, dizziness, headache

Gastrointestinal: Appetite increase, weight increase, nausea, diarrhea, abdominal pain, dry mouth

Genitourinary: Difficult urination, dysuria

Neuromuscular & skeletal: Arthralgia, weakness

Respiratory: Pharyngitis

Miscellaneous: Diaphoresis

<1%:

Cardiovascular: Edema, palpitations, hypotension

Central nervous system: Depression, sedation, dizziness, paradoxical excitement, fatigue, insomnia, convulsions, hallucinations

Dermatologic: Angioedema, rash
Genitourinary: Urinary retention
Hepatic: Hepatitis
Neuromuscular & skeletal: Myalgia paresthesia, tremor
Ocular: Photosensitivity, blurred vision
Respiratory: Bronchospasm, epistaxis, shortness of breath, troubled breathing

Brompheniramine and Phenylpropanolamine
(brome fen ir' a meen & fen il proe pa nole' a meen)

Brand Names Bromaline® Elixir [OTC]; Bromanate® Elixir [OTC]; Bromatapp® [OTC]; Bromphen® Tablet [OTC]; Cold & Allergy® Elixir [OTC]; Dimaphen® Elixir [OTC]; Dimaphen® Tablets [OTC]; Dimetapp® 4-Hour Liqui-Gel Capsule [OTC]; Dimetapp® Elixir [OTC]; Dimetapp® Tablet [OTC]; Dimetapp® Extentabs® [OTC]; Genatap® Elixir [OTC]; Myphetapp® [OTC]; Tamine® [OTC]; Vicks® DayQuil® Allergy Relief 4 Hour Tablet [OTC]

Therapeutic Category Antihistamine/Decongestant Combination

Synonyms Phenylpropanolamine and Brompheniramine

Use Temporary relief of nasal congestion, running nose, sneezing, and itchy, watery eyes

Local Anesthetic/Vasoconstrictor Precautions
Brompheniramine: No information available to require special precautions
Phenylpropanolamine: Use with caution since phenylpropanolamine is a sympathomimetic amine which could interact with epinephrine to cause a pressor response

Effects on Dental Treatment
Brompheniramine: Prolonged use may decrease salivary flow
Phenylpropanolamine: Up to 10% of patients could experience tachycardia, palpitations, and dry mouth; use vasoconstrictor with caution

Other Adverse Effects
>10%:
Cardiovascular: Tachycardia
Central nervous system: Slight to moderate drowsiness, nervousness, transient stimulation, insomnia
Respiratory: Thickening of bronchial secretions
1% to 10%:
Central nervous system: Headache, fatigue, nervousness, dizziness
Gastrointestinal: Appetite increase, weight increase, nausea, diarrhea, abdominal pain, dry mouth
Genitourinary: Difficult urination, dysuria
Respiratory: Pharyngitis
Neuromuscular & skeletal: Arthralgia, weakness
Miscellaneous: Diaphoresis
<1%:
Central nervous system: Depression, sedation, paradoxical excitement, convulsions, hallucinations
Cardiovascular: Edema, palpitations, hypotension
Dermatologic: Angioedema, rash
Genitourinary: Urinary retention
Hepatic: Hepatitis
Neuromuscular & skeletal: Myalgia, paresthesia, tremor
Ocular: Photosensitivity, blurred vision
Respiratory: Bronchospasm, epistaxis, shortness of breath, troubled breathing

Brompheniramine and Pseudoephedrine
(brome fen ir' a meen & soo doe e fed' rin)

Brand Names Brofed® Elixir [OTC]; Bromfed® Syrup [OTC]; Bromfed® Tablet [OTC]; Drixoral® Syrup [OTC]

Therapeutic Category Antihistamine/Decongestant Combination

Use Temporary relief of symptoms of seasonal and perennial allergic rhinitis, and vasomotor rhinitis, including nasal obstruction

Local Anesthetic/Vasoconstrictor Precautions Use with caution since pseudoephedrine is a sympathomimetic amine which could interact with epinephrine to cause a pressor response

Effects on Dental Treatment
Brompheniramine: Prolonged use may decrease salivary flow
Pseudoephedrine: Up to 10% of patients could experience tachycardia, palpitations, and dry mouth; use vasoconstrictor with caution
(Continued)

Brompheniramine and Pseudoephedrine *(Continued)*

Other Adverse Effects
>10%:
Cardiovascular: Tachycardia
Central nervous system: Slight to moderate drowsiness, nervousness, transient stimulation, insomnia
Respiratory: Thickening of bronchial secretions
1% to 10%:
Central nervous system: Headache, fatigue, nervousness, dizziness
Gastrointestinal: Appetite increase, weight increase, nausea, diarrhea, abdominal pain, dry mouth
Genitourinary: Difficult urination, dysuria
Respiratory: Pharyngitis
Neuromuscular & skeletal: Arthralgia, weakness
Miscellaneous: Diaphoresis
<1%:
Central nervous system: Depression, sedation, paradoxical excitement, convulsions, hallucinations
Cardiovascular: Edema, palpitations, hypotension
Dermatologic: Angioedema, rash
Genitourinary: Urinary retention
Hepatic: Hepatitis
Neuromuscular & skeletal: Myalgia, paresthesia, tremor
Ocular: Photosensitivity, blurred vision
Respiratory: Bronchospasm, epistaxis, shortness of breath, troubled breathing

Brompheniramine Maleate (brome fen ir' a meen mal' ee ate)

Brand Names Bromarest® [OTC]; Brombay® [OTC]; Bromphen® [OTC]; Brotane® [OTC]; Chlorphed® [OTC]; Codimal-A®; Cophene-B®; Dehist®; Diamine T.D.® [OTC]; Dimetane® [OTC]; Histaject®; Nasahist B®; ND-Stat®; Oraminic® II; Sinusol-B®; Veltane®

Therapeutic Category Antihistamine

Synonyms Bromofeniramina Maleato De (Mexico)

Use Perennial and seasonal allergic rhinitis and other allergic symptoms including urticaria

Usual Dosage
Oral:
Children:
≤6 years: 0.125 mg/kg/dose given every 6 hours; maximum: 6-8 mg/day
6-12 years: 2-4 mg every 6-8 hours; maximum: 12-16 mg/day
Adults: 4 mg every 4-6 hours or 8 mg of sustained release form every 8-12 hours or 12 mg of sustained release every 12 hours; maximum: 24 mg/day
Elderly: Initial: 4 mg once or twice daily. **Note:** Duration of action may be 36 hours or more, even when serum concentrations are low.
I.M., I.V., S.C.:
Children ≤12 years: 0.5 mg/kg/24 hours divided every 6-8 hours
Adults: 10 mg every 6-12 hours, maximum: 40 mg/24 hours

Mechanism of Action Competes with histamine for H_1-receptor sites on effector cells in the gastrointestinal tract, blood vessels, and respiratory tract

Local Anesthetic/Vasoconstrictor Precautions No information available to require special precautions

Effects on Dental Treatment Chronic use of antihistamines will inhibit salivary flow, particularly in elderly patients; this may contribute to periodontal disease and oral discomfort

Other Adverse Effects
>10%:
Central nervous system: Slight to moderate drowsiness (compared with other first generation antihistamines, brompheniramine is relatively nonsedating)
Respiratory: Thickening of bronchial secretions
1% to 10%:
Central nervous system: Headache, fatigue, nervousness, dizziness
Gastrointestinal: Appetite increase, weight increase, nausea, diarrhea, abdominal pain, dry mouth
Neuromuscular & skeletal: Arthralgia
Respiratory: Pharyngitis
<1%:
Cardiovascular: Palpitations
Central nervous system: Depression

Dermatologic: Photosensitivity, rash, angioedema
Hepatic: Hepatitis
Neuromuscular & skeletal: Myalgia, paresthesia
Respiratory: Bronchospasm, epistaxis
Drug Interactions Increased toxicity: CNS depressants, MAO inhibitors, alcohol, tricyclic antidepressants
Drug Uptake
Time to peak serum concentration: Oral: Within 2-5 hours
Duration: Varies with formulation
Serum half-life: 12-34 hours
Pregnancy Risk Factor C

Brompheniramine, Phenylpropanolamine, and Codeine (brome fen ir′ a meen, fen il proe pa nole′ a meen, & koe′ deen)
Brand Names Bromanate® DC; Bromphen® DC w/Codeine; Dimetane®-DC; Myphetane DC®; Poly-Histine CS®
Therapeutic Category Antihistamine/Decongestant Combination; Cough Preparation
Use Relief of coughs and upper respiratory symptoms, including nasal congestion, associated with allergy or the common cold
Local Anesthetic/Vasoconstrictor Precautions
Brompheniramine: No information available to require special precautions
Phenylpropanolamine: Use with caution since phenylpropanolamine is a sympathomimetic amine which could interact with epinephrine to cause a pressor response
Effects on Dental Treatment
Brompheniramine: Prolonged use may decrease salivary flow
Codeine: <1%: Dry mouth
Phenylpropanolamine: Up to 10% of patients could experience tachycardia, palpitations, and dry mouth; use vasoconstrictor with caution

Bromphen® Tablet [OTC] see Brompheniramine and Phenylpropanolamine on page 123

Bronchial® see Theophylline and Guaifenesin on page 836

Bronkephrine® Injection see Ethylnorepinephrine Hydrochloride on page 345

Bronkodyl® see Theophylline/Aminophylline on page 832

Bronkometer® see Isoetharine on page 470

Bronkosol® see Isoetharine on page 470

Brotane® [OTC] see Brompheniramine Maleate on previous page

BSS® Ophthalmic see Balanced Salt Solution on page 96

BTPABA see Bentiromide on page 101

Bucladin®-S Softab® see Buclizine Hydrochloride on this page

Buclizine Hydrochloride (byoo′ kli zeen hye droe klor′ ide)
Brand Names Bucladin®-S Softab®; Vibazine®
Therapeutic Category Antiemetic; Antihistamine
Use Prevention and treatment of motion sickness; symptomatic treatment of vertigo
Usual Dosage Adults: Oral:
Motion sickness (prophylaxis): 50 mg 30 minutes prior to traveling; may repeat 50 mg after 4-6 hours
Vertigo: 50 mg twice daily, up to 150 mg/day
Mechanism of Action Buclizine acts centrally to suppress nausea and vomiting. It is a piperazine antihistamine closely related to cyclizine and meclizine. It also has CNS depressant, anticholinergic, antispasmodic, and local anesthetic effects, and suppresses labyrinthine activity and conduction in vestibular-cerebellar nerve pathways.
Local Anesthetic/Vasoconstrictor Precautions No information available to require special precautions
Effects on Dental Treatment No effects or complications reported
Other Adverse Effects
>10%: Central nervous system: Drowsiness
<1%:
Cardiovascular: Hypotension, palpitations
Central nervous system: Sedation, dizziness, paradoxical excitement, fatigue, insomnia
Gastrointestinal: Nausea, vomiting
Genitourinary: Urinary retention
Neuromuscular & skeletal: Tremor
Ocular: Blurred vision
(Continued)

Buclizine Hydrochloride *(Continued)*

Drug Interactions Increased toxicity: CNS depressants, MAO inhibitors, tricyclic antidepressants
Pregnancy Risk Factor C

Budesonide *(byoo des' oh nide)*
Brand Names Rhinocort™
Canadian/Mexican Brand Names Entocort® (Canada); Pulmicort® (Canada)
Therapeutic Category Anti-inflammatory Agent; Corticosteroid, Inhalant; Glucocorticoid
Use Management of symptoms of seasonal or perennial rhinitis in adults and nonallergic perennial rhinitis in adults
Usual Dosage
Children <6 years: Not recommended
Children ≥6 years and Adults: 256 mcg/day, given as either 2 sprays in each nostril in the morning and evening or as 4 sprays in each nostril in the morning
Local Anesthetic/Vasoconstrictor Precautions No information available to require special precautions
Effects on Dental Treatment Localized infections with *Candida albicans* or *Aspergillus niger* have occurred frequently in the mouth and pharynx with repetitive use of oral inhaler of beclomethasone. Positive cultures for oral *Candida* may be present in up to 75% of patients. These infections may require treatment with appropriate antifungal therapy or discontinuance of treatment with beclomethasone inhaler.
Other Adverse Effects
>10%:
Cardiovascular: Pounding heartbeat, diaphoresis
Central nervous system: Nervousness, headache, dizziness
Dermatologic: Itching, skin rash
Gastrointestinal: GI irritation, bitter taste
Respiratory: Coughing, upper respiratory tract infection, bronchitis, hoarseness
Miscellaneous: Oral candidiasis, increased susceptibility to infections
1% to 10%:
Central nervous system: Insomnia
Dermatologic: Acne, hives
Endocrine & metabolic: Menstrual problems
Gastrointestinal: Anorexia, dry mouth/throat
Ocular: Cataracts
Miscellaneous: Loss of smell/taste, epistaxis, increase in appetite, psychic changes
< 1%:
Gastrointestinal: Abdominal fullness
Respiratory: Bronchospasm, shortness of breath
Drug Interactions No data reported
Pregnancy Risk Factor C

Bufferin® [OTC] *see Aspirin on page 78*
Bumetanida (Mexico) *see Bumetanide on this page*

Bumetanide *(byoo met' a nide)*
Related Information
Cardiovascular Diseases *on page 912*
Brand Names Bumex®
Canadian/Mexican Brand Names Burinex® (Canada); Bumedyl® (Mexico)
Therapeutic Category Diuretic, Loop
Synonyms Bumetanida (Mexico)
Use Management of edema secondary to congestive heart failure or hepatic or renal disease including nephrotic syndrome; may be used alone or in combination with antihypertensives in the treatment of hypertension; can be used in furosemide-allergic patients; (1 mg = 40 mg furosemide)
Usual Dosage
Children:
<6 months: Dose not established
>6 months:
Oral: Initial: 0.015 mg/kg/dose once daily or every other day; maximum dose: 0.1 mg/kg/day
I.M., I.V.: Dose not established

126

Adults:

Oral: 0.5-2 mg/dose 1-2 times/day; maximum: 10 mg/day

I.M., I.V.: 0.5-1 mg/dose; maximum: 10 mg/day

Continuous I.V. infusions of 0.9-1 mg/hour may be more effective than bolus dosing

Mechanism of Action Inhibits reabsorption of sodium and chloride in the ascending loop of Henle and proximal renal tubule, interfering with the chloride-binding cotransport system, thus causing increased excretion of water, sodium, chloride, magnesium, phosphate and calcium; it does not appear to act on the distal tubule

Local Anesthetic/Vasoconstrictor Precautions No information available to require special precautions

Effects on Dental Treatment No effects or complications reported

Other Adverse Effects

>10%:

Endocrine & metabolic: Hyperuricemia, hypochloremia, hypokalemia

Genitourinary: Azotemia

1% to 10%:

Central nervous system: Dizziness, encephalopathy, weakness, headache

Endocrine & metabolic: Hyponatremia

Neuromuscular & skeletal: Muscle cramps

<1%:

Cardiovascular: Hypotension

Dermatologic: Rash, pruritus

Endocrine & metabolic: Hyperglycemia, hyperuricemia

Gastrointestinal: Cramps, nausea, vomiting

Hepatic: Alteration of liver function test results

Otic: Hearing loss

Renal: Increased serum creatinine

Drug Interactions

Additive effect: Other antihypertensive agents

Decreased effect: Indomethacin and other NSAIDs, probenecid

Increased effect: Lithiums' excretion may be decreased

Drug Uptake

Onset of effect:

Oral, I.M.: 0.5-1 hour

I.V.: 2-3 minutes

Duration of action: 6 hours

Serum half-life:

Infants <6 months: Possibly 2.5 hours

Children and Adults: 1-1.5 hours

Pregnancy Risk Factor D

Bumex® *see* Bumetanide *on previous page*

Bupivacaine Hydrochloride (byoo piv' a kane hye droe klor' ide)
Related Information

Oral Pain *on page 940*

Brand Names Marcaine®; Sensorcaine®; Sensorcaine®-MPF

Canadian/Mexican Brand Names Buvacaina® (Mexico)

Therapeutic Category Dental/Local Anesthetics; Local Anesthetic, Injectable

Use Local anesthetic (injectable) for peripheral nerve block, infiltration, sympathetic block, caudal or epidural block, retrobulbar block

Usual Dosage Dose varies with procedure, depth of anesthesia, vascularity of tissues, duration of anesthesia and condition of patient. Metabisulfites (in epinephrine-containing injection); do not use solutions containing preservatives for caudal or epidural block.

Caudal block (with or without epinephrine):

Children: 1-3.7 mg/kg

Adults: 15-30 mL of 0.25% or 0.5%

Epidural block (other than caudal block):

Children: 1.25 mg/kg/dose

Adults: 10-20 mL of 0.25% or 0.5%

Peripheral nerve block: 5 mL dose of 0.25% or 0.5% (12.5-25 mg); maximum: 2.5 mg/kg (plain); 3 mg/kg (with epinephrine); up to a maximum of 400 mg/day

Sympathetic nerve block: 20-50 mL of 0.25% (no epinephrine) solution

Mechanism of Action Blocks both the initiation and conduction of nerve impulses by decreasing the neuronal membrane's permeability to sodium ions, (Continued)

Bupivacaine Hydrochloride (Continued)

which results in inhibition of depolarization with resultant blockade of conduction

Local Anesthetic/Vasoconstrictor Precautions No information available to require special precautions

Effects on Dental Treatment No effects or complications reported

Other Adverse Effects 1% to 10% (dose related):
Cardiovascular: Cardiac arrest, hypotension, bradycardia, palpitations
Central nervous system: Seizures, restlessness, anxiety, dizziness
Gastrointestinal: Nausea, vomiting
Neuromuscular & skeletal: Weakness
Ocular: Blurred vision
Otic: Tinnitus
Respiratory: Apnea

Contraindications Hypersensitivity to bupivacaine hydrochloride or any component, para-aminobenzoic acid or parabens

Warnings/Precautions Use with caution in patients with liver disease. Some commercially available formulations contain sodium metabisulfite, which may cause allergic-type reactions. Pending further data, should not be used in children <12 years of age and the solution for spinal anesthesia should not be used in children <18 years of age. **Do not use solutions containing preservatives for caudal or epidural block**; convulsions due to systemic toxicity leading to cardiac arrest have been reported, presumably following unintentional intravascular injection. 0.75% is **not** recommended for obstetrical anesthesia.

Drug Interactions
Increased effect: Hyaluronidase
Increased toxicity: Beta-blockers, ergot-type oxytocics, MAO inhibitors, TCAs, phenothiazines, vasopressors

Drug Uptake
Onset of anesthesia (dependent on route administered): Within 4-10 minutes generally
Duration of action: 1.5-8.5 hours
Serum half-life (age dependent):
Adults: 1.5-5.5 hours

Pregnancy Risk Factor C

Dosage Forms
Injection: 0.25% (10 mL, 20 mL, 30 mL, 50 mL); 0.5% (10 mL, 20 mL, 30 mL, 50 mL); 0.75% (2 mL, 10 mL, 20 mL, 30 mL)
Injection, with epinephrine (1:200,000): 0.25% (10 mL, 30 mL, 50 mL); 0.5% (1.8 mL, 3 mL, 5 mL, 10 mL, 30 mL, 50 mL); 0.75% (30 mL)

Generic Available Yes

Bupivacaine With Epinephrine

(byoo piv' a kane with ep i nef' rin)

Related Information
Oral Pain on page 940

Brand Names Marcaine® with Epinephrine

Canadian/Mexican Brand Names Sensorcaine® With Epinephrine (Canada); Buvacaina® (Mexico)

Therapeutic Category Dental/Local Anesthetics; Local Anesthetic, Injectable

Use Dental and Medical: Local anesthesia

Usual Dosage The lowest effective dose should be administered to provide anesthesia. Total dose spread out over a single dental appointment should not exceed 90 mg for adult (10 injections [1.8 mL] of bupivacaine 0.5% with epinephrine 1:200,000)

Mechanism of Action Local anesthetics bind selectively to the intracellular surface of sodium channels to block influx of sodium into the axon. As a result, depolarization necessary for action potential propagation and subsequent nerve function is prevented. The block at the sodium channel is reversible. When drug diffuses away from the axon, sodium channel function is restored and nerve propagation returns.

Epinephrine prolongs the duration of the anesthetic actions of bupivacaine by causing vasoconstriction (alpha adrenergic receptor agonist) of the vasculature surrounding the nerve axons. This prevents the diffusion of bupivacaine away from the nerves resulting in a longer retention in the axon

Local Anesthetic/Vasoconstrictor Precautions No information available to require special precautions

Effects on Dental Treatment No effects or complications reported

Other Adverse Effects Degree of adverse effects in the central nervous system and cardiovascular system are directly related to the blood levels of bupivacaine

Cardiovascular: Myocardial effects include a decrease in contraction force as well as a decrease in electrical excitability and myocardial conduction rate resulting in bradycardia and reduction in cardiac output.

Central nervous system: High blood levels result in anxiety, restlessness, disorientation, confusion, dizziness, tremors and seizures. This is followed by depression of CNS resulting in drowsiness, unconsciousness and possible respiratory arrest. Nausea and vomiting may also occur. In some cases, symptoms of CNS stimulation may be absent and the primary CNS effects are drowsiness and unconsciousness.

Hypersensitivity reactions: Extremely rare, but may be manifest as dermatologic reactions and edema at injection site. Asthmatic syndromes have occurred. Patients may exhibit hypersensitivity to bisulfites contained in local anesthetic solution to prevent oxidation of epinephrine. In general, patients reacting to bisulfites have a history of asthma and their airways are hyperreactive to asthmatic syndrome.

Psychogenic reactions: It is common to misinterpret psychogenic responses to local anesthetic injection as an allergic reaction. Intraoral injections are perceived by many patients as a stressful procedure in dentistry. Common symptoms to this stress are sweating, palpitations, hyperventilation, generalized pallor and a fainting feeling.

Oral manifestations: No data reported

Contraindications Hypersensitivity to bupivacaine

Warnings/Precautions Should be avoided in patients with uncontrolled hyperthyroidism

Drug Interactions Due to epinephrine component: With tricyclic antidepressants or MAO inhibitors could result in increased pressor response; with nonselective beta-blockers (ie, propranolol) could result in serious hypertension and reflex bradycardia

Drug Uptake
Onset of action: Infiltration and nerve block: 2-20 minutes
Duration:
Infiltration: 60 minutes
Nerve block: 5-7 hours
Serum half-life: 1.5-5.5 hours/adult

Pregnancy Risk Factor C

Breast-feeding Considerations Usual infiltration doses of bupivacaine with epinephrine given to nursing mothers has not been shown to affect the health of the nursing infant

Dosage Forms Injection: Bupivacaine hydrochloride 0.5% with epinephrine 1:200,000 (1.8 mL cartridges in boxes of 50)

Dietary Considerations No data reported

Selected Readings
Jastak JT and Yagiela JA, "Vasoconstrictors and Local Anesthesia: A Review and Rationale for Use," *J Am Dent Assoc*, 1983, 107(4):623-30.
MacKenzie TA and Young ER, "Local Anesthetic Update," *Anesth Prog*, 1993, 40(2):29-34.
Wynn RL, "Epinephrine Interactions With Beta-Blockers," *Gen Dent*, 1994, 42(1):16, 18.
Yagiela JA, "Local Anesthetics," *Anesth Prog*, 1991, 38(4-5):128-41.

Buprenex® *see* Buprenorphine Hydrochloride *on this page*
Buprenorfina (Mexico) *see* Buprenorphine Hydrochloride *on this page*

Buprenorphine Hydrochloride
(byoo pre nor' feen hye droe klor' ide)
Related Information
Narcotic Agonist Charts *on page 1019*
Brand Names Buprenex®
Canadian/Mexican Brand Names Temgesic® (Mexico)
Therapeutic Category Analgesic, Narcotic
Synonyms Buprenorfina (Mexico)
Use Management of moderate to severe pain
Usual Dosage I.M., slow I.V.:
Children ≥13 years and Adults: 0.3-0.6 mg every 6 hours as needed
Elderly: 0.15 mg every 6 hours; elderly patients are more likely to suffer from confusion and drowsiness compared to younger patients
Long-term use is not recommended
Mechanism of Action Opiate agonist/antagonist that produces analgesia by binding to kappa and mu opiate receptors in the CNS
(Continued)

Buprenorphine Hydrochloride *(Continued)*

Local Anesthetic/Vasoconstrictor Precautions No information available to require special precautions

Effects on Dental Treatment No effects or complications reported

Other Adverse Effects

>10%: Central nervous system: Drowsiness

1% to 10%:
  Cardiovascular: Hypotension
  Central nervous system: Respiratory depression, dizziness, headache
  Gastrointestinal: Vomiting, nausea

<1%:
  Central nervous system: Euphoria, slurred speech, malaise
  Dermatologic: Allergic dermatitis
  Genitourinary: Urinary retention
  Neuromuscular & skeletal: Paresthesia
  Ocular: Blurred vision

Drug Interactions Increased toxicity: Barbiturates, benzodiazepines (increase CNS and respiratory depression)

Drug Uptake
  Onset of analgesia: Within 10-30 minutes
  Absorption: I.M., S.C.: 30% to 40%
  Serum half-life: 2.2-3 hours

Pregnancy Risk Factor C

Bupropion (byoo proe' pee on)

Related Information
  Vasoconstrictor Interactions With Antidepressants *on page 1108*

Brand Names Wellbutrin®; Wellbutrin® SR

Therapeutic Category Antidepressant, Miscellaneous

Use Treatment of depression

Usual Dosage Oral:
  Adults: 100 mg 3 times/day; begin at 100 mg twice daily; may increase to a maximum dose of 450 mg/day
  Elderly: 50-100 mg/day, increase by 50-100 mg every 3-4 days as tolerated; there is evidence that the elderly respond at 150 mg/day in divided doses, but some may require a higher dose

Mechanism of Action Antidepressant structurally different from all other previously marketed antidepressants; like other antidepressants the mechanism of bupropion's activity is not fully understood; weak blocker of serotonin and norepinephrine re-uptake, inhibits neuronal dopamine re-uptake and is **not** a monoamine oxidase A or B inhibitor

Local Anesthetic/Vasoconstrictor Precautions None; this is not a tricyclic type antidepressant and will not enhance pressor response of epinephrine

Effects on Dental Treatment No effects or complications reported

Other Adverse Effects

>10%:
  Central nervous system: Agitation, insomnia, fever, headache, psychosis, confusion, anxiety, restlessness, dizziness, seizures, chills, akathisia
  Gastrointestinal: Nausea, vomiting, dry mouth, constipation, weight loss
  Genitourinary: Impotence
  Neuromuscular & skeletal: Tremor

1% to 10%:
  Central nervous system: Hallucinations, chills, tiredness
  Dermatologic: Skin rash
  Ocular: Blurred vision

<1%: Central nervous system: Fainting, drowsiness, seizures

Drug Interactions
  Decreased effects: Increased clearance: Carbamazepine, phenytoin, cimetidine, phenobarbital
  Increased effects: Levodopa, MAO inhibitors

Drug Uptake
  Absorption: Rapidly absorbed from GI tract
  Serum half-life: 14 hours
  Time to peak serum concentration: Oral: Within 3 hours

Pregnancy Risk Factor B

Burow's Otic *see* Aluminum Acetate and Acetic Acid *on page 39*

BuSpar® *see* Buspirone Hydrochloride *on next page*

Buspirona, Clorhidrato De (Mexico) *see* Buspirone Hydrochloride *on next page*

Buspirone Hydrochloride (byoo spye' rone hye droe klor' ide)
Related Information
   Patients Requiring Sedation *on page 965*
Brand Names BuSpar®
Canadian/Mexican Brand Names Neurosine® (Mexico)
Therapeutic Category Antianxiety Agent; Tranquilizer, Minor
Synonyms Buspirona, Clorhidrato De (Mexico)
Use Management of anxiety; has shown little potential for abuse
   Unlabeled use: Panic attacks
Usual Dosage Adults: Oral: 15 mg/day (5 mg 3 times/day); may increase in increments of 5 mg/day every 2-4 days to a maximum of 60 mg/day
Mechanism of Action Selectively antagonizes CNS serotonin 5-HT$_1$A receptors without affecting benzodiazepine-GABA receptors; may down-regulate postsynaptic 5-HT$_2$ receptors as do antidepressants
Local Anesthetic/Vasoconstrictor Precautions No information available to require special precautions
Effects on Dental Treatment No effects or complications reported
Other Adverse Effects
   >10%:
      Central nervous system: Dizziness, lightheadedness, headache, restlessness
      Gastrointestinal: Nausea
   1% to 10%: Central nervous system: Drowsiness
   <1%:
      Cardiovascular: Chest pain, tachycardia
      Central nervous system: Confusion, insomnia, nightmares, sedation, disorientation, excitement, fever, ataxia
      Dermatologic: Rash, urticaria
      Gastrointestinal: Dry mouth, vomiting, diarrhea, flatulence
      Hematologic: Leukopenia, eosinophilia
      Neuromuscular & skeletal: Muscle weakness
      Ocular: Blurred vision
      Otic: Tinnitus
Drug Interactions
   Increased effects: Cimetidine, food
   Increased toxicity: MAO inhibitors, phenothiazines, CNS depressants; increased toxicity of digoxin and haloperidol
Drug Uptake
   Serum half-life: 2-3 hours
   Time to peak serum concentration: Oral: Within 40-60 minutes
Pregnancy Risk Factor B
Dosage Forms Tablet: 5 mg, 10 mg
Dietary Considerations Food may decrease the absorption of buspirone, but it may also decrease the first-pass metabolism, thereby increasing the bioavailability of buspirone
Generic Available No

Busulfan (byoo sul' fan)
Brand Names Myleran®
Therapeutic Category Antineoplastic Agent, Alkylating Agent
Synonyms Busulfano (Mexico)
Use Chronic myelogenous leukemia and bone marrow disorders, such as polycythemia vera and myeloid metaplasia, conditioning regimens for bone marrow transplantation
Usual Dosage Oral (**refer to individual protocols**):
   Children:
      For remission induction of CML: 0.06-0.12 mg/kg/day **or** 1.8-4.6 mg/m^2/day; titrate dosage to maintain leukocyte count above 40,000/mm^3; reduce dosage by 50% if the leukocyte count reaches 30,000-40,000/mm^3; discontinue drug if counts fall to ≤20,000/mm^3
      BMT marrow-ablative conditioning regimen: 1 mg/kg/dose (ideal body weight) every 6 hours for 16 doses

   Adults:
      BMT marrow-ablative conditioning regimen: 1 mg/kg/dose (ideal body weight) every 6 hours for 16 doses
      Remission:
         Induction of CML: 4-8 mg/day (may be as high as 12 mg/day)
         Maintenance doses: Controversial, range from 1-4 mg/day to 2 mg/week; treatment is continued until WBC reaches 10,000-20,000 cells/mm^3 at

(Continued)

Busulfan (Continued)

which time drug is discontinued; when WBC reaches 50,000/mm^3, maintenance dose is resumed

Unapproved uses:

Polycythemia vera: 2-6 mg/day

Thrombocytosis: 4-6 mg/day

Mechanism of Action Reacts with N-7 position of guanosine and interferes with DNA replication and transcription of RNA. Busulfan has a more marked effect on myeloid cells (and is, therefore, useful in the treatment of CML) than on lymphoid cells. The drug is also very toxic to hematopoietic stem cells (thus its usefulness in high doses in BMT preparative regimens). Busulfan exhibits little immunosuppressive activity. Interferes with the normal function of DNA by alkylation and cross-linking the strands of DNA.

Local Anesthetic/Vasoconstrictor Precautions No information available to require special precautions

Effects on Dental Treatment No effects or complications reported

Other Adverse Effects Fertility/carcinogenesis: Sterility, ovarian suppression, amenorrhea, azoospermia, and testicular atrophy; malignant tumors have been reported in patients on busulfan therapy

>10%:

Hematologic: Severe pancytopenia, leukopenia, thrombocytopenia, anemia, and bone marrow suppression are common and patients should be monitored closely while on therapy. Since this is a delayed effect (busulfan affects the stem cells), the drug should be discontinued temporarily at the first sign of a large or rapid fall in any blood element. Some patients may develop bone marrow fibrosis or chronic aplasia which is probably due to the busulfan toxicity. In large doses, busulfan is myeloablative and is used for this reason in BMT.

Myelosuppressive:

WBC: Moderate

Platelets: Moderate

Onset (days): 7-10

Nadir (days): 14-21

Recovery (days): 28

1% to 10%:

Cardiovascular: Endocardial fibrosis

Central nervous system: Weakness

Dermatologic: Hyperpigmentation skin (busulfan tan), urticaria, erythema, alopecia

Endocrine & metabolic: Amenorrhea

Gastrointestinal: **Emetic potential:** Low (<10%); nausea, vomiting, diarrhea; drug has little effect on the GI mucosal lining

<1%:

Central nervous system: Generalized or myoclonic seizures and loss of consciousness have been associated with high-dose busulfan (4 mg/kg/day), blurred vision

Endocrine & metabolic: Adrenal suppression, gynecomastia, hyperuricemia

Genitourinary: Isolated cases of hemorrhagic cystitis have been reported

Hepatic: Hepatic dysfunction

Ocular: Cataracts

Respiratory: After long-term or high-dose therapy, a syndrome known as busulfan lung may occur. This syndrome is manifested by a diffuse interstitial pulmonary fibrosis and persistent cough, fever, rales, and dyspnea. May be relieved by corticosteroids.

Drug Interactions No data reported

Drug Uptake

Absorption: Rapidly and completely from the GI tract

Serum half-life:

After first dose: 3.4 hours

After last dose: 2.3 hours

Time to peak serum concentration:

Oral: Within 4 hours

I.V.: Within 5 minutes

Pregnancy Risk Factor D

Busulfano (Mexico) see Busulfan on previous page

Butabarbital Sodium (byoo ta bar' bi tal sow' dee um)

Brand Names Butalan®; Buticaps®; Butisol Sodium®

Therapeutic Category Barbiturate; Hypnotic; Sedative

Use Sedative, hypnotic

Usual Dosage Oral:
Children: Preop: 2-6 mg/kg/dose; maximum: 100 mg

Adults:
Sedative: 15-30 mg 3-4 times/day
Hypnotic: 50-100 mg
Preop: 50-100 mg 1-1½ hours before surgery

Mechanism of Action Interferes with transmission of impulses from the thalamus to the cortex of the brain resulting in an imbalance in central inhibitory and facilitatory mechanisms

Local Anesthetic/Vasoconstrictor Precautions No information available to require special precautions

Effects on Dental Treatment No effects or complications reported

Other Adverse Effects
>10%: Central nervous system: Dizziness, lightheadedness, drowsiness, "hangover" effect
1% to 10%:
Central nervous system: Confusion, mental depression, unusual excitement, nervousness, faint feeling, headache, insomnia, nightmares
Gastrointestinal: Constipation, nausea, vomiting
<1%:
Cardiovascular: Hypotension
Central nervous system: Hallucinations
Dermatologic: Skin rash, exfoliative dermatitis, Stevens-Johnson syndrome, angioedema
Hematologic: Agranulocytosis, megaloblastic anemia, thrombocytopenia
Local: Thrombophlebitis
Respiratory: Respiratory depression
Miscellaneous: Dependence

Drug Interactions
Barbiturates can induce hepatic microsomal enzymes resulting in increased metabolism and therefore decreased effects of anticoagulants, corticosteroids, doxycycline
Increased toxicity when combined with other CNS depressants or antidepressants, respiratory and CNS depression may be additive

Drug Uptake
Serum half-life: 40-140 hours
Time to peak serum concentration: Oral: Within 40-60 minutes

Pregnancy Risk Factor D

Butace® *see* Butalbital Compound *on this page*
Butalan® *see* Butabarbital Sodium *on previous page*

Butalbital Compound (byoo tal′ bi tal kom′ pound)

Brand Names Amaphen®; Anoquan®; Axotal®; B-A-C®; Bancap®; Butace®; Endolor®; Esgic®; Femcet®; Fiorgen PF®; Fioricet®; Fiorinal®; G-1®; Isollyl Improved®; Lanorinal®; Marnal®; Medigesic®; Phrenilin®; Phrenilin® Forte®; Repan®; Sedapap-10®; Triapin®; Two-Dyne®

Canadian/Mexican Brand Names Tecnal® (Canada)

Therapeutic Category Analgesic, Non-narcotic; Barbiturate

Use Relief of symptomatic complex of tension or muscle contraction headache

Usual Dosage Adults: Oral: 1-2 tablets or capsules every 4 hours; not to exceed 6/day

Mechanism of Action Butalbital, like other barbiturates, has a generalized depressant effect on the central nervous system (CNS). Barbiturates have little effect on peripheral nerves or muscle at usual therapeutic doses. However, at toxic doses serious effects on the cardiovascular system and other peripheral systems may be observed. These effects may result in hypotension or skeletal muscle weakness. While all areas of the central nervous system are acted on by barbiturates, the mesencephalic reticular activating system is extremely sensitive to their effects. Barbiturates act at synapses where gamma-amino-benzoic acid is a neurotransmitter, but they may act in other areas as well.

Local Anesthetic/Vasoconstrictor Precautions No information available to require special precautions

Effects on Dental Treatment No effects or complications reported

Other Adverse Effects
>10%:
Central nervous system: Dizziness, lightheadedness, drowsiness, "hangover" effect
Gastrointestinal: Nausea, heartburn, stomach pains, dyspepsia, epigastric discomfort
(Continued)

Butalbital Compound *(Continued)*

1% to 10%:
Central nervous system: Confusion, mental depression, unusual excitement, nervousness, faint feeling, headache, insomnia, nightmares, weakness, tiredness
Dermatologic: Skin rash
Gastrointestinal: Constipation, vomiting, gastrointestinal ulceration
Hematologic: Hemolytic anemia
Respiratory: Troubled breathing
Miscellaneous: Anaphylactic shock
<1%:
Cardiovascular: Hypotension
Central nervous system: Hallucinations, insomnia, nervousness, jitters
Dermatologic: Skin rash, exfoliative dermatitis, Stevens-Johnson syndrome
Hematologic: Agranulocytosis, megaloblastic anemia, occult bleeding, prolongation of bleeding time, leukopenia, thrombocytopenia, iron deficiency anemia
Hepatic: Hepatotoxicity
Local: Thrombophlebitis
Renal: Impaired renal function
Respiratory: Respiratory depression, bronchospasm

Drug Interactions
Decreased effect: Phenothiazines, haloperidol, quinidine, cyclosporine, tricyclic antidepressants, corticosteroids, theophylline, ethosuximide, warfarin, oral contraceptives, chloramphenicol, griseofulvin, doxycycline, beta-blockers
Increased effect/toxicity: Propoxyphene, benzodiazepines, CNS depressants, valproic acid, methylphenidate, chloramphenicol

Drug Uptake Half-life: 61 hours in healthy volunteers

Pregnancy Risk Factor D

Dosage Forms
Capsule, with acetaminophen:
Amaphen®, Anoquan®, Butace®, Endolor®, Esgic®, Femcet®, G-1®, Medigesic®, Repan®, Two-Dyne®: Butalbital 50 mg, caffeine 40 mg, and acetaminophen 325 mg
Bancap®, Triapin®: Butalbital 50 mg and acetaminophen 325 mg
Phrenilin Forte®: Butalbital 50 mg and acetaminophen 650 mg
Capsule, with aspirin: (Fiorgen PF®, Fiorinal®, Isollyl Improved®, Lanorinal®, Marnal®): Butalbital 50 mg, caffeine 40 mg, and aspirin 325 mg
Tablet, with acetaminophen:
Esgic®, Fioricet®, Repan®: Butalbital 50 mg, caffeine 40 mg, and acetaminophen 325 mg
Phrenilin®: Butalbital 50 mg and acetaminophen 325 mg
Sedapap-10®: Butalbital 50 mg and acetaminophen 650 mg
Tablet, with aspirin:
Axotal®: Butalbital 50 mg and aspirin 650 mg
B-A-C®: Butalbital 50 mg, caffeine 40 mg, and aspirin 650 mg
Fiorinal®, Isollyl Improved®, Lanorinal®, Marnal®: Butalbital 50 mg, caffeine 40 mg, and aspirin 325 mg

Generic Available Yes

Butalbital Compound and Codeine

(byoo tal' bi tal kom' pound & koe' deen)

Brand Names Fiorinal® With Codeine

Therapeutic Category Analgesic, Narcotic; Barbiturate

Synonyms Codeine and Butalbital Compound

Use Mild to moderate pain when sedation is needed

Local Anesthetic/Vasoconstrictor Precautions No information available to require special precautions

Effects on Dental Treatment <1%: Dry mouth

Other Adverse Effects
>10%:
Central nervous system: Dizziness, lightheadedness, drowsiness, "hangover" effect
Gastrointestinal: Nausea, heartburn, stomach pains, dyspepsia, epigastric discomfort
1% to 10%:
Central nervous system: Confusion, mental depression, unusual excitement, nervousness, faint feeling, headache, insomnia, nightmares, tiredness
Dermatologic: Skin rash

    Gastrointestinal: Constipation, vomiting, gastrointestinal ulceration
    Hematologic: Hemolytic anemia
    Neuromuscular & skeletal: Weakness
    Respiratory: Troubled breathing
    Miscellaneous: Anaphylactic shock
<1%:
    Cardiovascular: Hypotension
    Central nervous system: Hallucinations, nervousness, jitters
    Dermatologic: Skin rash, exfoliative dermatitis, Stevens-Johnson syndrome
    Hematologic: Agranulocytosis, megaloblastic anemia, thrombocytopenia, occult bleeding, prolongation of bleeding time, leukopenia, iron deficiency anemia
    Hepatic: Hepatotoxicity
    Local: Thrombophlebitis
    Renal: Impaired renal function
    Respiratory: Respiratory depression, bronchospasm
Comments Abrupt discontinuation after sustained use (generally >10 days) may cause withdrawal symptoms

Butenafine Hydrochloride
Brand Names Mentax®
Therapeutic Category Antifungal Agent, Topical
Use Topical treatment of tinea pedis (athlete's foot)
Usual Dosage Adults: Topical: Apply once daily for 4 weeks
Local Anesthetic/Vasoconstrictor Precautions No information available to require special precautions
Effects on Dental Treatment No effects or complications reported
Pregnancy Risk Factor B

Buticaps® *see* Butabarbital Sodium *on page 132*
Butisol Sodium® *see* Butabarbital Sodium *on page 132*

Butoconazole Nitrate (byoo toe koe' na zole nye' trate)
Brand Names Femstat®
Canadian/Mexican Brand Names Femstal® (Mexico)
Therapeutic Category Antifungal Agent, Vaginal
Synonyms Butoconazol (Mexico)
Use Local treatment of vulvovaginal candidiasis
Usual Dosage Adults:
    Nonpregnant: Insert 1 applicatorful (~5 g) intravaginally at bedtime for 3 days, may extend for up to 6 days if necessary
    Pregnant: **Use only during second or third trimesters**
Mechanism of Action Increases cell membrane permeability in susceptible fungi (*Candida*)
Local Anesthetic/Vasoconstrictor Precautions No information available to require special precautions
Effects on Dental Treatment No effects or complications reported
Other Adverse Effects
    1% to 10%: Genitourinary: Vulvar/vaginal burning
    <1%: Genitourinary: Vulvar itching, soreness, swelling, or discharge; urinary frequency
Drug Interactions No data reported
Drug Uptake
    Absorption: Following intravaginal application small amounts of drug are absorbed systemically (25%) within 2-8 hours
    Serum half-life: 21-24 hours
Pregnancy Risk Factor C (For use only in 2nd or 3rd trimester)
Dosage Forms Cream, vaginal: 2% with applicator (28 g)
Generic Available No

Butoconazol (Mexico) *see* Butoconazole Nitrate *on this page*
Butorfanol (Mexico) *see* Butorphanol Tartrate *on this page*

Butorphanol Tartrate (byoo tor' fa nole tar' trate)
Related Information
    Narcotic Agonist Charts *on page 1019*
Brand Names Stadol®; Stadol® NS
Therapeutic Category Analgesic, Narcotic
Synonyms Butorfanol (Mexico)
Use Management of moderate to severe pain
    (Continued)

Butorphanol Tartrate *(Continued)*

Usual Dosage Adults:

I.M.: 1-4 mg every 3-4 hours as needed

I.V.: 0.5-2 mg every 3-4 hours as needed

Nasal spray: Headache: 1 spray in 1 nostril; if adequate pain relief is not achieved within 60-90 minutes, an additional 1 spray in 1 nostril may be given (each spray gives ~1 mg of butorphanol)

Mechanism of Action Mixed narcotic agonist-antagonist with central analgesic actions; binds to opiate receptors in the CNS, causing inhibition of ascending pain pathways, altering the perception of and response to pain; produces generalized CNS depression

Local Anesthetic/Vasoconstrictor Precautions No information available to require special precautions

Effects on Dental Treatment No effects or complications reported

Other Adverse Effects

>10%: Central nervous system: Drowsiness

1% to 10%:

Cardiovascular: Flushing of the face, hypotension

Central nervous system: Dizziness, lightheadedness, headache

Gastrointestinal: Anorexia, nausea, vomiting

Genitourinary: Decreased urination

Miscellaneous: Increased sweating

<1%:

Cardiovascular: Bradycardia or tachycardia, hypertension

Central nervous system: Paradoxical CNS stimulation, confusion, hallucinations, mental depression, false sense of well being, malaise, restlessness, nightmares, weakness, CNS depression

Dermatologic: Skin rash

Gastrointestinal: Stomach cramps, constipation, dry mouth

Genitourinary: Painful urination

Ocular: Blurred vision

Otic: Tinnitus

Respiratory: Shortness of breath, troubled breathing, respiratory depression

Miscellaneous: Dependence with prolonged use

Drug Interactions Increased toxicity: CNS depressants, phenothiazines, barbiturates, skeletal muscle relaxants, alfentanil, guanabenz, MAO inhibitors

Drug Uptake

Absorption: Rapidly and well absorbed

Serum half-life: 2.5-4 hours

Pregnancy Risk Factor B (D if used for prolonged periods or in high doses at term)

Byclomine® *see Dicyclomine Hydrochloride on page 273*

C7E3 *see Abciximab on page 12*

C8-CCK *see Sincalide on page 789*

Cafatine® *see Ergotamine on page 319*

Cafergot® *see Ergotamine on page 319*

Cafetrate® *see Ergotamine on page 319*

Caffeine and Sodium Benzoate

(kaf' een & sow dee um ben' zoe ate)

Therapeutic Category Diuretic, Miscellaneous

Synonyms Sodium Benzoate and Caffeine

Use Emergency stimulant in acute circulatory failure; as a diuretic; and to relieve spinal puncture headache

Local Anesthetic/Vasoconstrictor Precautions No information available to require special precautions

Effects on Dental Treatment No effects or complications reported

Other Adverse Effects 1% to 10%:

Cardiovascular: Tachycardia, extrasystoles, palpitations

Central nervous system: Insomnia, restlessness, nervousness, mild delirium, headache, anxiety

Gastrointestinal: Nausea, vomiting, gastric irritation

Genitourinary: Diuresis

Neuromuscular & skeletal: Muscle tension following abrupt cessation of drug after regular consumption of 500-600 mg/day

Caffeine, Citrated (kaf' een, sit' rated)

Therapeutic Category Central Nervous System Stimulant, Nonamphetamine; Respiratory Stimulant

Use Central nervous system stimulant; used in the treatment of idiopathic apnea of prematurity

Local Anesthetic/Vasoconstrictor Precautions No information available to require special precautions

Effects on Dental Treatment No effects or complications reported

Comments Has several advantages over theophylline in the treatment of neonatal apnea, its half-life is about 3 times as long, allowing once daily dosing, drug levels do not need to be drawn at peak and trough; has a wider therapeutic window, allowing more room between an effective concentration and toxicity; 2 mg caffeine citrate = 1 mg caffeine base

Calan® *see* Verapamil Hydrochloride *on page 893*

Calan® SR *see* Verapamil Hydrochloride *on page 893*

Calcibind® *see* Cellulose Sodium Phosphate *on page 175*

Calci-Chew™ *see* Calcium Carbonate *on page 140*

Calcifediol (kal si fe dye′ ole)

Brand Names Calderol®

Therapeutic Category Vitamin D Analog

Use Treatment and management of metabolic bone disease associated with chronic renal failure

Usual Dosage Children and Adults: Hepatic osteodystrophy: Oral: 20-100 mcg/ day or every other day; titrate to obtain normal serum calcium/phosphate levels; increase dose at 4-week intervals

Mechanism of Action Vitamin D analog that (along with calcitonin and para-thyroid hormone) regulates serum calcium homeostasis by promoting absorp-tion of calcium and phosphorus in the small intestine; promotes renal tubule resorption of phosphate; increases rate of accretion and resorption in bone minerals

Local Anesthetic/Vasoconstrictor Precautions No information available to require special precautions

Effects on Dental Treatment No effects or complications reported

Other Adverse Effects

1% to 10%:
  Cardiovascular: Hypotension, cardiac arrhythmias, hypertension, irregular heartbeat
  Central nervous system: Irritability, headache
  Dermatologic: Pruritus
  Endocrine & metabolic: Polydipsia, hypermagnesemia
  Gastrointestinal: Nausea, vomiting, constipation, anorexia, pancreatitis
  Neuromuscular & skeletal: Muscle/bone pain
  Ocular: Conjunctivitis, photophobia
  Renal: Polyuria
  Miscellaneous: Metallic taste

<1%:
  Central nervous system: Overt psychosis, seizures
  Gastrointestinal: Weight loss
  Hepatic: Elevated AST/ALT
  Miscellaneous: Calcification

Drug Interactions

Cholestyramine reduces intestinal absorption of fat-soluble vitamins; may impair intestinal absorption of calcifediol

Magnesium-containing antacids and calcifediol should not be used concomi-tantly in patients on chronic renal dialysis due to potential for hypermagne-semia

Drug Uptake

Absorption: Rapid from the small intestines

Serum half-life: 12-22 days

Time to peak: Within 4 hours (oral)

Pregnancy Risk Factor A (D if used in doses above the recommended daily allowance)

Calciferol™ *see* Ergocalciferol *on page 317*

Calcijex™ *see* Calcitriol *on page 139*

Calcilac® [OTC] *see* Calcium Carbonate *on page 140*

Calcimar® *see* Calcitonin *on next page*

Calci-Mix™ *see* Calcium Carbonate *on page 140*

Calciparine® Injection *see* Heparin *on page 419*

Calcipotriene (kal si poe' try een)

Brand Names Dovonex®

Therapeutic Category Antipsoriatic Agent, Topical

Use Treatment of moderate plaque psoriasis

Usual Dosage Adults: Topical: Apply in a thin film to the affected skin twice daily and rub in gently and completely

Mechanism of Action Synthetic vitamin D_3 analog which regulates skin cell production and proliferation

Local Anesthetic/Vasoconstrictor Precautions No information available to require special precautions

Effects on Dental Treatment No effects or complications reported

Other Adverse Effects

>10%: Topical: Burning, itching, skin irritation, erythema, dry skin, peeling, rash, worsening of psoriasis

1% to 10%: Topical: Dermatitis

<1%:

Systemic: Hypercalcemia

Topical: Skin atrophy, hyperpigmentation, folliculitis

Drug Interactions No data reported

Pregnancy Risk Factor C

Calcitonin (kal si toe' nin)

Brand Names Calcimar®; Cibacalcin®; Miacalcin®

Canadian/Mexican Brand Names Caltine® (Canada)

Therapeutic Category Antidote, Hypercalcemia

Use

Calcitonin (salmon): Treatment of Paget's disease of bone and as adjunctive therapy for hypercalcemia; also used in postmenopausal osteoporosis

Calcitonin (human): Treatment of Paget's disease of bone

Usual Dosage

Children: Dosage not established

Adults:

Paget's disease:

Salmon calcitonin: I.M., S.C.: 100 units/day to start, 50 units/day or 50-100 units every 1-3 days maintenance dose; Intranasal: 200-400 units (1-2 sprays)/day

Human calcitonin: S.C.: Initial: 0.5 mg/day (maximum: 0.5 mg twice daily); maintenance: 0.5 mg 2-3 times/week or 0.25 mg/day

Hypercalcemia: Initial: Salmon calcitonin: I.M., S.C.: 4 units/kg every 12 hours; may increase up to 8 units/kg every 12 hours to a maximum of every 6 hours

Osteogenesis imperfecta: Salmon calcitonin: I.M., S.C.: 2 units/kg 3 times/week

Postmenopausal osteoporosis: Salmon calcitonin:

I.M., S.C.: 100 units/day

Intranasal: 200 units (1 spray)/day

Mechanism of Action Structurally similar to human calcitonin; it directly inhibits osteoclastic bone resorption; promotes the renal excretion of calcium, phosphate, sodium, magnesium and potassium by decreasing tubular reabsorption; increases the jejunal secretion of water, sodium, potassium, and chloride

Local Anesthetic/Vasoconstrictor Precautions No information available to require special precautions

Effects on Dental Treatment No effects or complications reported

Other Adverse Effects

>10%:

Gastrointestinal: Nausea, diarrhea, anorexia

Miscellaneous: Facial flushing, swelling at injection site

1% to 10%: Frequency of urination

<1%:

Central nervous system: Chills, headache, tingling of hands/feet, swelling, dizziness, weakness

Dermatologic: Skin rash, urticaria

Respiratory: Shortness of breath, nasal congestion, stuffy nose

Drug Interactions No data reported

Drug Uptake

Hypercalcemia:

Onset of reduction in calcium: 2 hours

Duration of effect: 6-8 hours

Serum half-life: S.C.: 1.2 hours

Pregnancy Risk Factor B

Calcitriol (kal si trye' ole)
Brand Names Calcijex™; Rocaltrol®
Therapeutic Category Vitamin D Analog
Use Management of hypocalcemia in patients on chronic renal dialysis; reduce elevated parathyroid hormone levels; decrease severity of psoriatic lesions in psoriatic vulgaris
Usual Dosage Individualize dosage to maintain calcium levels of 9-10 mg/dL
Renal failure:
Oral:
Children: Initial: 15 ng/kg/day; maintenance: 5-40 ng/kg/day
Adults: 0.25 mcg/day or every other day (may require 0.5-1 mcg/day)
I.V.: Adults: 0.5 mcg (0.01 mcg/kg) 3 times/week; most doses in the range of 0.5-3 mcg (0.01-0.05 mcg/kg) 3 times/week

Hypoparathyroidism/pseudohypoparathyroidism: Oral:
Children:
<1 year: 0.04-0.08 mcg/kg/day
1-6 years: Initial: 0.25 mcg/day, increase at 2- to 4-week intervals
Children >6 years and Adults: 0.5-2 mcg/day

Vitamin D-resistant rickets (familial hypophosphatemia): Oral: 2 mcg/day; initial: 15-20 ng/kg/day; maintenance: 30-60 ng/kg/day

Mechanism of Action Promotes absorption of calcium in the intestines and retention at the kidneys thereby increasing calcium levels in the serum; decreases excessive serum phosphatase levels, parathyroid hormone levels, and decreases bone resorption; increases renal tubule phosphate resorption
Local Anesthetic/Vasoconstrictor Precautions No information available to require special precautions
Effects on Dental Treatment No effects or complications reported
Other Adverse Effects
1% to 10%:
Cardiovascular: Hypotension, cardiac arrhythmias, hypertension, irregular heartbeat
Central nervous system: Irritability, headache
Dermatologic: Pruritus
Endocrine & metabolic: Polydipsia
Gastrointestinal: Nausea, vomiting, constipation, anorexia, pancreatitis, metallic taste
Neuromuscular & skeletal: Muscle/bone pain
Ocular: Conjunctivitis, photophobia
Renal: Polyuria
<1%:
Central nervous system: Overt psychosis, hyperthermia
Endocrine & metabolic: Hypercalcemia
Gastrointestinal: Weight loss
Hepatic: Increased LFTs
Respiratory: Rhinorrhea
Miscellaneous: Hypercholesterolemia
Drug Interactions
Cholestyramine reduces intestinal absorption of fat-soluble vitamins; may impair intestinal absorption of calcitriol
Magnesium-containing antacids and calcitriol should not be used concomitantly in patients on chronic renal dialysis due to potential for hypermagnesemia
Drug Uptake
Onset of action: ~2-6 hours
Duration: 3-5 days
Absorption: Oral: Rapid
Serum half-life: 3-8 hours
Pregnancy Risk Factor A (D if used in doses above the recommended daily allowance)

Calcium Acetate (kal' see um as' e tate)
Brand Names Phos-Ex®; PhosLo®
Therapeutic Category Calcium Salt
Use Control of hyperphosphatemia in end stage renal failure; calcium acetate binds phosphorus in the GI tract better than other calcium salts due to its lower solubility and subsequent reduced absorption and increased formation of calcium phosphate; calcium acetate does not promote aluminum absorption
(Continued)

Calcium Acetate *(Continued)*

Usual Dosage Adults: Oral: 2 tablets with each meal; dosage may be increased to bring serum phosphate value to <6 mg/dL; most patients require 3-4 tablets with each meal

Mechanism of Action Moderates nerve and muscle performance via action potential excitation threshold regulation; combines with dietary phosphate to form insoluble calcium phosphate which is excreted in feces

Local Anesthetic/Vasoconstrictor Precautions No information available to require special precautions

Effects on Dental Treatment No effects or complications reported

Other Adverse Effects
Mild hypercalcemia (calcium: >10.5 mg/dL) may be asymptomatic or manifest itself as constipation, anorexia, nausea, and vomiting
More severe hypercalcemia (calcium: >12 mg/dL) is associated with confusion, delirium, stupor, and coma

<1%:
Central nervous system: Headache
Endocrine & metabolic: Hypophosphatemia, hypercalcemia
Gastrointestinal: Nausea, anorexia, vomiting, abdominal pain, constipation
Miscellaneous: Thirst

Drug Interactions
Decreased effect:
Calcium may antagonize the effects of calcium channel blockers
May decrease the bioavailability of tetracyclines
Renders tetracycline antibiotics inactive
Increased toxicity: Administer cautiously to a digitalized patient, may precipitate arrhythmias

Drug Uptake
Absorption: Absorption from the GI tract requires vitamin D

Pregnancy Risk Factor C

Calcium Carbonate *(kal' see um kar' bun ate)*

Brand Names Alka-Mints® [OTC]; Amitone® [OTC]; Biocal® [OTC]; Calci-Chew™; Calcilac® [OTC]; Calci-Mix™; CalSup® [OTC]; Caltrate® [OTC]; Chooz® [OTC]; Dicarbosil® [OTC]; Glycate® [OTC]; Os-Cal® 250 [OTC]; Os-Cal® 500 [OTC]; Rolaids® Calcium Rich [OTC]; Suplical® [OTC]; Titralac® [OTC]; Tums® [OTC]

Canadian/Mexican Brand Names Apo-Cal® (Canada); Calcite-500® (Canada); Calsan® (Canada); Pharmacal® (Canada)

Therapeutic Category Antacid; Antidote, Hyperphosphatemia; Calcium Salt

Use Adjunct in prevention of postmenopausal osteoporosis, antacid, treatment and prevention of calcium depletion (osteoporosis, osteomalacia, etc); control of hyperphosphatemia in end stage renal disease

Usual Dosage Oral (dosage is in terms of elemental calcium):
Recommended daily allowance (RDA):
<6 months: 360 mg/day
6-12 months: 540 mg/day
1-10 years: 800 mg/day
10-18 years: 1200 mg/day
Adults: 800 mg/day

Hypocalcemia (dose depends on clinical condition and serum calcium level):
Children: 45-65 mg/kg/day in 4 divided doses
Adults: 1-2 g or more/day

Adults:
Dietary supplementation: 500 mg to 2 g divided 2-4 times/day
To reduce bone loss with aging/osteoporosis: 1000-1500 mg/day
Antacid: 2 tablets or 10 mL every 2 hours, up to 12 times/day

Mechanism of Action Moderates nerve and muscle performance via action potential excitation threshold regulation; combines with dietary phosphate to form insoluble calcium phosphate which is excreted in feces; may prevent negative calcium balance when used as a dietary supplement, or for calcium balance when used as a dietary supplement, or as treatment for osteoporosis

Local Anesthetic/Vasoconstrictor Precautions No information available to require special precautions

Effects on Dental Treatment No effects or complications reported

Other Adverse Effects
1% to 10%: Gastrointestinal: Constipation, flatulence
<1%:
Cardiovascular: Hypotension, bradycardia, cardiac arrhythmias

Central nervous system: Mood and mental changes, lethargy
Dermatologic: Erythema
Endocrine & metabolic: Hypercalcemia (with prolonged use), metastatic calcinosis, hypomagnesemia, hypophosphatemia, milk-alkali syndrome
Gastrointestinal: Laxative effect, acid rebound, nausea, vomiting, GI hemorrhage, fecal impaction
Hematologic: Elevated serum amylase
Neuromuscular & skeletal: Myalgia
Renal: Polyuria, renal calculi, renal dysfunction, hypercalciuria

Drug Interactions
Decreased effect:
Calcium may antagonize the effects of calcium channel blockers
May decrease the bioavailability of tetracyclines
Renders tetracycline antibiotics inactive
Increased toxicity: Administer cautiously to a digitalized patient, may precipitate arrhythmias

Drug Uptake
Absorption: From the GI tract requires vitamin D; calcium is absorbed in soluble, ionized form; solubility of calcium is increased in an acid environment

Pregnancy Risk Factor C

Calcium Carbonate and Simethicone
(kal' see um kar' bun ate & sye meth' i kone)
Brand Names Titralac® Plus Liquid [OTC]
Therapeutic Category Antacid
Synonyms Simethicone and Calcium Carbonate
Use Relief of acid indigestion, heartburn, peptic esophagitis, hiatal hernia, and gas
Local Anesthetic/Vasoconstrictor Precautions No information available to require special precautions
Effects on Dental Treatment Do not give tetracycline concomitantly

Calcium Channel Blockers & Gingival Hyperplasia *see page 1010*

Calcium Chloride (kal' see um klor' ide)
Brand Names Cal Plus®
Therapeutic Category Calcium Salt; Electrolyte Supplement, Parenteral
Use Cardiac resuscitation when epinephrine fails to improve myocardial contractions, cardiac disturbances of hyperkalemia, hypocalcemia, or calcium channel blocking agent toxicity; emergent treatment of hypocalcemic tetany, treatment of hypermagnesemia
Usual Dosage Note: Calcium chloride is 3 times as potent as calcium gluconate
Cardiac arrest in the presence of hyperkalemia or hypocalcemia, magnesium toxicity, or calcium antagonist toxicity: I.V.:
Children: 20 mg/kg; may repeat in 10 minutes if necessary
Adults: 2-4 mg/kg (10% solution), repeated every 10 minutes
Hypocalcemia: I.V.:
Children: 10-20 mg/kg/dose (children: 1-7 mEq), repeat every 4-6 hours if needed; doses may be repeated every 1-3 days if needed
Adults: 500 mg to 1 g (7-14 mEq), repeated at 1- to 3-day intervals if necessary
Hypocalcemic tetany: I.V.:
Children: 10 mg/kg (0.5-0.7 mEq/kg) over 5-10 minutes; may repeat after 6-8 hours or follow with an infusion with a maximum dose of 200 mg/kg/day
Adults: 4.5-16 mEq may be administered until response occurs
Hypocalcemia secondary to citrated blood transfusion give 0.45 mEq **elemental** calcium for each 100 mL citrated blood infused
Mechanism of Action Moderates nerve and muscle performance via action potential excitation threshold regulation
Local Anesthetic/Vasoconstrictor Precautions No information available to require special precautions
Effects on Dental Treatment No effects or complications reported
Other Adverse Effects <1%:
Cardiovascular: Vasodilation, hypotension, bradycardia, cardiac arrhythmias, ventricular fibrillation, syncope
Central nervous system: Lethargy, coma, mania
Dermatologic: Erythema
Endocrine & metabolic: Decreased serum magnesium, hypercalcemia
Hematologic: Elevated serum amylase
(Continued)

141

Calcium Chloride *(Continued)*

Local: Tissue necrosis
Neuromuscular & skeletal: Muscle weakness
Renal: Hypercalciuria

Drug Interactions
Decreased effect:
Calcium may antagonize the effects of calcium channel blockers
May decrease the bioavailability of tetracyclines
Renders tetracycline antibiotics inactive
Increased toxicity: Administer cautiously to a digitalized patient, may precipitate arrhythmias

Drug Uptake
Absorption: I.V. calcium salts are absorbed directly into the bloodstream

Pregnancy Risk Factor C

Calcium Citrate *(kal' see um si' trate)*

Brand Names Citracal® [OTC]

Therapeutic Category Calcium Salt

Use Adjunct in prevention of postmenopausal osteoporosis; treatment and prevention of calcium depletion

Usual Dosage Dosage is in terms of elemental calcium
Recommended daily allowance (RDA):
<6 months: 360 mg/day
6-12 months: 540 mg/day
1-10 years: 800 mg/day
10-18 years: 1200 mg/day
Adults: 800 mg/day
Adults: Oral: 1-2 g/day

Mechanism of Action Moderates nerve and muscle performance via action potential excitation threshold regulation

Local Anesthetic/Vasoconstrictor Precautions No information available to require special precautions

Effects on Dental Treatment No effects or complications reported

Other Adverse Effects <1%:
Central nervous system: Mental confusion, headache
Endocrine & metabolic: Hypercalcemia, milk-alkali syndrome, hypophosphatemia
Gastrointestinal: Constipation, vomiting, nausea

Drug Interactions
Decreased effect:
Calcium may antagonize the effects of calcium channel blockers
May decrease the bioavailability of tetracyclines
Renders tetracycline antibiotics inactive
Increased toxicity: Administer cautiously to a digitalized patient, may precipitate arrhythmias

Drug Uptake
Absorption: Absorption from the GI tract requires vitamin D

Pregnancy Risk Factor C

Calcium Glubionate *(kal' see um gloo bye' oh nate)*

Brand Names Neo-Calglucon® [OTC]

Therapeutic Category Calcium Salt

Use Adjunct in prevention of postmenopausal osteoporosis; treatment and prevention of calcium depletion

Usual Dosage Oral:
Recommended daily allowance (RDA) (in terms of elemental calcium):
<6 months: 360 mg/day
6-12 months: 540 mg/day
1-10 years: 800 mg/day
10-18 years: 1200 mg/day
Adults: 800 mg/day

Syrup is a hyperosmolar solution; dosage is in terms of calcium glubionate
Neonatal hypocalcemia: 1200 mg/kg/day in 4-6 divided doses
Maintenance: Children: 600-2000 mg/kg/day in 4 divided doses up to a maximum of 9 g/day

Adults: 6-18 g/day in divided doses

Mechanism of Action Moderates nerve and muscle performance via action potential excitation threshold regulation

Local Anesthetic/Vasoconstrictor Precautions No information available to require special precautions

Effects on Dental Treatment No effects or complications reported

Other Adverse Effects <1%:

Central nervous system: Dizziness, headache, mental confusion

Endocrine & metabolic: Hypercalcemia, hypomagnesemia, hypophosphatemia, milk-alkali syndrome

Gastrointestinal: GI irritation, diarrhea, constipation, dry mouth

Renal: Hypercalciuria

Drug Interactions

Decreased effect:

Calcium may antagonize the effects of calcium channel blockers

May decrease the bioavailability of tetracyclines

Renders tetracycline antibiotics inactive

Increased toxicity: Administer cautiously to a digitalized patient, may precipitate arrhythmias

Drug Uptake

Absorption: Absorption from the GI tract requires vitamin D

Pregnancy Risk Factor C

Calcium Gluceptate (kal′ see um gloo sep′ tate)

Therapeutic Category Calcium Salt

Use Treatment of cardiac disturbances of hyperkalemia, hypocalcemia, or calcium channel blocker toxicity; cardiac resuscitation when epinephrine fails to improve myocardial contractions; treatment of hypermagnesemia and hypocalcemia

Usual Dosage I.V. (dose expressed in mg of calcium gluceptate):

Cardiac resuscitation in the presence of hypocalcemia, hyperkalemia, magnesium toxicity, or calcium channel blocker toxicity:

Children: 110 mg/kg/dose

Adults: 1.1-1.5 g (5-7 mL)

Hypocalcemia:

Children: 200-500 mg/kg/day divided every 6 hours

Adults: 500 mg to 1.1 g/dose as needed

After citrated blood administration: Children and Adults: 0.4 mEq/100 mL blood infused

Mechanism of Action Moderates nerve and muscle performance via action potential excitation threshold regulation

Local Anesthetic/Vasoconstrictor Precautions No information available to require special precautions

Effects on Dental Treatment No effects or complications reported

Other Adverse Effects <1%:

Cardiovascular: Vasodilation, hypotension, bradycardia, cardiac arrhythmias, ventricular fibrillation, syncope, coma

Central nervous system: Lethargy, mania

Dermatologic: Erythema

Endocrine & metabolic: Hypomagnesemia, hypercalcemia

Hematologic: Elevated serum amylase

Local: Tissue necrosis

Neuromuscular & skeletal: Muscle weakness

Renal: Hypercalciuria

Drug Interactions

Decreased effect:

Calcium may antagonize the effects of calcium channel blockers

May decrease the bioavailability of tetracyclines

Renders tetracycline antibiotics inactive

Increased toxicity: Administer cautiously to digitalized patients, may precipitate arrhythmias

Drug Uptake

Absorption: I.M. and I.V. calcium salts are absorbed directly into the bloodstream

Pregnancy Risk Factor C

Calcium Gluconate (kal′ see um gloo′ koe nate)

Brand Names Kalcinate®

Therapeutic Category Calcium Salt

Use Treatment and prevention of hypocalcemia; treatment of tetany, cardiac disturbances of hyperkalemia, cardiac resuscitation when epinephrine fails to improve myocardial contractions, hypocalcemia, or calcium channel blocker toxicity; calcium supplementation

Usual Dosage Dosage is in terms of **elemental** calcium

(Continued)

Calcium Gluconate *(Continued)*

Recommended daily allowance (RDA):
  <6 months: 400 mg/day
  6-12 months: 600 mg/day
  1-10 years: 800 mg/day
  10-18 years: 1200 mg/day
  Adults: 800 mg/day
Calcium gluconate electrolyte requirement in newborn period:
  Premature: 200-1000 mg/kg/24 hours
  Term:
    0-24 hours: 0-500 mg/kg/24 hours
    24-48 hours: 200-500 mg/kg/24 hours
    48-72 hours: 200-600 mg/kg/24 hours
    >3 days: 200-800 mg/kg/24 hours
Hypocalcemia:
  Oral:
    Children: 200-500 mg/kg/day divided every 6 hours
    Adults: 500 mg to 2 g 2-4 times/day
  I.V.:
    Children: 200-500 mg/kg/day (children 1-7 mEq/day) as a continuous infusion or in 4 divided doses; doses may be repeated every 1-3 days if necessary
    Adults: 2-15 g/24 hours as a continuous infusion or in divided doses, which may be repeated every 1-3 days if necessary
Hypocalcemic tetany: I.V.:
  Children: 100-200 mg/kg/dose (0.5-0.7 mEq/kg/dose) over 5-10 minutes; may repeat every 6-8 hours **or** follow with an infusion of 500 mg/kg/day
  Adults: 1-3 g (4.5-16 mEq) may be administered until therapeutic response occurs
Osteoporosis/bone loss: Oral: 1000-1500 mg in divided doses/day
Calcium antagonist toxicity, magnesium intoxication, or cardiac arrest in the presence of hyperkalemia or hypocalcemia: I.V.:
  Children: Calcium chloride is recommended calcium salt; refer to calcium chloride monograph
  Adults: 5-8 mL/dose and repeated as necessary at 10-minute intervals, however, calcium chloride is recommended calcium salt; refer to Calcium Chloride monograph
Hypocalcemia secondary to citrated blood infusion: I.V.: Give 0.45 mEq **elemental** calcium for each 100 mL citrated blood infused
Exchange transfusion:
  Adults: 300 mg/100 mL of citrated blood exchanged
Maintenance electrolyte requirements for total parenteral nutrition: I.V.: Daily requirements: Adults: 8-16 mEq/1000 kcals/24 hours
Mechanism of Action Moderates nerve and muscle performance via action potential excitation threshold regulation
Local Anesthetic/Vasoconstrictor Precautions No information available to require special precautions
Effects on Dental Treatment No effects or complications reported
Other Adverse Effects <1%:
  Cardiovascular: Vasodilation, hypotension, bradycardia, cardiac arrhythmias, ventricular fibrillation, syncope, coma
  Central nervous system: Lethargy, mania
  Endocrine & metabolic: Decrease serum magnesium, hypercalcemia
  Hematologic: Erythema, elevated serum amylase
  Local: Tissue necrosis
  Neuromuscular & skeletal: Muscle weakness
  Renal: Hypercalciuria
Drug Interactions
  Decreased effect:
    Calcium may antagonize the effects of calcium channel blockers
    May decrease the bioavailability of tetracyclines
    Renders tetracycline antibiotics inactive
  Increased toxicity: Administer cautiously to a digitalized patient, may precipitate arrhythmias
Drug Uptake
  Absorption: I.M. and I.V. calcium salts are absorbed directly into the bloodstream; absorption from the GI tract requires vitamin D; calcium is absorbed in soluble, ionized form; solubility of calcium is increased in an acid environment (except calcium lactate)
Pregnancy Risk Factor C

Calcium Lactate (kal' see um lak' tate)

Therapeutic Category Calcium Salt

Use Adjunct in prevention of postmenopausal osteoporosis; treatment and prevention of calcium depletion

Usual Dosage Oral (in terms of calcium lactate)

Recommended daily allowance (RDA) (in terms of elemental calcium):

<6 months: 360 mg/day

6-12 months: 540 mg/day

1-10 years: 800 mg/day

10-18 years: 1200 mg/day

Adults: 800 mg/day

Children: 500 mg/kg/day divided every 6-8 hours

Maximum daily dose: 9 g

Adults: 1.5-3 g divided every 8 hours

Mechanism of Action Moderates nerve and muscle performance via action potential excitation threshold regulation

Local Anesthetic/Vasoconstrictor Precautions No information available to require special precautions

Effects on Dental Treatment No effects or complications reported

Other Adverse Effects <1%:

Central nervous system: Headache, mental confusion, dizziness

Endocrine & metabolic: Hypercalcemia, hypophosphatemia, hypomagnesemia, milk-alkali syndrome

Gastrointestinal: Constipation, nausea, dry mouth, vomiting

Renal: Hypercalciuria

Drug Interactions

Decreased effect:

Calcium may antagonize the effects of calcium channel blockers

May decrease the bioavailability of tetracyclines

Renders tetracycline antibiotics inactive

Increased toxicity: Administer cautiously to a digitalized patient, may precipitate arrhythmias

Drug Uptake

Absorption: Absorption from the GI tract requires vitamin D

Pregnancy Risk Factor C

Calcium Leucovorin see Leucovorin Calcium on page 491

Calcium Pantothenate see Pantothenic Acid on page 658

Calcium Phosphate, Tribasic (kal' see um fos' fate tri bay' sik)

Brand Names Posture® [OTC]

Therapeutic Category Calcium Salt

Use Adjunct in prevention of postmenopausal osteoporosis; treatment and prevention of calcium depletion

Usual Dosage Oral (all doses in terms of elemental calcium):

Recommended daily allowance (RDA) (elemental calcium):

<6 months: 360 mg/day

6-12 months: 540 mg/day

1-10 years: 800 mg/day

10-18 years: 1200 mg/day

Adults: 800 mg/day

Children: 45-65 mg/kg/day

Adults: 1-2 g/day

Mechanism of Action Moderates nerve and muscle performance via action potential excitation threshold regulation

Local Anesthetic/Vasoconstrictor Precautions No information available to require special precautions

Effects on Dental Treatment No effects or complications reported

Other Adverse Effects <1%:

Endocrine & metabolic: Hypercalcemia, milk-alkali syndrome, hypophosphatemia

Gastrointestinal: Constipation, nausea, dry mouth

Drug Interactions

Decreased effect:

Calcium may antagonize the effects of calcium channel blockers

May decrease the bioavailability of tetracyclines

Renders tetracycline antibiotics inactive

Increased toxicity: Administer cautiously to a digitalized patient, may precipitate arrhythmias

Pregnancy Risk Factor C

Calcium Polycarbophil (kal' see um pol i kar' boe fil)
Brand Names Equalactin® Chewable Tablet [OTC]; Fiberall® Chewable Tablet [OTC]; FiberCon® Tablet [OTC]; Fiber-Lax® Tablet [OTC]; Mitrolan® Chewable Tablet [OTC]

Therapeutic Category Antidiarrheal; Laxative, Bulk-Producing

Use Treatment of constipation or diarrhea; calcium polycarbophil is supplied as the approved substitute whenever a bulk-forming laxative is ordered in a tablet, capsule, wafer, or other oral solid dosage form

Usual Dosage Oral:

Children:

2-6 years: 500 mg (1 tablet) 1-2 times/day, up to 1.5 g/day

6-12 years: 500 mg (1 tablet) 1-3 times/day, up to 3 g/day

Adults: 1 g 4 times/day, up to 6 g/day

Mechanism of Action Restoring a more normal moisture level and providing bulk in the patient's intestinal tract

Local Anesthetic/Vasoconstrictor Precautions No information available to require special precautions

Effects on Dental Treatment Oral medication should be given at least 1 hour prior to taking the bulk-producing laxative in order to prevent decreased absorption of medication

Other Adverse Effects 1% to 10%: Abdominal fullness

Drug Interactions Decreased absorption of oral anticoagulants, digoxin, potassium-sparing diuretics, salicylates, tetracyclines

Pregnancy Risk Factor C

Calderol® see Calcifediol on page 137

Caldesene® Topical [OTC] see Undecylenic Acid and Derivatives on page 884

Calm-X® [OTC] see Dimenhydrinate on page 286

Cal Plus® see Calcium Chloride on page 141

CalSup® [OTC] see Calcium Carbonate on page 140

Caltrate® [OTC] see Calcium Carbonate on page 140

Cam-ap-es® see Hydralazine, Hydrochlorothiazide, and Reserpine on page 429

Campho-Phenique® [OTC] see Camphor and Phenol on this page

Camphor and Phenol (kam' for & fee' nole)
Brand Names Campho-Phenique® [OTC]

Therapeutic Category Topical Skin Product

Use Relief of pain and for minor infections

Local Anesthetic/Vasoconstrictor Precautions No information available to require special precautions

Effects on Dental Treatment No effects or complications reported

Camphor, Menthol, and Phenol (kam' for, men' thol, & fee' nole)
Brand Names Sarna [OTC]

Therapeutic Category Topical Skin Product

Use Relief of dry, itching skin

Local Anesthetic/Vasoconstrictor Precautions No information available to require special precautions

Effects on Dental Treatment No effects or complications reported

Other Adverse Effects 1% to 10%: Burning sensation, especially on broken skin

Camptosar® see Irinotecan on page 468

Cancer Chemotherapy Regimens see page 1011

Cankaid® [OTC] see Carbamide Peroxide on page 152

Cantharidin (kan thar' e din)
Brand Names Verr-Canth™

Therapeutic Category Keratolytic Agent

Use Removal of ordinary and periungual warts

Local Anesthetic/Vasoconstrictor Precautions No information available to require special precautions

Effects on Dental Treatment No effects or complications reported

Cantil® see Mepenzolate Bromide on page 538

Capastat® Sulfate see Capreomycin Sulfate on next page

Capital® and Codeine see Acetaminophen and Codeine on page 15

Capitrol® see Chloroxine on page 189

Capoten® see Captopril on page 148

Capozide® see Captopril and Hydrochlorothiazide on page 149

Capreomycin Sulfate (kap ree oh mye' sin sul' fate)
Related Information
Nonviral Infectious Diseases *on page 932*
Brand Names Capastat® Sulfate
Therapeutic Category Antibiotic, Miscellaneous; Antitubercular Agent
Use Treatment of tuberculosis in conjunction with at least one other anti-tuberculosis agent
Usual Dosage I.M.:
Children: 15-20 mg/kg/day, up to 1 g/day maximum
Adults: 15-30 mg/kg/day up to 1 g/day for 60-120 days, followed by 1 g 2-3 times/week
Mechanism of Action Capreomycin is a cyclic polypeptide antimicrobial. It is administered as a mixture of capreomycin IA and capreomycin IB. The mechanism of action of capreomycin is not well understood. Mycobacterial species that have become resistant to other agents are usually still sensitive to the action of capreomycin. However, significant cross-resistance with viomycin, kanamycin, and neomycin occurs.
Local Anesthetic/Vasoconstrictor Precautions No information available to require special precautions
Effects on Dental Treatment No effects or complications reported
Other Adverse Effects
>10%:
Otic: Ototoxicity
Renal: Nephrotoxicity
1% to 10%: Hematologic: Eosinophilia
<1%:
Central nervous system: Vertigo, fever, rash
Hematologic: Leukocytosis, thrombocytopenia
Local: Pain, induration, bleeding at injection site
Otic: Tinnitus
Drug Interactions Additive nephrotoxicity and ototoxicity with other aminoglycosides such as streptomycin
Drug Uptake
Absorption: Oral: Poor absorption necessitates parenteral administration
Serum half-life: Dependent upon renal function and varies with creatinine clearance; 4-6 hours
Time to peak serum concentration: I.M.: Within 1 hour
Pregnancy Risk Factor C

Capsaicin (kap say' sin)
Brand Names Zostrix®-HP [OTC]; Zostrix® [OTC]
Therapeutic Category Analgesic, Topical; Topical Skin Product
Use FDA approved for the topical treatment of pain associated with postherpetic neuralgia, rheumatoid arthritis, osteoarthritis, diabetic neuropathy, and post-surgical pain.

Unlabeled uses: Treatment of pain associated with psoriasis, chronic neuralgias unresponsive to other forms of therapy, and intractable pruritus
Usual Dosage Children ≥2 years and Adults: Topical: Apply to affected area at least 3-4 times/day; application frequency less than 3-4 times/day prevents the total depletion, inhibition of synthesis, and transport of substance P resulting in decreased clinical efficacy and increased local discomfort
Mechanism of Action Induces release of substance P, the principal chemomediator of pain impulses from the periphery to the CNS, from peripheral sensory neurons; after repeated application, capsaicin depletes the neuron of substance P and prevents reaccumulation
Local Anesthetic/Vasoconstrictor Precautions No information available to require special precautions
Effects on Dental Treatment No effects or complications reported
Other Adverse Effects
>10%: Local: ≥30%: Transient burning on application which usually diminishes with repeated use
1% to 10%:
Local: Itching, stinging sensation, erythema
Respiratory: Cough
Drug Interactions No data reported
Drug Uptake Data following the use of topical capsaicin in humans are lacking
Onset of action: Pain relief is usually seen within 14-28 days of regular topical application; maximal response may require 4-6 weeks of continuous therapy
Duration: Several hours
(Continued)

Capsaicin *(Continued)*
Pregnancy Risk Factor C

Captopril *(kap′ toe pril)*
Related Information
Cardiovascular Diseases *on page 912*
Brand Names Capoten®
Canadian/Mexican Brand Names Apo-Capto® (Canada); Novo-Captopril®
(Canada); Nu-Capto® (Canada); Syn-Captopril® (Canada); Capotena®
(Mexico); Capital® (Mexico); Cardipril® (Mexico); Cryopril® (Mexico);
Ecapresan® (Mexico); Ecaten® (Mexico); Kenolan® (Mexico); Lenpryl®
(Mexico); Precaptil® (Mexico)
Therapeutic Category Angiotensin-Converting Enzyme (ACE) Inhibitors
Use Management of hypertension and treatment of congestive heart failure

Unlabeled use: Hypertensive crisis, diabetic nephropathy, rheumatoid
arthritis, diagnosis of anatomic renal artery stenosis, hypertension secondary
to scleroderma renal crisis, diagnosis of aldosteronism, idiopathic edema,
Bartter's syndrome, postmyocardial infarction for prevention of ventricular
failure; increase circulation in Raynaud's phenomenon
Usual Dosage Note: Dosage must be titrated according to patient's response;
use lowest effective dose. Oral:
Children: Initial: 0.5 mg/kg/dose; titrate upward to maximum of 6 mg/kg/day in
2-4 divided doses
Older Children: Initial: 6.25-12.5 mg/dose every 12-24 hours; titrate upward to
maximum of 6 mg/kg/day
Adolescents: Initial: 12.5-25 mg/dose given every 8-12 hours; increase by 25
mg/dose to maximum of 450 mg/day
Adults:
Hypertension:
Initial dose: 12.5-25 mg 2-3 times/day; may increase by 12.5-25 mg/dose
at 1- to 2-week intervals up to 50 mg 3 times/day; add diuretic before
further dosage increases
Maximum dose: 150 mg 3 times/day
Congestive heart failure:
Initial dose: 6.25-12.5 mg 3 times/day in conjunction with cardiac glycoside
and diuretic therapy; initial dose depends upon patient's fluid/electrolyte
status
Target dose: 50 mg 3 times/day
Maximum dose: 100 mg 3 times/day
Mechanism of Action Competitive inhibitor of angiotensin-converting enzyme
(ACE); prevents conversion of angiotensin I to angiotensin II, a potent vaso-
constrictor; results in lower levels of angiotensin II which causes an increase in
plasma renin activity and a reduction in aldosterone secretion
Local Anesthetic/Vasoconstrictor Precautions No information available to
require special precautions
Effects on Dental Treatment No effects or complications reported

Drug-Drug Interactions With ACEIs

Precipitant Drug	Drug (Category) and Effect	Description
Antacids	ACE Inhibitors: decreased	Decreased bioavailability of ACEIs. May be more likely with captopril. Separate administration times by 1-2 hours.
NSAIDs (indomethacin)	ACEIs: decreased	Reduced hypotensive effects of ACEIs. More prominent in low renin or volume dependent hypertensive patients.
Phenothiazines	ACEIs: increased	Pharmacologic effects of ACEIs may be increased.
ACEIs	Allopurinol: increased	Higher risk of hypersensitivity reaction possible when given concurrently. Three case reports of Stevens-Johnson syndrome with captopril.
ACEIs	Digoxin: increased	Increased plasma digoxin levels.
ACEIs	Lithium: increased	Increased serum lithium levels and symptoms of toxicity may occur.
ACEIs	Potassium preps/ potassium sparing diuretics increased	Coadministration may result in elevated potassium levels.

Other Adverse Effects
1% to 10%:
Cardiovascular: Tachycardia, chest pain, palpitations
Central nervous system: Insomnia, headache, dizziness, fatigue, malaise
Dermatologic: Rash, pruritus, alopecia
Gastrointestinal: Abdominal pain, vomiting, nausea, diarrhea, anorexia, constipation, dysgeusia
Neuromuscular & skeletal: Paresthesias
Renal: Oliguria
Respiratory: Transient cough
<1%:
Cardiovascular: Hypotension
Dermatologic: Angioedema
Endocrine & metabolic: Hyperkalemia
Hematologic: Neutropenia, agranulocytosis
Renal: Proteinuria, increased BUN, serum creatinine
Miscellaneous: Loss of taste perception

Drug Interactions
Increased toxicity:
Probenecid increases blood levels of captopril
Captopril and diuretics have additive hypotensive effects; see table.
Increased serum lithium levels and symptoms of lithium toxicity have been reported in patients receiving concomitant lithium and ACE inhibitor therapy. These drugs should be coadministered with caution.

Drug Uptake
Onset of effect: Maximal decrease in blood pressure 1-1.5 hours after dose
Duration: Dose related, may require several weeks of therapy before full hypotensive effect is seen
Absorption: Oral: 60% to 75%
Serum half-life (dependent upon renal and cardiac function):
Adults, normal: 1.9 hours
Congestive heart failure: 2.06 hours
Anuria: 20-40 hours
Time to peak: Within 1-2 hours

Pregnancy Risk Factor D

Captopril and Hydrochlorothiazide
(kap' toe pril & hye droe klor oh thye' a zide)

Related Information
Cardiovascular Diseases on page 912

Brand Names Capozide®

Therapeutic Category Antihypertensive Agent, Combination

Use Management of hypertension and treatment of congestive heart failure

Usual Dosage Adults: Oral:
Hypertension: Initial: 25 mg 2-3 times/day; may increase at 1- to 2-week intervals up to 150 mg 3 times/day (captopril dosages)

Congestive heart failure: 6.25-25 mg 3 times/day (maximum: 450 mg/day) (captopril dosages)

Mechanism of Action Captopril is a competitive inhibitor of angiotensin-converting enzyme (ACE); prevents conversion of angiotensin I to angiotensin II, a potent vasoconstrictor. This results in lower levels of angiotensin II which causes an increase in plasma renin activity and a reduction in aldosterone secretion. Hydrochlorothiazide inhibits sodium reabsorption in the distal tubules causing increased excretion of sodium and water as well as potassium and hydrogen ions.

Local Anesthetic/Vasoconstrictor Precautions No information available to require special precautions

Effects on Dental Treatment No effects or complications reported

Other Adverse Effects
Captopril:
1% to 10%:
Cardiovascular: Tachycardia, chest pain, palpitations
Central nervous system: Insomnia, headache, dizziness, fatigue, malaise
Dermatologic: Rash, pruritus, alopecia
Gastrointestinal: Abdominal pain, vomiting, nausea, diarrhea, anorexia, constipation, dysgeusia
Neuromuscular & skeletal: Paresthesias
Renal: Oliguria
Respiratory: Transient cough
<1%:
Cardiovascular: Hypotension
(Continued)

149

Captopril and Hydrochlorothiazide *(Continued)*

    Dermatologic: Angioedema
    Endocrine & metabolic: Hyperkalemia
    Hematologic: Neutropenia, agranulocytosis
    Renal: Proteinuria, increased BUN, serum creatinine
    Miscellaneous: Loss of taste perception
  Hydrochlorothiazide:
    1% to 10%: Endocrine & metabolic: Hypokalemia
    <1%:
      Cardiovascular: Hypotension
      Dermatologic: Photosensitivity
      Endocrine & metabolic: Fluid and electrolyte imbalances (hypocalcemia, hypomagnesemia, hyponatremia), hyperglycemia
      Hematologic: Rarely blood dyscrasias
      Renal: Prerenal azotemia
Contraindications Hypersensitivity to captopril, hydrochlorothiazide or any component
Drug Interactions Probenecid increases blood levels of captopril. Increased serum lithium levels and symptoms of lithium toxicity have been reported in patients receiving concomitant lithium and ACE inhibitor therapy. Hydrochlorothiazide decreases antidiabetic drug efficacy. Hydrochlorothiazide has been reported to increase digoxin-related cardiac arrhythmias
Pregnancy Risk Factor C
Dosage Forms Tablet:
  25/15: Captopril 25 mg and hydrochlorothiazide 15 mg
  25/25: Captopril 25 mg and hydrochlorothiazide 25 mg
  50/15: Captopril 50 mg and hydrochlorothiazide 15 mg
  50/25: Captopril 50 mg and hydrochlorothiazide 25 mg
Generic Available No

Carafate® *see Sucralfate on page 804*

Caramiphen and Phenylpropanolamine
  (kar am′ i fen & fen il proe pa nole′ a meen)
Brand Names Ordrine AT® Extended Release Capsule; Rescaps-D® S.R. Capsule; Tuss-Allergine® Modified T.D. Capsule; Tuss-Genade® Modified Capsule; Tussogest® Extended Release Capsule; Tuss-Ornade® Liquid; Tuss-Ornade® Spansule®
Therapeutic Category Antihistamine/Decongestant Combination
Synonyms Phenylpropanolamine and Caramiphen
Use Symptomatic relief of cough and nasal congestion associated with the common cold
Local Anesthetic/Vasoconstrictor Precautions Use with caution since phenylpropanolamine is a sympathomimetic amine which could interact with epinephrine to cause a pressor response
Effects on Dental Treatment Up to 10% of patients could experience tachycardia, palpitations, and dry mouth; use vasoconstrictor with caution

Carampicillin Hydrochloride *see Bacampicillin Hydrochloride on page 92*

Carbachol (kar′ ba kole)
Brand Names Isopto® Carbachol; Miostat®
Therapeutic Category Antiglaucoma Agent; Cholinergic Agent, Ophthalmic; Ophthalmic Agent, Miotic
Use Lowers intraocular pressure in the treatment of glaucoma; cause miosis during surgery
Usual Dosage Adults:
  Ophthalmic: Instill 1-2 drops up to 3 times/day
  Intraocular: 0.5 mL instilled into anterior chamber before or after securing sutures
Mechanism of Action Synthetic direct-acting cholinergic agent that causes miosis by stimulating muscarinic receptors in the eye
Local Anesthetic/Vasoconstrictor Precautions No information available to require special precautions
Effects on Dental Treatment Ophthalmic use of carbachol has no effect on dental treatment
Other Adverse Effects
  1% to 10%: Ocular: Blurred vision, eye pain
  <1%:
    Cardiovascular: Transient fall in blood pressure
    Central nervous system: Headache

Gastrointestinal: Stomach cramps, diarrhea
Local: Ciliary spasm with temporary decrease of visual acuity
Ocular: Corneal clouding, persistent bullous keratopathy, postoperative keratitis, retinal detachment, transient ciliary and conjunctival injection
Respiratory: Asthma
Miscellaneous: Increased peristalsis

Drug Interactions No data reported

Drug Uptake
Ophthalmic instillation:
Onset of miosis: 10-20 minutes
Duration of reduction in intraocular pressure: 4-8 hours
Intraocular administration:
Onset of miosis: Within 2-5 minutes
Duration: 24 hours

Pregnancy Risk Factor C

Carbamazepine (kar ba maz' e peen)

Related Information
Dental Drug Interactions: Update on Drug Combinations Requiring Special Considerations *on page 1022*

Brand Names Epitol®; Tegretol®; Tegretol-XR®

Canadian/Mexican Brand Names Apo-Carbamazepine® (Canada); Mazepine® (Canada); Novo-Carbamaz® (Canada); Nu-Carbamazepine® (Canada); PMS-Carbamazepine® (Canada); Carbazep® (Mexico); Carbazina® (Mexico); Neugeron® (Mexico)

Therapeutic Category Anticonvulsant, Miscellaneous

Use
Dental: Used to relieve pain in trigeminal neuralgia
Medical: Prophylaxis of generalized tonic-clonic, partial (especially complex partial), and mixed partial or generalized seizure disorder

Unlabeled use: Treat bipolar disorders and other affective disorders; resistant schizophrenia, alcohol withdrawal, restless leg syndrome, and psychotic behavior associated with dementia; may be used to relieve pain in trigeminal neuralgia or diabetic neuropathy

Usual Dosage Oral (dosage must be adjusted according to patient's response and serum concentrations):
Children >12 years and Adults: 200 mg twice daily to start, increase by 200 mg/day at weekly intervals until therapeutic levels achieved; usual dose: 800-1200 mg/day in 3-4 divided doses; some patients have required up to 1.6-2.4 g/day; extended release tablet: 200 mg twice daily for epilepsy, initial dose: 100 mg for trigeminal neuralgia
Children <12 years: Not used in children for trigeminal neuralgia

Mechanism of Action In addition to anticonvulsant effects, carbamazepine has anticholinergic, antineuralgic, antidiuretic, muscle relaxant and antiarrhythmic properties; may depress activity in the nucleus ventralis of the thalamus or decrease synaptic transmission or decrease summation of temporal stimulation leading to neural discharge by limiting influx of sodium ions across cell membrane or other unknown mechanisms; stimulates the release of ADH and potentiates its action in promoting reabsorption of water; chemically related to tricyclic antidepressants

Local Anesthetic/Vasoconstrictor Precautions No information available to require special precautions

Effects on Dental Treatment No effects or complications reported

Other Adverse Effects
Dermatologic: Rash; but does not necessarily mean the drug should be stopped
>10%:
Central nervous system: Sedation, dizziness, fatigue, slurred speech, ataxia, clumsiness, confusion
Gastrointestinal: Nausea, vomiting
Ocular: Blurred vision, nystagmus

Oral manifestations: Sore throat, mouth ulcers

Contraindications Hypersensitivity to carbamazepine or any component; may have cross-sensitivity with tricyclic antidepressants; should not be used in any patient with bone marrow depression, or taking MAO inhibitors

Warnings/Precautions MAO inhibitors should be discontinued for a minimum of 14 days before carbamazepine is begun; administer with caution to patients with history of cardiac damage or hepatic disease; potentially fatal blood cell abnormalities have been reported following treatment; early detection of hematologic change is important; advise patients of early signs and symptoms
(Continued)

Carbamazepine *(Continued)*

including fever, sore throat, mouth ulcers, infections, easy bruising, petechial or purpuric hemorrhage; carbamazepine is not effective in absence, myoclonic or akinetic seizures; exacerbation of certain seizure types have been seen after initiation of carbamazepine therapy in children with mixed seizure disorders. Elderly may have increased risk of SIADH-like syndrome.

Drug Interactions Carbamazepine may induce the metabolism of warfarin, cyclosporine, doxycycline, oral contraceptives, phenytoin, theophylline, benzodiazepines, ethosuximide, valproic acid, corticosteroids, and thyroid hormones; erythromycin, isoniazid, propoxyphene, verapamil, danazol, isoniazid, diltiazem, and cimetidine may inhibit hepatic metabolism of carbamazepine with resultant increase of carbamazepine serum concentrations and toxicity

Drug Uptake

Absorption: Slowly absorbed from GI tract

Time to peak serum concentration: Unpredictable, within 4-8 hours

Serum half-life:

Initial: 18-55 hours

Multiple dosing:

Adults: 12-17 hours

Children: 8-14 hours

Pregnancy Risk Factor C

Breast-feeding Considerations May be taken while breast-feeding

Dosage Forms

Suspension, oral (citrus-vanilla flavor): 100 mg/5 mL (450 mL)

Tablet: 200 mg

Tablet, chewable: 100 mg

Tablet, extended release: 100 mg, 200 mg, 400 mg

Dietary Considerations Any food increases absorption

Generic Available Yes: Tablet

Carbamide Peroxide *(kar′ ba mide per ox′ ide)*

Related Information

Oral Rinse Products *on page 1067*

Brand Names Auro® Ear Drops [OTC]; Cankaid® [OTC]; Debrox® [OTC]; ERO Ear® [OTC]; Gly-Oxide® [OTC]; Murine® Ear Drops [OTC]; Orajel® Brace-Aid Rinse [OTC]; Proxigel® [OTC]

Canadian/Mexican Brand Names Clamurid® (Canada)

Therapeutic Category Anti-infective Agent, Oral; Otic Agent, Cerumenolytic

Use Relief of minor swelling of gums, oral mucosal surfaces, and lips including canker sores and dental irritation; emulsify and disperse ear wax

Usual Dosage Children and Adults:

Gel: Gently massage on affected area 4 times/day; do not drink or rinse mouth for 5 minutes after use

Oral solution (should not be used for >7 days): Oral preparation should not be used in children <3 years of age; apply several drops undiluted on affected area 4 times/day after meals and at bedtime; expectorate after 2-3 minutes **or** place 10 drops onto tongue, mix with saliva, swish for several minutes, expectorate

Otic solution (should not be used for >4 days): Tilt head sideways and instill 5-10 drops twice daily up to 4 days, tip of applicator should not enter ear canal; keep drops in ear for several minutes by keeping head tilted and placing cotton in ear

Mechanism of Action Carbamide peroxide releases hydrogen peroxide which serves as a source of nascent oxygen upon contact with catalase; deodorant action is probably due to inhibition of odor-causing bacteria; softens impacted cerumen due to its foaming action

Local Anesthetic/Vasoconstrictor Precautions No information available to require special precautions

Effects on Dental Treatment No effects or complications reported

Other Adverse Effects 1% to 10%: Local: Rash, irritation, superinfections, redness

Drug Interactions No data reported

Pregnancy Risk Factor C

Carbenicilina, Disodica (Mexico) *see* Carbenicillin *on next page*

Carbenicillin (kar ben i sil' in)
Brand Names Geocillin®
Canadian/Mexican Brand Names Geopen® (Canada); Carbecin® Inyectable (Mexico)
Therapeutic Category Antibiotic, Penicillin
Synonyms Carbenicilina, Disodica (Mexico)
Use Treatment of serious urinary tract infections and prostatitis caused by susceptible gram-negative aerobic bacilli or mixed aerobic-anaerobic bacterial infections excluding those secondary to *Klebsiella* sp and *Serratia marcescens*
Usual Dosage Oral:
Children: 30-50 mg/kg/day divided every 6 hours; maximum dose: 2-3 g/day

Adults: 1-2 tablets every 6 hours for urinary tract infections or 2 tablets every 6 hours for prostatitis
Mechanism of Action Interferes with bacterial cell wall synthesis during active multiplication
Local Anesthetic/Vasoconstrictor Precautions No information available to require special precautions
Effects on Dental Treatment Prolonged use of penicillins may lead to development of oral candidiasis
Other Adverse Effects
>10%: Gastrointestinal: Diarrhea
1% to 10%: Gastrointestinal: Nausea, bad taste, vomiting, flatulence, glossitis
<1%:
Central nervous system: Headache, hyperthermia
Dermatologic: Skin rash, urticaria
Endocrine & metabolic: Hypokalemia
Genitourinary: Vaginitis
Hematologic: Anemia, thrombocytopenia, leukopenia, neutropenia, eosinophilia
Hepatic: Elevated LFTs
Local: Thrombophlebitis
Ocular: Itchy eyes
Renal: Hematuria
Miscellaneous: Furry tongue
Drug Interactions
Decreased effect with administration of aminoglycosides within 1 hour; may inactivate both drugs
Increased duration of half-life with probenecid
Drug Uptake
Absorption: Oral: 30% to 40%
Serum half-life:
Children: 0.8-1.8 hours
Adults: 1-1.5 hours, prolonged to 10-20 hours with renal insufficiency
Time to peak serum concentration: Within 0.5-2 hours in patients with normal renal function; serum concentrations following oral absorption are inadequate for treatment of systemic infections
Pregnancy Risk Factor B

Carbidopa (kar bi doe' pa)
Brand Names Lodosyn®
Therapeutic Category Anti-Parkinson's Agent
Use Given with levodopa in the treatment of parkinsonism to enable a lower dosage of levodopa to be used and a more rapid response to be obtained and to decrease side-effects; for details of administration and dosage, see Levodopa; has no effect without levodopa
Usual Dosage Adults: Oral: 70-100 mg/day; maximum daily dose: 200 mg
Mechanism of Action Carbidopa is a peripheral decarboxylase inhibitor with little or no pharmacological activity when given alone in usual doses. It inhibits the peripheral decarboxylation of levodopa to dopamine; and as it does not cross the blood-brain barrier, unlike levodopa, effective brain concentrations of dopamine are produced with lower doses of levodopa. At the same time reduced peripheral formation of dopamine reduces peripheral side-effects, notably nausea and vomiting, and cardiac arrhythmias, although the dyskinesias and adverse mental effects associated with levodopa therapy tend to develop earlier.
Local Anesthetic/Vasoconstrictor Precautions No information available to require special precautions
Effects on Dental Treatment No effects or complications reported
Other Adverse Effects Adverse reactions are associated with concomitant administration with levodopa
(Continued)

Carbidopa *(Continued)*

>10%: Central nervous system: Anxiety, confusion, nervousness, mental depression

1% to 10%:

Cardiovascular: Orthostatic hypotension, palpitations, cardiac arrhythmias

Central nervous system: Memory loss, nervousness, insomnia, fatigue, hallucinations, ataxia, dystonic movements, blurred vision

Gastrointestinal: Nausea, vomiting, GI bleeding

<1%:

Cardiovascular: Hypertension

Gastrointestinal: Duodenal ulcer

Hematologic: Hemolytic anemia

Drug Interactions Reports of interaction with tricyclic antidepressants resulting in hypertension and dyskinesias

Drug Uptake

Absorption: Rapid but incomplete from GI tract

Pregnancy Risk Factor C

Carbinoxamine and Pseudoephedrine

(kar bi nox' a meen & soo doe e fed' rin)

Brand Names Carbiset® Tablet; Carbiset-TR® Tablet; Carbodec® Syrup; Carbodec® Tablet; Carbodec TR® Tablet; Cardec-S® Syrup; Rondec® Drops; Rondec® Filmtab®; Rondec® Syrup; Rondec-TR®

Therapeutic Category Antihistamine/Decongestant Combination

Use Temporary relief of nasal congestion, running nose, sneezing, itching of nose or throat, and itchy, watery eyes due to the common cold, hay fever, or other respiratory allergies

Usual Dosage Oral:

Children:

Drops: 1-18 months: 0.25-1 mL 4 times/day

Syrup:

18 months to 6 years: 2.5 mL 3-4 times/day

>6 years: 5 mL 2-4 times/day

Adults:

Liquid: 5 mL 4 times/day

Tablets: 1 tablet 4 times/day

Mechanism of Action Carbinoxamine competes with histamine for H_1-receptor sites on effector cells in the gastrointestinal tract, blood vessels, and respiratory tract

Local Anesthetic/Vasoconstrictor Precautions Pseudoephedrine is a sympathomimetic which has potential to enhance vasoconstrictor effects of epinephrine; use local anesthetic with vasoconstrictor with caution

Effects on Dental Treatment 1% to 10% of patients will experience dry mouth which disappears with cessation of drug therapy

Other Adverse Effects

>10%:

Central nervous system: Slight to moderate drowsiness

Miscellaneous: Thickening of bronchial secretions

1% to 10%:

Central nervous system: Headache, fatigue, nervousness, dizziness

Gastrointestinal: Appetite increase, weight increase, nausea, diarrhea, abdominal pain, dry mouth

Neuromuscular & skeletal: Arthralgia

Respiratory: Pharyngitis

<1%:

Cardiovascular: Edema, palpitations

Central nervous system: Depression

Dermatologic: Angioedema, photosensitivity, rash

Hepatic: Hepatitis

Neuromuscular & skeletal: Myalgia, paresthesia

Respiratory: Bronchospasm

Miscellaneous: Epistaxis

Drug Interactions May enhance the effects of barbiturates, TCAs, MAO inhibitors, ethanolamine antihistamines

Pregnancy Risk Factor C

Carbinoxamine, Pseudoephedrine, and Dextromethorphan
(kar bi nox' a meen, soo doe e fed' rin, & deks troe meth or' fan)

Brand Names Carbodec® DM; Cardec® DM; Pseudo-Car® DM; Rondamine®-DM Drops; Rondec®-DM; Tussafed® Drops

Therapeutic Category Antihistamine/Decongestant Combination; Cough Preparation

Use Relief of coughs and upper respiratory symptoms, including nasal congestion, associated with allergy or the common cold

Local Anesthetic/Vasoconstrictor Precautions Use with caution since pseudoephedrine is a sympathomimetic amine which could interact with epinephrine to cause a pressor response

Effects on Dental Treatment Up to 10% of patients could experience tachycardia, palpitations, and dry mouth; use vasoconstrictor with caution

Carbiset® Tablet *see* Carbinoxamine and Pseudoephedrine *on previous page*

Carbiset-TR® Tablet *see* Carbinoxamine and Pseudoephedrine *on previous page*

Carbocaine® 2% with Neo-Cobefrin® *see* Mepivacaine With Levonordefrin *on page 542*

Carbocaine® 3% *see* Mepivacaine Dental Anesthetic *on page 541*

Carbodec® DM *see* Carbinoxamine, Pseudoephedrine, and Dextromethorphan *on this page*

Carbodec® Syrup *see* Carbinoxamine and Pseudoephedrine *on previous page*

Carbodec® Tablet *see* Carbinoxamine and Pseudoephedrine *on previous page*

Carbodec TR® Tablet *see* Carbinoxamine and Pseudoephedrine *on previous page*

Carbol-Fuchsin Solution (kar bol fook' sin soe loo' shun)
Therapeutic Category Antifungal Agent, Topical

Synonyms Castellani Paint

Use Treatment of superficial mycotic infections

Local Anesthetic/Vasoconstrictor Precautions No information available to require special precautions

Effects on Dental Treatment No effects or complications reported

Carbolic Acid *see* Phenol *on page 682*

Carboplatin (kar' boe pla tin)
Brand Names Paraplatin®

Canadian/Mexican Brand Names Carboplat (Mexico); Blastocarb (Mexico)

Therapeutic Category Antineoplastic Agent, Alkylating Agent

Synonyms CBDCA

Use Palliative treatment of ovarian carcinoma; also used in the treatment of small cell lung cancer, squamous cell carcinoma of the esophagus; solid tumors of the bladder, cervix and testes; pediatric brain tumor, neuroblastoma

Usual Dosage IVPB, I.V. infusion, Intraperitoneal (**refer to individual protocols**):

Children:

Solid tumor: 560 mg/m^2 once every 4 weeks

Brain tumor: 175 mg/m^2 once weekly for 4 weeks with a 2-week recovery period between courses; dose is then adjusted on platelet count and neutrophil count values

Adults:

Ovarian cancer: Usual doses range from 360 mg/m^2 I.V. every 3 weeks single agent therapy to 300 mg/m^2 every 4 weeks as combination therapy

In general, however, single intermittent courses of carboplatin should not be repeated until the neutrophil count is at least 2000/mm^3 and the platelet count is at least 100,000/mm^3

Mechanism of Action Analogue of cisplatin which covalently binds to DNA; possible cross-linking and interference with the function of DNA

Local Anesthetic/Vasoconstrictor Precautions No information available to require special precautions

Effects on Dental Treatment No effects or complications reported

Other Adverse Effects

>10%: Asthenia, pain at injection site

Hepatic: Abnormal liver function tests

Hematologic: Neutropenia, leukopenia, thrombocytopenia (platelet count reaches a nadir between 14-21 days), anemia

Myelosuppressive: Dose-limiting toxicity; WBC: Severe (dose-dependent); Platelets: Severe; Nadir: 21-24 days; Recovery: 5-6 weeks

(Continued)

Carboplatin *(Continued)*

Endocrine & metabolic: Electrolyte abnormalities such as hypocalcemia, hypomagnesemia, hyponatremia, and hypokalemia

1% to 10%: Hemorrhagic complications
Central nervous system: Peripheral neuropathy, pain, asthenia
Dermatologic: Urticaria, rash, alopecia
Gastrointestinal: Emetogenic potential low (<10%), stomatitis, diarrhea, anorexia
Otic: Ototoxicity in 1% of patients

<1%: Blurred vision
Genitourinary: Nephrotoxicity (uncommon)
Miscellaneous: Neurotoxicity has only been noted in patients previously treated with cisplatin

Drug Uptake
Serum half-life, terminal: 22-40 hours

Pregnancy Risk Factor D

Carboprost Tromethamine (kar' boe prost tro meth' a meen)

Brand Names Hemabate™

Therapeutic Category Abortifacient; Prostaglandin

Use Termination of pregnancy

Usual Dosage Adults: I.M.:

Abortion: 250 mcg to start, 250 mcg at $1^1/_2$-hour to $3^1/_2$-hour intervals depending on uterine response; a 500 mcg dose may be given if uterine response is not adequate after several 250 mcg doses; do not exceed 12 mg total dose

Refractory postpartum uterine bleeding: Initial: 250 mcg; may repeat at 15- to 90-minute intervals to a total dose of 2 mg

Bladder irrigation for hemorrhagic cystitis (refer to individual protocols): [0.4-1.0 mg/dL as solution] 50 mL instilled into bladder 4 times/day for 1 hour

Mechanism of Action Carboprost tromethamine is a prostaglandin similar to prostaglandin F_2 alpha (dinoprost) except for the addition of a methyl group at the C-15 position. This substitution produces longer duration of activity than dinoprost; carboprost stimulates uterine contractility which usually results in expulsion of the products of conception and is used to induce abortion between 13-20 weeks of pregnancy. Hemostasis at the placentation site is achieved through the myometrial contractions produced by carboprost.

Local Anesthetic/Vasoconstrictor Precautions No information available to require special precautions

Effects on Dental Treatment No effects or complications reported

Other Adverse Effects
>10%: Gastrointestinal: Nausea
1% to 10%: Cardiovascular: Flushing
<1%:
Cardiovascular: Hypertension, hypotension
Central nervous system: Drowsiness, vertigo, nervousness, fever, headache, dystonia, vasovagal syndrome
Endocrine & metabolic: Breast tenderness
Gastrointestinal: Dry mouth, vomiting, diarrhea, hematemesis
Genitourinary: Bladder spasms
Neuromuscular & skeletal: Muscle pain
Ocular: Blurred vision
Respiratory: Coughing, asthma, respiratory distress
Miscellaneous: Taste alterations, septic shock, hiccups

Pregnancy Risk Factor X

Carbose D *see* Carboxymethylcellulose Sodium *on this page*

Carboxymethylcellulose Sodium

(kar box ee meth il sel' yoo lose sow' dee um)

Brand Names Cellufresh® [OTC]; Celluvisc® [OTC]

Therapeutic Category Ophthalmic Agent, Miscellaneous

Synonyms Carbose D

Use Preservative-free artificial tear substitute

Local Anesthetic/Vasoconstrictor Precautions No information available to require special precautions

Effects on Dental Treatment No effects or complications reported

Cardec® DM *see* Carbinoxamine, Pseudoephedrine, and Dextromethorphan *on previous page*

Cardec-S® Syrup *see* Carbinoxamine and Pseudoephedrine *on page 154*

Cardene® *see* Nicardipine Hydrochloride *on page 616*
Cardene® SR *see* Nicardipine Hydrochloride *on page 616*
Cardilate® *see* Erythrityl Tetranitrate *on page 320*
Cardio-Green® *see* Indocyanine Green *on page 457*
Cardioquin® *see* Quinidine *on page 759*
Cardiovascular Diseases *see page 912*
Cardizem® CD *see* Diltiazem *on page 284*
Cardizem® Injectable *see* Diltiazem *on page 284*
Cardizem® SR *see* Diltiazem *on page 284*
Cardizem® Tablet *see* Diltiazem *on page 284*
Cardura® *see* Doxazosin *on page 298*

Carisoprodol (kar eye soe proe' dole)
Brand Names Rela®; Sodol®; Soma®; Soma® Compound; Soprodol®; Soridol®
Canadian/Mexican Brand Names Dolaren® (Carisoprodol with Diclofenac) (Mexico); Naxodol® (Carisoprodol with Naproxen) (Mexico)
Therapeutic Category Muscle Relaxant; Skeletal Muscle Relaxant
Synonyms Isomeprobamate (Canada)
Use
Dental: Treatment of muscle spasm associated with acute temporomandibular joint pain
Medical: Skeletal muscle relaxant
Usual Dosage Adults: Oral: 350 mg 3-4 times/day; take last dose at bedtime; compound: 1-2 tablets 4 times/day
Mechanism of Action Precise mechanism is not yet clear, but many effects have been ascribed to its central depressant actions
Local Anesthetic/Vasoconstrictor Precautions No information available to require special precautions
Effects on Dental Treatment No effects or complications reported
Other Adverse Effects
>10%: Central nervous system: Drowsiness
1% to 10%: Central nervous system: Dizziness, lightheadedness

Oral manifestations: No data reported
Contraindications Acute intermittent porphyria, hypersensitivity to carisoprodol, meprobamate or any component
Warnings/Precautions Use with caution in renal and hepatic dysfunction
Drug Interactions Alcohol, CNS depressants, phenothiazines, clindamycin, MAO inhibitors
Drug Uptake
Onset of action: Within 30 minutes
Time to peak serum concentration: 4 hours
Duration: 4-6 hours
Serum half-life: 8 hours
Pregnancy Risk Factor C
Breast-feeding Considerations No data reported
Dosage Forms Tablet:
Rela®, Sodol®, Soma®, Soprodol®, Soridol®: 350 mg
Soma® Compound: Carisoprodol 200 mg and aspirin 325 mg
Dietary Considerations No data reported
Generic Available Yes

Carmol® [OTC] *see* Urea *on page 884*
Carmol-HC® Topical *see* Urea and Hydrocortisone *on page 885*

Carmustine (kar mus' teen)
Brand Names BiCNU®
Therapeutic Category Antineoplastic Agent, Alkylating Agent (Nitrosourea)
Synonyms BCNU

Use Brain tumors, multiple myeloma, Hodgkin's disease, and non-Hodgkin's lymphomas; some activity in malignant melanoma

Usual Dosage I.V. (**refer to individual protocols**):
Children: 200-250 mg/m^2 every 4-6 weeks as a single dose
Adults: 150-200 mg/m^2 every 6 weeks as a single dose or divided into daily injections on 2 successive days; next dose is to be determined based on hematologic response to the previous dose. See table.

Primary brain cancer: 150-200 mg/m^2 every 6-8 weeks

(Continued)

Carmustine *(Continued)*

Suggested Carmustine Dose Following Initial Dose

Nadir After Prior Dose		% of Prior Dose to Be Given
Leukocytes/mm³	Platelets/mm³	
>4000	>100,000	100
3000-3999	75,000-99,999	100
2000-2999	25,000-74,999	70
<2000	<25,000	50

Autologous BMT: All of the following doses are fatal without BMT
Combination therapy: Up to 300-900 mg/m²
Single agent therapy: Up to 1200 mg/m² (fatal necrosis is associated with doses >2 g/m²)

Mechanism of Action Interferes with the normal function of DNA by alkylation and cross-linking the strands of DNA, and by possible protein modification

Local Anesthetic/Vasoconstrictor Precautions No information available to require special precautions

Effects on Dental Treatment No effects or complications reported

Other Adverse Effects
>10%: Pain at injection site
Gastrointestinal: Nausea and vomiting occur within 2-4 hours after drug injection; dose-related
Emetic potential: <200 mg: Moderately high (60% to 90%); ≥200 mg: High (>90%)
1% to 10%: Anemia, stomatitis, facial flushing, alopecia, diarrhea, anorexia
<1%: Hyperpigmentation, dermatitis, hepatotoxicity, renal failure, facial flushing is probably due to the ethanol used in reconstitution
Hepatic: Reversible toxicity, increased LFTs in 20%
Myelosuppressive: Delayed, occurs 4-6 weeks after administration and is dose-related; usually persists for 1-2 weeks; thrombocytopenia is usually more severe than leukopenia. Myelofibrosis and preleukemic syndromes are being reported. WBC: Moderate; Platelets: Severe; Onset (days): 14; Nadir (days): 21-35; Recovery (days): 42-50
Pulmonary: Fibrosis occurs mostly in patients treated with prolonged total doses >1400 mg/m² or with bone marrow transplantation doses. Risk factors include a history of lung disease, concomitant bleomycin, or radiation therapy. PFTs should be conducted prior to therapy and monitored. Patients with predicted FVC or DL_co <70% are at a higher risk.
Renal: Azotemia, decrease in kidney size
Miscellaneous: Burning at injection site, hyperpigmentation of skin, ocular toxicity, and retinal hemorrhages, dizziness and ataxia

Drug Uptake
Absorption: Highly lipid soluble
Serum half-life (biphasic):
Initial: 1.4 minutes
Secondary: 20 minutes (active metabolites may persist for days and have a plasma half-life of 67 hours)

Pregnancy Risk Factor D

Carnitor® Injection *see Levocarnitine on page 494*
Carnitor® Oral *see Levocarnitine on page 494*

Carteolol Hydrochloride *(kar' tee oh lole hye droe klor' ide)*

Related Information
Cardiovascular Diseases *on page 912*

Brand Names Cartrol®; Ocupress®

Therapeutic Category Antianginal Agent; Antiglaucoma Agent; Beta-Adrenergic Blocker, Noncardioselective; Beta-Adrenergic Blocker, Ophthalmic

Use Management of hypertension; treatment of chronic open-angle glaucoma and intraocular hypertension

Usual Dosage Adults:
Oral: 2.5 mg as a single daily dose, with a maintenance dose normally 2.5-5 mg once every day; maximum daily dose: 10 mg; doses >10 mg do not increase response and may in fact decrease effect
Ophthalmic: Instill 1 drop in affected eye(s) twice daily; see Additional Information

Mechanism of Action Competitively blocks beta₁-adrenergic receptors with little or no effect on beta₂-receptors except at high doses; exhibits membrane stabilizing and intrinsic sympathomimetic activity

Local Anesthetic/Vasoconstrictor Precautions No information available to require special precautions

Effects on Dental Treatment Non-cardioselective beta-blockers (ie, propranolol, nadolol) enhance the pressor response to epinephrine, resulting in hypertension and bradycardia. This has not been reported for carteolol, a cardioselective beta-blocker. Therefore, local anesthetic with vasoconstrictor can be safely used in patients medicated with carteolol. Many nonsteroidal anti-inflammatory drugs such as ibuprofen and indomethacin can reduce the hypotensive effect of beta-blockers after 3 or more weeks of therapy with the NSAID. Short-term NSAID use (ie, 3 days) requires no special precautions in patients taking beta-blockers

Other Adverse Effects

1% to 10%:

Cardiovascular: Congestive heart failure, irregular heartbeat

Central nervous system: Mental depression, headache, dizziness

Neuromuscular & skeletal: Back pain, joint pain

<1%:

Cardiovascular: Bradycardia, chest pain, mesenteric arterial thrombosis, A-V block, persistent bradycardia, hypotension, edema, Raynaud's phenomena

Central nervous system: Fatigue, dizziness, headache, insomnia, lethargy, nightmares, depression, confusion

Dermatologic: Purpura

Endocrine & metabolic: Hyperglycemia

Gastrointestinal: Ischemic colitis, constipation, nausea, diarrhea

Genitourinary: Impotence

Hematologic: Thrombocytopenia

Respiratory: Bronchospasm

Miscellaneous: Cold extremities

Drug Interactions

Decreased effect of beta-blockers:

Barbiturates (increased liver metabolism of beta-blockers to result in lower serum levels)

NSAIDs (attenuate the hypotensive therapeutic effects of beta-blockers)

Rifampin (increased liver metabolism of beta-blockers to result in lower serum levels)

Increased effects of beta-blockers:

Calcium channel blockers (increased serum levels of beta-blockers by unknown mechanism to enhance hypotension)

Beta-blockers increase the effects of:

Epinephrine (vasoconstrictor; initial hypertensive episode followed by bradycardia) only from non-cardioselective type beta-blockers

Phenylephrine (Neosynephrine®; enhanced pressor response)

Theophylline (inhibit theophylline metabolism causing increase in serum concentrations)

Drug Uptake

Onset of effect: Oral: 1-1.5 hours

Peak effect: 2 hours

Duration: 12 hours

Absorption: Oral: 80%

Serum half-life: 6 hours

Pregnancy Risk Factor C

Selected Readings

Foster CA and Aston SJ, "Propranolol-Epinephrine Interaction: A Potential Disaster," *Plast Reconstr Surg*, 1983, 72(1):74-8.

Wong DG, Spence JD, Lamki L, et al, "Effect of Nonsteroidal Anti-Inflammatory Drugs on Control of Hypertension of Beta-Blockers and Diuretics," *Lancet*, 1986, 1(8488):997-1001.

Wynn RL, "Dental Nonsteroidal Anti-Inflammatory Drugs and Prostaglandin-Based Drug Interactions, Part Two," *Gen Dent*, 1992, 40(2):104, 106, 108.

Wynn RL, "Epinephrine Interactions With Beta-Blockers," *Gen Dent*, 1994, 42(1):16, 18.

Carter's Little Pills® [OTC] *see* Bisacodyl *on page 113*

Cartrol® *see* Carteolol Hydrochloride *on previous page*

Carvedilol (kar' ve dil ole)

Related Information

Cardiovascular Diseases *on page 912*

Brand Names Coreg®

Therapeutic Category Beta-Adrenergic Blocker, Noncardioselective

Use Management of hypertension; can be used alone or in combination with other agents, especially thiazide-type diuretics

Usual Dosage Adults: Oral:

(Continued)

Carvedilol (Continued)

Hypertension: 6.25 mg twice daily; if tolerated, dose should be maintained for 1-2 weeks, then increased to 12.5 mg twice daily; dosage may be increased to a maximum of 25 mg twice daily after 1-2 weeks; reduce dosage if heart rate drops <55 beats/minute

Congestive heart failure: 12.5-50 mg twice daily

Angina pectoris: 25-50 mg twice daily

Idiopathic cardiomyopathy: 6.25-25 mg twice daily

Mechanism of Action As a racemic mixture, carvedilol has nonselective beta-adrenoreceptor and alpha-adrenergic blocking activity at equal potency. No intrinsic sympathomimetic activity has been documented. Associated effects include reduction of cardiac output, exercise- or beta agonist-induced tachycardia, reduction of reflex orthostatic tachycardia, vasodilation, decreased peripheral vascular resistance (especially in standing position), decreased renal vascular resistance, reduced plasma renin activity, and increased levels of atrial natriuretic peptide.

Local Anesthetic/Vasoconstrictor Precautions No information available to require special precautions

Effects on Dental Treatment No effects or complications reported

Other Adverse Effects

1% to 10%:

Cardiovascular: Bradycardia, postural hypotension, edema

Central nervous system: Dizziness, somnolence, insomnia, fatigue

Gastrointestinal: Diarrhea, abdominal pain

Neuromuscular & skeletal: Back pain

Respiratory: Rhinitis, pharyngitis, dyspnea

<1%:

Cardiovascular: A-V block, extrasystoles, hypertension, hypotension, palpitations, peripheral ischemia, syncope

Central nervous system: Ataxia, vertigo, depression, nervousness, asthenia, malaise

Dermatologic: Pruritus, rash

Endocrine & metabolic: Decreased male libido, hypercholesterolemia, hyperglycemia, hyperuricemia

Gastrointestinal: Constipation, flatulence, dry mouth

Genitourinary: Impotence

Hematologic: Anemia, leukopenia

Hepatic: Hyperbilirubinemia, increased LFTs

Neuromuscular & skeletal: Paresthesia, myalgia

Ocular: Abnormal vision

Otic: Tinnitus

Respiratory: Asthma, cough

Miscellaneous: Increased sweating

Drug Uptake

Absorption: Rapid; food decreases the rate but not the extent of absorption; administration with food minimizes risks of orthostatic hypotension

Serum half-life: 7-10 hours

Casanthranol and Docusate see Docusate and Casanthranol on page 295

Cascara Sagrada (kas kar' a sah grah' dah)

Therapeutic Category Laxative, Stimulant

Use Temporary relief of constipation; sometimes used with milk of magnesia ("black and white" mixture)

Usual Dosage Note: Cascara sagrada fluid extract is 5 times more potent than cascara sagrada aromatic fluid extract.

Oral (aromatic fluid extract):

Children 2-11 years: 2.5 mL/day (range: 1-3 mL) as needed

Children ≥12 years and Adults: 5 mL/day (range: 2-6 mL) as needed at bedtime (1 tablet as needed at bedtime)

Mechanism of Action Direct chemical irritation of the intestinal mucosa resulting in an increased rate of colonic motility and change in fluid and electrolyte secretion

Local Anesthetic/Vasoconstrictor Precautions No information available to require special precautions

Effects on Dental Treatment No effects or complications reported

Other Adverse Effects 1% to 10%:

Central nervous system: Faintness

Endocrine & metabolic: Electrolyte and fluid imbalance

Gastrointestinal: Abdominal cramps, nausea, diarrhea

Miscellaneous: Discolors urine reddish pink or brown

Drug Interactions Decreased effect of oral anticoagulants
Drug Uptake
Onset of action: 6-10 hours
Pregnancy Risk Factor C

Casodex® *see* Bicalutamide *on page 113*
Castellani Paint *see* Carbol-Fuchsin Solution *on page 155*

Castor Oil (kas′ tor oyl)
Brand Names Alphamul® [OTC]; Emulsoil® [OTC]; Fleet® Flavored Castor Oil [OTC]; Neoloid® [OTC]; Purge® [OTC]
Therapeutic Category Laxative, Stimulant
Use Preparation for rectal or bowel examination or surgery; rarely used to relieve constipation; also applied to skin as emollient and protectant
Usual Dosage Oral:
Liquid:
Children 2-11 years: 5-15 mL as a single dose
Children ≥12 years and Adults: 15-60 mL as a single dose

Emulsified:
36.4%:
Children <2 years: 5-15 mL/dose
Children 2-11 years: 7.5-30 mL/dose
Children ≥12 years and Adults: 30-60 mL/dose
60% to 67%:
Children <2 years: 1.25-5 mL
Children 2-12 years: 5-15 mL
Adults: 15-45 mL
95%, mix with ¹/₂ to 1 full glass liquid:
Children: 5-10 mL
Adults: 15-60 mL

Mechanism of Action Acts primarily in the small intestine; hydrolyzed to ricinoleic acid which reduces net absorption of fluid and electrolytes and stimulates peristalsis
Local Anesthetic/Vasoconstrictor Precautions No information available to require special precautions
Effects on Dental Treatment No effects or complications reported
Other Adverse Effects
1% to 10%:
Central nervous system: Dizziness
Endocrine & metabolic: Electrolyte disturbance
Gastrointestinal: Abdominal cramps, nausea, diarrhea
<1%: Pelvic congestion
Drug Interactions No data reported
Drug Uptake Onset of action: Oral: 2-6 hours
Pregnancy Risk Factor X

Cataflam® *see* Diclofenac *on page 271*
Catapres® *see* Clonidine *on page 221*
Catapres-TTS® *see* Clonidine *on page 221*
Caverject® **Injection** *see* Alprostadil *on page 35*
CBDCA *see* Carboplatin *on page 155*
CCNU *see* Lomustine *on page 510*
2-CdA *see* Cladribine *on page 211*
CDDP *see* Cisplatin *on page 210*
Ceclor® *see* Cefaclor *on this page*
Ceclor® **CD** *see* Cefaclor *on this page*
Cecon® **[OTC]** *see* Ascorbic Acid *on page 76*
Cee-1000® **T.D. [OTC]** *see* Ascorbic Acid *on page 76*
CeeNU® **Oral** *see* Lomustine *on page 510*

Cefaclor (sef′ a klor)
Brand Names Ceclor®; Ceclor® CD
Therapeutic Category Antibiotic, Cephalosporin (Second Generation)
Use
Dental: An alternate antibiotic to treat orofacial infections in patients allergic to penicillins; susceptible bacteria including aerobic gram-positive bacteria and anaerobes
Medical: Infections in the medical patient caused by susceptible organisms including *Staphylococcus aureus* and *H. influenzae*; treatment of otitis
(Continued)

Cefaclor *(Continued)*

media, sinusitis, and infections involving the respiratory tract, skin and skin structure, bone and joint, and urinary tract

Usual Dosage Oral:

Children >1 month: 20-40 mg/kg/day divided every 8-12 hours; maximum dose: 2 g/day (twice daily option is for treatment of otitis media or pharyngitis)

Adults: 250-500 mg every 8 hours (or daily dose can be given in 2 divided doses) for at least 7 days

Mechanism of Action Inhibits bacterial cell wall synthesis by binding to one or more of the penicillin-binding proteins (PBPs) which in turn inhibits the final transpeptidation step of peptidoglycan synthesis in bacterial cell walls, thus inhibiting cell wall biosynthesis. Bacteria eventually lyse due to ongoing activity of cell wall autolytic enzymes (autolysins and murein hydrolases) while cell wall assembly is arrested.

Local Anesthetic/Vasoconstrictor Precautions No information available to require special precautions

Effects on Dental Treatment No effects or complications reported

Other Adverse Effects 1% to 10%: Gastrointestinal: Pseudomembranous colitis, diarrhea

Oral manifestations: No data reported

Contraindications Hypersensitivity to cefaclor, any component, or cephalosporins

Warnings/Precautions Modify dosage in patients with severe renal impairment; prolonged use may result in superinfection; a low incidence in cross-hypersensitivity to penicillins exists

Drug Interactions Probenecid may decrease cephalosporin elimination; furosemide, aminoglycosides may be a possible additive to nephrotoxicity

Drug Uptake

Absorption: Oral: Well absorbed, acid stable

Time to peak serum concentration:

Capsule: 60 minutes

Suspension: 45 minutes

Serum half-life: 0.5-1 hour

Influence of food: Decreases amount and slows rate of absorption

Pregnancy Risk Factor B

Breast-feeding Considerations Excreted into breast milk in small amounts like other cephalosporins

Dosage Forms

Capsule: 250 mg, 500 mg

Powder for oral suspension (strawberry flavor): 125 mg/5 mL (75 mL, 150 mL); 187 mg/5 mL (50 mL, 100 mL); 250 mg/5 mL (75 mL, 150 mL); 375 mg/5 mL (50 mL, 100 mL)

Tablet, extended release: 375 mg, 500 mg

Dietary Considerations May be taken with food, however, there is delayed absorption

Generic Available No

Comments Patients allergic to penicillins can use a cephalosporin; the incidence of cross-reactivity between penicillins and cephalosporins is 1% when the allergic reaction to penicillin is delayed. Cefaclor effective against anaerobic bacteria, but the sensitivity of alpha-hemolytic *Streptococcus* vary; approximately 10% of strains are resistant. Nearly 70% are intermediately sensitive. If the patient has a history of immediate reaction to penicillin, the incidence of cross-reactivity is 20%; cephalosporins are contraindicated in these patients.

Selected Readings

Saxon A, Beall GN, Kohr AS, et al, "Immediate Hypersensitivity Reactions to Beta-Lactam Antibiotics," *Ann Intern Med*, 1987, 107:204-15.

Cefadroxil Monohydrate *(sef a drox' il mon oh hye' drate)*

Brand Names Duricef®; Ultracef®

Canadian/Mexican Brand Names Cefamox® (Mexico); Duracef® (Mexico)

Therapeutic Category Antibiotic, Cephalosporin (First Generation)

Use Treatment of susceptible bacterial infections, including those caused by group A beta-hemolytic *Streptococcus*

Usual Dosage Oral:

Children: 30 mg/kg/day divided twice daily up to a maximum of 2 g/day

Adults: 1-2 g/day in 2 divided doses

Mechanism of Action Inhibits bacterial cell wall synthesis by binding to one or more of the penicillin-binding proteins (PBPs) which in turn inhibits the final transpeptidation step of peptidoglycan synthesis in bacterial cell walls, thus inhibiting cell wall biosynthesis. Bacteria eventually lyse due to ongoing activity of cell wall autolytic enzymes (autolysins and murein hydrolases) while cell wall assembly is arrested.

Local Anesthetic/Vasoconstrictor Precautions No information available to require special precautions

Effects on Dental Treatment No effects or complications reported

Other Adverse Effects

1% to 10%: Gastrointestinal: Diarrhea

<1%:

Central nervous system: Fatigue, chills

Dermatologic: Maculopapular and erythematous rash

Gastrointestinal: Dyspepsia, pseudomembranous colitis, nausea, vomiting, heartburn, gastritis, bloating

Hematologic: Neutropenia

Miscellaneous: Superinfections

Drug Interactions

Increased effect: High-dose probenecid decreases renal clearance of cephalosporins

Drug Uptake

Absorption: Oral: Rapid and well absorbed from GI tract

Serum half-life: 1-2 hours; 20-24 hours in renal failure

Serum time to peak serum concentration: Within 70-90 minutes

Pregnancy Risk Factor B

Cefadyl® see Cephapirin Sodium *on page 177*

Cefalotina Sal Sodica De (Mexico) *see* Cephalothin Sodium *on page 177*

Cefamandole Nafate (sef a man' dole naf' ate)

Brand Names Mandol®

Therapeutic Category Antibiotic, Cephalosporin (Second Generation)

Use Treatment of susceptible bacterial infection; mainly respiratory tract, skin and skin structure, bone and joint, urinary tract and gynecologic, as well as, septicemia

Usual Dosage I.M., I.V.:

Children: 100-150 mg/kg/day in divided doses every 4-6 hours

Adults: 4-12 g/24 hours divided every 4-6 hours or 500-1000 mg every 4-8 hours; maximum: 2 g/dose

Mechanism of Action Inhibits bacterial cell wall synthesis by binding to one or more of the penicillin-binding proteins (PBPs) which in turn inhibits the final transpeptidation step of peptidoglycan synthesis in bacterial cell walls, thus inhibiting cell wall biosynthesis. Bacteria eventually lyse due to ongoing activity of cell wall autolytic enzymes (autolysins and murein hydrolases) while cell wall assembly is arrested.

Local Anesthetic/Vasoconstrictor Precautions No information available to require special precautions

Effects on Dental Treatment No effects or complications reported

Other Adverse Effects

1% to 10%: Gastrointestinal: Diarrhea

<1%:

Central nervous system: CNS irritation, seizures, fever

Dermatologic: Rash, urticaria

Gastrointestinal: Abdominal cramps, pseudomembraneous colitis

Hematologic: Eosinophilia, hypoprothrombinemia, leukopenia, thrombocytopenia

Hepatic: Transient elevation of liver enzymes, cholestatic jaundice

Local: Pain at injection site

Miscellaneous: Superinfections

Drug Interactions

Disulfiram-like reaction has been reported when taken within 72 hours of alcohol consumption

Increased effect: High-dose probenecid decreases renal clearance of cephalosporins

Drug Uptake

Time to peak serum concentration:

I.M.: Within 1-2 hours

I.V.: Within 10 minutes

Serum half-life: 30-60 minutes

Pregnancy Risk Factor B

Cefanex® *see* Cephalexin Monohydrate *on page 176*

Cefazolina (Mexico) *see* Cefazolin Sodium *on this page*

Cefazolin Sodium (sef a' zoe lin sow' dee um)
Related Information
Animal and Human Bites Guidelines *on page 976*
Antimicrobial Prophylaxis in Surgical Patients *on page 1042*
Brand Names Ancef®; Kefzol®; Zolicef®
Canadian/Mexican Brand Names Cefamezin® (Mexico)
Therapeutic Category Antibiotic, Cephalosporin (First Generation)
Synonyms Cefazolina (Mexico)
Use Treatment of gram-positive bacilli and cocci (except enterococcus); some gram-negative bacilli including *E. coli*, *Proteus*, and *Klebsiella* may be susceptible
Usual Dosage I.M., I.V.:
Children >1 month: 50-100 mg/kg/day divided every 8 hours; maximum: 6 g/day
Adults: 1-2 g every 8 hours, depending on severity of infection; maximum dose: 12 g/day
Mechanism of Action Inhibits bacterial cell wall synthesis by binding to one or more of the penicillin-binding proteins (PBPs) which in turn inhibits the final transpeptidation step of peptidoglycan synthesis in bacterial cell walls, thus inhibiting cell wall biosynthesis. Bacteria eventually lyse due to ongoing activity of cell wall autolytic enzymes (autolysins and murein hydrolases) while cell wall assembly is arrested.
Local Anesthetic/Vasoconstrictor Precautions No information available to require special precautions
Effects on Dental Treatment No effects or complications reported
Other Adverse Effects
1% to 10%: Gastrointestinal: Diarrhea
<1%:
Central nervous system: CNS irritation, seizures, confusion, fever
Dermatologic: Rash, urticaria
Hematologic: Leukopenia, thrombocytopenia, neutropenia
Hepatic: Transient elevation of liver enzymes, cholestatic jaundice
Miscellaneous: Superinfections
Drug Interactions
Increased effect: High-dose probenecid decreases renal clearance of cephalosporins
Drug Uptake
Time to peak serum concentration:
I.M.: Within 0.5-2 hours
I.V.: Within 5 minutes
Serum half-life: 90-150 minutes (prolonged with renal impairment)
Pregnancy Risk Factor B

Cefepime (sef' e pim)
Brand Names Maxipime®
Therapeutic Category Antibiotic, Cephalosporin (Fourth Genration)
Use Treatment of respiratory tract infections (including bronchitis and pneumonia), cellulitis and other skin and soft tissue infections, and urinary tract infections; considered a fourth generation cephalosporin because it has good gram-negative coverage similar to third generation cephalosporins, but better gram-positive coverage
Usual Dosage I.V.:
Children: Unlabeled: 50 mg/kg every 8 hours; maximum dose: 2 g
Adults:
Most infections: 1-2 g every 12 hours for 5-10 days; higher doses or more frequent administration may be required in pseudomonal infections
Urinary tract infections, uncomplicated: 500 mg every 12 hours

Dosing adjustment in renal impairment:
Cl$_{cr}$ 10-30 mL/minute: Administer 500 mg every 24 hours
Cl$_{cr}$ <10 mL/minute: Administer 250 mg every 24 hours

Hemodialysis: Removed by dialysis; administer supplemental dose of 250 mg after each dialysis session

Peritoneal dialysis: Removed to a lesser extent than hemodialysis; administer 250 mg every 48 hours
Mechanism of Action Inhibits bacterial cell wall synthesis by binding to one or more of the penicillin-binding proteins (PBPs) which in turn inhibits the final transpeptidation step of peptidoglycan synthesis in bacterial cell walls, thus

inhibiting cell wall biosynthesis. Bacterial eventually lyse due to ongoing activity of cell wall autolytic enzymes (autolysis and murein hydrolases) while cell wall assembly is arrested.

Local Anesthetic/Vasoconstrictor Precautions No information available to require special precautions

Effects on Dental Treatment No effects or complications reported

Warnings/Precautions Modify dosage in patients with severe renal impairment; prolonged use may result in superinfection; a low incidence of cross-hypersensitivity to penicillins exists

Drug Interactions
Increased effect: High-dose probenecid decreases clearance
Increased toxicity: Aminoglycosides increase nephrotoxic potential

Drug Uptake
Absorption: I.M.: Rapid and complete; T_{max}: 0.5-1.5 hours
Half-life: 2 hours

Pregnancy Risk Factor C
Generic Available No

Cefixima (Mexico) see Cefixime on this page

Cefixime (sef ix' eem)
Related Information
Nonviral Infectious Diseases on page 932
Brand Names Suprax®
Canadian/Mexican Brand Names Denvar® (Mexico); Novacef® (Mexico)
Therapeutic Category Antibiotic, Cephalosporin (Third Generation)
Synonyms Cefixima (Mexico)
Use Treatment of urinary tract infections, otitis media, respiratory infections due to susceptible organisms including *S. pneumoniae* and *Pyogenes*, *H. influenzae* and many *Enterobacteriaceae*; documented poor compliance with other oral antimicrobials; outpatient therapy of serious soft tissue or skeletal infections due to susceptible organisms; single-dose oral treatment of uncomplicated cervical/urethral gonorrhea due to *N. gonorrhoeae*
Mechanism of Action Inhibits bacterial cell wall synthesis by binding to one or more of the penicillin-binding proteins (PBPs) which in turn inhibits the final transpeptidation step of peptidoglycan synthesis in bacterial cell walls, thus inhibiting cell wall biosynthesis. Bacteria eventually lyse due to ongoing activity of cell wall autolytic enzymes (autolysins and murein hydrolases) while cell wall assembly is arrested.
Local Anesthetic/Vasoconstrictor Precautions No information available to require special precautions
Effects on Dental Treatment No effects or complications reported
Other Adverse Effects
1% to 10%: Gastrointestinal: Diarrhea (up to 15% of children), abdominal pain, nausea, dyspepsia, flatulence, pseudomembranous colitis
<1%:
Central nervous system: Headache, dizziness, fever
Dermatologic: Rash, urticaria, pruritus
Genitourinary: Vaginitis
Hematologic: Thrombocytopenia, leukopenia, eosinophilia
Miscellaneous: Transient elevation of BUN or creatinine and LFTs
Drug Interactions
Increased effect: High-dose probenecid decreases renal clearance of cephalosporins
Pregnancy Risk Factor B

Cefizox® see Ceftizoxime on page 171

Cefmetazole Sodium (sef met' a zole sow' dee um)
Brand Names Zefazone®
Therapeutic Category Antibiotic, Cephalosporin (Second Generation)
Use Second generation cephalosporin with an antibacterial spectrum similar to cefoxitin, useful on many aerobic and anaerobic gram-positive and gram-negative bacteria
Usual Dosage Adults: I.V.:
Infections: 2 g every 6-12 hours for 5-14 days
Prophylaxis: 2 g 30-90 minutes before surgery **or** 1 g 30-90 minutes before surgery; repeat 8 and 16 hours later
Mechanism of Action Inhibits bacterial cell wall synthesis by binding to one or more of the penicillin-binding proteins (PBPs) which in turn inhibits the final transpeptidation step of peptidoglycan synthesis in bacterial cell walls, thus
(Continued)

Cefmetazole Sodium *(Continued)*

inhibiting cell wall biosynthesis. Bacteria eventually lyse due to ongoing activity of cell wall autolytic enzymes (autolysins and murein hydrolases) while cell wall assembly is arrested.

Local Anesthetic/Vasoconstrictor Precautions No information available to require special precautions

Effects on Dental Treatment No effects or complications reported

Other Adverse Effects

1% to 10%:
Dermatologic: Rash
Gastrointestinal: Diarrhea, nausea

<1%:
Cardiovascular: Shock, hypotension
Central nervous system: Headache, fever
Endocrine & metabolic: Hot flashes
Gastrointestinal: Epigastric pain, pseudomembraneous colitis
Genitourinary: Vaginitis
Hematologic: Bleeding
Local: Pain at injection site, phlebitis
Respiratory: Respiratory distress, dyspnea
Miscellaneous: Epistaxis, alteration of color, candidiasis

Drug Interactions
Increased effect: High-dose probenecid decreases renal clearance of cephalosporins

Drug Uptake
Serum half-life: 72 minutes

Pregnancy Risk Factor B

Cefobid® *see* Cefoperazone Sodium *on next page*
Cefol® Filmtab® *see* Vitamins, Multiple *on page 901*
Cefonicidid (Mexico) *see* Cefonicid Sodium *on this page*

Cefonicid Sodium (se fon' i sid sow' dee um)

Brand Names Monocid®
Canadian/Mexican Brand Names Monocidur® (Mexico)
Therapeutic Category Antibiotic, Cephalosporin (Second Generation)
Synonyms Cefonicidid (Mexico)
Use Treatment of susceptible bacterial infection; mainly respiratory tract, skin and skin structure, bone and joint, urinary tract and gynecologic, as well as, septicemia; second generation cephalosporin
Usual Dosage Adults: I.M., I.V.: 0.5-2 g every 24 hours
Prophylaxis: Preop: 1 g/hour
Mechanism of Action Inhibits bacterial cell wall synthesis by binding to one or more of the penicillin-binding proteins (PBPs) which in turn inhibits the final transpeptidation step of peptidoglycan synthesis in bacterial cell walls, thus inhibiting cell wall biosynthesis. Bacteria eventually lyse due to ongoing activity of cell wall autolytic enzymes (autolysins and murein hydrolases) while cell wall assembly is arrested.
Local Anesthetic/Vasoconstrictor Precautions No information available to require special precautions
Effects on Dental Treatment No effects or complications reported
Other Adverse Effects

1% to 10%:
Local: Pain at injection site
Hematologic: Increased platelets and eosinophils
Hepatic: Liver function alterations

<1%:
Central nervous system: Fever, headache
Dermatologic: Skin rash
Gastrointestinal: Nausea, diarrhea, abdominal pain, pseudomembranous colitis
Hematologic: Increased platelets and eosinophils
Miscellaneous: Transient elevations in liver enzymes, BUN, or creatinine

Drug Interactions
Increased effect: High-dose probenecid decreases renal clearance of cephalosporins

Drug Uptake
Serum half-life: 6-7 hours

Pregnancy Risk Factor B

Cefoperazona (Mexico) *see* Cefoperazone Sodium *on next page*

Cefoperazone Sodium (sef oh per' a zone sow' dee um)

Brand Names Cefobid®

Therapeutic Category Antibiotic, Cephalosporin (Third Generation)

Synonyms Cefoperazona (Mexico)

Use Treatment of susceptible bacterial infection; mainly respiratory tract, skin and skin structure, bone and joint, urinary tract and gynecologic, as well as, septicemia

Usual Dosage I.M., I.V.:

Children: 100-150 mg/kg/day divided every 8-12 hours; up to 12 g/day

Adults: 2-4 g/day in divided doses every 12 hours; up to 12 g/day

Mechanism of Action Inhibits bacterial cell wall synthesis by binding to one or more of the penicillin-binding proteins (PBPs) which in turn inhibits the final transpeptidation step of peptidoglycan synthesis in bacterial cell walls, thus inhibiting cell wall biosynthesis. Bacteria eventually lyse due to ongoing activity of cell wall autolytic enzymes (autolysins and murein hydrolases) while cell wall assembly is arrested.

Local Anesthetic/Vasoconstrictor Precautions No information available to require special precautions

Effects on Dental Treatment No effects or complications reported

Other Adverse Effects

1% to 10%: Gastrointestinal: Diarrhea

<1%:

Dermatologic: Maculopapular and erythematous rash

Gastrointestinal: Dyspepsia, pseudomembranous colitis, nausea, vomiting

Hematologic: Bleeding

Local: Pain and induration at injection site

Drug Interactions

Increased effect: High-dose probenecid decreases renal clearance of cephalosporins

Drug Uptake

Serum half-life: 2 hours, higher with hepatic disease or biliary obstruction

Time to peak serum concentration:

I.M.: Within 1-2 hours

I.V.: Within 15-20 minutes (serum levels 2-3 times the serum levels following I.M. administration)

Pregnancy Risk Factor B

Cefotan® *see* Cefotetan Disodium *on next page*

Cefotaxima (Mexico) *see* Cefotaxime Sodium *on this page*

Cefotaxime Sodium (sef oh taks' eem sow' dee um)

Brand Names Claforan®

Canadian/Mexican Brand Names Alfotax® (Mexico); Benaxima® (Mexico); Biosint® (Mexico); Cefaxim® (Mexico); Cefoclin® (Mexico); Fotexina® (Mexico); Taporin® (Mexico); Viken® (Mexico)

Therapeutic Category Antibiotic, Cephalosporin (Third Generation)

Synonyms Cefotaxima (Mexico)

Use Treatment of susceptible infection in respiratory tract, skin and skin structure, bone and joint, urinary tract, gynecologic as well as septicemia, and documented or suspected meningitis

Usual Dosage I.M., I.V.:

Children 1 month to 12 years:

<50 kg: 100-150 mg/kg/day in divided doses every 6-8 hours

Meningitis: 200 mg/kg/day in divided doses every 6 hours

>50 kg: Moderate to severe infection: 1-2 g every 6-8 hours; life-threatening infection: 2 g/dose every 4 hours; maximum dose: 12 g/day

Children >12 years and Adults: 1-2 g every 6-8 hours (up to 12 g/day)

Mechanism of Action Inhibits bacterial cell wall synthesis by binding to one or more of the penicillin-binding proteins (PBPs) which in turn inhibits the final transpeptidation step of peptidoglycan synthesis in bacterial cell walls, thus inhibiting cell wall biosynthesis. Bacteria eventually lyse due to ongoing activity of cell wall autolytic enzymes (autolysins and murein hydrolases) while cell wall assembly is arrested.

Local Anesthetic/Vasoconstrictor Precautions No information available to require special precautions

Effects on Dental Treatment No effects or complications reported

Other Adverse Effects

1% to 10%:

Central nervous system: Fever

Dermatologic: Rash, pruritus

(Continued)

Cefotaxime Sodium *(Continued)*

Gastrointestinal: Colitis, diarrhea, nausea, vomiting
Hematologic: Eosinophilia
Local: Pain at injection site
<1%:
Central nervous system: Headache
Gastrointestinal: Pseudomembranous colitis
Hematologic: Transient neutropenia, thrombocytopenia
Local: Phlebitis
Miscellaneous: Transient elevation of BUN, creatinine and liver enzymes

Drug Interactions
Increased effect: High-dose probenecid decreases renal clearance of cephalosporins

Drug Uptake
Serum half-life:
Cefotaxime:
Adults: 1-1.5 hours (prolonged with renal and/or hepatic impairment)
Desacetylcefotaxime: 1.5-1.9 hours (prolonged with renal impairment)
Time to peak serum concentration: I.M.: Within 30 minutes

Pregnancy Risk Factor B

Cefotetan Disodium (sef' oh tee tan dye' sow dee um)

Related Information
Animal and Human Bites Guidelines *on page 976*
Antimicrobial Prophylaxis in Surgical Patients *on page 1042*

Brand Names Cefotan®

Therapeutic Category Antibiotic, Cephalosporin (Second Generation)

Use Treatment of susceptible bacterial infection; mainly respiratory tract, skin and skin structure, bone and joint, urinary tract and gynecologic, as well as, septicemia, similar spectrum to cefoxitin

Usual Dosage I.M., I.V.:
Children: 20-40 mg/kg/dose every 12 hours

Adults: 1-6 g/day in divided doses every 12 hours, 1-2 g may be given every 24 hours for urinary tract infection

Mechanism of Action Inhibits bacterial cell wall synthesis by binding to one or more of the penicillin-binding proteins (PBPs) which in turn inhibits the final transpeptidation step of peptidoglycan synthesis in bacterial cell walls, thus inhibiting cell wall biosynthesis. Bacteria eventually lyse due to ongoing activity of cell wall autolytic enzymes (autolysins and murein hydrolases) while cell wall assembly is arrested.

Local Anesthetic/Vasoconstrictor Precautions No information available to require special precautions

Effects on Dental Treatment No effects or complications reported

Other Adverse Effects
1% to 10%:
Gastrointestinal: Diarrhea
Hepatic: Hepatic enzyme elevation
Miscellaneous: Hypersensitivity reactions
<1%:
Central nervous system: Fever
Dermatologic: Rash, pruritus
Gastrointestinal: Nausea, vomiting, antibiotic-associated colitis
Hematologic: Prolongation of bleeding time or prothrombin time, neutropenia, thrombocytopenia
Local: Phlebitis

Drug Interactions
Increased effect: High-dose probenecid decreases renal clearance of cephalosporins

Drug Uptake
Serum half-life: 1.5-3 hours
Time to peak serum concentration: I.M.: Within 1.5-3 hours

Pregnancy Risk Factor B

Cefoxitin Sodium (se fox' i tin sow' dee um)

Related Information
Antimicrobial Prophylaxis in Surgical Patients *on page 1042*

Brand Names Mefoxin®

Therapeutic Category Antibiotic, Cephalosporin (Second Generation)

Use Less active against staphylococci and streptococci than first generation cephalosporins, but active against anaerobes including *Bacteroides fragilis;*

active against gram-negative enteric bacilli including *E. coli*, *Klebsiella*, and *Proteus*; used predominantly for respiratory tract, skin and skin structure, bone and joint, urinary tract and gynecologic as well as septicemia; surgical prophylaxis; intra-abdominal infections and other mixed infections

Usual Dosage I.M., I.V.:

Children >3 months:
Mild-moderate infection: 80-100 mg/kg/day in divided doses every 4-6 hours
Severe infection: 100-160 mg/kg/day in divided doses every 4-6 hours
Maximum dose: 12 g/day

Adults: 1-2 g every 6-8 hours (I.M. injection is painful); up to 12 g/day

Mechanism of Action Inhibits bacterial cell wall synthesis by binding to one or more of the penicillin-binding proteins (PBPs) which in turn inhibits the final transpeptidation step of peptidoglycan synthesis in bacterial cell walls, thus inhibiting cell wall biosynthesis. Bacteria eventually lyse due to ongoing activity of cell wall autolytic enzymes (autolysins and murein hydrolases) while cell wall assembly is arrested.

Local Anesthetic/Vasoconstrictor Precautions No information available to require special precautions

Effects on Dental Treatment No effects or complications reported

Other Adverse Effects

1% to 10%: Gastrointestinal: Diarrhea
<1%:
Cardiovascular: Hypotension
Central nervous system: Fever
Dermatologic: Rash, exfoliative dermatitis
Gastrointestinal: Nausea, vomiting, pseudomembranous colitis
Hematologic: Transient leukopenia, thrombocytopenia, anemia, eosinophilia
Hepatic: Elevation in serum AST concentration
Local: Thrombophlebitis
Respiratory: Dyspnea
Miscellaneous: Elevations in serum creatinine and/or BUN

Drug Interactions
Increased effect: High-dose probenecid decreases renal clearance of cephalosporins

Drug Uptake
Serum half-life: 45-60 minutes, increases significantly with renal insufficiency
Time to peak serum concentration:
I.M.: Within 20-30 minutes
I.V.: Within 5 minutes

Pregnancy Risk Factor B

Cefpodoxime Proxetil (sef pode ox' eem prok' seh til)

Brand Names Vantin®

Therapeutic Category Antibiotic, Cephalosporin (Second Generation)

Use Treatment of susceptible acute, community-acquired pneumonia caused by *S. pneumoniae* or nonbeta-lactamase producing *H. influenzae*; acute uncomplicated gonorrhea caused by *N. gonorrhoeae*; uncomplicated skin and skin structure infections caused by *S. aureus* or *S. pyogenes*; acute otitis media caused by *S. pneumoniae*, *H. influenzae*, or *M. catarrhalis*; pharyngitis or tonsillitis; and uncomplicated urinary tract infections caused by *E. coli*, *Klebsiella*, and *Proteus*

Usual Dosage Oral:

Children >5 months to 12 years:
Acute otitis media: 10 mg/kg/day as a single dose or divided every 12 hours (400 mg/day)
Pharyngitis/tonsillitis: 10 mg/kg/day in 2 divided doses (maximum: 200 mg/day)

Children ≥13 years and Adults:
Acute community-acquired pneumonia and bacterial exacerbations of chronic bronchitis: 200 mg every 12 hours for 14 days and 10 days, respectively
Skin and skin structure: 400 mg every 12 hours for 7-14 days
Uncomplicated gonorrhea (male and female) and rectal gonococcal infections (female): 200 mg as a single dose
Pharyngitis/tonsillitis: 100 mg every 12 hours for 10 days
Uncomplicated urinary tract infection: 100 mg every 12 hours for 7 days

Mechanism of Action Inhibits bacterial cell wall synthesis by binding to one or more of the penicillin-binding proteins (PBPs) which in turn inhibits the final transpeptidation step of peptidoglycan synthesis in bacterial cell walls, thus inhibiting cell wall biosynthesis. Bacteria eventually lyse due to ongoing activity

(Continued)

169

Cefpodoxime Proxetil *(Continued)*

of cell wall autolytic enzymes (autolysins and murein hydrolases) while cell wall assembly is arrested.

Local Anesthetic/Vasoconstrictor Precautions No information available to require special precautions

Effects on Dental Treatment No effects or complications reported

Other Adverse Effects

1% to 10%: Gastrointestinal: Diarrhea

<1%:

Central nervous system: Headache

Dermatologic: Diaper rash

Gastrointestinal: Nausea, vomiting, abdominal pain, pseudomembranous colitis

Genitourinary: Vaginal fungal infections

Drug Interactions

Decreased effect: Antacids and H_2-receptor antagonists (reduce absorption and serum concentration of cefpodoxime)

Increased effect: Probenecid may decrease cephalosporin elimination

Drug Uptake

Absorption: Oral: Rapidly and well absorbed (50%), acid stable; enhanced in the presence of food or low gastric pH

Serum half-life: 2.2 hours (prolonged with renal impairment)

Pregnancy Risk Factor B

Dosage Forms

Granules for oral suspension (lemon creme flavor): 50 mg/5 mL (100 mL); 100 mg/5 mL (100 mL)

Tablet, film coated: 100 mg, 200 mg

Dietary Considerations May be taken with food, however, there is delayed absorption

Generic Available No

Cefprozil *(sef proe' zil)*

Brand Names Cefzil®

Therapeutic Category Antibiotic, Cephalosporin (Second Generation)

Use Infections causes by susceptible organisms including *S. pneumoniae*, *S. aureus*, *S. pyogenes*; treatment of otitis media and infections involving the respiratory tract and skin and skin structure

Usual Dosage Oral:

Children >6 months to 12 years: 7.5-15 mg/kg every 12 hours for 10 days

Pharyngitis/tonsillitis:

Children 2-12 years: 15 mg/kg/day divided every 12 hours; maximum: 1 g/day

Children >13 years and Adults: 250-500 mg every 12-24 hours for 10-14 days

Mechanism of Action Inhibits bacterial cell wall synthesis by binding to one or more of the penicillin-binding proteins (PBPs) which in turn inhibits the final transpeptidation step of peptidoglycan synthesis in bacterial cell walls, thus inhibiting cell wall biosynthesis. Bacteria eventually lyse due to ongoing activity of cell wall autolytic enzymes (autolysins and murein hydrolases) while cell wall assembly is arrested.

Local Anesthetic/Vasoconstrictor Precautions No information available to require special precautions

Effects on Dental Treatment No effects or complications reported

Other Adverse Effects

1% to 10%:

Central nervous system: Dizziness

Dermatologic: Diaper rash and superinfection, genital pruritus

Gastrointestinal: Diarrhea, nausea, vomiting, abdominal pain

Genitourinary: Vaginitis

Hematologic: Eosinophilia

Hepatic: Elevation of AST and ALT, elevation of alkaline phosphatase

<1%:

Central nervous system: Headache, insomnia, confusion

Dermatologic: Rash, urticaria

Hematologic: Prolonged PT

Hepatic: Cholestatic jaundice

Neuromuscular & skeletal: Arthralgia

Renal: Elevated BUN and serum creatinine

Drug Interactions

Increased effect: Probenecid may decrease cephalosporin elimination

Drug Uptake
Absorption: Oral: Well absorbed (94%)
Serum half-life, elimination: 1.3 hours (normal renal function)
Peak serum levels: 1.5 hours (fasting state)

Pregnancy Risk Factor B

Dosage Forms
Powder for oral suspension, as anhydrous: 125 mg/5 mL (50 mL, 75 mL, 100 mL); 250 mg/5 mL (50 mL, 75 mL, 100 mL)
Tablet, as anhydrous: 250 mg, 500 mg

Dietary Considerations May be taken with food, however, there is delayed absorption

Generic Available No

Cefradina (Mexico) *see* Cephradine *on page 178*
Ceftazidima (Mexico) *see* Ceftazidime *on this page*

Ceftazidime (sef' tay zi deem)

Brand Names Fortaz®; Tazicef®; Tazidime®
Canadian/Mexican Brand Names Ceptaz™ (Canada); Ceftazim® (Mexico); Fortum® (Mexico); Tagal® (Mexico); Taloken® (Mexico); Waytrax® (Mexico)
Therapeutic Category Antibiotic, Cephalosporin (Third Generation)
Synonyms Ceftazidima (Mexico)
Use Treatment of documented susceptible *Pseudomonas aeruginosa* infection; *Pseudomonas* infection in patients at risk of developing aminoglycoside-induced nephrotoxicity and/or ototoxicity; empiric therapy of febrile, granulo-cytopenic patients

Usual Dosage I.M., I.V.:
Children 1 month to 12 years: 30-50 mg/kg/dose every 8 hours; maximum dose: 6 g/day
Adults: 1-2 g every 8-12 hours
Urinary tract infections: 250-500 mg every 12 hours

Mechanism of Action Inhibits bacterial cell wall synthesis by binding to one or more of the penicillin-binding proteins (PBPs) which in turn inhibits the final transpeptidation step of peptidoglycan synthesis in bacterial cell walls, thus inhibiting cell wall biosynthesis. Bacteria eventually lyse due to ongoing activity of cell wall autolytic enzymes (autolysins and murein hydrolases) while cell wall assembly is arrested.

Local Anesthetic/Vasoconstrictor Precautions No information available to require special precautions

Effects on Dental Treatment No effects or complications reported

Other Adverse Effects
1% to 10%:
Gastrointestinal: Diarrhea
Local: Pain at injection site
<1%:
Central nervous system: Fever, headache, dizziness
Dermatologic: Rash, angioedema
Gastrointestinal: Nausea, vomiting, pseudomembranous colitis
Hematologic: Eosinophilia, thrombocytosis, transient leukopenia, hemolytic anemia
Local: Phlebitis
Neuromuscular & skeletal: Paresthesia
Miscellaneous: Transient elevation in liver enzymes, BUN and creatinine, candidiasis

Drug Interactions
Increased effect: High-dose probenecid decreases renal clearance of cephalosporins

Drug Uptake
Serum half-life: 1-2 hours (prolonged with renal impairment)
Time to peak serum concentration: I.M.: Within 1 hour

Pregnancy Risk Factor B

Ceftin® *see* Cefuroxime *on page 173*
Ceftizoxima (Mexico) *see* Ceftizoxime *on this page*

Ceftizoxime (sef ti zox' eem)

Brand Names Cefizox®
Canadian/Mexican Brand Names Ultracef® (Mexico)
Therapeutic Category Antibiotic, Cephalosporin (Third Generation)
Synonyms Ceftizoxima (Mexico)
(Continued)

Ceftizoxime *(Continued)*

Use Treatment of susceptible nonpseudomonal gram-negative rod infections or mixed gram-negative and anaerobic infections; predominantly respiratory tract, skin and skin structure, bone and joint, urinary tract and gynecologic, as well as septicemia

Usual Dosage I.M., I.V.:

Children ≥6 months: 150-200 mg/kg/day divided every 6-8 hours (maximum of 12 g/24 hours)

Adults: 1-2 g every 8-12 hours, up to 2 g every 4 hours or 4 g every 8 hours for life-threatening infections

Mechanism of Action Inhibits bacterial cell wall synthesis by binding to one or more of the penicillin-binding proteins (PBPs) which in turn inhibits the final transpeptidation step of peptidoglycan synthesis in bacterial cell walls, thus inhibiting cell wall biosynthesis. Bacteria eventually lyse due to ongoing activity of cell wall autolytic enzymes (autolysins and murein hydrolases) while cell wall assembly is arrested.

Local Anesthetic/Vasoconstrictor Precautions No information available to require special precautions

Effects on Dental Treatment No effects or complications reported

Other Adverse Effects

1% to 10%:

Central nervous system: Fever

Dermatologic: Rash, pruritus

Hematologic: Eosinophilia, thrombocytosis

Local: Pain, burning at injection site

Miscellaneous: Transient elevation of AST, ALT, and alkaline phosphatase

<1%:

Central nervous system: Numbness

Genitourinary: Vaginitis

Hematologic: Anemia, leukopenia, neutropenia, thrombocytopenia

Hepatic: Elevation of bilirubin

Renal: Transient elevations of BUN and creatinine

Drug Interactions

Increased effect: High-dose probenecid decreases renal clearance of cephalosporins

Drug Uptake

Serum half-life: 1.6 hours, increases to 25 hours when Cl_{cr} falls to <10 mL/minute

Time to peak serum concentration: I.M.: Within 0.5-1 hour

Pregnancy Risk Factor B

Ceftriaxona (Mexico) *see* Ceftriaxone Sodium *on this page*

Ceftriaxone Sodium *(sef try ak' sone sow' dee um)*

Related Information

Animal and Human Bites Guidelines *on page 976*

Nonviral Infectious Diseases *on page 932*

Brand Names Rocephin®

Canadian/Mexican Brand Names Benaxona® (Mexico); Cefaxona® (Mexico); Tacex® (Mexico); Triaken® (Mexico)

Therapeutic Category Antibiotic, Cephalosporin (Third Generation)

Synonyms Ceftriaxona (Mexico)

Use Treatment of lower respiratory tract infections, skin and skin structure infections, bone and joint infections, intra-abdominal and urinary tract infections, sepsis and meningitis due to susceptible organisms; documented or suspected infection due to susceptible organisms in home care patients and patients without I.V. line access; treatment of documented or suspected gonococcal infection or chancroid; emergency room management of patients at high risk for bacteremia, periorbital or buccal cellulitis, salmonellosis or shigellosis, and pneumonia of unestablished etiology (<5 years of age)

Usual Dosage I.M., I.V.:

Children: 50-75 mg/kg/day in 1-2 divided doses every 12-24 hours; maximum: 2 g/24 hours

Meningitis: 100 mg/kg/day divided every 12-24 hours, up to a maximum of 4 g/24 hours; loading dose of 75 mg/kg/dose may be given at start of therapy

Uncomplicated gonococcal infections, sexual assault, and STD prophylaxis: I.M.: 125 mg as a single dose

Complicated gonococcal infections:

<45 kg: 50 mg/kg/day once daily; maximum: 1 g/day; for ophthalmia, peritonitis, arthritis, or bacteremia: 50-100 mg/kg/day divided every 12-24 hours; maximum: 2 g/day for meningitis or endocarditis

>45 kg: 1 g/day once daily for disseminated gonococcal infections; 1-2 g dose every 12 hours for meningitis or endocarditis

Acute epididymitis: I.M.: 250 mg in a single dose

Adults: 1-2 g every 12-24 hours (depending on the type and severity of infection); maximum dose: 2 g every 12 hours for treatment of meningitis

Uncomplicated gonorrhea: I.M.: 250 mg as a single dose

Mechanism of Action Inhibits bacterial cell wall synthesis by binding to one or more of the penicillin-binding proteins (PBPs) which in turn inhibits the final transpeptidation step of peptidoglycan synthesis in bacterial cell walls, thus inhibiting cell wall biosynthesis. Bacteria eventually lyse due to ongoing activity of cell wall autolytic enzymes (autolysins and murein hydrolases) while cell wall assembly is arrested.

Local Anesthetic/Vasoconstrictor Precautions No information available to require special precautions

Effects on Dental Treatment No effects or complications reported

Other Adverse Effects

1% to 10%:
Dermatologic: Rash
Gastrointestinal: Diarrhea
Hematologic: Eosinophilia, thrombocytosis, leukopenia
Hepatic: Elevations of SGOT [AST], SGPT [ALT]
Local: Pain at injection site
Renal: Elevations of BUN

<1%:
Cardiovascular: Flushing
Central nervous system: Fever, chills, headache, dizziness
Dermatologic: Pruritus
Gastrointestinal: Nausea, vomiting, dysgeusia
Genitourinary: Presence of casts in urine, vaginitis
Hematologic: Anemia, hemolytic anemia, neutropenia, lymphopenia, thrombocytopenia
Local: Phlebitis
Renal: Elevation of creatinine
Miscellaneous: Elevations of alkaline phosphatase and bilirubin, moniliasis, diaphoresis

Drug Interactions
Increased effect: High-dose probenecid decreases renal clearance of cephalosporins

Drug Uptake
Serum half-life: Normal renal and hepatic function: 5-9 hours
Time to peak serum concentration:
I.M.: Within 1-2 hours
I.V.: Within minutes

Pregnancy Risk Factor B

Cefuroxima (Mexico) *see* Cefuroxime *on this page*

Cefuroxime (se fyoor ox' eem)

Brand Names Ceftin®; Kefurox®; Zinacef®
Canadian/Mexican Brand Names Froxal® (Mexico); Zinnat® (Mexico)
Therapeutic Category Antibiotic, Cephalosporin (Second Generation)
Synonyms Cefuroxima (Mexico)

Use Treatment of infections caused by staphylococci, group B streptococci, *H. influenzae* (type A and B), *E. coli*, *Enterobacter*, *Salmonella*, and *Klebsiella*; treatment of susceptible infections of the lower respiratory tract, otitis media, urinary tract, skin and soft tissue, bone and joint, sepsis and gonorrhea

Usual Dosage
Children:
Pharyngitis, tonsillitis: Oral:
Suspension: 20 mg/kg/day (maximum: 500 mg/day) in 2 divided doses
Tablet: 125 mg every 12 hours
Acute otitis media, impetigo: Oral:
Suspension: 30 mg/kg/day (maximum: 1 g/day) in 2 divided doses
Tablet: 250 mg every 12 hours
I.M., I.V.: 75-150 mg/kg/day divided every 8 hours; maximum dose: 6 g/day
Meningitis: Not recommended (doses of 200-240 mg/kg/day divided every 6-8 hours have been used); maximum dose: 9 g/day
Adults:
Oral: 250-500 mg twice daily; uncomplicated urinary tract infection: 125-250 mg every 12 hours
(Continued)

Cefuroxime *(Continued)*

    I.M., I.V.: 750 mg to 1.5 g/dose every 8 hours or 100-150 mg/kg/day in divided doses every 6-8 hours; maximum: 6 g/24 hours

Mechanism of Action Inhibits bacterial cell wall synthesis by binding to one or more of the penicillin-binding proteins (PBPs) which in turn inhibits the final transpeptidation step of peptidoglycan synthesis in bacterial cell walls, thus inhibiting cell wall biosynthesis. Bacteria eventually lyse due to ongoing activity of cell wall autolytic enzymes (autolysins and murein hydrolases) while cell wall assembly is arrested.

Local Anesthetic/Vasoconstrictor Precautions No information available to require special precautions

Effects on Dental Treatment No effects or complications reported

Other Adverse Effects

1% to 10%:
    Hematologic: Decreased hemoglobin and hematocrit, eosinophilia
    Local: Thrombophlebitis
    Miscellaneous: Transient rise in SGOT [AST]/SGPT [ALT] and alkaline phosphatase

<1%:
    Central nervous system: Dizziness, fever, headache
    Dermatologic: Rash
    Gastrointestinal: Nausea, vomiting, diarrhea, stomach cramps, colitis, GI bleeding
    Genitourinary: Vaginitis
    Hematologic: Transient neutropenia and leukopenia
    Hepatic: Transient increase in liver enzymes
    Local: Pain at the injection site
    Renal: Increase in creatinine and/or BUN

Drug Interactions
    Increased effect: High-dose probenecid decreases clearance of cefuroxime

Drug Uptake
    Absorption: Increased when given with or shortly after food or infant formula
    Serum half-life:
        Adults: 1-2 hours (prolonged in renal impairment)
            I.M.: Within 15-60 minutes
            I.V.: 2-3 minutes

Pregnancy Risk Factor B

Dosage Forms
    Infusion, premixed (frozen) (Zinacef®): 750 mg (50 mL); 1.5 g (50 mL)
    Powder for injection, as sodium (Kefurox®, Zinacef®): 750 mg, 1.5 g, 7.5 g
    Tablet, as axetil (Ceftin®): 125 mg, 250 mg, 500 mg

Dietary Considerations May be taken with food, however, bioavailability is increased with food

Generic Available No

Cefzil® *see* Cefprozil *on page 170*

Celestone® *see* Betamethasone *on page 109*

CellCept® *see* Mycophenolate Mofetil *on page 595*

Cellufresh® [OTC] *see* Carboxymethylcellulose Sodium *on page 156*

Cellulose, Oxidized *(sel' yoo lose, ok' si dyzed)*

Brand Names Oxycel®; Surgicel®

Therapeutic Category Hemostatic Agent

Use Temporary packing for the control of capillary, venous, or small arterial hemorrhage

Usual Dosage Minimal amounts of an appropriate size are laid on the bleeding site

Local Anesthetic/Vasoconstrictor Precautions No information available to require special precautions

Effects on Dental Treatment No effects or complications reported

Other Adverse Effects

1% to 10%:
    Central nervous system: Headache
    Respiratory: Nasal burning or stinging, sneezing (rhinological procedures)
    Miscellaneous: Encapsulation of fluid, foreign body reactions (with or without) infection

Oral manifestations: No data reported

Contraindications Do not apply as packing or wadding as a hemostatic agents; do not use for packing or implantation in fractures or laminectomies; do not use to control hemorrhage from large arteries or on nonhemorrhagic serous oozing surfaces

Warnings/Precautions By swelling, oxidized cellulose may cause nerve damage by pressure in bony confine (ie, optic nerve and chiasm); always remove from these sites of application or do not use at all (see contraindications); do not autoclave, do not moisten with water or saline (lessens hemostatic effect). Avoid wadding or packing tightly; do not use after application of $AgNO_3$ or other escharotic agents.

Drug Interactions No data reported

Pregnancy Risk Factor No data reported

Breast-feeding Considerations No data reported

Dosage Forms
Pad (Oxycel®): 3" x 3", 8 ply
Pledget (Oxycel®): 2" x 1" x 1"
Strip:
    Oxycel®:
        18" x 2", 4 ply
        5" x $1/2$", 4 ply
        36" x $1/2$", 4 ply
    Surgicel®:
        2" x 14"
        4" x 8"
        2" x 3"
        $1/2$" x 2"

Dietary Considerations No data reported

Generic Available No

Cellulose, Oxidized Regenerated
(sel' yoo lose, ok' si dyzed re jen' er aye ted)

Brand Names Surgicel® Absorbable Hemostat

Therapeutic Category Hemostatic Agent

Use
Dental: To control bleeding created during dental surgery
Medical: Hemostatic

Usual Dosage Minimal amounts of the fabric strip are laid on the bleeding site or held firmly against the tissues until hemostasis occurs

Mechanism of Action Cellulose, oxidized regenerated is saturated with blood at the bleeding site and swells into a brownish or black gelatinous mass which aids in the formation of a clot. When used in small amounts, it is absorbed from the sites of implantation with little or no tissue reaction.

Local Anesthetic/Vasoconstrictor Precautions No information available to require special precautions

Effects on Dental Treatment No effects or complications reported

Other Adverse Effects No data reported

    Oral manifestations: No data reported

Contraindications Not to be used as packing or wadding unless it is removed after hemostasis occurs; not to be used for implantation in bone defects

Warnings/Precautions Autoclaving causes physical breakdown of the product. Closing the material in a contaminated wound without drainage may lead to complications. The material should not be moistened before insertion since the hemostatic effect is greater when applied dry. The material should not be impregnated with anti-infective agents. Its hemostatic effect is not enhanced by the addition of thrombin. The material may be left in situ when necessary but it is advisable to remove it once hemostasis is achieved.

Drug Interactions No data reported

Breast-feeding Considerations No data reported

Dosage Forms Knitted fabric strips: Envelopes in a size of $1/2$" x 2"

Dietary Considerations No data reported

Comments Oxidized regenerated cellulose is prepared by the controlled oxidation of regenerated cellulose. The fabric is white with a pale yellow cast and has a faint, caramel-like aroma. A slight discoloration may occur with age but this does not effect its hemostatic actions.

Cellulose Sodium Phosphate
(sel' yoo lose sow' dee um fos' fate)

Brand Names Calcibind®

Therapeutic Category Urinary Tract Product

Synonyms CSP; Sodium Cellulose Phosphate

Use Adjunct to dietary restriction to reduce renal calculi formation in absorptive hypercalciuria type I

(Continued)

Cellulose Sodium Phosphate *(Continued)*

Local Anesthetic/Vasoconstrictor Precautions No information available to require special precautions

Effects on Dental Treatment No effects or complications reported

Celluvisc® [OTC] *see* Carboxymethylcellulose Sodium *on page 156*

Celontin® *see* Methsuximide *on page 564*

Cel-U-Jec® *see* Betamethasone *on page 109*

Cenafed® [OTC] *see* Pseudoephedrine *on page 749*

Cenafed® Plus [OTC] *see* Triprolidine and Pseudoephedrine *on page 878*

Cena-K® *see* Potassium Chloride *on page 708*

Cenolate® *see* Sodium Ascorbate *on page 791*

Centrax® *see* Prazepam *on page 715*

Cēpacol® Anesthetic Troches [OTC] *see* Cetylpyridinium Chloride and Benzocaine *on page 179*

Cēpastat® [OTC] *see* Phenol *on page 682*

Cephalexin Monohydrate (sef a lex' in mon oh hye' drate)
Related Information
Dental Drug Interactions: Update on Drug Combinations Requiring Special Considerations *on page 1022*
Oral Bacterial Infections *on page 945*

Brand Names Cefanex®; C-Lexin®; Entacef®; Keflet®; Keflex®; Keftab®

Canadian/Mexican Brand Names Apo-Cephalex® (Canada); Novo-Lexin® (Canada); Nu-Cephalex® (Canada); Ceporex® (Mexico)

Therapeutic Category Antibiotic, Cephalosporin (First Generation)

Use
Dental: An alternate antibiotic to treat orofacial infections in patients allergic to penicillins; susceptible bacteria including aerobic gram-positive bacteria and anaerobes

Medical: Treatment of susceptible bacterial infections in the medical patient, including those caused by group A beta-hemolytic *Streptococcus*, *Staphylococcus*, *Klebsiella pneumoniae*, *E. coli*, *Proteus mirabilis*, and *Shigella*; predominantly used for lower respiratory tract, urinary tract, skin and soft tissue, and bone and joint

Usual Dosage Oral:
Children: 25-50 mg/kg/day every 6 hours; severe infections: 50-100 mg/kg/day in divided doses every 6 hours; maximum: 3 g/24 hours
Adults: 250-1000 mg every 6 hours; maximum: 4 g/day

Mechanism of Action Inhibits bacterial cell wall synthesis by binding to one or more of the penicillin-binding proteins (PBPs) which in turn inhibits the final transpeptidation step of peptidoglycan synthesis in bacterial cell walls, thus inhibiting cell wall biosynthesis. Bacteria eventually lyse due to ongoing activity of cell wall autolytic enzymes (autolysins and murein hydrolases) while cell wall assembly is arrested.

Local Anesthetic/Vasoconstrictor Precautions No information available to require special precautions

Effects on Dental Treatment No effects or complications reported

Other Adverse Effects 1% to 10%: Gastrointestinal: Diarrhea

Oral manifestations: No data reported

Contraindications Hypersensitivity to cephalexin, any component, or cephalosporins

Warnings/Precautions Modify dosage in patients with severe renal impairment; prolonged use may result in superinfection; a low incidence of cross-hypersensitivity to penicillins exists

Drug Interactions High-dose probenecid increases clearance of cephalexin; aminoglycosides increase nephrotoxic potential

Drug Uptake
Absorption:
Adults: Rapid
Children: Delayed in young children
Time to peak serum concentration: Oral: Within 1 hour
Duration: 6 hours
Serum half-life: Adults: 0.5-1.2 hours (prolonged with renal impairment)
Influence of food: No effect

Pregnancy Risk Factor B

Breast-feeding Considerations Excreted into breast milk in small amounts like other cephalosporins

Dosage Forms
Capsule: 250 mg, 500 mg
Drops, pediatric: 100 mg/mL (10 mL)
Suspension: 125 mg/5 mL (5 mL unit dose, 60 mL, 100 mL, 200 mL); 250 mg/5 mL (5 mL unit dose, 100 mL, 200 mL)
Tablet: 250 mg, 500 mg, 1 g
Tablet, as hydrochloride (Keftab®): 250 mg, 500 mg

Dietary Considerations Should be taken on an empty stomach (ie, 1 hour prior to, or 2 hours after meals) to increase total absorption

Generic Available Yes

Comments Cephalexin is effective against anaerobic bacteria, but the sensitivity of alpha-hemolytic *Streptococcus* vary; approximately 10% of strains are resistant. Nearly 70% are intermediately sensitive. Patients allergic to penicillins can use a cephalosporin; the incidence of cross-reactivity between penicillins and cephalosporins is 1% when the allergic reaction to penicillin is delayed. If the patient has a history of immediate reaction to penicillin, the incidence of cross-reactivity is 20%; cephalosporins are contraindicated in these patients.

Selected Readings
Saxon A, Beall GN, Kohr AS, et al, "Immediate Hypersensitivity Reactions to Beta-Lactam Antibiotics," *Ann Intern Med*, 1987, 107:204-15.

Cephalothin Sodium (sef a′ loe thin sow′ dee um)
Brand Names Keflin®
Canadian/Mexican Brand Names Ceporacin® (Canada); Ceftina® (Mexico)
Therapeutic Category Antibiotic, Cephalosporin (First Generation)
Synonyms Cefalotina Sal Sodica De (Mexico)
Use Treatment of susceptible bacterial infections, including those caused by group A beta-hemolytic *Streptococcus*; respiratory, genitourinary, gastrointestinal, skin and soft tissue, bone and joint infections; septicemia; cephalexin is the oral equivalent

Usual Dosage I.M., I.V.:
Children: 75-125 mg/kg/day divided every 4-6 hours; maximum dose: 10 g in a 24-hour period
Adults: 500 mg to 2 g every 4-6 hours

Mechanism of Action Inhibits bacterial cell wall synthesis by binding to one or more of the penicillin-binding proteins (PBPs) which in turn inhibits the final transpeptidation step of peptidoglycan synthesis in bacterial cell walls, thus inhibiting cell wall biosynthesis. Bacteria eventually lyse due to ongoing activity of cell wall autolytic enzymes (autolysins and murein hydrolases) while cell wall assembly is arrested.

Local Anesthetic/Vasoconstrictor Precautions No information available to require special precautions

Effects on Dental Treatment No effects or complications reported

Other Adverse Effects
1% to 10%: Gastrointestinal: Nausea, vomiting, diarrhea
<1%:
Dermatologic: Maculopapular and erythematous rash
Gastrointestinal: Dyspepsia, pseudomembranous colitis
Hematologic: Bleeding
Local: Pain and induration at injection site

Drug Interactions
Increased effect: High-dose probenecid decreases renal clearance of cephalothin

Drug Uptake
Serum half-life: 30-60 minutes
Time to peak serum concentration:
I.M.: Within 30 minutes
I.V.: Within 15 minutes

Pregnancy Risk Factor B

Cephapirin Sodium (sef a pye′ rin sow′ dee um)
Brand Names Cefadyl®
Therapeutic Category Antibiotic, Cephalosporin (First Generation)
Use Treatment of infections when caused by susceptible strains including group A beta-hemolytic *Streptococcus*; used in serious respiratory, genitourinary, gastrointestinal, skin and soft tissue, bone and joint infections; septicemia; endocarditis; identical to cephalothin

Usual Dosage I.M., I.V.:
Children: 10-20 mg/kg/dose every 6 hours up to 4 g/24 hours
Adults: 500 mg to 1 g every 6 hours up to 12 g/day
(Continued)

Cephapirin Sodium (Continued)

Mechanism of Action Inhibits bacterial cell wall synthesis by binding to one or more of the penicillin-binding proteins (PBPs) which in turn inhibits the final transpeptidation step of peptidoglycan synthesis in bacterial cell walls, thus inhibiting cell wall biosynthesis. Bacteria eventually lyse due to ongoing activity of cell wall autolytic enzymes (autolysins and murein hydrolases) while cell wall assembly is arrested.

Local Anesthetic/Vasoconstrictor Precautions No information available to require special precautions

Effects on Dental Treatment No effects or complications reported

Other Adverse Effects

1% to 10%: Gastrointestinal: Diarrhea

<1%:

Central nervous system: CNS irritation, seizures, fever

Dermatologic: Rash, urticaria

Hematologic: Leukopenia, thrombocytopenia

Hepatic: Transient elevation of liver enzymes

Drug Interactions

Increased effect: High-dose probenecid decreases renal clearance of cephalosporins

Drug Uptake

Serum half-life: 36-60 minutes

Time to peak serum concentration:

I.M.: Within 30 minutes

I.V.: Within 5 minutes

Pregnancy Risk Factor B

Cephradine (sef' ra deen)

Brand Names Velosef®

Canadian/Mexican Brand Names Veracef® (Mexico)

Therapeutic Category Antibiotic, Cephalosporin (First Generation)

Synonyms Cefradina (Mexico)

Use Treatment of susceptible bacterial infections, including those caused by group A beta-hemolytic *Streptococcus*; used in in respiratory, genitourinary, gastrointestinal, skin and soft tissue, bone and joint infections

Usual Dosage Oral:

Children ≥9 months: 25-50 mg/kg/day in divided doses every 6 hours

Adults: 250-500 mg every 6-12 hours

Mechanism of Action Inhibits bacterial cell wall synthesis by binding to one or more of the penicillin-binding proteins (PBPs) which in turn inhibits the final transpeptidation step of peptidoglycan synthesis in bacterial cell walls, thus inhibiting cell wall biosynthesis. Bacteria eventually lyse due to ongoing activity of cell wall autolytic enzymes (autolysins and murein hydrolases) while cell wall assembly is arrested.

Local Anesthetic/Vasoconstrictor Precautions No information available to require special precautions

Effects on Dental Treatment No effects or complications reported

Other Adverse Effects

1% to 10%: Gastrointestinal: Diarrhea

<1%:

Dermatologic: Rash

Gastrointestinal: Nausea, vomiting, pseudomembranous colitis

Renal: Increased BUN and creatinine

Drug Interactions No data reported

Drug Uptake

Serum half-life: 1-2 hours

Time to peak serum concentration: Oral, I.M.: Within 1-2 hours

Pregnancy Risk Factor B

Cephulac® *see* Lactulose *on page 488*

Cerebyx® *see* Fosphenytoin *on page 389*

Ceredase® Injection *see* Alglucerase *on page 32*

Cerespan® *see* Papaverine Hydrochloride *on page 658*

Cerezyme® *see* Imglucerase *on page 450*

Cerose-DM® [OTC] *see* Chlorpheniramine, Phenylephrine, and Dextromethorphan *on page 193*

Cerubidine® *see* Daunorubicin Hydrochloride *on page 252*

Cerumenex® *see* Triethanolamine Polypeptide Oleate-Condensate *on page 868*

Cesamet® *see* Nabilone *on page 596*

Cetacaine® *see* Benzocaine, Butyl Aminobenzoate, Tetracaine, and Benzalkonium Chloride *on page 103*

Cetamide® *see* Sodium Sulfacetamide *on page 793*

Cetane® **[OTC]** *see* Ascorbic Acid *on page 76*

Cetapred® *see* Sodium Sulfacetamide and Prednisolone Acetate *on page 794*

Cetirizine Hydrochloride (se ti′ ra zeen hye droe klor′ ide)

Brand Names Zyrtec™

Therapeutic Category Antihistamine

Synonyms P-071; UCB-P071

Use Perennial and seasonal allergic rhinitis and other allergic symptoms including urticaria

Usual Dosage Children ≥12 years and Adults: Oral: 5-10 mg once daily, depending upon symptom severity

Dosing interval in hepatic or renal impairment:
Cl_{cr} ≤31 mL/minute: Administer 5 mg once daily

Mechanism of Action Competes with histamine for H_1-receptor sites on effector cells in the gastrointestinal tract, blood vessels, and respiratory tract

Local Anesthetic/Vasoconstrictor Precautions No information available to require special precautions

Effects on Dental Treatment No effects or complications reported

Other Adverse Effects
>10%: Central nervous system: Headache has been reported to occur in 10% to 12% of patients, drowsiness has been reported in as much as 26% of patients on high doses
1% to 10%:
Central nervous system: Somnolence, fatigue, dizziness
Gastrointestinal: Dry mouth
<1%: Central nervous system: Depression

Contraindications Hypersensitivity to cetirizine, hydroxyzine, or any component

Warnings/Precautions Cetirizine should be used cautiously in patients with hepatic or renal dysfunction, the elderly and in nursing mothers. Doses >10 mg/day may cause significant drowsiness

Drug Interactions Increased toxicity: CNS depressants, anticholinergics

Drug Uptake
Onset of effect: Within 15-30 minutes
Absorption: Oral: Rapid
Serum half-life: 8-11 hours
Time to peak serum concentration: Within 30-60 minutes

Pregnancy Risk Factor B

Generic Available No

Cetylpyridinium Chloride and Benzocaine

(see′ til peer i di′ nee um klor′ ide & ben′ zoe kane)

Brand Names Cēpacol® Anesthetic Troches [OTC]

Therapeutic Category Local Anesthetic, Oral

Synonyms Benzocaine and Cetylpyridinium Chloride

Use Symptomatic relief of sore throat

Local Anesthetic/Vasoconstrictor Precautions No information available to require special precautions

Effects on Dental Treatment No effects or complications reported

Cevalin® *see* Ascorbic Acid *on page 76*

Ce-Vi-Sol® **[OTC]** *see* Ascorbic Acid *on page 76*

Cevita® **[OTC]** *see* Ascorbic Acid *on page 76*

Cevitamic Acid (Canada) *see* Ascorbic Acid *on page 76*

Charcoaid® **[OTC]** *see* Charcoal *on this page*

Charcoal (char′ kole)

Brand Names Actidose-Aqua® [OTC]; Actidose® With Sorbitol [OTC]; Charcoaid® [OTC]; Charcocaps® [OTC]; Insta-Char® [OTC]; Liqui-Char® [OTC]; SuperChar® [OTC]

Therapeutic Category Antidiarrheal; Antidote, Adsorbent; Antiflatulent

Use Emergency treatment in poisoning by drugs and chemicals; repetitive doses for gastric dialysis in uremia to adsorb various waste products, and repetitive doses have proven useful to enhance the elimination of certain drugs (eg, theophylline, phenobarbital, and aspirin)
(Continued)

Charcoal *(Continued)*

Usual Dosage Oral:

Acute poisoning:

Charcoal with sorbitol: Single-dose:

Children 1-12 years: 1-2 g/kg/dose or 15-30 g or approximately 5-10 times the weight of the ingested poison; 1 g adsorbs 100-1000 mg of poison; the use of repeat oral charcoal with sorbitol doses is not recommended. In young children, sorbitol should be repeated no more than 1-2 times/day.

Adults: 30-100 g

Charcoal in water:

Single-dose:

Children 1-12 years: 15-30 g or 1-2 g/kg

Adults: 30-100 g or 1-2 g/kg

Multiple-dose:

Children 1-12 years: 20-60 g or 0.5-1 g/kg every 2-6 hours until clinical observations, serum drug concentration have returned to a subtherapeutic range, or charcoal stool apparent

Adults: 20-60 g or 0.5-1 g/kg every 2-6 hours

Gastric dialysis: Adults: 20-50 g every 6 hours for 1-2 days

Intestinal gas, diarrhea, GI distress: Adults: 520-975 mg after meals or at first sign of discomfort; repeat as needed to a maximum dose of 4.16 g/day

Mechanism of Action Adsorbs toxic substances or irritants, thus inhibiting GI absorption; adsorbs intestinal gas; the addition of sorbitol results in hyperosmotic laxative action causing catharsis

Local Anesthetic/Vasoconstrictor Precautions No information available to require special precautions

Effects on Dental Treatment No effects or complications reported

Other Adverse Effects

>10%:

Gastrointestinal: Emesis, vomiting, diarrhea with sorbitol, constipation

Miscellaneous: Stools will turn black

<1%: Swelling of abdomen

Drug Interactions Do not administer concomitantly with syrup of ipecac; do not mix with milk, ice cream, or sherbet

Drug Uptake

Absorption: Not absorbed from GI tract

Pregnancy Risk Factor C

Charcocaps® [OTC] *see Charcoal on previous page*

Chemical Dependency and Dental Practice *see page 971*

Cheracol® *see Guaifenesin and Codeine on page 408*

Cheracol D® [OTC] *see Guaifenesin and Dextromethorphan on page 408*

Chibroxin™ *see Norfloxacin on page 628*

Children's Hold® [OTC] *see Dextromethorphan on page 266*

Children's Kaopectate® [OTC] *see Attapulgite on page 86*

Chlo-Amine® [OTC] *see Chlorpheniramine Maleate on page 191*

Chlorafed® Liquid [OTC] *see Chlorpheniramine and Pseudoephedrine on page 191*

Chloral Hydrate *(klor' al hye' drate)*

Brand Names Aquachloral® Supprettes®; Noctec®; Somnos®

Canadian/Mexican Brand Names Novo-Chlorhydrate® (Canada); PMS®-Chloral Hydrate (Canada)

Therapeutic Category Hypnotic; Sedative

Use

Dental: Sedative/hypnotic for dental procedures

Medical: Short-term sedative and hypnotic (<2 weeks), sedative/hypnotic for diagnostic procedures; sedative prior to EEG evaluations

Usual Dosage

Children: Preoperative sedation: Oral: 50-75 mg/kg/dose 30-60 minutes prior to procedure; may repeat 30 minutes after initial dose if needed to a total maximum dose of 120 mg/kg or 1 g total

Adults: Very rarely used in adults as preoperative sedative in dentistry

Sedation, anxiety: 250 mg 3 times/day

Hypnotic: 500-1000 mg at bedtime or 30 minutes prior to procedure, not to exceed 2 g/24 hours

Mechanism of Action Central nervous system depressant effects are due to its active metabolite trichloroethanol, mechanism unknown

Local Anesthetic/Vasoconstrictor Precautions No information available to require special precautions

Effects on Dental Treatment No effects or complications reported

Other Adverse Effects

>10%: Gastrointestinal: Gastric irritation, nausea, vomiting, diarrhea

1% to 10%:

Central nervous system: Clumsiness, hallucinations, drowsiness, "hangover" effect

Dermatologic: Rash, urticaria

Oral manifestations: No data reported

Contraindications Hypersensitivity to chloral hydrate or any component; hepatic or renal impairment; gastritis or ulcers; severe cardiac disease

Warnings/Precautions Use with caution in patients with porphyria; use with caution in neonates, drug may accumulate with repeated use, prolonged use in neonates associated with hyperbilirubinemia; tolerance to hypnotic effect develops, therefore, not recommended for use >2 weeks; taper dosage to avoid withdrawal with prolonged use; trichloroethanol (TCE), a metabolite of chloral hydrate, is a carcinogen in mice; there is no data in humans. Chloral hydrate is considered a second line hypnotic agent in the elderly.

Drug Interactions May potentiate effects of warfarin, central nervous system depressants, alcohol; vasodilation reaction (flushing, tachycardia, etc) may occur with concurrent use of alcohol; concomitant use of furosemide (I.V.) may result in flushing, diaphoresis, and blood pressure changes

Drug Uptake

Absorption: Oral: Rapid

Time to peak serum concentration: Within 0.5-1 hour

Duration of effect: 4-8 hours

Serum half-life: Active metabolite: 8-11 hours

Pregnancy Risk Factor C

Breast-feeding Considerations May be taken while breast-feeding

Dosage Forms

Capsule: 250 mg, 500 mg

Suppository, rectal: 324 mg, 500 mg, 648 mg

Syrup: 250 mg/5 mL (10 mL); 500 mg/5 mL (5 mL, 10 mL, 480 mL)

Dietary Considerations May be taken with chilled liquid to mask taste

Generic Available Yes

Chlorambucil (klor am′ byoo sil)

Brand Names Leukeran®

Therapeutic Category Antineoplastic Agent, Alkylating Agent (Nitrogen Mustard)

Use Management of chronic lymphocytic leukemia (CLL), Hodgkin's and non-Hodgkin's lymphoma; breast and ovarian carcinoma, testicular carcinoma, choriocarcinoma; Waldenström's macroglobulinemia, and nephrotic syndrome unresponsive to conventional therapy

Usual Dosage Oral (**refer to individual protocols**):

Children:

General short courses: 0.1-0.2 mg/kg/day **or** 4.5 mg/m²/day for 3-6 weeks for remission induction (usual: 4-10 mg/day); maintenance therapy: 0.03-0.1 mg/kg/day (usual: 2-4 mg/day)

Nephrotic syndrome: 0.1-0.2 mg/kg/day every day for 5-15 weeks with low-dose prednisone

Chronic lymphocytic leukemia (CLL):

Biweekly regimen: Initial: 0.4 mg/kg/dose every 2 weeks; increase dose by 0.1 mg/kg every 2 weeks until a response occurs and/or myelosuppression occurs

Monthly regimen: Initial: 0.4 mg/kg, increase dose by 0.2 mg/kg every 4 weeks until a response occurs and/or myelosuppression occurs

Malignant lymphomas:

Non-Hodgkin's lymphoma: 0.1 mg/kg/day

Hodgkin's lymphoma: 0.2 mg/kg/day

Adults: 0.1-0.2 mg/kg/day **or** 3-6 mg/m²/day for 3-6 weeks, then adjust dose on basis of blood counts. Pulse dosing has been used in CLL as intermittent, biweekly, or monthly doses of 0.4 mg/kg and increased by 0.1 mg/kg until the disease is under control or toxicity ensues. An alternate regimen is 14 mg/m²/day for 5 days, repeated every 21-28 days.

Mechanism of Action Interferes with DNA replication and RNA transcription by alkylation and cross-linking the strands of DNA

Local Anesthetic/Vasoconstrictor Precautions No information available to require special precautions

(Continued)

Chlorambucil *(Continued)*

Effects on Dental Treatment No effects or complications reported

Other Adverse Effects

>10%:

Myelosuppressive: Use with caution when receiving radiation; bone marrow suppression frequently occurs and occasionally bone marrow failure has occurred; blood counts should be monitored closely while undergoing treatment; leukopenia, thrombocytopenia, anemia. WBC: Moderate; Platelets: Moderate; Onset (days): 7; Nadir (days): 10-14; Recovery (days): 28

Secondary malignancies: Increased incidence of AML

1% to 10%: Menstrual changes, skin rashes, hyperuricemia

Gastrointestinal: Diarrhea, oral ulceration are infrequent

Emetic potential: Low (<10%)

<1%: Drug fever, hepatic necrosis, weakness, rash, leukopenia, thrombocytopenia

Central nervous system: Tremors, muscular twitching, confusion, agitation, ataxia, hallucination; rarely generalized or focal seizures, peripheral neuropathy

Fertility impairment: Has caused chromosomal damage in man, oligospermia, both reversible and permanent sterility have occurred in both sexes; can produce amenorrhea in females, oligospermia

Miscellaneous: Pulmonary fibrosis, skin hypersensitivity, keratitis, hepatotoxicity

Drug Uptake

Absorption: 70% to 80%

Serum half-life: 90 minutes to 2 hours

Pregnancy Risk Factor D

Chloramphenicol (klor am fen' i kole)

Brand Names AK-Chlor®; Chloromycetin®; Chloroptic®; Ophthochlor®

Canadian/Mexican Brand Names Pentamycetin® (Canada); Diochloram® (Canada); Sopamycetin® (Canada); Cetina® (Mexico); Clorafen® (Mexico); Paraxin® (Mexico); Quemicetina® (Mexico)

Therapeutic Category Antibiotic, Ophthalmic; Antibiotic, Otic; Antibiotic, Miscellaneous

Synonyms Cloranfenicol (Mexico)

Use Treatment of serious infections due to organisms resistant to other less toxic antibiotics or when its penetrability into the site of infection is clinically superior to other antibiotics to which the organism is sensitive; useful in infections caused by *Bacteroides*, *H. influenzae*, *Neisseria meningitidis*, *Salmonella*, and *Rickettsia*

Usual Dosage

Meningitis: Oral, I.V.: Children: 75-100 mg/kg/day divided every 6 hours

Other infections: Oral, I.V.:

Children: 50-75 mg/kg/day divided every 6 hours; maximum daily dose: 4 g/day

Adults: 50-100 mg/kg/day in divided doses every 6 hours; maximum daily dose: 4 g/day

Ophthalmic: Children and Adults: Instill 1-2 drops or 1.25 cm (½" of ointment every 3-4 hours); increase interval between applications after 48 hours to 2-3 times/day

Otic solution: Instill 2-3 drops into ear 3 times/day

Topical: Gently rub into the affected area 1-4 times/day

Mechanism of Action Reversibly binds to 50S ribosomal subunits of susceptible organisms preventing amino acids from being transferred to growing peptide chains thus inhibiting protein synthesis

Local Anesthetic/Vasoconstrictor Precautions No information available to require special precautions

Effects on Dental Treatment No effects or complications reported

Other Adverse Effects

<1%:

Central nervous system: Nightmares, headache

Dermatologic: Rash

Gastrointestinal: Diarrhea, stomatitis, enterocolitis, nausea, vomiting

Hematologic: Bone marrow depression, aplastic anemia

Neuromuscular & skeletal: Peripheral neuropathy

Ocular: Optic neuritis

Miscellaneous: Gray baby syndrome

Three (3) major toxicities associated with chloramphenicol include:
Aplastic anemia, an idiosyncratic reaction which can occur with any route of administration; usually occurs 3 weeks to 12 months after initial exposure to chloramphenicol

Bone marrow suppression is thought to be dose-related with serum concentrations >25 μg/mL and reversible once chloramphenicol is discontinued; anemia and neutropenia may occur during the first week of therapy

Gray baby syndrome is characterized by circulatory collapse, cyanosis, acidosis, abdominal distention, myocardial depression, coma, and death; reaction appears to be associated with serum levels ≥50 μg/mL; may result from drug accumulation in patients with impaired hepatic or renal function

Drug Interactions
Decreased effect: Phenobarbital and rifampin may decrease concentration of chloramphenicol

Increased toxicity: Chloramphenicol inhibits the metabolism of chlorpropamide, phenytoin, oral anticoagulants

Drug Uptake
Serum half-life: (Prolonged with markedly reduced liver function or combined liver/kidney dysfunction):
Normal renal function: 1.6-3.3 hours
End stage renal disease: 3-7 hours
Cirrhosis: 10-12 hours
Time to peak serum concentration: Oral: Within 0.5-3 hours
Pregnancy Risk Factor C

Chloramphenicol and Prednisolone
(klor am fen' i kole & pred nis' oh lone)
Brand Names Chloroptic-P® Ophthalmic
Therapeutic Category Antibiotic, Ophthalmic; Corticosteroid, Ophthalmic
Use Topical anti-infective and corticosteroid for treatment of ocular infections
Local Anesthetic/Vasoconstrictor Precautions No information available to require special precautions
Effects on Dental Treatment No effects or complications reported

Chloramphenicol, Polymyxin B, and Hydrocortisone
(klor am fen' i kole, pol i mix' in bee, & hye droe kor' ti sone)
Brand Names Ophthocort® Ophthalmic
Therapeutic Category Antibiotic, Ophthalmic
Use Topical anti-infective and corticosteroid for treatment of ocular infections
Local Anesthetic/Vasoconstrictor Precautions No information available to require special precautions
Effects on Dental Treatment No effects or complications reported

Chloraseptic® Oral [OTC] see Phenol on page 682
Chlorate® [OTC] see Chlorpheniramine Maleate on page 191

Chlordiazepoxide (klor dye az e pox' ide)
Brand Names Libritabs®; Librium®; Mitran®; Reposans-10®
Canadian/Mexican Brand Names Apo-Chlordiazepoxide® (Canada); Corax® (Canada); Medilium® (Canada); Novo-Poxide® (Canada); Solium® (Canada)
Therapeutic Category Benzodiazepine; Hypnotic; Sedative
Synonyms Clorodiacepoxido (Mexico)
Use Approved for anxiety, may be useful for acute alcohol withdrawal symptoms
Usual Dosage
Children:
<6 years: Not recommended
>6 years: Anxiety: Oral, I.M.: 0.5 mg/kg/24 hours divided every 6-8 hours

Adults:
Anxiety:
Oral: 15-100 mg divided 3-4 times/day
I.M., I.V.: Initial: 50-100 mg followed by 25-50 mg 3-4 times/day as needed
Preoperative anxiety: I.M.: 50-100 mg prior to surgery
Alcohol withdrawal symptoms: Oral, I.V.: 50-100 mg to start, dose may be repeated in 2-4 hours as necessary to a maximum of 300 mg/24 hours
Mechanism of Action Benzodiazepines appear to potentiate the effects of GABA and other inhibitory transmitters by binding to specific benzodiazepine receptor sites; benzodiazepine anxiolytic sedative that produces CNS depression at the subcortical level, except at high doses, whereby it works at the cortical level
Local Anesthetic/Vasoconstrictor Precautions No information available to require special precautions
(Continued)

Chlordiazepoxide (Continued)

Effects on Dental Treatment Over 10% of patients will experience dry mouth which disappears with cessation of drug therapy

Other Adverse Effects

>10%:

Cardiovascular: Chest pain

Central nervous system: Drowsiness, fatigue, impaired coordination, light-headedness, memory impairment, insomnia, anxiety, depression, headache

Dermatologic: Skin eruptions, rash

Endocrine & metabolic: Decreased libido

Gastrointestinal: Nausea, constipation, vomiting, diarrhea, dry mouth, increased or decreased appetite

Neuromuscular & skeletal: Dysarthria

Ocular: Blurred vision

Miscellaneous: Decreased salivation, sweating

1% to 10%:

Cardiovascular: Hypotension, tachycardia, edema, syncope

Central nervous system: Drowsiness, ataxia, confusion, mental impairment, nervousness, dizziness, akathisia

Dermatologic: Dermatitis

Gastrointestinal: Nausea, vomiting, weight gain or loss

Neuromuscular & skeletal: Rigidity, tremor, muscle cramps

Ocular: Blurred vision

Otic: Tinnitus

Respiratory: Nasal congestion, hyperventilation

Miscellaneous: Increased salivation

<1%:

Endocrine & metabolic: Menstrual irregularities

Hematologic: Blood dyscrasias

Neuromuscular & skeletal: Depressed reflexes

Miscellaneous: Drug dependence

Drug Interactions Potentiation of chlordiazepoxide-induced sedation may occur with alcohol and sedative-hypnotics

Drug Uptake

Serum half-life: 6.6-25 hours

End stage renal disease: 5-30 hours

Cirrhosis: 30-63 hours

Time to peak serum concentration:

Oral: Within 2 hours

I.M.: Results in lower peak plasma levels than oral

Pregnancy Risk Factor D

Dosage Forms

Capsule, as hydrochloride: 5 mg, 10 mg, 25 mg

Powder for injection, as hydrochloride: 100 mg

Tablet: 5 mg, 10 mg, 25 mg

Generic Available Yes

Chlordiazepoxide and Amitriptyline see Amitriptyline and Chlordiazepoxide on page 49

Chlordiazepoxide and Clidinium see Clidinium and Chlordiazepoxide on page 214

Chloresium® [OTC] see Chlorophyll on next page

Chlorhexidine Gluconate (klor hex′ i deen gloo′ koe nate)

Related Information

Dentin Hypersensitivity; High Caries Index; Xerostomia on page 959

Oral Nonviral Soft Tissue Ulcerations or Erosions on page 955

Brand Names Dyna-Hex® [OTC]; Exidine® Scrub [OTC]; Hibiclens® [OTC]; Hibistat® [OTC]; Peridex®; PerioGard®

Therapeutic Category Antibacterial, Oral Rinse; Antibiotic, Topical; Antimicrobial Mouth Rinse; Antiplaque Agent

Use

Dental: Antibacterial dental rinse; chlorhexidine is active against gram-positive and gram-negative organisms, facultative anaerobes, aerobes, and yeast

Medical: Skin cleanser for surgical scrub, cleanser for skin wounds, germicidal hand rinse

Mechanism of Action The bactericidal effect of chlorhexidine is a result of the binding of this cationic molecule to negatively charged bacterial cell walls and extramicrobial complexes. At low concentrations, this causes an alteration of bacterial cell osmotic equilibrium and leakage of potassium and phosphorous resulting in a bacteriostatic effect. At high concentrations of chlorhexidine, the cytoplasmic contents of the bacterial cell precipitate and result in cell death.

Local Anesthetic/Vasoconstrictor Precautions No information available to require special precautions

Effects on Dental Treatment No effects or complications reported

Other Adverse Effects
>10%: Increase of tartar on teeth, changes in taste. Staining of oral surfaces (mucosa, teeth, dorsum of tongue) may be visible as soon as 1 week after therapy begins and is more pronounced when there is a heavy accumulation of unremoved plaque and when teeth fillings have rough surfaces. Stain does not have a clinically adverse effect but because removal may not be possible, patients with anterior restoration should be advised of the potential permanency of the stain.

1% to 10%: Tongue irritation, oral irritation

<1%: Respiratory: Nasal congestion, shortness of breath

Oral manifestations: Swelling of face has been reported

Drug Interactions No data reported

Pregnancy Risk Factor B

Breast-feeding Considerations No data reported

Dosage Forms
Liquid, topical:
Exidine® Skin Cleanser, Hibiclens® Skin Cleanser: 4% (15 mL, 120 mL, 240 mL, 480 mL, 960 mL, 4000 mL)
Dyna-Hex® Skin Cleanser: 2% (120 mL, 240 mL, 480 mL, 960 mL, 4000 mL); 4% (120 mL, 240 mL, 480 mL, 4000 mL)
Rinse, oral (mint flavor) (Peridex®, PerioGard®): 0.12% with alcohol 11.6% (480 mL)
Sponge/Brush (Hibiclens®): 4% with isopropyl alcohol 4% (22 mL)
Wipes (Hibistat®): 0.5% (50s)

Dietary Considerations No data reported

Generic Available No

2-Chlorodeoxyadenosine *see* Cladribine *on page 211*

Chloroethane *see* Ethyl Chloride *on page 344*

Chlorofon-F® *see* Chlorzoxazone *on page 200*

Chloromycetin® *see* Chloramphenicol *on page 182*

Chlorophylin *see* Chlorophyll *on this page*

Chlorophyll (klor' oh fil)

Brand Names Chloresium® [OTC]; Derifil® [OTC]; Nullo® [OTC]; PALS® [OTC]

Therapeutic Category Gastrointestinal Agent, Miscellaneous; Topical Skin Product

Synonyms Chlorophylin

Use Topically promotes normal healing, relieves pain and swelling, and reduces malodors in wounds, burns, surface ulcers, abrasions and skin irritations; used orally to control fecal and urinary odors in colostomy, ileostomy, or incontinence

Local Anesthetic/Vasoconstrictor Precautions No information available to require special precautions

Effects on Dental Treatment No effects or complications reported

Other Adverse Effects 1% to 10%: Mild diarrhea, green stools

Chloroprocaine Hydrochloride
(klor oh proe' kane hye droe klor' ide)

Related Information
Oral Pain *on page 940*

Brand Names Nesacaine®; Nesacaine®-MPF

Therapeutic Category Dental/Local Anesthetics; Local Anesthetic, Injectable

Use Infiltration anesthesia and peripheral and epidural anesthesia

Usual Dosage Dosage varies with anesthetic procedure, the area to be anesthetized, the vascularity of the tissues, depth of anesthesia required, degree of muscle relaxation required, and duration of anesthesia; range: 1.5-25 mL of 2% to 3% solution; single adult dose should not exceed 800 mg
Infiltration and peripheral nerve block: 1% to 2%
Infiltration, peripheral and central nerve block, including caudal and epidural block: 2% to 3%, without preservatives

Mechanism of Action Chloroprocaine HCl is benzoic acid, 4-amino-2-chloro-2-(diethylamino) ethyl ester monohydrochloride. Chloroprocaine is an ester-type local anesthetic, which stabilizes the neuronal membranes and prevents initiation and transmission of nerve impulses thereby affecting local anesthetic
(Continued)

Chloroprocaine Hydrochloride *(Continued)*

actions. Local anesthetics including chloroprocaine, reversibly prevent generation and conduction of electrical impulses in neurons by decreasing the transient increase in permeability to sodium. The differential sensitivity generally
depends on the size of the fiber; small fibers are more sensitive than larger
fibers and require a longer period for recovery. Sensory pain fibers are usually
blocked first, followed by fibers that transmit sensations of temperature, touch,
and deep pressure. High concentrations block sympathetic somatic sensory
and somatic motor fibers. The spread of anesthesia depends upon the distribution of the solution. This is primarily dependent on the volume of drug injected.

Local Anesthetic/Vasoconstrictor Precautions No information available to
require special precautions

Effects on Dental Treatment No effects or complications reported

Other Adverse Effects <1%:

Cardiovascular: Myocardial depression, hypotension, bradycardia, cardiovascular collapse, edema

Central nervous system: Anxiety, restlessness, disorientation, confusion,
seizures, drowsiness, unconsciousness, chills, shivering

Dermatologic: Urticaria

Gastrointestinal: Nausea, vomiting

Local: Transient stinging or burning at injection site

Neuromuscular & skeletal: Tremor

Ocular: Blurred vision

Otic: Tinnitus

Respiratory: Respiratory arrest

Miscellaneous: Anaphylactoid reactions

Drug Interactions PABA (from ester-type anesthetics) may inhibit sulfonamides

Drug Uptake

Onset of action: 6-12 minutes

Duration: 30-60 minutes

Pregnancy Risk Factor C

Dosage Forms Injection:

Preservative free (Nesacaine®-MPF): 2% (30 mL); 3% (30 mL)

With preservative (Nesacaine®): 1% (30 mL); 2% (30 mL)

Generic Available No

Chloroptic® *see Chloramphenicol on page 182*

Chloroptic-P® Ophthalmic *see Chloramphenicol and Prednisolone on
page 183*

Chloroquine and Primaquine *(klor' oh kwin & prim' a kween)*

Brand Names Aralen® Phosphate With Primaquine Phosphate

Therapeutic Category Antimalarial Agent

Use Prophylaxis of malaria, regardless of species, in all areas where the
disease is endemic

Usual Dosage Oral: Start at least 1 day before entering the endemic area;
continue for 8 weeks after leaving the endemic area

Children: For suggested weekly dosage (based on body weight), see table:

Weight		Chloroquine Base (mg)	Primaquine Base (mg)	Dose* (mL)
lb	kg			
10-15	4.5-6.8	20	3	2.5
16-25	7.3-11.4	40	6	5
26-35	11.8-15.9	60	9	7.5
36-45	16.4-20.5	80	12	10
46-55	20.9-25	100	15	12.5
56-100	25.4-45.4	150	22.5	½ tablet
100+	>45.4	300	45	1 tablet

*Dose based on liquid containing approximately 40 mg of chloroquine
base and 6 mg primaquine base per 5 mL, prepared from chloroquine
phosphate with primaquine phosphate tablets.

Adults: 1 tablet/week on the same day each week

Mechanism of Action Chloroquine concentrates within parasite acid vesicles
and raises internal pH resulting in inhibition of parasite growth; may involve
aggregates of ferriprotoporphyrin IX acting as chloroquine receptors causing

membrane damage; may also interfere with nucleoprotein synthesis. Primaquine eliminates the primary tissue exoerythrocytic forms of *P. falciparum*; disrupts mitochondria and binds to DNA.

Local Anesthetic/Vasoconstrictor Precautions No information available to require special precautions

Effects on Dental Treatment No effects or complications reported

Other Adverse Effects

1% to 10%: Gastrointestinal: Diarrhea, nausea

<1%:

Cardiovascular: Hypotension, EKG changes

Central nervous system: Fatigue, personality changes, headache

Dermatologic: Pruritus, hair bleaching

Gastrointestinal: Anorexia, vomiting, stomatitis

Hematologic: Blood dyscrasias

Ocular: Retinopathy, blurred vision

Drug Interactions

Decreased absorption if administered concomitantly with kaolin and magnesium trisilicate

Increased toxicity/levels with cimetidine

Drug Uptake

Absorption: Oral: Both drugs are readily absorbed

Pregnancy Risk Factor C

Chloroquine Phosphate (klor' oh kwin fos' fate)

Brand Names Aralen® Phosphate

Therapeutic Category Amebicide; Antimalarial Agent

Synonyms Cloroquina, Defosfato De (Mexico)

Use Suppression or chemoprophylaxis of malaria; treatment of uncomplicated or mild-moderate malaria; extraintestinal amebiasis; rheumatoid arthritis; discoid lupus erythematosus, scleroderma, pemphigus

Usual Dosage Oral **(dosage expressed in terms of mg of base):**

Suppression or prophylaxis of malaria:

Children: Administer 5 mg base/kg/week on the same day each week (not to exceed 300 mg base/dose); begin 1-2 weeks prior to exposure; continue for 4-6 weeks after leaving endemic area; if suppressive therapy is not begun prior to exposure, double the initial loading dose to 10 mg base/kg and give in 2 divided doses 6 hours apart, followed by the usual dosage regimen

Adults: 300 mg/week (base) on the same day each week; begin 1-2 weeks prior to exposure; continue for 4-6 weeks after leaving endemic area; if suppressive therapy is not begun prior to exposure, double the initial loading dose to 600 mg base and give in 2 divided doses 6 hours apart, followed by the usual dosage regimen

Acute attack:

Children: 10 mg/kg on day 1, followed by 5 mg/kg 6 hours later and 5 mg/kg on days 2 and 3

Adults: 600 mg on day 1, followed by 300 mg 6 hours later, followed by 300 mg on days 2 and 3

Extraintestinal amebiasis:

Children: 10 mg/kg once daily for 2-3 weeks (up to 300 mg base/day)

Adults: 600 mg base/day for 2 days followed by 300 mg base/day for at least 2-3 weeks

Mechanism of Action Binds to and inhibits DNA and RNA polymerase; interferes with metabolism and hemoglobin utilization by parasites; inhibits prostaglandin effects; chloroquine concentrates within parasite acid vesicles and raises internal pH resulting in inhibition of parasite growth; may involve aggregates of ferriprotoporphyrin IX acting as chloroquine receptors causing membrane damage; may also interfere with nucleoprotein synthesis

Local Anesthetic/Vasoconstrictor Precautions No information available to require special precautions

Effects on Dental Treatment No effects or complications reported

Other Adverse Effects

1% to 10%: Gastrointestinal: Nausea, diarrhea

<1%:

Cardiovascular: Hypotension, EKG changes

Central nervous system: Fatigue, personality changes, headache

Dermatologic: Pruritus, hair bleaching

Gastrointestinal: Anorexia, vomiting, stomatitis

Hematologic: Blood dyscrasias

Ocular: Retinopathy, blurred vision

(Continued)

Chloroquine Phosphate *(Continued)*

Drug Interactions
Decreased absorption if administered concomitantly with kaolin and magnesium trisilicate
Increased toxicity/levels with cimetidine

Drug Uptake
Absorption: Oral: Rapid (~89%)
Serum half-life: 3-5 days
Time to peak serum concentration: Within 1-2 hours

Pregnancy Risk Factor C

Chlorothiazide (klor oh thye' a zide)

Related Information
Cardiovascular Diseases *on page 912*

Brand Names Diurigen®; Diuril®

Therapeutic Category Diuretic, Thiazide Type

Use Management of mild to moderate hypertension, or edema associated with congestive heart failure, pregnancy, or nephrotic syndrome in patients unable to take oral hydrochlorothiazide, when a thiazide is the diuretic of choice

Usual Dosage I.V. form not recommended for children and should only be used in adults if unable to take oral in emergency situations:
Children >6 months:
Oral: 20 mg/kg/day in 2 divided doses
I.V.: 4 mg/kg/day
Adults:
Oral: 500 mg to 2 g/day divided in 1-2 doses
I.V.: 100-500 mg/day
Elderly: Oral: 500 mg once daily **or** 1 g 3 times/week

Mechanism of Action Inhibits sodium reabsorption in the distal tubules causing increased excretion of sodium and water as well as potassium and hydrogen ions, magnesium, phosphate, calcium

Local Anesthetic/Vasoconstrictor Precautions No information available to require special precautions

Effects on Dental Treatment No effects or complications reported

Other Adverse Effects
1% to 10%: Endocrine & metabolic: Hypokalemia, hyponatremia
<1%:
Cardiovascular: Irregular heartbeat, weak pulse, orthostatic hypotension
Central nervous system: Dizziness, vertigo, headache, fever
Dermatologic: Rash, photosensitivity
Endocrine & metabolic: Hypochloremic alkalosis, hyperglycemia, hyperlipidemia, hyperuricemia
Hematologic: Rarely blood dyscrasias, leukopenia, agranulocytosis, aplastic anemia
Neuromuscular & skeletal: Paresthesias
Renal: Prerenal azotemia

Drug Interactions
Decreased absorption of thiazides with cholestyramine resins; chlorothiazide causes a decreased effect of oral hypoglycemics
Increased toxicity: Digitalis glycosides, lithium (decreased clearance), probenecid

Drug Uptake
Absorption: Oral: Poor
Onset of diuresis: Oral: 2 hours
Duration of diuretic action:
Oral: 6-12 hours
I.V.: ~2 hours
Serum half-life: 1-2 hours

Pregnancy Risk Factor D

Chlorothiazide and Methyldopa
(klor oh thye' a zide & meth il doe' pa)

Brand Names Aldoclor®

Therapeutic Category Antihypertensive Agent, Combination

Synonyms Methyldopa and Chlorothiazide

Use Treatment of hypertension

Local Anesthetic/Vasoconstrictor Precautions No information available to require special precautions

Effects on Dental Treatment No effects or complications reported

Chlorothiazide and Reserpine
(klor oh thye' a zide & re ser' peen)
Brand Names Diupres-250®; Diupres-500®
Therapeutic Category Antihypertensive Agent, Combination
Synonyms Reserpine and Chlorothiazide
Use Management of hypertension
Local Anesthetic/Vasoconstrictor Precautions No information available to require special precautions
Effects on Dental Treatment No effects or complications reported

Chlorotrianisene (klor oh trye an' i seen)
Related Information
Endocrine Disorders & Pregnancy *on page 927*
Brand Names TACE®
Therapeutic Category Estrogen Derivative
Use Treat inoperable prostatic cancer; management of atrophic vaginitis, female hypogonadism, vasomotor symptoms of menopause
Usual Dosage Adults: Oral:
Atrophic vaginitis: 12-25 mg/day in 28-day cycles (21 days on and 7 days off)
Female hypogonadism: 12-25 mg cyclically for 21 days. May be followed by I.M. progesterone 100 mg or 5 days of oral progestin; next course may begin on day 5 of induced uterine bleeding.
Postpartum breast engorgement: 12 mg 4 times/day for 7 days or 50 mg every 6 hours for 6 doses; give first dose within 8 hours after delivery
Vasomotor symptoms associated with menopause: 12-25 mg cyclically for 30 days; one or more courses may be prescribed
Prostatic cancer (inoperable/progressing): 12-25 mg/day
Mechanism of Action Diethylstilbestrol derivative with similar estrogenic actions
Local Anesthetic/Vasoconstrictor Precautions No information available to require special precautions
Effects on Dental Treatment No effects or complications reported
Other Adverse Effects
>10%:
Endocrine & metabolic: Peripheral edema, enlargement of breasts (female and male), breast tenderness
Gastrointestinal: Nausea, anorexia, bloating
1% to 10%:
Central nervous system: Headache
Endocrine & metabolic: Increased libido (female), decreased libido (male)
Gastrointestinal: Vomiting, diarrhea
<1%:
Cardiovascular: Hypertension, thromboembolism, stroke, myocardial infarction, edema
Central nervous system: Depression, dizziness, anxiety
Dermatologic: Chloasma, melasma, rash
Endocrine & metabolic: Breast tumors, amenorrhea, alterations in frequency and flow of menses, decreased glucose tolerance, increased triglycerides and LDL
Gastrointestinal: Nausea, GI distress
Hepatic: Cholestatic jaundice
Ocular: Intolerance to contact lenses
Miscellaneous: Increased susceptibility to *Candida* infection
Drug Interactions No data reported
Drug Uptake
Onset of therapeutic effect: Commonly occurs within 14 days of therapy
Pregnancy Risk Factor X

Chloroxine (klor ox' een)
Brand Names Capitrol®
Therapeutic Category Antiseborrheic Agent, Topical; Shampoos
Use Treatment of dandruff or seborrheic dermatitis of the scalp
Local Anesthetic/Vasoconstrictor Precautions No information available to require special precautions
Effects on Dental Treatment No effects or complications reported

Chlorphed® [OTC] *see* Brompheniramine Maleate *on page 124*
Chlorphed®-LA Nasal Solution [OTC] *see* Oxymetazoline Hydrochloride *on page 649*

Chlorphenesin Carbamate (klor fen' e sin kar' ba mate)
Brand Names Maolate®
Therapeutic Category Muscle Relaxant; Skeletal Muscle Relaxant
Use Adjunctive treatment of discomfort in short-term, acute, painful musculo-skeletal conditions
Local Anesthetic/Vasoconstrictor Precautions No information available to require special precautions
Effects on Dental Treatment No effects or complications reported
Other Adverse Effects
>10%: Central nervous system: Drowsiness
1% to 10%:
  Cardiovascular: Tachycardia, flushing of face
  Central nervous system: Fainting, mental depression, allergic fever, dizzi-ness, lightheadedness, headache, paradoxical stimulation
  Dermatologic: Angioedema
  Gastrointestinal: Stomach cramps, hiccups, nausea, vomiting
  Respiratory: Shortness of breath, tightness in chest
  Ocular: Burning of eyes
  Neuromuscular & skeletal: Trembling
<1%:
  Central nervous system: Clumsiness
  Dermatologic: Skin rash, hives, erythema multiforme
  Hematologic: Aplastic anemia, leukopenia, eosinophilia
  Ocular: Blurred vision

Chlorpheniramine and Acetaminophen
(klor fen ir' a meen & a seet a min' oh fen)
Brand Names Coricidin® [OTC]
Therapeutic Category Analgesic, Non-narcotic; Antihistamine
Use Symptomatic relief of congestion, headache, aches and pains of colds and flu
Local Anesthetic/Vasoconstrictor Precautions No information available to require special precautions
Effects on Dental Treatment Chronic use of antihistamines will inhibit sali-vary flow, particularly in elderly patients; this may contribute to periodontal disease and oral discomfort

Chlorpheniramine and Phenylephrine
(klor fen ir' a meen & fen il ef' rin)
Brand Names Dallergy-D® Syrup; Ed A-Hist® Liquid; Histatab® Plus Tablet [OTC]; Histor-D® Syrup; Novahistine® Elixir [OTC]; Rolatuss® Plain Liquid; Ru-Tuss® Liquid
Therapeutic Category Antihistamine/Decongestant Combination
Synonyms Phenylephrine and Chlorpheniramine
Use Temporary relief of nasal congestion and eustachian tube congestion as well as runny nose, sneezing, itching of nose or throat, itchy and watery eyes
Local Anesthetic/Vasoconstrictor Precautions Use with caution since phenylephrine is a sympathomimetic amine which could interact with epineph-rine to cause a pressor response
Effects on Dental Treatment
  Chlorpheniramine: Prolonged use will cause significant xerostomia
  Phenylephrine: Up to 10% of patients could experience tachycardia, palpita-tions, and dry mouth; use vasoconstrictor with caution; prolonged use will cause significant xerostomia

Chlorpheniramine and Phenylpropanolamine
(klor fen ir' a meen & fen il proe pa nole' a meen)
Brand Names Allerest® 12 Hour Capsule [OTC]; A.R.M.® Caplet [OTC]; Chlor-Rest® Tablet [OTC]; Demazin® Syrup [OTC]; Genamin® Cold Syrup [OTC]; Ornade® Spansule®; Parhist SR®; Resaid®; Rescon Liquid [OTC]; Silaminic® Cold Syrup [OTC]; Temazin® Cold Syrup [OTC]; Thera-Hist® Syrup [OTC]; Triaminic® Cold Tablet [OTC]; Triaminic® Allergy Tablet [OTC]; Triaminic® Syrup [OTC]; Tri-Nefrin® Extra Strength Tablet [OTC]; Triphenyl® Syrup [OTC]
Therapeutic Category Antihistamine/Decongestant Combination
Synonyms Phenylpropanolamine and Chlorpheniramine
Use Symptomatic relief of nasal congestion, runny nose, sneezing, itchy nose or throat, and itchy or watery eyes due to the common cold or allergic rhinitis
Local Anesthetic/Vasoconstrictor Precautions Use with caution since phenylpropanolamine is a sympathomimetic amine which could interact with epinephrine to cause a pressor response

Effects on Dental Treatment

Chlorpheniramine: Prolonged use will cause significant xerostomia

Phenylpropanolamine: Up to 10% of patients could experience tachycardia, palpitations, and dry mouth; use vasoconstrictor with caution; prolonged use will cause significant xerostomia

Chlorpheniramine and Pseudoephedrine

(klor fen ir' a meen & soo doe e fed' rin)

Brand Names Allerest® Maximum Strength [OTC]; Anamine® Syrup [OTC]; Anaplex® Liquid [OTC]; Chlorafed® Liquid [OTC]; Chlor-Trimeton® 4 Hour Relief Tablet [OTC]; Co-Pyronil® 2 Pulvules® [OTC]; Deconamine® SR; Deconamine® Syrup [OTC]; Deconamine® Tablet [OTC]; Fedahist® Tablet [OTC]; Hayfebrol® Liquid [OTC]; Histalet® Syrup [OTC]; Klerist-D® Tablet [OTC]; Pseudo-Gest Plus® Tablet [OTC]; Rhinosyn® Liquid [OTC]; Rhinosyn-PD® Liquid [OTC]; Ryna® Liquid [OTC]; Sudafed® Plus Liquid [OTC]; Sudafed® Plus Tablet [OTC]

Therapeutic Category Antihistamine/Decongestant Combination

Synonyms Pseudoephedrine and Chlorpheniramine

Use Relief of nasal congestion associated with the common cold, hay fever, and other allergies, sinusitis, eustachian tube blockage, and vasomotor and allergic rhinitis

Local Anesthetic/Vasoconstrictor Precautions Use with caution since pseudoephedrine is a sympathomimetic amine which could interact with epinephrine to cause a pressor response

Effects on Dental Treatment

Chlorpheniramine: Prolonged use will cause significant xerostomia

Pseudoephedrine: Up to 10% of patients could experience tachycardia, palpitations, and dry mouth; use vasoconstrictor with caution; prolonged use will cause significant xerostomia

Chlorpheniramine, Ephedrine, Phenylephrine, and Carbetapentane

(klor fen ir' a meen, e fed' rin, fen il ef' rin, & kar bay ta pen' tane)

Brand Names Rentamine®; Rynatuss® Pediatric Suspension; Tri-Tannate® Plus

Therapeutic Category Antihistamine/Decongestant Combination

Use Symptomatic relief of cough

Local Anesthetic/Vasoconstrictor Precautions

Ephedrine: Use vasoconstrictors with caution since ephedrine may enhance cardiostimulation and vasopressor effects of sympathomimetics

Phenylephrine: Use with caution since phenylephrine is a sympathomimetic amine which could interact with epinephrine to cause a pressor response

Effects on Dental Treatment

Chlorpheniramine: Prolonged use will cause significant xerostomia

Ephedrine: No effects or complications reported

Phenylephrine: Up to 10% of patients could experience tachycardia, palpitations, and dry mouth; use vasoconstrictor with caution

Chlorpheniramine Maleate (klor fen ir' a meen mal' ee ate)

Related Information

Dentin Hypersensitivity; High Caries Index; Xerostomia *on page 959*

Oral Bacterial Infections *on page 945*

Brand Names Aller-Chlor® [OTC]; AL-R® [OTC]; Chlo-Amine® [OTC]; Chlorate® [OTC]; Chlor-Pro® [OTC]; Chlor-Trimeton® [OTC]; Kloromin® [OTC]; Phenetron®; Telachlor®; Teldrin® [OTC]

Canadian/Mexican Brand Names Chlor-Tripolon® (Canada)

Therapeutic Category Antihistamine

Synonyms Clorfeniramina, Maleato De (Mexico)

Use Perennial and seasonal allergic rhinitis and other allergic symptoms including urticaria

Usual Dosage

Children: Oral: 0.35 mg/kg/day in divided doses every 4-6 hours

2-6 years: 1 mg every 4-6 hours, not to exceed 6 mg in 24 hours

6-12 years: 2 mg every 4-6 hours, not to exceed 12 mg/day or sustained release 8 mg at bedtime

Children >12 years and Adults: Oral: 4 mg every 4-6 hours, not to exceed 24 mg/day or sustained release 8-12 mg every 8-12 hours, not to exceed 24 mg/day

Adults: Allergic reactions: I.M., I.V., S.C.: 10-20 mg as a single dose; maximum recommended dose: 40 mg/24 hours

(Continued)

Chlorpheniramine Maleate *(Continued)*

Elderly: 4 mg once or twice daily. **Note:** Duration of action may be 36 hours or more when serum concentrations are low.

Hemodialysis effects: Supplemental dose is not necessary

Mechanism of Action Competes with histamine for H_1-receptor sites on effector cells in the gastrointestinal tract, blood vessels, and respiratory tract

Local Anesthetic/Vasoconstrictor Precautions No information available to require special precautions

Effects on Dental Treatment Chronic use of antihistamines will inhibit salivary flow, particularly in elderly patients; this may contribute to periodontal disease and oral discomfort

Other Adverse Effects

Genitourinary: Polyuria, urinary retention

Ocular: Diplopia

>10%:

Central nervous system: Slight to moderate drowsiness

Respiratory: Thickening of bronchial secretions

1% to 10%:

Central nervous system: Weakness, headache, excitability, fatigue, nervousness, dizziness

Gastrointestinal: Nausea, dry mouth, diarrhea, abdominal pain, appetite increase, weight increase

Neuromuscular & skeletal: Arthralgia

Respiratory: Pharyngitis

<1%:

Cardiovascular: Palpitations

Central nervous system: Depression

Dermatologic: Dermatitis, photosensitivity, angioedema

Hepatic: Hepatitis

Neuromuscular & skeletal: Myalgia, paresthesia

Respiratory: Bronchospasm

Miscellaneous: Epistaxis

Drug Interactions Sedative effects of chlorpheniramine are enhanced by other CNS depressants, MAO inhibitors, alcohol, and tricyclic antidepressants

Drug Uptake

Serum half-life: 20-24 hours

Pregnancy Risk Factor B

Dosage Forms

Capsule: 12 mg

Capsule, timed release: 8 mg, 12 mg

Injection: 10 mg/mL (1 mL, 30 mL); 100 mg/mL (2 mL)

Syrup: 2 mg/5 mL (120 mL, 473 mL)

Tablet: 4 mg, 8 mg, 12 mg

Tablet:

Chewable: 2 mg

Timed release: 8 mg, 12 mg

Dietary Considerations May be taken with food or water

Generic Available Yes

Chlorpheniramine, Phenindamine, and Phenylpropanolamine

(klor fen ir′ a meen, fen in′ dah meen, & fen il proe pa nole′ a meen)

Brand Names Nolamine®

Therapeutic Category Antihistamine/Decongestant Combination

Use Upper respiratory and nasal congestion

Local Anesthetic/Vasoconstrictor Precautions Use with caution since phenylpropanolamine is a sympathomimetic amine which could interact with epinephrine to cause a pressor response

Effects on Dental Treatment

Chlorpheniramine: Prolonged use will cause significant xerostomia

Phenylpropanolamine: Up to 10% of patients could experience tachycardia, palpitations, and dry mouth; use vasoconstrictor with caution

Chlorpheniramine, Phenylephrine, and Codeine

(klor fen ir′ a meen, fen il ef′ rin, & koe′ deen)

Brand Names Pediacof®; Pedituss®

Therapeutic Category Antihistamine/Decongestant Combination; Cough Preparation

Use Symptomatic relief of rhinitis, nasal congestion and cough due to colds or allergy

Local Anesthetic/Vasoconstrictor Precautions Use with caution since phenylephrine is a sympathomimetic amine which could interact with epinephrine to cause a pressor response

Effects on Dental Treatment

Chlorpheniramine: Prolonged use will cause significant xerostomia

Codeine: <1%: Dry mouth

Phenylephrine: Up to 10% of patients could experience tachycardia, palpitations, and dry mouth; use vasoconstrictor with caution; prolonged use will cause significant xerostomia

Chlorpheniramine, Phenylephrine, and Dextromethorphan

(klor fen ir' a meen, fen il ef' rin, & deks troe meth or' fan)

Brand Names Cerose-DM® [OTC]

Therapeutic Category Antihistamine/Decongestant Combination; Cough Preparation

Use Temporary relief of cough due to minor throat and bronchial irritation; relieves nasal congestion, runny nose and sneezing

Local Anesthetic/Vasoconstrictor Precautions

Chlorpheniramine, Dextromethorphan: No information available to require special precautions

Phenylephrine: Use with caution since phenylephrine is a sympathomimetic amine which could interact with epinephrine to cause a pressor response

Effects on Dental Treatment

Chlorpheniramine: Prolonged use will cause significant xerostomia

Dextromethorphan: No effects or complications reported

Phenylephrine: Up to 10% of patients could experience tachycardia, palpitations, and dry mouth; use vasoconstrictor with caution; prolonged use will cause significant xerostomia

Chlorpheniramine, Phenylephrine, and Methscopolamine

(klor fen ir' a meen, fen il ef' rin, & meth skoe pol' a meen)

Brand Names Alersule Forte®; Dallergy®; Extendryl® SR; Histor-D® Timecelles®

Therapeutic Category Antihistamine/Decongestant Combination

Use Relieves nasal congestion, runny nose and sneezing

Local Anesthetic/Vasoconstrictor Precautions Use with caution since phenylephrine is a sympathomimetic amine which could interact with epinephrine to cause a pressor response

Effects on Dental Treatment

Chlorpheniramine: Prolonged use will cause significant xerostomia

Methscopolamine: Anticholinergic side effects can cause a reduction of saliva production or secretion contributes to discomfort and dental disease (ie, caries, oral candidiasis and periodontal disease)

Phenylephrine: Up to 10% of patients could experience tachycardia, palpitations, and dry mouth; use vasoconstrictor with caution

Chlorpheniramine, Phenylephrine, and Phenylpropanolamine

(klor fen ir' a meen, fen il ef' rin, & fen il proe pa nole' a meen)

Brand Names Hista-Vadrin® Tablet

Therapeutic Category Antihistamine/Decongestant Combination

Use Symptomatic relief of rhinitis and nasal congestion due to colds or allergy

Local Anesthetic/Vasoconstrictor Precautions Use with caution since phenylephrine and phenylpropanolamine are sympathomimetic amines which could interact with epinephrine to cause a pressor response

Effects on Dental Treatment Up to 10% of patients could experience tachycardia, palpitations, and dry mouth; use vasoconstrictor with caution; prolonged use will cause significant xerostomia

Chlorpheniramine, Phenylephrine, and Phenyltoloxamine

(klor fen ir' a meen, fen il ef' rin, & fen il tole lox' a meen)

Brand Names Comhist®; Comhist® LA

Therapeutic Category Antihistamine/Decongestant Combination

Use Symptomatic relief of rhinitis and nasal congestion due to colds or allergy

(Continued)

Chlorpheniramine, Phenylephrine, and Phenyltoloxamine *(Continued)*

Local Anesthetic/Vasoconstrictor Precautions Use with caution since phenylephrine is a sympathomimetic amine which could interact with epinephrine to cause a pressor response

Effects on Dental Treatment

Chlorpheniramine: Prolonged use will cause significant xerostomia

Phenylephrine: Up to 10% of patients could experience tachycardia, palpitations, and dry mouth; use vasoconstrictor with caution

Chlorpheniramine, Phenylpropanolamine, and Acetaminophen

(klor fen ir' a meen, fen il proe pa nole' a meen, & a seet a min' oh fen)

Brand Names BQ® Tablet [OTC]; Congestant® D [OTC]; Coricidin D® [OTC]; Dapacin® Cold Capsule [OTC]; Duadacin® Capsule [OTC]; Tylenol® Cold Effervescent Medication Tablet [OTC]

Therapeutic Category Analgesic, Non-narcotic; Antihistamine/Decongestant Combination

Use Symptomatic relief of nasal congestion and headache from colds/sinus congestion

Local Anesthetic/Vasoconstrictor Precautions Use with caution since phenylpropanolamine is a sympathomimetic amine which could interact with epinephrine to cause a pressor response

Effects on Dental Treatment

Acetaminophen: No effects or complications reported

Chlorpheniramine: Prolonged use will cause significant xerostomia

Phenylpropanolamine: Up to 10% of patients could experience tachycardia, palpitations, and dry mouth; use vasoconstrictor with caution

Chlorpheniramine, Phenylpropanolamine, and Dextromethorphan

(klor fen ir' a meen, fen il proe pa nole' a meen, & deks troe meth or' fan)

Brand Names Triaminicol® Multi-Symptom Cold Syrup [OTC]

Therapeutic Category Antihistamine/Decongestant Combination; Cough Preparation

Use Provides relief of runny nose, sneezing, suppresses cough, promotes nasal and sinus drainage

Local Anesthetic/Vasoconstrictor Precautions Use with caution since phenylpropanolamine is a sympathomimetic amine which could interact with epinephrine to cause a pressor response

Effects on Dental Treatment

Chlorpheniramine: Prolonged use will cause significant xerostomia

Dextromethorphan: No effects or complications reported

Phenylpropanolamine: Up to 10% of patients could experience tachycardia, palpitations, and dry mouth; use vasoconstrictor with caution; prolonged use will cause significant xerostomia

Comments Alcohol free

Chlorpheniramine, Phenyltoloxamine, Phenylpropanolamine, and Phenylephrine

(klor fen ir' a meen, fen il tole lox' a meen, fen il proe pa nole' a meen & fen il ef' rin)

Brand Names Naldecon®; Naldelate®; Nalgest®; Nalspan®; New Decongestant®; Par Decon®; Quadra-Hist®; Tri-Phen-Chlor®; Uni-Decon®

Therapeutic Category Antihistamine/Decongestant Combination

Use Symptomatic treatment of nasal and eustachian tube congestion associated with sinusitis and acute upper respiratory infection; symptomatic relief of perennial and allergic rhinitis

Local Anesthetic/Vasoconstrictor Precautions Use with caution since phenylpropanolamine & phenylephrine are sympathomimetic amines which could interact with epinephrine to cause a pressor response

Effects on Dental Treatment

Chlorpheniramine: Prolonged use will cause significant xerostomia

Phenylephrine, Phenylpropanolamine: Up to 10% of patients could experience tachycardia, palpitations, and dry mouth; use vasoconstrictor with caution

Chlorpheniramine, Pseudoephedrine, and Codeine
(klor fen ir' a meen, soo doe e fed' rin, & koe' deen)

Brand Names Codehist® DH; Decohistine® DH; Dihistine® DH; Novahistine® DH; Phen DH® w/Codeine; Ryna-C® Liquid

Therapeutic Category Antihistamine/Decongestant Combination; Cough Preparation

Use Temporary relief of cough associated with minor throat or bronchial irritation or nasal congestion due to common cold, allergic rhinitis, or sinusitis

Local Anesthetic/Vasoconstrictor Precautions Use with caution since pseudoephedrine is a sympathomimetic amine which could interact with epinephrine to cause a pressor response

Effects on Dental Treatment

Chlorpheniramine: Prolonged use will cause significant xerostomia

Codeine: <1%: Dry mouth

Pseudoephedrine: Up to 10% of patients could experience tachycardia, palpitations, and dry mouth; use vasoconstrictor with caution

Other Adverse Effects 1% to 10%:

Cardiovascular: Hypotension

Central nervous system: Sedation, dizziness, drowsiness, increased intracranial pressure

Gastrointestinal: Constipation, biliary/urinary tract spasm

Miscellaneous: Physical or psychological dependence with continued use

Chlorpheniramine, Pyrilamine, and Phenylephrine
(klor fen ir' a meen, pye ril' a meen, & fen il ef' rin)

Brand Names Rhinatate® Tablet; R-Tannamine® Tablet; R-Tannate® Tablet; Rynatan® Pediatric Suspension; Rynatan® Tablet; Tanoral® Tablet; Triotann® Tablet; Tri-Tannate® Tablet; Tritann® Pediatric; Tritan® Tablet

Therapeutic Category Antihistamine/Decongestant Combination

Use Symptomatic relief of nasal congestion associated with upper respiratory tract condition

Local Anesthetic/Vasoconstrictor Precautions Use with caution since phenylephrine is a sympathomimetic amine which could interact with epinephrine to cause a pressor response

Effects on Dental Treatment

Chlorpheniramine: Prolonged use will cause significant xerostomia

Phenylephrine: Up to 10% of patients could experience tachycardia, palpitations, and dry mouth; use vasoconstrictor with caution

Chlorpheniramine, Pyrilamine, Phenylephrine, and Phenylpropanolamine
(klor fen ir' a meen, pye ril' a meen, fen il ef' rin, & fen il proe pa nole' a meen)

Brand Names Histalet Forte® Tablet

Therapeutic Category Antihistamine/Decongestant Combination

Use Symptomatic relief of rhinitis and nasal congestion due to colds or allergy

Local Anesthetic/Vasoconstrictor Precautions Use with caution since phenylephrine & phenylpropanolamine are sympathomimetic amines which could interact with epinephrine to cause a pressor response

Effects on Dental Treatment

Chlorpheniramine: Prolonged use will cause significant xerostomia

Phenylephrine, Phenylpropanolamine: Up to 10% of patients could experience tachycardia, palpitations, and dry mouth; use vasoconstrictor with caution

Chlor-Pro® [OTC] *see* Chlorpheniramine Maleate *on page 191*

Chlorpromazine Hydrochloride
(klor proe' ma zeen hye droe klor' ide)

Brand Names Ormazine; Thorazine®

Canadian/Mexican Brand Names Largactil® (Canada); Apo-Chlorpromazine® (Canada); Chlorprom® (Canada); Chlorpromanyl® (Canada); Novo-Chlorpromazine® (Canada)

Therapeutic Category Antiemetic; Antipsychotic Agent; Phenothiazine Derivative

Use Treatment of psychoses, nausea and vomiting; Tourette's syndrome; mania; intractable hiccups (adults); behavioral problems (children)

(Continued)

Chlorpromazine Hydrochloride *(Continued)*

Usual Dosage

Children >6 months:

Psychosis:

Oral: 0.5-1 mg/kg/dose every 4-6 hours; older children may require 200 mg/day or higher

I.M., I.V.: 0.5-1 mg/kg/dose every 6-8 hours; maximum dose for <5 years (22.7 kg): 40 mg/day; maximum for 5-12 years (22.7-45.5 kg): 75 mg/day

Nausea and vomiting:

Oral: 0.5-1 mg/kg/dose every 4-6 hours as needed

I.M., I.V.: 0.5-1 mg/kg/dose every 6-8 hours; maximum dose for <5 years (22.7 kg): 40 mg/day; maximum for 5-12 years (22.7-45.5 kg): 75 mg/day

Rectal: 1 mg/kg/dose every 6-8 hours as needed

Adults:

Psychosis:

Oral: Range: 30-800 mg/day in 1-4 divided doses, initiate at lower doses and titrate as needed; usual dose: 200 mg/day; some patients may require 1-2 g/day

I.M., I.V.: Initial: 25 mg, may repeat (25-50 mg) in 1-4 hours, gradually increase to a maximum of 400 mg/dose every 4-6 hours until patient is controlled; usual dose: 300-800 mg/day

Intractable hiccups: Oral, I.M.: 25-50 mg 3-4 times/day

Nausea and vomiting:

Oral: 10-25 mg every 4-6 hours

I.M., I.V.: 25-50 mg every 4-6 hours

Rectal: 50-100 mg every 6-8 hours

Elderly (nonpsychotic patient; dementia behavior): Initial: 10-25 mg 1-2 times/day; increase at 4- to 7-day intervals by 10-25 mg/day. Increase dose intervals (bid, tid, etc) as necessary to control behavior response or side effects; maximum daily dose: 800 mg; gradual increases (titration) may prevent some side effects or decrease their severity.

Not dialyzable (0% to 5%)

Mechanism of Action Blocks postsynaptic mesolimbic dopaminergic receptors in the brain; exhibits a strong alpha-adrenergic blocking effect and depresses the release of hypothalamic and hypophyseal hormones; believed to depress the reticular-activating system, thus affecting basal metabolism, body temperature, wakefulness, vasomotor tone, and emesis

Local Anesthetic/Vasoconstrictor Precautions No information available to require special precautions

Effects on Dental Treatment Significant hypotension may occur, especially when the drug is administered parenterally; orthostatic hypotension is due to alpha-receptor blockade, the elderly are at greater risk for orthostatic hypotension

Tardive dyskinesia: Prevalence rate may be 40% in elderly; development of the syndrome and the irreversible nature are proportional to duration and total cumulative dose over time

Extrapyramidal reactions are more common in elderly with up to 50% developing these reactions after 60 years of age; drug-induced **Parkinson's syndrome** occurs often; **Akathisia** is the most common extrapyramidal reaction in elderly

Increased confusion, memory loss, psychotic behavior, and agitation frequently occur as a consequence of anticholinergic effects

Antipsychotic associated sedation in nonpsychotic patients is extremely unpleasant due to feelings of depersonalization, derealization, and dysphoria

Other Adverse Effects

>10%:

Cardiovascular: Hypotension (especially with I.V. use), tachycardia, arrhythmias, orthostatic hypotension

Central nervous system: Pseudoparkinsonism, akathisia, dystonias, tardive dyskinesia (persistent), dizziness

Gastrointestinal: Constipation

Ocular: Pigmentary retinopathy

Respiratory: Nasal congestion

Miscellaneous: Decreased sweating

1% to 10%:

Central nervous system: Dizziness, trembling of fingers

Dermatologic: Pruritus, rash, increased sensitivity to sun

Endocrine & metabolic: Amenorrhea, galactorrhea, gynecomastia, changes in libido

Gastrointestinal: GI upset, nausea, vomiting, stomach pain, weight gain, dry mouth, constipation

Genitourinary: Difficulty in urination, ejaculatory disturbances, urinary retention

Ocular: Blurred vision

Miscellaneous: Pain in breasts

<1%:

Central nervous system: Sedation, drowsiness, restlessness, anxiety, extrapyramidal reactions, seizures, altered central temperature regulation, lowering of seizures threshold, neuroleptic malignant syndrome (NMS)

Dermatologic: Discoloration of skin (blue-gray), photosensitivity

Endocrine & metabolic: Galactorrhea

Genitourinary: Priapism

Hematologic: Agranulocytosis (more often in women between 4th and 10th weeks of therapy), leukopenia (usually in patients with large doses for prolonged periods)

Hepatic: Cholestatic jaundice, hepatotoxicity

Ocular: Cornea and lens changes, pigmentary retinopathy

Miscellaneous: Anaphylactoid reactions

Warnings/Precautions Safety in children <6 months of age has not been established; use with caution in patients with seizures, bone marrow depression, or severe liver disease

Drug Interactions Increased toxicity: Additive effects with other CNS-depressants

Drug Uptake

Serum half-life, biphasic:

Initial: 2 hours

Terminal: 30 hours

Pregnancy Risk Factor C

Chlorpropamide (klor proe' pa mide)

Related Information

Endocrine Disorders & Pregnancy on page 927

Brand Names Diabinese®

Canadian/Mexican Brand Names Apo-Chlorpropamide® (Canada); Novo-Propamide® (Canada); Deavynfar® (Mexico); Insogen® (Mexico)

Therapeutic Category Antidiabetic Agent; Hypoglycemic Agent, Oral; Sulfonylurea Agent

Synonyms Clorpropamida (Mexico)

Use Control blood sugar in adult onset, noninsulin-dependent diabetes (type II); **unlabeled use:** Nephrogenic diabetes insipidus

Usual Dosage Oral: The dosage of chlorpropamide is variable and should be individualized based upon the patient's response

Initial dose:

Adults: 250 mg/day in mild to moderate diabetes in middle-aged, stable diabetic

Elderly: 100-125 mg/day in older patients

Maintenance dose: 100-250 mg/day; severe diabetics may require 500 mg/day; avoid doses >750 mg/day

Mechanism of Action Stimulates insulin release from the pancreatic beta cells; reduces glucose output from the liver; insulin sensitivity is increased at peripheral target sites

Local Anesthetic/Vasoconstrictor Precautions No information available to require special precautions

Effects on Dental Treatment Chlorpropamide-dependent diabetics (noninsulin dependent, Type II) should be appointed for dental treatment in morning in order to minimize chance of stress-induced hypoglycemia

Other Adverse Effects

>10%:

Central nervous system: Headache, dizziness

Gastrointestinal: Anorexia, constipation, heartburn, epigastric fullness, nausea, vomiting, diarrhea

1% to 10%: Dermatologic: Skin rash, hives, photosensitivity

<1%:

Cardiovascular: Edema

Endocrine & metabolic: Hypoglycemia, hyponatremia, SIADH

Hematologic: Blood dyscrasias, aplastic anemia, hemolytic anemia, bone marrow depression, thrombocytopenia, agranulocytosis

Hepatic: Cholestatic jaundice

(Continued)

Chlorpropamide *(Continued)*

Drug Interactions
Excessive ethanol intake may lead to hypoglycemia; "antabuse-like" reaction may occur in patients taking chlorpropamide

Salicylates may enhance the hypoglycemic response to chlorpropamide due to increased plasma levels of chlorpropamide by displacing from plasma proteins

Thiazide diuretics will increase blood glucose leading to increased requirements of chlorpropamide

Drug Uptake
Peak effect: Oral: Within 6-8 hours
Serum half-life: 30-42 hours; prolonged in the elderly or with renal disease
Time to peak serum concentration: Within 3-4 hours

Pregnancy Risk Factor C

Chlorprothixene *(klor proe thix' een)*

Brand Names Taractan®
Therapeutic Category Antipsychotic Agent; Thioxanthene Derivative
Use Management of psychotic disorders

Usual Dosage
Children >6 years: Oral: 10-25 mg 3-4 times/day

Adults:
Oral: 25-50 mg 3-4 times/day, to be increased as needed; doses exceeding 600 mg/day are rarely required
I.M.: 25-50 mg up to 3-4 times/day

Not dialyzable (0% to 5%)

Mechanism of Action The mechanism of action for chlorprothixene, like other thioxanthenes and phenothiazines, is not fully understood. The sites of action appear to be the reticular activating system of the midbrain, the limbic system, the hypothalamus, and the globus pallidus and corpus striatum. The mechanism appears to be one or more of a combination of postsynaptic blockade of adrenergic, dopaminergic, or serotonergic receptor sites, metabolic inhibition of oxidative phosphorylation, or decrease in the excitability of neuronal membranes.

Local Anesthetic/Vasoconstrictor Precautions No information available to require special precautions

Effects on Dental Treatment Over 10% of dental patients may experience tardive dyskinesia and Parkinson-like syndromes; orthostatic hypotension is induced by chlorprothixene in over 10% of patients

Other Adverse Effects
>10%:
Cardiovascular: Hypotension, orthostatic hypotension
Central nervous system: Pseudoparkinsonism, akathisia, dystonias, tardive dyskinesia (persistent), dizziness
Gastrointestinal: Constipation
Ocular: Pigmentary retinopathy
Respiratory: Nasal congestion
Miscellaneous: Decreased sweating

1% to 10%:
Dermatologic: Increased sensitivity to sun, skin rash
Endocrine & metabolic: Changes in menstrual cycle, ejaculatory disturbances, changes in libido, pain in breasts
Gastrointestinal: Weight gain, nausea, vomiting, stomach pain
Genitourinary: Difficulty in urination
Neuromuscular & skeletal: Trembling of fingers

<1%:
Central nervous system: Neuroleptic malignant syndrome (NMS)
Dermatologic: discoloration of skin (blue-gray)
Endocrine & metabolic: Galactorrhea
Genitourinary: Priapism
Hematologic: Agranulocytosis, leukopenia
Hepatic: Cholestatic jaundice, hepatotoxicity
Ocular: Cornea and lens changes, pigmentary retinopathy
Miscellaneous: Impairment of temperature regulation lowering of seizures threshold

Drug Interactions
Decreased effect of guanethidine
Increased effect/toxicity: Alcohol, CNS depressants

Pregnancy Risk Factor C

Chlor-Rest® Tablet [OTC] *see* Chlorpheniramine and Phenylpropanolamine *on page 190*

Chlortetracyline Hydrochloride
(klor tet ra sye' kleen hye droe klor' ide)

Brand Names Aureomycin®

Canadian/Mexican Brand Names Aureomicina® (Mexico)

Therapeutic Category Antibiotic, Ophthalmic; Antibiotic, Tetracycline Derivative

Synonyms Clortetraciclina (Mexico)

Use
Ophthalmic: Treatment of superficial ocular infections involving the conjunctiva or cornea due to strains of susceptible microorganisms
Topical: Treatment of superficial infections of the skin due to susceptible organisms, also infection prophylaxis in minor skin abrasions

Usual Dosage
Ophthalmic:
Acute infections: Instill ½" (1.25 cm) every 3-4 hours until improvement
Mild to moderate infections: Instill ½" (1.25 cm) 2-3 times/day

Topical: Apply 1-4 times/day, cover with sterile bandage if needed

Mechanism of Action Inhibits bacterial protein synthesis by binding with the 30S and possibly the 50S ribosomal subunit(s) of susceptible bacteria; may also cause alterations in the cytoplasmic membrane; usually bacteriostatic, may be bactericidal

Local Anesthetic/Vasoconstrictor Precautions No information available to require special precautions

Effects on Dental Treatment No effects or complications reported

Other Adverse Effects
1% to 10%: Dermatologic: Faint yellowing of skin
<1%: Dermatologic: Redness, swelling, irritation, photosensitivity

Drug Interactions No data reported

Pregnancy Risk Factor D

Dosage Forms Ointment:
Ophthalmic: 1% [10 mg/g] (3.5 g)
Topical: 3% (14.2 g, 30 g)

Generic Available Yes

Chlorthalidone (klor thal' i done)

Related Information
Cardiovascular Diseases *on page 912*

Brand Names Hygroton®; Thalitone®

Canadian/Mexican Brand Names Apo-Chlorthalidone® (Canada); Novo-Thalidone® (Canada); Uridon® (Canada); Higroton® 50 (Mexico)

Therapeutic Category Diuretic, Thiazide Type

Synonyms Clortalidona (Mexico)

Use Management of mild to moderate hypertension, used alone or in combination with other agents; treatment of edema associated with congestive heart failure, nephrotic syndrome, or pregnancy. Recent studies have found chlorthalidone effective in the treatment of isolated systolic hypertension in the elderly.

Usual Dosage Oral:
Children: 2 mg/kg/dose 3 times/week or 1-2 mg/kg/day
Adults: 25-100 mg/day or 100 mg 3 times/week
Elderly: Initial: 12.5-25 mg/day or every other day; there is little advantage to using doses >25 mg/day

Mechanism of Action Sulfonamide-derived diuretic that inhibits sodium and chloride reabsorption in the cortical-diluting segment of the ascending loop of Henle

Local Anesthetic/Vasoconstrictor Precautions No information available to require special precautions

Effects on Dental Treatment No effects or complications reported

Other Adverse Effects
1% to 10%: Endocrine & metabolic: Hypokalemia
<1%:
Cardiovascular: Hypotension
Dermatologic: Photosensitivity
Endocrine & metabolic: Fluid and electrolyte imbalances (hypocalcemia, hypomagnesemia, hyponatremia), hyperglycemia
Hematologic: Rarely blood dyscrasias
Renal: Prerenal azotemia
(Continued)

Chlorthalidone *(Continued)*

Drug Interactions
Decreased absorption of thiazides with cholestyramine resins; chlorthalidone may cause a decreased effect of oral hypoglycemics
Increased toxicity: Digitalis glycosides, lithium (decreased clearance), probenecid

Drug Uptake
Peak effect: 2-6 hours
Absorption: Oral: 65%
Serum half-life: 35-55 hours; may be prolonged with renal impairment, with anuria: 81 hours

Pregnancy Risk Factor D

Chlor-Trimeton® [OTC] *see* Chlorpheniramine Maleate *on page 191*

Chlor-Trimeton® 4 Hour Relief Tablet [OTC] *see* Chlorpheniramine and Pseudoephedrine *on page 191*

Chlorzoxazone (klor zox' a zone)

Related Information
Temporomandibular Dysfunction (TMD) *on page 963*

Brand Names Blanex®; Chlorofon-F®; Flexaphen®; Lobac®; Miflex®; Mus-Lac®; Paraflex®; Parafon Forte™ DSC; Pargen Fortified®; Polyflex®; Skelex®

Therapeutic Category Centrally Acting Skeletal Muscle Relaxant; Muscle Relaxant; Skeletal Muscle Relaxant

Use
Dental: Treatment of muscle spasm with acute temporomandibular joint pain
Medical: Treatment of muscle spasm associated with acute painful musculoskeletal conditions

Mechanism of Action Acts on the spinal cord and subcortical levels by depressing polysynaptic reflexes

Local Anesthetic/Vasoconstrictor Precautions No information available to require special precautions

Effects on Dental Treatment No effects or complications reported

Other Adverse Effects
>10%: Central nervous system: Drowsiness
1% to 10%:
Cardiovascular: Tachycardia, tightness in chest, flushing of face
Central nervous system: Fainting, mental depression, allergic fever, dizziness, lightheadedness, headache, paradoxical stimulation
Dermatologic: Angioedema
Gastrointestinal: Nausea, vomiting, stomach cramps
Neuromuscular & skeletal: Trembling
Ocular: Burning of eyes
Respiratory: Shortness of breath
Miscellaneous: Hiccups

Oral manifestations: No data reported

Drug Interactions Alcohol, CNS depressants

Drug Uptake
Onset of action: Within 1 hour

Pregnancy Risk Factor C

Breast-feeding Considerations No data reported

Dosage Forms
Caplet (Parafon Forte™ DSC): 500 mg
Capsule (Lobac®, Mus-Lac®): 250 mg with acetaminophen 300 mg
Tablet (Paraflex®): 250 mg

Dietary Considerations No data reported

Generic Available Yes

Cholac® *see* Lactulose *on page 488*

Cholan-HMB® *see* Dehydrocholic Acid *on page 254*

Cholecalciferol (kole e kal si' fer ole)

Brand Names Delta-D®

Therapeutic Category Vitamin D Analog

Synonyms D_3

Use Dietary supplement, treatment of vitamin D deficiency or prophylaxis of deficiency

Local Anesthetic/Vasoconstrictor Precautions No information available to require special precautions

Effects on Dental Treatment No effects or complications reported

Other Adverse Effects
1% to 10%:
Cardiovascular: Hypotension, cardiac arrhythmias, hypertension, irregular heart beat
Central nervous system: Irritability, headache
Dermatologic: Pruritus
Gastrointestinal: Nausea, vomiting, anorexia, pancreatitis, metallic taste
Genitourinary: Polyuria, polydipsia
Neuromuscular & skeletal: Bone pain, muscle pain
Ocular: Conjunctivitis, photophobia
<1%:
Central nervous system: Overt psychosis
Gastrointestinal: Weight loss
Comments Cholecalciferol 1 mg = 40,000 units of vitamin D activity

Choledyl® *see* Oxtriphylline *on page 645*

Cholera Vaccine (kol' er a vak seen')
Therapeutic Category Vaccine, Inactivated Bacteria
Use Primary immunization for cholera prophylaxis
Usual Dosage
Children:
6 months to 4 years: Two 0.2 mL doses I.M./S.C. 1 week to 1 month apart; booster doses (0.2 mL I.M./S.C.) every 6 months
5-10 years: Two 0.3 mL doses I.M./S.C. or two 0.2 mL intradermal doses 1 week to 1 month apart; booster doses (0.3 mL I.M./S.C. or 0.2 mL I.D.) every 6 months

Children ≥10 years and Adults: Two 0.5 mL doses given I.M./S.C. or two 0.2 mL doses I.D. 1 week to 1 month apart; booster doses (0.5 mL I.M. or S.C. or 0.2 mL I.D.) every 6 months
Mechanism of Action Inactivated vaccine producing active immunization
Local Anesthetic/Vasoconstrictor Precautions No information available to require special precautions
Effects on Dental Treatment No effects or complications reported
Other Adverse Effects >10%:
Cardiovascular: Swelling
Central nervous system: Malaise, fever, headache, pain
Dermatologic: Tenderness, erythema
Local: Induration at injection site
Pregnancy Risk Factor C
Comments Inactivated bacteria vaccine

Cholestyramine Resin (koe les' tir a meen rez' in)
Related Information
Cardiovascular Diseases *on page 912*
Brand Names Cholybar®; Questran®; Questran® Light
Canadian/Mexican Brand Names PMS-Cholestyramine® (Canada)
Therapeutic Category Lipid Lowering Drugs
Synonyms Colestiramina (Mexico)
Use Adjunct in the management of primary hypercholesterolemia; pruritus associated with elevated levels of bile acids; diarrhea associated with excess fecal bile acids; binding toxicologic agents; pseudomembraneous colitis
Usual Dosage Oral (dosages are expressed in terms of anhydrous resin):
Powder:
Children: 240 mg/kg/day in 3 divided doses; need to titrate dose depending on indication
Adults: 4 g 1-6 times/day to a maximum of 16-32 g/day
Tablet: Adults: Initial: 4 g once or twice daily; maintenance: 8-16 g/day in 2 divided doses

Not removed by hemo- or peritoneal dialysis; supplemental doses not necessary with dialysis or continuous arterio-venous or veno-venous hemofiltration effects
Mechanism of Action Forms a nonabsorbable complex with bile acids in the intestine, releasing chloride ions in the process; inhibits enterohepatic reuptake of intestinal bile salts and thereby increases the fecal loss of bile salt-bound low density lipoprotein cholesterol
Local Anesthetic/Vasoconstrictor Precautions No information available to require special precautions
Effects on Dental Treatment No effects or complications reported
(Continued)

Cholestyramine Resin *(Continued)*

Other Adverse Effects
1% to 10%: Gastrointestinal: Constipation

<1%:
Dermatologic: Rash, irritation of perianal area, skin, or tongue
Endocrine & metabolic: Hyperchloremic acidosis
Gastrointestinal: Nausea, vomiting, abdominal distention and pain, malabsorption of fat-soluble vitamins, intestinal obstruction, steatorrhea
Hematologic: Hypoprothrombinemia (secondary to Vitamin K deficiency)
Renal: Increased urinary calcium excretion

Drug Interactions Decreased effect: Decreased absorption (oral) of digitalis glycosides, warfarin, thyroid hormones, thiazide diuretics, propranolol, phenobarbital, amiodarone, methotrexate, NSAIDs, and other drugs by binding to the drug in the intestine

Drug Uptake
Peak effect: 21 days
Absorption: Not absorbed from the GI tract

Pregnancy Risk Factor C

Choline Magnesium Salicylate
(koe' leen mag nee' zhum sa lis' i late)

Related Information
Rheumatoid Arthritis, Osteoarthritis, and Joint Prostheses *on page 930*

Brand Names Trilisate®

Therapeutic Category Analgesic, Non-narcotic; Anti-inflammatory Agent; Nonsteroidal Anti-inflammatory Agent (NSAID), Oral; Salicylate

Use Management of osteoarthritis, rheumatoid arthritis, and other arthritis; salicylate salts may not inhibit platelet aggregation and, therefore, should not be substituted for aspirin in the prophylaxis of thrombosis

Usual Dosage Oral (based on total salicylate content):
Children <37 kg: 50 mg/kg/day given in 2 divided doses
Adults: 500 mg to 1.5 g 2-3 times/day; usual maintenance dose: 1-4.5 g/day

Mechanism of Action Inhibits prostaglandin synthesis; acts on the hypothalamus heat-regulating center to reduce fever; blocks the generation of pain impulses

Local Anesthetic/Vasoconstrictor Precautions No information available to require special precautions

Effects on Dental Treatment No effects or complications reported

Other Adverse Effects
>10%: Gastrointestinal: Nausea, heartburn, stomach pains, dyspepsia, epigastric discomfort

1% to 10%:
Central nervous system: Weakness, tiredness
Dermatologic: Skin rash
Gastrointestinal: Gastrointestinal ulceration
Hematologic: Hemolytic anemia
Respiratory: Troubled breathing
Miscellaneous: Anaphylactic shock

<1%:
Central nervous system: Insomnia, nervousness, jitters
Hematologic: Occult bleeding, prolongation of bleeding time, leukopenia, thrombocytopenia, iron deficiency anemia
Hepatic: Hepatotoxicity
Renal: Impaired renal function
Respiratory: Bronchospasm

Drug Interactions
Decreased effect with antacids
Increased effect of warfarin

Drug Uptake
Absorption: Absorbed from the stomach and small intestine
Serum half-life: Dose-dependent ranging from 2-3 hours at low doses to 30 hours at high doses
Time to peak serum concentration: ~2 hours

Pregnancy Risk Factor C

Choline Salicylate (koe' leen sa lis' i late)

Brand Names Arthropan® [OTC]
Canadian/Mexican Brand Names Teejel® (Canada)
Therapeutic Category Analgesic, Non-narcotic; Anti-inflammatory Agent; Nonsteroidal Anti-inflammatory Agent (NSAID), Oral; Salicylate

Use Temporary relief of pain of rheumatoid arthritis, rheumatic fever, osteoarthritis, and other conditions for which oral salicylates are recommended; useful in patients in which there is difficulty in administering doses in a tablet or capsule dosage form, because of the liquid dosage form

Usual Dosage

Children >12 years and Adults: Oral: 5 mL (870 mg) every 3-4 hours, if necessary, but not more than 6 doses in 24 hours

Rheumatoid arthritis: 870-1740 mg (5-10 mL) up to 4 times/day

Mechanism of Action Inhibits prostaglandin synthesis; acts on the hypothalamus heat-regulating center to reduce fever; blocks the generation of pain impulses

Local Anesthetic/Vasoconstrictor Precautions No information available to require special precautions

Effects on Dental Treatment No effects or complications reported

Other Adverse Effects

>10%: Gastrointestinal: Nausea, heartburn, stomach pains, dyspepsia, epigastric discomfort

1% to 10%:

Central nervous system: Weakness, tiredness

Dermatologic: Skin rash

Gastrointestinal: Gastrointestinal ulceration

Hematologic: Hemolytic anemia

Respiratory: Troubled breathing

Miscellaneous: Anaphylactic shock

<1%:

Central nervous system: Insomnia, nervousness, jitters

Hematologic: Occult bleeding, prolongation of bleeding time, leukopenia, thrombocytopenia, iron deficiency anemia

Hepatic: Hepatotoxicity

Renal: Impaired renal function

Respiratory: Bronchospasm

Drug Interactions

Decreased effect with antacids

Increased effect of warfarin

Drug Uptake

Absorption: From the stomach and small intestine within ~2 hours

Serum half-life: Dose-dependent ranging from 2-3 hours at low doses to 30 hours at high doses

Time to peak serum concentration: 1-2 hours

Pregnancy Risk Factor C

Choline Theophyllinate see Oxtriphylline on page 645

Choloxin® see Dextrothyroxine Sodium on page 266

Cholybar® see Cholestyramine Resin on page 201

Chondroitin Sulfate-Sodium Hyaluronate

(kon droy' tin sul' fate-sow' de um hye a loo roe' nate)

Brand Names Viscoat®

Therapeutic Category Ophthalmic Agent, Viscoeleastic

Synonyms Sodium Hyaluronate-Chrondroitin Sulfate

Use Surgical aid in anterior segment procedures, protects corneal endothelium and coats intraocular lens thus protecting it

Usual Dosage Carefully introduce (using a 27-gauge needle or cannula) into anterior chamber after thoroughly cleaning the chamber with a balanced salt solution

Mechanism of Action Functions as a tissue lubricant and is thought to play an important role in modulating the interactions between adjacent tissues

Local Anesthetic/Vasoconstrictor Precautions No information available to require special precautions

Effects on Dental Treatment No effects or complications reported

Other Adverse Effects 1% to 10%: Increased intraocular pressure (transient)

Drug Uptake

Absorption: Following intravitreous injection, diffusion occurs slowly

Pregnancy Risk Factor C

Chooz® [OTC] see Calcium Carbonate on page 140

Chorex® see Chorionic Gonadotropin on this page

Chorionic Gonadotropin (koe ree on' ik goe nad' oh troe pin)

Brand Names A.P.L.®; Chorex®; Choron®; Corgonject®; Follutein®; Glukor®; Gonic®; Pregnyl®; Profasi® HP

(Continued)

Chorionic Gonadotropin *(Continued)*

Therapeutic Category Gonadotropin; Ovulation Stimulator

Use Induces ovulation and pregnancy in anovulatory, infertile females; treatment of hypogonadotropic hypogonadism, prepubertal cryptorchidism

Usual Dosage I.M.:

Children:

Prepubertal cryptorchidism (not due to anatomical obstruction): 4000 units 3 times/week for 3 weeks

or

5000 units every other day for 4 injections

or

15 injections of 500-1000 units over a period of 6 weeks

or

500 units 3 times per week for 4-6 weeks. If unsuccessful, start another course 1 month later, giving 1000 units/injection.

Hypogonadotropic hypogonadism in males: 500-1000 units 3 times/week for 3 weeks, followed by the same dose twice weekly for 3 weeks

or

1000-2000 units 3 times/week

or

4000 units 3 times/week for 6-9 months; reduce dose to 2000 units 3 times/week for an additional 3 months

Adults:

Use with menotropins to stimulate spermatogenesis: 5000 units 3 times/week for 4-6 months. With the beginning of menotropins therapy, hCG dose is continued at 2000 2 times/week.

Induction of ovulation and pregnancy: 5000-10,000 units one day following last dose of menotropins

Mechanism of Action Stimulates production of gonadal steroid hormones by causing production of androgen by the testis; as a substitute for luteinizing hormone (LH) to stimulate ovulation

Local Anesthetic/Vasoconstrictor Precautions No information available to require special precautions

Effects on Dental Treatment No effects or complications reported

Other Adverse Effects

1% to 10%:

Central nervous system: Mental depression, tiredness

Endocrine & metabolic: Pelvic pain, ovarian cysts, enlargement of breasts, precocious puberty

Local: Pain at the injection site

Neuromuscular & skeletal: Premature closure of epiphyses

<1%:

Cardiovascular: Peripheral edema

Central nervous system: Irritability, restlessness, fatigue, headache

Endocrine & metabolic: Ovarian hyperstimulation syndrome, gynecomastia

Drug Interactions No data reported

Drug Uptake

Half-life, biphasic:

Initial: 11 hours

Terminal: 23 hours

Pregnancy Risk Factor C

Choron® *see* Chorionic Gonadotropin *on previous page*

Chromagen® OB [OTC] *see* Vitamins, Multiple *on page 901*

Chroma-Pak® *see* Trace Metals *on page 857*

Chromium *see* Trace Metals *on page 857*

Chronulac® *see* Lactulose *on page 488*

Chymex® *see* Bentiromide *on page 101*

Chymodiactin® *see* Chymopapain *on this page*

Chymopapain *(kye' moe pa pane)*

Brand Names Chymodiactin®; Discase®

Therapeutic Category Enzyme, Intradiscal; Enzyme, Proteolytic

Use Alternative to surgery in patients with herniated lumbar intervertebral disks

Usual Dosage Adults: 2000-4000 units/disc with a maximum cumulative dose not to exceed 8000 units for patients with multiple disc herniations

Mechanism of Action Chymopapain, when injected into the disc center, causes hydrolysis of the mucal mucopolysaccharide protein complex into acid polysaccharide, polypeptides, and amino acids. Subsequently, the water trapping properties of the nucleus pulposus are destroyed which permanently diminishes the pressure within the disc. The adjacent structures including the annulus fibrosus are not affected by chymopapain.

Local Anesthetic/Vasoconstrictor Precautions No information available to require special precautions

Effects on Dental Treatment No effects or complications reported

Other Adverse Effects
>10%: Neuromuscular & skeletal: Back pain
1% to 10%:
  Central nervous system: Dizziness, headache
  Gastrointestinal: Nausea
  Neuromuscular & skeletal: Weakness in legs
<1%:
  Central nervous system: CNS hemorrhage, seizures
  Dermatologic: Allergic dermatitis
  Gastrointestinal: Paralytic ileus
  Local: Thrombophlebitis
  Ocular: Conjunctivitis
  Respiratory: Runny nose, shortness of breath
  Miscellaneous: Anaphylaxis

Pregnancy Risk Factor C

Cianocobalamina (Mexico) *see* Cyanocobalamin *on page 237*

Cibacalcin® *see* Calcitonin *on page 138*

Cibalith-S® *see* Lithium *on page 508*

Ciclofosfamida (Mexico) *see* Cyclophosphamide *on page 240*

Ciclopirox Olamine (sye kloe peer' ox ole' a meen)
Brand Names Loprox®
Therapeutic Category Antifungal Agent, Topical
Use Treatment of tinea pedis (athlete's foot), tinea cruris (jock itch), tinea corporis (ringworm), cutaneous candidiasis, and tinea versicolor (pityriasis)
Usual Dosage Children >10 years and Adults: Apply twice daily, gently massage into affected areas; if no improvement after 4 weeks of treatment, re-evaluate the diagnosis
Mechanism of Action Inhibiting transport of essential elements in the fungal cell causing problems in synthesis of DNA, RNA, and protein
Local Anesthetic/Vasoconstrictor Precautions No information available to require special precautions
Effects on Dental Treatment No effects or complications reported
Other Adverse Effects 1% to 10%: Local: Irritation, redness, pain or burning; worsening of clinical condition
Drug Interactions No data reported
Drug Uptake
Absorption: <2% absorbed through intact skin
Serum half-life: 1.7 hours
Pregnancy Risk Factor B

Ciclosporina (Mexico) *see* Cyclosporine *on page 243*

Cidofovir (si dof' o veer)
Brand Names Vistide®
Therapeutic Category Antiviral Agent, Parenteral
Use Treatment of CMV retinitis in patients with acquired immunodeficiency syndrome (AIDS)
Usual Dosage
Induction treatment: 5 mg/kg once weekly for 2 consecutive weeks
Maintenance treatment: 5 mg/kg administered once every 2 weeks
Probenecid must be administered orally with each dose of cidofovir
Probenecid dose: 2 g 3 hours prior to cidofovir dose, 1 g 2 hours and 8 hours after completion of the infusion; patients should also receive 1 L of normal saline intravenously prior to each infusion of cidofovir; saline should be infused over 1-2 hours

Dosing adjustment in renal impairment:
Cl_{cr} 41-55 mL/minute:
  Induction (weekly x 2 doses): 2 mg/kg
  Maintenance (every other week): 2 mg/kg
Cl_{cr} 30-40 mL/minute:
  Induction (weekly x 2 doses): 1.5 mg/kg
  Maintenance (every other week): 1.5 mg/kg
Cl_{cr} 20-29 mL/minute:
  Induction (weekly x 2 doses): 1 mg/kg
(Continued)

Cidofovir *(Continued)*

    Maintenance (every other week): 1 mg/kg
    Cl_{cr} <19 mL/minute:
      Induction (weekly x 2 doses): 0.5 mg/kg
      Maintenance (every other week): 0.5 mg/kg

Patients with clinically significant changes in serum creatinine during therapy: Cidofovir dose should be reduced to 3 mg/kg and discontinued if creatinine rise is >0.5 mg/dL

Data unavailable in patients on dialysis

Mechanism of Action Cidofovir is converted to cidofovir diphosphate which is the active intracellular metabolite; cidofovir diphosphate suppresses CMV replication by selective inhibition of viral DNA synthesis. Incorporation of cidofovir into growing viral DNA chain results in reductions in the rate of viral DNA synthesis.

Local Anesthetic/Vasoconstrictor Precautions No information available to require special precautions

Effects on Dental Treatment No effects or complications reported

Other Adverse Effects

>10%:
    Central nervous system: Fever, asthenia, headache, chills
    Dermatologic: Rash, alopecia
    Gastrointestinal: Nausea, vomiting, diarrhea, anorexia, abdominal pain
    Hematologic: Neutropenia, anemia
    Ocular: Ocular hypotony
    Renal: Proteinuria, increased creatinine
    Respiratory: Dyspnea
    Miscellaneous: Infections

<10%:
    Cardiovascular: Hypotension, tachycardia
    Central nervous system: Anxiety, hallucinations, depression, convulsion, somnolence
    Dermatologic: Alopecia, acne, skin discoloration/dryness, rash, pruritus, urticaria
    Endocrine & metabolic: Hyperglycemia, hyperlipidemia, hypocalcemia, hypokalemia, dehydration
    Gastrointestinal: Colitis, GI distress, stomatitis
    Genitourinary: Urinary incontinence, glycosuria
    Hematologic: Thrombocytopenia
    Hepatic: Increased LFTs
    Neuromuscular & skeletal: Malaise, skeletal pain, myalgia, arthralgia, neuropathy
    Ocular: Ocular symptoms
    Renal: Hematuria
    Respiratory: respiratory symptoms
    Miscellaneous: Allergic reaction, sarcoma, sepsis

Warnings/Precautions Dose-dependent nephrotoxicity is a major dose-limiting toxicity related to cidofovir. Cidofovir is not recommended for use in patients with creatinine >1.5 mg/dL or creatinine clearance <55 mL/minute; in these benefits, consideration should be made of potential benefits vs risks. Dose adjustment or discontinuation may be required for changes in renal function while on therapy; renal function secondary to cidofovir is not always reversible. Neutropenia and metabolic acidosis (Fanconi syndrome) have been reported; administration of cidofovir must be accompanied by oral probenecid and intravenous saline prehydration.

Drug Interactions Probenecid may decrease metabolism or tubular excretion of drugs such as AZT, acyclovir, benzodiazepines, acetaminophen, ACE inhibitors, barbiturates, loop diuretics, famotidine, NSAIDs, and theophylline; avoid concomitant administration with other nephrotoxic agents

Drug Uptake The following pharmacokinetic data is based on a combination of cidofovir administered with probenecid:
    Serum half-life: ~2.6 hours (nonintracellular)

Pregnancy Risk Factor C

Generic Available No

Comments Cidofovir preparation should be performed in a class two laminar flow biologic safety cabinet and personnel should be wearing surgical gloves and a closed front surgical gown with knit cuffs; appropriate safety equipment is recommended for preparation, administration, and disposal of cidofovir. If cidofovir contacts skin, wash and flush thoroughly with water.

Selected Readings
Hitchcock MJ, Jaffe HS, Martin JC, et al, "Cidofovir, A New Agent With Potent Anti-Herpes Virus Activity," *Antiviral Chemistry and Chemotherapy*, 1996, 7:115-27.

Cimetidina (Mexico) *see* Cimetidine *on this page*

Cimetidine (sye met′ i deen)
Related Information
Dental Drug Interactions: Update on Drug Combinations Requiring Special Considerations *on page 1022*
Brand Names Tagamet®
Canadian/Mexican Brand Names Apo-Cimetidine® (Canada); Novo-Cimetidine® (Canada); Nu-Cimet® (Canada); Peptol® (Canada); Blocan® (Mexico); Cimetase® (Mexico); Cimetigal® (Mexico); Columina® (Mexico); Ulcedine® (Mexico); Zymerol® (Mexico)
Therapeutic Category Histamine-2 Antagonist
Synonyms Cimetidina (Mexico)
Use Short-term treatment of active duodenal ulcers and benign gastric ulcers; long-term prophylaxis of duodenal ulcer; gastric hypersecretory states; gastro-esophageal reflux; prevention of upper GI bleeding in critically ill patients.
Usual Dosage
Children: Oral, I.M., I.V.: 20-40 mg/kg/day in divided doses every 4 hours
Adults: Short-term treatment of active ulcers:
Oral: 300 mg 4 times/day or 800 mg at bedtime or 400 mg twice daily for up to 8 weeks
I.M., I.V.: 300 mg every 6 hours or 37.5 mg/hour by continuous infusion; I.V. dosage should be adjusted to maintain an intragastric pH ≥ 5

Patients with an active bleed: Give cimetidine as a continuous infusion (see above)
Duodenal ulcer prophylaxis: Oral: 400-800 mg at bedtime
Gastric hypersecretory conditions: Oral, I.M., I.V.: 300-600 mg every 6 hours; dosage not to exceed 2.4 g/day
Mechanism of Action Competitive inhibition of histamine at H_2-receptors of the gastric parietal cells resulting in reduced gastric acid secretion, gastric volume and hydrogen ion concentration reduced
Local Anesthetic/Vasoconstrictor Precautions No information available to require special precautions
Effects on Dental Treatment No effects or complications reported
Other Adverse Effects
1% to 10%:
Central nervous system: Dizziness, agitation, headache, drowsiness
Gastrointestinal: Diarrhea, nausea, vomiting
<1%:
Cardiovascular: Bradycardia, hypotension, tachycardia
Central nervous system: Confusion, fever
Dermatologic: Rash
Endocrine & metabolic: Gynecomastia, swelling of breasts
Genitourinary: Decreased sexual ability
Hematologic: Neutropenia, agranulocytosis, thrombocytopenia
Hepatic: Elevated creatinine, elevated AST and ALT
Neuromuscular & skeletal: Myalgia
Drug Interactions Inhibits liver metabolism of many drugs resulting in potential for increased toxicity of those drugs; these include warfarin anticoagulants, phenytoin, propranolol, nifedipine, diazepam, tricyclic antidepressants, theophylline, and metronidazole
Drug Uptake
Serum half-life:
Adults (with normal renal function): 2 hours
Time to peak serum concentration: Oral: Within 1-2 hours
Pregnancy Risk Factor B

Cinobac® Pulvules® *see* Cinoxacin *on this page*

Cinoxacin (sin ox′ a sin)
Brand Names Cinobac® Pulvules®
Canadian/Mexican Brand Names Gugecin® (Mexico)
Therapeutic Category Antibiotic, Quinolone
Synonyms Cinoxacino (Mexico)
Use Treatment of urinary tract infections
Usual Dosage Children >12 years and Adults: 1 g/day in 2-4 doses for 7-14 days
(Continued)

Cinoxacin *(Continued)*

Mechanism of Action Inhibits microbial synthesis of DNA with resultant problems in protein synthesis

Local Anesthetic/Vasoconstrictor Precautions No information available to require special precautions

Effects on Dental Treatment No effects or complications reported

Other Adverse Effects

1% to 10%:
   Central nervous system: Headache, dizziness
   Gastrointestinal: Heartburn, abdominal pain, GI bleeding, belching, flatulence, anorexia, nausea

<1%:
   Central nervous system: Insomnia, confusion
   Gastrointestinal: Diarrhea
   Hematologic: Thrombocytopenia
   Ocular: Photophobia
   Otic: Tinnitus

Drug Interactions

Decreased effect: Decreased urine levels with probenecid; decreased absorption with aluminum-, magnesium-, calcium-containing antacids

Drug Uptake

Absorption: Oral: Rapid and complete; food decreases peak levels by 30% but not total amount absorbed

Serum half-life: 1.5 hours, prolonged in renal impairment

Time to peak serum concentration: Oral: Within 2-3 hours

Pregnancy Risk Factor B

Cinoxacino (Mexico) *see* Cinoxacin *on previous page*

Cipro™ *see* Ciprofloxacin Hydrochloride *on this page*

Ciprofloxacin Hydrochloride (sip roe flox' a sin hye droe klor' ide)

Related Information

Nonviral Infectious Diseases *on page 932*

Brand Names Cipro™

Canadian/Mexican Brand Names Cimogal® (Mexico); Ciproflox® (Mexico); Ciproflur® (Mexico); Ciproxina® (Mexico); Eni® (Mexico); Italnik® (Mexico); Kenzoflex® (Mexico); Microrgan® (Mexico); Mitroken® (Mexico); Nivoflox® (Mexico); Sophixin® Ofteno (Mexico)

Therapeutic Category Antibiotic, Ophthalmic; Antibiotic, Quinolone

Use

Dental: In combination with rifampin, as an alternative to vancomycin in the treatment of orofacial infections involving methicillin-resistant staphylococci; useful as a single agent or in combination with metronidazole in the treatment of periodontitis associated with the presence of *Actinobacillus actinomycetemcomitans*, (AA) as well as enteric rods/pseudomonads

Medical: Treatment of documented or suspected pseudomonal infection (eg, home care patients); documented multidrug resistant gram-negative organisms; documented infectious diarrhea due to *Campylobacter jejuni*, *Shigella*, or *Salmonella*; osteomyelitis caused by susceptible organisms in which parenteral therapy is not feasible; used ophthalmically for superficial ocular infections (corneal ulcers, conjunctivitis) due to strains of microorganisms susceptible to ciprofloxacin

Usual Dosage Adults: Oral: 250-750 mg every 12 hours, depending on severity of infection and susceptibility; in treatment of periodontitis, ciprofloxacin and metronidazole 500 mg each twice daily for 8 days

Mechanism of Action Inhibits DNA-gyrase in susceptible organisms; inhibits relaxation of supercoiled DNA and promotes breakage of double-stranded DNA

Local Anesthetic/Vasoconstrictor Precautions No information available to require special precautions

Effects on Dental Treatment No effects or complications reported

Other Adverse Effects 1% to 10%:
   Central nervous system: Headache, restlessness
   Gastrointestinal: Nausea, diarrhea, vomiting, abdominal pain
   Dermatologic: Rash

   Oral manifestations: No data reported

Contraindications Hypersensitivity to ciprofloxacin, any component or other quinolones

Warnings/Precautions Not recommended in children <18 years of age; has caused transient arthropathy in children; CNS stimulation may occur (tremor,

208

restlessness, confusion, and very rarely hallucinations or seizures). Use with caution in patients with known or suspected CNS disorders.

Drug Interactions Decreased absorption with antacids containing aluminum, magnesium, and/or calcium (by up to 98% if given at the same time); quinolones cause increased levels of caffeine, warfarin, cyclosporine, and theophylline; azlocillin, cimetidine, probenecid increase quinolone levels

Drug Uptake
Absorption: Oral: Rapid
Time to peak serum concentration: Oral: Within 0.5-2 hours
Serum half-life: 3-5 hours in patients with normal renal function
Influence of food: Delayed but total absorption remains unchanged

Pregnancy Risk Factor C

Breast-feeding Considerations Not compatible; can resume breast-feeding 48 hours after the last dose

Dosage Forms
Infusion, in D_5W: 400 mg (200 mL)
Infusion, in NS or D_5W: 200 mg (100 mL)
Injection: 200 mg (20 mL); 400 mg (40 mL)
Tablet: 250 mg, 500 mg, 750 mg

Dietary Considerations Dairy foods decrease ciprofloxacin concentration, use caution with xanthine-containing foods and beverages

Generic Available No

Selected Readings
Rams TE and Slots J, "Antibiotics in Periodontal Therapy: An Update," *Compendium*, 1992, 13(12):1130, 1132, 1134.

Cisaprida (Mexico) *see* Cisapride *on this page*

Cisapride (sis′ a pride)

Related Information
Endocrine Disorders & Pregnancy *on page 927*

Brand Names Propulsid®

Canadian/Mexican Brand Names Prepulsid® (Canada); Enteropride® (Mexico); Kinestase® (Mexico); Unamol® (Mexico)

Therapeutic Category Antiemetic; Cholinergic Agent

Synonyms Cisaprida (Mexico)

Use Treatment of nocturnal symptoms of gastroesophageal reflux disease (GERD), also demonstrated effectiveness for gastroparesis, refractory constipation, and nonulcer dyspepsia

Usual Dosage Oral:
Children: 0.15-0.3 mg/kg/dose 3-4 times/day; maximum: 10 mg/dose
Adults: Initial: 10 mg 4 times/day at least 15 minutes before meals and at bedtime; in some patients the dosage will need to be increased to 20 mg to obtain a satisfactory result

Mechanism of Action Enhances the release of acetylcholine at the myenteric plexus. *In vitro* studies have shown cisapride to have serotonin-4 receptor agonistic properties which may increase gastrointestinal motility and cardiac rate; increases lower esophageal sphincter pressure and lower esophageal peristalsis; accelerates gastric emptying of both liquids and solids

Local Anesthetic/Vasoconstrictor Precautions No information available to require special precautions

Effects on Dental Treatment No effects or complications reported

Other Adverse Effects
>5%:
Central nervous system: Headache
Dermatologic: Rash
Gastrointestinal: Diarrhea, GI cramping, dyspepsia, flatulence, nausea, dry mouth
Respiratory: Rhinitis
<5%:
Cardiovascular: Tachycardia
Central nervous system: Extrapyramidal effects, somnolence, fatigue, seizures, insomnia, anxiety
Hematologic: Thrombocytopenia, increased LFTs, pancytopenia, leukopenia, granulocytopenia, aplastic anemia
Respiratory: Rhinitis, sinusitis, coughing, upper respiratory tract infection
Miscellaneous: Increased incidence of viral infection

Drug Interactions Cisapride accelerates gastric emptying; this could affect the absorption of other drugs given simultaneously

Drug Uptake
Onset of action: 0.5-1 hour
(Continued)

Cisapride *(Continued)*

Serum half-life: 6-12 hours
Pregnancy Risk Factor C

Cisplatin (sis´ pla tin)

Brand Names Platinol®; Platinol®-AQ
Canadian/Mexican Brand Names Blastolem (Mexico); Medsaplatin (Mexico); Niyaplat (Mexico)
Therapeutic Category Antineoplastic Agent, Alkylating Agent
Synonyms CDDP
Use Management of metastatic testicular or ovarian carcinoma, advanced bladder cancer, osteosarcoma, Hodgkin's and non-Hodgkin's lymphoma, head or neck cancer, cervical cancer, lung cancer, brain tumors, neuroblastoma; used alone or in combination with other agents
Usual Dosage I.V. **(refer to individual protocols):**

An estimated Cl_{cr} should be on all cisplatin chemotherapy orders along with other patient parameters (ie, patient's height, weight, and body surface area). Pharmacy and nursing staff should check the Cl_{cr} on the order and determine the appropriateness of cisplatin dosing.

It is recommended that a 24-hour urine creatinine clearance be checked prior to a patient's first dose of cisplatin and periodically thereafter (ie, after every 2-3 cycles of cisplatin)

Pretreatment hydration with 1-2 L of fluid is recommended prior to cisplatin administration; adequate hydration and urinary output (>100 mL/hour) should be maintained for 24 hours after administration

If the dose prescribed is a reduced dose, then this should be indicated on the chemotherapy order

Children: Various dosage schedules range from 30-100 mg/m² once every 2-3 weeks; may also dose similar to adult dosing

Osteogenic sarcoma or neuroblastoma: 90 mg/m² once every 3 weeks or 30 mg/m² once weekly

Recurrent brain tumors: 60 mg/m² once daily for 2 consecutive days every 3-4 weeks

Adults:

Head and neck cancer: 100-150 mg/m² every 3-4 weeks
Testicular cancer: 10-20 mg/m²/day for 5 days repeated every 3-4 weeks
Metastatic ovarian cancer: 50 mg/m² every 3 weeks
Intraperitoneal: cisplatin has been administered intraperitoneal with systemic sodium thiosulfate for ovarian cancer; doses up to 90-270 mg/m² have been administered and retained for 4 hours before draining

Mechanism of Action Inhibits DNA synthesis by the formation of DNA cross-links; denatures the double helix; covalently binds to DNA bases and disrupts DNA function; may also bind to proteins; the *cis*-isomer is 14 times more cytotoxic than the *trans*-isomer; both forms cross-link DNA but cis-platinum is less easily recognized by cell enzymes and, therefore, not repaired. Cisplatin can also bind two adjacent guanines on the same strand of DNA producing intrastrand cross-linking and breakage

Local Anesthetic/Vasoconstrictor Precautions No information available to require special precautions

Effects on Dental Treatment No effects or complications reported

Other Adverse Effects

>10%: Ototoxicity, manifested as high frequency hearing loss (especially pronounced in children), hyperuricemia

Gastrointestinal: Cisplatin is one of the most emetogenic agents used in cancer chemotherapy; nausea and vomiting occur in 76% to 100% of patients and is dose related. Prophylactic antiemetics should always be prescribed; nausea and vomiting may last up to 1 week after therapy

Emetic potential: <75 mg: Moderately high (60% to 90%); ≥75 mg: High (>90%)

Myelosuppressive effects: Mild with moderate doses, mild to moderate with high-dose therapy; WBC: Mild; Platelets: Mild; Onset (days): 10; Nadir (days): 14-23; Recovery (days): 21-39

Anaphylactic reaction occurs within minutes after administration and can be controlled with epinephrine, antihistamines, and steroids

Extravasation: May cause thrombophlebitis and tissue damage if infiltrated; may use sodium thiosulfate as antidote, but consult hospital policy for guidelines

Nephrotoxicity: Related to elimination, protein binding, and uptake of cisplatin. Two types of nephrotoxicity: Acute renal failure and chronic renal insufficiency.

Acute renal failure and azotemia is a dose-dependent process and can be minimized with proper administration and prophylaxis. Damage to the proximal tubules by the aquation products of cisplatin is suspected to cause the toxicity. It is manifested as increased BUN and creatinine, oliguria, protein wasting, and potassium, calcium, and magnesium wasting

Chronic renal dysfunction can develop in patients receiving multiple courses of cisplatin. This occurs with slow release of the platinum ion from tissues, which then accumulates in the distal tubules. Manifestations of this toxicity are varied and can include sodium and water wasting, nephropathy, decreased Cl_{cr}, and magnesium wasting

Recommendations for minimizing nephrotoxicity include:
Prepare cisplatin in saline-containing vehicles
Vigorous hydration (125-150 mL/hour) before, during, and after cisplatin administration
Simultaneous administration of either mannitol or furosemide
Avoid other nephrotoxic agents (aminoglycosides, amphotericin, etc)

1% to 10%: Anorexia, pain at injection site

<1%: Optic neuritis, blurred vision, mouth sores, SIADH, bradycardia, arrhythmias, phlebitis, mild alopecia, hypomagnesemia, hypocalcemia, hypokalemia, hypophosphatemia, elevation of liver enzymes, papilledema

Neurotoxicity: Peripheral neuropathy is dose- and duration-dependent. The mechanism is through axonal degeneration with subsequent damage to the long sensory nerves. Toxicity can first be noted at doses of 200 mg/m^2, with measurable toxicity at doses >350 mg/m^2. This process is irreversible and progressive with continued therapy. Baseline audiography should be performed.

Miscellaneous: Papilledema, bradycardia, arrhythmias, elevation of liver enzymes, hyperuricemia, mild alopecia

Drug Uptake
Serum half-life:
Initial: 20-30 minutes
Beta: 1 hour
Terminal: ~24 hours
Secondary half-life: 44-73 hours

Pregnancy Risk Factor D

Comments Sodium content (10 mg): 35.4 mg (1.54 mEq)

Citanest Forte® with Epinephrine see Prilocaine With Epinephrine on page 721

Citanest Plain 4% Injection see Prilocaine on page 721

Citracal® [OTC] see Calcium Citrate on page 142

Citrate of Magnesia see Magnesium Citrate on page 521

Citric Acid and d-gluconic Acid Irrigant see Citric Acid Bladder Mixture on this page

Citric Acid Bladder Mixture (si' trik as' id blad' dur miks' chur)
Brand Names Renacidin®
Therapeutic Category Irrigating Solution
Synonyms Citric Acid and d-gluconic Acid Irrigant; Hemiacidrin
Use Preparing solutions for irrigating indwelling urethral catheters; to dissolve or prevent formation of calcifications
Local Anesthetic/Vasoconstrictor Precautions No information available to require special precautions
Effects on Dental Treatment No effects or complications reported

Citrovorum Factor see Leucovorin Calcium on page 491

Citrucel® [OTC] see Methylcellulose on page 566

Cladribine (kla' dri been)
Brand Names Leustatin™
Therapeutic Category Antineoplastic Agent, Antimetabolite
Synonyms 2-CdA; 2-Chlorodeoxyadenosine
Use Hairy cell and chronic lymphocytic leukemias
Usual Dosage I.V.:
Children:
Acute leukemia:
The safety and effectiveness of cladribine in children have not been established; in a phase I study involving patients 1-21 years of age with relapsed acute leukemia, cladribine was administered by continuous
(Continued)

Cladribine *(Continued)*

intravenous infusion at doses ranging from 3-10.7 mg/m²/day for 5 days (0.5-2 times the dose recommended in HCL). Investigators reported beneficial responses in this study; the dose-limiting toxicity was severe myelosuppression with profound neutropenia and thrombocytopenia.
Continuous intravenous infusion: 15-18 mg/m²/day for 5 days

Adults:
Hairy cell leukemia:
Continuous intravenous infusion: 0.09-0.1 mg/kg/day continuous infusion for 7 consecutive days
Continuous intravenous infusion: 4 mg/m²/day for 7 days
Non-Hodgkin's lymphoma: Continuous intravenous infusion: 0.1 mg/kg/day for 7 days

Mechanism of Action A purine nucleoside analogue; prodrug which is activated via phosphorylation by deoxycytidine kinase to a 5'-triphosphate derivative. This active form incorporates into susceptible cells and into DNA to result in the breakage of DNA strand and shutdown of DNA synthesis and also results in a depletion of nicotinamide adenine dinucleotide and adenosine triphosphate (ATP). The induction of strand breaks results in a drop in the cofactor nicotinamide adenine dinucleotide and disruption of cell metabolism. ATP is depleted to deprive cells of an important source of energy. Cladribine is able to kill resting as well as dividing cells, unlike most other cytotoxic drugs.

Local Anesthetic/Vasoconstrictor Precautions No information available to require special precautions

Effects on Dental Treatment No effects or complications reported

Other Adverse Effects
>10%:
Bone marrow suppression: Commonly observed in patients treated with cladribine, especially at high doses; at the initiation of treatment, however, most patients in clinical studies had hematologic impairment as a result of HCL. During the first 2 weeks after treatment initiation, mean platelet counts decline and subsequently increased with normalization of mean counts by day 12. Absolute neutrophil counts and hemoglobin declined and subsequently increased with normalization of mean counts by week 5 and week 6.
Central nervous system: Fatigue, headache
Dermatologic: Rash
Fever: Temperature ≥101°F has been associated with the use of cladribine in approximately 66% of patients in the first month of therapy. Although 69% of patients developed fevers, less than 33% of febrile events were associated with documented infection.
Gastrointestinal: Nausea and vomiting are not severe with cladribine at any dose level. Most cases of nausea were mild, not accompanied by vomiting and did not require treatment with antiemetics. In patients requiring antiemetics, nausea was easily controlled most often by chlorpromazine.
Local: Injection site reactions
1% to 10%:
Cardiovascular: Edema, tachycardia
Central nervous system: Dizziness, insomnia, chills, asthenia, malaise, pain
Dermatologic: Pruritus, erythema
Gastrointestinal: Constipation, abdominal pain
Neuromuscular & skeletal: Arthralgia, myalgia
Miscellaneous: Diaphoresis, trunk pain

Drug Uptake
Serum half-life: Biphasic:
Alpha: 25 minutes
Beta: 6.7 hours
Terminal, mean (normal renal function): 5.4 hours

Pregnancy Risk Factor D

Claforan® *see* Cefotaxime Sodium *on page 167*

Clarithromycin *(kla rith' roe mye sin)*
Related Information
Respiratory Diseases *on page 924*
Brand Names Biaxin™ Filmtabs®
Canadian/Mexican Brand Names Klaricid® (Mexico)
Therapeutic Category Antibiotic, Macrolide
Use
Dental: Alternate antibiotic in the treatment of common orofacial infections caused by aerobic gram-positive cocci and susceptible anaerobes

Medical: Treatment against most respiratory pathogens (eg, *S. pyogenes, S. pneumoniae, S. agalactiae,* viridans *Streptococcus, M. catarrhalis, C. trachomatis, Legionella* sp, *Mycoplasma pneumoniae, S. aureus*). Clarithromycin is highly active (MICs ≤0.25 mcg/mL) against *H. influenzae,* the combination of clarithromycin and its metabolite demonstrate an additive effect. Additionally, clarithromycin has shown activity against *C. pneumoniae* (including strain TWAR) and *M. avium* infection.

Usual Dosage Oral:
Children: Safe use has not been established
Adults: 250-500 mg every 12 hours for 7 days

Mechanism of Action Exerts its antibacterial action by binding to 50S ribosomal subunit resulting in inhibition of protein synthesis. The 14-OH metabolite of clarithromycin is twice as active as the parent compound.

Local Anesthetic/Vasoconstrictor Precautions No information available to require special precautions

Effects on Dental Treatment No effects or complications reported

Other Adverse Effects 1% to 10%:
Central nervous system: Headache
Gastrointestinal: Diarrhea, nausea, abnormal taste, dyspepsia, abdominal pain

Oral manifestations: No data reported

Contraindications Hypersensitivity to clarithromycin, erythromycin, or any macrolide antibiotic; use with pimozide

Warnings/Precautions In presence of severe renal impairment with or without coexisting hepatic impairment, decreased dosage or prolonged dosing interval may be appropriate; antibiotic associated colitis has been reported with use of clarithromycin; elderly patients have experienced increased incidents of adverse effects due to known age-related decreases in renal function

Drug Interactions Clarithromycin increases serum theophylline levels by as much as 20% and significantly increases carbamazepine levels
Note: While other drug interactions (digoxin, anticoagulants, ergotamine, triazolam) known to occur with erythromycin have not been reported in clinical trials with clarithromycin, concurrent use of these drugs should be monitored closely

Drug Uptake
Absorption: Rapid; highly stable in the presence of gastric acid (unlike erythromycin)
Time to peak serum concentration: Oral: 2-4 hours
Serum half-life, elimination: 3-4 hours with a 250 mg dose; 5-7 hours with a 500 mg dose
Influence of food: Delays absorption; total absorption remains unchanged

Pregnancy Risk Factor C

Breast-feeding Considerations No data reported; however, erythromycins may be taken while breast-feeding

Dosage Forms Tablet, film coated: 250 mg, 500 mg

Dietary Considerations May be taken with or without meals; may be taken with milk

Generic Available No

Comments *Helicobacter pylori* induced gastric ulcers: Combination regimen with bismuth subsalicylate, tetracycline, clarithromycin, and an H_2 receptor antagonist; or combination of omeprazole and clarithromycin. Adult dosage: Oral: 250 mg twice daily to 500 mg 3 times/day

Selected Readings
"Pimozide (Orap) Contraindicated With Clarithromycin (Biaxin) and Other Macrolide Antibiotics," *FDA Medical Bulletin,* October 1996, 3.

Claritin® *see* Loratadine *on page 512*
Claritin-D® *see* Loratadine and Pseudoephedrine *on page 513*
Claritin-D 24-Hour® *see* Loratadine and Pseudoephedrine *on page 513*
Clearasil® [OTC] *see* Benzoyl Peroxide *on page 104*
ClearAway® *see* Salicylic Acid *on page 777*
Clear Eyes® [OTC] *see* Naphazoline Hydrochloride *on page 605*
Clemastina (Mexico) *see* Clemastine Fumarate *on next page*

Clemastine and Phenylpropanolamine
(klem' as teen & fen il proe pa nole' a meen)
Brand Names Tavist-D®
Therapeutic Category Antihistamine/Decongestant Combination
Use Symptomatic relief of allergic rhinitis; pruritus of the eyes, nose or throat, lacrimation and nasal congestion
Usual Dosage Children >12 years and Adults: Oral: 1 tablet every 12 hours
(Continued)

Clemastine and Phenylpropanolamine *(Continued)*

Local Anesthetic/Vasoconstrictor Precautions Use with caution since phenylpropanolamine is a sympathomimetic amine which could interact with epinephrine to cause a pressor response

Effects on Dental Treatment Up to 10% of patients could experience tachycardia, palpitations, and dry mouth; use vasoconstrictor with caution

Dosage Forms Tablet: Clemastine fumarate 1.34 mg and phenylpropanolamine hydrochloride 75 mg

Clemastine Fumarate (klem' as teen fyoo' ma rate)

Brand Names Tavist®

Therapeutic Category Antihistamine

Synonyms Clemastina (Mexico)

Use Perennial and seasonal allergic rhinitis and other allergic symptoms including urticaria

Usual Dosage Oral:

Children: <12 years: 0.4-1 mg twice daily

Children >12 years and Adults: 1.34 mg twice daily to 2.68 mg 3 times/day; do not exceed 8.04 mg/day; lower doses should be considered in patients >60 years

Mechanism of Action Competes with histamine for H_1-receptor sites on effector cells in the gastrointestinal tract, blood vessels, and respiratory tract

Local Anesthetic/Vasoconstrictor Precautions No information available to require special precautions

Effects on Dental Treatment No effects or complications reported

Other Adverse Effects

>10%:

Central nervous system: Slight to moderate drowsiness

Miscellaneous: Thickening of bronchial secretions

1% to 10%:

Central nervous system: Headache, fatigue, nervousness, increased dizziness

Gastrointestinal: Appetite increase, weight nausea, diarrhea, abdominal pain, dry mouth

Neuromuscular & skeletal: Arthralgia

Respiratory: Pharyngitis

<1%:

Cardiovascular: Edema, palpitations

Central nervous system: Depression

Dermatologic: Angioedema, photosensitivity, rash

Hepatic: Hepatitis

Neuromuscular & skeletal: Myalgia, paresthesia

Respiratory: Bronchospasm

Miscellaneous: Epistaxis

Drug Interactions May interact with other sedatives to cause drowsiness; these include alcohol and tranquilizers

Drug Uptake Absorption: Almost 100% from GI tract

Pregnancy Risk Factor C

Cleocin HCl® *see* Clindamycin *on this page*

Cleocin Pediatric® *see* Clindamycin *on this page*

Cleocin Phosphate® *see* Clindamycin *on this page*

C-Lexin® *see* Cephalexin Monohydrate *on page 176*

Clidinium and Chlordiazepoxide

(kli di' nee um & klor dye az e pox' ide)

Brand Names Clindex®; Clinoxide®; Clipoxide®; Librax®; Lidox®; Zebrax®

Therapeutic Category Antispasmodic Agent, Gastrointestinal

Synonyms Chlordiazepoxide and Clidinium

Use Adjunct treatment of peptic ulcer, treatment of irritable bowel syndrome

Local Anesthetic/Vasoconstrictor Precautions No information available to require special precautions

Effects on Dental Treatment No effects or complications reported

Comments After extended therapy, abrupt discontinuation should be avoided and a gradual dose tapering schedule followed

Clindamycin (klin da mye' sin)

Related Information

Animal and Human Bites Guidelines *on page 976*

Antimicrobial Prophylaxis in Surgical Patients *on page 1042*

Cardiovascular Diseases *on page 912*
Oral Bacterial Infections *on page 945*

Brand Names Cleocin HCl®; Cleocin Pediatric®; Cleocin Phosphate®

Canadian/Mexican Brand Names Dalacin® C [Hydrochloride] (Canada); Dalacin® C (Mexico); Galecin® (Mexico); Klyndaken® (Mexico)

Therapeutic Category Acne Products; Antibiotic, Anaerobic; Antibiotic, Miscellaneous

Use

Dental: Alternate antibiotic, when amoxicillin and erythromycin cannot be used, for the standard regimen for prevention of bacterial endocarditis in patients undergoing dental procedures; an alternative to penicillin VK and erythromycin for treating orofacial infections

Medical: Treatment against aerobic and anaerobic streptococci (except enterococci), most staphylococci, *Bacteroides* sp and *Actinomyces*; used topically in treatment of severe acne, vaginally for *Gardnerella vaginalis*, alternate treatment for toxoplasmosis

Usual Dosage

Children:

Initial prophylaxis: 10 mg/kg; follow-up dose is half the initial dose

Orofacial infections: 8-25 mg/kg in 3-4 equally divided doses

Adults:

Prevention of bacterial endocarditis in patients unable to take amoxicillin or erythromycin: Oral: 300 mg 1 hour before procedure, then 150 mg 6 hours after initial dose

Orofacial infections: 150-450 mg every 6 hours for at least 7 days; maximum dose: 1.8 g/day

Mechanism of Action Reversibly binds to 50S ribosomal subunits preventing peptide bond formation thus inhibiting bacterial protein synthesis; bacteriostatic or bactericidal depending on drug concentration, infection site, and organism

Local Anesthetic/Vasoconstrictor Precautions No information available to require special precautions

Effects on Dental Treatment No effects or complications reported

Other Adverse Effects

>10%: Gastrointestinal: Diarrhea

1% to 10%:

Dermatologic: Rashes

Gastrointestinal: Pseudomembranous colitis, nausea, vomiting

Oral manifestations: No data reported

Contraindications Hypersensitivity to clindamycin or any component; previous pseudomembranous colitis, hepatic impairment

Warnings/Precautions Dosage adjustment may be necessary in patients with severe hepatic dysfunction; no change necessary with renal insufficiency; can cause severe and possibly fatal colitis; use with caution in patients with a history of pseudomembranous colitis; discontinue drug if significant diarrhea, abdominal cramps, or passage of blood and mucus occurs

Drug Interactions Increased duration of neuromuscular blockade from tubocurarine, pancuronium

Drug Uptake

Absorption: 90% absorbed rapidly from GI tract following oral administration

Time to peak serum concentration: Oral: Within 60 minutes

Serum half-life: Adults: 1.6-5.3 hours, average: 2-3 hours

Influence of food: No change in absorption

Pregnancy Risk Factor B

Breast-feeding Considerations May be taken while breast-feeding

Dosage Forms

Capsule, as hydrochloride: 75 mg, 150 mg, 300 mg

Granules for oral solution, as palmitate: 75 mg/5 mL (100 mL)

Infusion, as phosphate, in D_5W: 300 mg (50 mL); 600 mg (50 mL)

Injection, as phosphate: 150 mg/mL (2 mL, 4 mL, 6 mL, 50 mL, 60 mL)

Dietary Considerations Peak concentrations may be delayed with food; may be taken with food

Generic Available Yes: Injection

Comments Clindamycin has not been shown to interfere with oral contraceptive activity; however, it reduces GI microflora, thus, oral contraceptive users should be advised to use additional methods of birth control. About 1% of clindamycin users develop pseudomembranous colitis. Symptoms may occur 2-9 days after initiation of therapy; however, it has never occurred with the 2-dose regimen of clindamycin used to prevent bacterial endocarditis.

(Continued)

Clindamycin *(Continued)*
Selected Readings
Council on Dental Therapeutics, American Heart Association, "Preventing Bacterial Endocarditis," *J Am Dent Assoc*, 1991, 122(2):87-92.

Dajani AS, Bisno AL, Chung KJ, et al, "Prevention of Bacterial Endocarditis. Recommendations by the American Heart Association," *JAMA*, 1990, 264(22): 2919-22.

Wynn RL and Bergman SA, "Antibiotics and Their Use in the Treatment of Orofacial Infections," *Gen Dent*, 1994, 42(Pt 1):398-402 and 42(Pt 2):498-502.

Wynn RL, "Clindamycin: An Often Forgotten but Important Antibiotic," *AGD Impact*, 1994, 22:10.

Clindex® *see* Clidinium and Chlordiazepoxide *on page 214*

Clinoril® *see* Sulindac *on page 813*

Clinoxide® *see* Clidinium and Chlordiazepoxide *on page 214*

Clioquinol and Hydrocortisone
(klye oh kwin' ole & hye droe kor' ti sone)

Brand Names Ala-Quin® Topical; Corque® Topical; Cortin® Topical; Hysone® Topical; Lanvisone® Topical; Pedi-Cort V® Topical; Racet® Topical; UAD® Topical

Therapeutic Category Antifungal Agent, Topical; Corticosteroid, Topical (Low Potency)

Synonyms Hydrocortisone and Clioquinol; Hydrocortisone and Iodochlorhydroxyquin; Iodochlorhydroxyquin and Hydrocortisone

Use Contact or atopic dermatitis; eczema; neurodermatitis; anogenital pruritus; mycotic dermatoses; moniliasis

Local Anesthetic/Vasoconstrictor Precautions No information available to require special precautions

Effects on Dental Treatment No effects or complications reported

Clipoxide® *see* Clidinium and Chlordiazepoxide *on page 214*

Clobetasol Propionate (kloe bay' ta sol pro pee oh' nate)
Related Information
Corticosteroids, Topical Comparison *on page 1018*
Oral Nonviral Soft Tissue Ulcerations or Erosions *on page 955*

Brand Names Temovate®

Canadian/Mexican Brand Names Dermasone® (Canada); Dermovate® (Canada); Gen-Clobetasol® (Canada); Novo-Clobetasol® (Canada); Dermatovate® (Mexico)

Therapeutic Category Corticosteroid, Topical (Very High Potency)

Synonyms Clobetasol, Propionato De (Mexico)

Use Short-term relief of inflammation of moderate to severe corticosteroid-responsive dermatosis (very high potency topical corticosteroid)

Usual Dosage Adults: Topical: Apply twice daily for up to 2 weeks with no more than 50 g/week

Mechanism of Action Stimulates the synthesis of enzymes needed to decrease inflammation, suppress mitotic activity, and cause vasoconstriction

Local Anesthetic/Vasoconstrictor Precautions No information available to require special precautions

Effects on Dental Treatment No effects or complications reported

Other Adverse Effects
1% to 10%: Local: Itching, burning, erythema, dryness, irritation, papular rashes

<1%: Local: Hypertrichosis, acneiform eruptions, hypopigmentation, perioral dermatitis, maceration of skin, skin atrophy, striae, miliaria

Drug Interactions No data reported

Drug Uptake
Absorption: Percutaneous absorption variable and dependent upon many factors including vehicle used, integrity of epidermis, dose, and use of occlusive dressings

Pregnancy Risk Factor C

Clobetasol, Propionato De (Mexico) *see* Clobetasol Propionate *on this page*

Clocortolone Pivalate (kloe kor' toe lone piv' ah late)
Related Information
Corticosteroids, Topical Comparison *on page 1018*

Brand Names Cloderm®

Therapeutic Category Corticosteroid, Topical (Medium Potency)

Use Inflammation of corticosteroid-responsive dermatoses (medium potency topical corticosteroid)

Usual Dosage Adults: Apply sparingly and gently; rub into affected area from 1-4 times/day

Mechanism of Action Stimulates the synthesis of enzymes needed to decrease inflammation, suppress mitotic activity, and cause vasoconstriction

Local Anesthetic/Vasoconstrictor Precautions No information available to require special precautions

Effects on Dental Treatment No effects or complications reported

Other Adverse Effects

1% to 10%: Local: Itching, burning, erythema, dryness, irritation, papular rashes

<1%: Local: Hypertrichosis, acneiform eruptions, hypopigmentation, perioral dermatitis, maceration of skin, skin atrophy, striae, miliaria

Drug Interactions No data reported

Drug Uptake

Absorption: Percutaneous absorption is variable and dependent upon many factors including vehicle used, integrity of epidermis, dose, and use of occlusive dressings

Pregnancy Risk Factor C

Cloderm® see Clocortolone Pivalate *on previous page*

Clofazimine Palmitate (kloe fa' zi meen palm' eh tate)

Brand Names Lamprene®

Therapeutic Category Antibiotic, Miscellaneous

Use Treatment of dapsone-resistant leprosy; multibacillary dapsone-sensitive leprosy; erythema nodosum leprosum; *Mycobacterium avium* - intracellular (MAI) infections

Usual Dosage Oral:

Children: Leprosy: 1 mg/kg/day every 24 hours in combination with dapsone and rifampin

Adults:

Dapsone-resistant leprosy: 100 mg/day in combination with one or more antileprosy drugs for 3 years; then alone 100 mg/day

Dapsone-sensitive multibacillary leprosy: 100 mg/day in combination with two or more antileprosy drugs for at least 2 years and continue until negative skin smears are obtained, then institute single drug therapy with appropriate agent

Erythema nodosum leprosum: 100-200 mg/day for up to 3 months or longer then taper dose to 100 mg/day when possible

Pyoderma gangrenosum: 300-400 mg/day for up to 12 months

Mechanism of Action Binds preferentially to mycobacterial DNA to inhibit mycobacterial growth; also has some anti-inflammatory activity through an unknown mechanism

Local Anesthetic/Vasoconstrictor Precautions No information available to require special precautions

Effects on Dental Treatment No effects or complications reported

Other Adverse Effects

>10%:

Dermatologic: Dry skin

Gastrointestinal: Abdominal pain, nausea, vomiting, diarrhea

Miscellaneous: Pink to brownish-black discoloration of the skin and conjunctiva

1% to 10%:

Dermatologic: Rash, pruritus

Endocrine & metabolic: Elevated blood sugar

Ocular: Irritation of the eyes

Miscellaneous: Discoloration of urine, feces, sputum, sweat

Drug Interactions No data reported

Drug Uptake

Absorption: Oral: 45% to 70% absorbed slowly

Serum half-life:

Terminal: 8 days

Tissue: 70 days

Time to peak serum concentration: 1-6 hours with chronic therapy

Pregnancy Risk Factor C

Clofibrate (kloe fye' brate)

Brand Names Atromid-S®

Canadian/Mexican Brand Names Claripex® (Canada); Novo-Fibrate® (Canada); Abitrate® (Canada)

Therapeutic Category Lipid Lowering Drugs

(Continued)

Clofibrate *(Continued)*

Use Adjunct to dietary therapy in the management of hyperlipidemias associated with high triglyceride levels (types III, IV, V); primarily lowers triglycerides and very low density lipoprotein

Usual Dosage Adults: Oral: 500 mg 4 times/day; some patients may respond to lower doses

Mechanism of Action Mechanism is unclear but thought to reduce cholesterol synthesis and triglyceride hepatic-vascular transference

Local Anesthetic/Vasoconstrictor Precautions No information available to require special precautions

Effects on Dental Treatment No effects or complications reported

Other Adverse Effects
>10%: Gastrointestinal: Nausea

1% to 10%: Gastrointestinal: Diarrhea, vomiting, dyspepsia, flatulence, abdominal distress

<1%:
Cardiovascular: Angina, cardiac arrhythmias
Central nervous system: Headache, dizziness, fatigue
Dermatologic: Skin rash, urticaria, pruritus, alopecia
Gastrointestinal: Gallstones
Genitourinary: Impotence
Hematologic: Leukopenia, anemia, eosinophilia, agranulocytosis
Hepatic: Increased liver function test
Neuromuscular & skeletal: Muscle cramping, aching, weakness, myalgia
Renal: Renal toxicity, rhabdomyolysis-induced renal failure
Miscellaneous: Dry, brittle hair

Drug Interactions
Increased effect: Effects of warfarin, insulin, and sulfonylureas may be increased

Increased toxicity/levels: Clofibrate's levels may be increased with probenecid

Drug Uptake
Absorption: Occurs completely; intestinal transformation is required to activate the drug

Serum half-life: 6-24 hours, increases significantly with reduced renal function; with anuria: 110 hours

Time to peak serum concentration: Within 3-6 hours

Pregnancy Risk Factor C

Clomid® *see* Clomiphene Citrate *on this page*

Clomifeno, Citrato De (Mexico) *see* Clomiphene Citrate *on this page*

Clomiphene Citrate *(kloe' mi feen sit' rate)*

Brand Names Clomid®; Serophene®

Canadian/Mexican Brand Names Omifin® (Mexico)

Therapeutic Category Ovulation Stimulator

Synonyms Clomifeno, Citrato De (Mexico)

Use Treatment of ovulatory failure in patients desiring pregnancy

Unlabeled use: Male infertility

Usual Dosage Adults: Oral:
Males (infertility): 25 mg/day for 25 days with 5 days rest, or 100 mg every Monday, Wednesday, Friday

Females (ovulatory failure): Oral: 50 mg/day for 5 days (first course); start the regimen on or about the fifth day of cycle; if ovulation occurs do not increase dosage; if not, increase next course to 100 mg/day for 5 days. Three courses of therapy are an adequate therapeutic trial. Further treatment is not recommended in patients who do not exhibit ovulation.

Mechanism of Action Induces ovulation by stimulating the release of pituitary gonadotropins

Local Anesthetic/Vasoconstrictor Precautions No information available to require special precautions

Effects on Dental Treatment No effects or complications reported

Other Adverse Effects
>10%: Endocrine & metabolic: Hot flashes, ovarian enlargement

1% to 10%:
Cardiovascular: Thromboembolism
Central nervous system: Mental depression, headache
Endocrine & metabolic: Breast enlargement (males), abnormal menstrual flow
Gastrointestinal: Distention, bloating, nausea, vomiting, hepatotoxicity

Ocular: Blurring of vision, diplopia, floaters, after-images, phosphenes, photophobia

<1%:

Central nervous system: Insomnia, fatigue

Dermatologic: Alopecia (reversible)

Gastrointestinal: Weight gain

Genitourinary: Increased urination

Drug Interactions No data reported

Drug Uptake

Serum half-life: 5-7 days

Pregnancy Risk Factor X

Clomipramine Hydrochloride

(kloe mi′ pra meen hye droe klor′ ide)

Brand Names Anafranil®

Canadian/Mexican Brand Names Apo-Clomipramine® (Canada)

Therapeutic Category Antidepressant, Tricyclic

Use Treatment of obsessive-compulsive disorder (OCD); may also relieve depression, panic attacks, and chronic pain

Usual Dosage Oral: Initial:

Children: 25 mg/day and gradually increase, as tolerated, to a maximum of 3 mg/kg/day or 200 mg/day, whichever is smaller

Adults: 25 mg/day and gradually increase, as tolerated, to 100 mg/day the first 2 weeks, may then be increased to a total of 250 mg/day maximum

Mechanism of Action Clomipramine appears to affect serotonin uptake while its active metabolite, desmethylclomipramine, affects norepinephrine uptake

Local Anesthetic/Vasoconstrictor Precautions Use with caution; epinephrine, norepinephrine and levonordefrin have been shown to have an increased pressor response in combination with TCAs

Effects on Dental Treatment Long-term treatment with TCAs such as amoxapine increases the risk of caries by reducing salivation and salivary buffer capacity

Other Adverse Effects

>10%:

Central nervous system: Dizziness, drowsiness, headache

Gastrointestinal: Dry mouth, constipation, increased appetite, nausea, weakness, unpleasant taste, weight gain

1% to 10%:

Cardiovascular: Arrhythmias, hypotension

Central nervous system: Confusion, delirium, hallucinations, nervousness, restlessness, parkinsonian syndrome, insomnia

Gastrointestinal: Diarrhea, heartburn

Genitourinary: Difficult urination, sexual function impairment

Neuromuscular & skeletal: Fine muscle tremors

Ocular: Blurred vision, eye pain

Miscellaneous: Excessive sweating

<1%:

Central nervous system: Anxiety, seizures

Dermatologic: Alopecia, photosensitivity

Endocrine & metabolic: Breast enlargement, galactorrhea, SIADH

Genitourinary: Testicular swelling

Hematologic: Agranulocytosis, leukopenia, eosinophilia

Hepatic: Cholestatic jaundice, increased liver enzymes

Ocular: Increased intraocular pressure

Otic: Tinnitus

Miscellaneous: Trouble with gums, decreased lower esophageal sphincter tone may cause GE reflux, allergic reactions

Drug Interactions

Decreased effect: Phenobarbital may increase the metabolism of clomipramine; clomipramine blocks the uptake of guanethidine and thus prevents the hypotensive effect of guanethidine

Increased toxicity: Clonidine causes hypertensive crisis; clomipramine may be additive with or may potentiate the action of other CNS depressants such as sedatives or hypnotics; with MAO inhibitors, hyperpyrexia, hypertension, tachycardia, confusion, and seizures. Clomipramine may increase the prothrombin time in patients stabilized on warfarin; clomipramine may potentiate the pressor and cardiac effects of sympathomimetic agents such as isoproterenol, epinephrine, etc; cimetidine and methylphenidate may decrease the metabolism of clomipramine

Additive anticholinergic effects seen with other anticholinergic agents

(Continued)

Clomipramine Hydrochloride *(Continued)*

Drug Uptake
Absorption: Oral: Rapid
Serum half-life: 20-30 hours

Pregnancy Risk Factor C

Selected Readings
Boakes AJ, Laurence DR, Teoh PC, et al, "Interactions Between Sympathomimetic Amines and Antidepressant Agents in Man," *Br Med J*, 1973, 1(849):311-5.
Jastak JT and Yagiela JA, "Vasoconstrictors and Local Anesthesia: A Review and Rationale for Use," *J Am Dent Assoc*, 1983, 107(4):623-30.
Larochelle P, Hamet P, and Enjalbert M, "Responses to Tyramine and Norepinephrine After Imipramine and Trazodone," *Clin Pharmacol Ther*, 1979, 26(1):24-30.
Mitchell JR, "Guanethidine and Related Agents. III Antagonism by Drugs Which Inhibit the Norepinephrine Pump in Man," *J Clin Invest*, 1970, 49(8):1596-604.
Rundegren J, van Dijken J, Mörnstad H, et al, "Oral Conditions in Patients Receiving Long-Term Treatment With Cyclic Antidepressant Drugs," *Swed Dent J*, 1985, 9(2):55-64.
Svedmyr N, "The Influence of a Tricyclic Antidepressive Agent (Protriptyline) on Some of the Circulatory Effects of Noradrenaline and Adrenaline® in Man," *Life Sci*, 1968, 7(1):77-84.

Clomycin® [OTC] *see* Bacitracin, Neomycin, Polymyxin B, and Lidocaine *on page 95*

Clonacepam (Mexico) *see* Clonazepam *on this page*

Clonazepam (kloe na' ze pam)

Brand Names Klonopin™

Canadian/Mexican Brand Names PMS-Clonazepam® (Canada); Rivotril® (Canada); Rivotril® (Mexico)

Therapeutic Category Anticonvulsant, Benzodiazepine

Synonyms Clonacepam (Mexico)

Use Prophylaxis of petit mal, petit mal variant (Lennox-Gastaut), akinetic, and myoclonic seizures

> **Unlabeled use:** Restless legs syndrome, neuralgia, multifocal tic disorder, parkinsonian dysarthria, acute manic episodes, and adjunct therapy for schizophrenia

Usual Dosage Oral:
Children <10 years or 30 kg:
Initial daily dose: 0.01-0.03 mg/kg/day (maximum: 0.05 mg/kg/day) given in 2-3 divided doses; increase by no more than 0.5 mg every third day until seizures are controlled or adverse effects seen
Usual maintenance dose: 0.1-0.2 mg/kg/day divided 3 times/day; not to exceed 0.2 mg/kg/day

Adults:
Initial daily dose not to exceed 1.5 mg given in 3 divided doses; may increase by 0.5-1 mg every third day until seizures are controlled or adverse effects seen
Usual maintenance dose: 0.05-0.2 mg/kg; do not exceed 20 mg/day

Hemodialysis effects: Supplemental dose is not necessary

Mechanism of Action Suppresses the spike-and-wave discharge in absence seizures by depressing nerve transmission in the motor cortex

Local Anesthetic/Vasoconstrictor Precautions No information available to require special precautions

Effects on Dental Treatment No effects or complications reported

Other Adverse Effects
>10%:
Cardiovascular: Tachycardia, chest pain
Central nervous system: Drowsiness, fatigue, impaired coordination, light-headedness, memory impairment, insomnia, anxiety, depression, headache
Dermatologic: Rash
Endocrine & metabolic: Decreased libido
Gastrointestinal: Dry mouth, constipation, diarrhea, nausea, increased or decreased appetite, vomiting
Neuromuscular & skeletal: Dysarthria
Ocular: Blurred vision
Miscellaneous: Decreased salivation sweating
1% to 10%:
Cardiovascular: Syncope, hypotension
Central nervous system: Confusion, nervousness, dizziness, akathisia
Dermatologic: Dermatitis
Gastrointestinal: Weight gain or loss
Neuromuscular & skeletal: Rigidity, tremor, muscle cramps
Otic: Tinnitus

Respiratory: Nasal congestion, hyperventilation
Miscellaneous: Increased salivation
<1%:
Central nervous system: Reflex slowing
Endocrine & metabolic: Menstrual irregularities
Hematologic: Blood dyscrasias
Miscellaneous: Drug dependence
Drug Interactions No significant interactions have been reported
Drug Uptake
Onset of effect: 20-60 minutes
Duration: Up to 6-8 hours in infants and young children, up to 12 hours in adults
Absorption: Oral: Well absorbed
Serum half-life:
Children: 22-33 hours
Adults: 19-50 hours
Time to peak serum concentration: Oral: 1-3 hours
Steady-state: 5-7 days
Pregnancy Risk Factor C

Clonidina (Mexico) *see Clonidine on this page*

Clonidine (kloe' ni deen)
Related Information
Cardiovascular Diseases *on page 912*
Brand Names Catapres®; Catapres-TTS®
Canadian/Mexican Brand Names Apo-Clonidine® (Canada); Dixarit® (Canada); Novo-Clonidine® (Canada); Nu-Clonidine® (Canada); Catapresan-100® (Mexico)
Therapeutic Category Alpha-Adrenergic Blockers - Peripheral-Acting (Alpha$_1$-Blockers); Antiglaucoma Agent
Synonyms Clonidina (Mexico)
Use Management of mild to moderate hypertension; either used alone or in combination with other antihypertensives; not recommended for first-line therapy for hypertension; also used for heroin withdrawal and in smoking cessation therapy; other uses may include prophylaxis of migraines, glaucoma, paralytic ileus, and diabetes-associated diarrhea
Usual Dosage
Oral:
Children: Initial: 5-10 mcg/kg/day in divided doses every 8-12 hours; increase gradually at 5- to 7-day intervals to 25 mcg/kg/day in divided doses every 6 hours; maximum: 0.9 mg/day
Clonidine tolerance test (test of growth hormone release from pituitary): 0.15 mg/m^2 or 4 mcg/kg as single dose
Adults: Initial dose: 0.1 mg twice daily, usual maintenance dose: 0.2-1.2 mg/day in 2-4 divided doses; maximum recommended dose: 2.4 mg/day
Nicotine withdrawal symptoms: 0.1 mg twice daily to maximum of 0.4 mg/day for 3-4 weeks
Elderly: Initial: 0.1 mg once daily at bedtime, increase gradually as needed
Transdermal: Apply once every 7 days; for initial therapy start with 0.1 mg and increase by 0.1 mg at 1- to 2-week intervals; dosages >0.6 mg do not improve efficacy
Mechanism of Action Stimulates alpha$_2$-adrenoreceptors in the brain stem, thus activating an inhibitory neuron, resulting in reduced sympathetic outflow, producing a decrease in vasomotor tone and heart rate
Local Anesthetic/Vasoconstrictor Precautions No information available to require special precautions
Effects on Dental Treatment No effects or complications reported
Other Adverse Effects
>10%:
Central nervous system: Drowsiness, dizziness
Gastrointestinal: Dry mouth, constipation
1% to 10%:
Cardiovascular: Orthostatic hypotension
Central nervous system: Nervousness, agitation, mental depression, headache, weakness, fatigue
Dermatologic: Rash
Endocrine & metabolic: Decreased sexual activity, impotence
Gastrointestinal: Nausea, vomiting
Genitourinary: Nocturia
Hepatic: Abnormal liver function tests
(Continued)

221

Clonidine *(Continued)*

    Miscellaneous: Loss of libido

    <1%:

        Cardiovascular: Palpitations, tachycardia, bradycardia, Raynaud's phenomenon, congestive heart failure

        Central nervous system: Insomnia, vivid dreams, delirium, fever

        Dermatologic: Pruritus, hives, urticaria, alopecia

        Endocrine & metabolic: Gynecomastia

        Gastrointestinal: Weight gain

        Genitourinary: Difficulty in micturition, urinary retention

        Ocular: Burning of the eyes, blurred vision

Drug Interactions

    Decreased effect: Tricyclic antidepressants antagonize hypotensive effects of clonidine

    Increased toxicity: Beta-blockers may potentiate bradycardia in patients receiving clonidine and may increase the rebound hypertension of withdrawal; discontinue beta-blocker several days before clonidine is tapered

Drug Uptake

    Onset of effect: Oral: 0.5-1 hour; T_{max}: 2-4 hours

    Duration: 6-10 hours

    Serum half-life: Adults:

        Normal renal function: 6-20 hours

        Renal impairment: 18-41 hours

Pregnancy Risk Factor C

Clonidine and Chlorthalidone (kloe' ni deen & klor thal' i done)

Brand Names Combipres®

Therapeutic Category Antihypertensive Agent, Combination

Use Management of mild to moderate hypertension

Local Anesthetic/Vasoconstrictor Precautions No information available to require special precautions

Effects on Dental Treatment No effects or complications reported

Clopra® *see* Metoclopramide *on page 572*

Cloracepato Dipotasico (Mexico) *see* Clorazepate Dipotassium *on this page*

Cloranfenicol (Mexico) *see* Chloramphenicol *on page 182*

Clorazepate Dipotassium (klor az' e pate dye poe tass' ee um)

Brand Names Gen-XENE®; Tranxene®

Canadian/Mexican Brand Names Apo-Clorazepate® (Canada); Novo-Clopate® (Canada)

Therapeutic Category Anticonvulsant, Benzodiazepine; Benzodiazepine; Sedative

Synonyms Cloracepato Dipotasico (Mexico)

Use Treatment of generalized anxiety and panic disorders; management of alcohol withdrawal; adjunct anticonvulsant in management of partial seizures

Usual Dosage Oral:

    Children 9-12 years: Anticonvulsant: Initial: 3.75-7.5 mg/dose twice daily; increase dose by 3.75 mg at weekly intervals, not to exceed 60 mg/day in 2-3 divided doses

    Children >12 years and Adults: Anticonvulsant: Initial: Up to 7.5 mg/dose 2-3 times/day; increase dose by 7.5 mg at weekly intervals; not to exceed 90 mg/day

    Adults:

        Anxiety: 7.5-15 mg 2-4 times/day, or given as single dose of 11.25 or 22.5 mg at bedtime

        Alcohol withdrawal: Initial: 30 mg, then 15 mg 2-4 times/day on first day; maximum daily dose: 90 mg; gradually decrease dose over subsequent days

Mechanism of Action Facilitates gamma aminobutyric acid (GABA)-mediated transmission inhibitory neurotransmitter action, depresses subcortical levels of CNS

Local Anesthetic/Vasoconstrictor Precautions No information available to require special precautions

Effects on Dental Treatment Many patients will experience drowsiness and dry mouth while taking clorazepate which will disappear with cessation of drug therapy; orthostatic hypotension is possible; it is suggested that narcotic analgesics not be given for pain control to patients taking clorazepate because of enhanced sedation

Other Adverse Effects
>10%:
Cardiovascular: Tachycardia, chest pain
Central nervous system: Drowsiness, fatigue, impaired coordination, light-headedness, memory impairment, insomnia, anxiety, headache, depression
Dermatologic: Rash
Endocrine & metabolic: Decreased libido
Gastrointestinal: Dry mouth, constipation, diarrhea, decreased salivation, nausea, vomiting, increased or decreased appetite
Neuromuscular & skeletal: Dysarthria
Ocular: Blurred vision
Miscellaneous: Sweating
1% to 10%:
Cardiovascular: Syncope, hypotension
Central nervous system: Confusion, nervousness, dizziness, akathisia
Dermatologic: Dermatitis
Gastrointestinal: Nausea, increased salivation, weight gain or loss
Neuromuscular & skeletal: Rigidity, tremor, muscle cramps
Otic: Tinnitus
Respiratory: Nasal congestion, hyperventilation
<1%:
Central nervous system: Reflex slowing
Endocrine & metabolic: Menstrual irregularities
Hematologic: Blood dyscrasias
Miscellaneous: Drug dependence, long-term use may also be associated with renal or hepatic injury and reduced hematocrit
Drug Interactions Increased effect: Cimetidine, CNS depressants, alcohol
Drug Uptake
Serum half-life: Adults:
Desmethyldiazepam: 48-96 hours
Oxazepam: 6-8 hours
Time to peak serum concentration: Oral: Within 1 hour
Pregnancy Risk Factor D

Clorfeniramina, Maleato De (Mexico) *see* Chlorpheniramine Maleate *on page 191*
Clorodiacepoxido (Mexico) *see* Chlordiazepoxide *on page 183*
Cloroquina, Defosfato De (Mexico) *see* Chloroquine Phosphate *on page 187*
Clorpactin® WCS-90 *see* Oxychlorosene Sodium *on page 646*
Clorpropamida (Mexico) *see* Chlorpropamide *on page 197*
Clortalidona (Mexico) *see* Chlorthalidone *on page 199*
Clortetraciclina (Mexico) *see* Chlortetracyline Hydrochloride *on page 199*

Clotrimazole (kloe trim' a zole)
Related Information
Oral Fungal Infections *on page 948*
Brand Names Mycelex® Troche
Therapeutic Category Antifungal Agent, Oral Nonabsorbed; Antifungal Agent, Topical; Antifungal Agent, Vaginal
Use
Dental: Treatment of susceptible fungal infections, including oropharyngeal candidiasis; limited data suggests that the use of clotrimazole troches may be effective for prophylaxis against oropharyngeal candidiasis in neutropenic patients
Medical: Treatment of susceptible fungal infections including dermatophytoses, superficial mycoses, and cutaneous candidiasis, as well as vulvovaginal candidiasis
Usual Dosage Children >3 years and Adults: 10 mg troche dissolved slowly 5 times/day for 14 consecutive days
Mechanism of Action Binds to phospholipids in the fungal cell membrane altering cell wall permeability resulting in loss of essential intracellular elements
Local Anesthetic/Vasoconstrictor Precautions No information available to require special precautions
Effects on Dental Treatment No effects or complications reported
Other Adverse Effects
>10%: Hepatic: Abnormal liver function tests
1% to 10%:
Gastrointestinal: Nausea and vomiting may occur in patients on clotrimazole troches
(Continued)

Clotrimazole (Continued)

Local: Mild burning, irritation, stinging to skin or vaginal area

Oral manifestations: No data reported

Contraindications Hypersensitivity to clotrimazole or any component

Warnings/Precautions Clotrimazole should not be used for treatment of systemic fungal infection; safety and effectiveness of clotrimazole lozenges (troches) in children <3 years of age have not been established

Drug Interactions Increased cyclosporine levels can occur; enhanced hypoglycemic effects with sulfonylureas

Drug Uptake
Absorption: Oral: Poor
Time to peak serum concentration: Oral topical administration: Salivary levels occur within 3 hours following 30 minutes of dissolution time in the mouth
Duration: Up to 3 hours

Pregnancy Risk Factor B/C (oral)

Breast-feeding Considerations No data reported

Dosage Forms Troche, oral (Mycelex®): 10 mg

Dietary Considerations No data reported

Generic Available No

Cloxacillin Sodium (klox a sil' in sow' dee um)

Brand Names Cloxapen®; Tegopen®

Canadian/Mexican Brand Names Apo-Cloxi® (Canada); Novo-Cloxin® (Canada); Nu-Cloxi® (Canada); Orbenin® (Canada); Taro-Cloxacillin® (Canada)

Therapeutic Category Antibiotic, Penicillin

Use
Dental: Treatment of susceptible orofacial infections, notably penicillinase-producing staphylococci
Medical: Treatment of susceptible bacterial infections in the medical patient, notably penicillinase-producing staphylococci causing respiratory tract, skin and skin structure, bone and joint, urinary tract infections, endocarditis, septicemia, and meningitis

Usual Dosage Oral:
Children <20 kg: 50-100 mg/kg/day in divided doses every 6 hours
Children >20 kg and Adults: 250-500 mg every 6 hours for at least 7 days

Mechanism of Action Inhibits bacterial cell wall synthesis by binding to one or more of the penicillin-binding proteins (PBPs) which in turn inhibits the final transpeptidation step of peptidoglycan synthesis in bacterial cell walls, thus inhibiting cell wall biosynthesis. Bacteria eventually lyse due to ongoing activity of cell wall autolytic enzymes (autolysins and murein hydrolases) while cell wall assembly is arrested.

Local Anesthetic/Vasoconstrictor Precautions No information available to require special precautions

Effects on Dental Treatment Prolonged use of penicillins may lead to development of oral candidiasis

Other Adverse Effects 1% to 10%:
Gastrointestinal: Nausea, diarrhea
Hematologic: Agranulocytosis
Hepatic: Elevations of AST and ALT
Renal: Hematuria
Miscellaneous: Serum sickness-like reactions

Oral manifestations: No data reported

Contraindications Hypersensitivity to cloxacillin or any component, or penicillins

Warnings/Precautions Monitor PTT if patient concurrently on warfarin, elimination of drug is slow in renally impaired; use with caution in patients allergic to cephalosporins due to a low incidence of cross-hypersensitivity

Drug Interactions Efficacy of oral contraceptives may be reduced; disulfiram, probenecid may increase cloxacillin levels; cloxacillin may increase the effect of anticoagulants

Drug Uptake
Absorption: Oral: ~50%
Time to peak serum concentration: Oral: Within 0.5-2 hours
Serum half-life: 0.5-1.5 hours

Pregnancy Risk Factor B

Breast-feeding Considerations No data reported; however, other penicillins may be taken while breast-feeding

Dosage Forms
Capsule: 250 mg, 500 mg
Powder for oral suspension: 125 mg/5 mL (100 mL, 200 mL)

Dietary Considerations Should be taken 1 hour before or 2 hours after meals with water

Generic Available Yes

Comments Although cloxacillin is a penicillin antibiotic indicated for infections caused by penicillinase-secreting staph, amoxicillin with clavulanic acid is considered the drug of choice for these types of orofacial infections

Cloxapen® see Cloxacillin Sodium on previous page

Clozapina (Mexico) see Clozapine on this page

Clozapine (kloe' za peen)

Brand Names Clozaril®
Canadian/Mexican Brand Names Leponex® (Mexico)
Therapeutic Category Antipsychotic Agent
Synonyms Clozapina (Mexico)
Use Management of schizophrenic patients
Usual Dosage Adults: Oral: 25 mg once or twice daily initially and increased, as tolerated to a target dose of 300-450 mg/day after 2 weeks, but may require doses as high as 600-900 mg/day
Mechanism of Action Clozapine is a weak $dopamine_1$ and $dopamine_2$ receptor blocker; in addition, it blocks the $serotonin_2$, alpha-adrenergic, and histamine H_1 central nervous system receptors
Local Anesthetic/Vasoconstrictor Precautions No information available to require special precautions
Effects on Dental Treatment Many patients may experience orthostatic hypotension with clozapine; precautions should be taken; do not use atropine-like drugs for xerostomia in patients taking clozapine because of significant potentiation

Other Adverse Effects
>10%:
Cardiovascular: Tachycardia, hypotension, orthostatic hypotension
Central nervous system: Fever, headache, drowsiness
Gastrointestinal: Constipation, nausea, vomiting, unusual weight gain
1% to 10%:
Cardiovascular: EKG changes, hypertension
Central nervous system: Agitation, akathisia
Gastrointestinal: Abdominal discomfort, heartburn, dry mouth
Ocular: Blurred vision
Miscellaneous: Increased sweating
<1%:
Central nervous system: Insomnia, seizures, tardive dyskinesia, neuroleptic malignant syndrome
Genitourinary: Difficult urination, impotence
Hematologic: Agranulocytosis, eosinophilia, granulocytopenia, leukopenia, thrombocytopenia
Neuromuscular & skeletal: Rigidity, tremor

Drug Interactions
Decreased effect with phenytoin
Increased effect of CNS depressants, guanabenz, anticholinergics
Increased toxicity with cimetidine, MAO inhibitors, neuroleptics, TCAs

Clozapine may significantly potentiate the hypotensive effects of antihypertensive drugs and the anticholinergic effects of atropine-type drugs. In medical emergencies, the administration of epinephrine should be avoided in the treatment of drug-induced hypotension because of a possible reverse epinephrine effect. There are no data to suggest any interaction between clozapine and the use of vasoconstrictors in local anesthesia.

Pregnancy Risk Factor B

Clozaril® see Clozapine on this page

Clysodrast® see Bisacodyl on page 113

Coal Tar (kole' tar)

Brand Names AquaTar® [OTC]; Denorex® [OTC]; DHS® Tar [OTC]; Duplex® T [OTC]; Estar® [OTC]; Fototar® [OTC]; Neutrogena® T/Derm; Pentrax® [OTC]; Polytar® [OTC]; psoriGel® [OTC]; T/Gel® [OTC]; Zetar® [OTC]
Therapeutic Category Antipsoriatic Agent, Topical; Antiseborrheic Agent, Topical
Synonyms Crude Coal Tar; LCD; Pix Carbonis
(Continued)

Coal Tar *(Continued)*

Use Topically for controlling dandruff, seborrheic dermatitis, or psoriasis

Local Anesthetic/Vasoconstrictor Precautions No information available to require special precautions

Effects on Dental Treatment No effects or complications reported

Other Adverse Effects 1% to 10%: Dermatitis, folliculitis

Comments Avoid exposure to sunlight for 24 hours after use; may stain clothing and skin

Coal Tar and Salicylic Acid (kole′ tar & sal i sil′ ik as′ id)

Brand Names X-seb® T [OTC]

Therapeutic Category Antipsoriatic Agent, Topical; Antiseborrheic Agent, Topical

Use Seborrheal dermatitis; dandruff

Local Anesthetic/Vasoconstrictor Precautions No information available to require special precautions

Effects on Dental Treatment No effects or complications reported

Coal Tar, Lanolin, and Mineral Oil

(kole′ tar, lan′ oh lin, & min′ er al oyl)

Brand Names Balnetar® [OTC]

Therapeutic Category Antipsoriatic Agent, Topical; Antiseborrheic Agent, Topical

Use Psoriasis; seborrheal dermatitis; atopic dermatitis; eczematoid dermatitis

Local Anesthetic/Vasoconstrictor Precautions No information available to require special precautions

Effects on Dental Treatment No effects or complications reported

Cobalamin (Canada) *see* Cyanocobalamin *on page 237*

Cobex® *see* Cyanocobalamin *on page 237*

Cocaine Hydrochloride (koe kane′ hye droe klor′ ide)

Therapeutic Category Local Anesthetic, Topical

Use Topical anesthesia (ester derivative) for mucous membranes

Usual Dosage Dosage depends on the area to be anesthetized, tissue vascularity, technique of anesthesia, and individual patient tolerance; use the lowest dose necessary to produce adequate anesthesia should be used, not to exceed 1 mg/kg. Use reduced dosages for children, elderly, or debilitated patients.

Topical application (ear, nose, throat, bronchoscopy): Concentrations of 1% to 4% are used; concentrations >4% are not recommended because of potential for increased incidence and severity of systemic toxic reactions

Mechanism of Action Blocks both the initiation and conduction of nerve impulses by decreasing the neuronal membrane's permeability to sodium ions, which results in inhibition of depolarization with resultant blockade of conduction; interferes with the uptake of norepinephrine by adrenergic nerve terminals producing vasoconstriction

Local Anesthetic/Vasoconstrictor Precautions No information available to require special precautions

Effects on Dental Treatment No effects or complications reported

Other Adverse Effects

>10%:
  Central nervous system: CNS stimulation
  Local: Loss of smell/taste, chronic rhinitis, stuffy nose

1% to 10%:
  Cardiovascular: Decreased heart rate with low doses, increased heart rate with moderate doses, hypertension, tachycardia, cardiac arrhythmias
  Central nervous system: Nervousness, restlessness, euphoria, excitement, hallucination, seizures
  Gastrointestinal: Vomiting
  Neuromuscular & skeletal: Tremors and clonic-tonic reactions
  Ocular: Sloughing of the corneal epithelium, ulceration of the cornea
  Respiratory: Tachypnea, respiratory failure

Drug Interactions Increased toxicity: MAO inhibitors

Drug Uptake Following topical administration to mucosa:
  Onset of action: Within 1 minute
  Peak action: Within 5 minutes
  Duration: ≥30 minutes, depending on dosage administered
  Absorption: Well absorbed through mucous membranes; limited by drug-induced vasoconstriction; enhanced by inflammation

Serum half-life: 75 minutes
Pregnancy Risk Factor C (X if nonmedicinal use)
Dosage Forms
Powder: 5 g, 25 g
Solution, topical: 4% [40 mg/mL] (4 mL, 10 mL); 10% [100 mg/mL] (4 mL, 10 mL)
Tablet, soluble, for topical solution: 135 mg
Generic Available Yes

Codafed® Expectorant *see* Guaifenesin, Pseudoephedrine, and Codeine *on page 410*

Codamine® *see* Hydrocodone and Phenylpropanolamine *on page 435*

Codamine® Pediatric *see* Hydrocodone and Phenylpropanolamine *on page 435*

Codehist® DH *see* Chlorpheniramine, Pseudoephedrine, and Codeine *on page 195*

Codeine (koe' deen)
Related Information
Dental Drug Interactions: Update on Drug Combinations Requiring Special Considerations *on page 1022*
Narcotic Agonist Charts *on page 1019*
Canadian/Mexican Brand Names Linctus Codeine Blac (Canada); Linctus With Codeine Phosphate (Canada); Paveral Stanley Syrup With Codeine Phosphate (Canada)
Therapeutic Category Analgesic, Narcotic; Antitussive
Synonyms Methylmorphine (Canada)
Use
Dental: Treatment of postoperative pain
Medical: Relief of pain
Usual Dosage Oral:
Children: Not recommended in pediatric dental patients
Adults: 30 mg/dose; range: 15-60 mg every 4-6 hours as needed; maximum: 360 mg/24 hours
Mechanism of Action Binds to opiate receptors (mu and kappa subtypes) in the CNS causing inhibition of ascending pain pathways, altering the perception of and response to pain
Local Anesthetic/Vasoconstrictor Precautions No information available to require special precautions
Effects on Dental Treatment No effects or complications reported
Other Adverse Effects
>10%:
Central nervous system: Lightheadedness, dizziness, sedation
Gastrointestinal: Nausea, vomiting
1% to 10%: Gastrointestinal: Constipation

Oral manifestations: <1%: Dry mouth
Contraindications Hypersensitivity to codeine
Warnings/Precautions Use with caution in patients with hypersensitivity reactions to other phenanthrene derivative opioid agonists (morphine, hydrocodone, hydromorphone, levorphanol, oxycodone, oxymorphone); respiratory diseases including asthma, emphysema, COPD, or severe liver or renal insufficiency; some preparations contain sulfites which may cause allergic reactions; may be habit-forming

Enhanced analgesia has been seen in elderly patients on therapeutic doses of narcotics; duration of action may be increased in the elderly; the elderly may be particularly susceptible to the CNS depressant and constipating effects of narcotics
Drug Interactions Increased toxicity of CNS depressants, phenothiazines, tricyclic antidepressants, guanabenz, MAO inhibitors (may also lead to a decrease in blood pressure)
Drug Uptake
Onset of effect: Analgesia: 30-45 minutes
Time to peak serum concentration: 1-2 hours
Duration of effect: 4-6 hours
Serum half-life: 2.5-3.5 hours
Pregnancy Risk Factor C (D if used for prolonged periods or in high doses at term)
Breast-feeding Considerations May be taken while breast-feeding
Dosage Forms
Tablet, as sulfate: 15 mg, 30 mg, 60 mg
(Continued)

Codeine *(Continued)*

Tablet, as phosphate, soluble: 30 mg, 60 mg
Tablet, as sulfate, soluble: 15 mg, 30 mg, 60 mg

Dietary Considerations May be taken with food or water to minimize GI distress

Generic Available Yes

Comments It is recommended that codeine not be used as the sole entity for analgesia because of moderate efficacy along with relatively high incidence of nausea, sedation, and constipation. In addition, codeine has some narcotic addiction liability. Codeine in combination with acetaminophen or aspirin is recommended. Maximum effective analgesic dose of codeine is 60 mg (1 grain). Beyond 60 mg increases respiratory depression only.

Selected Readings

Desjardins PJ, Cooper SA, Gallegos TL, et al, "The Relative Analgesic Efficacy of Propiram Fumarate, Codeine, Aspirin, and Placebo in Post-Impaction Dental Pain," *J Clin Pharmacol*, 1984, 24(1):35-42.

Forbes JA, Keller CK, Smith JW, et al, "Analgesic Effect of Naproxen Sodium, Codeine, a Naproxen-Codeine Combination and Aspirin on the Postoperative Pain of Oral Surgery," *Pharmacotherapy*, 1986, 6(5):211-8.

Codeine and Bromodiphenhydramine *see* Bromodiphenhydramine and Codeine *on page 122*

Codeine and Butalbital Compound *see* Butalbital Compound and Codeine *on page 134*

Codiclear® DH *see* Hydrocodone and Guaifenesin *on page 434*

Codimal-A® *see* Brompheniramine Maleate *on page 124*

Codoxy® *see* Oxycodone and Aspirin *on page 647*

Codroxomin® *see* Hydroxocobalamin *on page 439*

Cogentin® *see* Benztropine Mesylate *on page 106*

Co-Gesic® [5/500] *see* Hydrocodone and Acetaminophen *on page 431*

Cognex® *see* Tacrine Hydrochloride *on page 816*

Co-Hist® [OTC] *see* Acetaminophen, Chlorpheniramine, and Pseudoephedrine *on page 17*

Colace® [OTC] *see* Docusate *on page 295*

Co-Lav® *see* Polyethylene Glycol-Electrolyte Solution *on page 703*

Colax® [OTC] *see* Docusate and Phenolphthalein *on page 295*

ColBENEMID® *see* Colchicine and Probenecid *on next page*

Colchicina (Mexico) *see* Colchicine *on this page*

Colchicine *(kol′ chi seen)*

Canadian/Mexican Brand Names Colchiquim® (Mexico); Colchiquim-30® (Mexico)

Therapeutic Category Anti-inflammatory Agent; Uricosuric Agent

Synonyms Colchicina (Mexico)

Use Treat acute gouty arthritis attacks and to prevent recurrences of such attacks; management of familial Mediterranean fever

Usual Dosage

Prophylaxis of familial Mediterranean fever: Oral:
Children:
≤5 years: 0.5 mg/day
>5 years: 1-1.5 mg/day in 2-3 divided doses
Adults: 1-2 mg/day in 2-3 divided doses

Gouty arthritis, acute attacks: Adults:
Oral: Initial: 0.5-1.2 mg, then 0.5-0.6 mg every 1-2 hours or 1-1.2 mg every 2 hours until relief or GI side effects (nausea, vomiting, or diarrhea) occur to a maximum total dose of 8 mg; wait 3 days before initiating another course of therapy
I.V.: Initial: 1-3 mg, then 0.5 mg every 6 hours until response, not to exceed 4 mg/day; if pain recurs, it may be necessary to administer a daily dose of 1-2 mg for several days, however, do not give more colchicine by any route for at least 7 days after a full course of I.V. therapy (4 mg), transfer to oral colchicine in a dose similar to that being given I.V.

Gouty arthritis, prophylaxis of recurrent attacks: Adults: Oral: 0.5-0.6 mg/day or every other day

Mechanism of Action Decreases leukocyte motility, decreases phagocytosis in joints and lactic acid production, thereby reducing the deposition of urate crystals that perpetuates the inflammatory response

Local Anesthetic/Vasoconstrictor Precautions No information available to require special precautions

Effects on Dental Treatment No effects or complications reported

Other Adverse Effects
>10%: Gastrointestinal: Nausea, vomiting, diarrhea, abdominal pain
1% to 10%:
  Dermatologic: Alopecia
  Gastrointestinal: Anorexia
<1%:
  Central nervous system: Myopathy, peripheral neuritis
  Dermatologic: Rash
  Genitourinary: Azoospermia
  Hematologic: Bone marrow suppression, agranulocytosis, aplastic anemia
  Hepatic: Hepatotoxicity
Drug Interactions Decreased effect: Vitamin B_{12} absorption may be reduced
Drug Uptake
Onset of effect:
  Oral: Relief of pain and inflammation occurs after 24-48 hours
  I.V.: 6-12 hours
Serum half-life: 12-30 minutes
Time to peak serum concentration: Oral: Within 0.5-2 hours declining for the
  next 2 hours before increasing again due to enterohepatic recycling
Pregnancy Risk Factor C (oral)/D (parenteral)

Colchicine and Probenecid (kol' chi seen & proe ben' e sid)
Brand Names ColBENEMID®; Proben-C®
Therapeutic Category Uricosuric Agent
Synonyms Probenecid and Colchicine
Use Treatment of chronic gouty arthritis when complicated by frequent, recurrent acute attacks of gout
Local Anesthetic/Vasoconstrictor Precautions No information available to require special precautions
Effects on Dental Treatment No effects or complications reported
Other Adverse Effects 1% to 10%:
Cardiovascular: Flushing
Central nervous system: Headache, dizziness
Dermatologic: Rash, alopecia
Gastrointestinal: Anorexia, nausea, vomiting, diarrhea, abdominal pain
Genitourinary: Urinary frequency, uric acid stones
Hematologic: Anemia, leukopenia, aplastic anemia, agranulocytosis
Hepatic: Hepatic necrosis, hepatotoxicity
Neuromuscular & skeletal: Peripheral neuritis
Ocular: Myopathy
Renal: Nephrotic syndrome
Miscellaneous: Hypersensitivity reactions
Comments Do not initiate therapy until an acute gouty attack has subsided

Cold & Allergy® Elixir [OTC] see Brompheniramine and Phenylpropanolamine on page 123

Coldlac-LA® see Guaifenesin and Phenylpropanolamine on page 409

Coldloc® see Guaifenesin, Phenylpropanolamine, and Phenylephrine on page 410

Colestid® see Colestipol Hydrochloride on this page

Colestipol, Clorhidrato De (Mexico) see Colestipol Hydrochloride on this page

Colestipol Hydrochloride (koe les' ti pole hye droe klor' ide)
Related Information
Cardiovascular Diseases on page 912
Brand Names Colestid®
Therapeutic Category Lipid Lowering Drugs
Synonyms Colestipol, Clorhidrato De (Mexico)
Use Adjunct in management of primary hypercholesterolemia; regression of arteriolosclerosis; relief of pruritus associated with elevated levels of bile acids; possibly used to decrease plasma half-life of digoxin in toxicity
Usual Dosage Adults: Oral: 5-30 g/day in divided doses 2-4 times/day
Mechanism of Action Binds with bile acids to form an insoluble complex that is eliminated in feces; it thereby increases the fecal loss of bile acid-bound low density lipoprotein cholesterol
Local Anesthetic/Vasoconstrictor Precautions No information available to require special precautions
Effects on Dental Treatment No effects or complications reported
Other Adverse Effects
>10%: Gastrointestinal: Constipation
(Continued)

Colestipol Hydrochloride (Continued)

1% to 10%: Gastrointestinal: Abdominal pain and distention, belching, flatulence, nausea, vomiting, diarrhea

<1%:

Central nervous system: Headache, dizziness, anxiety, vertigo, drowsiness, fatigue

Dermatologic: Dermatitis, urticaria

Gastrointestinal: Peptic ulceration, GI irritation and bleeding, cholecystitis, anorexia

Hepatic: Cholelithiasis

Neuromuscular & skeletal: Joint pain, arthritis, weakness

Respiratory: Shortness of breath

Miscellaneous: Increased serum phosphorous and chloride with decrease of sodium and potassium

Drug Interactions Decreased absorption of tetracycline, penicillin G, vitamins A, D, E and K, digitalis glycosides, warfarin, thyroid hormones, thiazide diuretics, propranolol, phenobarbital, amiodarone, methotrexate, NSAIDs, and other drugs by binding to the drug in the intestine

Drug Uptake Absorption: Oral: Not absorbed

Pregnancy Risk Factor C

Colestiramina (Mexico) see Cholestyramine Resin on page 201

Colfosceril Palmitate (kole fos' er il palm' i tate)

Brand Names Exosurf® Neonatal™

Therapeutic Category Lung Surfactant

Synonyms Dipalmitoylphosphatidylcholine; DPPC; Synthetic Lung Surfactant

Use Neonatal respiratory distress syndrome (RDS):

Prophylactic therapy: Infants at risk for developing RDS with body weight <1350 g; infants with evidence of pulmonary immaturity with body weight >1350 g

Rescue therapy: Treatment of infants with RDS based on respiratory distress not attributable to any other causes and chest radiographic findings consistent with RDS

Usual Dosage For intratracheal use only

Prophylactic treatment: Give 5 mL/kg (as two 2.5 mL/kg half-doses) as soon as possible; the second and third doses should be administered at 12 and 24 hours later to those infants remaining on ventilators

Rescue treatment: Give 5 mL/kg (as two 2.5 mL/kg half-doses) as soon as the diagnosis of RDS is made; the second 5 mL/kg (as two 2.5 mL/kg half-doses) dose should be administered 12 hours later

Mechanism of Action Replaces deficient or ineffective endogenous lung surfactant in neonates with respiratory distress syndrome (RDS) or in neonates at risk of developing RDS; reduces surface tension and stabilizes the alveoli from collapsing

Local Anesthetic/Vasoconstrictor Precautions No information available to require special precautions

Effects on Dental Treatment No effects or complications reported

Other Adverse Effects 1% to 10%: Pulmonary hemorrhage, apnea, mucous plugging, decrease in transcutaneous O_2 of >20%

Drug Uptake

Absorption: Intratracheal: Absorbed from the alveolus

Colistimethate Sodium (koe lis ti meth' ate sow' dee um)

Brand Names Coly-Mycin® M Parenteral

Therapeutic Category Antibiotic, Miscellaneous

Use Treatment of infections due to sensitive strains of certain gram-negative bacilli

Local Anesthetic/Vasoconstrictor Precautions No information available to require special precautions

Effects on Dental Treatment No effects or complications reported

Other Adverse Effects 1% to 10%:

Central nervous system: Vertigo, slurring of speech

Dermatologic: Urticaria

Gastrointestinal: GI upset

Genitourinary: Decreased urine output

Respiratory: Respiratory arrest

Colistin, Neomycin, and Hydrocortisone
(koe lis' tin, nee oh mye' sin & hye droe kor' ti sone)
Brand Names Coly-Mycin® S Otic Drops
Therapeutic Category Antibiotic, Miscellaneous; Corticosteroid, Otic; Otic Agent, Anti-infective
Use Treatment of superficial and susceptible bacterial infections of the external auditory canal; for treatment of susceptible bacterial infections of mastoidectomy and fenestration cavities
Local Anesthetic/Vasoconstrictor Precautions No information available to require special precautions
Effects on Dental Treatment No effects or complications reported

Colistin Sulfate (koe lis' tin sul' fate)
Brand Names Coly-Mycin® S Oral
Therapeutic Category Antibiotic, Miscellaneous; Antidiarrheal
Synonyms Polymyxin E
Use Treat diarrhea in infants and children caused by susceptible organisms, especially *E. coli* and *Shigella*
Usual Dosage Diarrhea: Children: Oral: 5-15 mg/kg/day in 3 divided doses given every 8 hours
Mechanism of Action A polypeptide antibiotic that binds to and damages the bacterial cell membrane
Local Anesthetic/Vasoconstrictor Precautions No information available to require special precautions
Effects on Dental Treatment No effects or complications reported
Other Adverse Effects <1%:
Gastrointestinal: Nausea, vomiting
Neuromuscular & skeletal: Neuromuscular blockade
Renal: Nephrotoxicity
Respiratory: Respiratory arrest
Miscellaneous: Hypersensitivity reactions, superinfections
Drug Uptake
Absorption: Oral: Slightly absorbed from GI tract (adults); unpredictable absorption occurs in infants, can lead to significant serum levels
Serum half-life: 2.8-4.8 hours, prolonged in renal insufficiency; with anuria: 48-72 hours
Pregnancy Risk Factor C

CollaCote® *see* Collagen, Absorbable *on this page*

Collagen, Absorbable (kol' la jen, ab sorb' able)
Brand Names CollaCote®; CollaPlug®; CollaTape®
Therapeutic Category Hemostatic Agent
Use
Dental: To control bleeding created during dental surgery
Medical: Hemostatic
Usual Dosage Children and Adults: A sufficiently large dressing should be selected so as to completely cover the oral wound
Mechanism of Action The highly porous sponge structure absorbs blood and wound exudate. The collagen component causes aggregation of platelets which bind to collagen fibrils. The aggregated platelets degranulate, releasing coagulation factors that promote the formation of fibrin.
Local Anesthetic/Vasoconstrictor Precautions No information available to require special precautions
Effects on Dental Treatment No effects or complications reported
Other Adverse Effects No data reported

Oral manifestations: No data reported
Contraindications No data reported
Warnings/Precautions Should not be used on infected or contaminated wounds
Drug Interactions No data reported
Breast-feeding Considerations May be taken while breast-feeding
Dosage Forms Wound dressings: 1" x 3", $3/4$" x 1 $1/2$", $3/8$" x $3/4$"
Dietary Considerations No data reported
Comments The dressing should be applied over the wound and held in place with moderate pressure. The period of time necessary to apply pressure will vary with the degree of bleeding. In general, 2-5 minutes should be sufficient to achieve hemostasis. At the end of the procedure, the dressing can be removed, replaced or left in situ, any excess dressing should be removed prior to wound closure.

Collagenase (kol' la je nase)
Brand Names Santyl®
Therapeutic Category Enzyme, Topical Debridement
Use Promotes debridement of necrotic tissue in dermal ulcers and severe burns
Usual Dosage Topical: Apply once daily
Mechanism of Action Collagenase is an enzyme derived from the fermentation of *Clostridium histolyticum* and differs from other proteolytic enzymes in that its enzymatic action has a high specificity for native and denatured collagen. Collagenase will not attack collagen in healthy tissue or newly formed granulation tissue. In addition, it does not act on fat, fibrin, keratin, or muscle.
Local Anesthetic/Vasoconstrictor Precautions No information available to require special precautions
Effects on Dental Treatment No effects or complications reported
Other Adverse Effects
   1% to 10%: Local: Irritation
   <1%: Local: Pain and burning may occur at site of application
Drug Interactions Decreased effect: Enzymatic activity is inhibited by detergents, benzalkonium chloride, hexachlorophene, nitrofurazone, tincture of iodine, and heavy metal ions (silver and mercury)
Pregnancy Risk Factor C

CollaPlug® *see* Collagen, Absorbable *on previous page*

CollaTape® *see* Collagen, Absorbable *on previous page*

Collyrium Fresh® [OTC] *see* Tetrahydrozoline Hydrochloride *on page 831*

Colovage® *see* Polyethylene Glycol-Electrolyte Solution *on page 703*

Coly-Mycin® M Parenteral *see* Colistimethate Sodium *on page 230*

Coly-Mycin® S Oral *see* Colistin Sulfate *on previous page*

Coly-Mycin® S Otic Drops *see* Colistin, Neomycin, and Hydrocortisone *on previous page*

CoLyte® *see* Polyethylene Glycol-Electrolyte Solution *on page 703*

Combipres® *see* Clonidine and Chlorthalidone *on page 222*

Comfort® [OTC] *see* Naphazoline Hydrochloride *on page 605*

Comfort® Tears Solution [OTC] *see* Artificial Tears *on page 75*

Comhist® *see* Chlorpheniramine, Phenylephrine, and Phenyltoloxamine *on page 193*

Comhist® LA *see* Chlorpheniramine, Phenylephrine, and Phenyltoloxamine *on page 193*

Common Oral-Facial Infections and Antibiotics for Treatment *see page 1077*

Compazine® *see* Prochlorperazine *on page 728*

Compound W® [OTC] *see* Salicylic Acid *on page 777*

Compoz® [OTC] *see* Diphenhydramine Hydrochloride *on page 288*

Condylox® *see* Podofilox *on page 701*

Conex® [OTC] *see* Guaifenesin and Phenylpropanolamine *on page 409*

Congess® Jr *see* Guaifenesin and Pseudoephedrine *on page 409*

Congess® Sr *see* Guaifenesin and Pseudoephedrine *on page 409*

Congestac® *see* Guaifenesin and Pseudoephedrine *on page 409*

Congestant® D [OTC] *see* Chlorpheniramine, Phenylpropanolamine, and Acetaminophen *on page 194*

Constant-T® *see* Theophylline/Aminophylline *on page 832*

Constilac® *see* Lactulose *on page 488*

Constulose® *see* Lactulose *on page 488*

Contac® Cough Formula Liquid [OTC] *see* Guaifenesin and Dextromethorphan *on page 408*

Control® [OTC] *see* Phenylpropanolamine Hydrochloride *on page 687*

Control-L™ [OTC] *see* Pyrethrins *on page 753*

Controlled Substances *see page 1078*

Contuss® *see* Guaifenesin, Phenylpropanolamine, and Phenylephrine *on page 410*

Contuss® XT *see* Guaifenesin and Phenylpropanolamine *on page 409*

Cool Mint Listerine® Antiseptic [OTC] *see* Mouthwash, Antiseptic *on page 592*

Cophene-B® *see* Brompheniramine Maleate *on page 124*

Cophene XP® *see* Hydrocodone, Pseudoephedrine, and Guaifenesin *on page 435*

Copper *see* Trace Metals *on page 857*

Co-Pyronil® 2 Pulvules® [OTC] *see* Chlorpheniramine and Pseudoephedrine *on page 191*

Cordarone® *see* Amiodarone Hydrochloride *on page 48*

Cordran® *see* Flurandrenolide *on page 380*

Cordran® SP *see* Flurandrenolide *on page 380*

Coreg® *see* Carvedilol *on page 159*

Corgard® *see* Nadolol *on page 597*

Corgonject® *see* Chorionic Gonadotropin *on page 203*

Coricidin® [OTC] *see* Chlorpheniramine and Acetaminophen *on page 190*

Coricidin D® [OTC] *see* Chlorpheniramine, Phenylpropanolamine, and Acetaminophen *on page 194*

Corque® Topical *see* Clioquinol and Hydrocortisone *on page 216*

Correctol® [OTC] *see* Docusate and Phenolphthalein *on page 295*

Cortatrigen® Otic *see* Neomycin, Polymyxin B, and Hydrocortisone *on page 610*

Cortef® *see* Hydrocortisone *on page 436*

Corticaine® Topical *see* Dibucaine and Hydrocortisone *on page 270*

Corticosteroid Equivalencies Comparison *see page 1017*

Corticosteroids, Topical Comparison *see page 1018*

Corticotropin (kor ti koe troe' pin)
Brand Names ACTH®; Acthar®; H.P. Acthar® Gel

Therapeutic Category Adrenal Corticosteroid

Use Acute exacerbations of multiple sclerosis; diagnostic aid in adrenocortical insufficiency, severe muscle weakness in myasthenia gravis; cosyntropin is preferred over corticotropin for diagnostic test of adrenocortical insufficiency (cosyntropin is less allergenic and test is shorter in duration)

Mechanism of Action Stimulates the adrenal cortex to secrete adrenal steroids (including hydrocortisone, cortisone), androgenic substances, and a small amount of aldosterone

Local Anesthetic/Vasoconstrictor Precautions No information available to require special precautions

Effects on Dental Treatment No effects or complications reported

Other Adverse Effects
>10%:
  Central nervous system: Insomnia, nervousness
  Gastrointestinal: Increased appetite, indigestion
1% to 10%:
  Endocrine & metabolic: Diabetes mellitus
  Neuromuscular & skeletal: Joint pain
  Ocular: Cataracts
  Miscellaneous: Epistaxis
<1%:
  Central nervous system: Seizures, mood swings, headache, delirium, hallucinations, euphoria
  Dermatologic: Skin atrophy, bruising, hyperpigmentation, acne, hirsutism
  Endocrine & metabolic: Amenorrhea, sodium and water retention, Cushing's syndrome, hyperglycemia, bone growth suppression
  Gastrointestinal: Abdominal distention, ulcerative esophagitis, pancreatitis
  Neuromuscular & skeletal: Muscle wasting
  Sensitivity reactions: Hypersensitivity reactions

Drug Interactions Decreased effect: Spironolactone, hydrocortisone, cortisone; can antagonize the effects of anticholinesterases (eg, neostigmine)

Pregnancy Risk Factor C

Cortin® Topical *see* Clioquinol and Hydrocortisone *on page 216*

Cortisone Acetate (kor' ti sone as' eh tate)
Related Information
  Corticosteroid Equivalencies Comparison *on page 1017*
  Respiratory Diseases *on page 924*

Brand Names Cortone® Acetate

Therapeutic Category Adrenal Corticosteroid; Anti-inflammatory Agent; Corticosteroid, Systemic

Use Management of adrenocortical insufficiency

Usual Dosage If possible, administer glucocorticoids before 9 AM to minimize adrenocortical suppression; dosing depends upon the condition being treated and the response of the patient; supplemental doses may be warranted during times of stress in the course of withdrawing therapy

(Continued)

233

Cortisone Acetate *(Continued)*

Children:
  Anti-inflammatory or immunosuppressive:
    Oral: 2.5-10 mg/kg/day **or** 20-300 mg/m²/day in divided doses every 6-8 hours
    I.M.: 1-5 mg/kg/day **or** 14-375 mg/m²/day in divided doses every 12-24 hours
  Physiologic replacement:
    Oral: 0.5-0.75 mg/kg/day **or** 20-25 mg/m²/day in divided doses every 8 hours
    I.M.: 0.25-0.35 mg/kg/day once daily **or** 12.5 mg/m²/day
  Stress coverage for surgery: I.M.: 1 and 2 days before preanesthesia, and 1-3 days after surgery: 50-62.5 mg/m²/day; 4 days after surgery: 31-50 mg/m²/day; 5 days after surgery, resume presurgical corticosteroid dose.

Adults: Oral, I.M.: 25-300 mg/day in divided doses every 12-24 hours

Hemodialysis effects: Supplemental dose is not necessary

Mechanism of Action Decreases inflammation by suppression of migration of polymorphonuclear leukocytes and reversal of increased capillary permeability

Local Anesthetic/Vasoconstrictor Precautions No information available to require special precautions

Effects on Dental Treatment A compromised immune response may occur if patient has been taking systemic cortisone; the need for corticosteroid coverage in these patients should be considered before any dental treatment; consult with physician

Other Adverse Effects
>10%:
  Central nervous system: Insomnia, nervousness
  Gastrointestinal: Increased appetite, indigestion
1% to 10%:
  Endocrine & metabolic: Diabetes mellitus, hirsutism
  Gastrointestinal: Peptic ulcer, nausea, vomiting
  Neuromuscular & skeletal: Muscle weakness, osteoporosis, fractures, joint pain, epistaxis
  Ocular: Cataracts, glaucoma
<1%:
  Cardiovascular: Edema, hypertension
  Central nervous system: Mood swings, vertigo, seizures, headache, psychoses, pseudotumor cerebri, delirium, hallucinations, euphoria
  Dermatologic: Acne, skin atrophy, hyperpigmentation
  Endocrine & metabolic: Cushing's syndrome, pituitary-adrenal axis suppression, growth suppression, glucose intolerance, hypokalemia, alkalosis, amenorrhea, sodium and water retention, hyperglycemia
  Gastrointestinal: Abdominal distention, ulcerative esophagitis, pancreatitis
  Hematologic: Bruising
  Neuromuscular & skeletal: Muscle wasting
  Miscellaneous: Hypersensitivity reactions

Drug Interactions
Decreased effect:
  Barbiturates, phenytoin, rifampin causes decreased cortisone effects
  Cortisone causes decreased warfarin effects
  Cortisone causes decreased effects of salicylates
Increased effect: Estrogens (increased cortisone effects)
Increased toxicity:
  Cortisone + NSAIDs causes increased ulcerogenic potential
  Cortisone causes increased potassium deletion due to diuretics

Drug Uptake
Peak effect:
  Oral: Within 2 hours
  I.M.: Within 20-48 hours
Duration of action: 30-36 hours
Absorption: Slow rate of absorption
Serum half-life: 30 minutes to 2 hours
  End stage renal disease: 3.5 hours

Pregnancy Risk Factor D

Dosage Forms
Injection: 50 mg/mL (10 mL)
Tablet: 5 mg, 10 mg, 25 mg

Dietary Considerations Limit caffeine; may need diet with increased potassium, pyridoxine, vitamin C, vitamin D, folate, calcium, and phosphorus and decreased sodium; may be taken with food to decrease GI distress

Generic Available Yes

Cortisporin® Ophthalmic Ointment *see* Bacitracin, Neomycin, Polymyxin B, and Hydrocortisone *on page 95*

Cortisporin® Ophthalmic Suspension *see* Neomycin, Polymyxin B, and Hydrocortisone *on page 610*

Cortisporin® Otic *see* Neomycin, Polymyxin B, and Hydrocortisone *on page 610*

Cortisporin® Topical Cream *see* Neomycin, Polymyxin B, and Hydrocortisone *on page 610*

Cortisporin® Topical Ointment *see* Bacitracin, Neomycin, Polymyxin B, and Hydrocortisone *on page 95*

Cortone® Acetate *see* Cortisone Acetate *on page 233*

Cortrosyn® *see* Cosyntropin *on this page*

Cosmegen® *see* Dactinomycin *on page 248*

Cosyntropin (koe sin troe′ pin)
Brand Names Cortrosyn®
Therapeutic Category Adrenal Corticosteroid
Use Diagnostic test to differentiate primary adrenal from secondary (pituitary) adrenocortical insufficiency
Usual Dosage
Adrenocortical insufficiency: I.M., I.V. (over 2 minutes): Peak plasma cortisol concentrations usually occur 45-60 minutes after cosyntropin administration
Children <2 years: 0.125 mg
Children >2 years and Adults: 0.25 mg
When greater cortisol stimulation is needed, an I.V. infusion may be used:
Children >2 years and Adults: 0.25 mg administered at 0.04 mg/hour over 6 hours

Congenital adrenal hyperplasia evaluation: 1 mg/m^2/dose up to a maximum of 1 mg
Mechanism of Action Stimulates the adrenal cortex to secrete adrenal steroids (including hydrocortisone, cortisone), androgenic substances, and a small amount of aldosterone
Local Anesthetic/Vasoconstrictor Precautions No information available to require special precautions
Effects on Dental Treatment No effects or complications reported
Other Adverse Effects
1% to 10%:
Cardiovascular: Flushing
Central nervous system: Mild fever
Dermatologic: Pruritus
Gastrointestinal: Chronic pancreatitis
<1%: Hypersensitivity reactions
Drug Interactions No data reported
Drug Uptake
Time to peak serum concentration: Within 1 hour (plasma cortisol levels rise in healthy individuals within 5 minutes of administration I.M. or I.V. push)
Pregnancy Risk Factor C

Cotazym® *see* Pancrelipase *on page 657*

Cotazym-S® *see* Pancrelipase *on page 657*

Cotrim® *see* Trimethoprim and Sulfamethoxazole *on page 874*

Cotrim® DS *see* Trimethoprim and Sulfamethoxazole *on page 874*

Co-trimoxazole *see* Trimethoprim and Sulfamethoxazole *on page 874*

Coumadin® *see* Warfarin Sodium *on page 903*

Covera-HS® *see* Verapamil Hydrochloride *on page 893*

Cozaar® *see* Losartan Potassium *on page 515*

Creon® *see* Pancreatin *on page 656*

Creon® 10 *see* Pancrelipase *on page 657*

Creon® 20 *see* Pancrelipase *on page 657*

Cresylate® *see* m-Cresyl Acetate *on page 527*

Crixivan® *see* Indinavir *on page 456*

Cromoglicato Disodico (Mexico) *see* Cromolyn Sodium *on this page*

Cromolyn Sodium (kroe′ moe lin sow′ dee um)
Related Information
Respiratory Diseases *on page 924*
Brand Names Gastrocrom®; Intal®; Nasalcrom®
(Continued)

Cromolyn Sodium *(Continued)*

Canadian/Mexican Brand Names Novo-Cromolyn® (Canada); Opticrom® (Canada); PMS-Sodium Cromoglycate® (Canada); Rynacrom® (Canada)

Therapeutic Category Inhalation, Miscellaneous

Synonyms Cromoglicato Disodico (Mexico); Sodium Cromoglycate (Canada)

Use Adjunct in the prophylaxis of allergic disorders, including rhinitis, giant papillary conjunctivitis, and asthma; inhalation product may be used for prevention of exercise-induced bronchospasm; systemic mastocytosis, food allergy, and treatment of inflammatory bowel disease; **cromolyn is a prophylactic drug with no benefit for acute situations**

Usual Dosage Not effective for immediate relief of symptoms in acute asthmatic attacks; must be used at regular intervals for 2-4 weeks to be effective

Children:
Inhalation (taper frequency to the lowest effective dose, ie, 4 times/day → 3 times/day → twice daily):
Initial dose: Metered spray: >5 years: 2 inhalations 4 times/day by metered spray
Initial dose: Nebulization solution: >2 years: 20 mg 4 times/day
Prevention of exercise-induced bronchospasm: Metered spray: >5 years: Single dose of 2 inhalations (aerosol) just prior to (10 minutes to 1 hour) exercise
Nasal: >6 years: Instill 1 spray in each nostril 3-4 times/day
Children 2-12 years: Oral: 100 mg 4 times/day 15-20 minutes before meals, not to exceed 40 mg/kg/day
Children >12 years and Adults: Oral: 200 mg 4 times/day 15-20 minutes before meal, up to 400 mg 4 times/day
Adults:
Inhalation: Metered spray: 2 inhalations 4 times/day
Nasal: Instill 1 spray in each nostril 3-4 times/day
Ophthalmic: Instill 1-2 drops 4-6 times/day into each eye

Mechanism of Action Prevents the mast cell release of histamine, leukotrienes and slow-reacting substance of anaphylaxis by inhibiting degranulation after contact with antigens

Local Anesthetic/Vasoconstrictor Precautions No information available to require special precautions

Effects on Dental Treatment No effects or complications reported

Other Adverse Effects
>10%: Local: Hoarseness, coughing, unpleasant taste (inhalation aerosol)
1% to 10%:
Gastrointestinal: Dry mouth
Genitourinary: Dysuria
Respiratory: Sneezing, stuffy nose
Miscellaneous: Angioedema
<1%:
Central nervous system: Dizziness, headache
Dermatologic: Rash, urticaria
Gastrointestinal: Nausea, vomiting, diarrhea
Hypersensitivity: Anaphylactic reactions
Local: Nasal burning
Neuromuscular & skeletal: Joint pain
Ocular: Ocular stinging, lacrimation
Respiratory: Wheezing, throat irritation, eosinophilic pneumonia, pulmonary infiltrates

Drug Interactions No data reported

Drug Uptake
Absorption:
Inhalation: ~8% of dose reaches the lungs upon inhalation of the powder and is well absorbed
Oral: Only 0.5% to 2% of dose absorbed
Serum half-life: 80-90 minutes
Time to peak serum concentration: Inhalation: Within 15 minutes

Pregnancy Risk Factor B

Crotamiton *(kroe tam' i tonn)*

Brand Names Eurax®

Therapeutic Category Antipruritic, Topical; Scabicidal Agent

Synonyms Crotamiton (Mexico)

Use Treatment of scabies and symptomatic treatment of pruritus

Usual Dosage Topical:

Scabicide: Children and Adults: Wash thoroughly and scrub away loose scales, then towel dry; apply a thin layer and massage drug onto skin of the entire body from the neck to the toes (with special attention to skin folds, creases, and interdigital spaces). Repeat application in 24 hours. Take a cleansing bath 48 hours after the final application. Treatment may be repeated after 7-10 days if live mites are still present.

Pruritus: Massage into affected areas until medication is completely absorbed; repeat as necessary

Mechanism of Action Crotamiton has scabicidal activity against *Sarcoptes scabiei*; mechanism of action unknown

Local Anesthetic/Vasoconstrictor Precautions No information available to require special precautions

Effects on Dental Treatment No effects or complications reported

Other Adverse Effects <1%: Local: Pruritus, irritation, contact dermatitis, warm sensation

Drug Interactions No data reported

Pregnancy Risk Factor C

Crotamiton (Mexico) *see* Crotamiton *on previous page*

Crude Coal Tar *see* Coal Tar *on page 225*

Cruex® Topical [OTC] *see* Undecylenic Acid and Derivatives *on page 884*

Cryptenamine Tannates and Methyclothiazide *see* Methyclothiazide and Cryptenamine Tannates *on page 566*

Crystamine® *see* Cyanocobalamin *on this page*

Crysticillin® A.S. *see* Penicillin G Procaine *on page 667*

Crystodigin® *see* Digitoxin *on page 279*

CSP *see* Cellulose Sodium Phosphate *on page 175*

C-Span® [OTC] *see* Ascorbic Acid *on page 76*

Curretab® *see* Medroxyprogesterone Acetate *on page 533*

Cutivate™ *see* Fluticasone Propionate *on page 383*

Cyanocobalamin (sye an oh koe bal′ a min)

Brand Names Berubigen®; Cobex®; Crystamine®; Cyanoject®; Cyomin®; Ener-B® [OTC]; Kaybovite-1000®; Redisol®; Rubramin-PC®; Sytobex®

Canadian/Mexican Brand Names Rubramin® (Canada)

Therapeutic Category Vitamin, Water Soluble

Synonyms Cianocobalamina (Mexico); Cobalamin (Canada)

Use

Dental: Vitamin B_{12} deficiency

Medical: Treatment of pernicious anemia; increased B_{12} requirements due to pregnancy, thyrotoxicosis, hemorrhage, malignancy, liver or kidney disease

Usual Dosage I.M. or deep S.C. (oral is not generally recommended due to poor absorption and I.V. is not recommended due to more rapid elimination):

Recommended daily allowance (RDA):

Children: 0.3-2 mcg

Adults: 2 mcg

Pernicious anemia, congenital (if evidence of neurologic involvement): 1000 mcg/day for at least 2 weeks; maintenance: 50 mcg/month

Children: 30-50 mcg/day for 2 or more weeks (to a total dose of 1000-5000 mcg), then follow with 100 mcg month as maintenance dosage

Adults: 100 mcg/day for 6-7 days; if improvement, give same dose on alternate days for 7 doses; then every 3-4 days for 2-3 weeks; once hematologic values have returned to normal, maintenance dosage: 100 mcg/month. **Note:** Use only parenteral therapy as oral therapy is not dependable.

Vitamin B_{12} deficiency:

Children: 100 mcg/day for 10-15 days (total dose of 1-1.5 mg), then once or twice weekly for several months; may taper to 60 mcg every month

Adults: Initial: 30 mcg/day for 5-10 days; maintenance: 100-200 mcg/month

Mechanism of Action Coenzyme for various metabolic functions, including fat and carbohydrate metabolism and protein synthesis, used in cell replication and hematopoiesis

Local Anesthetic/Vasoconstrictor Precautions No information available to require special precautions

Effects on Dental Treatment No effects or complications reported

Other Adverse Effects 1% to 10%:

Dermatologic: Itching

Gastrointestinal: Diarrhea

(Continued)

237

Cyanocobalamin *(Continued)*

Contraindications Hypersensitivity to cyanocobalamin or any component, cobalt; patients with hereditary optic nerve atrophy

Warnings/Precautions I.M. route used to treat pernicious anemia; vitamin B_{12} deficiency for >3 months results in irreversible degenerative CNS lesions; treatment of vitamin B_{12} megaloblastic anemia may result in severe hypokalemia, sometimes, fatal, when anemia corrects due to cellular potassium requirements. B_{12} deficiency masks signs of polycythemia vera; vegetarian diets may result in B_{12} deficiency; pernicious anemia occurs more often in gastric carcinoma than in general population.

Drug Interactions

Aminosalicylic acid may reduce therapeutic action of vitamin B_{12}

Chloramphenicol may decrease the hematologic effect of vitamin B_{12} in patients with pernicious anemia

Colchicine and prolonged alcohol (>2 weeks) use may decrease absorption of vitamin B_{12}

Drug Uptake

Absorption: Absorbed from the terminal ileum in the presence of calcium; for absorption to occur gastric "intrinsic factor" must be present to transfer the compound across the intestinal mucosa

Pregnancy Risk Factor A (C if dose exceeds RDA recommendation)

Dosage Forms

Gel, nasal (Ener-B®): 400 mcg/0.1 mL

Injection: 30 mcg/mL (30 mL); 100 mcg/mL (1 mL, 10 mL, 30 mL); 1000 mcg/mL (1 mL, 10 mL, 30 mL)

Tablet [OTC]: 25 mcg, 50 mcg, 100 mcg, 250 mcg, 500 mcg, 1000 mcg

Generic Available Yes

Cyanoject® *see* Cyanocobalamin *on previous page*

Cyclan® *see* Cyclandelate *on this page*

Cyclandelate *(sye klan' de late)*

Brand Names Cyclan®; Cyclospasmol®

Therapeutic Category Vasodilator, Peripheral

Use Considered as "possibly effective" for adjunctive therapy in peripheral vascular disease and possibly senility due to cerebrovascular disease or multi-infarct dementia; migraine prophylaxis, vertigo, tinnitus, and visual disturbances secondary to cerebrovascular insufficiency and diabetic peripheral polyneuropathy

Usual Dosage Adults: Oral: Initial: 1.2-1.6 g/day in divided doses before meals and at bedtime until response; maintenance therapy: 400-800 mg/day in 2-4 divided doses; start with lowest dose in elderly due to hypotensive potential; decrease dose by 200 mg decrements to achieve minimal maintenance dose; improvement can usually be seen over weeks of therapy and prolonged use; short courses of therapy are usually ineffective and not recommended

Mechanism of Action Cyclandelate, 3,3,5-trimethylcyclohexyl mandelate is a vasodilator that exerts a direct, papaverine-like action on smooth muscles, particularly that found within the blood vessels. Animal data indicate that cyclandelate also has antispasmodic properties; exhibits no adrenergic stimulation or blocking action; action exceeds that of papaverine; mild calcium channel blocking agent, may benefit in mild hypercalcemia; calcium channel blocking activity may explain some of its pharmacologic effects (enhanced blood flow) and inhibition of platelet aggregation

Local Anesthetic/Vasoconstrictor Precautions No information available to require special precautions

Effects on Dental Treatment No effects or complications reported

Other Adverse Effects <1%:

Cardiovascular: Flushing of face, tachycardia

Central nervous system: Headache, pain, dizziness; tingling sensation in face, fingers, or toes

Gastrointestinal: Belching, heartburn

Neuromuscular & skeletal: Weakness

Drug Interactions No data reported

Pregnancy Risk Factor C

Cyclizine *(sye' kli zeen)*

Brand Names Marezine® [OTC]

Therapeutic Category Antiemetic; Antihistamine

Use Prevention and treatment of nausea, vomiting, and vertigo associated with motion sickness; control of postoperative nausea and vomiting

Usual Dosage
Children 6-12 years:
Oral: 25 mg up to 3 times/day
I.M.: Not recommended

Adults:
Oral: 50 mg taken 30 minutes before departure, may repeat in 4-6 hours if needed, up to 200 mg/day
I.M.: 50 mg every 4-6 hours as needed

Mechanism of Action Cyclizine is a piperazine derivative with properties of histamines. The precise mechanism of action in inhibiting the symptoms of motion sickness is not known. It may have effects directly on the labyrinthine apparatus and central actions on the labyrinthine apparatus and on the chemo-receptor trigger zone. Cyclizine exerts a central anticholinergic action.

Local Anesthetic/Vasoconstrictor Precautions No information available to require special precautions

Effects on Dental Treatment No effects or complications reported

Other Adverse Effects
>10%:
Central nervous system: Drowsiness
Gastrointestinal: Dry mouth
1% to 10%:
Central nervous system: Headache
Dermatologic: Dermatitis
Gastrointestinal: Nausea
Ocular: Diplopia
Renal: Polyuria, urinary retention

Drug Interactions Increased effect/toxicity with CNS depressants, alcohol

Pregnancy Risk Factor B

Cyclobenzaprine Hydrochloride
(sye kloe ben' za preen hye droe klor' ide)

Related Information
Temporomandibular Dysfunction (TMD) *on page 963*

Brand Names Cycoflex®; Flexeril®

Canadian/Mexican Brand Names Novo-Cycloprine® (Canada)

Therapeutic Category Muscle Relaxant; Skeletal Muscle Relaxant

Use
Dental: Treatment of muscle spasm associated with acute temporomandibular joint pain
Medical: Treatment of muscle spasm associated with acute painful musculo-skeletal conditions; supportive therapy in tetanus

Usual Dosage Oral: **Note:** Do not use longer than 2-3 weeks
Children: Dosage has not been established
Adults: 20-40 mg/day in 2-4 divided doses; maximum dose: 60 mg/day

Mechanism of Action Centrally acting skeletal muscle relaxant pharmacologi-cally related to tricyclic antidepressants; reduces tonic somatic motor activity influencing both alpha and gamma motor neurons

Local Anesthetic/Vasoconstrictor Precautions No information available to require special precautions

Effects on Dental Treatment No effects or complications reported

Other Adverse Effects
>10%: Central nervous system: Drowsiness, dizziness, lightheadedness
1% to 10%:
Cardiovascular: Swelling of face, lips, syncope
Gastrointestinal: Bloated feeling
Neuromuscular & skeletal: Problems in speaking, muscle weakness
Ocular: Blurred vision

Oral manifestations: >10%: Dry mouth

Contraindications Hypersensitivity to cyclobenzaprine or any component; do not use concomitantly or within 14 days of MAO inhibitors; hyperthyroidism, congestive heart failure, arrhythmias

Warnings/Precautions Cyclobenzaprine shares the toxic potentials of the tricyclic antidepressants and the usual precautions of tricyclic antidepressant therapy should be observed; use with caution in patients with urinary hesitancy or angle-closure glaucoma

Drug Interactions Do not use concomitantly or within 14 days after MAO inhibitors; because of chemical similarities to the tricyclic antidepressants, may have additive toxicities; because of cyclobenzaprine's anticholinergic action, use with caution in patients receiving these agents; alcohol, barbiturates, and other CNS depressants may be enhanced by cyclobenzaprine
(Continued)

Cyclobenzaprine Hydrochloride *(Continued)*

Drug Uptake
Absorption: Oral: Completely
Onset of action: Commonly occurs within 1 hour
Time to peak serum concentration: Within 3-8 hours
Duration: 12-24 hours
Serum half-life: 1-3 days
Pregnancy Risk Factor B
Breast-feeding Considerations No data reported
Dosage Forms Tablet: 10 mg
Dietary Considerations No data reported
Generic Available Yes

Cyclocort® *see* Amcinonide *on page 43*
Cyclogyl® *see* Cyclopentolate Hydrochloride *on this page*

Cyclopentolate Hydrochloride
(sye kloe pen′ toe late hye droe klor′ ide)
Brand Names AK-Pentolate®; Cyclogyl®; I-Pentolate®; Pentolair®
Therapeutic Category Anticholinergic Agent, Ophthalmic; Ophthalmic Agent, Mydriatic
Use Diagnostic procedures requiring mydriasis and cycloplegia
Usual Dosage
Children: Instill 1 drop of 0.5%, 1%, or 2% in eye followed by 1 drop of 0.5% or 1% in 5 minutes, if necessary
Adults: Instill 1 drop of 1% followed by another drop in 5 minutes; 2% solution in heavily pigmented iris
Mechanism of Action Prevents the muscle of the ciliary body and the sphincter muscle of the iris from responding to cholinergic stimulation, causing mydriasis and cycloplegia
Local Anesthetic/Vasoconstrictor Precautions No information available to require special precautions
Effects on Dental Treatment No effects or complications reported
Other Adverse Effects 1% to 10%:
Cardiovascular: Tachycardia
Central nervous system: Restlessness, hallucinations, psychosis, hyperactivity, seizures, incoherent speech, ataxia
Dermatologic: Burning sensation
Ocular: Increase in intraocular pressure, loss of visual accommodation
Miscellaneous: Allergic reaction
Drug Uptake
Peak effect:
Cycloplegia: 25-75 minutes
Mydriasis: 30-60 minutes
Duration: Recovery takes up to 24 hours
Pregnancy Risk Factor C
Comments Pilocarpine ophthalmic drops applied after the examination may reduce recovery time to 3-6 hours

Cyclophosphamide (sye kloe fos′ fa mide)
Brand Names Cytoxan®; Neosar®
Canadian/Mexican Brand Names Procytox® (Canada); Genoxal® (Mexico); Ledoxina® (Mexico)
Therapeutic Category Antineoplastic Agent, Alkylating Agent (Nitrogen Mustard)
Synonyms Ciclofosfamida (Mexico)
Use Treatment of Hodgkin's and non-Hodgkin's lymphoma, Burkitt's lymphoma, chronic lymphocytic leukemia, chronic granulocytic leukemia, AML, ALL, mycosis fungoides, breast cancer, multiple myeloma, neuroblastoma, retinoblastoma, rhabdomyosarcoma, Ewing's sarcoma; testicular, endometrium and ovarian, and lung cancer, and as a conditioning regimen for BMT; prophylaxis of rejection for kidney, heart, liver, and BMT transplants, severe rheumatoid disorders, nephrotic syndrome, Wegener's granulomatosis, idiopathic pulmonary hemosideroses, myasthenia gravis, multiple sclerosis, systemic lupus erythematosus, lupus nephritis, autoimmune hemolytic anemia, idiopathic thrombocytic purpura, macroglobulinemia, and antibody-induced pure red cell aplasia
Usual Dosage Refer to individual protocols
Patients with compromised bone marrow function may require a 33% to 50% reduction in initial loading dose

Children: I.V.:
Neuroblastomas/sarcomas: 3 g/m^2/day for 2 days or 2 g/m^2/day for 3 days
SLE: 500-750 mg/m^2 every month; maximum dose: 1 g/m^2
JRA/vasculitis: 10 mg/kg every 2 weeks

Children and Adults:
Oral: 50-100 mg/m^2/day as continuous therapy or 400-1000 mg/m^2 in divided doses over 4-5 days as intermittent therapy
I.V.:
Single doses: 400-1800 mg/m^2 (30-50 mg/kg) per treatment course (1-5 days) which can be repeated at 2- to 4-week intervals
Maximum single dose without BMT is 7 g/m^2 (190 mg/kg) single agent therapy
Continuous daily doses: 60-120 mg/m^2 (1-2.5 mg/kg) per day
Autologous BMT: IVPB: 50 mg/kg/dose for 4 days or 60 mg/kg/dose for 2 days; total dose is usually divided over 2-4 days

Nephrotic syndrome: Oral: 2-3 mg/kg/day every day for up to 12 weeks when corticosteroids are unsuccessful

Mechanism of Action Interferes with the normal function of DNA by alkylation and cross-linking the strands of DNA, and by possible protein modification; cyclophosphamide also possesses potent immunosuppressive activity; note that cyclophosphamide must be metabolized to its active form in the liver

Local Anesthetic/Vasoconstrictor Precautions No information available to require special precautions

Effects on Dental Treatment No effects or complications reported

Other Adverse Effects
>10%:
Dermatologic: Alopecia is frequent, but hair will regrow although it may be of a different color or texture. Hair loss usually occurs 3 weeks after therapy.
Fertility: May cause sterility; interferes with oogenesis and spermatogenesis; may be irreversible in some patients; gonadal suppression (amenorrhea)
Gastrointestinal: Nausea and vomiting occur more frequently with larger doses, usually beginning 6-10 hours after administration; also seen are anorexia, diarrhea, stomatitis; mucositis
Emetic potential:
Oral: Low (<10%)
<1 g: Moderate (30% to 60%)
≥1 g: High (>90%)
Hepatic: Jaundice seen occasionally
1% to 10%:
Central nervous system: Headache
Dermatologic: Skin rash, facial flushing
Myelosuppressive: Thrombocytopenia occurs less frequently than with mechlorethamine, anemia
WBC: Moderate
Platelets: Moderate
Onset (days): 7
Nadir (days): 10-14
Recovery (days): 21
<1%:
Cardiovascular: High-dose therapy may cause cardiac dysfunction manifested as congestive heart failure; cardiac necrosis or hemorrhagic myocarditis has occurred rarely, but is fatal. Cyclophosphamide may also potentiate the cardiac toxicity of anthracyclines.
Central nervous system: Dizziness
Dermatologic: Darkening of skin/fingernails
Endocrine & metabolic: Hyperglycemia, hypokalemia, distortion, hyperuricemia
Gastrointestinal: Stomatitis
Genitourinary: Acute hemorrhagic cystitis is believed to be a result of chemical irritation of the bladder by acrolein, a cyclophosphamide metabolite. Acute hemorrhagic cystitis occurs in 7% to 12% of patients, and has been reported in up to 40% of patients. Hemorrhagic cystitis can be severe and even fatal. Patients should be encouraged to drink plenty of fluids (3-4 L/ day) during therapy, void frequently, and avoid taking the drug at nighttime. If large I.V. doses are being administered, I.V. hydration should be given during therapy. The administration of mesna or continuous bladder irrigation may also be warranted.
Hepatic: Hepatic toxicity
Respiratory: Nasal stuffiness: Occurs when given in large I.V. doses; patients experience runny eyes, rhinorrhea, sinus congestion, and
(Continued)

Cyclophosphamide *(Continued)*

sneezing during or immediately after the infusion; interstitial pulmonary fibrosis with prolonged high dosage has occurred

Renal: SIADH has occurred with I.V. doses >50 mg/kg; renal tubular necrosis has also occurred, but usually resolves after the discontinuation of therapy

Secondary malignancy: Has developed with cyclophosphamide alone or in combination with other antineoplastics; both bladder carcinoma and acute leukemia are well documented

Drug Interactions

Decreased effect: Digoxin: Cyclophosphamide may reduce digoxin serum levels

Increased toxicity:

Allopurinol may cause an increase in bone marrow depression and may result in significant elevations of cyclophosphamide cytotoxic metabolites

Anesthetic agents: Cyclophosphamide reduces serum pseudocholinesterase concentrations and may prolong the neuromuscular blocking activity of succinylcholine; use with caution with halothane, nitrous oxide, and succinylcholine

Chloramphenicol results in prolonged cyclophosphamide half-life to increase toxicity

Cimetidine inhibits hepatic metabolism of drugs and may reduce the activation of cyclophosphamide

Doxorubicin: Cyclophosphamide may enhance cardiac toxicity of anthracyclines

Phenobarbital and phenytoin induce hepatic enzymes and cause a more rapid production of cyclophosphamide metabolites with a concurrent decrease in the serum half-life of the parent compound

Tetrahydrocannabinol results in enhanced immunosuppression in animal studies

Thiazide diuretics: Leukopenia may be prolonged

Pregnancy Risk Factor D

Cycloserine (sye kloe ser' een)

Related Information

Nonviral Infectious Diseases *on page 932*

Brand Names Seromycin® Pulvules®

Therapeutic Category Antibiotic, Miscellaneous; Antitubercular Agent

Use Adjunctive treatment in pulmonary or extrapulmonary tuberculosis; treatment of acute urinary tract infections caused by *E. coli* or *Enterobacter* sp when less toxic conventional therapy has failed or is contraindicated

Usual Dosage Some of the neurotoxic effects may be relieved or prevented by the concomitant administration of pyridoxine

Tuberculosis: Oral:

Children: 10-20 mg/kg/day in 2 divided doses up to 1000 mg/day for 18-24 months

Adults: Initial: 250 mg every 12 hours for 14 days, then give 500 mg to 1 g/day in 2 divided doses for 18-24 months (maximum daily dose: 1 g)

Mechanism of Action Inhibits bacterial cell wall synthesis by competing with amino acid (D-alanine) for incorporation into the bacterial cell wall; bacteriostatic or bactericidal

Local Anesthetic/Vasoconstrictor Precautions No information available to require special precautions

Effects on Dental Treatment No effects or complications reported

Other Adverse Effects

1% to 10%: Central nervous system: Drowsiness, headache

<1%:

Cardiovascular: Cardiac arrhythmias, coma

Central nervous system: Dizziness, vertigo, seizures, confusion, psychosis, paresis

Dermatologic: Rash

Hepatic: Elevated liver enzymes

Neuromuscular & skeletal: Tremor

Miscellaneous: Vitamin B_{12} deficiency, folate deficiency

Drug Interactions Increased toxicity: Alcohol, isoniazid, ethionamide increase toxicity of cycloserine; cycloserine inhibits the hepatic metabolism of phenytoin

Drug Uptake

Absorption: Oral: ~70% to 90% from the GI tract

Serum half-life: 10 hours in patients with normal renal function

Time to peak serum concentration: Oral: Within 3-4 hours

Pregnancy Risk Factor C

Cyclospasmol® *see* Cyclandelate *on page 238*

Cyclosporine (sye' kloe spor een)

Brand Names Sandimmune®

Canadian/Mexican Brand Names Consupren® (Mexico); Sandimmun® Neoral (Mexico)

Therapeutic Category Immunosuppressant Agent

Synonyms Ciclosporina (Mexico)

Use Immunosuppressant which may be used with azathioprine and/or corticosteroids to prolong organ and patient survival in kidney, liver, heart, and bone marrow transplants

Usual Dosage Children and Adults (oral dosage is ~3 times the I.V. dosage); dosage should be based on ideal body weight:

I.V.:
Initial: 5-6 mg/kg/day beginning 4-12 hours prior to organ transplantation; patients should be switched to oral cyclosporine as soon as possible; dose should be infused over 2-24 hours
Maintenance: 2-10 mg/kg/day in divided doses every 8-12 hours; dose should be adjusted to maintain whole blood HPLC trough concentrations in the reference range

Oral: Solution or soft gelatin capsule (Sandimmune®):
Initial: 14-18 mg/kg/day, beginning 4-12 hours prior to organ transplantation
Maintenance: 5-15 mg/kg/day divided every 12-24 hours; maintenance dose is usually tapered to 3-10 mg/kg/day
Focal segmental glomerulosclerosis: Initial: 3 mg/kg/day divided every 12 hours

Dosing considerations of cyclosporine, see table.

Cyclosporine

Condition	Cyclosporine
Switch from I.V. to oral therapy	Threefold increase in dose
T-tube clamping	Decrease dose; increase availability of bile facilitates absorption of CsA
Pediatric patients	About 2-3 times higher dose compared to adults
Liver dysfunction	Decrease I.V. dose; increase oral dose
Renal dysfunction	Decrease dose to decrease levels if renal dysfunction is related to the drug
Dialysis	Not removed
Inhibitors of hepatic metabolism	Decrease dose
Inducers of hepatic metabolism	Monitor drug level; may need to increase dose

Oral: Solution or soft gelatin capsule in a microemulsion (Neoral®): Based on the organ transplant population:
Initial: Same as the initial dose for solution or soft gelatin capsule (listed above)
or
Renal: 9 mg/kg/day (range: 6-12 mg/kg/day)
Liver: 8 mg/kg/day (range: 4-12 mg/kg/day)
Heart: 7 mg/kg/day (range: 4-10 mg/kg/day)

Note: A 1:1 ratio conversion from Sandimmune® to Neoral® has been recommended initially; however, lower doses of Neoral® may be required after conversion to prevent overdose. Total daily doses should be adjusted based on the cyclosporine trough blood concentration and clinical assessment of organ rejection. CsA blood trough levels should be determined prior to conversion. After conversion to Neoral®, CsA trough levels should be monitored every 4-7 days

Hemodialysis effects: Supplemental dose is not necessary
Peritoneal dialysis effects: Supplemental dose is not necessary

Mechanism of Action Inhibition of production and release of interleukin II and inhibits interleukin II-induced activation of resting T-lymphocytes

Local Anesthetic/Vasoconstrictor Precautions No information available to require special precautions

Effects on Dental Treatment No effects or complications reported
(Continued)

Cyclosporine *(Continued)*

Other Adverse Effects
>10%:
  Cardiovascular: Hypertension
  Dermatologic: Hirsutism
  Neuromuscular & skeletal: Tremor
  Renal: Nephrotoxicity
  Miscellaneous: Gingival hypertrophy
1% to 10%:
  Central nervous system: Seizure, headache
  Dermatologic: Acne
  Gastrointestinal: Abdominal discomfort, nausea, vomiting
  Neuromuscular & skeletal: Leg cramps
<1%:
  Cardiovascular: Hypotension, tachycardia, warmth, flushing
  Endocrine & metabolic: Hyperkalemia, hypomagnesemia, hyperuricemia
  Hepatic: Hepatotoxicity
  Neuromuscular & skeletal: Myositis, paresthesias
  Respiratory: Respiratory distress, sinusitis
  Miscellaneous: Anaphylaxis, pancreatitis, increased susceptibility to infection, and sensitivity to temperature extremes

Drug Interactions
Decreased effect: Rifampin, phenytoin, phenobarbital decreases plasma concentration of cyclosporine
Increased toxicity: Ketoconazole, fluconazole, and itraconazole increase plasma concentration of cyclosporine

Drug Uptake
Absorption: Oral:
  Solution or soft gelatin capsule (Sandimmune®): Erratically and incompletely absorbed; dependent on the presence of food, bile acids, and GI motility; larger oral doses of cyclosporine are needed in pediatric patients versus adults due to a shorter bowel length resulting in limited intestinal absorption
  Solution in microemulsion or soft gelatin capsule in a microemulsion are bioequivalent (Neoral®): Erratically and incompletely absorbed; increased absorption, up to 30% when compared to Sandimmune®; absorption is less dependent on food intake, bile, or GI motility when compared to Sandimmune®
Serum half-life:
  Solution or soft gelatin capsule (Sandimmune®): Biphasic, alpha phase: 1.4 hours and terminal phase 6-24 hours (prolonged in patients with hepatic dysfunction)
  Solution or soft gelatin capsule in a microemulsion (Neoral®): 8.4 hours, lower in pediatric patients versus adults due to the higher metabolism rate
Time to peak serum concentration:
  Oral solution or capsule (Sandimmune®): 2-6 hours; some patients have a second peak at 5-6 hours
  Oral solution or capsule in a microemulsion (Neoral®): 1.5-2 hours (in renal transplant patients)

Pregnancy Risk Factor C

Cycoflex® *see* Cyclobenzaprine Hydrochloride *on page 239*
Cycrin® *see* Medroxyprogesterone Acetate *on page 533*
Cyklokapron® Injection *see* Tranexamic Acid *on page 860*
Cyklokapron® Oral *see* Tranexamic Acid *on page 860*
Cylert® *see* Pemoline *on page 663*
Cyomin® *see* Cyanocobalamin *on page 237*

Cyproheptadine Hydrochloride
(si proe hep' ta deen hye droe klor' ide)
Brand Names Periactin®
Canadian/Mexican Brand Names PMS-Cyproheptadine® (Canada)
Therapeutic Category Antihistamine
Use Perennial and seasonal allergic rhinitis and other allergic symptoms including urticaria; its off-labeled uses have included appetite stimulation, blepharospasm, cluster headaches, migraine headaches, Nelson's syndrome, pruritus, schizophrenia, spinal cord damage associated spasticity, and tardive dyskinesia
Usual Dosage Oral:
Children: 0.25 mg/kg/day in 2-3 divided doses or 8 mg/m^2/day in 2-3 divided doses

2-6 years: 2 mg every 8-12 hours (not to exceed 12 mg/day)
7-14 years: 4 mg every 8-12 hours (not to exceed 16 mg/day)
Adults: 4-20 mg/day divided every 8 hours (not to exceed 0.5 mg/kg/day) in patients with significant hepatic dysfunction

Mechanism of Action A potent antihistamine and serotonin antagonist, competes with histamine for H_1-receptor sites on effector cells in the gastrointestinal tract, blood vessels, and respiratory tract

Local Anesthetic/Vasoconstrictor Precautions No information available to require special precautions

Effects on Dental Treatment No effects or complications reported

Other Adverse Effects

>10%:
  Central nervous system: Slight to moderate drowsiness
  Respiratory: Thickening of bronchial secretions

1% to 10%:
  Central nervous system: Headache, fatigue, nervousness, dizziness
  Gastrointestinal: Appetite stimulation, nausea, diarrhea, abdominal pain, dry mouth
  Neuromuscular & skeletal: Arthralgia
  Respiratory: Pharyngitis

<1%:
  Cardiovascular: Tachycardia, palpitations, edema
  Central nervous system: Sedation, CNS stimulation, seizures, depression
  Dermatologic: Photosensitivity, rash, angioedema
  Hematologic: Hemolytic anemia, leukopenia, thrombocytopenia
  Hepatic: Hepatitis
  Neuromuscular & skeletal: Myalgia, paresthesia
  Respiratory: Bronchospasm
  Miscellaneous: Epistaxis, allergic reactions

Drug Interactions Increased toxicity: MAO inhibitors cause hallucinations

Pregnancy Risk Factor B

Cystagon® *see* Cysteamine *on this page*

Cysteamine (sis tee' a meen)

Brand Names Cystagon®

Therapeutic Category Antiurolithic

Use Nephropathic cystinosis in children and adults

Usual Dosage Initiate therapy with $1/4$ to $1/8$ of maintenance dose; titrate slowly upward over 4-6 weeks
Children <12 years: Oral: Maintenance: 1.3 g/m^2/day divided into 4 doses
Children >12 years and Adults (>110 lbs): 2 g/day in 4 divided doses; dosage may in increased to 1.95 g/m^2/day if cystine levels are <1 nmol/$1/2$ cystine/mg protein, although intolerance and incidence of adverse events may be increased

Mechanism of Action Reacts with cystine in the lysosome to convert it to cysteine and to a cysteine-cysteamine mixed disulfide, both of which can then exit the lysosome in patients with cystinosis, an inherited defect of lysosomal transport

Local Anesthetic/Vasoconstrictor Precautions No information available to require special precautions

Effects on Dental Treatment No effects or complications reported

Other Adverse Effects

5% to 10%:
  Gastrointestinal: Vomiting, anorexia, diarrhea
  Central nervous system: Fever, lethargy
  Dermatologic: Rash

<5%:
  Cardiovascular: Hypertension
  Central nervous system: Somnolence, encephalopathy, headache, seizures, ataxia, confusion, dizziness, jitteriness, nervousness, impaired cognition, emotional changes, hallucinations, nightmares
  Dermatologic: Urticaria
  Endocrine & metabolic: Dehydration
  Gastrointestinal: Bad breath, abdominal pain, dyspepsia, constipation, gastroenteritis, duodenitis, duodenal ulceration
  Hematologic: Anemia, leukopenia
  Hepatic: Abnormal LFTs
  Neuromuscular & skeletal: Tremor, hyperkinesia
  Otic: Decreased hearing

Pregnancy Risk Factor C

Cysteine Hydrochloride (sis' teen hye droe klor' ide)
Therapeutic Category Nutritional Supplement
Use Total parenteral nutrition of infants as an additive to meet the I.V. amino acid requirements
Local Anesthetic/Vasoconstrictor Precautions No information available to require special precautions
Effects on Dental Treatment No effects or complications reported

Cystospaz® *see* Hyoscyamine Sulfate *on page 445*
Cystospaz-M® *see* Hyoscyamine Sulfate *on page 445*
Cytadren® *see* Aminoglutethimide *on page 46*

Cytarabine Hydrochloride (sye tare' a been hye droe klor' ide)
Brand Names Cytosar-U®
Therapeutic Category Antineoplastic Agent, Antimetabolite
Use Ara-C is one of the most active agents in leukemia; also active against lymphoma, meningeal leukemia, and meningeal lymphoma; has little use in the treatment of solid tumors
Usual Dosage I.V. bolus, IVPB, and continuous intravenous infusion doses of cytarabine are very different. Bolus doses are relatively well tolerated since the drug is rapidly metabolized; continuous infusion uniformly results in myelosuppression. Refer to individual protocols.
Children and Adults:
Induction remission:
    I.V.: 200 mg/m^2/day for 5 days at 2-week intervals
    100-200 mg/m^2/day for 5- to 10-day therapy course or every day until remission
    I.T.: 5-75 mg/m^2 every 2-7 days until CNS findings normalize
    or
    <1 year: 20 mg
    1-2 years: 30 mg
    2-3 years: 50 mg
    >3 years: 70 mg

Maintenance remission:
    I.V.: 70-200 mg/m^2/day for 2-5 days at monthly intervals
    I.M., S.C.: 1-1.5 mg/kg single dose for maintenance at 1- to 4-week intervals

High-dose therapies:
    Doses as high as 1-3 g/m^2 have been used for refractory or secondary leukemias or refractory non-Hodgkin's lymphoma
    Doses of 3 g/m^2 every 12 hours for up to 12 doses have been used
Bone marrow transplant: 1.5 g/m^2 continuous infusion over 48 hours
Mechanism of Action Inhibition of DNA synthesis; cell cycle-specific for the S phase of cell division; cytosine gains entry into cells by a carrier process, and then must be converted to its active compound; cytosine acts as an analog and is incorporated into DNA; however, the primary action is inhibition of DNA polymerase resulting in decreased DNA synthesis and repair; degree of its cytotoxicity correlates linearly with its incorporation into DNA; therefore, incorporation into the DNA is responsible for drug activity and toxicity
Local Anesthetic/Vasoconstrictor Precautions No information available to require special precautions
Effects on Dental Treatment No effects or complications reported
Other Adverse Effects
Central nervous system: Has produced seizures when given I.T.; cerebellar syndrome (or cerebellar toxicity), manifested as ataxia, dysarthria, and dysdiadochokinesia, has been reported to be dose-related. This may or may not be reversible.
High-dose therapy toxicities: Cerebellar toxicity, conjunctivitis (make sure the patient is on steroid eye drops during therapy), corneal keratitis, hyperbilirubinemia, pulmonary edema, pericarditis, and tamponade

>10%:
Central nervous system: Fever, rash
Dermatologic: Oral/anal ulceration
Gastrointestinal: Nausea, vomiting, diarrhea, and mucositis which subside quickly after discontinuing the drug; GI effects may be more pronounced with divided I.V. bolus doses than with continuous infusion
Emetic potential:
    ≤20 mg: Moderately low (10% to 30%)
    250 mg to 1 g: Moderately high (60% to 90%)
    >1 g: High (>90%)

Hematologic: Bleeding

Hepatic: Hepatic dysfunction, mild jaundice and acute increase in transaminases can be produced

Local: Thrombophlebitis

Myelosuppressive: Occurs within the first week of treatment and lasts for 10-14 days; primarily manifested as granulocytopenia, but anemia can also occur

WBC: Severe
Platelets: Severe
Onset (days): 4-7
Nadir (days): 14-18
Recovery (days): 21-28

1% to 10%:

Cardiovascular: Cardiomegaly

Central nervous system: Dizziness, headache, somnolence, confusion, neuritis, malaise

Dermatologic: Skin freckling, itching, alopecia, cellulitis at injection site

Genitourinary: Urinary retention

Neuromuscular & skeletal: Myalgia, bone pain, peripheral neuropathy

Respiratory: Syndrome of sudden respiratory distress progressing to pulmonary edema, pneumonia

Miscellaneous: Sepsis

Drug Interactions

Decreased effect of gentamicin, flucytosine; decreased digoxin oral tablet absorption

Increased toxicity: Alkylating agents and radiation; purine analogs; methotrexate

Drug Uptake

Absorption: Because high concentrations of cytidine deaminase are in the GI mucosa and liver, three- to tenfold higher doses than I.V. would need to be given orally; therefore, the oral route is not used

Serum half-life:
Initial: 7-20 minutes
Terminal: 0.5-2.6 hours

Pregnancy Risk Factor D

Cytomel® *see* Liothyronine Sodium *on page 504*

Cytosar-U® *see* Cytarabine Hydrochloride *on previous page*

Cytotec® *see* Misoprostol *on page 584*

Cytovene® *see* Ganciclovir *on page 393*

Cytoxan® *see* Cyclophosphamide *on page 240*

D$_3$ *see* Cholecalciferol *on page 200*

Dacarbazine (da kar' ba zeen)

Brand Names DTIC-Dome®

Therapeutic Category Antineoplastic Agent, Miscellaneous

Synonyms DIC; Dimethyl Triazeno Imidazol Carboxamide; DTIC; Imidazole Carboxamide

Use Singly or in various combination therapy to treat malignant melanoma, Hodgkin's disease, soft-tissue sarcomas (fibrosarcomas, rhabdomyosarcoma), islet cell carcinoma, medullary carcinoma of the thyroid, and neuroblastoma

Usual Dosage I.V. (**refer to individual protocols**):

Children:
Pediatric solid tumors: 200-470 mg/m^2/day over 5 days every 21-28 days
Pediatric neuroblastoma: 800-900 mg/m^2 as a single dose on day 1 of therapy every 3-4 weeks in combination therapy
Hodgkin's disease: 375 mg/m^2 on days 1 and 15 of treatment course, repeat every 28 days

Adults:
Malignant melanoma: 2-4.5 mg/kg/day for 10 days, repeat in 4 weeks **or** may use 250 mg/m^2/day for 5 days, repeat in 3 weeks
Hodgkin's disease: 150 mg/m^2/day for 5 days, repeat every 4 weeks **or** 375 mg/m^2 on day 1, repeat in 15 days of each 28-day cycle in combination with other agents **or** 375 mg/m^2 repeated in 15 days of each 28-day cycle

Mechanism of Action Alkylating agent which forms methylcarbonium ions that attack nucleophilic groups in DNA; cross-links strands of DNA resulting in the inhibition of DNA, RNA, and protein synthesis, but the exact mechanism of action is still unclear; originally developed as a purine antimetabolite, but it does not interfere with purine synthesis; metabolism by the host is necessary for activation of dacarbazine, then the methylated species acts by alkylation of nucleic acids; dacarbazine is active in all phases of the cell cycle

(Continued)

Dacarbazine (Continued)

Local Anesthetic/Vasoconstrictor Precautions No information available to require special precautions

Effects on Dental Treatment No effects or complications reported

Other Adverse Effects

>10%: Pain and burning at infusion site

Central nervous system: Weakness, polyneuropathy, blurred vision, headache, and seizures have been reported

Extravasation: Dacarbazine is a vesicant; may cause tissue necrosis after extravasation; apply ice and consult extravasation policy if this occurs

Gastrointestinal: Moderate to severe nausea and vomiting in 90% of patients and lasting up to 12 hours after administration; nausea and vomiting are dose-related and occur more frequently when given as a one-time dose, as opposed to a less intensive 5-day course; diarrhea may also occur

Emetic potential: <500 mg: Moderately high (60% to 90%); ≥500 mg: High (>90%)

Myelosuppressive effects: Mild to moderate is common and dose-related; leukopenia and thrombocytopenia may be delayed 2-3 weeks and may be the dose-limiting toxicity; WBC: Mild (primarily leukocytes); Platelets: Mild; Onset (days): 7; Nadir (days): 10-14; Recovery (days): 21-28

1% to 10%: Facial flushing, paresthesias, alopecia, rash, anorexia, metallic taste, myelosuppression

Flu-like effects: Fever, malaise, headache, myalgia, and sinus congestion may last up to several days after administration

<1%: Anaphylaxis, hepatotoxicity, stomatitis, photosensitivity reactions, diarrhea

Miscellaneous: Orthostatic hypotension, mild immunosuppression, elevated LFTs, alopecia, and anaphylaxis

Drug Uptake

Onset of action: I.V.: 18-24 days

Absorption: Oral administration demonstrates slow and variable absorption; preferable to administer by I.V. route

Serum half-life (biphasic):

Initial: 20-40 minutes

Terminal: 5 hours

Pregnancy Risk Factor C

Dacodyl® [OTC] see Bisacodyl on page 113

Dactinomycin (dak ti noe mye' sin)

Brand Names Cosmegen®

Therapeutic Category Antineoplastic Agent, Antibiotic

Synonyms ACT; Actinomycin D

Use Management, either alone or in combination with other treatment modalities of Wilms' tumor, rhabdomyosarcoma, neuroblastoma, retinoblastoma, Ewing's sarcoma, trophoblastic neoplasms, testicular carcinoma, and other malignancies

Usual Dosage Refer to individual protocols

Calculation of the dosage for obese or edematous patients should be on the basis of surface area in an effort to relate dosage to lean body mass

Children >6 months and Adults: I.V.:

15 mcg/kg/day **or** 400-600 mcg/m²/day (maximum: 500 mcg) for 5 days, may repeat every 3-6 weeks **or**

2.5 mg/m² given in divided doses over 1-week period and repeated at 2-week intervals **or**

0.75-2 mg/m² as a single dose given at intervals of 1-4 weeks have been used

Mechanism of Action Binds to the guanine portion of DNA intercalating between guanine and cytosine base pairs inhibiting DNA and RNA synthesis and protein synthesis; product of Streptomyces parvullus (a yeast species)

Local Anesthetic/Vasoconstrictor Precautions No information available to require special precautions

Effects on Dental Treatment No effects or complications reported

Other Adverse Effects

>10%: Alopecia (reversible), hyperpigmentation of skin, unusual tiredness, esophagitis

Extravasation: An irritant and should be administered through a rapidly running I.V. line; extravasation can lead to tissue necrosis, pain, and ulceration

248

Gastrointestinal: Severe nausea and vomiting occur in most patients and persist for up to 24 hours; stomatitis, anorexia, abdominal pain, and diarrhea

Myelosuppressive: Dose-limiting toxicity; anemia, aplastic anemia, agranulocytosis, pancytopenia
WBC: Moderate
Platelets: Moderate
Onset (days): 7
Nadir (days): 14-21
Recovery (days): 21-28

1% to 10%: Diarrhea, mucositis
<1%: Anaphylactoid reaction, hepatitis, liver function tests abnormalities, hyperuricemia
Miscellaneous effects: Skin eruptions, acne, fever, hypocalcemia

Drug Uptake
Serum half-life: 36 hours
Time to peak serum concentration: I.V.: Within 2-5 minutes

Pregnancy Risk Factor C

Dairy Ease® [OTC] *see* Lactase *on page 487*
Dakrina® Ophthalmic Solution [OTC] *see* Artificial Tears *on page 75*
Dalalone L.A.® *see* Dexamethasone *on page 260*
Dalgan® *see* Dezocine *on page 267*
Dallergy® *see* Chlorpheniramine, Phenylephrine, and Methscopolamine *on page 193*
Dallergy-D® Syrup *see* Chlorpheniramine and Phenylephrine *on page 190*
Dalmane® *see* Flurazepam Hydrochloride *on page 380*

Dalteparin (dal te′ pa rin)
Brand Names Fragmin®
Therapeutic Category Anticoagulant
Use Prevent deep vein thrombosis following abdominal surgery
Usual Dosage Adults: S.C.:
Low-moderate risk patients: 2500 units 1-2 hours prior to surgery, then once daily for 5-10 days postoperatively
High risk patients: 5000 units 1-2 hours prior to surgery and then once daily for 5-10 days postoperatively
Mechanism of Action Low molecular weight heparin analog with a molecular weight of 4000-6000 daltons; the commercial product contains 3% to 15% heparin with a molecular weight <3000 daltons, 65% to 78% with a molecular weight of 3000-8000 daltons and 14% to 26% with a molecular weight >8000 daltons; while dalteparin has been shown to inhibit both factor Xa and factor IIa (thrombin), the antithrombotic effect of dalteparin is characterized by a higher ratio of antifactor Xa to antifactor IIa activity (ratio = 4)
Local Anesthetic/Vasoconstrictor Precautions No information available to require special precautions
Effects on Dental Treatment No effects or complications reported
Other Adverse Effects 1% to 10%:
Dermatologic: Allergic reactions (eg, pruritus, rash, fever, injection site reaction, bullous eruption), anaphylactoid reactions and skin necrosis
Hematologic: Bleeding, wound hematoma, injection site hematoma, thrombocytopenia
Local: Pain at injection site

Damason-P® *see* Hydrocodone and Aspirin *on page 433*

Danazol (da′ na zole)
Brand Names Danocrine®
Canadian/Mexican Brand Names Cyclomen® (Canada); Ladogal® (Mexico); Zoldan-A® (Mexico)
Therapeutic Category Androgen
Use Treatment of endometriosis, fibrocystic breast disease, and hereditary angioedema
Usual Dosage Adults: Oral:
Endometriosis: 100-400 mg twice daily for 3-6 months (may extend to 9 months)
Fibrocystic breast disease: 50-200 mg twice daily for 2-6 months
Hereditary angioedema: 400-600 mg/day in 2-3 divided doses
Mechanism of Action Suppresses pituitary output of follicle-stimulating hormone and luteinizing hormone that causes regression and atrophy of normal and ectopic endometrial tissue; decreases rate of growth of abnormal
(Continued)

Danazol *(Continued)*

breast tissue; reduces attacks associated with hereditary angioedema by increasing levels of C4 component of complement

Local Anesthetic/Vasoconstrictor Precautions No information available to require special precautions

Effects on Dental Treatment No effects or complications reported

Other Adverse Effects

>10%:
Androgenic: Weight gain, oily skin, acne, hirsutism, voice deepening, breakthrough bleeding, irregular menstrual periods, decreased breast size
Cardiovascular: Fluid retention, edema
Hepatic: Hepatic impairment

1% to 10%:
Central nervous system: Weakness
Endocrine & metabolic: Virilization, androgenic effects, amenorrhea, hypoestrogenism

<1%:
Central nervous system: Dizziness, headache
Dermatologic: Skin rashes, photosensitivity
Genitourinary: Monilial vaginitis, testicular atrophy, enlarged clitoris
Hepatic: Cholestatic jaundice
Miscellaneous: Bleeding gums, carpal tunnel syndrome, benign intracranial hypertension, pancreatitis

Drug Interactions Danazol has prolonged the prothrombin times in patients taking warfarin; anticoagulant effects are enhanced; danazol has increased the serum concentrations of carbamazepine (Tegretol®) leading to dizziness, nausea, drowsiness, and ataxia

Drug Uptake
Onset of therapeutic effect: Within 4 weeks following daily doses
Serum half-life: 4.5 hours (variable)
Time to peak serum concentration: Within 2 hours

Pregnancy Risk Factor X

Danocrine® *see Danazol on previous page*

Dantrium® *see Dantrolene Sodium on this page*

Dantrolene Sodium (dan' troe leen sow' dee um)

Brand Names Dantrium®

Therapeutic Category Antidote, Malignant Hyperthermia; Hyperthermia, Treatment; Muscle Relaxant; Skeletal Muscle Relaxant

Use Treatment of spasticity associated with spinal cord injury, stroke, cerebral palsy, or multiple sclerosis; also used as treatment of malignant hyperthermia

Usual Dosage

Spasticity: Oral:
Children: Initial: 0.5 mg/kg/dose twice daily, increase frequency to 3-4 times/ day at 4- to 7-day intervals, then increase dose by 0.5 mg/kg to a maximum of 3 mg/kg/dose 2-4 times/day up to 400 mg/day
Adults: 25 mg/day to start, increase frequency to 2-4 times/day, then increase dose by 25 mg every 4-7 days to a maximum of 100 mg 2-4 times/day or 400 mg/day

Malignant hyperthermia: Children and Adults:
Oral: 4-8 mg/kg/day in 4 divided doses
Preoperative prophylaxis: Begin 1-2 days prior to surgery with last dose 3-4 hours prior to surgery
I.V.: 1 mg/kg; may repeat dose up to cumulative dose of 10 mg/kg (mean effective dose is 2.5 mg/kg), then switch to oral dosage
Preoperative: 2.5 mg/kg ~1¼ hours prior to anesthesia and infused over 1 hour with additional doses as needed and individualized

Mechanism of Action Acts directly on skeletal muscle by interfering with release of calcium ion from the sarcoplasmic reticulum; prevents or reduces the increase in myoplasmic calcium ion concentration that activates the acute catabolic processes associated with malignant hyperthermia

Local Anesthetic/Vasoconstrictor Precautions No information available to require special precautions

Effects on Dental Treatment No effects or complications reported

Other Adverse Effects

>10%:
Central nervous system: Drowsiness, dizziness, lightheadedness, fatigue, tiredness
Dermatologic: Rash

Gastrointestinal: Diarrhea (mild), nausea, vomiting
Neuromuscular & skeletal: Muscle weakness
1% to 10%:
Cardiovascular: Pleural effusion with pericarditis
Central nervous system: Chills, fever, headache, insomnia, nervousness, mental depression
Gastrointestinal: Diarrhea (severe), constipation, anorexia, stomach cramps
Ocular: Blurred vision
Respiratory: Respiratory depression
<1%:
Central nervous system: Seizures, confusion
Hepatic: Hepatitis
Drug Interactions When given simultaneously dantrolene has increased the toxicity of the following drugs: Estrogens (hepatotoxicity), CNS depressants (sedation), MAO inhibitors, phenothiazines, clindamycin (increased neuromuscular blockade), verapamil (hyperkalemia and cardiac depression), warfarin, clofibrate and tolbutamide
Drug Uptake
Absorption: Slow and incomplete from GI tract
Serum half-life: 8.7 hours
Pregnancy Risk Factor C

Dapa® [OTC] *see* Acetaminophen *on page 14*

Dapacin® Cold Capsule [OTC] *see* Chlorpheniramine, Phenylpropanolamine, and Acetaminophen *on page 194*

Dapiprazole Hydrochloride (da' pi pray zole hye droe klor' ide)
Brand Names Rēv-Eyes™
Therapeutic Category Alpha-Adrenergic Blocking Agent, Ophthalmic
Use Reverse dilation due to drugs (adrenergic or parasympathomimetic) after eye exams
Usual Dosage Adults: Administer 2 drops followed 5 minutes later by an additional 2 drops applied to the conjunctiva of each eye; should not be used more frequently than once a week in the same patient
Mechanism of Action Dapiprazole is a selective alpha-adrenergic blocking agent, exerting effects primarily on alpha$_1$-adrenoceptors. It induces miosis via relaxation of the smooth dilator (radial) muscle of the iris, which causes pupillary constriction. It is devoid of cholinergic effects. Dapiprazole also partially reverses the cycloplegia induced with parasympatholytic agents such as tropicamide. Although the drug has no significant effect on the ciliary muscle *per se*, it may increase accommodative amplitude, therefore relieving the symptoms of paralysis of accommodation.
Local Anesthetic/Vasoconstrictor Precautions No information available to require special precautions
Effects on Dental Treatment No effects or complications reported
Other Adverse Effects
>10%: Ophthalmic: Conjunctival injection, headache, burning sensation in the eyes, lid edema, ptosis, lid erythema, chemosis, itching, punctate keratitis, corneal edema, photophobia
1% to 10%: Ophthalmic: Dry eyes, blurring of vision, tearing of eye
Drug Interactions No data reported
Pregnancy Risk Factor B

Dapsone (dap' sone)
Brand Names Avlosulfon®
Therapeutic Category Antibiotic, Sulfone
Use Treatment of leprosy and dermatitis herpetiformis (infections caused by *Mycobacterium leprae*), alternative agent for *Pneumocystis carinii* pneumonia prophylaxis (given alone) and treatment (given with trimethoprim)
Usual Dosage Oral:
Leprosy:
Children: 1-2 mg/kg/24 hours, up to a maximum of 100 mg/day
Adults: 50-100 mg/day for 3-10 years
Dermatitis herpetiformis: Adults: Start at 50 mg/day, increase to 300 mg/day, or higher to achieve full control, reduce dosage to minimum level as soon as possible
Prophylaxis of *Pneumocystis carinii* pneumonia: Children >1 month: 1 mg/kg/day; maximum: 100 mg
Treatment of *Pneumocystis carinii* pneumonia: Adults: 100 mg/day in combination with trimethoprim (20 mg/kg/day) for 21 days
(Continued)

Dapsone *(Continued)*

Mechanism of Action Dapsone is a sulfone antimicrobial. The mechanism of action of the sulfones is similar to that of the sulfonamides. Sulfonamides are competitive antagonists of para-aminobenzoic acid (PABA) and prevent normal bacterial utilization of PABA for the synthesis of folic acid.

Local Anesthetic/Vasoconstrictor Precautions No information available to require special precautions

Effects on Dental Treatment No effects or complications reported

Other Adverse Effects

1% to 10%:
Hematologic: Dose-related hemolysis, methemoglobinemia with cyanosis
Miscellaneous: Reactional states

<1%:
Central nervous system: Peripheral neuropathy, insomnia, headache
Dermatologic: Exfoliative dermatitis
Gastrointestinal: Nausea, vomiting
Hematologic: Hemolytic anemia, methemoglobinemia, leukopenia, agranulo-
cytosis
Hepatic: Hepatitis, cholestatic jaundice
Ocular: Blurred vision
Otic: Tinnitus

Drug Interactions
Dapsone has decreased the effects of para-aminobenzoic acid and rifampin
Dapsone has increased the effects of folic acid antagonists

Drug Uptake
Absorption: Oral: Well absorbed
Serum half-life, elimination: 30 hours (range: 10-50 hours)

Pregnancy Risk Factor C

Daranide® *see* Dichlorphenamide *on page 271*

Daraprim® *see* Pyrimethamine *on page 754*

Daricon® *see* Oxyphencyclimine Hydrochloride *on page 652*

Darvocet-N® *see* Propoxyphene and Acetaminophen *on page 741*

Darvocet-N® 100 *see* Propoxyphene and Acetaminophen *on page 741*

Darvon® *see* Propoxyphene *on page 740*

Darvon® Compound-65 Pulvules® *see* Propoxyphene and Aspirin *on page 742*

Darvon-N® *see* Propoxyphene *on page 740*

Darvon®-N With ASA *see* Propoxyphene and Aspirin *on page 742*

Datril® [OTC] *see* Acetaminophen *on page 14*

Daunomycin *see* Daunorubicin Hydrochloride *on this page*

Daunorubicin Hydrochloride

(daw noe roo' bi sin hye droe klor' ide)

Brand Names Cerubidine®

Canadian/Mexican Brand Names Rubilem (Mexico); Trixilem (Mexico)

Therapeutic Category Antineoplastic Agent, Antibiotic

Synonyms Daunomycin; DNR; Rubidomycin Hydrochloride

Use In combination with other agents in the treatment of leukemias (ALL, AML)

Usual Dosage I.V. **(refer to individual protocols):**

Children:
ALL Combination therapy: Remission induction: 25-45 mg/m² on day 1 every week for 4 cycles **or** 30-45 mg/m²/day for 3 days
In children <2 years or <0.5 m², daunorubicin should be based on weight - mg/kg: 1 mg/kg per protocol with frequency dependent on regimen employed
Cumulative dose should not exceed 300 mg/m² in children >2 years or 10 mg/kg in children <2 years

Adults: 30-60 mg/m²/day for 3-5 days, repeat dose in 3-4 weeks
Single agent induction for AML: 60 mg/m²/day for 3 days; repeat every 3-4 weeks
Combination therapy induction for AML: 45 mg/m²/day for 3 days of the first course of induction therapy; subsequent courses: Every day for 2 days
ALL combination therapy: 45 mg/m²/day for 3 days
Cumulative dose should not exceed 400-600 mg/m²

Mechanism of Action Inhibition of DNA and RNA synthesis, by intercalating between DNA base pairs and by steric obstruction; is not cell cycle-specific for the S phase of cell division; daunomycin is preferred over doxorubicin for the treatment of ANLL because of its dose-limiting toxicity (myelosuppression) is not of concern in the therapy of this disease; has less mucositis associated with its use

Local Anesthetic/Vasoconstrictor Precautions No information available to require special precautions

Effects on Dental Treatment No effects or complications reported

Other Adverse Effects

>10%: Alopecia (reversible), discoloration of urine (red), stomatitis

Gastrointestinal: Mild nausea or vomiting occurs in 50% of patients within the first 24 hours; stomatitis may occur 3-7 days after administration, but is not as severe as that caused by doxorubicin

1% to 10%: GI ulceration, diarrhea, hyperuricemia, myelosuppression

Cardiac toxicity: Congestive heart failure; maximum lifetime dose: Refer to Warnings/Precautions

Extravasation: Daunorubicin is a vesicant; infiltration can cause severe inflammation, tissue necrosis, and ulceration; if the drug is infiltrated, consult institutional policy, apply ice to the area, and elevate the limb

Myelosuppressive: Dose-limiting toxicity, occurs in all patients; leukopenia is more significant than thrombocytopenia; WBC: Severe; Platelets: Severe; Onset (days): 7; Nadir (days): 14; Recovery (days): 21-28

<1%: Skin rash, pericarditis/myocarditis, pigmentation of nail beds, urticaria, elevation in serum bilirubin, AST, and alkaline phosphatase, chills

Miscellaneous: Fertility impairment, pigmentation changes in nailbeds, transient elevation of AST

Drug Uptake

Serum half-life: 14-20 hours

Pregnancy Risk Factor D

Daypro™ *see* Oxaprozin *on page 643*

Dayto Himbin® *see* Yohimbine Hydrochloride *on page 905*

DC 240® Softgels® [OTC] *see* Docusate *on page 295*

DCF *see* Pentostatin *on page 674*

DDAVP® *see* Desmopressin Acetate *on page 258*

Debrisan® [OTC] *see* Dextranomer *on page 264*

Debrox® [OTC] *see* Carbamide Peroxide *on page 152*

Decadron® *see* Dexamethasone *on page 260*

Decadron®-LA *see* Dexamethasone *on page 260*

Deca-Durabolin® *see* Nandrolone *on page 604*

Decaject-L.A.® *see* Dexamethasone *on page 260*

Decholin® *see* Dehydrocholic Acid *on next page*

Declomycin® *see* Demeclocycline Hydrochloride *on page 255*

Decofed® Syrup [OTC] *see* Pseudoephedrine *on page 749*

Decohistine® DH *see* Chlorpheniramine, Pseudoephedrine, and Codeine *on page 195*

Decohistine® Expectorant *see* Guaifenesin, Pseudoephedrine, and Codeine *on page 410*

Deconamine® SR *see* Chlorpheniramine and Pseudoephedrine *on page 191*

Deconamine® Syrup [OTC] *see* Chlorpheniramine and Pseudoephedrine *on page 191*

Deconamine® Tablet [OTC] *see* Chlorpheniramine and Pseudoephedrine *on page 191*

Deconsal® II *see* Guaifenesin and Pseudoephedrine *on page 409*

Defen-LA® *see* Guaifenesin and Pseudoephedrine *on page 409*

Deferoxamine Mesylate (de fer ox' a meen mes' i late)

Brand Names Desferal® Mesylate

Therapeutic Category Antidote, Aluminum Toxicity; Antidote, Iron Toxicity

Use Acute iron intoxication; chronic iron overload secondary to multiple transfusions; diagnostic test for iron overload; used investigationally in the treatment of aluminum accumulation in renal failure; iron overload secondary to congenital anemias; hemochromatosis; removal of corneal rust rings following surgical removal of foreign bodies

Usual Dosage

Children:

Acute iron intoxication (I.M. is preferred route for patients not in shock). Treat until urine is no longer pink salmon colored:

I.M.: 50 mg/kg/dose every 6 hours to a maximum of 6 g/day

I.V.: 15 mg/kg/hour; maximum: 6 g/day

Chronic iron overload:

I.M., I.V.: 50 mg/kg/dose to a maximum of 6 g/24 hours or 2 g/dose; do not exceed 15 mg/kg/hour I.V.

(Continued)

Deferoxamine Mesylate *(Continued)*

    S.C.: 20-40 mg/kg/day over 8-12 hours (via a portable, controlled infusion device)

    Aluminum-induced bone disease: 20-40 mg/kg every hemodialysis treatment, frequency dependent on clinical status of the patient

Adults:

    Acute iron intoxication: (I.M. is preferred route for patients not in shock). Treat until urine is no longer pink salmon colored:

        I.M., I.V.: 1 g stat, then 0.5 g every 4 hours for two doses, then 0.5 g every 4-12 hours up to 6 g/day; do not exceed 15 mg/kg/hour I.V.

    Chronic iron overload:

        I.M.: 0.5-1 g every day

        I.V.: 2 g after each unit of blood infusion at 15 mg/kg/hour

        S.C.: 1-2 g every day over 8-24 hours

Mechanism of Action Complexes with trivalent ions (ferric ions) to form ferrioxamine, which are removed by the kidneys

Local Anesthetic/Vasoconstrictor Precautions No information available to require special precautions

Effects on Dental Treatment No effects or complications reported

Other Adverse Effects

1% to 10%: Local: Pain and induration at injection site

<1%:

    Cardiovascular: Flushing, hypotension, tachycardia, shock, swelling

    Central nervous system: Fever

    Dermatologic: Erythema, urticaria, pruritus, rash, cutaneous wheal formation

    Gastrointestinal: Abdominal discomfort, diarrhea

    Neuromuscular & skeletal: Leg cramps

    Ocular: Blurred vision, cataracts

    Otic: Hearing loss

    Miscellaneous: Anaphylaxis

Drug Interactions No data reported

Drug Uptake

    Absorption: Oral: <15%

    Serum half-life:

        Parent drug: 6.1 hours

        Ferrioxamine: 5.8 hours

Pregnancy Risk Factor C

Deficol® [OTC] *see* Bisacodyl *on page 113*

Degest® 2 [OTC] *see* Naphazoline Hydrochloride *on page 605*

Dehist® *see* Brompheniramine Maleate *on page 124*

Dehydrocholic Acid *(dee hye droe koe′ lik as′ id)*

Brand Names Cholan-HMB®; Decholin®

Therapeutic Category Bile Acid; Laxative, Hydrocholeretic

Use Relief of constipation; adjunct to various biliary tract conditions

Local Anesthetic/Vasoconstrictor Precautions No information available to require special precautions

Effects on Dental Treatment No effects or complications reported

Other Adverse Effects 1% to 10%: Dehydration, diarrhea, abdominal cramps

Dekasol-L.A.® *see* Dexamethasone *on page 260*

Deladiol® *see* Estradiol *on page 325*

Deladumone® Injection *see* Estradiol and Testosterone *on page 326*

Delatest® *see* Testosterone *on page 825*

Delatestryl® *see* Testosterone *on page 825*

Delaxin® *see* Methocarbamol *on page 557*

Delestrogen® *see* Estradiol *on page 325*

Delfen® [OTC] *see* Nonoxynol 9 *on page 627*

Del-Mycin® Topical *see* Erythromycin, Topical *on page 324*

Delsym® [OTC] *see* Dextromethorphan *on page 266*

Delta-Cortef® *see* Prednisolone *on page 718*

Delta-D® *see* Cholecalciferol *on page 200*

Deltasone® *see* Prednisone *on page 719*

Delta-Tritex® *see* Triamcinolone *on page 862*

Demadex® *see* Torsemide *on page 856*

Demazin® Syrup [OTC] *see* Chlorpheniramine and Phenylpropanolamine *on page 190*

Demecarium Bromide (dem e kare' ee um broe' mide)

Brand Names Humorsol®

Therapeutic Category Antiglaucoma Agent; Cholinergic Agent, Ophthalmic; Ophthalmic Agent, Miotic

Use Management of chronic simple glaucoma, chronic and acute angle-closure glaucoma; strabismus

Usual Dosage Children and Adults: Ophthalmic:

Glaucoma: Instill 1 drop into eyes twice weekly to a maximum dosage of 1 or 2 drops twice daily for up to 4 months

Strabismus:

Diagnosis: Instill 1 drop daily for 2 weeks, then 1 drop every 2 days for 2-3 weeks. If eyes become straighter, an accommodative factor is demonstrated.

Therapy: Instill not more than 1 drop at a time in both eyes every day for 2-3 weeks. Then reduce dosage to 1 drop every other day for 3-4 weeks and re-evaluate. Continue at 1 drop every 2 days to 1 drop twice a week and evaluate the patient's condition every 4-12 weeks. If improvement continues, reduce dose to 1 drop once a week and eventually off of medication. Discontinue therapy after 4 months if control of the condition still requires 1 drop every 2 days.

Mechanism of Action Cholinesterase inhibitor (anticholinesterase) which causes acetylcholine to accumulate at cholinergic receptor sites and produces effects equivalent to excessive stimulation of cholinergic receptors. Demecarium mainly acts by inhibiting true (erythrocyte) cholinesterase and causes a reduction in intraocular pressure due to facilitation of outflow of aqueous humor; the reduction is likely to be particularly marked in eyes in which the pressure is elevated.

Local Anesthetic/Vasoconstrictor Precautions No information available to require special precautions

Effects on Dental Treatment No effects or complications reported

Other Adverse Effects

1% to 10%: Ophthalmic: Stinging, burning, myopia, visual blurring

<1%:

Cardiovascular: Bradycardia, hypotension, flushing

Gastrointestinal: Nausea, vomiting, diarrhea

Neuromuscular & skeletal: Muscle weakness

Ocular: Retinal detachment, miosis, twitching eyelids, watering eyes

Respiratory: Difficulty in breathing

Miscellaneous: Diaphoresis

Drug Interactions No data reported

Pregnancy Risk Factor C

Demeclociclina (Mexico) *see* Demeclocycline Hydrochloride *on this page*

Demeclocycline Hydrochloride

(dem e kloe sye' kleen hye droe klor' ide)

Brand Names Declomycin®

Canadian/Mexican Brand Names Ledermicina® (Mexico)

Therapeutic Category Antibiotic, Tetracycline Derivative

Synonyms Demeclociclina (Mexico)

Use Treatment of susceptible bacterial infections (acne, gonorrhea, pertussis and urinary tract infections) caused by both gram-negative and gram-positive organisms; used when penicillin is contraindicated (other agents are preferred); treatment of chronic syndrome of inappropriate secretion of antidiuretic hormone (SIADH)

Usual Dosage Oral:

Children ≥8 years: 8-12 mg/kg/day divided every 6-12 hours

Adults: 150 mg 4 times/day or 300 mg twice daily

Uncomplicated gonorrhea (penicillin sensitive): 600 mg stat, 300 mg every 12 hours for 4 days (3 g total)

SIADH: 900-1200 mg/day or 13-15 mg/kg/day divided every 6-8 hours initially, then decrease to 0.6-0.9 g/day

Mechanism of Action Inhibits protein synthesis by binding with the 30S and possibly the 50S ribosomal subunit(s) of susceptible bacteria; may also cause alterations in the cytoplasmic membrane

Local Anesthetic/Vasoconstrictor Precautions No information available to require special precautions

Effects on Dental Treatment Tetracycline's are not recommended for use during pregnancy or in children ≤8 years of age since they have been reported to cause enamel hypoplasia and permanent teeth discoloration. The use of (Continued)

Demeclocycline Hydrochloride *(Continued)*

tetracycline's should only be used in these patients if other agents are contra-indicated or alternative antimicrobials will not eradicate the organism. Long-term use associated with oral candidiasis.

Other Adverse Effects

1% to 10%:

Dermatologic: Photosensitivity

Gastrointestinal: Nausea, diarrhea

<1%:

Cardiovascular: Pericarditis

Central nervous system: Increased intracranial pressure, bulging fontanels in infants

Dermatologic: Dermatologic effects, pruritus, exfoliative dermatitis

Endocrine & metabolic: Diabetes insipidus syndrome

Gastrointestinal: Vomiting, esophagitis, anorexia, abdominal cramps

Neuromuscular & skeletal: Paresthesia

Renal: Acute renal failure, azotemia

Miscellaneous: Superinfections, anaphylaxis, pigmentation of nails

Drug Interactions

Decreased effect with antacids (aluminum, calcium, zinc, or magnesium), bismuth salts, sodium bicarbonate, barbiturates, carbamazepine, hydantoins

Decreased effect of oral contraceptives

Increased effect of warfarin

Drug Uptake

Onset of action for diuresis in SIADH: Several days

Absorption: ~50% to 80% from GI tract; food and dairy products reduce absorption

Serum half-life: Reduced renal function: 10-17 hours

Time to peak serum concentration: Oral: Within 3-6 hours

Pregnancy Risk Factor D

Dosage Forms

Capsule: 150 mg

Tablet: 150 mg, 300 mg

Dietary Considerations Should be taken 1 hour before or 2 hours after food or milk with plenty of fluid

Generic Available No

Demerol® *see* Meperidine Hydrochloride *on page 539*

4-demethoxydaunorubicin *see* Idarubicin *on page 448*

Demulen® *see* Ethinyl Estradiol and Ethynodiol Diacetate *on page 335*

Denavir® *see* Penciclovir *on page 664*

Denorex® [OTC] *see* Coal Tar *on page 225*

Dental Drug Interactions: Update on Drug Combinations Requiring Special Considerations *see page 1022*

Dental Office Emergencies *see page 984*

Dentifrice Products *see page 1051*

Dentin Hypersensitivity; High Caries Index; Xerostomia *see page 959*

Dentipatch® *see* Lidocaine Transoral *on page 502*

Denture Adhesive Products *see page 1060*

Denture Cleanser Products *see page 1062*

Deoxycoformycin *see* Pentostatin *on page 674*

2'-deoxycoformycin *see* Pentostatin *on page 674*

Depakene® *see* Valproic Acid and Derivatives *on page 888*

Depakote® *see* Valproic Acid and Derivatives *on page 888*

depAndrogyn® Injection *see* Estradiol and Testosterone *on page 326*

depGynogen® *see* Estradiol *on page 325*

depMedalone® *see* Methylprednisolone *on page 569*

Depo®-Estradiol *see* Estradiol *on page 325*

Depogen® *see* Estradiol *on page 325*

Depoject® *see* Methylprednisolone *on page 569*

Depo-Medrol® *see* Methylprednisolone *on page 569*

Deponit® *see* Nitroglycerin *on page 623*

Depopred® *see* Methylprednisolone *on page 569*

Depo-Provera® *see* Medroxyprogesterone Acetate *on page 533*

Depotest® *see* Testosterone *on page 825*

Depo-Testadiol® Injection *see* Estradiol and Testosterone *on page 326*

Depotestogen® Injection *see* Estradiol and Testosterone *on page 326*

Depo®-Testosterone *see* Testosterone *on page 825*

Deproist® Expectorant with Codeine *see* Guaifenesin, Pseudoephedrine, and Codeine *on page 410*

Derifil® [OTC] *see* Chlorophyll *on page 185*

Dermacomb® *see* Nystatin and Triamcinolone *on page 632*

Derma-Smoothe/FS® *see* Fluocinolone Acetonide *on page 372*

Dermatop® *see* Prednicarbate *on page 718*

Dermoxyl® [OTC] *see* Benzoyl Peroxide *on page 104*

Desferal® Mesylate *see* Deferoxamine Mesylate *on page 253*

Desipramina, Clorhidrato De (Mexico) *see* Desipramine Hydrochloride *on this page*

Desipramine Hydrochloride (des ip' ra meen hye droe klor' ide)

Brand Names Norpramin®; Pertofrane®

Canadian/Mexican Brand Names PMS-Desipramine® (Canada)

Therapeutic Category Antidepressant, Tricyclic

Synonyms Desipramina, Clorhidrato De (Mexico)

Use Treatment of various forms of depression, often in conjunction with psychotherapy; analgesic adjunct in chronic pain, peripheral neuropathies

Usual Dosage Oral:

Children 6-12 years: 10-30 mg/day or 1-5 mg/kg/day in divided doses; do not exceed 5 mg/kg/day

Adolescents: Initial: 25-50 mg/day; gradually increase to 100 mg/day in single or divided doses; maximum: 150 mg/day

Adults: Initial: 75 mg/day in divided doses; increase gradually to 150-200 mg/day in divided or single dose; maximum: 300 mg/day

Elderly: Initial dose: 10-25 mg/day; increase by 10-25 mg every 3 days for inpatients and every week for outpatients if tolerated; usual maintenance dose: 75-100 mg/day, but doses up to 300 mg/day may be necessary

Hemodialysis/peritoneal dialysis effects: Supplemental dose is not necessary

Mechanism of Action Traditionally believed to increase the synaptic concentration of norepinephrine in the central nervous system by inhibition of reuptake by the presynaptic neuronal membrane. However, additional receptor effects have been found including desensitization of adenyl cyclase, down regulation of beta-adrenergic receptors, and down regulation of serotonin receptors.

Local Anesthetic/Vasoconstrictor Precautions Use with caution; epinephrine, norepinephrine and levonordefrin have been shown to have an increased pressor response in combination TCAs

Effects on Dental Treatment Long-term treatment with TCAs such as amoxapine increases the risk of caries by reducing salivation and salivary buffer capacity

Other Adverse Effects

>10%:

Central nervous system: Dizziness, drowsiness, headache

Gastrointestinal: Dry mouth, constipation, increased appetite, nausea, weakness, unpleasant taste, weight gain

1% to 10%:

Cardiovascular: Arrhythmias, hypotension,

Central nervous system: Confusion, delirium, hallucinations, nervousness, restlessness, parkinsonian syndrome, insomnia

Gastrointestinal: Diarrhea, heartburn

Genitourinary: Difficult urination, sexual function impairment

Neuromuscular & skeletal: Fine muscle tremors

Ocular: Blurred vision, eye pain

Miscellaneous: Excessive sweating

<1%:

Central nervous system: Anxiety, seizures

Dermatologic: Alopecia

Endocrine & metabolic: Breast enlargement, galactorrhea, SIADH

Genitourinary: Testicular swelling

Hematologic: Agranulocytosis, leukopenia, eosinophilia

Hepatic: Cholestatic jaundice, increased liver enzymes

Ocular: Photosensitivity, increased intraocular pressure

Otic: Tinnitus

Miscellaneous: Trouble with gums, decreased lower esophageal sphincter tone may cause GE reflux, allergic reactions

(Continued)

Desipramine Hydrochloride *(Continued)*

Drug Interactions

Decreased effect: Phenobarbital may increase the metabolism, of desipramine; desipramine blocks the uptake of guanethidine and thus prevents the hypotensive effect of guanethidine

Increased toxicity: Clonidine causes hypertensive crisis; desipramine may be additive with or may potentiate the action of other CNS depressants such as sedatives or hypnotics; with MAO inhibitors, hyperpyrexia, hypertension, tachycardia, confusion, and seizures. Desipramine may increase the prothrombin time in patients stabilized on warfarin; desipramine may potentiate the pressor and cardiac effects of sympathomimetic agents such as isoproterenol, epinephrine, etc; cimetidine and methylphenidate may decrease the metabolism of desipramine

Additive anticholinergic effects seen with other anticholinergic agents

Drug Uptake

Onset of action: 1-3 weeks (maximum antidepressant effects: after >2 weeks)

Absorption: Well absorbed (90%) from GI tract

Serum half-life: Adults: 12-57 hours

Pregnancy Risk Factor C

Selected Readings

Boakes AJ, Laurence DR, Teoh PC, et al, "Interactions Between Sympathomimetic Amines and Antidepressant Agents in Man," *Br Med J*, 1973, 1(849):311-5.

Jastak JT and Yagiela JA, "Vasoconstrictors and Local Anesthesia: A Review and Rationale for Use," *J Am Dent Assoc*, 1983, 107(4):623-30.

Larochelle P, Hamet P, and Enjalbert M, "Responses to Tyramine and Norepinephrine After Imipramine and Trazodone," *Clin Pharmacol Ther*, 1979, 26(1):24-30.

Mitchell JR, "Guanethidine and Related Agents. III Antagonism by Drugs Which Inhibit the Norepinephrine Pump in Man," *J Clin Invest*, 1970, 49(8):1596-604.

Rundegren J, van Dijken J, Mörnstad H, et al, "Oral Conditions in Patients Receiving Long-Term Treatment With Cyclic Antidepressant Drugs," *Swed Dent J*, 1985, 9(2):55-64.

Svedmyr N, "The Influence of a Tricyclic Antidepressive Agent (Protriptyline) on Some of the Circulatory Effects of Noradrenaline and Adrenalin® in Man," *Life Sci*, 1968, 7(1):77-84.

Desitin® Topical [OTC] *see* Zinc Oxide, Cod Liver Oil, and Talc *on page 909*

Desmopressin Acetate (des moe press' in as' e tate)

Brand Names DDAVP®; Stimate™

Canadian/Mexican Brand Names Octostim® (Canada)

Therapeutic Category Antihemophilic Agent; Hemostatic Agent; Vasopressin Analog, Synthetic

Use Treatment of diabetes insipidus and controlling bleeding in mild hemophilia, von Willebrand's disease, and thrombocytopenia (eg, uremia)

Usual Dosage Dilute I.V. dose in 50 mL 0.9% sodium chloride and infuse over 15-30 minutes

Children:

Diabetes insipidus: 3 months to 12 years: Intranasal: Initial: 5 mcg/day divided 1-2 times/day; range: 5-30 mcg/day divided 1-2 times/day

Von Willebrand disease, thrombocytopathies, hemophilia: >3 months:

Intranasal: 2-4 mcg/kg/dose

I.V.: 0.3 mcg/kg by slow infusion over 15-30 minutes; usually tachyphylaxis occurs after 2-3 doses in 24 hours, recovery of response may take 48-72 hours

Nocturnal enuresis: ≥6 years: Intranasal: Initial: 20 mcg at bedtime; range: 10-40 mcg

Adults:

Diabetes insipidus: I.V., S.C.: 2-4 mcg/day in 2 divided doses or ¹/₁₀ of the maintenance intranasal dose; intranasal: 5-40 mcg/day 1-3 times/day

Von Willebrand disease, thrombocytopathies, hemophilia:

Intranasal: 2-4 mcg/kg/dose

I.V.: 0.3 mcg/kg by slow infusion over 15-30 minutes; usually tachyphylaxis occurs after 2-3 doses in 24 hours; recovery of responsiveness may take 48-72 hours

Oral: Begin therapy 12 hours after the last intranasal dose for patients previously on intranasal therapy

Children: Initial: 0.05 mg; fluid restrictions required in children to prevent hyponatremia and water intoxication

Adults: 0.05 mg twice daily; adjust individually to optimal therapeutic dose. Total daily dose should be increased or decreased (range: 0.1-1.2 mg divided 2-3 times/day) as needed to obtain adequate antidiuresis.

Mechanism of Action Enhances reabsorption of water in the kidneys by increasing cellular permeability of the collecting ducts; possibly causes smooth muscle constriction with resultant vasoconstriction; raises plasma levels of von Willebrand's factor and factor VIII

Local Anesthetic/Vasoconstrictor Precautions No information available to require special precautions

Effects on Dental Treatment No effects or complications reported

Other Adverse Effects
1% to 10%:
  Cardiovascular: Facial flushing
  Central nervous system: Headache, dizziness
  Gastrointestinal: Nausea, abdominal cramps
  Genitourinary: Vulval pain
  Local: Pain at the injection site, nasal congestion
<1%:
  Cardiovascular: Increase in blood pressure
  Endocrine & metabolic: Hyponatremia
  Genitourinary: Water intoxication

Drug Interactions No data reported

Drug Uptake
Intranasal administration:
  Onset of ADH effects: Within 1 hour
  Peak effect: Within 1-5 hours
  Duration: 5-21 hours
I.V. infusion:
  Onset of increased factor VIII activity: Within 15-30 minutes
  Peak effect: 90 minutes to 3 hours
Absorption: Nasal: Slow; 10% to 20%
Serum half-life: Elimination (terminal): 75 minutes

Pregnancy Risk Factor B

Desogen® *see* Ethinyl Estradiol and Desogestrel *on page 335*

Desogestrel and Ethinyl Estradiol *see* Ethinyl Estradiol and Desogestrel *on page 335*

Desonide (des' oh nide)

Brand Names DesOwen®; Tridesilon®
Canadian/Mexican Brand Names Desocort® (Canada)
Therapeutic Category Corticosteroid, Topical (Low Potency)
Use Adjunctive therapy for inflammation in acute and chronic corticosteroid responsive dermatosis (low potency corticosteroid)
Usual Dosage Children and Adults: Topical: Apply 2-4 times/day sparingly
Mechanism of Action Stimulates the synthesis of enzymes needed to decrease inflammation, suppress mitotic activity, and cause vasoconstriction
Local Anesthetic/Vasoconstrictor Precautions No information available to require special precautions
Effects on Dental Treatment No effects or complications reported
Other Adverse Effects <1%: Topical: Burning, itching, irritation, dryness, folliculitis, hypertrichosis, acneiform eruptions, hypopigmentation, perioral dermatitis, allergic contact dermatitis, skin maceration, secondary infection, skin atrophy, striae, miliaria
Drug Interactions No data reported
Drug Uptake
Onset of effect: Commonly noted within 7 days of continued therapy
Absorption: Topical absorption extensive from the scalp, face, axilla and scrotum; adequate through epidermis on appendages; absorption can be increased with occlusion or the addition of penetrants (eg, urea, DMSO)
Pregnancy Risk Factor C

DesOwen® *see* Desonide *on this page*

Desoximetasone (des ox i met' a sone)

Related Information
Corticosteroids, Topical Comparison *on page 1018*
Brand Names Topicort®; Topicort®-LP
Therapeutic Category Corticosteroid, Topical (High Potency)
Use Relieves inflammation and pruritic symptoms of corticosteroid-responsive dermatosis [medium to high potency topical corticosteroid]
Usual Dosage Topical:
Children: Apply sparingly in a very thin film to affected area 1-2 times/day
Adults: Apply sparingly in a thin film twice daily
Mechanism of Action Stimulates the synthesis of enzymes needed to decrease inflammation, suppress mitotic activity, and cause vasoconstriction
(Continued)

Desoximetasone *(Continued)*

Local Anesthetic/Vasoconstrictor Precautions No information available to require special precautions

Effects on Dental Treatment No effects or complications reported

Other Adverse Effects <1%: Topical: Burning, itching, irritation, dryness, folliculitis, hypertrichosis, acneiform eruptions, hypopigmentation, perioral dermatitis, allergic contact dermatitis, skin maceration, secondary infection, skin atrophy, striae, miliaria

Drug Interactions No data reported

Drug Uptake Topical:

Absorption: Extensive from the scalp, face, axilla, and scrotum and adequate through epidermis on appendages; absorption can be increased with occlusion or the addition of penetrants

Pregnancy Risk Factor C

Desoxyn® *see* Methamphetamine Hydrochloride *on page 553*

Desoxyribonuclease and Fibrinolysin *see* Fibrinolysin and Desoxyribonuclease *on page 362*

Despec® Liquid *see* Guaifenesin, Phenylpropanolamine, and Phenylephrine *on page 410*

Desquam-E® *see* Benzoyl Peroxide *on page 104*

Desquam-X® *see* Benzoyl Peroxide *on page 104*

Desyrel® *see* Trazodone *on page 861*

Detussin® Expectorant *see* Hydrocodone, Pseudoephedrine, and Guaifenesin *on page 435*

Devrom® (subgallate) [OTC] *see* Bismuth *on page 114*

Dexacidin® *see* Neomycin, Polymyxin B, and Dexamethasone *on page 610*

Dex-A-Diet® [OTC] *see* Phenylpropanolamine Hydrochloride *on page 687*

Dexamethasone *(dex a meth′ a sone)*

Related Information

Corticosteroid Equivalencies Comparison *on page 1017*
Corticosteroids, Topical Comparison *on page 1018*
Oral Nonviral Soft Tissue Ulcerations or Erosions *on page 955*
Respiratory Diseases *on page 924*

Brand Names Dalalone L.A.®; Decadron®; Decadron®-LA; Decaject-L.A.®; Dekasol-L.A.®; Dexasone L.A.®; Dexone®; Dexone L.A.®; Hexadrol®; I-Methasone®; Solurex L.A.®

Canadian/Mexican Brand Names Alin® (Mexico); Alin® Depot (Mexico); Decadronal® (Mexico); Decorex® (Mexico); Dibasona® (Mexico)

Therapeutic Category Antiemetic; Anti-inflammatory Agent; Corticosteroid, Inhalant; Corticosteroid, Ophthalmic; Corticosteroid, Systemic; Corticosteroid, Topical (Low Potency)

Use

Dental: Treatment of a variety of oral diseases of allergic, inflammatory or autoimmune origin

Medical: Systemically and locally for chronic swelling, allergic, hematologic, neoplastic, and autoimmune diseases; may be used in management of cerebral edema, septic shock, as a diagnostic agent, antiemetic

Usual Dosage

Children: Anti-inflammatory immunosuppressant: Oral, I.M., I.V. (injections should be given as sodium phosphate): 0.08-0.3 mg/kg/day or 2.5-10 mg/m^2/day in divided doses every 6-12 hours

Adults: Anti-inflammatory:

Oral, I.M., I.V. (injections should be given as sodium phosphate): 0.5-9 mg/day in divided doses every 6-12 hours

I.M. (as acetate): 8-16 mg; may repeat in 1-3 weeks

Intralesional (as acetate): 0.8-1.6 mg

Mechanism of Action Decreases inflammation by suppression of migration of polymorphonuclear leukocytes and reversal of increased capillary permeability; suppresses normal immune response

Local Anesthetic/Vasoconstrictor Precautions No information available to require special precautions

Effects on Dental Treatment No effects or complications reported

Other Adverse Effects >10%:

Central nervous system: Insomnia, nervousness

Gastrointestinal: Increased appetite, indigestion

Oral manifestations: No data reported

Contraindications Active untreated infections; viral, fungal, or tuberculosis; diseases of the eye

Warnings/Precautions Fatalities have occurred due to adrenal insufficiency in asthmatic patients during and after transfer from systemic corticosteroids to aerosol steroids; aerosol steroids do **not** provide the systemic steroid needed to treat patients having trauma, surgery, or infections; use with caution in patients with hypothyroidism, cirrhosis, hypertension, congestive heart failure, ulcerative colitis, thromboembolic disorders. Because of the risk of adverse effects, systemic corticosteroids should be used cautiously in the elderly in the smallest possible dose and for the shortest possible time.

Drug Interactions Barbiturates, phenytoin, rifampin cause decrease in dexamethasone effects; dexamethasone decreases effect of salicylates, vaccines, toxoids

Drug Uptake
Absorption: Rapid and complete
Time to peak serum concentration:
Oral: Within 1-2 hours
I.M.: Within 8 hours
Duration of metabolic effect: Can last for 72 hours; acetate is a long-acting repository preparation with a prompt onset of action
Serum half-life:
Normal renal function: 1.8-3.5 hours
Biological half-life: 36-54 hours

Pregnancy Risk Factor C

Breast-feeding Considerations No data reported

Dosage Forms
Elixir: 0.5 mg/5 mL (5 mL, 20 mL, 100 mL, 120 mL, 237 mL, 240 mL, 500 mL)
Injection, as acetate suspension: 8 mg/mL (1 mL, 5 mL); 16 mg/mL (1 mL, 5 mL)
Injection, as sodium phosphate: 4 mg/mL (1 mL, 5 mL, 10 mL, 25 mL, 30 mL); 10 mg/mL (1 mL, 10 mL); 20 mg/mL (5 mL); 24 mg/mL (5 mL, 10 mL)
Solution, oral:
Concentrate: 0.5 mg/0.5 mL (30 mL) (30% alcohol)
Oral: 0.5 mg/5 mL (5 mL, 20 mL, 500 mL)
Tablet: 0.25 mg, 0.5 mg, 0.75 mg, 1 mg, 1.5 mg, 2 mg, 4 mg, 6 mg
Tablet, therapeutic pack: 6 x 1.5 mg; 8 x 0.75 mg

Dietary Considerations May be taken with meals to decrease GI upset; limit caffeine; may need diet with increased potassium, pyridoxine, vitamin C, vitamin D, folate, calcium, and phosphorus

Generic Available Yes

Dexamethasone and Neomycin *see* Neomycin and Dexamethasone *on page 609*

Dexasone L.A.® *see* Dexamethasone *on previous page*

Dexasporin® *see* Neomycin, Polymyxin B, and Dexamethasone *on page 610*

Dexatrim® **[OTC]** *see* Phenylpropanolamine Hydrochloride *on page 687*

Dexbrompheniramine and Pseudoephedrine
(deks brom fen eer' a meen & soo doe e fed' rin)

Brand Names Disobrom® [OTC]; Disophrol® Chrontabs® [OTC]; Disophrol® Tablet [OTC]; Drixoral® [OTC]; Histrodrix® [OTC]; Resporal® [OTC]

Therapeutic Category Antihistamine/Decongestant Combination

Synonyms Pseudoephedrine and Dexbrompheniramine

Use Relief of symptoms of upper respiratory mucosal congestion in seasonal and perennial nasal allergies, acute rhinitis, rhinosinusitis and eustachian tube blockage

Local Anesthetic/Vasoconstrictor Precautions Use with caution since pseudoephedrine is a sympathomimetic amine which could interact with epinephrine to cause a pressor response

Effects on Dental Treatment Up to 10% of patients could experience tachycardia, palpitations, and dry mouth; use vasoconstrictor with caution

Dexchlor® *see* Dexchlorpheniramine Maleate *on this page*

Dexchlorpheniramine Maleate
(deks klor fen eer' a meen mal' ee ate)

Brand Names Dexchlor®; Poladex®; Polaramine®; Polargen®

Therapeutic Category Antihistamine

Synonyms Dextroclorofeniramina (Mexico)

Use Perennial and seasonal allergic rhinitis and other allergic symptoms including urticaria
(Continued)

Dexchlorpheniramine Maleate *(Continued)*

Usual Dosage Oral:

Children:

2-5 years: 0.5 mg every 4-6 hours (do not use timed release)

6-11 years: 1 mg every 4-6 hours or 4 mg timed release at bedtime

Adults: 2 mg every 4-6 hours or 4-6 mg timed release at bedtime or every 8-10 hours

Mechanism of Action Competes with histamine for H_1-receptor sites on effector cells in the gastrointestinal tract, blood vessels, and respiratory tract

Local Anesthetic/Vasoconstrictor Precautions No information available to require special precautions

Effects on Dental Treatment Up to 10% of patients will complain of significant dry mouth and drowsiness. This will disappear with cessation of drug therapy.

Other Adverse Effects

>10%:

Central nervous system: Slight to moderate drowsiness

Miscellaneous: Thickening of bronchial secretions

1% to 10%:

Central nervous system: Headache, fatigue, nervousness, dizziness

Gastrointestinal: Appetite increase, weight increase, nausea, diarrhea, abdominal pain, dry mouth

Neuromuscular & skeletal: Arthralgia

Respiratory: Pharyngitis

<1%:

Cardiovascular: Edema, palpitations

Central nervous system: Depression, epistaxis

Dermatologic: Angioedema, photosensitivity, rash

Hepatic: Hepatitis

Neuromuscular & skeletal: Myalgia, paresthesia

Respiratory: Bronchospasm

Drug Interactions Alcohol and other sedative drugs will potentiate the sedative effects of dexchlorpheniramine

Drug Uptake

Duration: 3-6 hours

Absorption: Well absorbed from GI tract

Pregnancy Risk Factor B

Dexedrine® *see Dextroamphetamine Sulfate* *on page 265*

Dexfenfluramine Hydrochloride

Brand Names Redux®

Therapeutic Category Anorexiant

Synonyms S5614

Use Management of obesity (initial body mass >30 kg/m² or >27 kg/m² with other risk factors such as hypertension, diabetes, or hyperlipidemia); given as an adjunct to dietary restriction

Usual Dosage Oral: Adults: 15 mg 2 times/day with meals

Local Anesthetic/Vasoconstrictor Precautions Use vasoconstrictor with caution in patients taking fenfluramine; amphetamine like drugs enhance the sympathomimetic response of epinephrine and norepinephrine leading to potential hypertension and cardiotoxicity.

Effects on Dental Treatment No effects or complications reported

Contraindications Hypersensitivity to dexfenfluramine or fenfluramine, glaucoma, pulmonary hypertension or use of monoamine oxidase inhibitors within 2 weeks of dexfenfluramine; children, pregnancy, or nursing women

Warnings/Precautions Use with caution in patients with cardiac disease, renal or hepatic insufficiency, porphyria, drug abuse, psychiatric disorder, or organic causes for obesity

Drug Uptake

Peak serum levels: 2-4 hours

Serum half-life:

18 hours (dexfenfluramine)

30 hours (d-norfenfluramine)

Dosage Forms Capsule: 15 mg

Dexone® *see Dexamethasone* *on page 260*

Dexone L.A.® *see Dexamethasone* *on page 260*

Dexpanthenol (deks pan' the nole)
Brand Names Ilopan®; Ilopan-Choline®; Panthoderm® [OTC]
Therapeutic Category Gastrointestinal Agent, Stimulant
Use Prophylactic use to minimize paralytic ileus, treatment of postoperative distention
Usual Dosage
  Children and Adults: Relief of itching and aid in skin healing: Topical: Apply to affected area 1-2 times/day
  Adults:
    Relief of gas retention: Oral: 2-3 tablets 3 times/day
    Prevention of postoperative ileus: I.M.: 250-500 mg stat, repeat in 2 hours, followed by doses every 6 hours until danger passes
    Paralyzed ileus: I.M.: 500 mg stat, repeat in 2 hours, followed by doses every 6 hours, if needed
Mechanism of Action A pantothenic acid B vitamin analog that is converted to coenzyme A internally; coenzyme A is essential to normal fatty acid synthesis, amino acid synthesis and acetylation of choline in the production of the neurotransmitter, acetylcholine
Local Anesthetic/Vasoconstrictor Precautions No information available to require special precautions
Effects on Dental Treatment No effects or complications reported
Other Adverse Effects <1%:
  Cardiovascular: Slight drop in blood pressure
  Central nervous system: Tingling
  Dermatologic: Dermatitis, urticaria
  Gastrointestinal: Vomiting, diarrhea, hyperperistalsis
  Hematologic: Prolonged bleeding time
  Local: Irritation
  Respiratory: Dyspnea
Drug Interactions Increased/prolonged effect of succinylcholine (do not administer within 1 hour)
Drug Uptake
  Absorption: Well absorbed
Pregnancy Risk Factor C

Dexrazoxane (deks ray zoks' ane)
Brand Names Zinecard®
Therapeutic Category Cardioprotective Agent
Use Prevention of cardiomyopathy associated with doxorubicin administration
Usual Dosage Adults: I.V.: The recommended dosage ratio of dexrazoxane:doxorubicin is 10:1 (eg, 500 mg/m^2 dexrazoxane:50 mg/m^2 doxorubicin). Administer the reconstituted solution by slow I.V. push or rapid IV infusion from a bag. After completing the infusion, and prior to a total elapsed time of 30 minutes (from the beginning of the dexrazoxane infusion), give the I.V. injection of doxorubicin.
Mechanism of Action As the D(+)-isomer of razoxane and a cyclic piperazine EDTA derivative, dexrazoxane is believed to exhibit cardioprotective effects secondary to its antioxidant activity; it inhibits free radical formation by chelating iron, thus reducing the cardiotoxicity of doxorubicin without affecting antitumor activity. Some data suggest that it has its own antitumor activity by blocking the entry of phytohemagglutinin-synchronized human lymphocytes into mitosis, thereby causing a phase-specific inhibition of cell growth and a cytostatic effect. It may additionally act as an alkylating agent, itself.
Local Anesthetic/Vasoconstrictor Precautions No information available to require special precautions
Effects on Dental Treatment No effects or complications reported
Drug Uptake
  Serum half-life: 2.1-2.5 hours
Pregnancy Risk Factor C

Dextran (deks' tran)
Brand Names Gentran®; LMD®; Macrodex®; Rheomacrodex®
Canadian/Mexican Brand Names Alpha-Dextrano"40" (Mexico)
Therapeutic Category Plasma Volume Expander
Synonyms Dextran 40; Dextran 70; Dextran, High Molecular Weight; Dextran, Low Molecular Weight
Use Fluid replacement and blood volume expander used in the treatment of hypovolemia, shock, or near shock states
Usual Dosage I.V.: (requires an infusion pump):
  Children: Total dose should not be >20 mL/kg during first 24 hours
(Continued)

Dextran *(Continued)*

Adults: 500-1000 mL at rate of 20-40 mL/minute; if therapy continues beyond 24 hours, total daily dosage should not exceed 10 mL/kg and therapy should not continue beyond 5 days

Mechanism of Action Produces plasma volume expansion by virtue of its highly colloidal starch structure, similar to albumin

Local Anesthetic/Vasoconstrictor Precautions No information available to require special precautions

Effects on Dental Treatment No effects or complications reported

Other Adverse Effects <1%:
Cardiovascular: Mild hypotension, tightness of chest
Central nervous system: Fever
Dermatologic: Urticaria
Gastrointestinal: Nausea, vomiting
Neuromuscular & skeletal: Arthralgia
Respiratory: Nasal congestion, wheezing
Miscellaneous: Anaphylaxis

Drug Uptake
Onset of action: I.V.: Within minutes to 1 hour (depending upon the molecular weight polysaccharide administered), infusion volume expansion occurs

Pregnancy Risk Factor C

Comments Dextran 40 is known as low molecular weight dextran (LMD) and has an average molecular weight of 40,000; dextran 75 has an average molecular weight of 75,000

Dextran 1 (deks' tran won)

Brand Names Promit®

Therapeutic Category Plasma Volume Expander

Use Prophylaxis of serious anaphylactic reactions to I.V. infusion of dextran

Usual Dosage I.V. (time between dextran 1 and dextran solution should not exceed 15 minutes):
Children: 0.3 mL/kg 1-2 minutes before I.V. infusion of dextran
Adults: 20 mL 1-2 minutes before I.V. infusion of dextran

Mechanism of Action Binds to dextran-reactive immunoglobulin without bridge formation and no formation of large immune complexes

Local Anesthetic/Vasoconstrictor Precautions No information available to require special precautions

Effects on Dental Treatment No effects or complications reported

Other Adverse Effects <1%:
Cardiovascular: Mild hypotension, tightness of chest
Central nervous system: Fever
Dermatologic: Urticaria
Gastrointestinal: Nausea, vomiting
Local: Cutaneous reactions
Neuromuscular & skeletal: Arthralgia
Respiratory: Nasal congestion, wheezing

Pregnancy Risk Factor C

Dextran 40 *see Dextran on previous page*

Dextran 70 *see Dextran on previous page*

Dextran, High Molecular Weight *see Dextran on previous page*

Dextran, Low Molecular Weight *see Dextran on previous page*

Dextranomer (deks tran' oh mer)

Brand Names Debrisan® [OTC]

Therapeutic Category Topical Skin Product

Use Clean exudative wounds; no controlled studies have found dextranomer to be more effective than conventional therapy

Usual Dosage Debride and clean wound prior to application; apply to affected area every 12 hours or more frequent as needed; removal should be done by irrigation

Mechanism of Action Dextranomer is a network of dextran-sucrose beads possessing a great many exposed hydroxy groups; when this network is applied to an exudative wound surface, the exudate is drawn by capillary forces generated by the swelling of the beads, with vacuum forces producing an upward flow of exudate into the network

Local Anesthetic/Vasoconstrictor Precautions No information available to require special precautions

Effects on Dental Treatment No effects or complications reported

Other Adverse Effects 1% to 10%: Local: Maceration may occur, transitory pain, bleeding, blistering, erythema
Drug Interactions No data reported
Pregnancy Risk Factor C

Dextroamphetamine Sulfate (deks troe am fet′ a meen sul′ fate)

Brand Names Dexedrine®; Ferndex; Oxydess® II; Spancap® No. 1
Therapeutic Category Amphetamine; Anorexiant; Central Nervous System Stimulant, Amphetamine
Use Narcolepsy, exogenous obesity, abnormal behavioral syndrome in children (minimal brain dysfunction), attention deficit hyperactive disorder (ADHD)
Usual Dosage Oral:
Children:
Narcolepsy: 6-12 years: Initial: 5 mg/day, may increase at 5 mg increments in weekly intervals until side effects appear; maximum dose: 60 mg/day
Attention deficit disorder:
3-5 years: Initial: 2.5 mg/day given every morning; increase by 2.5 mg/day in weekly intervals until optimal response is obtained, usual range: 0.1-0.5 mg/kg/dose every morning with maximum of 40 mg/day
≥6 years: 5 mg once or twice daily; increase in increments of 5 mg/day at weekly intervals until optimal response is reached, usual range: 0.1-0.5 mg/kg/dose every morning (5-20 mg/day) with maximum of 40 mg/day
Children >12 years and Adults:
Narcolepsy: Initial: 10 mg/day, may increase at 10 mg increments in weekly intervals until side effects appear; maximum: 60 mg/day
Exogenous obesity: 5-30 mg/day in divided doses of 5-10 mg 30-60 minutes before meals
Mechanism of Action Blocks reuptake of dopamine and norepinephrine from the synapse, thus increases the amount of circulating dopamine and norepinephrine in cerebral cortex to reticular activating system; inhibits the action of monoamine oxidase and causes catecholamines to be released
Local Anesthetic/Vasoconstrictor Precautions Use vasoconstriction with caution in patients taking dextroamphetamine. Amphetamines enhance the sympathomimetic response of epinephrine and norepinephrine leading to potential hypertension and cardiotoxicity.
Effects on Dental Treatment Up to 10% of patients taking dextroamphetamines may present with hypertension. The use of local anesthetic without vasoconstrictor is recommended in these patients.
Other Adverse Effects
>10%:
Cardiovascular: Irregular heartbeat
Central nervous system: False feeling of well being, nervousness, restlessness, insomnia
1% to 10%:
Cardiovascular: Hypertension
Central nervous system: Mood or mental changes, dizziness, lightheadedness, headache
Endocrine & metabolic: Changes in libido
Gastrointestinal: Diarrhea, nausea, vomiting, stomach cramps, constipation, anorexia, weight loss, dry mouth
Ocular: Blurred vision
Miscellaneous: Increased sweating
<1%:
Cardiovascular: Chest pain
Central nervous system: CNS stimulation (severe), Tourette's syndrome, hyperthermia, seizures, paranoia
Dermatologic: Skin rash, hives
Miscellaneous: Tolerance and withdrawal with prolonged use
Drug Interactions
Adrenergic blockers are inhibited by amphetamines
Amphetamines enhance the activity of tricyclic or sympathomimetic agents
MAO Inhibitors slow the metabolism of amphetamines
Amphetamines will counteract the sedative effects of antihistamines
Amphetamines potentiate the analgesic effects of meperidine
Drug Uptake
Onset of action: 1-1.5 hours
Serum half-life: Adults: 34 hours (pH dependent)
Time to peak serum concentration: Oral: Within 3 hours
Pregnancy Risk Factor C

Dextroclorofeniramina (Mexico) see Dexchlorpheniramine Maleate on page 261

Dextromethorphan (deks troe meth or' fan)

Brand Names Benylin® DM [OTC]; Children's Hold® [OTC]; Delsym® [OTC]; Hold® DM [OTC]; Pertussin® CS [OTC]; Pertussin® ES [OTC]; Robitussin® Cough Calmers [OTC]; Robitussin® Pediatric [OTC]; Scot-Tussin® DM Cough Chasers [OTC]; St. Joseph® Cough Suppressant [OTC]; Sucrets® Cough Calmers [OTC]; Suppress® [OTC]; Trocal® [OTC]; Vicks Formula 44® [OTC]; Vicks Formula 44® Pediatric Formula [OTC]

Canadian/Mexican Brand Names Balminil-DM® (Canada)

Therapeutic Category Antitussive

Synonyms Dextrometorfano (Mexico)

Use Symptomatic relief of coughs caused by minor viral upper respiratory tract infections or inhaled irritants; most effective for a chronic nonproductive cough

Usual Dosage Oral:

Children:

<2 years: Use only as directed by a physician

2-6 years (syrup): 2.5-7.5 mg every 4-8 hours; extended release is 15 mg twice daily (maximum: 30 mg/24 hours)

6-12 years: 5-10 mg every 4 hours or 15 mg every 6-8 hours; extended release is 30 mg twice daily (maximum: 60 mg/24 hours)

Children >12 years and Adults: 10-30 mg every 4-8 hours or 30 mg every 6-8 hours; extended release is 60 mg twice daily (maximum: 120 mg/24 hours)

Mechanism of Action Chemical relative of morphine lacking narcotic properties except in overdose; controls cough by depressing the medullary cough center

Local Anesthetic/Vasoconstrictor Precautions No information available to require special precautions

Effects on Dental Treatment No effects or complications reported

Other Adverse Effects <1%:

Central nervous system: Drowsiness, dizziness, coma, respiratory depression

Gastrointestinal: Nausea, GI upset, constipation, abdominal discomfort

Drug Interactions No data reported

Drug Uptake

Onset of antitussive action: Within 15-30 minutes

Duration: Up to 6 hours

Pregnancy Risk Factor C

Dextrometorfano (Mexico) see Dextromethorphan on this page

Dextrose, Levulose and Phosphoric Acid see Phosphorated Carbohydrate Solution on page 690

Dextrothyroxine Sodium (deks troe thye rox' een sow' dee um)

Brand Names Choloxin®

Therapeutic Category Lipid Lowering Drugs

Use Reduction of elevated serum cholesterol

Usual Dosage Oral:

Children: 0.05 mg/kg/day, increase at 1-month intervals by 0.05 mg/kg/day to a maximum of 0.4 mg/kg/day or 4 mg/day

Adults: 1-2 mg/day, increase at 1-2 mg at intervals of 4 weeks, up to a maximum of 8 mg/day

Mechanism of Action Unclear mechanism, thought to increase the liver breakdown of cholesterol

Local Anesthetic/Vasoconstrictor Precautions No information available to require special precautions

Effects on Dental Treatment No effects or complications reported

Other Adverse Effects <1%:

Cardiovascular: Myocardial infarction, angina, arrhythmias

Central nervous system: Insomnia, headache

Dermatologic: Hair loss, skin rash

Gastrointestinal: Weight loss

Neuromuscular & skeletal: Tremor, paresthesia

Ocular: Visual disturbances

Otic: Tinnitus

Miscellaneous: Sweating

Drug Interactions

Decreased effect of beta-blockers, digitalis, hypoglycemics; decreased effect with cholestyramine

Increased effect of anticoagulants

Drug Uptake

Absorption: Poorly absorbed from GI tract (25%)

Serum half-life: 18 hours

Pregnancy Risk Factor C

Dey-Dose® Isoproterenol *see* Isoproterenol *on page 472*

Dey-Dose® Metaproterenol *see* Metaproterenol Sulfate *on page 550*

Dey-Lute® Isoetharine *see* Isoetharine *on page 470*

Dezocine (dez' oh seen)

Related Information
Narcotic Agonist Charts *on page 1019*

Brand Names Dalgan®

Therapeutic Category Analgesic, Narcotic

Use Relief of moderate to severe postoperative, acute renal and ureteral colic, and cancer pain

Usual Dosage Adults (not recommended for patients <18 years):
I.M.: Initial: 5-20 mg; may be repeated every 3-6 hours as needed; maximum: 120 mg/day and 20 mg/dose
I.V.: Initial: 2.5-10 mg; may be repeated every 2-4 hours as needed

Mechanism of Action Binds to opiate receptors in the CNS, causing inhibition of ascending pain pathways, altering the perception of and response to pain; produces generalized CNS depression; it is a mixed agonist-antagonist that appears to bind selectively to CNS μ and Δ opiate receptors

Local Anesthetic/Vasoconstrictor Precautions No information available to require special precautions

Effects on Dental Treatment No effects or complications reported

Other Adverse Effects
1% to 10%:
Central nervous system: Sedation, dizziness, vertigo
Gastrointestinal: Nausea, vomiting
Local: Injection site reactions
<1%:
Cardiovascular: Hypotension, palpitations, bradycardia, peripheral vasodilation
Central nervous system: Increased intracranial pressure, CNS depression, drowsiness
Endocrine & metabolic: Antidiuretic hormone release
Gastrointestinal: Constipation
Ocular: Miosis
Respiratory: Respiratory depression
Miscellaneous: Biliary or urinary tract spasm, histamine release, physical and psychological dependence with prolonged use

Drug Interactions Increased effect with CNS depressants

Drug Uptake
Onset of analgesia: Within 15-30 minutes
Duration of analgesia: 4-6 hours
Serum half-life: 2.6-2.8 hours

Pregnancy Risk Factor C

DHAD *see* Mitoxantrone Hydrochloride *on page 586*

DHC Plus® *see* Dihydrocodeine, Acetaminophen, and Aspirin *on page 281*

D.H.E. 45® *see* Dihydroergotamine Mesylate *on page 283*

DHS® Tar [OTC] *see* Coal Tar *on page 225*

DHS Zinc® [OTC] *see* Pyrithione Zinc *on page 755*

DHT™ *see* Dihydrotachysterol *on page 283*

Diaβeta® *see* Glyburide *on page 401*

Diabetic Tussin® DM [OTC] *see* Guaifenesin and Dextromethorphan *on page 408*

Diabinese® *see* Chlorpropamide *on page 197*

Dialose® [OTC] *see* Docusate *on page 295*

Dialose® Plus Capsule [OTC] *see* Docusate and Casanthranol *on page 295*

Dialose® Plus Tablet [OTC] *see* Docusate and Phenolphthalein *on page 295*

Dialume® [OTC] *see* Aluminum Hydroxide *on page 39*

Diamine T.D.® [OTC] *see* Brompheniramine Maleate *on page 124*

Diamox® *see* Acetazolamide *on page 18*

Diamox® Sequels® *see* Acetazolamide *on page 18*

Diaparene® [OTC] *see* Methylbenzethonium Chloride *on page 566*

Diapid® *see* Lypressin *on page 519*

Diasorb® [OTC] *see* Attapulgite *on page 86*

Diazepam (dye az' e pam)

Related Information
Dental Drug Interactions: Update on Drug Combinations Requiring Special Considerations *on page 1022*
Patients Requiring Sedation *on page 965*
Temporomandibular Dysfunction (TMD) *on page 963*

Brand Names Valium®; Valrelease®; Zetran® Injection

Canadian/Mexican Brand Names Apo-Diazepam® (Canada); Diazemuls® (Canada); E Pam® (Canada); Meval® (Canada); Novo-Dipam® (Canada); PMS®-Diazepam (Canada); Vivol® (Canada)

Therapeutic Category Antianxiety Agent; Anticonvulsant, Benzodiazepine; Muscle Relaxant; Sedative; Skeletal Muscle Relaxant; Tranquilizer, Minor

Use
Dental: Oral medication for preoperative dental anxiety; sedative component in I.V. conscious sedation in oral surgery patients; skeletal muscle relaxant
Medical: In medicine, management of general anxiety disorders, panic disorders, and provide preoperative sedation, light anesthesia, and amnesia; treatment of status epilepticus, alcohol withdrawal symptoms; used as a skeletal muscle relaxant

Usual Dosage
Children: Oral:
Conscious sedation for procedures: 0.2-0.3 mg/kg (maximum: 10 mg) 45-60 minutes prior to procedure
Sedation or muscle relaxation or anxiety: 0.12-0.8 mg/kg/day in divided doses every 6-8 hours the day before the procedure
Adults:
Oral: Preop sedation/antianxiety: 2-10 mg 2 times/day the day before the procedure; 2-10 mg morning of procedure if needed
I.V.: Conscious sedation: 5-15 mg titrated slowly to effect

Mechanism of Action Depresses all levels of the CNS, including the limbic and reticular formation, probably through the increased action of gamma-aminobutyric acid (GABA), which is a major inhibitory neurotransmitter in the brain

Local Anesthetic/Vasoconstrictor Precautions No information available to require special precautions

Effects on Dental Treatment No effects or complications reported

Other Adverse Effects
>10%:
Central nervous system: Drowsiness, ataxia, amnesia, slurred speech, lightheadedness
Local: Phlebitis, pain with injection
1% to 10%: Central nervous system: Confusion, dizziness

Oral manifestations: >10%: Dry mouth, changes in salivation

Contraindications Hypersensitivity to diazepam or any component; there may be a cross-sensitivity with other benzodiazepines; do not use in a comatose patient, in those with pre-existing CNS depression, respiratory depression, narrow-angle glaucoma, or severe uncontrolled pain; do not use in pregnant women

Warnings/Precautions Use with caution in patients receiving other CNS depressants, patients with low albumin, hepatic dysfunction, and in the elderly and young infants. Due to its long-acting metabolite, diazepam is not considered a drug of choice in the elderly; long-acting benzodiazepines have been associated with falls in the elderly.

Drug Interactions Enzyme inducers may increase the metabolism of diazepam; CNS depressants (alcohol, barbiturates, opioids) may enhance sedation and respiratory depression; cimetidine may decrease the metabolism of diazepam; cisapride can significantly increase diazepam levels; valproic acid may displace diazepam from binding sites which may result in an increase in sedative effects; selective serotonin reuptake inhibitors (eg, fluoxetine, sertraline, paroxetine) have greatly increased diazepam levels by altering its clearance

Drug Uptake
Absorption: Oral: 85% to 100%, more reliable than I.M.
Time to peak serum concentration: 0.5-2 hours
Serum half-life:
Parent drug: Adults: 20-50 hours, increased half-life in neonates, elderly, and those with severe hepatic disorders
Active major metabolite (desmethyldiazepam): 50-100 hours, can be prolonged in neonates

Pregnancy Risk Factor D

Breast-feeding Considerations Not compatible
Dosage Forms
Capsule, sustained release (Valrelease®): 15 mg
Injection: 5 mg/mL (1 mL, 2 mL, 5 mL, 10 mL)
Solution, oral (wintergreen-spice flavor): 5 mg/5 mL (5 mL, 10 mL, 500 mL)
Solution, oral concentrate: 5 mg/mL (30 mL)
Tablet: 2 mg, 5 mg, 10 mg
Dietary Considerations May be taken with food or water
Generic Available Yes

Diazoxide (dye az ox′ ide)
Brand Names Hyperstat® I.V.; Proglycem®
Canadian/Mexican Brand Names Sefulken® (Mexico)
Therapeutic Category Antihypertensive; Antihypoglycemic Agent
Synonyms Diazoxido (Mexico)
Use
Oral: Hypoglycemia related to islet cell adenoma, carcinoma, hyperplasia, or adenomatosis, nesidioblastosis, leucine sensitivity, or extrapancreatic malignancy
I.V.: Emergency lowering of blood pressure
Usual Dosage
Hypertension: Children and Adults: I.V.: 1-3 mg/kg up to a maximum of 150 mg in a single injection; repeat dose in 5-15 minutes until blood pressure adequately reduced; repeat administration at intervals of 4-24 hours; monitor the blood pressure closely; do not use longer than 10 days
Hyperinsulinemic hypoglycemia: Oral: **Note:** Use lower dose listed as initial dose
Children and Adults: 3-8 mg/kg/day in divided doses every 8-12 hours
Mechanism of Action Inhibits insulin release from the pancreas; produces direct smooth muscle relaxation of the peripheral arterioles which results in decrease in blood pressure and reflex increase in heart rate and cardiac output
Local Anesthetic/Vasoconstrictor Precautions No information available to require special precautions
Effects on Dental Treatment No effects or complications reported
Other Adverse Effects
1% to 10%:
Cardiovascular: Hypotension
Central nervous system: Dizziness
Gastrointestinal: Nausea, vomiting
Neuromuscular & skeletal: Weakness
<1%:
Cardiovascular: Tachycardia, flushing
Central nervous system: Seizures, headache, extrapyramidal symptoms and development of abnormal facies with chronic oral use
Dermatologic: Rash, hirsutism
Endocrine & metabolic: Hyperglycemia, ketoacidosis, sodium and water retention, hyperuricemia
Gastrointestinal: Anorexia, constipation
Hematologic: Leukopenia, thrombocytopenia
Local: Pain, burning, cellulitis/phlebitis upon extravasation
Miscellaneous: Inhibition of labor
Drug Interactions
Decreased effect: Diazoxide may increase phenytoin metabolism or free fraction
Increased toxicity:
Diuretics and hypotensive agents may potentiate diazoxide adverse effects
Diazoxide may decrease warfarin protein binding
Drug Uptake
Hyperglycemic effect: Oral:
Onset of action: Within 1 hour
Duration (normal renal function): 8 hours
Hypotensive effect: I.V.:
Peak: Within 5 minutes
Duration: Usually 3-12 hours
Serum half-life:
Children: 9-24 hours
Adults: 20-36 hours
End stage renal disease: >30 hours
Pregnancy Risk Factor C

Diazoxido (Mexico) *see* Diazoxide *on this page*

Dibent® *see* Dicyclomine Hydrochloride *on page 273*
Dibenzyline® *see* Phenoxybenzamine Hydrochloride *on page 682*

Dibucaine (dye´ byoo kane)
Brand Names Nupercainal® [OTC]
Therapeutic Category Local Anesthetic, Topical
Use
Dental: Amide derivative local anesthetic for minor skin conditions
Medical: Fast, temporary relief of pain and itching due to hemorrhoids, minor burns
Usual Dosage Children and Adults: Topical: Apply gently to the affected areas; no more than 30 g for adults or 7.5 g for children should be used in any 24-hour period
Mechanism of Action Local anesthetics bind selectively to the intracellular surface of sodium channels to block influx of sodium into the axon. As a result, depolarization necessary for action potential propagation and subsequent nerve function is prevented. The block at the sodium channel is reversible. When drug diffuses away from the axon, sodium channel function is restored and nerve propagation returns.
Local Anesthetic/Vasoconstrictor Precautions No information available to require special precautions
Effects on Dental Treatment No effects or complications reported
Other Adverse Effects 1% to 10%:
Local: Burning
Dermatologic: Angioedema, contact dermatitis

Oral manifestations: No data reported
Contraindications Known hypersensitivity to amide-type anesthetics, ophthalmic use
Warnings/Precautions Avoid use in sensitive individuals
Drug Interactions No data reported
Drug Uptake
Absorption: Poor through intact skin, but well absorbed through mucous membranes and excoriated skin
Onset of action: Within 15 minutes
Duration: 2-4 hours
Pregnancy Risk Factor C
Breast-feeding Considerations No data reported; however, topical administration is probably compatible
Dosage Forms
Cream, topical: 0.5% (45 g)
Ointment, topical: 1% (30 g, 60 g, 454 g)
Dietary Considerations No data reported
Generic Available Yes

Dibucaine and Hydrocortisone
(dye´ byoo kane & hye droe kor´ ti sone)
Brand Names Corticaine® Topical
Therapeutic Category Corticosteroid, Topical (Low Potency); Local Anesthetic, Topical
Synonyms Hydrocortisone and Dibucaine
Use Relief of the inflammatory and pruritic manifestations of corticosteroid-responsive dermatoses and for external anal itching
Local Anesthetic/Vasoconstrictor Precautions No information available to require special precautions
Effects on Dental Treatment No effects or complications reported

DIC *see* Dacarbazine *on page 247*
Dicarbosil® [OTC] *see* Calcium Carbonate *on page 140*

Dichlorodifluoromethane and Trichloromonofluoromethane
(dye klor oh dye flor oh meth´ ane & tri klor oh mon oh flor oh meth´ ane)
Related Information
Temporomandibular Dysfunction (TMD) *on page 963*
Brand Names Fluori-Methane®
Therapeutic Category Local Anesthetic, Topical
Use
Dental: Topical application in the management of myofascial pain, restricted motion, and muscle spasm
Medical: For the control of pain associated with injections

Usual Dosage Invert bottle over treatment area approximately 12" away from site of application; open dispenseal spring valve completely, allowing liquid to flow in a stream from the bottle. The rate of spraying is approximately 10 cm/second and should be continued until entire muscle has been covered.

Local Anesthetic/Vasoconstrictor Precautions No information available to require special precautions

Effects on Dental Treatment No effects or complications reported

Other Adverse Effects No data reported

Oral manifestations: No data reported

Contraindications In individuals with a history of hypersensitivity to dichlorofluoromethane and/or trichloromonofluoromethane; should not be used on patients having vascular impairment of the extremities

Warnings/Precautions For external use only; care should be taken to minimize inhalation of vapors, especially with application to head and neck; avoid contact with eyes; should not be applied to the point of frost formation

Drug Interactions No data reported

Drug Uptake No data reported

Breast-feeding Considerations No data reported

Dosage Forms Spray: 4 oz amber glass bottles; calibrated fine spray and calibrated medium spray

Dietary Considerations No data reported

Generic Available No

Comments Dichlorodifluoromethane and trichloromonofluoromethane are not classified as carcinogens; based on animal studies and human experience, these fluorocarbons pose no hazard to man relative to systemic toxicity, carcinogenicity, mutagenicity, or teratogenicity when occupational exposures are <1000 ppm over an 8-hour time weighted average.

Dichlorotetrafluoroethane and Ethyl Chloride see Ethyl Chloride and Dichlorotetrafluoroethane on page 344

Dichlorphenamide (dye klor fen' a mide)
Brand Names Daranide®

Therapeutic Category Antiglaucoma Agent; Carbonic Anhydrase Inhibitor; Diuretic, Carbonic Anhydrase Inhibitor

Synonyms Diclofenamide

Use Adjunct in treatment of open-angle glaucoma and perioperative treatment for angle-closure glaucoma

Local Anesthetic/Vasoconstrictor Precautions No information available to require special precautions

Effects on Dental Treatment No effects or complications reported

Other Adverse Effects
>10%:
Central nervous system: Tiredness, malaise
Gastrointestinal: Diarrhea, anorexia, metallic taste
Genitourinary: Increased urination
1% to 10%:
Central nervous system: Mental depression, drowsiness
Renal: Renal calculi
<1%:
Central nervous system: Fever, fatigue
Dermatologic: Rash
Endocrine & metabolic: Hyperchloremic metabolic acidosis, hypokalemia,
Gastrointestinal: Black stools, GI irritation, dryness of the mouth
Genitourinary: Dysuria
Hematologic: Blood dyscrasias, elevation of blood glucose, bone marrow suppression
Neuromuscular & skeletal: Paresthesias
Ocular: Myopia

Diclofenac (dye kloe' fen ak)
Related Information
Nonsteroidal Anti-Inflammatory Agents, Comparative Dosages, and Pharmacokinetics on page 1021
Rheumatoid Arthritis, Osteoarthritis, and Joint Prostheses on page 930

Brand Names Cataflam®; Voltaren®

Canadian/Mexican Brand Names Apo-Diclo® (Canada); Novo-Difenac® (Canada); Novo-Difenac-SR® (Canada); Nu-Diclo® (Canada); Artrenac® (Mexico); Clonodifen® (Mexico); Dolo Pangavit D® (Mexico); Fustaren® Retard (Mexico); Galedol® (Mexico); Liroken® (Mexico)
(Continued)

Diclofenac *(Continued)*

Therapeutic Category Analgesic, Non-narcotic; Anti-inflammatory Agent; Nonsteroidal Anti-Inflammatory Agent (NSAID), Ophthalmic; Nonsteroidal Anti-inflammatory Agent (NSAID), Oral

Synonyms Diclofenaco (Mexico)

Use Acute treatment of mild to moderate pain; acute and chronic treatment of rheumatoid arthritis, ankylosing spondylitis, and osteoarthritis; used for juvenile rheumatoid arthritis, gout, dysmenorrhea; ophthalmic solution for the treatment of postoperative swelling in patients who have undergone cataract extraction and for the treatment of photophobia in patients undergoing incisional refractive surgery

Usual Dosage Adults:

Oral:

Analgesia (Cataflam®): Starting dose: 50 mg 3 times/day

Rheumatoid arthritis: 150-200 mg/day in 2-4 divided doses (100 mg/day of sustained release product)

Osteoarthritis: 100-150 mg/day in 2-3 divided doses (100-200 mg/day of sustained release product)

Ankylosing spondylitis: 100-125 mg/day in 4-5 divided doses

Ophthalmic: Instill 1 drop into affected eye 4 times/day beginning 24 hours after cataract surgery and continuing for 2 weeks

Mechanism of Action Inhibits prostaglandin synthesis by decreasing the activity of the enzyme, cyclo-oxygenase, which results in decreased formation of prostaglandin precursors

Local Anesthetic/Vasoconstrictor Precautions No information available to require special precautions

Effects on Dental Treatment No effects or complications reported

Other Adverse Effects

>10%:

Dermatologic: Skin rash

Gastrointestinal: Abdominal cramps, heartburn, indigestion, nausea

1% to 10%:

Cardiovascular: Angina pectoris, arrhythmias

Central nervous system: Dizziness, nervousness

Dermatologic: Skin rash, itching

Gastrointestinal: GI ulceration, vomiting

Genitourinary: Vaginal bleeding

Otic: Tinnitus

<1%:

Cardiovascular: Chest pain, congestive heart failure, hypertension, tachycardia

Central nervous system: Epistaxis, convulsions, forgetfulness, mental depression, drowsiness, nervousness, insomnia, weakness

Dermatologic: Hives, exfoliative dermatitis, erythema multiforme, Stevens-Johnson syndrome, angioedema

Gastrointestinal: Stomatitis

Genitourinary: Cystitis

Hematologic: Agranulocytosis, anemia, pancytopenia, leukopenia, thrombocytopenia

Hepatic: Hepatitis

Neuromuscular & skeletal: Peripheral neuropathy, trembling

Ocular: Blurred vision, change in vision

Otic: Decreased hearing

Renal: Interstitial nephritis, nephrotic syndrome, renal impairment

Respiratory: Wheezing, laryngeal edema, shortness of breath

Miscellaneous: Anaphylaxis, increased sweating

Drug Interactions

Decreased effect with aspirin; decreased effect of thiazides, furosemide

Increased toxicity of digoxin, methotrexate, cyclosporine, lithium, insulin, sulfonylureas, potassium-sparing diuretics, aspirin

Drug Uptake

Onset of action: Cataflam® has a more rapid onset of action than does the sodium salt (Voltaren®), because it is absorbed in the stomach instead of the duodenum

Serum half-life: 2 hours

Time to peak serum concentration:

Cataflam®: Within 1 hour

Voltaren®: Within 2 hours

Pregnancy Risk Factor B

Dosage Forms
Solution, ophthalmic, as sodium: 0.1% (2.5 mL, 5 mL)
Tablet, enteric coated, as sodium: 25 mg, 50 mg, 75 mg
Tablet, as potassium: 50 mg
Dietary Considerations May be taken with food to decrease GI distress
Generic Available No

Diclofenaco (Mexico) *see* Diclofenac *on page 271*
Diclofenamide *see* Dichlorphenamide *on page 271*

Dicloxacillin Sodium (dye klox a sil′ in sow′ dee um)
Related Information
Oral Bacterial Infections *on page 945*
Brand Names Dycill®; Dynapen®; Pathocil®
Canadian/Mexican Brand Names Brispen® (Mexico); Posipen® (Mexico)
Therapeutic Category Antibiotic, Penicillin
Use
Dental: Treatment of susceptible orofacial infections, notably penicillinase-producing staph
Medical: Treatment of systemic infections in the medical patient such as pneumonia, skin and soft tissue infections, and osteomyelitis caused by penicillinase-producing staphylococci
Usual Dosage Oral:
Children >40 kg and Adults: 250-500 mg every 6 hours for at least 7 days
Children <40 kg: 125-150 mg/kg/day divided every 6 hours
Mechanism of Action Interferes with bacterial cell wall synthesis during active multiplication, causing cell wall death and resultant bactericidal activity against susceptible bacteria
Local Anesthetic/Vasoconstrictor Precautions No information available to require special precautions
Effects on Dental Treatment Prolonged use of penicillins may lead to development of oral candidiasis
Other Adverse Effects 1% to 10%: Gastrointestinal: Diarrhea

Oral manifestations: No data reported
Contraindications Known hypersensitivity to dicloxacillin, penicillin, or any components
Warnings/Precautions Monitor PT if patient concurrently on warfarin; elimination of drug is slow in neonates; use with caution in patients allergic to cephalosporins; bad taste of suspension may make compliance difficult
Drug Interactions Efficacy of oral contraceptives may be reduced; disulfiram, probenecid causes increased penicillin levels; increased effect of anticoagulants
Drug Uptake
Absorption: 35% to 76% from GI tract; food decreases rate and extent of absorption
Time to peak serum concentration: Within 0.5-2 hours
Serum half-life: 0.6-0.8 hours
Pregnancy Risk Factor B
Breast-feeding Considerations No data reported; however, other penicillins may be taken while breast-feeding
Dosage Forms
Capsule: 125 mg, 250 mg, 500 mg
Powder for oral suspension: 62.5 mg/5 mL (80 mL, 100 mL, 200 mL)
Dietary Considerations Should be taken with water 1 hour before or 2 hours after meals on an empty stomach
Generic Available Yes
Comments Although dicloxacillin is a penicillin antibiotic indicated for infections caused by penicillinase secreting staph, amoxicillin with clavulanic acid is considered the drug of choice for these types of orofacial infections

Dicyclomine Hydrochloride
(dye sye′ kloe meen hye droe klor′ ide)
Brand Names Antispas®; Bemote®; Bentyl® Hydrochloride; Byclomine®; Dibent®; Di-Spaz®; Neoquess®; Or-Tyl®; Spasmoject®
Canadian/Mexican Brand Names Bentylol® (Canada)
Therapeutic Category Antispasmodic Agent, Gastrointestinal
Synonyms Dicycloverine Hydrochloride
Use Treatment of functional disturbances of GI motility such as irritable bowel syndrome

Unlabeled use: Urinary incontinence
(Continued)

273

Dicyclomine Hydrochloride *(Continued)*

Usual Dosage
Oral:
 Children: 10 mg/dose 3-4 times/day
 Adults: Begin with 80 mg/day in 4 equally divided doses, then increase up to 160 mg/day
 I.M. **(should not be used I.V.)**: Adults: 80 mg/day in 4 divided doses (20 mg/dose)

Mechanism of Action Blocks the action of acetylcholine at parasympathetic sites in smooth muscle, secretory glands and the CNS

Local Anesthetic/Vasoconstrictor Precautions No information available to require special precautions

Effects on Dental Treatment No effects or complications reported

Other Adverse Effects
>10%:
 Gastrointestinal: Constipation
 Local: Injection site reactions
 Miscellaneous: Decreased sweating; dry mouth, nose, throat, or skin
1% to 10%: Decreased flow of breast milk, difficulty in swallowing, blurred vision, increased sensitivity to light
<1%:
 Cardiovascular: Orthostatic hypotension, tachycardia, palpitations
 Central nervous system: Confusion, drowsiness, headache, lightheadedness, loss of memory, weakness, tiredness, seizures, coma, nervousness, excitement, insomnia
 Dermatologic: Skin rash
 Gastrointestinal: Bloated feeling, nausea, vomiting
 Genitourinary: Difficult urination, urinary retention
 Neuromuscular & skeletal: Muscular hypotonia
 Ocular: Increased intraocular pain
 Respiratory: Asphyxia, respiratory distress

Drug Interactions
Decreased effect: Phenothiazines, anti-Parkinson's drugs, haloperidol, sustained release dosage forms; decreased effect with antacids
Increased toxicity: Anticholinergics, amantadine, narcotic analgesics, type I antiarrhythmics, antihistamines, phenothiazines, TCAs

Drug Uptake
Onset of effect: 1-2 hours
Duration: Up to 4 hours
Absorption: Oral: Well absorbed
Serum half-life:
 Initial phase: 1.8 hours
 Terminal phase: 9-10 hours

Pregnancy Risk Factor B

Dicycloverine Hydrochloride see Dicyclomine Hydrochloride *on previous page*
Didanosina (Mexico) see Didanosine *on this page*

Didanosine (dye dan' oh seen)
Related Information
Systemic Viral Diseases *on page 934*

Brand Names Videx®
Therapeutic Category Antiviral Agent, Oral
Synonyms Didanosina (Mexico)
Use Treatment of advanced HIV infection in patients who are intolerant of zidovudine therapy or who have demonstrated significant clinical or immunologic deterioration during zidovudine therapy
Usual Dosage Oral (administer on an empty stomach):
 Children: 180 mg/m^2/day divided every 12 hours **or** dosing is based on body surface area (m^2): See table.

Didanosine — Pediatric Dosing

Body Surface Area (m^2)	Dosing (Tablets) (mg bid)
≤0.4	25
0.5-0.7	50
0.8-1	75
1.1-1.4	100

Adults: Dosing is based on patient weight: See table.

Didanosine — Adult Dosing

Patient Weight (kg)	Dosing (Tablets) (mg bid)
35-49	125
50-74	200
≥75	300

Note: Children >1 year and Adults should receive 2 tablets per dose and children <1 year should receive 1 tablet per dose for adequate buffering and absorption; tablets should be chewed

Mechanism of Action Didanosine, a purine nucleoside analogue and the deamination product of dideoxyadenosine (ddA), inhibits HIV replication *in vitro* in both T cells and monocytes. Didanosine is converted within the cell to the mono-, di-, and triphosphates of ddA. These ddA triphosphates act as substrate and inhibitor of HIV reverse transcriptase substrate and inhibitor of HIV reverse transcriptase thereby blocking viral DNA synthesis and suppressing HIV replication.

Local Anesthetic/Vasoconstrictor Precautions No information available to require special precautions

Effects on Dental Treatment No effects or complications reported

Other Adverse Effects

>10%:
  Central nervous system: Anxiety, headache, irritability, insomnia, restlessness
  Gastrointestinal: Abdominal pain, nausea, diarrhea
  Neuromuscular & skeletal: Peripheral neuropathy

1% to 10%:
  Central nervous system: Depression
  Dermatologic: Rash, pruritus
  Gastrointestinal: Pancreatitis

<1%:
  Central nervous system: Seizures
  Hematologic: Anemia, granulocytopenia, leukopenia, thrombocytopenia
  Hepatic: Hepatitis
  Ocular: Retinal depigmentation
  Renal: Renal impairment
  Miscellaneous: Hypersensitivity

Drug Interactions Drugs whose absorption depends on the level of acidity in the stomach such as ketoconazole, itraconazole, and dapsone should be administered at least 2 hours prior to didanosine

Decreased effect: Didanosine may decrease absorption of quinolones or tetracyclines, didanosine should be held during PCP treatment with pentamidine

Increased toxicity: Concomitant administration of other drugs which have the potential to cause peripheral neuropathy or pancreatitis may increase the risk of these toxicities

Drug Uptake

Absorption: Subject to degradation by the acidic pH of the stomach; buffered to resist the acidic pH; as much as 50% reduction in the peak plasma concentration is observed in the presence of food

Serum half-life:
  Children and Adolescents: 0.8 hour
  Adults:
    Normal renal function: 1.5 hours; however, its active metabolite ddATP has an intracellular half-life >12 hours *in vitro*; this permits the drug to be dosed at 12-hour intervals; total body clearance averages 800 mL/minute
    Impaired renal function: Half-life is increased, with values ranging from 2.5-5 hours

Pregnancy Risk Factor B

Didrex® *see* Benzphetamine Hydrochloride *on page 105*

Didronel® *see* Etidronate Disodium *on page 346*

Dienestrol (dye en es' trole)

Brand Names DV® Cream; Ortho® Dienestrol

Therapeutic Category Estrogen Derivative

Use Symptomatic management of atrophic vaginitis or kraurosis vulvae in postmenopausal women

(Continued)

Dienestrol *(Continued)*

Usual Dosage Adults: Vaginal: Insert 1 applicatorful once or twice daily for 1-2 weeks and then $1/2$ of that dose for 1-2 weeks; maintenance dose: 1 applicatorful 1-3 times/week for 3-6 months

Mechanism of Action Increases the synthesis of DNA, RNA, and various proteins in target tissues; reduces the release of gonadotropin-releasing hormone from the hypothalamus; reduces FSH and LH release from the pituitary

Local Anesthetic/Vasoconstrictor Precautions No information available to require special precautions

Effects on Dental Treatment No effects or complications reported

Other Adverse Effects

1% to 10%:
Cardiovascular: Peripheral edema
Endocrine & metabolic: Breast tenderness, breast enlargement
Gastrointestinal: Anorexia, abdominal cramping

<1%:
Cardiovascular: Hypertension, thromboembolism, myocardial infarction
Central nervous system: Stroke, migraine, dizziness, anxiety, depression, headache
Dermatologic: Chloasma, melasma, rash
Endocrine & metabolic: Decreased glucose tolerance, alterations in frequency and flow of menses, breast tenderness or enlargement, increased triglycerides and LDL
Gastrointestinal: Nausea, GI distress
Hepatic: Cholestatic jaundice
Miscellaneous: Increased susceptibility to *Candida* infection

Drug Interactions No data reported

Drug Uptake

Time to peak serum concentration: Topical: Within 3-4 hours

Pregnancy Risk Factor X

Diethylpropion Hydrochloride

(dye eth il proe' pee on hye droe klor' ide)

Brand Names Tenuate®; Tenuate® Dospan®; Tepanil®

Canadian/Mexican Brand Names Nobesine® (Canada)

Therapeutic Category Anorexiant

Synonyms Amfepramone (Canada)

Use Short-term adjunct in exogenous obesity

Usual Dosage Adults: Oral:
Tablet: 25 mg 3 times/day before meals or food
Tablet, controlled release: 75 mg at midmorning

Mechanism of Action Diethylpropion is used as an anorexiant agent possessing pharmacological and chemical properties similar to those of amphetamines. The mechanism of action of diethylpropion in reducing appetite appears to be secondary to CNS effects, specifically stimulation of the hypothalamus to release catecholamines into the central nervous system; anorexiant effects are mediated via norepinephrine and dopamine metabolism. An increase in physical activity and metabolic effects (inhibition of lipogenesis and enhancement of lipolysis) may also contribute to weight loss.

Local Anesthetic/Vasoconstrictor Precautions Use vasoconstrictor with caution in patients taking diethylpropion. Amphetamine-like drugs such as diethylpropion enhance the sympathomimetic response of epinephrine and norepinephrine leading to potential hypertension and cardiotoxicity.

Effects on Dental Treatment Up to 10% of patients may present with hypertension. The use of local anesthetic without vasoconstrictor is recommended in these patients.

Other Adverse Effects

>10%:
Cardiovascular: Hypertension
Central nervous system: Euphoria, nervousness, insomnia

1% to 10%:
Central nervous system: Confusion, mental depression
Endocrine & metabolic: Changes in libido
Gastrointestinal: Nausea, vomiting, restlessness, constipation
Hematologic: Blood dyscrasias
Neuromuscular & skeletal: Tremor
Ocular: Blurred vision

<1%:
Cardiovascular: Tachycardia, arrhythmias

Central nervous system: Depression, headache
Dermatologic: Alopecia
Gastrointestinal: Diarrhea, abdominal cramps
Neuromuscular & skeletal: Myalgia, tremor
Renal: Dysuria, polyuria
Respiratory: Dyspnea
Miscellaneous: Increased sweating
Drug Interactions
Decreased effect of guanethidine; decreased effect with phenothiazines
Increased effect/toxicity with MAO inhibitors (hypertensive crisis), CNS depressants, general anesthetics (arrhythmias), sympathomimetics
Pregnancy Risk Factor B

Diethylstilbestrol (dye eth il stil bes' trole)
Brand Names Stilphostrol®
Canadian/Mexican Brand Names Honvol® (Canada)
Therapeutic Category Estrogen Derivative
Use Palliative treatment of inoperable metastatic prostatic carcinoma and post-menopausal inoperable, progressing breast cancer
Usual Dosage Adults:
Male:
Prostate carcinoma (inoperable, progressing): Oral: 1-3 mg/day
Diphosphate: Inoperable progressing prostate cancer:
Oral: 50 mg 3 times/day; increase up to 200 mg or more 3 times/day; maximum daily dose: 1 g
I.V.: Give 0.5 g, dissolved in 250 mL of saline or D_5W, administer slowly the first 10-15 minutes then adjust rate so that the entire amount is given in 1 hour; repeat for ≥5 days depending on patient response, then repeat 0.25-0.5 g 1-2 times for one week or change to oral therapy
Female: Postmenopausal inoperable, progressing breast carcinoma: Oral: 15 mg/day
Mechanism of Action Competes with estrogenic and androgenic compounds for binding onto tumor cells and thereby inhibits their effects on tumor growth
Local Anesthetic/Vasoconstrictor Precautions No information available to require special precautions
Effects on Dental Treatment No effects or complications reported
Other Adverse Effects
>10%:
Cardiovascular: Peripheral edema
Endocrine & metabolic: Enlargement of breasts (female and male), breast tenderness
Gastrointestinal: Nausea, anorexia, bloating
1% to 10%:
Central nervous system: Headache
Endocrine & metabolic: Increased libido (female), decreased libido (male)
Gastrointestinal: Vomiting, diarrhea
<1%:
Cardiovascular: Hypertension, thromboembolism, myocardial infarction, edema
Central nervous system: Stroke, depression, dizziness, anxiety
Dermatologic: Chloasma, melasma, rash
Endocrine & metabolic: Breast tumors, amenorrhea, alterations in frequency and flow of menses
Gastrointestinal: Nausea, GI distress
Hepatic: Increased triglycerides and LDL, cholestatic jaundice
Miscellaneous: Intolerance to contact lenses, decreased glucose tolerance, increased susceptibility to *Candida* infection
Drug Interactions No data reported
Pregnancy Risk Factor X

Difenoxin and Atropine (dye fen ox' in & a' troe peen)
Brand Names Motofen®
Therapeutic Category Antidiarrheal
Use Treatment of diarrhea
Local Anesthetic/Vasoconstrictor Precautions No information available to require special precautions
Effects on Dental Treatment No effects or complications reported
Other Adverse Effects
1% to 10%:
Central nervous system: Dizziness, drowsiness, lightheadedness, headache
Gastrointestinal: Nausea, vomiting, dry mouth, epigastric distress
(Continued)

Difenoxin and Atropine *(Continued)*

<1%:
Central nervous system: Confusion
Gastrointestinal: Constipation
Ocular: Blurred vision

Differin® *see* Adapalene *on page 25*

Diflorasone Diacetate (dye flor' a sone dye as' e tate)
Related Information
Corticosteroids, Topical Comparison *on page 1018*
Brand Names Florone®; Florone® E; Maxiflor®; Psorcon™
Therapeutic Category Corticosteroid, Topical (High Potency)
Use Relieves inflammation and pruritic symptoms of corticosteroid-responsive dermatosis [high to very high potency topical corticosteroid]
Usual Dosage Topical: Apply ointment sparingly 1-3 times/day; apply cream sparingly 2-4 times/day
Mechanism of Action Decreases inflammation by suppression of migration of polymorphonuclear leukocytes and reversal of increased capillary permeability
Local Anesthetic/Vasoconstrictor Precautions No information available to require special precautions
Effects on Dental Treatment No effects or complications reported
Other Adverse Effects <1%:
Local: Burning, itching, folliculitis, dryness, maceration
Neuromuscular & skeletal: Muscle atrophy, arthralgia
Miscellaneous: Secondary infection
Drug Interactions No data reported
Drug Uptake
Absorption: Topical: Negligible, around 1% reaches dermal layers or systemic circulation; occlusive dressings increase absorption percutaneously
Pregnancy Risk Factor C

Diflucan® *see* Fluconazole *on page 367*

Diflunisal (dye floo' ni sal)
Related Information
Dental Drug Interactions: Update on Drug Combinations Requiring Special Considerations *on page 1022*
Oral Pain *on page 940*
Rheumatoid Arthritis, Osteoarthritis, and Joint Prostheses *on page 930*
Brand Names Dolobid®
Canadian/Mexican Brand Names Apo-Diflunisal® (Canada); Novo-Diflu-nisal® (Canada); Nu-Diflunisal® (Canada)
Therapeutic Category Analgesic, Non-narcotic; Nonsteroidal Anti-inflamma-tory Agent (NSAID)
Use
Dental: Treatment of postoperative pain
Medical: Management of pain and inflammatory disorders usually including rheumatoid arthritis and osteoarthritis
Usual Dosage Adults: Oral: 500-1000 mg followed by 250-500 mg every 8-12 hours; maximum daily dose: 1.5 g
Mechanism of Action Inhibits prostaglandin synthesis by decreasing the activity of the enzyme, cyclo-oxygenase, which results in decreased formation of prostaglandin precursors
Local Anesthetic/Vasoconstrictor Precautions No information available to require special precautions
Effects on Dental Treatment No effects or complications reported
Other Adverse Effects
>10%:
Cardiovascular: Fluid retention
Central nervous system: Headache
1% to 10%: Gastrointestinal: GI ulceration

Oral manifestations: No data reported
Contraindications Hypersensitivity to diflunisal or any component, may be a cross-sensitivity with other nonsteroidal anti-inflammatory agents including aspirin; should not be used in patients with active GI bleeding
Warnings/Precautions Peptic ulceration and GI bleeding have been reported; platelet function and bleeding time are inhibited; ophthalmologic effects; impaired renal function, use lower dosage; peripheral edema; possibility of Reye's syndrome; may cause elevated liver function tests

Drug Interactions Decreased effect with antacids; increased effect/toxicity of digoxin, methotrexate, anticoagulants, phenytoin, sulfonylureas, sulfonamides, lithium, indomethacin, hydrochlorothiazide, acetaminophen

Drug Uptake
Absorption: Rapid and complete
Onset of effect: Within 1 hour
Time to peak serum concentration: Within 2-3 hours
Duration of effect: 8-12 hours
Serum half-life: 8-12 hours

Pregnancy Risk Factor C (D if used in the 3rd trimester)

Breast-feeding Considerations Diflunisal is excreted in breast milk, however, there is no specific data regarding use during lactation

Dosage Forms Tablet: 250 mg, 500 mg

Dietary Considerations Should be taken with food to decrease GI distress

Generic Available No

Comments The advantage of diflunisal as a pain reliever is its 12-hour duration of effect. In many cases, this long effect will ensure a full night sleep during the postoperative pain period.

Selected Readings
Brooks PM and Day RO, "Nonsteroidal Anti-inflammatory Drugs-Differences and Similarities," *N Engl J Med*, 1991, 324(24):1716-25.
Dionne RA, "New Approaches to Preventing and Treating Postoperative Pain," *J Am Dent Assoc*, 1992, 123(6):26-34.
Forbes JA, Butterworth GA, Burchfield WH, et al, "A 12-Hour Evaluation of the Analgesic Efficacy of Diflunisal, Zomepirac Sodium, Aspirin, and Placebo in Postoperative Oral Surgery Pain," *Pharmacotherapy*, 1983, 3(2 Pt 2):38S-46S.
Forbes JA, Calderazzo JP, Bowser MW, et al, "A 12-Hour Evaluation of the Analgesic Efficacy of Diflunisal, Aspirin, and Placebo in Postoperative Dental Pain," *J Clin Pharmacol*, 1982, 22(2-3):89-96.
Gobetti JP, "Controlling Dental Pain," *J Am Dent Assoc*, 1992, 123(6):47-52.

Di-Gel® [OTC] *see Aluminum Hydroxide, Magnesium Hydroxide, and Simethicone on page 41*

Digepepsin® *see Pancreatin on page 656*

Digitoxin (di ji tox′ in)

Related Information
Cardiovascular Diseases *on page 912*

Brand Names Crystodigin®

Canadian/Mexican Brand Names Digitaline® (Canada)

Therapeutic Category Antiarrhythmic Agent (Supraventricular); Antiarrhythmic Agent, Miscellaneous; Cardiac Glycoside

Use Treatment of congestive heart failure, atrial fibrillation, atrial flutter, paroxysmal atrial tachycardia, and cardiogenic shock

Usual Dosage Oral:
Children: Doses are very individualized; **when recommended**, digitalizing dose is as follows:
<1 year: 0.045 mg/kg
1-2 years: 0.04 mg/kg
>2 years: 0.03 mg/kg which is equivalent to 0.75 mg/mm^2
Maintenance: Approximately $^1/_{10}$ of the digitalizing dose
Adults: Oral:
Rapid loading dose: Initial: 0.6 mg followed by 0.4 mg and then 0.2 mg at intervals of 4-6 hours
Slow loading dose: 0.2 mg twice daily for a period of 4 days followed by a maintenance dose
Maintenance: 0.05-0.3 mg/day
Most common dose: 0.15 mg/day

Mechanism of Action Digitalis binds to and inhibits magnesium and adenosine triphosphate dependent sodium and potassium ATPase thereby increasing the influx of calcium ions, from extracellular to intracellular cytoplasm due to the inhibition of sodium and potassium ion movement across the myocardial membranes; this increase in calcium ions results in a potentiation of the activity of the contractile heart muscle fibers and an increase in the force of myocardial contraction (positive inotropic effect); digitalis may also increase intracellular entry of calcium via slow calcium channel influx; stimulates release and blocks re-uptake of norepinephrine; decreases conduction through the S-A and A-V nodes

Local Anesthetic/Vasoconstrictor Precautions Use vasoconstrictor with caution due to risk of cardiac arrhythmias with digitoxin

Effects on Dental Treatment Sensitive gag reflex may cause difficulty in taking a dental impression
(Continued)

Digitoxin *(Continued)*

Other Adverse Effects
1% to 10%: Gastrointestinal: Anorexia, nausea, vomiting

<1%:

Cardiovascular: Sinus bradycardia, A-V block, S-A block, atrial or nodal ectopic beats, ventricular arrhythmias, bigeminy, trigeminy, atrial tachycardia with A-V block

Central nervous system: Drowsiness, headache, fatigue, lethargy, neuralgia, vertigo, disorientation

Endocrine & metabolic: Hyperkalemia with acute toxicity

Gastrointestinal: Feeding intolerance, abdominal pain, diarrhea

Ocular: Blurred vision, halos, yellow or green vision, diplopia, photophobia, flashing lights

Drug Interactions
Decreased effect/levels of digitoxin/digoxin: Antacids (magnesium, aluminum), cholestyramine, colestipol, kaolin/pectin, aminosalicylic acid, metoclopramide, sulfasalazine

Decreased effect/levels of digitoxin only (eg, increased metabolism): Aminoglutethimide, barbiturates, hydantoins, rifampin, phenylbutazone, thyroid replacement

Increased effect/toxicity/levels of digitoxin/digoxin: Amiodarone, nifedipine, quinidine, quinine, verapamil, nondepolarizing muscle relaxants, succinylcholine, potassium-losing diuretics

Concomitant use of digitoxin and sympathomimetics increases the risk of cardiac arrhythmias

Drug Uptake
Absorption: 90% to 100%

Time to peak: 8-12 hours

Serum half-life: 7-8 days

Pregnancy Risk Factor C

Digoxin (di jox' in)

Related Information
Cardiovascular Diseases *on page 912*

Brand Names Lanoxicaps®; Lanoxin®

Canadian/Mexican Brand Names Novo-Digoxin® (Canada); Mapluxin® (Mexico)

Therapeutic Category Antiarrhythmic Agent (Supraventricular); Antiarrhythmic Agent, Miscellaneous; Cardiac Glycoside

Synonyms Digoxina (Mexico)

Use Treatment of congestive heart failure and to slow the ventricular rate in tachyarrhythmias such as atrial fibrillation, atrial flutter, and supraventricular tachycardia (paroxysmal atrial tachycardia); cardiogenic shock

Usual Dosage When changing from oral (tablets or liquid) or I.M. to I.V. therapy, dosage should be reduced by 20% to 25%. See table.

Dosage Recommendations for Digoxin

Age	Total Digitalizing Dose† (mcg/kg)*		Daily Maintenance Dose‡ (mcg/kg*)	
	P.O.	I.V. or I.M.	P.O.	I.V. or I.M.
Preterm infant*	20-30	15-25	5-7.5	4-6
Full-term infant*	25-35	20-30	6-10	5-8
1 mo - 2 y*	35-60	30-50	10-15	7.5-12
2-5 y*	30-40	25-35	7.5-10	6-9
5-10 y*	20-35	15-30	5-10	4-8
>10 y*	10-15	8-12	2.5-5	2-3
Adults	0.75-1.5 mg	0.5-1 mg	0.125-0.5 mg	0.1-0.4 mg

†Give one-half of the total digitalizing dose (TDD) in the initial dose, then give one-quarter of the TDD in each of two subsequent doses at 8- to 12-hour intervals. Obtain EKG 6 hours after each dose to assess potential toxicity.

*Based on lean body weight and normal renal function for age. Decrease dose in patients with ↓ renal function; digitalizing dose often not recommended in infants and children.

‡Divided every 12 hours in infants and children <10 years of age. Given once daily to children >10 years of age and adults.

Mechanism of Action

Congestive heart failure: Inhibition of the sodium/potassium ATPase pump which acts to increase the intracellular sodium-calcium exchange to increase intracellular calcium leading to increased contractility

Supraventricular arrhythmias: Direct suppression of the A-V node conduction to increase effective refractory period and decrease conduction velocity - positive inotropic effect, enhanced vagal tone, and decreased ventricular rate to fast atrial arrhythmias. Atrial fibrillation may decrease sensitivity and increase tolerance to higher serum digoxin concentrations.

Local Anesthetic/Vasoconstrictor Precautions Use vasoconstrictor with caution due to risk of cardiac arrhythmias with digoxin

Effects on Dental Treatment Sensitive gag reflex may cause difficulty in taking a dental impression

Other Adverse Effects

1% to 10%: Gastrointestinal: Anorexia, nausea, vomiting

<1%:

Cardiovascular: Sinus bradycardia, A-V block, S-A block, atrial or nodal ectopic beats, ventricular arrhythmias, bigeminy, trigeminy, atrial tachycardia with A-V block

Central nervous system: Drowsiness, headache, fatigue, lethargy, neuralgia, vertigo, disorientation

Endocrine & metabolic: Hyperkalemia with acute toxicity

Gastrointestinal: Feeding intolerance, abdominal pain, diarrhea

Ocular: Blurred vision, halos, yellow or green vision, diplopia, photophobia, flashing lights

Drug Interactions

Decreased effect/levels of digitoxin/digoxin: Antacids (magnesium, aluminum), cholestyramine, colestipol, kaolin/pectin, aminosalicylic acid, metoclopramide, sulfasalazine

Decreased effect/levels of digitoxin only (eg, increased metabolism): Aminoglutethimide, barbiturates, hydantoins, rifampin, phenylbutazone, thyroid replacement

Increased effect/toxicity/levels of digitoxin/digoxin: Amiodarone, nifedipine, quinidine, quinine, verapamil, nondepolarizing muscle relaxants, succinylcholine, potassium-losing diuretics

Concomitant use of digitoxin and sympathomimetics increase the risk of cardiac arrhythmias

Drug Uptake

Onset of action:

Oral: 1-2 hours

I.V.: 5-30 minutes

Peak effect:

Oral: 2-8 hours

I.V.: 1-4 hours

Duration: Adults: 3-4 days both forms

Absorption: By passive nonsaturable diffusion in the upper small intestine; food may delay, but does not affect extent of digoxin absorption

Serum half-life: Dependent upon age, renal and cardiac function:

Children: 35 hours

Adults: 38-48 hours

Adults, anephric: 4-6 days

Time to peak serum concentration: Oral: Within 1 hour

Pregnancy Risk Factor C

Digoxina (Mexico) see Digoxin on previous page

Dihidroergotamina (Mexico) see Dihydroergotamine Mesylate on page 283

Dihistine® DH see Chlorpheniramine, Pseudoephedrine, and Codeine on page 195

Dihistine® Expectorant see Guaifenesin, Pseudoephedrine, and Codeine on page 410

Dihydrocodeine, Acetaminophen, and Aspirin

(dye hye droe koe' deen, a seet a min' oh fen, & as' pir in)

Related Information

Oral Pain on page 940

Brand Names DHC Plus®; Synalgos®-DC

Therapeutic Category Analgesic, Narcotic

Use

Dental: Management of postoperative pain

Medical: Management of mild to moderate pain from medical conditions

(Continued)

Dihydrocodeine, Acetaminophen, and Aspirin
(Continued)

Usual Dosage Oral:

Children: Not recommended

Adults: 1-2 capsules every 4-6 hours as needed for pain; maximum dose: 12 capsules/day

Mechanism of Action Dihydrocodeine binds to opiate receptors (mu and kappa subtypes) in the CNS causing inhibition of ascending pain pathways, altering the perception of and response to pain; produces generalized CNS depression; causes cough suppression by direct central action in the medulla; produces generalized CNS depression

Acetaminophen inhibits the synthesis of prostaglandins in the CNS and peripherally blocks pain impulse generation; produces antipyresis from inhibition of hypothalamic heat-regulating center

Aspirin inhibits prostaglandin synthesis by decreasing the activity of the enzyme, cyclo-oxygenase, which results in decreased formation of prostaglandin precursors acts on the hypothalamic heat-regulating center to reduce fever, blocks thromboxane synthetase action which prevents formation of the platelet-aggregating substance thromboxane A_2

Local Anesthetic/Vasoconstrictor Precautions No information available to require special precautions

Effects on Dental Treatment Use with caution in patients with platelet and bleeding disorders, renal dysfunction, erosive gastritis, or peptic ulcer disease, previous nonreaction does not guarantee future safe taking of medication; do not use aspirin in children <16 years of age for chickenpox or flu symptoms due to the association with Reye's syndrome

Avoid aspirin if possible, for 1 week prior to surgery because of the possibility of postoperative bleeding; use with caution in impaired hepatic function

Elderly are a high-risk population for adverse effects from nonsteroidal anti-inflammatory agents. As much as 60% of elderly with GI complications to NSAIDs can develop peptic ulceration and/or hemorrhage asymptomatically. Also, concomitant disease and drug use contribute to the risk for GI adverse effects. Use lowest effective dose for shortest period possible. Consider renal function decline with age. Use with caution in patients with history of asthma

Other Adverse Effects

>10%:

Central nervous system: Lightheadedness, dizziness, sedation

Gastrointestinal: Nausea, heartburn, stomach pains, dyspepsia, vomiting

1% to 10%: Gastrointestinal: Ulceration, constipation

Oral manifestations: No data reported

Contraindications Hypersensitivity to acetaminophen or aspirin; hypersensitivity to other phenanthrene derivative opioid agonists (morphine, hydrocodone, hydromorphone, levorphanol, oxycodone, oxymorphone)

Warnings/Precautions Respiratory diseases including asthma, emphysema, COPD, or severe liver or renal insufficiency; some preparations contain sulfites which may cause allergic reactions; may be habit-forming; dextromethorphan has equivalent antitussive activity but has much lower toxicity in accidental overdose

Enhanced analgesia has been seen in elderly patients on therapeutic doses of narcotics; duration of action may be increased in the elderly; the elderly may be particularly susceptible to the CNS depressant and constipating effects of narcotics

Drug Interactions

Dihydrocodeine component: MAO inhibitors cause increased adverse symptoms

Acetaminophen component: Refer to Acetaminophen monograph

Aspirin component: Refer to Aspirin monograph

Drug Uptake

Onset of action: 10-30 minutes

Time to peak serum concentration: 30-60 minutes

Duration: Oral: 4-6 hours

Serum half-life: 3.8 hours

Pregnancy Risk Factor B (D if used for prolonged periods or in high doses at term)

Breast-feeding Considerations

Acetaminophen: May be taken while breast-feeding

Aspirin: Use cautiously due to potential adverse effects in nursing infants

Dihydrocodeine: No data reported

Dosage Forms Capsule:
DHC Plus®: Dihydrocodeine bitartrate 16 mg, acetaminophen 356.4 mg, and caffeine 30 mg
Synalgos®-DC: Dihydrocodeine bitartrate 16 mg, aspirin 356.4 mg, and caffeine 30 mg

Dietary Considerations Should be taken with food

Generic Available Yes

Comments Dihydrocodeine products, as with other narcotic analgesics, are recommended only for acute dosing (ie, 3 days or less). The most common adverse effect you will see in your dental patients from dihydrocodeine is nausea, followed by sedation and constipation. Dihydrocodeine has narcotic addiction liability, especially when given long term. Dihydrocodeine with aspirin could have anticoagulant effects and could possibly affect bleeding times. Dihydrocodeine with acetaminophen should be used with caution in patients with alcoholic liver disease.

Dihydroergotamine Mesylate
(dye hye droe er got' a meen mes' i late)
Brand Names D.H.E. 45®
Therapeutic Category Ergot Alkaloid and Derivative
Synonyms Dihidroergotamina (Mexico)
Use Aborts or prevents vascular headaches; also as an adjunct for DVT prophylaxis for hip surgery, for orthostatic hypotension, xerostomia secondary to antidepressant use, and pelvic congestion with pain
Usual Dosage Adults:
I.M.: 1 mg at first sign of headache; repeat hourly to a maximum dose of 3 mg total
I.V.: Up to 2 mg maximum dose for faster effects; maximum dose: 6 mg/week
Mechanism of Action Ergot alkaloid alpha-adrenergic blocker directly stimulates vascular smooth muscle to vasoconstrict peripheral and cerebral vessels; also has effects on serotonin receptors
Local Anesthetic/Vasoconstrictor Precautions No information available to require special precautions
Effects on Dental Treatment No effects or complications reported
Other Adverse Effects
>10%:
Cardiovascular: Localized edema, peripheral vascular effects (numbness and tingling of fingers and toes)
Central nervous system: Drowsiness, dizziness
Gastrointestinal: Dry mouth, diarrhea, nausea, vomiting
1% to 10%:
Cardiovascular: Precordial distress and pain, transient tachycardia or bradycardia
Neuromuscular & skeletal: Muscle pain in the extremities, weakness in the legs
Drug Interactions
Increased effect of heparin
Increased toxicity with erythromycin, clarithromycin, nitroglycerin, propranolol, troleandomycin
Drug Uptake
Onset of action: Within 15-30 minutes
Duration: 3-4 hours
Serum half-life: 1.3-3.9 hours
Time to peak serum concentration: I.M.: Within 15-30 minutes
Pregnancy Risk Factor X

Dihydrotachysterol (dye hye droe tak is' ter ole)
Brand Names DHT™; Hytakerol®
Therapeutic Category Vitamin D Analog
Use Treatment of hypocalcemia associated with hypoparathyroidism; prophylaxis of hypocalcemic tetany following thyroid surgery
Usual Dosage Oral:
Hypoparathyroidism:
Young Children: Initial: 1-5 mg/day for 4 days, then 0.1-0.5 mg/day
Older Children and Adults: Initial: 0.8-2.4 mg/day for several days followed by maintenance doses of 0.2-1 mg/day
Nutritional rickets: 0.5 mg as a single dose or 13-50 mcg/day until healing occurs
Renal osteodystrophy: Maintenance: 0.25-0.6 mg/24 hours adjusted as necessary to achieve normal serum calcium levels and promote bone healing
(Continued)

Dihydrotachysterol *(Continued)*

Mechanism of Action Synthetic analogue of vitamin D with a faster onset of action; stimulates calcium and phosphate absorption from the small intestine, promotes secretion of calcium from bone to blood; promotes renal tubule resorption of phosphate

Local Anesthetic/Vasoconstrictor Precautions No information available to require special precautions

Effects on Dental Treatment No effects or complications reported

Other Adverse Effects

>10%:
  Endocrine & metabolic: Hypercalcemia, hypercalciuria
  Renal: Elevated serum creatinine

<1%:
  Central nervous system: Convulsions
  Endocrine & metabolic: Polydipsia
  Gastrointestinal: Nausea, vomiting, anorexia, weight loss
  Hematologic: Anemia
  Neuromuscular & skeletal: Weakness, metastatic calcification
  Renal: Renal damage, polyuria

Drug Interactions
  Decreased effect/levels of vitamin D: Cholestyramine, colestipol, mineral oil
  Increased toxicity: Thiazide diuretics increase calcium

Drug Uptake
  Peak hypercalcemic effect: Within 2-4 weeks
  Duration: Can be as long as 9 weeks
  Absorption: Well absorbed from the GI tract

Pregnancy Risk Factor A (D if used in doses above the recommended daily allowance)

Dihydroxypropyl Theophylline *see Dyphylline on page 305*

Dilacor™ XR *see Diltiazem on this page*

Dilantin® *see Phenytoin on page 688*

Dilantin® With Phenobarbital *see Phenytoin With Phenobarbital on page 689*

Dilatrate®-SR *see Isosorbide Dinitrate on page 474*

Dilaudid® *see Hydromorphone Hydrochloride on page 438*

Dilaudid-HP® *see Hydromorphone Hydrochloride on page 438*

Dilocaine® *see Lidocaine Hydrochloride on page 502*

Dilor® *see Dyphylline on page 305*

Diltiazem *(dil tye' a zem)*

Related Information
  Calcium Channel Blockers & Gingival Hyperplasia *on page 1010*
  Cardiovascular Diseases *on page 912*

Brand Names Cardizem® CD; Cardizem® Injectable; Cardizem® SR; Cardizem® Tablet; Dilacor™ XR

Canadian/Mexican Brand Names Apo-Diltiaz® (Canada); Novo-Diltiazem® (Canada); Nu-Diltiaz® (Canada); Syn-Diltiazem® (Canada); Angiotrofen® (Mexico); Angiotrofen A.P.® (Mexico); Angiotrofen® Retard (Mexico); Presoken® (Mexico); Presoquim® (Mexico); Tilazem® (Mexico)

Therapeutic Category Antianginal Agent; Calcium Channel Blocker

Synonyms Diltiazem, Clorhidrato De (Mexico)

Use
  Capsule: Hypertension (alone or in combination); chronic stable angina or angina from coronary artery spasm
  Injection: Atrial fibrillation or atrial flutter; paroxysmal supraventricular tachycardias (PSVT)

Usual Dosage Adults:
  Oral: 30-120 mg 3-4 times/day; dosage should be increased gradually, at 1- to 2-day intervals until optimum response is obtained; usual maintenance dose: 240-360 mg/day
  Sustained-release capsules:
  Cardizem SR®: Initial: 60-12 mg twice daily; adjust to maximum antihypertensive effect (usually within 14 days); usual range: 240-360 mg/day
  Cardizem® CD, Tiazac®: Hypertension: Total daily dose of short-acting administered once daily or initially 180 or 240 mg once daily; adjust to maximum effect (usually within 14 days); maximum: 360 mg/day; usual range: 240-360 mg/day
  Cardizem® CD: Angina: Initial: 120-180 mg once daily; maximum: 480 mg once/day

Dilacor™ XR:
　　Hypertension: 180-240 mg once daily; maximum: 540 mg/day; usual range: 180-480 mg/day; use lower dose in elderly
　　Angina: Initial: 120 mg/day; titrate slowly over 7-14 days up to 480 mg/day, as needed
　Note: Hypertensive or anginal patients treated with other formulations of diltiazem sustained release can be safely switched to Dilacor™ XR at the nearest equivalent total daily dose; subsequent titration may be needed
I.V. (requires an infusion pump): See table.

Diltiazem — I.V. Dosage and Administration

Initial Bolus Dose	0.25 mg/kg actual body weight over 2 min (average adult dose: 20 mg)
Repeat Bolus Dose may be administered after 15 min if the response is inadequate	0.35 mg/kg actual body weight over 2 min (average adult dose: 25 mg)
Continuous Infusion Infusions >24 h or infusion rates >15 mg/h are not recommended due to potential accumulation of metabolites and increased toxicity	Initial infusion rate of 10 mg/h; rate may be increased in 5 mg/h increments up to 15 mg/h as needed; some patients may respond to an initial rate of 5 mg/h

If Cardizem® injectable is administered by continuous infusion for >24 hours, the possibility of decreased diltiazem clearance, prolonged elimination half-life, and increased diltiazem and/or diltiazem metabolite plasma concentrations should be considered

Conversion from I.V. diltiazem to oral diltiazem: Start oral approximately 3 hours after bolus dose

Oral dose (mg/day) is approximately equal to [rate (mg/hour) x 3 + 3] x 10

　　3 mg/hour = 120 mg/day
　　5 mg/hour = 180 mg/day
　　7 mg/hour = 240 mg/day
　　11 mg/hour = 360 mg/day (maximum recommended dose)

Mechanism of Action Inhibits calcium ion from entering the "slow channels" or select voltage-sensitive areas of vascular smooth muscle and myocardium during depolarization, producing a relaxation of coronary vascular smooth muscle and coronary vasodilation; increases myocardial oxygen delivery in patients with vasospastic angina

Local Anesthetic/Vasoconstrictor Precautions No information available to require special precautions

Effects on Dental Treatment Calcium channel blockers cause gingival hyperplasia in approximately 1% of patients. There have been fewer reports with diltiazem than with other CCBs. The hyperplasia will disappear with cessation of drug therapy. Consultation with physician is suggested.

Other Adverse Effects
>10%: Headache
1% to 10%:
　Cardiovascular: Bradycardia, A-V block (first degree), edema, EKG abnormality
　Central nervous system: Dizziness, asthenia
　Gastrointestinal: Nausea, vomiting
<1%:
　Cardiovascular: A-V block (second degree), angina
　Central nervous system: Abnormal dreams, amnesia, depression, gait abnormality, insomnia, nervousness
　Dermatologic: Urticaria, photosensitivity, alopecia, purpura
　Gastrointestinal: Anorexia, constipation, diarrhea, dysgeusia, dyspepsia
　Hematologic: Hemolytic anemia, leukopenia thrombocytopenia
　Neuromuscular & skeletal: Paresthesia, tremor
　Ocular: Amblyopia, retinopathy
　Respiratory: Pharyngitis, cough increase
　Miscellaneous: Flu syndrome

Drug Interactions Increased toxicity/effect/levels:
H$_2$-blockers cause increased bioavailability of diltiazem
Beta-blockers cause increased cardiac depressant effects on A-V conduction
Diltiazem increases serum levels and effects/toxicity of carbamazepine, cyclosporin, digitalis, quinidine, and theophylline

Drug Uptake
Onset of action: Oral: 30-60 minutes (including sustained release)
Absorption: 80% to 90%
(Continued)

Diltiazem *(Continued)*

Time to peak serum concentration:
Short-acting tablets: Within 2-3 hours
Sustained release: 6-11 hours

Pregnancy Risk Factor C

Diltiazem, Clorhidrato De (Mexico) *see* Diltiazem *on page 284*

Dimaphen® Elixir [OTC] *see* Brompheniramine and Phenylpropanolamine *on page 123*

Dimaphen® Tablets [OTC] *see* Brompheniramine and Phenylpropanolamine *on page 123*

Dimenhidrinato (Mexico) *see* Dimenhydrinate *on this page*

Dimenhydrinate *(dye men hye' dri nate)*

Brand Names Calm-X® [OTC]; Dimetabs®; Dinate®; Dramamine® [OTC]; Dramilin®; Hydrate®; Marmine® [OTC]; Tega-Cert® [OTC]; TripTone® Caplets® [OTC]; Wehamine®

Canadian/Mexican Brand Names Apo-Dimenhydrinate® (Canada); Gravol® (Canada); PMS-Dimenhydrinate® (Canada); Travel Aid® (Canada); Travel Tabs® (Canada); Vomisen® (Mexico)

Therapeutic Category Antiemetic; Antihistamine

Synonyms Dimenhidrinato (Mexico)

Use Treatment and prevention of nausea, vertigo, and vomiting associated with motion sickness

Usual Dosage
Children:
Oral:
2-5 years: 12.5-25 mg every 6-8 hours, maximum: 75 mg/day
6-12 years: 25-50 mg every 6-8 hours, maximum: 150 mg/day
I.M.: 1.25 mg/kg or 37.5 mg/m^2 4 times/day, not to exceed 300 mg/day

Adults: Oral, I.M., I.V.: 50-100 mg every 4-6 hours, not to exceed 400 mg/day

Mechanism of Action Competes with histamine for H_1-receptor sites on effector cells in the gastrointestinal tract, blood vessels, and respiratory tract; blocks chemoreceptor trigger zone, diminishes vestibular stimulation, and depresses labyrinthine function through its central anticholinergic activity

Local Anesthetic/Vasoconstrictor Precautions No information available to require special precautions

Effects on Dental Treatment Up to 10% of patients will complain of significant dry mouth and drowsiness. This will disappear with cessation of drug therapy.

Other Adverse Effects
>10%:
Central nervous system: Slight to moderate drowsiness
Miscellaneous: Thickening of bronchial secretions
1% to 10%:
Central nervous system: Headache, fatigue, nervousness, dizziness
Gastrointestinal: Appetite increase, weight increase, nausea, diarrhea, abdominal pain, dry mouth
Neuromuscular & skeletal: Arthralgia
Respiratory: Pharyngitis
<1%:
Cardiovascular: Edema, palpitations, hypotension
Central nervous system: Depression, drowsiness, paradoxical CNS stimulation
Dermatologic: Angioedema, photosensitivity, rash
Gastrointestinal: Anorexia
Genitourinary: Urinary frequency
Hepatic: Hepatitis,
Local: Pain at the injection site
Neuromuscular & skeletal: Myalgia, paresthesia
Ocular: Blurred vision
Otic: Tinnitus
Respiratory: Bronchospasm
Miscellaneous: Epistaxis

Drug Interactions
Increased effect/toxicity with CNS depressants, anticholinergics, TCAs, MAO inhibitors
Increased toxicity of antibiotics, especially aminoglycosides (ototoxicity)

Drug Uptake
Onset of action: Oral: Within 15-30 minutes

Absorption: Well absorbed from GI tract
Pregnancy Risk Factor B

Dimercaprol (dye mer kap' role)
Brand Names BAL in Oil®
Therapeutic Category Antidote, Arsenic Toxicity; Antidote, Gold Toxicity; Antidote, Lead Toxicity; Antidote, Mercury Toxicity
Use Antidote to gold, arsenic, and mercury poisoning; adjunct to edetate calcium disodium in lead poisoning
Usual Dosage Children and Adults: Deep I.M.:
Mild arsenic and gold poisoning: 2.5 mg/kg/dose every 6 hours for 2 days, then every 12 hours on the third day, and once daily thereafter for 10 days
Severe arsenic and gold poisoning: 3 mg/kg/dose every 4 hours for 2 days then every 6 hours on the third day, then every 12 hours thereafter for 10 days
Mercury poisoning: Initial: 5 mg/kg followed by 2.5 mg/kg/dose 1-2 times/day for 10 days
Lead poisoning (use with edetate calcium disodium):
Mild: 3 mg/kg/dose every 4 hours for 5-7 days
Severe and acute encephalopathy: 4 mg/kg/dose initially alone then every 4 hours in combination of edetate calcium disodium
Mechanism of Action Sulfhydryl group combines with ions of various heavy metals to form relatively stable, nontoxic, soluble chelates which are excreted in urine
Local Anesthetic/Vasoconstrictor Precautions No information available to require special precautions
Effects on Dental Treatment No effects or complications reported
Other Adverse Effects
>10%:
Cardiovascular: Hypertension, tachycardia
Central nervous system: Convulsions
1% to 10%: Gastrointestinal: Nausea, vomiting
<1%:
Central nervous system: Nervousness, fever, headache
Gastrointestinal: Salivation
Hematologic: Transient neutropenia
Local: Pain at the injection site
Ocular: Blepharospasm
Renal: Nephrotoxicity
Miscellaneous: Burning sensation of the lips, mouth, throat, eyes, and penis
Drug Interactions Toxic complexes with iron, cadmium, selenium, or uranium
Drug Uptake
Time to peak serum concentration: 0.5-1 hour
Pregnancy Risk Factor C

Dimetabs® see Dimenhydrinate on previous page
Dimetane® [OTC] see Brompheniramine Maleate on page 124
Dimetane®-DC see Brompheniramine, Phenylpropanolamine, and Codeine on page 125
Dimetane® Decongestant Elixir [OTC] see Brompheniramine and Phenylephrine on page 122
Dimetapp® 4-Hour Liqui-Gel Capsule [OTC] see Brompheniramine and Phenyl-propanolamine on page 123
Dimetapp® Elixir [OTC] see Brompheniramine and Phenylpropanolamine on page 123
Dimetapp® Extentabs® [OTC] see Brompheniramine and Phenylpropanolamine on page 123
Dimetapp® Sinus Caplets [OTC] see Pseudoephedrine and Ibuprofen on page 750
Dimetapp® Tablet [OTC] see Brompheniramine and Phenylpropanolamine on page 123
Dimethyl Triazeno Imidazol Carboxamide see Dacarbazine on page 247
Dinate® see Dimenhydrinate on previous page
Diocto® [OTC] see Docusate on page 295
Diocto C® [OTC] see Docusate and Casanthranol on page 295
Diocto-K® [OTC] see Docusate on page 295
Diocto-K Plus® [OTC] see Docusate and Casanthranol on page 295
Dioctolose Plus® [OTC] see Docusate and Casanthranol on page 295
Dioeze® [OTC] see Docusate on page 295
Dioval® see Estradiol on page 325

Dipalmitoylphosphatidylcholine *see* Colfosceril Palmitate *on page 230*
Dipentum® *see* Olsalazine Sodium *on page 635*
Diphen® Cough [OTC] *see* Diphenhydramine Hydrochloride *on this page*

Diphenhydramine Hydrochloride
(dye fen hye' dra meen hye droe klor' ide)

Related Information
Oral Nonviral Soft Tissue Ulcerations or Erosions *on page 955*
Oral Viral Infections *on page 951*
Patients Undergoing Cancer Therapy *on page 967*

Brand Names AllerMax® [OTC]; Banophen® [OTC]; Beldin® [OTC]; Belix®
[OTC]; Benadryl® [OTC]; Benylin® Cough Syrup [OTC]; Compoz® [OTC];
Diphen® Cough [OTC]; Genahist®; Nidryl® [OTC]; Nordryl®; Nytol® [OTC];
Tusstat®

Canadian/Mexican Brand Names Allerdryl® (Canada); Allernix® (Canada)

Therapeutic Category Antidote, Hypersensitivity Reactions; Antihistamine;
Sedative

Use
Dental: Symptomatic relief of allergic symptoms caused by histamine release
which include nasal allergies and allergic dermatosis; also to produce local
anesthesia through infiltration of mucous membranes
Medical: Can be used for mild nighttime sedation; prevention of motion sickness and as an antitussive; has antinauseant and topical anesthetic properties; treatment of phenothiazine-induced dystonic reactions

Usual Dosage Oral:
Children >10 kg: 12.5-25 mg 3-4 times/day; maximum daily dose: 300 mg
Adults: 25-50 mg every 6-8 hours

Mechanism of Action Competes with histamine for H_1-receptor sites on
effector cells in the gastrointestinal tract, blood vessels, and respiratory tract

Local Anesthetic/Vasoconstrictor Precautions No information available to
require special precautions

Effects on Dental Treatment Chronic use of antihistamines will inhibit salivary flow, particularly in elderly patients; this may contribute to periodontal
disease and oral discomfort

Other Adverse Effects >10%: Central nervous system: Slight to moderate
drowsiness

Oral manifestations: 1% to 10%: Dry mouth

Contraindications Hypersensitivity to diphenhydramine or any component;
should not be used in acute attacks of asthma

Warnings/Precautions Use with caution in patients with angle-closure glaucoma, peptic ulcer, urinary tract obstruction, hyperthyroidism; some preparations contain sodium bisulfite; syrup contains alcohol; diphenhydramine has
high sedative and anticholinergic properties, so it may not be considered the
antihistamine of choice for prolonged use in the elderly

Drug Interactions CNS depressants worsens CNS and respiratory depression, monoamine oxidase inhibitors may cause increased anticholinergic
effects; syrup should not be given to patients taking drugs that can cause
disulfiram reactions (ie, metronidazole, chlorpropamide) due to high alcohol
content

Drug Uptake
Absorption: Oral: 40% to 60% reaches systemic circulation due to first-pass
metabolism
Maximum sedative effect: 1-3 hours
Time to peak serum concentration: 2-4 hours
Duration of action: 4-7 hours
Serum half-life:
Elderly: 13.5 hours
Adults: 2-8 hours

Pregnancy Risk Factor C

Breast-feeding Considerations No data reported

Dosage Forms
Capsule: 25 mg, 50 mg
Elixir: 12.5 mg/5 mL (5 mL, 10 mL, 20 mL, 120 mL, 480 mL, 3780 mL)
Injection: 10 mg/mL (10 mL, 30 mL); 50 mg/mL (1 mL, 10 mL)
Syrup: 12.5 mg/5 mL (5 mL, 120 mL, 240 mL, 480 mL, 3780 mL)
Tablet: 25 mg, 50 mg

Dietary Considerations May be taken with food or water

Generic Available Yes

Comments 25-50 mg of diphenhydramine orally every 4-6 hours can be used
to treat mild dermatologic manifestations of allergic reactions to penicillin and

other antibiotics; used as local anesthetic in patients allergic to all other local anesthetics; used for infiltration only; should never be used for block anesthesia because of irritative qualities of vehicle

Diphenidol Hydrochloride (dye fen' i dole hye droe klor' ide)
Brand Names Vontrol®
Therapeutic Category Antiemetic
Use Control of nausea and vomiting; peripheral vertigo and associated nausea and vomiting, Ménière's disease, and middle and inner ear surgery
Local Anesthetic/Vasoconstrictor Precautions No information available to require special precautions
Effects on Dental Treatment No effects or complications reported
Other Adverse Effects
>10%: Central nervous system: Drowsiness
1% to 10%:
Central nervous system: Dizziness, headache, nervousness, insomnia, weakness
Gastrointestinal: Dry mouth, heartburn
Ocular: Blurred vision
<1%: Central nervous system: Confusion, hallucinations

Diphenoxylate and Atropine (dye fen ox' i late & at' roe peen)
Brand Names Lofene®; Logen®; Lomanate®; Lomodix®; Lomotil®; Lonox®; Low-Quel®
Therapeutic Category Antidiarrheal
Use Treatment of diarrhea
Usual Dosage Oral:
Children (use with caution in young children due to variable responses): Liquid: 0.3-0.4 mg of diphenoxylate/kg/day in 2-4 divided doses **or**
<2 years: Not recommended
2-5 years: 2 mg of diphenoxylate 3 times/day
5-8 years: 2 mg of diphenoxylate 4 times/day
8-12 years: 2 mg of diphenoxylate 5 times/day
Adults: 15-20 mg/day of diphenoxylate in 3-4 divided doses; maintenance: 5-15 mg/day in 2-3 divided doses
Mechanism of Action Diphenoxylate inhibits excessive GI motility and GI propulsion; commercial preparations contain a subtherapeutic amount of atropine to discourage abuse
Local Anesthetic/Vasoconstrictor Precautions No information available to require special precautions
Effects on Dental Treatment Up to 10% of patients will complain of significant dry mouth and drowsiness. This will disappear with cessation of drug therapy.
Other Adverse Effects
1% to 10%:
Central nervous system: Nervousness, restlessness, dizziness, drowsiness, headache, mental depression
Gastrointestinal: Paralytic ileus, dry mouth
Genitourinary: Urinary retention and difficult urination
Ocular: Blurred vision
Respiratory: Respiratory depression
<1%:
Cardiovascular: Tachycardia
Central nervous system: Sedation, euphoria, weakness
Dermatologic: Pruritus, urticaria
Gastrointestinal: Nausea, vomiting, abdominal discomfort, pancreatitis, stomach cramps
Neuromuscular & skeletal: Muscle cramps
Miscellaneous: Hyperthermia, increased sweating
Drug Interactions Increased toxicity: MAO inhibitors (hypertensive crisis), CNS depressants, antimuscarinics (paralytic ileus); may prolong half-life of drugs metabolized in liver
Drug Uptake
Onset of action: Within 45-60 minutes
Duration: 3-4 hours
Absorption: Oral: Well absorbed
Serum half-life: Diphenoxylate: 2.5 hours
Time to peak serum concentration: 2 hours
Pregnancy Risk Factor C

Diphenylan Sodium® *see* Phenytoin *on page 688*

Diphtheria CRM$_{197}$ Protein Conjugate *see Haemophilus* b Conjugate Vaccine *on page 414*

Diphtheria Toxoid Conjugate *see Haemophilus* b Conjugate Vaccine *on page 414*

Dipiridamol (Mexico) *see Dipyridamole on this page*

Dipivefrin (dye pi' ve frin)

Brand Names Propine®

Therapeutic Category Adrenergic Agonist Agent, Ophthalmic; Antiglaucoma Agent; Ophthalmic Agent, Vasoconstrictor

Use Reduces elevated intraocular pressure in chronic open-angle glaucoma; also used to treat ocular hypertension, low tension, and secondary glaucomas

Usual Dosage Adults: Ophthalmic: Instill 1 drop every 12 hours into the eyes

Mechanism of Action Dipivefrin is a prodrug of epinephrine which is the active agent that stimulates alpha- and/or beta-adrenergic receptors increasing aqueous humor outflow

Local Anesthetic/Vasoconstrictor Precautions No information available to require special precautions

Effects on Dental Treatment No effects or complications reported

Other Adverse Effects
1% to 10%:
Central nervous system: Headache
Local: Burning, stinging
Ocular: Ocular congestion, photophobia, mydriasis, blurred vision, ocular pain, bulbar conjunctival follicles, blepharoconjunctivitis, cystoid macular edema
<1%: Cardiovascular: Arrhythmias, hypertension

Drug Interactions Increased or synergistic effect when used with other agents to lower intraocular pressure

Drug Uptake
Ocular pressure effect:
Onset of action: Within 30 minutes
Duration: ≥12 hours
Mydriasis:
Onset of action: May occur within 30 minutes
Duration: Several hours
Absorption: Rapid into the aqueous humor

Pregnancy Risk Factor B

Diprivan® Injection *see Propofol on page 738*

Diprolene® *see Betamethasone on page 109*

Diprolene® AF *see Betamethasone on page 109*

Diprosone® *see Betamethasone on page 109*

Dipyridamole (dye peer id' a mole)

Brand Names Persantine®

Canadian/Mexican Brand Names Apo-Dipyridamole® FC (Canada); Apo-Dipyridamole® SC (Canada); Novo-Dipiradol® (Canada); Dirinol® (Mexico); Lodimol® (Mexico); Trompersantin® (Mexico)

Therapeutic Category Antiplatelet Agent

Synonyms Dipiridamol (Mexico)

Use Maintains patency after surgical grafting procedures including coronary artery bypass; used with warfarin to decrease thrombosis in patients after artificial heart valve replacement; used with aspirin to prevent coronary artery thrombosis; in combination with aspirin or warfarin to prevent other thrombo-embolic disorders. Dipyridamole may also be given 2 days prior to open heart surgery to prevent platelet activation by extracorporeal bypass pump and as a diagnostic agent in CAD.

Usual Dosage
Oral:
Children: 3-6 mg/kg/day in 3 divided doses
Doses of 4-10 mg/kg/day have been used investigationally to treat proteinuria in pediatric renal disease
Adults: 75-400 mg/day in 3-4 divided doses
I.V.: 0.14 mg/kg/minute for 4 minutes; maximum dose: 60 mg

Mechanism of Action Inhibits the activity of adenosine deaminase and phosphodiesterase, which causes an accumulation of adenosine, adenine nucleotides, and cyclic AMP; these mediators then inhibit platelet aggregation and may cause vasodilation; may also stimulate release of prostacyclin or PGD$_2$; causes coronary vasodilation

Local Anesthetic/Vasoconstrictor Precautions No information available to require special precautions

Effects on Dental Treatment No effects or complications reported

Other Adverse Effects

>10%:
  Cardiovascular: Exacerbation of angina pectoris
  Central nervous system: Dizziness

1% to 10%:
  Cardiovascular: Hypotension, hypertension, tachycardia
  Central nervous system: Headache
  Dermatologic: Rash
  Gastrointestinal: Abdominal distress
  Respiratory: Dyspnea

<1%:
  Cardiovascular: Vasodilatation, flushing, syncope, edema
  Central nervous system: Migraine
  Neuromuscular & skeletal: Weakness, hypertonia
  Respiratory: Rhinitis, hyperventilation
  Miscellaneous: Allergic reaction, pleural pain

Drug Interactions No data reported

Drug Uptake

Absorption: Readily absorbed from GI tract but variable
Serum half-life, terminal: 10-12 hours
Time to peak serum concentration: 2-2.5 hours

Pregnancy Risk Factor C

Dirithromycin (dye rith' roe mye sin)

Brand Names Dynabac®

Therapeutic Category Antibiotic, Macrolide

Use Treatment of mild to moderate upper and lower respiratory tract infections, infections of the skin and skin structure, and sexually transmitted diseases due to susceptible strains

Usual Dosage Adults: Oral: 500 mg once daily for 7-14 days (14 days required for treatment of community-acquired pneumonia due to *Legionella*, *Mycoplasma*, or *S. pneumoniae*; 10 days is recommended for treatment of *S. pyogenes* pharyngitis/tonsillitis)

Mechanism of Action After being converted during intestinal absorption to its active form, erthromycylamine, dirithromycin inhibits protein synthesis by binding to the 50S ribosomal subunits of susceptible microorganisms

Local Anesthetic/Vasoconstrictor Precautions No information available to require special precautions

Effects on Dental Treatment No effects or complications reported

Other Adverse Effects

Central nervous system: Headache, dizziness, asthenia
Dermatologic: Skin rash, urticaria
Gastrointestinal: Abdominal pain, nausea, diarrhea, vomiting, dyspepsia, flatulence
Hepatic: Increased LFTs, alkaline phosphatase
Renal: Nephrotoxicity

Contraindications Hypersensitivity to any macrolide or component of dirithromycin; use with pimozide

Warnings/Precautions Contrary to potential serious consequences with other macrolides (eg, cardiac arrhythmias), the combination of terfenadine and dirithromycin has not shown alteration of terfenadine metabolism; however, caution should be taken during coadministration of dirithromycin and terfenadine; pseudomembranous colitis has been reported and should be considered in patients presenting with diarrhea subsequent to therapy with dirithromycin

Drug Interactions

Increased effect: Absorption of dirithromycin is slightly enhanced with concomitant antacids and H_2 antagonists; dirithromycin may, like erythromycin, increase the effect of alfentanil, anticoagulants, bromocriptine, carbamazepine, cyclosporine, digoxin, disopyramide, ergots, methylprednisolone, and triazolam

Note: Interactions with nonsedating antihistamines (eg, terfenadine) and theophylline are not known to occur, however, caution is advised with coadministration

Drug Uptake

Absorption: Rapidly absorbed and nonenzymatically hydrolyzed to erythromycylamine; T_{max}: 4 hours
Serum half-life: 8 hours (range: 2-36 hours)

Pregnancy Risk Factor C

(Continued)

Dirithromycin (Continued)

Dosage Forms Tablet, enteric coated: 250 mg

Generic Available No

Selected Readings
"Pimozide (Orap) Contraindicated With Clarithromycin (Biaxin) and Other Macrolide Antibiotics," *FDA Medical Bulletin*, October 1996, 3.

Disalcid® *see* Salsalate *on page 779*

Disanthrol® [OTC] *see* Docusate and Casanthranol *on page 295*

Discase® *see* Chymopapain *on page 204*

Disobrom® [OTC] *see* Dexbrompheniramine and Pseudoephedrine *on page 261*

Disolan® [OTC] *see* Docusate and Phenolphthalein *on page 295*

Disonate® [OTC] *see* Docusate *on page 295*

Disophrol® Chrontabs® [OTC] *see* Dexbrompheniramine and Pseudoephedrine *on page 261*

Disophrol® Tablet [OTC] *see* Dexbrompheniramine and Pseudoephedrine *on page 261*

Disopiramida (Mexico) *see* Disopyramide Phosphate *on this page*

Disopyramide Phosphate (dye soe peer' a mide fos' fate)

Related Information
Cardiovascular Diseases *on page 912*

Brand Names Norpace®

Canadian/Mexican Brand Names Dimodan® (Mexico)

Therapeutic Category Antiarrhythmic Agent, Class I-A; Antiarrhythmic Agent (Supraventricular & Ventricular)

Synonyms Disopiramida (Mexico)

Use Suppression and prevention of unifocal and multifocal premature, ventricular premature complexes, coupled ventricular tachycardia; effective in the conversion of atrial fibrillation, atrial flutter, and paroxysmal atrial tachycardia to normal sinus rhythm and prevention of the reoccurrence of these arrhythmias after conversion by other methods

Usual Dosage Oral:
Children:
<1 year: 10-30 mg/kg/24 hours in 4 divided doses
1-4 years: 10-20 mg/kg/24 hours in 4 divided doses
4-12 years: 10-15 mg/kg/24 hours in 4 divided doses
12-18 years: 6-15 mg/kg/24 hours in 4 divided doses
Adults:
<50 kg: 100 mg every 6 hours or 200 mg every 12 hours (controlled release)
>50 kg: 150 mg every 6 hours or 300 mg every 12 hours (controlled release); if no response, may increase to 200 mg every 6 hours; maximum dose required for patients with severe refractory ventricular tachycardia is 400 mg every 6 hours

Mechanism of Action Class IA antiarrhythmic: Decreases myocardial excitability and conduction velocity; reduces disparity in refractory between normal and infarcted myocardium; possesses anticholinergic, peripheral vasoconstrictive, and negative inotropic effects

Local Anesthetic/Vasoconstrictor Precautions No information available to require special precautions

Effects on Dental Treatment No effects or complications reported

Other Adverse Effects
>10%: Genitourinary: Urinary retention/hesitancy
1% to 10%:
Cardiovascular: Chest pains, congestive heart failure, hypotension
Endocrine & metabolic: Hypokalemia
Gastrointestinal: Stomach pain, bloating, dry mouth
Neuromuscular & skeletal: Muscle weakness
Ocular: Blurred vision
<1%:
Cardiovascular: Syncope and conduction disturbances including A-V block, widening QRS complex and lengthening of Q-T interval
Central nervous system: Fatigue, malaise, nervousness, acute psychosis, depression, dizziness, headache, pain
Dermatologic: Generalized rashes
Endocrine & metabolic: Hypoglycemia, may initiate contractions of pregnant uterus, hyperkalemia may enhance toxicities, increased cholesterol and triglycerides
Gastrointestinal: Constipation, nausea, vomiting, diarrhea, gas, anorexia, weight gain

Hepatic: Hepatic cholestasis, elevated liver enzymes
Neuromuscular & skeletal: Weakness
Respiratory: Dyspnea
Miscellaneous: Dry nose, eyes, and throat

Drug Interactions
Decreased effect with hepatic microsomal enzyme-inducing agents (ie, phenytoin, phenobarbital, rifampin)
Increased effect/levels/toxicity with erythromycin; increased levels of digoxin

Drug Uptake
Onset of action: 0.5-3.5 hours
Duration of effect: 1.5-8.5 hours
Absorption: 60% to 83%
Serum half-life: Adults: 4-10 hours, increased half-life with hepatic or renal disease

Pregnancy Risk Factor C

Di-Spaz® *see* Dicyclomine Hydrochloride *on page 273*

Dispos-a-Med® Isoproterenol *see* Isoproterenol *on page 472*

Disulfiram (dye sul' fi ram)

Brand Names Antabuse®

Therapeutic Category Aldehyde Dehydrogenase Inhibitor Agent; Antialcoholic Agent

Use Management of chronic alcoholism

Usual Dosage Adults: Oral: Do not administer until the patient has abstained from alcohol for at least 12 hours
Initial: 500 mg/day as a single dose for 1-2 weeks; maximum daily dose is 500 mg
Average maintenance dose: 250 mg/day; range: 125-500 mg; duration of therapy is to continue until the patient is fully recovered socially and a basis for permanent self control has been established; maintenance therapy may be required for months or even years

Mechanism of Action Disulfiram is a thiuram derivative which interferes with aldehyde dehydrogenase. When taken concomitantly with alcohol, there is an increase in serum acetaldehyde levels. High acetaldehyde causes uncomfortable symptoms including flushing, nausea, thirst, palpitations, chest pain, vertigo, and hypotension. This reaction is the basis for disulfiram use in postwithdrawal long-term care of alcoholism.

Local Anesthetic/Vasoconstrictor Precautions No information available to require special precautions

Effects on Dental Treatment No effects or complications reported

Other Adverse Effects
>10%: Central nervous system: Drowsiness
1% to 10%:
Central nervous system: Headache, tiredness, mood changes, neurotoxicity
Miscellaneous: Impotence, metallic or garlic-like aftertaste, skin rash
<1%:
Hepatic: Hepatitis, encephalopathy
Disulfiram reaction with alcohol: Flushing, sweating, cardiovascular collapse, myocardial infarction, vertigo, seizures, headache, nausea, vomiting, dyspnea, chest pain, death

Drug Interactions
Increased effect: Diazepam, chlordiazepoxide
Increased toxicity:
Alcohol and disulfiram: Antabuse® reaction
Tricyclic antidepressants, metronidazole, isoniazid: Encephalopathy
Disulfiram has caused increases in serum levels of phenytoin and warfarin leading to phenytoin toxicity and enhanced anticoagulation

Drug Uptake
Absorption: Rapid from GI tract
Full effect: 12 hours
Duration: May persist for 1-2 weeks after last dose

Pregnancy Risk Factor C

Ditropan® *see* Oxybutynin Chloride *on page 645*

Diucardin® *see* Hydroflumethiazide *on page 437*

Diupres-250® *see* Chlorothiazide and Reserpine *on page 189*

Diupres-500® *see* Chlorothiazide and Reserpine *on page 189*

Diurigen® *see* Chlorothiazide *on page 188*

Diuril® *see* Chlorothiazide *on page 188*

Diutensin® *see* Methyclothiazide and Cryptenamine Tannates *on page 566*

Dizmiss® [OTC] *see* Meclizine Hydrochloride *on page 530*

DNR *see* Daunorubicin Hydrochloride *on page 252*

Dobutamina, Clorhidrato De (Mexico) *see* Dobutamine Hydrochloride *on this page*

Dobutamine Hydrochloride (doe byoo' ta meen hye droe klor' ide)

Brand Names Dobutrex®

Canadian/Mexican Brand Names Dobuject® (Mexico); Oxiken® (Mexico)

Therapeutic Category Adrenergic Agonist Agent

Synonyms Dobutamina, Clorhidrato De (Mexico)

Use Short-term management of patients with cardiac decompensation

Usual Dosage I.V. infusion:

Children: 2.5-15 mcg/kg/minute, titrate to desired response

Adults: 2.5-15 mcg/kg/minute; maximum: 40 mcg/kg/minute, titrate to desired response

Infusion Rates of Various Dilutions of Dobutamine

Desired Delivery Rate (mcg/kg/min)	Infusion Rate (mL/kg/min)	
	500 mcg/mL*	1000 mcg/mL†
2.5	0.005	0.0025
5.0	0.01	0.005
7.5	0.015	0.0075
10.0	0.02	0.01
12.5	0.025	0.0125
15.0	0.03	0.015

* 500 mg per liter or 250 mg per 500 mL of diluent.

†1000 mg per liter or 250 mg per 250 mL of diluent.

Mechanism of Action Stimulates beta$_1$-adrenergic receptors, causing increased contractility and heart rate, with little effect on beta$_2$- or alpha-receptors

Local Anesthetic/Vasoconstrictor Precautions No information available to require special precautions

Effects on Dental Treatment No effects or complications reported

Other Adverse Effects

>10%:

Cardiovascular: Ectopic heartbeats, increased heart rate, chest pain, angina, palpitations, elevation in blood pressure; in higher doses ventricular tachycardia or arrhythmias may be seen; patients with atrial fibrillation or flutter are at risk of developing a rapid ventricular response

1% to 10%:

Cardiovascular: Premature ventricular beats, chest pain, angina, palpitations, shortness of breath

Central nervous system: Tingling sensation, headache

Gastrointestinal: Nausea, vomiting

Neuromuscular & skeletal: Mild leg cramps, paresthesia

Respiratory: Dyspnea

Drug Interactions

Decreased effect: Beta-adrenergic blockers (increased peripheral resistance)

Increased toxicity: General anesthetics (ie, halothane or cyclopropane) and usual doses of dobutamine have resulted in ventricular arrhythmias in animals

Drug Uptake

Onset of action: I.V.: 1-10 minutes

Serum half-life: 2 minutes

Pregnancy Risk Factor C

Dobutrex® *see* Dobutamine Hydrochloride *on this page*

Docetaxel (doe se tax' el)

Brand Names Taxotere®

Therapeutic Category Antineoplastic Agent, Miscellaneous

Use Treatment of breast cancer

Usual Dosage Adults: I.V.: 60-100 mg/m^2 administered over 1 hour every 3 weeks

Local Anesthetic/Vasoconstrictor Precautions No information available to require special precautions

Effects on Dental Treatment No effects or complications reported

Pregnancy Risk Factor D

Generic Available No

Docucal-P® [OTC] *see* Docusate and Phenolphthalein *on this page*

Docusate (dok′ yoo sate)

Brand Names Colace® [OTC]; DC 240® Softgels® [OTC]; Dialose® [OTC]; Diocto® [OTC]; Diocto-K® [OTC]; Dioeze® [OTC]; Disonate® [OTC]; DOK® [OTC]; DOS® Softgel® [OTC]; Doxinate® [OTC]; D-S-S® [OTC]; Kasof® [OTC]; Modane® Soft [OTC]; Pro-Cal-Sof® [OTC]; Pro-Sof® [OTC]; Regulax SS® [OTC]; Regutol® [OTC]; Sulfalax® [OTC]; Surfak® [OTC]

Canadian/Mexican Brand Names Colax-C® (Canada); Albert Docusate® (Canada); PMS-Docusate Calcium® (Canada)

Therapeutic Category Laxative, Surfactant; Stool Softener

Use Stool softener in patients who should avoid straining during defecation and constipation associated with hard, dry stools; prophylaxis for straining (Valsalva) following myocardial infarction. A safe agent to be used in elderly; some evidence that doses <200 mg are ineffective; stool softeners are unnecessary if stool is well hydrated or "mushy" and soft; shown to be ineffective used long-term.

Usual Dosage Docusate salts are interchangeable; the amount of sodium, calcium, or potassium per dosage unit is clinically insignificant

Children <3 years: Oral: 10-40 mg/day in 1-4 divided doses
Children: Oral:
    3-6 years: 20-60 mg/day in 1-4 divided doses
    6-12 years: 40-150 mg/day in 1-4 divided doses
Adolescents and Adults: Oral: 50-500 mg/day in 1-4 divided doses
Older Children and Adults: Rectal: Add 50-100 mg of docusate liquid to enema fluid (saline or water); give as retention or flushing enema

Mechanism of Action Reduces surface tension of the oil-water interface of the stool resulting in enhanced incorporation of water and fat allowing for stool softening

Local Anesthetic/Vasoconstrictor Precautions No information available to require special precautions

Effects on Dental Treatment No effects or complications reported

Other Adverse Effects 1% to 10%: Gastrointestinal: Intestinal obstruction, diarrhea, abdominal cramping, throat irritation

Drug Interactions
Decreased effect of Coumadin®, aspirin
Increased toxicity with mineral oil, phenolphthalein

Drug Uptake Onset of action: 12-72 hours

Pregnancy Risk Factor C

Docusate and Casanthranol (dok′ yoo sate & ka san′ thra nole)

Brand Names Dialose® Plus Capsule [OTC]; Diocto C® [OTC]; Diocto-K Plus® [OTC]; Dioctolose Plus® [OTC]; Disanthrol® [OTC]; DSMC Plus® [OTC]; D-S-S Plus® [OTC]; Genasoft® Plus [OTC]; Peri-Colace® [OTC]; Pro-Sof® Plus [OTC]; Regulace® [OTC]; Silace-C® [OTC]

Therapeutic Category Laxative, Surfactant; Stool Softener

Synonyms Casanthranol and Docusate; DSS With Casanthranol

Use Treatment of constipation generally associated with dry, hard stools and decreased intestinal motility

Local Anesthetic/Vasoconstrictor Precautions No information available to require special precautions

Effects on Dental Treatment No effects or complications reported

Other Adverse Effects 1% to 10%:
Dermatologic: Rash
Gastrointestinal: Intestinal obstruction, diarrhea, abdominal cramping, throat irritation

Docusate and Phenolphthalein
(dok′ yoo sate & fee nole thay′ leen)

Brand Names Colax® [OTC]; Correctol® [OTC]; Dialose® Plus Tablet [OTC]; Disolan® [OTC]; Docucal-P® [OTC]; Doxidan® [OTC]; Ex-Lax®, Extra Gentle Pills [OTC]; Feen-a-Mint® Pills [OTC]; Femilax® [OTC]; Modane® Plus [OTC]; Phillips′® LaxCaps® [OTC]; Unilax® [OTC]

Therapeutic Category Laxative, Stimulant; Laxative, Surfactant; Stool Softener

Use Management of chronic functional constipation

Local Anesthetic/Vasoconstrictor Precautions No information available to require special precautions

Effects on Dental Treatment No effects or complications reported

ALPHABETICAL LISTING OF DRUGS

DOK® [OTC] *see* Docusate *on previous page*

Doktors® Nasal Solution [OTC] *see* Phenylephrine Hydrochloride *on page 685*

Dolacet® [5/500] *see* Hydrocodone and Acetaminophen *on page 431*

Dolene® *see* Propoxyphene *on page 740*

Dolobid® *see* Diflunisal *on page 278*

Dolophine® *see* Methadone Hydrochloride *on page 552*

Domeboro® Topical [OTC] *see* Aluminum Sulfate and Calcium Acetate *on page 41*

Dome Paste Bandage *see* Zinc Gelatin *on page 908*

Donnamor® *see* Hyoscyamine, Atropine, Scopolamine, and Phenobarbital *on page 444*

Donnapectolin-PG® *see* Hyoscyamine, Atropine, Scopolamine, Kaolin, Pectin, and Opium *on page 445*

Donnapine® *see* Hyoscyamine, Atropine, Scopolamine, and Phenobarbital *on page 444*

Donna-Sed® *see* Hyoscyamine, Atropine, Scopolamine, and Phenobarbital *on page 444*

Donnatal® *see* Hyoscyamine, Atropine, Scopolamine, and Phenobarbital *on page 444*

Donnazyme® *see* Pancreatin *on page 656*

Donphen® *see* Hyoscyamine, Atropine, Scopolamine, and Phenobarbital *on page 444*

Dopar® *see* Levodopa *on page 495*

Dopram® Injection *see* Doxapram Hydrochloride *on next page*

Doral® *see* Quazepam *on page 755*

Dorcol® [OTC] *see* Acetaminophen *on page 14*

Dornase Alfa (door' nace al' fa)
Brand Names Pulmozyme®
Therapeutic Category Enzyme
Use Management of cystic fibrosis patients to reduce the frequency of respiratory infections that require parenteral antibiotics, and to improve pulmonary function
Usual Dosage Children >5 years and Adults: Inhalation: 2.5 mg once daily through selected nebulizers in conjunction with a Pulmo-Aide® or a Pari-Proneb® compressor
Mechanism of Action The hallmark of cystic fibrosis lung disease is the presence of abundant, purulent airway secretions composed primarily of highly polymerized DNA. The principal source of this DNA is the nuclei of degenerating neutrophils, which is present in large concentrations in infected lung secretions. The presence of this DNA produces a viscous mucous that may contribute to the decreased mucocilliary transport and persistent infections that are commonly seen in this population. Dornase alfa is a deoxyribonuclease (DNA) enzyme produced by recombinant gene technology. Dornase selectively cleaves DNA, thus reducing mucous viscosity and as a result, airflow in the lung is improved and the risk of bacterial infection may be decreased.
Local Anesthetic/Vasoconstrictor Precautions No information available to require special precautions
Effects on Dental Treatment No effects or complications reported
Other Adverse Effects
>10%: Voice alteration, pharyngitis
1% to 10%:
Cardiovascular: Chest pain
Dermatologic: Rash
Ocular: Conjunctivitis
Respiratory: Laryngitis, cough, dyspnea, hemoptysis, rhinitis, hoarse throat, wheezing
Drug Interactions No data reported
Drug Uptake Following nebulization, enzyme levels are measurable in the sputum within 15 minutes and decline rapidly thereafter
Pregnancy Risk Factor B

Doryx® *see* Doxycycline *on page 301*

Dorzolamide Hydrochloride (dor zole' a mide hye droe klor' ide)
Brand Names Trusopt®
Therapeutic Category Antiglaucoma Agent; Carbonic Anhydrase Inhibitor
Use Lower intraocular pressure to treat glaucoma

Usual Dosage Adults: Glaucoma: Instill 1 drop in the affected eye(s) 3 times/
day

Local Anesthetic/Vasoconstrictor Precautions No information available to
require special precautions

Effects on Dental Treatment No effects or complications reported

Other Adverse Effects
Central nervous system: Headache
Dermatologic: Rash
Gastrointestinal: Bitter taste (~25%), nausea, asthenia/fatigue (infrequent)
Genitourinary: Urolithiasis
Ocular: Burning, stinging, or discomfort immediately following administration
(~33%); iridocyclitis (rare); superficial punctate keratitis (10% to 15%); signs
and symptoms of ocular allergic reaction (~10%); blurred vision, tearing,
dryness (1% to 5%); photophobia (~1% to 5%)

Drug Uptake
Peak effect: 2 hours
Duration: 8-12 hours
Absorption: Systemically absorbed, however, detailed absorption characteris-
tics and pharmacokinetic data are unavailable
Serum half-life: Terminal RBC half-life of 147 days

DOS® Softgel® [OTC] see Docusate *on page 295*

Dovonex® see Calcipotriene *on page 138*

Doxapram Hydrochloride (dox′ a pram hye droe klor′ ide)
Brand Names Dopram® Injection

Therapeutic Category Central Nervous System Stimulant, Nonamphetamine;
Respiratory Stimulant

Use Respiratory and CNS stimulant; idiopathic apnea of prematurity refractory
to xanthines

Usual Dosage Not for use in newborns since doxapram contains a significant
amount of benzyl alcohol (0.9%)

Neonatal apnea (apnea of prematurity): I.V.:
Initial: 1-1.5 mg/kg/hour
Maintenance: 0.5-2.5 mg/kg/hour, titrated to the lowest rate at which apnea
is controlled

Adults: Respiratory depression following anesthesia: I.V.:
Initial: 0.5-1 mg/kg; may repeat at 5-minute intervals; maximum total dose: 2
mg/kg
I.V. infusion: Initial: 5 mg/minute until adequate response or adverse effects
seen; decrease to 1-3 mg/minute; usual total dose: 0.5-4 mg/kg; maximum:
300 mg

Not dialyzable

Mechanism of Action Stimulates respiration through action on respiratory
center in medulla or indirectly on peripheral carotid chemoreceptors

Local Anesthetic/Vasoconstrictor Precautions No information available to
require special precautions

Effects on Dental Treatment No effects or complications reported

Other Adverse Effects
1% to 10%:
Cardiovascular: Ectopic beats, hypotension, vasoconstriction, tachycardia,
anginal pain, palpitations
Central nervous system: Headache
Gastrointestinal: Nausea, vomiting
Respiratory: Dyspnea
<1%:
Cardiovascular: Hypertension (dose related), arrhythmias, flushing
Central nervous system: CNS stimulation, restlessness, lightheadedness,
jitters, hallucinations, irritability, seizures, hyperpyrexia
Gastrointestinal: Abdominal distension, retching
Hematologic: Hemolysis
Local: Phlebitis
Neuromuscular & skeletal: Tremor, hyperreflexia
Ocular: Mydriasis, lacrimation
Respiratory: Coughing, laryngospasm
Miscellaneous: Sweating, feeling of warmth

Drug Uptake
Onset of action (respiratory stimulation): I.V.: Within 20-40 seconds
Peak effect: Within 1-2 minutes
Duration: 5-12 minutes
(Continued)

Doxapram Hydrochloride *(Continued)*

Serum half-life:
  Adults: 3.4 hours (mean half-life)

Pregnancy Risk Factor B

Comments Initial studies suggest a therapeutic range of at least 1.5 mg/L; toxicity becomes frequent at serum levels >5 mg/L

Doxazosin *(dox aye' zoe sin)*

Related Information
  Cardiovascular Diseases *on page 912*

Brand Names Cardura®

Therapeutic Category Alpha-Adrenergic Blockers - Peripheral-Acting (Alpha$_1$-Blockers)

Use Treatment of hypertension, severe congestive heart failure (in conjunction with diuretics and cardiac glycosides)

Unlabeled use: Symptoms of benign prostatic hypertrophy

Usual Dosage Oral:
  Adults: 1 mg once daily in morning or evening; may be increased to 2 mg once daily; thereafter titrate upwards, if needed, over several weeks, balancing therapeutic benefit with doxazosin-induced postural hypotension; maximum dose for hypertension: 16 mg/day, for BPH: 8 mg/day
  Elderly: Initial: 0.5 mg once daily

Mechanism of Action Competitively inhibits postsynaptic alpha-adrenergic receptors which results in vasodilation of veins and arterioles and a decrease in total peripheral resistance and blood pressure; approximately 50% as potent on a weight by weight basis as prazosin

Local Anesthetic/Vasoconstrictor Precautions No information available to require special precautions

Effects on Dental Treatment No effects or complications reported

Other Adverse Effects
  >10%: Central nervous system: Dizziness
  1% to 10%:
    Cardiovascular: Palpitations, arrhythmia
    Central nervous system: Vertigo, nervousness, somnolence, anxiety
    Endocrine & metabolic: Decreased libido
    Gastrointestinal: Nausea, vomiting, dry mouth, diarrhea, constipation
    Neuromuscular & skeletal: Shoulder, neck, back pain
    Ocular: Abnormal vision
    Respiratory: Rhinitis
  <1%:
    Cardiovascular: Hypotension, tachycardia
    Central nervous system: Depression
    Gastrointestinal: Abdominal discomfort, flatulence
    Genitourinary: Incontinence
    Ocular: Conjunctivitis
    Otic: Tinnitus
    Renal: Polyuria
    Respiratory: Dyspnea, sinusitis
    Miscellaneous: Epistaxis

Drug Interactions Increased effect with diuretics and antihypertensive medications (especially beta-blockers)

Pregnancy Risk Factor B

Doxepin Hydrochloride *(dox' e pin hye droe klor' ide)*

Brand Names Adapin®; Sinequan®

Canadian/Mexican Brand Names Apo-Doxepin® (Canada); Novo-Doxepin® (Canada); Triadapin® (Canada)

Therapeutic Category Antianxiety Agent; Antidepressant, Tricyclic; Tranquilizer, Minor

Use Treatment of various forms of depression, usually in conjunction with psychotherapy; treatment of anxiety disorders; analgesic for certain chronic and neuropathic pain

Usual Dosage
  Oral (entire daily dose may be given at bedtime):
    Adolescents: Initial: 25-50 mg/day in single or divided doses; gradually increase to 100 mg/day
    Adults: Initial: 30-150 mg/day at bedtime or in 2-3 divided doses; may gradually increase up to 300 mg/day; single dose should not exceed 150 mg; select patients may respond to 25-50 mg/day

Mechanism of Action Increases the synaptic concentration of serotonin and/ or norepinephrine in the central nervous system by inhibition of their reuptake by the presynaptic neuronal membrane

Local Anesthetic/Vasoconstrictor Precautions Use with caution; epinephrine, norepinephrine and levonordefrin have been shown to have an increased pressor response in combination with TCAs

Effects on Dental Treatment Long-term treatment with TCAs such as amoxapine increases the risk of caries by reducing salivation and salivary buffer capacity

Other Adverse Effects

>10%:

Central nervous system: Sedation, drowsiness, dizziness, headache

Gastrointestinal: Dry mouth, constipation, increased appetite, nausea, weakness, unpleasant taste, weight gain

1% to 10%:

Cardiovascular: Hypotension, arrhythmias

Central nervous system: Confusion, delirium, hallucinations, nervousness, restlessness, parkinsonian syndrome, insomnia

Gastrointestinal: Difficult urination, diarrhea, heartburn

Genitourinary: Sexual function impairment

Neuromuscular & skeletal: Fine muscle tremors

Ocular: Blurred vision, eye pain

Miscellaneous: Excessive sweating

<1%:

Central nervous system: Anxiety, seizures

Dermatologic: Alopecia, dermal photosensitivity

Endocrine & metabolic: Breast enlargement, galactorrhea

Genitourinary: Urinary retention, testicular swelling, SIADH

Hematologic: Agranulocytosis, leukopenia, eosinophilia

Hepatic: Hepatitis, cholestatic jaundice and increased liver enzymes

Ocular: Increased intraocular pressure, photosensitivity

Otic: Tinnitus

Miscellaneous: Trouble with gums, decreased lower esophageal sphincter tone may cause GE reflux, allergic reactions

Drug Interactions

Decreased effect: Phenobarbital may increase the metabolism of doxepin; doxepin blocks the uptake of guanethidine and thus prevents the hypotensive effect of guanethidine

Increased toxicity: Clonidine causes hypertensive crisis; doxepin may be additive with or may potentiate the action of other CNS depressants such as sedatives or hypnotics; with MAO inhibitors, hyperpyrexia, hypertension, tachycardia, confusion, and seizures. Doxepin may increase the prothrombin time in patients stabilized on warfarin; doxepin may potentiate the pressor and cardiac effects of sympathomimetic agents such as isoproterenol, epinephrine, etc; cimetidine and methylphenidate may decrease the metabolism of doxepin

Additive anticholinergic effects seen with other anticholinergic agents

Drug Uptake

Serum half-life: Adults: 6-8 hours

Pregnancy Risk Factor C

Selected Readings

Boakes AJ, Laurence DR, Teoh PC, et al, "Interactions Between Sympathomimetic Amines and Antidepressant Agents in Man," *Br Med J*, 1973, 1(849):311-5.

Jastak JT and Yagiela JA, "Vasoconstrictors and Local Anesthesia: A Review and Rationale for Use," *J Am Dent Assoc*, 1983, 107(4):623-30.

Larochelle P, Hamet P, and Enjalbert M, "Responses to Tyramine and Norepinephrine After Imipramine and Trazodone," *Clin Pharmacol Ther*, 1979, 26(1):24-30.

Mitchell JR, "Guanethidine and Related Agents. III Antagonism by Drugs Which Inhibit the Norepinephrine Pump in Man," *J Clin Invest*, 1970, 49(8):1596-604.

Rundgren J, van Dijken J, Mörnstad H, et al, "Oral Conditions in Patients Receiving Long-Term Treatment With Cyclic Antidepressant Drugs," *Swed Dent J*, 1985, 9(2):55-64.

Svedmyr N, "The Influence of a Tricyclic Antidepressive Agent (Protriptyline) on Some of the Circulatory Effects of Noradrenaline and Adrenalin® in Man," *Life Sci*, 1968, 7(1):77-84.

Doxidan® [OTC] *see* Docusate and Phenolphthalein *on page 295*

Doxil® Injection *see* Doxorubicin Hydrochloride *on this page*

Doxinate® [OTC] *see* Docusate *on page 295*

Doxorubicin Hydrochloride (dox oh roo' bi sin hye droe klor' ide)

Brand Names Adriamycin® PFS; Adriamycin® RDF; Doxil® Injection; Rubex®

Canadian/Mexican Brand Names Doxolem (Mexico)

Therapeutic Category Antineoplastic Agent, Antibiotic

Synonyms ADR; Hydroxydaunomycin Hydrochloride

(Continued)

Doxorubicin Hydrochloride (Continued)

Use Treatment of various solid tumors including ovarian, breast, and bladder tumors; various lymphomas and leukemias (ANL, ALL), soft tissue sarcomas, neuroblastoma, osteosarcoma

Usual Dosage Refer to individual protocols

I.V. (patient's ideal weight should be used to calculate body surface area):
Children: 35-75 mg/m^2 as a single dose, repeat every 21 days; **or** 20-30 mg/m^2 once weekly; **OR** 60-90 mg/m^2 given as a continuous infusion over 96 hours every 3-4 weeks

Adults: 60-75 mg/m^2 as a single dose, repeat every 21 days **or** other dosage regimens like 20-30 mg/m^2/day for 2-3 days, repeat in 4 weeks **or** 20 mg/m^2 once weekly

The lower dose regimen should be given to patients with decreased bone marrow reserve, prior therapy or marrow infiltration with malignant cells

Currently the maximum cumulative dose is 550 mg/m^2 or 450 mg/m^2 in patients who have received RT to the mediastinal areas; a baseline MUGA should be performed prior to initiating treatment. If the LVEF is <30% to 40%, therapy should not be instituted; LVEF should be monitored during therapy.

Doxorubicin has also been administered intraperitoneal (phase I in refractory ovarian cancer patients) and intra-arterially.

Mechanism of Action Doxorubicin works through inhibition of topoisomerase-II at the point of DNA cleavage. A second mechanism of action is the production of free radicals (the hydroxy radical OH) by doxorubicin, which in turn can destroy DNA and cancerous cells. Doxorubicin is also a very powerful iron chelator, equal to deferoxamine. The iron-doxorubicin complex can bind DNA and cell membranes rapidly and produce free radicals that immediately cleave the DNA and cell membranes. Inhibits DNA and RNA synthesis by intercalating between DNA base pairs and by steric obstruction; active throughout entire cell cycle.

Local Anesthetic/Vasoconstrictor Precautions No information available to require special precautions

Effects on Dental Treatment No effects or complications reported

Other Adverse Effects

>10%: Alopecia

Gastrointestinal: Acute nausea and vomiting may be seen in 21% to 55% of patients; mucositis, ulceration, and necrosis of the colon, anorexia, and diarrhea

Emetic potential:
≤20 mg: Moderately low (10% to 30%)
>20 mg or <75 mg: Moderate (30% to 60%)
≥75 mg: Moderately high (60% to 90%)

Myelosuppressive: 60% to 80% of patients will have leukopenia; dose-limiting toxicity; WBC: Moderate; Platelets: Moderate; Onset (days): 7; Nadir (days): 10-14; Recovery (days): 21-28

Radiation recall: Noticed in patients who have had prior irradiation; reactions include redness, warmth, erythema, and dermatitis in the radiation port. Can progress to severe desquamation and ulceration. Occurs 5-7 days after doxorubicin administration; local therapy with topical corticosteroids and cooling have given the best relief.

Extravasation: Doxorubicin is one of the most notorious vesicants. Infiltration can cause severe inflammation, tissue necrosis, and ulceration. If the drug is infiltrated, consult institutional policy, apply ice to the area, and elevate the limb. Can have ongoing tissue destruction secondary to propagation of free radicals; may require debridement.

1% to 10%: Erythematous streaking along the vein if administered too rapidly

Cardiac toxicity: Dose-limiting and related to cumulative dose; usually a maximum total lifetime dose of 450-550 mg/m^2 is administered; although, it has been demonstrated that if given by continuous infusion in breast cancer patients, higher doses may be tolerated. Cardiac tissue seems to be very sensitive to damage by free radicals produced by doxorubicin. Patients may present with acute toxicity (arrhythmias, heart block, pericarditis-myocarditis) which may be fatal. More commonly, chronic toxicity is seen, in which patients present with signs of congestive heart failure. Several methods of monitoring cardiac toxicity have been utilized, including myocardial biopsy (expensive and hazardous procedure).

<1%: Allergic reaction, anaphylaxis

Miscellaneous: Fever, chills, urticaria, conjunctivitis

Drug Uptake

Absorption: Oral: Poor, <50%

Serum half-life, triphasic:
Primary: 30 minutes
Secondary: 3-3.5 hours for metabolites
Terminal: 17-30 hours for doxorubicin and its metabolites
Pregnancy Risk Factor D

Doxy® *see Doxycycline on this page*

Doxychel® *see Doxycycline on this page*

Doxycycline (dox i sye′ kleen)
Related Information
Animal and Human Bites Guidelines *on page 976*
Antimicrobial Prophylaxis in Surgical Patients *on page 1042*
Nonviral Infectious Diseases *on page 932*
Brand Names Doryx®; Doxy®; Doxychel®; Vibramycin®; Vibra-Tabs®
Canadian/Mexican Brand Names Apo-Doxy® (Canada); Apo-Doxy® Tabs (Canada); Doxycin® (Canada); Doxytec® (Canada); Novo-Doxylin® (Canada); Nu-Doxycycline® (Canada); Vibramicina® (Mexico)
Therapeutic Category Antibiotic, Tetracycline Derivative
Use
Dental: Treatment of periodontitis associated with presence of *Actinobacillus actinomycetemcomitans* (AA)
Medical: In medicine, principally in the treatment of infections caused by susceptible *Rickettsia*, *Chlamydia*, and *Mycoplasma* along with uncommon susceptible gram-negative and gram-positive organisms; alternative to mefloquine for malaria prophylaxis
Unapproved use: Treatment for syphilis in penicillin-allergic patients; sclerosing agent for pleural effusions
Usual Dosage Adults: 100 mg/day for 21 days or until improvement
Mechanism of Action Inhibits protein synthesis by binding with the 30S and possibly the 50S ribosomal subunit(s) of susceptible bacteria; may also cause alterations in the cytoplasmic membrane
Local Anesthetic/Vasoconstrictor Precautions No information available to require special precautions
Effects on Dental Treatment Tetracycline's are not recommended for use during pregnancy or in children ≤8 years of age since they have been reported to cause enamel hypoplasia and permanent teeth discoloration. The use of tetracycline's should only be used in these patients if other agents are contraindicated or alternative antimicrobials will not eradicate the organism. Long-term use associated with oral candidiasis.
Other Adverse Effects
>10%: Miscellaneous: Discoloration of teeth in children
<1%: Gastrointestinal: Nausea, diarrhea
Oral manifestations: Opportunistic "superinfection" with *Candida albicans*
Contraindications Hypersensitivity to doxycycline, tetracycline or any component; children <8 years of age; severe hepatic dysfunction
Warnings/Precautions Use of tetracyclines during tooth development may cause permanent discoloration of the teeth and enamel hypoplasia; prolonged use may result in superinfection; photosensitivity reaction may occur with this drug; avoid prolonged exposure to sunlight or tanning equipment
Drug Interactions Iron and bismuth subsalicylate may decrease doxycycline bioavailability; barbiturates, phenytoin, and carbamazepine decrease doxycycline's half-life; increased effect of warfarin
Drug Uptake
Absorption: Oral: 90% to 100%
Time to peak serum concentration: Within 1.5-4 hours
Serum half-life: 12-15 hours (usually increases to 22-24 hours with multiple dosing)
Pregnancy Risk Factor D
Breast-feeding Considerations May be taken while breast-feeding
Dosage Forms
Capsule, as hyclate:
Doxychel®, Vibramycin®: 50 mg
Doxy®, Doxychel®, Vibramycin®: 100 mg
Capsule, coated pellets, as hyclate (Doryx®): 100 mg
Powder for injection, as hyclate (Doxy®, Doxychel®, Vibramycin® IV): 100 mg, 200 mg
Powder for oral suspension, as monohydrate (raspberry flavor) (Vibramycin®): 25 mg/5 mL (60 mL)
(Continued)

Doxycycline *(Continued)*

Syrup, as calcium (raspberry-apple flavor) (Vibramycin®): 50 mg/5 mL (30 mL, 473 mL)

Tablet, as hyclate
Doxychel®: 50 mg
Doxychel®, Vibra-Tabs®: 100 mg

Dietary Considerations May be taken with food, milk, or water

Generic Available Yes

Selected Readings

Rams TE and Slots J, "Antibiotics in Periodontal Therapy: An Update," *Compendium*, 1992, 13(12):1130, 1132, 1134.

DPPC *see* Colfosceril Palmitate *on page 230*

Dramamine® [OTC] *see* Dimenhydrinate *on page 286*

Dramilin® *see* Dimenhydrinate *on page 286*

Dri-Ear® Otic [OTC] *see* Boric Acid *on page 118*

Drisdol® *see* Ergocalciferol *on page 317*

Dristan® Long Lasting Nasal Solution [OTC] *see* Oxymetazoline Hydrochloride *on page 649*

Dristan® Sinus Caplets [OTC] *see* Pseudoephedrine and Ibuprofen *on page 750*

Drithocreme® *see* Anthralin *on page 68*

Drithocreme® HP 1% *see* Anthralin *on page 68*

Dritho-Scalp® *see* Anthralin *on page 68*

Drixoral® [OTC] *see* Dexbrompheniramine and Pseudoephedrine *on page 261*

Drixoral® Cough & Congestion Liquid Caps [OTC] *see* Pseudoephedrine and Dextromethorphan *on page 750*

Drixoral® Cough & Sore Throat Liquid Caps [OTC] *see* Acetaminophen and Dextromethorphan *on page 16*

Drixoral® Non-Drowsy [OTC] *see* Pseudoephedrine *on page 749*

Drixoral® Syrup [OTC] *see* Brompheniramine and Pseudoephedrine *on page 123*

Dronabinol *(droe nab′ i nol)*

Related Information

Chemical Dependency and Dental Practice *on page 971*

Brand Names Marinol®

Therapeutic Category Antiemetic

Use When conventional antiemetics fail to relieve the nausea and vomiting associated with cancer chemotherapy, AIDS-related anorexia

Usual Dosage Oral:

Children: NCI protocol recommends 5 mg/m^2 starting 6-8 hours before chemotherapy and every 4-6 hours after to be continued for 12 hours after chemotherapy is discontinued

Adults: 5 mg/m^2 1-3 hours before chemotherapy, then give 5 mg/m^2/dose every 2-4 hours after chemotherapy for a total of 4-6 doses/day; dose may be increased up to a maximum of 15 mg/m^2/dose if needed (dosage may be increased by 2.5 mg/m^2 increments)

Appetite stimulant (AIDS-related): Initial: 2.5 mg twice daily (before lunch and dinner); titrate up to a maximum of 20 mg/day

Mechanism of Action Not well defined, probably inhibits the vomiting center in the medulla oblongata

Local Anesthetic/Vasoconstrictor Precautions No information available to require special precautions

Effects on Dental Treatment No effects or complications reported

Other Adverse Effects

>10%: Central nervous system: Drowsiness, dizziness, detachment, anxiety, difficulty concentrating, mood change

1% to 10%:
Cardiovascular: Orthostatic hypotension, tachycardia
Central nervous system: Coordination impairment, depression, weakness, headache, vertigo, hallucinations, memory lapse, ataxia
Gastrointestinal: Dry mouth
Neuromuscular & skeletal: Paresthesia

<1%:
Cardiovascular: Syncope
Central nervous system: Nightmares, speech difficulties
Gastrointestinal: Diarrhea
Neuromuscular & skeletal: Muscular pains
Otic: Tinnitus

Miscellaneous: Sweating

Drug Interactions Increased toxicity (drowsiness) with alcohol, barbiturates, benzodiazepines

Drug Uptake
Absorption: Oral: Erratic
Serum half-life: 19-24 hours
Time to peak serum concentration: Within 2-3 hours

Pregnancy Risk Factor B

Droperidol (droe per' i dole)

Brand Names Inapsine®

Canadian/Mexican Brand Names Dehydrobenzperidol® (Mexico)

Therapeutic Category Antiemetic; Antipsychotic Agent

Use Tranquilizer and antiemetic in surgical and diagnostic procedures; antiemetic for cancer chemotherapy; preoperative medication; has good antiemetic effect as well as sedative and antianxiety effects

Usual Dosage Titrate carefully to desired effect
Children 2-12 years:
Premedication: I.M.: 0.1-0.15 mg/kg; smaller doses may be sufficient for control of nausea or vomiting
Adjunct to general anesthesia: I.V. induction: 0.088-0.165 mg/kg
Nausea and vomiting: I.M., I.V.: 0.05-0.06 mg/kg/dose every 4-6 hours as needed
Adults:
Premedication: I.M.: 2.5-10 mg 30 minutes to 1 hour preoperatively
Adjunct to general anesthesia: I.V. induction: 0.22-0.275 mg/kg; maintenance: 1.25-2.5 mg/dose
Alone in diagnostic procedures: I.M.: Initial: 2.5-10 mg 30 minutes to 1 hour before; then 1.25-2.5 mg if needed
Nausea and vomiting: I.M., I.V.: 2.5-5 mg/dose every 3-4 hours as needed

Mechanism of Action Alters the action of dopamine in the CNS, at subcortical levels, to produce sedation; reduces emesis by blocking dopamine stimulation of the chemotrigger zone

Local Anesthetic/Vasoconstrictor Precautions No information available to require special precautions

Effects on Dental Treatment Significant hypotension may occur, especially when the drug is administered parenterally; orthostatic hypotension is due to alpha-receptor blockade, the elderly are at greater risk for orthostatic hypotension

Tardive dyskinesia: Prevalence rate may be 40% in elderly; development of the syndrome and the irreversible nature are proportional to duration and total cumulative dose over time

Extrapyramidal reactions are more common in elderly with up to 50% developing these reactions after 60 years of age; drug-induced **Parkinson's syndrome** occurs often; **akathisia** is the most common extrapyramidal reaction in elderly

Increased confusion, memory loss, psychotic behavior, and agitation frequently occur as a consequence of anticholinergic effects

Antipsychotic associated sedation in nonpsychotic patients is extremely unpleasant due to feelings of depersonalization, derealization, and dysphoria

Other Adverse Effects
>10%:
Cardiovascular: Mild to moderate hypotension, tachycardia
Central nervous system: Postoperative drowsiness
1% to 10%:
Cardiovascular: Hypertension
Central nervous system: Extrapyramidal reactions
Respiratory: Respiratory depression
<1%:
Central nervous system: Dizziness, chills, shivering, postoperative hallucinations
Respiratory: Laryngospasm, bronchospasm

Drug Interactions Increased toxicity: CNS depressants, fentanyl and other analgesics increased blood pressure; conduction anesthesia decreased blood pressure; epinephrine decreased blood pressure; atropine, lithium

Drug Uptake
Following parenteral administration:
Duration: 2-4 hours, may extend to 12 hours
Serum half-life: Adults: 2.3 hours
(Continued)

Droperidol *(Continued)*

Pregnancy Risk Factor C

Drotic® Otic see Neomycin, Polymyxin B, and Hydrocortisone *on page 610*

Drugs Associated With Adverse Hematologic Effects *see page 1079*

Dry Eyes® Solution [OTC] see Artificial Tears *on page 75*

Dry Eye® Therapy Solution [OTC] see Artificial Tears *on page 75*

Dryox® [OTC] see Benzoyl Peroxide *on page 104*

DSMC Plus® [OTC] see Docusate and Casanthranol *on page 295*

D-S-S® [OTC] see Docusate *on page 295*

D-S-S Plus® [OTC] see Docusate and Casanthranol *on page 295*

DSS With Casanthranol see Docusate and Casanthranol *on page 295*

DTIC see Dacarbazine *on page 247*

DTIC-Dome® see Dacarbazine *on page 247*

Duadacin® Capsule [OTC] see Chlorpheniramine, Phenylpropanolamine, and Acetaminophen *on page 194*

Dulcolax® [OTC] see Bisacodyl *on page 113*

DuoCet™ [5/500] see Hydrocodone and Acetaminophen *on page 431*

Duo-Cyp® Injection see Estradiol and Testosterone *on page 326*

Duofilm® Solution see Salicylic Acid and Lactic Acid *on page 778*

Duo-Medihaler® Aerosol see Isoproterenol and Phenylephrine *on page 473*

Duo-Trach® see Lidocaine Hydrochloride *on page 502*

Duotrate® see Pentaerythritol Tetranitrate *on page 669*

DuP 753 see Losartan Potassium *on page 515*

Duphalac® see Lactulose *on page 488*

Duplex® T [OTC] see Coal Tar *on page 225*

Durabolin® see Nandrolone *on page 604*

Duradyne DHC® [5/500] see Hydrocodone and Acetaminophen *on page 431*

Dura-Estrin® see Estradiol *on page 325*

Duragen® see Estradiol *on page 325*

Duragesic™ see Fentanyl *on page 357*

Dura-Gest® see Guaifenesin, Phenylpropanolamine, and Phenylephrine *on page 410*

Duralone® see Methylprednisolone *on page 569*

Duralutin® see Hydroxyprogesterone Caproate *on page 441*

Duramorph® Injection see Morphine Sulfate *on page 590*

Duranest® with Epinephrine see Etidocaine Hydrochloride (With Epinephrine) *on page 345*

Duraphyl™ see Theophylline/Aminophylline *on page 832*

Duratest® see Testosterone *on page 825*

Duratestrin® Injection see Estradiol and Testosterone *on page 326*

Durathate® see Testosterone *on page 825*

Duration® Nasal Solution [OTC] see Oxymetazoline Hydrochloride *on page 649*

Dura-Vent® see Guaifenesin and Phenylpropanolamine *on page 409*

Duricef® see Cefadroxil Monohydrate *on page 162*

Durrax® see Hydroxyzine *on page 443*

Duvoid® see Bethanechol Chloride *on page 112*

DV® Cream see Dienestrol *on page 275*

Dwelle® Ophthalmic Solution [OTC] see Artificial Tears *on page 75*

Dyazide® see Triamterene and Hydrochlorothiazide *on page 865*

Dycill® see Dicloxacillin Sodium *on page 273*

Dyclone® see Dyclonine Hydrochloride *on this page*

Dyclonine Hydrochloride *(dye' kloe neen)*

Related Information

Oral Viral Infections *on page 951*

Brand Names Dyclone®

Therapeutic Category Local Anesthetic, Oral

Use

Dental: Use topically for temporary relief of pain associated with oral mucosa or anogenital lesions

Medical: Local anesthetic prior to laryngoscopy, bronchoscopy, or endotracheal intubation

Mechanism of Action Blocks impulses at peripheral nerve endings in skin and mucous membranes by altering cell membrane permeability to ionic transfer

Local Anesthetic/Vasoconstrictor Precautions No information available to require special precautions

Effects on Dental Treatment No effects or complications reported

Other Adverse Effects <1%:
Cardiovascular: Hypotension, bradycardia, respiratory arrest, cardiac arrest
Central nervous system: Excitation, drowsiness, nervousness, dizziness, seizures
Local: Slight irritation and stinging may occur when applied
Ocular: Blurred vision
Sensitivity reactions: Allergic reactions

Oral manifestations: No data reported

Drug Interactions No data reported

Pregnancy Risk Factor C

Breast-feeding Considerations No data reported

Dietary Considerations No data reported

Dyflex® *see* Dyphylline *on this page*

Dymelor® *see* Acetohexamide *on page 19*

Dynabac® *see* Dirithromycin *on page 291*

DynaCirc® *see* Isradipine *on page 476*

Dyna-Hex® [OTC] *see* Chlorhexidine Gluconate *on page 184*

Dynapen® *see* Dicloxacillin Sodium *on page 273*

Dyphylline (dye' fi lin)

Brand Names Dilor®; Dyflex®; Lufyllin®; Neothylline®

Therapeutic Category Bronchodilator; Theophylline Derivative

Synonyms Dihydroxypropyl Theophylline

Use Bronchodilator in reversible airway obstruction due to asthma or COPD

Local Anesthetic/Vasoconstrictor Precautions No information available to require special precautions

Effects on Dental Treatment Do not prescribe any erythromycin product to patients taking theophylline products. Erythromycin will delay the normal metabolic inactivation of theophyllines leading to increased blood levels; this has resulted in nausea, vomiting and CNS restlessness

Other Adverse Effects
Uncommon at serum theophylline concentrations ≤20 mcg/mL
1% to 10%:
Cardiovascular: Tachycardia
Central nervous system: Nervousness, restlessness
Gastrointestinal: Nausea, vomiting
<1%:
Central nervous system: Insomnia, irritability, seizures
Dermatologic: Skin rash
Gastrointestinal: Gastric irritation
Neuromuscular & skeletal: Tremor
Miscellaneous: Allergic reactions

Comments This drug is rarely used today. Requires a special laboratory measuring procedure rather than the standard theophylline assay. Saliva levels are approximately equal to 60% of plasma levels; charcoal-broiled foods may increase elimination, reducing half-life by 50%; cigarette smoking may require an increase of dosage by 50% to 100%. Because different salts of theophylline have different theophylline content, various salts are not equivalent.

Dyrenium® *see* Triamterene *on page 865*

7E3 *see* Abciximab *on page 12*

Easprin® *see* Aspirin *on page 78*

Echothiophate Iodide (ek oh thye' oh fate eye' oh dide)

Brand Names Phospholine Iodide®

Therapeutic Category Antiglaucoma Agent; Ophthalmic Agent, Miotic

Use Reverses toxic CNS effects caused by anticholinergic drugs; used as miotic in treatment of glaucoma; accommodative esotropia

Usual Dosage Adults:
Ophthalmic: Glaucoma: Instill 1 drop twice daily into eyes with 1 dose just prior to bedtime; some patients have been treated with 1 dose daily or every other day
Accommodative esotropia:
Diagnosis: Instill 1 drop of 0.125% once daily into both eyes at bedtime for 2-3 weeks

(Continued)

Echothiophate Iodide (Continued)

Treatment: Use lowest concentration and frequency which gives satisfactory response, with a maximum dose of 0.125% once daily, although more intensive therapy may be used for short periods of time

Mechanism of Action Produces miosis and changes in accommodation by inhibiting cholinesterase, thereby preventing the breakdown of acetylcholine; acetylcholine is, therefore, allowed to continuously stimulate the iris and ciliary muscles of the eye

Local Anesthetic/Vasoconstrictor Precautions No information available to require special precautions

Effects on Dental Treatment No effects or complications reported

Other Adverse Effects

1% to 10%: Ocular: Stinging, burning, myopia, visual blurring

<1%:

Cardiovascular: Bradycardia, hypotension, flushing

Gastrointestinal: Nausea, vomiting, diarrhea

Ocular: Retinal detachment, diaphoresis, muscle weakness, browache, miosis, twitching eyelids, watering eyes

Respiratory: Difficulty in breathing

Drug Interactions Increased toxicity: Carbamate or organophosphate insecticides and pesticides; succinylcholine; systemic acetylcholinesterases may increase neuromuscular effects

Drug Uptake

Onset of action:

Miosis: 10-30 minutes

Intraocular pressure decrease: 4-8 hours

Peak intraocular pressure decrease: 24 hours

Duration: Up to 1-4 weeks

Pregnancy Risk Factor C

E-Complex-600® [OTC] *see* Vitamin E *on page 900*

Econazole Nitrate (e kone' a zole nye' trate)

Brand Names Spectazole™

Canadian/Mexican Brand Names Ecostatin® (Canada); Micostyl® (Mexico)

Therapeutic Category Antifungal Agent, Topical

Use Topical treatment of tinea pedis (athlete's foot), tinea cruris (jock itch), tinea corporis (ringworm), tinea versicolor, and cutaneous candidiasis

Usual Dosage Children and Adults: Topical:

Tinea pedis, tinea cruris, tinea corporis, tinea versicolor: Apply sufficient amount to cover affected areas once daily

Cutaneous candidiasis: Apply sufficient quantity twice daily (morning and evening)

Duration of treatment: Candidal infections and tinea cruris, versicolor, and corporis should be treated for 2 weeks and tinea pedis for 1 month; occasionally, longer treatment periods may be required

Mechanism of Action Alters fungal cell wall membrane permeability; may interfere with RNA and protein synthesis, and lipid metabolism

Local Anesthetic/Vasoconstrictor Precautions No information available to require special precautions

Effects on Dental Treatment No effects or complications reported

Other Adverse Effects 1% to 10%: Local: Pruritus, erythema, burning, stinging

Drug Interactions No data reported

Drug Uptake

Absorption: Topical: <10%

Pregnancy Risk Factor C

Dosage Forms Cream: 1% in water miscible base (15 g, 30 g, 85 g)

Generic Available No

Econopred® *see* Prednisolone *on page 718*

Econopred® Plus *see* Prednisolone *on page 718*

Ecotrin® [OTC] *see* Aspirin *on page 78*

Ectasule® *see* Ephedrine Sulfate *on page 310*

Ed A-Hist® Liquid *see* Chlorpheniramine and Phenylephrine *on page 190*

Edecrin® *see* Ethacrynic Acid *on page 331*

E.E.S.® *see* Erythromycin *on page 321*

Efedrina (Mexico) *see* Ephedrine Sulfate *on page 310*

Efedron® *see* Ephedrine Sulfate *on page 310*

Effer-K™ *see* Potassium Bicarbonate and Potassium Citrate, Effervescent *on page 707*

Effer-Syllium® [OTC] *see* Psyllium *on page 750*

Effexor® *see* Venlafaxine *on page 892*

Efidac/24® [OTC] *see* Pseudoephedrine *on page 749*

Efodine® [OTC] *see* Povidone-Iodine *on page 713*

Efudex® Topical *see* Fluorouracil *on page 376*

Elase-Chloromycetin® Topical *see* Fibrinolysin and Desoxyribonuclease *on page 362*

Elase® Topical *see* Fibrinolysin and Desoxyribonuclease *on page 362*

Elavil® *see* Amitriptyline Hydrochloride *on page 51*

Eldepryl® *see* Selegiline Hydrochloride *on page 784*

Eldercaps® [OTC] *see* Vitamins, Multiple *on page 901*

Eldopaque® [OTC] *see* Hydroquinone *on page 439*

Eldopaque Forte® *see* Hydroquinone *on page 439*

Eldoquin® [OTC] *see* Hydroquinone *on page 439*

Eldoquin Forte® *see* Hydroquinone *on page 439*

Electrolyte Lavage Solution *see* Polyethylene Glycol-Electrolyte Solution *on page 703*

Elimite™ *see* Permethrin *on page 676*

Elixophyllin® *see* Theophylline/Aminophylline *on page 832*

Elixophyllin® SR *see* Theophylline/Aminophylline *on page 832*

Elmiron® *see* Pentosan Polysulfate Sodium *on page 674*

Elocon® *see* Mometasone Furoate *on page 589*

E-Lor® *see* Propoxyphene and Acetaminophen *on page 741*

Elspar® *see* Asparaginase *on page 77*

Eltroxin™ *see* Levothyroxine Sodium *on page 498*

Emcyt® *see* Estramustine Phosphate Sodium *on page 326*

Emecheck® [OTC] *see* Phosphorated Carbohydrate Solution *on page 690*

Emetrol® [OTC] *see* Phosphorated Carbohydrate Solution *on page 690*

Emgel™ Topical *see* Erythromycin, Topical *on page 324*

Eminase® *see* Anistreplase *on page 67*

Emko® [OTC] *see* Nonoxynol 9 *on page 627*

EMLA® *see* Lidocaine and Prilocaine *on page 501*

Empirin® [OTC] *see* Aspirin *on page 78*

Empirin® With Codeine *see* Aspirin and Codeine *on page 80*

Emulsoil® [OTC] *see* Castor Oil *on page 161*

E-Mycin® *see* Erythromycin *on page 321*

Enalapril (e nal' a pril)

Related Information
Cardiovascular Diseases *on page 912*

Brand Names Vasotec®

Canadian/Mexican Brand Names Apo-Enalapril® (Canada); Enaladil® (Mexico); Glioten® (Mexico); Renitec® (Mexico)

Therapeutic Category Angiotensin-Converting Enzyme (ACE) Inhibitors

Use Management of mild to severe hypertension and congestive heart failure

Unlabeled use: Hypertensive crisis, diabetic nephropathy, rheumatoid arthritis, diagnosis of anatomic renal artery stenosis, hypertension secondary to scleroderma renal crisis, diagnosis of aldosteronism, idiopathic edema, Bartter's syndrome, postmyocardial infarction for prevention of ventricular failure

Usual Dosage Use lower listed initial dose in patients with hyponatremia, hypovolemia, severe congestive heart failure, decreased renal function, or in those receiving diuretics

Children:
Investigational initial oral doses of **enalapril**: 0.1 mg/kg/day increasing as needed over 2 weeks to 0.5 mg/kg/day have been used to treat severe congestive heart failure in infants
Investigational I.V. doses of **enalaprilat**: 5-10 mcg/kg/dose administered every 8-24 hours have been used for the treatment of neonatal hypertension; monitor patients carefully; select patients may require higher doses

Adults:
Oral: **Enalapril**
Hypertension: 2.5-5 mg/day then increase as required, usual therapeutic dose for hypertension: 10-40 mg/day in 1-2 divided doses; usual therapeutic dose for heart failure: 5-20 mg/day

(Continued)

Enalapril *(Continued)*

Heart failure: As adjunct with diuretics and digitalis, initiate with 2.5 mg once or twice daily (usual range: 5-20 mg/day in 2 divided doses; maximum: 40 mg)

Asymptomatic left ventricular dysfunction: 2.5 mg twice daily, titrated as tolerated to 20 mg/day

I.V.: Enalaprilat

Hypertension: 1.25 mg/dose, given over 5 minutes every 6 hours; doses as high as 5 mg/dose every 6 hours have been tolerated for up to 36 hours. **Note:** If patients are concomitantly receiving diuretic therapy, begin with 0.625 mg I.V. over 5 minutes; if the effect is not adequate after 1 hour, repeat the dose and administer 1.25 mg at 6-hour intervals thereafter; if adequate, administer 0.625 mg I.V. every 6 hours

Conversion from I.V. to oral therapy if not concurrently on diuretics: 5 mg once daily; subsequent titration as needed; if concurrently receiving diuretics and responding to 0.625 mg I.V. every 6 hours, initiate with 2.5 mg/day

Mechanism of Action Competitive inhibitor of angiotensin-converting enzyme (ACE); prevents conversion of angiotensin I to angiotensin II, a potent vasoconstrictor; results in lower levels of angiotensin II which causes an increase in plasma renin activity and a reduction in aldosterone secretion

Local Anesthetic/Vasoconstrictor Precautions No information available to require special precautions

Effects on Dental Treatment No effects or complications reported

Other Adverse Effects

1% to 10%:

Cardiovascular: Chest pain, palpitations, tachycardia, syncope

Central nervous system: Insomnia, headache dizziness, fatigue, malaise, asthenia

Dermatologic: Rash

Gastrointestinal: Dysgeusia, abdominal pain, vomiting, nausea, diarrhea, anorexia, constipation

Neuromuscular & skeletal: Paresthesia

Respiratory: Bronchitis, cough, dyspnea

<1%:

Cardiovascular: Angina pectoris, flushing

Dermatologic: Alopecia, erythema multiforme, pruritus, Stevens-Johnson syndrome, urticaria, angioedema

Endocrine & metabolic: Hypoglycemia, hyperkalemia

Genitourinary: Impotence

Hematologic: Agranulocytosis, neutropenia, anemia

Neuromuscular & skeletal: Myalgia

Ocular: Blurred vision

Otic: Tinnitus

Renal: Oliguria

Respiratory: Asthma, bronchospasm

Miscellaneous: Sweating

Drug-Drug Interactions With ACEIs

Precipitant Drug	Drug (Category) and Effect	Description
Antacids	ACE Inhibitors: decreased	Decreased bioavailability of ACEIs. May be more likely with captopril. Separate administration times by 1-2 hours.
NSAIDs (indomethacin)	ACEIs: decreased	Reduced hypotensive effects of ACEIs. More prominent in low renin or volume dependent hypertensive patients.
Phenothiazines	ACEIs: increased	Pharmacologic effects of ACEIs may be increased.
ACEIs	Allopurinol: increased	Higher risk of hypersensitivity reaction possible when given concurrently. Three case reports of Stevens-Johnson syndrome with captopril.
ACEIs	Digoxin: increased	Increased plasma digoxin levels.
ACEIs	Lithium: increased	Increased serum lithium levels and symptoms of toxicity may occur.
ACEIs	Potassium preps/ potassium sparing diuretics increased	Coadministration may result in elevated potassium levels.

Drug Interactions See table.
Drug Uptake
Oral:
Onset of action: ~1 hour
Duration: 12-24 hours
Absorption: Oral: 55% to 75%
Serum half-life:
Enalapril: Adults:
Healthy: 2 hours
With congestive heart failure: 3.4-5.8 hours
Enalaprilat:
Infants 6 weeks to 8 months: 6-10 hours
Adults: 35-38 hours
Time to peak serum concentration: Oral:
Enalapril: Within 0.5-1.5 hours
Enalaprilat (active): Within 3-4.5 hours
Pregnancy Risk Factor D

Enalapril and Hydrochlorothiazide
Related Information
Cardiovascular Diseases *on page 912*
Brand Names Vaseretic® 5-12.5; Vaseretic® 10-25
Therapeutic Category Antihypertensive Agent, Combination
Use Treatment of hypertension
Usual Dosage Oral: Dose is individualized
Local Anesthetic/Vasoconstrictor Precautions No information available to require special precautions
Effects on Dental Treatment No effects or complications reported

Encainide Hydrochloride (en kay' nide hye droe klor' ide)
Related Information
Cardiovascular Diseases *on page 912*
Brand Names Enkaid®
Therapeutic Category Antiarrhythmic Agent, Class I-C; Antiarrhythmic Agent (Supraventricular & Ventricular)
Use Ventricular arrhythmias; supraventricular arrhythmias
Local Anesthetic/Vasoconstrictor Precautions No information available to require special precautions
Effects on Dental Treatment No effects or complications reported
Other Adverse Effects
>10%:
Central nervous system: Dizziness
Ocular: Blurred vision
1% to 10%:
Central nervous system: Asthenia, headache
Cardiovascular: Chest pain congestive heart failure, ventricular tachycardia
Gastrointestinal: Vomiting
Otic: Tinnitus
<1%: Neuromuscular & skeletal: Tremor
Comments Based on adverse outcomes noted with encainide in the CAST trial, the FDA recommends that use of encainide be limited to patients with life-threatening ventricular arrhythmias

Encare® [OTC] *see* Nonoxynol 9 *on page 627*
Endep® *see* Amitriptyline Hydrochloride *on page 51*
End Lice® [OTC] *see* Pyrethrins *on page 753*
Endocrine Disorders & Pregnancy *see page 927*
Endolor® *see* Butalbital Compound *on page 133*
Enduron® *see* Methyclothiazide *on page 565*
Enduronyl® *see* Methyclothiazide and Deserpidine *on page 566*
Enduronyl® Forte *see* Methyclothiazide and Deserpidine *on page 566*
Ener-B® [OTC] *see* Cyanocobalamin *on page 237*
Engerix-B® *see* Hepatitis B Vaccine *on page 422*
Enhanced-potency Inactivated Poliovirus Vaccine *see* Poliovirus Vaccine, Inactivated *on page 702*
Enisyl® [OTC] *see* L-Lysine Hydrochloride *on page 509*
Enkaid® *see* Encainide Hydrochloride *on this page*
Enomine® *see* Guaifenesin, Phenylpropanolamine, and Phenylephrine *on page 410*

Enovid® see Mestranol and Norethynodrel *on page 549*
Enovil® see Amitriptyline Hydrochloride *on page 51*

Enoxacin (en ox´ a sin)
Brand Names Penetrex™
Canadian/Mexican Brand Names Comprecin® (Mexico)
Therapeutic Category Antibiotic, Quinolone
Synonyms Enoxacina (Mexico)
Use Treatment of complicated and uncomplicated urinary tract infections caused by susceptible gram-negative and gram-positive bacteria
Usual Dosage Adults: Oral: 400 mg twice daily
  Dosing adjustment in renal impairment:
    Cl_cr <50 mL/minute: Administer 50% of dose
Mechanism of Action Exerts a broad spectrum antimicrobial effect. The primary target of the fluoroquinolones is DNA gyrase (topoisomerase II) an essential bacterial enzyme that maintains the superhelical structure of DNA. DNA gyrase is required for DNA replication and transcription, DNA repair, recombination, and transposition.
Local Anesthetic/Vasoconstrictor Precautions No information available to require special precautions
Effects on Dental Treatment No effects or complications reported
Other Adverse Effects
  1% to 10%: Gastrointestinal: Nausea, vomiting
  <1%:
    Central nervous system: Restlessness, dizziness, confusion, seizures, headache
    Dermatologic: Rash
    Gastrointestinal: Diarrhea, GI bleeding
    Hematologic: Anemia
    Hepatic: Increased liver enzymes
    Neuromuscular & skeletal: Tremor, arthralgia
    Renal: Increased serum creatinine and BUN, acute renal failure
Drug Interactions
  Decreased effect with antacids (magnesium, aluminum), iron and zinc salts, sucralfate, bismuth salts
  Increased toxicity/levels of warfarin, cyclosporine, digoxin, caffeine; increased levels with cimetidine
Drug Uptake
  Absorption: 98%
  Serum half-life: 3-6 hours (average)
Pregnancy Risk Factor C

Enoxacina (Mexico) see Enoxacin *on this page*
Entacef® see Cephalexin Monohydrate *on page 176*
Entex® see Guaifenesin, Phenylpropanolamine, and Phenylephrine *on page 410*
Entex® LA see Guaifenesin and Phenylpropanolamine *on page 409*
Entex® PSE see Guaifenesin and Pseudoephedrine *on page 409*
Enulose® see Lactulose *on page 488*
Enzone® see Pramoxine and Hydrocortisone *on page 714*

Ephedrine Sulfate (e fed´ rin sul´ fate)
Brand Names Ectasule®; Efedron®; Ephedsol®; Vicks Vatronol®
Therapeutic Category Adrenergic Agonist Agent
Synonyms Efedrina (Mexico)
Use Treatment of bronchial asthma, nasal congestion, acute bronchospasm, idiopathic orthostatic hypotension
Usual Dosage
  Children:
    Oral, S.C.: 3 mg/kg/day or 25-100 mg/m²/day in 4-6 divided doses every 4-6 hours
    I.M., slow I.V. push: 0.2-0.3 mg/kg/dose every 4-6 hours
  Adults:
    Oral: 25-50 mg every 3-4 hours as needed
    I.M., S.C.: 25-50 mg, parenteral adult dose should not exceed 150 mg in 24 hours
    I.V.: 5-25 mg/dose slow I.V. push repeated after 5-10 minutes as needed, then every 3-4 hours not to exceed 150 mg/24 hours
Mechanism of Action Releases tissue stores of epinephrine and thereby produces an alpha- and beta-adrenergic stimulation; longer acting and less potent than epinephrine

Local Anesthetic/Vasoconstrictor Precautions Use vasoconstrictors with caution since ephedrine may enhance cardiostimulation and vasopressor effects of sympathomimetics such as epinephrine

Effects on Dental Treatment No effects or complications reported

Other Adverse Effects

>10%: Central nervous system: CNS stimulating effects, nervousness, anxiety, apprehension, fear, tension, agitation, excitation, restlessness, irritability, insomnia, hyperactivity

1% to 10%:

Cardiovascular: Hypertension, tachycardia, palpitations, elevation or depression of blood pressure

Central nervous system: Dizziness, headache, weakness

Gastrointestinal: Dry mouth, nausea, anorexia, GI upset, vomiting

Genitourinary: Painful urination

Neuromuscular & skeletal: Trembling, tremor (more common in the elderly)

Miscellaneous: Increased sweating, unusual paleness

<1%:

Cardiovascular: Chest pain, arrhythmias

Central nervous system: Anxiety, apprehension, fear, tension, agitation, excitation, restlessness, irritability

Neuromuscular & skeletal: Tremor

Respiratory: Difficulty in breathing

Drug Interactions

Decreased effect: Alpha- and beta-adrenergic blocking agents decrease ephedrine vasopressor effects

Increased toxicity: Additive cardiostimulation with other sympathomimetic agents; theophylline leads to cardiostimulation; MAO inhibitors or atropine lead to increased blood pressure; cardiac glycosides or general anesthetics lead to increased cardiac stimulation

Drug Uptake

Oral:

Duration of action: 3-6 hours

Serum half-life: 2.5-3.6 hours

Pregnancy Risk Factor C

Ephedrine, Theophylline and Phenobarbital *see* Theophylline, Ephedrine, and Phenobarbital *on page 836*

Ephedsol® *see* Ephedrine Sulfate *on previous page*

E-Pilo-x® Ophthalmic *see* Pilocarpine and Epinephrine *on page 693*

Epinal® *see* Epinephryl Borate *on page 315*

Epinephrine (ep i nef′ rin)

Related Information

Dental Drug Interactions: Update on Drug Combinations Requiring Special Considerations *on page 1022*

Respiratory Diseases *on page 924*

Therapeutic Category Adrenergic Agonist Agent; Antidote, Hypersensitivity Reactions; Antiglaucoma Agent; Bronchodilator

Use Treatment of bronchospasms, anaphylactic reactions, cardiac arrest, management of open-angle (chronic simple) glaucoma

Usual Dosage

Bronchodilator:

Children: S.C.: 10 mcg/kg (0.01 mL/kg of 1:1000) (single doses not to exceed 0.5 mg); injection suspension (1:200): 0.005 mL/kg/dose (0.025 mg/kg/dose) to a maximum of 0.15 mL (0.75 mg for single dose) every 8-12 hours

Adults:

I.M., S.C. (1:1000): 0.1-0.5 mg every 10-15 minutes to 4 hours

Suspension (1:200) S.C.: 0.1-0.3 mL (0.5-1.5 mg)

I.V.: 0.1-0.25 mg (single dose maximum: 1 mg)

Cardiac arrest:

Children: Asystole or pulseless arrest:

I.V., intraosseous: First dose: 0.01 mg/kg (0.1 mL/kg of a 1:10,000 solution); subsequent doses: 0.1 mg/kg (0.1 mL/kg of a 1:1000 solution); doses as high as 0.2 mg/kg may be effective; repeat every 3-5 minutes

Intratracheal: 0.1 mg/kg (0.1 mL/kg of a 1:1000 solution); doses as high as 0.2 mg/kg may be effective

Adults: Asystole:

I.V.: 1 mg every 3-5 minutes; if this approach fails, alternative regimens include: Intermediate: 2-5 mg every 3-5 minutes; Escalating: 1 mg, 3 mg, 5 mg at 3-minute intervals; High: 0.1 mg/kg every 3-5 minutes

(Continued)

311

Epinephrine *(Continued)*

Intratracheal: Although optimal dose is unknown, doses of 2-2.5 times the I.V. dose may be needed

Bradycardia: Children:
I.V.: 0.01 mg/kg (0.1 mL/kg of 1:10,000 solution) every 3-5 minutes as needed (maximum: 1 mg/10 mL)
Intratracheal: 0.1 mg/kg (0.1 mL/kg of 1:1000 solution every 3-5 minutes); doses as high as 0.2 mg/kg may be effective

Refractory hypotension (refractory to dopamine/dobutamine): I.V. infusion administration requires the use of an infusion pump:
Children: Infusion rate 0.1-4 mcg/kg/minute
Adults: I.V. infusion: 1 mg in 250 mL NS/D_5W at 0.1-1 mcg/kg/minute; titrate to desired effect

Hypersensitivity reaction:
Children: S.C.: 0.01 mg/kg every 15 minutes for 2 doses then every 4 hours as needed (single doses not to exceed 0.5 mg)
Adults: I.M., S.C.: 0.2-0.5 mg every 20 minutes to 4 hours (single dose maximum: 1 mg)

Nebulization:
Children <2 years: 0.25 mL of 1:1000 diluted in 3 mL NS with treatments ordered individually
Children >2 years and Adolescents: 0.5 mL of 1:1000 concentration diluted in 3 mL NS
Children >2 years and Adults (racemic epinephrine):
<10 kg: 2 mL of 1:8 dilution over 15 minutes every 1-4 hours
10-15 kg: 2 mL of 1:6 dilution over 15 minutes every 1-4 hours
15-20 kg: 2 mL of 1:4 dilution over 15 minutes every 1-4 hours
>20 kg: 2 mL of 1:3 dilution over 15 minutes every 1-4 hours
Adults: Instill 8-15 drops into nebulizer reservoirs; administer 1-3 inhalations 4-6 times/day

Ophthalmic: Instill 1-2 drops in eye(s) once or twice daily

Intranasal: Children ≥6 years and Adults: Apply locally as drops or spray or with sterile swab

Mechanism of Action Stimulates alpha-, beta$_1$-, and beta$_2$-adrenergic receptors resulting in relaxation of smooth muscle of the bronchial tree, cardiac stimulation, and dilation of skeletal muscle vasculature; small doses can cause vasodilation via beta$_2$-vascular receptors; large doses may produce constriction of skeletal and vascular smooth muscle; decreases production of aqueous humor and increases aqueous outflow; dilates the pupil by contracting the dilator muscle

Local Anesthetic/Vasoconstrictor Precautions No information available to require special precautions

Effects on Dental Treatment No effects or complications reported

Other Adverse Effects
>10%:
Cardiovascular: Tachycardia (parenteral), pounding heartbeat
Central nervous system: Nervousness, restlessness
1% to 10%:
Cardiovascular: Flushing, hypertension
Central nervous system: Headache, dizziness, lightheadedness, insomnia
Gastrointestinal: Nausea, vomiting
Neuromuscular & skeletal: Weakness, trembling
Miscellaneous: Increased sweating, unusual paleness

Contraindications Hypersensitivity to epinephrine or any component; cardiac arrhythmias, angle-closure glaucoma

Warnings/Precautions Use with caution in elderly patients, patients with diabetes mellitus, cardiovascular diseases (angina, tachycardia, myocardial infarction), thyroid disease, or cerebral arteriosclerosis, Parkinson's; some products contain sulfites as antioxidants. Rapid I.V. infusion may cause death from cerebrovascular hemorrhage or cardiac arrhythmias. Oral inhalation of epinephrine is **not** the preferred route of administration.

Drug Interactions Increased cardiac irritability if administered concurrently with halogenated inhalational anesthetics, beta-blocking agents, alpha-blocking agents

Drug Uptake
Onset of bronchodilation:
Subcutaneous: Within 5-10 minutes
Inhalation: Within 1 minute

Conjunctival instillation:
  Onset of effect: Intraocular pressures fall within 1 hour
  Peak effect: Within 4-8 hours
  Duration of ocular effect: 12-24 hours
  Absorption: Orally ingested doses are rapidly metabolized in the GI tract and liver; pharmacologically active concentrations are not achieved

Pregnancy Risk Factor C

Breast-feeding Considerations No data reported

Dosage Forms
  Aerosol, oral:
    Bitartrate (AsthmaHaler®, Bronitin®, Medihaler-Epi®, Primatene® Suspension): 0.3 mg/spray [epinephrine base 0.16 mg/spray] (10 mL, 15 mL, 22.5 mL)
    Bronkaid®: 0.5% (10 mL, 15 mL, 22.5 mL)
    Primatene®: 0.2 mg/spray (15 mL, 22.5 mL)
  Auto-injector:
    EpiPen®: Delivers 0.3 mg I.M. of epinephrine 1:1000 (2 mL)
    EpiPen® Jr.: Delivers 0.15 mg I.M. of epinephrine 1:2000 (2 mL)
  Injection (Adrenalin®): 0.01 mg/mL [1:100,000] (5 mL); 0.1 mg/mL [1:10,000] (3 mL, 10 mL); 1 mg/mL [1:1000] (1 mL, 2 mL, 30 mL)
  Solution:
    Inhalation:
      Adrenalin®: 1% [10 mg/mL, 1:100] (7.5 mL)
      AsthmaNefrin®, microNefrin®, Nephron®: Racepinephrine 2% [epinephrine base 1.125%] (7.5 mL, 15 mL, 30 mL)
      Vaponefrin®: Racepinephrine 2% [epinephrine base 1%] (15 mL, 30 mL)
    Nasal (Adrenalin®): 0.1% [1 mg/mL, 1:1000] (30 mL)
    Ophthalmic, as base (Epifrin®): 0.5% (15 mL); 1% (15 mL); 2% (15 mL)
    Ophthalmic, as hydrochloride: 0.1% (1 mL)
      Glaucon®: 1% (10 mL); 2% (10 mL)
    Topical (Adrenalin®): 0.1% [1 mg/mL, 1:1000] (30 mL, 10 mL)
  Suspension for injection (Sus-Phrine®): 5 mg/mL [1:200] (0.3 mL, 5 mL)

Dietary Considerations No data reported

Generic Available Yes

Epinephrine (Dental) (ep i nef' rin)

Related Information
  Dental Drug Interactions: Update on Drug Combinations Requiring Special Considerations *on page 1022*
  Respiratory Diseases *on page 924*

Brand Names Adrenalin®; Sus-Phrine®

Therapeutic Category Adrenergic Agonist Agent; Antidote, Hypersensitivity Reactions; Bronchodilator

Use
  Dental: Emergency drug for treatment of anaphylactic reactions; used as vasoconstrictor to prolong local anesthesia

Usual Dosage
  Hypersensitivity reaction:
    Children: S.C.: 0.01 mg/kg every 15 minutes for 2 doses then every 4 hours as needed (single doses not to exceed 0.5 mg)
    Adults: I.M., S.C.: 0.2-0.5 mg every 20 minutes to 4 hours (single dose maximum: 1 mg)

Mechanism of Action Stimulates alpha-, beta$_1$-, and beta$_2$-adrenergic receptors resulting in relaxation of smooth muscle of the bronchial tree, cardiac stimulation, and dilation of skeletal muscle vasculature; small doses can cause vasodilation via beta$_2$-vascular receptors; large doses may produce constriction of skeletal and vascular smooth muscle; decreases production of aqueous humor and increases aqueous outflow; dilates the pupil by contracting the dilator muscle

Local Anesthetic/Vasoconstrictor Precautions No information available to require special precautions

Effects on Dental Treatment No effects or complications reported

Other Adverse Effects
  Oral manifestations: No data reported

Contraindications Hypersensitivity to epinephrine or any component; cardiac arrhythmias, angle-closure glaucoma

Warnings/Precautions Use with caution in elderly patients, patients with diabetes mellitus, cardiovascular diseases (angina, tachycardia, myocardial infarction), thyroid disease, or cerebral arteriosclerosis, Parkinson's; some products contain sulfites as antioxidants. Rapid I.V. infusion may cause death
(Continued)

313

Epinephrine (Dental) *(Continued)*

from cerebrovascular hemorrhage or cardiac arrhythmias. Oral inhalation of epinephrine is **not** the preferred route of administration.

Drug Interactions Increased cardiac irritability if administered concurrently with halogenated inhalational anesthetics, beta-blocking agents, alpha-blocking agents

Drug Uptake
Absorption: Not absorbed orally

Pregnancy Risk Factor C

Breast-feeding Considerations Usual infiltration doses of epinephrine given to nursing mothers has not been shown to affect the health of the nursing infant

Dosage Forms
Injection:
Adrenalin®: 0.01 mg/mL [1:100,000] (5 mL); 0.1 mg/mL [1:10,000] (3 mL, 10 mL); 1 mg/mL [1:1000] (1 mL, 2 mL, 30 mL)
Suspension (Sus-Phrine®): 5 mg/mL [1:200] (0.3 mL, 5 mL)
Solution, topical (Adrenalin®): 0.1% [1 mg/mL, 1:1000] (30 mL, 10 mL)

Dietary Considerations No data reported

Generic Available Yes

Epinephrine, Racemic *(ep i nef′ rin, ra se′ mik)*

Brand Names AsthmaNefrin®; microNefrin®; Nephron®; S-2®; Vaponefrin®

Therapeutic Category Vasoconstrictor

Local Anesthetic/Vasoconstrictor Precautions No information available to require special precautions

Effects on Dental Treatment No effects or complications reported

Other Adverse Effects No data reported

Oral manifestations: No data reported

Drug Interactions No data reported

Drug Uptake
Absorption: Not absorbed orally
Onset of bronchodilation:
Subcutaneous: Within 5-10 minutes
Inhalation: Within 1 minute

Breast-feeding Considerations No data reported

Dosage Forms
Solution, inhalation:
AsthmaNefrin®, microNefrin®, Nephron®, S-2®: Racepinephrine 2.25% [epinephrine base 1.125%] (7.5 mL, 15 mL, 30 mL)
Vaponefrin®: Racepinephrine 2% [epinephrine base 1%] (15 mL, 30 mL)

Dietary Considerations No data reported

Epinephrine, Racemic and Aluminum Potassium Sulfate

(ep i nef′ rin, ra se′ mik and a loo′ mi num poe tass′ y um sul′ fate)

Brand Names Van R Gingibraid®

Therapeutic Category Astringent; Vasoconstrictor

Use
Dental: Gingival retraction
Medical: None

Usual Dosage Pass the impregnated yarn around the neck of the tooth and place into gingival sulcus; normal tissue moisture, water, or gingival retraction solutions activate impregnated yarn. Limit use to one quadrant of the mouth at a time; recommended use is for 3-8 minutes in the mouth.

Mechanism of Action Epinephrine stimulates alpha$_1$ adrenergic receptors to cause vasoconstriction in blood vessels in gingiva; aluminum potassium sulfate, precipitates tissue and blood proteins

Local Anesthetic/Vasoconstrictor Precautions No information available to require special precautions

Effects on Dental Treatment No effects or complications reported

Other Adverse Effects None reported
Oral manifestations: Tissue retraction around base of the tooth (therapeutic effect)

Contraindications Patients with cardiovascular disease, hyperthyroidism, or diabetes; patients sensitive to epinephrine; do not apply to areas of heavy or deep bleeding or over exposed bone

Warnings/Precautions Caution should be exercised whenever using gingival retraction cords with epinephrine since it delivers vasoconstrictor doses of

314

racemic epinephrine to patients; the general medical history should be thoroughly evaluated before using in any patient

Drug Interactions No data reported

Drug Uptake No data reported

Breast-feeding Considerations No data reported

Dosage Forms Yarn, saturated in solution of 8% racemic epinephrine and 7% aluminum potassium sulfate; yarn labeled type "0e" contains 0.20±0.10 mg epinephrine per inch; "1e" contains 0.40±0.20 mg per inch; "2e" contains 0.60±0.20 mg per inch

Dietary Considerations No data reported

Epinephryl Borate (ep i nef' ril bor' ate)

Brand Names Epinal®

Therapeutic Category Adrenergic Agonist Agent, Ophthalmic; Antiglaucoma Agent; Ophthalmic Agent, Vasoconstrictor

Use Reduces elevated intraocular pressure in chronic open-angle glaucoma

Local Anesthetic/Vasoconstrictor Precautions No information available to require special precautions

Effects on Dental Treatment No effects or complications reported

Epitol® see Carbamazepine on page 151

Epivir® see Lamivudine on page 489

EPO see Epoetin Alfa on this page

Epoetin Alfa (e poe' e tin al' fa)

Brand Names Epogen®; Procrit®

Canadian/Mexican Brand Names Eprex® (Mexico)

Therapeutic Category Recombinant Human Erythropoietin

Synonyms EPO; Erythropoietin; rHuEPO-α

Use Anemia associated with end stage renal disease; anemia related to therapy with AZT-treated HIV-infected patients; anemia in cancer patients receiving chemotherapy; anemia of prematurity

Usual Dosage

Individuals with anemia due to iron deficiency, sickle cell disease, autoimmune hemolytic anemia, and bleeding, generally have appropriate endogenous EPO levels to drive erythropoiesis and would not ordinarily be candidates for EPO therapy.

In patients on dialysis, epoetin alfa usually has been administered as an IVP 3 times/week. While the administration is independent of the dialysis procedure, it may be administered into the venous line at the end of the dialysis procedure to obviate the need for additional venous access; in patients with CRF not on dialysis, epoetin alfa may be given either as an IVP or S.C. injection.

Children and Adults: Dosing recommendations:

Dosing schedules need to be individualized and careful monitoring of patients receiving the drug is mandatory

rHuEPO-α may be ineffective if other factors such as iron or B_{12}/folate deficiency limit marrow response

IVP, S.C.:

Chronic renal failure patients:

Initial dose: 50-100 units/kg 3 times/week

Dose should be reduced when the hematocrit reaches the target range of 30% to 36% or a hematocrit increase >4% points over any 2-week period

Dose should be held if the hematocrit exceeds 36% and until the hematocrit decreases to the target range (30% to 36%).

Dose should be increased not more frequently than once a month, unless clinically indicated. After any dose adjustment, the hematocrit should be determined twice weekly for at least 2-6 weeks. If a hematocrit increase of 5-6 points is not achieved after a 8-week period and iron stores are adequate, the dose may be incrementally increased. Further increases may be made at 4-6 week intervals until the desired response is obtained.

Maintenance dose: Should be individualized to maintain the hematocrit within the 30% to 33% target range. The median maintenance dose in phase III studies in chronic renal failure patients on dialysis was 75 units/kg 3 times/week (range 12.5-525 units/kg 3 times/week).

Epoetin doses of 75-150 units/kg/week have been shown to maintain hematocrits of 36% to 38% for up to 6 months in patients with chronic renal failure not requiring dialysis

(Continued)

Epoetin Alfa *(Continued)*

Zidovudine-treated HIV patients: Prior to beginning epoetin alfa, serum erythropoietin levels should be determined. Available evidence suggest that patients receiving zidovudine with endogenous serum erythropoietin levels >500 mIU/mL are unlikely to respond to therapy with epoetin alfa.

Initial dose: For patients with serum erythropoietin levels <500 mIU/mL who are receiving a dose of zidovudine ≤4,200 mg/week: 100 units/kg 3 times/week for 8 weeks.

Dose should be held if the hematocrit is >40% until the hematocrit drops to 36%. The dose should be reduced by 25% when the treatment is resumed and then titrated to maintain the desired hematocrit.

Dose should be reduced if the initial dose of epoetin alfa includes a rapid rise in hematocrit (>4% points in any 2-week period).

Increase dose by 50-100 units/kg if the response is not satisfactory in terms of reducing transfusion requirements or increasing hematocrit after 8 weeks of therapy. Response should be evaluated every 4-8 weeks thereafter and the dose adjusted and the dose adjusted accordingly by 50-100 units/kg increments 3 times/week. If patients have not responded satisfactorily to a dose of 300 units/kg 3 times/week, it is unlikely that they will respond to higher doses.

Maintenance dose: Dose should be titrated to maintain target hematocrit range: 36% to 40%

Cancer patients on chemotherapy: Although no specific serum erythropoietin level can be stipulated above which patients would be unlikely to respond to epoetin alfa therapy, treatment of patients with grossly elevated serum erythropoietin levels (>200 mIU/mL) is not recommended

Initial dose: 150 units/kg 3 times/week

Increase dose: Response should be evaluated every 8 weeks thereafter and the dose adjusted and the dose adjusted accordingly by 50-100 units/kg increments 3 times/week up to 300 units/kg 3 times/week if the response is not satisfactory. If patients have not responded satisfactorily to a dose of 300 units/kg 3 times/week, it is unlikely that they will respond to higher doses.

Dose should be held if the hematocrit is >40% until the hematocrit drops to 36%. The dose should be reduced by 25% when the treatment is resumed and then titrated to maintain the desired hematocrit.

Dose should be reduced if the initial dose of epoetin alfa includes a rapid rise in hematocrit (>4% points in any 2-week period), the dose should be reduced

Maintenance dose: Dose should be titrated to maintain target hematocrit range: 36% to 40%

Mechanism of Action Induces erythropoiesis by stimulating the division and differentiation of committed erythroid progenitor cells; induces the release of reticulocytes from the bone marrow into the blood stream, where they mature to erythrocytes. There is a dose response relationship with this effect. This results in an increase in reticulocyte counts followed by a rise in hematocrit and hemoglobin levels.

Local Anesthetic/Vasoconstrictor Precautions No information available to require special precautions

Effects on Dental Treatment No effects or complications reported

Other Adverse Effects

1% to 10%:
 Cardiovascular: Hypertension, chest pain, edema
 Central nervous system: Fatigue, headache, asthenia, dizziness, seizures
 Dermatologic: Rash
 Gastrointestinal: Nausea, vomiting, diarrhea
 Hematologic: Clotted access
 Neuromuscular & skeletal: Arthralgias

<1%:
 Cardiovascular: Myocardial infarction, CVA/TIA
 Sensitivity reactions: Hypersensitivity reactions

Drug Uptake

Onset of action: Several days

Peak effect: 2-3 weeks

Serum half-life: Circulating: 4-13 hours in patients with chronic renal failure; 20% shorter in patients with normal renal function

Time to peak serum concentrations: S.C.: 2-8 hours

Pregnancy Risk Factor C

Comments Epogen® reimbursement hotline number for information regarding coverage of epoetin alfa is 1-800-2-PAY-EPO. ProCrit™ reimbursement hotline is 1-800-441-1366.

Epogen® *see* Epoetin Alfa *on page 315*

Epoprostenol Sodium (e poe prost′ en ole sow′ dee um)
Brand Names Flolan® Injection
Therapeutic Category Plasma Volume Expander, Colloidal
Use Long-term intravenous treatment of primary pulmonary hypertension (PPH)
Usual Dosage I.V.: The drug is administered by continuous intravenous infusion via a central venous catheter using an ambulatory infusion pump; during dose ranging it may be administered peripherally
  Acute dose ranging: The initial infusion rate should be 2 ng/kg/minute by continuous I.V. and increased in increments of 2 ng/kg/minute every 15 minutes or longer until dose-limiting effects are elicited (such as chest pain, anxiety, dizziness, changes in heart rate, dyspnea, nausea, vomiting, headache, hypotension and/or flushing)
  Continuous chronic infusion: Initial: 4 ng/kg/minute **less** than the maximum-tolerated infusion rate determined during acute dose ranging.
  If maximum-tolerated infusion rate is <5 ng/kg/minute the chronic infusion rate should be ½ the maximum-tolerated acute infusion rate
  Dosage adjustments: Dose adjustments in the chronic infusion rate should be based on persistence, recurrence or worsening of patient symptoms of pulmonary hypertension
  If symptoms persist or recur after improving, the infusion rate should be increased by 1-2 ng/kg/minute increments, every 15 minutes or greater; following establishment of a new chronic infusion rate, the patient should be observed and vital signs monitored.

Preparation of Infusion

To make 100 mL of solution with concentration:	Directions:
3000 ng/mL	Dissolve one 0.5 mg vial with 6 mL supplied diluent, withdraw 3 mL and add to sufficient diluent to make a total of 100 mL
5000 ng/mL	Dissolve one 0.5 mg vial with 5 mL supplied diluent, withdraw entire vial contents and add a sufficient volume of diluent to make a total of 100 mL
10,000 ng/mL	Dissolve two 0.5 mg vials each with 5 mL supplied diluent, withdraw entire vial contents and add a sufficient volume of diluent to make a total of 100 mL
15,000 ng/mL	Dissolve one 1.5 mg vial with 5 mL supplied diluent, withdraw entire vial contents and add a sufficient volume of diluent to make a total of 100 mL

Local Anesthetic/Vasoconstrictor Precautions No information available to require special precautions
Effects on Dental Treatment No effects or complications reported
Drug Uptake
  Steady state levels are reached in about 15 minutes with continuous infusions
  Serum half-life: 2.7-6 minutes

Epsom Salts *see* Magnesium Sulfate *on page 524*
EPT *see* Teniposide *on page 820*
Equagesic® *see* Aspirin and Meprobamate *on page 81*
Equalactin® Chewable Tablet [OTC] *see* Calcium Polycarbophil *on page 146*
Equanil® *see* Meprobamate *on page 543*
Ercaf® *see* Ergotamine *on page 319*
Ergamisol® *see* Levamisole Hydrochloride *on page 493*

Ergocalciferol (er goe kal sif′ e role)
Brand Names Calciferol™; Drisdol®
Canadian/Mexican Brand Names Ostoforte®(Canada); Radiostol® (Canada)
Therapeutic Category Vitamin D Analog
Synonyms Ergocalciferol (Mexico)
Use Treatment of refractory rickets, hypophosphatemia, hypoparathyroidism
(Continued)

Ergocalciferol *(Continued)*

Usual Dosage Oral dosing is preferred

Dietary supplementation (each mcg = 40 USP units):
Healthy Children: 10 mcg/day (400 units)
Adults: 10 mcg/day (400 units)

Renal failure:
Children: 100-1000 mcg/day (4000-40,000 units)
Adults: 500 mcg/day (20,000 units)

Hypoparathyroidism:
Children: 1.25-5 mg/day (50,000-200,000 units) and calcium supplements
Adults: 625 mcg to 5 mg/day (25,000-200,000 units) and calcium supplements

Vitamin D-dependent rickets:
Children: 75-125 mcg/day (3000-5000 units); maximum: 1500 mcg/day
Adults: 250 mcg to 1.5 mg/day (10,000-60,000 units)

Nutritional rickets and osteomalacia:
Children and Adults (with normal absorption): 25-125 mcg/day (1000-5000 units)
Children with malabsorption: 250-625 mcg/day (10,000-25,000 units)
Adults with malabsorption: 250-7500 mcg (10,000-300,000 units)

Vitamin D-resistant rickets:
Children: Initial: 1000-2000 mcg/day (400,000-800,000 units) with phosphate supplements; daily dosage is increased at 3- to 4-month intervals in 250-500 mcg (10,000-20,000 units) increments
Adults: 250-1500 mcg/day (10,000-60,000 units) with phosphate supplements

Mechanism of Action Stimulates calcium and phosphate absorption from the small intestine, promotes secretion of calcium from bone to blood; promotes renal tubule phosphate resorption

Local Anesthetic/Vasoconstrictor Precautions No information available to require special precautions

Effects on Dental Treatment No effects or complications reported

Other Adverse Effects

1% to 10%:
Cardiovascular: Hypotension, cardiac arrhythmias, hypertension, irregular heartbeat
Central nervous system: Irritability, headache
Gastrointestinal: Nausea, vomiting, anorexia, pancreatitis, metallic taste
Dermatologic: Pruritus
Endocrine & metabolic: Polydipsia
Neuromuscular & skeletal: Bone pain, muscle pain
Ocular: Conjunctivitis, photophobia
Renal: Polyuria

<1%:
Central nervous system: Overt psychosis
Gastrointestinal: Weight loss

Drug Interactions

Decreased effect: Cholestyramine, colestipol, mineral oil causes decreased oral absorption
Increased effect: Thiazide diuretics causes increased vitamin D effects
Increased toxicity: Cardiac glycosides causes increased toxicity

Drug Uptake

Peak effect: In ~1 month following daily doses
Absorption: Readily absorbed from GI tract; absorption requires intestinal presence of bile

Pregnancy Risk Factor A (C if dose exceeds RDA recommendation)

Ergocalciferol (Mexico) *see* Ergocalciferol *on previous page*

Ergoloid Mesylates *(er' goe loid mes' i lates)*

Brand Names Germinal®; Hydergine®; Hydergine® LC; Hydro-Ergoloid®; Niloric®

Therapeutic Category Ergot Alkaloid and Derivative

Use Treatment of cerebrovascular insufficiency in primary progressive dementia, Alzheimer's dementia, and senile onset

Usual Dosage Adults: Oral: 1 mg 3 times/day up to 4.5-12 mg/day; up to 6 months of therapy may be necessary

Mechanism of Action Ergot alkaloid alpha-adrenergic agonist directly stimulates vascular smooth muscle to vasoconstrict peripheral and cerebral vessels; may also have antagonist effects on serotonin

Local Anesthetic/Vasoconstrictor Precautions No information available to require special precautions

Effects on Dental Treatment No effects or complications reported

Other Adverse Effects
1% to 10%:
  Gastrointestinal: Transient nausea
  Miscellaneous: Sublingual irritation
<1%:
  Cardiovascular: Bradycardia, orthostatic hypotension
  Central nervous system: Fainting, flushing, headache
  Dermatologic: Skin rash
  Gastrointestinal: Anorexia, nausea, vomiting, stomach cramps
  Ocular: Blurred vision
  Respiratory: Stuffy nose

Drug Interactions Increased toxicity with dopamine

Drug Uptake
Absorption: Rapid yet incomplete
Serum half-life: 3.5 hours
Time to peak serum concentration: Within 1 hour

Pregnancy Risk Factor C

Ergometrine Maleate (Canada) see Ergonovine Maleate on this page

Ergonovina (Mexico) see Ergonovine Maleate on this page

Ergonovine Maleate (er goe noe' veen mal' ee ate)
Brand Names Ergotrate® Maleate
Therapeutic Category Ergot Alkaloid and Derivative
Synonyms Ergometrine Maleate (Canada); Ergonovina (Mexico)
Use Prevention and treatment of postpartum and postabortion hemorrhage caused by uterine atony or subinvolution

Usual Dosage Adults:
Oral: 1-2 tablets (0.2-0.4 mg) every 6-12 hours for up to 48 hours
I.M., I.V. (I.V. should be reserved for emergency use only): 0.2 mg, repeat dose in 2-4 hours as needed

Mechanism of Action Ergot alkaloid alpha-adrenergic agonist directly stimulates vascular smooth muscle to vasoconstrict peripheral and cerebral vessels; may also have antagonist effects on serotonin

Local Anesthetic/Vasoconstrictor Precautions No information available to require special precautions

Effects on Dental Treatment No effects or complications reported

Other Adverse Effects
1% to 10%: Gastrointestinal: Nausea, vomiting
<1%:
  Cardiovascular: Palpitations, bradycardia, transient chest pain, hypertension, cerebrovascular accidents
  Central nervous system: Seizures, dizziness, headache
  Local: Thrombophlebitis
  Otic: Tinnitus
  Respiratory: Dyspnea
  Miscellaneous: Diaphoresis

Drug Interactions No data reported

Drug Uptake
Onset of effect:
  Oral: Within 5-15 minutes
  I.M.: Within 2-5 minutes
Duration: Uterine effects persist for 3 hours, except when given I.V., then effects persist for ~45 minutes

Pregnancy Risk Factor X

Ergostat® see Ergotamine on this page

Ergotamina Tartrato De (Mexico) see Ergotamine on this page

Ergotamine (er got' a meen)
Brand Names Cafatine®; Cafergot®; Cafetrate®; Ercaf®; Ergostat®; Wigraine®
Canadian/Mexican Brand Names Ergomar® (Canada); Gynergen® (Canada); Ergocaf® (Mexico); Sydolil® (Mexico)
Therapeutic Category Adrenergic Blocking Agent; Ergot Alkaloid and Derivative
Synonyms Ergotamina Tartrato De (Mexico)
Use Abort or prevent vascular headaches, such as migraine or cluster
(Continued)

Ergotamine *(Continued)*

Usual Dosage Adults:

Oral:

Cafergot®: 2 tablets at onset of attack; then 1 tablet every 30 minutes as needed; maximum: 6 tablets per attack; do not exceed 10 tablets/week

Ergostat®: 1 tablet under tongue at first sign, then 1 tablet every 30 minutes, 3 tablets/24 hours, 5 tablets/week

Rectal (Cafergot® suppositories, Wigraine® suppositories, Cafatine® suppositories): 1 at first sign of an attack; follow with second dose after 1 hour, if needed; maximum dose: 2 per attack; do not exceed 5/week

Inhalation: Initial: 1 inhalation, followed by repeat inhalations 5 minutes apart to a maximum of 6 inhalations/24 hours or 15 inhalations/1 week

Mechanism of Action Ergot alkaloid alpha-adrenergic blocker directly stimulates vascular smooth muscle to vasoconstrict peripheral and cerebral vessels; also has antagonist effects on serotonin

Local Anesthetic/Vasoconstrictor Precautions No information available to require special precautions

Effects on Dental Treatment No effects or complications reported

Other Adverse Effects

>10%:

Cardiovascular: Tachycardia, bradycardia, arterial spasm, claudication and vasoconstriction; rebound headache may occur with sudden withdrawal of the drug in patients on prolonged therapy; localized edema, peripheral vascular effects (numbness and tingling of fingers and toes)

Central nervous system: Drowsiness, dizziness

Gastrointestinal: Nausea, vomiting, diarrhea, dry mouth

1% to 10%:

Cardiovascular: Transient tachycardia or bradycardia, precordial distress and pain

Neuromuscular & skeletal: Weakness in the legs, abdominal or muscle pain, muscle pains in the extremities, paresthesia

Drug Interactions Increased toxicity:

Propranolol: One case of severe vasoconstriction with pain and cyanosis has been reported

Erythromycin, troleandomycin and other macrolide antibiotics: Monitor for signs of ergot toxicity

Drug Uptake

Absorption: Oral, rectal: Erratic; enhanced by caffeine coadministration

Time to peak serum concentration: Within 0.5-3 hours following co-administration with caffeine

Pregnancy Risk Factor X

Ergotrate® Maleate *see* Ergonovine Maleate *on previous page*

Eridium® *see* Phenazopyridine Hydrochloride *on page 679*

Eritromicina y Sulfisoxasol (Mexico) *see* Erythromycin and Sulfisoxazole *on page 323*

ERO Ear® [OTC] *see* Carbamide Peroxide *on page 152*

Eryc® *see* Erythromycin *on next page*

Erycette® Topical *see* Erythromycin, Topical *on page 324*

EryDerm® Topical *see* Erythromycin, Topical *on page 324*

Erygel® Topical *see* Erythromycin, Topical *on page 324*

Erymax® Topical *see* Erythromycin, Topical *on page 324*

EryPed® *see* Erythromycin *on next page*

Ery-sol® Topical *see* Erythromycin, Topical *on page 324*

Ery-Tab® *see* Erythromycin *on next page*

Erythrityl Tetranitrate *(e ri' thri til te tra nye' trate)*

Related Information

Cardiovascular Diseases *on page 912*

Brand Names Cardilate®

Therapeutic Category Antianginal Agent; Nitrate; Vasodilator, Coronary

Use Prophylaxis and long-term treatment of frequent or recurrent anginal pain and reduced exercise tolerance associated with angina pectoris

Usual Dosage Adults: Oral: 5 mg under the tongue or in the buccal pouch 3 times/day or 10 mg before meals or food, chewed 3 times/day, increasing in 2-3 days if needed; dosages of up to 100 mg/day are tolerated; some patients may need bedtime doses if they experience nocturnal symptoms

Mechanism of Action Erythrityl tetranitrate, like other organic nitrates, induces vasodilation by dephosphorylation of the myosin light chain in smooth muscles. This is accomplished by activation of guanylate cyclase, which eventually stimulates a cyclic GMP-dependent protein kinase that alters the phosphoryla-tion of the myosin. Venodilation causes peripheral blood pooling, which decreases venous return to the heart, central venous pressure, and pulmonary capillary wedge pressure. A reduction in pulmonary vascular resistance occurs secondary to pulmonary arteriolar dilation and afterload may be decreased by a lowering of systemic arterial pressure.

Local Anesthetic/Vasoconstrictor Precautions No information available to require special precautions

Effects on Dental Treatment No effects or complications reported

Other Adverse Effects
>10%: Central nervous system: Headache
1% to 10%: Cardiovascular: Tachycardia, hypotension, flushing
<1%:
Central nervous system: Restlessness, dizziness
Gastrointestinal: Nausea, vomiting, diarrhea
Hematologic: Methemoglobinemia
Neuromuscular & skeletal: Weakness

Pregnancy Risk Factor C

Comments Doses up to 100 mg are generally well tolerated; headache may occur when increasing doses; should headache occur, reduce dose for 2-3 days; may use analgesics to treat headache

Erythrocin® see Erythromycin on this page

Erythromycin (er ith roe mye' sin)

Related Information
Antimicrobial Prophylaxis in Surgical Patients on page 1042
Cardiovascular Diseases on page 912
Dental Drug Interactions: Update on Drug Combinations Requiring Special Considerations on page 1022
Oral Bacterial Infections on page 945
Oral Viral Infections on page 951
Respiratory Diseases on page 924

Brand Names E.E.S.®; E-Mycin®; Eryc®; EryPed®; Ery-Tab®; Erythrocin®; Ilosone®; PCE®; Wyamycin® S

Canadian/Mexican Brand Names Apo-Erythro® E-C (Canada); Diomycin® (Canada); Erybid® (Canada); Erythro-Base® (Canada); Novo-Rythro® Encap (Canada); PMS®-Erythromycin (Canada); Eritroquim® (Mexico); Latotryd® (Mexico); Lauricin® (Mexico); Luritran® (Mexico); Lederpax® (Mexico); Pantomicina® (Mexico); Tromigal® (Mexico)

Therapeutic Category Antibiotic, Macrolide; Antibiotic, Ophthalmic

Use
Dental: Alternate antibiotic, in penicillin-allergic patients, for the standard regimen for prevention of bacterial endocarditis in patients undergoing dental procedures; an alternative to penicillin VK for treating orofacial infections
Medical: Treatment of susceptible bacterial infections in the medical patient including *M. pneumoniae*, *Legionella pneumophila*, diphtheria, pertussis, chancroid, *Chlamydia*, and *Campylobacter* gastroenteritis; used in conjunc-tion with neomycin for decontaminating the bowel
Unlabeled use: Gastroparesis

Usual Dosage
Adults:
Prevention of bacterial endocarditis in patients allergic to penicillin:
Stearate or base: Oral: 1 g 2 hours before procedure, then 500 mg 6 hours after initial dose
Ethylsuccinate: 800 mg 2 hours before procedure, then 400 mg 6 hours after initial dose
Orofacial infections:
Stearate or base: 250-500 mg every 6 hours for at least 7 days
Ethylsuccinate: 400-800 mg every 6 hours for at least 7 days

Children:
Prophylaxis: Stearate or ethylsuccinate: 20 mg/kg; follow-up dose is half the initial dose
Orofacial infections: Base and ethylsuccinate: 30-50 mg/kg/day divided every 6-8 hours; do not exceed 2 g/day

Mechanism of Action Inhibits RNA-dependent protein synthesis at the chain elongation step; binds to the 50S ribosomal subunit resulting in blockage of transpeptidation

Local Anesthetic/Vasoconstrictor Precautions No information available to require special precautions

Effects on Dental Treatment No effects or complications reported
(Continued)

Erythromycin *(Continued)*

Other Adverse Effects
>10%: Gastrointestinal: Abdominal pain, cramping, nausea, vomiting
1% to 10%:
Gastrointestinal: Oral candidiasis
Hepatic: Cholestatic jaundice
Local: Phlebitis at the injection site
Miscellaneous: Hypersensitivity reactions

Oral manifestations: 1% to 10%: Oral candidiasis

Contraindications Hepatic impairment, known hypersensitivity to erythromycin or its components; use with pimozide

Warnings/Precautions Hepatic impairment with or without jaundice has occurred, it may be accompanied by malaise, nausea, vomiting, abdominal colic, and fever; discontinue use if these occur; avoid using erythromycin lactobionate in neonates since formulations may contain benzyl alcohol which is associated with toxicity in neonates

Drug Interactions Cytochrome P-450 IIIA enzyme inhibitor
Increased toxicity:
Erythromycin decreases clearance of carbamazepine, cyclosporine, and triazolam
Erythromycin may decrease theophylline clearance and increase theophylline's half-life by up to 60% (patients on high-dose theophylline and erythromycin or who have received erythromycin for >5 days may be at higher risk)
Terfenadine increases Q-T interval
May potentiate anticoagulant effect of warfarin
Concurrent use of erythromycin and lovastatin may result in rhabdomyolysis

Drug Uptake
Absorption: Variable but better with salt forms than with base form; 18% to 45% absorbed orally; due to differences in absorption, **200 mg erythromycin ethylsuccinate produces the same serum levels as 125 mg of erythromycin base**
Time to peak serum concentration: 4 hours for the base, 30 minutes to 2.5 hours for the ethylsuccinate
Serum half-life: 1.5-2 hours (peak)
Influence of food: Ethylsuccinate may be better absorbed with food

Pregnancy Risk Factor B

Breast-feeding Considerations May be taken while breast-feeding

Dosage Forms
Capsule, as estolate: 250 mg
Granules, for oral suspension, ethylsuccinate: 400 mg/5 mL (60 mL, 100 mL, 200 mL)
Injection, lactobionate: 500 mg, 1 g
Suspension:
Estolate: 125 mg/5 mL (480 mL); 250 mg/5 mL (480 mL)
Ethylsuccinate: 200 mg/5 mL (480 mL); 400 mg/5 mL (480 mL)
Suspension, drops, as ethylsuccinate: 100 mg/2.5 mL (50 mL)
Tablet:
Chewable, as ethylsuccinate: 200 mg
Delayed release, as base: 250 mg, 333 mg, 500 mg
Estolate: 500 mg
Ethylsuccinate: 400 mg
Film coated: 250 mg, 500 mg
Film coated, stearate: 250 mg, 500 mg
Polymer coated particles, as base: 333 mg, 500 mg

Dietary Considerations Decreased absorption with food; avoid milk and acidic beverages 1 hour before or after a dose; ethylsuccinate, estolate, and enteric coated products are **not** affected by food

Generic Available Yes

Comments Many patients cannot tolerate erythromycin because of abdominal pain and nausea; the mechanism of this adverse effect appears to be the motilin agonistic properties of erythromycin in the GI tract. For these patients, clindamycin is indicated as the alternative antibiotic for both prevention of bacterial endocarditis and treatment of orofacial infections.

Erythromycin has been used as a prokinetic agent to improve gastric emptying time and intestinal motility. In adults, 200 mg was infused I.V. initially followed by 250 mg orally 3 times/day 30 minutes before meals. In children, erythromycin 3 mg/kg I.V. has been infused over 60 minutes initially followed by 20 mg/kg/day orally in 3-4 divided doses before meals or before meals and at bedtime.

Selected Readings

Council on Dental Therapeutics, American Heart Association, "Preventing Bacterial Endocarditis," *J Am Dent Assoc*, 1991, 122(2):87-92.

Dajani AS, Bisno AL, Chung KJ, et al, "Prevention of Bacterial Endocarditis. Recommendations by the American Heart Association," *JAMA*, 1990, 264(22):2919-22.

"Pimozide (Orap) Contraindicated With Clarithromycin (Biaxin) and Other Macrolide Antibiotics," *FDA Medical Bulletin*, October 1996, 3.

Wynn RL and Bergman SA, "Antibiotics and Their Use in the Treatment of Orofacial Infections," *Gen Dent*, 1994, 42(Pt 1):398-402 and 42(Pt 2):498-502.

Wynn RL, "Current Concepts of the Erythromycins," *Gen Dent*, 1991, 39(6):408,10-1.

Erythromycin and Benzoyl Peroxide

(er ith roe mye' sin & ben' zoe il per ox' ide)

Brand Names Benzamycin®

Therapeutic Category Acne Products

Use Topical control of acne vulgaris

Local Anesthetic/Vasoconstrictor Precautions No information available to require special precautions

Effects on Dental Treatment No effects or complications reported

Erythromycin and Sulfisoxazole

(er ith roe mye' sin & sul fi sox' a zole)

Brand Names Eryzole®; Pediazole®

Therapeutic Category Antibiotic, Macrolide; Antibiotic, Sulfonamide Derivative

Synonyms Eritromicina y Sulfisoxasol (Mexico)

Use Treatment of susceptible bacterial infections of the upper and lower respiratory tract, otitis media in children caused by susceptible strains of *Haemophilus influenzae*, and other infections in patients allergic to penicillin

Usual Dosage Oral (dosage recommendation is based on the product's erythromycin content):

Children ≥2 months: 50 mg/kg/day erythromycin and 150 mg/kg/day sulfisoxazole in divided doses every 6 hours; not to exceed 2 g erythromycin/day or 6 g sulfisoxazole/day for 10 days

Adults: 400 mg erythromycin and 1200 mg sulfisoxazole every 6 hours

Mechanism of Action Erythromycin inhibits bacterial protein synthesis; sulfisoxazole competitively inhibits bacterial synthesis of folic acid from paraaminobenzoic acid

Local Anesthetic/Vasoconstrictor Precautions No information available to require special precautions

Effects on Dental Treatment No effects or complications reported

Other Adverse Effects

>10%: Gastrointestinal: Abdominal pain, cramping, nausea, vomiting

1% to 10%:

Gastrointestinal: Oral candidiasis

Hepatic: Cholestatic jaundice

Local: Phlebitis at the injection site

Miscellaneous: Hypersensitivity reactions

<1%:

Cardiovascular: Ventricular arrhythmias

Central nervous system: Fever, headache

Dermatologic: Skin rash, Stevens-Johnson syndrome, toxic epidermal necrolysis

Gastrointestinal: Hypertrophic pyloric stenosis, diarrhea

Hematologic: Eosinophilia, agranulocytosis, aplastic anemia

Hepatic: Hepatic necrosis

Local: Thrombophlebitis

Renal: Toxic nephrosis, crystalluria

Drug Interactions Increased effect/toxicity/levels of alfentanil, anticoagulants, astemizole, terfenadine, loratadine, bromocriptine, carbamazepine, cyclosporine, digoxin, disopyramide, theophylline, triazolam, and warfarin

Drug Uptake

Erythromycin ethylsuccinate:

Absorption: Well absorbed from GI tract

Serum half-life: 1-1.5 hours

Sulfisoxazole acetyl:

Absorption: Readily absorbed

Serum half-life: 6 hours, prolonged in renal impairment

Pregnancy Risk Factor C

Erythromycin, Topical (er ith roe mye' sin top' i kal)
Brand Names Akne-Mycin® Topical; A/T/S® Topical; Del-Mycin® Topical; Emgel™ Topical; Erycette® Topical; EryDerm® Topical; Erygel® Topical; Erymax® Topical; Ery-sol® Topical; E-Solve-2® Topical; ETS-2%® Topical; Ilotycin® Ophthalmic; Staticin® Topical; T-Stat® Topical
Therapeutic Category Acne Products; Antibiotic, Topical
Use Topical treatment of acne vulgaris
Local Anesthetic/Vasoconstrictor Precautions No information available to require special precautions
Effects on Dental Treatment No effects or complications reported
Other Adverse Effects 1% to 10%: Erythema, desquamation, dryness, pruritus

Erythropoietin see Epoetin Alfa on page 315

Eryzole® see Erythromycin and Sulfisoxazole on previous page

Esgic® see Butalbital Compound on page 133

Esidrix® see Hydrochlorothiazide on page 430

Eskalith® see Lithium on page 508

E-Solve-2® Topical see Erythromycin, Topical on this page

Esoterica® Facial [OTC] see Hydroquinone on page 439

Esoterica® Regular [OTC] see Hydroquinone on page 439

Esoterica® Sensitive Skin Formula [OTC] see Hydroquinone on page 439

Esoterica® Sunscreen [OTC] see Hydroquinone on page 439

Espotabs® [OTC] see Phenolphthalein on page 682

Estar® [OTC] see Coal Tar on page 225

Estazolam (es ta' zoe lam)
Brand Names ProSom™
Canadian/Mexican Brand Names Tasedan® (Mexico)
Therapeutic Category Benzodiazepine; Hypnotic; Sedative
Use Short-term management of insomnia; there has been little experience with this drug in the elderly, but because of its lack of active metabolites, it is a reasonable choice when a benzodiazepine hypnotic is indicated
Usual Dosage Adults: Oral: 1 mg at bedtime, some patients may require 2 mg; start at doses of 0.5 mg in debilitated or small elderly patients
Mechanism of Action Benzodiazepines may exert their pharmacologic effect through potentiation of the inhibitory activity of GABA. Benzodiazepines do not alter the synthesis, release, reuptake, or enzymatic degradation of GABA.
Local Anesthetic/Vasoconstrictor Precautions No information available to require special precautions
Effects on Dental Treatment Significant xerostomia occurs in up to 10% of patients. Disappears with cessation of drug therapy.
Other Adverse Effects
>10%:
  Cardiovascular: Tachycardia, chest pain
  Central nervous system: Drowsiness, fatigue, impaired coordination, light-headedness, memory impairment, insomnia, anxiety, depression, headache
  Dermatologic: Rash
  Endocrine & metabolic: Decreased libido
  Gastrointestinal: Dry mouth, constipation, decreased salivation, nausea, vomiting, diarrhea, increased or decreased appetite
  Neuromuscular & skeletal: Dysarthria
  Ocular: Blurred vision
  Miscellaneous: Sweating
1% to 10%:
  Cardiovascular: Syncope hypotension
  Central nervous system: Confusion, nervousness, dizziness, akathisia
  Dermatologic: Dermatitis
  Gastrointestinal: Weight gain or loss, increased salivation
  Neuromuscular & skeletal: Rigidity, tremor, muscle cramps
  Otic: Tinnitus
  Respiratory: Nasal congestion, hyperventilation
<1%:
  Central nervous system: Reflex slowing
  Endocrine & metabolic: Menstrual irregularities
  Hematologic: Blood dyscrasias
  Miscellaneous: Drug dependence

Drug Interactions

Decreased effect: Enzyme inducers may increase the metabolism of estazolam

Increased toxicity: CNS depressants may increase CNS adverse effects; cimetidine may decrease metabolism of estazolam

Pregnancy Risk Factor X

Estinyl® see Ethinyl Estradiol on page 334

Estivin® II [OTC] see Naphazoline Hydrochloride on page 605

Estrace® see Estradiol on this page

Estra-D® see Estradiol on this page

Estraderm® see Estradiol on this page

Estradiol (es tra dye' ole)

Related Information

Endocrine Disorders & Pregnancy on page 927

Brand Names Deladiol®; Delestrogen®; depGynogen®; Depo®-Estradiol; Depogen®; Dioval®; Dura-Estrin®; Duragen®; Estrace®; Estra-D®; Estraderm®; Estra-L®; Estro-Cyp®; Estroject-L.A.®; Gynogen L.A.®; Valergen®

Canadian/Mexican Brand Names Ginedisc® (Mexico); Oestrogel® (Mexico); Systen® (Mexico)

Therapeutic Category Estrogen Derivative

Use Treatment of atrophic vaginitis, atrophic dystrophy of vulva, menopausal symptoms, female hypogonadism, ovariectomy, primary ovarian failure, inoperable breast cancer, inoperable prostatic cancer, mild to severe vasomotor symptoms associated with menopause

Usual Dosage Adults (all dosage needs to be adjusted based upon the patient's response):

Male:

Prostate cancer: Valerate: I.M.: ≥30 mg or more every 1-2 weeks

Prostate cancer (androgen-dependent, inoperable, progressing): Oral: 10 mg 3 times/day for at least 3 months

Female:

Breast cancer (inoperable, progressing): Oral: 10 mg 3 times/day for at least 3 months

Osteoporosis prevention: Oral: 0.5 mg/day in a cyclic regimen (3 weeks on and 1 week off of drug)

Hypogonadism, moderate to severe vasomotor symptoms:

Oral: 1-2 mg/day in a cyclic regimen for 3 weeks on drug, then 1 week off drug

Moderate to severe vasomotor symptoms:

I.M.: Cypionate: 1-5 mg every 3-4 weeks

I.M.: Valerate: 10-20 mg every 4 weeks

Postpartum breast engorgement: I.M.: Valerate: 10-25 mg at end of first stage of labor

Transdermal: Apply 0.05 mg patch initially (titrate dosage to response) applied twice weekly in a cyclic regimen, for 3 weeks on drug and 1 week off drug in patients with an intact uterus and continuously in patients without a uterus

Atrophic vaginitis, kraurosis vulvae: Vaginal: Insert 2-4 g/day for 2 weeks then gradually reduce to 1/2 the initial dose for 2 weeks followed by a maintenance dose of 1 g 1-3 times/week

Mechanism of Action Increases the synthesis of DNA, RNA, and various proteins in target tissues; reduces the release of gonadotropin-releasing hormone from the hypothalamus; reduces FSH and LH release from the pituitary

Local Anesthetic/Vasoconstrictor Precautions No information available to require special precautions

Effects on Dental Treatment No effects or complications reported

Other Adverse Effects

>10%:

Cardiovascular: Peripheral edema

Endocrine & metabolic: Enlargement of breasts (female and male), breast tenderness, bloating

Gastrointestinal: Nausea, anorexia

1% to 10%:

Central nervous system: Headache

Endocrine & metabolic: Increased libido (female), decreased libido (male)

Gastrointestinal: Vomiting, diarrhea

(Continued)

Estradiol *(Continued)*

<1%:
  Cardiovascular: Increase in blood pressure, edema, thromboembolic disorders, myocardial infarction
  Central nervous system: Depression, dizziness, anxiety, stroke
  Dermatologic: Chloasma, melasma, rash
  Endocrine & metabolic: Hypercalcemia, folate deficiency, change in menstrual flow, breast tumors, amenorrhea, decreased glucose tolerance, increased triglycerides and LDL
  Gastrointestinal: Nausea, GI distress
  Hepatic: Cholestatic jaundice
  Local: Pain at injection site
  Miscellaneous: Intolerance to contact lenses, increased susceptibility to *Candida* infection

Drug Interactions
  Decreased effect: Rifampin decreases estrogen serum concentrations
  Increased toxicity: Hydrocortisone increases corticosteroid toxic potential; increases potential for thromboembolic events with anticoagulants

Drug Uptake
  Absorption: Readily absorbed through skin and GI tract; reabsorbed from bile in GI tract and enterohepatically recycled
  Serum half-life: 50-60 minutes

Pregnancy Risk Factor X

Estradiol and Testosterone (es tra dye' ole & tes tos' ter one)

Brand Names Andro®/Fem Injection; Deladumone® Injection; depAndrogyn® Injection; Depo-Testadiol® Injection; Depotestogen® Injection; Duo-Cyp® Injection; Duratestrin® Injection; Estra-Testrin® Injection; Valertest No.1® Injection

Therapeutic Category Estrogen and Androgen Combination

Synonyms Testosterone and Estradiol

Use Vasomotor symptoms associated with menopause; postpartum breast engorgement

Local Anesthetic/Vasoconstrictor Precautions No information available to require special precautions

Effects on Dental Treatment No effects or complications reported

Estradurin® *see* Polyestradiol Phosphate *on page 702*

Estra-L® *see* Estradiol *on previous page*

Estramustine Phosphate Sodium
(es tra mus' teen fos' fate sow' dee um)

Brand Names Emcyt®

Therapeutic Category Antineoplastic Agent, Hormone (Estrogen/Nitrogen Mustard)

Use Palliative treatment of prostatic carcinoma (progressive or metastatic)

Usual Dosage Adults: Oral: 14 mg/kg/day (range: 10-16 mg/kg/day) in 3-4 divided doses for 30-90 days; some patients have been maintained for >3 years on therapy

Mechanism of Action Mechanism is not completely clear, thought to act as an alkylating agent and as estrogen

Local Anesthetic/Vasoconstrictor Precautions No information available to require special precautions

Effects on Dental Treatment No effects or complications reported

Other Adverse Effects
>10%:
  Cardiovascular: Edema
  Gastrointestinal: Diarrhea, nausea, mild increases in AST (SGOT) or LDH
  Endocrine & metabolic: Decreased libido, breast tenderness, breast enlargement
  Respiratory: Dyspnea
1% to 10%:
  Cardiovascular: Myocardial infarction
  Central nervous system: Insomnia, lethargy
  Gastrointestinal: Anorexia, flatulence
  Hematologic: Leukopenia
  Local: Thrombophlebitis
  Neuromuscular & skeletal: Leg cramps
  Respiratory: Pulmonary embolism
<1%:
  Cardiovascular: Cardiac arrest
  Central nervous system: Night sweats, depression

Dermatologic: Pigment changes
Endocrine & metabolic: Hypercalcemia, hot flashes
Otic: Tinnitus
Drug Interactions Decreased effect: Milk products and calcium-rich foods/drugs may impair the oral absorption of estramustine phosphate sodium
Drug Uptake
Absorption: Oral: Well absorbed (75%)
Serum half-life: 20 hours
Time to peak serum concentration: Within 2-3 hours
Pregnancy Risk Factor C

Estratab® *see* Estrogens, Esterified *on next page*

Estratest® H.S. Oral *see* Estrogens With Methyltestosterone *on page 329*

Estratest® Oral *see* Estrogens With Methyltestosterone *on page 329*

Estra-Testrin® Injection *see* Estradiol and Testosterone *on previous page*

Estro-Cyp® *see* Estradiol *on page 325*

Estrogenos Conjugados (Mexico) *see* Estrogens, Conjugated *on this page*

Estrogens and Medroxyprogesterone
(es' troe jenz & me drox' ee proe jes' te rone)
Related Information
Endocrine Disorders & Pregnancy *on page 927*
Brand Names Premphase™; Prempro™
Therapeutic Category Estrogen and Androgen Combination
Use Women with an intact uterus for the treatment of moderate to severe vasomotor symptoms associated with the menopause; treatment of atrophic vaginitis; primary ovarian failure; osteoporosis prophylactic
Local Anesthetic/Vasoconstrictor Precautions No information available to require special precautions
Effects on Dental Treatment No effects or complications reported
Other Adverse Effects
>10%:
Cardiovascular: Peripheral edema
Endocrine & metabolic: Changes in menstrual flow, amenorrhea, enlargement of breasts, breast tenderness
Gastrointestinal: Anorexia, edema, weakness, nausea, bloating
Hematologic: Breakthrough bleeding, spotting
Local: Pain at injection site
1% to 10%:
Cardiovascular: Edema
Central nervous system: Mental depression, fever, insomnia, headache
Dermatologic: Melasma or chloasma, allergic rash with or without pruritus
Endocrine & metabolic: Changes in cervical erosion and secretions, increased breast tenderness, increased libido
Gastrointestinal: Weight gain or loss, vomiting, diarrhea
Hepatic: Cholestatic jaundice
Local: Thrombophlebitis, pain at injection site
Respiratory: Central thrombosis and embolism
<1%:
Cardiovascular: Hypertension, thromboembolism, stroke, myocardial infarction, edema
Central nervous system: Depression, dizziness, anxiety
Dermatologic: Chloasma, melasma, rash
Endocrine & metabolic: Breast tumors, amenorrhea, alterations in frequency and flow of menses, decreased glucose tolerance, increased triglycerides and LDL
Gastrointestinal: GI distress
Hepatic: Cholestatic jaundice
Ocular: Intolerance to contact lenses
Miscellaneous: Increased susceptibility to *Candida* infection

Estrogens, Conjugated (es' troe jenz, kon' ju gate ed)
Related Information
Dental Drug Interactions: Update on Drug Combinations Requiring Special Considerations *on page 1022*
Endocrine Disorders & Pregnancy *on page 927*
Brand Names Premarin®
Canadian/Mexican Brand Names C.E.S.® (Canada); Congest® (Canada)
Therapeutic Category Estrogen Derivative
Synonyms Estrogenos Conjugados (Mexico)
(Continued)

Estrogens, Conjugated (Continued)

Use Atrophic vaginitis; hypogonadism; primary ovarian failure; vasomotor symptoms of menopause; prostatic carcinoma; osteoporosis prophylactic

Usual Dosage Adults:

Male: Prostate cancer: Oral: 1.25-2.5 mg 3 times/day

Female:

Hypogonadism: Oral: 2.5-7.5 mg/day for 20 days, off 10 days and repeat until menses occur

Abnormal uterine bleeding:

Oral: 2.5-5 mg/day for 7-10 days; then decrease to 1.25 mg/day for 2 weeks

I.M., I.V.: 25 mg every 6-12 hours until bleeding stops

Moderate to severe vasomotor symptoms: Oral: 0.625-1.25 mg/day

Postpartum breast engorgement: Oral: 3.75 mg every 4 hours for 5 doses, then 1.25 mg every 4 hours for 5 days

Atrophic vaginitis, kraurosis vulvae: Vaginal: 2-4 g instilled/day 3 weeks on and 1 week off

Osteoporosis: Oral: 0.625 mg/day chronically

Uremic bleeding: I.V.: 0.6 mg/kg/dose daily for 5 days

Mechanism of Action Increases the synthesis of DNA, RNA, and various proteins in target tissues; reduces the release of gonadotropin-releasing hormone from the hypothalamus; reduces FSH and LH release from the pituitary

Local Anesthetic/Vasoconstrictor Precautions No information available to require special precautions

Effects on Dental Treatment No effects or complications reported

Other Adverse Effects

>10%:

Cardiovascular: Peripheral edema

Endocrine & metabolic: Breast tenderness, hypercalcemia, enlargement of breasts

Gastrointestinal: Nausea, anorexia, bloating

1% to 10%:

Central nervous system: Headache

Endocrine & metabolic: Increased libido

Gastrointestinal: Vomiting, diarrhea

Local: Pain at injection site

<1%:

Cardiovascular: Increase in blood pressure, edema, thromboembolic disorder, myocardial infarction, stroke, hypertension

Central nervous system: Depression, dizziness, anxiety

Dermatologic: Chloasma, melasma, rash

Endocrine & metabolic: Breast tumors, amenorrhea, alterations in frequency and flow of menses, decreased glucose tolerance, increased triglycerides and LDL

Gastrointestinal: Vomiting, GI distress

Hepatic: Cholestatic jaundice

Miscellaneous: Intolerance to contact lenses, increased susceptibility to *Candida* infection

Drug Interactions

Decreased effect: Rifampin decreases estrogen serum concentrations

Increased toxicity:

Anticoagulants: Increases potential for thromboembolic events with anticoagulants

Drug Uptake

Absorption: Readily absorbed from GI tract

Pregnancy Risk Factor X

Estrogens, Esterified (es' troe jenz, es ter' i fied)

Related Information

Dental Drug Interactions: Update on Drug Combinations Requiring Special Considerations *on page 1022*

Endocrine Disorders & Pregnancy *on page 927*

Brand Names Estratab®; Menest®

Canadian/Mexican Brand Names Neo-Estrone® (Canada)

Therapeutic Category Estrogen Derivative

Use Atrophic vaginitis; hypogonadism; primary ovarian failure; vasomotor symptoms of menopause; prostatic carcinoma; osteoporosis prophylactic

Usual Dosage Adults: Oral:

Male: Prostate cancer (inoperable, progressing): 1.25-2.5 mg 3 times/day

Female:

Hypogonadism: 2.5-7.5 mg/day for 20 days, off 10 days and repeat until menses occur

Moderate to severe vasomotor symptoms: 0.3-1.25 mg/day

Breast cancer (inoperable, progressing): 10 mg 3 times/day for at least 3 months

Mechanism of Action Primary effects on the interphase DNA-protein complex (chromatin) by binding to a receptor (usually located in the cytoplasm of a target cell) and initiating translocation of the hormone-receptor complex to the nucleus

Local Anesthetic/Vasoconstrictor Precautions No information available to require special precautions

Effects on Dental Treatment No effects or complications reported

Other Adverse Effects

>10%:

Cardiovascular: Peripheral edema

Endocrine & metabolic: Enlargement of breasts, breast tenderness, bloating

Gastrointestinal: Nausea, anorexia

1% to 10%:

Central nervous system: Headache

Endocrine & metabolic: Increased libido

Gastrointestinal: Vomiting, diarrhea

<1%:

Cardiovascular: Hypertension, thromboembolism, myocardial infarction, edema

Central nervous system: Stroke, depression, dizziness, anxiety

Dermatologic: Chloasma, melasma, rash

Endocrine & metabolic: Breast tumors, amenorrhea, alterations in frequency and flow of menses, decreased glucose tolerance, increased triglycerides and LDL

Gastrointestinal: GI distress

Hepatic: Cholestatic jaundice

Miscellaneous: Intolerance to contact lenses, increased susceptibility to *Candida* infection

Drug Interactions

Decreased effect: Rifampin decreases estrogen serum concentrations

Increased toxicity:

Anticoagulants: Increases potential for thromboembolic events with anticoagulants

Drug Uptake

Absorption: Readily absorbed from GI tract

Pregnancy Risk Factor X

Estrogens With Methyltestosterone

(es' troe jenz with meth il tes tos' te rone)

Related Information

Endocrine Disorders & Pregnancy *on page 927*

Brand Names Estratest® H.S. Oral; Estratest® Oral; Premarin® With Methyltestosterone Oral

Therapeutic Category Estrogen and Androgen Combination

Use Atrophic vaginitis; hypogonadism; primary ovarian failure; vasomotor symptoms of menopause; prostatic carcinoma; osteoporosis prophylactic

Local Anesthetic/Vasoconstrictor Precautions No information available to require special precautions

Effects on Dental Treatment No effects or complications reported

Estroject-L.A.® *see Estradiol on page 325*

Estrone (es' trone)

Related Information

Endocrine Disorders & Pregnancy *on page 927*

Brand Names Estronol®; Kestrone®; Theelin®

Canadian/Mexican Brand Names Femogen® (Canada); Neo-Estrone® (Canada); Oestrillin® (Canada)

Therapeutic Category Estrogen Derivative

Use Hypogonadism; primary ovarian failure; vasomotor symptoms of menopause; prostatic carcinoma; inoperable breast cancer, kraurosis vulvae, abnormal uterine bleeding due to hormone imbalance

Usual Dosage Adults: I.M.:

Male: Prostatic carcinoma: 2-4 mg 2-3 times/week

(Continued)

Estrone *(Continued)*

Female:

Senile vaginitis and kraurosis vulvae: 0.1-0.5 mg 2-3 times/week

Breast cancer (inoperable, progressing): 5 mg 3 or more times/week

Primary ovarian failure, hypogonadism: 0.1-1 mg/week, up to 2 mg/week in single or divided doses

Abnormal uterine bleeding: 2.5 mg/day for several days

Mechanism of Action Estrone is a natural ovarian estrogenic hormone that is available as an aqueous mixture of water insoluble estrone and water soluble estrone potassium sulfate; all estrogens, including estrone, act in a similar manner; there is no evidence that there are biological differences among various estrogen preparations other than their ability to bind to cellular receptors inside the target cells

Local Anesthetic/Vasoconstrictor Precautions No information available to require special precautions

Effects on Dental Treatment No effects or complications reported

Other Adverse Effects

>10%:

Cardiovascular: Peripheral edema

Endocrine & metabolic: Enlargement of breasts, breast tenderness, bloating

Gastrointestinal: Nausea, anorexia

1% to 10%:

Central nervous system: Headache

Endocrine & metabolic: Increased libido

Gastrointestinal: Vomiting, diarrhea

<1%:

Cardiovascular: Hypertension, thromboembolism, myocardial infarction, edema

Central nervous system: Stroke, depression, dizziness, anxiety

Dermatologic: Chloasma, melasma, rash

Endocrine & metabolic: Breast tumors, amenorrhea, alterations in frequency and flow of menses, decreased glucose tolerance, increased triglycerides and LDL

Gastrointestinal: GI distress

Hepatic: Cholestatic jaundice

Miscellaneous: Intolerance to contact lenses, increased susceptibility to *Candida* infection

Drug Interactions

Decreased effect: Rifampin decreases estrogen serum concentrations

Increased toxicity:

Anticoagulants: Increases potential for thromboembolic events with anticoagulants

Pregnancy Risk Factor X

Estronol® *see* Estrone *on previous page*

Estropipate *(es' troe pih pate)*

Related Information

Endocrine Disorders & Pregnancy *on page 927*

Brand Names Ogen®; Ortho-Est®

Canadian/Mexican Brand Names Estrouis® (Canada)

Therapeutic Category Estrogen Derivative

Use Atrophic vaginitis; hypogonadism; primary ovarian failure; vasomotor symptoms of menopause; osteoporosis prophylactic

Usual Dosage Adults: Female:

Moderate to severe vasomotor symptoms: Oral: 0.625-5 mg/day

Hypogonadism or primary ovarian failure: Oral: 1.25-7.5 mg/day for 3 weeks followed by an 8- to 10-day rest period

Osteoporosis prevention: Oral: 0.625 mg/day for 25 days of a 31-day cycle

Atrophic vaginitis or kraurosis vulvae: Vaginal: Instill 2-4 g/day 3 weeks on and 1 week off

Mechanism of Action Crystalline estrone that has been solubilized as the sulfate and stabilized with piperazine. Primary effects on the interphase DNA-protein complex (chromatin) by binding to a receptor (usually located in the cytoplasm of a target cell) and initiating translocation of the hormone receptor complex to the nucleus.

Local Anesthetic/Vasoconstrictor Precautions No information available to require special precautions

Effects on Dental Treatment No effects or complications reported

Other Adverse Effects
>10%:
  Cardiovascular: Peripheral edema
  Endocrine & metabolic: Enlargement of breasts, breast tenderness, bloating
  Gastrointestinal: Nausea, anorexia
1% to 10%:
  Central nervous system: Headache
  Endocrine & metabolic: Increased libido
  Gastrointestinal: Vomiting, diarrhea
<1%:
  Cardiovascular: Hypertension, thromboembolism, myocardial infarction, edema
  Central nervous system: Stroke, depression, dizziness, anxiety
  Dermatologic: Chloasma, melasma, rash
  Endocrine & metabolic: Breast tumors, amenorrhea, alterations in frequency and flow of menses, decreased glucose tolerance, increased triglycerides and LDL
  Gastrointestinal: GI distress
  Hepatic: Cholestatic jaundice
  Miscellaneous: Intolerance to contact lenses, increased susceptibility to *Candida* infection

Drug Interactions
Decreased effect: Rifampin decreases estrogen serum concentrations
Increased toxicity:
  Anticoagulants: Increases potential for thromboembolic events with anticoagulants

Pregnancy Risk Factor X

Estrovis® *see* Quinestrol *on page 757*

Ethacrynic Acid (eth a krin' ik as' id)
Related Information
Cardiovascular Diseases *on page 912*
Brand Names Edecrin®
Therapeutic Category Diuretic, Loop
Use Management of edema associated with congestive heart failure; hepatic cirrhosis or renal disease; short-term management of ascites due to malignancy, idiopathic edema, and lymphedema
Usual Dosage I.V. formulation should be diluted in D₅W or NS (1 mg/mL) and infused over several minutes

Children:
  Oral: 1 mg/kg/dose once daily; increase at intervals of 2-3 days as needed, to a maximum of 3 mg/kg/day
  I.V.: 1 mg/kg/dose, (maximum: 50 mg/dose); repeat doses not routinely recommended; however, if indicated, repeat doses every 8-12 hours
Adults:
  Oral: 50-100 mg/day in 1-2 divided doses; may increase in increments of 25-50 mg at intervals of several days to a maximum of 400 mg/24 hours
  I.V.: 0.5-1 mg/kg/dose (maximum: 100 mg/dose); repeat doses not routinely recommended; however, if indicated, repeat doses every 8-12 hours

Mechanism of Action Inhibits reabsorption of sodium and chloride in the ascending loop of Henle and distal renal tubule, interfering with the chloride-binding cotransport system, thus causing increased excretion of water, sodium, chloride, magnesium, and calcium

Local Anesthetic/Vasoconstrictor Precautions No information available to require special precautions
Effects on Dental Treatment No effects or complications reported
Other Adverse Effects
>10%: Diarrhea
1% to 10%:
  Central nervous system: Headache
  Endocrine & metabolic: Hyponatremia, hypochloremic alkalosis, hypokalemia
  Gastrointestinal: Loss of appetite
  Neuromuscular & skeletal: Orthostatic hypotension
  Ocular: Blurred vision
  Otic: Ototoxicity
<1%:
  Central nervous system: Nervousness
  Dermatologic: Skin rash
  Endocrine & metabolic: Hyperuricemia, gout
(Continued)

331

Ethacrynic Acid *(Continued)*

    Gastrointestinal: Gastrointestinal bleeding, pancreatitis, stomach cramps
    Hepatic: Hepatic dysfunction, abnormal LFTs
    Hematologic: Leukopenia, agranulocytosis, thrombocytopenia
    Local: Local irritation
    Renal: Renal injury, hematuria

Drug Interactions
  Increased effect:
    Hypotensive agents causes additive decrease in blood pressure
    Drugs affected by or causing potassium depletion cause additive decrease in potassium
    Increased nephrotoxic potential with aminoglycosides
    Digoxin increases cardiotoxic potential leading to arrhythmias
    Increased warfarin anticoagulant effects; increased lithium levels
  Decreased effect:
    Probenecid decreases diuretic effects
    Decreased effectiveness of antidiabetic agents

Drug Uptake
  Onset of diuretic effect:
    Oral: Within 30 minutes
    I.V.: 5 minutes
  Peak effect:
    Oral: 2 hours
    I.V.: 30 minutes
  Duration of action:
    Oral: 12 hours
    I.V.: 2 hours
  Absorption: Oral: Rapid
  Serum half-life: Normal renal function: 2-4 hours

Pregnancy Risk Factor B

Ethambutol Hydrochloride (e tham' byoo tole hye droe klor' ide)

Related Information
  Nonviral Infectious Diseases *on page 932*
Brand Names Myambutol®
Canadian/Mexican Brand Names Etibl® (Canada)
Therapeutic Category Antitubercular Agent
Use Treatment of tuberculosis and other mycobacterial diseases in conjunction with other antituberculosis agents; only indicated when patients are from areas where drug-resistant M. tuberculosis is endemic, in HIV-infected elderly patients, and when drug-resistant M. tuberculosis is suspected

Usual Dosage Oral:
  Ethambutol is generally not recommended in children whose visual acuity cannot be monitored (<6 years of age). However, ethambutol should be considered for all children with organisms resistant to other drugs, when susceptibility to ethambutol has been demonstrated, or susceptibility is likely.
  Note: A four-drug regimen (isoniazid, rifampin, pyrazinamide, and either streptomycin or ethambutol) is preferred for the initial, empiric treatment of TB. When the drug susceptibility results are available, the regimen should be altered as appropriate.

  Patients with tuberculosis and without HIV infection:
    OPTION 1: Isoniazid resistance rate <4%: Administer daily isoniazid, rifampin, and pyrazinamide for 8 weeks followed by isoniazid and rifampin daily or directly observed therapy (DOT) 2-3 times/week for 16 weeks. If isoniazid resistance rate is not documented, ethambutol or streptomycin should also be administered until susceptibility to isoniazid or rifampin is demonstrated. Continue treatment for at least 6 months or 3 months beyond culture conversion.
    OPTION 2: Administer daily isoniazid, rifampin, pyrazinamide, and either streptomycin or ethambutol for 2 weeks followed by DOT 2 times/week administration of the same drugs for 6 weeks, and subsequently, with isoniazid and rifampin DOT 2 times/week administration for 16 weeks
    OPTION 3: Administer isoniazid, rifampin, pyrazinamide, and either ethambutol or streptomycin by DOT 3 times/week for 6 months

  Patients with TB and with HIV infection: Administer any of the above OPTIONS 1, 2 or 3; however, treatment should be continued for a total of 9 months and at least 6 months beyond culture conversion

Note: Some experts recommend that the duration of therapy should be extended to 9 months for patients with disseminated disease, miliary disease, disease involving the bones or joints, or tuberculosis lymphadenitis

Children (>6 years) and Adults:
Daily therapy: 15-25 mg/kg/day (maximum: 2.5 g/day)
Directly observed therapy (DOT): Twice weekly: 50 mg/kg (maximum: 2.5 g)
DOT: 3 times/week: 25-30 mg/kg (maximum: 2.5 g)

Mechanism of Action Suppresses mycobacteria multiplication by interfering with RNA synthesis

Local Anesthetic/Vasoconstrictor Precautions No information available to require special precautions

Effects on Dental Treatment No effects or complications reported

Other Adverse Effects
1% to 10%:
Central nervous system: Headache, confusion, disorientation
Endocrine & metabolic: Acute gout or hyperuricemia
Gastrointestinal: Abdominal pain, anorexia, nausea, vomiting
<1%:
Central nervous system: Malaise, peripheral neuritis, mental confusion, fever
Dermatologic: Rash, pruritus
Hepatic: Abnormal liver function tests
Ocular: Optic neuritis
Miscellaneous: Anaphylaxis

Drug Interactions Decreased absorption with aluminum salts

Drug Uptake
Absorption: Oral: ~80%
Serum half-life: 2.5-3.6 hours
End stage renal disease: 7-15 hours
Time to peak serum concentration: 2-4 hours

Pregnancy Risk Factor B

Ethamolin® *see* Ethanolamine Oleate *on this page*

ETH and C *see* Terpin Hydrate and Codeine *on page 825*

Ethanolamine Oleate (eth′ a nol a meen oh′ lee ate)
Brand Names Ethamolin®
Therapeutic Category Sclerosing Agent
Synonyms Monoethanolamine (Canada)
Use Mild sclerosing agent used for bleeding esophageal varices
Usual Dosage Adults: 1.5-5 mL per varix, up to 20 mL total or 0.4 mL/kg; patients with severe hepatic dysfunction should receive less than recommended maximum dose
Mechanism of Action Derived from oleic acid and similar in physical properties to sodium morrhuate; however, the exact mechanism of the hemostatic effect used in endoscopic injection sclerotherapy is not known. Intravenously injected ethanolamine oleate produces a sterile inflammatory response resulting in fibrosis and occlusion of the vein; a dose-related extravascular inflammatory reaction occurs when the drug diffuses through the venous wall. Autopsy results indicate that variceal obliteration occurs secondary to mural necrosis and fibrosis. Thrombosis appears to be a transient reaction.
Local Anesthetic/Vasoconstrictor Precautions No information available to require special precautions
Effects on Dental Treatment No effects or complications reported
Other Adverse Effects
1% to 10%:
Central nervous system: Pyrexia
Gastrointestinal: Esophageal ulcer, esophageal stricture
Respiratory: Pleural effusion, pneumonia
Miscellaneous: Retrosternal pain
<1%:
Local: Injection necrosis
Renal: Acute renal failure
Miscellaneous: Aspiration, anaphylaxis
Drug Interactions No data reported
Pregnancy Risk Factor C

Ethaquin® *see* Ethaverine Hydrochloride *on next page*
Ethatab® *see* Ethaverine Hydrochloride *on next page*

Ethaverine Hydrochloride (eth av′ er een hye dro klor′ ide)
Brand Names Ethaquin®; Ethatab®; Ethavex-100®; Isovex®
Therapeutic Category Vasodilator
Use Peripheral and cerebral vascular insufficiency associated with arterial spasm
Local Anesthetic/Vasoconstrictor Precautions No information available to require special precautions
Effects on Dental Treatment No effects or complications reported
Other Adverse Effects <1%:
Cardiovascular: Flushing of the face, tachycardia, hypotension
Central nervous system: Depression, dizziness, vertigo, drowsiness, sedation, lethargy, headache
Dermatologic: Pruritus
Gastrointestinal: Dry mouth, nausea, constipation
Hepatic: Hepatic hypersensitivity
Miscellaneous: Sweating

Ethavex-100® see Ethaverine Hydrochloride *on this page*

Ethchlorvynol (eth klor vi′ nole)
Brand Names Placidyl®
Therapeutic Category Hypnotic; Sedative
Use Short-term management of insomnia
Usual Dosage Adults: Oral: 500-1000 mg at bedtime
Dosing adjustment in renal impairment: Cl_{cr} <50 mL/minute: Avoid use
Mechanism of Action Causes nonspecific depression of the reticular activating system
Local Anesthetic/Vasoconstrictor Precautions No information available to require special precautions
Effects on Dental Treatment No effects or complications reported
Other Adverse Effects
>10%:
Central nervous system: Dizziness, weakness
Gastrointestinal: Indigestion, nausea, stomach pain, unpleasant aftertaste
Ocular: Blurred vision
1% to 10%:
Central nervous system: Nervousness, excitement, clumsiness, confusion, drowsiness (daytime)
Dermatologic: Skin rash
<1%:
Cardiovascular: Bradycardia
Central nervous system: Hyperthermia, weakness (severe), slurred speech
Hepatic: Cholestatic jaundice
Neuromuscular & skeletal: Trembling
Respiratory: Shortness of breath
Drug Interactions
Decreased effect of oral anticoagulants
Increased toxicity (CNS depression) with alcohol, CNS depressants, MAO inhibitors, TCAs (delirium)
Drug Uptake
Onset of action: 15-60 minutes
Duration: 5 hours
Absorption: Rapid from GI tract
Serum half-life: 10-20 hours
Time to peak serum concentration: 2 hours
Pregnancy Risk Factor C

Ethinyl Estradiol (eth′ in il es tra dye′ ole)
Related Information
Endocrine Disorders & Pregnancy *on page 927*
Brand Names Estinyl®
Therapeutic Category Estrogen Derivative
Synonyms Etinilestradiol (Mexico)
Use Hypogonadism; primary ovarian failure; vasomotor symptoms of menopause; prostatic carcinoma; breast cancer
Usual Dosage Adults: Oral:
Male: Prostatic cancer (inoperable, progressing): 0.15-2 mg/day for palliation
Female:
Hypogonadism: 0.05 mg 1-3 times/day for 2 weeks of a theoretical menstrual cycle followed by progesterone for 3-6 months
Vasomotor symptoms: 0.02-0.05 mg for 21 days, off 7 days and repeat

Breast cancer (inoperable, progressing): 1 mg 3 times/day for palliation

Mechanism of Action Increases the synthesis of DNA, RNA, and various proteins in target tissues; reduces the release of gonadotropin-releasing hormone from the hypothalamus; reduces FSH and LH release from the pituitary

Local Anesthetic/Vasoconstrictor Precautions No information available to require special precautions

Effects on Dental Treatment No effects or complications reported

Other Adverse Effects
>10%:
  Cardiovascular: Peripheral edema
  Endocrine & metabolic: Enlargement of breasts, breast tenderness, bloating
  Gastrointestinal: Nausea, anorexia
1% to 10%:
  Central nervous system: Headache
  Endocrine & metabolic: Increased libido
  Gastrointestinal: Vomiting, diarrhea
<1%:
  Cardiovascular: Hypertension, thromboembolism, myocardial infarction, edema
  Central nervous system: Stroke, depression, dizziness, anxiety
  Dermatologic: Chloasma, melasma, rash
  Endocrine & metabolic: Breast tumors, amenorrhea, alterations in frequency and flow of menses, decreased glucose tolerance, increased triglycerides and LDL
  Gastrointestinal: GI distress
  Hepatic: Cholestatic jaundice
  Miscellaneous: Intolerance to contact lenses, increased susceptibility to *Candida* infection

Drug Interactions
Decreased effect: Rifampin decreases estrogen serum concentrations
Increased toxicity:
  Anticoagulants: Increases potential for thromboembolic events with anticoagulants

Drug Uptake
Absorption: Absorbed well from GI tract

Pregnancy Risk Factor X

Ethinyl Estradiol and Desogestrel
(eth' in il es tra dye' ole & des oh jes' trel)
Brand Names Desogen®; Ortho-Cept®
Therapeutic Category Contraceptive, Oral
Synonyms Desogestrel and Ethinyl Estradiol
Use Prevention of pregnancy
Local Anesthetic/Vasoconstrictor Precautions No information available to require special precautions
Effects on Dental Treatment When prescribing antibiotics, patient must be warned to use supplemental methods of birth control if on oral contraceptives

Ethinyl Estradiol and Ethynodiol Diacetate
(eth' in il es tra dye' ole & e thye noe dye' ole dye as' e tate)
Related Information
Endocrine Disorders & Pregnancy *on page 927*
Brand Names Demulen®
Therapeutic Category Contraceptive, Oral
Use Prevention of pregnancy; treatment of hypermenorrhea, endometriosis, female hypogonadism
Usual Dosage Adults: Female: Oral:
For 21-tablet cycle packs, with 21 active tablets (28-day packs have 21 active tablets and 7 inert tablets): Take 1 tablet daily starting on the fifth day of menstrual cycle, with day 1 being the first day of menstruation; begin taking a new cycle pack on the eighth day after taking the last tablet from the previous pack

With 28-tablet packages, dosage is 1 tablet daily without interruption; extra tablets are placebos or contain iron. If next menstrual period does not begin on schedule, rule out pregnancy before starting new dosing cycle. If menstrual period begins, start new dosing cycle 7 days after last tablet was taken. If all doses have been taken on schedule and one menstrual period is missed, continue dosing cycle. If two consecutive menstrual periods are missed, pregnancy test is required before new dosing cycle is started.
(Continued)

335

Ethinyl Estradiol and Ethynodiol Diacetate *(Continued)*

One dose missed: Take as soon as remembered or take 2 tablets next day

Two doses missed: Take 2 tablets as soon as remembered or 2 tablets next 2 days

Three doses missed: Begin new compact of tablets starting on day 1 of next cycle

Mechanism of Action Combination oral contraceptives inhibit ovulation via a negative feedback mechanism on the hypothalamus, which alters the normal pattern of gonadotropin secretion of a follicle-stimulating hormone (FSH) and luteinizing hormone by the anterior pituitary. The follicular phase FSH and midcycle surge of gonadotropins are inhibited. In addition, oral contraceptives produce alterations in the genital tract, including changes in the cervical mucus, rendering it unfavorable for sperm penetration even if ovulation occurs. Changes in the endometrium may also occur, producing an unfavorable environment for nidation. Oral contraceptive drugs may alter the tubal transport of the ova through the fallopian tubes. Progestational agents may also alter sperm fertility.

Local Anesthetic/Vasoconstrictor Precautions No information available to require special precautions

Effects on Dental Treatment When prescribing antibiotics, patient must be warned to use supplemental methods of birth control if on oral contraceptives

Other Adverse Effects

>10%:

Cardiovascular: Peripheral edema

Endocrine & metabolic: Enlargement of breasts, breast tenderness, bloating

Gastrointestinal: Nausea, anorexia

1% to 10%:

Central nervous system: Headache

Endocrine & metabolic: Increased libido

Gastrointestinal: Vomiting, diarrhea

<1%:

Cardiovascular: Hypertension, thromboembolism, stroke, myocardial infarction, edema

Central nervous system: Depression, dizziness, anxiety

Dermatologic: Chloasma, melasma, rash

Endocrine & metabolic: Decreased glucose tolerance, breast tumors, amenorrhea, alterations in frequency and flow of menses, increased triglycerides and LDL

Gastrointestinal: GI distress

Hepatic: Cholestatic jaundice

Miscellaneous: Intolerance to contact lenses, increased susceptibility to *Candida* infection

See tables.

Drug Interactions

Decreased effect of oral contraceptives with barbiturates, hydantoins - phenytoin, rifampin, antibiotics - penicillins, tetracyclines, griseofulvin

Increased toxicity of acetaminophen, anticoagulants, benzodiazepines, caffeine, corticosteroids, metoprolol, theophylline, tricyclic antidepressants

Drug Uptake

Ethinyl estradiol:

Absorption: Absorbed well from GI tract

Serum half-life, terminal: 5-14 hours

Pregnancy Risk Factor X

Pharmacological Effects of Progestins Used in Oral Contraceptives

	Progestin	Estrogen	Antiestrogen	Androgen
Norgestrel/levonorgestrel	+++	0	++	+++
Ethynodiol diacetate	++	+*	+*	+
Norethindrone acetate	+	+	+++	+
Norethindrone	+	+*	+*	+
Norethynodrel	+	+++	0	0

*Has estrogenic effect at low doses; may have antiestrogenic effect at higher doses.

+++ = pronounced effect

++ = moderate effect

+ = slight effect

0 = moderate effect

Achieving Proper Hormonal Balance in an Oral Contraceptive

Estrogen		Progestin	
Excess	**Deficiency**	**Excess**	**Deficiency**
Nausea, bloating	Early or midcycle	Increased appetite	Late breakthrough
Cervical mucorrhea,	breakthrough	Weight gain	bleeding
polyposis	bleeding	Tiredness, fatigue	Amenorrhea
Melasma	Increased spotting	Hypomenorrhea	Hypermenorrhea
Migraine headache	Hypomenorrhea	Acne, oily scalp*	
Breast fullness or		Hair loss,	
		hirsutism*	
tenderness		Depression	
Edema		Monilial vaginitis	
Hypertension		Breast regression	

*Result of androgenic activity of progestins.

Ethinyl Estradiol and Fluoxymesterone
(eth i nil es tra dye′ ole & floo ox i mes′ te rone)
Therapeutic Category Androgen; Estrogen Derivative
Synonyms Fluoxymesterone and Estradiol
Use Moderate to severe vasomotor symptoms of menopause, postpartum breast engorgement
Local Anesthetic/Vasoconstrictor Precautions No information available to require special precautions
Effects on Dental Treatment When prescribing antibiotics, patient must be warned to use supplemental methods of birth control if on oral contraceptives
Other Adverse Effects 1% to 10%:
Cardiovascular: Stroke, hypertension, thromboembolism, myocardial infarction, edema
Central nervous system: Depression, migraine, dizziness, anxiety, headache
Dermatologic: Chloasma, melasma, rash
Endocrine & metabolic: Decreased glucose tolerance, alterations in frequency and flow of menses, breast tenderness or enlargement
Gastrointestinal: Nausea, GI distress
Hepatic: Increased triglycerides and LDL, cholestatic jaundice
Miscellaneous: Increased susceptibility to *Candida* infection

Ethinyl Estradiol and Levonorgestrel
(eth′ in il es tra dye′ ole & lee′ voe nor jes trel)
Related Information
Endocrine Disorders & Pregnancy *on page 927*
Brand Names Levlen®; Levora®; Nordette®; Tri-Levlen®; Triphasil®
Canadian/Mexican Brand Names Microgynon® (Mexico); Nordet® (Mexico); Nordiol® (Mexico)
Therapeutic Category Contraceptive, Oral
Use Prevention of pregnancy; treatment of hypermenorrhea, endometriosis, female hypogonadism
Usual Dosage Adults: Female: Oral:
Contraception: 1 tablet daily, beginning on day 5 of menstrual cycle (first day of menstrual flow is day 1). With 20-tablet and 21-tablet packages, new dosing cycle begins 7 days after last tablet taken. With 28-tablet packages, dosage is 1 tablet daily without interruption; extra tablets are placebos or contain iron. If next menstrual period does not begin on schedule, rule out pregnancy before starting new dosing cycle. If menstrual period begins, start new dosing cycle 7 days after last tablet was taken. If all doses have been taken on schedule and one menstrual period is missed, continue dosing cycle. If two consecutive menstrual periods are missed, pregnancy test is required before new dosing cycle is started.
One dose missed: Take as soon as remembered or take 2 tablets next day
Two doses missed: Take 2 tablets as soon as remembered or 2 tablets next 2 days
Three doses missed: Begin new compact of tablets starting on day 1 of next cycle
Triphasic oral contraceptive (Tri-Levlen®, Triphasil®): 1 tablet/day in the sequence specified by the manufacturer
Mechanism of Action Combination oral contraceptives inhibit ovulation via a negative feedback mechanism on the hypothalamus, which alters the normal pattern of gonadotropin secretion of a follicle-stimulating hormone (FSH) and
(Continued)

Ethinyl Estradiol and Levonorgestrel *(Continued)*

luteinizing hormone by the anterior pituitary. The follicular phase FSH and midcycle surge of gonadotropins are inhibited. In addition, oral contraceptives produce alterations in the genital tract, including changes in the cervical mucus, rendering it unfavorable for sperm penetration even if ovulation occurs. Changes in the endometrium may also occur, producing an unfavorable environment for nidation. Oral contraceptive drugs may alter the tubal transport of the ova through the fallopian tubes. Progestational agents may also alter sperm fertility.

Local Anesthetic/Vasoconstrictor Precautions No information available to require special precautions

Effects on Dental Treatment When prescribing antibiotics, patient must be warned to use supplemental methods of birth control if on oral contraceptives

Other Adverse Effects

>10%:
Cardiovascular: Peripheral edema
Endocrine & metabolic: Enlargement of breasts, breast tenderness, bloating
Gastrointestinal: Nausea, anorexia

1% to 10%:
Central nervous system: Headache
Endocrine & metabolic: Increased libido
Gastrointestinal: Vomiting, diarrhea

<1%:
Cardiovascular: Hypertension, thromboembolism, stroke, myocardial infarction, edema
Central nervous system: Depression, dizziness, anxiety
Dermatologic: Chloasma, melasma, rash
Endocrine & metabolic: Decreased glucose tolerance, breast tumors, amenorrhea, alterations in frequency and flow of menses, increased triglycerides and LDL
Gastrointestinal: GI distress
Hepatic: Cholestatic jaundice
Miscellaneous: Intolerance to contact lenses, increased susceptibility to *Candida* infection

See tables.

Achieving Proper Hormonal Balance in an Oral Contraceptive

Estrogen		Progestin	
Excess	**Deficiency**	**Excess**	**Deficiency**
Nausea, bloating	Early or midcycle breakthrough bleeding	Increased appetite	Late breakthrough bleeding
Cervical mucorrhea, polyposis		Weight gain	
		Tiredness, fatigue	Amenorrhea
Melasma	Increased spotting	Hypomenorrhea	Hypermenorrhea
Migraine headache	Hypomenorrhea	Acne, oily scalp*	
Breast fullness or		Hair loss, hirsutism*	
tenderness		Depression	
Edema		Monilial vaginitis	
Hypertension		Breast regression	

*Result of androgenic activity of progestins.

Pharmacological Effects of Progestins Used in Oral Contraceptives

	Progestin	Estrogen	Antiestrogen	Androgen
Norgestrel/levonorgestrel	+++	0	++	+++
Ethynodiol diacetate	++	+*	+*	+
Norethindrone acetate	+	+	+++	+
Norethindrone	+	+*	+*	+
Norethynodrel	+	+++	0	0

*Has estrogenic effect at low doses; may have antiestrogenic effect at higher doses.

+++ = pronounced effect

++ = moderate effect

+ = slight effect

0 = moderate effect

Drug Interactions
Decreased effect of oral contraceptives with barbiturates, hydantoins - phenytoin, rifampin, antibiotics - penicillins, tetracyclines, griseofulvin
Increased toxicity of acetaminophen, anticoagulants, benzodiazepines, caffeine, corticosteroids, metoprolol, theophylline, tricyclic antidepressants

Drug Uptake
Ethinyl estradiol:
Absorption: Absorbed well from GI tract
Levonorgestrel:
Time to peak: 0.5-2 hours
Serum half-life, terminal: 11-45 hours

Pregnancy Risk Factor X

Ethinyl Estradiol and Norethindrone
(eth′ in il es tra dye′ ole & nor eth in′ drone)

Related Information
Endocrine Disorders & Pregnancy *on page 927*

Brand Names Brevicon®; Genora® 0.5/35; Genora® 1/35; Jenest-28™; Loestrin®; Modicon™; N.E.E.® 1/35; Nelova™ 0.5/35E; Nelova™ 10/11; Norethin™ 1/35E; Norinyl® 1+35; Ortho-Novum™ 1/35; Ortho-Novum™ 7/7/7; Ortho-Novum™ 10/11; Ovcon® 35; Ovcon 50; Tri-Norinyl®

Canadian/Mexican Brand Names Synphasic® (Canada); Ortho®0.5/35 (Canada); Trinovum® (Mexico)

Therapeutic Category Contraceptive, Oral

Synonyms Etinilestradiol and Noretindrona (Mexico)

Use Prevention of pregnancy; treatment of hypermenorrhea, endometriosis, female hypogonadism

Usual Dosage Adults: Female: Oral:
For 21-tablet cycle packs, with 21 active tablets (28-day packs have 21 active tablets and 7 inert tablets): Take 1 tablet daily starting on the fifth day of menstrual cycle, with day 1 being the first day of menstruation; begin taking a new cycle pack on the eighth day after taking the last tablet from the previous pack

With 28-tablet packages, dosage is 1 tablet daily without interruption; extra tablets are placebos or contain iron. If next menstrual period does not begin on schedule, rule out pregnancy before starting new dosing cycle. If menstrual period begins, start new dosing cycle 7 days after last tablet was taken. If all doses have been taken on schedule and one menstrual period is missed, continue dosing cycle. If two consecutive menstrual periods are missed, pregnancy test is required before new dosing cycle is started.

One dose missed: Take as soon as remembered or take 2 tablets next day
Two doses missed: Take 2 tablets as soon as remembered or 2 tablets next 2 days

Three doses missed: Begin new compact of tablets starting on day 1 of next cycle

Biphasic oral contraceptive (Jenest™-28, Ortho-Novum™ 10/11, Nelova™ 10/11): 1 color tablet/day for 10 days, then next color tablet for 11 days

Triphasic oral contraceptive (Ortho-Novum™ 7/7/7, Tri-Norinyl®, Triphasil®): 1 tablet/day in the sequence specified by the manufacturer

Mechanism of Action Combination oral contraceptives inhibit ovulation via a negative feedback mechanism on the hypothalamus, which alters the normal pattern of gonadotropin secretion of a follicle-stimulating hormone (FSH) and luteinizing hormone by the anterior pituitary. The follicular phase FSH and midcycle surge of gonadotropins are inhibited. In addition, oral contraceptives produce alterations in the genital tract, including changes in the cervical mucus, rendering it unfavorable for sperm penetration even if ovulation occurs. Changes in the endometrium may also occur, producing an unfavorable environment for nidation. Oral contraceptive drugs may alter the tubal transport of the ova through the fallopian tubes. Progestational agents may also alter sperm fertility.

Local Anesthetic/Vasoconstrictor Precautions No information available to require special precautions

Effects on Dental Treatment When prescribing antibiotics, patient must be warned to use supplemental methods of birth control if on oral contraceptives

Other Adverse Effects
>10%:
Cardiovascular: Peripheral edema
Endocrine & metabolic: Enlargement of breasts, breast tenderness, bloating
Gastrointestinal: Nausea, anorexia
1% to 10%:
Central nervous system: Headache
(Continued)

Ethinyl Estradiol and Norethindrone *(Continued)*

Endocrine & metabolic: Increased libido

Gastrointestinal: Vomiting, diarrhea

<1%:

Cardiovascular: Hypertension, thromboembolism, stroke, myocardial infarction, edema

Central nervous system: Depression, dizziness, anxiety

Dermatologic: Chloasma, melasma, rash

Endocrine & metabolic: Decreased glucose tolerance, breast tumors, amenorrhea, alterations in frequency and flow of menses, increased triglycerides and LDL

Gastrointestinal: GI distress

Hepatic: Cholestatic jaundice

Miscellaneous: Intolerance to contact lenses, increased susceptibility to *Candida* infection

See tables.

Achieving Proper Hormonal Balance in an Oral Contraceptive

Estrogen		Progestin	
Excess	**Deficiency**	**Excess**	**Deficiency**
Nausea, bloating	Early or midcycle	Increased appetite	Late breakthrough
Cervical mucorrhea,	breakthrough	Weight gain	bleeding
polyposis	bleeding	Tiredness, fatigue	Amenorrhea
Melasma	Increased spotting	Hypomenorrhea	Hypermenorrhea
Migraine headache	Hypomenorrhea	Acne, oily scalp*	
Breast fullness or		Hair loss, hirsutism*	
tenderness		Depression	
Edema		Monilial vaginitis	
Hypertension		Breast regression	

*Result of androgenic activity of progestins.

Pharmacological Effects of Progestins Used in Oral Contraceptives

	Progestin	Estrogen	Antiestrogen	Androgen
Norgestrel/levonorgestrel	+++	0	++	+++
Ethynodiol diacetate	++	+*	+*	+
Norethindrone acetate	+	+	+++	+
Norethindrone	+	+*	+*	+
Norethynodrel	+	+++	0	0

*Has estrogenic effect at low doses; may have antiestrogenic effect at higher doses.

+++ = pronounced effect

++ = moderate effect

+ = slight effect

0 = moderate effect

Drug Interactions

Decreased effect of oral contraceptives with barbiturates, hydantoins - phenytoin, rifampin, antibiotics - penicillins, tetracyclines, griseofulvin

Increased toxicity of acetaminophen, anticoagulants, benzodiazepines, caffeine, corticosteroids, metoprolol, theophylline, tricyclic antidepressants

Drug Uptake

Ethinyl estradiol:

Absorption: Absorbed well from GI tract

Norethindrone:

Time to peak: Oral: 0.5-4 hours

Serum half-life, terminal: 5-14 hours

Pregnancy Risk Factor X

Ethinyl Estradiol and Norgestimate

(eth' in il es tra dye' ole & nor jes' ti mate)

Brand Names Ortho-Cyclen®; Ortho Tri-Cyclen®

Therapeutic Category Contraceptive, Oral

Synonyms Norgestimate and Ethinyl Estradiol

Use Prevention of pregnancy

Local Anesthetic/Vasoconstrictor Precautions No information available to require special precautions

Effects on Dental Treatment When prescribing antibiotics, patient must be warned to use supplemental methods of birth control if on oral contraceptives

Ethinyl Estradiol and Norgestrel

(eth' in il es tra dye' ole & nor jes' trel)

Brand Names Lo/Ovral®; Ovral®

Therapeutic Category Contraceptive, Oral

Use Prevention of pregnancy; treatment of hypermenorrhea, endometriosis, female hypogonadism; postcoital contraception

Usual Dosage Adults: Female: Oral: Contraception: 1 tablet daily, beginning on day 5 of menstrual cycle (first day of menstrual flow is day 1). With 20-tablet and 21-tablet packages, new dosing cycle begins 7 days after last tablet taken; with 28-tablet packages, dosage is 1 tablet daily without interruption; extra tablets are placebos or contain iron. If next menstrual period does not begin on schedule, rule out pregnancy before starting new dosing cycle; if menstrual period begins, start new dosing cycle 7 days after last tablet was taken; if all doses have been taken on schedule and one menstrual period is missed, continue dosing cycle; if two consecutive menstrual periods are missed, pregnancy test is required before new dosing cycle is started.

One dose missed: Take as soon as remembered or take 2 tablets next day

Two doses missed: Take 2 tablets as soon as remembered or 2 tablets next 2 days

Three doses missed: Begin new compact of tablets starting on day 1 of next cycle

"Morning After" pill: Postcoital contraception (Ovral®): 2 tablets at initial visit and 2 tablets 12 hours later

Mechanism of Action Combination oral contraceptives inhibit ovulation via a negative feedback mechanism on the hypothalamus, which alters the normal pattern of gonadotropin secretion of a follicle-stimulating hormone (FSH) and luteinizing hormone by the anterior pituitary. The follicular phase FSH and midcycle surge of gonadotropins are inhibited. In addition, oral contraceptives produce alterations in the genital tract, including changes in the cervical mucus, rendering it unfavorable for sperm penetration even if ovulation occurs. Changes in the endometrium may also occur, producing an unfavorable environment for nidation. Oral contraceptive drugs may alter the tubal transport of the ova through the fallopian tubes. Progestational agents may also alter sperm fertility.

Local Anesthetic/Vasoconstrictor Precautions No information available to require special precautions

Effects on Dental Treatment When prescribing antibiotics, patient must be warned to use supplemental methods of birth control if on oral contraceptives

Other Adverse Effects

>10%:
Cardiovascular: Peripheral edema
Endocrine & metabolic: Enlargement of breasts, breast tenderness, bloating
Gastrointestinal: Nausea, anorexia

1% to 10%:
Central nervous system: Headache
Endocrine & metabolic: Increased libido
Gastrointestinal: Vomiting, diarrhea

<1%:
Cardiovascular: Hypertension, thromboembolism, stroke, myocardial infarction, edema
Central nervous system: Depression, dizziness, anxiety
Dermatologic: Chloasma, melasma, rash
Endocrine & metabolic: Decreased glucose tolerance, breast tumors, amenorrhea, alterations in frequency and flow of menses, increased triglycerides and LDL
Gastrointestinal: GI distress
Hepatic: Cholestatic jaundice
Miscellaneous: Intolerance to contact lenses, increased susceptibility to *Candida* infection

See tables.

(Continued)

Ethinyl Estradiol and Norgestrel *(Continued)*
Achieving Proper Hormonal Balance in an Oral Contraceptive

Estrogen		Progestin	
Excess	**Deficiency**	**Excess**	**Deficiency**
Nausea, bloating	Early or midcycle breakthrough bleeding	Increased appetite	Late breakthrough bleeding
Cervical mucorrhea, polyposis		Weight gain	Amenorrhea
Melasma	Increased spotting	Tiredness, fatigue	Hypermenorrhea
Migraine headache	Hypomenorrhea	Hypomenorrhea	
Breast fullness or		Acne, oily scalp*	
tenderness		Hair loss, hirsutism*	
Edema		Depression	
Hypertension		Monilial vaginitis	
		Breast regression	

*Result of androgenic activity of progestins.

Pharmacological Effects of Progestins Used in Oral Contraceptives

	Progestin	Estrogen	Antiestrogen	Androgen
Norgestrel/levonorgestrel	+++	0	++	+++
Ethynodiol diacetate	++	+*	+*	+
Norethindrone acetate	+	+	+++	+
Norethindrone	+	+*	+*	+
Norethynodrel	+	+++	0	0

*Has estrogenic effect at low doses; may have antiestrogenic effect at higher doses.

+++ = pronounced effect   + = slight effect

++ = moderate effect   0 = moderate effect

Drug Interactions
Decreased effect of oral contraceptives with barbiturates, hydantoins - phenytoin, rifampin, antibiotics - penicillins, tetracyclines, griseofulvin

Increased toxicity of acetaminophen, anticoagulants, benzodiazepines, caffeine, corticosteroids, metoprolol, theophylline, tricyclic antidepressants

Drug Uptake
Ethinyl estradiol:
  Absorption: Absorbed well from GI tract
Norgestrel:
  Time to peak: 0.5-2 hours
  Serum half-life, terminal: 11-45 hours

Pregnancy Risk Factor X

Ethionamide (e thye on am' ide)
Related Information
Nonviral Infectious Diseases *on page 932*

Brand Names Trecator®-SC

Therapeutic Category Antitubercular Agent

Use Treatment of tuberculosis and other mycobacterial diseases, in conjunction with other antituberculosis agents, when first-line agents have failed or resistance has been demonstrated

Usual Dosage Oral:
Children: 15-20 mg/kg/day in 2 divided doses, not to exceed 1 g/day
Adults: 500-1000 mg/day in 1-3 divided doses

Mechanism of Action Inhibits peptide synthesis

Local Anesthetic/Vasoconstrictor Precautions No information available to require special precautions

Effects on Dental Treatment No effects or complications reported

Other Adverse Effects
>10%: Gastrointestinal: Anorexia, nausea, vomiting
1% to 10%:
  Cardiovascular: Postural hypotension
  Central nervous system: Peripheral neuritis, psychiatric disturbances
  Gastrointestinal: Metallic taste
  Hepatic: Hepatitis, jaundice
<1%:
  Central nervous system: Drowsiness, dizziness, seizures, headache
  Dermatologic: Rash
  Endocrine & metabolic: Hypothyroidism or goiter, hypoglycemia, gynecomastia

Gastrointestinal: Stomatitis, abdominal pain, diarrhea
Hematologic: Thrombocytopenia
Ocular: Optic neuritis
Drug Interactions No data reported
Drug Uptake
Serum half-life: 2-3 hours
Time to peak serum concentration: Oral: Within 3 hours
Pregnancy Risk Factor C

Ethmozine® *see Moricizine Hydrochloride on page 589*

Ethopropazine Hydrochloride
(eth oh proe′ pa zeen hye droe klor′ ide)
Brand Names Parsidol®
Therapeutic Category Anti-Parkinson's Agent
Use Treatment of Parkinsonism, drug induced extrapyramidal reactions, and congenital athetosis
Local Anesthetic/Vasoconstrictor Precautions No information available to require special precautions
Effects on Dental Treatment Dry mouth
Other Adverse Effects
>10%:
Gastrointestinal: Constipation
Miscellaneous: Decreased sweating; dry mouth, nose, throat, or skin
1% to 10%:
Endocrine & metabolic: Decreased flow of breast milk
Gastrointestinal: Difficulty in swallowing
Ocular: Increased sensitivity to light
<1%:
Dermatologic: Skin rash
Cardiovascular: Orthostatic hypotension, ventricular fibrillation, tachycardia, palpitations
Central nervous system: Confusion, drowsiness, headache, loss of memory, tiredness, ataxia
Gastrointestinal: Bloated feeling, nausea, vomiting
Genitourinary: Difficult urination
Ocular: Increased intraocular pain, blurred vision
Neuromuscular & skeletal: Weakness
Comments Prominent anticholinergic effects; less effective than the synthetic anticholinergic agents; high doses are relatively well tolerated in adults

Ethosuximide (eth oh sux′ i mide)
Brand Names Zarontin®
Therapeutic Category Anticonvulsant, Succinimide
Use Management of absence (petit mal) seizures, myoclonic seizures, and akinetic epilepsy; considered to be drug of choice for simple absence seizures
Usual Dosage Oral:
Children 3-6 years: Initial: 250 mg/day (or 15 mg/kg/day) in 2 divided doses; increase every 4-7 days; usual maintenance dose: 15-40 mg/kg/day in 2 divided doses
Children >6 years and Adults: Initial: 250 mg twice daily; increase by 250 mg as needed every 4-7 days up to 1.5 g/day in 2 divided doses; usual maintenance dose: 20-40 mg/kg/day in 2 divided doses
Mechanism of Action Increases the seizure threshold and suppresses paroxysmal spike-and-wave pattern in absence seizures; depresses nerve transmission in the motor cortex
Local Anesthetic/Vasoconstrictor Precautions No information available to require special precautions
Effects on Dental Treatment No effects or complications reported
Other Adverse Effects
>10%:
Central nervous system: Ataxia, drowsiness, sedation, dizziness, lethargy, euphoria, hallucinations, insomnia, agitation, behavioral changes, headache
Dermatologic: Stevens-Johnson syndrome
Gastrointestinal: Weight loss
Gastrointestinal: Nausea, vomiting, anorexia, abdominal pain
Miscellaneous: Hiccups, SLE
1% to 10%: Central nervous system: Aggressiveness, mental depression, nightmares, weakness, tiredness
(Continued)

343

Ethosuximide *(Continued)*

<1%:
  Central nervous system: Paranoid psychosis
  Dermatologic: Rashes, urticaria, exfoliative dermatitis
  Hematologic: Leukopenia, aplastic anemia, thrombocytopenia, agranulocytosis, pancytopenia

Drug Interactions
Decreased effect: Phenytoin, carbamazepine, primidone, phenobarbital may increase the hepatic metabolism of ethosuximide
Increased toxicity: Isoniazid may inhibit hepatic metabolism with a resultant increase in ethosuximide serum concentrations

Drug Uptake
Time to peak serum concentration:
  Capsule: Within 2-4 hours
  Syrup: <2-4 hours
Serum half-life:
  Children: 30 hours
  Adults: 50-60 hours

Pregnancy Risk Factor C

Ethotoin (eth´ oh toyn)

Brand Names Peganone®
Therapeutic Category Anticonvulsant, Hydantoin
Synonyms Ethylphenylhydantoin
Use Generalized tonic-clonic or complex-partial seizures
Local Anesthetic/Vasoconstrictor Precautions No information available to require special precautions
Effects on Dental Treatment No effects or complications reported
Other Adverse Effects
>10%:
  Central nervous system: Psychiatric changes, slurred speech, drowsiness
  Gastrointestinal: Constipation, nausea, vomiting, dizziness
  Neuromuscular & skeletal: Trembling
1% to 10%:
  Central nervous system: Drowsiness, headache, insomnia
  Dermatologic: Skin rash
  Gastrointestinal: Anorexia, weight loss
  Hematologic: Leukopenia
  Hepatic: Hepatitis
  Renal: Increase in serum creatinine
<1%:
  Cardiovascular: Hypotension, bradycardia, cardiac arrhythmias, cardiovascular collapse
  Central nervous system: Confusion, fever, ataxia
  Dermatologic: Stevens-Johnson syndrome or SLE-like syndrome
  Gastrointestinal: Gingival hyperplasia
  Hematologic: Blood dyscrasias, venous irritation and pain
  Local: Thrombophlebitis
  Neuromuscular & skeletal: Paresthesia, peripheral neuropathy
  Ocular: Diplopia, nystagmus, blurred vision
  Miscellaneous: Lymphadenopathy

Ethyl Chloride (eth´ il klor´ ide)

Therapeutic Category Local Anesthetic, Topical
Synonyms Chloroethane
Use Local anesthetic in minor operative procedures and to relieve pain caused by insect stings and burns, and irritation caused by myofascial and visceral pain syndromes
Local Anesthetic/Vasoconstrictor Precautions No information available to require special precautions
Effects on Dental Treatment No effects or complications reported
Other Adverse Effects 1% to 10%: Mucous membrane irritation, freezing may alter skin pigment
Comments Spray for a few seconds to the point of frost formation when the tissue becomes white; avoid prolonged spraying of skin beyond this point

Ethyl Chloride and Dichlorotetrafluoroethane
(eth´ il klor´ ide & dye klor oh te tra floo or oh eth´ ane)
Brand Names Fluro-Ethyl® Aerosol
Therapeutic Category Local Anesthetic, Topical

Synonyms Dichlorotetrafluoroethane and Ethyl Chloride

Use Topical refrigerant anesthetic to control pain associated with minor surgical procedures, dermabrasion, injections, contusions, and minor strains

Local Anesthetic/Vasoconstrictor Precautions No information available to require special precautions

Effects on Dental Treatment No effects or complications reported

Ethylnorepinephrine Hydrochloride
(eth il nor ep i nef′ rin hye droe klor′ ide)

Brand Names Bronkephrine® Injection

Therapeutic Category Adrenergic Agonist Agent; Bronchodilator

Use Bronchial asthma and reversible bronchospasm

Local Anesthetic/Vasoconstrictor Precautions No information available to require special precautions

Effects on Dental Treatment No effects or complications reported

Other Adverse Effects

>10%:
Cardiovascular: Tachycardia, pounding heart beat
Central nervous system: Nervousness
Gastrointestinal: Nausea
Neuromuscular & skeletal: Trembling, tremor

1% to 10%:
Cardiovascular: Flushing of face, hypertension or hypotension
Central nervous system: Dizziness, lightheadedness, drowsiness, headache, insomnia
Gastrointestinal: Dry mouth, heartburn, vomiting, unusual taste
Genitourinary: Difficult urination
Neuromuscular & skeletal: Muscle cramping, weakness
Respiratory: Coughing
Miscellaneous: Increased sweating

<1%:
Cardiovascular: Chest pain, vasoconstriction, hypertension, cerebral hemorrhage, cardiac arrhythmias, palpitations, angina, cardiac arrest, flushing, sudden death
Central nervous system: Fainting, fear, anxiety, restlessness, insomnia, confusion, irritability, psychotic states, headache
Endocrine & metabolic: Altered glucose metabolism
Gastrointestinal: Loss of appetite, hypersalivation
Genitourinary: Difficulty in micturition, urinary retention
Respiratory: Paradoxical bronchospasm, pulmonary edema, dyspnea
Miscellaneous: Unusual paleness, sweating, extravasation results in tissue necrosis

Ethylphenylhydantoin *see Ethotoin on previous page*

Etidocaine Hydrochloride (With Epinephrine)
(e ti′ doe kane hye droe klor′ ide) (with ep i nef′ rin)

Related Information

Oral Pain *on page 940*

Brand Names Duranest® with Epinephrine

Therapeutic Category Dental/Local Anesthetics; Local Anesthetic, Injectable

Use Dental: An amide-type local anesthetic for local infiltration anesthesia; injection near nerve trunks to produce nerve block

Usual Dosage In maxillary infiltration and/or inferior alveolar nerve block, initial dosages of 1.0-5.0 mL ($1/2$-$2^1/_2$ cartridges) of 1.5% with epinephrine 1:200,000 are usually effective. The maximum dose as a single injection should not exceed 400 mg with epinephrine 1:200,000.

Mechanism of Action Local anesthetics bind selectively to the intracellular surface of sodium channels to block influx of sodium into the axon. As a result, depolarization necessary for action potential propagation and subsequent nerve function is prevented. The block at the sodium channel is reversible. When drug diffuses away from the axon, sodium channel function is restored and nerve propagation is subsequently restored.

Epinephrine prolongs the duration of the anesthetic actions of etidocaine by causing vasoconstriction (alpha adrenergic receptor agonist) of the vasculature surrounding the nerve axons. This prevents the diffusion of lidocaine away from the nerves resulting in a longer retention in the axon.

Local Anesthetic/Vasoconstrictor Precautions No information available to require special precautions

Effects on Dental Treatment No effects or complications reported

(Continued)

Etidocaine Hydrochloride (With Epinephrine)
(Continued)

Other Adverse Effects Degree of adverse effects in the central nervous system and cardiovascular system are directly related to the blood levels of etidocaine. The effects below are more likely to occur after systemic administration rather than infiltration.

Cardiovascular: Myocardial effects include a decrease in contraction force as well as a decrease in electrical excitability and myocardial conduction rate resulting in bradycardia and reduction in cardiac output.

Central nervous system: High blood levels result in anxiety, restlessness, disorientation, confusion, dizziness, tremors and seizures. This is followed by depression of CNS resulting in drowsiness, unconsciousness and possible respiratory arrest. Nausea and vomiting may also occur. In some cases, symptoms of CNS stimulation may be absent and the primary CNS effects are drowsiness and unconsciousness.

Hypersensitivity reactions: Extremely rare, but may be manifest as dermatologic reactions and edema at injection site. Asthmatic syndromes have occurred. Patients may exhibit hypersensitivity to bisulfites contained in local anesthetic solution to prevent oxidation of epinephrine. In general, patients reacting to bisulfites have a history of asthma and their airways are hyperreactive to asthmatic syndrome

Psychogenic reactions: It is common to misinterpret psychogenic responses to local anesthetic injection as an allergic reaction. Intraoral injections are perceived by many patients as a stressful procedure in dentistry. Common symptoms to this stress are sweating, palpitations, hyperventilation, generalized pallor and a fainting feeling.

Oral manifestations: No data reported

Contraindications Hypersensitivity to local anesthetics of the amide-type

Warnings/Precautions Should be avoided in patients with uncontrolled hyperthyroidism. Should be used in minimal amounts in patients with significant cardiovascular problems (because of epinephrine component). Aspirate the syringe after tissue penetration and before injection to minimize chance of direct vascular injection.

Drug Interactions Due to epinephrine component, use with tricyclic antidepressants or MAO inhibitors could result in increased pressor response; use with nonselective beta-blockers (ie, propranolol) could result in serious hypertension and reflex bradycardia

Drug Uptake
Onset of action: Maxillary infiltration and inferior alveolar nerve block: 3-5 minutes
Duration after infiltration or nerve block: 5-10 hours
Serum half-life: 2.7 hours

Pregnancy Risk Factor B

Breast-feeding Considerations Usual infiltration doses of etidocaine hydrochloride with epinephrine given to nursing mothers has not been shown to affect the health of the nursing infant

Dosage Forms Etidocaine Hydrochloride 1.5% with epinephrine 1:200,000 cartridges, 1.8 mL, in 100 cartridge boxes

Dietary Considerations No data reported

Generic Available No

Selected Readings
Jastak JT and Yagiela JA, "Vasoconstrictors and Local Anesthesia: A Review and Rationale for Use," *J Am Dent Assoc*, 1983, 107(4):623-30.
MacKenzie TA and Young ER, "Local Anesthetic Update," *Anesth Prog*, 1993, 40(2):29-34.
Wynn RL, "Epinephrine Interactions With Beta-Blockers," *Gen Dent*, 1994, 42(1):16, 18.
Yagiela JA, "Local Anesthetics," *Anesth Prog*, 1991, 38(4-5):128-41.

Etidronate Disodium (e ti droe' nate dye sow' dee um)
Brand Names Didronel®

Therapeutic Category Antidote, Hypercalcemia; Biphosphonate Derivative

Use Symptomatic treatment of Paget's disease and heterotopic ossification due to spinal cord injury or after total hip replacement, hypercalcemia associated with malignancy

Usual Dosage Adults:
Paget's disease: Oral: 5 mg/kg/day given every day for no more than 6 months; may give 10 mg/kg/day for up to 3 months; daily dose may be divided if adverse GI effects occur
Heterotopic ossification with spinal cord injury: 20 mg/kg/day for 2 weeks, then 10 mg/kg/day for 10 weeks (this dosage has been used in children, however, treatment >1 year has been associated with a rachitic syndrome)

Hypercalcemia associated with malignancy:
  I.V. (Dilute dose in at least 250 mL NS): 7.5 mg/kg/day for 3 days; there
    should be at least 7 days between courses of treatment
  Oral: Start 20 mg/kg/day on the last day of infusion and continue for 30-90
    days

Mechanism of Action Decreases bone resorption by inhibiting osteocystic
osteolysis; decreases mineral release and matrix or collagen breakdown in
bone

Local Anesthetic/Vasoconstrictor Precautions No information available to
require special precautions

Effects on Dental Treatment No effects or complications reported

Other Adverse Effects
  1% to 10%:
    Central nervous system: Fever, convulsions
    Endocrine & metabolic: Hypophosphatemia, hypomagnesemia, fluid over-
      load
    Neuromuscular & skeletal: Bone pain
    Respiratory: Dyspnea
  <1%:
    Dermatologic: Angioedema, skin rash
    Gastrointestinal: Occult blood in stools, altered taste
    Hypersensitivity: Hypersensitivity reactions
    Renal: Nephrotoxicity
    Miscellaneous: Pain, increased risk of fractures

Drug Interactions No data reported

Drug Uptake
  Onset of therapeutic effect: Within 1-3 months of therapy
  Duration: Can persist for 12 months without continuous therapy
  Absorption: Dependent upon dose administered

Pregnancy Risk Factor B (oral)/C (parenteral)

Etinilestradiol and Noretindrona (Mexico) *see* Ethinyl Estradiol and Norethindrone *on page 339*

Etinilestradiol (Mexico) *see* Ethinyl Estradiol *on page 334*

Etodolac (ee toe doe′ lak)
  Related Information
    Nonsteroidal Anti-Inflammatory Agents, Comparative Dosages, and Pharma-
      cokinetics *on page 1021*
    Rheumatoid Arthritis, Osteoarthritis, and Joint Prostheses *on page 930*
  Brand Names Lodine®; Lodine® XL
  Canadian/Mexican Brand Names Lodine® Retard (Mexico)
  Therapeutic Category Analgesic, Non-narcotic; Nonsteroidal Anti-inflamma-
    tory Agent (NSAID)
  Use
    Dental: Management of postoperative pain
    Medical: Acute and long-term use in the management of signs and symptoms
      of osteoarthritis and management of pain, not approved for use in rheuma-
      toid arthritis
  Usual Dosage Adults: Oral: Single dose of 76-100 mg is comparable to the
    analgesic effect of aspirin 650 mg; in patients ≥65 years, no substantial differ-
    ences in the pharmacokinetics or side-effects profile were seen compared with
    the general population

    Acute pain: 200-400 mg every 6-8 hours, as needed, not to exceed total daily
      doses of 1200 mg; for patients weighing <60 kg, total daily dose should not
      exceed 20 mg/kg/day; extended release dose: one tablet daily
  Mechanism of Action Inhibits prostaglandin synthesis by decreasing the
    activity of the enzyme, cyclo-oxygenase, which results in decreased formation
    of prostaglandin precursors
  Local Anesthetic/Vasoconstrictor Precautions No information available to
    require special precautions
  Effects on Dental Treatment No effects or complications reported
  Other Adverse Effects >10%:
    Central nervous system: Dizziness
    Dermatologic: Rash
    Gastrointestinal: Abdominal cramps, heartburn, indigestion, nausea

    Oral manifestations: No data reported
  Contraindications Hypersensitivity to etodolac, aspirin, or other NSAIDs
    (Continued)

Etodolac *(Continued)*

Warnings/Precautions Use with caution in patients with congestive heart failure, hypertension, decreased renal or hepatic function, history of GI disease, or those receiving anticoagulants

Drug Interactions Decreased effect with aspirin; increased effect/toxicity with aspirin (GI irritation), probenecid; increased effect/toxicity of lithium (nausea), methotrexate, digoxin, cyclosporin (nephrotoxicity), warfarin (bleeding)

Drug Uptake
Onset of effect: 0.5 hours following single dose of 200-400 mg
Time to peak serum concentration: 1 hour
Duration of effect: 4-6 hours
Serum half-life: 7 hours

Pregnancy Risk Factor C

Breast-feeding Considerations No data reported

Dosage Forms
Capsule: 200 mg, 300 mg
Tablet: 400 mg
Tablet, extended release: 400 mg, 600 mg

Dietary Considerations May be taken with food to decrease GI distress

Generic Available No

Selected Readings
Brooks PM and Day RO, "Nonsteroidal Anti-inflammatory Drugs-Differences and Similarities," *N Engl J Med*, 1991, 324(24):1716-25.

Etoposide (e toe poe' side)

Brand Names VePesid®

Canadian/Mexican Brand Names Etopos® (Mexico); Medsaposide® (Mexico); Serozide® (Mexico)

Therapeutic Category Antineoplastic Agent, Mitotic Inhibitor

Use Treatment of lymphomas, ANLL, lung, testicular, bladder, and prostate carcinoma, hepatoma, rhabdomyosarcoma, uterine carcinoma, neuroblastoma, mycosis fungoides, Kaposi's sarcoma, histiocytosis, gestational trophoblastic disease, Ewing's sarcoma, Wilms' tumor, and brain tumors

Usual Dosage Refer to individual protocols
Oral: Twice the I.V. dose rounded to the nearest 50 mg given once daily if total dose ≤400 mg or in divided doses if >400 mg

Children: I.V.: 60-120 mg/m^2/day for 3-5 days every 3-6 weeks
AML:
Remission induction: 150 mg/m^2/day for 2-3 days for 2-3 cycles
Intensification or consolidation: 250 mg/m^2/day for 3 days, courses 2-5
Conditioning regimen for allogeneic BMT: 60 mg/kg/dose as a single dose

Adults:
Small cell lung cancer:
Oral: Twice the I.V. dose rounded to the nearest 50 mg given once daily if
I.V.: 35 mg/m^2/day for 4 days or 50 mg/m^2/day for 5 days every 3-4 weeks total dose ≤400 mg/day or in divided doses if >400 mg/day
IVPB: 200-250 mg/m^2 repeated every 7 weeks
Continuous intravenous infusion: 500 mg/m^2 over 24 hours every 3 weeks
Testicular cancer:
IVPB: 50-100 mg/m^2/day for 5 days repeated every 3-4 weeks
I.V.: 100 mg/m^2 every other day for 3 doses repeated every 3-4 weeks
BMT/relapsed leukemia: I.V.: 2.4-3.5 g/m^2 or 25-70 mg/kg administered over 4-36 hours

Mechanism of Action Inhibits mitotic activity; inhibits cells from entering prophase; inhibits DNA synthesis. Initially thought to be mitotic inhibitors similar to podophyllotoxin, but actually have no effect on microtubule assembly. However, later shown to induce DNA strand breakage and inhibition of topoisomerase II (an enzyme which breaks and repairs DNA); etoposide acts in late S or early G2 phases.

Local Anesthetic/Vasoconstrictor Precautions No information available to require special precautions

Effects on Dental Treatment No effects or complications reported

Other Adverse Effects
>10%:
Gastrointestinal: Occasional diarrhea and infrequent nausea and vomiting at standard doses; severe mucositis occurs with high (BMT) doses
Emetic potential: Moderately low (10% to 30%)
Miscellaneous: Alopecia (reversible), anorexia
Myelosuppressive: Principal dose-limiting toxicity of VP-16. White blood cell count nadir is 5-15 days after administration and is more frequent than

thrombocytopenia. Recovery is usually within 24-28 days and cumulative toxicity has not been noted with VP-16 as a single agent. No difference in toxicity is seen when VP-16 is administered over a 24-hour period or over 2 hours on 5 consecutive days.

    WBC: Mild to severe

    Platelets: Mild

    Onset (days): 10

    Nadir (days): 14-16

    Recovery (days): 21-28

1% to 10%:

    Central nervous system: Unusual tiredness

    Gastrointestinal: Stomatitis, diarrhea, abdominal pain, hepatitic dysfunction

    Hypotension: Related to drug infusion time; may be related to vehicle used in the I.V. preparation (polysorbate 80 plus polyethylene glycol). Best to administer the drug over 1 hour.

<1%:

    Cardiovascular: Tachycardia

    Central nervous system: Neurotoxicity, somnolence, fatigue, fever, headache, peripheral neuropathy

    Irritant chemotherapy; thrombophlebitis has been reported

    Hepatic: Toxic hepatitis (with high-dose therapy)

    Hypersensitivity: Reports of flushing or bronchospasm, which did not reoccur in one report if patients were pretreated with corticosteroids and antihistamines

Drug Interactions Increased toxicity:

    Warfarin may cause increases prothrombin time with concurrent use

    Methotrexate: Alteration of MTX transport has been found as a slow efflux of MTX and its polyglutamated form out of the cell, leading to intercellular accumulation of MTX

    Calcium antagonists: Increases the rate of VP-16-induced DNA damage and cytotoxicity *in vitro*

    Carmustine: Reports of frequent hepatic dysfunction with hyperbilirubinemia, ascites, and thrombocytopenia

    Cyclosporine: Additive cytotoxic effects on tumor cells

Drug Uptake

    Absorption: Oral: 32% to 57%

    Serum half-life: Terminal: 4-15 hours

        Children: 6-8 hours with normal renal and hepatic function

    Time to peak serum concentration: Oral: 1-1.5 hours

Pregnancy Risk Factor D

Etrafon® *see* Amitriptyline and Perphenazine *on page 50*

Etretinate (e tret′ i nate)

Brand Names Tegison®

Therapeutic Category Antipsoriatic Agent, Systemic

Use Treatment of severe recalcitrant psoriasis in patients intolerant of or unresponsive to standard therapies

Usual Dosage Adults: Oral: Individualized; Initial: 0.75-1 mg/kg/day in divided doses, increase by 0.25 mg/kg/day at weekly intervals up to 1.5 mg/kg/day; maintenance dose established after 8-10 weeks of therapy 0.5-0.75 mg/kg/day

Mechanism of Action Unknown; related to retinoic acid and retinol (vitamin A)

Local Anesthetic/Vasoconstrictor Precautions No information available to require special precautions

Effects on Dental Treatment No effects or complications reported

Other Adverse Effects

>10%:

    Central nervous system: Fatigue, headache, fever, epistaxis

    Dermatologic: Chapped lips, alopecia

    Endocrine & metabolic: Hypercholesterolemia, hypertriglyceridemia

    Gastrointestinal: Nausea, appetite change, dry mouth, sore tongue

    Neuromuscular & skeletal: Hyperostosis, Bone and joint pain

    Ocular: Eye irritation

1% to 10%:

    Cardiovascular: Edema

    Central nervous system: Dizziness, lethargy

    Hepatic: Hepatitis

    Neuromuscular & skeletal: Myalgia

    Ocular: Blurred vision

    Otic: Otitis externa

    Respiratory: Dyspnea

(Continued)

349

Etretinate *(Continued)*

<1%:

Cardiovascular: Syncope

Central nervous system: Amnesia, confusion, pseudotumor cerebri, depression

Dermatologic: Urticaria

Gastrointestinal: Mouth ulcers, diarrhea, constipation, flatulence, weight loss, gingival bleeding

Endocrine & metabolic: Gout

Local: Phlebitis

Neuromuscular & skeletal: Hyperkinesia, hypertonia

Ocular: Photophobia

Otic: Ear infection

Renal: Polyuria, dysuria, kidney stones

Miscellaneous: Runny nose

Drug Interactions

Increased effect: Milk increases absorption of etretinate

Increased toxicity: Additive toxicity with vitamin A

Drug Uptake

Absorption: Oral: Absorbed from small intestine; absorption enhanced when coadministered with whole milk or a high lipid meal (highly lipophilic)

Serum half-life: 4-8 days (with multiple doses)

Pregnancy Risk Factor X

ETS-2%® Topical *see* Erythromycin, Topical *on page 324*

Eudal-SR® *see* Guaifenesin and Pseudoephedrine *on page 409*

Eulexin® *see* Flutamide *on page 382*

Eurax® *see* Crotamiton *on page 236*

Euthroid® *see* Liotrix *on page 505*

Eutron® *see* Methyclothiazide and Pargyline *on page 566*

Evac-Q-Mag® [OTC] *see* Magnesium Citrate *on page 521*

Evac-U-Gen® [OTC] *see* Phenolphthalein *on page 682*

Evac-U-Lax® [OTC] *see* Phenolphthalein *on page 682*

Evalose® *see* Lactulose *on page 488*

Everone® *see* Testosterone *on page 825*

E-Vista® *see* Hydroxyzine *on page 443*

E-Vitamin® [OTC] *see* Vitamin E *on page 900*

Excedrin®, Extra Strength [OTC] *see* Acetaminophen, Aspirin, and Caffeine *on page 17*

Excedrin® IB [OTC] *see* Ibuprofen *on page 447*

Excedrin® P.M. [OTC] *see* Acetaminophen and Diphenhydramine *on page 16*

Exelderm® *see* Sulconazole Nitrate *on page 806*

Exidine® Scrub [OTC] *see* Chlorhexidine Gluconate *on page 184*

Ex-Lax® [OTC] *see* Phenolphthalein *on page 682*

Ex-Lax®, Extra Gentle Pills [OTC] *see* Docusate and Phenolphthalein *on page 295*

Exna® *see* Benzthiazide *on page 105*

Exosurf® Neonatal™ *see* Colfosceril Palmitate *on page 230*

Exsel® *see* Selenium Sulfide *on page 785*

Extendryl® SR *see* Chlorpheniramine, Phenylephrine, and Methscopolamine *on page 193*

Extra Action Cough Syrup [OTC] *see* Guaifenesin and Dextromethorphan *on page 408*

Eye-Lube-A® Solution [OTC] *see* Artificial Tears *on page 75*

Eye-Sed® [OTC] *see* Zinc Supplements *on page 909*

Eye-Zine® [OTC] *see* Tetrahydrozoline Hydrochloride *on page 831*

Ezide® *see* Hydrochlorothiazide *on page 430*

Factor IX Complex (Human) *(fak' ter nyne kom' pleks hyu' min)*

Brand Names AlphaNine®; Konȳne® 80; Mononine®; Profilnine® Heat-Treated; Proplex® T

Therapeutic Category Antihemophilic Agent; Blood Product Derivative

Use To control bleeding in patients with Factor IX deficiency (Hemophilia B or Christmas Disease); prevention/control of bleeding in hemophilia A patients with inhibitors to factor VIII; Proplex® T is indicated to prevent or control bleeding due to factor VII deficiency

Usual Dosage Children and Adults: Dosage is expressed in units of factor IX activity and must be individualized. I.V. only:

Factor VII deficiency: Highly individualized

0.5 unit/kg x body weight (kg) x desired increase (%)

For example, for a 70 kg adult to increase level by 25%:

0.5 unit/kg x 70 kg x 25 = 875 units

Factor IX deficiency: Highly individualized

1 unit/kg x body weight (in kg) x desired increase (%)

For example, to increase the level by 25% in a 70 kg adult:

1 unit x 70 kg x 25 = 1,750 units

Formula for units required to raise blood level %:

Total blood volume (mL blood/kg) = 70 mL/kg (adults), 80 mL/kg (children)

Plasma volume = total blood volume (mL) x [1 - Hct (in decimals)]

For example, for a 70 kg adult with a Hct = 40%: Plasma volume = [70 kg x 70 mL/kg] x [1 - 0.4] = 2940 mL

To calculate number of units needed to increase level to desired range (highly individualized and dependent on patient's condition):

Number of units = desired level increase [desired level - actual level] x plasma volume (in mL)

For example, for a 100% level in the above patient who has an actual level of 20%: Number of units needed = [1 (for a 100% level) - 0.2] x 2940 mL = 2,352 units

As a general rule, the level of factor IX required for treatment of different conditions is shown in the table.

	Minor Spontaneous Hemorrhage, Prophylaxis	Major Trauma or Surgery
Desired levels of factor IX for hemostasis	15%-25%	25%-50%
Initial loading dose to achieve desired level	<20-30 units/kg	<75 units/kg
Frequency of dosing	Once; repeated in 24 h if necessary	q18-30h, depending on half-life and measured factor IX levels
Duration of treatment	Once; repeated if necessary	Up to 10 days, depending upon nature of insult

Factor VIII inhibitor patients: 75 units/kg/dose; may be given every 6-12 hours

Anticoagulant overdosage: I.V.: 15 units/kg

Mechanism of Action Replaces deficient clotting factor including factor X; hemophilia B, or Christmas disease, is an X-linked recessively inherited disorder of blood coagulation characterized by insufficient or abnormal synthesis of the clotting protein factor IX. Factor IX is a vitamin K-dependent coagulation factor which is synthesized in the liver. Factor IX is activated by factor XIa in the intrinsic coagulation pathway. Activated factor IX (IXa), in combination with factor VII:C activates factor X to Xa, resulting ultimately in the conversion of prothrombin to thrombin and the formation of a fibrin clot. The infusion of exogenous factor IX to replace the deficiency present in hemophilia B temporarily restores hemostasis.

Local Anesthetic/Vasoconstrictor Precautions No information available to require special precautions

Effects on Dental Treatment No effects or complications reported

Other Adverse Effects

1% to 10%: Following rapid administration: Transient fever, chills, headache, flushing, tingling

<1%: DIC, thrombosis following high dosages in hemophilia B patients, somnolence, urticaria, tightness in chest and neck

Drug Uptake

Serum half-life:

VII component: Cleared rapidly from the serum in two phases; initial: 4-6 hours; terminal: 22.5 hours

IX component: 24 hours

Pregnancy Risk Factor C

Comments Factor VII and IX units are listed per vial and per lot to lot variation

Factor VIII see Antihemophilic Factor (Human) on page 68

Factor VIII Recombinant see Antihemophilic Factor (Recombinant) on page 70

Famciclovir (fam sye' kloe veer)

Related Information

Systemic Viral Diseases *on page 934*

Brand Names Famvir™

Therapeutic Category Antiviral Agent, Oral

Use Management of acute herpes zoster (shingles)

Usual Dosage Adults: Oral:

Acute herpes zoster: 500 mg every 8 hours for 7 days

Recurrent herpes simplex in immunocompetent patients: 125 mg twice daily for 5 days

Mechanism of Action After undergoing rapid biotransformation to the active compound, penciclovir, famciclovir is phosphorylated by viral thymidine kinase in HSV-1, HSV-2, and VZV-infected cells to a monophosphate form; this is then converted to penciclovir triphosphate and competes with deoxyguanosine triphosphate to inhibit HSV-2 polymerase (ie, herpes viral DNA synthesis/replication is selectively inhibited)

Local Anesthetic/Vasoconstrictor Precautions No information available to require special precautions

Effects on Dental Treatment No effects or complications reported

Other Adverse Effects

>10%:

Central nervous system: Headache

Gastrointestinal: Nausea

1% to 10%:

Central nervous system: Fatigue, fever, dizziness, somnolence

Gastrointestinal: Diarrhea, vomiting, constipation, anorexia, abdominal pain

Neuromuscular & skeletal: Rigors, paresthesia

Drug Interactions No data reported

Drug Uptake

Absorption: Food decreases the maximum peak concentration and delays the time to peak; AUC remains the same

Serum half-life: Penciclovir: 2-3 hours (10, 20, and 7 hours in HSV-1, HSV-2, and VZV-infected cells); linearly decreased with reductions in renal failure

Pregnancy Risk Factor B

Dosage Forms Tablet: 500 mg

Dietary Considerations May be taken with food or on an empty stomach

Generic Available No

Famotidina (Mexico) *see* Famotidine *on this page*

Famotidine (fa moe' ti deen)

Brand Names Pepcid® [OTC]

Canadian/Mexican Brand Names Apo-Famotidine® (Canada); Novo-Famotidine® (Canada); Nu-Famotidine® (Canada); Durater® (Mexico); Famoxal® (Mexico); Farmotex® (Mexico); Pepcidine® (Mexico); Sigafam® (Mexico)

Therapeutic Category Histamine-2 Antagonist

Synonyms Famotidina (Mexico)

Use Therapy and treatment of duodenal ulcer, gastric ulcer, control gastric pH in critically ill patients, symptomatic relief in gastritis, gastroesophageal reflux, active benign ulcer, and pathological hypersecretory conditions

Usual Dosage

Children: Oral, I.V.: Doses of 1-2 mg/kg/day have been used; maximum dose: 40 mg

Adults:

Oral:

Duodenal ulcer, gastric ulcer: 40 mg/day at bedtime for 4-8 weeks

Hypersecretory conditions: Initial: 20 mg every 6 hours, may increase up to 160 mg every 6 hours

GERD: 20 mg twice daily for 6 weeks

I.V.: 20 mg every 12 hours

Mechanism of Action Competitive inhibition of histamine at H_2 receptors of the gastric parietal cells, which inhibits gastric acid secretion

Local Anesthetic/Vasoconstrictor Precautions No information available to require special precautions

Effects on Dental Treatment No effects or complications reported

Other Adverse Effects

1% to 10%:

Central nervous system: Dizziness, headache

Gastrointestinal: Constipation, diarrhea

<1%:
 Cardiovascular: Bradycardia, tachycardia, palpitations, hypertension
 Central nervous system: Fever, dizziness, weakness, fatigue, seizures, insomnia, drowsiness
 Dermatologic: Acne, pruritus, urticaria, dry skin
 Gastrointestinal: Abdominal discomfort, flatulence, belching, anorexia
 Hematologic: Agranulocytosis, neutropenia, thrombocytopenia
 Hepatic: Increases in AST, ALT
 Neuromuscular & skeletal: Paresthesia
 Renal: Increases in BUN, creatinine, proteinuria
 Respiratory: Bronchospasm
 Miscellaneous: Allergic reaction

Drug Interactions Decreased effect of ketoconazole, itraconazole

Drug Uptake
 Onset of GI effect: Oral: Within 1 hour
 Duration: 10-12 hours
 Serum half-life: 2.5-3.5 hours; increases with renal impairment, oliguric patients: 20 hours
 Time to peak serum concentration: Oral: Within 1-3 hours

Pregnancy Risk Factor B

Famvir™ see Famciclovir on previous page

Fansidar® see Sulfadoxine and Pyrimethamine on page 808

Fastin® see Phentermine Hydrochloride on page 683

Fat Emulsion (fat e mul′ shun)

Brand Names Intralipid®; Liposyn®

Canadian/Mexican Brand Names Emulsan 20% (Mexico); Lyposyn (Mexico); Lipocin (Mexico)

Therapeutic Category Caloric Agent; Intravenous Nutritional Therapy

Synonyms Intravenous Fat Emulsion

Use Source of calories and essential fatty acids for patients requiring parenteral nutrition of extended duration

Usual Dosage Fat emulsion should not exceed 60% of the total daily calories
 Children: Initial dose: 0.5-1 g/kg/day, increase by 0.5 g/kg/day to a maximum of 3-4 g/kg/day; maximum rate of infusion: 0.25 g/kg/hour (1.25 mL/kg/hour of 20% solution)
 Adolescents and Adults: Initial dose: 1 g/kg/day, increase by 0.5-1 g/kg/day to a maximum of 2.5 g/kg/day of 10% and 3 g/kg/day of 20%; maximum rate of infusion: 0.25 g/kg/hour (1.25 mL/kg/hour of 20% solution); do not exceed 50 mL/hour (20%) or 100 mL/hour (10%)
 Note: At the onset of therapy, the patient should be observed for any immediate allergic reactions such as dyspnea, cyanosis, and fever. Slower initial rates of infusion may be used for the first 10-15 minutes of the infusion (eg, 0.1 mL/minute of 10% or 0.05 mL/minute of 20% solution).

 Prevention of fatty acid deficiency (8% to 10% of total caloric intake): 0.5-1 g/kg/24 hours
 Children: 5-10 mL/kg/day at 0.1 mL/minute then up to 100 mL/hour
 Adults: 500 mL twice weekly at rate of 1 mL/minute for 30 minutes, then increase to 500 mL over 4-6 hours

 Can be used in both children and adults on a daily basis as a caloric source in TPN

Mechanism of Action Essential for normal structure and function of cell membranes

Local Anesthetic/Vasoconstrictor Precautions No information available to require special precautions

Effects on Dental Treatment No effects or complications reported

Other Adverse Effects
 >10%: Local: Thrombophlebitis
 1% to 10%: Endocrine & metabolic: Hyperlipemia
 <1%:
 Cardiovascular: Cyanosis, flushing, chest pain
 Gastrointestinal: Nausea, vomiting, diarrhea
 Hepatic: Hepatomegaly
 Respiratory: Dyspnea
 Miscellaneous: Sepsis

Drug Uptake
 Serum half-life: 0.5-1 hour

Pregnancy Risk Factor B/C

Fedahist® Expectorant [OTC] *see* Guaifenesin and Pseudoephedrine *on page 409*

Fedahist® Tablet [OTC] *see* Chlorpheniramine and Pseudoephedrine *on page 191*

Feen-a-Mint® [OTC] *see* Phenolphthalein *on page 682*

Feen-a-Mint® Pills [OTC] *see* Docusate and Phenolphthalein *on page 295*

Feiba VH Immuno® *see* Anti-Inhibitor Coagulant Complex *on page 70*

Felbamate (fel′ ba mate)
Brand Names Felbatol™

Therapeutic Category Anticonvulsant, Miscellaneous

Use Not a first-line agent; reserved for patients who do not adequately respond to alternative agents and whose epilepsy is so severe that benefit outweighs risk of liver failure or aplastic anemia; used as monotherapy and adjunctive therapy in patients ≥14 years of age with partial seizures with and without secondary generalization; adjunctive therapy in children ≥2 years of age who have partial and generalized seizures associated with Lennox-Gastaut syndrome

Local Anesthetic/Vasoconstrictor Precautions No information available to require special precautions

Effects on Dental Treatment No effects or complications reported

Other Adverse Effects
>10%:
Gastrointestinal: Nausea, diarrhea, anorexia, vomiting, constipation
Central nervous system: Anxiety, headache, fatigue, dizziness
Respiratory: Cough
1% to 10%:
Central nervous system: Drowsiness, insomnia, clumsiness, depression or behavior changes, clouded sensorium, lethargy, slurred speech
Gastrointestinal: Weight gain,
Neuromuscular & skeletal: Muscle twitches
Ocular: Blurred or double vision, uncontrollable eye movements
Dermatologic: Acne, skin rash
<1%:
Dermatologic: Alopecia
Gastrointestinal: Gum bleeding or hyperplasia

Comments Monotherapy has not been associated with gingival hyperplasia, impaired concentration, weight gain, or abnormal thinking

Felbatol™ *see* Felbamate *on this page*

Feldene® *see* Piroxicam *on page 699*

Felodipina (Mexico) *see* Felodipine *on this page*

Felodipine (fe loe′ di peen)
Related Information
Calcium Channel Blockers & Gingival Hyperplasia *on page 1010*
Cardiovascular Diseases *on page 912*

Brand Names Plendil®

Canadian/Mexican Brand Names Renedil® (Canada); Munobal® (Mexico)

Therapeutic Category Calcium Channel Blocker

Synonyms Felodipina (Mexico)

Use Treatment of hypertension, congestive heart failure

Usual Dosage Adults: Oral: 5-10 mg once daily; increase by 5 mg at 2-week intervals, as needed, to a maximum of 20 mg/day (Elderly: Begin with 2.5 mg/day)

Mechanism of Action Inhibits calcium ions from entering the select voltage-sensitive areas or "slow channels" of vascular smooth muscle and myocardium during depolarization, producing a relaxation of coronary vascular smooth muscle and coronary vasodilation; increases myocardial oxygen delivery in patients with vasospastic angina

Local Anesthetic/Vasoconstrictor Precautions No information available to require special precautions

Effects on Dental Treatment Calcium channel blockers cause gingival hyperplasia in approximately 1% of patients. There have been fewer reports with felodipine than with other CCBs. The hyperplasia will disappear with cessation of drug therapy. Consultation with physician is suggested.

Other Adverse Effects
>10%: Cardiovascular: Peripheral edema
1% to 10%:
Cardiovascular: Chest pain, tachycardia
Central nervous system: Dizziness, lightheadedness

Dermatologic: Skin rash
Gastrointestinal: Constipation, diarrhea
<1%:
Cardiovascular: Hypotension, arrhythmia, bradycardia, palpitations
Central nervous system: Mental depression, dizziness, headache
Dermatologic: Rash
Gastrointestinal: Gingival hyperplasia, dry mouth, nausea
Hepatic: Marked elevations in liver function tests
Ocular: Blurred vision
Respiratory: Shortness of breath
Drug Interactions Increased toxicity/effect/levels:
Calcium channel blockers (CCB) and H_2-blockers such as cimetidine cause increased bioavailability CCB
Beta-blockers cause increased depressant effects on A-V conduction
Drug Uptake
Onset of effect: 2-5 hours
Duration: 16-24 hours
Absorption: 100%; absolute: 20% due to first-pass effect
Serum half-life: 11-16 hours
Pregnancy Risk Factor C

Femcet® see Butalbital Compound on page 133
Femilax® [OTC] see Docusate and Phenolphthalein on page 295
Femiron® [OTC] see Ferrous Fumarate on page 359
Femstat® see Butoconazole Nitrate on page 135
Fenazopiridina (Mexico) see Phenazopyridine Hydrochloride on page 679
Fenesin™ see Guaifenesin on page 407

Fenfluramine Hydrochloride (fen flure' a meen hye droe klor' ide)
Brand Names Pondimin®
Canadian/Mexican Brand Names Ponderal® (Canada)
Therapeutic Category Adrenergic Agonist Agent; Anorexiant
Use Short-term adjunct in exogenous obesity
Usual Dosage Adults: Oral: 20 mg 3 times/day before meals or food, up to 40 mg 3 times/day; maximum daily dose: 120 mg
Mechanism of Action Fenfluramine hydrochloride is a phenethylamine structurally related to amphetamine; central nervous system depression is more common than stimulation, which makes fenfluramine pharmacologically different from amphetamine. Fenfluramine's exact mechanism of action is not well understood; the drug's appetite suppressing action may be due to the stimulation of the hypothalamus; the anorectic effect may also be due to delayed gastric emptying.
Local Anesthetic/Vasoconstrictor Precautions Use vasoconstrictor with caution in patients taking fenfluramine; amphetamine like drugs enhance the sympathomimetic response of epinephrine and norepinephrine leading to potential hypertension and cardiotoxicity.
Effects on Dental Treatment Up to 10% of patients may present with hypertension. The use of local anesthetic without vasoconstrictor is recommended in these patients.
Other Adverse Effects
>10%:
Cardiovascular: Hypertension
Central nervous system: Euphoria, nervousness, insomnia
1% to 10%:
Central nervous system: Confusion, mental depression, restlessness
Endocrine & metabolic: Changes in libido
Gastrointestinal: Nausea, vomiting, constipation
Hematologic: Blood dyscrasias
Neuromuscular & skeletal: Tremor
Ocular: Blurred vision
<1%:
Cardiovascular: Tachycardia, arrhythmias
Central nervous system: Restlessness, depression, headache
Dermatologic: Alopecia
Gastrointestinal: Diarrhea, abdominal cramps
Neuromuscular & skeletal: Myalgia
Renal: Dysuria, polyuria
Respiratory: Dyspnea
Miscellaneous: Increased sweating
Drug Interactions
Adrenergic blockers are inhibited by amphetamines
(Continued)

Fenfluramine Hydrochloride *(Continued)*

Amphetamines enhance the activity of tricyclic or sympathomimetic agents
MAO inhibitors slow the metabolism of amphetamines
Amphetamines will counteract the sedative effects of antihistamines
Amphetamines potentiate the analgesic effects of meperidine
Pregnancy Risk Factor C

Fenilefrina (Mexico) *see* Phenylephrine Hydrochloride *on page 685*

Fenilpropanolamina (Mexico) *see* Phenylpropanolamine Hydrochloride *on page 687*

Fenobarbital (Mexico) *see* Phenobarbital *on page 680*

Fenofibrate *(fen oh fye' brate)*
Brand Names Lipidil®
Canadian/Mexican Brand Names Controlip® (Mexico)
Therapeutic Category Lipid Lowering Drugs
Synonyms Fenofibrato (Mexico)
Use Adjunct to dietary therapy for the treatment of adults with very high elevations of serum triglyceride levels (types IV and V hyperlipidemia) who are at risk of pancreatitis and who do not respond adequately to a determined dietary effort; its efficacy can be enhanced by combination with other hypolipidemic agents that have a different mechanism of action; safety and efficacy may be greater than that of clofibrate
Usual Dosage Oral:
Children >10 years: 5 mg/kg/day
Adults: 100 mg 3 times/day with meals or 200 mg in the morning and 100 mg in the evening
Mechanism of Action Fenofibric acid is believed to increase VLDL catabolism by enhancing the synthesis of lipoprotein lipase; as a result of a decrease in VLDL levels, total plasma triglycerides are reduced by 30% to 60% (VLDL contains ~60% triglycerides and 10% to 15% cholesterol); apolipoprotein B, which stabilizes the structure of VLDL and LDL, decreases in a parallel fashion and plasma cholesterol levels decrease by fenofibrate's effect on LDL levels and cholesterol synthesis; modest increase in HDL occurs in some hypertriglyceridemic patients since it is involved in the storage and transport of cholesterol ester and apolipoproteins
Local Anesthetic/Vasoconstrictor Precautions No information available to require special precautions
Effects on Dental Treatment No effects or complications reported
Other Adverse Effects
>10%: Gastrointestinal: Nausea, gastric discomfort
1% to 10%:
Dermatologic: Skin reactions
Gastrointestinal: Constipation, diarrhea
<1%:
Central nervous system: Dizziness, headache, fatigue, insomnia
Hepatic: Transient increases in LFTs
Neuromuscular & skeletal: Arthralgia, myalgia
Drug Interactions
Increased hypolipidemic effect: Cholestyramine, colestipol will add to the hypolipidemic effect of fenofibrate
Drug Uptake
Peak effect: 4-6 hours
Absorption: 60% to 90% when given with meals
Serum half-life: Fenofibrate: 21 hours (30 hours in elderly, 44-54 hours in hepatic impairment)
Pregnancy Risk Factor C

Fenofibrato (Mexico) *see* Fenofibrate *on this page*

Fenoprofen Calcium *(fen oh proe' fen kal' see um)*
Related Information
Nonsteroidal Anti-Inflammatory Agents, Comparative Dosages, and Pharmacokinetics *on page 1021*
Rheumatoid Arthritis, Osteoarthritis, and Joint Prostheses *on page 930*
Brand Names Nalfon®
Therapeutic Category Analgesic, Non-narcotic; Anti-inflammatory Agent; Nonsteroidal Anti-inflammatory Agent (NSAID), Oral
Synonyms Fenoprofeno Calcico (Mexico)
Use Symptomatic treatment of acute and chronic rheumatoid arthritis and osteoarthritis; relief of mild to moderate pain

Usual Dosage Adults: Oral:
Rheumatoid arthritis: 300-600 mg 3-4 times/day up to 3.2 g/day
Mild to moderate pain: 200 mg every 4-6 hours as needed

Mechanism of Action Inhibits prostaglandin synthesis by decreasing the activity of the enzyme, cyclo-oxygenase, which results in decreased formation of prostaglandin precursors

Local Anesthetic/Vasoconstrictor Precautions No information available to require special precautions

Effects on Dental Treatment No effects or complications reported

Other Adverse Effects
>10%:
  Central nervous system: Dizziness
  Dermatologic: Skin rash
  Gastrointestinal: Abdominal cramps, heartburn, indigestion, nausea
1% to 10%:
  Cardiovascular: Fluid retention
  Central nervous system: Headache, nervousness
  Dermatologic: Itching
  Gastrointestinal: Vomiting
  Otic: Ringing in ears
<1%:
  Cardiovascular: Congestive heart failure, hypertension, arrhythmias, tachycardia, hot flushes
  Central nervous system: Confusion, hallucinations, aseptic meningitis, mental depression, drowsiness, insomnia
  Dermatologic: Hives, erythema multiforme, toxic epidermal necrolysis, Stevens-Johnson syndrome, angioedema
  Endocrine & metabolic: Polydipsia
  Gastrointestinal: Gastritis, GI ulceration
  Genitourinary: Cystitis
  Hematologic: Agranulocytosis, anemia, hemolytic anemia, bone marrow depression, leukopenia, thrombocytopenia
  Hepatic: Hepatitis
  Neuromuscular & skeletal: Peripheral neuropathy
  Ocular: Toxic amblyopia, blurred vision, conjunctivitis, dry eyes
  Otic: Decreased hearing
  Renal: Polyuria, acute renal failure
  Respiratory: Allergic rhinitis, shortness of breath
  Miscellaneous: Epistaxis

Drug Interactions
Decreased effect with phenobarbital
Increased effect/toxicity of phenytoin, sulfonamides, sulfonylureas
Increased toxicity with salicylates, oral anticoagulants

Drug Uptake
Absorption: Rapid (to 80%) from upper GI tract
Half-life: 2.5-3 hours
Time to peak serum concentration: Within 2 hours

Pregnancy Risk Factor B (D if used in the 3rd trimester or near delivery)

Fenoprofeno Calcico (Mexico) see Fenoprofen Calcium *on previous page*

Fentanyl (fen' ta nil)
Related Information
Narcotic Agonist Charts *on page 1019*

Brand Names Duragesic™; Fentanyl Oralet®; Sublimaze®

Canadian/Mexican Brand Names Durogesic® (Mexico); Fentanest® (Mexico)

Therapeutic Category Analgesic, Narcotic; General Anesthetic, Intravenous

Use
Dental: Adjunct in preoperative intravenous conscious sedation in patients undergoing dental surgery
Medical: In medicine, adjunct to general or regional anesthesia; management of chronic pain (transdermal product)

Usual Dosage
Children 1-12 years:
  Sedation for minor procedures/analgesia:
    I.M., I.V.: 1-2 mcg/kg/dose
    Transmucosal (lozenge): 5 mcg/kg if child is not fearful; fearful children and some younger children may require doses of 5-15 mcg/kg (which also carries an increased risk of hypoventilation); drug effect begins within 10 minutes, with sedation beginning shortly thereafter

(Continued)

Fentanyl *(Continued)*

Children >12 years and Adults:

Sedation for minor procedures/analgesia:

I.M., I.V.: 0.5-1 mcg/kg/dose; higher doses are used for major procedures

Transmucosal (lozenge): 5 mcg/kg, suck on lozenge vigorously approximately 20-40 minutes before the start of procedure, drug effect begins within 10 minutes, with sedation beginning shortly thereafter

Preoperative sedation: I.M., I.V.: 50-100 mcg/dose

Pain control: Transdermal fentanyl is not to be used for acute dosing in treatment of dental pain

Mechanism of Action Binds to opiate receptors (mu and kappa subtypes) in the CNS causing inhibition of ascending pain pathways, altering the perception of and response to pain; produces generalized CNS depression

Local Anesthetic/Vasoconstrictor Precautions No information available to require special precautions

Effects on Dental Treatment No effects or complications reported

Other Adverse Effects >10%:

Cardiovascular: Hypotension, bradycardia

Central nervous system: CNS depression, drowsiness, sedation

Gastrointestinal: Nausea, vomiting, constipation

Respiratory: Respiratory depression

Oral manifestations: No data reported

Contraindications Hypersensitivity to fentanyl or any component; increased intracranial pressure; severe respiratory depression; severe liver or renal insufficiency;

Transmucosal is contraindicated in unmonitored settings where a risk of unrecognized hypoventilation exists or in treating acute or chronic pain

Warnings/Precautions Fentanyl shares the toxic potentials of opiate agonists, and precautions of opiate agonist therapy should be observed; use with caution in patients with bradycardia; rapid I.V. infusion may result in skeletal muscle and chest wall rigidity → impaired ventilation → respiratory distress → apnea, bronchoconstriction, laryngospasm; inject slowly over 3-5 minutes; nondepolarizing skeletal muscle relaxant may be required.

Enhanced analgesia has been seen in elderly patients on therapeutic doses of narcotics; duration of action may be increased in the elderly; the elderly may be particularly susceptible to the CNS depressant and constipating effects of narcotics

Drug Interactions Increased toxicity of CNS depressants, phenothiazines, tricyclic antidepressants may potentiate fentanyl's adverse effects

Drug Uptake

Onset of effect (respiratory depressant effect may last longer than analgesic effect):

I.M.: Analgesia: 7-15 minutes

I.V.: Analgesia: Almost immediate

Transmucosal (lozenge): 5-15 minutes with a maximum reduction in activity/apprehension

Duration of effect:

I.M.: 1-2 hours

I.V.: 0.5-1 hour

Transmucosal: Related to blood level of drug

Serum half-life: 2-4 hours; transmucosal: 5-15 hours

Influence of food: No effect

Pregnancy Risk Factor B (D if used for prolonged periods or in high doses at term)

Breast-feeding Considerations Not contraindicated

Dosage Forms

Injection, as citrate: 0.05 mg/mL (2 mL, 5 mL, 10 mL, 20 mL, 50 mL)

Lozenge, oral transmucosal (raspberry flavored): 200 mcg, 300 mcg, 400 mcg

Transdermal system: 25 mcg/hour [10 cm^2]; 50 mcg/hour [20 cm^2]; 75 mcg/hour [30 cm^2]; 100 mcg/hour [40 cm^2] (all available in 5s)

Dietary Considerations No data reported

Generic Available No

Comments Transdermal fentanyl should not be used as a pain reliever in dentistry due to danger of hypoventilation

Fentanyl Oralet® *see Fentanyl on previous page*

Fentermina (Mexico) *see Phentermine Hydrochloride on page 683*

Feosol® [OTC] *see Ferrous Sulfate on page 360*

Feostat® [OTC] *see Ferrous Fumarate on next page*

Ferancee® [OTC] *see Ferrous Sulfate and Ascorbic Acid on page 361*

Feratab® [OTC] *see Ferrous Sulfate on next page*

Fergon® [OTC] *see Ferrous Gluconate on next page*

Fer-In-Sol® [OTC] *see Ferrous Sulfate on next page*

Fer-Iron® [OTC] *see Ferrous Sulfate on next page*

Ferndex *see Dextroamphetamine Sulfate on page 265*

Fero-Grad 500® [OTC] *see Ferrous Sulfate and Ascorbic Acid on page 361*

Fero-Gradumet® [OTC] *see Ferrous Sulfate on next page*

Ferospace® [OTC] *see Ferrous Sulfate on next page*

Ferralet® [OTC] *see Ferrous Gluconate on next page*

Ferralyn® Lanacaps® [OTC] *see Ferrous Sulfate on next page*

Ferra-TD® [OTC] *see Ferrous Sulfate on next page*

Ferromar® [OTC] *see Ferrous Sulfate and Ascorbic Acid on page 361*

Ferro-Sequels® [OTC] *see Ferrous Fumarate on this page*

Ferrous Fumarate (fer' us fyoo' ma rate)

Brand Names Femiron® [OTC]; Feostat® [OTC]; Ferro-Sequels® [OTC]; Fumasorb® [OTC]; Fumerin® [OTC]; Hemocyte® [OTC]; Ircon® [OTC]; Nephro-Fer™ [OTC]; Span-FF® [OTC]

Canadian/Mexican Brand Names Palafer® (Canada); Ferval® Ferroso (Mexico)

Therapeutic Category Iron Salt

Use Prevention and treatment of iron deficiency anemias

Usual Dosage Oral **(dose expressed in terms of elemental iron):**
Children:
Severe iron deficiency anemia: 4-6 mg Fe/kg/day in 3 divided doses
Mild to moderate iron deficiency anemia: 3 mg Fe/kg/day in 1-2 divided doses
Prophylaxis: 1-2 mg Fe/kg/day
Adults:
Iron deficiency: 60-100 mg twice daily up to 60 mg 2 times/day
Prophylaxis: 60-100 mg/day
To avoid GI upset, start with a single daily dose and increase by 1 tablet/day each week or as tolerated until desired daily dose is achieved
Elderly: 200 mg 3-4 times/day

Mechanism of Action Replaces iron found in hemoglobin, myoglobin, and enzymes; allows the transportation of oxygen via hemoglobin

Local Anesthetic/Vasoconstrictor Precautions No information available to require special precautions

Effects on Dental Treatment Do not prescribe tetracyclines simultaneously with iron since GI tract absorption of both tetracycline and iron may be inhibited

Other Adverse Effects
>10%: Gastrointestinal: Stomach cramping, constipation, nausea, vomiting, dark stools
1% to 10%:
Gastrointestinal: Heartburn, diarrhea
Miscellaneous; Discolored urine, staining of teeth
<1%: Ocular: Contact irritation

Drug Interactions
Decreased effect: Absorption of oral preparation of iron and tetracyclines are decreased when both of these drugs are given together; concurrent administration of antacids may decrease iron absorption; iron may decrease absorption of penicillamine when given at the same time; response to iron therapy may be delayed in patients receiving chloramphenicol
Milk may decrease absorption of iron
Increased effect: Current administration of ≥200 mg vitamin C per 30 mg elemental iron increases absorption of oral iron

Drug Uptake
Onset of hematologic response (essentially the same to either oral or parenteral iron salts): Red blood cell form and color changes within 3-10 days
Peak reticulocytosis: Within 5-10 days; hemoglobin values increase within 2-4 weeks
Absorption: Iron is absorbed in the duodenum and upper jejunum; in persons with normal iron stores 10% of an oral dose is absorbed, this is increased to 20% to 30% in persons with inadequate iron stores; food and achlorhydria will decrease absorption

Pregnancy Risk Factor A

Ferrous Gluconate (fer' us gloo' koe nate)

Brand Names Fergon® [OTC]; Ferralet® [OTC]; Simron® [OTC]

Canadian/Mexican Brand Names Apo-Ferrous® Gluconate (Canada)

Therapeutic Category Iron Salt

Use Prevention and treatment of iron deficiency anemias

Usual Dosage Oral (dose expressed in terms of elemental iron):

Children:

Severe iron deficiency anemia: 4-6 mg Fe/kg/day in 3 divided doses

Mild to moderate iron deficiency anemia: 3 mg Fe/kg/day in 1-2 divided doses

Prophylaxis: 1-2 mg Fe/kg/day

Adults:

Iron deficiency: 60 mg twice daily up to 60 mg 4 times/day

Prophylaxis: 60 mg/day

Mechanism of Action Replaces iron found in hemoglobin, myoglobin, and enzymes; allows the transportation of oxygen via hemoglobin

Local Anesthetic/Vasoconstrictor Precautions No information available to require special precautions

Effects on Dental Treatment Do not prescribe tetracyclines simultaneously with iron since GI tract absorption of both tetracycline and iron may be inhibited

Other Adverse Effects

>10%: Gastrointestinal: Stomach cramping, constipation, nausea, vomiting, dark stools

1% to 10%:

Gastrointestinal: Heartburn, diarrhea

Miscellaneous: Discolored urine, staining of teeth

<1%: Ocular: Contact irritation

Drug Interactions Absorption of oral preparation of iron and tetracyclines is decreased when both of these drugs are given together; concurrent administration of antacids may decrease iron absorption; iron may decrease absorption of penicillamine when given at the same time. Response to iron therapy may be delayed in patients receiving chloramphenicol. Concurrent administration of ≥ 200 mg vitamin C/30 mg elemental iron increases absorption of oral iron; milk may decrease absorption of iron.

Drug Uptake Onset of hematologic response (essentially the same to either oral or parenteral iron salts): Red blood cells form and color changes within 3-10 days, peak reticulocytosis occurs in 5-10 days, and hemoglobin values increase within 2-4 weeks

Pregnancy Risk Factor A

Ferrous Sulfate (fer' us sul' fate)

Brand Names Feosol® [OTC]; Feratab® [OTC]; Fer-In-Sol® [OTC]; Fer-Iron® [OTC]; Fero-Gradumet® [OTC]; Ferospace® [OTC]; Ferralyn® Lanacaps® [OTC]; Ferra-TD® [OTC]; Mol-Iron® [OTC]; Slow FE® [OTC]

Canadian/Mexican Brand Names Apo-Ferrous® Sulfate (Canada); PMS-Ferrous® Sulfate (Canada); Hemobion® 200 (Mexico); Hemobion® 400 (Mexico); Orafer® (Mexico)

Therapeutic Category Iron Salt

Use Prevention and treatment of iron deficiency anemias

Usual Dosage Oral:

Children (dose expressed in terms of elemental iron):

Severe iron deficiency anemia: 4-6 mg Fe/kg/day in 3 divided doses

Mild to moderate iron deficiency anemia: 3 mg Fe/kg/day in 1-2 divided doses

Prophylaxis: 1-2 mg Fe/kg/day up to a maximum of 15 mg/day

Adults (dose expressed in terms of ferrous sulfate):

Iron deficiency: 300 mg twice daily up to 300 mg 4 times/day or 250 mg (extended release) 1-2 times/day

Prophylaxis: 300 mg/day

Mechanism of Action Replaces iron, found in hemoglobin, myoglobin, and other enzymes; allows the transportation of oxygen via hemoglobin

Local Anesthetic/Vasoconstrictor Precautions No information available to require special precautions

Effects on Dental Treatment Do not prescribe tetracyclines simultaneously with iron since GI tract absorption of both tetracycline and iron may be inhibited

Other Adverse Effects

>10%: Gastrointestinal: GI irritation, epigastric pain, nausea, dark stool, vomiting, stomach cramping, constipation

1% to 10%:

Gastrointestinal: Heartburn, diarrhea

Miscellaneous: Liquid preparations may temporarily stain the teeth, discolored urine

<1%: Ocular: Contact irritation

Drug Interactions

Decreased effect: Absorption of oral preparation of iron and tetracyclines are decreased when both of these drugs are given together; concurrent administration of antacids may decrease iron absorption; iron may decrease absorption of penicillamine when given at the same time; response to iron therapy may be delayed in patients receiving chloramphenicol; milk may decrease absorption of iron

Increased effect: Concurrent administration of ≥200 mg vitamin C per 30 mg elemental Fe increases absorption of oral iron

Drug Uptake

Onset of hematologic response (essentially the same to either oral or parenteral iron salts): Red blood cell form and color changes within 3-10 days

Peak reticulocytosis: Occurs in 5-10 days, and hemoglobin values increase within 2-4 weeks

Absorption: Iron is absorbed in the duodenum and upper jejunum; in persons with normal serum iron stores, 10% of an oral dose is absorbed; this is increased to 20% to 30% in persons with inadequate iron stores. Food and achlorhydria will decrease absorption

Pregnancy Risk Factor A

Ferrous Sulfate and Ascorbic Acid

(fer' us sul' fate & a skor' bik as' id)

Brand Names Ferancee® [OTC]; Fero-Grad 500® [OTC]; Ferromar® [OTC]

Therapeutic Category Iron Salt; Vitamin

Synonyms Ascorbic Acid and Ferrous Sulfate

Use Treatment of iron deficiency in nonpregnant adults; treatment and prevention of iron deficiency in pregnant adults

Local Anesthetic/Vasoconstrictor Precautions No information available to require special precautions

Effects on Dental Treatment Do not prescribe tetracyclines simultaneously with iron since GI tract absorption of both tetracycline and iron may be inhibited

Ferrous Sulfate, Ascorbic Acid, and Vitamin B-Complex

(fer' us sul' fate, a skor' bik as' id, & vye' ta min bee kom' pleks)

Brand Names Iberet®-Liquid [OTC]

Therapeutic Category Iron Salt; Vitamin

Use Conditions of iron deficiency with an increased needed for B-complex vitamins and vitamin C

Local Anesthetic/Vasoconstrictor Precautions No information available to require special precautions

Effects on Dental Treatment Do not prescribe tetracyclines simultaneously with iron since GI tract absorption of both tetracycline and iron may be inhibited

Ferrous Sulfate, Ascorbic Acid, Vitamin B-Complex, and Folic Acid

(fer' us sul' fate, a skor' bik as' id, vye' ta min bee kom' pleks, & foe' lik as' id)

Brand Names Iberet-Folic-500®

Therapeutic Category Iron Salt; Vitamin

Use Treatment of iron deficiency and prevention of concomitant folic acid deficiency where there is an associated deficient intake or increased need for B-complex vitamins

Local Anesthetic/Vasoconstrictor Precautions No information available to require special precautions

Effects on Dental Treatment Do not prescribe tetracyclines simultaneously with iron since GI tract absorption of both tetracycline and iron may be inhibited

Feverall™ [OTC] *see Acetaminophen* *on page 14*

Fexofenadine Hydrochloride

Brand Names Allegra®

Therapeutic Category Antihistamine

Use A nonsedating antihistamine indicated for the relief of seasonal allergic rhinitis in patients age 12 and over

Usual Dosage

Adults: Oral: One 60-mg capsule twice a day

(Continued)

Fexofenadine Hydrochloride *(Continued)*

Reanl impairment dose: 60 mg once daily

Local Anesthetic/Vasoconstrictor Precautions No information available to require special precautions

Effects on Dental Treatment No effects or complications reported

Pregnancy Risk Factor C

Generic Available No

Comments Fexofenadine (Allegra®) is a metabolite of terfenadine (Seldane®) which has been chemically manipulated to eliminate the potentially fatal cardiovascular drug interactions associated with Seldane®. Seldane®, when administered with erythromycin or ketoconazole (Nizoral®) has resulted in Q-T interval prolongation and ventricular arrhythmias. However, when fexofenadine (Allegra®) has been given with erythromycin or ketoconazole (Nizoral®), these cardiovascular effects have not occurred.

Fiberall® [OTC] *see* Psyllium *on page 750*

Fiberall® Chewable Tablet [OTC] *see* Calcium Polycarbophil *on page 146*

FiberCon® Tablet [OTC] *see* Calcium Polycarbophil *on page 146*

Fiber-Lax® Tablet [OTC] *see* Calcium Polycarbophil *on page 146*

Fibrinolysin and Desoxyribonuclease

(fye brin oh lye' sin & des ox i rye boo noo' klee ase)

Brand Names Elase-Chloromycetin® Topical; Elase® Topical

Therapeutic Category Enzyme, Topical Debridement

Synonyms Desoxyribonuclease and Fibrinolysin

Use Debriding agent; cervicitis; and irrigating agent in infected wounds

Local Anesthetic/Vasoconstrictor Precautions No information available to require special precautions

Effects on Dental Treatment No effects or complications reported

Filgrastim *(fil gra' stim)*

Brand Names Neupogen® Injection

Therapeutic Category Colony Stimulating Factor

Synonyms G-CSF; Granulocyte Colony Stimulating Factor

Use To reduce the duration of neutropenia and the associated risk of infection in patients with nonmyeloid malignancies receiving myelosuppressive chemotherapeutic regimens associated with a significant incidence of severe neutropenia with fever; it has also been used in AIDS patients on zidovudine and in patients with noncancer chemotherapy-induced neutropenia

Usual Dosage Children and Adults: administered S.C. or I.V. as a single daily infusion over 20-30 minutes

Myelosuppressive chemotherapy 5 mcg/kg/day S.C. or I.V.

Doses may be increased in increments of 5 mcg/kg for each chemotherapy cycle, according to the duration and severity of the absolute neutrophil count (ANC) nadir. In phase III trials, efficacy was observed at doses of 4-6 mcg/kg/day. Discontinue therapy if the ANC count is >10,000/mm^3 after the ANC nadir has occurred following the expected chemotherapy-induced neutrophil nadir. Some cancer centers are stopping therapy at an ANC of 2500. Duration of therapy needed to attenuate chemotherapy-induced neutropenia may be dependent on the myelosuppressive potential of the chemotherapy regimen employed. Duration of therapy in clinical studies has ranged from 2 weeks to 3 years.

Bone marrow transplant patients

Bone marrow transplant patients: 10 mcg/kg/day as an I.V. infusion of 4 or 24 hours or as continuous 24-hour S.C. infusion. Administer first dose at least 24 hours after cytotoxic chemotherapy and at least 24 hours after bone marrow infusion.

Filgrastim Dose Based on Neutrophil Response

Absolute Neutrophil Count	Filgrastim Dose Adjustment
When ANC >1000/mm^3 for 3 consecutive days	Reduce to 5 mcg/kg/day
If ANC remains >1000/mm^3 for 3 more consecutive days	Discontinue filgrastim
If ANC decreases to <1000/mm^3	Resume at 5 mcg/kg/day

Severe chronic neutropenia:

Congenital neutropenia: 6 mcg/kg twice daily S.C.

Idiopathic/cyclic neutropenia: 5 mcg/kg/day S.C.

Chronic daily administration is required to maintain clinical benefit. Adjust dose based on the patients' clinical course as well as ANC. In phase III studies, the target ANC was 1,500-10,000/mm^3. Reduce the dose of the ANC is persistently >10,000/mm^3.

Premature discontinuation of G-CSF therapy prior to the time of recovery from the expected neutrophil is generally not recommended. A transient increase in neutrophil counts is typically seen 1-2 days after initiation of therapy.

Mechanism of Action Stimulates the production, maturation, and activation of neutrophils, G-CSF activates neutrophils to increase both their migration and cytotoxicity. Natural proteins which stimulate hematopoietic stem cells to proliferate, prolong cell survival, stimulate cell differentiation, and stimulate functional activity of mature cells. CSFs are produced by a wide variety of cell types. Specific mechanisms of action are not yet fully understood, but possibly work by a second-messenger pathway with resultant protein production. See table.

Proliferation/Differentiation	G-CSF (Filgrastim)	GM-CSF (Sargramostim)
Neutrophils	Yes	Yes
Eosinophils	No	Yes
Macrophages	No	Yes
Neutrophil migration	Enhanced	Inhibited

Local Anesthetic/Vasoconstrictor Precautions No information available to require special precautions

Effects on Dental Treatment No effects or complications reported

Other Adverse Effects Effects are generally mild and dose related

>10%:
Central nervous system: Neutropenic fever, fever
Dermatologic: Alopecia
Gastrointestinal: Nausea, vomiting, diarrhea, mucositis
Medullary bone pain (24% incidence): This occurs most commonly in lower back pain, posterior iliac crest, and sternum and is controlled with nonnarcotic analgesics
Splenomegaly: This occurs more commonly in patients with cyclic neutropenia/congenital agranulocytosis who received S.C. injections for a prolonged (>14 days) period of time; ~33% of these patients experience subclinical splenomegaly (detected by MRI or CT scan); ~3% of these patients experience clinical splenomegaly

1% to 10%:
Cardiovascular: Chest pain
Central nervous system: Headache
Dermatologic: Rash
Endocrine & metabolic: Fluid retention
Gastrointestinal: Anorexia, stomatitis, constipation, sore throat
Local: Pain at injection site
Hematologic: Leukocytosis
Neuromuscular & skeletal: Weakness
Respiratory: Dyspnea, cough

<1%:
Cardiovascular: Transient supraventricular arrhythmia, pericarditis
Local: Thrombophlebitis
Hypersensitivity: Anaphylactic reaction

Drug Uptake
Onset of action: Rapid elevation in neutrophil counts within the first 24 hours, reaching a plateau in 3-5 days
Duration: ANC decreases by 50% within 2 days after discontinuing G-CSF; white counts return to the normal range in 4-7 days
Absorption: S.C.: 100% absorbed; peak plasma levels can be maintained for up to 12 hours
Serum half-life: 1.8-3.5 hours
Time to peak serum concentration: S.C.: Within 2-6 hours

Pregnancy Risk Factor C

Comments Reimbursement hotline: 1-800-28-AMGEN

Filibon® [OTC] *see* Vitamins, Multiple *on page 901*

Finasteride (fi nas' teer ide)

Brand Names Proscar®

Therapeutic Category Antiandrogen; Urinary Tract Product

(Continued)

Finasteride *(Continued)*

Use Early data indicate that finasteride is useful in the treatment of symptomatic benign prostatic hyperplasia (BPH)

Unlabeled use: Adjuvant monotherapy after radical prostatectomy in the treatment of prostatic cancer

Usual Dosage Adults: Male: Benign prostatic hyperplasia: Oral: 5 mg/day as a single dose; clinical responses occur within 12 weeks to 6 months of initiation of therapy; long-term administration is recommended for maximal response

Mechanism of Action Finasteride is a 4-azo analog of testosterone and is a competitive inhibitor of both tissue and hepatic 5-alpha reductase. This results in inhibition of the conversion of testosterone to dihydrotestosterone and markedly suppresses serum dihydrotestosterone levels; depending on dose and duration, serum testosterone concentrations may or may not increase. Testosterone-dependent processes such as fertility, muscle strength, potency, and libido are not affected by finasteride.

Local Anesthetic/Vasoconstrictor Precautions No information available to require special precautions

Effects on Dental Treatment No effects or complications reported

Other Adverse Effects 1% to 10%:
Endocrine & metabolic: Decreased libido
Genitourinary: <4% incidence of impotence, decreased volume of ejaculate

Drug Interactions No data reported

Drug Uptake
Onset of clinical effect: Within 12 weeks to 6 months of ongoing therapy
Duration of action:
After a single oral dose as small as 0.5 mg: 65% depression of plasma dihydrotestosterone levels persists 5-7 days
After 6 months of treatment with 5 mg/day: Circulating dihydrotestosterone levels are reduced to castrate levels without significant effects on circulating testosterone; levels return to normal within 14 days of discontinuation of treatment
Absorption: Oral: Extent may be reduced if administered with food
Time to peak serum concentration: Oral: 2-6 hours
Serum half-life, serum: Parent drug: ~5-17 hours (mean: 1.9 fasting, 4.2 with breakfast)
Serum half-life:
Elderly: 8 hours
Adults: 6 hours (3-16)

Pregnancy Risk Factor X

Fiorgen PF® *see* Butalbital Compound *on page 133*

Fioricet® *see* Butalbital Compound *on page 133*

Fiorinal® *see* Butalbital Compound *on page 133*

Fiorinal® **With Codeine** *see* Butalbital Compound and Codeine *on page 134*

Flagyl® *see* Metronidazole *on page 576*

Flarex® *see* Fluorometholone *on page 375*

Flatulex® **[OTC]** *see* Simethicone *on page 788*

Flavorcee® **[OTC]** *see* Ascorbic Acid *on page 76*

Flavoxate *(fla vox' ate)*

Brand Names Urispas®

Therapeutic Category Antispasmodic Agent, Urinary

Use Antispasmodic used to provide symptomatic relief of dysuria, nocturia, suprapubic pain, urgency, and incontinence

Usual Dosage Children >12 years and Adults: Oral: 100-200 mg 3-4 times/day; reduce the dose when symptoms improve

Mechanism of Action Synthetic antispasmotic with similar actions to that of propantheline; it exerts a direct relaxant effect on smooth muscles via phosphodiesterase inhibition, providing relief to a variety of smooth muscle spasms; it is especially useful for the treatment of bladder spasticity, whereby it produces an increase in urinary capacity

Local Anesthetic/Vasoconstrictor Precautions No information available to require special precautions

Effects on Dental Treatment No effects or complications reported

Other Adverse Effects
>10%:
Central nervous system: Drowsiness
Gastrointestinal: Dry mouth/throat

1% to 10%:
  Cardiovascular: Tachycardia, palpitations,
  Central nervous system: Nervousness, fatigue, vertigo, headache, drowsiness, hyperpyrexia
  Gastrointestinal: Constipation, nausea, vomiting
<1%:
  Central nervous system: Confusion (especially in the elderly)
  Dermatologic: Skin rash
  Hematologic: Leukopenia
  Ophthalmic: Increased intraocular pressure
Drug Interactions No data reported
Drug Uptake
  Onset of action: 55-60 minutes
Pregnancy Risk Factor B

Flecainida, Acetato De (Mexico) see Flecainide Acetate on this page

Flecainide Acetate (fle kay' nide)

Related Information
  Cardiovascular Diseases on page 912
Brand Names Tambocor™
Therapeutic Category Antiarrhythmic Agent, Class I-C; Antiarrhythmic Agent (Supraventricular & Ventricular)
Synonyms Flecainida, Acetato De (Mexico)
Use Prevention and suppression of documented life-threatening ventricular arrhythmias (ie, sustained ventricular tachycardia); controlling symptomatic, disabling supraventricular tachycardias in patients without structural heart disease in whom other agents fail
Usual Dosage Oral:
  Children:
    Initial: 3 mg/kg/day or 50-100 mg/m²/day in 3 divided doses
    Usual: 3-6 mg/kg/day or 100-150 mg/m²/day in 3 divided doses; up to 11 mg/kg/day or 200 mg/m²/day for uncontrolled patients with subtherapeutic levels
  Adults:
    Life-threatening ventricular arrhythmias:
      Initial: 100 mg every 12 hours
      Increase by 50-100 mg/day (given in 2 doses/day) every 4 days; maximum: 400 mg/day
      For patients receiving 400 mg/day who are not controlled and have trough concentrations <0.6 µg/mL, dosage may be increased to 600 mg/day
    Prevention of paroxysmal supraventricular arrhythmias in patients with disabling symptoms but no structural heart disease:
      Initial: 50 mg every 12 hours
      Increase by 50 mg twice daily at 4-day intervals; maximum: 300 mg/day
Mechanism of Action Class IC antiarrhythmic; slows conduction in cardiac tissue by altering transport of ions across cell membranes; causes slight prolongation of refractory periods; decreases the rate of rise of the action potential without affecting its duration; increases electrical stimulation threshold of ventricle, HIS-Purkinje system; possesses local anesthetic and moderate negative inotropic effects
Local Anesthetic/Vasoconstrictor Precautions No information available to require special precautions
Effects on Dental Treatment No effects or complications reported
Other Adverse Effects
  >10%:
    Central nervous system: Dizziness
    Ocular: Visual disturbances
    Respiratory: Dyspnea
  1% to 10%:
    Cardiovascular: Palpitations, chest pain, edema, tachycardia
    Central nervous system: Headache, fatigue, asthenia, fever
    Dermatologic: Rash
    Gastrointestinal: Nausea, constipation, abdominal pain
    Neuromuscular & skeletal: Tremor
  <1%:
    Cardiovascular: Bradycardia, heart block, increased P-R, QRS duration, worsening ventricular arrhythmias, congestive heart failure
    Central nervous system: Nervousness, hypoesthesia
    Dermatologic: Alopecia
    Hematologic: Blood dyscrasias
(Continued)

Flecainide Acetate *(Continued)*

Hepatic: Possible hepatic dysfunction
Neuromuscular & skeletal: Paresthesia

Drug Interactions
Increased toxicity:
Alkalinizing agents (high dose antacids, cimetidine, carbonic anhydrase inhibitors or sodium bicarbonate) may decrease flecainide clearance
Beta-adrenergic blockers, disopyramide, verapamil (possible additive negative inotropic effects)
Digoxin, amiodarone (increased plasma concentrations)
Decreased toxicity: Smoking and acid urine (increases flecainide clearance)

Drug Uptake
Absorption: Oral: Rapid
Serum half-life:
Children: 8 hours
Adults: 7-22 hours, increased with congestive heart failure or renal dysfunction
End stage renal disease: 19-26 hours
Time to peak serum concentration: Within 1.5-3 hours

Pregnancy Risk Factor C

Fleet® Babylax® Rectal [OTC] *see* Glycerin *on page 402*

Fleet® Enema [OTC] *see* Sodium Phosphates *on page 792*

Fleet® Flavored Castor Oil [OTC] *see* Castor Oil *on page 161*

Fleet® Laxative [OTC] *see* Bisacodyl *on page 113*

Fleet® Phospho®-Soda [OTC] *see* Sodium Phosphates *on page 792*

Flexaphen® *see* Chlorzoxazone *on page 200*

Flexeril® *see* Cyclobenzaprine Hydrochloride *on page 239*

Flolan® Injection *see* Epoprostenol Sodium *on page 317*

Flonase™ *see* Fluticasone Propionate *on page 383*

Florinef® Acetate *see* Fludrocortisone Acetate *on page 369*

Florone® *see* Diflorasone Diacetate *on page 278*

Florone® E *see* Diflorasone Diacetate *on page 278*

Floropryl® *see* Isoflurophate *on page 470*

Florvite® *see* Vitamins, Multiple *on page 901*

Flosequinan *(floe se′ kwi nan)*

Brand Names Manoplax®
Therapeutic Category Vasodilator, Peripheral
Use Management of congestive heart failure (CHF) in patients not responding to diuretics, with or without digitalis, who cannot tolerate an angiotensin-converting enzyme (ACE) inhibitor or who have not responded to a regimen including an ACE inhibitor
Local Anesthetic/Vasoconstrictor Precautions No information available to require special precautions
Effects on Dental Treatment No effects or complications reported

Floxin® *see* Ofloxacin *on page 634*

Floxuridine *(flox yoor′ i deen)*

Brand Names FUDR®
Therapeutic Category Antineoplastic Agent, Antimetabolite
Synonyms Fluorodeoxyuridine
Use Palliative management of carcinomas of head, neck, and brain as well as liver, gallbladder, and bile ducts
Usual Dosage Adults (refer to individual protocols):
Intra-arterial: Primarily by an implantable pump: 0.1-0.6 mg/kg/day continuous intra-arterial administration for 14 days then heparinized saline is given for 14 days; toxicity requires dose reduction
I.V.: 0.5-1 mg/kg/day for 6-15 days
Mechanism of Action Mechanism of action and pharmacokinetics are very similar to 5-FU; FUDR® is the deoxyribonucleotide of 5-FU. Inhibits DNA and RNA synthesis via formation of carbonium ions; cross-links strands of DNA, causing an imbalance of growth and cell death
Local Anesthetic/Vasoconstrictor Precautions No information available to require special
Effects on Dental Treatment No effects or complications reported
Other Adverse Effects
>10%: Gastrointestinal: GI hemorrhage, stomatitis, esophagopharyngitis, diarrhea, gastritis

1% to 10%:
  Gastrointestinal: Anorexia, glossitis
  Dermatologic: Alopecia, dermatitis, rash
<1%:
  Cardiovascular: Myocardial ischemia, angina
  Central nervous system: Lethargy, weakness, acute cerebellar syndrome, confusion, euphoria, fever
  Hematologic: Severe hematologic toxicity, leukopenia, thrombocytopenia, pancytopenia, agranulocytosis
  Ocular: Photophobia
  Miscellaneous: Anaphylaxis
Pregnancy Risk Factor D

Fluconazole (floo koe' na zole)
Related Information
  Oral Fungal Infections *on page 948*
Brand Names Diflucan®
Canadian/Mexican Brand Names Oxifungol® (Mexico); Zonal® (Mexico)
Therapeutic Category Antifungal Agent, Systemic
Use Oral fluconazole should be used in persons able to tolerate oral medications; parenteral fluconazole should be reserved for patients who are both unable to take oral medications and are unable to tolerate amphotericin B (eg, due to hypersensitivity or renal insufficiency)

  Dental: Treatment of susceptible fungal infections in the oral cavity including candidiasis, oral thrush, and chronic mucocutaneous candidiasis; treatment of esophageal and oropharyngeal candidiasis caused by *Candida* species; treatment of severe, chronic mucocutaneous candidiasis caused by *Candida* species
  Medical: Vaginal candidiasis unresponsive to nystatin or clotrimazole; treatment of hepatosplenic candidiasis; treatment of other *Candida* infections in persons unable to tolerate amphotericin B; treatment of cryptococcal infections; secondary prophylaxis for cryptococcal meningitis in persons with AIDS; antifungal prophylaxis in allogeneic bone marrow transplant recipients
Usual Dosage The daily dose of fluconazole is the same for oral and I.V. administration
  Children: Efficacy of fluconazole has not been established in children; a small number of patients from 3-13 years of age have been treated with fluconazole using doses of 3-6 mg/kg/day once daily. Doses as high as 12 mg/kg/day once daily have been used to treat candidiasis in immunocompromised children; 10-12 mg/kg/day has been used prophylactically against fungal infections in pediatric bone marrow transplant patients.

  Adults: Oral, I.V.: See table for once daily dosing.

Indication	Day 1	Daily Therapy	Minimum Duration of Therapy
Oropharyngeal candidiasis	200 mg	100 mg	14 d
Esophageal candidiasis	200 mg	100 mg	21 d
Systemic candidiasis	400 mg	200 mg	28 d
Cryptococcal meningitis			10-12 wk after CSF culture becomes negative
acute	400 mg	200 mg	
relapse	200 mg	200 mg	

Mechanism of Action Interferes with cytochrome P-450 activity, decreasing ergosterol synthesis (principal sterol in fungal cell membrane) and inhibiting cell membrane formation
Local Anesthetic/Vasoconstrictor Precautions No information available to require special precautions
Effects on Dental Treatment No effects or complications reported
Other Adverse Effects 1% to 10%:
  Central nervous system: Headache
  Dermatologic: Skin rash
  Gastrointestinal: Nausea, vomiting, abdominal pain, diarrhea

  Oral manifestations: No data reported
Contraindications Known hypersensitivity to fluconazole or other azoles
Warnings/Precautions Should be used with caution in patients with renal and hepatic dysfunction or previous hepatotoxicity from other azole derivatives. Patients who develop abnormal liver function tests during fluconazole therapy should be monitored closely and discontinued if symptoms consistent with liver disease develop.
(Continued)

Fluconazole *(Continued)*

Drug Interactions Cytochrome P-450 IIIA4 enzyme inhibitor and cytochrome P-450 IIC enzyme inhibitor

Rifampin decreases concentrations of fluconazole; fluconazole may increase cyclosporine levels when high doses used; may increase phenytoin serum concentration; fluconazole may also inhibit warfarin metabolism

Drug Uptake

Absorption: >90%

Time to peak serum concentration: Oral: Within 2-4 hours

Serum half-life: 25-30 hours with normal renal function

Pregnancy Risk Factor C

Breast-feeding Considerations Probably safe (not absorbed orally)

Dosage Forms

Injection: 2 mg/mL (100 mL, 200 mL)

Tablet: 50 mg, 100 mg, 200 mg

Dietary Considerations No data reported

Generic Available No

Flucytosine *(floo sye′ toe seen)*

Brand Names Ancobon®

Canadian/Mexican Brand Names Ancotil® (Canada)

Therapeutic Category Antifungal Agent, Systemic

Synonyms 5-Flurocytosine

Use Adjunctive treatment of susceptible fungal infections (usually *Candida* or *Cryptococcus*); in combination with amphotericin B, fluconazole, or itraconazole; synergy with amphotericin B for fungal infections (*Aspergillus*)

Usual Dosage Children and Adults: Oral: 50-150 mg/kg/day in divided doses every 6 hours

Mechanism of Action Penetrates fungal cells and is converted to fluorouracil which competes with uracil interfering with fungal RNA and protein synthesis

Local Anesthetic/Vasoconstrictor Precautions No information available to require special precautions

Effects on Dental Treatment No effects or complications reported

Other Adverse Effects

1% to 10%:

Dermatologic: Skin rash

Gastrointestinal: Abdominal pain, diarrhea, loss of appetite, nausea, vomiting

Hematologic: Anemia, leukopenia, thrombocytopenia

Hepatic: Hepatitis, jaundice

<1%:

Cardiovascular: Cardiac arrest

Central nervous system: Confusion, hallucinations, dizziness, drowsiness, headache, parkinsonism, psychosis, ataxia

Dermatologic: Photosensitivity

Endocrine & metabolic: Temporary growth failure, hypoglycemia, hypokalemia

Hematologic: Bone marrow depression

Hepatic: Elevated liver enzymes

Neuromuscular & skeletal: Paresthesia

Otic: Hearing loss

Respiratory: Respiratory arrest

Drug Interactions Increased effect/toxicity (enterocolitis) with concurrent amphotericin administration

Drug Uptake

Absorption: Oral: 75% to 90%

Serum half-life: 3-8 hours

Anuria: May be as long as 200 hours

End stage renal disease: 75-200 hours

Time to peak serum concentration: Within 2-6 hours

Pregnancy Risk Factor C

Fludara® *see* Fludarabine Phosphate *on this page*

Fludarabine Phosphate *(floo dare′ a been fos′ fate)*

Brand Names Fludara®

Therapeutic Category Antineoplastic Agent, Antimetabolite

Use Treatment of B-cell chronic lymphocytic leukemia unresponsive to previous therapy with an alkylating agent containing regimen. Fludarabine has been tested in patients with refractory acute lymphocytic leukemia and acute nonlymphocytic leukemia, but required a highly toxic dose to achieve response.

Usual Dosage I.V.:

Children:

Acute leukemia: 10 mg/m² bolus over 15 minutes followed by continuous infusion of 30.5 mg/m²/day over 5 days **or**

10.5 mg/m² bolus over 15 minutes followed by 30.5 mg/m²/day over 48 hours followed by cytarabine has been used in clinical trials

Solid tumors: 9 mg/m² bolus followed by 27 mg/m²/day continuous infusion over 5 days

Adults:

Chronic lymphocytic leukemia: 20-25 mg/m²/day over a 30-minute period for 5 days; 5-day courses are repeated every 28-35 days days

Non-Hodgkin's lymphoma: Loading dose: 20 mg/m² followed by 30 mg/m²/day for 48 hours

Mechanism of Action Fludarabine is analogous to that of Ara-C and Ara-A. Following systemic administration, FAMP is rapidly dephosphorylated to 2-fluoro-Ara-A. 2-Fluoro-Ara-A enters the cell by a carrier-mediated transport process, then is phosphorylated intracellularly by deoxycytidine kinase to form the active metabolite 2-fluoro-Ara-ATP. 2-Fluoro-Ara-ATP inhibits DNA synthesis by inhibition of DNA polymerase and ribonucleotide reductase.

Local Anesthetic/Vasoconstrictor Precautions No information available to require special precautions

Effects on Dental Treatment No effects or complications reported

Other Adverse Effects

>10%:

Cardiovascular: Edema

Central nervous system: Fever, chills, fatigue, pain

Dermatologic: Rash

Gastrointestinal: Mild nausea, vomiting, diarrhea, stomatitis, GI bleeding

Genitourinary: Urinary infection

Myelosuppression: Dose-limiting toxicity; myelosuppression may not be related to cumulative dose

Granulocyte nadir: 13 days (3-25)

Platelet nadir: 16 days (2-32)

WBC nadir: 8 days

Recovery: 5-7 weeks

Neuromuscular & skeletal: Paresthesia, myalgia, weakness

Respiratory: Manifested as dyspnea and a nonproductive cough; lung biopsy has shown pneumonitis in some patients, pneumonia

Miscellaneous: Infection

1% to 10%:

Cardiovascular: Congestive heart failure

Central nervous system: Malaise, headache

Dermatologic: Alopecia

Endocrine & metabolic: Hyperglycemia

Gastrointestinal: Anorexia

Otic: Hearing loss

<1%:

Central nervous system: Reported with higher dose levels; most patients shown to have CNS demyelination; somnolence also noted; severe neurotoxicity

Endocrine & metabolic: Metabolic acidosis

Gastrointestinal: Metallic taste

Hepatic: Reversible hepatotoxicity

Renal: Renal failure, hematuria, increased serum creatinine

Respiratory: Interstitial pneumonitis

Miscellaneous: Tumor lysis syndrome

Drug Uptake

Absorption: Oral preparation is under study

Serum half-life, elimination: 2-fluoro-vidarabine: 9 hours

Pregnancy Risk Factor D

Fludrocortisone Acetate (floo droe kor' ti sone as' e tate)

Brand Names Florinef® Acetate

Therapeutic Category Mineralocorticoid

Use Partial replacement therapy for primary and secondary adrenocortical insufficiency in Addison's disease; treatment of salt-losing adrenogenital syndrome

Usual Dosage Adults: Oral: 0.1-0.2 mg/day with ranges of 0.1 mg 3 times/week to 0.2 mg/day

(Continued)

Fludrocortisone Acetate *(Continued)*

Mechanism of Action Promotes increased reabsorption of sodium and loss of potassium from renal distal tubules

Local Anesthetic/Vasoconstrictor Precautions No information available to require special precautions

Effects on Dental Treatment No effects or complications reported

Other Adverse Effects 1% to 10%:
Cardiovascular: Hypertension, edema, congestive heart failure
Central nervous system: Convulsions, headache, sweating, dizziness
Dermatologic: Acne, rash
Endocrine & metabolic: Hypokalemic alkalosis, suppression of growth, hyperglycemia, HPA suppression
Gastrointestinal: Peptic ulcer
Hematologic: Bruising
Neuromuscular & skeletal: Muscle weakness
Ocular: Cataracts

Drug Interactions
Decreased corticosteroid effects by rifampin, barbiturates, and hydantoins

Drug Uptake
Absorption: Rapid and complete from GI tract, partially absorbed through skin
Serum half-life:
Plasma: 30-35 minutes
Biological: 18-36 hours
Time to peak serum concentration: Within 1.7 hours

Pregnancy Risk Factor C

Flufenacina (Mexico) *see* Fluphenazine *on page 379*
Flu-Imune® *see* Influenza Virus Vaccine *on page 458*
Flumadine® *see* Rimantadine Hydrochloride *on page 771*

Flumazenil (floo′ may ze nil)

Brand Names Romazicon™

Canadian/Mexican Brand Names Anexate® (Canada); Lanexat® (Mexico)

Therapeutic Category Antidote, Benzodiazepine

Use Benzodiazepine antagonist - reverses sedative effects of benzodiazepines used in general anesthesia; for management of benzodiazepine overdose; flumazenil does **not** antagonize the CNS effects of other GABA agonists (such as ethanol, barbiturates, or general anesthetics), **does not** reverse narcotics

Usual Dosage See table.
Resedation: Repeated doses may be given at 20-minute intervals as needed; repeat treatment doses of 1 mg (at a rate of 0.5 mg/minute) should be given at any time and no more than 3 mg should be given in any hour. After intoxication with high doses of benzodiazepines, the duration of a single dose of flumazenil is not expected to exceed 1 hour; if desired, the period of wakefulness may be prolonged with repeated low intravenous doses of flumazenil, or by an infusion of 0.1-0.4 mg/hour. Most patients with benzodiazepine overdose will respond to a cumulative dose of 1-3 mg and doses >3 mg do not reliably produce additional effects. Rarely, patients with a partial response at 3 mg may require additional titration up to a total dose of 5 mg. **If a patient has not responded 5 minutes after receiving a cumulative dose of 5 mg, the major cause of sedation is not likely to be due to benzodiazepines.**

Mechanism of Action Antagonizes the effect of benzodiazepines on the GABA/benzodiazepine receptor complex. Flumazenil is benzodiazepine specific and does not antagonize other nonbenzodiazepine GABA agonists (including ethanol, barbiturates, general anesthetics); flumazenil does not reverse the effects of opiates

Local Anesthetic/Vasoconstrictor Precautions No information available to require special precautions

Effects on Dental Treatment No effects or complications reported

Other Adverse Effects
>10%:
Central nervous system: Dizziness
Gastrointestinal: Vomiting, nausea
1% to 10%:
Central nervous system: Headache, asthenia, malaise, anxiety, nervousness, insomnia, abnormal crying, euphoria, depression, increased sweating disorders
Endocrine & metabolic: Hot flushes
Gastrointestinal: Dry mouth

Local: Pain at injection site
Neuromuscular & skeletal: Tremor
Respiratory: Dyspnea, hyperventilation
<1%:
Cardiovascular: Bradycardia, tachycardia, chest pain, hypertension, ventricular extrasystoles, altered blood pressure (increases and decreases)
Central nervous system: Anxiety and sensation of coldness, generalized convulsions, withdrawal syndrome, shivering, somnolence
Otic: Abnormal hearing
Miscellaneous: Thick tongue, hiccups

Flumazenil

Pediatric Dosage	
Further studies are needed	
Pediatric dosage for **reversal of conscious sedation:** Intravenously through a freely running intravenous infusion into a large vein to minimize pain at the injection site	
Initial dose	0.01 mg/kg over 15 seconds (maximum dose of 0.2 mg)
Repeat doses	0.005-0.01 mg/kg (maximum dose of 0.2 mg) repeated at 1-minute intervals
Maximum total cumulative dose	1 mg
Pediatric dosage for **management of benzodiazepine overdose** Intravenously through a freely running intravenous infusion into a large vein to minimize pain at the injection site	
Initial dose	0.01 mg/kg (maximum dose: 2 mg)
Repeat doses	0.01 mg/kg (maximum dose of 0.2 mg) repeated at 1-minute intervals
Maximum total cumulative dose	1 mg
In place of repeat bolus doses, follow-up continuous infusions of 0.005-0.01 mg/kg/hour have been used; further studies are needed	

Adult Dosage	
Adult dosage for **reversal of conscious sedation:** Intravenously through a freely running intravenous infusion into a large vein to minimize pain at the injection site	
Initial dose	0.2 mg intravenously over 15 seconds
Repeat doses	If desired level of consciousness is not obtained, 0.2 mg may be repeated at 1-minute intervals
Maximum total cumulative dose	1 mg (usual dose 0.6-1 mg) **In the event of resedation:** repeat doses may be given at 20-minute intervals with maximum of 1 mg/dose and 3 mg/hour
Adult dosage for **suspected benzodiazepine overdose:** Intravenously through a freely running intravenous infusion into a large vein to minimize pain at the injection site	
Initial dose	0.2 mg intravenously over 30 seconds
Repeat doses	0.5 mg over 30 seconds repeated at 1-minute intervals
Maximum total cumulative dose	3 mg (usual dose 1-3 mg) Patients with a partial response at 3 mg may require additional titration up to a total dose of 5 mg. If a patient has not responded 5 minutes after cumulative dose of 5 mg, the major cause of sedation is not likely due to benzodiazepines. **In the event of resedation:** may repeat doses at 20-minute intervals with maximum of 1 mg/dose and 3 mg/hour

Drug Interactions Increased toxicity:
Use with caution in overdosage involving mixed drug overdose
Toxic effects may emerge (especially with cyclic antidepressants) with the reversal of the benzodiazepine effect by flumazenil
Drug Uptake
Onset of action: 1-3 minutes; 80% response within 3 minutes
(Continued)

Flumazenil *(Continued)*

Peak effect: 6-10 minutes

Duration: Resedation occurs usually within 1 hour; duration is related to dose given and benzodiazepine plasma concentrations; reversal effects of flumazenil may wear off before effects of benzodiazepine

Serum half-life, adults:

Alpha: 7-15 minutes

Terminal: 41-79 minutes

Pregnancy Risk Factor C

Dosage Forms Injection: 0.1 mg/mL (5 mL, 10 mL)

Generic Available No

Flunisolide (floo nis' oh lide)

Related Information

Respiratory Diseases *on page 924*

Brand Names AeroBid®; AeroBid-M®; Nasalide®

Canadian/Mexican Brand Names Bronalide® (Canada); Rhinalar® (Canada); Rhinaris-F® (Canada); Syn-Flunisolide® (Canada)

Therapeutic Category Anti-inflammatory Agent; Corticosteroid, Inhalant

Use Steroid-dependent asthma; nasal solution is used for seasonal or perennial rhinitis

Usual Dosage

Children >6 years:

Oral inhalation: 2 inhalations twice daily (morning and evening) up to 4 inhalations/day

Nasal: 1 spray each nostril twice daily (morning and evening), not to exceed 4 sprays/day each nostril

Adults:

Oral inhalation: 2 inhalations twice daily (morning and evening) up to 8 inhalations/day maximum

Nasal: 2 sprays each nostril twice daily (morning and evening); maximum dose: 8 sprays/day in each nostril

Mechanism of Action Decreases inflammation by suppression of migration of polymorphonuclear leukocytes and reversal of increased capillary permeability; does not depress hypothalamus

Local Anesthetic/Vasoconstrictor Precautions No information available to require special precautions

Effects on Dental Treatment No effects or complications reported

Other Adverse Effects

>10%:

Cardiovascular: Pounding heartbeat

Central nervous system: Dizziness, headache, nervousness

Dermatologic: Itching, skin rash

Endocrine & metabolic: Adrenal suppression, menstrual problems

Gastrointestinal: GI irritation, anorexia

Local: Nasal burning, nasal congestion, nasal dryness, sore throat, bitter taste, *Candida* infections of the nose or pharynx, atrophic rhinitis

Respiratory: Sneezing, coughing, upper respiratory tract infection, bronchitis

Miscellaneous: Increased susceptibility to infections

1% to 10%:

Central nervous system: Insomnia, psychic changes

Dermatologic: Acne, hives

Gastrointestinal: Increase in appetite, dry mouth/throat

Ocular: Cataracts

Miscellaneous: Epistaxis, diaphoresis, loss of smell/taste

<1%:

Gastrointestinal: Abdominal fullness

Respiratory: Bronchospasm, shortness of breath

Drug Interactions No data reported

Drug Uptake

Absorption: Nasal inhalation: ~50%

Serum half-life: 1.8 hours

Pregnancy Risk Factor C

Fluocinolona, Acetonido De (Mexico) *see* Fluocinolone Acetonide *on this page*

Fluocinolone Acetonide (floo oh sin' oh lone a set' oh nide)

Related Information

Corticosteroids, Topical Comparison *on page 1018*

Brand Names Derma-Smoothe/FS®; Fluonid®; Flurosyn®; FS Shampoo®; Synalar®; Synalar-HP®; Synemol®

Canadian/Mexican Brand Names Lidemol® (Canada); Cremisona® (Mexico); Synalar® Simple (Mexico)

Therapeutic Category Corticosteroid, Topical (Medium Potency)

Synonyms Fluocinolona, Acetonido De (Mexico)

Use Relief of susceptible inflammatory dermatosis [low, medium, high potency topical corticosteroid]

Usual Dosage Children and Adults: Topical: Apply a thin layer to affected area 2-4 times/day

Mechanism of Action A synthetic corticosteroid which differs structurally from triamcinolone acetonide in the presence of an additional fluorine atom in the 6-alpha position on the steroid nucleus. The mechanism of action for all topical corticosteroids is not well defined, however, is believed to be a combination of three important properties: anti-inflammatory activity, immunosuppressive properties, and antiproliferative actions.

Local Anesthetic/Vasoconstrictor Precautions No information available to require special precautions

Effects on Dental Treatment No effects or complications reported

Other Adverse Effects <1%:
Dermatologic: Acne, hypopigmentation, allergic dermatitis, maceration of the skin, skin atrophy, folliculitis, hypertrichosis
Endocrine & metabolic: HPA suppression, Cushing's syndrome, growth retardation
Local: Burning, itching, irritation, dryness
Miscellaneous: Secondary infection

Drug Interactions No data reported

Drug Uptake
Absorption: Dependent on strength of preparation, amount applied,and nature of skin at application site; ranges from ~1% in thick stratum corneum areas (palms, soles, elbows, etc) to 36% in areas of thinnest stratum corneum (face, eyelids, etc); increased absorption in areas of skin damage, inflammation, or occlusion

Pregnancy Risk Factor C

Fluocinonide (floo oh sin' oh nide)
Related Information
Corticosteroids, Topical Comparison *on page 1018*
Oral Nonviral Soft Tissue Ulcerations or Erosions *on page 955*

Brand Names Fluonex®; Lidex®; Lidex-E®

Canadian/Mexican Brand Names Lyderm® (Canada); Topactin® (Canada); Topsyn® (Canada); Gelisyn® (Mexico)

Therapeutic Category Corticosteroid, Topical (High Potency)

Synonyms Fluocinonido (Mexico)

Use Anti-inflammatory, antipruritic, relief of inflammatory and pruritic manifestations [high potency topical corticosteroid]

Usual Dosage Children and Adults: Topical: Apply thin layer to affected area 2-4 times/day depending on the severity of the condition

Mechanism of Action Not well defined for all topical corticosteroids; however, is felt to be a combination of three important properties: anti-inflammatory activity, immunosuppressive properties, and antiproliferative actions.

Local Anesthetic/Vasoconstrictor Precautions No information available to require special precautions

Effects on Dental Treatment No effects or complications reported

Other Adverse Effects <1%:
Central nervous system: Intracranial hypertension
Dermatologic: Acne, hypopigmentation, allergic dermatitis, maceration of the skin, skin atrophy
Endocrine & metabolic: HPA suppression, Cushing's syndrome, growth retardation
Local: Burning, itching, irritation, dryness, folliculitis, hypertrichosis
Miscellaneous: Secondary infection

Drug Interactions No data reported

Drug Uptake
Absorption: Dependent on amount applied and nature of skin at application site; ranges from ~1% in areas of thick stratum corneum (palms, soles, elbows, etc) to 36% in areas of thin stratum corneum (face, eyelids, etc); absorption is increased in areas of skin damage, inflammation, or occlusion

Pregnancy Risk Factor C

Dosage Forms Ointment, topical (Lidex®): 0.05% (15 g, 30 g, 60 g, 120 g)

Fluocinonido (Mexico) *see Fluocinonide on previous page*
Fluogen® *see Influenza Virus Vaccine on page 458*
Fluonex® *see Fluocinonide on previous page*
Fluonid® *see Fluocinolone Acetonide on page 372*
Fluoracaine® *see Proparacaine and Fluorescein on page 736*

Fluoride (flur′ ide)

Related Information
Dentin Hypersensitivity; High Caries Index; Xerostomia *on page 959*
Patients Undergoing Cancer Therapy *on page 967*

Brand Names ACT® [OTC]; Fluorigard® [OTC]; Fluorinse®; Fluoritab®; Flura®; Flura-Drops®; Flura-Loz®; Gel Kam®; Gel-Tin® [OTC]; Karidium®; Karigel®; Karigel®-N; Listermint® with Fluoride [OTC]; Luride®; Luride® Lozi-Tab®; Luride®-SF Lozi-Tab®; Minute-Gel®; Pediaflor®; Pharmaflur®; Phos-Flur®; Point-Two®; PreviDent®; Stop® [OTC]; Thera-Flur®; Thera-Flur-N®

Therapeutic Category Fluoride; Mineral, Oral; Mineral, Oral Topical

Synonyms Acidulated Phosphate Fluoride; Sodium Fluoride; Stannous Fluoride

Use
Dental: Prevention of dental caries

Usual Dosage Oral:
Recommended daily fluoride supplement (2.2 mg of sodium fluoride is equivalent to 1 mg of fluoride ion): See table.

Fluoride Ion

Fluoride Content of Drinking Water	Daily Dose, Oral (mg)
<0.3 ppm	
Birth - 6 mo	None
6 mo - 3 y	0.25
3-6 y	0.5
6 y	1.0
0.3-0.7 ppm	
Birth - 6 mo	0
6 mo - 3 y	0.125
3-6 y	0.25
6 y	0.5

Dental rinse or gel:
Adults: 10 mL rinse or apply to teeth and spit daily after brushing
Children 6-12 years: 5-10 mL rinse or apply to teeth and spit daily after brushing

Mechanism of Action Promotes remineralization of decalcified enamel; inhibits the cariogenic microbial process in dental plaque; increases tooth resistance to acid dissolution

Local Anesthetic/Vasoconstrictor Precautions No information available to require special precautions

Effects on Dental Treatment No effects or complications reported

Other Adverse Effects <1%:
Dermatologic: Rash
Gastrointestinal: Nausea, vomiting
Miscellaneous: Products containing stannous fluoride may stain the teeth

Oral manifestations: No data reported

Contraindications Hypersensitivity to fluoride or any component, or when fluoride content of drinking water exceeds 0.7 ppm

Warnings/Precautions Prolonged ingestion with excessive doses may result in dental fluorosis and osseous changes; do **not** exceed recommended dosage; some products contain tartrazine

Drug Interactions Decreased effect/absorption with magnesium-, aluminum-, and calcium-containing products

Drug Uptake
Absorption: Rapid and complete from GI tract; calcium, iron, or magnesium may delay absorption
Time to peak serum concentration: 30-60 minutes

Pregnancy Risk Factor C

Breast-feeding Considerations No data reported

Dosage Forms Fluoride ion content listed in brackets

Drops, oral, as sodium:
  Fluoritab®, Flura-Drops®: 0.55 mg/drop [0.25 mg/drop] (22.8 mL, 24 mL)
  Karidium®, Luride®: 0.275 mg/drop [0.125 mg/drop] (30 mL, 60 mL)
  Pediaflor®: 1.1 mg/mL [0.5 mg/mL] (50 mL)
Gel, topical:
  Acidulated phosphate fluoride (Minute-Gel®): 1.23% (480 mL)
  Sodium fluoride (Karigel®, Karigel®-N, PreviDent®): 1.1% [0.5%] (24 g, 30 g, 60 g, 120 g, 130 g, 250 g)
  Stannous fluoride (Gel Kam®, Gel-Tin®, Stop®): 0.4% [0.1%] (60 g, 65 g, 105 g, 120 g)
Lozenge, as sodium (Flura-Loz®) (raspberry flavor): 2.2 mg [1 mg]
Rinse, topical, as sodium:
  ACT®, Fluorigard®: 0.05% [0.02%] (90 mL, 180 mL, 300 mL, 360 mL, 480 mL)
  Fluorinse®, Point-Two®: 0.2% [0.09%] (240 mL, 480 mL, 3780 mL)
  Listermint® with Fluoride: 0.02% [0.01%] (180 mL, 300 mL, 360 mL, 480 mL, 540 mL, 720 mL, 960 mL, 1740 mL)
Solution, oral, as sodium (Phos-Flur®): 0.44 mg/mL [0.2 mg/mL] (250 mL, 500 mL, 3780 mL)
Tablet, as sodium:
  Chewable:
    Fluoritab®, Luride® Lozi-Tab®, Pharmaflur®: 1.1 mg [0.5 mg]
    Fluoritab®, Karidium®, Luride® Lozi-Tab®, Luride®-SF Lozi-Tab®, Pharmaflur®: 2.2 mg [1 mg]
  Oral: Flura®, Karidium®: 2.2 mg [1 mg]

Dietary Considerations Do not administer with milk; do **not** allow eating or drinking for 30 minutes after use

Generic Available Yes

Comments Neutral pH fluoride preparations are preferred in patients with oral mucositis to reduce tissue irritation; long-term use of acidulated fluorides has been associated with enamel demineralization and damage to porcelain crowns

Fluorigard® [OTC] see Fluoride on previous page

Fluori-Methane® see Dichlorodifluoromethane and Trichloromonofluoromethane on page 270

Fluorinse® see Fluoride on previous page

Fluoritab® see Fluoride on previous page

Fluorodeoxyuridine see Floxuridine on page 366

Fluorometholone (flure oh meth' oh lone)
Related Information
  Corticosteroids, Topical Comparison on page 1018
Brand Names Flarex®; Fluor-Op®; FML®; FML® Forte
Therapeutic Category Anti-inflammatory Agent, Ophthalmic; Corticosteroid, Ophthalmic
Use Inflammatory conditions of the eye, including keratitis, iritis, cyclitis, and conjunctivitis
Usual Dosage Children >2 years and Adults: Ophthalmic:
  Ointment: May be applied every 4 hours in severe cases; 1-3 times/day in mild to moderate cases
  Solution: Instill 1-2 drops into conjunctival sac every hour during day, every 2 hours at night until favorable response is obtained, then use 1 drop every 4 hours; for mild to moderate inflammation, instill 1-2 drops into conjunctival sac 2-4 times/day
Mechanism of Action Decreases inflammation by suppression of migration of polymorphonuclear leukocytes and reversal of increased capillary permeability
Local Anesthetic/Vasoconstrictor Precautions No information available to require special precautions
Effects on Dental Treatment No effects or complications reported
Other Adverse Effects
  1% to 10%: Ophthalmic: Blurred vision
  <1%: Ophthalmic: Stinging, burning, increased intraocular pressure, open-angle glaucoma, defect in visual acuity and field of vision, cataracts
Drug Interactions No data reported
Drug Uptake Absorption: Into aqueous humor with slight systemic absorption
Pregnancy Risk Factor C

Fluor-Op® see Fluorometholone on this page

Fluoroplex® Topical see Fluorouracil on next page

Fluorouracil (flure oh yoor' a sil)

Brand Names Adrucil® Injection; Efudex® Topical; Fluoroplex® Topical

Canadian/Mexican Brand Names Efudix® (Mexico); Fluoro-uracil® (Mexico)

Therapeutic Category Antineoplastic Agent, Antimetabolite

Synonyms 5-Fluorouracil; 5-FU

Use Treatment of carcinoma of stomach, colon, rectum, breast, and pancreas; also used topically for management of multiple actinic keratoses and superficial basal cell carcinomas

Usual Dosage Refer to individual protocols

All dosages are based on the patient's actual weight. However, the estimated lean body mass (dry weight) is used if the patient is obese or if there has been a spurious weight gain due to edema, ascites or other forms of abnormal fluid retention.

Children and Adults:

I.V.: Initial: 400-500 mg/m^2/day (12 mg/kg/day; maximum: 800 mg/day) for 4-5 days either as a single daily I.V. push or 4-day continuous intravenous infusion

I.V.: Maintenance dose regimens:

200-250 mg/m^2 (6 mg/kg) every other day for 4 days repeated in 4 weeks

500-600 mg/m^2 (15 mg/kg) weekly as a continuous intravenous infusion or I.V. push

I.V.: Concomitant with leucovorin:

370 mg/m^2/day for 5 days

500-1000 mg/m^2 every 2 weeks

600 mg/m^2/week for 6 weeks

Although the manufacturer recommends no daily dose >800 mg, higher doses of up to 2 g/day are routinely administered by continuous intravenous infusion; by continuous intravenous infusion, higher daily doses have been successfully used

Hemodialysis: Administer dose posthemodialysis

Dosing adjustment/comments in hepatic impairment: Bilirubin >5 mg/dL: Omit use

Topical:

Actinic or solar keratosis: Apply twice daily for 2-6 weeks

Superficial basal cell carcinomas: Apply 5% twice daily for at least 3-6 weeks and up to 10-12 weeks

Mechanism of Action A pyrimidine antimetabolite that interferes with DNA synthesis by blocking the methylation of deoxyuricytic acid; 5-FU rapidly enters the cell and is activated to the nucleotide level; there it inhibits thymidylate synthetase (TS), or is incorporated into RNA (most evident during the GI phase of the cell cycle). The reduced folate cofactor is required for tight binding to occur between the 5-FdUMP and TS.

Local Anesthetic/Vasoconstrictor Precautions No information available to require special precautions

Effects on Dental Treatment No effects or complications reported

Other Adverse Effects Toxicity depends on route and duration of infusion

Irritant chemotherapy

>10%:

Dermatologic: Dermatitis, alopecia

Gastrointestinal (route and schedule dependent): Heartburn, stomatitis, nausea, vomiting, esophagitis, anorexia, and diarrhea; bolus dosing produces milder GI problems, while continuous infusion tends to produce severe mucositis and diarrhea; emesis is moderate, occurring in 30% to 60% of patients, and responds well to phenothiazines and dexamethasone

Emetic potential:

<1000 mg: Moderately low (10% to 30%)

≥1000 mg: Moderate (30% to 60%)

1% to 10%:

Dermatologic: Dry skin

Gastrointestinal: GI ulceration

Myelosuppressive: Granulocytopenia occurs around 9-14 days after 5-FU and thrombocytopenia around 7-17 days. The marrow recovers after 22 days. Myelosuppression tends to be more pronounced in patients receiving bolus dosing of 5-FU.

WBC: Mild to moderate

Platelets: Mild

Onset (days): 7-10

Nadir (days): 14

Recovery (days): 21

<1%:

Cardiovascular: Chest pain, EKG changes similar to ischemic changes, and possibly cardiac enzyme abnormalities. Usually occurs within the first 2 days of therapy, and may resolve with nitroglycerin and calcium channel blockers. May be due to coronary vessel vasospasm induced by 5-FU.

Central nervous system: Headache, cerebellar ataxia, tingling of hands; somnolence, ataxia are seen primarily in intracarotid arterial infusions for head and neck tumors; this is believed to be caused by fluorocitrate, a neurotoxic metabolite of the parent compound

Dermatologic: Alopecia, hyperpigmentation of nailbeds, face, hands, and veins used in infusion; photosensitization with UV light; palmar-plantar syndrome; hand-foot syndrome, pruritic maculopapular rash

Hematologic: Coagulopathy

Hepatic: Hepatotoxicity

Ocular: Conjunctivitis, tear duct stenosis, excessive lacrimation, visual disturbances

Respiratory: Shortness of breath

Drug Uptake

Absorption: Oral: Erratic and rarely used

Serum half-life (biphasic): Initial: 6-20 minutes; doses of 400-600 mg/m^2 produce drug concentrations above the threshold for cytotoxicity for normal tissue and remain there for 6 hours; 2 metabolites, FdUMP and FUTP, have prolonged half-lives depending on the type of tissue; the clinical effect of these metabolites has not been determined

Pregnancy Risk Factor D (injection); X (topical)

Comments Myelosuppressive effects:

WBC: Mild

Platelets: Mild

Onset (days): 7-10

Nadir (days): 9-14

Recovery (days): 21

5-Fluorouracil see Fluorouracil on previous page

Fluoxetina Clorhidrato De (Mexico) see Fluoxetine Hydrochloride on this page

Fluoxetine Hydrochloride (floo ox' e teen hye droe klor' ide)

Related Information

Vasoconstrictor Interactions With Antidepressants on page 1108

Brand Names Prozac®

Canadian/Mexican Brand Names Fluoxac® (Mexico)

Therapeutic Category Antidepressant, Selective Serotonin Reuptake Inhibitor

Synonyms Fluoxetina Clorhidrato De (Mexico)

Use Treatment of major depression

Usual Dosage Oral:

Children <18 years: Dose and safety not established; preliminary experience in children 6-14 years using initial doses of 20 mg/day have been reported

Adults: 20 mg/day in the morning; may increase after several weeks by 20 mg/day increments; maximum: 80 mg/day; doses >20 mg should be divided into morning and noon doses

Usual dosage range:

20-80 mg/day for depression and OCD

20-60 mg/day for obesity

60-80 mg/day for bulimia nervosa

Note: Lower doses of 5 mg/day have been used for initial treatment

Elderly: Some patients may require an initial dose of 10 mg/day with dosage increases of 10 and 20 mg every several weeks as tolerated; should not be taken at night unless patient experiences sedation

Mechanism of Action Inhibits CNS neuron serotonin uptake; minimal or no effect on reuptake of norepinephrine or dopamine; does not significantly bind to alpha-adrenergic, histamine or cholinergic receptors; may therefore be useful in patients at risk from sedation, hypotension, and anticholinergic effects of tricyclic antidepressants

Local Anesthetic/Vasoconstrictor Precautions Although caution should be used in patients taking tricyclic antidepressants, no interactions have been reported with vasoconstrictors and fluoxetine, a nontricyclic antidepressant which acts to increase serotonin

Effects on Dental Treatment No effects or complications reported

Other Adverse Effects Predominant adverse effects are CNS and GI

(Continued)

Fluoxetine Hydrochloride *(Continued)*

>10%:
 Central nervous system: Headache, nervousness, insomnia, drowsiness
 Gastrointestinal: Nausea, diarrhea, dry mouth

1% to 10%:
 Central nervous system: Anxiety, dizziness, fatigue, sedation
 Dermatologic: Rash, pruritus
 Endocrine & metabolic: SIADH, hypoglycemia, hyponatremia (elderly or volume-depleted patients)
 Gastrointestinal: Anorexia, dyspepsia, constipation
 Neuromuscular & skeletal: Tremor
 Miscellaneous: Excessive sweating

<1%:
 Central nervous system: Extrapyramidal reactions (rare)
 Ocular: Visual disturbances
 Miscellaneous: Anaphylactoid reactions, allergies, suicidal ideation

Drug Interactions
 Increased/decreased effect of lithium (both increases and decreases level has been reported)
 Increased toxicity of diazepam, trazodone via decreased clearance; increased toxicity with MAO inhibitors (hyperpyrexia, tremors, seizures, delirium, coma)
 Displace protein bound drugs

Drug Uptake
 Peak antidepressant effect: After >4 weeks
 Absorption: Oral: Well absorbed
 Serum half-life: Adults: 2-3 days; due to long half-life, resolution of adverse reactions after discontinuation may be slow
 Time to peak serum concentration: Within 4-8 hours

Pregnancy Risk Factor B

Fluoximesterona (Mexico) *see* Fluoxymesterone *on this page*

Fluoxymesterone (floo ox i mes' te rone)

Brand Names Halotestin®
Canadian/Mexican Brand Names Stenox® (Mexico)
Therapeutic Category Androgen
Synonyms Fluoximesterona (Mexico)
Use Replacement of endogenous testicular hormone; in female used as palliative treatment of breast cancer, postpartum breast engorgement

Usual Dosage Adults: Oral:
 Male:
  Hypogonadism: 5-20 mg/day
  Delayed puberty: 2.5-20 mg/day for 4-6 months
 Female:
  Inoperable breast carcinoma: 10-40 mg/day in divided doses for 1-3 months
  Breast engorgement: 2.5 mg after delivery, 5-10 mg/day in divided doses for 4-5 days

Mechanism of Action Synthetic androgenic anabolic hormone responsible for the normal growth and development of male sex organs and maintenance of secondary sex characteristics; stimulates RNA polymerase activity resulting in an increase in protein production; increases bone development

Local Anesthetic/Vasoconstrictor Precautions No information available to require special precautions

Effects on Dental Treatment No effects or complications reported

Other Adverse Effects
 >10%:
  Males: Priapism
  Females: Menstrual problems (amenorrhea), virilism, breast soreness
  Dermatologic: Edema, acne

 1% to 10%:
  Males: Prostatic carcinoma, hirsutism (increase in pubic hair growth), impotence, testicular atrophy
  Dermatologic: Edema
  Gastrointestinal: GI irritation, nausea, vomiting, prostatic hypertrophy
  Hepatic: Hepatic dysfunction

 <1%:
  Males: Gynecomastia
  Females: Amenorrhea
  Endocrine & metabolic: Hypercalcemia
  Hematologic: Leukopenia, polycythemia
  Hepatic: Hepatic necrosis, cholestatic hepatitis

Miscellaneous: Hypersensitivity reactions
Drug Interactions
Decreased blood glucose concentrations and insulin requirements in patients with diabetes
Increased effect of oral anticoagulants
Drug Uptake
Absorption: Oral: Rapid
Serum half-life: 10-100 minutes
Pregnancy Risk Factor X

Fluoxymesterone and Estradiol *see* Ethinyl Estradiol and Fluoxymesterone *on page 337*

Fluphenazine (floo fen' a zeen)

Brand Names Permitil®; Prolixin®; Prolixin Decanoate®; Prolixin Enanthate®
Canadian/Mexican Brand Names Modecate® [Fluphenazine Decanoate] (Canada); Modecate® Enanthate [Fluphenazine Enanthate] (Canada); Apo-Fluphenazine® [Hydrochloride] (Canada); Moditen® Hydrochloride (Canada); PMS-Fluphenazine® [Hydrochloride] (Canada)
Therapeutic Category Antipsychotic Agent; Phenothiazine Derivative
Synonyms Flufenacina (Mexico)
Use Management of manifestations of psychotic disorders
Usual Dosage Adults:
Oral: 0.5-10 mg/day in divided doses at 6- to 8-hour intervals; some patients may require up to 40 mg/day
I.M.: 2.5-10 mg/day in divided doses at 6- to 8-hour intervals (parenteral dose is $\frac{1}{3}$ to $\frac{1}{2}$ the oral dose for the hydrochloride salts)
I.M., S.C. (decanoate): 12.5 mg every 3 weeks
Conversion from hydrochloride to decanoate I.M. 0.5 mL (12.5 mg) decanoate every 3 weeks is approximately equivalent to 10 mg hydrochloride/day
I.M., S.C. (enanthate): 12.5-25 mg every 3 weeks

Not dialyzable (0% to 5%)

Mechanism of Action Blocks postsynaptic mesolimbic dopaminergic D_1 and D_2 receptors in the brain; exhibits a strong alpha-adrenergic blocking and anticholinergic effect, depresses the release of hypothalamic and hypophyseal hormones; believed to depress the reticular activating system thus affecting basal metabolism, body temperature, wakefulness, vasomotor tone, and emesis
Local Anesthetic/Vasoconstrictor Precautions No information available to require special precautions
Effects on Dental Treatment Orthostatic hypotension and nasal congestion possible in dental patients. Since the drug is a dopamine antagonist, extrapyramidal symptoms of the TMJ a possibility.
Other Adverse Effects
>10%:
Cardiovascular: Orthostatic hypotension, hypotension, tachycardia, arrhythmias
Central nervous system: Parkinsonian symptoms, akathisia, dystonias, tardive dyskinesia (persistent), dizziness
Gastrointestinal: Constipation
Ocular: Pigmentary retinopathy
Respiratory: Nasal congestion
Miscellaneous: Decreased sweating
1% to 10%:
Central nervous system: Dizziness
Dermatologic: Increased sensitivity to sun, skin rash
Endocrine & metabolic: Changes in menstrual cycle pain in breasts, amenorrhea, galactorrhea, gynecomastia, changes in libido
Gastrointestinal: Weight gain, nausea, vomiting, stomach pain
Genitourinary: Difficulty in urination, ejaculatory disturbances
Neuromuscular & skeletal: Trembling of fingers
<1%:
Central nervous system: Sedation, drowsiness, restlessness, anxiety, extrapyramidal reactions, pseudoparkinsonian signs and symptoms, seizures, altered central temperature regulation
Dermatologic: Photosensitivity, hyperpigmentation, pruritus, rash, discoloration of skin (blue-gray)
Endocrine & metabolic: Galactorrhea
Gastrointestinal: GI upset, dry mouth, constipation
Genitourinary: Priapism, urinary retention
(Continued)

Fluphenazine *(Continued)*

Hematologic: Agranulocytosis (more often in women between 4th and 10th weeks of therapy); leukopenia (usually in patients with large doses for prolonged periods)

Hepatic: Cholestatic jaundice, hepatotoxicity

Ocular: Retinal pigmentation, cornea and lens changes, blurred vision

Drug Interactions

Decreased effect: Barbiturate levels and decreased fluphenazine effectiveness when given together

Increased toxicity: With ethanol, effects of both drugs may be increased; EPSEs and other CNS effects may be increased when coadministered with lithium; may potentiate the effects of narcotics including respiratory depression

Drug Uptake

Following I.M. or S.C. administration (derivative dependent):

Decanoate (lasts the longest and requires more time for onset):

Onset of action: 24-72 hours

Hydrochloride salt (acts quickly and persists briefly):

Onset of action: Within 1 hour

Duration: 6-8 hours

Serum half-life: Derivative dependent:

Enanthate: 84-96 hours

Hydrochloride: 33 hours

Decanoate: 163-232 hours

Pregnancy Risk Factor C

Flura® *see Fluoride on page 374*

Flura-Drops® *see Fluoride on page 374*

Flura-Loz® *see Fluoride on page 374*

Flurandrenolide *(flure an dren' oh lide)*

Related Information

Corticosteroids, Topical Comparison *on page 1018*

Brand Names Cordran®; Cordran® SP

Canadian/Mexican Brand Names Drenison® (Canada)

Therapeutic Category Corticosteroid, Topical (Medium Potency)

Use Inflammation of corticosteroid-responsive dermatoses [medium potency topical corticosteroid]

Usual Dosage Topical:

Children:

Ointment, cream: Apply sparingly 1-2 times/day

Tape: Apply once daily

Adults: Cream, lotion, ointment: Apply sparingly 2-3 times/day

Mechanism of Action Decreases inflammation by suppression of migration of polymorphonuclear leukocytes and reversal of increased capillary permeability

Local Anesthetic/Vasoconstrictor Precautions No information available to require special precautions

Effects on Dental Treatment No effects or complications reported

Other Adverse Effects <1%:

Systemic: HPA suppression, Cushing's syndrome, growth retardation, burning, secondary infection

Topical: Burning, itching, irritation, dryness, folliculitis, hypertrichosis, acneiform eruptions, hypopigmentation, perioral dermatitis, allergic contact dermatitis, skin atrophy, striae, miliaria; intracranial hypertension, acne, maceration of the skin

Drug Interactions No data reported

Drug Uptake

Absorption: Adequate with intact skin

Pregnancy Risk Factor C

Flurazepam Hydrochloride *(flure az' e pam hye droe klor' ide)*

Brand Names Dalmane®

Canadian/Mexican Brand Names Apo-Flurazepam® (Canada); Somnol® (Canada); Som Pam® (Canada); Novo-Flupam® (Canada); PMS-Flupam® (Canada)

Therapeutic Category Benzodiazepine; Hypnotic; Sedative

Use Short-term treatment of insomnia

Usual Dosage Oral:

Children:

<15 years: Dose not established

>15 years: 15 mg at bedtime
Adults: 15-30 mg at bedtime

Mechanism of Action Depresses all levels of the CNS, including the limbic and reticular formation, probably through the increased action of gamma-aminobutyric acid (GABA), which is a major inhibitory neurotransmitter in the brain

Local Anesthetic/Vasoconstrictor Precautions No information available to require special precautions

Effects on Dental Treatment No effects or complications reported

Other Adverse Effects
>10%:
Cardiovascular: Tachycardia, chest pain
Central nervous system: Drowsiness, fatigue, impaired coordination, light-headedness, memory impairment, insomnia, anxiety, depression, headache,
Dermatologic: Rash
Endocrine & metabolic: Decreased libido
Gastrointestinal: Dry mouth, constipation, decreased salivation, nausea, vomiting, diarrhea, increased or decreased appetite
Neuromuscular & skeletal: Dysarthria
Ocular: Blurred vision
Miscellaneous: Sweating
1% to 10%:
Cardiovascular: Syncope, hypotension
Central nervous system: Confusion, nervousness, dizziness, akathisia,
Dermatologic: Dermatitis
Gastrointestinal: Weight gain or loss, increased salivation
Neuromuscular & skeletal: Rigidity, tremor, muscle cramps
Otic: Tinnitus
Respiratory: Hyperventilation, nasal congestion
<1%:
Central nervous system: Reflex slowing
Endocrine & metabolic: Menstrual irregularities
Hematologic: Blood dyscrasias
Miscellaneous: Drug dependence

Drug Interactions
Decreased effect with enzyme inducers
Increased toxicity with other CNS depressants and cimetidine

Drug Uptake
Onset of hypnotic effect: 15-20 minutes
Peak: 3-6 hours
Duration of action: 7-8 hours
Serum half-life: Adults: 40-114 hours

Pregnancy Risk Factor X

Flurbiprofen Sodium (flure bi′ proe fen sow′ dee um)

Related Information
Dental Drug Interactions: Update on Drug Combinations Requiring Special Considerations *on page 1022*
Nonsteroidal Anti-Inflammatory Agents, Comparative Dosages, and Pharmacokinetics *on page 1021*
Rheumatoid Arthritis, Osteoarthritis, and Joint Prostheses *on page 930*
Temporomandibular Dysfunction (TMD) *on page 963*

Brand Names Ansaid®

Canadian/Mexican Brand Names Apro-Flurbiprofen® (Canada); Froben® (Canada); Froben-SR® (Canada); Novo-Flurprofen® (Canada); Nu-Flurprofen® (Canada)

Therapeutic Category Analgesic, Non-narcotic; Nonsteroidal Anti-inflammatory Agent (NSAID)

Use
Dental: Management of postoperative pain
Medical: Acute or long-term treatment of signs and symptoms of rheumatoid arthritis and osteoarthritis; ophthalmic preparation indicated for inhibition of intraoperative miosis

Usual Dosage Adults: Oral: 200-300 mg/day in 2, 3, or 4 divided doses

Mechanism of Action Inhibits prostaglandin synthesis by decreasing the activity of the enzyme, cyclo-oxygenase, which results in decreased formation of prostaglandin precursors

Local Anesthetic/Vasoconstrictor Precautions No information available to require special precautions

Effects on Dental Treatment No effects or complications reported
(Continued)

Flurbiprofen Sodium *(Continued)*

Other Adverse Effects >10%:
Central nervous system: Dizziness
Dermatologic: Rash
Gastrointestinal: Abdominal cramps, heartburn, indigestion, nausea

Oral manifestations: <1%: Dry mouth

Contraindications Hypersensitivity to flurbiprofen or any component

Warnings/Precautions Should be used with caution in patients affected by inhibition of platelet aggregation

Drug Interactions Has caused bleeding in combination with anticoagulants; when given concurrently with aspirin, has resulted in 50% lower serum levels of flurbiprofen

Drug Uptake
Absorption: Rapid and nearly complete
Onset of effect: Within 1 hour
Time to peak serum concentration: 1.5 hours
Duration of effect: 6-8 hours
Serum half-life: 6.5 hours
Influence of food: Food alters rate of absorption but not amount

Pregnancy Risk Factor B

Breast-feeding Considerations No data reported

Dosage Forms Tablet (Ansaid®): 50 mg, 100 mg

Dietary Considerations Can be taken with food, milk, or antacid to decrease GI effects

Generic Available Yes

Comments Flurbiprofen is a chiral NSAID with the S-(+) enantiomer possessing most of the beneficial anti-inflammatory activity; both the S-(+) and R-(-) enantiomers possess analgesic activity. All flurbiprofen preparations are marketed as the racemic mixture (equal parts of each enantiomer). Flurbiprofen may be effective in the treatment of periodontal disease. Animal studies have shown flurbiprofen in topical form to be effective in reducing loss of attachment and bone loss. Flurbiprofen as with other NSAIDs can be administered preoperatively in the patient undergoing dental surgery in order to delay the onset and severity of postoperative pain. Doses which have been used are 100 mg twice daily the day before procedure, and 50-100 mg 30 minutes before the procedure.

Selected Readings
Cooper SA, Mardirossian G, and Miles M, "Analgesic Relative Potency Assay Comparing Flurbiprofen 50, 100, and 150 mg, Aspirin 600 mg, and Placebo in Postsurgical Dental Pain," *Clin J Pain*, 1988, 4:175-81.

Dionne RA, "Suppression of Dental Pain by the Preoperative Administration of Flurbiprofen," *Am J Med*, 1986, 80(3A):41-9.

Forbes JA, Yorio CC, Selinger LR, et al, "An Evaluation of Flurbiprofen, Aspirin, and Placebo in Postoperative Oral Surgery Pain," *Pharmacotherapy*, 1989, 9(2):66-73.

Malmberg AB and Yaksh TL, "Antinociception Produced by Spinal Delivery of the S and R Enantiomers of Flurbiprofen in the Formalin Test," *Eur J Pharmacol*, 1994, 256(2):205-9.

5-Flurocytosine *see Flucytosine on page 368*

Fluro-Ethyl® Aerosol *see Ethyl Chloride and Dichlorotetrafluoroethane on page 344*

Flurosyn® *see Fluocinolone Acetonide on page 372*

Flutamide *(floo' ta mide)*

Brand Names Eulexin®

Canadian/Mexican Brand Names Fluken® (Mexico); Eulexin® (Mexico); Flulem (Mexico)

Therapeutic Category Antiandrogen

Use In combination with LHRH agonistic analogs for the treatment of metastatic prostatic carcinoma

Usual Dosage Adults: Oral: 2 capsules every 8 hours for a total daily dose of 750 mg

Mechanism of Action Nonsteroidal antiandrogen that inhibits androgen uptake or inhibits binding of androgen in target tissues

Local Anesthetic/Vasoconstrictor Precautions No information available to require special precautions

Effects on Dental Treatment No effects or complications reported

Other Adverse Effects
>10%:
Gastrointestinal: Nausea, vomiting, diarrhea
Genitourinary: Impotence
Endocrine & metabolic: Loss of libido, hot flashes

1% to 10%:
   Endocrine & metabolic: Gynecomastia
   Gastrointestinal: Anorexia
   Neuromuscular & skeletal: Numbness in extremities
<1%:
   Cardiovascular: Hypertension, edema
   Central nervous system: Drowsiness, nervousness, confusion
   Hepatic: Hepatitis
Drug Uptake
   Absorption: Rapid and complete
   Serum half-life: 5-6 hours
Pregnancy Risk Factor D
Comments To achieve benefit to combination therapy, both drugs need to be started simultaneously

Fluticasone Propionate (floo tik' a sone pro' pee oh nate)
Brand Names Cutivate™; Flonase™
Therapeutic Category Corticosteroid, Topical (Medium Potency)
Use
   Intranasal: Management of seasonal and perennial allergic rhinitis in patients ≥12 years of age
   Topical: Relief of inflammation and pruritus associated with corticosteroid-responsive dermatoses [medium potency topical corticosteroid]
Usual Dosage
   Adolescents:
      Topical: Apply sparingly in a thin film twice daily
      Intranasal: Initially 1 spray (50 mcg/spray) per nostril once daily. Patients not adequately responding or patients with more severe symptoms may use 2 sprays (200 mcg) per nostril. Depending on response, dosage may be reduced to 100 mcg daily. Total daily dosage should not exceed 4 sprays (200 mcg)/day.

   Adults:
      Topical: Apply sparingly in a thin film twice daily
      Intranasal: Initially 2 sprays (50 mcg/spray) per nostril once daily. After the first few days, dosage may be reduced to 1 spray per nostril once daily for maintenance therapy. Maximum total daily dose should not exceed 4 sprays (200 mcg)/day.

Mechanism of Action Fluticasone belongs to a new group of corticosteroids which utilizes a fluorocarbothioate ester linkage at the 17 carbon position; extremely potent vasoconstrictive and anti-inflammatory activity; has a weak hypothalamic -pituitary- adrenocortical axis (HPA) inhibitory potency when applied topically, which gives the drug a high therapeutic index. The mechanism of action for all topical corticosteroids is not well defined, however, is believed to be a combination of three important properties: anti-inflammatory activity, immunosuppressive properties, and antiproliferative actions.
Local Anesthetic/Vasoconstrictor Precautions No information available to require special precautions
Effects on Dental Treatment No effects or complications reported
Other Adverse Effects <1%:
   Dermatologic: Acne, hypopigmentation, allergic dermatitis, maceration of the skin, skin atrophy, folliculitis, hypertrichosis
   Endocrine & metabolic: HPA suppression, Cushing's syndrome, growth retardation
   Local: Burning, itching, irritation, dryness
   Miscellaneous: Secondary infection
Drug Interactions No data reported
Pregnancy Risk Factor C
Dosage Forms
   Spray, intranasal: 50 mcg/actuation (9 g = 60 actuations, 16 g = 120 actuations)
   Topical:
      Cream: 0.05% (15 g, 30 g, 60 g)
      Ointment, topical: 0.005% (15 g, 60 g)
Generic Available No

Fluvastatin (floo' va sta tin)
Related Information
   Cardiovascular Diseases on page 912
Brand Names Lescol®
Therapeutic Category HMG-CoA Reductase Inhibitor; Lipid Lowering Drugs
(Continued)

Fluvastatin (Continued)

Use Adjunct to dietary therapy to decrease elevated serum total and LDL cholesterol concentrations in primary hypercholesterolemia

Usual Dosage Adults: Oral:
Initial dose: 20 mg at bedtime
Usual dose: 20-40 mg at bedtime
Note: Splitting the 40 mg dose into a twice/daily regimen may provide a modest improvement in LDL response; maximum response occurs within 4-6 weeks; decrease dose and monitor effects carefully in patients with hepatic insufficiency

Mechanism of Action Acts by competitively inhibiting 3-hydroxy-3-methylglutaryl-coenzyme A (HMG-CoA) reductase, the enzyme that catalyzes the reduction of HMG-CoA to mevalonate; this is an early rate-limiting step in cholesterol biosynthesis. HDL is increased while total, LDL and VLDL cholesterols, apolipoprotein B, and plasma triglycerides are decreased

Local Anesthetic/Vasoconstrictor Precautions No information available to require special precautions

Effects on Dental Treatment No effects or complications reported

Other Adverse Effects 1% to 1%:
Central nervous system: Headache, dizziness, insomnia
Dermatologic: Rash
Gastrointestinal: Dyspepsia, diarrhea, nausea, vomiting, constipation, flatulence
Neuromuscular & skeletal: Back pain, abdominal and other muscle pain, arthropathy
Miscellaneous: Cold symptoms

Drug Interactions
Anticoagulant effect of warfarin may be increased
Concurrent use of erythromycin and HMG-CoA reductase inhibitors may result in rhabdomyolysis

Drug Uptake
Serum half-life: 1.2 hours

Pregnancy Risk Factor X

Fluvoxamine (floo vox′ ah meen)

Brand Names Luvox®

Therapeutic Category Antidepressant, Selective Serotonin Reuptake Inhibitor

Use Treatment of obsessive-compulsive disorder (OCD); effective in the treatment of major depression; may be useful for the treatment of panic disorder

Usual Dosage
Adults: Initial: 50 mg at bedtime; adjust in 50 mg increments at 4- to 7-day intervals; usual dose range: 100-300 mg/day; divide total daily dose into 2 doses; give larger portion at bedtime
Elderly or hepatic impairment: Reduce dose, titrate slowly

Mechanism of Action Inhibits CNS neuron serotonin uptake; minimal or no effect on reuptake of norepinephrine or dopamine; does not significantly bind to alpha-adrenergic, histamine or cholinergic receptors

Local Anesthetic/Vasoconstrictor Precautions Although caution should be used in patients taking tricyclic antidepressants, no interactions have been reported with vasoconstrictors and fluvoxamine, a nontricyclic antidepressant which acts to increase serotonin

Effects on Dental Treatment No effects or complications reported

Other Adverse Effects
>10%: Gastrointestinal: Nausea
1% to 10%:
Cardiovascular: Palpitations
Central nervous system: Somnolence, asthenia, headache, insomnia, dizziness, nervousness, mania, hypomania, vertigo, abnormal thinking, agitation, anxiety, malaise, amnesia
Endocrine & metabolic: Decreased libido
Gastrointestinal: Dry mouth, abdominal pain, vomiting, dyspepsia, constipation, diarrhea, dysgeusia, anorexia
Neuromuscular & skeletal: Tremors
Miscellaneous: Sweating
<1%:
Central nervous system: Seizures
Dermatologic: Toxic epidermal necrolysis
Hematologic: Thrombocytopenia, increases in serum creatinine
Hepatic: Hepatic dysfunction

Miscellaneous: Extrapyramidal reactions

Drug Interactions Because fluvoxamine inhibits cytochrome P-450 isozymes IA2, IIC9, IIIA4, and possibly IID6, it is associated with numerous significant drug interactions

Increased toxicity: Terfenadine and astemizole are both metabolized by the cytochrome P-450 IIIA4 isozyme, increased levels of these drugs have been associated with prolongation of the Q-T interval and potentially fatal, torsade de pointes ventricular arrhythmias. Since fluvoxamine inhibits the enzyme responsible for their clearance, the concomitant use of these agents is contraindicated.

Potentiates triazolam and alprazolam (dose should be reduced by at least 50%), hypertensive crisis with MAO inhibitors, theophylline (doses should be reduced by $1/3$ and plasma levels monitored), warfarin (reduce its dose and monitor PT/INR), carbamazepine (monitor levels), tricyclic antidepressants (monitor effects and reduce doses accordingly), methadone, beta-blockers (reduce dose of propranolol or metoprolol), diltiazem. Caution with other benzodiazepines, phenytoin, lithium, clozapine, alcohol, other CNS drugs, quinidine, ketoconazole.

Pregnancy Risk Factor C

Fluzone® see Influenza Virus Vaccine on page 458

FML® see Fluorometholone on page 375

FML® Forte see Fluorometholone on page 375

FML-S® Ophthalmic Suspension see Sodium Sulfacetamide and Fluorometholone on page 794

Folbesyn® see Vitamin B Complex With Vitamin C and Folic Acid on page 900

Folex® see Methotrexate on page 559

Folic Acid (foe′ lik as′ id)

Brand Names Folvite®

Canadian/Mexican Brand Names Apo-Folic® (Canada); Flodine® (Canada); Novo-Folacid® (Canada); Dalisol® (Mexico); Folitab® (Mexico); A.F. Valdecasas® (Mexico)

Therapeutic Category Vitamin, Water Soluble

Synonyms Folico Acido (Mexico)

Use

Dental: Treatment of megaloblastic and macrocytic anemias due to folate deficiency

Medical: Dietary supplement to prevent neural tube defects

Usual Dosage Oral, I.M., I.V., S.C.:

Children: Initial: 1 mg/day

Deficiency: 0.5-1 mg/day

Maintenance dose:

<4 years: Up to 0.3 mg/day

>4 years: 0.4 mg/day

Adults: Initial: 1 mg/day

Deficiency: 1-3 mg/day

Maintenance dose: 0.5 mg/day

Women of childbearing age, pregnant, and lactating women: 0.8 mg/day

Mechanism of Action Folic acid is necessary for formation of a number of coenzymes in many metabolic systems, particularly for purine and pyrimidine synthesis; required for nucleoprotein synthesis and maintenance in erythropoiesis; stimulates WBC and platelet production in folate deficiency anemia

Local Anesthetic/Vasoconstrictor Precautions No information available to require special precautions

Effects on Dental Treatment No effects or complications reported

Other Adverse Effects <1%:

Cardiovascular: Slight flushing

Central nervous system: General malaise

Dermatologic: Pruritus, rash

Respiratory: Bronchospasm

Miscellaneous: Allergic reaction

Contraindications Pernicious, aplastic, or normocytic anemias

Warnings/Precautions Doses <0.1 mg/day may obscure pernicious anemia with continuing irreversible nerve damage progression. Resistance to treatment may occur with depressed hematopoiesis, alcoholism, deficiencies of other vitamins. Injection contains benzyl alcohol (1.5%) as preservative (use care in administration to neonates).

(Continued)

Folic Acid *(Continued)*

Drug Interactions
Decreased effect: In folate-deficient patients, folic acid therapy may increase phenytoin metabolism. Phenytoin, primidone, para-aminosalicylic acid, and sulfasalazine may decrease serum folate concentrations and cause deficiency. Oral contraceptives may also impair folate metabolism producing depletion, but the effect is unlikely to cause anemia or megaloblastic changes. Concurrent administration of chloramphenicol and folic acid may result in antagonism of the hematopoietic response to folic acid.

Drug Uptake
Peak effect: Oral: Within 0.5-1 hour

Absorption: In the proximal part of the small intestine

Pregnancy Risk Factor A (C if dose exceeds RDA recommendation)

Breast-feeding Considerations May be taken while breast-feeding

Dosage Forms
Injection, as sodium folate: 5 mg/mL (10 mL); 10 mg/mL (10 mL)

Folvite®: 5 mg/mL (10 mL)

Tablet: 0.1 mg, 0.4 mg, 0.8 mg, 1 mg

Folvite®: 1 mg

Generic Available Yes

Folico Acido (Mexico) *see* Folic Acid *on previous page*

Folinic Acid *see* Leucovorin Calcium *on page 491*

Follutein® *see* Chorionic Gonadotropin *on page 203*

Folvite® *see* Folic Acid *on previous page*

Footwork® [OTC] *see* Tolnaftate *on page 855*

Formula Q® [OTC] *see* Quinine Sulfate *on page 760*

5-Formyl Tetrahydrofolate *see* Leucovorin Calcium *on page 491*

Fortaz® *see* Ceftazidime *on page 171*

Fosamax® *see* Alendronate Sodium *on page 30*

Foscarnet (fos kar' net)
Related Information
Systemic Viral Diseases *on page 934*

Brand Names Foscavir®

Dose Adjustment for Renal Impairment

The induction dose of foscarnet should be adjusted according to creatinine clearance as follows:

Creatinine Clearance (mL/min/kg)	Foscarnet Induction Dose (mg/kg q8h)
1.6	60
1.5	57
1.4	53
1.3	49
1.2	46
1.1	42
1	39
0.9	35
0.8	32
0.7	28
0.6	25
0.5	21
0.4	18

The maintenance dose of foscarnet should be adjusted according to creatinine clearance as follows:

Creatinine Clearance (mL/min/kg)	Foscarnet Maintenance Dose (mg/kg/day)
1.4	90-120
1.2-1.4	78-104
1-1.2	75-100
0.8-1	71-94
0.6-0.8	63-84
0.4-0.6	57-75

Therapeutic Category Antiviral Agent, Parenteral

Use Approved indications in adult patients:

Herpesvirus infections suspected to be caused by acyclovir (HSV, VZV) or ganciclovir (CMV) resistant strains (this occurs almost exclusively in persons with advanced AIDS who have received prolonged treatment for a herpesvirus infection)

CMV retinitis in persons with AIDS

Other CMV infections in persons unable to tolerate ganciclovir

Usual Dosage

Adolescents and Adults: I.V.:

Induction treatment: 60 mg/kg/dose every 8 hours for 14-21 days

Maintenance therapy: 90-120 mg/kg/day as a single infusion

See table.

Mechanism of Action Pyrophosphate analogue which acts as a noncompetitive inhibitor of many viral RNA and DNA polymerases as well as HIV reverse transcriptase. Inhibitory effects occur at concentrations which do not affect host cellular DNA polymerases; however, some human cell growth suppression has been observed with high *in vitro* concentrations. Similar to ganciclovir, foscarnet is a virostatic agent. Foscarnet does not require activation by thymidine kinase.

Local Anesthetic/Vasoconstrictor Precautions No information available to require special precautions

Effects on Dental Treatment No effects or complications reported

Other Adverse Effects

>10%:

Central nervous system: Fever, headache, seizures

Gastrointestinal: Nausea, diarrhea, vomiting

Hematologic: Anemia

Renal: Abnormal renal function, decreased creatinine clearance

1% to 10%:

Central nervous system: Fatigue, rigors, asthenia, malaise, dizziness, hypoesthesia, neuropathy, depression, confusion, anxiety

Dermatologic: Rash

Endocrine & metabolic: Electrolyte imbalance

Gastrointestinal: Anorexia

Hematologic: Granulocytopenia, leukopenia

Local: Injection site pain

Neuromuscular & skeletal: Paresthesia, involuntary muscle contractions

Ocular: Vision abnormalities

Renal: Decreased creatinine clearance

Respiratory: Coughing, dyspnea

Miscellaneous: Sepsis, increased sweating

<1%:

Cardiovascular: Cardiac failure, bradycardia, arrhythmias, cerebral edema, leg edema, peripheral edema, syncope, coma

Central nervous system: Hypothermia, abnormal crying, malignant hyperpyrexia, vertigo

Endocrine & metabolic: Gynecomastia, decreased gonadotropins

Hepatic: Cholecystitis, cholelithiasis, hepatitis, hepatosplenomegaly, ascites

Neuromuscular & skeletal: Abnormal gait, dyskinesia

Ocular: Nystagmus

Miscellaneous: Substernal chest pain, hypertonia, vocal cord paralysis, speech disorders

Drug Interactions No data reported

Drug Uptake

Absorption: Oral: Poorly absorbed; I.V. therapy is needed for the treatment of viral infections in AIDS patients

Serum half-life: ~3 hours

Pregnancy Risk Factor C

Foscavir® see Foscarnet *on previous page*

Fosinopril (foe sin' oh pril)

Related Information

Cardiovascular Diseases *on page 912*

Brand Names Monopril®

Therapeutic Category Angiotensin-Converting Enzyme (ACE) Inhibitors

Synonyms Fosinopril Sodico (Mexico)

Use Treatment of hypertension, either alone or in combination with other antihypertensive agents; congestive heart failure

Usual Dosage Adults: Oral:

(Continued)

Fosinopril (Continued)

Hypertension: Initial: 10 mg/day; increase to a maximum dose of 80 mg/day; most patients are maintained on 20-40 mg/day; may need to divide the dose into two if trough effect is inadequate; discontinue the diuretic, if possible 2-3 days before initiation of therapy; resume diuretic therapy carefully, if needed.

Heart failure: Initial: 10 mg/day (5 mg if renal dysfunction present) and increase, as needed, to a maximum of 40 mg once daily over several weeks; usual dose: 20-40 mg/day; if hypotension, orthostasis, or azotemia occur during titration, consider decreasing concomitant diuretic dose, if any

Mechanism of Action Competitive inhibitor of angiotensin-converting enzyme (ACE); prevents conversion of angiotensin I to angiotensin II, a potent vasoconstrictor; results in lower levels of angiotensin II which causes an increase in plasma renin activity and a reduction in aldosterone secretion; a CNS mechanism may also be involved in hypotensive effect as angiotensin II increases adrenergic outflow from CNS; vasoactive kallikreins may be decreased in conversion to active hormones by ACE inhibitors, thus reducing blood pressure

Local Anesthetic/Vasoconstrictor Precautions No information available to require special precautions

Effects on Dental Treatment No effects or complications reported

Other Adverse Effects

1% to 10%:
Cardiovascular: Orthostatic hypotension
Central nervous system: Headache, dizziness, fatigue
Endocrine & metabolic: Sexual dysfunction
Gastrointestinal: Diarrhea, nausea, vomiting
Respiratory: Cough

<1%:
Cardiovascular: Syncope
Central nervous system: Vertigo, insomnia
Dermatologic: Angioedema, rash
Endocrine & metabolic: Hypoglycemia, hyperkalemia
Genitourinary: Impotence
Hematologic: Neutropenia, agranulocytosis, anemia
Neuromuscular & skeletal: Muscle cramps
Renal: Deterioration in renal function
Miscellaneous: Loss of taste perception

Drug Interactions

Fosinopril and diuretics have additive hypotensive effects; see table.

Drug-Drug Interactions With ACEIs

Precipitant Drug	Drug (Category) and Effect	Description
Antacids	ACE Inhibitors: decreased	Decreased bioavailability of ACEIs. May be more likely with captopril. Separate administration times by 1-2 hours.
NSAIDs (indomethacin)	ACEIs: decreased	Reduced hypotensive effects of ACEIs. More prominent in low renin or volume dependent hypertensive patients.
Phenothiazines	ACEIs: increased	Pharmacologic effects of ACEIs may be increased.
ACEIs	Allopurinol: increased	Higher risk of hypersensitivity reaction possible when given concurrently. Three case reports of Stevens-Johnson syndrome with captopril.
ACEIs	Digoxin: increased	Increased plasma digoxin levels.
ACEIs	Lithium: increased	Increased serum lithium levels and symptoms of toxicity may occur.
ACEIs	Potassium preps/ potassium sparing diuretics increased	Coadministration may result in elevated potassium levels.

Drug Uptake
Absorption: 36%
Serum half-life, serum (fosinoprilat): 12 hours
Time to peak serum concentration: ~3 hours

Pregnancy Risk Factor D

Fosinopril Sodico (Mexico) see Fosinopril on previous page

Fosphenytoin (fos' fen i toyn)

Brand Names Cerebyx®

Therapeutic Category Anticonvulsant, Hydantoin

Use Indicated for short-term parenteral administration when other means of phenytoin administration are unavailable, inappropriate or deemed less advantageous; the safety and effectiveness of fosphenytoin in this use has not been systematically evaluated for more than 5 days; may be used for the control of generalized convulsive status epilepticus and prevention and treatment of seizures occurring during neurosurgery

Usual Dosage The dose, concentration in solutions, and infusion rates for fosphenytoin are expressed as phenytoin sodium equivalents; fosphenytoin should always be prescribed and dispensed in phenytoin sodium equivalents

Status epilepticus: I.V.: Adults: Loading dose: Phenytoin equivalent 15-20 mg/kg I.V. administered at 100-150 mg/minute

Nonemergent loading and maintenance dosing: I.V. or I.M.: Adults:
Loading dose: Phenytoin equivalent 10-20 mg/kg I.V. or I.M. (max I.V. rate 150 mg/minute)
Initial daily maintenance dose: Phenytoin equivalent 4-6 mg/kg/day I.V. or I.M.

I.M. or I.V. substitution for oral phenytoin therapy: May be substituted for oral phenytoin sodium at the same total daily dose, however, Dilantin® capsules are ~90% bioavailable by the oral route; phenytoin, supplied as fosphenytoin, is 100% bioavailable by both the I.M. and I.V. routes; for this reason, plasma phenytoin concentrations may increase when I.M. or I.V. fosphenytoin is substituted for oral phenytoin sodium therapy; in clinical trials I.M. fosphenytoin was administered as a single daily dose utilizing either 1 or 2 injection sites; some patients may require more frequent dosing

Dosing adjustments in renal and hepatic impairment: Phenytoin clearance may be substantially reduced in cirrhosis and plasma level monitoring with dose adjustment advisable; free phenytoin levels should be monitored closely in patients with renal or hepatic disease or in those with hypoalbumineria; furthermore fosphenytoin clearance to phenytoin may be increased without a similar increase in phenytoin in these patients leading to increase frequency and severity of adverse events

Local Anesthetic/Vasoconstrictor Precautions No information available to require special precautions

Effects on Dental Treatment No effects or complications reported

Other Adverse Effects

I.V. administration (maximum dose/rate):
Body as whole: Pelvic pain (4.4%), asthenia (2.2%), back pain (2.2%), headache (2.2%)
Cardiovascular: I.V.: Hypotension (7.7%), vasodilation (5.6%), tachycardia (2.2%)
Central nervous system: Dizziness (31%), somnolence (20%), ataxia (11%), stupor (7.7%), incoordination (4.4%), extrapyramidal syndrome (4.4%), agitation (3.3%), hypesthesia (2.2%), vertigo (2.2%), brain edema (2.2%)
Dermatologic: Pruritus (48.9%)
Gastrointestinal: Nausea (8.9%), tongue disorder (4.4%), dry mouth (4.4%), vomiting (2.2%), taste perversion (3.3%)
Neuromuscular & skeletal: Paresthesia (4.4%), dysarthria (2.2%), tremor (3.3%)
Ocular: Diplopia (3.3%), amblyopia (2.2%), nystagmus (44%)
Otic: Tinnitus (8.9%), deafness (2.2%)

I.M. administration (substitute for oral phenytoin):
Body as a whole: Headache (8.9%), asthenia (3.9%), accidental injury (3.4%)
Central nervous system: Ataxia (8.4%), incoordination (7.8%), somnolence (6.7%), dizziness (5%), reflexes decreased (2.8%)
Dermatologic: Pruritus (2.8%)
Gastrointestinal: Nausea (4.5%), vomiting (2.8%)
Dermatologic: Ecchymosis (7.3%)
Neuromuscular & skeletal: Tremor (9.5%), paresthesia (3.9%)
Ocular: Nystagmus (15%)

Other ≤1%:
Cardiovascular: Hypertension, cardiac arrest, migraine, syncope, cerebral hemorrhage, palpitations, sinus bradycardia, atrial flutter, bundle branch block, cardiomegaly, cerebral infarct, postural hypotension, pulmonary

(Continued)

Fosphenytoin *(Continued)*

embolus, QT interval prolongation, thrombophlebitis, ventricular extrasystoles, congestive heart failure

Dermatologic: Rash, maculopapular rash, urticaria, sweating, skin discoloration, contact dermatitis, pustular rash, skin nodule

Endocrine & metabolic: Hypokalemia, hyperglycemia, hypophosphatemia, alkalosis, acidosis, dehydration, hyperkalemia, ketosis

Hematologic/lymphatic: Thrombocytopenia, anemia, leukocytosis, cyanosis, hypochromic anemia, leukopenia, lymphadenopathy, petechia

Hepatic: Acute hepatotoxicity, acute hepatic failure

Warnings/Precautions Doses of fosphenytoin are expressed as their phenytoin sodium equivalent; antiepileptic drugs should not be abruptly discontinued; hypotension may occur, especially after I.V. administration at high doses and high rates of administration, administration of phenytoin has been associated with atrial and ventricular conduction depression and ventricular fibrillation, careful cardiac monitoring is needed when administering I.V. loading doses of fosphenytoin; use with caution in patients with hypotension and severe myocardial insufficiency; discontinue if skin rash or lymphadenopathy occurs; acute hepatotoxicity associated with a hypersensitivity syndrome characterized by fever, skin eruptions and lymphadenopathy has been reported to occur within the first 2 months of treatment

Drug Interactions No drugs are known to interfere with the conversion of fosphenytoin to phenytoin; phenytoin may decrease the serum concentration or effectiveness of valproic acid, ethosuximide, felbamate, benzodiazepines, carbamazepine, lamotrigine, primidone, warfarin, oral contraceptives, corticosteroids, cyclosporine, theophylline, chloramphenicol, rifampin, doxycycline, quinidine, mexiletine, disopyramide, dopamine, or nondepolarizing skeletal muscle relaxants; phenytoin may increase phenobarbital and primidone levels; protein binding of phenytoin can be affected by valproic acid or salicylates; serum phenytoin concentrations may be increased by cimetidine, felbamate, ethosuximide, methsuximide, chloramphenicol, disulfiram, fluconazole, omeprazole, isoniazid, trimethoprim, or sulfonamides and decreased by rifampin, cisplatin, vinblastine, bleomycin, folic acid

Drug Uptake

Fosphenytoin is a prodrug of phenytoin and its anticonvulsant effects are attributable to phenytoin

Conversion to phenytoin: Following I.V. administration conversion half-life is 15 minutes; following I.M. administration peak phenytoin levels are reached in 3 hours

Pregnancy Risk Factor D

Generic Available No

Fostex® [OTC] *see* Sulfur and Salicylic Acid *on page 813*

Fostex® BPO [OTC] *see* Benzoyl Peroxide *on page 104*

Fototar® [OTC] *see* Coal Tar *on page 225*

Fragmin® *see* Dalteparin *on page 249*

Fresh Burst Listerine® Antiseptic [OTC] *see* Mouthwash, Antiseptic *on page 592*

FS Shampoo® *see* Fluocinolone Acetonide *on page 372*

5-FU *see* Fluorouracil *on page 376*

FUDR® *see* Floxuridine *on page 366*

Fulvicin® P/G *see* Griseofulvin *on page 406*

Fulvicin-U/F® *see* Griseofulvin *on page 406*

Fumasorb® [OTC] *see* Ferrous Fumarate *on page 359*

Fumerin® [OTC] *see* Ferrous Fumarate *on page 359*

Fungatin® [OTC] *see* Tolnaftate *on page 855*

Fungizone® *see* Amphotericin B *on page 60*

Fungoid® *see* Triacetin *on page 862*

Fungoid® Topical Solution *see* Undecylenic Acid and Derivatives *on page 884*

Furacin® *see* Nitrofurazone *on page 623*

Furadantin® *see* Nitrofurantoin *on page 622*

Furalan® *see* Nitrofurantoin *on page 622*

Furan® *see* Nitrofurantoin *on page 622*

Furanite® *see* Nitrofurantoin *on page 622*

Furazolidona (Mexico) *see* Furazolidone *on next page*

Furazolidone (fyoor a zoe′ li done)
Brand Names Furoxone®
Canadian/Mexican Brand Names Furoxona® Gotas (Mexico); Furoxona® Tabletas (Mexico); Fuxol® (Mexico)
Therapeutic Category Antibiotic, Miscellaneous; Antidiarrheal; Antiprotozoal
Synonyms Furazolidona (Mexico)
Use Treatment of bacterial or protozoal diarrhea and enteritis caused by susceptible organisms *Giardia lamblia* and *Vibrio cholerae*
Usual Dosage Oral:
    Children >1 month: 5-8 mg/kg/day in 4 divided doses for 7 days, not to exceed 400 mg/day or 8.8 mg/kg/day
    Adults: 100 mg 4 times/day for 7 days
Mechanism of Action Inhibits several vital enzymatic reactions causing antibacterial and antiprotozoal action
Local Anesthetic/Vasoconstrictor Precautions No information available to require special precautions
Effects on Dental Treatment No effects or complications reported
Other Adverse Effects
    >10%: Miscellaneous: Dark yellow to brown discoloration of urine
    1% to 10%:
        Central nervous system: Headache
        Gastrointestinal: Abdominal pain, diarrhea, nausea, vomiting
    <1%:
        Cardiovascular: Orthostatic hypotension
        Central nervous system: Fever, dizziness, drowsiness, malaise
        Dermatologic: Skin rash
        Endocrine & metabolic: Hypoglycemia, disulfiram-like reaction after alcohol ingestion, leukopenia
        Hematologic: Agranulocytosis, hemolysis in patients with G-6-PD deficiency
        Neuromuscular & skeletal: Joint pain
Drug Interactions
    Increased effect with indirectly acting sympathomimetic amines such as ephedrine and phenylephrine, tricyclic antidepressants, tyramine-containing foods, MAO inhibitors, meperidine, anorexiants, dextromethorphan, fluoxetine, paroxetine, sertraline, trazodone
    Increased effect/toxicity of levodopa
    Disulfiram-like reaction with alcohol
Drug Uptake
    Absorption: Oral: Poor
Pregnancy Risk Factor C

Furosemida (Mexico) *see* Furosemide *on this page*

Furosemide (fyoor oh′ se mide)
Related Information
    Cardiovascular Diseases *on page 912*
Brand Names Lasix®
Canadian/Mexican Brand Names Apo-Furosemide® (Canada); Furoside® (Canada); Novo-Semide® (Canada); Uritol® (Canada); Edenol® (Mexico); Henexal® (Mexico)
Therapeutic Category Diuretic, Loop
Synonyms Furosemida (Mexico); Fursemide (Canada)
Use Management of edema associated with congestive heart failure and hepatic or renal disease; used alone or in combination with antihypertensives in treatment of hypertension
Usual Dosage
    Children:
        Oral: 1-2 mg/kg/dose increased in increments of 1 mg/kg/dose with each succeeding dose until a satisfactory effect is achieved to a maximum of 6 mg/kg/dose no more frequently than 6 hours
        I.M., I.V.: 1 mg/kg/dose, increasing by each succeeding dose at 1 mg/kg/dose at intervals of 6-12 hours until a satisfactory response up to 6 mg/kg/dose
    Adults:
        Oral: 20-80 mg/dose initially increased in increments of 20-40 mg/dose at intervals of 6-8 hours; usual maintenance dose interval is twice daily or every day
        I.M., I.V.: 20-40 mg/dose, may be repeated in 1-2 hours as needed and increased by 20 mg/dose with each succeeding dose up to 1000 mg/day; usual dosing interval: 6-12 hours
(Continued)

Furosemide *(Continued)*

Continuous I.V. infusion: Initial I.V. bolus dose of 0.1 mg/kg followed by continuous I.V. infusion doses of 0.1 mg/kg/hour doubled every 2 hours to a maximum of 0.4 mg/kg/hour if urine output is <1 mL/kg/hour have been found to be effective and result in a lower daily requirement of furosemide than with intermittent dosing. Other studies have used 20-160 mg/hour continuous I.V. infusion

Elderly: Oral, I.M., I.V.: Initial: 20 mg/day; increase slowly to desired response

Mechanism of Action Inhibits reabsorption of sodium and chloride in the ascending loop of Henle and distal renal tubule, interfering with the chloride-binding cotransport system, thus causing increased excretion of water, sodium, chloride, magnesium, and calcium

Local Anesthetic/Vasoconstrictor Precautions No information available to require special precautions

Effects on Dental Treatment No effects or complications reported

Other Adverse Effects

>10%:
 Cardiovascular: Orthostatic hypotension
 Central nervous system: Dizziness

1% to 10%:
 Central nervous system: Headache
 Dermatologic: Photosensitivity
 Endocrine & metabolic: Electrolyte imbalance (hypokalemia, hyponatremia, hypochloremia, hypercalciuria, hyperuricemia), alkalosis, dehydration
 Gastrointestinal: Diarrhea, loss of appetite, stomach cramps or pain
 Ocular: Blurred vision

<1%:
 Dermatologic: Skin rash
 Gastrointestinal: Pancreatitis, nausea
 Genitourinary: Prerenal azotemia
 Hepatic: Hepatic dysfunction
 Hematologic: Agranulocytosis, leukopenia, anemia, thrombocytopenia
 Local: Redness at injection site
 Neuromuscular & skeletal: Gout
 Ocular: Xanthopsia
 Otic: Ototoxicity
 Renal: Nephrocalcinosis, interstitial nephritis

Drug Interactions

Decreased effect:
 Furosemide interferes with hypoglycemic effect of antidiabetic agents
 Indomethacin may reduce natriuretic and hypotensive effects of furosemide

Increased effect: Effects of antihypertensive agents may be enhanced by furosemide

Increased toxicity:
 Furosemide inhibits renal clearance of lithium resulting in risk of lithium toxicity
 Concomitant use of furosemide with aminoglycoside antibiotics or other ototoxic drugs should be avoided

Drug Uptake

Onset of diuresis:
 Oral: Within 30-60 minutes
 I.M.: 30 minutes
 I.V.: Within 5 minutes

Peak effect: Oral: Within 1-2 hours

Duration:
 Oral: 6-8 hours
 I.V.: 2 hours

Absorption: Oral: 60% to 67%

Serum half-life:
 Normal renal function: 0.5-1.1 hours
 End stage renal disease: 9 hours

Pregnancy Risk Factor C

Furoxone® *see* Furazolidone *on previous page*

Fursemide (Canada) *see* Furosemide *on previous page*

G-1® *see* Butalbital Compound *on page 133*

Gabapentin *(ga′ ba pen tin)*

Brand Names Neurontin®

Therapeutic Category Anticonvulsant, Miscellaneous

Use Adjunct for treatment of drug-refractory partial and secondarily generalized seizures in adults with epilepsy; not effective for absence seizures

Usual Dosage If gabapentin is discontinued or if another anticonvulsant is added to therapy, it should be done slowly over a minimum of 1 week

Children >12 years and Adults: Oral:

Initial: 300 mg on day 1 (at bedtime to minimize sedation), then 300 mg twice daily on day 2, and then 300 mg 3 times/day on day 3

Total daily dosage range: 900-1800 mg/day administered in 3 divided doses at 8-hour intervals

Mechanism of Action Exact mechanism of action is not known, but does have properties in common with other anticonvulsants; although structurally related to GABA, it does not interact with GABA receptors

Local Anesthetic/Vasoconstrictor Precautions No information available to require special precautions

Effects on Dental Treatment No effects or complications reported

Other Adverse Effects

>10%: Central nervous system: Somnolence, dizziness, ataxia, fatigue

1% to 10%:

Cardiovascular: Peripheral edema

Central nervous system: Nervousness, amnesia, depression, anxiety, abnormal coordination

Dermatologic: Pruritus

Gastrointestinal: Dyspepsia, dry mouth/throat, nausea, constipation, appetite stimulation (weight gain)

Genitourinary: Impotence

Hematologic: Leukopenia

Neuromuscular & skeletal: Back pain, myalgia, dysarthria, tremor

Ocular: Diplopia, blurred vision, nystagmus

Respiratory: Rhinitis, bronchospasm

Miscellaneous: Hiccups

Drug Interactions

Gabapentin does not modify plasma concentrations of standard anticonvulsant medications (ie, valproic acid, carbamazepine, phenytoin, or phenobarbital)

Decreased effect: Antacids reduce the bioavailability of gabapentin by 20%

Increased toxicity: Cimetidine may decrease clearance of gabapentin; gabapentin may increase levels of norethindrone by 13%

Drug Uptake

Absorption: Oral: 50% to 60%

Serum half-life: 5-6 hours

Pregnancy Risk Factor C

Gamastan® see Immune Globulin, Intramuscular *on page 453*
Gamimune® N see Immune Globulin, Intravenous *on page 454*
Gammagard® see Immune Globulin, Intravenous *on page 454*
Gammagard® S/D see Immune Globulin, Intravenous *on page 454*
Gammar® see Immune Globulin, Intramuscular *on page 453*

Ganciclovir (gan sye' kloe veer)

Related Information

Systemic Viral Diseases *on page 934*

Brand Names Cytovene®

Canadian/Mexican Brand Names Cymevene® (Mexico)

Therapeutic Category Antiviral Agent, Parenteral

Synonyms Ganciclovir Sodico (Mexico)

Use Treatment of CMV retinitis in immunocompromised individuals, including patients with acquired immunodeficiency syndrome; treatment of CMV pneumonia in marrow transplant recipients AIDS patients and organ transplant recipients with CMV colitis, pneumonitis, and multiorgan involvement; bone marrow transplant patients when given in combination with IVIG or CMV hyperimmune globulin

Oral: Alternative to the I.V. formulation for maintenance treatment of CMV retinitis in immunocompromised patients, including patients with AIDS, in whom retinitis is stable following appropriate induction therapy and for whom the risk of more rapid progression is balanced by the benefit associated with avoiding daily I.V. infusions

Usual Dosage

Slow I.V. infusion (dosing is based on total body weight):

Children >3 months and Adults:

Induction therapy: 5 mg/kg/dose every 12 hours for 14-21 days followed by maintenance therapy

(Continued)

Ganciclovir *(Continued)*

Maintenance therapy: 5 mg/kg/day as a single daily dose for 7 days/week or 6 mg/kg/day for 5 days/week

Oral: 1000 mg 3 times/day with food **or** 500 mg 6 times/day with food

Mechanism of Action Ganciclovir is phosphorylated to a substrate which competitively inhibits the binding of deoxyguanosine triphosphate to DNA polymerase resulting in inhibition of viral DNA synthesis

Local Anesthetic/Vasoconstrictor Precautions No information available to require special precautions

Effects on Dental Treatment No effects or complications reported

Other Adverse Effects

>10%:

Central nervous system: Headache

Hematologic: Granulocytopenia, thrombocytopenia

1% to 10%:

Central nervous system: Confusion, fever

Dermatologic: Rash

Hematologic: Anemia

Hepatic: Abnormal liver function values

Miscellaneous: Sepsis

<1%:

Cardiovascular: Arrhythmia, hypertension, hypotension, coma, edema

Central nervous system: Ataxia, dizziness, nervousness, psychosis, malaise

Dermatologic: Alopecia, pruritus, urticaria

Gastrointestinal: Nausea, vomiting, diarrhea, abdominal pain

Hematologic: Eosinophilia, hemorrhage

Local: Inflammation or pain at injection site

Neuromuscular & skeletal: Paresthesia, tremor

Ocular: Retinal detachment

Respiratory: Dyspnea

Drug Interactions

Increased toxicity:

Zidovudine, immunosuppressive agents leads to increased hematologic toxicity

Imipenem/cilastatin leads to increased seizure potential

Probenecid: The renal clearance of ganciclovir is decreased in the presence of probenecid

Drug Uptake

Absorption: Oral: Absolute bioavailability under fasting conditions: 5% and following food: 6% to 9%; following fatty meal: 28% to 31%

Serum half-life: 1.7-5.8 hours; increases with impaired renal function

End stage renal disease: 3.6 hours

Pregnancy Risk Factor C

Ganciclovir Sodico (Mexico) *see* Ganciclovir *on previous page*

Gantanol® *see* Sulfamethoxazole *on page 809*

Gantrisin® *see* Sulfisoxazole *on page 811*

Garamycin® *see* Gentamicin Sulfate *on page 396*

Gas-Ban DS® [OTC] *see* Aluminum Hydroxide, Magnesium Hydroxide, and Simethicone *on page 41*

Gas Relief® [OTC] *see* Simethicone *on page 788*

Gastrocrom® *see* Cromolyn Sodium *on page 235*

Gastrosed™ *see* Hyoscyamine Sulfate *on page 445*

Gas-X® [OTC] *see* Simethicone *on page 788*

Gaviscon®-2 Tablet [OTC] *see* Aluminum Hydroxide and Magnesium Trisilicate *on page 41*

Gaviscon® Liquid [OTC] *see* Aluminum Hydroxide and Magnesium Carbonate *on page 40*

Gaviscon® Tablet [OTC] *see* Aluminum Hydroxide and Magnesium Trisilicate *on page 41*

G-CSF *see* Filgrastim *on page 362*

Gee Gee® [OTC] *see* Guaifenesin *on page 407*

Gelatin, Absorbable *(jell′ a tin ab sorb′ able)*

Brand Names Gelfoam® Topical

Canadian/Mexican Brand Names Gelafundin® (Mexico); Haemaccel® (Mexico)

Therapeutic Category Hemostatic Agent

Synonyms Gelatina Desdoblada Pulimerizado De (Mexico)

Use
Dental: Adjunct to provide hemostasis in oral and dental surgery
Medical: In medicine, adjunct to provide hemostasis in surgery; open prostatic surgery

Usual Dosage Hemostasis: Apply packs or sponges dry or saturated with sodium chloride. When applied dry, hold in place with moderate pressure. When applied wet, squeeze to remove air bubbles. The powder is applied as a paste prepared by adding approximately 4 mL of sterile saline solution to the powder.

Local Anesthetic/Vasoconstrictor Precautions No information available to require special precautions

Effects on Dental Treatment No effects or complications reported

Other Adverse Effects 1% to 10%: Local: Infection and abscess formation

Oral manifestations: No data reported

Contraindications Should not be used in closure of skin incisions since they may interfere with the healing of skin edges

Warnings/Precautions Do not sterilize by heat; do not use in the presence of infection

Drug Interactions No data reported

Pregnancy Risk Factor No data reported

Breast-feeding Considerations No data reported

Dosage Forms
Packs:
Size 2 cm (40 cm x 2 cm) (1s)
Size 6 cm (40 cm x 6 cm) (6s)
Packs, dental:
Size 2 (10 mm x 20 mm x 7 mm) (15s)
Size 4 (20 mm x 20 mm x 7 mm) (15s)

Dietary Considerations No data reported

Generic Available No

Gelatina Desdoblada Pulimerizado De (Mexico) *see* Gelatin, Absorbable *on previous page*

Gelatin, Pectin, and Methylcellulose
(jel′ a tin, pek′ tin, & meth il sel′ yoo lose)
Brand Names Orabase® Plain [OTC]
Therapeutic Category Protectant, Topical
Use Temporary relief from minor oral irritations
Local Anesthetic/Vasoconstrictor Precautions No information available to require special precautions
Effects on Dental Treatment No effects or complications reported

Gelfoam® Topical *see* Gelatin, Absorbable *on previous page*

Gel Kam® *see* Fluoride *on page 374*

Gelpirin® [OTC] *see* Acetaminophen, Aspirin, and Caffeine *on page 17*

Gel-Tin® [OTC] *see* Fluoride *on page 374*

Gelucast® *see* Zinc Gelatin *on page 908*

Gelusil® [OTC] *see* Aluminum Hydroxide, Magnesium Hydroxide, and Simethicone *on page 41*

Gemfibrozil (jem fi′ broe zil)
Related Information
Cardiovascular Diseases *on page 912*
Brand Names Lopid®
Canadian/Mexican Brand Names Apo-Gemfibrozil® (Canada); Nu-Gemfi-brozil® (Canada)
Therapeutic Category Lipid Lowering Drugs
Use Treatment of hypertriglyceridemia in types IV and V hyperlipidemia for patients who are at greater risk for pancreatitis and who have not responded to dietary intervention; reduction of coronary heart disease in type IIB patients who have low HDL cholesterol, increased LDL cholesterol, and increased triglycerides

Usual Dosage Adults: Oral: 1200 mg/day in 2 divided doses, 30 minutes before breakfast and dinner
Hemodialysis effects: Not removed by hemodialysis; supplemental dose is not necessary

Mechanism of Action The exact mechanism of action of gemfibrozil is unknown, however, several theories exist regarding the VLDL effect; it can inhibit lipolysis and decrease subsequent hepatic fatty acid uptake as well as inhibit hepatic secretion of VLDL; together these actions decrease serum (Continued)

Gemfibrozil *(Continued)*

VLDL levels; increases HDL cholesterol; the mechanism behind HDL elevation is currently unknown

Local Anesthetic/Vasoconstrictor Precautions No information available to require special precautions

Effects on Dental Treatment No effects or complications reported

Other Adverse Effects

>10%:
Gastrointestinal: Dyspepsia, abdominal pain
Hepatic: Cholelithiasis

1% to 10%:
Central nervous system: Fatigue, vertigo, headache
Dermatologic: Eczema, rash
Gastrointestinal: Diarrhea, nausea, vomiting, constipation, acute appendicitis

<1%:
Cardiovascular: Atrial fibrillation
Central nervous system: Hypesthesia, dizziness, drowsiness, somnolence, mental depression
Gastrointestinal: Flatulence
Neuromuscular & skeletal: Paresthesia
Ocular: Blurred vision

Drug Interactions

Increased toxicity:
Gemfibrozil may potentiate the effects of warfarin
Manufacturer warns against the use of gemfibrozil with concomitant lovastatin therapy

Drug Uptake

Absorption: Well absorbed
Serum half-life: 1.4 hours
Time to peak serum concentration: Within 1-2 hours

Pregnancy Risk Factor B

Genabid® *see* Papaverine Hydrochloride *on page 658*

Genac® [OTC] *see* Triprolidine and Pseudoephedrine *on page 878*

Genagesic® *see* Propoxyphene and Acetaminophen *on page 741*

Genahist® *see* Diphenhydramine Hydrochloride *on page 288*

Genamin® Cold Syrup [OTC] *see* Chlorpheniramine and Phenylpropanolamine *on page 190*

Genamin® Expectorant [OTC] *see* Guaifenesin and Phenylpropanolamine *on page 409*

Genapap® [OTC] *see* Acetaminophen *on page 14*

Genasoft® Plus [OTC] *see* Docusate and Casanthranol *on page 295*

Genaspor® [OTC] *see* Tolnaftate *on page 855*

Genatap® Elixir [OTC] *see* Brompheniramine and Phenylpropanolamine *on page 123*

Genatuss® [OTC] *see* Guaifenesin *on page 407*

Genatuss DM® [OTC] *see* Guaifenesin and Dextromethorphan *on page 408*

Gen-K® *see* Potassium Chloride *on page 708*

Genora® 0.5/35 *see* Ethinyl Estradiol and Norethindrone *on page 339*

Genora® 1/35 *see* Ethinyl Estradiol and Norethindrone *on page 339*

Genora® 1/50 *see* Mestranol and Norethindrone *on page 547*

Genpril® [OTC] *see* Ibuprofen *on page 447*

Gentab-LA® *see* Guaifenesin and Phenylpropanolamine *on page 409*

Gentamicin and Prednisolone *see* Prednisolone and Gentamicin *on page 719*

Gentamicin Sulfate *(jen ta mye' sin sul' fate)*

Related Information

Antimicrobial Prophylaxis in Surgical Patients *on page 1042*
Cardiovascular Diseases *on page 912*

Brand Names Garamycin®

Canadian/Mexican Brand Names Garalen® (Mexico); Garamicina® (Mexico); Genenicina® (Mexico); Genkova® (Mexico); Genrex® (Mexico); Gentarim® (Mexico); Nozolon® (Mexico); Quilagen® (Mexico); Yectamicina® (Mexico)

Therapeutic Category Antibiotic, Aminoglycoside; Antibiotic, Ophthalmic; Antibiotic, Topical

Use

Dental: An alternate antibiotic for the prevention of bacterial endocarditis in patients undergoing dental procedures; it is to be used in those patients considered high risk and not candidates for the standard regimen of prevention of bacterial endocarditis

Medical: Treatment of susceptible bacterial infections, normally gram-negative organisms including *Pseudomonas*, *Proteus*, *Serratia*, and gram-positive *Staphylococcus*; treatment of bone infections, respiratory tract infections, skin and soft tissue infections, as well as abdominal and urinary tract infections, endocarditis, and septicemia; used topically to treat superficial infections of the skin or ophthalmic infections caused by susceptible bacteria

Usual Dosage

Children: 2 mg/kg with total dose not exceeding total adult dose

Adults; I.M., I.V.: 2 g plus gentamicin 1.5 mg/kg (not to exceed 80 mg) 30 minutes before the procedure, followed by amoxicillin 1.5 g orally 6 hours after initial dose; alternatively, the parenteral regimen may be repeated 8 hours after initial dose

Mechanism of Action Interferes with bacterial protein synthesis by binding to 30S and 50S ribosomal subunits resulting in a defective bacterial cell membrane

Local Anesthetic/Vasoconstrictor Precautions No information available to require special precautions

Effects on Dental Treatment No effects or complications reported

Other Adverse Effects

>10%:

Central nervous system: Neurotoxicity (vertigo, ataxia, gait instability)

Otic: Ototoxicity (auditory), ototoxicity (vestibular)

Renal: Nephrotoxicity, decreased creatinine clearance

1% to 10%: Dermatologic: Itching, redness, rash, swelling

Oral manifestations: Increased salivation

Contraindications Hypersensitivity to gentamicin or other aminoglycosides

Warnings/Precautions

Not intended for long-term therapy due to toxic hazards associated with extended administration; pre-existing renal insufficiency, vestibular or cochlear impairment, myasthenia gravis, hypocalcemia, conditions which depress neuromuscular transmission

Parenteral aminoglycosides are associated with significant nephrotoxicity or ototoxicity; the ototoxicity may be directly proportional to the amount of drug given and the duration of treatment; tinnitus or vertigo are indications of vestibular injury and impending hearing loss; renal damage is usually reversible

Drug Interactions Penicillins, cephalosporins, amphotericin B, loop diuretics may increase nephrotoxic potential; neuromuscular blocking agents may increase neuromuscular blockade

Drug Uptake

Absorption: Oral: Not absorbed

Time to peak serum concentration:

I.M.: Within 30-90 minutes

I.V.: 30 minutes after a 30-minute infusion

Serum half-life: Adults: 1.5-3 hours

Pregnancy Risk Factor C

Breast-feeding Considerations No data reported; however, gentamicin is not absorbed orally and other aminoglycosides may be taken while breast-feeding

Dosage Forms

Injection: 40 mg/mL (1 mL, 2 mL, 10 mL, 20 mL)

Injection, pediatric: 10 mg/mL (2 mL)

Dietary Considerations No data reported

Generic Available Yes

Selected Readings

Council on Dental Therapeutics, American Heart Association, "Preventing Bacterial Endocarditis," *J Am Dent Assoc*, 1991, 122(2):87-92.

Dajani AS, Bisno AL, Chung KJ, et al, "Prevention of Bacterial Endocarditis, Recommendations by the American Heart Association," *JAMA*, 1990, 264(22):2919-22.

Wynn RL, "Gentamicin for Prophylaxis of Bacterial Endocarditis: A Review for the Dentist," *Oral Surg Oral Med Oral Pathol*, 1985, 60(2):159-65.

Gentian Violet (jen' shun vye' oh let)

Therapeutic Category Antibacterial, Topical; Antifungal Agent, Topical

Use Treatment of cutaneous or mucocutaneous infections caused by *Candida albicans* and other superficial skin infections - antibacterial and antifungal dye

Usual Dosage Children and Adults: Topical: Apply 0.5% to 2% locally with cotton to lesion 2-3 times/day for 3 days, do not swallow and avoid contact with eyes

(Continued)

Gentian Violet *(Continued)*

Mechanism of Action Topical antiseptic/germicide effective against some vegetative gram-positive bacteria, particularly *Staphylococcus* sp, and some yeast; it is much less effective against gram-negative bacteria and is ineffective against acid-fast bacteria

Local Anesthetic/Vasoconstrictor Precautions No information available to require special precautions

Effects on Dental Treatment No effects or complications reported

Other Adverse Effects 1% to 10%:

Local: Esophagitis, burning, irritation, vesicle formation, ulceration of mucous membranes

Systemic: Sensitivity reactions, laryngitis, tracheitis, laryngeal obstruction

Drug Interactions No data reported

Pregnancy Risk Factor C

Gentran® *see* Dextran *on page 263*

Gen-XENE® *see* Clorazepate Dipotassium *on page 222*

Geocillin® *see* Carbenicillin *on page 153*

Geref® Injection *see* Sermorelin Acetate *on page 786*

Geridium® *see* Phenazopyridine Hydrochloride *on page 679*

German Measles Vaccine *see* Rubella Virus Vaccine, Live *on page 776*

Germinal® *see* Ergoloid Mesylates *on page 318*

Gesterol® *see* Progesterone *on page 731*

Gesterol® L.A. *see* Hydroxyprogesterone Caproate *on page 441*

Gevrabon® [OTC] *see* Vitamin B Complex *on page 899*

GG-Cen® [OTC] *see* Guaifenesin *on page 407*

Gingi-Aid® Gingival Retraction Cord *see* Aluminum Chloride *on page 39*

Gingi-Aid® Solution *see* Aluminum Chloride *on page 39*

Glandosane® Spray [OTC] *see* Saliva Substitute *on page 778*

Glibenclamida (Mexico) *see* Glyburide *on page 401*

Glimepiride *(glye' me pye ride)*

Related Information

Endocrine Disorders & Pregnancy *on page 927*

Brand Names Amaryl®

Therapeutic Category Antidiabetic Agent; Hypoglycemic Agent, Oral; Sulfonylurea Agent

Use

Management of noninsulin-dependent diabetes mellitus (type II) as an adjunct to diet and exercise to lower blood glucose

Use in combination with insulin to lower blood glucose in patients whose hyperglycemia cannot be controlled by diet and exercise in conjunction with an oral hypoglycemic agent

Usual Dosage Oral (allow several days between dose titrations):

Adults: Initial: 1-2 mg once daily, administered with breakfast or the first main meal; usual maintenance dose: 1-4 mg once daily; after a dose of 2 mg once daily, increase in increments of 2 mg at 1- to 2-week intervals based upon the patient's blood glucose response to a maximum of 8 mg once daily

Elderly: Initial: 1 mg/day

Combination with insulin therapy (fasting glucose level for instituting combination therapy is in the range of >150 mg/dL in plasma or serum depending on the patient): 8 mg once daily with the first main meal

After starting with low-dose insulin, upward adjustments of insulin can be done approximately weekly as guided by frequent measurements of fasting blood glucose. Once stable, combination-therapy patients should monitor their capillary blood glucose on an ongoing basis, preferably daily.

Dosing adjustment/comments in renal impairment: Cl_{cr} <22 mL/minute: Initial starting dose should be 1 mg and dosage increments should be based on fasting blood glucose levels

Dosing adjustment in hepatic impairment: No data available

Mechanism of Action Stimulates insulin release from the pancreatic beta cells; reduces glucose output from the liver; insulin sensitivity is increased at peripheral target sites

Local Anesthetic/Vasoconstrictor Precautions No information available to require special precautions

Effects on Dental Treatment Glipizide-dependent diabetics (noninsulin dependent, Type II) should be appointed for dental treatment in morning in order to minimize chance of stress-induced hypoglycemia

Contraindications Hypersensitivity to glimepiride or any component, other sulfonamides; diabetic ketoacidosis (with or without coma)

Warnings/Precautions

The administration of oral hypoglycemic drugs (ie, tolbutamide) has been reported to be associated with increased cardiovascular mortality as compared to treatment with diet alone or diet plus insulin

All sulfonylurea drugs are capable of producing severe hypoglycemia. Hypoglycemia is more likely to occur when caloric intake is deficient, after severe or prolonged exercise, when alcohol is ingested, or when more than one glucose-lowering drug is used.

Drug Interactions

Decreased effects: Beta-blockers, cholestyramine, hydantoins, rifampin, thiazide diuretics, urinary alkalines, charcoal

Increased effects: H_2 antagonists, anticoagulants, androgens, fluconazole, salicylates, gemfibrozil, sulfonamides, tricyclic antidepressants, probenecid, MAO inhibitors, methyldopa, digitalis glycosides, urinary acidifiers

Increased toxicity: Cimetidine → ↑ hypoglycemic effects

Drug Uptake

Duration of action: 24 hours

Peak blood glucose reductions: Within 2-3 hours

Absorption: 100% absorbed; delayed when given with food

Serum half-life: 5-9 hours

Pregnancy Risk Factor C

Generic Available No

Glipicida (Mexico) *see* Glipizide *on this page*
Glipizida (Mexico) *see* Glipizide *on this page*

Glipizide (glip′ i zide)

Related Information

Endocrine Disorders & Pregnancy *on page 927*

Brand Names Glucotrol®; Glucotrol® XL

Canadian/Mexican Brand Names Minodiab® (Mexico)

Therapeutic Category Antidiabetic Agent; Hypoglycemic Agent, Oral; Sulfonylurea Agent

Synonyms Glipicida (Mexico); Glipizida (Mexico)

Use Management of noninsulin-dependent diabetes mellitus (type II)

Usual Dosage Oral (allow several days between dose titrations):

Adults: 2.5-40 mg/day; doses >15-20 mg/day should be divided and given twice daily

Elderly: Initial: 2.5-5 mg/day; increase by 2.5-5 mg/day at 1- to 2-week intervals

Mechanism of Action Stimulates insulin release from the pancreatic beta cells; reduces glucose output from the liver; insulin sensitivity is increased at peripheral target sites

Local Anesthetic/Vasoconstrictor Precautions No information available to require special precautions

Effects on Dental Treatment Glipizide-dependent diabetics (noninsulin dependent, Type II) should be appointed for dental treatment in morning in order to minimize chance of stress-induced hypoglycemia

Other Adverse Effects

>10%:

Central nervous system: Headache

Gastrointestinal: Anorexia, nausea, vomiting, diarrhea, epigastric fullness, constipation, heartburn

1% to 10%: Dermatologic: Rash, hives, photosensitivity

<1%:

Cardiovascular: Edema

Endocrine & metabolic: Hypoglycemia, hyponatremia, hypoglycemia

Genitourinary: Diuretic effect

Hematologic: Blood dyscrasias, aplastic anemia, hemolytic anemia, bone marrow depression, thrombocytopenia, agranulocytosis

Hepatic: Cholestatic jaundice

Drug Interactions

Salicylates may enhance the hypoglycemic response to glipizide due to increased plasma levels of glipizide by displacing from plasma proteins

Thiazide diuretics will increase blood glucose leading to increased requirements of glipizide

Drug Uptake

Duration of action: 12-24 hours

Peak blood glucose reductions: Within 1.5-2 hours

(Continued)

Glipizide *(Continued)*

Absorption: Delayed when given with food
Serum half-life: 2-4 hours
Pregnancy Risk Factor C

Glucagon (gloo' ka gon)

Therapeutic Category Antihypoglycemic Agent
Use Hypoglycemia; diagnostic aid in the radiologic examination of GI tract when a hypotonic state is needed; used with some success as a cardiac stimulant in management of severe cases of beta-adrenergic blocking agent overdosage
Usual Dosage
Hypoglycemia or insulin shock therapy: I.M., I.V., S.C.:
Children: 0.025-0.1 mg/kg/dose, not to exceed 1 mg/dose, repeated in 20 minutes as needed
Adults: 0.5-1 mg, may repeat in 20 minutes as needed
If patient fails to respond to glucagon, I.V. dextrose must be given
Diagnostic aid: Adults: I.M., I.V.: 0.25-2 mg 10 minutes prior to procedure
Mechanism of Action Stimulates adenylate cyclase to produce increased cyclic AMP, which promotes hepatic glycogenolysis and gluconeogenesis, causing a raise in blood glucose levels
Local Anesthetic/Vasoconstrictor Precautions No information available to require special precautions
Effects on Dental Treatment No effects or complications reported
Other Adverse Effects 1% to 10%:
Cardiovascular: Hypotension
Dermatologic: Urticaria
Gastrointestinal: Nausea, vomiting
Respiratory: Respiratory distress
Drug Uptake
Peak effect on blood glucose levels: Parenteral: Within 5-20 minutes
Duration of action: 60-90 minutes
Serum half-life, plasma: 3-10 minutes
Pregnancy Risk Factor B
Comments 1 unit = 1 mg

Glucocerebrosidase *see* Alglucerase *on page 32*

Glucophage® *see* Metformin Hydrochloride *on page 551*

Glucose (gloo' kose)

Brand Names B-D Glucose® [OTC]; Glutose® [OTC]; Insta-Glucose® [OTC]
Therapeutic Category Antihypoglycemic Agent
Use Management of hypoglycemia
Local Anesthetic/Vasoconstrictor Precautions No information available to require special precautions
Effects on Dental Treatment No effects or complications reported
Other Adverse Effects 1% to 10%:
Central nervous system: Fainting
Gastrointestinal: Nausea, vomiting, diarrhea
Comments 4 calories/g

Glucose Polymers (gloo' kose pol' i merz)

Brand Names Moducal® [OTC]; Polycose® [OTC]; Sumacal® [OTC]
Therapeutic Category Nutritional Supplement
Use Supplies calories for those persons not able to meet the caloric requirement with usual food intake
Local Anesthetic/Vasoconstrictor Precautions No information available to require special precautions
Effects on Dental Treatment No effects or complications reported

Glucotrol® *see* Glipizide *on previous page*

Glucotrol® XL *see* Glipizide *on previous page*

Glukor® *see* Chorionic Gonadotropin *on page 203*

Glutamic Acid (gloo tam' ik as' id)

Therapeutic Category Gastrointestinal Agent, Miscellaneous
Use Treatment of hypochlorhydria and achlorhydria
Local Anesthetic/Vasoconstrictor Precautions No information available to require special precautions
Effects on Dental Treatment No effects or complications reported

Other Adverse Effects Systemic acidosis may occur with massive overdosage

Glutethimide (gloo teth' i mide)
Therapeutic Category Hypnotic; Sedative
Use Short-term treatment of insomnia
Local Anesthetic/Vasoconstrictor Precautions No information available to require special precautions
Effects on Dental Treatment No effects or complications reported
Other Adverse Effects
>10%: Central nervous system: Daytime drowsiness
1% to 10%:
Central nervous system: Confusion, headache
Dermatologic: Skin rash
Gastrointestinal: Nausea, vomiting
Ocular: Blurred vision
<1%:
Hematologic: Blood dyscrasias
Cardiovascular: Bradycardia
Central nervous system: Paradoxical reaction, convulsions, fever

Glutose® [OTC] see Glucose on previous page

Glyate® [OTC] see Guaifenesin on page 407

Glyburide (glye' byoor ide)
Related Information
Endocrine Disorders & Pregnancy on page 927
Brand Names Diaβeta®; Glynase™ PresTab™; Micronase®
Canadian/Mexican Brand Names Albert® Glyburide (Canada); Apo-Glyburide® (Canada); Euglucon® (Canada); Gen-Glybe® (Canada); Novo-Glyburide® (Canada); Nu-Glyburide® (Canada); Daonil® (Mexico); Euglucon® (Mexico); Glibenil® (Mexico); Glucal® (Mexico); Norboral® (Mexico)
Therapeutic Category Antidiabetic Agent; Hypoglycemic Agent, Oral; Sulfonylurea Agent
Synonyms Glibenclamida (Mexico)
Use Management of noninsulin-dependent diabetes mellitus (type II)
Usual Dosage Oral:
Adults: 1.25-5 mg to start then increase at weekly intervals to 1.25-20 mg maintenance dose/day divided in 1-2 doses
Elderly: Initial: 1.25-2.5 mg/day, increase by 1.25-2.5 mg/day every 1-3 weeks
Prestab™: Initial: 0.75-3 mg/day, increase by 1.5 mg/day in weekly intervals, maximum: 12 mg/day
Mechanism of Action Stimulates insulin release from the pancreatic beta cells; reduces glucose output from the liver; insulin sensitivity is increased at peripheral target sites
Local Anesthetic/Vasoconstrictor Precautions No information available to require special precautions
Effects on Dental Treatment Glyburide-dependent diabetics (noninsulin dependent, Type II) should be appointed for dental treatment in morning in order to minimize chance of stress-induced hypoglycemia
Other Adverse Effects
>10%:
Central nervous system: Headache, dizziness
Gastrointestinal: Nausea, epigastric fullness, heartburn, constipation, diarrhea, anorexia
1% to 10%:
Dermatologic: Pruritus, rash, hives
Sensitivity reactions: Photosensitivity reaction
<1%:
Endocrine & metabolic: Hypoglycemia
Genitourinary: Nocturia, diuretic effect
Hematologic: Leukopenia, thrombocytopenia, hemolytic anemia, aplastic anemia, bone marrow depression, agranulocytosis
Hepatic: Cholestatic jaundice
Neuromuscular & skeletal: Joint pain, paresthesia
Drug Interactions
Salicylates may enhance the hypoglycemic response to glyburide due to increased plasma levels of glyburide by displacing from plasma proteins
Thiazide diuretics will increase blood glucose leading to increased requirements of glyburide
(Continued)

Glyburide *(Continued)*

Drug Uptake
Onset of action: Oral: Insulin levels in the serum begin to increase within 15-60 minutes after a single dose
Duration: Up to 24 hours
Serum half-life: 5-16 hours; may be prolonged with renal insufficiency or hepatic insufficiency
Time to peak serum concentration: Adults: Within 2-4 hours

Pregnancy Risk Factor D

Glycate® [OTC] *see* Calcium Carbonate *on page 140*

Glycerin (glis′ er in)

Brand Names Fleet® Babylax® Rectal [OTC]; Ophthalgan® Ophthalmic; Osmoglyn® Ophthalmic; Sani-Supp® Suppository [OTC]
Therapeutic Category Laxative, Hyperosmolar
Synonyms Glycerol
Use Constipation; reduction of intraocular pressure; reduction of corneal edema; glycerin has been administered orally to reduce intracranial pressure
Usual Dosage
Constipation: Rectal:
Children <6 years: 1 infant suppository 1-2 times/day as needed or 2-5 mL as an enema
Children >6 years and Adults: 1 adult suppository 1-2 times/day as needed or 5-15 mL as an enema
Children and Adults:
Reduction of intraocular pressure: Oral: 1-1.8 g/kg 1-1½ hours preoperatively; additional doses may be administered at 5-hour intervals
Reduction of intracranial pressure: Oral: 1.5 g/kg/day divided every 4 hours; 1 g/kg/dose every 6 hours has also been used
Reduction of corneal edema: Ophthalmic solution: Instill 1-2 drops in eye(s) prior to examination OR for lubricant effect, instill 1-2 drops in eye(s) every 3-4 hours
Mechanism of Action Osmotic dehydrating agent which increases osmotic pressure; draws fluid into colon and thus stimulates evacuation
Local Anesthetic/Vasoconstrictor Precautions No information available to require special precautions
Effects on Dental Treatment No effects or complications reported
Other Adverse Effects
>10%:
Central nervous system: Headache
Gastrointestinal: Nausea, vomiting
1% to 10%:
Central nervous system: Confusion, dizziness
Gastrointestinal: Diarrhea, dry mouth
Genitourinary: Polydipsia
<1%:
Cardiovascular: Arrhythmias
Endocrine & metabolic: Hyperglycemia
Gastrointestinal: Tenesmus, rectal irritation, cramping pain
Drug Uptake
Absorption:
Oral: Well absorbed
Rectal: Poorly absorbed
Decrease in intraocular pressure: Oral:
Onset of action: Within 10-30 minutes
Peak effect: Within 60-90 minutes
Duration: 4-8 hours
Reduction of intracranial pressure: Oral:
Onset of action: Within 10-60 minutes
Peak effect: Within 60-90 minutes
Duration: ~2-3 hours
Constipation: Suppository: Onset of action: 15-30 minutes
Serum half-life: 30-45 minutes

Pregnancy Risk Factor C

Glycerin, Lanolin, and Peanut Oil

(glis′ er in, lan′ oh lin, & pee′ nut oyl)
Brand Names Massé® Breast Cream [OTC]
Therapeutic Category Topical Skin Product
Use Nipple care of pregnant and nursing women

Local Anesthetic/Vasoconstrictor Precautions No information available to require special precautions

Effects on Dental Treatment No effects or complications reported

Glycerol see Glycerin on previous page

Glycerol-T® see Theophylline and Guaifenesin on page 836

Glycerol Triacetate see Triacetin on page 862

Glycofed® see Guaifenesin and Pseudoephedrine on page 409

Glycopyrrolate (glye koe pye' roe late)

Brand Names Robinul®; Robinul® Forte

Therapeutic Category Anticholinergic Agent; Antispasmodic Agent, Gastrointestinal

Use Adjunct in treatment of peptic ulcer disease; inhibit salivation and excessive secretions of the respiratory tract preoperatively; reversal of neuromuscular blockade; control of upper airway secretions

Usual Dosage

Children:

Control of secretions:

Oral: 40-100 mcg/kg/dose 3-4 times/day

I.M., I.V.: 4-10 mcg/kg/dose every 3-4 hours; maximum: 0.2 mg/dose or 0.8 mg/24 hours

Intraoperative: I.V.: 4 mcg/kg not to exceed 0.1 mg; repeat at 2- to 3-minute intervals as needed

Preoperative: I.M.:

<2 years: 4.4-8.8 mcg/kg 30-60 minutes before procedure

>2 years: 4.4 mcg/kg 30-60 minutes before procedure

Children and Adults: Reverse neuromuscular blockade: I.V.: 0.2 mg for each 1 mg of neostigmine or 5 mg of pyridostigmine administered

Adults:

Intraoperative: I.V.: 0.1 mg repeated as needed at 2- to 3-minute intervals

Preoperative: I.M.: 4.4 mcg/kg 30-60 minutes before procedure

Peptic ulcer:

Oral: 1-2 mg 2-3 times/day

I.M., I.V.: 0.1-0.2 mg 3-4 times/day

Mechanism of Action Blocks the action of acetylcholine at parasympathetic sites in smooth muscle, secretory glands, and the CNS

Local Anesthetic/Vasoconstrictor Precautions No information available to require special precautions

Effects on Dental Treatment Over 10% of patients will experience significant dry mouth (reversible with cessation of drug therapy)

Other Adverse Effects

>10%:

Gastrointestinal: Constipation, dry mouth

Local: Irritation at injection site

Miscellaneous: Decreased sweating; dry nose, throat, or skin

1% to 10%: Decreased flow of breast milk, difficulty in swallowing, increased sensitivity to light

<1%:

Cardiovascular: Orthostatic hypotension, ventricular fibrillation, tachycardia, palpitations

Central nervous system: Confusion, drowsiness, headache, loss of memory, weakness, tiredness, ataxia

Dermatologic: Skin rash

Gastrointestinal: Bloated feeling, nausea, vomiting

Genitourinary: Difficult urination

Ocular: Increased intraocular pain, blurred vision

Drug Interactions

Decreased effect of levodopa

Increased toxicity with amantadine

Drug Uptake

Oral:

Onset of action: Within 50 minutes

I.M.: Onset of action: 20-40 minutes

I.V.: Onset of action: 10-15 minutes

Absorption: Oral: Poor and erratic

Pregnancy Risk Factor B

Glycotuss® [OTC] see Guaifenesin on page 407

Glycotuss-DM® [OTC] see Guaifenesin and Dextromethorphan on page 408

Glynase™ PresTab™ see Glyburide on page 401

Gly-Oxide® [OTC] *see* Carbamide Peroxide *on page 152*

Glytuss® [OTC] *see* Guaifenesin *on page 407*

GM-CSF *see* Sargramostim *on page 780*

Go-Evac® *see* Polyethylene Glycol-Electrolyte Solution *on page 703*

Gold Sodium Thiomalate (gold sow' dee um thye oh mal' ate)
Brand Names Auralate®; Myochrysine®
Therapeutic Category Gold Compound
Use Treatment of progressive rheumatoid arthritis
Usual Dosage I.M.:
   Children: Initial: Test dose of 10 mg is recommended, followed by 1 mg/kg/
   week for 20 weeks; maintenance: 1 mg/kg/dose at 2- to 4-week intervals
   thereafter for as long as therapy is clinically beneficial and toxicity does not
   develop. Administration for 2-4 months is usually required before clinical
   improvement is observed.
   Adults: 10 mg first week; 25 mg second week; then 25-50 mg/week until 1 g
   cumulative dose has been given; if improvement occurs without adverse
   reactions, give 25-50 mg every 2-3 weeks for 2-20 weeks, then every 3-4
   weeks indefinitely
Mechanism of Action Unknown, may decrease prostaglandin synthesis or
   may alter cellular mechanisms by inhibiting sulfhydryl systems
Local Anesthetic/Vasoconstrictor Precautions No information available to
   require special precautions
Effects on Dental Treatment No effects or complications reported
Other Adverse Effects
   >10%:
      Dermatologic: Itching, skin rash
      Gastrointestinal: Stomatitis, gingivitis, glossitis
      Ocular: Conjunctivitis
   1% to 10%:
      Dermatologic: Hives, alopecia
      Hematologic: Eosinophilia, leukopenia, thrombocytopenia
      Renal: Hematuria, proteinuria
   <1%:
      Dermatologic: Angioedema, gray-to-blue pigmentation
      Gastrointestinal: Difficulty in swallowing, ulcerative enterocolitis, GI hemor-
         rhage, metallic taste
      Hematologic: Agranulocytosis, anemia, aplastic anemia
      Hepatic: Hepatotoxicity
      Neuromuscular & skeletal: Peripheral neuropathy
      Respiratory: Interstitial pneumonitis
Drug Uptake
   Serum half-life: 5 days; may lengthen with multiple doses
   Time to peak serum concentration: Within 4-6 hours
Pregnancy Risk Factor C
Comments Approximately 50% gold

GoLYTELY® *see* Polyethylene Glycol-Electrolyte Solution *on page 703*

Gonak™ [OTC] *see* Hydroxypropyl Methylcellulose *on page 442*

Gonic® *see* Chorionic Gonadotropin *on page 203*

Gonioscopic Ophthalmic Solution *see* Hydroxypropyl Methylcellulose *on
   page 442*

Goniosol® [OTC] *see* Hydroxypropyl Methylcellulose *on page 442*

Goody's® Headache Powders *see* Acetaminophen, Aspirin, and Caffeine *on
   page 17*

Goserelin Acetate (goe' se rel in as' e tate)
Brand Names Zoladex® Implant
Canadian/Mexican Brand Names Prozoladex® (Mexico)
Therapeutic Category Gonadotropin Releasing Hormone Analog
Use Palliative treatment of advanced prostate cancer
Usual Dosage
   Adults: S.C.: 3.6 mg injected into upper abdomen every 28 days; do not try to
   aspirate with the goserelin syringe, if the needle is in a large vessel, blood
   will immediately appear in syringe chamber
   Prostate carcinoma: Intended for long-term administration
   Endometriosis: Recommended duration is 6 months; retreatment is not recom-
   mended since safety data is not available
Mechanism of Action LHRH synthetic analog of luteinizing hormone-
   releasing hormone also known as gonadotropin-releasing hormone (GnRH)

incorporated into a biodegradable depot material which allows for continuous slow release over 28 days; mechanism of action is similar to leuprolide

Local Anesthetic/Vasoconstrictor Precautions No information available to require special precautions

Effects on Dental Treatment No effects or complications reported

Other Adverse Effects

General: Worsening of signs and symptoms may occur during the first few weeks of therapy and are usually manifested by an increase in bone pain, increased difficulty in urinating, hot flashes, injection site irritation, and weakness; this will subside, but patients should be aware

>10%:

Endocrine & metabolic: Gynecomastia, postmenopausal symptoms, sexual dysfunction, loss of libido, hot flashes

Genitourinary: Impotence, decreased erection

1% to 10%:

Cardiovascular: Edema

Central nervous system: Headache, spinal cord compression (possible result of tumor flare), lethargy, dizziness, insomnia

Dermatologic: Rash

Endocrine & metabolic: Breast tenderness/enlargement

Gastrointestinal: Nausea and vomiting, anorexia, diarrhea, weight gain

Genitourinary: Vaginal spotting and breakthrough bleeding

Local: Pain on injection

Neuromuscular & skeletal: Bone loss, increased bone pain

Miscellaneous: Sweating

Drug Uptake

Absorption:

Oral: Inactive when administered orally

S.C.: Rapid and can be detected in the serum in 10 minutes

Time to peak serum concentration: S.C.: 12-15 days

Serum half-life: Following a bolus S.C. dose: 5 hours

Pregnancy Risk Factor X

Granisetron (gra ni' se tron)

Brand Names Kytril®

Therapeutic Category Antiemetic

Use Prophylaxis and treatment of chemotherapy-related emesis; may be prescribed for patients who are refractory to or have severe adverse reactions to standard antiemetic therapy. Granisetron may be prescribed for young patients (ie, <45 years of age who are more likely to develop extrapyramidal reactions to high-dose metoclopramide) who are to receive highly emetogenic chemotherapeutic agents as listed:

Agents with high emetogenic potential (>90%) (dose/m^2):

Carmustine ≥200 mg

Cisplatin ≥75 mg

Cyclophosphamide ≥1000 mg

Cytarabine ≥1000 mg

Dacarbazine ≥500 mg

Ifosfamide ≥1000 mg

Lomustine ≥60 mg

Mechlorethamine

Pentostatin

Streptozocin

or two agents classified as having high or moderately high emetogenic potential as listed:

Agents with moderately high emetogenic potential (60% to 90%) (dose/m^2):

Carmustine <200 mg

Cisplatin <75 mg

Cyclophosphamide 1000 mg

Cytarabine 250-1000 mg

Dacarbazine <500 mg

Doxorubicin ≥75 mg

Ifosfamide

Lomustine <60 mg

Methotrexate ≥250 mg

Mitomycin

Mitoxantrone

Procarbazine

(Continued)

Granisetron (Continued)

Granisetron should not be prescribed for chemotherapeutic agents with a low emetogenic potential (eg, bleomycin, busulfan, cyclophosphamide <1000 mg, etoposide, 5-fluorouracil, vinblastine, vincristine)

Usual Dosage

I.V.: Children and Adults: 10 mcg/kg for 1-3 doses. Doses should be administered as a single IVPB over 5 minutes to 1 hour, given just prior to chemotherapy (15-60 minutes before); as intervention therapy for breakthrough nausea and vomiting, during the first 24 hours following chemotherapy, 2 or 3 repeat infusions (same dose) have been administered, separated by at least 10 minutes

Oral: Adults: 1 mg twice daily; the first 1 mg dose should be given up to 1 hour before chemotherapy, and the second tablet, 12 hours after the first

Note: Granisetron should only be given on the day(s) of chemotherapy

Mechanism of Action Selective 5-HT$_3$ receptor antagonist, blocking serotonin, both peripherally on vagal nerve terminals and centrally in the chemoreceptor trigger zone

Local Anesthetic/Vasoconstrictor Precautions No information available to require special precautions

Effects on Dental Treatment No effects or complications reported

Other Adverse Effects

>10%: Central nervous system: Headache

1% to 10%:

Central nervous system: Asthenia, dizziness, insomnia, anxiety

Gastrointestinal: Constipation, abdominal pain, diarrhea

Hematologic: Transient blood pressure changes

<1%:

Cardiovascular: Arrhythmias

Central nervous system: Somnolence, agitation, weakness

Endocrine & metabolic: Hot flashes

Hepatic: Liver enzyme elevations

Drug Interactions No data reported

Drug Uptake

Onset of action: Commonly controls emesis within 1-3 minutes of administration

Duration: Effects generally last no more than 24 hours maximum

Serum half-life:

Cancer patients: 10-12 hours

Healthy volunteers: 3-4 hours

Pregnancy Risk Factor B

Granulex see Trypsin, Balsam Peru, and Castor Oil on page 881

Granulocyte Colony Stimulating Factor see Filgrastim on page 362

Granulocyte-Macrophage Colony Stimulating Factor see Sargramostim on page 780

Grifulvin® V see Griseofulvin on this page

Grisactin® see Griseofulvin on this page

Grisactin® Ultra see Griseofulvin on this page

Griseofulvin (gri see oh ful' vin)

Brand Names Fulvicin® P/G; Fulvicin-U/F®; Grifulvin® V; Grisactin®; Grisactin® Ultra; Gris-PEG®

Canadian/Mexican Brand Names Grisovin-FP® (Canada); Fulvina® P/G (Mexico); Grisovin-FP® (Mexico)

Therapeutic Category Antifungal Agent, Systemic

Synonyms Griseofulvina (Mexico)

Use Treatment of susceptible tinea infections of the skin, hair, and nails

Usual Dosage Oral:

Children:

Microsize: 10-15 mg/kg/day in single or divided doses

Ultramicrosize: >2 months: 5.5-7.3 mg/kg/day in single or divided doses

Adults:

Microsize: 500-1000 mg/day in single or divided doses

Ultramicrosize: 330-375 mg/day in single or divided doses; doses up to 750 mg/day have been used for infections more difficult to eradicate such as tinea unguium and tinea pedis

Duration of therapy depends on the site of infection:

Tinea corporis: 2-4 weeks

Tinea capitis: 4-6 weeks or longer

Tinea pedis: 4-8 weeks

Tinea unguium: 4-6 months

Mechanism of Action Inhibits fungal cell mitosis at metaphase; binds to human keratin making it resistant to fungal invasion

Local Anesthetic/Vasoconstrictor Precautions No information available to require special precautions

Effects on Dental Treatment Griseofulvin may cause soreness or irritation of mouth or tongue

Other Adverse Effects

>10%: Dermatologic: Skin rash, urticaria

1% to 10%:

Central nervous system: Headache, fatigue, dizziness, insomnia, mental confusion

Dermatologic: Photosensitivity

Gastrointestinal: Nausea, vomiting, epigastric distress, diarrhea

Miscellaneous: Oral thrush

<1%:

Endocrine & metabolic: Menstrual toxicity

Gastrointestinal: GI bleeding

Hematologic: Leukopenia

Hepatic: Hepatic toxicity

Renal: Proteinuria, nephrosis

Miscellaneous: Angioneurotic edema

Drug Interactions

Decreased effect:

Barbiturates leads to decreased levels of griseofulvin

Decreased warfarin activity

Decreased oral contraceptive effectiveness

Increased toxicity: With alcohol causes tachycardia and flushing

Drug Uptake

Absorption: Ultramicrosize griseofulvin absorption is almost complete; absorption of microsize griseofulvin is variable (25% to 70% of an oral dose); absorption is enhanced by ingestion of a fatty meal

Serum half-life: 9-22 hours

Pregnancy Risk Factor C

Griseofulvina (Mexico) see Griseofulvin on previous page

Gris-PEG® see Griseofulvin on previous page

Guaifed® [OTC] see Guaifenesin and Pseudoephedrine on page 409

Guaifed-PD® see Guaifenesin and Pseudoephedrine on page 409

Guaifenesin (gwye fen' e sin)

Brand Names Amonidrin® [OTC]; Anti-Tuss® Expectorant [OTC]; Breonesin® [OTC]; Fenesin™; Gee Gee® [OTC]; Genatuss® [OTC]; GG-Cen® [OTC]; Glyate® [OTC]; Glycotuss® [OTC]; Glytuss® [OTC]; Guiatuss® [OTC]; Halotussin® [OTC]; Humibid® L.A.; Humibid® Sprinkle; Hytuss-2X® [OTC]; Hytuss® [OTC]; Malotuss® [OTC]; Mytussin® [OTC]; Naldecon® Senior EX [OTC]; Robitussin® [OTC]; Scot-Tussin® [OTC]; Sinumist®-SR Capsulets®; Uni-Tussin® [OTC]

Canadian/Mexican Brand Names Balminil® Expectorant (Canada); Calmylin® Expectorant (Canada)

Therapeutic Category Expectorant

Synonyms Guaifenesina (Mexico)

Use Temporary control of cough due to minor throat and bronchial irritation

Usual Dosage Oral:

Children:

<2 years: 12 mg/kg/day in 6 divided doses

2-5 years: 50-100 mg every 4 hours, not to exceed 600 mg/day

6-11 years: 100-200 mg every 4 hours, not to exceed 1.2 g/day

Children >12 years and Adults: 200-400 mg every 4 hours to a maximum of 2.4 g/day

Mechanism of Action Thought to act as an expectorant by irritating the gastric mucosa and stimulating respiratory tract secretions, thereby increasing respiratory fluid volumes and decreasing phlegm viscosity

Local Anesthetic/Vasoconstrictor Precautions No information available to require special precautions

Effects on Dental Treatment No effects or complications reported

Other Adverse Effects 1% to 10%:

Central nervous system: Drowsiness, headache

Dermatologic: Rash

Gastrointestinal: Nausea, vomiting, stomach pain

Drug Interactions No data reported

(Continued)

Guaifenesin *(Continued)*

Drug Uptake
Absorption: Well absorbed from GI tract
Pregnancy Risk Factor C

Guaifenesina Dextrometorfano (Mexico) *see* Guaifenesin and Dextromethorphan *on this page*

Guaifenesina (Mexico) *see* Guaifenesin *on previous page*

Guaifenesin and Codeine (gwye fen' e sin & koe' deen)

Brand Names Cheracol®; Guaituss AC®; Guiatussin® with Codeine; Halotussin® AC; Mytussin® AC; Robafen® AC; Robitussin® A-C
Therapeutic Category Antitussive; Cough Preparation; Expectorant
Use Temporary control of cough due to minor throat and bronchial irritation
Usual Dosage Oral:
Children:
2-6 years: 1-1.5 mg/kg codeine/day divided into 4 doses administered every 4-6 hours (maximum: 30 mg/24 hours)
6-12 years: 5 mL every 4 hours, not to exceed 30 mL/24 hours
Children >12 years and Adults: 5-10 mL every 4-8 hours not to exceed 60 mL/24 hours
Mechanism of Action
Guaifenesin is thought to act as an expectorant by irritating the gastric mucosa and stimulating respiratory tract secretions, thereby increasing respiratory fluid volumes and decreasing phlegm viscosity
Codeine is an antitussive that controls cough by depressing the medullary cough center
Local Anesthetic/Vasoconstrictor Precautions No information available to require special precautions
Effects on Dental Treatment No effects or complications reported
Other Adverse Effects
Codeine:
>10%:
Central nervous system: Drowsiness
Gastrointestinal: Constipation
1% to 10%:
Cardiovascular: Hypotension, palpitations, tachycardia or bradycardia, peripheral vasodilation
Central nervous system: CNS depression, drowsiness, sedation, confusion, headache, increased intracranial pressure, dizziness, lightheadedness, false feeling of well being, restlessness, paradoxical CNS stimulation, weakness, malaise
Dermatologic: Skin rash, hives
Endocrine & metabolic: Antidiuretic hormone release
Gastrointestinal: Nausea, vomiting, anorexia, dry mouth
Genitourinary: Decreased urination
Ocular: Miosis, blurred vision
Respiratory: Respiratory depression, shortness of breath, troubled breathing
Miscellaneous: Histamine release, physical and psychological dependence with prolonged use, biliary or urinary tract spasm
<1%:
Central nervous system: Convulsions, hallucinations, mental depression, nightmares, insomnia
Gastrointestinal: Biliary spasm, stomach cramps, paralytic ileus
Neuromuscular & skeletal: Trembling, muscle rigidity
Guaifenesin:
1% to 10%:
Central nervous system: Drowsiness, headache
Dermatologic: Rash
Gastrointestinal: Nausea, vomiting, stomach pain
Drug Interactions Increased toxicity: CNS depressant medications produce additive sedative properties
Pregnancy Risk Factor C

Guaifenesin and Dextromethorphan
(gwye fen' e sin & deks troe meth or' fan)
Brand Names Benylin® Expectorant [OTC]; Cheracol D® [OTC]; Contac® Cough Formula Liquid [OTC]; Diabetic Tussin® DM [OTC]; Extra Action Cough Syrup [OTC]; Genatuss DM® [OTC]; Glycotuss-DM® [OTC]; GuiaCough® [OTC]; Guiatuss DM® [OTC]; Halotussin® DM [OTC]; Humibid® DM [OTC];

Iophen DM® [OTC]; Kolephrin® GG/DM [OTC]; Mytussin® DM [OTC]; Naldecon® Senior DX [OTC]; Rhinosyn-DMX® [OTC]; Robafen DM® [OTC]; Robitussin®-DM [OTC]; Safe Tussin 30 Liquid® [OTC]; Syracol-CF® [OTC]; Tolu-Sed® DM [OTC]; Tuss-DM® [OTC]; Uni-tussin® DM [OTC]

Therapeutic Category Antitussive; Cough Preparation; Expectorant

Synonyms Guaifenesina Dextrometorfano (Mexico)

Use Temporary control of cough due to minor throat and bronchial irritation

Usual Dosage Oral:

Children: Dextromethorphan: 1-2 mg/kg/24 hours divided 3-4 times/day

Children >12 years and Adults: 5 mL every 4 hours or 10 mL every 6-8 hours not to exceed 40 mL/24 hours

Mechanism of Action

Guaifenesin is thought to act as an expectorant by irritating the gastric mucosa and stimulating respiratory tract secretions, thereby increasing respiratory fluid volumes and decreasing phlegm viscosity

Dextromethorphan is a chemical relative of morphine lacking narcotic properties except in overdose; controls cough by depressing the medullary cough center

Local Anesthetic/Vasoconstrictor Precautions No information available to require special precautions

Effects on Dental Treatment No effects or complications reported

Other Adverse Effects 1% to 10%:

Central nervous system: Drowsiness, headache

Dermatologic: Rash

Gastrointestinal: Nausea, vomiting

Drug Interactions No data reported

Drug Uptake

Onset of action: Exerts its antitussive effect in 15-30 minutes after oral administration

Pregnancy Risk Factor C

Guaifenesin and Hydrocodone see Hydrocodone and Guaifenesin on page 434

Guaifenesin and Phenylpropanolamine

(gwye fen' e sin & fen il proe pa nole' a meen)

Brand Names Ami-Tex LA®; Coldlac-LA®; Conex® [OTC]; Contuss® XT; Dura-Vent®; Entex® LA; Genamin® Expectorant [OTC]; Gentab-LA®; Guaifenex® PPA 75; Guaipax®; Myminic® Expectorant [OTC]; Naldecon-EX® Children's Syrup [OTC]; Nolex® LA; Partuss® LA; Phenylfenesin® L.A.; Profen II®; Profen LA®; Rymed-TR®; Silaminic® Expectorant [OTC]; Sildicon-E® [OTC]; Snaplets-EX® [OTC]; Theramin® Expectorant [OTC]; Triaminic® Expectorant [OTC]; Tri-Clear® Expectorant [OTC]; Triphenyl® Expectorant [OTC]; ULR-LA®; Vanex-LA®; Vicks® DayQuil® Sinus Pressure & Congestion Relief [OTC]

Therapeutic Category Decongestant; Expectorant

Synonyms Phenylpropanolamine and Guaifenesin

Use Symptomatic relief of those respiratory conditions where tenacious mucous plugs and congestion complicate the problem such as sinusitis, pharyngitis, bronchitis, asthma, and as an adjunctive therapy in serous otitis media

Local Anesthetic/Vasoconstrictor Precautions Use with caution since phenylpropanolamine is a sympathomimetic amine which could interact with epinephrine to cause a pressor response

Effects on Dental Treatment

Guaifenesin: No effects or complications reported

Phenylpropanolamine: Up to 10% of patients could experience tachycardia, palpitations, and dry mouth; use vasoconstrictor with caution

Guaifenesin and Pseudoephedrine

(gwye fen' e sin & soo doe e fed' rin)

Brand Names Congess® Jr; Congess® Sr; Congestac®; Deconsal® II; Defen-LA®; Entex® PSE; Eudal-SR®; Fedahist® Expectorant [OTC]; Glycofed®; Guaifed® [OTC]; Guaifed-PD®; Guaifenex PSE®; GuaiMax-D®; Guaitab®; Guai-Vent/PSE®; Guiatuss PE® [OTC]; Halotussin® PE [OTC]; Histalet X®; Nasabid™; Respa-1st®; Respaire®-60 SR; Respaire®-120 SR; Robitussin-PE® [OTC]; Robitussin® Severe Congestion Liqui-Gels [OTC]; Ru-Tuss® DE; Rymed®; Sinufed® Timecelles®; Sudex®; Touro LA®; Tuss-LA®; V-Dec-M®; Versacaps®; Zephrex®; Zephrex LA®

Therapeutic Category Decongestant; Expectorant

Synonyms Pseudoephedrine and Guaifenesin

Use Enhance the output of respiratory tract fluid and reduce mucosal congestion and edema in the nasal passage

(Continued)

Guaifenesin and Pseudoephedrine *(Continued)*

Local Anesthetic/Vasoconstrictor Precautions Use with caution since pseudoephedrine is a sympathomimetic amine which could interact with epinephrine to cause a pressor response

Effects on Dental Treatment
Guaifenesin: No effects or complications reported
Pseudoephedrine: Up to 10% of patients could experience tachycardia, palpitations, and dry mouth; use vasoconstrictor with caution

Guaifenesin, Phenylpropanolamine, and Dextromethorphan

(gwye fen' e sin, fen il proe pa nole' a meen, & deks troe meth or' fan)

Brand Names Anatuss® [OTC]; Guiatuss CF® [OTC]; Naldecon® DX Adult Liquid [OTC]; Robafen® CF [OTC]; Robitussin-CF® [OTC]; Siltussin-CF® [OTC]

Therapeutic Category Cough Preparation; Decongestant; Expectorant

Use Temporarily relieves nasal congestion and controls cough due to minor throat and bronchial irritation; helps loosen phlegm and thin bronchial secretions to make coughs more productive

Local Anesthetic/Vasoconstrictor Precautions Use with caution since phenylpropanolamine is a sympathomimetic amine which could interact with epinephrine to cause a pressor response

Effects on Dental Treatment
Dextromethorphan, Guaifenesin: No effects or complications reported
Phenylpropanolamine: Up to 10% of patients could experience tachycardia, palpitations, and dry mouth; use vasoconstrictor with caution

Guaifenesin, Phenylpropanolamine, and Phenylephrine

(gwye fen' e sin, fen il proe pa nole' a meen, & fen il ef' rin)

Brand Names Coldloc®; Contuss®; Despec® Liquid; Dura-Gest®; Enomine®; Entex®; Guaifenex®; Guiatex®; Respinol-G®; ULR®

Therapeutic Category Decongestant; Expectorant

Use Temporary relief of nasal congestion, running nose, sneezing, itching of nose and throat, and itchy, watery eyes due to common cold, hay fever, or other upper respiratory allergies

Local Anesthetic/Vasoconstrictor Precautions Use with caution since phenylpropanolamine and phenylephrine are sympathomimetic amines which could interact with epinephrine to cause a pressor response

Effects on Dental Treatment
Guaifenesin: No effects or complications reported
Phenylephrine, Phenylpropanolamine: Up to 10% of patients could experience tachycardia, palpitations, and dry mouth; use vasoconstrictor with caution

Guaifenesin, Pseudoephedrine, and Codeine

(gwye fen' e sin, soo doe e fed' rin, & koe' deen)

Brand Names Codafed® Expectorant; Decohistine® Expectorant; Deproist® Expectorant with Codeine; Dihistine® Expectorant; Guiatuss DAC®; Guiatussin® DAC; Halotussin® DAC; Isoclor® Expectorant; Mytussin® DAC; Novahistine® Expectorant; Nucofed®; Nucofed® Pediatric Expectorant; Nucotuss®; Phenhist® Expectorant; Robitussin®-DAC; Ryna-CX®; Tussar® SF Syrup

Therapeutic Category Cough Preparation; Decongestant; Expectorant

Use Temporarily relieves nasal congestion and controls cough due to minor throat and bronchial irritation; helps loosen phlegm and thin bronchial secretions to make coughs more productive

Local Anesthetic/Vasoconstrictor Precautions Use with caution since pseudoephedrine is a sympathomimetic amine which could interact with epinephrine to cause a pressor response

Effects on Dental Treatment
Codeine: <1%: Dry mouth
Guaifenesin: No effects or complications reported
Pseudoephedrine: Up to 10% of patients could experience tachycardia, palpitations, and dry mouth; use vasoconstrictor with caution

Guaifenex® *see* Guaifenesin, Phenylpropanolamine, and Phenylephrine *on this page*

Guaifenex® PPA 75 *see* Guaifenesin and Phenylpropanolamine *on previous page*

Guaifenex PSE® *see* Guaifenesin and Pseudoephedrine *on previous page*

GuaiMax-D® *see* Guaifenesin and Pseudoephedrine *on previous page*

Guaipax® *see* Guaifenesin and Phenylpropanolamine *on previous page*

Guaitab® *see* Guaifenesin and Pseudoephedrine *on page 409*
Guaituss AC® *see* Guaifenesin and Codeine *on page 408*
Guai-Vent/PSE® *see* Guaifenesin and Pseudoephedrine *on page 409*

Guanabenz Acetate (gwahn′ a benz as′ e tate)
Related Information
Cardiovascular Diseases *on page 912*
Brand Names Wytensin®
Therapeutic Category Alpha-Adrenergic Blockers - Peripheral-Acting (Alpha$_1$-Blockers)
Use Management of hypertension
Usual Dosage Adults: Oral: Initial: 4 mg twice daily, increase in increments of 4-8 mg/day every 1-2 weeks to a maximum of 32 mg twice daily
Mechanism of Action Stimulates alpha$_2$-adrenoreceptors in the brain stem, thus activating an inhibitory neuron, resulting in reduced sympathetic outflow, producing a decrease in vasomotor tone and heart rate
Local Anesthetic/Vasoconstrictor Precautions No information available to require special precautions
Effects on Dental Treatment Over 10% of patients will experience significant dry mouth; normal salivation occurs with cessation of drug therapy
Other Adverse Effects
>10%:
  Central nervous system: Drowsiness or sedation, dizziness
  Gastrointestinal: Dry mouth
  Neuromuscular & skeletal: Weakness
1% to 10%:
  Cardiovascular: Chest pain, edema
  Central nervous system: Headache
  Endocrine & metabolic: Decreased sexual ability
  Gastrointestinal: Nausea
<1%:
  Cardiovascular: Arrhythmias, palpitations
  Central nervous system: Anxiety, ataxia, depression, sleep disturbances
  Dermatologic: Rash, pruritus
  Endocrine & metabolic: Disturbances of sexual function, gynecomastia
  Gastrointestinal: Diarrhea, vomiting, constipation
  Genitourinary: Urinary frequency
  Neuromuscular & skeletal: Muscle aches
  Ocular: Blurring of vision
  Respiratory: Nasal congestion, dyspnea
  Miscellaneous: Taste disorders
Drug Interactions
Decreased hypotensive effect of guanabenz with tricyclic antidepressants
Increased effect: Other hypotensive agents
Drug Uptake
Onset of antihypertensive effect: Within 1 hour
Absorption: ~75%
Serum half-life: 7-10 hours
Pregnancy Risk Factor C

Guanadrel Sulfate (gwahn′ a drel sul′ fate)
Related Information
Cardiovascular Diseases *on page 912*
Brand Names Hylorel®
Therapeutic Category Alpha-Adrenergic Blockers - Peripheral-Acting (Alpha$_1$-Blockers)
Use Considered a second line agent in the treatment of hypertension, usually with a diuretic
Usual Dosage
Adults: Oral: Initial: 10 mg/day (5 mg twice daily); adjust dosage until blood pressure is controlled, usual dosage: 20-75 mg/day, given twice daily
Elderly: Initial: 5 mg once daily
Mechanism of Action Acts as a false neurotransmitter that blocks the adrenergic actions of norepinephrine; it displaces norepinephrine from its presynaptic storage granules and thus exposes it to degradation; it thereby produces a reduction in total peripheral resistance and, therefore, blood pressure
Local Anesthetic/Vasoconstrictor Precautions No information available to require special precautions
Effects on Dental Treatment No effects or complications reported
(Continued)

Guanadrel Sulfate *(Continued)*

Other Adverse Effects
>10%:
Cardiovascular: Palpitations, chest pain, peripheral edema
Central nervous system: Fatigue, headache, faintness, drowsiness, confusion
Gastrointestinal: Increased bowel movements, gas pain, constipation, anorexia, weight gain/loss
Genitourinary: Nocturia, urinary frequency, ejaculation disturbances
Neuromuscular & skeletal: Paresthesia, aching limbs, leg cramps, backache, joint pain
Ocular: Visual disturbances
Respiratory: Shortness of breath, coughing
1% to 10%:
Cardiovascular: Orthostatic hypotension
Central nervous system: Psychological problems, depression, sleep disorders
Gastrointestinal: Increased bowel movements, glossitis, nausea, vomiting, dry mouth
Genitourinary: Impotence
Renal: Hematuria
<1%: Cardiovascular: Syncope, angina

Drug Interactions
Decreased effect with tricyclic antidepressants, indirect-acting amines (ephedrine, phenylpropanolamine), phenothiazines
Increased toxicity of direct-acting amines (epinephrine, norepinephrine)
Increased effect of beta-blockers, vasodilators

Drug Uptake
Peak effect: Within 4-6 hours
Duration: 4-14 hours
Absorption: Oral: Rapid
Serum half-life, biphasic:
Initial: 1-4 hours
Terminal: 5-45 hours
Time to peak serum concentration: Within 1.5-2 hour

Pregnancy Risk Factor B

Guanethidine Sulfate (gwahn eth' i deen mon' oh sul' fate)

Related Information
Cardiovascular Diseases *on page 912*

Brand Names Ismelin®

Canadian/Mexican Brand Names Apo-Guanethidine® (Canada)

Therapeutic Category Alpha-Adrenergic Blockers - Peripheral-Acting (Alpha$_1$-Blockers)

Use Treatment of moderate to severe hypertension

Usual Dosage Oral:
Children: Initial: 0.2 mg/kg/day, increase by 0.2 mg/kg/day at 7- to 10-day intervals to a maximum of 3 mg/kg/day
Adults:
Ambulatory patients: Initial: 10 mg/day, increase at 5- to 7-day intervals to a maximum of 25-50 mg/day
Hospitalized patients: Initial: 25-50 mg/day, increase by 25-50 mg/day or every other day to desired therapeutic response
Elderly: Initial: 5 mg once daily

Mechanism of Action Acts as a false neurotransmitter that blocks the adrenergic actions of norepinephrine; it displaces norepinephrine from its presynaptic storage granules and thus exposes it to degradation; it thereby produces a reduction in total peripheral resistance and, therefore, blood pressure

Local Anesthetic/Vasoconstrictor Precautions No information available to require special precautions

Effects on Dental Treatment No effects or complications reported

Other Adverse Effects
>10%:
Cardiovascular: Palpitations, chest pain, peripheral edema
Central nervous system: Fatigue, headache, faintness, drowsiness, confusion
Endocrine & metabolic: Ejaculation disturbances
Gastrointestinal: Increased bowel movements, gas pain, constipation, anorexia, weight gain/loss
Genitourinary: Nocturia, urinary frequency, impotence

Neuromuscular & skeletal: Paresthesia, aching limbs, leg cramps, backache, joint pain

Ocular: Visual disturbances

Respiratory: Shortness of breath, coughing

1% to 10%:

Cardiovascular: Orthostatic hypotension

Central nervous system: Psychological problems, depression, sleep disorders

Gastrointestinal: Increased bowel movements, glossitis, nausea, vomiting, dry mouth

Renal: Hematuria

<1%: Cardiovascular: Syncope, angina

Drug Interactions

Decreased effect with tricyclic antidepressants, indirect-acting amines (ephedrine, phenylpropanolamine)

Increased toxicity of direct-acting amines (epinephrine, norepinephrine)

Drug Uptake

Onset of effect: Within 0.5-2 hours

Peak antihypertensive effect: Within 6-8 hours

Duration: 24-48 hours

Absorption: Irregular (3% to 55%)

Serum half-life: 5-10 days

Pregnancy Risk Factor C

Guanfacine Hydrochloride (gwahn' fa seen hye droe klor' ide)

Related Information

Cardiovascular Diseases *on page 912*

Brand Names Tenex®

Therapeutic Category Alpha-Adrenergic Blockers - Peripheral-Acting (Alpha$_1$-Blockers)

Use Management of hypertension

Usual Dosage Adults: Oral: 1 mg usually at bedtime, may increase if needed at 3- to 4-week intervals to a maximum of 3 mg/day; 1 mg/day is most common dose

Mechanism of Action Stimulates alpha$_2$-adrenoreceptors in the brain stem, thus activating an inhibitory neuron, resulting in reduced sympathetic outflow, producing a decrease in vasomotor tone and heart rate

Local Anesthetic/Vasoconstrictor Precautions No information available to require special precautions

Effects on Dental Treatment Guanfacine may inhibit salivary flow

Other Adverse Effects

>10%:

Central nervous system: Somnolence, dizziness

Gastrointestinal: Dry mouth, constipation

1% to 10%:

Central nervous system: Fatigue, headache, insomnia

Endocrine & metabolic: Decreased sexual ability

Gastrointestinal: Nausea, vomiting

Ocular: Conjunctivitis

<1%:

Cardiovascular: Bradycardia, palpitations

Central nervous system: Amnesia, confusion, depression, malaise

Dermatologic: Dermatitis, pruritus, purpura

Gastrointestinal: Abdominal pain, diarrhea, dyspepsia, dysphagia, taste perversion

Genitourinary: Testicular disorder, urinary incontinence

Neuromuscular & skeletal: Leg cramps, hypokinesia, paresthesia

Otic: Tinnitus

Respiratory: Rhinitis, dyspnea

Miscellaneous: Substernal pain, sweating

Drug Interactions

Decreased hypotensive effect of guanfacine with tricyclic antidepressants

Increased effect: Other hypotensive agents

Drug Uptake

Peak effect: Within 8-11 hours

Duration: 24 hours following a single dose

Serum half-life: 17 hours

Time to peak serum concentration: Within 1-4 hours

Pregnancy Risk Factor B

GuiaCough® [OTC] *see* Guaifenesin and Dextromethorphan *on page 408*

Guiatex® *see* Guaifenesin, Phenylpropanolamine, and Phenylephrine *on page 410*

Guiatuss® [OTC] *see* Guaifenesin *on page 407*

Guiatuss CF® [OTC] *see* Guaifenesin, Phenylpropanolamine, and Dextromethorphan *on page 410*

Guiatuss DAC® *see* Guaifenesin, Pseudoephedrine, and Codeine *on page 410*

Guiatuss DM® [OTC] *see* Guaifenesin and Dextromethorphan *on page 408*

Guiatussin® DAC *see* Guaifenesin, Pseudoephedrine, and Codeine *on page 410*

Guiatussin® with Codeine *see* Guaifenesin and Codeine *on page 408*

Guiatuss PE® [OTC] *see* Guaifenesin and Pseudoephedrine *on page 409*

Gum Benjamin *see* Benzoin *on page 104*

G-well® *see* Lindane *on page 504*

Gyne-Sulf® *see* Sulfabenzamide, Sulfacetamide, and Sulfathiazole *on page 806*

Gynogen L.A.® *see* Estradiol *on page 325*

Gynol II® [OTC] *see* Nonoxynol 9 *on page 627*

Habitrol™ *see* Nicotine *on page 617*

Haemophilus b Conjugate Vaccine

(he mof' i lus bee kon' joo gate vak seen')

Brand Names HibTITER®; OmniHIB®; PedvaxHIB™; ProHIBiT®

Therapeutic Category Vaccine, Inactivated Bacteria

Synonyms Diphtheria CRM$_{197}$ Protein Conjugate; Diphtheria Toxoid Conjugate; *Haemophilus* b Oligosaccharide Conjugate Vaccine; *Haemophilus* b Polysaccharide Vaccine; HbCV; Hib Polysaccharide Conjugate; PRP-D

Use Immunization of children 24 months to 6 years of age against diseases caused by *H. influenzae* type b

Usual Dosage Children: I.M.: 0.5 mL as a single dose should be administered according to one of the following "brand-specific" schedules; do not inject I.V.

Vaccination Schedule for Haemophilus b Conjugate Vaccines

Age at 1st Dose (mo)	HibTITER® Primary Series	HibTITER® Booster	PedvaxHIB® Primary Series	PedvaxHIB® Booster	ProHIBiT® Primary Series	ProHIBiT® Booster
2-6*	3 doses, 2 months apart	15 mo†	2 doses, 2 months apart	12 mo†		
7-11	2 doses, 2 months apart	15 mo†	2 doses, 2 months apart	15 mo†		
12-14	1 dose	15 mo†	1 dose	15 mo†		
15-60	1 dose	—	1 dose	—	1 dose	—

*It is not currently recommended that the various Haemophilus b conjugate vaccines be interchanged (ie, the same brand should be used throughout the entire vaccination series). If the health care provider does not know which vaccine was previously used, it is prudent that an infant, 2-6 months of age, be given a primary series of three doses.

†At least 2 months after previous dose.

Mechanism of Action Stimulates production of anticapsular antibodies and provides active immunity to *Haemophilus influenzae*; Hib conjugate vaccines use covalent binding of capsular polysaccharide of *Haemophilus influenzae* type b to diphtheria CRM 197 (HibTITER®) to produce an antigen which is postulated to convert a T-independent antigen into a T-dependent antigen to result in enhanced antibody response and on immunologic memory

Local Anesthetic/Vasoconstrictor Precautions No information available to require special precautions

Effects on Dental Treatment No effects or complications reported

Other Adverse Effects When administered during the same visit that DTP vaccine is given, the rates of systemic reactions do not differ from those observed only when DTP vaccine is administered

25%:
Cardiovascular: Swelling
Dermatologic: Local erythema
Local: Increased risk of *Haemophilus* b infections in the week after vaccination
Miscellaneous: Warmth

>10%: Acute febrile reactions

1% to 10%:
Central nervous system: Fever (up to 102.2°F), irritability, lethargy

Gastrointestinal: Anorexia, diarrhea
Local: Irritation at injection site
<1%:
Central nervous system: Convulsions, fever >102.2°F
Gastrointestinal: Vomiting
Neuromuscular & skeletal: Weakness
Miscellaneous: Allergic or anaphylactic reactions (difficulty in breathing, hives, itching, swelling of eyes, face, unusual tiredness)

Drug Uptake
The seroconversion following one dose of Hib vaccine for children 18 months or 24 months of age or older is 75% to 90% respectively
Onset of serum antibody responses: 1-2 weeks after vaccination
Duration: Immunity appears to last 1.5 years

Pregnancy Risk Factor C

Comments Federal law requires that the date of administration, the vaccine manufacturer, lot number of vaccine, and the administering person's name, title and address be entered into the patient's permanent medical record

Haemophilus b Oligosaccharide Conjugate Vaccine see *Haemophilus* b Conjugate Vaccine *on previous page*

Haemophilus b Polysaccharide Vaccine see *Haemophilus* b Conjugate Vaccine *on previous page*

Halazepam (hal az' e pam)
Brand Names Paxipam®
Therapeutic Category Benzodiazepine
Use Management of anxiety disorders; short-term relief of the symptoms of anxiety
Local Anesthetic/Vasoconstrictor Precautions No information available to require special precautions
Effects on Dental Treatment Significant dry mouth will occur in over 10% of patients; normal salivary flow occurs with cessation of drug therapy
Other Adverse Effects
>10%:
Cardiovascular: Chest pain
Central nervous system: Drowsiness, fatigue, impaired coordination, lightheadedness, memory impairment, insomnia, anxiety, depression, headache
Dermatologic: Rash
Endocrine & metabolic: Decreased libido
Gastrointestinal: Dry mouth, constipation, diarrhea, decreased salivation, nausea, vomiting, increased or decreased appetite
Neuromuscular & skeletal: Dysarthria
Miscellaneous: Sweating
1% to 10%:
Central nervous system: Confusion, nervousness, dizziness, akathisia
Cardiovascular: Syncope, tachycardia, hypotension
Ocular: Blurred vision
Neuromuscular & skeletal: Rigidity, tremor, muscle cramps
Dermatologic: Dermatitis
Respiratory: Nasal congestion, hyperventilation
Gastrointestinal: Weight gain or loss, increased salivation
Otic: Tinnitus
<1%:
Central nervous system: Reflex slowing
Endocrine & metabolic: Menstrual irregularities
Hematologic: Blood dyscrasias
Miscellaneous: Drug dependence

Comments Halazepam offers no significant advantage over other benzodiazepines

Halcinonida (Mexico) see Halcinonide *on this page*

Halcinonide (hal sin' oh nide)
Related Information
Corticosteroids, Topical Comparison *on page 1018*
Brand Names Halog®; Halog®-E
Canadian/Mexican Brand Names Dermalog® Simple (Mexico)
Therapeutic Category Corticosteroid, Topical (High Potency)
Synonyms Halcinonida (Mexico)
Use Inflammation of corticosteroid-responsive dermatoses [high potency topical corticosteroid]
(Continued)

Halcinonide (Continued)

Usual Dosage Children and Adults: Topical: Apply sparingly 1-3 times/day, occlusive dressing may be used for severe or resistant dermatoses; a thin film of cream or ointment is effective; do not overuse

Mechanism of Action Decreases inflammation by suppression of migration of polymorphonuclear leukocytes and reversal of increased capillary permeability

Local Anesthetic/Vasoconstrictor Precautions No information available to require special precautions

Effects on Dental Treatment No effects or complications reported

Other Adverse Effects <1%: Topical: Burning, itching, irritation, dryness, folliculitis, hypertrichosis, acneiform eruptions, hypopigmentation, perioral dermatitis, allergic contact dermatitis, skin maceration, secondary infection, skin atrophy, striae, miliaria

Drug Interactions No data reported

Drug Uptake
Absorption: Percutaneous absorption varies by location of topical application and the use of occlusive dressings

Pregnancy Risk Factor C

Halcion® *see* Triazolam *on page 866*

Haldol® *see* Haloperidol *on next page*

Haldol® Decanoate *see* Haloperidol *on next page*

Haldrone® *see* Paramethasone Acetate *on page 659*

Halenol® [OTC] *see* Acetaminophen *on page 14*

Haley's M-O® [OTC] *see* Magnesium Hydroxide and Mineral Oil Emulsion *on page 523*

Halfan® *see* Halofantrine *on this page*

Halobetasol Propionate (hal oh bay' ta sol pro' pee oh nate)

Brand Names Ultravate™

Therapeutic Category Corticosteroid, Topical (Very High Potency)

Use Relief of inflammatory and pruritic manifestations of corticosteroid-response dermatoses [very high potency topical corticosteroid]

Usual Dosage Children and Adults: Topical: Apply sparingly to skin twice daily, rub in gently and completely; treatment should not exceed 2 consecutive weeks and total dosage should not exceed 50 g/week

Mechanism of Action Corticosteroids inhibit the initial manifestations of the inflammatory process (ie, capillary dilation and edema, fibrin deposition, and migration and diapedesis of leukocytes into the inflamed site) as well as later sequelae (angiogenesis, fibroblast proliferation)

Local Anesthetic/Vasoconstrictor Precautions No information available to require special precautions

Effects on Dental Treatment No effects or complications reported

Other Adverse Effects <1%: Topical: Burning, itching, irritation, dryness, folliculitis, hypertrichosis, acneiform eruptions, hypopigmentation, perioral dermatitis, allergic contact dermatitis, skin maceration, secondary infection, skin atrophy, striae, miliaria

Drug Interactions No data reported

Drug Uptake
Absorption: Percutaneous absorption varies by location of topical application and the use of occlusive dressings; ~3% of a topically applied dose of ointment enters the circulation within 96 hours

Pregnancy Risk Factor C

Halofantrine (ha loe fan' trin)

Brand Names Halfan®

Therapeutic Category Antimalarial Agent

Use Treatment of mild to moderate acute malaria caused by susceptible strains of *Plasmodium falciparum* and *Plasmodium vivax*

Usual Dosage Oral:
Children <40 kg: 8 mg/kg every 6 hours for 3 doses
Adults: 500 mg every 6 hours for 3 doses

Mechanism of Action Similar to mefloquine; destruction of asexual blood forms, possible inhibition of proton pump

Local Anesthetic/Vasoconstrictor Precautions No information available to require special precautions

Effects on Dental Treatment No effects or complications reported

Other Adverse Effects
>10%: Dermatologic: Pruritus

1% to 10%:
  Cardiovascular: Edema
  Central nervous system: Malaise, headache
  Gastrointestinal: Nausea, vomiting
  Hematologic: Leukocytosis
  Hepatic: Elevated LFTs
  Local: Tenderness
  Neuromuscular & skeletal: Myalgia
  Respiratory: Cough
  Miscellaneous: Lymphadenopathy
<1%:
  Cardiovascular: Tachycardia, hypotension
  Dermatologic: Urticaria
  Endocrine & metabolic: Hypoglycemia
  Local: Sterile abscesses
  Respiratory: Asthma
  Miscellaneous: Anaphylactic shock
Drug Interactions No data reported
Drug Uptake
  Mean time to parasite clearance: 40-84 hours
  Absorption: Erratic and variable; serum levels are proportional to dose up to 1000 mg; doses greater than this should be divided; may be increased 60% with high fat meals
  Serum half-life: 23 hours; metabolite: 82 hours; may be increased in active disease

Pregnancy Risk Factor X

Halog® *see* Halcinonide *on page 415*
Halog®-E *see* Halcinonide *on page 415*

Haloperidol (ha loe per' i dole)
Brand Names Haldol®; Haldol® Decanoate
Canadian/Mexican Brand Names Haloperil® (Mexico)
Therapeutic Category Antipsychotic Agent
Use Treatment of psychoses, Tourette's disorder, and severe behavioral problems in children; may be used for the emergency sedation of severely agitated or delirious patients
Usual Dosage
  Children: 3-12 years (15-40 kg): Oral:
    Initial: 0.05 mg/kg/day or 0.25-0.5 mg/day given in 2-3 divided doses; increase by 0.25-0.5 mg every 5-7 days; maximum: 0.15 mg/kg/day
    Usual maintenance:
      Agitation or hyperkinesia: 0.01-0.03 mg/kg/day once daily
      Nonpsychotic disorders: 0.05-0.075 mg/kg/day in 2-3 divided doses
      Psychotic disorders: 0.05-0.15 mg/kg/day in 2-3 divided doses
  Children 6-12 years: I.M. (as lactate): 1-3 mg/dose every 4-8 hours to a maximum of 0.15 mg/kg/day; change over to oral therapy as soon as able
  Adults:
    Oral: 0.5-5 mg 2-3 times/day; usual maximum: 30 mg/day; some patients may require up to 100 mg/day
    I.M. (as lactate): 2-5 mg every 4-8 hours as needed
    I.M. (as decanoate): Initial: 10-15 times the daily oral dose administered at 3- to 4-week intervals
  Sedation in the Intensive Care Unit:
    I.M./IVP/IVPB: May repeat bolus doses after 30 minutes until calm achieved then administer 50% of the maximum dose every 6 hours
      Mild agitation: 0.5-2 mg
      Moderate agitation: 2-5 mg
      Severe agitation: 10-20 mg
    Continuous intravenous infusion (100 mg/100 mL D_5W): Rates of 1-40 mg/hour have been used

  Elderly (nonpsychotic patients, dementia behavior):
    Initial: Oral: 0.25-0.5 mg 1-2 times/day; increase dose at 4- to 7-day intervals by 0.25-0.5 mg/day; increase dosing intervals (twice daily, 3 times/day, etc) as necessary to control response or side effects
    Maximum daily dose: 50 mg; gradual increases (titration) may prevent side effects or decrease their severity

  Hemodialysis/peritoneal dialysis effects: Supplemental dose is not necessary
Mechanism of Action Blocks postsynaptic mesolimbic dopaminergic D_1 and D_2 receptors in the brain; exhibits a strong alpha-adrenergic blocking and anticholinergic effect, depresses the release of hypothalamic and hypophyseal
(Continued)

Haloperidol *(Continued)*

hormones; believed to depress the reticular activating system thus affecting basal metabolism, body temperature, wakefulness, vasomotor tone, and emesis

Local Anesthetic/Vasoconstrictor Precautions No information available to require special precautions

Effects on Dental Treatment Orthostatic hypotension and nasal congestion possible in dental patients. Since the drug is a dopamine antagonist, extrapyramidal symptoms of the TMJ a possibility.

Other Adverse Effects Sedation and anticholinergic effects are more pronounced than extrapyramidal effects; EKG changes, retinal pigmentation are more common than with chlorpromazine

>10%:

Central nervous system: Sedation, drowsiness, restlessness, anxiety, extrapyramidal reactions, dystonic reactions, pseudoparkinsonian signs and symptoms, tardive dyskinesia, neuroleptic malignant syndrome, seizures, altered central temperature regulation, akathisia

Endocrine & metabolic: Swelling of breasts

Gastrointestinal: Weight gain, constipation

1% to 10%:

Cardiovascular: Hypotension (especially orthostatic), tachycardia, arrhythmias, abnormal T waves with prolonged ventricular repolarization

Central nervous system: Hallucinations, persistent tardive dyskinesia, drowsiness

Gastrointestinal: Nausea, vomiting

Genitourinary: Difficult urination

<1%:

Central nervous system: Tardive dystonia, neuroleptic malignant syndrome (NMS)

Dermatologic: Hyperpigmentation, pruritus, rash, contact dermatitis, alopecia, photosensitivity (rare)

Endocrine & metabolic: Amenorrhea, galactorrhea, gynecomastia

Gastrointestinal: Adynamic ileus, GI upset, dry mouth (problem for denture user)

Genitourinary: Urinary retention, overflow incontinence, priapism, sexual dysfunction

Hematologic: Agranulocytosis, leukopenia (usually inpatients with large doses for prolonged periods)

Hepatic: Cholestatic jaundice

Ocular: Blurred vision, retinal pigmentation, decreased visual acuity (may be irreversible)

Respiratory: Laryngospasm, respiratory depression

Miscellaneous: Heat stroke, obstructive jaundice, altered central temperature regulation

Drug Interactions Cytochrome P-450 IID6 enzyme inhibitor

Decreased effect: Carbamazepine and phenobarbital may increase metabolism and decreased effectiveness of haloperidol

Increased toxicity: CNS depressants may increase adverse effects; epinephrine may cause hypotension; haloperidol and anticholinergic agents cause increased intraocular pressure; concurrent use with lithium has occasionally caused acute encephalopathy-like syndrome

Drug Uptake

Onset of sedation: I.V.: Within 1 hour

Duration of action: ~3 weeks for decanoate form

Serum half-life: 20 hours

Time to peak serum concentration: 20 minutes

Pregnancy Risk Factor C

Haloprogin *(ha loe proe' jin)*

Brand Names Halotex®

Therapeutic Category Antifungal Agent, Topical

Use Topical treatment of tinea pedis (athlete's foot), tinea cruris (jock itch), tinea corporis (ring worm), tinea manuum caused by *Trichophyton rubrum*, *Trichophyton tonsurans*, *Trichophyton mentagrophytes*, *Microsporum canis*, or *Epidermophyton floccosum*. Topical treatment of *Malassezia furfur*.

Usual Dosage Topical: Children and Adults: Apply liberally twice daily for 2-3 weeks; intertriginous areas may require up to 4 weeks of treatment

Mechanism of Action Interferes with fungal DNA replication to inhibit yeast cell respiration and disrupt its cell membrane

Local Anesthetic/Vasoconstrictor Precautions No information available to require special precautions

Effects on Dental Treatment No effects or complications reported

Other Adverse Effects <1%: Topical: Pruritus, folliculitis, irritation, burning sensation, vesicle formation, erythema

Drug Interactions No data reported

Drug Uptake
Absorption: Poorly through the skin (~11%)

Pregnancy Risk Factor B

Halotestin® *see* Fluoxymesterone *on page 378*

Halotex® *see* Haloprogin *on previous page*

Halotussin® [OTC] *see* Guaifenesin *on page 407*

Halotussin® AC *see* Guaifenesin and Codeine *on page 408*

Halotussin® DAC *see* Guaifenesin, Pseudoephedrine, and Codeine *on page 410*

Halotussin® DM [OTC] *see* Guaifenesin and Dextromethorphan *on page 408*

Halotussin® PE [OTC] *see* Guaifenesin and Pseudoephedrine *on page 409*

Haltran® [OTC] *see* Ibuprofen *on page 447*

Havrix® *see* Hepatitis A Vaccine *on page 421*

Hayfebrol® Liquid [OTC] *see* Chlorpheniramine and Pseudoephedrine *on page 191*

HbCV *see* Haemophilus b Conjugate Vaccine *on page 414*

H-BIG® *see* Hepatitis B Immune Globulin *on page 422*

Head & Shoulders® [OTC] *see* Pyrithione Zinc *on page 755*

Healon® *see* Sodium Hyaluronate *on page 791*

Healon® GV *see* Sodium Hyaluronate *on page 791*

Healon® Yellow *see* Sodium Hyaluronate *on page 791*

Helidac® Combination *see* Metronidazole *on page 576*

Hemabate™ *see* Carboprost Tromethamine *on page 156*

Hemiacidin *see* Citric Acid Bladder Mixture *on page 211*

Hemin (hee' min)

Brand Names Panhematin®

Therapeutic Category Blood Modifiers

Use Treatment of recurrent attacks of acute intermittent porphyria (AIP) only after an appropriate period of alternate therapy has been tried

Local Anesthetic/Vasoconstrictor Precautions No information available to require special precautions

Effects on Dental Treatment No effects or complications reported

Other Adverse Effects 1% to 10%:
Central nervous system: Mild pyrexia
Hematologic: Leukocytosis
Local: Phlebitis

Hemocyte® [OTC] *see* Ferrous Fumarate *on page 359*

Hemodent® Gingival Retraction Cord *see* Aluminum Chloride *on page 39*

Hemofil® M *see* Antihemophilic Factor (Human) *on page 68*

Hepalac® *see* Lactulose *on page 488*

Heparin (hep' a rin)

Brand Names Calciparine® Injection; Hep-Lock® Injection; Liquaemin® Injection

Canadian/Mexican Brand Names Dixaparine® (Mexico); Fraxiparine® (Mexico); Helberina (Mexico); Inhepar (Mexico)

Therapeutic Category Anticoagulant

Synonyms Heparin Lock Flush; Heparin Sodium, Heparin Calcium

Use Prophylaxis and treatment of thromboembolic disorders

Usual Dosage
Line flushing: When using daily flushes of heparin to maintain patency of single and double lumen central catheters, 10 units/mL is commonly used for younger infants (eg, <10 kg) while 100 units/mL is used for older infants, children, and adults. Capped PVC catheters and peripheral heparin locks require flushing more frequently (eg, every 6-8 hours). Volume of heparin flush is usually similar to volume of catheter (or slightly greater). Additional flushes should be given when stagnant blood is observed in catheter, after catheter is used for drug or blood administration, and after blood withdrawal from catheter.

(Continued)

Heparin *(Continued)*

Addition of heparin (0.5-1 unit/mL) to peripheral and central TPN has been shown to increase duration of line patency. The final concentration of heparin used for TPN solutions may need to be decreased to 0.5 units/mL in small infants receiving larger amounts of volume in order to avoid approaching therapeutic amounts. Arterial lines are heparinized with a final concentration of 1 unit/mL.

Children:

Intermittent I.V.: Initial: 50-100 units/kg, then 50-100 units/kg every 4 hours

I.V. infusion: Initial: 50 units/kg, then 15-25 units/kg/hour; increase dose by 2-4 units/kg/hour every 6-8 hours as required

Adults:

Prophylaxis (low-dose heparin): S.C.: 5000 units every 8-12 hours

Intermittent I.V.: Initial: 10,000 units, then 50-70 units/kg (5000-10,000 units) every 4-6 hours

I.V. infusion: 50 units/kg to start, then 15-25 units/kg/hour as continuous infusion; increase dose by 5 units/kg/hour every 4 hours as required according to PTT results, usual range: 10-30 units/hour

Weight-based protocol: 80 units/kg I.V. push followed by continuous infusion of 18 units/kg/hour. See table.

Standard Heparin Solution
(25,000 units/500 mL D$_5$ W)

To Administer a Dose of	Set Infusion Rate at
400 units/h	8 mL/h
500 units/h	10 mL/h
600 units/h	12 mL/h
700 units/h	14 mL/h
800 units/h	16 mL/h
900 units/h	18 mL/h
1000 units/h	20 mL/h
1100 units/h	22 mL/h
1200 units/h	24 mL/h
1300 units/h	26 mL/h
1400 units/h	28 mL/h
1500 units/h	30 mL/h
1600 units/h	32 mL/h
1700 units/h	34 mL/h
1800 units/h	36 mL/h
1900 units/h	38 mL/h
2000 units/h	40 mL/h

Mechanism of Action Potentiates the action of antithrombin III and thereby inactivates thrombin (as well as activated coagulation factors IX, X, XI, XII, and plasmin) and prevents the conversion of fibrinogen to fibrin; heparin also stimulates release of lipoprotein lipase (lipoprotein lipase hydrolyzes triglycerides to glycerol and free fatty acids)

Local Anesthetic/Vasoconstrictor Precautions No information available to require special precautions

Effects on Dental Treatment No effects or complications reported

Other Adverse Effects

>10%:

Gastrointestinal: Constipation, vomiting of blood

Hematologic: Hemorrhage, blood in urine, bleeding from gums

Miscellaneous: Unexplained bruising

1% to 10%:

Cardiovascular: Chest pain

Genitourinary: Frequent or persistent erection

Neuromuscular & skeletal: Peripheral neuropathy

Miscellaneous: Allergic reactions

<1%:

Central nervous system: Fever, headache, chills

Dermatologic: Urticaria

Gastrointestinal: Nausea, vomiting

Hematologic: Thrombocytopenia (heparin-associated thrombocytopenia occurs in <1% of patients, immune thrombocytopenia occurs with progressive fall in platelet counts and, in some cases, thromboembolic complications; daily platelet counts for 5-7 days at initiation of therapy may help detect the onset of this complication)

Hepatic: Elevated liver enzymes

Local: Irritation, ulceration, cutaneous necrosis have been rarely reported with deep S.C. injections

Neuromuscular & skeletal: Osteoporosis (chronic therapy effect)

Drug Uptake

Onset of anticoagulation:
I.V.: Immediate with use
S.C.: Within 20-30 minutes
Absorption: Oral, rectal, sublingual, I.M.: Erratic
Serum half-life:
Mean: 1.5 hours
Range: 1-2 hours; affected by obesity, renal function, hepatic function, malignancy, presence of pulmonary embolism, and infections

Pregnancy Risk Factor C

Comments Heparin does not possess fibrinolytic activity and, therefore, cannot lyse established thrombi; discontinue heparin if hemorrhage occurs; severe hemorrhage or overdosage may require protamine; monitor platelet counts, signs of bleeding, PTT.

When using daily flushes of heparin to maintain patency of single and double lumen central catheters, 10 units/mL is commonly used for younger infants (eg, <10 kg) while 100 units/mL is used for older infants and children (eg, ≥10 kg). Capped PVC catheters and peripheral heparin locks require flushing more frequently (eg, every 6-8 hours). Volume of heparin flush is usually similar to volume of catheter (or slightly greater) or may be standardized according to specific hospital's policy (eg, 2-5 mL/flush). Dose of heparin flush used should not approach therapeutic per kg dose. Additional flushes should be given when stagnant blood is observed in catheter, after catheter is used for drug or blood administration, and after blood withdrawal from catheter.

Heparin 1 unit/mL (final concentration) may be added to TPN solutions, both central and peripheral. (Addition of heparin to peripheral TPN has been shown to increase duration of line patency.) The final concentration of heparin used for TPN solutions may need to be decreased to 0.5 units/mL in small infants receiving larger amounts of volume in order to avoid approaching therapeutic amounts.

Arterial lines are heparinized with a final concentration of 1 unit/mL.

Heparin Cofactor I see Antithrombin III on page 71
Heparin Lock Flush see Heparin on page 419
Heparin Sodium, Heparin Calcium see Heparin on page 419

Hepatitis A Vaccine (hep a tye' tis aye vak seen')
Related Information
Systemic Viral Diseases on page 934
Brand Names Havrix®
Therapeutic Category Vaccine, Inactivated Virus
Use For populations desiring protection against hepatitis A or for populations at high risk of exposure to hepatitis A virus (travelers to developing countries, household and sexual contacts of persons infected with hepatitis A), child day care employees, illicit drug users, male homosexuals, institutional workers (eg, institutions for the mentally and physically handicapped persons, prisons, etc), and healthcare workers who may be exposed to hepatitis A virus (eg, laboratory employees)
Usual Dosage I.M.:
Children: 0.5 mL (360 units) on days 1 and 30, with a booster dose 6-12 months later (completion of the first 2 doses [ie, the primary series] should be accomplished at least 2 weeks before anticipated exposure to hepatitis A)
Adults: 1 mL (1440 units), with a booster dose at 6-12 months
Mechanism of Action As an inactivated virus vaccine, hepatitis A vaccine offers active immunization against hepatitis A virus infection at an effective immune response rate in up to 99% of subjects
Local Anesthetic/Vasoconstrictor Precautions No information available to require special precautions
Effects on Dental Treatment No effects or complications reported
(Continued)

421

Hepatitis A Vaccine *(Continued)*

Other Adverse Effects
Central nervous system: Headache, fatigue, fever (rare)
Hepatic: Transient liver function test abnormalities
Local: Cutaneous reactions at the injection site (pain, soreness, tenderness, swelling, warmth, and redness)

Drug Interactions No interference of immunogenicity was reported when mixed with hepatitis B vaccine

Drug Uptake
Onset of action (protection): 3 weeks after a single dose
Duration: Neutralizing antibodies have persisted for >3 years; unconfirmed evidence indicates that antibody levels may persist for 5-10 years

Pregnancy Risk Factor C

Hepatitis B Immune Globulin
(hep a tye' tis bee i myun' glob' yoo lin)

Related Information
Occupational Exposure to Bloodborne Pathogens (Universal Precautions) *on page 1030*
Systemic Viral Diseases *on page 934*

Brand Names H-BIG®; Hep-B-Gammagee®; HyperHep®

Therapeutic Category Immune Globulin

Use Provide prophylactic passive immunity to hepatitis B infection to those individuals exposed; newborns of mothers known to be hepatitis B surface antigen positive; hepatitis B immune globulin is not indicated for treatment of active hepatitis B infections and is ineffective in the treatment of chronic active hepatitis B infection

Usual Dosage I.M.:
Newborns: Hepatitis B: 0.5 mL as soon after birth as possible (within 12 hours)
Adults: Postexposure prophylaxis: 0.06 mL/kg; usual dose: 3-5 mL; maximum dose: 5 mL as soon as possible after exposure (within 96 hours); repeat at 28-30 days after exposure

Mechanism of Action Hepatitis B immune globulin (HBIG) is a nonpyrogenic sterile solution containing 10% to 18% protein of which at least 80% is monomeric immunoglobulin G (IgG). HBIG differs from immune globulin in the amount of anti-HBs. Immune globulin is prepared from plasma that is not preselected for anti-HBs content. HBIG is prepared from plasma preselected for high titer anti-HBs. In the U.S., HBIG has an anti-HBs high titer of higher than 1:100,000 by IRA. There is no evidence that the causative agent of AIDS (HTLV-III/LAV) is transmitted by HBIG.

Local Anesthetic/Vasoconstrictor Precautions No information available to require special precautions

Effects on Dental Treatment No effects or complications reported

Other Adverse Effects
1% to 10%:
Central nervous system: Dizziness, malaise,
Dermatologic: Urticaria, angioedema, rash, erythema
Local: Pain and tenderness at injection site
Neuromuscular & skeletal: Joint pains
<1%: Miscellaneous: Anaphylaxis

Drug Interactions Increased toxicity: Live virus vaccines

Drug Uptake
Absorption: Slow
Time to peak serum concentration: 1-6 days

Pregnancy Risk Factor C

Hepatitis B Vaccine (hep a tye' tis bee vak seen')

Related Information
Systemic Viral Diseases *on page 934*

Brand Names Engerix-B®; Recombivax HB®

Therapeutic Category Vaccine, Inactivated Virus

Use Immunization against infection caused by all known subtypes of hepatitis B virus in individuals considered at high risk of potential exposure to hepatitis B virus or HB$_s$Ag-positive materials

Usual Dosage See tables.

Immunization Regimen of Three I.M. Hepatitis B Vaccine Doses

Age	Initial		1 mo		6 mo	
	Recom-bivax HB® (mL)	Enger-ix-B® (mL)	Recom-bivax HB® (mL)	Enger-ix-B® (mL)	Recom-bivax HB® (mL)	Enger-ix-B® (mL)
Birth* - 10 y	0.25	0.5	0.25	0.5	0.25	0.5
11-19 y	0.5	1	0.5	1	0.5	1
≥20 y	1	1	1	1	1	1
Dialysis or immuno-compromised patients	2†		2†		2†	

*Infants born of HB$_s$Ag negative mothers.   †Two 1 mL doses given at different sites.

Recommended Dosage for Infants Born to HB$_s$Ag Positive Mothers

Treatment	Birth	Within 7 d	1 mo	6 mo
Engerix-B® (pediatric dose 10 mcg/0.5 mL)	*	0.5 mL*	0.5 mL	0.5 mL
Recombivax HB® (pediatric dose 5 mcg/0.5 mL)	*	0.5 mL*	0.5 mL	0.5 mL
Hepatitis B immune globulin	0.5 mL	—	—	—

*The first dose may be given at birth at the same time as HBIG, but give in the opposite anterolateral thigh. This may better ensure vaccine absorption.

Mechanism of Action Recombinant hepatitis B vaccine is a noninfectious subunit viral vaccine. The vaccine is derived from hepatitis B surface antigen (HB$_s$Ag) produced through recombinant DNA techniques from yeast cells. The portion of the hepatitis B gene which codes for HB$_s$Ag is cloned into yeast which is then cultured to produce hepatitis B vaccine.

Local Anesthetic/Vasoconstrictor Precautions No information available to require special precautions

Effects on Dental Treatment No effects or complications reported

Other Adverse Effects
>10%:
  Central nervous system: Fever, malaise, fatigue, headache
  Local: Mild local tenderness, local inflammatory reaction
1% to 10%:
  Gastrointestinal: Nausea, diarrhea
  Respiratory: Pharyngitis
<1%:
  Cardiovascular: Tachycardia, hypotension, sensation of warmth, flushing,
  Central nervous system: Lightheadedness, chills, somnolence, insomnia, irritability, agitation
  Dermatologic: Pruritus, rash, erythema, urticaria
  Gastrointestinal: Vomiting, GI disturbances, constipation, abdominal cramps, dyspepsia, anorexia
  Neuromuscular & skeletal: Arthralgia, myalgia, stiffness in back/neck/arm or shoulder
  Otic: Earache
  Renal: Dysuria
  Respiratory: Rhinitis, cough, nosebleed
  Miscellaneous: Sweating

Drug Interactions Decreased effect: Immunosuppressive agents

Drug Uptake Duration of action: Following all 3 doses of hepatitis B vaccine, immunity will last approximately 5-7 years

Pregnancy Risk Factor C

Hep-B-Gammagee® see Hepatitis B Immune Globulin on previous page
Hep-Lock® Injection see Heparin on page 419
Herbal Medicines see page 1081
Herplex® see Idoxuridine on page 449
Hespan® see Hetastarch on this page

Hetastarch (het′ a starch)
Brand Names Hespan®
Therapeutic Category Plasma Volume Expander
Synonyms HES; Hydroxyethyl Starch
Use Blood volume expander used in treatment of shock or impending shock when blood or blood products are not available; does not have oxygen-carrying capacity and is not a substitute for blood or plasma; an adjunct in leukapheresis to enhance the yield of granulocytes by centrifugal means
(Continued)

Hetastarch *(Continued)*

Usual Dosage I.V. infusion (requires an infusion pump):
Children: Safety and efficacy have not been established
Adults: 500-1000 mL (up to 1500 mL/day) or 20 mL/kg/day (up to 1500 mL/day); larger volumes (15,000 mL/24 hours) have been used safely in small numbers of patients

Mechanism of Action Produces plasma volume expansion by virtue of its highly colloidal starch structure, similar to albumin

Local Anesthetic/Vasoconstrictor Precautions No information available to require special precautions

Effects on Dental Treatment No effects or complications reported

Other Adverse Effects <1%:
Cardiovascular: Peripheral edema, heart failure, circulatory overload
Central nervous system: Fever, chills, headaches
Dermatologic: Itching, pruritus
Gastrointestinal: Vomiting
Hematologic: Bleeding, prolongation of PT, PTT, clotting time, and bleeding time
Neuromuscular & skeletal: Muscle pains
Miscellaneous: Hypersensitivity

Drug Uptake
Onset of volume expansion: I.V.: Within 30 minutes
Duration: 24-36 hours

Pregnancy Risk Factor C

Comments Does not have oxygen-carrying capacity and is not a substitute for blood or plasma; large volumes may interfere with platelet function and prolong PT and PTT times; safety and efficacy in children have not been established; hetastarch is a synthetic polymer derived from a waxy starch composed of amylopectin; average molecular weight = 450,000

Hexachlorophene *(hex a klor' oh feen)*

Brand Names pHisoHex®; pHiso® Scrub; Septisol®

Therapeutic Category Antibacterial, Topical; Soap

Use Surgical scrub and as a bacteriostatic skin cleanser; control an outbreak of gram-positive infection when other procedures have been unsuccessful

Usual Dosage Children and Adults: Topical: Apply 5 mL cleanser and water to area to be cleansed; lather and rinse thoroughly under running water

Mechanism of Action Bacteriostatic polychlorinated biphenyl which inhibits membrane-bound enzymes and disrupts the cell membrane

Local Anesthetic/Vasoconstrictor Precautions No information available to require special precautions

Effects on Dental Treatment No effects or complications reported

Other Adverse Effects <1%:
Central nervous system: CNS injury, seizures, irritability
Dermatologic: Photosensitity, dermatitis, redness, dry skin

Drug Interactions No data reported

Drug Uptake
Absorption: Percutaneously through inflamed, excoriated, and intact skin
Serum half-life: Infants: 6.1-44.2 hours

Pregnancy Risk Factor C

Hexadrol® *see* Dexamethasone *on page 260*

Hexalen® *see* Altretamine *on page 38*

Hexlixate® *see* Antihemophilic Factor (Recombinant) *on page 70*

H.H.R.® *see* Hydralazine, Hydrochlorothiazide, and Reserpine *on page 429*

Hibiclens® [OTC] *see* Chlorhexidine Gluconate *on page 184*

Hibistat® [OTC] *see* Chlorhexidine Gluconate *on page 184*

Hib Polysaccharide Conjugate *see* Haemophilus b Conjugate Vaccine *on page 414*

HibTITER® *see* Haemophilus b Conjugate Vaccine *on page 414*

Hidralacina Clorhidrato De (Mexico) *see* Hydralazine Hydrochloride *on page 428*

Hidroclorotiacida (Mexico) *see* Hydrochlorothiazide *on page 430*

Hidroquinona (Mexico) *see* Hydroquinone *on page 439*

Hidroxicloroquina Sulfato De (Mexico) *see* Hydroxychloroquine Sulfate *on page 440*

Hidroxiprogesterona Caproato De (Mexico) *see* Hydroxyprogesterone Caproate *on page 441*

Hidroxocobalamina (Mexico) *see* Hydroxocobalamin *on page 439*

Hiprex® *see* Methenamine *on page 555*

Hismanal® *see* Astemizole *on page 82*

Histaject® *see* Brompheniramine Maleate *on page 124*

Histalet Forte® Tablet *see* Chlorpheniramine, Pyrilamine, Phenylephrine, and Phenylpropanolamine *on page 195*

Histalet® Syrup [OTC] *see* Chlorpheniramine and Pseudoephedrine *on page 191*

Histalet X® *see* Guaifenesin and Pseudoephedrine *on page 409*

Histatab® Plus Tablet [OTC] *see* Chlorpheniramine and Phenylephrine *on page 190*

Hista-Vadrin® Tablet *see* Chlorpheniramine, Phenylephrine, and Phenylpropanolamine *on page 193*

Histerone® *see* Testosterone *on page 825*

Histolyn-CYL® Injection *see* Histoplasmin *on this page*

Histoplasmin (hiss toe plaz′ min)
Brand Names Histolyn-CYL® Injection
Therapeutic Category Diagnostic Agent, Skin Test
Synonyms Histoplasmosis Skin Test Antigen
Use Diagnosing histoplasmosis; to assess cell-mediated immunity
Local Anesthetic/Vasoconstrictor Precautions No information available to require special precautions
Effects on Dental Treatment No effects or complications reported
Other Adverse Effects 1% to 10%:
   Dermatologic: Pruritus, urticaria
   Local: Ulceration or necrosis may occur at test site
   Respiratory: Shortness of breath

Histoplasmosis Skin Test Antigen *see* Histoplasmin *on this page*

Histor-D® Syrup *see* Chlorpheniramine and Phenylephrine *on page 190*

Histor-D® Timecelles® *see* Chlorpheniramine, Phenylephrine, and Methscopolamine *on page 193*

Histrelin (his trel′ in)
Brand Names Supprelin™
Therapeutic Category Gonadotropin Releasing Hormone Analog
Use Treatment of central idiopathic precocious puberty; treatment of estrogen-associated gynecological disorders such as acute intermittent porphyria, endometriosis, leiomyomata uteri, and premenstrual syndrome
Usual Dosage
   Central idiopathic precocious puberty: S.C.: Usual dose is 10 mcg/kg/day given as a single daily dose at the same time each day
   Acute intermittent porphyria in women: S.C.: 5 mcg/day
   Endometriosis: S.C.: 100 mcg/day
   Leiomyomata uteri: S.C.: 20-50 mcg/day or 4 mcg/kg/day
Mechanism of Action Histrelin is a synthetic long-acting gonadotropin-releasing hormone analog; with daily administration, it desensitizes the pituitary to endogenous gonadotropin-releasing hormone (ie, suppresses gonadotropin release by causing down regulation of the pituitary); this results in a decrease in gonadal sex steroid production which stops the secondary sexual development
Local Anesthetic/Vasoconstrictor Precautions No information available to require special precautions
Effects on Dental Treatment No effects or complications reported
Other Adverse Effects
   >10%:
      Cardiovascular: Vasodilation
      Central nervous system: Headache
      Gastrointestinal: Abdominal pain
      Genitourinary: Vaginal bleeding, vaginal dryness
      Local: Skin reaction at injection site
   1% to 10%:
      Central nervous system: Mood swings, headache
      Dermatologic: Skin rashes, hives
      Endocrine & metabolic: Breast tenderness, hot flashes
      Gastrointestinal: Nausea, vomiting
      Genitourinary: Increased urinary calcium excretion
      Neuromuscular & skeletal: Joint stiffness, pain
Drug Interactions No data reported
(Continued)

Histrelin *(Continued)*

Drug Uptake
Precocious puberty: Onset of hormonal responses: Within 3 months of initiation of therapy

Acute intermittent porphyria associated with menses: Amelioration of symptoms: After 1-2 months of therapy

Treatment of endometriosis or leiomyomata uteri: Onset of responses: After 3-6 months of treatment

Pregnancy Risk Factor X

Histrodrix® [OTC] *see* Dexbrompheniramine and Pseudoephedrine *on page 261*

Hi-Vegi-Lip® *see* Pancreatin *on page 656*

Hivid® *see* Zalcitabine *on page 906*

HMS Liquifilm® Ophthalmic *see* Medrysone *on page 533*

Hold® DM [OTC] *see* Dextromethorphan *on page 266*

Homatropine and Hydrocodone *see* Hydrocodone and Homatropine *on page 434*

Homatropine Hydrobromide
(hoe ma′ troe peen hye droe broe′ mide)

Brand Names AK-Homatropine® Ophthalmic; Isopto® Homatropine Ophthalmic

Therapeutic Category Anticholinergic Agent, Ophthalmic; Ophthalmic Agent, Mydriatic

Use Producing cycloplegia and mydriasis for refraction; treatment of acute inflammatory conditions of the uveal tract

Usual Dosage
Children:
Mydriasis and cycloplegia for refraction: Instill 1 drop of 2% solution immediately before the procedure; repeat at 10-minute intervals as needed
Uveitis: Instill 1 drop of 2% solution 2-3 times/day

Adults:
Mydriasis and cycloplegia for refraction: Instill 1-2 drops of 2% solution or 1 drop of 5% solution before the procedure; repeat at 5- to 10-minute intervals as needed
Uveitis: Instill 1-2 drops of 2% or 5% 2-3 times/day up to every 3-4 hours as needed

Mechanism of Action Blocks response of iris sphincter muscle and the accommodative muscle of the ciliary body to cholinergic stimulation resulting in dilation and loss of accommodation

Local Anesthetic/Vasoconstrictor Precautions No information available to require special precautions

Effects on Dental Treatment No effects or complications reported

Other Adverse Effects
>10%: Ocular: Blurred vision, photophobia
1% to 10%:
Local: Stinging, local irritation
Ocular: Increased intraocular pressure
Respiratory: Congestion
<1%:
Cardiovascular: Vascular congestion, edema
Central nervous system: Drowsiness
Dermatologic: Exudate, eczematoid dermatitis
Ocular: Follicular conjunctivitis

Drug Uptake
Onset of accommodation and pupil effect: Ophthalmic:
Maximum mydriatic effect: Within 10-30 minutes
Maximum cycloplegic effect: Within 30-90 minutes
Duration:
Mydriasis: 6 hours to 4 days
Cycloplegia: 10-48 hours

Pregnancy Risk Factor C

Horse Anti-human Thymocyte Gamma Globulin *see* Lymphocyte Immune Globulin, Anti-thymocyte Globulin (Equine) *on page 518*

H.P. Acthar® Gel *see* Corticotropin *on page 233*

Humalog® *see* Insulin Preparations *on page 459*

Human Growth Hormone (hyu′ min grothe hor′ mon)
Brand Names Humatrope®; Nutropin®; Protropin®
Therapeutic Category Growth Hormone

Use
Long-term treatment of growth failure from lack of adequate endogenous growth hormone secretion

Nutropin®: Treatment of children who have growth failure associated with chronic renal insufficiency up until the time of renal transplantation

Usual Dosage Children (individualize dose):

Somatrem (Protropin®): I.M., S.C.: Up to 0.1 mg (0.26 units)/kg/dose 3 times/week

Somatropin (Humatrope®): I.M., S.C.: Up to 0.06 mg (0.16 units)/kg/dose 3 times/week

Somatropin (Nutropin®): S.C.:

Growth hormone inadequacy: Weekly dosage of 0.3 mg/kg (0.78 units/kg) administered daily

Chronic renal insufficiency: Weekly dosage of 0.35 mg/kg (0.91 units/kg) administered daily

Therapy should be discontinued when patient has reached satisfactory adult height, when epiphyses have fused, or when the patient ceases to respond

Growth of 5 cm/year or more is expected, if growth rate does not exceed 2.5 cm in a 6-month period, double the dose for the next 6 months, if there is still no satisfactory response, discontinue therapy

Mechanism of Action Somatrem and somatropin are purified polypeptide hormones of recombinant DNA origin; somatrem contains the identical sequence of amino acids found in human growth hormone while somatropin's amino acid sequence is identical plus an additional amino acid, methionine; human growth hormone stimulates growth of linear bone, skeletal muscle, and organs; stimulates erythropoietin which increases red blood cell mass; exerts both insulin-like and diabetogenic effects

Local Anesthetic/Vasoconstrictor Precautions No information available to require special precautions

Effects on Dental Treatment No effects or complications reported

Other Adverse Effects S.C. administration can cause local lipoatrophy or lipodystrophy and may enhance the development of neutralizing antibodies
1% to 10%: Endocrine & metabolism: Hypothyroidism
<1%:
Dermatologic: Skin rash, itching
Endocrine & metabolic: Hypoglycemia
Local: Pain at injection site
Miscellaneous: Small risk for developing leukemia, pain in hip/knee

Drug Interactions Decreased effect: Glucocorticoid therapy may inhibit growth-promoting effects.

Drug Uptake Somatrem and somatropin have equivalent pharmacokinetic properties
Duration of action: Maintains supraphysiologic levels for 18-20 hours
Absorption: I.M.: Well absorbed
Serum half-life: 15-50 minutes

Pregnancy Risk Factor C

Humate-P® *see* Antihemophilic Factor (Human) *on page 68*

Humatin® *see* Paromomycin Sulfate *on page 660*

Humatrope® *see* Human Growth Hormone *on previous page*

Humibid® DM [OTC] *see* Guaifenesin and Dextromethorphan *on page 408*

Humibid® L.A. *see* Guaifenesin *on page 407*

Humibid® Sprinkle *see* Guaifenesin *on page 407*

Humorsol® *see* Demecarium Bromide *on page 255*

Humulin® 50/50 *see* Insulin Preparations *on page 459*

Humulin® 70/30 *see* Insulin Preparations *on page 459*

Humulin® L *see* Insulin Preparations *on page 459*

Humulin® N *see* Insulin Preparations *on page 459*

Humulin® R *see* Insulin Preparations *on page 459*

Humulin® U *see* Insulin Preparations *on page 459*

Hurricaine® [OTC] *see* Benzocaine *on page 102*

Hyaluronic Acid *see* Sodium Hyaluronate *on page 791*

Hyaluronidase (hye al yoor on' i dase)

Brand Names Wydase® Injection

Therapeutic Category Antidote, Extravasation

Use Increase the dispersion and absorption of other drugs; increase rate of absorption of parenteral fluids administered by hypodermoclysis; management of I.V. extravasations

(Continued)

Hyaluronidase *(Continued)*

Usual Dosage

Children:

Management of I.V. extravasation: Reconstitute the 150 unit vial of lyophilized powder with 1 mL normal saline; take 0.1 mL of this solution and dilute with 0.9 mL normal saline to yield 15 units/mL; using a 25- or 26-gauge needle, five 0.2 mL injections are made subcutaneously or intradermally into the extravasation site at the leading edge, changing the needle after each injection

Hypodermoclysis:

S.C.: 1 mL (150 units) is added to 1000 mL of infusion fluid and 0.5 mL (75 units) in injected into each clysis site at the initiation of the infusion

I.V.: 15 units is added to each 100 mL of I.V. fluid to be administered

Adults: Absorption and dispersion of drugs: 150 units are added to the vehicle containing the drug

Mechanism of Action Modifies the permeability of connective tissue through hydrolysis of hyaluronic acid, one of the chief ingredients of tissue cement which offers resistance to diffusion of liquids through tissues

Local Anesthetic/Vasoconstrictor Precautions No information available to require special precautions

Effects on Dental Treatment No effects or complications reported

Other Adverse Effects <1%:

Cardiovascular: Tachycardia, hypotension

Central nervous system: Dizziness, chills

Dermatologic: Urticaria, erythema

Gastrointestinal: Nausea, vomiting

Drug Uptake

Onset of action: Immediate by the subcutaneous or intradermal routes for the treatment of extravasation

Duration: 24-48 hours

Pregnancy Risk Factor C

Comments The USP hyaluronidase unit is equivalent to the turbidity-reducing (TR) unit and the International Unit; each unit is defined as being the activity contained in 100 mcg of the International Standard Preparation

Hyate®:C *see* Antihemophilic Factor (Porcine) *on page 69*

Hybalamin® *see* Hydroxocobalamin *on page 439*

Hybolin™ Decanoate *see* Nandrolone *on page 604*

Hybolin™ Improved *see* Nandrolone *on page 604*

Hycamptamine *see* Topotecan Hydrochloride *on page 855*

Hycamtin® *see* Topotecan Hydrochloride *on page 855*

HycoClear Tuss® *see* Hydrocodone and Guaifenesin *on page 434*

Hycodan® *see* Hydrocodone and Homatropine *on page 434*

Hycomine® *see* Hydrocodone and Phenylpropanolamine *on page 435*

Hycomine® Compound *see* Hydrocodone, Chlorpheniramine, Phenylephrine, Acetaminophen and Caffeine *on page 435*

Hycomine® Pediatric *see* Hydrocodone and Phenylpropanolamine *on page 435*

Hycotuss® Expectorant Liquid *see* Hydrocodone and Guaifenesin *on page 434*

Hydeltrasol® *see* Prednisolone *on page 718*

Hydeltra-T.B.A.® *see* Prednisolone *on page 718*

Hydergine® *see* Ergoloid Mesylates *on page 318*

Hydergine® LC *see* Ergoloid Mesylates *on page 318*

Hydralazine and Hydrochlorothiazide (hye dral' a zeen & hye droe klor oh thye' a zide)

Brand Names Apresazide®; Hydrazide®; Hy-Zide®

Therapeutic Category Antihypertensive Agent, Combination

Synonyms Hydrochlorothiazide and Hydralazine

Use Management of moderate to severe hypertension and treatment of congestive heart failure

Local Anesthetic/Vasoconstrictor Precautions No information available to require special precautions

Effects on Dental Treatment No effects or complications reported

Hydralazine Hydrochloride (hye dral' a zeen hye droe klor' ide)

Related Information

Cardiovascular Diseases *on page 912*

Brand Names Apresoline®

Canadian/Mexican Brand Names Apo-Hydralazine® (Canada); Novo-Hylazin® (Canada); Nu-Hydral® (Canada); Apresolina® (Mexico)

Therapeutic Category Vasodilator

Synonyms Hidralacina Clorhidrato De (Mexico)

Use Management of moderate to severe hypertension, congestive heart failure, hypertension secondary to pre-eclampsia/eclampsia; also used to treat primary pulmonary hypertension

Usual Dosage
Children:
Oral: Initial: 0.75-1 mg/kg/day in 2-4 divided doses, not to exceed 25 mg/dose; increase over 3-4 weeks to maximum of 7.5 mg/kg/day in 2-4 divided doses; maximum daily dose: 200 mg/day
I.M., I.V.: 0.1-0.2 mg/kg/dose (not to exceed 20 mg) every 4-6 hours as needed, up to 1.7-3.5 mg/kg/day in 4-6 divided doses

Adults:
Oral: Hypertension:
Initial dose: 10 mg 4 times/day
Increase by 10-25 mg/dose every 2-5 days
Maximum dose: 300 mg/day
Oral: Congestive heart failure:
Initial dose: 10-25 mg TID
Target dose: 75 mg TID
Maximum dose: 100 mg TID
I.M., I.V.:
Hypertensive Initial: 10-20 mg/dose every 4-6 hours as needed, may increase to 40 mg/dose; change to oral therapy as soon as possible
Pre-eclampsia/eclampsia: 5 mg/dose then 5-10 mg every 20-30 minutes as needed

Elderly: Oral: Initial: 10 mg 2-3 times/day; increase by 10-25 mg/day every 2-5 days

Mechanism of Action Direct vasodilation of arterioles (with little effect on veins) with decreased systemic resistance

Local Anesthetic/Vasoconstrictor Precautions No information available to require special precautions

Effects on Dental Treatment No effects or complications reported

Other Adverse Effects
>10%:
Cardiovascular: Palpitations, flushing, tachycardia, angina pectoris
Central nervous system: Headache
Gastrointestinal: Nausea, vomiting, diarrhea, anorexia
1% to 10%:
Cardiovascular: Hypotension, redness or flushing of face
Gastrointestinal: Constipation
Ocular: Lacrimation
Respiratory: Dyspnea, nasal congestion
<1%:
Central nervous system: Malaise, peripheral neuritis, fever, dizziness
Dermatologic: Rash, edema
Neuromuscular & skeletal: Arthralgias, weakness

Drug Interactions Increased toxicity: Concomitant administration of MAO inhibitors causes significant decrease in blood pressure; indomethacin leads to decreased hypotensive effects

Drug Uptake
Onset of action:
Oral: 20-30 minutes
I.V.: 5-20 minutes
Duration:
Oral: 2-4 hours
I.V.: 2-6 hours
Serum half-life:
Normal renal function: 2-8 hours
End stage renal disease: 7-16 hours

Pregnancy Risk Factor C

Hydralazine, Hydrochlorothiazide, and Reserpine
(hye dral′ a zeen, hye droe klor oh thye′ a zide, & re ser′ peen)

Brand Names Cam-ap-es®; H.H.R.®; Hydrap-ES®; Marpres®; Ser-A-Gen®; Ser-Ap-Es®; Serathide®; Tri-Hydroserpine®; Unipres®

Therapeutic Category Antihypertensive Agent, Combination

Use Hypertensive disorders

(Continued)

Hydralazine, Hydrochlorothiazide, and Reserpine
(Continued)

Local Anesthetic/Vasoconstrictor Precautions No information available to require special precautions

Effects on Dental Treatment No effects or complications reported

Hydrap-ES® *see* Hydralazine, Hydrochlorothiazide, and Reserpine *on previous page*

Hydrate® *see* Dimenhydrinate *on page 286*

Hydrazide® *see* Hydralazine and Hydrochlorothiazide *on page 428*

Hydrea® *see* Hydroxyurea *on page 442*

Hydrex® *see* Benzthiazide *on page 105*

Hydrisalic™ *see* Salicylic Acid *on page 777*

Hydrobexan® *see* Hydroxocobalamin *on page 439*

Hydrocet® **[5/500]** *see* Hydrocodone and Acetaminophen *on next page*

Hydrochlorothiazide (hye droe klor oh thye' a zide)

Related Information
  Cardiovascular Diseases *on page 912*

Brand Names Esidrix®; Ezide®; HydroDIURIL®; Hydro-Par®; Oretic®

Canadian/Mexican Brand Names Apo-Hydro® (Canada); Diuchlor® (Canada); Neo-Codema® (Canada); Novo-Hydrazide® (Canada); Urozide® (Canada); Diclotride® (Mexico)

Therapeutic Category Diuretic, Thiazide Type

Synonyms Hidroclorotiacida (Mexico)

Use Management of mild to moderate hypertension; treatment of edema in congestive heart failure and nephrotic syndrome

Usual Dosage Oral (effect of drug may be decreased when used every day):
  Children (In pediatric patients, chlorothiazide may be preferred over hydrochlorothiazide as there are more dosage formulations (eg, suspension) available):
    <6 months: 2-3 mg/kg/day in 2 divided doses
    >6 months: 2 mg/kg/day in 2 divided doses
  Adults: 25-100 mg/day in 1-2 doses
    Maximum: 200 mg/day
  Elderly: 12.5-25 mg once daily
  Minimal increase in response and more electrolyte disturbances are seen with doses >50 mg/day

Mechanism of Action Inhibits sodium reabsorption in the distal tubules causing increased excretion of sodium and water as well as potassium and hydrogen ions

Local Anesthetic/Vasoconstrictor Precautions No information available to require special precautions

Effects on Dental Treatment No effects or complications reported

Other Adverse Effects
  1% to 10%: Endocrine & metabolic: Hypokalemia
  <1%:
    Cardiovascular: Hypotension
    Dermatologic: Photosensitivity
    Endocrine & metabolic: Fluid and electrolyte imbalances (hypocalcemia, hypomagnesemia, hyponatremia), hyperglycemia
    Hematologic: Rarely blood dyscrasias
    Renal: Prerenal azotemia

Drug Interactions
  Decreased effect: Decreased antidiabetic drug efficacy
  Increased toxicity:
    Hypotensive agents cause increased hypotensive potential
    Increased digoxin related arrhythmias when given with digoxin
    Increased lithium levels due to reduced lithium clearance

Drug Uptake
  Onset of diuretic action: Oral: Within 2 hours
  Peak effect: 4 hours
  Duration: 6-12 hours
  Absorption: Oral: ~60% to 80%

Pregnancy Risk Factor D

Hydrochlorothiazide and Amiloride *see* Amiloride and Hydrochlorothiazide *on page 45*

Hydrochlorothiazide and Hydralazine *see* Hydralazine and Hydrochlorothiazide *on page 428*

Hydrochlorothiazide and Methyldopa *see* Methyldopa and Hydrochlorothiazide on page 567

Hydrochlorothiazide and Reserpine

(hye droe klor oh thye' a zide & re ser' peen)
Brand Names Hydropres®; Hydro-Serp®; Hydroserpine®
Therapeutic Category Antihypertensive Agent, Combination
Synonyms Reserpine and Hydrochlorothiazide
Use Management of mild to moderate hypertension; treatment of edema in congestive heart failure and nephrotic syndrome
Local Anesthetic/Vasoconstrictor Precautions No information available to require special precautions
Effects on Dental Treatment No effects or complications reported

Hydrochlorothiazide and Spironolactone

(hye droe klor oh thye' a zide & speer on oh lak' tone)
Related Information
Cardiovascular Diseases *on page 912*
Brand Names Alazide®; Aldactazide®; Spironazide®; Spirozide®
Therapeutic Category Antihypertensive Agent, Combination; Diuretic, Combination
Synonyms Spironolactone and Hydrochlorothiazide
Use Management of mild to moderate hypertension; treatment of edema in congestive heart failure and nephrotic syndrome
Usual Dosage Oral:
Children: 1.66-3.3 mg/kg/day (of spironolactone) in 2-4 divided doses
Adults: 1-8 tablets in 1-2 divided doses
Local Anesthetic/Vasoconstrictor Precautions No information available to require special precautions
Effects on Dental Treatment No effects or complications reported
Other Adverse Effects 1% to 10%:
Central nervous system: Headache, lethargy
Dermatology: Rash
Endocrine & metabolic: Hyperkalemia, gynecomastia, hyperchloremic metabolic acidosis (in decompensated hepatic cirrhosis), dehydration, hyponatremia
Gastrointestinal: Anorexia, nausea, vomiting, diarrhea
Contraindications Anuria, hyperkalemia, renal or hepatic failure, hypersensitivity to hydrochlorothiazide, spironolactone, or any component
Dosage Forms Tablet:
25/25: Hydrochlorothiazide 25 mg and spironolactone 25 mg
50/50: Hydrochlorothiazide 50 mg and spironolactone 50 mg

Hydrocil® [OTC] *see* Psyllium *on page 750*
Hydro-Cobex® *see* Hydroxocobalamin *on page 439*

Hydrocodone and Acetaminophen

(hye droe koe' done & a seet a min' oh fen)
Related Information
Dental Drug Interactions: Update on Drug Combinations Requiring Special Considerations *on page 1022*
Narcotic Agonist Charts *on page 1019*
Oral Pain *on page 940*
Brand Names Anexsia® 5/500; Anexsia® 7.5/650; Anexsia® 10/660; Anodynos-DHC® [5/500]; Bancap HC® [5/500]; Co-Gesic® [5/500]; Dolacet® [5/500]; DuoCet™ [5/500]; Duradyne DHC® [5/500]; Hydrocet® [5/500]; Hydrogesic® [5/500]; Hy-Phen® [5/500]; Lorcet® [5/500]; Lorcet®-HD [5/500]; Lorcet® Plus [7.5/650]; Lortab® 2.5/500; Lortab® 5/500; Lortab® 7.5/500; Lortab® 10/500; Lortab® 10/650; Lortab® Elixir; Lortab® Solution; Margesic® H [5/500]; Norcet® [5/500]; Stagesic® [5/500]; T-Gesic® [5/500]; Vicodin® [5/500]; Vicodin® ES [7.5/750]; Zydone® [5/500]
Canadian/Mexican Brand Names Vapocet® (Canada)
Therapeutic Category Analgesic, Narcotic
Use
Dental: Treatment of postoperative pain
Medical: Relief of pain
Usual Dosage Oral:
Children: Not recommended in pediatric dental patients
Adults: Analgesic: 1-2 tablets or capsules every 4-6 hours or 5-10 mL solution every 4-6 hours as needed for pain; maximum dose: 12 tablets or capsules/day
(Continued)

Hydrocodone and Acetaminophen *(Continued)*

Mechanism of Action

Hydrocodone, as with other narcotic (opiate) analgesics, blocks pain perception in the cerebral cortex by binding to specific receptor molecules (opiate receptors) within the neuronal membranes of synpases. This binding results in a decreased synaptic chemical transmission throughout the CNS thus inhibiting the flow of pain sensations into the higher centers. Mu and kappa are the two subtypes of the opiate receptor which hydrocodone binds to to cause analgesia.

Acetaminophen inhibits the synthesis of prostaglandins in the CNS and peripherally blocks pain impulse generation; produces antipyresis from inhibition of hypothalamic heat-regulating center.

Local Anesthetic/Vasoconstrictor Precautions No information available to require special precautions

Effects on Dental Treatment No effects or complications reported

Other Adverse Effects

>10%:

Cardiovascular: Hypotension

Central nervous system: Lightheadedness, dizziness, sedation

1% to 10%: Gastrointestinal: Nausea

Oral manifestations: <1%: Dry mouth

Contraindications Patients with known G-6-PD deficiency; hypersensitivity to acetaminophen; hypersensitivity to hydrocodone

Warnings/Precautions Use with caution in patients with hypersensitivity reactions to other phenanthrene derivative opioid agonists (morphine, codeine, levorphanol, oxycodone, oxymorphone); respiratory diseases including asthma, emphysema, COPD, or severe liver or renal insufficiency; some preparations contain sulfites which may cause allergic reactions; may be habit-forming

Drug Interactions The use of MAO inhibitors or tricyclic antidepressants with hydrocodone may **increase** the effect of either the antidepressant or hydrocodone; concurrent use of hydrocodone with anticholinergics may cause paralytic ileus; patients taking other narcotic agents, antipsychotics, antianxiety agents or other CNS depressants (including alcohol) with hydrocodone and aspirin may experience an additive CNS depression

Drug Uptake

Onset of effect: Narcotic analgesia: Within 10-20 minutes

Duration of effect: 3-6 hours

Serum half-life: 3.8 hours

Pregnancy Risk Factor C

Breast-feeding Considerations

Hydrocodone: No data reported

Acetaminophen: May be taken while breast-feeding

Dosage Forms

Capsule:

Bancap HC®, Dolacet®, Hydrocet®, Hydrogesic®, Lorcet®-HD, Margesic® H, Medipain 5®, Norcet®, Stagesic®, T-Gesic®, Zydone®: Hydrocodone bitartrate 5 mg and acetaminophen 500 mg

Elixir (tropical fruit punch flavor) (Lortab®): Hydrocodone bitartrate 2.5 mg and acetaminophen 167 mg per 5 mL with alcohol 7% (480 mL)

Solution, oral (tropical fruit punch flavor) (Lortab®): Hydrocodone bitartrate 2.5 mg and acetaminophen 167 mg per 5 mL with alcohol 7% (480 mL)

Tablet:

Lortab® 2.5/500: Hydrocodone bitartrate 2.5 mg and acetaminophen 500 mg

Anexsia® 5/500, Anodynos-DHC®, Co-Gesic®, DuoCet™, Duradyne DHC®, Hy-Phen®, Lorcet®, Lortab®® 5/500, Vicodin®: Hydrocodone bitartrate 5 mg and acetaminophen 500 mg

Lortab® 7.5/500: Hydrocodone bitartrate 7.5 mg and acetaminophen 500 mg

Anexsia® 7.5/650, Lorcet® Plus: Hydrocodone bitartrate 7.5 mg and acetaminophen 650 mg

Vicodin® ES: Hydrocodone bitartrate 7.5 mg and acetaminophen 750 mg

Lortab® 10/500: Hydrocodone bitartrate 10 mg and acetaminophen 500 mg

Lortab® 10/650: Hydrocodone bitartrate 10 mg and acetaminophen 650 mg

Anexsia® 10/660, Vicodin® HP: Hydrocodone bitartrate 10 mg and acetaminophen 660 mg

Dietary Considerations No data reported

Generic Available Yes

Comments Neither hydrocodone nor acetaminophen elicit anti-inflammatory effects. Because of addiction liability of opiate analgesics, the use of hydrocodone should be limited to 2-3 days postoperatively for treatment of dental pain.

Nausea is the most common adverse effect seen after use in dental patients; sedation and constipation are second. Nausea elicited by narcotic analgesics is centrally mediated and the presence or absence of food will not affect the degree nor incidence of nausea.

Selected Readings

Dionne RA, "New Approaches to Preventing and Treating Postoperative Pain," *J Am Dent Assoc*, 1992, 123(6):26-34.

Gobetti JP, "Controlling Dental Pain," *J Am Dent Assoc*, 1992, 123(6):47-52.

Hydrocodone and Aspirin (hye droe koe' done & as' pir in)

Related Information

Dental Drug Interactions: Update on Drug Combinations Requiring Special Considerations *on page 1022*

Narcotic Agonist Charts *on page 1019*

Brand Names Azdone®; Damason-P®; Lortab® ASA

Therapeutic Category Analgesic, Narcotic

Use

Dental: Treatment of postoperative pain

Medical: Relief of pain

Usual Dosage Oral:

Children: Not recommended in pediatric dental patients

Adults: 1-2 tablets every 4-6 hours as needed for pain

Mechanism of Action Hydrocodone, as with other narcotic (opiate) analgesics, blocks pain perception in the cerebral cortex by binding to specific receptor molecules (opiate receptors) within the neuronal membranes of synapsis. This binding results in a decreased synaptic chemical transmission throughout the CNS thus inhibiting the flow of pain sensations into the higher centers. Mu and kappa are the two subtypes of the opiate receptor which hydrocodone binds to to cause analgesia.

Aspirin inhibits prostaglandin synthesis by decreasing the activity of the enzyme, cyclo-oxygenase, which results in decreased formation of prostaglandin precursors, acts on the hypothalamic heat-regulating center to reduce fever, blocks thromboxane synthetase action which prevents formation of the platelet-aggregating substance thromboxane A_2

Local Anesthetic/Vasoconstrictor Precautions No information available to require special precautions

Effects on Dental Treatment Use with caution in patients with platelet and bleeding disorders, renal dysfunction, erosive gastritis, or peptic ulcer disease, previous nonreaction does not guarantee future safe taking of medication; do not use aspirin in children <16 years of age for chickenpox or flu symptoms due to the association with Reye's syndrome

Avoid aspirin if possible, for 1 week prior to surgery because of the possibility of postoperative bleeding; use with caution in impaired hepatic function

Elderly are a high-risk population for adverse effects from nonsteroidal anti-inflammatory agents. As much as 60% of elderly with GI complications to NSAIDs can develop peptic ulceration and/or hemorrhage asymptomatically. Also, concomitant disease and drug use contribute to the risk for GI adverse effects. Use lowest effective dose for shortest period possible. Consider renal function decline with age. Use with caution in patients with history of asthma

Other Adverse Effects

>10%:

Central nervous system: Lightheadedness, dizziness, sedation

Gastrointestinal: Nausea, heartburn, stomach pains, dyspepsia

1% to 10%: Gastrointestinal: Gastrointestinal ulceration

Oral manifestations: <1%: Dry mouth

Warnings/Precautions Because of aspirin component, use with caution in patients with impaired renal function, erosive gastritis, or peptic ulcer disease; children and teenagers should not use for chickenpox or flu symptoms before a physician is consulted about Reye's syndrome

Drug Interactions The use of MAO inhibitors or tricyclic antidepressants with hydrocodone may **increase** the effect of either the antidepressant or hydrocodone; concurrent use of hydrocodone with anticholinergics may cause paralytic ileus; patients taking other narcotic agents, antipsychotic, antianxiety agents or other CNS depressants (including alcohol) with hydrocodone and aspirin may experience an additive CNS depression; aspirin interacts with warfarin to cause bleeding

Drug Uptake

Onset of effect: Onset of narcotic analgesia: Within 10-20 minutes

Duration of effect: 3-6 hours

Serum half-life: 3.8 hours

(Continued)

Hydrocodone and Aspirin *(Continued)*

Pregnancy Risk Factor D
Breast-feeding Considerations
Hydrocodone: No data reported
Aspirin: Cautious use due to potential adverse effects in nursing infants
Dosage Forms Tablet: Hydrocodone bitartrate 5 mg and aspirin 500 mg
Dietary Considerations May be taken with food or milk to minimize GI distress
Generic Available Yes
Comments Because of addiction liability of opiate analgesics, the use of hydrocodone should be limited to 2-3 days postoperatively for treatment of dental pain; nausea is the most common adverse effect seen after use in dental patients; sedation and constipation are second; aspirin component affects bleeding times and could influence time of wound healing
Selected Readings
Dionne RA, "New Approaches to Preventing and Treating Postoperative Pain," *J Am Dent Assoc,* 1992, 123(6):26-34.
Gobetti JP, "Controlling Dental Pain," *J Am Dent Assoc,* 1992, 123(6):47-52.

Hydrocodone and Chlorpheniramine

(hye droe koe' done & klor fen ir' a meen)
Brand Names Tussionex®
Therapeutic Category Antitussive; Cough Preparation
Use Symptomatic relief of cough
Local Anesthetic/Vasoconstrictor Precautions No information available to require special precautions
Effects on Dental Treatment Prolonged use will cause significant xerostomia

Hydrocodone and Guaifenesin

(hye droe koe' done & gwye fen' e sin)
Brand Names Codiclear® DH; HycoClear Tuss®; Hycotuss® Expectorant Liquid; Kwelcof®
Therapeutic Category Antitussive; Cough Preparation
Synonyms Guaifenesin and Hydrocodone
Use Symptomatic relief of nonproductive coughs associated with upper and lower respiratory tract congestion
Local Anesthetic/Vasoconstrictor Precautions No information available to require special precautions
Effects on Dental Treatment No effects or complications reported

Hydrocodone and Homatropine

(hye droe koe' done & hoe ma' troe peen)
Brand Names Hycodan®; Hydromet®; Hydropane®; Hydrotropine®; Tussigon®
Therapeutic Category Antitussive; Cough Preparation
Synonyms Homatropine and Hydrocodone
Use Symptomatic relief of cough
Usual Dosage Oral (based on hydrocodone component):
Children: 0.6 mg/kg/day in 3-4 divided doses; do not administer more frequently than every 4 hours
A single dose should not exceed 1.25 mg in children <2 years of age, 5 mg in children 2-12 years, and 10 mg in children >12 years
Adults: 5-10 mg every 4-6 hours, a single dose should not exceed 15 mg; do not administer more frequently than every 4 hours
Local Anesthetic/Vasoconstrictor Precautions No information available to require special precautions
Effects on Dental Treatment Dry mouth
Other Adverse Effects
>10%:
Cardiovascular: Hypotension
Central nervous system: Lightheadedness, dizziness, sedation, drowsiness, tiredness
Neuromuscular & skeletal: Weakness
1% to 10%:
Cardiovascular: Bradycardia, tachycardia
Central nervous system: Confusion
Gastrointestinal: Nausea, vomiting
Genitourinary: Decreased urination
Respiratory: Shortness of breath, troubled breathing
<1%:
Cardiovascular: Hypertension

Central nervous system: Hallucinations
Gastrointestinal: Dry mouth, anorexia, biliary spasm, impaired GI motility
Genitourinary: Urinary tract spasm
Ocular: Miosis, mydriasis, blurred vision, double vision
Miscellaneous: Histamine release, physical and psychological dependence with prolonged use; dry hot skin
Pregnancy Risk Factor C

Hydrocodone and Phenylpropanolamine
(hye droe koe' done & fen il proe pa nole' a meen)
Brand Names Codamine®; Codamine® Pediatric; Hycomine®; Hycomine® Pediatric
Therapeutic Category Cough Preparation; Decongestant
Synonyms Phenylpropanolamine and Hydrocodone
Use Symptomatic relief of cough and nasal congestion
Local Anesthetic/Vasoconstrictor Precautions Use with caution since phenylpropanolamine is a sympathomimetic amine which could interact with epinephrine to cause a pressor response
Effects on Dental Treatment Up to 10% of patients could experience tachycardia, palpitations, and dry mouth; use vasoconstrictor with caution

Hydrocodone, Chlorpheniramine, Phenylephrine, Acetaminophen and Caffeine
(hye droe koe' done, klor fen ir' a meen, fen il ef' rin, a seet a min' oh fen, & kaf' een)
Brand Names Hycomine® Compound
Therapeutic Category Antitussive; Cough Preparation
Use Symptomatic relief of cough and symptoms of upper respiratory infections
Local Anesthetic/Vasoconstrictor Precautions Use with caution since phenylephrine is a sympathomimetic amine which could interact with epinephrine to cause a pressor response
Effects on Dental Treatment
Acetaminophen: No effects or complications reported
Chlorpheniramine: Prolonged use will cause significant xerostomia
Phenylephrine: Up to 10% of patients could experience tachycardia, palpitations, and dry mouth; use vasoconstrictor with caution
Selected Readings
Barker JD Jr, de Carle DJ, and Anuras S, "Chronic Excessive Acetaminophen Use in Liver Damage," *Ann Intern Med*, 1977, 87(3):299-301.
Dionne RA, Campbell RA, Cooper SA, et al, "Suppression of Postoperative Pain by Preoperative Administration of Ibuprofen in Comparison to Placebo, Acetaminophen, and Acetaminophen Plus Codeine," *J Clin Pharmacol*, 1983, 23(1):37-43.
Licht H, Seeff LB, and Zimmerman HJ, "Apparent Potentiation of Acetaminophen Hepatotoxicity by Alcohol," *Ann Intern Med*, 1980, 92(4):511.

Hydrocodone, Phenylephrine, Pyrilamine, Phenindamine, Chlorpheniramine, and Ammonium Chloride
(hye droe koe' done, fen il ef' rin, peer il' a meen, fen in' da meen, klor fen ir' a meen, & a moe' nee um klor' ide)
Brand Names P-V-Tussin®
Therapeutic Category Antihistamine/Decongestant Combination; Cough Preparation
Use Symptomatic relief of cough and nasal congestion
Local Anesthetic/Vasoconstrictor Precautions Use with caution since phenylephrine is a sympathomimetic amine which could interact with epinephrine to cause a pressor response
Effects on Dental Treatment
Chlorpheniramine: Prolonged use will cause significant xerostomia
Phenylephrine: Up to 10% of patients could experience tachycardia, palpitations, and dry mouth; use vasoconstrictor with caution

Hydrocodone, Pseudoephedrine, and Guaifenesin
(hye droe koe' done, soo doe e fed' rin & gwye fen' e sin)
Brand Names Cophene XP®; Detussin® Expectorant; SRC® Expectorant; Tussafin® Expectorant
Therapeutic Category Cough Preparation; Decongestant; Expectorant
Use Symptomatic relief of irritating, nonproductive cough associated with respiratory conditions such as bronchitis, bronchial asthma, tracheobronchitis, and the common cold
(Continued)

Hydrocodone, Pseudoephedrine, and Guaifenesin
(Continued)

Local Anesthetic/Vasoconstrictor Precautions Use with caution since pseudoephedrine is a sympathomimetic amine which could interact with epinephrine to cause a pressor response

Effects on Dental Treatment
Guaifenesin: No effects or complications reported
Pseudoephedrine: Up to 10% of patients could experience tachycardia, palpitations, and dry mouth; use vasoconstrictor with caution

Hydrocortisone (hye droe kor' ti sone)
Related Information
Corticosteroid Equivalencies Comparison *on page 1017*
Corticosteroids, Topical Comparison *on page 1018*

Brand Names Cortef®; Hydrocortone® Acetate; Hydrocortone® Phosphate; Orabase® HCA; Solu-Cortef®

Canadian/Mexican Brand Names Flebocortid® [Sodium Succinate] (Mexico); Nositrol® [Sodium Succinate] (Mexico)

Therapeutic Category Anti-inflammatory Agent; Corticosteroid, Systemic; Corticosteroid, Topical (Low Potency)

Use
Dental: Treatment of a variety of oral diseases of allergic, inflammatory or autoimmune origin
Medical: Management of adrenocortical insufficiency; relief of inflammation of corticosteroid-responsive dermatoses (low and medium potency topical corticosteroid); adjunctive treatment of ulcerative colitis

Usual Dosage Adults: Anti-inflammatory or immunosuppressive:
Oral: 20-240 mg/day in 2-4 divided doses;
I.M., I.V.: Succinate: 100-500 mg every 2-10 hours
I.M., I.V., S.C.: Sodium phosphate: Initially 15-240 mg/day (approximately 1/3 to 1/2 of the oral dose) in divided doses every 12 hours. In acute diseases, doses higher than 240 mg may be required.

Mechanism of Action Decreases inflammation by suppression of migration of polymorphonuclear leukocytes and reversal of increased capillary permeability

Local Anesthetic/Vasoconstrictor Precautions No information available to require special precautions

Effects on Dental Treatment No effects or complications reported

Other Adverse Effects >10%:
Central nervous system: Insomnia, nervousness
Gastrointestinal: Increased appetite, indigestion

Oral manifestations: No data reported

Contraindications Serious infections, except septic shock or tuberculous meningitis; known hypersensitivity to hydrocortisone; viral, fungal, or tubercular skin lesions

Warnings/Precautions
Use with caution in patients with hyperthyroidism, cirrhosis, nonspecific ulcerative colitis, hypertension, osteoporosis, thromboembolic tendencies, CHF, convulsive disorders, myasthenia gravis, thrombophlebitis, peptic ulcer, diabetes

Acute adrenal insufficiency may occur with abrupt withdrawal after long-term therapy or with stress; young pediatric patients may be more susceptible to adrenal axis suppression from topical therapy

Because of the risk of adverse effects, systemic corticosteroids should be used cautiously in the elderly, in the smallest possible dose, and for the shortest possible time

Drug Interactions Insulin decreases hypoglycemic effect; phenytoin, phenobarbital, ephedrine, and rifampin have caused increased metabolism of hydrocortisone and decreased steroid blood level; oral anticoagulants change prothrombin time; potassium- depleting diuretics increase risk of hypokalemia; cardiac glucosides increase risk of arrhythmias or digitalis toxicity secondary to hypokalemia

Drug Uptake
Hydrocortisone acetate salt has a slow onset but long duration of action when compared with more soluble preparations
Hydrocortisone sodium phosphate salt is a water soluble salt with a rapid onset but short duration of action
Hydrocortisone sodium succinate salt is a water soluble salt with is rapidly active
Absorption: Rapid by all routes, except rectally

Serum half-life, biologic: 8-12 hours

Pregnancy Risk Factor C

Breast-feeding Considerations No data reported

Dosage Forms

Hydrocortisone acetate: Injection, suspension: 25 mg/mL (5 mL, 10 mL); 50 mg/mL (5 mL, 10 mL)

Hydrocortisone base: Tablet, oral: 5 mg, 10 mg, 20 mg

Hydrocortisone cypionate: Suspension, oral: 10 mg/5 mL (120 mL)

Hydrocortisone sodium phosphate: Injection, IM/IV/SC: 50 mg/mL (2 mL, 10 mL)

Hydrocortisone sodium succinate: Injection, IM/IV: 100 mg, 250 mg, 500 mg, 1000 mg

Dietary Considerations May be taken with meals to decrease GI upset; limit caffeine; need diet rich in pyridoxine, vitamin C, vitamin D, folate, calcium, and phosphorus

Generic Available Yes

Hydrocortisone and Clioquinol *see* Clioquinol and Hydrocortisone *on page 216*

Hydrocortisone and Dibucaine *see* Dibucaine and Hydrocortisone *on page 270*

Hydrocortisone and Iodochlorhydroxyquin *see* Clioquinol and Hydrocortisone *on page 216*

Hydrocortisone and Pramoxine *see* Pramoxine and Hydrocortisone *on page 714*

Hydrocortisone and Urea *see* Urea and Hydrocortisone *on page 885*

Hydrocortone® Acetate *see* Hydrocortisone *on previous page*

Hydrocortone® Phosphate *see* Hydrocortisone *on previous page*

Hydro-Crysti-12® *see* Hydroxocobalamin *on page 439*

HydroDIURIL® *see* Hydrochlorothiazide *on page 430*

Hydro-Ergoloid® *see* Ergoloid Mesylates *on page 318*

Hydroflumethiazide (hye droe floo meth eye' a zide)

Related Information

Cardiovascular Diseases *on page 912*

Brand Names Diucardin®; Saluron®

Therapeutic Category Diuretic, Thiazide Type

Use Management of mild to moderate hypertension; treatment of edema in congestive heart failure and nephrotic syndrome

Usual Dosage Oral:

Children: 1 mg/kg/24 hours

Adults: 50-200 mg/day

Mechanism of Action The diuretic mechanism of action is primarily inhibition of sodium, chloride, and water reabsorption in the renal distal tubules, thereby producing diuresis with a resultant reduction in plasma volume

Local Anesthetic/Vasoconstrictor Precautions No information available to require special precautions

Effects on Dental Treatment No effects or complications reported

Other Adverse Effects

1% to 10%: Endocrine & metabolic: Hypokalemia

<1%:

Cardiovascular: Hypotension

Central nervous system: Drowsiness

Dermatologic: Photosensitivity, rash

Endocrine & metabolic: Fluid and electrolyte imbalances (hypocalcemia, hypomagnesemia, hyponatremia), hyperglycemia

Gastrointestinal: Anorexia

Genitourinary: Uremia

Hematologic: Aplastic anemia, hemolytic anemia, leukopenia, agranulocytosis, thrombocytopenia, rarely blood dyscrasias

Hepatic: Hepatitis

Neuromuscular & skeletal: Paresthesia

Renal: Polyuria, prerenal azotemia

Drug Interactions

Decreased effect of oral hypoglycemics; decreased absorption with cholestyramine and colestipol

Increased effect with furosemide and other loop diuretics

Increased toxicity/levels of lithium

Drug Uptake

Onset of diuretic effect: Within ~2 hours

Peak effect: Within ~4 hours

(Continued)

Hydroflumethiazide *(Continued)*
Duration of action: 12-24 hours
Pregnancy Risk Factor D

Hydroflumethiazide and Reserpine
(hye droe floo meth eye′ a zide & re ser′ peen)
Brand Names Hydro-Fluserpine®; Salutensin®; Salutensin-Demi®
Therapeutic Category Antihypertensive Agent, Combination
Use Management of hypertension
Local Anesthetic/Vasoconstrictor Precautions No information available to require special precautions
Effects on Dental Treatment No effects or complications reported

Hydro-Fluserpine® see Hydroflumethiazide and Reserpine *on this page*
Hydrogesic® [5/500] *see* Hydrocodone and Acetaminophen *on page 431*
Hydromagnesium aluminate *see* Magaldrate *on page 520*
Hydromet® *see* Hydrocodone and Homatropine *on page 434*

Hydromorphone Hydrochloride
(hye droe mor′ fone hye droe klor′ ide)
Related Information
Narcotic Agonist Charts *on page 1019*
Brand Names Dilaudid®; Dilaudid-HP®
Canadian/Mexican Brand Names PMS-Hydromorphone® (Canada)
Therapeutic Category Analgesic, Narcotic; Antitussive
Use Management of moderate to severe pain; antitussive at lower doses
Usual Dosage
Doses should be titrated to appropriate analgesic effects; when changing routes of administration, note that oral doses are less than half as effective as parenteral doses (may be only one-fifth as effective)

Pain: Older Children and Adults:
Oral, I.M., I.V., S.C.: 1-4 mg/dose every 4-6 hours as needed; usual adult dose: 2 mg/dose
Rectal: 3 mg every 6-8 hours

Antitussive: Oral:
Children 6-12 years: 0.5 mg every 3-4 hours as needed
Children >12 years and Adults: 1 mg every 3-4 hours as needed
Mechanism of Action Binds to opiate receptors in the CNS, causing inhibition of ascending pain pathways, altering the perception of and response to pain; causes cough supression by direct central action in the medulla; produces generalized CNS depression
Local Anesthetic/Vasoconstrictor Precautions No information available to require special precautions
Effects on Dental Treatment Dry mouth and nausea in 10% of patients
Other Adverse Effects
Endocrine & metabolic: Antidiuretic hormone release
Ocular: Miosis
Sensitivity reactions: Histamine release
Miscellaneous: Physical and psychological dependence, biliary or urinary tract spasm

>10%:
Cardiovascular: Palpitations, hypotension, peripheral vasodilation
Central nervous system: Dizziness, lightheadedness, drowsiness
Gastrointestinal: Anorexia
1% to 10%:
Cardiovascular: Tachycardia, bradycardia, flushing of face
Central nervous system: CNS depression, increased intracranial pressure, weakness, tiredness, headache, nervousness, restlessness
Gastrointestinal: Nausea, vomiting, constipation, stomach cramps, dry mouth
Genitourinary: Decreased urination, ureteral spasm
Neuromuscular & skeletal: Trembling
Respiratory: Respiratory depression, troubled breathing, shortness of breath
<1%:
Central nervous system: Hallucinations, mental depression, paralytic ileus
Dermatologic: Pruritus, skin rash, hives
Drug Interactions Increased toxicity: CNS depressants, phenothiazines, tricyclic antidepressants may potentiate the adverse effects of hydromorphone

Drug Uptake
Onset of analgesic effect: Within 15-30 minutes
Duration: 4-5 hours
Serum half-life: 1-3 hours
Pregnancy Risk Factor B (D if used for prolonged periods or in high doses at term)

Hydromox® see Quinethazone on page 758
Hydropane® see Hydrocodone and Homatropine on page 434
Hydro-Par® see Hydrochlorothiazide on page 430
Hydrophen® see Theophylline, Ephedrine, and Hydroxyzine on page 836
Hydropres® see Hydrochlorothiazide and Reserpine on page 431

Hydroquinone (hye' droe kwin one)
Brand Names Eldopaque® [OTC]; Eldopaque Forte®; Eldoquin® [OTC]; Eldoquin Forte®; Esoterica® Facial [OTC]; Esoterica® Regular [OTC]; Esoterica® Sensitive Skin Formula [OTC]; Esoterica® Sunscreen [OTC]; Melanex®; Porcelana® [OTC]; Solaquin® [OTC]; Solaquin Forte®
Canadian/Mexican Brand Names Neostrata® HQ (Canada); Ultraquin® (Canada); Crema Blanca Bustillos (Mexico)
Therapeutic Category Depigmenting Agent
Synonyms Hidroquinona (Mexico)
Use Gradual bleaching of hyperpigmented skin conditions
Usual Dosage Children >12 years and Adults: Topical: Apply thin layer and rub in twice daily
Mechanism of Action Produces reversible depigmentation of the skin by suppression of melanocyte metabolic processes, in particular the inhibition of the enzymatic oxidation of tyrosine to DOPA (3,4-dihydroxyphenylalanine); sun exposure reverses this effect and will cause repigmentation.
Local Anesthetic/Vasoconstrictor Precautions No information available to require special precautions
Effects on Dental Treatment No effects or complications reported
Other Adverse Effects 1% to 10%: Dermatologic: Dermatitis, dryness, erythema, stinging, irritation, inflammatory reaction, sensitization
Drug Interactions No data reported
Drug Uptake Onset and duration of depigmentation produced by hydroquinone varies among individuals
Pregnancy Risk Factor C

Hydro-Serp® see Hydrochlorothiazide and Reserpine on page 431
Hydroserpine® see Hydrochlorothiazide and Reserpine on page 431
Hydrotropine® see Hydrocodone and Homatropine on page 434
Hydroxacen® see Hydroxyzine on page 443

Hydroxocobalamin (hye drox oh koe bal' a min)
Brand Names Alphamin®; Codroxomin®; Hybalamin®; Hydrobexan®; Hydro-Cobex®; Hydro-Crysti-12®; LA-12®
Canadian/Mexican Brand Names Acti-B$_{12}$® (Canada); Duradoce® (Mexico)
Therapeutic Category Vitamin, Water Soluble
Synonyms Hidroxocobalamina (Mexico)
Use Treatment of pernicious anemia, vitamin B$_{12}$ deficiency, increased B$_{12}$ requirements due to pregnancy, thyrotoxicosis, hemorrhage, malignancy, liver or kidney disease
Usual Dosage Vitamin B$_{12}$ deficiency: I.M.:
Children: 1-5 mg given in single doses of 100 mcg over 2 or more weeks, followed by 30-50 mcg/month
Adults: 30 mcg/day for 5-10 days, followed by 100-200 mcg/month
Mechanism of Action Coenzyme for various metabolic functions, including fat and carbohydrate metabolism and protein synthesis, used in cell replication and hematopoiesis
Local Anesthetic/Vasoconstrictor Precautions No information available to require special precautions
Effects on Dental Treatment No effects or complications reported
Other Adverse Effects
1% to 10%:
Dermatologic: Itching
Gastrointestinal: Diarrhea
<1%:
Cardiovascular: Peripheral vascular thrombosis
Dermatologic: Urticaria
Miscellaneous: Anaphylaxis
(Continued)

Hydroxocobalamin *(Continued)*
Drug Interactions No data reported
Pregnancy Risk Factor C

Hydroxyamphetamine and Tropicamide
(hye drox ee am fet′ a meen & troe pik′ a mide)
Brand Names Paremyd® Ophthalmic
Therapeutic Category Ophthalmic Agent, Mydriatic
Use Mydriasis with cycloplegia
Local Anesthetic/Vasoconstrictor Precautions No information available to require special precautions
Effects on Dental Treatment No effects or complications reported

Hydroxyamphetamine Hydrobromide
(hye drox ee am fet′ a meen hye droe broe′ mide)
Brand Names Paredrine®
Therapeutic Category Ophthalmic Agent, Mydriatic
Use Produce mydriasis in diagnostic eye examination
Local Anesthetic/Vasoconstrictor Precautions No information available to require special precautions
Effects on Dental Treatment No effects or complications reported

Hydroxycarbamide *see* Hydroxyurea *on page 442*

Hydroxychloroquine Sulfate (hye drox ee klor′ oh kwin sul′ fate)
Related Information
  Rheumatoid Arthritis, Osteoarthritis, and Joint Prostheses *on page 930*
Brand Names Plaquenil®
Therapeutic Category Antimalarial Agent
Synonyms Hidroxicloroquina Sulfato De (Mexico)
Use Suppresses and treats acute attacks of malaria; treatment of systemic lupus erythematosus and rheumatoid arthritis
Usual Dosage Oral:
  Children:
    Chemoprophylaxis of malaria: 5 mg/kg (base) once weekly; should not exceed the recommended adult dose; begin 2 weeks before exposure; continue for 4-6 weeks after leaving endemic area
    Acute attack: 10 mg/kg (base) initial dose; followed by 5 mg/kg at 6, 24, and 48 hours
    JRA or SLE: 3-5 mg/kg/day divided 1-2 times/day to a maximum of 400 mg/day; not to exceed 7 mg/kg/day
  Adults:
    Chemoprophylaxis of malaria: 2 tablets weekly on same day each week; begin 2 weeks before exposure; continue for 4-6 weeks after leaving endemic area
    Acute attack: 4 tablets first dose day 1; 2 tablets in 6 hours day 1; 2 tablets in 1 dose day 2; and 2 tablets in 1 dose on day 3
    Rheumatoid arthritis: 2-3 tablets/day to start taken with food or milk; increase dose until optimum response level is reached; usually after 4-12 weeks dose should be reduced by ½ and a maintenance dose of 1-2 tablets/day given
    Lupus erythematosus: 2 tablets every day or twice daily for several weeks depending on response; 1-2 tablets/day for prolonged maintenance therapy
Mechanism of Action Interferes with digestive vacuole function within sensitive malarial parasites by increasing the pH and interfering with lysosomal degradation of hemoglobin; inhibits locomotion of neutrophils and chemotaxis of eosinophils; impairs complement-dependent antigen-antibody reactions
Local Anesthetic/Vasoconstrictor Precautions No information available to require special precautions
Effects on Dental Treatment No effects or complications reported
Other Adverse Effects
  >10%:
    Central nervous system: Headache
    Dermatologic: Itching
    Gastrointestinal: Diarrhea, loss of appetite, nausea, stomach cramps, vomiting
    Ocular: Ciliary muscle dysfunction

1% to 10%:
  Central nervous system: Dizziness, lightheadedness, nervousness, restlessness
  Dermatologic: Bleaching of hair, skin rash blue-black discoloration of skin
  Ocular: Ocular toxicity, keratopathy, retinopathy
<1%:
  Central nervous system: Emotional changes, seizures
  Hematologic: Agranulocytosis, aplastic anemia, neutropenia, thrombocytopenia
  Neuromuscular & skeletal: Neuromyopathy
  Otic: Ototoxicity
Drug Interactions No data reported
Drug Uptake
  Absorption: Oral: Complete
Pregnancy Risk Factor C

Hydroxydaunomycin Hydrochloride *see* Doxorubicin Hydrochloride *on page 299*

Hydroxyethylcellulose *see* Artificial Tears *on page 75*

Hydroxyethyl Starch *see* Hetastarch *on page 423*

Hydroxyprogesterone Caproate
(hye drox ee proe jess' te rone kap' roe ate)
Brand Names Duralutin®; Gesterol® L.A.; Hy-Gestrone®; Hylutin®; Hyprogest®
Canadian/Mexican Brand Names Primolut® Depot (Mexico)
Therapeutic Category Progestin Derivative
Synonyms Hidroxiprogesterona Caproato De (Mexico)
Use Treatment of amenorrhea, abnormal uterine bleeding, endometriosis, uterine carcinoma
Usual Dosage Adults: Female: I.M.:
  Amenorrhea: 375 mg; if no bleeding, begin cyclic treatment with estradiol valerate
  Production of secretory endometrium and desquamation: (Medical D and C): 125-250 mg administered on day 10 of cycle; repeat every 7 days until supression is no longer desired.
  Uterine carcinoma: 1 g one or more times/day (1-7 g/week) for up to 12 weeks
Mechanism of Action Natural steroid hormone that induces secretory changes in the endometrium, promotes mammary gland development, relaxes uterine smooth muscle, blocks follicular maturation and ovulation and maintains pregnancy
Local Anesthetic/Vasoconstrictor Precautions No information available to require special precautions
Effects on Dental Treatment No effects or complications reported
Other Adverse Effects
  >10%:
    Cardiovascular: Edema
    Central nervous system: Weakness
    Endocrine & metabolic: Breakthrough bleeding, spotting, changes in menstrual flow, amenorrhea
    Gastrointestinal: Anorexia
    Local: Pain at injection site
  1% to 10%:
    Cardiovascular: Edema
    Central nervous system: Mental depression, insomnia, fever
    Dermatologic: Melasma or chloasma, allergic rash with or without pruritus
    Gastrointestinal: Weight gain or loss
    Genitourinary: Changes in cervical erosion and secretions, increased breast tenderness
    Hepatic: Cholestatic jaundice
Drug Interactions Decreased effect: Rifampin causes an increased clearance of hydroxyprogesterone
Drug Uptake
  Peak serum concentration: I.M.: 3-7 days; concentrations are measurable for 3-4 weeks after injection
Pregnancy Risk Factor D

Hydroxypropyl Cellulose (hye drox ee proe' pil sel' yoo lose)
Brand Names Lacrisert®
Therapeutic Category Ophthalmic Agent, Miscellaneous
Use Dry eyes
(Continued)

Hydroxypropyl Cellulose *(Continued)*

Local Anesthetic/Vasoconstrictor Precautions No information available to require special precautions
Effects on Dental Treatment No effects or complications reported
Other Adverse Effects 1% to 10%: Local irritation

Hydroxypropyl Methylcellulose
(hye drox ee proe′ pil meth il sel′ yoo lose)

Brand Names Gonak™ [OTC]; Goniosol® [OTC]; Occucoat™
Therapeutic Category Ophthalmic Agent, Miscellaneous
Synonyms Gonioscopic Ophthalmic Solution
Use Ophthalmic surgical aid in cataract extraction and intraocular implantation; gonioscopic examinations
Local Anesthetic/Vasoconstrictor Precautions No information available to require special precautions
Effects on Dental Treatment No effects or complications reported
Other Adverse Effects 1% to 10%: Local irritation

Hydroxyurea (hye drox ee yoor ee′ a)

Brand Names Hydrea®
Therapeutic Category Antineoplastic Agent, Miscellaneous
Synonyms Hydroxycarbamide
Use Treatment of chronic myelocytic leukemia (CML), melanoma, and ovarian carcinomas; also used with radiation in treatment of tumors of the head and neck; adjunct in the management of sickle cell patients
Usual Dosage Oral (**refer to individual protocols**):
Children:
No FDA-approved dosage regimens have been established. Dosages of 1500-3000 mg/m^2 as a single dose in combination with other agents every 4-6 weeks have been used in the treatment of pediatric astrocytoma, medulloblastoma and primitive neuroectodermal tumors.
CML: Initial: 10-20 mg/kg/day once daily; adjust dose according to hematologic response

Adults: Dose should always be titrated to patient response and WBC counts; usual oral doses range from 10-30 mg/kg/day or 500-3000 mg/day; if WBC count falls <2500 cells/mm^3, or the platelet count <100,000/mm^3, therapy should be stopped for at least 3 days and resumed when values rise toward normal
Solid tumors:
Intermittent therapy: 80 mg/kg as a single dose every third day
Continuous therapy: 20-30 mg/kg/day given as a single dose/day
Concomitant therapy with irradiation: 80 mg/kg as a single dose every third day starting at least 7 days before initiation of irradiation
Resistant chronic myelocytic leukemia: 20-30 mg/kg/day divided daily
Sickle cell anemia (moderate/severe disease): Hydroxyurea administration in adults (age range: 22-42 years) has produced beneficial effects in several small studies
Initial: 15 mg/kg/day, increased by 5 mg/kg every 12 weeks unless toxicity is observed or the maximum tolerated dose of 35 mg/kg/day is achieved.
Monitor for toxicity every 2 weeks. If toxicity occurs, stop treatment until the bone marrow recovers. Restart at 2.5 mg/kg/day less than the dose at which toxicity occurs. If no toxicity occurs over the next 12 weeks, then the subsequent dose should be increased by 2.5 mg/kg/day. Reduced dosage of hydroxyurea alternating with erythropoietin may decrease myelotoxicity and increase levels of fetal hemoglobin in patients who have not been helped by hydroxyurea alone
Mechanism of Action Interferes with synthesis of DNA, during the S phase of cell division, without interfering with RNA synthesis; inhibits ribonucleoside diphosphate reductase, preventing conversion of ribonucleotides to deoxyribonucleotides; cell-cycle specific for the S phase and may hold other cells in the G$_1$ phase of the cell cycle.
Local Anesthetic/Vasoconstrictor Precautions No information available to require special precautions
Effects on Dental Treatment No effects or complications reported
Other Adverse Effects
>10%:
Central nervous system: Drowsiness
Gastrointestinal: Mild to moderate nausea and vomiting may occur, as well as diarrhea, constipation, mucositis, ulceration of the GI tract, anorexia, and stomatitis

Myelosuppression: Dose-limiting toxicity, causes a rapid drop in leukocyte count (seen in 4-5 days in nonhematologic malignancy and more rapidly in leukemia). Thrombocytopenia and anemia occur less often; reversal of WBC count occurs rapidly, but the platelet count may take 7-10 days to recover.

1% to 10%:
Dermatologic: Dermatologic changes (hyperpigmentation, erythema of the hands and face, maculopapular rash, or dry skin), alopecia
Hepatic: Abnormal LFTs and hepatitis
Renal: Increased BUN/creatinine
Miscellaneous: Carcinogenic potential

<1%:
Central nervous system: Neurotoxicity, renal tubular function impairment, dizziness, disorientation, hallucination, seizures, headache
Dermatologic: Facial erythema
Endocrine & metabolic: Hyperuricemia
Genitourinary: Dysuria
Hepatic: Elevation of hepatic enzymes

Drug Uptake
Absorption: Readily absorbed from GI tract (≥80%)
Serum half-life: 3-4 hours
Time to peak serum concentration: Within 2 hours

Pregnancy Risk Factor D

Hydroxyzine (hye drox' i zeen)
Related Information
Patients Requiring Sedation *on page 965*
Brand Names Anxanil®; Atarax®; Atozine®; Durrax®; E-Vista®; Hydroxacen®; Hy-Pam®; Hyzine-50®; Neucalm®; Quiess®; Vamate®; Vistacon-50®; Vistaject-25®; Vistaject-50®; Vistaquel®; Vistaril®; Vistazine®
Canadian/Mexican Brand Names Apo-Hydroxyzine® (Canada); Multipax® (Canada); Novo-Hydroxyzine® (Canada); PMS®-Hydroxyzine (Canada)
Therapeutic Category Antianxiety Agent; Antiemetic; Antihistamine; Sedative; Tranquilizer, Minor
Use
Dental: Treatment of anxiety, as a preoperative sedative in pediatric dentistry
Medical: Antipruritic, antiemetic, and in alcohol withdrawal symptoms
Usual Dosage
Children:
>6 years:
Oral: 25-50 mg 1 hour before procedure or 0.6 mg/kg/dose every 6 hours
I.M.: 0.5-1 mg/kg/dose every 4-6 hours as needed
<6 years: Oral: 12.5-25 mg 1 hours before procedure
Adults: Very rarely used in adults as preoperative sedative
Oral: 50-100 mg 1 hour before procedure
I.M.: 25-100 mg 1 hour before procedure
Mechanism of Action Competes with histamine for H_1-receptor sites on effector cells in the gastrointestinal tract, blood vessels, and respiratory tract
Local Anesthetic/Vasoconstrictor Precautions No information available to require special precautions
Effects on Dental Treatment No effects or complications reported
Other Adverse Effects
>10%:
Central nervous system: Slight to moderate drowsiness
Respiratory: Thickening of bronchial secretions
1% to 10%:
Central nervous system: Headache, fatigue, nervousness, dizziness
Gastrointestinal: Appetite increase, weight increase, nausea, diarrhea, abdominal pain
Neuromuscular & skeletal: Arthralgia
Respiratory: Pharyngitis

Oral manifestations: 1% to 10%: Dry mouth
Contraindications Hypersensitivity to hydroxyzine or any component
Warnings/Precautions S.C., intra-arterial and I.V. administration **not** recommended since thrombosis and digital gangrene can occur; extravasation can result in sterile abscess and marked tissue induration; should be used with caution in patients with narrow-angle glaucoma, prostatic hypertrophy, and bladder neck obstruction; should also be used with caution in patients with asthma or COPD
(Continued)

443

Hydroxyzine *(Continued)*

Anticholinergic effects are not well tolerated in the elderly. Hydroxyzine may be useful as a short-term antipruritic, but it is not recommended for use as a sedative or anxiolytic in the elderly.

Drug Interactions Increased toxicity with CNS depressants, anticholinergics

Drug Uptake
Absorption: Oral: Rapid
Onset of effect: Within 15-30 minutes
Duration: 4-6 hours
Serum half-life: 3-7 hours

Pregnancy Risk Factor C

Breast-feeding Considerations No data reported

Dosage Forms
Hydroxyzine hydrochloride:
Injection:
Vistaject-25®, Vistaril®: 25 mg/mL (1 mL, 2 mL, 10 mL)
E-Vista®, Hydroxacen®, Hyzine-50®, Neucalm®, Quiess®, Vistacon-50®, Vistaject-50®, Vistaquel®, Vistaril®, Vistazine®: 50 mg/mL (1 mL, 2 mL, 10 mL)
Syrup (Atarax®): 10 mg/5 mL (120 mL, 480 mL, 4000 mL)
Tablet:
Anxanil®: 25 mg
Atarax®: 10 mg, 25 mg, 50 mg, 100 mg
Atozine®: 10 mg, 25 mg, 50 mg
Durrax®: 10 mg, 25 mg
Hydroxyzine pamoate:
Capsule:
Hy-Pam®: 25 mg, 50 mg
Vamate®: 25 mg, 50 mg, 100 mg
Vistaril®: 25 mg, 50 mg, 100 mg
Suspension, oral (Vistaril®:) 25 mg/5 mL (120 mL, 480 mL)

Dietary Considerations No data reported

Generic Available Yes

Hy-Gestrone® *see* Hydroxyprogesterone Caproate *on page 441*

Hygroton® *see* Chlorthalidone *on page 199*

Hylorel® *see* Guanadrel Sulfate *on page 411*

Hylutin® *see* Hydroxyprogesterone Caproate *on page 441*

Hyoscyamine, Atropine, Scopolamine, and Phenobarbital

(hye oh sye' a meen, a' troe peen, skoe pol' a meen & fee noe bar' bi tal)

Brand Names Barbidonna®; Barophen®; Donnamor®; Donnapine®; Donna-Sed®; Donnatal®; Donphen®; Hyosophen®; Kinesed®; Malatal®; Relaxadon®; Spaslin®; Spasmolin®; Spasmophen®; Spasquid®; Susano®

Therapeutic Category Anticholinergic Agent; Antispasmodic Agent, Gastrointestinal

Use Adjunct in treatment of peptic ulcer disease, irritable bowel, spastic colitis, spastic bladder, and renal colic

Usual Dosage Oral:
Children 2-12 years: Kinesed® dose: ½ to 1 tablet 3-4 times/day

Children: Donnatal® elixir: 0.1 mL/kg/dose every 4 hours; maximum dose: 5 mL **or** see table for alternative.

Weight (kg)	Dose (mL)	
	q4h	q6h
4.5	0.5	0.75
10	1	1.5
14	1.5	2
23	2.5	3.8
34	3.8	5
≥45	5	7.5

Adults: 1-2 capsules or tablets 3-4 times/day; or 1 Donnatal® Extentab® in sustained release form every 12 hours; or 5-10 mL elixir 3-4 times/day or every 8 hours

Mechanism of Action Refer to individual agents

Local Anesthetic/Vasoconstrictor Precautions No information available to require special precautions

Effects on Dental Treatment Dry mouth in >10% of patients (normal salivary flow returns with cessation of drug therapy)

Other Adverse Effects

>10%:

Gastrointestinal: Constipation, dry mouth

Local: Irritation at injection site

Miscellaneous: Decreased sweating; dry nose, throat, or skin

1% to 10%: Decreased flow of breast milk, difficulty in swallowing, increased sensitivity to light

<1%:

Cardiovascular: Orthostatic hypotension, ventricular fibrillation, tachycardia, palpitations

Central nervous system: Confusion, drowsiness, headache, loss of memory, tiredness, ataxia

Dermatologic: Skin rash

Gastrointestinal: Bloated feeling, nausea, vomiting

Genitourinary: Difficult urination

Ocular: Increased intraocular pain, blurred vision

Drug Interactions The following drugs may cause enhanced effects of this preparation: CNS depressants, amantadine, antihistamine, phenothiazines, corticosteroids, digitalis, griseofulvin, anticonvulsants, MAO inhibitors, tricyclic antidepressants

Drug Uptake Absorption: Well absorbed from GI tract

Pregnancy Risk Factor C

Hyoscyamine, Atropine, Scopolamine, Kaolin, and Pectin

(hye oh sye' a meen, a' troe peen, skoe pol' a meen, kay' oh lin & pek' tin)

Therapeutic Category Antidiarrheal

Use Antidiarrheal; also used in gastritis, enteritis, colitis, and acute gastrointestinal upsets, and nausea which may accompany any of these conditions

Local Anesthetic/Vasoconstrictor Precautions No information available to require special precautions

Effects on Dental Treatment Dry mouth in >10% of patients (normal salivary flow returns with cessation of drug therapy)

Comments Hyoscyamine is dialyzable

Hyoscyamine, Atropine, Scopolamine, Kaolin, Pectin, and Opium

(hye oh sye' a meen, a' troe peen, skoe pol' a meen, kay' oh lin, pek' tin, & oh' pee um)

Brand Names Donnapectolin-PG®; Kapectolin PG®

Therapeutic Category Antidiarrheal

Use Treatment of diarrhea

Local Anesthetic/Vasoconstrictor Precautions No information available to require special precautions

Effects on Dental Treatment Dry mouth in >10% of patients (normal salivary flow returns with cessation of drug therapy)

Hyoscyamine Sulfate (hye oh sye' a meen sul' fate)

Brand Names Anaspaz®; Cystospaz®; Cystospaz-M®; Gastrosed™; Levsin®; Levsinex®

Therapeutic Category Anticholinergic Agent; Antispasmodic Agent, Gastrointestinal

Use Treatment of GI tract disorders caused by spasm, adjunctive therapy for peptic ulcers

Usual Dosage

Children: Oral, S.L.: Dose as per table repeated every 4 hours as needed

Adults:

Oral or S.L.: 0.125-0.25 mg 3-4 times/day before meals or food and at bedtime

Oral: 0.375-0.75 mg (timed release) every 12 hours

I.M., I.V., S.C.: 0.25-0.5 mg every 6 hours

(Continued)

445

Hyoscyamine

Weight (kg)	Dose (mcg)	Maximum 24-Hour Dose (mcg)
Children <2 y		
2.3	12.5	75
3.4	16.7	100
5	20.8	125
7	25	150
10	31.3-33.3	200
15	45.8	275
Children 2-10 y		
10	31.3-33.3	
20	62.5	Do not exceed
40	93.8	0.75 mg
50	125	

Mechanism of Action Blocks the action of acetylcholine at parasympathetic sites in smooth muscle, secretory glands and the CNS; increases cardiac output, dries secretions, antagonizes histamine and serotonin

Local Anesthetic/Vasoconstrictor Precautions No information available to require special precautions

Effects on Dental Treatment Dry mouth in >10% of patients (normal salivary flow returns with cessation of drug therapy)

Other Adverse Effects
>10%:
  Gastrointestinal: Dry mouth
  Local: Irritation at injection site
  Miscellaneous: Decreased sweating; Dry nose, throat, or skin
1% to 10%:
  Dermatologic: Photosensitivity
  Gastrointestinal: Constipation
  Ocular: Blurred vision, mydriasis
  Miscellaneous: Difficulty in swallowing
<1%:
  Cardiovascular: Palpitations, orthostatic hypotension
  Central nervous system: Headache, lightheadedness, memory loss, fatigue, delirium, restlessness, ataxia
  Dermatologic: Skin rash
  Genitourinary: Difficult urination
  Neuromuscular & skeletal: Tremor
  Ocular: Increased intraocular pressure

Drug Interactions
  Decreased effect with antacids
  Increased toxicity with amantadine, antimuscarinics, haloperidol, phenothiazines, TCAs, MAO inhibitors

Drug Uptake
  Onset of effect: 2-3 minutes
  Duration: 4-6 hours
  Absorption: Oral: Absorbed well
  Serum half-life: 13% to 38%

Pregnancy Risk Factor C

Hyosophen® see Hyoscyamine, Atropine, Scopolamine, and Phenobarbital on page 444

Hy-Pam® see Hydroxyzine on page 443

Hyperab® see Rabies Immune Globulin, Human on page 761

HyperHep® see Hepatitis B Immune Globulin on page 422

Hyperstat® I.V. see Diazoxide on page 269

Hyper-Tet® see Tetanus Immune Globulin, Human on page 826

Hy-Phen® [5/500] see Hydrocodone and Acetaminophen on page 431

HypoTears PF Solution [OTC] see Artificial Tears on page 75

HypoTears Solution [OTC] see Artificial Tears on page 75

HypRho®-D see Rh₀(D) Immune Globulin on page 767

HypRho®-D Mini-Dose see Rh₀(D) Immune Globulin on page 767

Hyprogest® see Hydroxyprogesterone Caproate on page 441

Hysone® Topical see Clioquinol and Hydrocortisone on page 216

Hytakerol® see Dihydrotachysterol on page 283

Hytinic® **[OTC]** *see* Polysaccharide-Iron Complex *on page 705*

Hytrin® *see* Terazosin *on page 821*

Hytuss® **[OTC]** *see* Guaifenesin *on page 407*

Hytuss-2X® **[OTC]** *see* Guaifenesin *on page 407*

Hyzaar® *see* Losartan and Hydrochlorothiazide *on page 515*

Hy-Zide® *see* Hydralazine and Hydrochlorothiazide *on page 428*

Hyzine-50® *see* Hydroxyzine *on page 443*

Iberet-Folic-500® *see* Ferrous Sulfate, Ascorbic Acid, Vitamin B-Complex, and Folic Acid *on page 361*

Iberet®-Liquid [OTC] *see* Ferrous Sulfate, Ascorbic Acid, and Vitamin B-Complex *on page 361*

Ibuprin® **[OTC]** *see* Ibuprofen *on this page*

Ibuprofen (eye byoo proe' fen)
Related Information
Dental Drug Interactions: Update on Drug Combinations Requiring Special Considerations *on page 1022*

Nonsteroidal Anti-Inflammatory Agents, Comparative Dosages, and Pharmacokinetics *on page 1021*

Oral Pain *on page 940*

Rheumatoid Arthritis, Osteoarthritis, and Joint Prostheses *on page 930*

Temporomandibular Dysfunction (TMD) *on page 963*

Brand Names Aches-N-Pain® [OTC]; Advil® [OTC]; Excedrin® IB [OTC]; Genpril® [OTC]; Haltran® [OTC]; Ibuprin® [OTC]; Ibuprohm® [OTC]; Ibu-Tab®; Medipren® [OTC]; Menadol® [OTC]; Midol® 200 [OTC]; Motrin®; Motrin® IB [OTC]; Nuprin® [OTC]; Pamprin IB® [OTC]; PediaProfen™; Rufen®; Saleto-200® [OTC]; Saleto-400®; Trendar® [OTC]; Uni-Pro® [OTC]

Canadian/Mexican Brand Names Actiprofen® (Canada); Apo-Ibuprofen® (Canada); Novo-Profen® (Canada); Nu-Ibuprofen® (Canada); Butacortelone® (Mexico); Dibufen® (Mexico); Kedvil® (Mexico); proartinal® (Mexico); Quadrax® (Mexico); Tabalon® (Mexico)

Therapeutic Category Analgesic, Non-narcotic; Anti-inflammatory Agent; Nonsteroidal Anti-inflammatory Agent (NSAID)

Use
Dental: Management of pain and swelling

Medical: Inflammatory diseases and rheumatoid disorders including juvenile rheumatoid arthritis, mild to moderate pain, fever, dysmenorrhea, gout, ankylosing spondylitis, acute migraine headache

Usual Dosage Oral:
Children: Analgesic: 4-10 mg/kg/dose every 6-8 hours

Adults: 400-800 mg/dose 3-4 times/day; maximum daily dose: 3.2 (3200 mg) g/day

Mechanism of Action Inhibits prostaglandin synthesis by decreasing the activity of the enzyme, cyclo-oxygenase, which results in decreased formation of prostaglandin precursors

Local Anesthetic/Vasoconstrictor Precautions No information available to require special precautions

Effects on Dental Treatment Use with caution in patients taking anticoagulants

Other Adverse Effects
>10%: Gastrointestinal: Indigestion, nausea

1% to 10%: Gastrointestinal: Abdominal pain

Oral manifestations: <1%: Dry mouth

Contraindications Hypersensitivity to ibuprofen, any component, aspirin, or other nonsteroidal anti-inflammatory drugs (NSAIDs)

Warnings/Precautions Do not exceed 3200 mg/day; use with caution in patients with congestive heart failure, hypertension, decreased renal or hepatic function, history of GI disease (bleeding or ulcers), or those receiving anticoagulants; safety and efficacy in children <6 months of age have not yet been established; elderly are a high-risk population for adverse effects from nonsteroidal anti-inflammatory agents. As much as 60% of elderly can develop peptic ulceration and/or hemorrhage asymptomatically.

Use lowest effective dose for shortest period possible. CNS adverse effects such as confusion, agitation, and hallucination are generally seen in overdose or high dose situations; but elderly may demonstrate these adverse effects at lower doses than younger adults.

Drug Interactions Aspirin may decrease ibuprofen serum concentrations; may increase digoxin, methotrexate, and lithium serum concentrations; other nonsteroidal anti-inflammatories may increase adverse gastrointestinal effects (Continued)

Ibuprofen *(Continued)*

Drug Uptake
Absorption: Rapid
Onset of effect: 30-60 minutes
Time to peak serum concentration: Within 1-2 hours
Duration of effect: 4-6 hours
Serum half-life: 2-4 hours
Influence of food: Rate is decreased but extent remains the same

Pregnancy Risk Factor B (D if used in the 3rd trimester)

Breast-feeding Considerations May be taken while breast-feeding

Dosage Forms
Suspension, oral: 100 mg/5 mL (120 mL, 480 mL)
Tablet: 200 mg [OTC], 300 mg, 400 mg, 600 mg, 800 mg

Dietary Considerations May be taken with food or milk to decrease GI adverse effects

Generic Available Yes: Tablet

Comments Preoperative use of ibuprofen at a dose of 400-600 mg every 6 hours 24 hours before the appointment decreases postoperative edema and hastens healing time

Selected Readings
Brooks PM and Day RO, "Nonsteroidal Anti-inflammatory Drugs-Differences and Similarities," *N Engl J Med*, 1991, 324(24):1716-25.
Dionne RA, "New Approaches to Preventing and Treating Postoperative Pain," *J Am Dent Assoc*, 1992, 123(6):26-34.
Gobetti JP, "Controlling Dental Pain," *J Am Dent Assoc*, 1992, 123(6):47-52.
Winter L Jr, Bass E, Recant B, et al, "Analgesic Activity of Ibuprofen (Motrin®) in Postoperative Oral Surgical Pain," *Oral Surg Oral Med Oral Pathol*, 1978, 45(2):159-66.

Ibuprohm® [OTC] *see* Ibuprofen *on previous page*

Ibu-Tab® *see* Ibuprofen *on previous page*

Idamycin® *see* Idarubicin *on this page*

Idarubicin *(eye da roo′ bi sin)*

Brand Names Idamycin®

Therapeutic Category Antineoplastic Agent, Antibiotic

Synonyms 4-demethoxydaunorubicin; IDR

Use In combination with other antineoplastic agents for treatment of acute myelogenous leukemia (AML) in adults and acute lymphocytic leukemia (ALL) in children

Usual Dosage I.V.:
Children:
Leukemia: 10-12 mg/m² once daily for 3 days and repeat every 3 weeks
Solid tumors: 5 mg/m² once daily for 3 days and repeat every 3 weeks

Adults: 12 mg/m²/day for 3 days in combination with Ara-C or 25 mg/m² bolus

Mechanism of Action Similar to daunorubicin, idarubicin exhibits inhibitory effects on DNA and RNA polymerase *in vitro*. Idarubicin has an affinity for DNA similar to daunorubicin and somewhat higher efficacy in stabilizing the DNA double helix against heat denaturation. Idarubicin has been as active or more active than daunorubicin in inhibiting 3H-TdR uptake by DNA or RNA of mouse embryo fibroblasts.

Local Anesthetic/Vasoconstrictor Precautions No information available to require special precautions

Effects on Dental Treatment No effects or complications reported

Other Adverse Effects
>10%:
Central nervous system: Headache, fever
Gastrointestinal: Mucositis
Genitourinary: Discoloration of urine (red)
Hematologic: Hemorrhage
Miscellaneous: Infection
Local: Tissue necrosis upon extravasation, erythematous streaking
Vesicant chemotherapy
Dermatologic: Alopecia, rash, urticaria
Gastrointestinal: Nausea, vomiting, diarrhea, stomatitis
Hematologic:
Leukopenia (nadir: 8-29 days)
Thrombocytopenia (nadir: 10-15 days)
Anemia
1% to 10%:
Central nervous system: Seizures
Neuromuscular & skeletal: Peripheral neuropathy

Miscellaneous: Pulmonary allergy
<1%:
Cardiovascular: Arrhythmias, EKG changes, cardiomyopathy, congestive heart failure, myocardial toxicity, acute life-threatening arrhythmias
Endocrine & metabolic: Hyperuricemia
Hepatic: Elevations in liver enzymes or bilirubin
Drug Uptake
Absorption: Oral: Rapid but erratic (20% to 30%) from GI tract
Serum half-life, elimination:
Oral: 14-35 hours
I.V.: 12-27 hours
Time to peak serum concentration: Within 2-4 hours and varies considerably
Pregnancy Risk Factor D
Comments Discoloration of urine may persist for 48 hours

Idoxuridina (Mexico) *see* Idoxuridine *on this page*

Idoxuridine (eye dox yoor' i deen)
Brand Names Herplex®
Therapeutic Category Antiviral Agent, Ophthalmic
Synonyms Idoxuridina (Mexico)
Use Treatment of herpes simplex keratitis
Usual Dosage Adults: Ophthalmic:
Ointment: Instill 5 times/day (every 4 hours) in the conjunctival sac with last dose at bedtime; continue therapy for 5-7 days after healing appears complete
Solution: Instill 1 drop in eye(s) every hour during day and every 2 hours at night, continue until definite improvement is noted, then reduce daytime dose to 1 drop every 2 hours and every 4 hours at night; continue for 5-7 days after healing appears complete
Alternative dosing schedule: Instill 1 drop every minute for 5 minutes; repeat every 4 hours day and night
Mechanism of Action Incorporated into viral DNA in place of thymidine resulting in mutations and inhibition of viral replication
Local Anesthetic/Vasoconstrictor Precautions No information available to require special precautions
Effects on Dental Treatment No effects or complications reported
Other Adverse Effects
1% to 10%:
Dermatologic: Pruritus, follicular conjunctivitis
Local: Irritation, pain, inflammation, mild edema of the eyelids and cornea
Ocular: Visual haze, corneal clouding, photophobia, small punctate defects on the corneal epithelium
<1%: Ocular: Small punctate defects on the corneal epithelium
Drug Interactions Increased toxicity: Do not coadminister with boric acid containing solutions
Drug Uptake
Absorption: Ophthalmic: Poorly absorbed following instillation; tissue uptake is a function of cellular metabolism, which is inhibited by high concentrations of the drug (absorption decreases as the concentration of drug increases)
Pregnancy Risk Factor C

IDR *see* Idarubicin *on previous page*
Ifex® Injection *see* Ifosfamide *on this page*

Ifosfamide (eye foss' fa mide)
Brand Names Ifex® Injection
Canadian/Mexican Brand Names Ifoxan® (Mexico)
Therapeutic Category Antineoplastic Agent, Alkylating Agent
Use In combination with other antineoplastics in treatment of lung cancer, Hodgkin's and non-Hodgkin's lymphoma, breast cancer, acute and chronic lymphocytic leukemia, ovarian cancer, testicular cancer, and sarcomas
Usual Dosage I.V. (**refer to individual protocols**):
Children: 1200-1800 mg/m^2/day for 3-5 days every 21-28 days **or** 5 g/m^2 as a single 24-hour infusion **or** 3 g/m^2/day for 2 days

Adults:
Doses may be given as 50 mg/kg/day **or** 700-2000 mg/m^2/day for 5 days
Alternatives include 2400 mg/m^2/day for 3 days **or** 5000 mg/m^2 as a single dose
Doses of 700-900 mg/m^2/day for 5 days may be given IVP; courses may be repeated every 3-4 weeks
(Continued)

Ifosfamide *(Continued)*

To prevent bladder toxicity, ifosfamide should be given with extensive hydration consisting of at least 2 L of oral or I.V. fluid per day. A protector, such as mesna, should also be used to prevent hemorrhagic cystitis. The dose-limiting toxicity is hemorrhagic cystitis and ifosfamide should be used in conjunction with a uroprotective agent.

Mechanism of Action Causes cross-linking of strands of DNA by binding with nucleic acids and other intracellular structures; inhibits protein synthesis and DNA synthesis; an analogue of cyclophosphamide, and like cyclophosphamide, it undergoes activation by microsomal enzymes in the liver. Ifosfamide is metabolized to active compounds, ifosfamide mustard, and acrolein

Local Anesthetic/Vasoconstrictor Precautions No information available to require special precautions

Effects on Dental Treatment No effects or complications reported

Other Adverse Effects

>10%:

Alopecia: Occurs in 50% to 83% of patients 2-4 weeks after initiation of therapy; may be as high as 100% in combination therapy

Gastrointestinal: Nausea and vomiting in 58% of patients is dose and schedule related (more common with higher doses and after bolus regimens); nausea and vomiting can persist up to 3 days after therapy; also anorexia, diarrhea, constipation, transient increase in LFTs and stomatitis noted.

Emetic potential: Moderate (58%)

Genitourinary toxicity: Hemorrhagic cystitis has been frequently associated with the use of ifosfamide. A urinalysis prior to each dose should be obtained. **Ifosfamide should never be administered without a uroprotective agent (MESNA).** Hematuria has been reported in 6% to 92% of patients. Renal toxicity occurs in 6% of patients and is manifested as an increase in BUN or serum creatinine and is most likely related to tubular damage. Metabolic acidosis may occur in up to 31% of patients.

1% to 10%: Phlebitis, stomatitis, elevated liver enzymes, polyneuropathy

Myelosuppression: Less of a problem than with cyclophosphamide if used alone. Leukopenia is mild to moderate, thrombocytopenia and anemia are rare. However, myelosuppression can be severe when used with other chemotherapeutic agents. Be cautious with patients with compromised bone marrow reserve. WBC: Moderate; Platelets: Mild; Onset (days): 7; Nadir (days): 10-14; Recovery (days): 21

Neurologic: Somnolence, confusion, hallucinations in 12% and coma (rare) have occurred and are usually reversible; usually occur with higher doses; depressive psychoses

Miscellaneous: Phlebitis, nasal stuffiness, SIADH, immunosuppression, sterility, skin hyperpigmentation, pulmonary fibrosis, cardiotoxicity, dermatitis, nail ridging, possible secondary malignancy, impaired wound healing, and allergic reactions

<1%: Cardiotoxicity, stomatitis, pulmonary toxicity

Drug Uptake Pharmacokinetics are dose-dependent

Absorption: Oral: Peak plasma levels occur within 1 hour

Serum half-life: Beta phase: 11-15 hours with high-dose ($3800\text{-}5000$ mg/m^2) or 4-7 hours with lower doses (1800 mg/m^2)

Pregnancy Risk Factor D

Comments Usually used in combination with mesna, a prophylactic agent for hemorrhagic cystitis

IL-2 *see* Aldesleukin *on page 29*

Ilopan® *see* Dexpanthenol *on page 263*

Ilopan-Choline® *see* Dexpanthenol *on page 263*

Ilosone® *see* Erythromycin *on page 321*

Ilotycin® Ophthalmic *see* Erythromycin, Topical *on page 324*

Ilozyme® *see* Pancrelipase *on page 657*

Imdur™ *see* Isosorbide Mononitrate *on page 474*

I-Methasone® *see* Dexamethasone *on page 260*

Imglucerase *(im gloo′ ser ase)*

Brand Names Cerezyme®

Therapeutic Category Enzyme, Glucocerebrosidase

Use Long-term enzyme replacement therapy for patients with Type 1 Gaucher's disease

Local Anesthetic/Vasoconstrictor Precautions No information available to require special precautions

Effects on Dental Treatment No effects or complications reported

Imidazole Carboxamide *see Dacarbazine on page 247*

Imipenem/Cilastatin (i mi pen' em/sye la stat' in)
Related Information
Animal and Human Bites Guidelines *on page 976*
Brand Names Primaxin®
Canadian/Mexican Brand Names Tienam® (Mexico)
Therapeutic Category Antibiotic, Miscellaneous
Use Treatment of documented multidrug resistant gram-negative infection due to organisms proven or suspected to be susceptible to imipenem/cilastatin; treatment of multiple organism infection in which other agents have an insufficient spectrum of activity or are contraindicated due to toxic potential; Antibacterial activity includes resistant gram-negative bacilli (*Pseudomonas aeruginosa* and *Enterococcus* sp.), gram-positive bacteria (methicillin-sensitive *Staphylococcus aureus* and *Enterococcus* sp.) and anaerobes
Usual Dosage I.M. and I.V. (dosing based on imipenem component):
Children: I.V.: 60-100 mg/kg/24 hours divided every 6 hours (maximum: 4 g/day)
Adults: I.V.: 500 mg every 6-8 hours (1 g every 6-8 hours for severe *Pseudomonas* infection); infuse each 250-500 mg dose over 20-30 minutes; infuse each 1 g dose over 40-60 minutes
Mild to moderate infection **only**: I.M.: 500-750 mg every 12 hours (**Note:** 750 mg is recommended for intra-abdominal and more severe respiratory, dermatologic, or gynecologic infections; total daily I.M. dosages >1500 mg are not recommended; deep I.M. injection should be carefully made into a large muscle mass only)
Mechanism of Action
A carbapenem with broad-spectrum antibacterial activity including resistant gram-negative bacilli (*Pseudomonas aeruginosa* and *Enterococcus* sp.), gram-positive bacteria (methicillin-sensitive *Staphylococcus aureus* and *Enterococcus* sp.) and anaerobes
Inhibits cell wall synthesis by binding to penicillin-binding proteins on the bacterial outer membrane; cilastatin prevents renal metabolism of imipenem by competitive inhibition of dehydropeptidase along the brush border of the proximal renal tubules
Local Anesthetic/Vasoconstrictor Precautions No information available to require special precautions
Effects on Dental Treatment No effects or complications reported
Other Adverse Effects
1% to 10%:
Gastrointestinal: Nausea, diarrhea, vomiting
Local: Phlebitis
<1%:
Cardiovascular: Hypotension, palpitations
Central nervous system: Seizures
Dermatologic: Rash
Gastrointestinal: Pseudomembranous colitis
Hematologic: Neutropenia, eosinophilia
Local: Pain at injection site
Miscellaneous: Emergence of resistant strains of *P. aeruginosa*
Drug Interactions Increased toxicity: Probenecid causes increased toxic potential
Drug Uptake
Imipenem:
Serum half-life: 1 hour, extended with renal insufficiency

Cilastatin:
Serum half-life: 1 hour, extended with renal insufficiency
Pregnancy Risk Factor C

Imipramine (im ip' ra meen)
Brand Names Janimine®; Tofranil®; Tofranil-PM®
Canadian/Mexican Brand Names Apo-Imipramine® (Canada); Novo-Pramine® (Canada); PMS-Imipramine® (Canada); Talpramin® (Mexico)
Therapeutic Category Antidepressant, Tricyclic
Use Treatment of various forms of depression, often in conjunction with psychotherapy; enuresis in children; analgesic for certain chronic and neuropathic pain
Usual Dosage Maximum antidepressant effect may not be seen for 2 or more weeks after initiation of therapy.
(Continued)

451

Imipramine (Continued)

Children: Oral:

Depression: 1.5 mg/kg/day with dosage increments of 1 mg/kg every 3-4 days to a maximum dose of 5 mg/kg/day in 1-4 divided doses; monitor carefully especially with doses ≥3.5 mg/kg/day

Enuresis: ≥6 years: Initial: 10-25 mg at bedtime, if inadequate response still seen after 1 week of therapy, increase by 25 mg/day; dose should not exceed 2.5 mg/kg/day or 50 mg at bedtime if 6-12 years of age or 75 mg at bedtime if ≥12 years of age

Adjunct in the treatment of cancer pain: Initial: 0.2-0.4 mg/kg at bedtime; dose may be increased by 50% every 2-3 days up to 1-3 mg/kg/dose at bedtime

Adolescents: Oral: Initial: 25-50 mg/day; increase gradually; maximum: 100 mg/day in single or divided doses

Adults:

Oral: Initial: 25 mg 3-4 times/day, increase dose gradually, total dose may be given at bedtime; maximum: 300 mg/day

I.M.: Initial: Up to 100 mg/day in divided doses; change to oral as soon as possible

Elderly: Initial: 10-25 mg at bedtime; increase by 10-25 mg every 3 days for inpatients and weekly for outpatients if tolerated; average daily dose to achieve a therapeutic concentration: 100 mg/day; range: 50-150 mg/day

Mechanism of Action Traditionally believed to increase the synaptic concentration of serotonin and/or norepinephrine in the central nervous system by inhibition of their reuptake by the presynaptic neuronal membrane. However, additional receptor effects have been found including desensitization of adenyl cyclase, down regulation of beta-adrenergic receptors, and down regulation of serotonin receptors.

Local Anesthetic/Vasoconstrictor Precautions Use with caution; epinephrine, norepinephrine and levonordefrin have been shown to have an increased pressor response in combination with TCAs

Effects on Dental Treatment Long-term treatment with TCAs such as imipramine increases the risk of caries by reducing salivation and salivary buffer capacity. In a study by Rundergren, et al, pathological alterations were observed in the oral mucosa of 72% of 58 patients; 55% had new carious lesions after taking TCAs for a median of 5½ years. Current research is investigating the use of the salivary stimulant pilocarpine to overcome the xerostomia from imipramine.

Other Adverse Effects Less sedation and anticholinergic effects than amitriptyline

>10%:

Central nervous system: Dizziness, drowsiness, headache

Gastrointestinal: Increased appetite, nausea, weakness, unpleasant taste, weight gain, dry mouth, constipation

Genitourinary: Urinary retention

1% to 10%:

Cardiovascular: Postural hypotension, arrhythmias, tachycardia, sudden death

Central nervous system: Confusion, delirium, hallucinations, nervousness, restlessness, parkinsonian syndrome, insomnia

Gastrointestinal: Diarrhea, heartburn

Genitourinary: Difficult urination, sexual dysfunction

Neuromuscular & skeletal: Fine muscle tremors

Ocular: Blurred vision, eye pain

Miscellaneous: Excessive sweating

<1%:

Central nervous system: Anxiety, seizures

Dermatologic: Alopecia, photosensitivity

Endocrine & metabolic: Breast enlargement, galactorrhea, SIADH

Genitourinary: Testicular swelling

Hematologic: Leukopenia, eosinophilia, rarely agranulocytosis

Hepatic: Increased liver enzymes, cholestatic jaundice

Ocular: Increased intraocular pressure

Otic: Tinnitus

Miscellaneous: Allergic reactions, trouble with gums, decreased lower esophageal sphincter tone may cause GE reflux, allergic reactions, has been associated with falls

Drug Interactions

Decreased effect: Phenobarbital may increase the metabolism of imipramine; imipramine blocks the uptake of guanethidine and thus prevents the hypotensive effect of guanethidine

Increased toxicity: Clonidine may increase hypertensive crisis; imipramine may be additive with or may potentiate the action of other CNS depressants such as sedatives or hypnotics; with MAO inhibitors, hyperpyrexia, hypertension, tachycardia, confusion, and seizures. Imipramine may increase the prothrombin time in patients stabilized on warfarin; imipramine potentiates the pressor and cardiac effects of sympathomimetic agents such as isoproterenol, epinephrine, etc; cimetidine and methylphenidate may decrease the metabolism of imipramine

Additive anticholinergic effects seen with other anticholinergic agents

Drug Uptake

Peak antidepressant effect: Usually after ≥2 weeks

Absorption: Oral: Well absorbed

Serum half-life: 6-18 hours

Pregnancy Risk Factor D

Selected Readings

Boakes AJ, Laurence DR, Teoh PC, et al, "Interactions Between Sympathomimetic Amines and Antidepressant Agents in Man," *Br Med J*, 1973, 1(849):311-5.

Jastak JT and Yagiela JA, "Vasoconstrictors and Local Anesthesia: A Review and Rationale for Use," *J Am Dent Assoc*, 1983, 107(4):623-30.

Larochelle P, Hamet P, and Enjalbert M, "Responses to Tyramine and Norepinephrine After Imipramine and Trazodone," *Clin Pharmacol Ther*, 1979, 26(1):24-30.

Mitchell JR, "Guanethidine and Related Agents. III Antagonism by Drugs Which Inhibit the Norepinephrine Pump in Man," *J Clin Invest*, 1970, 49(8):1596-604.

Rundegren J, van Dijken J, Mörnstad H, et al, "Oral Conditions in Patients Receiving Long-Term Treatment With Cyclic Antidepressant Drugs," *Swed Dent J*, 1985, 9(2):55-64.

Svedmyr N, "The Influence of a Tricyclic Antidepressive Agent (Protriptyline) on Some of the Circulatory Effects of Noradrenaline and Adrenaline in Man," *Life Sci*, 1968, 7(1):77-84.

Imitrex® *see* Sumatriptan Succinate *on page 814*

Immune Globulin, Intramuscular

(i myun' glob' yoo lin, in' tra mus' kyoo ler)

Related Information

Systemic Viral Diseases *on page 934*

Brand Names Gamastan®; Gammar®

Canadian/Mexican Brand Names Gammabulin Immuno (Canada); Iveegam® (Canada)

Therapeutic Category Immune Globulin

Use Household and sexual contacts of persons with hepatitis A, measles, varicella, and possibly rubella; travelers to high-risk areas outside tourist routes; staff, attendees, and patients of diapered attendees in day-care center outbreaks

For travelers, IG is not an alternative to careful selection of foods and water; immune globulin can interfere with the antibody response to parenterally administered live virus vaccines. Frequent travelers should be tested for hepatitis A antibody, immune hemolytic anemia, and neutropenia (with ITP, I.V. route is usually used).

Usual Dosage I.M.:

Hepatitis A:

Pre-exposure prophylaxis upon travel into endemic areas:

0.02 mL/kg for anticipated risk 1-3 months

0.06 mL/kg for anticipated risk >3 months

Repeat approximate dose every 4-6 months if exposure continues

Postexposure prophylaxis: 0.02 mL/kg given within 2 weeks of exposure

Measles:

Prophylaxis: 0.25 mL/kg/dose (maximum dose: 15 mL) given within 6 days of exposure followed by live attenuated measles vaccine in 3 months or at 15 months of age (whichever is later)

For patients with leukemia, lymphoma, immunodeficiency disorders, generalized malignancy, or receiving immunosuppressive therapy: 0.5 mL/kg (maximum dose: 15 mL)

Poliomyelitis: Prophylaxis: 0.3 mL/kg/dose as a single dose

Rubella: Prophylaxis: 0.55 mL/kg/dose within 72 hours of exposure

Varicella:: Prophylaxis: 0.6-1.2 mL/kg (varicella zoster immune globulin preferred) within 72 hours of exposure

IgG deficiency: 1.3 mL/kg, then 0.66 mL/kg in 3-4 weeks

Hepatitis B: Prophylaxis: 0.06 mL/kg/dose (HBIG preferred)

Mechanism of Action Provides passive immunity by increasing the antibody titer and antigen-antibody reaction potential

(Continued)

Immune Globulin, Intramuscular *(Continued)*

Local Anesthetic/Vasoconstrictor Precautions No information available to require special precautions

Effects on Dental Treatment No effects or complications reported

Other Adverse Effects

>10%: Local: Pain, tenderness, muscle stiffness at I.M. site

1% to 10%:
Cardiovascular: Flushing
Central nervous system: Chills
Gastrointestinal: Nausea

<1%:
Central nervous system: Lethargy, fever
Dermatologic: Urticaria, angioedema, erythema
Gastrointestinal: Emesis
Neuromuscular & skeletal: Myalgia
Miscellaneous: Hypersensitivity reactions

Drug Interactions Increased toxicity: Live virus, vaccines (measles, mumps, rubella); do not administer within 3 months after administration of these vaccines

Drug Uptake
Duration of immune effect: Usually 3-4 weeks
Serum half-life: 23 days
Time to peak serum concentration: I.M.: Within 24-48 hours

Pregnancy Risk Factor C

Immune Globulin, Intravenous

(i myun' glob' yoo lin, in' tra vee' nus)

Related Information

Systemic Viral Diseases *on page 934*

Brand Names Gamimune® N; Gammagard®; Gammagard® S/D; Polygam®; Polygam® S/D; Sandoglobulin®; Venoglobulin®-I; Venoglobulin®-S

Canadian/Mexican Brand Names Citax (Mexico); Intacglobin® (Mexico); Sandoglubolina® (Mexico)

Therapeutic Category Immune Globulin

Synonyms IVIG

Use Immunodeficiency syndrome, idiopathic thrombocytopenic purpura (ITP) and B-cell chronic lymphocytic leukemia (CLL); used in conjunction with appropriate anti-infective therapy to prevent or modify acute bacterial or viral infections in patients with iatrogenically-induced or disease-associated immunodepression; autoimmune neutropenia, bone marrow transplantation patients, Kawasaki disease, Guillain-Barré syndrome, demyelinating polyneuropathies

Usual Dosage Children and Adults: I.V.:

Dosages should be based on ideal body weight and not actual body weight in morbidly obese patients

Primary immunodeficiency disorders: 200-400 mg/kg every 4 weeks or as per monitored serum IgG concentrations

Chronic lymphocytic leukemia (CLL): 400 mg/kg/dose every 3 weeks

Idiopathic thrombocytopenic purpura (ITP): Maintenance dose:
400 mg/kg/day for 5 consecutive days
800 mg/kg/day for 2 consecutive days

Chronic ITP: 400-1000 mg/kg/dose every 7 or 14 days

Kawasaki disease:
400 mg/kg/day for 4 days within 10 days of onset of fever
800 mg/kg/day for 1-2 days within 10 days of onset of fever
2 g/kg for one dose only

Acquired immunodeficiency syndrome (patients must be symptomatic):
200-250 mg/kg/dose every 2 weeks
400-500 mg/kg/dose every month or every 4 weeks

Autoimmune hemolytic anemia and neutropenia: 1000 mg/kg/dose for 2-3 days

Autoimmune diseases: 400 mg/kg/day for 4 days

Post allogeneic bone marrow transplant: 500 mg/kg/week for 4 months post-transplant

Adjuvant to severe cytomegalovirus infections: 500 mg/kg/dose every other day for 7 doses

Severe systemic viral and bacterial infections:
Children: 500-1000 mg/kg/week

Prevention of gastroenteritis: Children: Oral: 50 mg/kg/day divided every 6 hours

Guillain-Barré syndrome:
  400 mg/kg/day for 4 days
  1000 mg/kg/day for 2 days
  2000 mg/kg/day for one day
Refractory dermatomyositis: 2 g/kg/dose every month x 3-4 doses
Refractory polymyositis: 1 g/kg/day x 2 days every month x 4 doses
Chronic inflammatory demyelinating polyneuropathy:
  400 mg/kg/day for 5 doses once each month
  800 mg/kg/day for 3 doses once each month
  1000 mg/kg/day for 2 days once each month

Mechanism of Action Replacement therapy for primary and secondary immunodeficiencies; interference with F_c receptors on the cells of the reticuloendothelial system for autoimmune cytopenias and ITP; possible role of contained antiviral-type antibodies

Local Anesthetic/Vasoconstrictor Precautions No information available to require special precautions

Effects on Dental Treatment No effects or complications reported

Other Adverse Effects
1% to 10%:
  Cardiovascular: Flushing of the face, tachycardia
  Central nervous system: Chills
  Gastrointestinal: Nausea
  Respiratory: Dyspnea
<1%:
  Cardiovascular: Hypotension, tightness in the chest
  Central nervous system: Dizziness, fever, headache
  Miscellaneous: Diaphoresis, hypersensitivity reactions

Drug Uptake I.V. provides immediate antibody levels
  Half-life: 21-24 days

Pregnancy Risk Factor C

Comments Gammagard®, Polygam®, or Iveegam® have low titers of IgA and may be used in patients with IgA deficiency

Imodium® see Loperamide Hydrochloride on page 511

Imodium® A-D [OTC] see Loperamide Hydrochloride on page 511

Imogam® see Rabies Immune Globulin, Human on page 761

Imovax® Rabies I.D. Vaccine see Rabies Virus Vaccine on page 761

Imovax® Rabies Vaccine see Rabies Virus Vaccine on page 761

Imuran® see Azathioprine on page 89

I-Naphline® see Naphazoline Hydrochloride on page 605

Inapsine® see Droperidol on page 303

Indapamide (in dap' a mide)

Related Information
  Cardiovascular Diseases on page 912

Brand Names Lozol®

Canadian/Mexican Brand Names Lozide® (Canada)

Therapeutic Category Diuretic, Thiazide Type

Use Management of mild to moderate hypertension; treatment of edema in congestive heart failure and nephrotic syndrome

Usual Dosage Adults: Oral: 2.5-5 mg/day. **Note:** There is little therapeutic benefit to increasing the dose >5 mg/day; there is, however, an increased risk of electrolyte disturbances.

Mechanism of Action Diuretic effect is localized at the proximal segment of the distal tubule of the nephron; it does not appear to have significant effect on glomerular filtration rate nor renal blood flow; like other diuretics, it enhances sodium, chloride, and water excretion by interfering with the transport of sodium ions across the renal tubular epithelium

Local Anesthetic/Vasoconstrictor Precautions No information available to require special precautions

Effects on Dental Treatment No effects or complications reported

Other Adverse Effects
1% to 10%: Endocrine & metabolic: Hypokalemia
<1%:
  Cardiovascular: Irregular heartbeats, weak pulse, hypotension
  Central nervous system: Mood changes
  Dermatologic: Photosensitivity
  Endocrine & metabolic: Fluid and electrolyte imbalances (hypocalcemia, hypomagnesemia, hyponatremia), hyperglycemia
  Gastrointestinal: Dry mouth
(Continued)

455

Indapamide *(Continued)*

Hematologic: Rarely blood dyscrasias
Neuromuscular & skeletal: Numbness or tingling in hands, feet or lips, muscle cramps or pain, unusual weakness
Renal: Prerenal azotemia
Respiratory: Shortness of breath
Miscellaneous: Increased thirst

Drug Interactions
Decreased effect of oral hypoglycemics; decreased absorption with cholestyramine and colestipol
Increased effect with furosemide and other loop diuretics
Increased toxicity/levels of lithium; when given with digoxin, diuretic-induced hypokalemia increases the risk of digoxin toxicity

Drug Uptake
Absorption: Completely from GI tract
Serum half-life: 14-18 hours
Time to peak serum concentration: 2-2.5 hours

Pregnancy Risk Factor D

Inderal® *see* Propranolol Hydrochloride *on page 743*

Inderal® LA *see* Propranolol Hydrochloride *on page 743*

Inderide® *see* Propranolol and Hydrochlorothiazide *on page 743*

Indinavir (in din' a veer)

Related Information
Systemic Viral Diseases *on page 934*

Brand Names Crixivan®

Therapeutic Category Antiviral Agent, Oral; Protease Inhibitor

Use Treatment of HIV infection, especially advanced disease; usually administered as part of a three-drug regimen (two nucleosides plus a protease inhibitor) or double therapy (one nucleoside plus a protease inhibitor)

Usual Dosage Adults: Oral: 800 mg every 8 hours
Dosage adjustment in hepatic impairment: 600 mg every 8 hours with mild/medium impairment due to cirrhosis or with ketoconazole coadministration

Mechanism of Action Indinavir is a protease inhibitor which prevents cleavage of protein precursors essential for HIV infection of new cells and viral replication. Some patients with advanced HIV infection have significantly improved clinically with the use of a protease inhibitor; resistant strains are cross-resistant to ritonavir and saquinavir.

Local Anesthetic/Vasoconstrictor Precautions No information available to require special precautions

Effects on Dental Treatment No effects or complications reported

Other Adverse Effects 1% to 10%:
Gastrointestinal: Mild elevation of indirect bilirubin (10%)
Renal: Kidney stones (2% to 3%)

Contraindications Hypersensitivity to the drug or its components; avoid use with terfenadine, astemizole, cisapride, or benzodiazepines

Warnings/Precautions Use caution in patients with hepatic insufficiency; dosage reduction may be needed; nephrolithiasis may occur with use; if signs and symptoms of nephrolithiasis occur, interrupt therapy for 1-3 days; ensure adequate hydration

Drug Interactions
Decreased effect: Concurrent use of rifampin and rifabutin may decrease the effectiveness of indinavir; dosage decreases of rifampin/rifabutin is recommended
Increase toxicity: Gastric pH is lowered and absorption may be decreased when didanosine and indinavir are taken <1 hour apart; a reduction of dose is often required when coadministered with ketoconazole; terfenadine, astemizole, cisapride, and benzodiazepines should be avoided with indinavir due to a potentially serious toxicity

Drug Uptake
Bioavailability: Oral: Good; T_{max}: 0.8 ± 0.3 hour
Half-life: 1.8 ± 0.4 hour

Pregnancy Risk Factor C

Dosage Forms Capsule: 400 mg

Comments One study of previously untreated patients with a mean CD4-cell count of 250 cell/mm³ found that indinavir plus zidovudine lowered serum HIV below detectable levels in 56% of 52 patients treated for 24 weeks. Other studies show similar results. Indinavir alone has suppressed serum HIV below detectable levels in 40% to 60% of patients treated up to 48 weeks.

Indochron E-R® *see* Indomethacin *on this page*
Indocin® *see* Indomethacin *on this page*
Indocin® I.V. *see* Indomethacin *on this page*
Indocin® SR *see* Indomethacin *on this page*

Indocyanine Green (in doe sye′ a neen green)
Brand Names Cardio-Green®
Therapeutic Category Diagnostic Agent, Cardiac Function
Use Determining hepatic function, cardiac output and liver blood flow and for ophthalmic angiography
Local Anesthetic/Vasoconstrictor Precautions No information available to require special precautions
Effects on Dental Treatment No effects or complications reported
Other Adverse Effects 1% to 10%:
Central nervous system: Headache
Dermatologic: Pruritus, skin discoloration
Miscellaneous: Diaphoresis, anaphylactoid reactions

Indometacina (Mexico) *see* Indomethacin *on this page*

Indomethacin (in doe meth′ a sin)
Related Information
Nonsteroidal Anti-Inflammatory Agents, Comparative Dosages, and Pharma-cokinetics *on page 1021*
Rheumatoid Arthritis, Osteoarthritis, and Joint Prostheses *on page 930*
Brand Names Indochron E-R®; Indocin®; Indocin® I.V.; Indocin® SR
Canadian/Mexican Brand Names Apo-Indomethacin® (Canada); Indocid® (Canada); Indocid-SR® (Canada); Novo-Methacin® (Canada); Nu-Indo® (Canada); Pro-Indo® (Canada); Antalgin® Dialicels (Mexico); Indocid® (Mexico); Malival® y Malival® AP (Mexico)
Therapeutic Category Analgesic, Non-narcotic; Anti-inflammatory Agent; Nonsteroidal Anti-inflammatory Agent (NSAID), Oral; Nonsteroidal Anti-Inflam-matory Agent (NSAID), Parenteral
Synonyms Indometacina (Mexico)
Use Management of inflammatory diseases and rheumatoid disorders; moderate pain; acute gouty arthritis; I.V. form used as alternative to surgery for closure of patent ductus arteriosus in neonates
Usual Dosage
Patent ductus arteriosus:
Neonates: I.V.: Initial: 0.2 mg/kg; followed with: 2 doses of 0.1 mg/kg at 12- to 24-hour intervals if age <48 hours at time of first dose; 0.2 mg/kg 2 times if 2-7 days old at time of first dose; or 0.25 mg/kg 2 times if over 7 days at time of first dose; discontinue if significant adverse effects occur. Dose should be withheld if patient has anuria or oliguria.
Analgesia:
Children: Oral: Initial: 1-2 mg/kg/day in 2-4 divided doses; maximum: 4 mg/kg/day; not to exceed 150-200 mg/day
Adults: Oral, rectal: 25-50 mg/dose 2-3 times/day; maximum dose: 200 mg/day; extended release capsule should be given on a 1-2 times/day schedule
Mechanism of Action Inhibits prostaglandin synthesis by decreasing the activity of the enzyme, cyclo-oxygenase, which results in decreased formation of prostaglandin precursors
Local Anesthetic/Vasoconstrictor Precautions No information available to require special precautions
Effects on Dental Treatment No effects or complications reported
Other Adverse Effects
>10%:
Central nervous system: Dizziness
Dermatologic: Rash
Gastrointestinal: Nausea, epigastric pain, abdominal pain, anorexia, GI bleeding, ulcers, perforation, abdominal cramps, heartburn, indigestion
1% to 10%:
Central nervous system: Headache, nervousness
Dermatologic: Itching
Gastrointestinal: Vomiting
Otic: Tinnitus
Miscellaneous: Fluid retention
<1%:
Cardiovascular: Hypertension, congestive heart failure, arrhythmias, tachy-cardia
(Continued)

457

Indomethacin *(Continued)*

Central nervous system: Somnolence, fatigue, depression, confusion, drowsiness, hallucinations

Dermatologic: Hives, erythema multiforme, toxic epidermal necrolysis, Stevens-Johnson syndrome, angioedema

Endocrine & metabolic: Hyperkalemia, dilutional hyponatremia (I.V.), oliguria, hypoglycemia (I.V.), hot flushes, polydipsia

Gastrointestinal; Gastritis, GI ulceration

Genitourinary: Renal failure, cystitis

Hematologic: Hemolytic anemia, bone marrow depression, agranulocytosis, thrombocytopenia, inhibition of platelet aggregation, anemia, leukopenia

Hepatic: Hepatitis

Neuromuscular & skeletal: Peripheral neuropathy

Ocular: Corneal opacities, blurred vision, conjunctivitis, dry eyes, toxic amblyopia

Otic: Decreased hearing

Renal: Polyuria

Respiratory: Shortness of breath, allergic rhinitis

Miscellaneous: Epistaxis, aseptic meningitis, hypersensitivity reactions

Drug Interactions

Decreased effect: May decrease antihypertensive effects of beta-blockers, hydralazine and captopril

Increased toxicity: May increase serum potassium with potassium-sparing diuretics; probenecid may increase indomethacin serum concentrations; other NSAIDs may increase GI adverse effects; may increase nephrotoxicity of cyclosporin

Indomethacin may increase serum concentrations of digoxin, methotrexate, lithium, and aminoglycosides (reported with I.V. use in neonates)

Drug Uptake

Onset of action: Within 30 minutes

Duration: 4-6 hours

Absorption: Prompt and extensive

Serum half-life: 4.5 hours

Time to peak serum concentration: Oral: Within 3-4 hours

Pregnancy Risk Factor B (D if used longer than 48 hours or after 34-week gestation)

Infectious Disease - Antimicrobial Activity Against Selected Organisms *see* *page 1034*

InFed™ Injection *see* Iron Dextran Complex *on page 468*

Inflamase® *see* Prednisolone *on page 718*

Inflamase® Mild *see* Prednisolone *on page 718*

Influenza Virus Vaccine (in floo en' za vye' rus vak' seen)

Brand Names Flu-Imune®; Fluogen®; Fluzone®

Canadian/Mexican Brand Names Fluviral® (Canada)

Therapeutic Category Vaccine, Inactivated Virus

Use Provide active immunity to influenza virus strains contained in the vaccine; for high risk persons, previous year vaccines should not be to prevent present year influenza

Those at risk for influenza injection:

Persons ≥65 years of age

Institutionalized patients

Persons of any age with chronic disorders of pulmonary and/or cardiovascular system

Persons who have required medical follow-up following hospitalization for other chronic diseases such as diabetes, renal disease, immunodepressive disorders, etc

Travelers, especially those at risk (above)

Usual Dosage Adults: I.M.: 0.5 mL each year of appropriate vaccine for the year, one dose is all that is necessary; administer in late fall to allow maximum titers to develop by peak epidemic periods usually occurring in early December

Local Anesthetic/Vasoconstrictor Precautions No information available to require special precautions

Effects on Dental Treatment No effects or complications reported

Other Adverse Effects

1% to 10%:

Central nervous system: Fever, malaise

Local: Tenderness, redness, or induration at the site of injection

<1%:
   Central nervous system: Guillain-Barré syndrome, fever
   Dermatologic: Hives, angioedema
   Neuromuscular & skeletal: Myalgia
   Respiratory: Asthma
   Miscellaneous: Anaphylactoid reactions (most likely to residual egg protein),
      allergic reactions
Drug Interactions
   Decreased effect with immunosuppressive agents; do not administer within 7
      days after administration of diphtheria and tetanus toxoids and pertussis
      vaccine adsorbed (DTP)
   Increased effect/toxicity of theophylline and warfarin
Pregnancy Risk Factor C

Infumorph™ Injection *see* Morphine Sulfate *on page 590*
INH™ *see* Isoniazid *on page 471*
Inocor® *see* Amrinone Lactate *on page 65*

Insect Sting Kit (in′ sekt sting kit)
Brand Names Ana-Kit®
Therapeutic Category Antidote, Insect Sting
Use Anaphylaxis emergency treatment of insect bites or stings by the sensitive
   patient that may occur within minutes of insect sting or exposure to an allergic
   substance
Local Anesthetic/Vasoconstrictor Precautions No information available to
   require special precautions
Effects on Dental Treatment No effects or complications reported
Comments Not intended for I.V. use (I.M. or S.C. only)

Insta-Char® [OTC] *see* Charcoal *on page 179*
Insta-Glucose® [OTC] *see* Glucose *on page 400*
Insulina (Mexico) *see* Insulin Preparations *on this page*

Insulin Preparations (in′ su lin prep a ray′ shuns)
Related Information
   Endocrine Disorders & Pregnancy *on page 927*
Brand Names Humalog®; Humulin® 50/50; Humulin® 70/30; Humulin® L;
   Humulin® N; Humulin® R; Humulin® U; Lente® Iletin I; Lente® Iletin II; Lente®
   Insulin; Lente® L; Novolin® 70/30; Novolin® L; Novolin® N; Novolin® R; NPH
   Iletin® I; NPH Insulin; NPH-N; Pork NPH Iletin® II; Pork Regular Iletin® II;
   Regular (Concentrated) Iletin® II U-500; Regular Iletin® I; Regular Insulin;
   Regular Purified Pork Insulin; Velosulin® Human
Canadian/Mexican Brand Names Insulina Lenta® (Mexico); Insulina NPH®
   (Mexico); Insulina Regular® (Mexico)
Therapeutic Category Antidiabetic Agent
Synonyms Insulina (Mexico)
Use Treatment of insulin-dependent diabetes mellitus, also noninsulin-
   dependent diabetes mellitus unresponsive to treatment with diet and/or oral
   hypoglycemics; to assure proper utilization of glucose and reduce glucosuria in
   nondiabetic patients receiving parenteral nutrition whose glucosuria cannot be
   adequately controlled with infusion rate adjustments or those who require
   assistance in achieving optimal caloric intakes; hyperkalemia (use with glucose
   to shift potassium into cells to lower serum potassium levels)
Usual Dosage Dose requires continuous medical supervision; may administer
   I.V. (regular), I.M., S.C.

Diabetes mellitus:
   Children and Adults: 0.5-1 unit/kg/day in divided doses
   Adolescents (growth spurts): 0.8-1.2 units/kg/day in divided doses
   Adjust dose to maintain premeal and bedtime blood glucose of 80-140 mg/dL
      (children <5 years: 100-200 mg/dL)

Hyperkalemia: Give calcium gluconate and $NaHCO_3$ first then 50% dextrose at
   0.5-1 mL/kg and insulin 1 unit for every 4-5 g dextrose given

Diabetic ketoacidosis: Children and Adults: I.V. loading dose: 0.1 unit/kg, then
   maintenance continuous infusion: 0.1 unit/kg/hour (range: 0.05-0.2 units/kg/
   hour depending upon the rate of decrease of serum glucose - too rapid
   decrease of serum glucose may lead to cerebral edema).
   Optimum rate of decrease (serum glucose): 80-100 mg/dL/hour
   Note: Newly diagnosed patients with IDDM presenting in DKA and patients
      with blood sugars <800 mg/dL may be relatively "sensitive" to insulin and
(Continued)

Insulin Preparations *(Continued)*

should receive loading and initial maintenance doses approximately ¹/₂ of those indicated above.

Mechanism of Action Replacement therapy for persons unable to produce the hormone naturally or in insufficient amounts to maintain glycemic control

Local Anesthetic/Vasoconstrictor Precautions No information available to require special precautions

Effects on Dental Treatment Insulin-dependent diabetics (juvenile onset, type I) should be appointed for dental treatment in the morning in order to minimize chance of stress-induced hypoglycemia

Other Adverse Effects 1% to 10%:

Cardiovascular: Perspiration, palpitation, tachycardia

Central nervous system: Fatigue, tingling of fingers, mental confusion, loss of consciousness, headache

Dermatologic: Urticaria, anaphylaxis

Endocrine & metabolic: Hypoglycemia, hypothermia

Gastrointestinal: Hunger, pallor, nausea, numbness of mouth

Local: Itching, redness, swelling, stinging, or warmth at injection site, atrophy or hypertrophy of S.C. fat tissue

Neuromuscular & skeletal: Muscle weakness, tremor

Ocular: Transient presbyopia or blurred vision

Drug Interactions See table.

Drug Interactions With Insulin Injection

Decrease Hypoglycemic Effect of Insulin	Increase Hypoglycemic Effect of Insulin
Contraceptives, oral	Alcohol
Corticosteroids	Alpha blockers
Dextrothyroxine	Anabolic steroids
Diltiazem	Beta-blockers*
Dobutamine	Clofibrate
Epinephrine	Fenfluramine
Smoking	Guanethidine
Thiazide diuretics	MAO inhibitors
Thyroid hormone	Pentamidine
Niacin	Phenylbutazone
	Salicylates
	Sulfinpyrazone
	Tetracyclines

*Nonselective beta-blockers may delay recovery from hypoglycemic episodes and mask signs/symptoms of hypoglycemia. Cardioselective agents may be alternatives.

Drug Uptake

Onset and duration of hypoglycemic effects depend upon preparation administered. See table.

Pharmacokinetics/Pharmacodynamics: Onset and Duration of Hypoglycemic Effects Depend Upon Preparation Administered

	Onset (h)	Peak (h)	Duration (h)
Insulin, regular (Novolin® R)	0.5–1	2-3	5–7
Prompt insulin zinc suspension (Semilente®)	0.5–1	4–7	18–24
Insulin zinc suspension (NPH) (Novolin® N)	1–1.5	4–12	18–24
Isophane insulin suspension (Lente®)	1–2.5	8–12	18–24
Isophane insulin suspension and regular insulin injection (Novolin® 70/30)	0.5	4–8	24
Prompt zinc insulin suspension (PZI)	4-8	14-24	36
Extended insulin zinc suspension (Ultralente®)	4-8	16–18	>36

Onset and duration: Biosynthetic NPH human insulin shows a more rapid onset and shorter duration of action than corresponding porcine insulins; human insulin and purified porcine regular insulin are similarly efficacious following S.C. administration. The duration of action of highly purified porcine insulins is shorter than that of conventional insulin equivalents. Duration depends on type of preparation and route of administration as well as patient related variables. In general, the larger the dose of insulin, the longer the duration of activity.

Absorption: Biosynthetic regular human insulin is absorbed from the S.C. injection site more rapidly than insulins of animal origin (60-90 minutes peak vs 120-150 minutes peak respectively) and lowers the initial blood glucose much faster. Human Ultralente® insulin is absorbed about twice as quickly as its bovine equivalent, and bioavailability is also improved. Human Lente® insulin preparations are also absorbed more quickly than their animal equivalents.

Pregnancy Risk Factor B

Intal® see Cromolyn Sodium on page 235
Intercept™ [OTC] see Nonoxynol 9 on page 627

Interferon Alfa-2a (in ter feer' on al' fa too aye)
Related Information
Systemic Viral Diseases on page 934
Brand Names Roferon-A®
Therapeutic Category Antineoplastic Agent, Miscellaneous; Interferon
Use FDA approved: Patients >18 years of age: Hairy cell leukemia, AIDS related Kaposi's sarcoma; multiple **unlabeled uses**; indications and dosage regimens are specific for a particular brand of interferon
Usual Dosage Refer to individual protocols
Children: Hemangiomas of infancy, pulmonary hemangiomatosis: S.C.: 1-3 million units/m²/day once daily
Adults >18 years: I.M., S.C.:
Hairy cell leukemia:
Induction: 3 million units/day for 16-24 weeks.
Maintenance: 3 million units 3 times/week (may be treated for up to 20 consecutive weeks)
AIDS-related Kaposi's sarcoma:
Induction: 36 million units/day for 10-12 weeks
Maintenance: 36 million units 3 times/week (may begin with dose escalation from 3-9-18 million units each day over 3 consecutive days followed by 36 million units/day for the remainder of the 10-12 weeks of induction)
If severe adverse reactions occur, modify dosage (50% reduction) or temporarily discontinue therapy until adverse reactions abate

Local Anesthetic/Vasoconstrictor Precautions No information available to require special precautions
Effects on Dental Treatment Significant dry mouth, metallic taste in >10% of patients
Other Adverse Effects
>10%:
Central nervous system: Dizziness, tiredness, fatigue, malaise, fever (usually within 4-6 hours), chills
Dermatologic: Skin rash
Gastrointestinal: Dry mouth, sweating, nausea, vomiting, diarrhea, dizziness, abdominal cramps, weight loss, metallic taste
Hematologic: Mildly myelosuppressive and well tolerated if used without adjunct antineoplastic agents; thrombocytosis has been reported, leukopenia (mainly neutropenia), anemia, thrombocytopenia, decreased hemoglobin, hematocrit, platelets
Neuromuscular & skeletal: Rigors, arthralgia
Miscellaneous: Flu-like syndrome
1% to 10%:
Central nervous system: Headache, delirium, somnolence neurotoxicity
Dermatologic: alopecia, dry skin
Gastrointestinal: Anorexia, stomatitis
Hepatic: Hepatotoxicity
Neuromuscular & skeletal: Peripheral neuropathy, leg cramps
Ocular: Blurred vision
Miscellaneous: Diaphoresis
<1%:
Cardiovascular: Tachycardia, arrhythmias, chest pain, hypotension, SVT, edema
(Continued)

461

Interferon Alfa-2a *(Continued)*

Central nervous system: Confusion, sensory neuropathy, fever, headache, psychiatric effects, EEG abnormalities, depression, chills
Dermatologic: Partial alopecia, rash
Gastrointestinal: Weight loss, change in taste
Hematologic: Decreased hemoglobin, hematocrit, platelets
Hepatic: Increased hepatic transaminase
Neuromuscular & skeletal: Myalgia, arthralgia, rigors
Ocular: Blurred vision, visual disturbances
Renal: Proteinuria, increased uric acid level, increased Cr, increased BUN
Respiratory: Coughing, chest pain, dyspnea, nasal congestion
Miscellaneous: Hypothyroidism, neutralizing antibodies, local sensitivity to injection; usually patient can build up a tolerance to side effects

Drug Interactions
Increased effect:
Cimetidine: May augment the antitumor effects of interferon in melanoma
Theophylline: Clearance has been reported to be decreased in hepatitis patients receiving interferon
Increased toxicity: Vinblastine: Enhances interferon toxicity in several patients; increased incidence of paresthesia has also been noted

Drug Uptake
Absorption: Filtered and absorbed at the renal tubule
Serum half-life: Elimination:
I.M., I.V.: 2 hours after administration
S.C.: 3 hours
Time to peak serum concentration: I.M., S.C.: ~6-8 hours

Pregnancy Risk Factor C

Interferon Alfa-2b (in ter feer' on al' fa too bee)

Related Information
Systemic Viral Diseases *on page 934*

Brand Names Intron® A

Therapeutic Category Antineoplastic Agent, Miscellaneous; Biological Response Modulator; Interferon

Use FDA approved: Patients >18 years of age: Hairy cell leukemia, condylomata acuminata, AIDS-related Kaposi's sarcoma, chronic hepatitis non-A, non-B(C), chronic hepatitis B; indications and dosage regimens are specific for a particular brand of interferon

Usual Dosage Adults (**refer to individual protocols**):
Hairy cell leukemia: I.M., S.C.: 2 million units/m^2 3 times/week for 2 to ≥6 months of therapy
AIDS-related Kaposi's sarcoma: I.M., S.C. (use 50 million unit vial): 30 million units/m^2 3 times/week
Condylomata acuminata: Intralesionally (use 10 million unit vial): 1 million units/lesion 3 times/week for 4-8 weeks; not to exceed 5 million units per treatment (maximum: 5 lesions at one time)
Chronic hepatitis C (non-A/non-B): I.M., S.C.: 3 million units 3 times/week for approximately a 6-month course
Chronic hepatitis B: I.M., S.C.: 5 million units/day or 10 million units 3 times/week for 16 weeks; if severe adverse reactions occur, reduce dosage 50% or temporarily discontinue therapy until adverse reactions abate; when platelet/granulocyte count returns to normal, reinstitute therapy

Mechanism of Action Alpha interferons are a family of proteins, produced by nucleated cells, that have antiviral, antiproliferative, and immune-regulating activity. There are 16 known subtypes of alpha interferons. Interferons interact with cells through high affinity cell surface receptors. Following activation, multiple effects can be detected including induction of gene transcription. Inhibits cellular growth, alters the state of cellular differentiation, interferes with oncogene expression, alters cell surface antigen expression, increases phagocytic activity of macrophages, and augments cytotoxicity of lymphocytes for target cells

Local Anesthetic/Vasoconstrictor Precautions No information available to require special precautions

Effects on Dental Treatment Significant dry mouth, metallic taste in >10% of patients

Other Adverse Effects
>10%:
Central nervous system: Dizziness, tiredness, fatigue, malaise, fever (usually within 4-6 hours). chills
Dermatologic: Skin rash

Gastrointestinal: Dry mouth, sweating, nausea, vomiting, diarrhea, dizziness, abdominal cramps, weight loss, metallic taste, anorexia

Hematologic: Mildly myelosuppressive and well tolerated if used without adjunct antineoplastic agents; thrombocytosis has been reported, leukopenia (mainly neutropenia), anemia, thrombocytopenia, decreased hemoglobin, hematocrit, platelets

Neuromuscular & skeletal: Rigors, arthralgia

Miscellaneous: Flu-like syndrome

1% to 10%:

Central nervous system: Neurotoxicity

Dermatologic: Dry skin, alopecia

Gastrointestinal: Stomatitis

Hepatic: Hepatotoxicity

Neuromuscular & skeletal: Peripheral neuropathy, leg cramps

Ocular: Blurred vision

Miscellaneous: Diaphoresis

<1%:

Cardiovascular: Cardiotoxicity, tachycardia, arrhythmias, hypotension, SVT, arrhythmias, chest pain, edema

Central nervous system: EEG abnormalities, confusion, sensory neuropathy, fever, headache, psychiatric effects, delirium, somnolence, chills

Dermatologic: Partial alopecia, rash

Gastrointestinal: Weight loss, change in taste

Hematologic: Decreased hemoglobin, hematocrit, platelets

Hepatic: Increased hepatic transaminase, increased ALT and AST

Neuromuscular & skeletal: Myalgia, rigors

Ocular: Visual disturbances, blurred vision

Renal: Proteinuria, increased uric acid level, increased Cr, increased BUN

Respiratory: Coughing, dyspnea, nasal congestion

Miscellaneous: Local sensitivity to injection, hypothyroidism, neutralizing antibodies; usually patient can build up a tolerance to side effects

Drug Interactions

Increased effect: Cimetidine: May augment the antitumor effects of interferon in melanoma

Increased toxicity:

Theophylline: Clearance has been reported to be decreased in hepatitis patients receiving interferon

Vinblastine: Enhances interferon toxicity in several patients; increased incidence of paresthesia has also been noted

Drug Uptake

Absorption: Filtered and absorbed at the renal tubule

Serum half-life: Elimination:

I.M., I.V.: 2 hours

S.C.: 3 hours

Time to peak serum concentration: I.M., S.C.: ~6-8 hours

Pregnancy Risk Factor C

Interferon Alfa-N3 (in ter feer' on al' fa en three)

Related Information

Systemic Viral Diseases *on page 934*

Brand Names Alferon® N

Therapeutic Category Antineoplastic Agent, Miscellaneous; Interferon

Use FDA approved: Patients ≥18 years of age: Condylomata acuminata, intralesional treatment of refractory or recurring genital or venereal warts; useful in patients who do not respond or are not candidates for usual treatments; indications and dosage regimens are specific for a particular brand of interferon

Usual Dosage Adults: Inject 250,000 units (0.05 mL) in each wart twice weekly for a maximum of 8 weeks; therapy should not be repeated for at least 3 months after the initial 8-week course of therapy

Mechanism of Action Interferons interact with cells through high affinity cell surface receptors. Following activation, multiple effects can be detected including induction of gene transcription. Inhibits cellular growth, alters the state of cellular differentiation, interferes with oncogene expression, alters cell surface antigen expression, increases phagocytic activity of macrophages, and augments cytotoxicity of lymphocytes for target cells

Local Anesthetic/Vasoconstrictor Precautions No information available to require special precautions

Effects on Dental Treatment Significant dry mouth, metallic taste in >10% of patients

(Continued)

Interferon Alfa-N3 *(Continued)*

Other Adverse Effects

>10%:

Central nervous system: Fatigue, malaise, fever (usually within 4-6 hours), rigors, chills, tiredness

Dermatologic: Skin rash

Gastrointestinal: Dry mouth, sweating, nausea, vomiting, diarrhea, dizziness, abdominal cramps, weight loss, metallic tastes, anorexia

Hematologic: Mildly myelosuppressive and well tolerated if used without adjunct antineoplastic agents; thrombocytosis has been reported, leukopenia (mainly neutropenia), anemia, thrombocytopenia, decreased hemoglobin, hematocrit, platelets

Neuromuscular & skeletal: Arthralgia

Miscellaneous: Flu-like syndrome

1% to 10%:

Central nervous system: Headache, delirium, somnolence, neurotoxicity

Dermatologic: Alopecia, dry skin

Gastrointestinal: Stomatitis, hepatotoxicity

Neuromuscular & skeletal: Peripheral neuropathy

Miscellaneous: Diaphoresis, leg cramps, blurred vision

<1%:

Cardiovascular: Tachycardia, arrhythmias, chest pain, hypotension, SVT, edema

Central nervous system: EEG abnormalities, confusion, sensory neuropathy, fever, headache, confusion, psychiatric effects, depression, chills

Dermatologic: Rash, partial alopecia, local sensitivity to injection

Gastrointestinal: Weight loss, change in taste

Hematologic: Decreased hemoglobin, hematocrit, platelets

Hepatic: Increased hepatic transaminase, increased ALT and AST

Neuromuscular & skeletal: Arthralgia, rigors, myalgia

Ocular: Visual disturbances, blurred vision

Renal: Proteinuria, increased uric acid level, increased Cr, increased BUN, proteinuria

Respiratory: Coughing, chest pain, dyspnea, cough, nasal congestion

Miscellaneous: Hypothyroidism, neutralizing antibodies, usually patient can build up a tolerance to side effects

Drug Interactions

Increased effect: Cimetidine: May augment the antitumor effects of interferon in melanoma

Increased toxicity:

Vinblastine: Enhances interferon toxicity in several patients; increased incidence of paresthesia has also been noted

Theophylline: Clearance has been reported to be decreased in hepatitis patients receiving interferon

Pregnancy Risk Factor C

Interferon Beta-1b (in ter feer' on bay' ta won bee)

Brand Names Betaseron®

Therapeutic Category Interferon

Use Reduces the frequency of clinical exacerbations in ambulatory patients with relapsing-remitting multiple sclerosis (MS)

Usual Dosage S.C.:

Children <18 years: Not recommended

Adults >18 years: 0.25 mg (8 million units) every other day

Mechanism of Action Interferon beta-1b differs from naturally occurring human protein by a single amino acid substitution and the lack of carbohydrate side chains; alters the expression and response to surface antigens and can enhance immune cell activities. Properties of interferon beta-1b that modify biologic responses are mediated by cell surface receptor interactions; mechanism in the treatment of MS is unknown.

Local Anesthetic/Vasoconstrictor Precautions No information available to require special precautions

Effects on Dental Treatment No effects or complications reported

Other Adverse Effects Due to the pivotal position of interferon in the immune system, toxicities can affect nearly every organ system. Injection site reactions, injection site necrosis, flu-like symptoms, menstrual disorders, depression (with suicidal ideations), somnolence, palpitations, peripheral vascular disorders, hypertension, blood dyscrasias, dyspnea, laryngitis, cystitis, gastrointestinal complaints

Drug Interactions No data reported

Pregnancy Risk Factor C

Interferon Gamma-1B (in ter feer' on gam' ah won bee)
Brand Names Actimmune®
Therapeutic Category Biological Response Modulator; Interferon
Use Reduce the frequency and severity of serious infections associated with chronic granulomatous disease
Local Anesthetic/Vasoconstrictor Precautions No information available to require special precautions
Effects on Dental Treatment No effects or complications reported
Other Adverse Effects
>10%:
Central nervous system: Fever, headache, chills, fatigue
Dermatologic: Rash
Gastrointestinal: Diarrhea, vomiting, nausea
1% to 10%:
Central nervous system: Myalgia depression
Gastrointestinal: Abdominal pain, weight loss, anorexia
Neuromuscular & skeletal: Arthralgia, back pain
Comments More heat- and acid-labile than alfa interferons

Interleukin-2 see Aldesleukin on page 29
Intralipid® see Fat Emulsion on page 353
Intravenous Fat Emulsion see Fat Emulsion on page 353
Intron® A see Interferon Alfa-2b on page 462
Inversine® see Mecamylamine Hydrochloride on page 530
Invirase® see Saquinavir Mesylate on page 780
Iodex® Regular see Povidone-Iodine on page 713

Iodinated Glycerol (eye' oh di nay ted gli' ser ole)
Brand Names Iophen®; Organidin®; Par Glycerol®; R-Gen®
Therapeutic Category Expectorant
Use Mucolytic expectorant in adjunctive treatment of bronchitis, bronchial asthma, pulmonary emphysema, cystic fibrosis, or chronic sinusitis
Mechanism of Action Increases respiratory tract secretions by decreasing surface tension and thereby decreases the viscosity of mucus, which aids in removal of the mucus
Local Anesthetic/Vasoconstrictor Precautions No information available to require special precautions
Effects on Dental Treatment No effects or complications reported
Other Adverse Effects
1% to 10%: Gastrointestinal: Diarrhea, nausea, vomiting
<1%:
Central nervous system: Headache
Dermatologic: Acne, dermatitis
Endocrine & metabolic: Acute parotitis
Gastrointestinal: GI irritation
Respiratory: Pulmonary edema
Miscellaneous: Thyroid gland enlargement, swelling of the eyelids, hypersensitivity
Drug Interactions Increased toxicity: Disulfiram, metronidazole, procarbazine, MAO inhibitors, CNS depressants, lithium
Pregnancy Risk Factor X

Iodine (eye' oh din)
Therapeutic Category Topical Skin Product
Use Used topically as an antiseptic in the management of minor, superficial skin wounds and has been used to disinfect the skin preoperatively
Local Anesthetic/Vasoconstrictor Precautions No information available to require special precautions
Effects on Dental Treatment No effects or complications reported
Other Adverse Effects 1% to 10%:
Central nervous system: Fever, headache
Dermatologic: Skin rash, angioedema, mucosal hemorrhage, urticaria, acne
Gastrointestinal: Metallic taste, diarrhea
Endocrine & metabolic: Hypothyroidism
Hematologic: Eosinophilia
Neuromuscular & skeletal: Arthralgia
Respiratory: Pulmonary edema
Miscellaneous: Lymph node enlargement, swelling of eyelids
(Continued)

Iodine (Continued)

Comments Sodium thiosulfate inactivates iodine and is an effective chemical antidote for codeine poisoning; solutions of sodium thiosulfate may be used to remove iodine stains from skin and clothing

Iodine *see* Trace Metals *on page 857*

Iodochlorhydroxyquin (eye oh doe klor' hye drox ee kwin)

Brand Names Vioform® [OTC]

Canadian/Mexican Brand Names Clioquinol® (Canada)

Therapeutic Category Antifungal Agent, Topical

Use Used topically in the treatment of tinea pedis, tinea cruris, and skin infections caused by dermatophytic fungi (ring worm)

Usual Dosage Children and Adults: Topical: Apply 2-3 times/day; do not use for longer than 7 days

Mechanism of Action Chelates bacterial surface and trace metals needed for bacterial growth

Local Anesthetic/Vasoconstrictor Precautions No information available to require special precautions

Effects on Dental Treatment No effects or complications reported

Other Adverse Effects 1% to 10%:

Dermatologic: Skin irritation, rash

Neuromuscular & skeletal: Peripheral neuropathy

Ocular: Optic atrophy

Drug Interactions No data reported

Drug Uptake

Absorption: With an occlusive dressing, up to 40% of dose can be absorbed systemically during a 12-hour period; absorption is enhanced when applied under diapers

Serum half-life: 11-14 hours

Pregnancy Risk Factor C

Iodochlorhydroxyquin and Hydrocortisone *see* Clioquinol and Hydrocortisone *on page 216*

Iodopen® *see* Trace Metals *on page 857*

Iodoquinol (eye oh doe kwin' ole)

Brand Names Sebaquin® [OTC]; Yodoxin®

Canadian/Mexican Brand Names Diodoquin® (Canada)

Therapeutic Category Amebicide

Use Treatment of acute and chronic intestinal amebiasis; asymptomatic cyst passers; *Blastocystis hominis* infections; ineffective for amebic hepatitis or hepatic abscess

Usual Dosage Oral:

Children: 30-40 mg/kg/day (maximum: 650 mg/dose) in 3 divided doses for 20 days; not to exceed 1.95 g/day

Adults: 650 mg 3 times/day after meals for 20 days; not to exceed 2 g/day

Mechanism of Action Contact amebicide that works in the lumen of the intestine by an unknown mechanism

Local Anesthetic/Vasoconstrictor Precautions No information available to require special precautions

Effects on Dental Treatment No effects or complications reported

Other Adverse Effects

>10%: Gastrointestinal: Diarrhea, nausea, vomiting, stomach pain

1% to 10%:

Central nervous system: Fever, chills, agitation, retrograde amnesia, headache

Dermatologic: Skin rash, hives

Endocrine & metabolic: Thyroid gland enlargement

Neuromuscular & skeletal: Peripheral neuropathy, weakness

Ocular: Optic neuritis, optic atrophy, visual impairment

Miscellaneous: Itching of rectal area

Drug Interactions No data reported

Drug Uptake

Absorption: Oral: Poor and irregular

Pregnancy Risk Factor C

Iodoquinol and Hydrocortisone
(eye oh doe kwin' ole & hye droe kor' ti sone)

Brand Names Vytone® Topical

Therapeutic Category Antifungal Agent, Topical; Corticosteroid, Topical (Low Potency)

Use Treatment of eczema; infectious dermatitis; chronic eczematoid otitis externa; mycotic dermatoses

Local Anesthetic/Vasoconstrictor Precautions No information available to require special precautions

Effects on Dental Treatment No effects or complications reported

Ionamin® *see* Phentermine Hydrochloride *on page 683*

Ionil® [OTC] *see* Salicylic Acid *on page 777*

Iophen® *see* Iodinated Glycerol *on page 465*

Iophen DM® [OTC] *see* Guaifenesin and Dextromethorphan *on page 408*

Iopidine® *see* Apraclonidine Hydrochloride *on page 72*

Iosat® *see* Potassium Iodide *on page 711*

I-Paracaine® *see* Proparacaine Hydrochloride *on page 737*

I-Parescein® *see* Proparacaine and Fluorescein *on page 736*

Ipecac Syrup (ip' e kak sir' up)

Therapeutic Category Antidote, Emetic

Use Treatment of acute oral drug overdosage and certain poisonings

Usual Dosage Oral:

Children:

6-12 months: 5-10 mL followed by 10-20 mL/kg of water; repeat dose one time if vomiting does not occur within 20 minutes

1-12 years: 15 mL followed by 10-20 mL/kg of water; repeat dose one time if vomiting does not occur within 20 minutes

If emesis does not occur within 30 minutes after second dose, ipecac must be removed from stomach by gastric lavage

Adults: 15-30 mL followed by 200-300 mL of water; repeat dose one time if vomiting does not occur within 20 minutes

Mechanism of Action Irritates the gastric mucosa and stimulates the medullary chemoreceptor trigger zone to induce vomiting

Local Anesthetic/Vasoconstrictor Precautions No information available to require special precautions

Effects on Dental Treatment No effects or complications reported

Other Adverse Effects 1% to 10%:

Cardiovascular: Cardiotoxicity

Central nervous system: Lethargy

Gastrointestinal: Protracted vomiting, diarrhea

Ocular: Myopathy

Drug Uptake

Onset of action: Within 15-30 minutes

Duration: 20-25 minutes; can last longer, 60 minutes in some cases

Absorption: Significant amounts, mainly when it does not produce emesis

Pregnancy Risk Factor C

I-Pentolate® *see* Cyclopentolate Hydrochloride *on page 240*

I-Phrine® Ophthalmic Solution *see* Phenylephrine Hydrochloride *on page 685*

I-Picamide® Ophthalmic *see* Tropicamide *on page 881*

IPOL™ *see* Poliovirus Vaccine, Inactivated *on page 702*

Ipratropium Bromide (i pra troe' pee um broe' mide)

Related Information

Respiratory Diseases *on page 924*

Brand Names Atrovent®

Therapeutic Category Anticholinergic Agent; Bronchodilator

Use Anticholinergic bronchodilator in bronchospasm associated with COPD, bronchitis, and emphysema

Usual Dosage

Children:

<2 years: Nebulization: 250 mcg 3 times/day

3-14 years: Metered dose inhaler: 1-2 inhalations 3 times/day, up to 6 inhalations/24 hours

Children >12 years and Adults: Nebulization: 500 mcg (1 unit-dose vial) administered 3-4 times/day by oral nebulization, with doses 6-8 hours apart

Children >14 years and Adults: Metered dose inhaler: 2 inhalations 4 times/day every 4-6 hours up to 12 inhalations in 24 hours

(Continued)

Ipratropium Bromide *(Continued)*

Mechanism of Action Blocks the action of acetylcholine at parasympathetic sites in bronchial smooth muscle causing bronchodilation

Local Anesthetic/Vasoconstrictor Precautions No information available to require special precautions

Effects on Dental Treatment Dry mouth in >10% of patients

Other Adverse Effects Note: Ipratropium is poorly absorbed from the lung, so systemic effects are rare

>10%:
  Central nervous system: Nervousness, dizziness, fatigue, headache
  Gastrointestinal: Nausea, dry mouth, stomach upset
  Respiratory: Cough

1% to 10%:
  Cardiovascular: Palpitations, hypotension
  Central nervous system: Insomnia
  Genitourinary: Urinary retention
  Neuromuscular & skeletal: Trembling
  Ocular: Blurred vision
  Respiratory: Nasal congestion

<1%:
  Dermatologic: Skin rash, hives
  Gastrointestinal: Stomatitis

Drug Interactions
Increased effect with albuterol
Increased toxicity with anticholinergics or drugs with anticholinergic properties, dronabinol

Drug Uptake
Onset of bronchodilation: 1-3 minutes after administration
Duration: Up to 4-6 hours
Absorption: Not readily absorbed into the systemic circulation from the surface of the lung or from the GI tract

Pregnancy Risk Factor B

IPV *see* Poliovirus Vaccine, Inactivated *on page 702*

Ircon® [OTC] *see* Ferrous Fumarate *on page 359*

Irinotecan *(eye rye no tee' kan)*

Brand Names Camptosar®

Therapeutic Category Antineoplastic Agent, Miscellaneous

Use For the treatment of patients with metastatic carcinoma of the colon or rectum whose disease has progressed following 5-FU based therapy

Usual Dosage Adults: I.V.: Starting dose is 125 mg/m² administered over 90 min, once a week for 4 weeks; repeated every 6 weeks (4 weeks on, 2 weeks off); dose is adjusted depending on individual tolerance to as high as 150 mg/m² or as low as 50 mg/m²

Local Anesthetic/Vasoconstrictor Precautions No information available to require special precautions

Effects on Dental Treatment No effects or complications reported

Pregnancy Risk Factor D

Generic Available No

Iron Dextran Complex *(eye' ern deks' tran kom' pleks)*

Brand Names InFed™ Injection

Canadian/Mexican Brand Names Driken® (Mexico)

Therapeutic Category Iron Salt

Use Treatment of microcytic, hypochromic anemia resulting from iron deficiency when oral iron administration is infeasible or ineffective

Usual Dosage I.M. (Z-track method should be used for I.M. injection), I.V.:
A 0.5 mL test dose (0.25 mL in infants) should be given prior to starting iron dextran therapy; total dose should be divided into a daily schedule for I.M., total dose may be given as a single continuous infusion

Iron deficiency anemia: Dose (mL) = 0.0476 x wt (kg) x (normal hemoglobin - observed hemoglobin) + (1 mL/5 kg) to maximum of 14 mL for iron stores

Iron replacement therapy for blood loss: Replacement iron (mg) = blood loss (mL) x hematocrit

Maximum daily dose (can give total dose at one time I.V.):
  Children:
    5-10 kg: 50 mg iron (1 mL)
    10-50 kg: 100 mg iron (2 mL)

Adults >50 kg: 100 mg iron (2 mL)

Mechanism of Action The released iron, from the plasma, eventually replenishes the depleted iron stores in the bone marrow where it is incorporated into hemoglobin

Local Anesthetic/Vasoconstrictor Precautions No information available to require special precautions

Effects on Dental Treatment No effects or complications reported

Other Adverse Effects
>10%:
Central nervous system: Chills, fever, sweating, headache
Dermatologic: Staining of skin at the site of I.M. injection
Gastrointestinal: Metallic taste, nausea, vomiting
Local: Pain at injection site
1% to 10%:
Gastrointestinal: Diarrhea
Genitourinary: Discolored urine
<1%:
Cardiovascular: Flushing
Local: Phlebitis
Neuromuscular & skeletal: Arthralgia
Respiratory: Respiratory difficulty
Miscellaneous: Lymphadenopathy

Drug Uptake
Absorption:
I.M.: 50% to 90% is promptly absorbed, the balance is slowly absorbed over month
I.V.: Uptake of iron by the reticuloendothelial system appears to be constant at about 10-20 mg/hour

Pregnancy Risk Factor C

Comments 2 mL of undiluted iron dextran is the maximum recommended daily dose; epinephrine should be immediately available in the event of acute hypersensitivity reaction

Ismelin® *see* Guanethidine Sulfate *on page 412*

Ismo™ *see* Isosorbide Mononitrate *on page 474*

Ismotic® *see* Isosorbide *on page 473*

Iso-Bid® *see* Isosorbide Dinitrate *on page 474*

Isocaine® HCl 2% *see* Mepivacaine With Levonordefrin *on page 542*

Isocaine® HCl 3% *see* Mepivacaine Dental Anesthetic *on page 541*

Isocarboxazid (eye soe kar box' a zid)

Brand Names Marplan®

Therapeutic Category Antidepressant, Monoamine Oxidase Inhibitor

Use Symptomatic treatment of atypical, nonendogenous or neurotic depression

Usual Dosage Adults: Oral: 10 mg 3 times/day; reduce to 10-20 mg/day in divided doses when condition improves

Mechanism of Action Thought to act by increasing endogenous concentrations of epinephrine, norepinephrine, dopamine, and serotonin through inhibition of the enzyme (monoamine oxidase) responsible for the breakdown of these neurotransmitters

Local Anesthetic/Vasoconstrictor Precautions Attempts should be made to avoid use of vasoconstrictor due to possibility of hypertensive episodes with monoamine oxidase inhibitors

Effects on Dental Treatment Orthostatic hypotension in >10% of patients; meperidine should be avoided as an analgesic due to toxic reactions with MAO inhibitors

Other Adverse Effects
>10%:
Cardiovascular: Orthostatic hypotension
Central nervous system: Drowsiness, weakness
Endocrine & metabolic: Decreased sexual ability
Neuromuscular & skeletal: Trembling
Ocular: Blurred vision
1% to 10%:
Cardiovascular: Tachycardia, peripheral edema
Central nervous system: Nervousness, chills
Gastrointestinal: Diarrhea, anorexia, dry mouth, constipation
<1%:
Central nervous system: Parkinsonian syndrome
Hematologic: Leukopenia
Hepatic: Hepatitis
(Continued)

Isocarboxazid *(Continued)*

Drug Interactions
Decreased effect of antihypertensives
Increased toxicity with disulfiram (possible seizures), fluoxetine (and other serotonin active agents), TCAs (cardiovascular instability), meperidine (cardiovascular instability), phenothiazines (hyperpyretic crisis), levodopa, sympathomimetics (hypertensive crisis), barbiturates, rauwolfia alkaloids (eg, reserpine), dextroamphetamine (psychoses), foods containing tyramine

Pregnancy Risk Factor C

Isoclor® Expectorant *see* Guaifenesin, Pseudoephedrine, and Codeine *on page 410*

Isodine® [OTC] *see* Povidone-Iodine *on page 713*

Isoetharine *(eye soe eth' a reen)*

Related Information
Respiratory Diseases *on page 924*

Brand Names Arm-a-Med® Isoetharine; Beta-2®; Bronkometer®; Bronkosol®; Dey-Lute® Isoetharine

Therapeutic Category Adrenergic Agonist Agent; Antiasthmatic; Bronchodilator

Use Bronchodilator in bronchial asthma and for reversible bronchospasm occurring with bronchitis and emphysema

Usual Dosage Treatments are usually not repeated more often than every 4 hours, except in severe cases

Nebulizer: Children: 0.01 mL/kg; minimum dose 0.1 mL; maximum dose: 0.5 mL diluted in 2-3 mL normal saline
Inhalation: Oral: Adults: 1-2 inhalations every 4 hours as needed

Mechanism of Action Relaxes bronchial smooth muscle by action on beta$_2$-receptors with very little effect on heart rate

Local Anesthetic/Vasoconstrictor Precautions Isoetharine is selective for beta-adrenergic receptors and not alpha receptors; therefore, there is no precaution in the use of vasoconstrictor

Effects on Dental Treatment Dry mouth in 1% to 10% of patients

Other Adverse Effects
1% to 10%:
Cardiovascular: Tachycardia, hypertension, pounding heartbeat
Central nervous system: Dizziness, lightheadedness, headache, nervousness, insomnia, weakness
Gastrointestinal: Dry mouth, nausea, vomiting
Neuromuscular & skeletal: Trembling
<1%: Respiratory: Paradoxical bronchospasm

Drug Interactions
Decreased effect with beta-blockers
Increased toxicity with other sympathomimetics (eg, epinephrine)

Drug Uptake Duration: 1-4 hours

Pregnancy Risk Factor C

Isoflurophate *(eye soe flure' oh fate)*

Brand Names Floropryl®

Therapeutic Category Antiglaucoma Agent; Cholinergic Agent, Ophthalmic; Ophthalmic Agent, Miotic

Use Treat primary open-angle glaucoma and conditions that obstruct aqueous outflow and to treat accommodative convergent strabismus

Usual Dosage Adults: Ophthalmic:
Glaucoma: Instill 0.25" strip in eye every 8-72 hours
Strabismus: Instill 0.25" strip to each eye every night for 2 weeks then reduce to 0.25" every other night to once weekly for 2 months

Mechanism of Action Cholinesterase inhibitor that causes contraction of the iris and ciliary muscles producing miosis, reduced intraocular pressure, and increased aqueous humor outflow

Local Anesthetic/Vasoconstrictor Precautions No information available to require special precautions

Effects on Dental Treatment No effects or complications reported

Other Adverse Effects
1% to 10%: Ocular: Stinging, burning, myopia, visual blurring
<1%:
Cardiovascular: Bradycardia, hypotension, flushing
Gastrointestinal: Nausea, vomiting, diarrhea
Neuromuscular & skeletal: Muscle weakness

Ocular: Retinal detachment, browache, miosis, twitching eyelids, watering eyes
Respiratory: Difficulty in breathing
Miscellaneous: Diaphoresis

Drug Interactions Increased toxicity: Succinylcholine, systemic anticholinesterases, carbamate or organic phosphate insecticides, cause decrease in cholinesterase levels

Drug Uptake
Peak IOP reduction: 24 hours
Duration: 1 week
Onset of miosis: Within 5-10 minutes
Duration: Up to 4 weeks

Pregnancy Risk Factor X

Isollyl Improved® *see* Butalbital Compound *on page 133*

Isomeprobamate (Canada) *see* Carisoprodol *on page 157*

Isonate® *see* Isosorbide Dinitrate *on page 474*

Isoniazid (eye soe nye' a zid)
Related Information
Nonviral Infectious Diseases *on page 932*
Brand Names INH™; Laniazid®; Nydrazid®
Canadian/Mexican Brand Names PMS-Isoniazid® (Canada)
Therapeutic Category Antitubercular Agent
Use Treatment of susceptible tuberculosis infections and prophylactically to those individuals exposed to tuberculosis
Usual Dosage Oral, I.M. (recommendations often change due to resistant strains and newly developed information; consult *MMWR* for current CDC recommendations):

Children: 10-20 mg/kg/day in 1-2 divided doses (maximum: 300 mg total dose)
Prophylaxis: 10 mg/kg/day given daily (up to 300 mg total dose) for 6 months

Adults: 5 mg/kg/day given daily (usual dose is 300 mg)
Disseminated disease: 10 mg/kg/day in 1-2 divided doses
Treatment should be continued for 9 months with rifampin or for 6 months with rifampin and pyrazinamide
Prophylaxis: 300 mg/day given daily for 6 months

American Thoracic Society and CDC currently recommend twice weekly therapy as part of a short-course regimen which follows 1-2 months of daily treatment for uncomplicated pulmonary tuberculosis in compliant patients
Children: 20-40 mg/kg/dose (up to 900 mg) twice weekly
Adults: 15 mg/kg/dose (up to 900 mg) twice weekly

Mechanism of Action Unknown, but may include the inhibition of myocolic acid synthesis resulting in disruption of the bacterial cell wall
Local Anesthetic/Vasoconstrictor Precautions No information available to require special precautions
Effects on Dental Treatment No effects or complications reported
Other Adverse Effects
>10%:
Central nervous system: Peripheral neuritis
Gastrointestinal: Loss of appetite, nausea, vomiting, stomach pain
Hepatic: Hepatitis
Neuromuscular & skeletal: Weakness
1% to 10%:
Central nervous system: Dizziness, slurred speech, lethargy
Neuromuscular & skeletal: Hyperreflexia
<1%:
Central nervous system: Fever, seizures, mental depression, psychosis
Dermatologic: Skin rash
Hematologic: Blood dyscrasias
Neuromuscular & skeletal: Arthralgia
Ocular: Blurred vision, loss of vision
Drug Interactions
Decreased effect/levels of isoniazid with aluminum salts
Increased toxicity/levels of oral anticoagulants, carbamazepines, cycloserine, hydantoins, hepatically metabolized benzodiazepines; reaction with disulfiram
Drug Uptake
Absorption: Oral, I.M.: Rapid and complete; rate can be slowed when orally administered with food
(Continued)

Isoniazid *(Continued)*

Serum half-life:
  Fast acetylators: 30-100 minutes
  Slow acetylators: 2-5 hours; half-life may be prolonged in patients with impaired hepatic function or severe renal impairment
Time to peak serum concentration: Within 1-2 hours
Pregnancy Risk Factor C

Isonipecaine (Canada) *see* Meperidine Hydrochloride *on page 539*

Isopro® *see* Isoproterenol *on this page*

Isoproterenol *(eye soe proe ter' e nole)*

Related Information
Cardiovascular Diseases *on page 912*

Brand Names Arm-a-Med® Isoproterenol; Dey-Dose® Isoproterenol; Dispos-a-Med® Isoproterenol; Isopro®; Isuprel®; Medihaler-Iso®; Norisodrine®; Vapo-Iso®

Therapeutic Category Adrenergic Agonist Agent; Bronchodilator

Use Treatment of reversible airway obstruction as in asthma or COPD; used parenterally in ventricular arrhythmias due to A-V nodal block; hemodynamically compromised bradyarrhythmias or atropine-resistant bradyarrhythmias; temporary use in third degree A-V block until pacemaker insertion; low cardiac output; vasoconstrictive shock states

Usual Dosage
Children:
  Bronchodilation: Inhalation: Metered dose inhaler: 1-2 metered doses up to 5 times/day
  Bronchodilation (using 1:200 inhalation solution) 0.01 mL/kg/dose every 4 hours as needed (maximum: 0.05 mL/dose) diluted with NS to 2 mL
  Sublingual: 5-10 mg every 3-4 hours, not to exceed 30 mg/day
  Cardiac arrhythmias: I.V.: Start 0.1 mcg/kg/minute (usual effective dose 0.2-2 mcg/kg/minute)

Adults:
  Bronchodilation: Inhalation: Metered dose inhaler: 1-2 metered doses 4-6 times/day
  Bronchodilation: 1-2 inhalations of a 0.25% solution, no more than 2 inhalations at any one time (1-5 minutes between inhalations); no more than 6 inhalations in any hour during a 24-hour period; maintenance therapy: 1-2 inhalations 4-6 times/day. Alternatively: 0.5% solution via hand bulb nebulizer is 5-15 deep inhalations repeated once in 5-10 minutes if necessary; treatments may be repeated up to 5 times/day.
  Sublingual: 10-20 mg every 3-4 hours; not to exceed 60 mg/day
  Cardiac arrhythmias: I.V.: 5 mcg/minute initially, titrate to patient response (2-20 mcg/minute)
  Shock: I.V.: 0.5-5 mcg/minute; adjust according to response

Mechanism of Action Stimulates beta$_1$- and beta$_2$-receptors resulting in relaxation of bronchial, GI, and uterine smooth muscle, increased heart rate and contractility, vasodilation of peripheral vasculature

Local Anesthetic/Vasoconstrictor Precautions Isoproterenol is selective for beta-adrenergic receptors and not alpha receptors; therefore, there is no precaution in the use of vasoconstrictor such as epinephrine

Effects on Dental Treatment Significant dry mouth in >10% of patients

Other Adverse Effects
>10%:
  Central nervous system: Insomnia, restlessness
  Gastrointestinal: Dry mouth or throat
  Miscellaneous: Discoloration of saliva (pinkish-red)
1% to 10%:
  Cardiovascular: Sweating, flushing of the face or skin, ventricular arrhythmias, tachycardias, profound hypotension, hypertension
  Central nervous system: Nervousness, anxiety, dizziness, headache, weakness, lightheadedness
  Gastrointestinal: Vomiting, nausea
  Neuromuscular & skeletal: Trembling, tremor
<1%:
  Cardiovascular: Arrhythmias, chest pain
  Respiratory: Paradoxical bronchospasm

Drug Interactions Increased toxicity: Sympathomimetic agents lead to headaches; general anesthetics lead to arrhythmias

Drug Uptake
  Onset of bronchodilation: Oral inhalation: Immediately
  Time to peak serum concentration: Oral: Within 1-2 hours
  Duration:
    Oral inhalation: 1 hour
    S.C.: Up to 2 hours
  Serum half-life: 2.5-5 minutes
Pregnancy Risk Factor C

Isoproterenol and Phenylephrine
(eye soe proe ter' e nole & fen il ef' rin)
Brand Names Duo-Medihaler® Aerosol
Therapeutic Category Adrenergic Agonist Agent
Use Treatment of bronchospasm associated with acute and chronic bronchial asthma, bronchitis, pulmonary emphysema, and bronchiectasis
Local Anesthetic/Vasoconstrictor Precautions No information available to require special precautions
Effects on Dental Treatment No effects or complications reported

Isoptin® see Verapamil Hydrochloride on page 893

Isoptin® SR see Verapamil Hydrochloride on page 893

Isopto® Carbachol see Carbachol on page 150

Isopto® Carpine® see Pilocarpine on page 691

Isopto® Eserine® see Physostigmine on page 690

Isopto® Frin Ophthalmic Solution see Phenylephrine Hydrochloride on page 685

Isopto® Homatropine Ophthalmic see Homatropine Hydrobromide on page 426

Isopto® Hyoscine see Scopolamine on page 781

Isopto® Plain Solution [OTC] see Artificial Tears on page 75

Isopto® Tears Solution [OTC] see Artificial Tears on page 75

Isordil® see Isosorbide Dinitrate on next page

Isosorbide (eye soe sor' bide)
Brand Names Ismotic®
Therapeutic Category Antiglaucoma Agent; Diuretic, Osmotic; Ophthalmic Agent, Osmotic
Use Short-term emergency treatment of acute angle-closure glaucoma and short-term reduction of intraocular pressure prior to and following intraocular surgery; may be used to interrupt an acute glaucoma attack; preferred agent when need to avoid nausea and vomiting
Usual Dosage Adults: Oral: Initial: 1.5 g/kg with a usual range of 1-3 g/kg 2-4 times/day as needed
Mechanism of Action Elevates osmolarity of glomerular filtrate to hinder the tubular resorption of water and increase excretion of sodium and chloride to result in diuresis; creates an osmotic gradient between plasma and ocular fluids
Local Anesthetic/Vasoconstrictor Precautions No information available to require special precautions
Effects on Dental Treatment No effects or complications reported
Other Adverse Effects
  1% to 10%:
    Central nervous system: Headache, confusion, disorientation
    Gastrointestinal: Vomiting
  <1%:
    Cardiovascular: Syncope
    Central nervous system: Lethargy, vertigo, dizziness, lightheadedness, irritability
    Dermatologic: Rash
    Endocrine & metabolic: Hypernatremia, hyperosmolarity, thirst
    Gastrointestinal: Nausea, abdominal/gastric discomfort (infrequently), anorexia
    Miscellaneous: Hiccups
Drug Interactions No data reported
Drug Uptake
  Onset of action: Within 10-30 minutes
  Peak action: 1-1.5 hours
  Duration: 5-6 hours
  Serum half-life: 5-9.5 hours
Pregnancy Risk Factor B

Isosorbide Dinitrate (eye soe sor' bide dye nye' trate)

Related Information
  Cardiovascular Diseases *on page 912*
Brand Names Dilatate®-SR; Iso-Bid®; Isonate®; Isordil®; Isotrate®; Sorbitrate®
Canadian/Mexican Brand Names Apo-ISDN® (Canada); Cedocard-SR® (Canada); Coradur® (Canada); Isoket® (Mexico); Isorbid® (Mexico)
Therapeutic Category Antianginal Agent; Nitrate; Vasodilator, Coronary
Use Prevention and treatment of angina pectoris; for congestive heart failure; to relieve pain, dysphagia, and spasm in esophageal spasm with GE reflux
Usual Dosage Adults (elderly should be given lowest recommended daily doses initially and titrate upward):
  Oral: Angina: 5-40 mg 4 times/day or 40 mg every 8-12 hours in sustained released dosage form
  Oral: Congestive heart failure:
    Initial dose: 10 mg 3 times/day
    Target dose: 40 mg 3 times/day
    Maximum dose: 80 mg 3 times/day
  Sublingual: 2.5-10 mg every 4-6 hours
  Chew: 5-10 mg every 2-3 hours
  Tolerance to nitrate effects develops with chronic exposure
  Dose escalation does not overcome this effect. Tolerance can only be overcome by short periods of nitrate absence from the body. Short periods (10-12 hours) or nitrate withdrawal help minimize tolerance.

  Hemodialysis: During hemodialysis, administer dose postdialysis or administer supplemental 10-20 mg dose; during peritoneal dialysis, supplemental dose is not necessary
Mechanism of Action Stimulation of intracellular cyclic-GMP results in vascular smooth muscle relaxation of both arterial and venous vasculature. Increased venous pooling decreases left ventricular pressure (preload) and arterial dilatation decreases arterial resistance (afterload). Therefore, this reduces cardiac oxygen demand by decreasing left ventricular pressure and systemic vascular resistance by dilating arteries. Additionally, coronary artery dilation improves collateral flow to ischemic regions; esophageal smooth muscle is relaxed via the same mechanism.
Local Anesthetic/Vasoconstrictor Precautions No information available to require special precautions
Effects on Dental Treatment No effects or complications reported
Other Adverse Effects
  >10%:
    Cardiovascular: Flushing, postural hypotension
    Central nervous system: Headache, lightheadedness, dizziness
    Neuromuscular & skeletal: Weakness
  1% to 10%: Dermatologic: Drug rash, exfoliative dermatitis
  <1%:
    Gastrointestinal: Nausea, vomiting
    Hematologic: Methemoglobinemia (overdose)
Drug Interactions No data reported
Drug Uptake
  Serum half-life:
    Parent drug: 1-4 hours
    Metabolite (5-mononitrate): 4 hours
Pregnancy Risk Factor C

Isosorbide Mononitrate (eye' soe sor bide mon oh nye' trate)

Related Information
  Cardiovascular Diseases *on page 912*
Brand Names Imdur™; Ismo™; Monoket®
Canadian/Mexican Brand Names Elantan® (Mexico); Mono-Mack® (Mexico)
Therapeutic Category Antianginal Agent; Vasodilator, Coronary
Use Long-acting metabolite of the vasodilator isosorbide dinitrate used for the prophylactic treatment of angina pectoris
Usual Dosage Adults: Oral:
  Regular tablet: 20 mg twice daily separated by 7 hours; maintenance doses as high as 120 mg have been used
  Extended release tablet (Imdur™): Initial: 30-60 mg once daily; after several days the dosage may be increased to 120 mg/day (given as two 60 mg tablets); daily dose should be taken in the morning upon arising; maximum: 240 mg/day
  Asymmetrical dosing regimen of 7 AM and 3 PM or 9 AM and 5 PM to allow for a nitrate-free dosing interval to minimize nitrate tolerance

Mechanism of Action Prevailing mechanism of action for nitroglycerin (and other nitrates) is systemic venodilation, decreasing preload as measured by pulmonary capillary wedge pressure and left ventricular end diastolic volume and pressure; the average reduction in LVEDV is 25% at rest, with a corresponding increase in ejection fractions of 50% to 60%. This effect improves congestive symptoms in heart failure and improves the myocardial perfusion gradient in patients with coronary artery disease.

Local Anesthetic/Vasoconstrictor Precautions No information available to require special precautions

Effects on Dental Treatment No effects or complications reported

Other Adverse Effects

>10%: Central nervous system: Headache

1% to 10%: Gastrointestinal: Dizziness, nausea, vomiting

<1%:

Cardiovascular: Angina pectoris, arrhythmias, atrial fibrillation, hypotension, palpitations, postural hypotension, premature ventricular contractions, supraventricular tachycardia, syncope, edema

Central nervous system: Asthenia, malaise, agitation, anxiety, confusion, hypoesthesia, insomnia, nervousness, nightmares

Dermatologic: Pruritus, rash

Gastrointestinal: Abdominal pain, diarrhea, dyspepsia, tenesmus, increased appetite

Genitourinary: Impotence, urinary frequency

Hematologic: Methemoglobinemia (rarely)

Neuromuscular & skeletal: Neck stiffness, rigors, arthralgia, dyscoordination

Ocular: Blurred vision, diplopia

Renal: Dysuria

Respiratory: Bronchitis, pneumonia, upper respiratory tract infection

Miscellaneous: Tooth disorder, cold sweat

Drug Interactions No data reported

Drug Uptake

Absorption: Oral: Nearly complete and low intersubject variability in its pharmacokinetic parameters and plasma concentrations

Pregnancy Risk Factor C

Isotrate® *see* Isosorbide Dinitrate *on previous page*

Isotretinoin (eye soe tret' i noyn)

Brand Names Accutane®

Canadian/Mexican Brand Names Isotrex® (Canada)

Therapeutic Category Acne Products; Retinoic Acid Derivative; Vitamin A Derivative

Use Treatment of severe recalcitrant cystic and/or conglobate acne unresponsive to conventional therapy; used investigationally for the treatment of children with metastatic neuroblastoma or leukemia that does not respond to conventional therapy

Usual Dosage Oral:

Children: Maintenance therapy for neuroblastoma: 100-250 mg/m²/day in 2 divided doses has been used investigationally

Children and Adults: 0.5-2 mg/kg/day in 2 divided doses (dosages as low as 0.05 mg/kg/day have been reported to be beneficial) for 15-20 weeks or until the total cyst count decreases by 70%, whichever is sooner

Mechanism of Action Reduces sebaceous gland size and reduces sebum production; regulates cell proliferation and differentiation

Local Anesthetic/Vasoconstrictor Precautions No information available to require special precautions

Effects on Dental Treatment No effects or complications reported

Other Adverse Effects

>10%:

Cardiovascular: Epistaxis

Dermatologic: Burning, redness, itching of eye, cheilitis, inflammation of lips, dry skin, pruritus, photosensitivity

Endocrine/metabolic: Increased serum concentration of triglycerides

Gastrointestinal: Dry mouth

Neuromuscular & skeletal: Bone or joint pain, muscle aches, myalgia

Respiratory: Dry nose

1% to 10%:

Central nervous system: Fatigue, headache, mental depression, tiredness

Dermatologic: Skin peeling on hands or soles of feet, skin rash

Gastrointestinal: Stomach upset

Ocular: Dry eyes, photophobia

(Continued)

Isotretinoin *(Continued)*

<1%:
Central nervous system: Mood changes, pseudomotor cerebri
Dermatologic: Hair loss, pruritus
Endocrine & metabolic: Hyperuricemia
Gastrointestinal: Xerostomia, anorexia, nausea, vomiting, inflammatory bowel syndrome, bleeding of gums
Hematologic: Increase in erythrocyte sedimentation rate, decrease in hemoglobin and hematocrit
Hepatic: Hepatitis
Ocular: Conjunctivitis, corneal opacities, optic neuritis, cataracts

Note: **Not to be used in women of childbearing potential** unless woman is capable of complying with effective contraceptive measures; therapy is normally begun on the second or third day of next normal menstrual period; effective contraception must be used for at least 1 month before beginning therapy, during therapy, and for 1 month after discontinuation of therapy. Because of the high likelihood of teratogenic effects (~20%), physicians do not prescribe isotretinoin for women who are or who are likely to become pregnant while using the drug.

Drug Interactions
Increased effect: Increased clearance of carbamazepine
Increased toxicity: Avoid other vitamin A products; may interfere with medications used to treat hypertriglyceridemia

Drug Uptake
Absorption: Oral: Demonstrates biphasic absorption
Serum half-life, terminal:
Parent drug: 10-20 hours
Time to peak serum concentration: Within 3 hours

Pregnancy Risk Factor X

Isovex® *see* Ethaverine Hydrochloride *on page 334*

Isoxsuprine Hydrochloride *(eye sox' syoo preen hye droe klor' ide)*

Brand Names Vasodilan®
Canadian/Mexican Brand Names Vadosilan® (Mexico); Vadosilan® 20 (Mexico)
Therapeutic Category Vasodilator
Use Treatment of peripheral vascular diseases, such as arteriosclerosis obliterans and Raynaud's disease
Usual Dosage Adults: 10-20 mg 3-4 times/day; start with lower dose in elderly due to potential hypotension
Mechanism of Action In studies on normal human subjects, isoxsuprine increases muscle blood flow, but skin blood flow is usually unaffected. Rather than increasing muscle blood flow by beta-receptor stimulation, isoxsuprine probably has a direct action on vascular smooth muscle. The generally accepted mechanism of action of isoxsuprine on the uterus is beta-adrenergic stimulation. Isoxsuprine was shown to inhibit prostaglandin synthetase at high serum concentrations, with low concentrations there was an increase in the P-G synthesis.
Local Anesthetic/Vasoconstrictor Precautions No information available to require special precautions
Effects on Dental Treatment No effects or complications reported
Other Adverse Effects
1% to 10%: Gastrointestinal: Nausea, vomiting
<1%:
Cardiovascular: Chest pain, hypotension
Dermatologic: Rash
Respiratory: Pulmonary edema
Drug Interactions No data reported
Drug Uptake
Absorption: Nearly complete
Serum half-life, serum: 1.25 hours mean
Time to peak serum concentration: Oral, I.M.: Within 1 hour
Pregnancy Risk Factor C

Isradipine *(iz ra' di peen)*

Related Information
Calcium Channel Blockers & Gingival Hyperplasia *on page 1010*
Cardiovascular Diseases *on page 912*
Brand Names DynaCirc®

Canadian/Mexican Brand Names DynaCirc SRO® (Mexico)

Therapeutic Category Calcium Channel Blocker

Use Treatment of hypertension, congestive heart failure, migraine prophylaxis

Usual Dosage Adults: 2.5 mg twice daily; antihypertensive response seen in 2-3 hours; maximal response in 2-4 weeks; increase dose at 2- to 4-week intervals at 2.5-5 mg increments; usual dose range: 5-20 mg/day. **Note:** Most patients show no improvement with doses >10 mg/day except adverse reaction rate increases; therefore, maximal dose in elderly should be 10 mg/day.

Mechanism of Action Inhibits calcium ion from entering the "slow channels" or select voltage-sensitive areas of vascular smooth muscle and myocardium during depolarization, producing a relaxation of coronary vascular smooth muscle and coronary vasodilation; increases myocardial oxygen delivery in patients with vasospastic angina

Local Anesthetic/Vasoconstrictor Precautions No information available to require special precautions

Effects on Dental Treatment Other drugs of this class can cause gingival hyperplasia (ie, nifedipine) but there have been no reports for amlodipine

Other Adverse Effects

>10%: Headache

1% to 10%:

Cardiovascular: Edema, palpitations, flushing, chest pain, tachycardia, hypotension

Central nervous system: Dizziness, fatigue, weakness

Dermatologic: Rash

Gastrointestinal: Nausea, abdominal discomfort, vomiting, diarrhea

Respiratory: Dyspnea

<1%:

Cardiovascular: Heart failure, atrial and ventricular fibrillation, TIAs, A-V block, myocardial infarction, abnormal EKG

Central nervous system: Disturbed sleep

Dermatologic: Pruritus, urticaria, rash

Gastrointestinal: Dry mouth

Genitourinary: Nocturia

Hematologic: Leukopenia

Neuromuscular & skeletal: Foot cramps, paresthesia, numbness

Ocular: Visual disturbance

Respiratory: Cough

Drug Interactions Increased toxicity/effect/levels: H_2-blockers cause increased bioavailability of isradipine

Severe hypotension has been reported during fentanyl anesthesia with concomitant use of beta-blockers and calcium channel blockers; even though such interactions have not been seen specifically with isradipine, caution is suggested in using isradipine with fentanyl

Drug Uptake

Absorption: Oral: 90% to 95%

Serum half-life: 8 hours

Time to peak: Serum concentration: 1-1.5 hours

Pregnancy Risk Factor C

Isuprel® *see* Isoproterenol *on page 472*

Itch-X® **[OTC]** *see* Pramoxine Hydrochloride *on page 714*

Itraconazole (i tra koe' na zole)

Related Information

Oral Fungal Infections *on page 948*

Brand Names Sporanox®

Canadian/Mexican Brand Names Isox® (Mexico); Itranax® (Mexico)

Therapeutic Category Antifungal Agent, Systemic

Use

Dental: Treatment of susceptible fungal infections in immunocompromised and immunocompetent patients including blastomycosis and histoplasmosis; also has activity against *Aspergillus, Candida, Coccidioides, Cryptococcus, Sporothrix* and chromomycosis

Medical: Treatment of susceptible fungal infection as described for dental use

Usual Dosage Oral (absorption is best if taken with food, therefore, it is best to administer itraconazole after meals):

Children: Efficacy and safety have not been established; a small number of patients 3-16 years of age have been treated with 100 mg/day for systemic fungal infections with no serious adverse effects reported

(Continued)

Itraconazole *(Continued)*

Adults: 200 mg once daily, if obvious improvement or there is evidence of progressive fungal disease, increase the dose in 100 mg increments to a maximum of 400 mg/day; doses >200 mg/day are given in 2 divided doses

Mechanism of Action Inhibits fungal cytochrome P-450-dependent enzymes (cytochrome P-450 3A4 and cytochrome P-450 2C); this blocks the synthesis of ergosterol which is the vital component in the fungal cell membrane. Triazoles contain three nitrogen atoms in the five-membered azole ring; the triazole ring increases tissue penetration, prolongs half-life, and enhances efficacy while decreasing toxicity compared with the imidazoles.

Local Anesthetic/Vasoconstrictor Precautions No information available to require special precautions

Effects on Dental Treatment No effects or complications reported

Other Adverse Effects

>10%: Gastrointestinal: Nausea

1% to 10%:
Central nervous system: Headache
Dermatologic: Rash
Gastrointestinal: Abdominal pain, vomiting

Oral manifestations: No data reported

Contraindications Known hypersensitivity to itraconazole or other azoles; terfenadine

Warnings/Precautions Rare cases of serious cardiovascular adverse event, including death, ventricular tachycardia and torsade de pointes have been observed due to increased terfenadine concentrations induced by itraconazole; patients who develop abnormal liver function tests during fluconazole therapy should be monitored and therapy discontinued if symptoms of liver disease develop

Drug Interactions Decreased serum levels with isoniazid and phenytoin; decreased/undetectable serum levels with rifampin - **should not be administered concomitantly with rifampin**; absorption requires gastric acidity, therefore, antacids, H$_2$ antagonists (cimetidine and ranitidine), omeprazole, and sucralfate significantly reduce bioavailability resulting in treatment failures and should not be administered concomitantly; amphotericin B or fluconazole should be used instead. May increase cyclosporine levels (by 50%) when high doses are used; may increase phenytoin serum concentration; may inhibit warfarins metabolism; may increase digoxin serum levels; may increase terfenadine levels - **concomitant administration is not recommended**.

Drug Uptake

Absorption: Oral: ~55%
Time to peak serum concentration: 1-2 hours
Serum half-life: After single 200 mg dose: 21±5 hours
Influence of food: Absorption enhanced by food and requires gastric acidity

Pregnancy Risk Factor C

Breast-feeding Considerations No data reported

Dosage Forms Capsule: 100 mg

Dietary Considerations No data reported

Generic Available No

IVIG *see* Immune Globulin, Intravenous *on page 454*

Janimine® *see* Imipramine *on page 451*

Japanese Encephalitis Virus Vaccine, Inactivated

(jap a neese' en sef a lye' tis vye' rus vak seen', in ak ti vay' ted)

Brand Names JE-VAX®

Therapeutic Category Vaccine, Live Virus

Use Active immunization against Japanese encephalitis for persons spending a month or longer in endemic areas, especially if travel will include rural areas

Local Anesthetic/Vasoconstrictor Precautions No information available to require special precautions

Effects on Dental Treatment No effects or complications reported

Other Adverse Effects

1% to 10%:
Cardiovascular: Hypotension
Central nervous system: Fever, headache, malaise, chills, dizziness
Dermatologic: Rash, urticaria, itching with or without accompanying rash
Gastrointestinal: Nausea, vomiting, abdominal pain
Local: Tenderness, redness, and swelling at injection site
Neuromuscular & skeletal: Myalgia

<1%:
  Central nervous system: Encephalitis, encephalopathy, seizure
  Dermatologic: Erythema multiforme, erythema nodosum, angioedema
  Neuromuscular & skeletal: Peripheral neuropathy
  Respiratory: Dyspnea
  Miscellaneous: Anaphylactic reaction, joint swelling

Report allergic or unusual adverse reactions to the Vaccine Adverse Event Reporting System (VAERS 1-800-822-7967)

Comments Japanese encephalitis vaccine is currently available only from the Centers for Disease Control. Contact Centers for Disease Control at (404) 639-6370 (Mon-Fri) or (404) 639-2888 (nights, weekends, or holidays).

Jenest-28™ *see* Ethinyl Estradiol and Norethindrone *on page 339*

JE-VAX® *see* Japanese Encephalitis Virus Vaccine, Inactivated *on previous page*

Just Tears® Solution [OTC] *see* Artificial Tears *on page 75*

K⁺8® *see* Potassium Chloride *on page 708*

Kabikinase® *see* Streptokinase *on page 801*

Kadian® Capsule *see* Morphine Sulfate *on page 590*

Kalcinate® *see* Calcium Gluconate *on page 143*

Kanamycin Sulfate (kan a mye' sin sul' fate)
Related Information
  Nonviral Infectious Diseases *on page 932*
Brand Names Kantrex®
Canadian/Mexican Brand Names Randikan® (Mexico)
Therapeutic Category Antibiotic, Aminoglycoside
Use
  Oral: Preoperative bowel preparation in the prophylaxis of infections and adjunctive treatment of hepatic coma (oral kanamycin is not indicated in the treatment of systemic infections); treatment of susceptible bacterial infection including gram-negative aerobes, gram-positive *Bacillus* as well as some mycobacteria
  Parenteral: Rarely used in antibiotic irrigations during surgery
Usual Dosage
  Children:
    Infections: I.M., I.V.: 15-30 mg/kg/day in divided doses every 8 hours
    Suppression of bowel flora: Oral: 150-250 mg/kg/day in divided doses administered every 1-6 hours
  Adults:
    Infections: I.M., I.V.: 5-7.5 mg/kg/dose in divided doses every 8-12 hours
    Preoperative intestinal antisepsis: Oral: 1 g every 4-6 hours for 36-72 hours
    Hepatic coma: Oral: 8-12 g/day in divided doses
Mechanism of Action Interferes with protein synthesis in bacterial cell by binding to ribosomal subunit
Local Anesthetic/Vasoconstrictor Precautions No information available to require special precautions
Effects on Dental Treatment No effects or complications reported
Other Adverse Effects
  >10%: Renal: Nephrotoxicity
  1% to 10%:
    Cardiovascular: Swelling
    Central nervous system: Neurotoxicity
    Dermatologic: Skin itching, redness, rash
    Otic: Ototoxicity (auditory), ototoxicity (vestibular)
  <1%:
    Central nervous system: Drowsiness, headache, pseudomotor cerebri
    Dermatologic: Photosensitivity, erythema
    Gastrointestinal: Anorexia, nausea, vomiting, weight loss, increased salivation, enterocolitis
    Hematologic: Granulocytopenia, agranulocytosis, thrombocytopenia
    Local: Burning, stinging
    Neuromuscular & skeletal: Weakness, tremors, muscle cramps
    Respiratory: Difficulty in breathing
Drug Interactions
  Increased toxicity:
    Penicillins, cephalosporins, amphotericin B, diuretics cause increased nephrotoxicity of kanamycin
    Neuromuscular blocking agents cause increased neuromuscular blockade of kanamycin
  (Continued)

Kanamycin Sulfate *(Continued)*

Drug Uptake
Absorption: Oral: Not absorbed following administration
Serum half-life: 2-4 hours, increases in anuria to 80 hours
  End stage renal disease: 40-96 hours
Time to peak serum concentration: I.M.: 1-2 hours

Pregnancy Risk Factor D

Kantrex® *see* Kanamycin Sulfate *on previous page*

Kaochlor-Eff® *see* Potassium Bicarbonate, Potassium Chloride, and Potassium Citrate *on page 708*

Kaochlor® S-F *see* Potassium Chloride *on page 708*

Kaodene® [OTC] *see* Kaolin and Pectin *on this page*

Kaolin and Pectin (kay' oh lin & pek' tin)

Brand Names Kaodene® [OTC]; Kao-Spen® [OTC]; Kapectolin® [OTC]
Therapeutic Category Antidiarrheal
Synonyms Pectin and Kaolin
Use Treatment of uncomplicated diarrhea
Local Anesthetic/Vasoconstrictor Precautions No information available to require special precautions
Effects on Dental Treatment No effects or complications reported
Other Adverse Effects 1% to 10%: Constipation, fecal impaction

Kaolin and Pectin With Opium
(kay' oh lin & pek' tin with oh' pee um)
Brand Names Parepectolin®
Therapeutic Category Antidiarrheal
Use Symptomatic relief of diarrhea
Local Anesthetic/Vasoconstrictor Precautions No information available to require special precautions
Effects on Dental Treatment No effects or complications reported

Kaon® *see* Potassium Gluconate *on page 710*

Kaon-CL® *see* Potassium Chloride *on page 708*

Kaopectate® Advanced Formula [OTC] *see* Attapulgite *on page 86*

Kaopectate® II [OTC] *see* Loperamide Hydrochloride *on page 511*

Kaopectate® Maximum Strength Caplets *see* Attapulgite *on page 86*

Kao-Spen® [OTC] *see* Kaolin and Pectin *on this page*

Kapectolin® [OTC] *see* Kaolin and Pectin *on this page*

Kapectolin PG® *see* Hyoscyamine, Atropine, Scopolamine, Kaolin, Pectin, and Opium *on page 445*

Karidium® *see* Fluoride *on page 374*

Karigel® *see* Fluoride *on page 374*

Karigel®-N *see* Fluoride *on page 374*

Kasof® [OTC] *see* Docusate *on page 295*

Kato® *see* Potassium Chloride *on page 708*

Kaybovite-1000® *see* Cyanocobalamin *on page 237*

Kaylixir® *see* Potassium Gluconate *on page 710*

K+ Care® Effervescent *see* Potassium Bicarbonate *on page 707*

K-Dur® *see* Potassium Chloride *on page 708*

Keflet® *see* Cephalexin Monohydrate *on page 176*

Keflex® *see* Cephalexin Monohydrate *on page 176*

Keflin® *see* Cephalothin Sodium *on page 177*

Keftab® *see* Cephalexin Monohydrate *on page 176*

Kefurox® *see* Cefuroxime *on page 173*

Kefzol® *see* Cefazolin Sodium *on page 164*

K-Electrolyte® Effervescent *see* Potassium Bicarbonate *on page 707*

Kemadrin® *see* Procyclidine Hydrochloride *on page 730*

Kenacort® Syrup *see* Triamcinolone *on page 862*

Kenacort® Tablet *see* Triamcinolone *on page 862*

Kenalog® Injection *see* Triamcinolone *on page 862*

Kenalog® in Orabase® *see* Triamcinolone Acetonide Dental Paste *on page 864*

Kenonel® *see* Triamcinolone *on page 862*

Keralyt® *see* Salicylic Acid *on page 777*

Keralyt® Gel *see* Salicylic Acid and Propylene Glycol *on page 778*

Kerlone® *see* Betaxolol Hydrochloride *on page 111*

Kestrone® *see* Estrone *on page 329*
Ketalar® *see* Ketamine Hydrochloride *on this page*

Ketamine Hydrochloride (keet' a meen hye droe klor' ide)
Brand Names Ketalar®
Canadian/Mexican Brand Names Ketalin® (Mexico)
Therapeutic Category General Anesthetic, Intravenous
Use Induction of anesthesia; short surgical procedures; dressing changes
Usual Dosage Used in combination with anticholinergic agents to ↓ hypersalivation

Children: Initial induction:
Oral: 6-10 mg/kg for 1 dose (mixed in 0.2-0.3 mL/kg of cola or other beverage) given 30 minutes before the procedure
I.M.: 3-7 mg/kg
I.V.: Range: 0.5-2 mg/kg, use smaller doses (0.5-1 mg/kg) for sedation for minor procedures; usual induction dosage: 1-2 mg/kg
Continuous I.V. infusion: Sedation: 5-20 mcg/kg/minute

Adults: Initial induction:
I.M.: 3-8 mg/kg
I.V.: Range: 1-4.5 mg/kg; usual induction dosage: 1-2 mg/kg

Children and Adults: Maintenance: Supplemental doses of ¹/₂ to the full induction dose; repeat as needed

Mechanism of Action Produces dissociative anesthesia by direct action on the cortex and limbic system

Local Anesthetic/Vasoconstrictor Precautions No information available to require special precautions

Effects on Dental Treatment No effects or complications reported
Other Adverse Effects
>10%:
Cardiovascular: Hypertension, tachycardia, increased cardiac output, paradoxical direct myocardial depression
Central nervous system: Increased intracranial pressure, vivid dreams, visual hallucinations
Neuromuscular & skeletal: Tonic-clonic movements, tremors
Miscellaneous: Emergence reactions, vocalization

1% to 10%:
Cardiovascular: Bradycardia, hypotension
Dermatologic: Pain at injection site, skin rash
Gastrointestinal: Vomiting, anorexia, nausea
Ocular: Nystagmus, diplopia
Respiratory: Respiratory depression

<1%:
Cardiovascular: Cardiac arrhythmias, myocardial depression
Central nervous system: Increased intracranial pressure, increases in cerebral blood, fasciculations
Endocrine & metabolic: Increased metabolic rate, increased intraocular pressure
Neuromuscular & skeletal: Increased skeletal muscle tone
Ocular: Increased intraocular pressure
Respiratory: Increased airway resistance, cough reflex may be depressed, decreased bronchospasm, respiratory depression or apnea with large doses or rapid infusions, laryngospasm
Miscellaneous: Hypersalivation

Drug Interactions
Increased toxicity:
Barbiturates, narcotics, hydroxyzine increase prolonged recovery from ketamine
Muscle relaxants, thyroid hormones cause increased blood pressure and heart rate in combination with ketamine
Halothane causes decreased blood pressure in combination with ketamine

Drug Uptake Duration of action (following a single dose):
Unconsciousness: 10-15 minutes
Analgesia: 30-40 minutes
Amnesia: May persist for 1-2 hours
Pregnancy Risk Factor D

Ketoconazole (kee toe koe' na zole)
Related Information
Dental Drug Interactions: Update on Drug Combinations Requiring Special Considerations *on page 1022*
Oral Fungal Infections *on page 948*
(Continued)

Ketoconazole (Continued)

Respiratory Diseases on page 924

Brand Names Nizoral®

Canadian/Mexican Brand Names Akorazol® (Mexico)

Therapeutic Category Antifungal Agent, Systemic; Antifungal Agent, Topical

Use

Dental: Treatment of susceptible fungal infections in the oral cavity including candidiasis, oral thrush, and chronic mucocutaneous candidiasis

Medical: Treatment of susceptible fungal infections including blastomycosis, histoplasmosis, paracoccidioidomycosis, as well as certain recalcitrant cutaneous dermatophytosis; used topically for treatment of tinea corporis, tinea cruris, tinea versicolor, and cutaneous candidiasis, seborrheic dermatitis

Usual Dosage

Children >2 years:

Oral: 5-10 mg/kg/day divided every 12-24 hours for 2-4 weeks

Topical: Rub gently to affected area 1-2 times/day

Adults:

Oral: 200-400 mg/day as a single daily dose

Topical: Rub gently to affected area 1-2 times/day

Mechanism of Action Alters the permeability of the cell wall; inhibits biosynthesis of triglycerides and phospholipids by fungi; inhibits several fungal enzymes that results in a build-up of toxic concentrations of hydrogen peroxide

Local Anesthetic/Vasoconstrictor Precautions No information available to require special precautions

Effects on Dental Treatment No effects or complications reported

Other Adverse Effects

Oral: 1% to 10%:

Dermatologic: Pruritus

Gastrointestinal: Nausea, vomiting, abdominal pain, diarrhea

Cream: Severe irritation, pruritus, stinging (~5%)

Shampoo: Increases in normal hair loss, irritation (<1%), abnormal hair texture, scalp pustules, mild dryness of skin, itching, oiliness/dryness of hair

Oral manifestations: No data reported

Contraindications Hypersensitivity to ketoconazole or any component; CNS fungal infections (due to poor CNS penetration); coadministration with terfenadine is contraindicated

Warnings/Precautions Rare cases of serious cardiovascular adverse event, including death, ventricular tachycardia and torsade de pointes have been observed due to increased terfenadine concentrations induced by ketoconazole. Use with caution in patients with impaired hepatic function; has been associated with hepatotoxicity, including some fatalities; perform periodic liver function tests; high doses of ketoconazole may depress adrenocortical function.

Drug Interactions Decreased serum levels with isoniazid and phenytoin; decreased/undetectable serum levels with rifampin - **should not be administered concomitantly with rifampin**; absorption requires gastric acidity, therefore, antacids, H_2 antagonists (cimetidine and ranitidine), omeprazole, and sucralfate significantly reduce bioavailability resulting in treatment failures and should not be administered concomitantly; amphotericin B or fluconazole should be used instead. May increase cyclosporine levels (by 50%) when high doses are used; may increase phenytoin serum concentration; may inhibit warfarins metabolism; may increase digoxin serum levels; may increase terfenadine levels - **concomitant administration is not recommended**.

Drug Uptake

Time to peak serum concentration: 1-2 hours

Serum half-life: Biphasic: Initial: 2 hours; terminal: 8 hours

Pregnancy Risk Factor C

Breast-feeding Considerations No data reported

Dosage Forms

Cream: 2% (15 g, 30 g, 60 g)

Shampoo: 2% (120 mL)

Tablet: 200 mg

Dietary Considerations May be taken with food or milk to decrease GI adverse effects

Generic Available No

Selected Readings

Wynn RL, "Erythromycin and Ketoconazole (Nizoral®) Associated With Terfenadine (Seldane®)-Induced Ventricular Arrhythmias," *Gen Dent*, 1993, 41:27-9.

Ketoprofen (kee toe proe' fen)

Related Information

Nonsteroidal Anti-Inflammatory Agents, Comparative Dosages, and Pharmacokinetics *on page 1021*

Oral Pain *on page 940*

Rheumatoid Arthritis, Osteoarthritis, and Joint Prostheses *on page 930*

Brand Names Orudis®; Orudis KT® [OTC]; Oruvail®

Canadian/Mexican Brand Names Apo-Keto® (Canada); Apo-Keto-E® (Canada); Novo-Keto-EC® (Canada); Nu-Ketoprofen® (Canada); Nu-Ketoprofen-E® (Canada); Rhodis® (Canada); Rhodis-EC® (Canada); PMS-Ketoprofen® (Canada); Keduril® (Mexico); K-Profen® (Mexico); Pro-Fenid® (Mexico); Profenid® 200 (Mexico); Profenid-IM® (Mexico)

Therapeutic Category Analgesic, Non-narcotic; Anti-inflammatory Agent; Nonsteroidal Anti-inflammatory Agent (NSAID), Oral

Synonyms Ketoprofeno (Mexico)

Use

Dental: Management of pain and swelling

Medical: Acute and long-term treatment of rheumatoid arthritis and osteoarthritis; primary dysmenorrhea; mild to moderate pain

Usual Dosage Oral:

Children: Not recommended

Adults: 25-50 mg every 6-8 hours as necessary; daily doses >300 mg are not recommended

Mechanism of Action Inhibits prostaglandin synthesis by decreasing the activity of the enzyme, cyclo-oxygenase, which results in decreased formation of prostaglandin precursors

Local Anesthetic/Vasoconstrictor Precautions No information available to require special precautions

Effects on Dental Treatment Use with caution in patients taking anticoagulants

Other Adverse Effects >10%:

Central nervous system: Dizziness

Dermatologic: Skin rash

Gastrointestinal: Cramps, heartburn, nausea

Oral manifestations: None reported

Contraindications Ketoprofen is contraindicated in patients who have known hypersensitivity to it; should not be given to patients in whom aspirin or other nonsteroidal anti-inflammatory drugs induce asthma, urticaria, or other allergic-type reactions because severe, rarely fatal, anaphylactic reactions to ketoprofen have been reported in such patients

Warnings/Precautions Use lowest effective dose for shortest period possible; use with caution in patients with a history of GI disease (bleeding or ulcers)

Drug Interactions Probenecid increases both free and bound ketoprofen by reducing the plasma clearance of ketoprofen to about one-third, as well as decreasing its protein-binding; the combination of ketoprofen and probenecid is not recommended; coadministration of ketoprofen and methotrexate should be avoided because increased toxicity due to displacement of protein-bound methotrexate has been reported to occur

Drug Uptake

Absorption: Rapid and complete

Onset of effect: 30-60 minutes

Time to peak serum concentration: 0.5-2 hours

Serum half-life: 2-4 hours

Influence of food: Rate of absorption is slowed resulting in delayed and reduced peak serum concentrations

Pregnancy Risk Factor B

Breast-feeding Considerations May be taken while breast-feeding

Dosage Forms

Caplet (Orudis KT®) [OTC]: 12.5 mg

Capsule (Orudis®): 25 mg, 50 mg, 75 mg

Capsule, extended release (Oruvail®): 100 mg, 200 mg

Dietary Considerations In order to minimize gastrointestinal effects, ketoprofen can be prescribed to be taken with food or milk; although food affects the bioavailability of ketoprofen, analgesic efficacy is not significantly diminished

Generic Available No

Selected Readings

Brooks PM and Day RO, "Nonsteroidal Anti-Inflammatory Drugs-Differences and Similarities," *N Engl J Med*, 1991, 324(24):1716-25.

Ketoprofeno (Mexico) *see* Ketoprofen *on previous page*

Ketorolac Tromethamine (kee′ toe role ak trow meth′ a meen)

Related Information
Dental Drug Interactions: Update on Drug Combinations Requiring Special Considerations *on page 1022*
Nonsteroidal Anti-Inflammatory Agents, Comparative Dosages, and Pharma-cokinetics *on page 1021*

Brand Names Toradol®

Canadian/Mexican Brand Names Dolac® Oral (Mexico); Dolac® Inyectable (Mexico)

Therapeutic Category Analgesic, Non-narcotic; Anti-inflammatory Agent; Nonsteroidal Anti-inflammatory Agent (NSAID)

Use
Dental: Short-term (<5 days) management of pain
Medical: First parenteral NSAID for analgesia; 30 mg I.M. provides the analgesia comparable to 12 mg of morphine or 100 mg of meperidine

Usual Dosage Adults: Treatment of acute postsurgical pain:
Manufacturer recommendation: I.M.: 30 mg followed by an oral dose (10 mg) as needed, then 10 mg every 4-6 hours as needed thereafter; total time for drug administration should be no longer than 5 days; maximum oral daily dose: 40 mg (or 120 mg combined oral and I.M.)
I.M.: Initial: 30-60 mg, then 15-30 mg every 6 hours as needed for up to 5 days maximum; maximum dose in the first 24 hours: 150 mg with 120 mg/24 hours for up to 5 days total

Mechanism of Action Inhibits prostaglandin synthesis by decreasing the activity of the enzyme, cyclo-oxygenase, which results in decreased formation of prostaglandin precursors

Local Anesthetic/Vasoconstrictor Precautions No information available to require special precautions

Effects on Dental Treatment No effects or complications reported

Other Adverse Effects 1% to 10%: Gastrointestinal: Abdominal pain, nausea, gastric ulcers

Oral manifestations: No data reported

Contraindications In patients who have developed nasal polyps, angioedema, or bronchospastic reactions to other NSAIDs, active peptic ulcer disease, recent GI bleeding or perforation, patients with advanced renal disease or risk of renal failure, labor and delivery, nursing mothers, patients with hypersensitivity to ketorolac, aspirin, or other NSAIDs, **prophylaxis before major surgery**, suspected or confirmed cerebrovascular bleeding, hemorrhagic diathesis, concurrent aspirin or other NSAIDs, epidural or intrathecal administration, concomitant probenecid

Warnings/Precautions Use extra caution and reduce dosages in the elderly because it is cleared renally somewhat slower, and the elderly are also more sensitive to the renal effects of NSAIDs; use with caution in patients with congestive heart failure, hypertension, decreased renal or hepatic function, history of GI disease (bleeding or ulcers), or those receiving anticoagulants

Drug Interactions High dose salicylates may increase plasma levels of ketorolac by displacing from plasma proteins; coadministration with probenecid reduces renal excretion of ketorolac causing increased plasma levels; ketorolac reduces diuretic effect of furosemide; some NSAIDs may prevent renal excretion of lithium; effect of ketorolac on lithium is unknown

Drug Uptake
Absorption: Oral: Rapid and complete
Onset of effect: I.M.: Within 10 minutes
Time to peak serum concentration: I.M.: 30-60 minutes
Duration of effect: 6-8 hours
Serum half-life: 2-8 hours
Influence of food: Rate is decreased but extent remains the same

Pregnancy Risk Factor B (D if used in the 3rd trimester)

Breast-feeding Considerations No data reported

Dosage Forms
Injection: 15 mg/mL (1 mL); 30 mg/mL (1 mL, 2 mL)
Solution, ophthalmic: 0.5% (5 mL)
Tablet: 10 mg

Dietary Considerations May be taken with food to decrease GI distress

Generic Available No

Comments According to the manufacturer, ketorolac has been used inappropriately by physicians in the past. The drug had been prescribed to NSAID-sensitive patients, patients with GI bleeding, and for long-term use; a warning

has been issued regarding increased incidence and severity of GI complications with increasing doses and duration of use. Labeling now includes the statement that ketorolac inhibits platelet function and is indicated for up to 5 days use only.

Selected Readings

Brown CR, Moodie JE, Evans SE, et al, "Efficacy of Intramuscular (I.M.) Ketorolac and Meperidine in Pain Following Major Oral Surgery," *Clin Pharmacol Ther*, 1988, 43:161 (abstract).

Forbes JA, Butterworth GA, Burchfield WH, et al, "Evaluation of Ketorolac, Aspirin, and an Acetaminophen-Codeine Combination in Postoperative Oral Surgery Pain," *Pharmacotherapy*, 1990, 10(6 Pt 2): 77S-93S.

Forbes JA, Kehm CJ, Grodin CD, et al, "Evaluation of Ketorolac, Ibuprofen, Acetaminophen, and an Acetaminophen-Codeine Combination in Postoperative Oral Surgery Pain," *Pharmacotherapy*, 1990, 10(6 Pt 2):94S-105S.

Fricke J and Angelocci D, "The Analgesic Efficacy of I.M. Ketorolac and Meperidine for the Control of Postoperative Dental Pain," *Clin Pharmacol Ther*, 1987, 41:181.

Fricke JR Jr, Angelocci D, Fox K, et al, "Comparison of the Efficacy and Safety of Ketorolac and Meperidine in the Relief of Dental Pain," *J Clin Pharmacol*, 1992, 32(4):376-84.

Gannon R, "Focus on Ketorolac: A Nonsteroidal, Anti-Inflammatory Agent for the Treatment of Moderate to Severe Pain," *Hosp Formul*, 1989, 24:695-702.

Wynn RL, "Ketorolac (Toradol®) for Dental Pain," *Gen Dent*, 1992, 40(6):476-9.

Key-Pred® *see* Prednisolone *on page 718*

Key-Pred-SP® *see* Prednisolone *on page 718*

K-G® Elixir *see* Potassium Gluconate *on page 710*

K-Gen® Effervescent *see* Potassium Bicarbonate *on page 707*

Kinesed® *see* Hyoscyamine, Atropine, Scopolamine, and Phenobarbital *on page 444*

Kinevac® *see* Sincalide *on page 789*

Klerist-D® Tablet [OTC] *see* Chlorpheniramine and Pseudoephedrine *on page 191*

Klonopin™ *see* Clonazepam *on page 220*

K-Lor™ *see* Potassium Chloride *on page 708*

Klor-con® *see* Potassium Chloride *on page 708*

Klor-Con®/EF *see* Potassium Bicarbonate and Potassium Citrate, Effervescent *on page 707*

Kloromin® [OTC] *see* Chlorpheniramine Maleate *on page 191*

Klorvess® *see* Potassium Chloride *on page 708*

Klorvess® Effervescent *see* Potassium Bicarbonate and Potassium Chloride, Effervescent *on page 707*

Klotrix® *see* Potassium Chloride *on page 708*

K-Lyte® *see* Potassium Bicarbonate and Potassium Citrate, Effervescent *on page 707*

K-Lyte/CL® *see* Potassium Bicarbonate and Potassium Chloride, Effervescent *on page 707*

K-Lyte® Effervescent *see* Potassium Bicarbonate *on page 707*

Kōate®-HP *see* Antihemophilic Factor (Human) *on page 68*

Kōate®-HS *see* Antihemophilic Factor (Human) *on page 68*

KoGENate® *see* Antihemophilic Factor (Human) *on page 68*

Kolephrin® GG/DM [OTC] *see* Guaifenesin and Dextromethorphan *on page 408*

Kolyum® *see* Potassium Chloride and Potassium Gluconate *on page 709*

Konakion® *see* Phytonadione *on page 690*

Konsyl® [OTC] *see* Psyllium *on page 750*

Konsyl-D® [OTC] *see* Psyllium *on page 750*

Konȳne® 80 *see* Factor IX Complex (Human) *on page 350*

Koromex® [OTC] *see* Nonoxynol 9 *on page 627*

K-Phos® Neutral *see* Potassium Phosphate and Sodium Phosphate *on page 713*

K-Phos® Original *see* Potassium Acid Phosphate *on page 707*

K-Tab® *see* Potassium Chloride *on page 708*

Ku-Zyme® HP *see* Pancrelipase *on page 657*

K-Vescent® *see* Potassium Bicarbonate and Potassium Citrate, Effervescent *on page 707*

Kwelcof® *see* Hydrocodone and Guaifenesin *on page 434*

Kwell® *see* Lindane *on page 504*

Kytril® *see* Granisetron *on page 405*

LA-12® *see* Hydroxocobalamin *on page 439*

Labetalol Hydrochloride (la bet' a lole hye droe klor' ide)

Related Information

Cardiovascular Diseases *on page 912*

Brand Names Normodyne®; Trandate®

Canadian/Mexican Brand Names Midotens® (Mexico)

Therapeutic Category Alpha-/Beta- Adrenergic Blocker

Use Treatment of mild to severe hypertension; I.V. for hypertensive emergencies

Usual Dosage Due to limited documentation of its use, labetalol should be initiated cautiously in pediatric patients with careful dosage adjustment and blood pressure monitoring

Children:

Oral: Limited information regarding labetalol use in pediatric patients is currently available in literature. Some centers recommend initial oral doses of 4 mg/kg/day in 2 divided doses. Reported oral doses have started at 3 mg/kg/day and 20 mg/kg/day and have increased up to 40 mg/kg/day.

I.V., intermittent bolus doses of 0.3-1 mg/kg/dose have been reported

For treatment of pediatric hypertensive emergencies, initial continuous infusions of 0.4-1 mg/kg/hour with a maximum of 3 mg/kg/hour have been used; administration requires the use of an infusion pump

Adults:

Oral: Initial: 100 mg twice daily, may increase as needed every 2-3 days by 100 mg until desired response is obtained; usual dose: 200-400 mg twice daily; not to exceed 2.4 g/day

I.V.: 20 mg or 1-2 mg/kg whichever is lower, IVP over 2 minutes, may give 40-80 mg at 10-minute intervals, up to 300 mg total dose

I.V. infusion: Initial: 2 mg/minute; titrate to response up to 300 mg total dose; administration requires the use of an infusion pump

I.V. infusion (500 mg/250 mL D_5) rates:

1 mg/minute: 30 mL/hour

2 mg/minute: 60 mL/hour

3 mg/minute: 90 mL/hour

4 mg/minute: 120 mL/hour

5 mg/minute: 150 mL/hour

6 mg/minute: 180 mL/hour

Not removed by hemo- or peritoneal dialysis; supplemental dose is not necessary

Mechanism of Action Blocks alpha-, beta$_1$-, and beta$_2$-adrenergic receptor sites; elevated renins are reduced

Local Anesthetic/Vasoconstrictor Precautions Use with caution; epinephrine has interacted with nonselective beta-blockers to result in initial hypertensive episode followed by bradycardia

Effects on Dental Treatment Non-cardioselective beta-blockers (ie, propranolol, nadolol) enhance the pressor response to epinephrine, resulting in hypertension and bradycardia. Many nonsteroidal anti-inflammatory drugs such as ibuprofen and indomethacin can reduce the hypotensive effect of beta-blockers after 3 or more weeks of therapy with the NSAID. Short-term NSAID use (ie, 3 days) requires no special precautions in patients taking beta-blockers.

Other Adverse Effects

1% to 10%:

Cardiovascular: Congestive heart failure, irregular heartbeat, reduced peripheral circulation, orthostatic hypotension

Central nervous system: Mental depression, dizziness, drowsiness

Dermatologic: Itching, numbness of skin

Endocrine & metabolic: Decreased sexual ability

Gastrointestinal: Nausea, vomiting, stomach discomfort

Neuromuscular & skeletal: Weakness

Respiratory: Breathing difficulty, stuffy nose

Miscellaneous: Changes in taste

<1%:

Cardiovascular: Bradycardia, chest pain

Dermatologic: Skin rash

Gastrointestinal: Diarrhea

Hepatic: Hepatotoxicity

Neuromuscular & skeletal: Joint pain

Ocular: Dry eyes

Drug Interactions

Decreased effect of beta-blockers:

Barbiturates (increased liver metabolism of beta-blockers to result in lower serum levels)

NSAIDs (attenuate the hypotensive therapeutic effects of beta-blockers)

Rifampin (increased liver metabolism of beta-blockers to result in lower serum levels)

Increased effects of beta-blockers:

Calcium channel blockers (increase serum levels of beta-blockers by unknown mechanism to enhance hypotension)

Beta-blockers increase the effects of:

Epinephrine (vasoconstrictor; initial hypertensive episode followed by bradycardia) only from non-cardioselective type beta-blockers

Phenylephrine (Neosynephrine®; enhanced pressor response)

Theophylline (inhibit theophylline metabolism causing increase in serum concentrations)

Drug Uptake

Onset of action:

Oral: 20 minutes to 2 hours

I.V.: 2-5 minutes

Peak effect:

Oral: 1-4 hours

I.V.: 5-15 minutes

Duration:

Oral: 8-24 hours (dose-dependent)

I.V.: 2-4 hours

Serum half-life, normal renal function: 6-8 hours

Pregnancy Risk Factor C

LaBID® *see* Theophylline/Aminophylline *on page 832*

Lac-Hydrin® *see* Lactic Acid With Ammonium Hydroxide *on this page*

Lacril® Ophthalmic Solution [OTC] *see* Artificial Tears *on page 75*

Lacrisert® *see* Hydroxypropyl Cellulose *on page 441*

Lactaid® [OTC] *see* Lactase *on this page*

Lactase (lak' tase)

Brand Names Dairy Ease® [OTC]; Lactaid® [OTC]; Lactrase® [OTC]

Therapeutic Category Nutritional Supplement

Use Help digest lactose in milk for patients with lactose intolerance

Local Anesthetic/Vasoconstrictor Precautions No information available to require special precautions

Effects on Dental Treatment No effects or complications reported

Lactic Acid and Salicylic Acid *see* Salicylic Acid and Lactic Acid *on page 778*

Lactic Acid and Sodium-PCA

(lak' tik as' id & sow' dee um-pee see aye)

Brand Names LactiCare® [OTC]

Therapeutic Category Topical Skin Product

Synonyms Sodium-PCA and Lactic Acid

Use Lubricate and moisturize the skin counteracting dryness and itching

Local Anesthetic/Vasoconstrictor Precautions No information available to require special precautions

Effects on Dental Treatment No effects or complications reported

Lactic Acid With Ammonium Hydroxide

(lak' tik as' id with a moe' nee um hye drok' side)

Brand Names Lac-Hydrin®

Therapeutic Category Topical Skin Product

Synonyms Ammonium Lactate

Use Treatment of moderate to severe xerosis and ichthyosis vulgaris

Local Anesthetic/Vasoconstrictor Precautions No information available to require special precautions

Effects on Dental Treatment No effects or complications reported

LactiCare® [OTC] *see* Lactic Acid and Sodium-PCA *on this page*

Lactinex® [OTC] *see* Lactobacillus acidophilus and Lactobacillus bulgaricus *on next page*

ALPHABETICAL LISTING OF DRUGS

Lactobacillus acidophilus and *Lactobacillus bulgaricus*
(lak toe ba sil' us as i dof' fil us & lak toe ba sil' us bul gar' i cus)

Related Information
Oral Nonviral Soft Tissue Ulcerations or Erosions *on page 955*

Brand Names Bacid® [OTC]; Lactinex® [OTC]; More-Dophilus® [OTC]

Canadian/Mexican Brand Names Fermalac® (Canada); Lacteol® Fort (Mexico); Sinuberase® (Mexico)

Therapeutic Category Antidiarrheal

Use Treatment of uncomplicated diarrhea particularly that caused by antibiotic therapy; re-establish normal physiologic and bacterial flora of the intestinal tract

Usual Dosage Children >3 years and Adults: Oral:
Capsules: 2 capsules 2-4 times/day
Granules: 1 packet added to or taken with cereal, food, milk, fruit juice, or water, 3-4 times/day
Powder: 1 teaspoonful daily with liquid
Tablet, chewable: 4 tablets 3-4 times/day; may follow each dose with a small amount of milk, fruit juice, or water

Mechanism of Action Creates an environment unfavorable to potentially pathogenic fungi or bacteria through the production of lactic acid, and favors establishment of an aciduric flora, thereby suppressing the growth of pathogenic microorganisms; helps re-establish normal intestinal flora

Local Anesthetic/Vasoconstrictor Precautions No information available to require special precautions

Effects on Dental Treatment No effects or complications reported

Other Adverse Effects 1% to 10%: Intestinal flatus

Drug Interactions No data reported

Drug Uptake Absorption: Oral: Not absorbed

Pregnancy Risk Factor No rating

Lactrase® [OTC] *see Lactase on previous page*

Lactulose (lak' tyoo lose)
Brand Names Cephulac®; Cholac®; Chronulac®; Constilac®; Constulose®; Duphalac®; Enulose®; Evalose®; Hepalac®; Lactulose PSE®

Therapeutic Category Ammonium Detoxicant; Laxative, Miscellaneous

Use Adjunct in the prevention and treatment of portal-systemic encephalopathy (PSE); treatment of chronic constipation

Usual Dosage Diarrhea may indicate overdosage and responds to dose reduction
Prevention of portal systemic encephalopathy (PSE): Oral:
Older Children: Daily dose of 40-90 mL divided 3-4 times/day; if initial dose causes diarrhea, then reduce it immediately; adjust dosage to produce 2-3 stools/day
Constipation:
Children: 5 g/day (7.5 mL) after breakfast

Adults:
Acute PSE:
Oral: 20-30 g (30-45 mL) every 1-2 hours to induce rapid laxation; adjust dosage daily to produce 2-3 soft stools; doses of 30-45 mL may be given hourly to cause rapid laxation, then reduce to recommended dose; usual daily dose: 60-100 g or 20-30 g (30-45 mL), 3-4 times/day
Rectal administration: 200 g (300 mL) diluted with 700 mL of H_2O or NS; administer rectally via rectal balloon catheter and retain 30-60 minutes every 4-6 hours
Constipation: Oral: 15-30 mL/day increased to 60 mL/day if necessary

Mechanism of Action The bacterial degradation of lactulose resulting in an acidic pH inhibits the diffusion of NH_3 into the blood by causing the conversion of NH_3 to NH_4+; also enhances the diffusion of NH_3 from the blood into the gut where conversion to NH_4+ occurs; produces an osmotic effect in the colon with resultant distention promoting peristalsis

Local Anesthetic/Vasoconstrictor Precautions No information available to require special precautions

Effects on Dental Treatment No effects or complications reported

Other Adverse Effects
>10%: Gastrointestinal: Flatulence, diarrhea (excessive dose)
1% to 10%: Gastrointestinal: Abdominal discomfort, nausea, vomiting

488

Drug Uptake
Absorption: Oral: Not absorbed appreciably following administration; this is desirable since the intended site of action is within the colon
Pregnancy Risk Factor C

Lactulose PSE® see Lactulose *on previous page*
Ladakamycin see Azacitidine *on page 88*
Lamictal® see Lamotrigine *on this page*
Lamisil® see Terbinafine *on page 822*

Lamivudine (la mi′ vyoo deen)
Related Information
Systemic Viral Diseases *on page 934*
Brand Names Epivir®
Therapeutic Category Antiviral Agent, Oral
Synonyms 3TC
Use In combination with zidovudine for treatment of HIV infection when therapy is warranted based on clinical and/or immunological evidence of disease progression
Usual Dosage Oral:
Children 3 months to 12 years: 4 mg/kg twice daily (maximum: 150 mg twice daily) with zidovudine
Adolescents 12-16 years and Adults: 150 mg twice daily with zidovudine
Adults <50 kg: 2 mg/kg twice daily with zidovudine
Local Anesthetic/Vasoconstrictor Precautions No information available to require special precautions
Effects on Dental Treatment No effects or complications reported
Drug Uptake
Absorption: Oral: Rapid in HIV-infected patients
Serum half-life:
Children: 2 hours
Adults: 5-7 hours

Lamotrigina (Mexico) see Lamotrigine *on this page*

Lamotrigine (la moe′ tri jeen)
Brand Names Lamictal®
Therapeutic Category Anticonvulsant, Miscellaneous
Synonyms Lamotrigina (Mexico)
Use Partial/secondary generalized seizures in adults; childhood epilepsy (not approved for use in children <16 years of age)
Usual Dosage Oral:
Children: 2-15 mg/kg/day in 2 divided doses
Adults: Initial dose: 50-100 mg/day then titrate to daily maintenance dose of 100-400 mg/day in 1-2 divided daily doses
With concomitant valproic acid therapy: Start initial dose at 25 mg/day then titrate to maintenance dose of 50-200 mg/day in 1-2 divided daily doses
Mechanism of Action A triazine derivative which inhibits release of glutamate (an excitatory amino acid) and inhibits voltage-sensitive sodium channels, which stabilizes neuronal membranes
Local Anesthetic/Vasoconstrictor Precautions No information available to require special precautions
Effects on Dental Treatment No effects or complications reported
Other Adverse Effects 1% to 10%:
Central nervous system: Dizziness, sedation, ataxia
Dermatologic: Hypersensitivity rash, Stevens-Johnson syndrome, angioedema
Ocular: Nystagmus, diplopia
Renal: Hematuria
Drug Interactions
Decreased effect: Acetaminophen (increases renal clearance); carbamazepine, phenobarbital, and phenytoin (increases metabolic clearance)
Increased effect: Valproic acid increases half-life of lamotrigine (decreased metabolic clearance)
Drug Uptake
Serum half-life: 24 hours; increases to 59 hours with concomitant valproic acid therapy; decreases with concomitant phenytoin or carbamazepine therapy to 15 hours
Pregnancy Risk Factor C

Lamprene® see Clofazimine Palmitate *on page 217*
Laniazid® see Isoniazid *on page 471*

Lanolin, Cetyl Alcohol, Glycerin, and Petrolatum
(lan' oh lin, see' til al' koe hol, glis' er in, & pe troe lay' tum)
Brand Names Lubriderm® [OTC]
Therapeutic Category Topical Skin Product
Use Treatment of dry skin
Local Anesthetic/Vasoconstrictor Precautions No information available to require special precautions
Effects on Dental Treatment No effects or complications reported
Other Adverse Effects 1% to 10%: Local irritation

Lanophyllin-GG® *see* Theophylline and Guaifenesin *on page 836*

Lanorinal® *see* Butalbital Compound *on page 133*

Lanoxicaps® *see* Digoxin *on page 280*

Lanoxin® *see* Digoxin *on page 280*

Lansoprazole (lan soe' pra zole)
Brand Names Prevacid®
Therapeutic Category Gastric Acid Secretion Inhibitor
Use Short-term treatment (up to 4 weeks) for healing and symptom relief of active duodenal ulcers (should not be used for maintenance therapy of duodenal ulcers); up to 8 weeks of treatment for all grades of erosive esophagitis (8 additional weeks can be given for incompletely healed esophageal erosions or for recurrence); and long-term treatment of pathological hypersecretory conditions, including Zollinger-Ellison syndrome
Usual Dosage
Duodenal or gastric ulcer: 30 mg once daily for 4-8 weeks
Erosive esophagitis: 30 mg once daily for 4-8 weeks
Hypersecretory conditions: 30-180 mg once daily, titrated to reduce acid secretion to <10 mEq/hour (5 mEq/hour in patients with prior gastric surgery)
Local Anesthetic/Vasoconstrictor Precautions No information available to require special precautions
Effects on Dental Treatment No effects or complications reported
Other Adverse Effects
1% to 10%:
Central nervous system: Fatigue, dizziness, headache
Gastrointestinal: Abdominal pain, diarrhea, nausea, increased appetite, hypergastrinoma
<1%:
Dermatologic: Rash
Otic: Tinnitus
Renal: Proteinuria
Pregnancy Risk Factor B

Lanvisone® Topical *see* Clioquinol and Hydrocortisone *on page 216*

Largon® Injection *see* Propiomazine Hydrochloride *on page 737*

Lariam® *see* Mefloquine Hydrochloride *on page 535*

Larodopa® *see* Levodopa *on page 495*

Larotid® *see* Amoxicillin Trihydrate *on page 58*

Lasan™ *see* Anthralin *on page 68*

Lasan HP-1™ *see* Anthralin *on page 68*

Lasix® *see* Furosemide *on page 391*

L-asparaginase *see* Asparaginase *on page 77*

Lassar's Zinc Paste *see* Zinc Oxide *on page 908*

Latanoprost
Brand Names Xalatan®
Therapeutic Category Ophthalmic Agent, Miscellaneous
Use Prostaglandin analog to reduce intraocular pressure that occurs in patients with glaucoma who cannot tolerate or have not responded to any other available treatments
Usual Dosage Adults: Ophthalmic: One drop in affected eye(s) once daily in the evening
Local Anesthetic/Vasoconstrictor Precautions No information available to require special precautions
Effects on Dental Treatment No effects or complications reported
Pregnancy Risk Factor C
Generic Available No

Lax-Pills® [OTC] *see* Phenolphthalein *on page 682*

LazerSporin-C® Otic *see* Neomycin, Polymyxin B, and Hydrocortisone *on page 610*

L-Carnitine *see* Levocarnitine *on page 494*

LCD *see* Coal Tar *on page 225*

LCR *see* Vincristine Sulfate *on page 896*

Ledercillin® VK *see* Penicillin V Potassium *on page 668*

Lederplex® [OTC] *see* Vitamin B Complex *on page 899*

Legatrin® [OTC] *see* Quinine Sulfate *on page 760*

Lente® Iletin® I *see* Insulin Preparations *on page 459*

Lente® Iletin® II *see* Insulin Preparations *on page 459*

Lente® Insulin *see* Insulin Preparations *on page 459*

Lente® L *see* Insulin Preparations *on page 459*

Lescol® *see* Fluvastatin *on page 383*

Leucovorin Calcium (loo koe vor' in kal' see um)

Brand Names Wellcovorin® Injection; Wellcovorin® Oral

Canadian/Mexican Brand Names Dalisol (Mexico); Medasavorin (Mexico)

Therapeutic Category Antidote, Methotrexate; Folic Acid Derivative

Synonyms Calcium Leucovorin; Citrovorum Factor; Folinic Acid; 5-Formyl Tetrahydrofolate

Use Antidote for folic acid antagonists; treatment of folate deficient megaloblastic anemias of infancy, sprue, pregnancy; nutritional deficiency when oral folate therapy is not possible

Usual Dosage Children and Adults:

Treatment of folic acid antagonist overdosage (eg, pyrimethamine or trimethoprim): Oral: 2-15 mg/day for 3 days or until blood counts are normal or 5 mg every 3 days; doses of 6 mg/day are needed for patients with platelet counts <100,000/mm^3

Folate-deficient megaloblastic anemia: I.M.: 1 mg/day

Megaloblastic anemia secondary to congenital deficiency of dihydrofolate reductase: I.M.: 3-6 mg/day

Rescue dose (rescue therapy should start within 24 hours of MTX therapy): I.V.: 10 mg/m^2 to start, then 10 mg/m^2 every 6 hours orally for 72 hours until serum MTX concentration is <10^{-8} molar; if serum creatinine 24 hours after methotrexate is elevated 50% or more above the pre-MTX serum creatinine **or** the serum MTX concentration is >5 x 10^{-6} molar (see graph), increase dose to 100 mg/m^2/dose every 3 hours until serum methotrexate level is <1 x 10^{-8} molar

Investigational: Post I.T. methotrexate: Oral, I.V.: 12 mg/m^2 as a single dose; post high-dose methotrexate: 100-1000 mg/m^2/dose until the serum methotrexate level is less than 1 x 10^{-7} molar

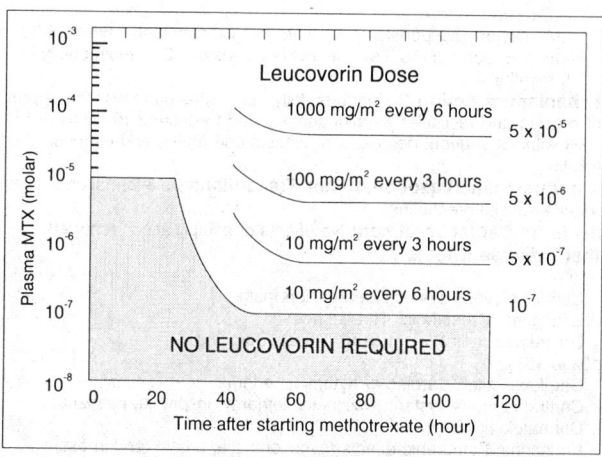

The drug should be given parenterally instead of orally in patients with GI toxicity, nausea, vomiting, and when individual doses are >25 mg
(Continued)

Leucovorin Calcium *(Continued)*

Mechanism of Action A reduced form of folic acid, but does not require a reduction reaction by an enzyme for activation, allows for purine and thymidine synthesis, a necessity for normal erythropoiesis; leucovorin supplies the necessary cofactor blocked by MTX, enters the cells via the same active transport system as MTX

Local Anesthetic/Vasoconstrictor Precautions No information available to require special precautions

Effects on Dental Treatment No effects or complications reported

Other Adverse Effects <1%:
Dermatologic: Rash, pruritus, erythema, urticaria
Hematologic: Thrombocytosis
Respiratory: Wheezing

Drug Uptake
Onset of activity:
Oral: Within 30 minutes
I.V.: Within 5 minutes
Absorption: Oral, I.M.: Rapid
Serum half-life:
Leucovorin: 15 minutes
5MTHF: 33-35 minutes

Pregnancy Risk Factor C

Comments Drug should be given parenterally instead of orally in patients with GI toxicity, nausea, vomiting, and when individual doses are >25 mg

Leukeran® *see* Chlorambucil *on page 181*

Leukine™ *see* Sargramostim *on page 780*

Leuprolide Acetate *(loo proe' lide as' e tate)*

Brand Names Lupron®; Lupron® Depot; Lupron® Depot-Ped

Canadian/Mexican Brand Names Lucrin (Mexico); Lucrin Depot (Mexico)

Therapeutic Category Antineoplastic Agent, Hormone (Gonadotropin Hormone-Releasing Antigen); Gonadotropin Releasing Hormone Analog

Synonyms Leuprorelin Acetate

Use Treatment of precocious puberty; palliative treatment of advanced prostate carcinoma

Usual Dosage Requires parenteral administration
Children: Precocious puberty:
S.C.: 20-45 mcg/kg/day
I.M. (Depot®) formulation: 0.3 mg/kg/dose given every 28 days
≤25 kg: 7.5 mg
>25-37.5 kg: 11.25 mg
>37.5 kg: 15 mg
Adults:
Male: Advanced prostatic carcinoma:
S.C.: 1 mg/day **or**
I.M., Depot® (suspension): 7.5 mg/dose given monthly (every 28-33 days)
Female: Endometriosis: I.M., Depot® (suspension): 3.75 mg monthly for up to 6 months

Mechanism of Action Continuous daily administration results in suppression of ovarian and testicular steroidogenesis due to decreased levels of LH and FSH with subsequent decrease in testosterone (male) and estrogen (female) levels

Local Anesthetic/Vasoconstrictor Precautions No information available to require special precautions

Effects on Dental Treatment No effects or complications reported

Other Adverse Effects
>10%:
Central nervous system: Depression, pain
Endocrine & metabolic: Hot flashes
Gastrointestinal: Weight gain, nausea, vomiting
1% to 10%:
Cardiovascular: Cardiac arrhythmias, edema
Central nervous system: Dizziness, lethargy, insomnia, headache
Dermatologic: Rash
Endocrine: Estrogenic effects (gynecomastia, breast tenderness)
Gastrointestinal: Nausea, vomiting, diarrhea, GI bleed
Hematologic: Decreased hemoglobin and hematocrit
Neuromuscular & skeletal: Paresthesia, myalgia
Ocular: Blurred vision

<1%:
Cardiovascular: Myocardial infarction
Local: Thrombophlebitis
Respiratory: Pulmonary embolism

Drug Uptake
Onset of action: Serum testosterone levels first increase within 3 days of therapy
Duration: Levels decrease after 2-4 weeks with continued therapy
Serum half-life: 3-4.25 hours

Pregnancy Risk Factor X

Comments Has the advantage of not increasing risk of atherosclerotic vascular disease, causing swelling of breasts, fluid retention, and thromboembolism as compared to estrogen therapy

Leuprorelin Acetate see Leuprolide Acetate on previous page

Leurocristine see Vincristine Sulfate on page 896

Leustatin™ see Cladribine on page 211

Levamisole Hydrochloride (lee vam' i sole hye droe klor' ide)
Brand Names Ergamisol®
Therapeutic Category Immune Modulator
Use Adjuvant treatment with fluorouracil in Dukes stage C colon cancer
Usual Dosage Adults: Oral: Initial: 50 mg every 8 hours for 3 days, then 50 mg every 8 hours for 3 days every 2 weeks (fluorouracil is always given concomitantly)

Mechanism of Action Clinically, combined therapy with levamisole and 5-fluorouracil has been effective in treating colon cancer patients, whereas demonstrable activity has been. Due to the broad range of pharmacologic activities of levamisole, it has been suggested that the drug may act as a biochemical modulator (of fluorouracil, for example, in colon cancer), an effect entirely independent of immune modulation. Further studies are needed to evaluate the mechanisms of action of the drug in cancer patients.

Local Anesthetic/Vasoconstrictor Precautions No information available to require special precautions

Effects on Dental Treatment No effects or complications reported

Other Adverse Effects
>10%: Gastrointestinal: Nausea, diarrhea
1% to 10%:
Cardiovascular: Edema
Central nervous system: Fatigue, fever, dizziness, headache, somnolence, depression, nervousness, insomnia
Dermatologic: Dermatitis, alopecia
Gastrointestinal: Stomatitis, vomiting, anorexia, abdominal pain, constipation, taste perversion
Hematologic: Leukopenia
Neuromuscular & skeletal: Rigors, arthralgia, myalgia, paresthesia
Miscellaneous: Infection
<1%:
Cardiovascular: Chest pain
Central nervous system: Anxiety
Dermatologic: Pruritus, urticaria
Gastrointestinal: Flatulence, dyspepsia
Hematologic: Thrombocytopenia, anemia, granulocytopenia
Ocular: Abnormal tearing, blurred vision, conjunctivitis
Respiratory: Epistaxis
Miscellaneous: Altered sense of smell

Drug Uptake
Absorption: Well absorbed
Half-life, elimination: 2-6 hours
Time to peak serum concentration: 1-2 hours

Pregnancy Risk Factor C

Comments Should not be used at dose exceeding the recommended dose or frequency due to increasing adverse reactions

Levatol® see Penbutolol Sulfate on page 664

Levlen® see Ethinyl Estradiol and Levonorgestrel on page 337

Levobunolol Hydrochloride
(lee voe byoo' noe lole hye droe klor' ide)
Brand Names AKBeta®; Betagan®
Therapeutic Category Antiglaucoma Agent; Beta-Adrenergic Blocker, Ophthalmic
(Continued)

Levobunolol Hydrochloride *(Continued)*

Use To lower intraocular pressure in chronic open-angle glaucoma or ocular hypertension

Usual Dosage Adults: Instill 1 drop in the affected eye(s) 1-2 times/day

Mechanism of Action A nonselective beta-adrenergic blocking agent that lowers intraocular pressure by reducing aqueous humor production and possibly increases the outflow of aqueous humor

Local Anesthetic/Vasoconstrictor Precautions No information available to require special precautions

Effects on Dental Treatment No effects or complications reported

Other Adverse Effects
>10%: Ocular: Stinging/burning of eye
1% to 10%:
  Cardiovascular: Bradycardia, arrhythmia, hypotension
  Central nervous system: Dizziness, headache
  Dermatologic: Alopecia, erythema
  Local: Stinging, burning
  Ocular: Blepharoconjunctivitis, conjunctivitis
  Respiratory: Bronchospasm
<1%:
  Dermatologic: Skin rash
  Local: Itching
  Ocular: Visual disturbances, keratitis, decreased visual acuity

Drug Interactions
  Increased toxicity:
  Systemic beta-adrenergic blocking agents
  Ophthalmic epinephrine (increased blood pressure/loss of IOP effect)
  Quinidine (sinus bradycardia)
  Verapamil (bradycardia and asystole have been reported)

Drug Uptake
  Onset of action: Decreases in intraocular pressure (IOP) can be noted within 1 hour
  Peak effect: 2-6 hours
  Duration: 1-7 days

Pregnancy Risk Factor C

Levocabastine Hydrochloride

(lee' voe kab as teen hye droe klor' ide)

Brand Names Livostin®

Canadian/Mexican Brand Names Livostin® Nasal (Mexico); Livostin® Oftalmico (Mexico)

Therapeutic Category Ophthalmic Agent, Miscellaneous

Use Treatment of allergic conjunctivitis

Usual Dosage Children >12 years and Adults: Instill 1 drop in affected eye(s) 4 times/day for up to 2 weeks

Mechanism of Action Potent, selective histamine H_1-receptor antagonist for topical ophthalmic use

Local Anesthetic/Vasoconstrictor Precautions No information available to require special precautions

Effects on Dental Treatment No effects or complications reported

Other Adverse Effects
>10%: Local: Transient burning, stinging, discomfort
1% to 10%:
  Central nervous system: Headache, somnolence, fatigue
  Dermatologic: Rash
  Gastrointestinal: Dry mouth
  Ocular: Blurred vision, eye pain, somnolence, red eyes, eyelid edema
  Respiratory: Dyspnea

Drug Interactions No data reported

Drug Uptake Absorption: Topical: Systemically absorbed

Pregnancy Risk Factor B

Levocarnitine (lee voe kar' ni teen)

Brand Names Carnitor® Injection; Carnitor® Oral; Vitacarn® Oral

Therapeutic Category Dietary Supplement

Synonyms L-Carnitine

Use Treatment of primary or secondary carnitine deficiency

Local Anesthetic/Vasoconstrictor Precautions No information available to require special precautions

Effects on Dental Treatment No effects or complications reported
Comments Tolerance may be improved by mixing the product with liquids or food and spacing doses evenly throughout the day with meals

Levodopa (lee voe doe' pa)
Brand Names Dopar®; Larodopa®
Therapeutic Category Anti-Parkinson's Agent
Use Treatment of Parkinson's disease; used as a diagnostic agent for growth hormone deficiency
Usual Dosage Oral:
Children (give as a single dose to evaluate growth hormone deficiency):
0.5 g/m² **or**
<30 lbs: 125 mg
30-70 lbs: 250 mg
>70 lbs: 500 mg

Adults: 500-1000 mg/day in divided doses every 6-12 hours; increase by 100-750 mg/day every 3-7 days until response or total dose of 8,000 mg is reached

A significant therapeutic response may not be obtained for 6 months
Mechanism of Action Increases dopamine levels in the brain, then stimulates dopaminergic receptors in the basal ganglia to improve the balance between cholinergic and dopaminergic activity
Local Anesthetic/Vasoconstrictor Precautions No information available to require special precautions
Effects on Dental Treatment No effects or complications reported
Other Adverse Effects
>10%:
Cardiovascular: Orthostatic hypotension, arrhythmias
Central nervous system: Choreiform and involuntary movements, dizziness, anxiety, confusion, nightmares
Gastrointestinal: Anorexia, nausea, vomiting, constipation
Ocular: Blepharospasm
Renal: Difficult urination
1% to 10%:
Central nervous system: Headache
Gastrointestinal: Anorexia, diarrhea, dry mouth
Neuromuscular & skeletal: Muscle twitching
Ocular: Eyelid spasms
Renal: Discoloration of urine/sweat
<1%:
Cardiovascular: Hypertension
Gastrointestinal: Duodenal ulcer, GI bleeding
Hematologic: Hemolytic anemia
Ocular: Blurred vision
Drug Interactions
Decreased effect:
Hydantoins cause decreased effectiveness of levodopa
Phenothiazines and hypotensive agents cause decreased effect of levodopa
Pyridoxine causes increased peripheral conversion, causing decreased levodopa effectiveness
Increased toxicity:
Monoamine oxidase inhibitors may increase hypertensive reactions
Antacids cause increased levodopa
Drug Uptake
Time to peak serum concentration: Oral: 1-2 hours
Serum half-life: 1.2-2.3 hours
Pregnancy Risk Factor C

Levodopa and Carbidopa (lee voe doe' pa & kar bi doe' pa)
Brand Names Sinemet®
Canadian/Mexican Brand Names Racovel® (Mexico)
Therapeutic Category Anti-Parkinson's Agent
Use Treatment of parkinsonian syndrome; 50-100 mg/day of carbidopa is needed to block the peripheral conversion of levodopa to dopamine. "On-off" can be managed by giving smaller, more frequent doses of Sinemet® or adding a dopamine agonist or selegiline; when adding a new agent, doses of Sinemet® should usually be decreased.
Usual Dosage Oral:
Adults: Initial: 25/100 2-4 times/day, increase as necessary to a maximum of 200/2000 mg/day
(Continued)

Levodopa and Carbidopa *(Continued)*

Elderly: Initial: 25/100 twice daily, increase as necessary

Conversion from Sinemet® to Sinemet® CR (50/200): (Sinemet® [total daily dose of levodopa] / Sinemet® CR)

300-400 mg / 1 tablet twice daily

500-600 mg / 1½ tablets twice daily or one 3 times/day

700-800 mg / 4 tablets in 3 or more divided doses

900-1000 mg / 5 tablets in 3 or more divided doses

Intervals between doses of Sinemet® CR should be 4-8 hours while awake

Mechanism of Action Parkinson's symptoms are due to a lack of striatal dopamine; levodopa circulates in the plasma to the blood-brain-barrier (BBB), where it crosses, to be converted by striatal enzymes to dopamine; carbidopa inhibits the peripheral plasma breakdown of levodopa by inhibiting its decarboxylation, and thereby increases available levodopa at the BBB

Local Anesthetic/Vasoconstrictor Precautions No information available to require special precautions

Effects on Dental Treatment No effects or complications reported

Other Adverse Effects

>10%:

Cardiovascular: Orthostatic hypotension, palpitations, cardiac arrhythmias

Central nervous system: Confusion, nightmares, dizziness, anxiety

Gastrointestinal: Nausea, vomiting, anorexia, constipation

Neuromuscular & skeletal: Dystonic movements, "on-off", choreiform and involuntary movements

Ocular: Blepharospasm

Renal: Difficult urination

1% to 10%:

Central nervous system: Headache, muscle twitching

Gastrointestinal: Anorexia, diarrhea, dry mouth

Ocular: Eyelid spasms

Miscellaneous: Discoloration of urine/sweat

<1%:

Cardiovascular: Hypertension

Central nervous system: Memory loss, nervousness, anxiety, insomnia, fatigue, hallucinations, ataxia

Gastrointestinal: Duodenal ulcer, GI bleeding

Hematologic: Hemolytic anemia

Ocular: Blurred vision

Drug Interactions

Decreased effect:

Hydantoins cause decreased effectiveness

Phenothiazines and hypotensive agents cause decreased effect of levodopa

Increased toxicity: Monoamine oxidase inhibitors may increase hypertensive reactions

Drug Uptake

Carbidopa:

Absorption: Oral: 40% to 70%

Serum half-life: 1-2 hours

Levodopa:

Absorption: May be decreased if given with a high protein meal

Serum half-life: 1.2-2.3 hours

Pregnancy Risk Factor C

Levo-Dromoran® *see* Levorphanol Tartrate *on next page*

Levomepromazine *see* Methotrimeprazine Hydrochloride *on page 562*

Levomethadyl Acetate Hydrochloride

(lee voe meth' a dil as' e tate hye droe klor' ide)

Brand Names ORLAAM®

Therapeutic Category Analgesic, Narcotic

Use Management of opiate dependence

Usual Dosage Adults: Oral: 20-40 mg 3 times/week, with ranges of 10 mg to as high as 140 mg 3 times/week; always dilute before administration and mix with diluent prior to dispensing

Local Anesthetic/Vasoconstrictor Precautions No information available to require special precautions

Effects on Dental Treatment No effects or complications reported

Other Adverse Effects

>10%:

Cardiovascular: Bradycardia, hypotension

Central nervous system: Drowsiness
Gastrointestinal: Nausea, vomiting
Respiratory: Respiratory depression
1% to 10%:
Cardiovascular: Peripheral vasodilation, orthostatic hypotension, increased intracranial pressure
Central nervous system: Dizziness/vertigo, CNS depression, confusion, sedation
Endocrine & metabolic: Antidiuretic hormone release
Gastrointestinal: Constipation
Ocular: Miosis, blurred vision
Miscellaneous: Biliary or urinary tract spasm
Drug Interactions Decreased effect/levels with phenobarbital
Pregnancy Risk Factor C

Levonorgestrel (lee' voe nor jes trel)
Related Information
Endocrine Disorders & Pregnancy *on page 927*
Brand Names Norplant®
Canadian/Mexican Brand Names Microlut® (Mexico)
Therapeutic Category Contraceptive, Implant (Progestin); Contraceptive, Progestin Only; Progestin Derivative
Use Prevention of pregnancy. The net cumulative 5 year pregnancy rate for levonorgestrel implant use has been reported to be from 1.5-3.9 pregnancies/100 users. Norplant® is a very efficient, yet reversible, method of contraception. The long duration of action may be particularly advantageous in women who desire an extended period of contraceptive protection without sacrificing the possibility of future fertility.
Usual Dosage Total administration doses (implanted): 216 mg in 6 capsules which should be implanted during the first 7 days of onset of menses subdermally in the upper arm; each Norplant® silastic capsule releases 80 mcg of drug/day for 6-18 months, following which a rate of release of 25-30 mcg/day is maintained for ≤5 years; capsules should be removed by end of 5th year
Mechanism of Action Ovulation is inhibited in about 50% to 60% of implant users from a negative feedback mechanism on the hypothalamus, leading to reduced secretion of follicle stimulating hormone (FSH) and luteinizing hormone (LH). An insufficient luteal phase has also been demonstrated with levonorgestrel administration and may result from defective gonadotropin stimulation of the ovary or from a direct effect of the drug on progesterone synthesis by the corpora lutea.
Local Anesthetic/Vasoconstrictor Precautions No information available to require special precautions
Effects on Dental Treatment No precaution is necessary in using antibiotics in Norplant® users since there is no estrogen component in Norplant®
Other Adverse Effects
>10%: Hormonal: Prolonged menstrual flow, spotting
1% to 10%:
Central nervous system: Headache, nervousness, dizziness
Dermatologic: Dermatitis, acne
Endocrine & metabolic: Amenorrhea, irregular menstrual cycles, scanty bleeding, breast discharge
Gastrointestinal: Nausea, change in appetite, weight gain
Genitourinary: Vaginitis, leukorrhea
Neuromuscular & skeletal: Myalgia
Miscellaneous: Pain or itching at implant site
<1%: Miscellaneous: Infection at implant site
Drug Interactions Decreased effect: Carbamazepine/phenytoin
Drug Uptake
Serum half-life, terminal: 11-45 hours
Pregnancy Risk Factor X

Levoprome® *see* Methotrimeprazine Hydrochloride *on page 562*
Levora® *see* Ethinyl Estradiol and Levonorgestrel *on page 337*

Levorphanol Tartrate (lee vor' fa nole tar' trate)
Related Information
Narcotic Agonist Charts *on page 1019*
Brand Names Levo-Dromoran®
Therapeutic Category Analgesic, Narcotic
(Continued)

Levorphanol Tartrate *(Continued)*

Use Relief of moderate to severe pain; also used parenterally for preoperative sedation and an adjunct to nitrous oxide/oxygen anesthesia; 2 mg levorphanol produces analgesia comparable to that produced by 10 mg of morphine

Usual Dosage Adults:

Oral: 2 mg every 6-24 hours as needed

S.C.: 2 mg, up to 3 mg if necessary, every 6-8 hours

Mechanism of Action Levorphanol tartrate is a synthetic opioid agonist that is classified as a morphinan derivative. Opioids interact with stereospecific opioid receptors in various parts of the central nervous system and other tissues. Analgesic potency parallels the affinity for these binding sites. These drugs do not alter the threshold or responsiveness to pain, but the perception of pain.

Local Anesthetic/Vasoconstrictor Precautions No information available to require special precautions

Effects on Dental Treatment Dry mouth in about 10% of patients (will disappear with cessation of therapy)

Other Adverse Effects

>10%:

Cardiovascular: Palpitations, hypotension, bradycardia, peripheral vasodilation

Central nervous system: CNS depression, weakness, tiredness, drowsiness, dizziness

Dermatologic: Pruritus

Gastrointestinal: Nausea, vomiting

1% to 10%:

Central nervous system: Nervousness, headache, restlessness, anorexia, malaise, confusion

Endocrine & metabolic: Antidiuretic hormone release

Gastrointestinal: Stomach cramps, dry mouth, constipation

Genitourinary: Decreased urination

Local: Pain at injection site

Ocular: Miosis

Respiratory: Respiratory depression

Miscellaneous: Biliary or urinary tract spasm

<1%:

Central nervous system: Paralytic ileus, mental depression, histamine release, hallucinations, paradoxical CNS stimulation

Dermatologic: Skin rash, hives

Sensitivity reactions: Histamine release

Miscellaneous: Increased intracranial pressure, physical and psychological dependence

Drug Interactions Increased toxicity: CNS depressants increased CNS depression

Pregnancy Risk Factor B (D if used for prolonged periods or in high doses at term)

Levo-T™ *see* Levothyroxine Sodium *on this page*

Levothroid® *see* Levothyroxine Sodium *on this page*

Levothyroxine Sodium (lee voe thye rox' een sow' dee um)

Related Information

Endocrine Disorders & Pregnancy *on page 927*

Brand Names Eltroxin™; Levo-T™; Levothroid®; Levoxyl™; Synthroid®

Canadian/Mexican Brand Names Eltroxin® (Canada); PMS-Levothyroxine® Sodium (Canada); Eutirox® (Mexico); Tiroidine® (Mexico)

Therapeutic Category Thyroid Product

Synonyms Levotiroxina (Mexico)

Use Replacement or supplemental therapy in hypothyroidism; some clinicians suggest levothyroxine is the drug of choice for replacement therapy

Usual Dosage

Children:

Oral:

0-6 months: 8-10 mcg/kg/day **or** 25-50 mcg/day

6-12 months: 6-8 mcg/kg/day **or** 50-75 mcg/day

1-5 years: 5-6 mcg/kg/day **or** 75-100 mcg/day

6-12 years: 4-5 mcg/kg/day **or** 100-150 mcg/day

>12 years: 2-3 mcg/kg/day **or** ≥150 mcg/day

I.M., I.V.: 50% to 75% of the oral dose

Adults:
Oral: 12.5-50 mcg/day to start, then increase by 25-50 mcg/day at intervals of 2-4 weeks; average adult dose: 100-200 mcg/day
I.M., I.V.: 50% of the oral dose

Myxedema coma or stupor: I.V.: 200-500 mcg one time, then 100-300 mcg the next day if necessary
Thyroid suppression therapy: Oral: 2-6 mcg/kg/day for 7-10 days

Mechanism of Action Exact mechanism of action is unknown; however, it is believed the thyroid hormone exerts its many metabolic effects through control of DNA transcription and protein synthesis; involved in normal metabolism, growth, and development; promotes gluconeogenesis, increases utilization and mobilization of glycogen stores, and stimulates protein synthesis, increases basal metabolic rate

Local Anesthetic/Vasoconstrictor Precautions No precautions with vasoconstrictor are necessary if patient is well controlled with levothyroxine

Effects on Dental Treatment No effects or complications reported

Other Adverse Effects <1%:
Cardiovascular: Palpitations, cardiac arrhythmias, tachycardia, chest pain
Central nervous system: Nervousness, sweating, headache, insomnia, fever, clumsiness
Dermatologic: Hair loss
Endocrine: Changes in menstrual cycle
Gastrointestinal: Weight loss, increased appetite, diarrhea, abdominal cramps, constipation
Neuromuscular & skeletal: Muscle aches, hand tremors, tremor
Respiratory: Shortness of breath

Drug Interactions
Decreased effect:
Phenytoin may decreased levothyroxine levels
Cholestyramine may decreased absorption of levothyroxine
Increases oral hypoglycemic requirements
Increased effect: Increased effects of oral anticoagulants
Increased toxicity: Tricyclic antidepressants cause increased toxic potential of both drugs

Drug Uptake
Onset of therapeutic effect:
Oral: 3-5 days
I.V. Within 6-8 hours
Peak effect: I.V.: Within 24 hours
Absorption: Oral: Erratic
Time to peak serum concentration: 2-4 hours

Pregnancy Risk Factor A

Levotiroxina (Mexico) see Levothyroxine Sodium on previous page

Levoxyl™ see Levothyroxine Sodium on previous page

Levsin® see Hyoscyamine Sulfate on page 445

Levsinex® see Hyoscyamine Sulfate on page 445

Levulose, Dextrose and Phosphoric Acid see Phosphorated Carbohydrate Solution on page 690

Librax® see Clidinium and Chlordiazepoxide on page 214

Libritabs® see Chlordiazepoxide on page 183

Librium® see Chlordiazepoxide on page 183

Lida-Mantle HC® Topical see Lidocaine and Hydrocortisone on page 501

Lidex® see Fluocinonide on page 373

Lidex-E® see Fluocinonide on page 373

Lidocaine and Epinephrine (lye' doe kane & ep i nef' rin)
Related Information
Oral Pain on page 940
Brand Names Octocaine® 50; Octocaine® 100; Xylocaine® With Epinephrine
Canadian/Mexican Brand Names Pisacaina® (Mexico); Uvega® (Mexico); Xylocaina® (Mexico)
Therapeutic Category Dental/Local Anesthetics; Local Anesthetic, Injectable
Use Dental: Amide-type anesthetic used for local infiltration anesthesia; injection near nerve trunks to produce nerve block
Usual Dosage
Children <10 years: It is rarely necessary to administer more than one-half cartridge/procedure to achieve anesthesia for a procedure involving a single tooth.
(Continued)

Lidocaine and Epinephrine (Continued)

Children >10 years and Adults: Dosage requirements should be determined on an individual basis. The least volume of solution that results in effective local anesthesia should be administered. For most routine dental procedures, lidocaine hydrochloride injection 2% with epinephrine 1:100,000 is preferred. When a more pronounced hemostasis is required, a 1:50,000 epinephrine concentration should be used

Mechanism of Action Local anesthetics bind selectively to the intracellular surface of sodium channels to block influx of sodium into the axon. As a result, depolarization necessary for action potential propagation and subsequent nerve function is prevented. The block at the sodium channel is reversible. When drug diffuses away from the axon, sodium channel function is restored and nerve propagation returns.

Epinephrine prolongs the duration of the anesthetic actions of lidocaine by causing vasoconstriction (alpha adrenergic receptor agonist) of the vasculature surrounding the nerve axons. This prevents the diffusion of lidocaine away from the nerves resulting in a longer retention in the axon.

Local Anesthetic/Vasoconstrictor Precautions No information available to require special precautions

Effects on Dental Treatment No effects or complications reported

Other Adverse Effects Degree of adverse effects in the central nervous system and cardiovascular system are directly related to the blood levels of lidocaine. The effects below are more likely to occur after systemic administration rather than infiltration.

Cardiovascular: Myocardial effects include a decrease in contraction force as well as a decrease in electrical excitability and myocardial conduction rate resulting in bradycardia and reduction in cardiac output.

Central nervous system: High blood levels result in anxiety, restlessness, disorientation, confusion, dizziness, tremors and seizures. This is followed by depression of CNS resulting in drowsiness, unconsciousness and possible respiratory arrest. Nausea and vomiting may also occur. In some cases, symptoms of CNS stimulation may be absent and the primary CNS effects are drowsiness and unconsciousness.

Hypersensitivity reactions: Extremely rare, but may be manifest as dermatologic reactions and edema at injection site. Asthmatic syndromes have occurred. Patients may exhibit hypersensitivity to bisulfites contained in local anesthetic solution to prevent oxidation of epinephrine. In general, patients reacting to bisulfites have a history of asthma and their airways are hyperreactive to asthmatic syndrome.

Psychogenic reactions: It is common to misinterpret psychogenic responses to local anesthetic injection as an allergic reaction. Intraoral injections are perceived by many patients as a stressful procedure in dentistry. Common symptoms to this stress are sweating, palpitations, hyperventilation, generalized pallor and a fainting feeling

Oral manifestations: No data reported

Contraindications Hypersensitivity to local anesthetics of the amide-type

Warnings/Precautions Should be avoided in patients with uncontrolled hyperthyroidism. Should be used in minimal amounts in patients with significant cardiovascular problems (because of epinephrine component). Aspirate the syringe after tissue penetration and before injection to minimize chance of direct vascular injection.

Drug Interactions Due to epinephrine component, use with tricyclic antidepressants or MAO inhibitors could result in increased pressor response; use with nonselective beta-blockers (ie, propranolol) could result in serious hypertension and reflex bradycardia

Drug Uptake
Onset of action: Infiltration less than 2 minutes; nerve block 2-4 minutes
Duration after infiltration: Soft tissue anesthesia ~2.5 hours; pulp anesthesia <60 minutes
Duration after nerve block: Soft tissue anesthesia ~3.25 hours; pulp anesthesia at least 90 minutes

Pregnancy Risk Factor B

Breast-feeding Considerations Usual infiltration doses of lidocaine with epinephrine given to nursing mothers has not been shown to affect the health of the nursing infant

Dosage Forms Injection:
Lidocaine Hydrochloride 2% with epinephrine 1:100,000 (Octocaine® 100, Xylocaine®): (1.8 mL dental cartridges)

Lidocaine Hydrochloride 2% with epinephrine 1:50,000 (Octocaine® 50, Xylo-caine®): (1.8 mL dental cartridges)

Dietary Considerations No data reported

Generic Available Yes

Selected Readings

Jastak JT and Yagiela JA, "Vasoconstrictors and Local Anesthesia: A Review and Rationale for Use," *J Am Dent Assoc*, 1983, 107(4):623-30.

MacKenzie TA and Young ER, "Local Anesthetic Update," *Anesth Prog*, 1993, 40(2):29-34.

Wynn RL, "Epinephrine Interactions With Beta-Blockers," *Gen Dent*, 1994, 42(1):16, 18.

Yagiela JA, "Local Anesthetics," *Anesth Prog*, 1991, 38(4-5):128-41.

Lidocaine and Hydrocortisone

(lye' doe kane & hye droe kor' ti sone)

Brand Names Lida-Mantle HC® Topical

Therapeutic Category Corticosteroid, Topical (Low Potency); Local Anesthetic, Topical

Use Topical anti-inflammatory and anesthetic for skin disorders

Local Anesthetic/Vasoconstrictor Precautions No information available to require special precautions

Effects on Dental Treatment No effects or complications reported

Lidocaine and Prilocaine (lye' doe kane & pril' oh kane)

Brand Names EMLA®

Therapeutic Category Analgesic, Topical; Antipruritic, Topical; Local Anesthetic, Topical

Use

Dental: Amide-type topical anesthetic for use on normal intact skin to provide local analgesia for minor procedures such as I.V. cannulation or venipuncture

Medical: Has also been used for painful procedures such as lumbar puncture and skin graft harvesting

Mechanism of Action Local anesthetics bind selectively to the intracellular surface of sodium channels to block influx of sodium into the axon. As a result, depolarization necessary for action potential propagation and subsequent nerve function is prevented. The block at the sodium channel is reversible. When drug diffuses away from the axon, sodium channel function is restored and nerve propagation returns.

Local Anesthetic/Vasoconstrictor Precautions No information available to require special precautions

Effects on Dental Treatment No effects or complications reported

Other Adverse Effects 1% to 10%:

Dermatologic: Angioedema, contact dermatitis

Local: Burning, stinging

Oral manifestations: No data reported

Contraindications Known hypersensitivity to lidocaine, prilocaine, any component or local anesthetics of the amide type; patients with congenital or idiopathic methemoglobinemia, infants <1 month of age, infants <12 months of age who are receiving concurrent treatment with methemoglobin-inducing agents (ie, sulfas, acetaminophen, benzocaine, chloroquine, dapsone, nitrofurantoin, nitroglycerin, nitroprusside, phenobarbital, phenytoin)

Warnings/Precautions Use with caution in patients receiving class I antiarrhythmic drugs, since systemic absorption occurs and synergistic toxicity is possible

Drug Interactions Increased toxicity with Class I antiarrhythmic drugs (tocainide, mexiletine) - effects are additive and potentially synergistic and with drugs known to induce methemoglobinemia

Drug Uptake

Absorption: Related to the duration of application and to the area over which it is applied

3-hour application: 3.6% lidocaine and 6.1% prilocaine were absorbed

24-hour application: 16.2% lidocaine and 33.5% prilocaine were absorbed

Onset of action: 1 hour for sufficient dermal analgesia

Peak effect: 2-3 hours

Duration: 1-2 hours after removal of the cream

Serum half-life:

Lidocaine: 65-150 minutes, prolonged with cardiac or hepatic dysfunction

Prilocaine: 10-150 minutes, prolonged in hepatic or renal dysfunction

Pregnancy Risk Factor B

Breast-feeding Considerations Usual infiltration doses of lidocaine and prilocaine given to nursing mothers has not been shown to affect the health of the nursing infant

(Continued)

Lidocaine and Prilocaine *(Continued)*

Dosage Forms Cream: Lidocaine 2.5% and prilocaine 2.5% [2 Tegaderm® dressings] (5 g, 30 g)

Dietary Considerations No data reported

Lidocaine Hydrochloride (lye' doe kane hye droe klor' ide)

Related Information
Cardiovascular Diseases *on page 912*
Oral Pain *on page 940*
Oral Viral Infections *on page 951*
Patients Undergoing Cancer Therapy *on page 967*

Brand Names Dilocaine®; Duo-Trach®; Nervocaine®; Octocaine®; Xylocaine®

Canadian/Mexican Brand Names PMS®-Lidocaine Viscous (Canada); Xylocard® (Canada); Pisacina® (Mexico); Xylocaina® (Mexico)

Therapeutic Category Antiarrhythmic Agent (Supraventricular & Ventricular); Dental/Local Anesthetics; Local Anesthetic, Injectable

Use
Dental: Amide-type injectable local anesthetic and topical local anesthetic; Patch: Production of mild topical anesthesia of accessible mucous membranes of the mouth prior to superficial dental procedures
Medical: Drug of choice for ventricular ectopy, ventricular tachycardia, ventricular fibrillation; for pulseless VT or VF preferably give **after** defibrillation and epinephrine; control of premature ventricular contractions, wide-complex PSVT

Usual Dosage Injectable local anesthetic: Varies with procedure, degree of anesthesia needed, vascularity of tissue, duration of anesthesia required, and physical condition of patient; maximum: 4.5 mg/kg/dose; do not repeat within 2 hours

Mechanism of Action Class IB antiarrhythmic; local anesthetics bind selectively to the intracellular surface of sodium channels to block influx of sodium into the axon. As a result, depolarization necessary for action potential propagation and subsequent nerve function is prevented. The block at the sodium channel is reversible. When drug diffuses away from the axon, sodium channel function is restored and nerve propagation returns.

Local Anesthetic/Vasoconstrictor Precautions No information available to require special precautions

Effects on Dental Treatment No effects or complications reported

Other Adverse Effects No data reported

Oral manifestations: No data reported

Contraindications Known hypersensitivity to amide-type local anesthetics; patients with Adams-Stokes syndrome or with severe degree of S-A, A-V, or intraventricular heart block (without a pacemaker)

Drug Interactions No data reported

Pregnancy Risk Factor C

Breast-feeding Considerations May be taken while breast-feeding

Dosage Forms
Injection: 0.5% [5 mg/mL] (50 mL); 1% [10 mg/mL] (2 mL, 5 mL, 10 mL, 20 mL, 30 mL, 50 mL); 1.5% [15 mg/mL] (20 mL); 2% [20 mg/mL] (2 mL, 5 mL, 10 mL, 20 mL, 30 mL, 50 mL); 4% [40 mg/mL] (5 mL)
Liquid, viscous: 2% (20 mL, 100 mL)

Dietary Considerations No data reported

Generic Available Yes

Comments Lidocaine without epinephrine is not marketed as a dental 1.8 mL carpule and as such is not used as a dental local anesthetic

Lidocaine Transoral (lye' doe kane)

Related Information
Oral Pain *on page 940*

Brand Names Dentipatch®

Therapeutic Category Local Anesthetic, Transoral

Use Local anesthesia of the oral mucosa prior to oral injections and soft-tissue dental procedures

Usual Dosage One patch on selected area of oral mucosa

Mechanism of Action Blocks both the initiation and conduction of nerve impulses by decreasing the neuronal membrane's permeability to sodium ions, which results in inhibition of depolarization with resultant blockade of conduction

Local Anesthetic/Vasoconstrictor Precautions No information available to require special precautions

Effects on Dental Treatment No effects or complications reported
Other Adverse Effects Oral manifestations: No data reported
Contraindications Known hypersensitivity to any of its components
Drug Uptake
  Onset of action: 2 minutes
  Duration of anesthesia after patch application: 45 minutes
Dosage Forms Patch: 23 mg/2 cm^2, 46.1 mg/2 cm^2 (50s, 100s)
Generic Available No
Comments The manufacturer claims Dentipatch® is safe, with "negligible systemic absorption" of lidocaine. The agent is "clinically proven to prevent injection pain from 25-gauge needles that are inserted to the level of the bone."
Selected Readings Hersh EV, Houpt MI, Cooper SA, et al, "Analgesic Efficacy and Safety of an Intraoral Lidocaine Patch," *JADA*, 1996, 127:1626-34.

Lidox® *see* Clidinium and Chlordiazepoxide *on page 214*
Limbitrol® *see* Amitriptyline and Chlordiazepoxide *on page 49*
Lincocin® *see* Lincomycin *on this page*
Lincomicina (Mexico) *see* Lincomycin *on this page*

Lincomycin (lin koe mye′ sin)
Brand Names Lincocin®
Canadian/Mexican Brand Names Princol® (Mexico)
Therapeutic Category Antibiotic, Macrolide
Synonyms Lincomicina (Mexico)
Use Treatment of susceptible bacterial infections, mainly those caused by streptococci and staphylococci resistant to other agents
Usual Dosage
  Children >1 month:
    Oral: 30-60 mg/kg/day in divided doses every 8 hours
    I.M.: 10 mg/kg every 8-12 hours
    I.V.: 10-20 mg/kg/day in divided doses every 8-12 hours

  Adults:
    Oral: 500 mg every 6-8 hours
    I.M.: 600 mg every 12-24 hours
    I.V.: 600-1 g every 8-12 hours up to 8 g/day
Mechanism of Action Lincosamide antibiotic which was isolated from a strain of *Streptomyces lincolnensis*; lincomycin, like clindamycin, inhibits bacterial protein synthesis by specifically binding on the 50S subunit and affecting the process of peptide chain initiation. Other macrolide antibiotics (erythromycin) also bind to the 50S subunit. Since only one molecule of antibiotic can bind to a single ribosome, the concomitant use of erythromycin and lincomycin is not recommended.
Local Anesthetic/Vasoconstrictor Precautions No information available to require special precautions
Effects on Dental Treatment No effects or complications reported
Other Adverse Effects
  1% to 10%: Gastrointestinal: Nausea, vomiting, diarrhea
  <1%:
    Cardiovascular: Hypotension
    Central nervous system: Vertigo
    Dermatologic: Urticaria, rash, Stevens-Johnson syndrome
    Gastrointestinal: Pseudomembranous colitis, glossitis, stomatitis, pruritus
    Genitourinary: Vaginitis
    Hematologic: Granulocytopenia, thrombocytopenia, pancytopenia
    Hepatic: Elevation of liver enzymes
    Local: Sterile abscess at I.M. injection site, thrombophlebitis
    Otic: Tinnitus
Drug Interactions
  Decreased effect with erythromycin
  Increased activity/toxicity of neuromuscular blocking agents
Drug Uptake
  Absorption: Oral: ~20% to 30%
  Serum half-life, elimination: 2-11.5 hours
  Time to peak serum concentration:
    Oral: 2-4 hours
    I.M.: 1 hour
Pregnancy Risk Factor B

ALPHABETICAL LISTING OF DRUGS

Lindane (lin′ dane)
Brand Names G-well®; Kwell®; Scabene®
Canadian/Mexican Brand Names Hexit® (Canada); Kwellada® (Canada); PMS-Lindane® (Canada); Herklin® (Mexico); Scabisan® Shampoo (Mexico)
Therapeutic Category Antiparasitic Agent, Topical; Pediculocide; Scabicidal Agent; Shampoos
Synonyms Lindano (Mexico)
Use Treatment of scabies (*Sarcoptes scabiei*), *Pediculus capitis* (head lice), and *Pediculus pubis* (crab lice)
Usual Dosage Children and Adults: Topical:
Scabies: Apply a thin layer of lotion or cream and massage it on skin from the neck to the toes (head to toe in infants). For adults, bathe and remove the drug after 8-12 hours; for children, wash off 6-8 hours after application (for infants, wash off 6 hours after application); repeat treatment in 7 days if lice or nits are still present
Pediculosis, capitis and pubis: 15-30 mL of shampoo is applied and lathered for 4-5 minutes; rinse hair thoroughly and comb with a fine tooth comb to remove nits; repeat treatment in 7 days if lice or nits are still present
Mechanism of Action Directly absorbed by parasites and ova through the exoskeleton; stimulates the nervous system resulting in seizures and death of parasitic arthropods
Local Anesthetic/Vasoconstrictor Precautions No information available to require special precautions
Effects on Dental Treatment No effects or complications reported
Other Adverse Effects <1%:
Cardiovascular: Cardiac arrhythmia
Central nervous system: Dizziness, restlessness, seizures, headache, ataxia
Dermatologic: Eczematous eruptions, contact dermatitis, skin and adipose tissue may act as repositories
Gastrointestinal: Nausea, vomiting
Hematologic: Aplastic anemia
Hepatic: Hepatitis
Local: Burning and stinging
Neuromuscular & skeletal: Ataxia
Renal: Hematuria
Respiratory: Pulmonary edema
Drug Interactions Increased toxicity: Oil-based hair dressing may increase toxic potential
Drug Uptake
Absorption: Systemic absorption of up to 13% may occur
Serum half-life: Children: 17-22 hours
Time to peak serum concentration: Topical: Children: 6 hours
Pregnancy Risk Factor B

Lindano (Mexico) *see* Lindane *on this page*
Lioresal® *see* Baclofen *on page 95*

Liothyronine Sodium (lye oh thye′ roe neen sow′ dee um)
Related Information
Endocrine Disorders & Pregnancy *on page 927*
Brand Names Cytomel®; Triostat™
Therapeutic Category Thyroid Product
Use Replacement or supplemental therapy in hypothyroidism, management of nontoxic goiter, chronic lymphocytic thyroiditis, as an adjunct in thyrotoxicosis and as a diagnostic aid; **levothyroxine is recommended for chronic therapy**
Usual Dosage
Congenital hypothyroidism: Children: Oral: 5 mcg/day increase by 5 mcg every 3 days to 20 mcg/day for infants, 50 mcg/day for children 1-3 years of age, and give adult dose for children >3 years.

Hypothyroidism: Oral:
Adults: 25 mcg/day increase by 12.5-25 mcg/day every 1-2 weeks to a maximum of 100 mcg/day
Elderly: Initial: 5 mcg/day, increase by 5 mcg/day every 1-2 weeks; usual maintenance dose: 25-75 mcg/day

T_3 suppression test: Oral: 75-100 mcg/day for 7 days; use lowest dose for elderly

Myxedema coma: I.V.: 25-50 mcg
Patients with known or suspected cardiovascular disease: 10-20 mcg
Note: Normally, at least 4 hours should be allowed between doses to adequately assess therapeutic response and no more than 12 hours

should elapse between doses to avoid fluctuations in hormone levels. Oral therapy should be resumed as soon as the clinical situation has been stabilized and the patient is able to take oral medication. If levothyroxine rather than liothyronine sodium is used in initiating oral therapy, the physician should bear in mind that there is a delay of several days in the onset of levothyroxine activity and that I.V. therapy should be discontinued gradually.

Mechanism of Action Primary active compound is T_3 (tri-iodothyronine), which may be converted from T_4 (thyroxine) and then circulates throughout the body to influence growth and maturation of various tissues; exact mechanism of action is unknown; however, it is believed the thyroid hormone exerts its many metabolic effects through control of DNA transcription and protein synthesis; involved in normal metabolism, growth, and development; promotes gluconeogenesis, increases utilization and mobilization of glycogen stores, and stimulates protein synthesis, increases basal metabolic rate

Local Anesthetic/Vasoconstrictor Precautions No precautions with vasoconstrictor are necessary if patient is well controlled with liothyronine

Effects on Dental Treatment No effects or complications reported

Other Adverse Effects <1%:

Cardiovascular: Palpitations, sweating, tachycardia, cardiac arrhythmias, chest pain

Central nervous system: Nervousness, insomnia, fever, headache, insomnia, clumsiness

Dermatologic: Hair loss

Endocrine & metabolic: Changes in menstrual cycle

Gastrointestinal: Weight loss, increased appetite, diarrhea, abdominal cramps, constipation

Neuromuscular & skeletal: Muscle aches, hand tremors, tremor

Respiratory: Shortness of breath

Drug Interactions

Decreased effect:
Cholestyramine resin causes decreased absorption of liothyronine
Antidiabetic drug requirements are increased
Estrogens cause increased thyroid requirements

Increased effect: Increased oral anticoagulant effects

Drug Uptake

Onset of effect: Within 24-72 hours

Duration: Up to 72 hours

Absorption: Oral: Well absorbed (~85% to 90%)

Serum half-life: 16-49 hours

Pregnancy Risk Factor A

Liotrix (lye' oh trix)

Related Information

Endocrine Disorders & Pregnancy on page 927

Brand Names Euthroid®; Thyrolar®

Therapeutic Category Thyroid Product

Use Replacement or supplemental therapy in hypothyroidism (uniform mixture of T_4:T_3 in 4:1 ratio by weight); little advantage to this product exists and cost is not justified

Usual Dosage Oral:

Congenital hypothyroidism:

Children (dose of T_4 or levothyroxine/day):
0-6 months: 8-10 mcg/kg or 25-50 mcg/day
6-12 months: 6-8 mcg/kg or 50-75 mcg/day
1-5 years: 5-6 mcg/kg or 75-100 mcg/day
6-12 years: 4-5 mcg/kg or 100-150 mcg/day
>12 years: 2-3 mcg/kg or >150 mcg/day

Hypothyroidism (dose of thyroid equivalent):
Adults: 30 mg/day, increasing by 15 mg/day at 2- to 3-week intervals to a maximum of 180 mg/day (usual maintenance dose: 60-120 mg/day)
Elderly: Initial: 15 mg, adjust dose at 2- to 4-week intervals by increments of 15 mg

Mechanism of Action The primary active compound is T_3 (tri-iodothyronine), which may be converted from T_4 (thyroxine) and then circulates throughout the body to influence growth and maturation of various tissues. Liotrix is uniform mixture of synthetic T_4 and T_3 in 4:1 ratio; exact mechanism of action is unknown; however, it is believed the thyroid hormone exerts its many metabolic effects through control of DNA transcription and protein synthesis; (Continued)

Liotrix *(Continued)*

involved in normal metabolism, growth, and development; promotes gluconeogenesis, increases utilization and mobilization of glycogen stores and stimulates protein synthesis, increases basal metabolic rate

Local Anesthetic/Vasoconstrictor Precautions No precautions with vasoconstrictor are necessary if patient is well controlled with liotrix

Effects on Dental Treatment No effects or complications reported

Other Adverse Effects <1%:

Cardiovascular: Palpitations, tachycardia, cardiac arrhythmias, chest pain

Central nervous system: Nervousness, sweating, headache, insomnia, fever, clumsiness

Dermatologic: Hair loss

Endocrine & metabolic: Excessive bone loss with overtreatment (excess thyroid replacement), heat intolerance, changes in menstrual cycle

Gastrointestinal: Weight loss, increased appetite, diarrhea, abdominal cramps, vomiting, constipation

Neuromuscular & skeletal: Tremor, muscle aches, hand tremors

Respiratory: Shortness of breath

Drug Interactions

Decreased effect:

Thyroid hormones increase hypoglycemic drug requirements

Phenytoin may decrease clinical lymphothyroidism

Cholestyramine causes decreased drug absorption of liotrix

Increased effect: Increased oral anticoagulant effect

Increased toxicity: Tricyclic antidepressants cause increased potential of both drugs

Drug Uptake

Absorption: 50% to 95% from GI tract

Time to peak serum concentration: 12-48 hours

Serum half-life: 6-7 days

Pregnancy Risk Factor A

Lipancreatin *see* Pancrelipase *on page 657*

Lipidil® *see* Fenofibrate *on page 356*

Liposyn® *see* Fat Emulsion *on page 353*

Lipovite® [OTC] *see* Vitamin B Complex *on page 899*

Liquaemin® Injection *see* Heparin *on page 419*

Liqui-Char® [OTC] *see* Charcoal *on page 179*

Liquid Pred® *see* Prednisone *on page 719*

Liqui-E® *see* Tocophersolan *on page 852*

Liquifilm® Forte Solution [OTC] *see* Artificial Tears *on page 75*

Liquifilm® Tears Solution [OTC] *see* Artificial Tears *on page 75*

Lisinopril *(lyse in' oh pril)*

Related Information

Cardiovascular Diseases *on page 912*

Brand Names Prinivil®; Zestril®

Therapeutic Category Angiotensin-Converting Enzyme (ACE) Inhibitors

Use Treatment of hypertension, either alone or in combination with other antihypertensive agents; adjunctive therapy in treatment of CHF (afterload reduction)

Usual Dosage

Adults: Initial: 10 mg/day; increase doses 5-10 mg/day at 1- to 2-week intervals; maximum daily dose: 40 mg

Elderly: Initial: 2.5-5 mg/day; increase doses 2.5-5 mg/day at 1- to 2-week intervals; maximum daily dose: 40 mg

Patients taking diuretics should have them discontinued 2-3 days prior to initiating lisinopril if possible; restart diuretic after blood pressure is stable if needed; in patients with hyponatremia (<130 mEq/L), start dose at 2.5 mg/day

Acute myocardial infarction (within 24 hours in hemodynamically stable patients): Oral: 5 mg immediately, then 5 mg at 24 hours, 10 mg at 48 hours, and 10 mg every day thereafter for 6 weeks; patients should continue to receive standard treatments such as thrombolytics, aspirin, and beta-blockers

Mechanism of Action Competitive inhibitor of angiotensin-converting enzyme (ACE); prevents conversion of angiotensin I to angiotensin II, a potent vasoconstrictor; results in lower levels of angiotensin II which causes an increase in plasma renin activity and a reduction in aldosterone secretion; a CNS mechanism may also be involved in hypotensive effect as angiotensin II increases adrenergic outflow from CNS; vasoactive kallikreins may be decreased in conversion to active hormones by ACE inhibitors, thus reducing blood pressure

Local Anesthetic/Vasoconstrictor Precautions No information available to require special precautions

Effects on Dental Treatment No effects or complications reported

Other Adverse Effects

1% to 10%:
Cardiovascular: Hypotension
Central nervous system: Dizziness, headache, fatigue
Gastrointestinal: Diarrhea
Renal: Increased BUN and serum creatinine
Respiratory: Upper respiratory symptoms, cough

<1%:
Cardiovascular: Chest discomfort, flushing, myocardial infarction, angina pectoris, orthostatic hypotension, rhythm disturbances, tachycardia, peripheral edema, vasculitis, palpitations, syncope
Central nervous system: Fever, malaise, depression, somnolence, insomnia
Dermatologic: Urticaria, pruritus, angioedema
Endocrine & metabolic: Gout
Gastrointestinal: Pancreatitis, abdominal pain, anorexia, constipation, flatulence, dry mouth
Hematologic: Neutropenia, bone marrow depression
Hepatic: Hepatitis
Neuromuscular & skeletal: Joint pain, shoulder pain
Ocular: Blurred vision
Respiratory: Bronchitis, sinusitis, pharyngeal pain
Miscellaneous: Diaphoresis

Drug Interactions See table.

Drug-Drug Interactions With ACEIs

Precipitant Drug	Drug (Category) and Effect	Description
Antacids	ACE Inhibitors: decreased	Decreased bioavailability of ACEIs. May be more likely with captopril. Separate administration times by 1-2 hours.
NSAIDs (indomethacin)	ACEIs: decreased	Reduced hypotensive effects of ACEIs. More prominent in low renin or volume dependent hypertensive patients.
Phenothiazines	ACEIs: increased	Pharmacologic effects of ACEIs may be increased.
ACEIs	Allopurinol: increased	Higher risk of hypersensitivity reaction possible when given concurrently. Three case reports of Stevens-Johnson syndrome with captopril.
ACEIs	Digoxin: increased	Increased plasma digoxin levels.
ACEIs	Lithium: increased	Increased serum lithium levels and symptoms of toxicity may occur.
ACEIs	Potassium preps/ potassium sparing diuretics increased	Coadministration may result in elevated potassium levels.

Increased toxicity: Lisinopril and diuretics have additive hypotensive effects

Drug Uptake
Peak hypotensive effect: Oral: Within 6 hours
Absorption: Well absorbed; unaffected by food
Serum half-life: 11-12 hours

Pregnancy Risk Factor D

Lisinopril and Hydrochlorothiazide

(lyse in' oh pril & hye droe klor oh thye' a zide)

Related Information
Cardiovascular Diseases on page 912

Brand Names Prinzide®; Zestoretic®

Therapeutic Category Antihypertensive

Use Treatment of hypertension

Local Anesthetic/Vasoconstrictor Precautions No information available to require special precautions

Effects on Dental Treatment No effects or complications reported

ALPHABETICAL LISTING OF DRUGS

Listerine® Antiseptic [OTC] *see Mouthwash, Antiseptic on page 592*
Listermint® with Fluoride [OTC] *see Fluoride on page 374*
Lithane® *see Lithium on this page*

Lithium (lith′ ee um)
Related Information
Dental Drug Interactions: Update on Drug Combinations Requiring Special Considerations *on page 1022*
Brand Names Cibalith-S®; Eskalith®; Lithane®; Lithobid®; Lithonate®; Lithotabs®
Canadian/Mexican Brand Names Carbolit® (Mexico); Lithellm® 300 (Mexico)
Therapeutic Category Antimanic Agent
Synonyms Lito Carbonato De (Mexico)
Use Management of acute manic episodes, bipolar disorders, and depression
Usual Dosage Oral: Monitor serum concentrations and clinical response (efficacy and toxicity) to determine proper dose
Children 6-12 years: 15-60 mg/kg/day in 3-4 divided doses; dose not to exceed usual adult dosage
Adults: 300-600 mg 3-4 times/day; usual maximum maintenance dose: 2.4 g/day or 450-900 mg of sustained release twice daily
Elderly: Initial dose: 300 mg twice daily; increase weekly in increments of 300 mg/day, monitoring levels; rarely need to go >900-1200 mg/day
Mechanism of Action Alters cation transport across cell membrane in nerve and muscle cells and influences reuptake of serotonin and/or norepinephrine
Local Anesthetic/Vasoconstrictor Precautions No information available to require special precautions
Effects on Dental Treatment Avoid NSAIDs if analgesics are required since lithium toxicity has been reported with concomitant administration; acetaminophen products (ie, singly or with narcotics) are recommended
Other Adverse Effects
>10%:
Endocrine & metabolic: Polydipsia, stress
Gastrointestinal: Nausea, diarrhea, impaired taste
Neuromuscular & skeletal: Trembling
1% to 10%:
Central nervous system: Weakness, tiredness
Dermatologic: Skin rash
Gastrointestinal: Bloated feeling, weight gain
Neuromuscular: Muscle twitching
<1%:
Central nervous system: Lethargy, fatigue, dizziness, vertigo, pseudotumor cerebri
Dermatologic: Eruptions
Endocrine & metabolic: Hypothyroidism, goiter, acneiform
Gastrointestinal: Anorexia, dry mouth
Genitourinary: Diabetes insipidus, nonspecific nephron atrophy, renal tubular acidosis
Hematologic: Leukocytosis
Neuromuscular & skeletal: Muscle weakness, cogwheel rigidity, chronic movements of the limbs, tremor
Ocular: Vision problems
Miscellaneous: Discoloration of fingers and toes
Drug Interactions
Decreased effect with xanthines (eg, theophylline, caffeine)
Increased effect/toxicity of CNS depressants, alfentanil, iodide salts increased hypothyroid effect
Increased toxicity with thiazide diuretics (dose may need to be reduced by 30%), NSAIDs, haloperidol, phenothiazines (neurotoxicity), neuromuscular blockers, carbamazepine, fluoxetine, ACE inhibitors
Drug Uptake
Serum half-life: 18-24 hours; can increase to more than 36 hours in elderly or patients with renal impairment
Time to peak serum concentration (nonsustained release product): Within 0.5-2 hours following oral absorption
Pregnancy Risk Factor D

Lithobid® *see Lithium on this page*
Lithonate® *see Lithium on this page*
Lithostat® *see Acetohydroxamic Acid on page 20*
Lithotabs® *see Lithium on this page*
Lito Carbonato De (Mexico) *see Lithium on this page*

Livostin® *see* Levocabastine Hydrochloride *on page 494*
LKV-Drops® **[OTC]** *see* Vitamins, Multiple *on page 901*

L-Lysine Hydrochloride (el lye' seen hye droe klor' ide)
Brand Names Enisyl® [OTC]; Lycolan® Elixir [OTC]
Therapeutic Category Dietary Supplement
Use Improves utilization of vegetable proteins
Local Anesthetic/Vasoconstrictor Precautions No information available to require special precautions
Effects on Dental Treatment No effects or complications reported

LMD® *see* Dextran *on page 263*
Lobac® *see* Chlorzoxazone *on page 200*
Lodine® *see* Etodolac *on page 347*
Lodine® **XL** *see* Etodolac *on page 347*
Lodosyn® *see* Carbidopa *on page 153*

Lodoxamide Tromethamine (loe dox' a mide troe meth' a meen)
Brand Names Alomide®
Therapeutic Category Ophthalmic Agent, Miscellaneous
Use Treatment of vernal keratoconjunctivitis, vernal conjunctivitis, and vernal keratitis
Usual Dosage Children >2 years and Adults: Instill 1-2 drops in eye(s) 4 times/day for up to 3 months
Mechanism of Action Mast cell stabilizer that inhibits the *in vivo* type I immediate hypersensitivity reaction to increase cutaneous vascular permeability associated with IgE and antigen-mediated reactions
Local Anesthetic/Vasoconstrictor Precautions No information available to require special precautions
Effects on Dental Treatment No effects or complications reported
Other Adverse Effects
>10%: Local: Transient burning, stinging, discomfort
1% to 10%:
  Central nervous system: Headache
  Ocular: Blurred vision, corneal erosion/ulcer, eye pain, corneal abrasion, blepharitis
<1%:
  Central nervous system: Dizziness, somnolence
  Dermatologic: Rash
  Gastrointestinal: Nausea, stomach discomfort
  Ocular: Blepharitis
  Respiratory: Sneezing
  Miscellaneous: Dry nose
Drug Interactions No data reported
Drug Uptake Absorption: Topical: Very small and undetectable
Pregnancy Risk Factor B

Loestrin® *see* Ethinyl Estradiol and Norethindrone *on page 339*
Lofene® *see* Diphenoxylate and Atropine *on page 289*
Logen® *see* Diphenoxylate and Atropine *on page 289*
Lomanate® *see* Diphenoxylate and Atropine *on page 289*

Lomefloxacin Hydrochloride (loe me flox' a sin hye droe klor' ide)
Brand Names Maxaquin®
Therapeutic Category Antibiotic, Quinolone
Synonyms Lomefloxacino Clorhidato De (Mexico)
Use Quinolone antibiotic for skin and skin structure, lower respiratory and urinary tract infections, and sexually transmitted diseases
Usual Dosage Oral: Adults: 400 mg once daily for 10-14 days
Mechanism of Action Inhibits DNA-gyrase in susceptible organisms thereby inhibits relaxation of supercoiled DNA and promotes breakage of DNA strands. DNA gyrase (topoisomerase II), is an essential bacterial enzyme that maintains the superhelical structure of DNA and is required for DNA replication and transcription, DNA repair, recombination, and transposition.
Local Anesthetic/Vasoconstrictor Precautions No information available to require special precautions
Effects on Dental Treatment No effects or complications reported
Other Adverse Effects
1% to 10%:
  Central nervous system: Headache, dizziness
  Dermatologic: Photosensitivity
(Continued)

Lomefloxacin Hydrochloride *(Continued)*

Gastrointestinal: Nausea, dizziness

<1%:

Cardiovascular: Flushing, chest pain, hypotension, hypertension, edema, syncope, tachycardia, bradycardia, arrhythmia, extrasystoles, cyanosis, cardiac failure, angina pectoris, myocardial infarction, coma

Central nervous system: Fatigue, malaise, asthenia, chills, convulsions, vertigo

Dermatologic: Purpura, rash

Endocrine & metabolic: Gout, hypoglycemia

Gastrointestinal: Abdominal pain, vomiting, flatulence, constipation, dry mouth

Genitourinary: Micturition disorder

Hematologic: Thrombocytopenia

Neuromuscular & skeletal: Back pain, hyperkinesia, tremor, paresthesias, leg cramps, myalgia

Otic: Earache

Renal: Dysuria, hematuria, anuria

Respiratory: Dyspnea, cough

Miscellaneous: Increased sweating, allergic reaction, face edema, flu-like symptoms, decreased heat tolerance, tongue discoloration, increased fibrinolysis, thirst, epistaxis, taste perversion

Drug Interactions

Decreased effect: Decreased absorption with antacids containing aluminum, magnesium, and/or calcium (by up to 98% if given at the same time)

Increased toxicity/serum levels: Quinolones cause increased levels of caffeine, warfarin, cyclosporine, and theophylline; azlocillin, cimetidine, probenecid increase quinolone levels

Drug Uptake

Absorption: Well absorbed

Serum half-life, elimination: 5-7.5 hours

Pregnancy Risk Factor C

Lomefloxacino Clorhidato De (Mexico) *see* Lomefloxacin Hydrochloride *on previous page*

Lomodix® *see* Diphenoxylate and Atropine *on page 289*

Lomotil® *see* Diphenoxylate and Atropine *on page 289*

Lomustine *(loe mus' teen)*

Brand Names CeeNU® Oral

Therapeutic Category Antineoplastic Agent, Alkylating Agent (Nitrosourea)

Synonyms CCNU

Use Treatment of brain tumors, Hodgkin's and non-Hodgkin's lymphomas, melanoma, renal carcinoma, lung cancer, colon cancer

Usual Dosage Oral (**refer to individual protocols**):

Children: 75-150 mg/m^2 as a single dose every 6 weeks. Subsequent doses are readjusted after initial treatment according to platelet and leukocyte counts.

Adults: 100-130 mg/m^2 as a single dose every 6 weeks; readjust after initial treatment according to platelet and leukocyte counts

With compromised marrow function: Initial dose: 100 mg/m^2 as a single dose every 6 weeks

Subsequent dosing adjustment based on nadir:

Leukocytes 2000-2900/mm^3, platelets 25,000-74,999/mm^3: Administer 70% of prior dose

Leukocytes <2000/mm^3, platelets <25,000/mm^3: Administer 50% of prior dose

Mechanism of Action Inhibits DNA and RNA synthesis via carbamylation of DNA polymerase, alkylation of DNA, and alteration of RNA, proteins, and enzymes

Local Anesthetic/Vasoconstrictor Precautions No information available to require special precautions

Effects on Dental Treatment No effects or complications reported

Other Adverse Effects

>10%:

Gastrointestinal: Nausea and vomiting occur 3-6 hours after oral administration; this is due to a centrally mediated mechanism, not a direct effect on the GI lining; if vomiting occurs, it is not necessary to replace the dose unless it occurs immediately after drug administration

Myelosuppression: Anemia; effects occur 4-6 weeks after a dose and may persist for 1-2 weeks

1% to 10%:
Central nervous system: Neurotoxicity
Dermatologic: Rash
Gastrointestinal: Stomatitis, diarrhea
Hematologic: Anemia

<1%:
Central nervous system: Disorientation, lethargy, ataxia, dysarthria
Dermatologic: Alopecia
Hepatic: Hepatotoxicity
Renal: Renal failure
Respiratory: Pulmonary fibrosis with cumulative doses >600 mg

Drug Uptake
Absorption: Complete from GI tract; appears in plasma within 3 minutes after administration
Serum half-life: Parent drug: 16-72 hours
Active metabolite: Terminal half-life: 1.3-2 days
Time to peak serum concentration: Active metabolite: Within 3 hours

Pregnancy Risk Factor D

Comments Myelosuppression is delayed about 4-6 weeks after a dose

Loniten® see Minoxidil on page 583

Lonox® see Diphenoxylate and Atropine on page 289

Lo/Ovral® see Ethinyl Estradiol and Norgestrel on page 341

Loperamide Hydrochloride (loe per' a mide hye droe klor' ide)

Brand Names Imodium®; Imodium® A-D [OTC]; Kaopectate® II [OTC]; Pepto® Diarrhea Control [OTC

Canadian/Mexican Brand Names PMS-Loperamine® (Canada); Acanol® (Mexico); Pramidal® (Mexico); Raxedin® (Mexico)

Therapeutic Category Antidiarrheal

Use Treatment of acute diarrhea and chronic diarrhea associated with inflammatory bowel disease; chronic functional diarrhea (idiopathic), chronic diarrhea caused by bowel resection or organic lesions; to decrease the volume of ileostomy discharge

Unlabeled use: Treatment of traveler's diarrhea in combination with trimethoprim-sulfamethoxazole (co-trimoxazole) (3 days therapy)

Usual Dosage Oral:
Children:
Acute diarrhea: Initial doses (in first 24 hours):
2-6 years: 1 mg three times/day
6-8 years: 2 mg twice daily
8-12 years: 2 mg three times/day
Maintenance: After initial dosing, 0.1 mg/kg doses after each loose stool, but not exceeding initial dosage
Chronic diarrhea: 0.08-0.24 mg/kg/day divided 2-3 times/day, maximum: 2 mg/dose
Adults: Initial: 4 mg (2 capsules), followed by 2 mg after each loose stool, up to 16 mg/day (8 capsules)

Mechanism of Action Acts directly on intestinal muscles to inhibit peristalsis and prolongs transit time enhancing fluid and electrolyte movement through intestinal mucosa; reduces fecal volume, increases viscosity, and diminishes fluid and electrolyte loss; demonstrates antisecretory activity; exhibits peripheral action

Local Anesthetic/Vasoconstrictor Precautions No information available to require special precautions

Effects on Dental Treatment No effects or complications reported

Other Adverse Effects
Central nervous system: Sedation, fatigue, dizziness, drowsiness
Dermatologic: Rash
Gastrointestinal: Nausea, vomiting, constipation, abdominal cramping, dry mouth, abdominal distention

Drug Interactions Increased toxicity: CNS depressants, phenothiazines, tricyclic antidepressants may potentiate the adverse effects of loperamide

Drug Uptake
Onset of action: Oral: Within 0.5-1 hour
Absorption: Oral: <40%; levels in breast milk expected to be very low
Serum half-life: 7-14 hours

Pregnancy Risk Factor B

Lopid® *see* Gemfibrozil *on page 395*
Lopremone *see* Protirelin *on page 747*
Lopressor® [Tartrate] *see* Metoprolol *on page 574*
Loprox® *see* Ciclopirox Olamine *on page 205*
Lorabid™ *see* Loracarbef *on this page*

Loracarbef (lor a kar' bef)
Brand Names Lorabid™
Canadian/Mexican Brand Names Carbac® (Mexico)
Therapeutic Category Antibiotic, Carbacephem
Use Infections caused by susceptible organisms involving the respiratory tract, acute otitis media, sinusitis, skin and skin structure, bone and joint, and urinary tract and gynecologic
Usual Dosage Oral:
Children:
Acute otitis media: 15 mg/kg twice daily for 10 days
Pharyngitis: 7.5-15 mg/kg twice daily for 10 days
Adults: Women:
Uncomplicated urinary tract infections: 200 mg once daily for 7 days
Skin and soft tissue: 200-400 mg every 12-24 hours
Uncomplicated pyelonephritis: 400 mg every 12 hours for 14 days
Mechanism of Action Inhibits bacterial cell wall synthesis by binding to one or more of the penicillin binding proteins (PBPs); inhibits the final transpeptidation step of peptidoglycan synthesis in bacterial cell walls, thus inhibiting cell wall biosynthesis. It is thought that beta-lactam antibiotics inactivate transpeptidase via acylation of the enzyme with cleavage of the CO-N bond of the beta-lactam ring. Upon exposure to beta-lactam antibiotics, bacteria eventually lyse due to ongoing activity of cell wall autolytic enzymes (autolysins and murein hydrolases) while cell wall assembly is arrested.
Local Anesthetic/Vasoconstrictor Precautions No information available to require special precautions
Effects on Dental Treatment No effects or complications reported
Other Adverse Effects
1% to 10%:
Central nervous system: Headache
Dermatologic: Skin rashes
Gastrointestinal: Diarrhea, nausea, vomiting, abdominal pain, anorexia
Genitourinary: Vaginitis, vaginal moniliasis
<1%:
Cardiovascular: Vasodilation
Central nervous system: Somnolence, nervousness, dizziness
Hematologic: Transient thrombocytopenia, leukopenia, and eosinophilia
Miscellaneous: Transient elevations of ALT, AST, alkaline phosphatase and BUN, creatinine
Drug Interactions Increased serum levels with probenecid
Drug Uptake
Absorption: Oral: Rapid
Serum half-life, elimination: ~1 hour
Time to peak serum concentration: Oral: Within 1 hour
Pregnancy Risk Factor B

Loracepam (Mexico) *see* Lorazepam *on next page*
Loratadina (Mexico) *see* Loratadine *on this page*

Loratadine (lor at' a deen)
Brand Names Claritin®
Canadian/Mexican Brand Names Clarityne® (Mexico); Lertamine® (Mexico); Lowadina® (Mexico)
Therapeutic Category Antihistamine
Synonyms Loratadina (Mexico)
Use Relief of nasal and non-nasal symptoms of seasonal allergic rhinitis
Usual Dosage Children >12 years and Adults: Oral: 10 mg/day on an empty stomach
Mechanism of Action Long-acting tricyclic antihistamine with selective peripheral histamine H_1 receptor antagonistic properties
Local Anesthetic/Vasoconstrictor Precautions No information available to require special precautions
Effects on Dental Treatment Over 10% of patients may experience dry mouth which will disappear with cessation of drug therapy

Other Adverse Effects
>10%:
  Central nervous system: Headache, somnolence, fatigue
  Gastrointestinal: Dry mouth
1% to 10%:
  Cardiovascular: Hypotension, hypertension, palpitations, tachycardia
  Central nervous system: Anxiety, depression
  Endocrine & metabolic: Breast pain
  Neuromuscular & skeletal: Hyperkinesia, arthralgias
  Respiratory: Nasal dryness, pharyngitis, dyspnea
  Miscellaneous: Sweating

Drug Interactions
Increased plasma concentrations of loratadine and its active metabolite with ketoconazole; erythromycin increases the AUC of loratadine and its active metabolite; no change in Q-T$_c$ interval was seen
Increased toxicity: Procarbazine, other antihistamines, alcohol

Drug Uptake
Onset of action: Within 1-3 hours
Peak effect: 8-12 hours
Duration: >24 hours
Absorption: Rapid
Serum half-life: 12-15 hours

Pregnancy Risk Factor B
Dosage Forms Tablet: 10 mg

Loratadine and Pseudoephedrine
(lor at' a deen & soo doe e fed' rin)
Related Information
Oral Bacterial Infections *on page 945*
Brand Names Claritin-D®; Claritin-D 24-Hour®
Therapeutic Category Antihistamine/Decongestant Combination
Use Temporary relief of symptoms of seasonal and perennial allergic rhinitis, and vasomotor rhinitis, including nasal obstruction
Local Anesthetic/Vasoconstrictor Precautions Use with caution since pseudoephedrine is a sympathomimetic amine which could interact with epinephrine to cause a pressor response
Effects on Dental Treatment Up to 10% of patients could experience tachycardia, palpitations, and dry mouth; use vasoconstrictor with caution; over 10% of patients may experience dry mouth which will disappear with cessation of drug therapy

Other Adverse Effects
>10%:
  Cardiovascular: Tachycardia
  Central nervous system: Slight to moderate drowsiness, nervousness, transient stimulation, insomnia
  Respiratory: Thickening of bronchial secretions
1% to 10%:
  Central nervous system: Headache, fatigue, nervousness, dizziness
  Gastrointestinal: Appetite increase, weight increase, nausea, diarrhea, abdominal pain, dry mouth
  Genitourinary: Difficult urination, dysuria
  Neuromuscular & skeletal: Weakness, arthralgia
  Respiratory: Pharyngitis
  Miscellaneous: Diaphoresis
<1%:
  Cardiovascular: Edema, palpitations, hypotension, shortness of breath
  Central nervous system: Depression, sedation, paradoxical excitement, insomnia, convulsions, hallucinations
  Dermatologic: Angioedema, rash
  Genitourinary: Urinary retention
  Hepatic: Hepatitis
  Neuromuscular & skeletal: Myalgia, paresthesia, tremor
  Ocular: Photosensitivity, blurred vision
  Respiratory: Bronchospasm, epistaxis, troubled breathing

Lorazepam (lor a' ze pam)
Related Information
Patients Requiring Sedation *on page 965*
Temporomandibular Dysfunction (TMD) *on page 963*
Brand Names Ativan®
(Continued)

Lorazepam *(Continued)*

Canadian/Mexican Brand Names Apo-Lorazepam® (Canada); Novo-Lora-zepam® (Canada); Nu-Loraz® (Canada); PMS-Lorazepam® (Canada); Pro-Lorazepam® (Canada)

Therapeutic Category Antianxiety Agent; Benzodiazepine; Hypnotic; Sedative; Tranquilizer, Minor

Synonyms Loracepam (Mexico)

Use Management of anxiety, status epilepticus, preoperative sedation, for desired amnesia, and as an antiemetic adjunct

Unapproved uses: Alcohol detoxification, insomnia, psychogenic catatonia, partial complex seizures

Usual Dosage

Antiemetic:
Children 2-15 years: I.V.: 0.05 mg/kg (up to 2 mg/dose) prior to chemotherapy
Adults: Oral, I.V.: 0.5-2 mg every 4-6 hours as needed

Anxiety and sedation:
Children: Oral, I.V.: Usual: 0.05 mg/kg/dose (range: 0.02-0.09 mg/kg) every 4-8 hours
Adults: Oral: 1-10 mg/day in 2-3 divided doses; usual dose: 2-6 mg/day in divided doses

Insomnia: Adults: Oral: 2-4 mg at bedtime

Preoperative: Adults:
I.M.: 0.05 mg/kg administered 2 hours before surgery; maximum: 4 mg/dose
I.V.: 0.044 mg/kg 15-20 minutes before surgery; usual maximum: 2 mg/dose

Operative amnesia: Adults: I.V.: up to 0.05 mg/kg; maximum: 4 mg/dose

Status epilepticus: I.V.:
Children: 0.1 mg/kg slow I.V. over 2-5 minutes, do not exceed 4 mg/single dose; may repeat second dose of 0.05 mg/kg slow I.V. in 10-15 minutes if needed
Adolescents: 0.07 mg/kg slow I.V. over 2-5 minutes; maximum: 4 mg/dose; may repeat in 10-15 minutes
Adults: 4 mg/dose given slowly over 2-5 minutes; may repeat in 10-15 minutes; usual maximum dose: 8 mg

Mechanism of Action Depresses all levels of the CNS, including the limbic and reticular formation, probably through the increased action of gamma-aminobutyric acid (GABA), which is a major inhibitory neurotransmitter in the brain

Local Anesthetic/Vasoconstrictor Precautions No information available to require special precautions

Effects on Dental Treatment Significant dry mouth will occur in over 10% of patients; normal salivary flow occurs with cessation of drug therapy

Other Adverse Effects

Respiratory: Decrease in respiratory rate, apnea, laryngospasm

>10%:
Cardiovascular: Tachycardia, chest pain
Central nervous system: Drowsiness, confusion, ataxia, amnesia, slurred speech, paradoxical excitement, rage, headache, depression, anxiety, fatigue, lightheadedness, insomnia
Dermatologic: Rash
Endocrine & metabolic: Decreased libido
Gastrointestinal: Dry mouth, constipation, diarrhea, nausea, vomiting, increased or decreased appetite
Local: Phlebitis, pain with injection
Neuromuscular & skeletal: Impaired coordination, dysarthria
Ocular: Blurred vision, diplopia
Miscellaneous: Decreased salivation, sweating

1% to 10%:
Cardiovascular: Cardiac arrest, hypotension, bradycardia, cardiovascular collapse, syncope
Central nervous system: Confusion, nervousness, dizziness, akathisia
Neuromuscular & skeletal: Rigidity, tremor, muscle cramps
Dermatologic: Dermatitis
Gastrointestinal: Weight gain or loss
Otic: Tinnitus
Respiratory: Nasal congestion, hyperventilation

<1%:
Endocrine & metabolic: Menstrual irregularities

Hematologic: Blood dyscrasias
Miscellaneous: Reflex slowing, physical and psychological dependence with prolonged use, increased salivation

Drug Interactions
Decreased effect with oral contraceptives (combination products), cigarette smoking; decreased effect of levodopa
Increased effect with morphine
Increased toxicity with alcohol, CNS depressants, MAO inhibitors, loxapine, tricyclic antidepressants

Drug Uptake
Onset of hypnosis: I.M.: 20-30 minutes
Duration: 6-8 hours
Absorption: Oral, I.M.: Prompt following administration
Serum half-life:
Older Children: 10.5 hours
Adults: 12.9 hours
Elderly: 15.9 hours
End stage renal disease: 32-70 hours

Pregnancy Risk Factor D
Dosage Forms
Injection: 2 mg/mL (1 mL, 10 mL); 4 mg/mL (1 mL, 10 mL)
Solution, oral concentrated: 2 mg/mL (30 mL)
Tablet: 0.5 mg, 1 mg, 2 mg
Generic Available Yes

Lorcet® [5/500] *see* Hydrocodone and Acetaminophen *on page 431*

Lorcet®-HD [5/500] *see* Hydrocodone and Acetaminophen *on page 431*

Lorcet® Plus [7.5/650] *see* Hydrocodone and Acetaminophen *on page 431*

Lorelco® *see* Probucol *on page 725*

Loroxide® [OTC] *see* Benzoyl Peroxide *on page 104*

Lortab® 2.5/500 *see* Hydrocodone and Acetaminophen *on page 431*

Lortab® 5/500 *see* Hydrocodone and Acetaminophen *on page 431*

Lortab® 7.5/500 *see* Hydrocodone and Acetaminophen *on page 431*

Lortab® 10/500 *see* Hydrocodone and Acetaminophen *on page 431*

Lortab® 10/650 *see* Hydrocodone and Acetaminophen *on page 431*

Lortab® ASA *see* Hydrocodone and Aspirin *on page 433*

Lortab® Elixir *see* Hydrocodone and Acetaminophen *on page 431*

Lortab® Solution *see* Hydrocodone and Acetaminophen *on page 431*

Losartan and Hydrochlorothiazide
(loe sar' tan & hye droe klor oh thye' a zide)
Brand Names Hyzaar®
Therapeutic Category Angiotensin II Antagonist; Diuretic, Thiazide Type
Use Treatment of hypertension
Local Anesthetic/Vasoconstrictor Precautions No information available to require special precautions
Effects on Dental Treatment No effects or complications reported

Losartan Potassium (loe sar' tan poe tass' ee um)
Related Information
Cardiovascular Diseases *on page 912*
Brand Names Cozaar®
Therapeutic Category Angiotensin II Antagonist
Synonyms DuP 753; MK594
Use Treatment of hypertension alone or in combination with other antihypertensives; in considering the use of monotherapy with Cozaar®, it should be noted that in controlled trials Cozaar® had an effect on blood pressure that was notably less in black patients than in nonblacks, a finding similar to the small effect of ACE inhibitors in blacks
Usual Dosage
Oral: 25-100 mg once or twice daily (adjust dosage at weekly intervals; maximum effect may not be apparent for 3-6 weeks)
Usual initial doses in patients receiving diuretics or those with intravascular volume depletion: 25 mg
Patients not receiving diuretics: 50 mg
Mechanism of Action As a selective and competitive, nonpeptide angiotensin II receptor antagonist, losartan blocks the vasoconstrictor and aldosterone-secreting effects of angiotensin II; losartan interacts reversibly at the AT1 and AT2 receptors of many tissues and has slow dissociation kinetics; its affinity for the AT1 receptor is 1000 times greater than the AT2 receptor. Angiotensin II
(Continued)

Losartan Potassium *(Continued)*

receptor antagonists may induce a more complete inhibition of the renin-angiotensin system than ACE inhibitors, they do not affect the response to bradykinin, and are less likely to be associated with nonrenin-angiotensin effects (eg, cough and angioedema). Losartan increases urinary flow rate and in addition to being natriuretic and kaliuretic, increases excretion of chloride, magnesium, uric acid, calcium, and phosphate.

Local Anesthetic/Vasoconstrictor Precautions No information available to require special precautions

Effects on Dental Treatment No effects or complications reported

Other Adverse Effects

1% to 10%:

Cardiovascular: Hypotension without reflex tachycardia

Central nervous system: Dizziness, insomnia

Endocrine & metabolic: Hyperkalemia

Gastrointestinal: Diarrhea, dyspepsia

Hematologic: Slight decreases in hemoglobin and hematocrit

Neuromuscular & skeletal: Back, leg, and muscle pain

Renal: Hypouricemia (with large doses)

Respiratory: Cough (less than ACE inhibitors), nasal congestion, sinus disorders, sinusitis

<1%:

Cardiovascular: Orthostatic effects, angina, second degree A-V block, CVA, palpitations, sinus bradycardia, tachycardia, flushing

Central nervous system: Anxiety, ataxia, confusion, depression, dream abnormality, migraine headache, sleep disorders, vertigo, fever

Dermatologic: Alopecia, dermatitis, dry skin, ecchymosis, erythema, photosensitivity, pruritus, rash, urticaria, facial edema

Endocrine & metabolic: Gout

Gastrointestinal: Anorexia, constipation, flatulence, vomiting, taste alteration, gastritis

Genitourinary: Impotence, decreased libido, urinary frequency, nocturia

Hepatic: Slight elevations of LFTs and bilirubin

Neuromuscular & skeletal: Paresthesia, tremor; arm, hip, shoulder, and knee pain, joint swelling, fibromyalgia, muscle weakness

Ocular: Blurred vision, burning and stinging eyes, conjunctivitis, decreased visual acuity

Otic: Tinnitus

Renal: Urinary tract infection, nocturia, mild increases in BUN/creatinine

Respiratory: Dyspnea, bronchitis, pharyngeal discomfort, epistaxis, rhinitis, respiratory congestion

Miscellaneous: Sweating

Drug Uptake

Onset of effect: 6 hours

Serum half-life:

Losartan: 1.5-2 hours

E-3174: 6-9 hours

Time to peak: Peak serum levels of losartan: 1 hour; metabolite, E-3174: 3-4 hours

Pregnancy Risk Factor D (1st trimester); C (2nd and 3rd trimesters)

Comments Cozaar® may be administered with other antihypertensive agents

Lotensin® *see Benazepril Hydrochloride on page 99*

Lotrel™ *see Amlodipine and Benazepril on page 54*

Lotrisone® *see Betamethasone and Clotrimazole on page 111*

Lovastatin *(loe' va sta tin)*

Related Information

Cardiovascular Diseases *on page 912*

Brand Names Mevacor®

Therapeutic Category HMG-CoA Reductase Inhibitor; Lipid Lowering Drugs

Synonyms Lovastatina (Mexico)

Use Adjunct to dietary therapy to decrease elevated serum total and LDL cholesterol concentrations in primary hypercholesterolemia

Usual Dosage Adults: Oral: Initial: 20 mg with evening meal, then adjust at 4-week intervals; maximum dose: 80 mg/day; before initiation of therapy, patients should be placed on a standard cholesterol-lowering diet for 3-6 months and the diet should be continued during drug therapy

Mechanism of Action Lovastatin acts by competitively inhibiting 3-hydroxyl-3-methylglutaryl-coenzyme A (HMG-CoA) reductase, the enzyme that catalyzes the rate-limiting step in cholesterol biosynthesis

Local Anesthetic/Vasoconstrictor Precautions No information available to require special precautions

Effects on Dental Treatment No effects or complications reported

Other Adverse Effects

Endocrine & metabolic: Gynecomastia

1% to 10%: Elevated creatine phosphokinase (CPK)
Central nervous system: Headache, dizziness
Dermatologic: Rash, pruritus
Gastrointestinal: Flatulence, abdominal pain, cramps, diarrhea, pancreatitis, constipation, nausea, dyspepsia, heartburn
Neuromuscular & skeletal: Myalgia

<1%:
Gastrointestinal: Dysgeusia
Ocular: Blurred vision, myositis, lenticular opacities

Drug Interactions

Increased toxicity: Gemfibrozil (musculoskeletal effects such as myopathy, myalgia and/or muscle weakness accompanied by markedly elevated CK concentrations, rash and/or pruritus); clofibrate, niacin (myopathy), erythromycin, cyclosporine, oral anticoagulants (elevated PT)

Increased effect/toxicity of levothyroxine

Concurrent use of erythromycin and lovastatin may result in rhabdomyolysis

Drug Uptake

Onset of effect: 3 days of therapy required for LDL cholesterol concentration reductions

Absorption: Oral: 30%

Serum half-life: 1.1-1.7 hours

Time to peak serum concentration: Oral: 2-4 hours

Pregnancy Risk Factor X

Lovastatina (Mexico) *see* Lovastatin *on previous page*

Low-Quel® *see* Diphenoxylate and Atropine *on page 289*

Loxapine (lox´ a peen)

Brand Names Loxitane®

Canadian/Mexican Brand Names Loxapac® (Canada)

Therapeutic Category Antiemetic; Antipsychotic Agent; Phenothiazine Derivative

Use Treatment of psychoses, nausea and vomiting; Tourette's syndrome; mania; intractable hiccups (adults); behavioral problems (children)

Usual Dosage Adults:

Oral: 10 mg twice daily, increase dose until psychotic symptoms are controlled; usual dose range: 60-100 mg/day in divided doses 2-4 times/day; dosages >250 mg/day are not recommended

I.M.: 12.5-50 mg every 4-6 hours or longer as needed and change to oral therapy as soon as possible

Mechanism of Action Blocks postsynaptic mesolimbic dopaminergic receptors in the brain; exhibits a strong alpha-adrenergic blocking effect and depresses the release of hypothalamic and hypophyseal hormones; believed to depress the reticular-activating system, thus affecting basal metabolism, body temperatures, wakefulness, vasomotor tone, and emesis

Local Anesthetic/Vasoconstrictor Precautions No information available to require special precautions

Effects on Dental Treatment Significant hypotension may occur, especially when the drug is administered parenterally; orthostatic hypotension is due to alpha-receptor blockade, the elderly are at greater risk for orthostatic hypotension

Tardive dyskinesia: Prevalence rate may be 40% in elderly; development of the syndrome and the irreversible nature are proportional to duration and total cumulative dose over time

Extrapyramidal reactions are more common in elderly with up to 50% developing these reactions after 60 years of age; drug-induced **Parkinson's syndrome** occurs often; **Akathisia** is the most common extrapyramidal reaction in elderly

Increased confusion, memory loss, psychotic behavior, and agitation frequently occur as a consequence of anticholinergic effects

Antipsychotic associated sedation in nonpsychotic patients is extremely unpleasant due to feelings of depersonalization, derealization, and dysphoria

(Continued)

Loxapine *(Continued)*

Other Adverse Effects

>10%:

Cardiovascular: Orthostatic hypotension

Central nervous system: Drowsiness, extrapyramidal effects (parkinsonian), confusion, persistent tardive dyskinesia

Gastrointestinal: Dry mouth

Ocular: Blurred vision

1% to 10%:

Dermatologic: Skin rash

Endocrine & metabolic: Enlargement of breasts

Gastrointestinal: Constipation, nausea, vomiting

<1%:

Cardiovascular: Tachycardia, arrhythmias, abnormal T-waves with prolonged ventricular repolarization

Central nervous system: Neuroleptic malignant syndrome (NMS), sedation, drowsiness, restlessness, anxiety, seizures

Dermatologic: Hyperpigmentation, pruritus, rash, photosensitivity

Endocrine & metabolic: Galactorrhea, amenorrhea, galactorrhea, gynecomastia

Gastrointestinal: Weight gain, adynamic ileus

Genitourinary: Urinary retention, overflow incontinence, priapism, sexual dysfunction

Hematologic: Agranulocytosis (more often in women between fourth and tenth week of therapy), leukopenia (usually in patients with large doses for prolonged periods)

Hepatic: Cholestatic jaundice

Ocular: Retinal pigmentation

Miscellaneous: Altered central temperature regulation

Drug Interactions

Decreased effect of guanethidine, phenytoin

Increased toxicity with CNS depressants, metrizamide (increased seizure potential), guanabenz, MAO inhibitors

Drug Uptake

Onset of neuroleptic effect: Oral: Within 20-30 minutes

Peak effect: 1.5-3 hours

Duration: ~12 hours

Serum half-life, biphasic:

Initial: 5 hours

Terminal: 12-19 hours

Pregnancy Risk Factor C

Loxitane® *see* Loxapine *on previous page*

Lozol® *see* Indapamide *on page 455*

L-PAM *see* Melphalan *on page 536*

L-Sarcolysin *see* Melphalan *on page 536*

Lubriderm® [OTC] *see* Lanolin, Cetyl Alcohol, Glycerin, and Petrolatum *on page 490*

LubriTears® Solution [OTC] *see* Artificial Tears *on page 75*

Ludiomil® *see* Maprotiline Hydrochloride *on page 525*

Lufyllin® *see* Dyphylline *on page 305*

Luminal® *see* Phenobarbital *on page 680*

Lupron® *see* Leuprolide Acetate *on page 492*

Lupron® Depot *see* Leuprolide Acetate *on page 492*

Lupron® Depot-Ped *see* Leuprolide Acetate *on page 492*

Luride® *see* Fluoride *on page 374*

Luride® Lozi-Tab® *see* Fluoride *on page 374*

Luride®-SF Lozi-Tab® *see* Fluoride *on page 374*

Luvox® *see* Fluvoxamine *on page 384*

Lycolan® Elixir [OTC] *see* L-Lysine Hydrochloride *on page 509*

Lymphocyte Immune Globulin, Anti-thymocyte Globulin (Equine)

(lim' foe site i myun' glob' yoo lin, an tee thye' moe site glob' yoo lin ee' kwine)

Brand Names Atgam®

Therapeutic Category Immunosuppressant Agent

Synonyms Antithymocyte Globulin (Equine); Antithymocyte Immunoglobulin; ATG; Horse Anti-human Thymocyte Gamma Globulin

Use Prevention and treatment of acute allograft rejection; treatment of moderate to severe aplastic anemia in patients not considered suitable candidates for bone marrow transplantation; prevention of graft-vs-host disease following bone marrow transplantation

Usual Dosage An intradermal skin test is recommended prior to administration of the initial dose of ATG; use 0.1 mL of a 1:1000 dilution of ATG in normal saline

Children: I.V.:
Aplastic anemia protocol: 10-20 mg/kg/day for 8-14 days, then give every other day for 7 more doses
Cardiac allograft: 10 mg/kg/day for 7 days
Renal allograft: 5-25 mg/kg/day

Adults: I.V.:
Aplastic anemia protocol: 10-20 mg/kg/day for 8-14 days, then give every other day for 7 more doses **or** 40 mg/kg/day for 4 days
Rejection prevention: 15 mg/kg/day for 14 days, then give every other day for 7 more doses for a total of 21 doses in 28 days; initial dose should be administered within 24 hours before or after transplantation
Rejection treatment: 10-15 mg/kg/day for 14 days, then give every other day for 7 more doses

Mechanism of Action May involve elimination of antigen-reactive T-lymphocytes (killer cells) in peripheral blood or alteration of T-cell function

Local Anesthetic/Vasoconstrictor Precautions No information available to require special precautions

Effects on Dental Treatment No effects or complications reported

Other Adverse Effects
>10%:
Central nervous system: Fever, chills
Dermatologic: Rash
Hematologic: Leukopenia, thrombocytopenia
Miscellaneous: Systemic infection
1% to 10%:
Cardiovascular: Hypotension, hypertension, tachycardia, edema, chest pain
Central nervous system: Headache, malaise
Gastrointestinal: Diarrhea, nausea, stomatitis, GI bleeding
Respiratory: Dyspnea
Local: Pain, swelling or redness at injection site, thrombophlebitis
Neuromuscular & skeletal: Myalgia, back pain
Renal: Abnormal renal function tests
Sensitivity reactions: Anaphylaxis may be indicated by hypotension, respiratory distress, serum sickness
Miscellaneous: Viral infection
<1%:
Central nervous system: Seizures
Dermatologic: Pruritus, urticaria
Hematologic: Hemolysis, anemia
Neuromuscular & skeletal: Arthralgia, weakness
Renal: Acute renal failure
Miscellaneous: Lymphadenopathy

Drug Uptake
Serum half-life, plasma: 1.5-12 days

Pregnancy Risk Factor C

Comments Do not dilute with D_5W (may cause precipitation). The use of highly acidic infusion solutions is not recommended because of possible physical instability. When the dose of corticosteroids and other immunosuppressants is being reduced, some previously masked reaction to Atgam® may appear.

Lyphocin® *see* Vancomycin Hydrochloride *on page 889*

Lypressin (lye press' in)
Brand Names Diapid®
Therapeutic Category Antidiuretic Hormone Analog
Use Controls or prevents signs and complications of neurogenic diabetes insipidus
Usual Dosage Children and Adults: Instill 1-2 sprays into one or both nostrils whenever frequency of urination increases or significant thirst develops; usual dosage is 1-2 sprays 4 times/day; range: 1 spray/day at bedtime to 10 sprays each nostril every 3-4 hours
Mechanism of Action Increases cyclic adenosine monophosphate (cAMP) which increases water permeability at the renal tubule resulting in decreased
(Continued)

Lypressin (Continued)

urine volume and increased osmolality; causes peristalsis by directly stimulating the smooth muscle in the GI tract

Local Anesthetic/Vasoconstrictor Precautions No information available to require special precautions

Effects on Dental Treatment No effects or complications reported

Other Adverse Effects

1% to 10%:
Central nervous system: Dizziness, headache
Gastrointestinal: Abdominal cramping, increased bowel movements
Local: Rhinorrhea, nasal congestion, irritation or burning
Respiratory: Chest tightness, coughing, dyspnea
<1%: Miscellaneous: Water intoxication, inadvertent inhalation

Drug Interactions Increased effect: Chlorpropamide, clofibrate, carbamazepine causes prolongation of antidiuretic effects

Drug Uptake

Onset of antidiuretic effect: Intranasal spray: Within 0.5-2 hours
Duration: 3-8 hours
Serum half-life: 15-20 minutes

Pregnancy Risk Factor C

Lysodren® see Mitotane on page 585

Maalox® [OTC] see Aluminum Hydroxide and Magnesium Hydroxide on page 40

Maalox® Plus [OTC] see Aluminum Hydroxide, Magnesium Hydroxide, and Simethicone on page 41

Maalox® Therapeutic Concentrate [OTC] see Aluminum Hydroxide and Magnesium Hydroxide on page 40

Macrobid® see Nitrofurantoin on page 622

Macrodantin® see Nitrofurantoin on page 622

Macrodex® see Dextran on page 263

Mafenide Acetate (ma' fe nide as' e tate)

Brand Names Sulfamylon®

Therapeutic Category Antibacterial, Topical; Antibiotic, Topical

Use Adjunct in the treatment of second and third degree burns to prevent septicemia caused by susceptible organisms such as Pseudomonas aeruginosa; prevention of graft loss of meshed autografts on excised burn wounds

Usual Dosage Children and Adults: Topical: Apply once or twice daily with a sterile gloved hand; apply to a thickness of approximately 16 mm; the burned area should be covered with cream at all times

Mechanism of Action Interferes with bacterial folic acid synthesis through competitive inhibition of para-aminobenzoic acid

Local Anesthetic/Vasoconstrictor Precautions No information available to require special precautions

Effects on Dental Treatment No effects or complications reported

Other Adverse Effects

>10%: Local: Burning sensation, excoriation, pain
1% to 10%:
Dermatologic: Skin rash
Miscellaneous: Swelling of face, troubled breathing
<1%:
Dermatologic: Erythema
Endocrine & metabolic: Hyperchloremia, metabolic acidosis
Hematologic: Bone marrow suppression, hemolytic anemia, bleeding
Hepatic: Porphyria
Respiratory: Hyperventilation, tachypnea
Sensitivity reactions: Hypersensitivity

Drug Interactions No data reported

Drug Uptake

Absorption: Diffuses through devascularized areas and is rapidly absorbed from burned surface
Time to peak serum concentration: Topical: 2-4 hours

Pregnancy Risk Factor C

Magaldrate (mag' al drate)

Brand Names Riopan® [OTC]

Therapeutic Category Antacid

Synonyms Hydromagnesium aluminate

Use Symptomatic relief of hyperacidity associated with peptic ulcer, gastritis, peptic esophagitis and hiatal hernia

Local Anesthetic/Vasoconstrictor Precautions No information available to require special precautions

Effects on Dental Treatment No effects or complications reported

Other Adverse Effects

>10%: Gastrointestinal: Constipation, chalky taste, stomach cramps, fecal impaction

1% to 10%: Gastrointestinal: Nausea, vomiting, discoloration of feces (white speckles)

<1%: Endocrine & metabolic: Hypophosphatemia, hypomagnesemia

Comments Chemical entity known as hydroxy magnesium aluminate equivalent to magnesium oxide and aluminum oxide; unlike other magnesium-containing antacids, Riopan® is safe to use in renal patients

Magaldrate and Simethicone (mag' al drate & sye meth' i kone)

Brand Names Riopan Plus® [OTC]

Therapeutic Category Antacid; Antiflatulent

Synonyms Simethicone and Magaldrate

Use Relief of hyperacidity associated with peptic ulcer, gastritis, peptic esophagitis and hiatal hernia which are accompanied by symptoms of gas

Local Anesthetic/Vasoconstrictor Precautions No information available to require special precautions

Effects on Dental Treatment No effects or complications reported

Comments Chemical entity known as hydroxy magnesium aluminate equivalent to magnesium oxide and aluminum oxide; unlike other magnesium containing antacids, Riopan® is safe to use in renal patients if used cautiously

Magalox Plus® [OTC] see Aluminum Hydroxide, Magnesium Hydroxide, and Simethicone on page 41

Magnesio, Hidroxido De (Mexico) see Magnesium Hydroxide on next page

Magnesio, Oxide De (Mexico) see Magnesium Oxide on page 523

Magnesium Chloride (mag nee' zhum klor' ide)

Brand Names Slow-Mag® [OTC]

Therapeutic Category Magnesium Salt

Use Correct or prevent hypomagnesemia

Local Anesthetic/Vasoconstrictor Precautions No information available to require special precautions

Effects on Dental Treatment Magnesium products may prevent gastrointestinal absorption of tetracyclines by forming a large ionized chelated molecule with the tetracyclines in the stomach. Tetracyclines should be given at least 1 hour before magnesium.

Other Adverse Effects 1% to 10%:

Cardiovascular: Flushing

Central nervous system: Depressed CNS, somnolence

Gastrointestinal: Diarrhea

Neuromuscular & skeletal: Blocked peripheral neuromuscular transmission, deep tendon reflexes

Respiratory: Respiratory paralysis

Magnesium Citrate (mag nee' zhum sit' rate)

Brand Names Evac-Q-Mag® [OTC]

Therapeutic Category Laxative, Saline

Synonyms Citrate of Magnesia

Use To evacuate bowel prior to certain surgical and diagnostic procedures

Usual Dosage Cathartic: Oral:

Children:

<6 years: 0.5 mL/kg up to a maximum of 200 mL repeated every 4-6 hours until stools are clear

6-12 years: 100-150 mL

Adults ≥12 years: 1/2 to 1 full bottle (120-300 mL)

Mechanism of Action Promotes bowel evacuation by causing osmotic retention of fluid which distends the colon with increased peristaltic activity

Local Anesthetic/Vasoconstrictor Precautions No information available to require special precautions

Effects on Dental Treatment Magnesium products may prevent gastrointestinal absorption of tetracyclines by forming a large ionized chelated molecule with the tetracyclines in the stomach. Tetracyclines should be given at least 1 hour before magnesium.

(Continued)

Magnesium Citrate *(Continued)*

Other Adverse Effects 1% to 10%:
Cardiovascular: Hypotension
Endocrine & metabolic: Hypermagnesemia
Gastrointestinal: Abdominal cramps, diarrhea, gas formation
Respiratory: Respiratory depression
Drug Uptake
Absorption: Oral: 15% to 30%
Pregnancy Risk Factor B
Comments Magnesium content of 5 mL: 3.85-4.71 mEq

Magnesium Gluconate *(mag nee' zhum gloo' koe nate)*

Brand Names Magonate® [OTC]
Therapeutic Category Magnesium Salt
Use Dietary supplement for treatment of magnesium deficiencies
Usual Dosage The recommended dietary allowance (RDA) of magnesium is 4.5 mg/kg which is a total daily allowance of 350-400 mg for adult men and 280-300 mg for adult women. During pregnancy the RDA is 300 mg and during lactation the RDA is 355 mg. Average daily intakes of dietary magnesium have declined in recent years due to processing of food. The latest estimate of the average American dietary intake was 349 mg/day.

Dietary supplement: Oral:
Children: 3-6 mg/kg/day in divided doses 3-4 times/day; maximum: 400 mg/day
Adults: 27-54 mg 2-3 times/day or 100 mg 4 times/day
Mechanism of Action Magnesium is important as a cofactor in many enzymatic reactions in the body involving protein synthesis and carbohydrate metabolism, (at least 300 enzymatic reactions require magnesium). Actions on lipoprotein lipase have been found to be important in reducing serum cholesterol and on sodium/potassium ATPase in promoting polarization (ie, neuromuscular functioning).
Local Anesthetic/Vasoconstrictor Precautions No information available to require special precautions
Effects on Dental Treatment Magnesium products may prevent gastrointestinal absorption of tetracyclines by forming a large ionized chelated molecule with the tetracyclines in the stomach. Tetracyclines should be given at least 1 hour before magnesium.
Other Adverse Effects
1% to 10%: Gastrointestinal: Diarrhea (excessive dose)
<1%:
Endocrine & metabolic: Hypotension, hypermagnesemia
Gastrointestinal: Abdominal cramps
Neuromuscular & skeletal: Muscle weakness
Respiratory: Respiratory depression
Drug Uptake
Absorption: Oral: 15% to 30%
Comments Magnesium content of 500 mg: 27 mg

Magnesium Hydroxide *(mag nee' zhum hye drok' side)*

Brand Names Phillips'® Milk of Magnesia [OTC]
Canadian/Mexican Brand Names Leche De Magnesia Normex (Mexico)
Therapeutic Category Antacid; Laxative, Saline; Magnesium Salt
Synonyms Magnesio, Hidroxido De (Mexico)
Use Short-term treatment of occasional constipation and symptoms of hyperacidity, magnesium replacement therapy
Usual Dosage Oral:
Laxative:
<2 years: 0.5 mL/kg/dose
2-5 years: 5-15 mL/day or in divided doses
6-12 years: 15-30 mL/day or in divided doses
≥12 years: 30-60 mL/day or in divided doses

Antacid:
Children: 2.5-5 mL as needed up to 4 times/day
Adults: 5-15 mL or 650 mg to 1.3 g tablets up to 4 times/day as needed
Mechanism of Action Promotes bowel evacuation by causing osmotic retention of fluid which distends the colon with increased peristaltic activity; reacts with hydrochloric acid in stomach to form magnesium chloride
Local Anesthetic/Vasoconstrictor Precautions No information available to require special precautions

Effects on Dental Treatment Magnesium products may prevent gastrointestinal absorption of tetracyclines by forming a large ionized chelated molecule with the tetracyclines in the stomach. Tetracyclines should be given at least 1 hour before magnesium.

Other Adverse Effects
>10%: Diarrhea
1% to 10%:
   Cardiovascular: Hypotension
   Endocrine & metabolic: Hypermagnesemia
   Gastrointestinal: Abdominal cramps
   Neuromuscular & skeletal: Muscle weakness
   Respiratory: Respiratory depression

Drug Interactions Decreased effect: Decreased absorption of tetracyclines, digoxin, indomethacin, or iron salts

Drug Uptake Onset of laxative action: 4-8 hours

Pregnancy Risk Factor B

Magnesium Hydroxide and Aluminum Hydroxide see Aluminum Hydroxide and Magnesium Hydroxide on page 40

Magnesium Hydroxide and Mineral Oil Emulsion
(mag nee' zhum hye drok' side & min' er al oyl e mul' shun)
Brand Names Haley's M-O® [OTC]
Therapeutic Category Laxative, Lubricant; Laxative, Saline
Synonyms MOM/Mineral Oil Emulsion
Use Short-term treatment of occasional constipation
Local Anesthetic/Vasoconstrictor Precautions No information available to require special precautions
Effects on Dental Treatment Magnesium products may prevent gastrointestinal absorption of tetracyclines by forming a large ionized chelated molecule with the tetracyclines in the stomach. Tetracyclines should be given at least 1 hour before magnesium.

Magnesium Oxide (mag nee' zhum ok' side)
Brand Names Maox®
Therapeutic Category Antacid
Synonyms Magnesio, Oxide De (Mexico)
Use Short-term treatment of occasional constipation and symptoms of hyperacidity
Usual Dosage Magnesium RDA: 4.5 mg/kg, which is a total daily allowance of 350 mg for adult men and 280-300 mg for adult women. During pregnancy, the RDA is 200 mg and during lactation it is 355 mg. Average daily intakes of dietary magnesium have declined in recent years due to processing of food. The latest estimate of the average American dietary intake was 349 mg/day.

Adults: Oral:
   Dietary supplement: 27-54 mEq (1-2 tablets) 2-3 times
   Antacid: $\frac{1}{2}$ to 3 tablets (0.21-1.68 g) with water or milk 4 times/day after meals and at bedtime
   Laxative: 2-4 g at bedtime with full glass of water

Mechanism of Action Promotes bowel evacuation by causing osmotic retention of fluid which distends the colon with increased peristaltic activity
Local Anesthetic/Vasoconstrictor Precautions No information available to require special precautions
Effects on Dental Treatment Magnesium products may prevent gastrointestinal absorption of tetracyclines by forming a large ionized chelated molecule with the tetracyclines in the stomach. Tetracyclines should be given at least 1 hour before magnesium.

Other Adverse Effects
>10%: Diarrhea
1% to 10%:
   Cardiovascular: Hypotension, EKG changes
   Central nervous system: Mental depression, coma
   Gastrointestinal: Nausea, vomiting
   Respiratory: Respiratory depression

Drug Interactions Decreased effect: Tetracyclines, digoxin, indomethacin, iron salts, isoniazid, quinolones

Drug Uptake Onset of laxative action: 4-8 hours

Pregnancy Risk Factor B

Magnesium Sulfate (mag nee' zhum sul' fate)

Therapeutic Category Anticonvulsant, Miscellaneous; Electrolyte Supplement, Parenteral; Laxative, Saline; Magnesium Salt

Synonyms Epsom Salts

Use Treatment and prevention of hypomagnesemia; hypertension; encephalopathy and seizures associated with acute nephritis in children; also used as a cathartic

Usual Dosage The recommended dietary allowance (RDA) of magnesium is 4.5 mg/kg which is a total daily allowance of 350-400 mg for adult men and 280-300 mg for adult women. During pregnancy the RDA is 300 mg and during lactation the RDA is 355 mg. Average daily intakes of dietary magnesium have declined in recent years due to processing of food. The latest estimate of the average American dietary intake was 349 mg/day. Dose represented as $MgSO_4$ unless stated otherwise.

Note: Serum magnesium is poor reflection of repletional status as the majority of magnesium is intracellular; serum levels may be transiently normal for a few hours after a dose is given, therefore, aim for consistently high normal serum levels in patients with normal renal function for most efficient repletion

Hypomagnesemia:

Children: I.M., I.V.: 25-50 mg/kg/dose (0.2-0.4 mEq/kg/dose) every 4-6 hours for 3-4 doses, maximum single dose: 2000 mg (16 mEq), may repeat if hypomagnesemia persists (higher dosage up to 100 mg/kg/dose $MgSO_4$ I.V. has been used); maintenance: I.V.: 30-60 mg/kg/day (0.25-0.5 mEq/kg/day)

Management of seizures and hypertension:

Children:

Oral: 100-200 mg/kg/dose 4 times/day

I.M., I.V.: 20-100 mg/kg/dose every 4-6 hours as needed; in severe cases doses as high as 200 mg/kg/dose have been used

Adults:

Oral: 3 g every 6 hours for 4 doses as needed

I.M., I.V.: 1 g every 6 hours for 4 doses; for severe hypomagnesemia: 8-12 g $MgSO_4$/day in divided doses has been used

Eclampsia, pre-eclampsia: Adults:

I.M.: 1-4 g every 4 hours

I.V.: Initial: 4 g, then switch to I.M. or 1-4 g/hour by continuous infusion

Maximum dose should not exceed 30-40 g/day; maximum rate of infusion: 1-2 g/hour

Maintenance electrolyte requirements:

Daily requirements: 0.2-0.5 mEq/kg/24 hours or 3-10 mEq/1000 kcal/24 hours

Maximum: 8-16 mEq/24 hours

Cathartic: Oral:

Children: 0.25 g/kg every 4-6 hours

Adults: 10-15 g in a glass of water

Mechanism of Action Promotes bowel evacuation by causing osmotic retention of fluid which distends the colon with increased peristaltic activity when taken orally; parenterally, decreases acetylcholine in motor nerve terminals and acts on myocardium by slowing rate of S-A node impulse formation and prolonging conduction time

Local Anesthetic/Vasoconstrictor Precautions No information available to require special precautions

Effects on Dental Treatment Magnesium products may prevent gastrointestinal absorption of tetracyclines by forming a large ionized chelated molecule with the tetracyclines in the stomach. Tetracyclines should be given at least 1 hour before magnesium.

Other Adverse Effects

1% to 10%:

Serum magnesium levels >3 mg/dL:

Central nervous system: Depressed CNS

Gastrointestinal: Diarrhea

Neuromuscular & skeletal: Blocked peripheral neuromuscular transmission leading to anticonvulsant effects

Serum magnesium levels >5 mg/dL:

Cardiovascular: Flushing

Central nervous system: Somnolence

Serum magnesium levels >12.5 mg/dL:

Cardiovascular: Complete heart block

Respiratory: Respiratory paralysis

Drug Uptake
Oral: Onset of cathartic action: Within 1-2 hours
I.M.:
Onset of action: 1 hour
Duration: 3-4 hours
I.V.:
Onset of action: Immediate
Duration: 30 minutes

Pregnancy Risk Factor B

Comments $MgSO_4$ 500 mg = magnesium 4.06 mEq = elemental magnesium 49.3 mg

Magonate® [OTC] *see* Magnesium Gluconate *on page 522*

Maigret-50 *see* Phenylpropanolamine Hydrochloride *on page 687*

Malatal® *see* Hyoscyamine, Atropine, Scopolamine, and Phenobarbital *on page 444*

Mallergan-VC® With Codeine *see* Promethazine, Phenylephrine, and Codeine *on page 734*

Malotuss® [OTC] *see* Guaifenesin *on page 407*

Malt Soup Extract (malt soop eks′ trakt)
Brand Names Maltsupex® [OTC]
Therapeutic Category Laxative, Bulk-Producing
Use Short-term treatment of constipation
Local Anesthetic/Vasoconstrictor Precautions No information available to require special precautions
Effects on Dental Treatment No effects or complications reported
Other Adverse Effects 1% to 10%: Gastrointestinal: Abdominal cramps, diarrhea, rectal obstruction

Maltsupex® [OTC] *see* Malt Soup Extract *on this page*

Mandelamine® *see* Methenamine *on page 555*

Mandol® *see* Cefamandole Nafate *on page 163*

Manganese *see* Trace Metals *on page 857*

Manoplax® *see* Flosequinan *on page 366*

Mantoux *see* Tuberculin Purified Protein Derivative *on page 882*

Maolate® *see* Chlorphenesin Carbamate *on page 190*

Maox® *see* Magnesium Oxide *on page 523*

Maprotilina, Clorhidrato De (Mexico) *see* Maprotiline Hydrochloride *on this page*

Maprotiline Hydrochloride (ma proe′ ti leen hye droe klor′ ide)
Related Information
Vasoconstrictor Interactions With Antidepressants *on page 1108*
Brand Names Ludiomil®
Therapeutic Category Antidepressant, Tetracyclic
Synonyms Maprotilina, Clorhidrato De (Mexico)
Use Treatment of depression and anxiety associated with depression
Usual Dosage Oral:
Children 6-14 years: 10 mg/day, increase to a maximum daily dose of 75 mg
Adults: 75 mg/day to start, increase by 25 mg every 2 weeks up to 150-225 mg/day; given in 3 divided doses or in a single daily dose
Elderly: Initial: 25 mg at bedtime, increase by 25 mg every 3 days for inpatients and weekly for outpatients if tolerated; usual maintenance dose: 50-75 mg/day, higher doses may be necessary in nonresponders

Mechanism of Action Traditionally believed to increase the synaptic concentration of norepinephrine in the central nervous system by inhibition of their reuptake by the presynaptic neuronal membrane. However, additional receptor effects have been found including desensitization of adenyl cyclase, down regulation of beta-adrenergic receptors, and down regulation of serotonin receptors.

Local Anesthetic/Vasoconstrictor Precautions Use with caution; epinephrine, norepinephrine and levonordefrin have been shown to have an increased pressor response in combination with TCAs

Effects on Dental Treatment Long-term treatment with TCAs such as amoxapine increases the risk of caries by reducing salivation and salivary buffer capacity

Other Adverse Effects
>10%:
Cardiovascular: Orthostatic hypotension
(Continued)

Maprotiline Hydrochloride (Continued)

Central nervous system: Drowsiness, weakness
Dermatologic: Skin rash
Gastrointestinal: Dry mouth
Genitourinary: Urinary retention
1% to 10%:
Central nervous system: Insomnia
Gastrointestinal: Constipation, nausea, vomiting, increased appetite and weight gain, weight loss
Neuromuscular & skeletal: Trembling
<1%:
Central nervous system: Confusion
Endocrine & metabolic: Breast enlargement
Genitourinary: Swelling of testicles
Hepatic: Cholestatic hepatitis
Ocular: Blurred vision, increased intraocular pressure
Otic: Tinnitus

Drug Interactions
Decreased effect: Phenobarbital may increase the metabolism of maprotiline; maprotiline blocks the uptake of guanethidine and thus prevents the hypotensive effect of guanethidine
Increased toxicity: Clonidine causes hypertensive crisis; maprotiline may be additive with or may potentiate the action of other CNS depressants such as sedatives or hypnotics; with MAO inhibitors, hyperpyrexia, hypertension, tachycardia, confusion, and seizures. Maprotiline may increase the prothrombin time in patients stabilized on warfarin; maprotiline potentiate the pressor and cardiac effects of sympathomimetic agents such as isoproterenol, epinephrine, etc; cimetidine and methylphenidate may decrease the metabolism of maprotiline
Additive anticholinergic effects seen with other anticholinergic agents

Drug Uptake
Absorption: Slow
Serum half-life: 27-58 hours (mean, 43 hours)
Time to peak serum concentration: Within 12 hours

Pregnancy Risk Factor B

Selected Readings
Boakes AJ, Laurence DR, Teoh PC, et al, "Interactions Between Sympathomimetic Amines and Antidepressant Agents in Man," Br Med J, 1973, 1(849):311-5.
Jastak JT and Yagiela JA, "Vasoconstrictors and Local Anesthesia: A Review and Rationale for Use," J Am Dent Assoc, 1983, 107(4):623-30.
Larochelle P, Hamet P, and Enjalbert M, "Responses to Tyramine and Norepinephrine After Imipramine and Trazodone," Clin Pharmacol Ther, 1979, 26(1):24-30.
Mitchell JR, "Guanethidine and Related Agents. III Antagonism by Drugs Which Inhibit the Norepinephrine Pump in Man," J Clin Invest, 1970, 49(8):1596-604.
Rundegren J, van Dijken J, Mörnstad H, et al, "Oral Conditions in Patients Receiving Long-Term Treatment With Cyclic Antidepressant Drugs," Swed Dent J, 1985, 9(2):55-64.
Svedmyr N, "The Influence of a Tricyclic Antidepressive Agent (Protriptyline) on Some of the Circulatory Effects of Noradrenaline and Adrenaline in Man," Life Sci, 1968, 7(1):77-84.

Marax® see Theophylline, Ephedrine, and Hydroxyzine on page 836
Marazide® see Benzthiazide on page 105
Marbaxin® see Methocarbamol on page 557
Marcaine® see Bupivacaine Hydrochloride on page 127
Marcaine® with Epinephrine see Bupivacaine With Epinephrine on page 128
Marezine® [OTC] see Cyclizine on page 238
Margesic® H [5/500] see Hydrocodone and Acetaminophen on page 431
Marinol® see Dronabinol on page 302
Marmine® [OTC] see Dimenhydrinate on page 286
Marnal® see Butalbital Compound on page 133
Marplan® see Isocarboxazid on page 469
Marpres® see Hydralazine, Hydrochlorothiazide, and Reserpine on page 429

Masoprocol (ma soe' pro kole)

Brand Names Actinex®
Therapeutic Category Topical Skin Product
Use Treatment of actinic keratosis
Usual Dosage Adults: Topical: Wash and dry area; gently massage into affected area every morning and evening for 28 days
Mechanism of Action Antiproliferative activity against keratinocytes
Local Anesthetic/Vasoconstrictor Precautions No information available to require special precautions
Effects on Dental Treatment No effects or complications reported

Other Adverse Effects
>10%: Dermatologic: Erythema, flaking, dryness, burning, itching
1% to 10%: Soreness, eye irritation, rash, tingling
<1%: Blistering, excoriation, skin roughness, wrinkling
Drug Interactions No data reported
Drug Uptake Absorption: Topical: <1% to 2%
Pregnancy Risk Factor B

Massé® Breast Cream [OTC] *see* Glycerin, Lanolin, and Peanut Oil *on page 402*

Matulane® *see* Procarbazine Hydrochloride *on page 727*

Mavik® *see* Trandolapril *on page 858*

Maxair™ *see* Pirbuterol Acetate *on page 698*

Maxaquin® *see* Lomefloxacin Hydrochloride *on page 509*

Max-Caro® [OTC] *see* Beta-Carotene *on page 109*

Maxiflor® *see* Diflorasone Diacetate *on page 278*

Maximum Strength Anbesol® [OTC] *see* Benzocaine *on page 102*

Maximum Strength Orajel® [OTC] *see* Benzocaine *on page 102*

Maxipime® *see* Cefepime *on page 164*

Maxitrol® *see* Neomycin, Polymyxin B, and Dexamethasone *on page 610*

Maxivate® *see* Betamethasone *on page 109*

Maxolon® *see* Metoclopramide *on page 572*

Maxzide® *see* Triamterene and Hydrochlorothiazide *on page 865*

Mazanor® *see* Mazindol *on this page*

Mazindol (may' zin dole)
Brand Names Mazanor®; Sanorex®
Therapeutic Category Anorexiant
Use Short-term adjunct in exogenous obesity
Local Anesthetic/Vasoconstrictor Precautions No information available to require special precautions
Effects on Dental Treatment No effects or complications reported
Other Adverse Effects
>10%:
Cardiovascular: Hypertension
Central nervous system: Euphoria, nervousness, insomnia
1% to 10%:
Central nervous system: Confusion, mental depression, restlessness
Endocrine & metabolic: Changes in libido
Gastrointestinal: Nausea, vomiting, constipation
Hematologic: Blood dyscrasias
Neuromuscular & skeletal: Tremor
Ocular: Blurred vision
<1%:
Cardiovascular: Tachycardia, arrhythmias
Central nervous system: Restlessness, depression, headache
Dermatologic: Alopecia
Gastrointestinal: Diarrhea, abdominal cramps
Genitourinary: Dysuria, testicular pain
Respiratory: Dyspnea
Neuromuscular & skeletal: Myalgia
Renal: Polyuria
Miscellaneous: Increased sweating

m-Cresyl Acetate (em-kree' sil as' e tate)
Brand Names Cresylate®
Therapeutic Category Otic Agent, Anti-infective
Use Provides an acid medium; for external otitis infections caused by susceptible bacteria or fungus
Local Anesthetic/Vasoconstrictor Precautions No information available to require special precautions
Effects on Dental Treatment No effects or complications reported

MCT Oil® [OTC] *see* Medium Chain Triglycerides *on page 532*

Measles and Rubella Vaccines, Combined
(mee' zels & roo bel' a vak seens' kom bined')
Brand Names M-R-VAX® II
Therapeutic Category Vaccine, Live Virus
Synonyms Rubella and Measles Vaccines, Combined
(Continued)

Measles and Rubella Vaccines, Combined *(Continued)*

Use Simultaneous immunization against measles and rubella

Usual Dosage Children at 15 months and Adults: S.C.: Inject 0.5 mL into outer aspect of upper arm; no routine booster for rubella

Local Anesthetic/Vasoconstrictor Precautions No information available to require special precautions

Effects on Dental Treatment No effects or complications reported

Other Adverse Effects All serious adverse reactions must be reported to the FDA

>10%:
  Central nervous system: Fever <100°F
  Dermatologic: Urticaria, rash, local erythema
  Local: Burning at injection site, local tenderness
  Neuromuscular & skeletal: Arthralgias

1% to 10%:
  Central nervous system: Fever between 100°F and 103°F, malaise, head-ache
  Gastrointestinal: Sore throat
  Miscellaneous: Allergic reaction (delayed type), lymphadenopathy

<1%:
  Central nervous system: Tiredness, convulsions, encephalitis, confusion, severe headache, fever >103°F (prolonged)
  Dermatologic: Hives, itching, reddening of skin (especially around ears and eyes)
  Gastrointestinal: Vomiting
  Hematologic: Thrombocytopenic purpura
  Neuromuscular & skeletal: Stiff neck
  Ocular: Diplopia, optic neuritis
  Respiratory: Difficulty of breathing
  Miscellaneous: Hypersensitivity

The chance of a child having a convulsion after receiving the measles vaccine is small. The risk is up to 5 times greater if the child has ever had a convulsion before or if the child's brother, sister, or parent has ever had a convulsion.

Pregnancy Risk Factor X

Comments Federal law requires that the date of administration, the vaccine manufacturer, lot number of vaccine, and the administering person's name, title and address be entered into the patient's permanent medical record

Measles, Mumps, and Rubella Vaccines, Combined

(mee' zels, mumpz & roo bel' a vak seens' kom bined')

Brand Names M-M-R® II

Therapeutic Category Vaccine, Live Virus

Synonyms MMR; Mumps, Measles and Rubella Vaccines, Combined; Rubella, Measles and Mumps Vaccines, Combined

Use Measles, mumps, and rubella prophylaxis

Usual Dosage
  Infants <12 months: If there is risk of exposure to measles, single-antigen measles vaccine should be administered at 6-11 months of age with a second dose (of MMR) at >12 months of age
  Give S.C. in outer aspect of the upper arm to children ≥15 months of age:
    0.5 mL at 15 months of age and then repeated at 4-6 years• of age
    In some areas, MMR vaccine may be given at 12 months
    •Many experts recommend that this dose of MMR be given at entry to middle school or junior high school

Local Anesthetic/Vasoconstrictor Precautions No information available to require special precautions

Effects on Dental Treatment No effects or complications reported

Other Adverse Effects All serious adverse reactions must be reported to the FDA

1% to 10%:
  Dermatologic: Transient rash, tenderness erythema and swelling
  Gastrointestinal: Sore throat
  Miscellaneous: Allergic reactions

<1%: Central nervous system: Seizures, malaise, fever

The chance of a child having a convulsion after receiving the measles vaccine is small. The risk is up to 5 times greater if the child has ever had a convulsion before or if the child's brother, sister, or parent has ever had a convulsion.

Pregnancy Risk Factor X

Comments Federal law requires that the date of administration, the vaccine manufacturer, lot number of vaccine, and the administering person's name, title and address be entered into the patient's permanent medical record

Measles Virus Vaccine, Live (mee' zels vye' rus vak seen', live)
Brand Names Attenuvax®
Canadian/Mexican Brand Names Ervevax (Mexico)
Therapeutic Category Vaccine, Live Virus
Synonyms More Attenuated Enders Strain; Rubeola Vaccine
Use Immunization against measles (rubeola) in persons ≥15 months of age
Usual Dosage Children >15 months and Adults: S.C.: 0.5 mL in outer aspect of the upper arm, no routine boosters
Local Anesthetic/Vasoconstrictor Precautions No information available to require special precautions
Effects on Dental Treatment No effects or complications reported
Other Adverse Effects All serious adverse reactions must be reported to the FDA
Central nervous system: Rarely encephalitis, fever, headache
Dermatologic: Rarely urticaria, erythema

>10%:
  Cardiovascular: Swelling
  Central nervous system: Fever <100°F
  Local: Burning or stinging, induration
1% to 10%:
  Central nervous system: Fever between 100°F and 103°F
  Miscellaneous: Allergic reaction (delayed type)
<1%:
  Dermatologic: Hives, itching, reddening of skin (especially around ears and eyes)
  Central nervous system: Tiredness, convulsions, encephalitis, confusion, severe headache, fever >103°F (prolonged)
  Gastrointestinal: Vomiting, sore throat
  Hematologic: Thrombocytopenic purpura
  Ocular: Diplopia
  Neuromuscular & skeletal: Stiff neck
  Respiratory: Difficulty of breathing
  Miscellaneous: Lymphadenopathy, coryza
Pregnancy Risk Factor X
Comments Federal law requires that the date of administration, the vaccine manufacturer, lot number of vaccine, and the administering person's name, title and address be entered into the patient's permanent medical record

Measurin® [OTC] see Aspirin on page 78
Mebaral® see Mephobarbital on page 540

Mebendazole (me ben' da zole)
Brand Names Vermox®
Canadian/Mexican Brand Names Helminzole® (Mexico); Mebensole® (Mexico); Revapol® (Mexico); Soltric® (Mexico); Vermicol® (Mexico)
Therapeutic Category Anthelmintic
Use Treatment of pinworms, whipworms, roundworms, and hookworms
Usual Dosage Children and Adults: Oral:
Pinworms: 100 mg as a single dose; may need to repeat after 2 weeks; treatment should include family members in close contact with patient
Whipworms, roundworms, hookworms: One tablet twice daily, morning and evening on 3 consecutive days; if patient is not cured within 3-4 weeks, a second course of treatment may be administered
Capillariasis: 200 mg twice daily for 20 days
Mechanism of Action Selectively and irreversibly blocks glucose uptake and other nutrients in susceptible adult intestine-dwelling helminths
Local Anesthetic/Vasoconstrictor Precautions No information available to require special precautions
Effects on Dental Treatment No effects or complications reported
Other Adverse Effects
1% to 10%: Gastrointestinal: Abdominal pain, diarrhea, nausea, vomiting
<1%:
  Central nervous system: Fever, dizziness, headache
  Dermatologic: Skin rash, itching, alopecia (with high dose)
  Hematologic: Neutropenia (sore throat, unusual tiredness and weakness)
Drug Interactions Decreased effect: Anticonvulsants such as carbamazepine and phenytoin may increase metabolism of mebendazole
(Continued)

Mebendazole *(Continued)*

Drug Uptake
Absorption: Only 2% to 10%
Serum half-life: 1-11.5 hours
Time to peak serum concentration: Within 2-4 hours
Pregnancy Risk Factor C

Mecamylamine Hydrochloride
(mek a mil' a meen hye droe klor' ide)
Brand Names Inversine®
Therapeutic Category Ganglionic Blocking Agent
Use Treatment of moderately severe to severe hypertension and in uncomplicated malignant hypertension
Usual Dosage Adults: Oral: 2.5 mg twice daily after meals for 2 days; increased by increments of 2.5 mg at intervals ≥2 days until desired blood pressure response is achieved; average daily dose: 25 mg
Mechanism of Action Mecamylamine is a ganglionic blocker. This agent inhibits acetylcholine at the autonomic ganglia, causing a decrease in blood pressure. Mecamylamine also blocks central nicotinic cholinergic receptors, which inhibits the effects of nicotine and may suppress the desire to smoke.
Local Anesthetic/Vasoconstrictor Precautions No information available to require special precautions
Effects on Dental Treatment No effects or complications reported
Other Adverse Effects
>10%:
Cardiovascular: Postural hypotension
Central nervous system: Drowsiness
Endocrine & metabolic: Decreased sexual ability
Gastrointestinal: Dry mouth
Ocular: Blurred vision, enlarged pupils
1% to 10%:
Gastrointestinal: Loss of appetite, nausea, vomiting
Renal: Difficult urination
<1%:
Central nervous system: Convulsions, confusion, mental depression
Gastrointestinal: Bloating, frequent stools, followed by severe constipation
Neuromuscular & skeletal: Uncontrolled movements of hands, arms, legs, or face, trembling
Respiratory: Shortness of breath
Pregnancy Risk Factor C

Meclan® *see* Meclocycline Sulfosalicylate *on next page*

Meclizine Hydrochloride (mek' li zeen hye droe klor' ide)
Brand Names Antivert®; Antrizine®; Bonine® [OTC]; Dizmiss® [OTC]; Meni-D®; Ru-Vert-M®; Vergon® [OTC]
Therapeutic Category Antiemetic; Antihistamine
Synonyms Meclozina, Clorhidrato De (Mexico)
Use Prevention and treatment of symptoms of motion sickness; management of vertigo with diseases affecting the vestibular system
Usual Dosage Children >12 years and Adults: Oral:
Motion sickness: 12.5-25 mg 1 hour before travel, repeat dose every 12-24 hours if needed; doses up to 50 mg may be needed
Vertigo: 25-100 mg/day in divided doses
Mechanism of Action Has central anticholinergic action by blocking chemoreceptor trigger zone; decreases excitability of the middle ear labyrinth and blocks conduction in the middle ear vestibular-cerebellar pathways
Local Anesthetic/Vasoconstrictor Precautions No information available to require special precautions
Effects on Dental Treatment Up to 10% of patients will have significant dry mouth which will disappear with cessation of drug therapy
Other Adverse Effects
>10%:
Central nervous system: Slight to moderate drowsiness
Respiratory: Thickening of bronchial secretions
1% to 10%:
Central nervous system: Headache, fatigue, nervousness, dizziness
Gastrointestinal: Appetite increase, weight increase, nausea, diarrhea, abdominal pain, dry mouth
Neuromuscular & skeletal: Arthralgia
Respiratory: Pharyngitis

<1%:
  Cardiovascular: Palpitations, hypotension
  Central nervous system: Depression, sedation
  Dermatologic: Photosensitivity, rash, angioedema
  Genitourinary: Urinary retention
  Hepatic: Hepatitis
  Neuromuscular & skeletal: Myalgia, tremor, paresthesia
  Ocular: Blurred vision
  Respiratory: Bronchospasm
  Miscellaneous: Epistaxis
Drug Interactions Increased toxicity: CNS depressants, neuroleptics, anticholinergics
Drug Uptake
  Onset of action: Oral: Within 1 hour
  Duration: 8-24 hours
  Serum half-life: 6 hours
Pregnancy Risk Factor B

Meclocycline Sulfosalicylate
  (me kloe sye' kleen sul foe sa lis' i late)
Brand Names Meclan®
Therapeutic Category Antibiotic, Topical; Topical Skin Product, Acne
Use Topical treatment of inflammatory acne vulgaris
Usual Dosage Children >11 years and Adults: Topical: Apply generously to affected areas twice daily
Mechanism of Action Inhibits bacterial protein synthesis by binding with the 30S and possibly the 50S ribosomal subunit(s) of susceptible bacteria; may also cause alterations in the cytoplasmic membrane
Local Anesthetic/Vasoconstrictor Precautions No information available to require special precautions
Effects on Dental Treatment No effects or complications reported
Other Adverse Effects
  >10%: Topical: Follicular staining, yellowing of the skin, burning/stinging feeling
  1% to 10%: Topical: Pain, redness, skin irritation, dermatitis
Drug Interactions No data reported
Drug Uptake Absorption: Topical: Very little
Pregnancy Risk Factor B

Meclofenamate Sodium (me kloe fen am' ate sow' dee um)
Related Information
  Nonsteroidal Anti-Inflammatory Agents, Comparative Dosages, and Pharmacokinetics *on page 1021*
  Rheumatoid Arthritis, Osteoarthritis, and Joint Prostheses *on page 930*
Brand Names Meclomen®
Therapeutic Category Analgesic, Non-narcotic; Anti-inflammatory Agent; Nonsteroidal Anti-inflammatory Agent (NSAID), Oral
Use Treatment of inflammatory disorders
Usual Dosage Children >14 years and Adults: Oral:
  Mild to moderate pain: 50 mg every 4-6 hours, not to exceed 400 mg/day
  Rheumatoid arthritis/osteoarthritis: 200-400 mg/day in 3-4 equal doses
Mechanism of Action Inhibits prostaglandin synthesis by decreasing the activity of the enzyme, cyclo-oxygenase, which results in decreased formation of prostaglandin precursors
Local Anesthetic/Vasoconstrictor Precautions No information available to require special precautions
Effects on Dental Treatment Caution is recommended in dental patients requiring surgery since most NSAIDs inhibit platelet aggregation and prolong bleeding time. Recovery of platelet function usually occurs 1-2 days after discontinuation of NSAIDs.
Other Adverse Effects
  >10%:
    Central nervous system: Dizziness
    Dermatologic: Skin rash
    Gastrointestinal: Abdominal cramps, heartburn, indigestion, nausea
  1% to 10%:
    Cardiovascular: Fluid retention
    Central nervous system: Headache, nervousness
    Dermatologic: Itching
    Gastrointestinal: Vomiting
(Continued)

Meclofenamate Sodium *(Continued)*

Otic: Ringing in ears

<1%:

Cardiovascular: Congestive heart failure, hypertension, arrhythmia, hot flushes, tachycardia

Central nervous system: Epistaxis, confusion, hallucinations, aseptic meningitis, mental depression, drowsiness, insomnia

Dermatologic: Hives, erythema multiforme, toxic epidermal necrolysis, Stevens-Johnson syndrome, angioedema

Endocrine & metabolic: Polydipsia

Gastrointestinal: Gastritis, GI ulceration

Genitourinary: Cystitis

Hematologic: Agranulocytosis, anemia, hemolytic anemia, bone marrow depression, leukopenia, thrombocytopenia

Hepatic: Hepatitis

Neuromuscular & skeletal: Peripheral neuropathy

Ocular: Toxic amblyopia, blurred vision, conjunctivitis, dry eyes

Otic: Decreased hearing

Renal: Polyuria, acute renal failure

Respiratory: Allergic rhinitis, shortness of breath

Drug Interactions

Decreased effect with aspirin; decreased effect of diuretics, antihypertensives

Increased effect/toxicity of warfarin, methotrexate

Drug Uptake

Duration of action: 2-4 hours

Serum half-life: 2-3.3 hours

Time to peak serum concentration: Within 0.5-1.5 hours

Pregnancy Risk Factor B (D if used in the 3rd trimester)

Meclomen® *see* Meclofenamate Sodium *on previous page*

Meclozina, Clorhidrato De (Mexico) *see* Meclizine Hydrochloride *on page 530*

Medigesic® *see* Butalbital Compound *on page 133*

Medihaler-Iso® *see* Isoproterenol *on page 472*

Medilax® [OTC] *see* Phenolphthalein *on page 682*

Medipren® [OTC] *see* Ibuprofen *on page 447*

Medi-Quick® *see* Bacitracin, Neomycin, and Polymyxin B *on page 94*

Medium Chain Triglycerides

(mee dee' um chane trye glis' er ides)

Brand Names MCT Oil® [OTC]

Therapeutic Category Nutritional Supplement

Synonyms Triglycerides, Medium Chain

Use Dietary supplement for those who cannot digest long chain fats; malabsorption associated with disorders such as pancreatic insufficiency, bile salt deficiency, and bacterial overgrowth of the small bowel; induce ketosis as a prevention for seizures (akinetic, clonic, and petit mal)

Local Anesthetic/Vasoconstrictor Precautions No information available to require special precautions

Effects on Dental Treatment No effects or complications reported

Other Adverse Effects

CNS effects: May result in **narcosis** and **coma** in cirrhotic patients due to high levels of medium chain fatty acids in the serum which then enter the cerebral spinal fluid; electroencephalogram effects include slowing of the alpha wave (can occur during infusion of fatty acids of 2-6 carbon lengths)

Endocrine & metabolic effects:

MCT therapy does not produce recognized metabolic side effects of any clinical importance, nor do they interfere with the metabolism of other food stuffs or with the absorption of drugs; when administered in the form of a mixed diet with carbohydrates and protein, there is no clinical evidence of **hyperketonemia**; hyperketonemia may occur in normal or diabetic subjects in the absence of carbohydrates; has been reported that MCT may increase hepatic free fatty acid synthesis and reduce ketone clearance

Fecal water, sodium and potassium excretion are decreased in patients with steatorrhea who are treated with MCT; enhanced calcium absorption has been demonstrated in patients with steatorrhea who are given MCT

Gastrointestinal effects: Nausea, occasional vomiting, abdominal discomfort and distention, diarrhea, and borborygmi are common adverse reactions occurring in about 10% of the patients receiving supplements or diets

532

containing MCT; these symptoms may be related to rapid hydrolysis of MCT, high concentrations of free fatty acids in the stomach and small intestine, hyperosmolarity causing influx of large amounts of fluid, and lactose intolerance; abdominal cramps, nausea and vomiting occurred despite cautionary administration of MCT in small sips throughout meals, but subsided with continued administration

Comments Does not provide any essential fatty acids; only saturated fats are contained; supplementation with safflower, corn oil, or other polyunsaturated vegetable oil must be given to provide the patient with the essential fatty acids. The minimum daily requirement has not been established for oral intake, but 10-15 mL of safflower oil (60% to 70% linoleic acid) appears to be satisfactory. Contains 7.7 kcal/mL

Medralone® *see* Methylprednisolone *on page 569*

Medrol® *see* Methylprednisolone *on page 569*

Medroxyprogesterone Acetate
(me drox' ee proe jes' te rone as' e tate)
Related Information
Endocrine Disorders & Pregnancy *on page 927*
Brand Names Amen®; Curretab®; Cycrin®; Depo-Provera®; Provera®
Therapeutic Category Contraceptive, Progestin Only; Progestin Derivative
Use Endometrial carcinoma or renal carcinoma as well as secondary amenorrhea or abnormal uterine bleeding due to hormonal imbalance; prevention of pregnancy
Usual Dosage
Adolescents and Adults: Oral:
Amenorrhea: 5-10 mg/day for 5-10 days or 2.5 mg/day
Abnormal uterine bleeding: 5-10 mg for 5-10 days starting on day 16 or 21 of cycle
Accompanying cyclic estrogen therapy, postmenopausal: 2.5-10 mg the last 10-13 days of estrogen dosing each month
Adults: I.M.:
Endometrial or renal carcinoma: 400-1000 mg/week
Contraception: 150 mg every 3 months or 450 mg every 6 months
Mechanism of Action Inhibits secretion of pituitary gonadotropins, which prevents follicular maturation and ovulation, stimulates growth of mammary tissue
Local Anesthetic/Vasoconstrictor Precautions No information available to require special precautions
Effects on Dental Treatment Caution is not required in prescribing antibiotics to female dental patients taking Depo-Provera® since there is no interaction with the progesterone ingredient
Other Adverse Effects
>10%:
Cardiovascular: Edema
Central nervous system: Weakness
Endocrine & metabolic: Breakthrough bleeding, spotting, changes in menstrual flow, amenorrhea
Gastrointestinal: Anorexia
Local: Pain at injection site
1% to 10%:
Cardiovascular: Embolism, central thrombosis
Central nervous system: Mental depression, fever, insomnia
Dermatologic: Melasma or chloasma, allergic rash with or without pruritus
Endocrine & metabolic: Changes in cervical erosion and secretions, weight gain or loss, increased breast tenderness
Hepatic: Cholestatic jaundice
Local: Thrombophlebitis
Drug Interactions Decreased effect: Aminoglutethimide may decrease effects by increasing hepatic metabolism
Drug Uptake
Absorption: I.M.: Slow
Pregnancy Risk Factor X

Medrysone (me' dri sone)
Brand Names HMS Liquifilm® Ophthalmic
Therapeutic Category Anti-inflammatory Agent, Ophthalmic; Corticosteroid, Ophthalmic
Use Treatment of allergic conjunctivitis, vernal conjunctivitis, episcleritis, ophthalmic epinephrine sensitivity reaction
(Continued)

Medrysone (Continued)

Usual Dosage Children and Adults: Ophthalmic: Instill 1 drop in conjunctival sac 2-4 times/day up to every 4 hours; may use every 1-2 hours during first 1-2 days

Mechanism of Action Decreases inflammation by suppression of migration of polymorphonuclear leukocytes and reversal of increased capillary permeability

Local Anesthetic/Vasoconstrictor Precautions No information available to require special precautions

Effects on Dental Treatment No effects or complications reported

Other Adverse Effects

1% to 10%: Ocular: Temporary mild blurred vision

<1%: Ocular: Stinging, burning eyes, corneal thinning, increased intraocular pressure, glaucoma, damage to the optic nerve, defects in visual activity, cataracts, secondary ocular infection

Drug Uptake

Absorption: Through aqueous humor

Pregnancy Risk Factor C

Comments Medrysone is a synthetic corticosteroid; structurally related to progesterone; if no improvement after several days of treatment, discontinue medrysone and institute other therapy; duration of therapy: 3-4 days to several weeks dependent on type and severity of disease; taper dose to avoid disease exacerbation

Mefenamic Acid (me fe nam' ik as' id)

Related Information

Nonsteroidal Anti-Inflammatory Agents, Comparative Dosages, and Pharma-cokinetics *on page 1021*

Brand Names Ponstel®

Canadian/Mexican Brand Names Ponstan® (Canada); Ponstan-500® (Mexico)

Therapeutic Category Analgesic, Non-narcotic; Nonsteroidal Anti-inflamma-tory Agent (NSAID), Oral

Synonyms Mefenamico, Acido (Mexico)

Use Short-term relief of mild to moderate pain including primary dysmenorrhea

Usual Dosage Children >14 years and Adults: Oral: 500 mg to start then 250 mg every 4 hours as needed; maximum therapy: 1 week

Mechanism of Action Inhibits prostaglandin synthesis by decreasing the activity of the enzyme, cyclo-oxygenase, which results in decreased formation of prostaglandin precursors

Local Anesthetic/Vasoconstrictor Precautions No information available to require special precautions

Effects on Dental Treatment Caution is recommended in dental patients requiring surgery since most NSAIDs inhibit platelet aggregation and prolong bleeding time. Recovery of platelet function usually occurs 1-2 days after discontinuation of NSAIDs.

Other Adverse Effects

>10%:
Central nervous system: Dizziness
Dermatologic: Skin rash
Gastrointestinal: Abdominal cramps, heartburn, indigestion, nausea

1% to 10%:
Cardiovascular: Fluid retention
Central nervous system: Headache, nervousness
Dermatologic: Itching
Gastrointestinal: Vomiting
Otic: Ringing in ears

<1%:
Cardiovascular: Congestive heart failure, hypertension, arrhythmias, tachy-cardia, hot flushes
Central nervous system: Epistaxis, confusion, hallucinations, aseptic menin-gitis, mental depression, drowsiness, insomnia
Dermatologic: Hives, erythema multiforme, toxic epidermal necrolysis, Stevens-Johnson syndrome, angioedema
Endocrine & metabolic: Polydipsia
Gastrointestinal: Gastritis, GI ulceration
Genitourinary: Cystitis
Hematologic: Agranulocytosis, anemia, hemolytic anemia, bone marrow depression, leukopenia, thrombocytopenia
Hepatic: Hepatitis
Neuromuscular & skeletal: Peripheral neuropathy

Ocular: Toxic amblyopia, blurred vision, conjunctivitis, dry eyes
Otic: Decreased hearing
Renal: Polyuria, acute renal failure
Respiratory: Shortness of breath, allergic rhinitis
Drug Interactions
Decreased effect of diuretics, antihypertensives; decreased effect with aspirin
Increased effect/toxicity with oral anticoagulants, methotrexate
Drug Uptake
Duration of action: Up to 6 hours
Serum half-life: 3.5 hours
Pregnancy Risk Factor C

Mefenamico, Acido (Mexico) see Mefenamic Acid on previous page

Mefloquine Hydrochloride (me' floe kwin hye droe klor' ide)
Brand Names Lariam®
Therapeutic Category Antimalarial Agent
Use Treatment of acute malarial infections and prevention of malaria
Usual Dosage Oral:
Children: Malaria prophylaxis:
15-19 kg: ¼ tablet
20-30 kg: ½ tablet
31-45 kg: ¾ tablet
>45 kg: 1 tablet
Administer weekly starting 1 week before travel, continuing weekly during travel and for 4 weeks after leaving endemic area

Adults:
Treatment of mild to moderate malaria infection: 5 tablets (1250 mg) as a single dose with at least 8 oz of water
Malaria prophylaxis: 1 tablet (250 mg) once weekly for 4 weeks, then 1 tablet every other week; start treatment 1 week prior to departure to an endemic area; to avoid development of malaria after return from an endemic area, continue prophylaxis for 4 additional weeks; for prolonged stays in an endemic area, this prophylaxis can be achieved by continuing the recommended dosage schedule once weekly for 4 weeks, then once every other week, until traveler has taken 3 doses following return to a malaria-free area
Mechanism of Action Mefloquine is a quinoline-methanol compound structurally similar to quinine; mefloquine's effectiveness in the treatment and prophylaxis of malaria is due to the destruction of the asexual blood forms of the malarial pathogens that affect humans, Plasmodium falciparum, P. vivax, P. malariae, P. ovale
Local Anesthetic/Vasoconstrictor Precautions No information available to require special precautions
Effects on Dental Treatment No effects or complications reported
Other Adverse Effects
1% to 10%:
Central nervous system: Difficulty concentrating, headache, insomnia, lightheadedness, vertigo
Gastrointestinal: Vomiting, diarrhea, stomach pain, nausea
Ocular: Visual disturbances
Otic: Tinnitus
<1%:
Cardiovascular: Bradicardia, extrasystoles, syncope
Central nervous system: Anxiety, dizziness, confusion, seizures, hallucinations, mental depression, psychosis
Drug Uptake
Absorption: Oral: Well absorbed
Serum half-life: 21-22 days
Pregnancy Risk Factor C
Comments To avoid relapse after initial treatment with mefloquine, patients should subsequently be treated with an 8-aminoquinolone (eg, primaquine)

Mefoxin® see Cefoxitin Sodium on page 168
Mega-B® [OTC] see Vitamin B Complex on page 899
Megace® see Megestrol Acetate on this page
Megaton™ [OTC] see Vitamin B Complex on page 899

Megestrol Acetate (me jes' trole as' e tate)
Brand Names Megace®
Therapeutic Category Antineoplastic Agent, Hormone; Progestin Derivative
(Continued)

Megestrol Acetate *(Continued)*

Use Palliative treatment of breast and endometrial carcinomas, appetite stimulation, and promotion of weight gain in cachexia

Usual Dosage Adults: Oral (**refer to individual protocols**):

Female:

Breast carcinoma: 40 mg 4 times/day

Endometrial: 40-320 mg/day in divided doses; use for 2 months to determine efficacy; maximum doses used have been up to 800 mg/day

Uterine bleeding: 40 mg 2-4 times/day

Male and Female: HIV-related cachexia: Initial dose: 800 mg/day; daily doses of 400 and 800 mg/day were found to be clinically effective

Mechanism of Action Megestrol is an antineoplastic progestin thought to act through an antileutenizing effect mediated via the pituitary

Local Anesthetic/Vasoconstrictor Precautions No information available to require special precautions

Effects on Dental Treatment No effects or complications reported

Other Adverse Effects

>10%:

Cardiovascular: Edema

Central nervous system: Weakness

Endocrine & metabolic: Breakthrough bleeding and amenorrhea, spotting, changes in menstrual flow

1% to 10%:

Central nervous system: Insomnia, depression, fever, headache

Dermatologic: Allergic rash with or without pruritus, melasma or chloasma, skin rash, and rarely alopecia

Endocrine & metabolic: Changes in cervical erosion and secretions, increased breast tenderness, amenorrhea, changes in vaginal bleeding pattern, edema, fluid retention, hyperglycemia

Gastrointestinal: Weight gain (not attributed to edema or fluid retention), nausea, vomiting, stomach cramps

Hepatic: Cholestatic jaundice, hepatotoxicity

Myelosuppressive:

WBC: None

Platelets: None

Local: Thrombophlebitis

Miscellaneous: Hyperpnea, carpal tunnel syndrome

Drug Interactions No data reported

Drug Uptake

Onset of action: At least 2 months of continuous therapy is necessary

Absorption: Oral: Well absorbed

Time to peak serum concentration: Oral: Within 1-3 hours

Serum half-life, elimination: 15-20 hours

Pregnancy Risk Factor X

Melanex® *see* Hydroquinone *on page 439*

Mellaril® *see* Thioridazine *on page 840*

Mellaril-S® *see* Thioridazine *on page 840*

Melphalan *(mel' fa lan)*

Brand Names Alkeran®

Therapeutic Category Antineoplastic Agent, Alkylating Agent (Nitrogen Mustard)

Synonyms L-PAM; L-Sarcolysin; Phenylalanine Mustard

Use Palliative treatment of multiple myeloma and nonresectable epithelial ovarian carcinoma; neuroblastoma, rhabdomyosarcoma, breast cancer, sarcoma; I.V. formulation: Use in patients in whom oral therapy is not appropriate

Usual Dosage

Oral (refer to individual protocols); dose should always be adjusted to patient response and weekly blood counts:

Children: 4-20 mg/m^2/day for 1-21 days

Adults:

Multiple myeloma: 6 mg/day initially adjusted as indicated **or** 0.15 mg/kg/day for 7 days **or** 0.25 mg/kg/day for 4 days; repeat at 4- to 6-week intervals

Ovarian carcinoma: 0.2 mg/kg/day for 5 days, repeat every 4-5 weeks

I.V. (refer to individual protocols):

Children:

Pediatric rhabdomyosarcoma: 10-35 mg/m^2/dose every 21-28 days

High-dose melphalan with bone marrow transplantation for neuroblastoma: 70-100 mg/m^2/day on day 7 and 6 before BMT; **or** 140-220 mg/m^2 single dose before BMT **or** 50 mg/m^2/day for 4 days; **or** 70 mg/m^2/day for 3 days

Adults: Multiple myeloma: 16 mg/m^2 administered at 2-week intervals for 4 doses, then repeat monthly as per protocol for multiple myeloma

Mechanism of Action Alkylating agent which is a derivative of mechloretha-mine that inhibits DNA and RNA synthesis via formation of carbonium ions; cross-links strands of DNA

Local Anesthetic/Vasoconstrictor Precautions No information available to require special precautions

Effects on Dental Treatment No effects or complications reported

Other Adverse Effects

>10%:

Myelosuppressive: Leukopenia and thrombocytopenia are the most common effects of melphalan. Irreversible bone marrow failure has been reported. WBC: Moderate; Platelets: Moderate; Onset (days): 7; Nadir (days): 8-10 and 27-32; Recovery (days): 42-50

Second malignancies: Reported are melphalan more frequently

Miscellaneous: SIADH, sterility and amenorrhea, pulmonary fibrosis, intersti-tial pneumonitis, alopecia, hypersensitivity, anemia, agranulocytosis, hemolytic anemia, pruritus, rash

1% to 10%: Vasculitis, alopecia, rash, pruritus, leukopenia, thrombocytopenia, anemia, agranulocytosis, hemolytic anemia, vesiculation of skin, bladder irritation, hemorrhagic cystitis, pulmonary fibrosis

Gastrointestinal: Nausea and vomiting are mild; stomatitis and diarrhea are infrequent

Drug Uptake

Absorption: Oral: Variable and incomplete from the GI tract; food interferes with absorption

Serum half-life, terminal: 1.5 hours

Time to peak serum concentration: Reportedly within 2 hours

Pregnancy Risk Factor D

Menadol® [OTC] see Ibuprofen on page 447

Menest® see Estrogens, Esterified on page 328

Meni-D® see Meclizine Hydrochloride on page 530

Meningococcal Polysaccharide Vaccine, Groups A, C, Y, and W-135

(me nin' joe kok al pol i sak' a ride vak seen' groops aye, see, why & dubl yoo won thur tee fyve)

Brand Names Menomune®-A/C/Y/W-135

Therapeutic Category Vaccine, Live Bacteria

Use Immunization against infection caused by *Neisseria meningitidis* groups A,C,Y, and W-135 in persons ≥2 years

Usual Dosage One dose I.M. (0.5 mL); the need for booster is unknown

Mechanism of Action Induces the formation of bactericidal antibodies to meningococcal antigens; the presence of these antibodies is strongly corre-lated with immunity to meningococcal disease caused by *Neisseria meningi-tidis* groups A, C, Y and W-135.

Local Anesthetic/Vasoconstrictor Precautions No information available to require special precautions

Effects on Dental Treatment No effects or complications reported

Other Adverse Effects

>10%:

Central nervous system: Pain

Dermatologic: Erythema and induration

Local: Tenderness

1% to 10%: Central nervous system: Headache, malaise, fever, chills

Drug Uptake

Onset: Antibody levels are achieved within 10-14 days after administration

Duration: Antibodies against group A and C polysaccharides decline markedly (to prevaccination levels) over the first 3 years following a single dose of vaccine, especially in children <4 years of age

Pregnancy Risk Factor C

Menomune®-A/C/Y/W-135 see Meningococcal Polysaccharide Vaccine, Groups A, C, Y, and W-135 on this page

Menotropins (men oh troe' pins)
Brand Names Pergonal®
Therapeutic Category Gonadotropin; Ovulation Stimulator
Use Sequentially with hCG to induce ovulation and pregnancy in the infertile woman with functional anovulation; used with hCG in men to stimulate spermatogenesis in those with primary hypogonadotropic hypogonadism
Usual Dosage Adults: I.M.:
   Male: Following pretreatment with hCG, 1 ampul 3 times/week and hCG 2000 units twice weekly until sperm is detected in the ejaculate (4-6 months) then may be increased to 2 ampuls of menotropins (150 units FSH/150 units LH) 3 times/week
   Female: 1 ampul/day (75 units of FSH and LH) for 9-12 days followed by 10,000 units hCG 1 day after the last dose; repeated at least twice at same level before increasing dosage to 2 ampuls (150 units FSH/150 units LH)
Mechanism of Action Actions occur as a result of both follicle stimulating hormone (FSH) effects and luteinizing hormone (LH) effects; menotropins stimulate the development and maturation of the ovarian follicle (FSH), cause ovulation (LH), and stimulate the development of the corpus luteum (LH); in males it stimulates spermatogenesis (LH)
Local Anesthetic/Vasoconstrictor Precautions No information available to require special precautions
Effects on Dental Treatment No effects or complications reported
Other Adverse Effects
   Male:
      >10%: Gynecomastia
      1% to 10%: Erythrocytosis (shortness of breath, dizziness, anorexia, fainting, epistaxis)
   Female:
      >10%: Ovarian enlargement, abdominal distention, pain/rash at injection site
      1% to 10%: Ovarian hyperstimulation syndrome
      <1%: Thromboembolism, pain, febrile reactions
Drug Interactions No data reported
Pregnancy Risk Factor X

Mentax® see Butenafine Hydrochloride on page 135

Mepenzolate Bromide (me pen' zoe late broe' mide)
Brand Names Cantil®
Therapeutic Category Anticholinergic Agent; Antispasmodic Agent, Gastrointestinal
Use Management of peptic ulcer disease; inhibit salivation and excessive secretions in respiratory tract preoperatively
Local Anesthetic/Vasoconstrictor Precautions No information available to require special precautions
Effects on Dental Treatment No effects or complications reported
Other Adverse Effects
   >10%:
      Gastrointestinal: Constipation
      Miscellaneous: Decreased sweating; dry mouth, skin, nose, or throat
   1% to 10%: Gastrointestinal: Difficulty in swallowing
   <1%:
      Dermatologic: Rash
      Central nervous system: Confusion, headache, loss of memory, tiredness, drowsiness, nervousness, insomnia
      Ocular: Increased intraocular pressure, blurred vision
      Gastrointestinal: Bloated feeling, nausea, vomiting
      Neuromuscular & skeletal: Weakness
      Genitourinary: Urinary retention
      Cardiovascular: Tachycardia

Mepergan® see Meperidine and Promethazine on this page

Meperidine and Promethazine
   (me per' i deen & proe meth' a zeen)
Brand Names Mepergan®
Therapeutic Category Analgesic, Narcotic
Use Management of moderate to severe pain
Local Anesthetic/Vasoconstrictor Precautions No information available to require special precautions
Effects on Dental Treatment Causes dry mouth in 1% to 10% of patients

Meperidine Hydrochloride (me per' i deen hye droe klor' ide)
Related Information
Dental Drug Interactions: Update on Drug Combinations Requiring Special Considerations *on page 1022*
Narcotic Agonist Charts *on page 1019*
Oral Pain *on page 940*
Brand Names Demerol®
Therapeutic Category Analgesic, Narcotic
Synonyms Isonipecaine (Canada); Pethidine Hydrochloride (Canada)
Use
Dental: Adjunct in preoperative intravenous conscious sedation in patients undergoing dental surgery; alternate oral narcotic in patients allergic to codeine to treat moderate to moderate-severe pain
Medical: Management of moderate to severe pain
Usual Dosage
Children: Oral: 25-50 mg every 4-6 hours as needed for pain
Adults:
I.V.: 50-100 mg titrated as a single dose to produce sedation
Oral: 50-100 mg every 4-6 hours as needed for pain
Mechanism of Action Binds to opiate receptors in the CNS, causing inhibition of ascending pain pathways, altering the perception of and response to pain; produces generalized CNS depression
Local Anesthetic/Vasoconstrictor Precautions No information available to require special precautions
Effects on Dental Treatment No effects or complications reported
Other Adverse Effects >10%:
Cardiovascular: Hypotension
Central nervous system: Weakness, tiredness, drowsiness, dizziness
Gastrointestinal: Nausea, vomiting, constipation
Miscellaneous: Histamine release

Oral manifestations: 1% to 10%: Dry mouth
Contraindications Hypersensitivity to meperidine or any component; patients receiving MAO inhibitors presently or in the past 14 days
Warnings/Precautions Use with caution in patients with pulmonary, hepatic, renal disorders, or increased intracranial pressure; use with caution in patients with renal failure or seizure disorders or those receiving high-dose meperidine; normeperidine (an active metabolite and CNS stimulant) may accumulate and precipitate twitches, tremors, or seizures; some preparations contain sulfites which may cause allergic reaction

Enhanced analgesia has been seen in elderly patients on therapeutic doses of narcotics; duration of action may be increased in the elderly; the elderly may be particularly susceptible to the CNS depressant and constipating effects of narcotics
Drug Interactions Phenytoin may decrease the analgesic effects of meperidine; meperidine may aggravate the adverse effects of isoniazid; MAO inhibitors, fluoxetine, and other serotonin uptake inhibitors greatly potentiate the effects of meperidine; acute opioid overdosage symptoms can be seen, including severe toxic reactions; CNS depressants, tricyclic antidepressants, phenothiazines may potentiate the effects of meperidine
Drug Uptake
Onset of effect: I.V.: Within 5 minutes
Time to peak serum concentration: Oral: 90-120 minutes
Duration: 4-6 hours
Serum half-life:
Parent drug, terminal phase:
Adults: 2.5-4 hours
Adults with liver disease: 7-11 hours
Normeperidine (active metabolite): 15-30 hours; dependent on renal function and can accumulate with higher doses or in patients with decreased renal function
Pregnancy Risk Factor B (D if used for prolonged periods or in high doses at term)
Breast-feeding Considerations Considered compatible by AAO in 1983 statement; however, not included in the 1989 statement
Dosage Forms
Syrup: 50 mg/5 mL (500 mL)
Tablet: 50 mg, 100 mg
Dietary Considerations No data reported
Generic Available Yes
(Continued)

Meperidine Hydrochloride *(Continued)*

Comments Meperidine is not to be used as the narcotic drug of first choice. It is recommended only to be used in codeine-allergic patients when a narcotic analgesic is indicated. Meperidine is not an anti-inflammatory agent. Meperidine, as with other narcotic analgesics, is recommended only for limited acute dosing (ie, 3 days or less); common adverse effects in the dental patient are nausea, sedation, and constipation. Meperidine has a significant addiction liability, especially when given long term.

Mephenytoin *(me fen' i toyn)*
Brand Names Mesantoin®
Therapeutic Category Anticonvulsant, Hydantoin
Use Treatment of tonic-clonic and partial seizures in patients who are uncontrolled with less toxic anticonvulsants
Mechanism of Action Stabilizes neuronal membranes and decreases seizure activity by increasing efflux or decreasing influx of sodium ions across cell membranes in the motor cortex during generation of nerve impulses; prolongs effective refractory period and suppresses ventricular pacemaker automaticity, shortens action potential in the heart
Local Anesthetic/Vasoconstrictor Precautions No information available to require special precautions
Effects on Dental Treatment Mephenytoin, like phenytoin, causes gingival hyperplasia. Usually starts during the first 6 months of dental treatment as gingivitis. The incidence is higher in patients under 20 years of age. To minimize severity and growth rate of gingival tissue begin a program of professional cleaning and patient plaque control within 10 days of starting anticonvulsant therapy. GH induced by mephenytoin disappears with cessation of drug therapy.
Other Adverse Effects
>10%:
  Central nervous system: Psychiatric changes, slurred speech, dizziness, drowsiness
  Gastrointestinal: Constipation, nausea, vomiting
  Neuromuscular & skeletal: Trembling
1% to 10%:
  Central nervous system: Drowsiness, headache, insomnia
  Dermatologic: Skin rash
  Gastrointestinal: Anorexia, weight loss
  Hematologic: Leukopenia
  Hepatic: Hepatitis
  Miscellaneous: Increase in serum creatinine
<1%:
  Cardiovascular: Hypotension, bradycardia, cardiac arrhythmias, cardiovascular collapse
  Central nervous system: Confusion, fever, ataxia
  Dermatologic: Stevens-Johnson syndrome or SLE-like syndrome
  Gastrointestinal: Gingival hyperplasia
  Hematologic: Blood dyscrasias
  Hepatic: Hepatitis
  Local: Venous irritation and pain, thrombophlebitis
  Neuromuscular & skeletal: Paresthesia, peripheral neuropathy
  Ocular: Diplopia, nystagmus, blurred vision, photophobia
  Miscellaneous: Lymphadenopathy, Hodgkin's disease-like syndrome, serum sickness
Drug Interactions
  Decreased effect with carbamazepine, TCAs, calcium antacids; decreased effect of oral anticoagulants, oral contraceptives, steroids, quinidine, vitamin D, vitamin K, doxycycline, furosemide, TCAs
  Increased effect/toxicity with alcohol, sulfonamides, chloramphenicol, cimetidine, isoniazid, disulfiram, phenothiazines, benzodiazepines
Pregnancy Risk Factor C

Mephobarbital *(me foe bar' bi tal)*
Brand Names Mebaral®
Therapeutic Category Anticonvulsant, Barbiturate
Use Sedative; treatment of grand mal and petit mal epilepsy
Usual Dosage Oral:
  Epilepsy:
    Children: 6-12 mg/kg/day in 2-4 divided doses
    Adults: 200-600 mg/day in 2-4 divided doses

Sedation:
Children:
<5 years: 16-32 mg 3-4 times/day
>5 years: 32-64 mg 3-4 times/day
Adults: 32-100 mg 3-4 times/day

Mechanism of Action Increases seizure threshold in the motor cortex; depresses monosynaptic and polysynaptic transmission in the CNS

Local Anesthetic/Vasoconstrictor Precautions No information available to require special precautions

Effects on Dental Treatment No effects or complications reported

Other Adverse Effects
>10%: Central nervous system: Dizziness, lightheadedness, drowsiness, "hangover" effect
1% to 10%:
Central nervous system: Confusion, mental depression, unusual excitement, nervousness, faint feeling, headache, insomnia, nightmares
Gastrointestinal: Constipation, nausea, vomiting
<1%:
Cardiovascular: Hypotension
Central nervous system: Hallucinations
Dermatologic: Skin rash, exfoliative dermatitis, Stevens-Johnson syndrome, angioedema
Hematologic: Agranulocytosis, megaloblastic anemia, thrombocytopenia
Local: Thrombophlebitis
Respiratory: Respiratory depression
Miscellaneous: Dependence

Drug Interactions
Mephobarbital causes decreased effects of the following drugs: Phenothiazines, haloperidol, quinidine, cyclosporine, TCAs, corticosteroids, theophylline, ethosuximide, warfarin, oral contraceptives, chloramphenicol, griseofulvin, doxycycline, beta-blockers
The following drugs enhance the CNS effects of mephobarbital: Propoxyphene, benzodiazepines, CNS depressants, valproic acid, methylphenidate, chloramphenicol

Drug Uptake
Onset of action: 20-60 minutes
Duration: 6-8 hours
Absorption: Oral: ~50%
Serum half-life: 34 hours

Pregnancy Risk Factor D

Mephyton® see Phytonadione on page 690

Mepivacaine Dental Anesthetic
(me piv' a kane den' tal an es the' tik)

Related Information
Oral Pain on page 940

Brand Names Carbocaine® 3%; Isocaine® HCl 3%; Polocaine® 3%

Canadian/Mexican Brand Names Polocaine® (Canada)

Therapeutic Category Dental/Local Anesthetics; Local Anesthetic, Injectable

Use Dental: Amide-type anesthetic used for local infiltration anesthesia; injection near nerve trunks to produce nerve block

Usual Dosage The lowest dose needed to provide effective anesthesia should be administered. For infiltration and block injections in the upper and lower jaw, the average dose of one cartridge is usually effective. Each cartridge contains 54 mg (3% of 1.8 mL solution); five cartridges (270 mg of 3% solution) are usually adequate to affect anesthesia of the entire oral cavity. Total dose for all injected sites should not exceed 400 mg in adults.

Mechanism of Action Local anesthetics bind selectively to the intracellular surface of sodium channels to block influx of sodium into the axon. As a result, depolarization necessary for action potential propagation and subsequent nerve function is prevented. The block at the sodium channel is reversible. When drug diffuses away from the axon, sodium channel function is restored and nerve propagation returns.

Local Anesthetic/Vasoconstrictor Precautions No information available to require special precautions

Effects on Dental Treatment No effects or complications reported

Other Adverse Effects Degree of adverse effects in the CNS and cardiovascular system are directly related to the blood levels of local anesthetic.
(Continued)

Mepivacaine Dental Anesthetic *(Continued)*

Cardiovascular: Myocardial effects include a decrease in contraction force as well as a decrease in electrical excitability and myocardial conduction rate resulting in bradycardia and reduction in cardiac output

Central nervous system: High blood levels result in anxiety, restlessness, disorientation, confusion, dizziness, tremors and seizures. This is followed by depression of CNS resulting in drowsiness, unconsciousness and possible respiratory arrest. Nausea and vomiting may also occur. In some cases, symptoms of CNS stimulation may be absent and the primary CNS effects are drowsiness and unconsciousness.

Hypersensitivity reactions: May be manifest as dermatologic reactions and edema at injection site. Asthmatic syndromes have occurred.

Psychogenic reactions: It is common to misinterpret psychogenic responses to local anesthetic injection as an allergic reaction. Intraoral injections is perceived by many patients as a stressful procedure in dentistry. Common symptoms to this stress are sweating, palpitations, hyperventilation, generalized pallor and a fainting feeling.

Oral manifestations: No data reported

Contraindications Hypersensitivity to local anesthetics of the amide type

Warnings/Precautions Aspirate the syringe after tissue penetration and before injection to minimize chance of direct vascular injection

Drug Interactions No data reported

Drug Uptake

Onset of action: 30-120 seconds in upper jaw; 1-4 minutes in lower jaw

Duration: 20 minutes in upper jaw; 40 minutes in lower jaw

Serum half-life: 1.9 hours

Pregnancy Risk Factor C

Breast-feeding Considerations Usual infiltration doses of mepivacaine dental anesthetic given to nursing mothers has not been shown to affect the health of the nursing infant

Dosage Forms Injection: Mepivacaine hydrochloride 3% (1.8 mL dental cartridges)

Dietary Considerations No data reported

Generic Available Yes

Mepivacaine With Levonordefrin

(me piv' a kane with lee voe nor def' rin)

Related Information

Oral Pain *on page 940*

Brand Names Carbocaine® 2% with Neo-Cobefrin®; Isocaine® HCl 2%; Polocaine® 2%

Canadian/Mexican Brand Names Polocaine® and Levonordefrin (Canada)

Therapeutic Category Dental/Local Anesthetics; Local Anesthetic, Injectable

Use Dental: Amide-type anesthetic used for local infiltration anesthesia; injection near nerve trunks to produce nerve block

Usual Dosage The lowest dose needed to provide effective anesthesia should be administered. For infiltration and block injections in the upper and lower jaw, an average dose of one cartridge usually provides effective anesthesia. Each cartridge contains 1.8 mL (36 mg of 2%). Five cartridges (180 mg of the 2% solution) are usually adequate to affect anesthesia of the entire oral cavity.

Mechanism of Action Local anesthetics bind selectively to the intracellular surface of sodium channels to block influx of sodium into the axon. As a result, depolarization necessary for action potential propagation and subsequent nerve function is prevented. The block at the sodium channel is reversible. When drug diffuses away from the axon, sodium channel function is restored and nerve propagation returns.

Levonordefrin prolongs the duration of the anesthetic actions of mepivacaine by causing vasoconstriction (alpha adrenergic receptor agonist) of the vasculature surrounding the nerve axons. This prevents the diffusion of mepivacaine away from the nerves resulting in a longer retention in the axon.

Local Anesthetic/Vasoconstrictor Precautions No information available to require special precautions

Effects on Dental Treatment No effects or complications reported

Other Adverse Effects Degree of adverse effects in the CNS and cardiovascular system are directly related to the blood levels of mepivacaine. The effects below are more likely to occur after systemic administration rather than infiltration.

Central nervous system: High blood levels result in anxiety, restlessness, disorientation, confusion, dizziness, tremors and seizures. This is followed by depression of CNS resulting in drowsiness, unconsciousness and possible respiratory arrest. Nausea and vomiting may also occur. In some cases, symptoms of CNS stimulation may be absent and the primary CNS effects are drowsiness and unconsciousness.

Cardiovascular: Myocardial effects include a decrease in contraction force as well as a decrease in electrical excitability and myocardial conduction rate resulting in bradycardia and reduction in cardiac output.

Hypersensitivity reactions: Extremely rare, but may be manifest as dermatologic reactions and edema at injection site. Asthmatic syndromes have occurred. Patients may exhibit hypersensitivity to bisulfites contained in local anesthetic solution to prevent oxidation of levonordefrin. In general, patients reacting to bisulfites have a history of asthma and their airways are hyperreactive to asthmatic syndrome.

Psychogenic reactions: It is common to misinterpret psychogenic responses to local anesthetic injection as an allergic reaction. Intraoral injections are perceived by many patients as a stressful procedure in dentistry. Common symptoms to this stress are sweating, palpitations, hyperventilation, generalized pallor and a fainting feeling.

Oral manifestations: No data reported

Contraindications Hypersensitivity to local anesthetics of the amide-type

Warnings/Precautions Should be avoided in patients with uncontrolled hyperthyroidism. Should be used in minimal amounts in patients with significant cardiovascular problems (because of levonordefrin component). Aspirate the syringe after tissue penetration and before injection to minimize chance of direct vascular injection.

Drug Interactions Due to levonordefrin component, use with tricyclic antidepressants or MAO inhibitors could result in increased pressor response; use with nonselective beta-blockers (ie, propranolol) could result in serious hypertension and reflex bradycardia

Drug Uptake
Duration: 1-2.5 hours in upper jaw and 2.5-5.5 hours in lower jaw
Infiltration: 50 minutes
Inferior alveolar block: 60-75 minutes

Pregnancy Risk Factor C

Breast-feeding Considerations Usual infiltration doses of mepivacaine with levonordefrin given to nursing mothers has not been shown to affect the health of the nursing infant

Dosage Forms Injection: Mepivacaine hydrochloride 2% with levonordefrin 1:20,000 (1.8 mL dental cartridges)

Dietary Considerations No data reported

Selected Readings
Jastak JT and Yagiela JA, "Vasoconstrictors and Local Anesthesia: A Review and Rationale for Use," *J Am Dent Assoc*, 1983, 107(4):623-30.
MacKenzie TA and Young ER, "Local Anesthetic Update," *Anesth Prog*, 1993, 40(2):29-34.
Wynn RL, "Epinephrine Interactions With Beta-Blockers," *Gen Dent*, 1994, 42(1):16, 18.
Yagiela JA, "Local Anesthetics," *Anesth Prog*, 1991, 38(4-5):128-41.

Meprobamate (me proe ba' mate)

Brand Names Equanil®; Meprospan®; Miltown®; Neuramate®

Canadian/Mexican Brand Names Apo-Meprobamate® (Canada); Meditran® (Canada); Novo-Mepro® (Canada)

Therapeutic Category Antianxiety Agent; Muscle Relaxant; Skeletal Muscle Relaxant; Tranquilizer, Minor

Use
Dental: Treatment of muscle spasm associated with acute temporomandibular joint pain; management of dental anxiety disorders
Unlabeled use: Demonstrated value for muscle contraction, headache, premenstrual tension, external sphincter spasticity, muscle rigidity, opisthotonos-associated with tetanus

Usual Dosage Oral:
Children 6-12 years: 100-200 mg 2-3 times/day
Sustained release: 200 mg twice daily
Adults: 400 mg 3-4 times/day, up to 2400 mg/day
Sustained release: 400-800 mg twice daily

Mechanism of Action Precise mechanism is not yet clear, but many effects have been ascribed to its central depressant actions

Local Anesthetic/Vasoconstrictor Precautions No information available to require special precautions

Effects on Dental Treatment No effects or complications reported

Other Adverse Effects
>10%: Central nervous system: Drowsiness, ataxia, loss of motor coordination
(Continued)

Meprobamate *(Continued)*

1% to 10%: Central nervous system: Dizziness

Oral manifestations: <1%: Stomatitis

Contraindications Acute intermittent porphyria; hypersensitivity to meprobamate or any component; do not use in patients with pre-existing CNS depression, narrow-angle glaucoma, or severe uncontrolled pain

Warnings/Precautions Physical and psychological dependence and abuse may occur; not recommended in children <6 years of age; allergic reaction may occur in patients with history of dermatological condition (usually by fourth dose); use with caution in patients with renal or hepatic impairment, or with a history of seizures

Drug Interactions CNS depressants cause increased CNS depression

Drug Uptake

Absorption: Oral: Rapid and nearly complete

Onset of sedation: Oral: Within 1 hour

Serum half-life: 10 hours

Pregnancy Risk Factor D

Breast-feeding Considerations Milk concentrations are higher then plasma; effects unknown; not recommended

Dosage Forms

Capsule, sustained release: 200 mg, 400 mg

Tablet: 200 mg, 400 mg, 600 mg

Dietary Considerations No data reported

Generic Available Yes

Meprobamate and Aspirin *see Aspirin and Meprobamate on page 81*

Mepron™ *see Atovaquone on page 84*

Meprospan® *see Meprobamate on previous page*

Merbromin *(mer broe' min)*

Brand Names Mercurochrome®

Therapeutic Category Topical Skin Product

Use Topical antiseptic

Local Anesthetic/Vasoconstrictor Precautions No information available to require special precautions

Effects on Dental Treatment No effects or complications reported

Mercaptopurine *(mer kap toe pyoor' een)*

Brand Names Purinethol®

Therapeutic Category Antineoplastic Agent, Antimetabolite; Antineoplastic Agent, Purine

Synonyms 6-Mercaptopurine; 6-MP

Use Treatment of acute leukemias (ALL, CML)

Usual Dosage Oral (**refer to individual protocols**):

Children:

Induction: 2.5-5 mg/kg/day given once daily

Maintenance: 1.5-2.5 mg/kg/day given once daily **or** 70-100 mg/m^2/day once daily

Adults:

Induction: 2.5-5 mg/kg/day (100-200 mg)

Maintenance: 1.5-2.5 mg/kg/day **or** 80-100 mg/m^2/day given once daily

Elderly: Due to renal decline with age, start with lower recommended doses for adults

Mechanism of Action Purine antagonist which inhibits DNA and RNA synthesis; acts as false metabolite and is incorporated into DNA and RNA, eventually inhibiting their synthesis. 6-MP is substituted for hypoxanthine; must be metabolized to active nucleotides once inside the cell.

Local Anesthetic/Vasoconstrictor Precautions No information available to require special precautions

Effects on Dental Treatment No effects or complications reported

Other Adverse Effects

>10%:

Hepatic: 6-MP can cause an intrahepatic cholestasis and focal centralobular necrosis manifested as hyperbilirubinemia, increased alkaline phosphatase, and increased AST. This may be dose related, occurring more frequently at doses >2.5 mg/kg/day; jaundice is noted 1-2 months into therapy, but has ranged from 1 week to 8 years.

1% to 10%: Renal toxicity, drug fever, hyperpigmentation, rash, weakness, hyperuricemia

Gastrointestinal: Nausea, vomiting, diarrhea, stomatitis, anorexia, stomach pain, and mucositis may require parenteral nutrition and dose reduction; 6-TG is less GI toxic than 6-MP

Hematologic: Leukopenia, thrombocytopenia, anemia may occur at high doses

Myelosuppressive: WBC: Moderate; Platelets: Moderate; Onset (days): 7-10; Nadir (days): 14; Recovery (days): 21

<1%: Glossitis, tarry stools

Miscellaneous: 6-MP can cause a dry, scaling rash, drug fever, eosinophilia, renal toxicity

Drug Uptake

Absorption: Variable and incomplete (16% to 50%)

Serum half-life (age-dependent):

Children: 21 minutes

Adults: 47 minutes

Time to peak serum concentration: Within 2 hours

Pregnancy Risk Factor D

6-Mercaptopurine *see* Mercaptopurine *on previous page*

Mercuric Oxide (mer kyoor' ik ok' side)

Therapeutic Category Antibiotic, Ophthalmic

Synonyms Yellow Mercuric Oxide

Use Treatment of irritation and minor infections of the eyelids

Local Anesthetic/Vasoconstrictor Precautions No information available to require special precautions

Effects on Dental Treatment No effects or complications reported

Mercurochrome® *see* Merbromin *on previous page*

Merlenate® Topical [OTC] *see* Undecylenic Acid and Derivatives *on page 884*

Meronem® *see* Meropenem *on this page*

Meropenem (mer oh pen' em)

Brand Names Meronem®; Merrem® I.V.

Therapeutic Category Antibiotic, Carbacephem

Use Meropenem is indicated as single agent therapy for the treatment of intra-abdominal infections including complicated appendicitis and peritonitis in adults and bacterial meningitis in pediatric patients >3 months of age caused by *S. pneumoniae, H. influenzae,* and *N. meningitidis* (penicillin-resistant pneumococci have not been studied in clinical trials); it is better tolerated than imipenem and highly effective against a broad range of bacteria

Usual Dosage

Children:

Intra-abdominal infections: 20 mg/kg every 8 hours (maximum dose: 1 g every 8 hours)

Meningitis: 40 mg/kg every 8 hours (maximum dose: 2 g every 8 hours)

Adults: 1 g every 8 hours (see Administration)

Dosing adjustment in renal impairment: Adults:

Cl_{cr} 26-50 mL/minute: Administer 1 g every 12 hours

Cl_{cr} 10-25 mL/minute: Administer 500 mg every 12 hours

Cl_{cr} <10 mL/minute: Administer 500 mg every 24 hours

Meropenem and its metabolites are readily dialyzable

Mechanism of Action Inhibits bacterial cell wall synthesis by binding to several of the penicillin-binding proteins, which in turn inhibit the final transpeptidation step of peptidoglycan synthesis in bacterial cell walls, thus inhibiting cell wall biosynthesis; bacteria eventually lyse due to ongoing activity of cell wall autolytic enzymes (autolysins and murein hydrolases) while cell wall assembly is arrested

Local Anesthetic/Vasoconstrictor Precautions No information available to require special precautions

Effects on Dental Treatment 1% to 10% of patients will experience oral moniliasis and glossitis

Other Adverse Effects

1% to 10%:

Central nervous system: Headache

Dermatologic: Rash, pruritus

Gastrointestinal: Diarrhea, nausea/vomiting, constipation, oral moniliasis, glossitis

Local: Injection site reaction/thrombophlebitis

Respiratory: Apnea

(Continued)

Meropenem *(Continued)*

<1%:
Cardiovascular: Heart failure, other cardiac symptoms including myocardial infarction and arrhythmias, edema
Central nervous system: Pain, fever, agitation/delirium, dizziness, seizure, hallucinations
Dermatologic: Urticaria
Gastrointestinal: Anorexia, flatulence
Hematologic: Bleeding event, anemia, hematologic effects both increase and decrease in cell counts
Hepatic: Hepatic failure, hepatic effects, increased LFTs
Renal: Kidney failure
Respiratory: Dyspnea
Miscellaneous: Sweating

Warnings/Precautions Do not administer to patients with serious hypersensitivity reactions to beta-lactam agents. Seizures and other CNS events have been reported during treatment with meropenem; these experiences have occurred most commonly in patients with pre-existing CNS disorders, with bacterial meningitis, and/or decreased renal function; may cause pseudomembranous colitis

Drug Interactions Probenecid interferes with renal excretion of meropenem

Drug Uptake
Serum half-life: ~1 hours

Pregnancy Risk Factor B

Generic Available No

Comments 1 g of meropenem contains 90.2 mg of sodium as sodium carbonate (3.92 mEq)

Selected Readings
Wiseman LR, Wagstaff AJ, Brogden RN, et al, "Meropenem: A Review of Its Antibacterial Activity, Pharmacokinetic Properties, and Clinical Efficacy," *Drugs*, 1995, 50:73-101.

Merrem® I.V. *see* Meropenem *on previous page*

Mersol® [OTC] *see* Thimerosal *on page 838*

Merthiolate® [OTC] *see* Thimerosal *on page 838*

Meruvax® II *see* Rubella Virus Vaccine, Live *on page 776*

Mesalamine *(me sal′ a meen)*

Brand Names Asacol®; Pentasa®; Rowasa®

Therapeutic Category 5-Aminosalicylic Acid Derivative; Anti-inflammatory Agent, Rectal

Use Treatment of ulcerative colitis, proctosigmoiditis, and proctitis

Usual Dosage Adults (usual course of therapy is 3-6 weeks):
Oral:
Capsule: 1 g 4 times/day
Tablet: 800 mg 3 times/day
Retention enema: 60 mL (4 g) at bedtime, retained overnight, approximately 8 hours
Rectal suppository: Insert 1 suppository in rectum twice daily
Some patients may require rectal and oral therapy concurrently

Mechanism of Action Mesalamine (5-aminosalicylic acid) is the active component of sulfasalazine; the specific mechanism of action of mesalamine is unknown; however, it is thought that it modulates local chemical mediators of the inflammatory response, especially leukotrienes; action appears topical rather than systemic

Local Anesthetic/Vasoconstrictor Precautions No information available to require special precautions

Effects on Dental Treatment No effects or complications reported

Other Adverse Effects
>10%:
Central nervous system: Headache, malaise
Gastrointestinal: Abdominal pain, cramps, flatulence, gas
1% to 10%: Dermatologic: Alopecia, rash
<1%: Anal irritation, acute intolerance syndrome (bloody diarrhea, severe abdominal cramps, severe headache)

Drug Interactions Decreased effect: Decreased digoxin bioavailability

Drug Uptake
Absorption: Rectal: ~15%; variable and dependent upon retention time, underlying GI disease, and colonic pH
Serum half-life:
5-ASA: 0.5-1.5 hours
Acetyl 5-ASA: 5-10 hours

Time to peak serum concentration: Within 4-7 hours
Pregnancy Risk Factor B

Mesantoin® *see* Mephenytoin *on page 540*

Mesoridazine Besylate (mez oh rid′ a zeen bes′ i late)

Brand Names Serentil®
Therapeutic Category Antipsychotic Agent; Phenothiazine Derivative
Use Symptomatic management of psychotic disorders, including schizophrenia, behavioral problems, alcoholism as well as reducing anxiety and tension occurring in neurosis
Usual Dosage Concentrate may be diluted just prior to administration with distilled water, acidified tap water, orange or grape juice; do not prepare and store bulk dilutions

Adults:
Oral: 25-50 mg 3 times/day; maximum: 100-400 mg/day
I.M.: 25 mg initially, repeat in 30-60 minutes as needed; optimal dosage range: 25-200 mg/day

Not dialyzable (0% to 5%)
Mechanism of Action Blockade of postsynaptic CNS dopamine receptors
Local Anesthetic/Vasoconstrictor Precautions No information available to require special precautions
Effects on Dental Treatment No effects or complications reported
Other Adverse Effects
>10%:
Cardiovascular: Hypotension, orthostatic hypotension
Central nervous system: Pseudoparkinsonism, akathisia, dystonias, tardive dyskinesia (persistent), dizziness
Gastrointestinal: Constipation
Ocular: Pigmentary retinopathy
Respiratory: Nasal congestion
Miscellaneous: Decreased sweating
1% to 10%:
Dermatologic: Increased sensitivity to sun, skin rash
Endocrine & metabolic: Changes in menstrual cycle, changes in libido, pain in breasts
Gastrointestinal: Weight gain, nausea, vomiting, stomach pain
Genitourinary: Difficulty in urination, ejaculatory disturbances
Neuromuscular & skeletal: Trembling of fingers
<1%:
Central nervous system: Neuroleptic malignant syndrome (NMS)
Dermatologic: Discoloration of skin (blue-gray)
Endocrine & metabolic: Galactorrhea
Genitourinary: Priapism
Hematologic: Agranulocytosis, leukopenia
Hepatic: Cholestatic jaundice, hepatotoxicity
Ocular: Cornea and lens changes, pigmentary retinopathy
Miscellaneous: Impairment of temperature regulation, lowering of seizures threshold
Drug Interactions
Decreased effect with anticonvulsants, anticholinergics
Increased toxicity with CNS depressants, metrizamide (increased seizures), propranolol
Drug Uptake
Duration of action: 4-6 hours
Absorption: Very erratic with oral tablet; oral liquids much more dependable
Serum half-life: 24-48 hours
Time to peak serum concentration: 2-4 hours
Pregnancy Risk Factor C

Mestranol and Norethindrone (mes′ tra nole & nor eth in′ drone)

Related Information
Endocrine Disorders & Pregnancy *on page 927*
Brand Names Genora® 1/50; Nelova™ 1/50M; Norethin™ 1/50M; Norinyl® 1+50; Ortho-Novum™ 1/50
Therapeutic Category Contraceptive, Low Estrogen/Progestin; Contraceptive, Monophasic; Contraceptive, Oral; Progestin Derivative
Use Prevention of pregnancy; treatment of hypermenorrhea, endometriosis, female hypogonadism [monophasic oral contraceptive]
Usual Dosage Adults: Female: Oral:
(Continued)

Mestranol and Norethindrone *(Continued)*

Contraception: 1 tablet daily, beginning on day 5 of menstrual cycle (first day of menstrual flow is day 1). With 20-tablet and 21-tablet packages, new dosing cycle begins 7 days after last tablet taken. With 28-tablet packages, dosage is 1 tablet daily without interruption; extra tablets are placebos or contain iron. If next menstrual period does not begin on schedule, rule out pregnancy before starting new dosing cycle. If menstrual period begins, start new dosing cycle 7 days after last tablet was taken. If all doses have been taken on schedule and one menstrual period is missed, continue dosing cycle. If two consecutive menstrual periods are missed, pregnancy test is required before new dosing cycle is started.

One dose missed: Take as soon as remembered or take 2 tablets next day

Two doses missed: Take 2 tablets as soon as remembered or 2 tablets next 2 days

Three doses missed: Begin new compact of tablets starting on day 1 of next cycle

Mechanism of Action Inhibits ovulation via a negative feedback mechanism on the hypothalamus, which alters the normal pattern of gonadotropin secretion of a follicle-stimulating hormone (FSH) and luteinizing hormone by the anterior pituitary. Follicular phase FSH and midcycle surge of gonadotropins are inhibited. Produces alterations in the genital tract, including changes in the cervical mucus, rendering it unfavorable for sperm penetration even if ovulation occurs. Changes in the endometrium may also occur, producing an unfavorable environment for nidation. May alter the tubal transport of the ova through the fallopian tubes. Progestational agents may also alter sperm fertility.

Local Anesthetic/Vasoconstrictor Precautions No information available to require special precautions

Effects on Dental Treatment When prescribing antibiotics, patients must be advised to use additional methods of birth control when taking oral contraceptives

Other Adverse Effects

>10%:

Cardiovascular: Peripheral edema

Central nervous system: Headache

Endocrine: Enlargement of breasts, breast tenderness, bloating, increased libido

Gastrointestinal: Nausea, anorexia

1% to 10%: Gastrointestinal: Vomiting, diarrhea

<1%:

Cardiovascular: Hypertension, thromboembolism, edema, stroke, myocardial infarction

Central nervous system: Depression, dizziness, anxiety

Dermatologic: Chloasma, melasma, rash

Endocrine: Decreased glucose tolerance, breast tumors, amenorrhea, alterations in frequency and flow of menses, increased triglycerides and LDL

Gastrointestinal: GI distress

Hepatic: Cholestatic jaundice

Miscellaneous: Intolerance to contact lenses, increased susceptibility to *Candida* infection

See tables.

Achieving Proper Hormonal Balance in an Oral Contraceptive

Estrogen		Progestin	
Excess	**Deficiency**	**Excess**	**Deficiency**
Nausea, bloating	Early or midcycle	Increased appetite	Late breakthrough
Cervical mucorrhea,	breakthrough	Weight gain	bleeding
polyposis	bleeding	Tiredness, fatigue	Amenorrhea
Melasma	Increased spotting	Hypomenorrhea	Hypermenorrhea
Migraine headache	Hypomenorrhea	Acne, oily scalp*	
Breast fullness or		Hair loss, hirsutism*	
tenderness		Depression	
Edema		Monilial vaginitis	
Hypertension		Breast regression	

*Result of androgenic activity of progestins.

Pharmacological Effects of Progestins Used in Oral Contraceptives

	Progestin	Estrogen	Antiestrogen	Androgen
Norgestrel/levonorgestrel	+++	0	++	+++
Ethynodiol diacetate	++	+*	+*	+
Norethindrone acetate	+	+	+++	+
Norethindrone	+	+*	+*	+
Norethynodrel	+	+++	0	0

*Has estrogenic effect at low doses; may have antiestrogenic effect at higher doses.

+++ = pronounced effect

++ = moderate effect

+ = slight effect

0 = moderate effect

Drug Interactions

Decreased effect of oral contraceptives with barbiturates, hydantoins - phenytoin, rifampin, antibiotics - penicillins, tetracyclines, erythromycins, clindamycin, griseofulvin

Increased toxicity of acetaminophen, anticoagulants, benzodiazepines, caffeine, corticosteroids, metoprolol, theophylline, tricyclic antidepressants

Pregnancy Risk Factor X

Mestranol and Norethynodrel

(mes' tra nole & nor e thye' noe drel)

Related Information

Endocrine Disorders & Pregnancy *on page 927*

Brand Names Enovid®

Therapeutic Category Contraceptive, Oral

Use Treatment of hypermenorrhea, endometriosis, female hypogonadism

Usual Dosage Adults: Female: Oral:

Endometriosis: 5-10 mg/day for 2 weeks beginning on day 5 of menstrual cycle; increase by 5-10 mg increments at 2-week intervals up to 20 mg/day for 6-9 months

Hypermenorrhea: 20-30 mg/day until bleeding is controlled, then reduce to 10 mg/day and continue through day 24 of cycle; administer 5-10 mg/day from day 5 through day 24 of next 2-3 cycles

Mechanism of Action Inhibits ovulation via a negative feedback mechanism on the hypothalamus, which alters the normal pattern of gonadotropin secretion of a follicle-stimulating hormone (FSH) and luteinizing hormone by the anterior pituitary. The follicular phase FSH and midcycle surge of gonadotropins are inhibited. Oral contraceptives produce alterations in the genital tract, including changes in the cervical mucus, rendering it unfavorable for sperm penetration even if ovulation occurs. Changes in the endometrium may also occur, producing an unfavorable environment for nidation. May alter the tubal transport of the ova through the fallopian tubes. Progestational agents may also alter sperm fertility.

Local Anesthetic/Vasoconstrictor Precautions No information available to require special precautions

Effects on Dental Treatment When prescribing antibiotics, patients must be advised to use additional methods of birth control when taking oral contraceptives

Other Adverse Effects

>10%:

Cardiovascular: Peripheral edema

Endocrine & metabolic: Enlargement of breasts, breast tenderness, bloating

Gastrointestinal: Nausea, anorexia

1% to 10%:

Central nervous system: Headache

Endocrine & metabolic: Increased libido

Gastrointestinal: Vomiting, diarrhea

<1%:

Cardiovascular: Hypertension, thromboembolism, stroke, myocardial infarction, edema

Central nervous system: Depression, dizziness, anxiety

Dermatologic: Chloasma, melasma, rash

Endocrine & metabolic: Decreased glucose tolerance, breast tumors, amenorrhea, alterations in frequency and flow of menses, increased triglycerides and LDL

Gastrointestinal: GI distress

(Continued)

Mestranol and Norethynodrel *(Continued)*

Hepatic: Cholestatic jaundice

Miscellaneous: Intolerance to contact lenses, increased susceptibility to *Candida* infection

Drug Interactions

Decreased effect with barbiturates, hydantoins - phenytoin, rifampin, antibiotics - penicillins, tetracyclines, erythromycins, clindamycin, griseofulvin

Increased toxicity of acetaminophen, anticoagulants, benzodiazepines, caffeine, corticosteroids, metoprolol, theophylline, tricyclic antidepressants

Drug Uptake

Mestranol:

Demethylated to ethinyl estradiol

Serum half-life: 6-20 hours

Norethynodrel:

Serum half-life, terminal: 5-14 hours

Pregnancy Risk Factor X

Methydrin® *see* Trichlormethiazide *on page 867*

Metamucil® [OTC] *see* Psyllium *on page 750*

Metamucil® Instant Mix [OTC] *see* Psyllium *on page 750*

Metandren® *see* Methyltestosterone *on page 570*

Metaprel® *see* Metaproterenol Sulfate *on this page*

Metaproterenol Sulfate (met a proe ter' e nol sul' fate)

Related Information

Respiratory Diseases *on page 924*

Brand Names Alupent®; Arm-a-Med® Metaproterenol; Dey-Dose® Metaproterenol; Metaprel®; Prometa®

Therapeutic Category Adrenergic Agonist Agent; Antiasthmatic; Beta-2-Adrenergic Agonist Agent; Bronchodilator

Use Bronchodilator in reversible airway obstruction due to asthma or COPD; because of its delayed onset of action (one hour) and prolonged effect (4 or more hours), this may not be the drug of choice for assessing response to a bronchodilator

Usual Dosage

Oral:

Children:

<2 years: 0.4 mg/kg/dose given 3-4 times/day; in infants, the dose can be given every 8-12 hours

2-6 years: 1-2.6 mg/kg/day divided every 6 hours

6-9 years: 10 mg/dose 3-4 times/day

Children >9 years and Adults: 20 mg 3-4 times/day

Elderly: Initial: 10 mg 3-4 times/day, increasing as necessary up to 20 mg 3-4 times/day

Inhalation: Children >12 years and Adults: 2-3 inhalations every 3-4 hours, up to 12 inhalations in 24 hours

Nebulizer:

Children: 0.01-0.02 mL/kg of 5% solution; minimum dose: 0.1 mL; maximum dose: 0.3 mL diluted in 2-3 mL normal saline every 4-6 hours (may be given more frequently according to need)

Adolescents and Adults: 5-20 breaths of full strength 5% metaproterenol **or** 0.2 to 0.3 mL 5% metaproterenol in 2.5-3 mL normal saline until nebulized every 4-6 hours (can be given more frequently according to need)

Mechanism of Action Relaxes bronchial smooth muscle by action on beta$_2$-receptors with very little effect on heart rate

Local Anesthetic/Vasoconstrictor Precautions No information available to require special precautions

Effects on Dental Treatment No effects or complications reported

Other Adverse Effects

>10%:

Central nervous system: Nervousness

Neuromuscular & skeletal: Tremor

1% to 10%:

Cardiovascular: Tachycardia, palpitations, hypertension

Central nervous system: Weakness, headache, dizziness

Gastrointestinal: Nausea, vomiting, bad taste

Neuromuscular & skeletal: Trembling, muscle cramps

Respiratory: Coughing

Miscellaneous: Increased sweating

<1%: Paradoxical bronchospasm

Drug Interactions
Decreased effect: Beta-blockers
Increased toxicity: Sympathomimetics, TCAs, MAO inhibitors
Drug Uptake
Oral:
Onset of bronchodilation: Within 15 minutes
Peak effect: Within 1 hour
Duration of action: ~1-5 hours
Inhalation:
Onset of effects: Within 60 seconds
Duration of action: Similar (~1-5 hours) regardless of route administered
Pregnancy Risk Factor C

Metasep® [OTC] *see* Parachlorometaxylenol *on page 659*

Metaxalone (me tax' a lone)
Brand Names Skelaxin®
Therapeutic Category Muscle Relaxant; Skeletal Muscle Relaxant
Use Relief of discomfort associated with acute, painful musculoskeletal conditions
Usual Dosage Children >12 years and Adults: Oral: 800 mg 3-4 times/day
Mechanism of Action Does not have a direct effect on skeletal muscle; most of its therapeutic effect comes from actions on the central nervous system
Local Anesthetic/Vasoconstrictor Precautions No information available to require special precautions
Effects on Dental Treatment No effects or complications reported
Other Adverse Effects
>10%:
Central nervous system: Paradoxical stimulation, headache, drowsiness, dizziness
Gastrointestinal: Nausea, vomiting, stomach cramps
<1%:
Dermatologic: Allergic dermatitis
Hematologic: Leukopenia, hemolytic anemia
Hepatic: Hepatotoxicity
Miscellaneous: Anaphylaxis
Drug Interactions Increased effect of alcohol, CNS depressants
Drug Uptake
Onset of action: ~1 hour
Duration: ~4-6 hours
Serum half-life: 2-3 hours
Pregnancy Risk Factor C

Metforma (Mexico) *see* Metformin Hydrochloride *on this page*

Metformin Hydrochloride (met for' min hye droe klor' ide)
Related Information
Endocrine Disorders & Pregnancy *on page 927*
Brand Names Glucophage®
Canadian/Mexican Brand Names Novo-Metformin® (Canada); Glucophage® Forte (Mexico)
Therapeutic Category Hypoglycemic Agent, Oral
Synonyms Metforma (Mexico)
Use Management of noninsulin-dependent diabetes mellitus (type II) as monotherapy when hyperglycemia cannot be managed on diet alone. May be used concomitantly with a sulfonylurea when diet and metformin or sulfonylurea alone do not result in adequate glycemic control.
Usual Dosage Oral (allow 1-2 weeks between dose titrations):
Adults:
500 mg tablets: Initial: 500 mg twice daily (given with the morning and evening meals). Dosage increases should be made in increments of one tablet every week, given in divided doses, up to a maximum of 2,500 mg/day. Doses of up to 2000 mg/day may be given twice daily. If a dose of 2,500 mg/day is required, it may be better tolerated 3 times/day (with meals).
850 mg tablets: Initial: 850 mg once daily (given with the morning meal). Dosage increases should be made in increments of one tablet every OTHER week, given in divided doses, up to a maximum of 2550 mg/day. The usual maintenance dose is 850 mg twice daily (with the morning and evening meals). Some patients may be given 850 mg 3 times/day (with meals).
(Continued)

Metformin Hydrochloride *(Continued)*

Elderly patients: The initial and maintenance dosing should be conservative, due to the potential for decreased renal function. Generally, elderly patients should not be titrated to the maximum dose of metformin.

Transfer from other antidiabetic agents: No transition period is generally necessary except when transferring from chlorpropamide. When transferring from chlorpropamide, care should be exercised during the first 2 weeks because of the prolonged retention of chlorpropamide in the body, leading to overlapping drug effects and possible hypoglycemia.

Concomitant metformin and oral sulfonylurea therapy: If patients have not responded to 4 weeks of the maximum dose of metformin monotherapy, consideration to a gradually addition of an oral sulfonylurea while continuing metformin at the maximum dose, even if prior primary or secondary failure to a sulfonylurea has occurred.

Mechanism of Action Decreases hepatic glucose production, decreasing intestinal absorption of glucose and improves insulin sensitivity (increases peripheral glucose uptake and utilization)

Local Anesthetic/Vasoconstrictor Precautions No information available to require special precautions

Effects on Dental Treatment Metformin-dependent diabetics (noninsulin dependent, Type II) should be appointed for dental treatment in morning in order to minimize chance of stress-induced hypoglycemia

Other Adverse Effects

>10%: Gastrointestinal: Anorexia, nausea, vomiting, diarrhea, epigastric fullness, constipation, heartburn

1% to 10%:
Dermatologic: Rash, hives, photosensitivity
Miscellaneous: Decreased vitamin B_{12} levels

<1%: Hematologic: Blood dyscrasias, aplastic anemia, hemolytic anemia, bone marrow depression, thrombocytopenia, agranulocytosis

Drug Interactions

Decreased effects: Drugs which tend to produce hyperglycemia (eg, diuretics, corticosteroids, phenothiazines, thyroid products, estrogens, oral contraceptives, phenytoin, nicotinic acid, sympathomimetics, calcium channel blocking drugs, isoniazid) may lead to a loss of glycemic control

Increased toxicity:
Cationic drugs (eg, amiloride, digoxin, morphine, procainamide, quinidine, quinine, ranitidine, triamterene, trimethoprim, and vancomycin) which are eliminated by renal tubular secretion could have the potential for interaction with metformin by competing for common renal tubular transport systems
Cimetidine increases (by 60%) peak metformin plasma and whole blood concentrations

Drug Uptake
Serum half-life, plasma elimination: 6.2 hours

Pregnancy Risk Factor B

Methadone Hydrochloride *(meth′ a done hye droe klor′ ide)*

Related Information
Narcotic Agonist Charts *on page 1019*

Brand Names Dolophine®

Canadian/Mexican Brand Names Methadose® (Canada)

Therapeutic Category Analgesic, Narcotic

Use Management of severe pain, used in narcotic detoxification maintenance programs

Usual Dosage Doses should be titrated to appropriate effects
Children: Analgesia:
Oral, I.M., S.C.: 0.7 mg/kg/24 hours divided every 4-6 hours as needed or 0.1-0.2 mg/kg every 4-12 hours as needed; maximum: 10 mg/dose
I.V.: 0.1 mg/kg every 4 hours initially for 2-3 doses, then every 6-12 hours as needed; maximum: 10 mg/dose
Adults:
Analgesia: Oral, I.M., I.V., S.C.: 2.5-10 mg every 3-8 hours as needed, up to 5-20 mg every 6-8 hours
Detoxification: Oral: 15-40 mg/day; should not exceed 21 days and may not be repeated earlier than 4 weeks after completion of preceding course
Maintenance of opiate dependence: Oral: 20-120 mg/day

Mechanism of Action Binds to opiate receptors in the CNS, causing inhibition of ascending pain pathways, altering the perception of and response to pain; produces generalized CNS depression

Local Anesthetic/Vasoconstrictor Precautions No information available to require special precautions

Effects on Dental Treatment Up to 10% of patients will experience significant dry mouth which will disappear with cessation of drug therapy

Other Adverse Effects

Central nervous system: CNS depression

Endocrine & metabolic: Antidiuretic hormone release

Ocular: Miosis

Respiratory: Respiratory depression

>10%:

Cardiovascular: Palpitations, hypotension, bradycardia, peripheral vasodilation

Central nervous system: Weakness, tiredness, drowsiness, dizziness

Gastrointestinal: Nausea, vomiting, constipation

Miscellaneous: Histamine release

1% to 10%:

Central nervous system: Nervousness, headache, restlessness, anorexia, malaise, confusion, increased intracranial pressure

Gastrointestinal: Stomach cramps, dry mouth

Genitourinary: Decreased urination

Local: Pain at injection site

Respiratory: Troubled breathing, shortness of breath

Miscellaneous: Biliary or urinary tract spasm

<1%:

Central nervous system: Mental depression, hallucinations, paradoxical CNS stimulation

Dermatologic: Pruritus, skin rash, hives

Gastrointestinal: Paralytic ileus

Miscellaneous: Physical and psychological dependence

Drug Interactions

Decreased effect: Phenytoin, pentazocine and rifampin may increase the metabolism of methadone and may precipitate withdrawal

Increased toxicity: CNS depressants, phenothiazines, tricyclic antidepressants, MAO inhibitors may potentiate the adverse effects of methadone

Drug Uptake

Oral:

Onset of analgesia: Within 0.5-1 hour

Duration: 6-8 hours, increases to 22-48 hours with repeated doses

Parenteral:

Onset of effect: Within 10-20 minutes

Peak effect: Within 1-2 hours

Serum half-life: 15-29 hours, may be prolonged with alkaline pH

Pregnancy Risk Factor B (D if used for prolonged periods or in high doses at term)

Methamphetamine Hydrochloride

(meth am fet' a meen hye droe klor' ide)

Brand Names Desoxyn®

Therapeutic Category Amphetamine; Central Nervous System Stimulant, Amphetamine

Use Treatment of narcolepsy, exogenous obesity, abnormal behavioral syndrome in children (minimal brain dysfunction)

Usual Dosage

Attention deficit disorder: Children >6 years: 2.5-5 mg 1-2 times/day, may increase by 5 mg increments weekly until optimum response is achieved, usually 20-25 mg/day

Exogenous obesity: Children >12 years and Adults: 5 mg, 30 minutes before each meal; long-acting formulation: 10-15 mg in morning; treatment duration should not exceed a few weeks

Local Anesthetic/Vasoconstrictor Precautions Use vasoconstriction with caution in patients taking methamphetamine. Amphetamines enhance the sympathomimetic response of epinephrine and norepinephrine leading to potential hypertension and cardiotoxicity.

Effects on Dental Treatment Up to 10% of patients taking dextroamphetamines may present with hypertension. The use of local anesthetic without vasoconstrictor is recommended in these patients.

Other Adverse Effects

>10%:

Cardiovascular: Irregular heartbeat

(Continued)

Methamphetamine Hydrochloride *(Continued)*

Central nervous system: False feeling of well being, nervousness, restlessness, insomnia

1% to 10%:

Cardiovascular: Hypertension

Central nervous system: Mood or mental changes, dizziness, lightheadedness, headache

Endocrine & metabolic: Changes in libido

Gastrointestinal: Diarrhea, nausea, vomiting, stomach cramps, constipation, anorexia, weight loss dry mouth

Ocular: Blurred vision

Miscellaneous: Increased sweating

<1%:

Cardiovascular: Chest pain

Central nervous system: CNS stimulation (severe), Tourette's syndrome, hyperthermia, seizures, paranoia

Dermatologic: Skin rash, hives

Miscellaneous: Tolerance and withdrawal with prolonged use

Drug Interactions Increased toxicity with MAO inhibitors (hypertensive crisis)

Pregnancy Risk Factor C

Methantheline Bromide *(meth an' tha leen broe' mide)*

Brand Names Banthine®

Therapeutic Category Anticholinergic Agent; Antispasmodic Agent, Gastrointestinal

Synonyms Methanthelinium Bromide

Use Adjunctive treatment of peptic ulcer, irritable bowel syndrome, pancreatitis, ureteral and urinary bladder spasm; to reduce duodenal motility during diagnostic radiologic procedures and treatment of an uninhibited neurogenic bladder

Local Anesthetic/Vasoconstrictor Precautions No information available to require special precautions

Effects on Dental Treatment Dry mouth in 1% to 10% of patients

Other Adverse Effects

>10%:

Gastrointestinal: Constipation

Miscellaneous: Decreased sweating; dry mouth, skin, nose, or throat

1% to 10%: Gastrointestinal: Difficulty in swallowing

<1%:

Cardiovascular: Tachycardia

Central nervous system: Confusion, headache, loss of memory, tiredness, drowsiness, nervousness, insomnia

Dermatologic: Rash

Gastrointestinal: Bloated feeling, nausea, vomiting

Genitourinary: Urinary retention

Neuromuscular & skeletal: Weakness

Ocular: Increased intraocular pressure, blurred vision

Methanthelinium Bromide *see* Methantheline Bromide *on this page*

Methazolamide *(meth a zoe' la mide)*

Brand Names Neptazane®

Therapeutic Category Antiglaucoma Agent; Carbonic Anhydrase Inhibitor; Diuretic, Carbonic Anhydrase Inhibitor

Use Adjunctive treatment of open-angle or secondary glaucoma; short-term therapy of narrow-angle glaucoma when delay of surgery is desired

Usual Dosage Adults: Oral: 50-100 mg 2-3 times/day

Mechanism of Action Noncompetitive inhibition of the enzyme carbonic anhydrase; thought that carbonic anhydrase is located at the luminal border of cells of the proximal tubule. When the enzyme is inhibited, there is an increase in urine volume and a change to an alkaline pH with a subsequent decrease in the excretion of titratable acid and ammonia.

Local Anesthetic/Vasoconstrictor Precautions No information available to require special precautions

Effects on Dental Treatment No effects or complications reported

Other Adverse Effects

>10%:

Central nervous system: Malaise, weakness

Gastrointestinal: Metallic taste, anorexia

Renal: Increased urination

1% to 10%:
    Central nervous system: Mental depression, drowsiness, dizziness
    Renal: Crystalluria

<1%:
    Central nervous system: Fever, headache, seizures, unsteadiness, fatigue
    Dermatologic: Rash, sulfonamide rash, Stevens-Johnson syndrome
    Endocrine & metabolic: Hyperchloremic metabolic acidosis, hypokalemia, elevation of blood glucose
    Gastrointestinal: GI irritation, constipation, anorexia, dry mouth, black tarry stools
    Hematologic: Bone marrow suppression
    Neuromuscular & skeletal: Paresthesia, trembling
    Ocular: Myopia
    Otic: Tinnitus
    Renal: Dysuria
    Miscellaneous: Loss of smell, hypersensitivity

Drug Interactions
Increased toxicity:
    May induce hypokalemia which would sensitize a patient to digitalis toxicity
    May increase the potential for salicylate toxicity
    Hypokalemia may be compounded with concurrent diuretic use or steroids
    Primidone absorption may be delayed
Decreased effect: Increased lithium excretion and altered excretion of other drugs by alkalinization of the urine, such as amphetamines, quinidine, procainamide, methenamine, phenobarbital, salicylates

Drug Uptake
Onset of action: Slow in comparison with acetazolamide (2-4 hours)
Peak effect: 6-8 hours
Duration: 10-18 hours
Absorption: Slowly from GI tract
Serum half-life: ~14 hours

Pregnancy Risk Factor C

Methenamine (meth en' a meen)

Brand Names Hiprex®; Mandelamine®; Urex®; Urised®
Canadian/Mexican Brand Names Hip-Rex® (Canada); Dehydral® (Canada); Urasal® (Canada)
Therapeutic Category Antibiotic, Miscellaneous
Use Prophylaxis or suppression of recurrent urinary tract infections; urinary tract discomfort secondary to hypermotility; should not be used to treat infections outside of urinary tract
Usual Dosage Oral:
Children: 6-12 years:
    Hippurate: 25-50 mg/kg/day divided every 12 hours
    Mandelate: 50-75 mg/kg/day divided every 6 hours

Children >12 years and Adults:
    Hippurate: 1 g twice daily
    Mandelate: 1 g 4 times/day after meals and at bedtime
Mechanism of Action Methenamine is hydrolyzed to formaldehyde and ammonia in acidic urine; formaldehyde has nonspecific bactericidal action
Local Anesthetic/Vasoconstrictor Precautions No information available to require special precautions
Effects on Dental Treatment No effects or complications reported
Other Adverse Effects
1% to 10%:
    Dermatologic: Skin rash
    Gastrointestinal: Nausea, vomiting, diarrhea, anorexia, abdominal cramping
<1%:
    Central nervous system: Headache
    Genitourinary: Bladder irritation
    Hepatic: Elevation in AST and ALT
    Renal: Hematuria, dysuria, crystalluria
Drug Interactions
Decreased effect: Sodium bicarbonate and acetazolamide will decrease effect secondary to alkalinization of urine
Increased toxicity: Sulfonamides (may precipitate)
Drug Uptake
Absorption: Readily absorbed from GI tract
Serum half-life: 3-6 hours
Pregnancy Risk Factor C

Methergine® *see* Methylergonovine Maleate *on page 567*

Methicillin Sodium (meth i sil' in sow' dee um)
Brand Names Staphcillin®
Therapeutic Category Antibiotic, Penicillin
Use Treatment of susceptible bacterial infections such as osteomyelitis, septicemia, endocarditis, and CNS infections due to penicillinase-producing strains of *Staphylococcus*; other antistaphylococcal penicillins are usually preferred
Usual Dosage I.M., I.V.:
Children: 150-200 mg/kg/day divided every 6 hours; 200-400 mg/kg/day divided every 4-6 hours has been used for treatment of severe infections; maximum dose: 12 g/day
Adults: 4-12 g/day in divided doses every 4-6 hours
Mechanism of Action Inhibits bacterial cell wall synthesis by binding to one or more of the penicillin binding proteins (PBPs); which in turn inhibits the final transpeptidation step of peptidoglycan synthesis in bacterial cell walls, thus inhibiting cell wall biosynthesis. Bacteria eventually lyse due to ongoing activity of cell wall autolytic enzymes (autolysins and murein hydrolases) while cell wall assembly is arrested.
Local Anesthetic/Vasoconstrictor Precautions No information available to require special precautions
Effects on Dental Treatment Prolonged use of penicillins may lead to development of oral candidiasis
Other Adverse Effects
1% to 10%:
Dermatologic: Skin rash
Renal: Acute interstitial nephritis
<1%:
Central nervous system: Fever
Dermatologic: Rash
Hematologic: Eosinophilia, anemia, leukopenia, neutropenia, thrombocytopenia
Local: Phlebitis
Renal: Hemorrhagic cystitis
Miscellaneous: Serum sickness-like reactions
Drug Interactions
Decreased effect: Efficacy of oral contraceptives may be reduced
Increased effect: Disulfiram, probenecid may increase penicillin levels, increased effect of anticoagulants
Drug Uptake
Serum half-life (with normal renal function):
Children 2-16 years: 0.8 hour
Adults: 0.4-0.5 hour
Time to peak serum concentration:
I.M.: 0.5-1 hour
I.V. infusion: Within 5 minutes
Pregnancy Risk Factor B

Methimazole (meth im' a zole)
Related Information
Endocrine Disorders & Pregnancy *on page 927*
Brand Names Tapazole®
Therapeutic Category Antithyroid Agent
Use Palliative treatment of hyperthyroidism, return the hyperthyroid patient to a normal metabolic state prior to thyroidectomy, and to control thyrotoxic crisis that may accompany thyroidectomy. The use of antithyroid thioamides is as effective in elderly as they are in younger adults; however, the expense, potential adverse effects, and inconvenience (compliance, monitoring) make them undesirable. The use of radioiodine due to ease of administration and less concern for long-term side effects and reproduction problems (some older males) makes it a more appropriate therapy.
Usual Dosage Oral: Administer in 3 equally divided doses at approximately 8-hour intervals
Children: Initial: 0.4 mg/kg/day in 3 divided doses; maintenance: 0.2 mg/kg/day in 3 divided doses up to 30 mg/24 hours maximum
Adults: Initial: 5 mg every 8 hours; maintenance dose: 5-15 mg/day up to 60 mg/day for severe hyperthyroidism
Adjust dosage as required to achieve and maintain serum T_3, T_4, and TSH levels in the normal range. An elevated T_3 may be the sole indicator of inadequate treatment. An elevated TSH indicates excessive antithyroid treatment.

Mechanism of Action Inhibits the synthesis of thyroid hormones by blocking the oxidation of iodine in the thyroid gland, blocking iodine's ability to combine with tyrosine to form thyroxine and triiodothyronine (T_3), does not inactivate circulating T_4 and T_3

Local Anesthetic/Vasoconstrictor Precautions No information available to require special precautions

Effects on Dental Treatment No effects or complications reported

Other Adverse Effects
>10%:
  Central nervous system: Fever
  Dermatologic: Skin rash
  Hematologic: Leukopenia
1% to 10%:
  Central nervous system: Dizziness
  Gastrointestinal: Nausea, vomiting, stomach pain, loss of taste
  Hematologic: Agranulocytosis
  Miscellaneous: SLE-like syndrome
<1%:
  Cardiovascular: Edema
  Central nervous system: Drowsiness, vertigo, headache
  Dermatologic: Rash, urticaria, pruritus, hair loss
  Endocrine & metabolic: Goiter
  Gastrointestinal: Constipation, weight gain
  Genitourinary: Nephrotic syndrome
  Hematologic: Thrombocytopenia, aplastic anemia
  Hepatic: Cholestatic jaundice
  Neuromuscular & skeletal: Arthralgia, paresthesia
  Miscellaneous: Swollen salivary glands

Drug Interactions Increased toxicity: Iodinated glycerol, lithium, potassium iodide; anticoagulant activity increased

Drug Uptake
Onset of antithyroid effect: Oral: Within 30-40 minutes
Duration: 2-4 hours
Serum half-life: 4-13 hours

Pregnancy Risk Factor D

Methionine (me thye' oh neen)

Brand Names Pedameth®

Therapeutic Category Dietary Supplement

Use Treatment of diaper rash and control of odor, dermatitis and ulceration caused by ammoniacal urine

Local Anesthetic/Vasoconstrictor Precautions No information available to require special precautions

Effects on Dental Treatment No effects or complications reported

Methocarbamol (meth oh kar' ba mole)

Related Information
Temporomandibular Dysfunction (TMD) *on page 963*

Brand Names Delaxin®; Marbaxin®; Robaxin®; Robomol®

Therapeutic Category Muscle Relaxant; Skeletal Muscle Relaxant

Use
Dental: Treatment of muscle spasm associated with acute temporomandibular joint pain
Medical: Treatment of muscle spasm associated with acute painful musculoskeletal conditions, supportive therapy in tetanus

Usual Dosage Adults: Muscle spasm: Oral: 1.5 g 4 times/day for 2-3 days, then decrease to 4-4.5 g/day in 3-6 divided doses

Mechanism of Action Causes skeletal muscle relaxation by reducing the transmission of impulses from the spinal cord to skeletal muscle

Local Anesthetic/Vasoconstrictor Precautions No information available to require special precautions

Effects on Dental Treatment No effects or complications reported

Other Adverse Effects >10%: Central nervous system: Drowsiness, dizziness, lightheadedness

Oral manifestations: No data reported

Contraindications Renal impairment, hypersensitivity to methocarbamol or any component

Warnings/Precautions Rate of injection should not exceed 3 mL/minute; solution is hypertonic; avoid extravasation; use with caution in patients with a history of seizures

(Continued)

557

Methocarbamol *(Continued)*

Drug Interactions Increased effect/toxicity with CNS depressants

Drug Uptake
Absorption: Rapid
Onset of muscle relaxation: Oral: Within 30 minutes
Time to peak serum concentration: Oral: ~2 hours
Serum half-life: 1-2 hours

Pregnancy Risk Factor C

Breast-feeding Considerations May be taken while breast-feeding

Dosage Forms
Injection: 100 mg/mL in polyethylene glycol 50% (10 mL)
Tablet: 500 mg, 750 mg

Dietary Considerations Tablets may be crushed and mixed with food or liquid if needed

Generic Available Yes

Methocarbamol and Aspirin *(meth oh kar′ ba mole & as′ pir in)*

Brand Names Robaxisal®

Therapeutic Category Muscle Relaxant; Skeletal Muscle Relaxant

Use
Dental: Treatment of muscle spasm associated with acute temporomandibular joint pain
Medical: Treatment of muscle spasm associated with acute painful musculo-skeletal conditions, supportive therapy in tetanus

Usual Dosage Children >12 years and Adults: Oral: 2 tablets 4 times/day

Mechanism of Action Causes skeletal muscle relaxation by reducing the transmission of impulses from the spinal cord to skeletal muscle

Local Anesthetic/Vasoconstrictor Precautions No information available to require special precautions

Effects on Dental Treatment Use with caution in patients with platelet and bleeding disorders, renal dysfunction, erosive gastritis, or peptic ulcer disease, previous nonreaction does not guarantee future safe taking of medication; do not use aspirin in children <16 years of age for chickenpox or flu symptoms due to the association with Reye's syndrome

Avoid aspirin if possible, for 1 week prior to surgery because of the possibility of postoperative bleeding; use with caution in impaired hepatic function

Elderly are a high-risk population for adverse effects from nonsteroidal anti-inflammatory agents. As much as 60% of elderly with GI complications to NSAIDs can develop peptic ulceration and/or hemorrhage asymptomatically. Also, concomitant disease and drug use contribute to the risk for GI adverse effects. Use lowest effective dose for shortest period possible. Consider renal function decline with age. Use with caution in patients with history of asthma

Other Adverse Effects
Methocarbamol: >10%: Central nervous system: Drowsiness, dizziness, light-headedness

Aspirin:
>10%: Gastrointestinal: Nausea, vomiting, dyspepsia, epigastric discomfort, heartburn, stomach pains
1% to 10%: Gastrointestinal: Ulceration

Oral manifestations: No data reported

Contraindications
Methocarbamol: Renal impairment, hypersensitivity to methocarbamol or any component
Aspirin: Bleeding disorders (factor VII or IX deficiencies), hypersensitivity to salicylates or other NSAIDs, tartrazine dye and asthma

Warnings/Precautions Use aspirin with caution in patients with platelet and bleeding disorders, renal dysfunction, erosive gastritis, or peptic ulcer disease, previous nonreaction does not guarantee future safe taking of medication; do not use aspirin in children <16 years of age for chickenpox or flu symptoms due to the association with Reye's syndrome

Avoid aspirin if possible, for 1 week prior to surgery because of the possibility of postoperative bleeding; use with caution in impaired hepatic function

Elderly are a high-risk population for adverse effects from nonsteroidal anti-inflammatory agents. As much as 60% of elderly with GI complications to NSAIDs can develop peptic ulceration and/or hemorrhage asymptomatically. Also, concomitant disease and drug use contribute to the risk for GI adverse effects. Use lowest effective dose for shortest period possible. Consider renal function decline with age. Use with caution in patients with history of asthma

Drug Interactions
Methocarbamol: Increased effect/toxicity with CNS depressants

Aspirin: Concomitant use of aspirin may result in possible decreased serum concentration of NSAIDs; aspirin may antagonize effects of probenecid; aspirin may increase methotrexate serum levels. Aspirin may displace valproic acid from binding sites which can result in toxicity; warfarin and aspirin result in increased bleeding; NSAIDs and aspirin result in increased GI adverse effects.

Drug Uptake
Methocarbamol:

Absorption: Rapid

Onset of muscle relaxation: Oral: Within 30 minutes

Time to peak serum concentration: Oral: ~2 hours

Serum half-life: 1-2 hours

Aspirin:

Absorption: Rapid

Time to peak serum concentration: ~1-2 hours

Serum half-life:

Parent drug: 15-20 minutes

Salicylates (dose-dependent): From 3 hours at lower doses (300-600 mg), to 5-6 hours (after 1 g) to 10 hours with higher doses

Influence of food: Decreases rate but not extent of absorption (oral)

Pregnancy Risk Factor C

Breast-feeding Considerations Use cautiously due to potential adverse effects in nursing infants

Dosage Forms Tablet: Methocarbamol 400 mg and aspirin 325 mg

Generic Available Yes

Methohexital Sodium (meth oh hex′ i tal sow′ dee um)
Brand Names Brevital® Sodium

Canadian/Mexican Brand Names Brietal® Sodium (Canada)

Therapeutic Category Barbiturate; General Anesthetic, Intravenous; Sedative

Use

Dental: I.V. induction and maintenance of general anesthesia for short periods

Medical: None

Usual Dosage I.V.:

Children: 1-2 mg/kg/dose

Adults: 50-120 mg to start; 20-40 mg every 4-7 minutes

Mechanism of Action Ultrashort-acting I.V. barbiturate anesthetic; acts as agonist within the multisubunit $GABA_A$ receptor ion chloride-channel complex in central nervous system neurons; this leads to inhibition of many brain functions resulting in loss of consciousness. May also dissolve in neuronal membranes to cause stabilization and eventual loss of action potentials which also leads to inhibition of brain function.

Local Anesthetic/Vasoconstrictor Precautions No information available to require special precautions

Effects on Dental Treatment No effects or complications reported

Other Adverse Effects >10%: Local: Pain on I.M. injection

Oral manifestations: No data reported

Contraindications Porphyria, hypersensitivity to methohexital or any component

Warnings/Precautions Use with extreme caution in patients with liver impairment, asthma, cardiovascular instability

Drug Interactions CNS depressants worsen CNS depression

Drug Uptake

Onset of effect: Immediately after I.V. injection

Duration of effect: 10-20 minutes after a single dose

Pregnancy Risk Factor C

Breast-feeding Considerations No data reported

Dosage Forms Injection: 500 mg, 2.5 g, 5 g

Dietary Considerations Should not be given to patients with food in stomach because of danger of vomiting during anesthesia

Generic Available No

Methotrexate (meth oh trex′ ate)
Related Information

Rheumatoid Arthritis, Osteoarthritis, and Joint Prostheses *on page 930*

Brand Names Folex®; Rheumatrex®

Canadian/Mexican Brand Names Ledertrexate® (Mexico)

(Continued)

Methotrexate *(Continued)*

Therapeutic Category Antineoplastic Agent, Antimetabolite

Synonyms Metotrexato (Mexico)

Use Treatment of trophoblastic neoplasms; leukemias; psoriasis; rheumatoid arthritis; breast, head, and lung carcinomas; osteosarcoma; sarcomas; carcinoma of gastric, esophagus, testes; lymphomas

Usual Dosage Refer to individual protocols. May be administered orally, I.M., intra-arterially, intrathecally, I.V., or S.C.

Leucovorin may be administered concomitantly or within 24 hours of methotrexate

Children:

Juvenile rheumatoid arthritis: Oral, I.M.: 5-15 mg/m^2/week as a single dose **or** as 3 divided doses given 12 hours apart

Antineoplastic dosage range:

Oral, I.M.: 7.5-30 mg/m^2/week **or** every 2 weeks

I.V.: 10-33,000 mg/m^2 bolus dosing **or** continuous infusion over 6-42 hours

Methotrexate Dosing Schedules

	Dose	Route	Frequency
Conventional dose	15-20 mg/m^2 30-50 mg/m^2 15 mg/day for 5 days	Oral Oral, I.V. Oral, I.M.	Twice weekly Weekly Every 2-3 weeks
Intermediate dose	50-150 mg/m^2 240 mg/m^{2*} 0.5-1 g/m^{2*}	I.V. push I.V. infusion I.V. infusion	Every 2-3 weeks Every 4-7 days Every 2-3 weeks
High dose	1-12 g/m^{2*}	I.V. infusion	Every 1-3 weeks

Pediatric solid tumors: I.V.:

<12 years: 12 g/m^2 (dosage range: 12-18 g)

≥ 12 years: 8 g/m^2 (maximum: 18 g)

Meningeal leukemia: I.V.: Loading dose: 6 g/m^2 followed by I.V. continuous infusion of 1.2 g/m^2/hour for 23 hours

Acute lymphocytic leukemia (high dose): I.V.: Loading: 200 mg/m^2 followed by a 24-hour infusion of 1200 mg/m^2/day

ANLL: I.V.: 7.5 mg/m^2/day on days 1-5

Resistant ANLL: I.V.: 100 mg/m^2/dose on day 1

Hodgkin's lymphoma: I.V.: 200-500 mg/m^2; repeat every 28 days

Induction of remission in acute lymphoblastic leukemias: Oral: 3.3 mg/m^2/day for 4-6 weeks; remission maintenance: Oral, I.M.: 20-30 mg/m^2 twice weekly

Meningeal leukemia: I.T.: 10-15 mg/m^2 (maximum dose: 15 mg)

or

≤3 months: 3 mg/dose

4-11 months: 6 mg/dose

1 year: 8 mg/dose

2 years: 10 mg/dose

≥3 years: 12 mg/dose

I.T. doses are prepared with preservative-free MTX **only**. Hydrocortisone may be added to the I.T. preparation; total volume should range from 3-6 mL. Doses should be repeated at 2- to 5-day intervals until CSF counts return to normal followed by a dose once weekly for 2 weeks then monthly thereafter.

Adults: I.V.: Range is wide from 30-40 mg/m^2/week to 100-7500 mg/m^2 with leucovorin rescue

Doses not requiring leucovorin rescue range from 30-40 mg/m^2 I.V. or I.M. repeated weekly, or oral regimens of 10 mg/m^2 twice weekly

High-dose MTX is considered to be >100 mg/m^2 and can be as high as 1500-7500 mg/m^2. These doses require leucovorin rescue. Patients receiving doses ≥1000 mg/m^2 should have their urine alkalinized with bicarbonate or Bicitra® prior to and following MTX therapy.

Trophoblastic neoplasms: Oral, I.M.: 15-30 mg/day for 5 days; repeat in 7 days for 3-5 courses

Head and neck cancer: Oral, I.M., I.V.: 25-50 mg/m^2 once weekly

Rheumatoid arthritis: Oral: 7.5 mg once weekly **or** 2.5 mg every 12 hours for 3 doses/week; not to exceed 20 mg/week

Psoriasis: Oral: 2.5-5 mg/dose every 12 hours for 3 doses given once weekly

or

Oral, I.M.: 10-25 mg/dose given once weekly

Elderly: Rheumatoid arthritis/psoriasis: Oral:
  Initial: 5 mg once weekly
  If nausea occurs, split dose to 2.5 mg every 12 hours for the day of administration
  Dose may be increased to 7.5 mg/week based on response, not to exceed 20 mg/week

Ectopic pregnancy: I.M./I.V.: 50 mg/m^2 single-dose without leucovorin rescue

Mechanism of Action Antimetabolite that inhibits DNA synthesis and cell reproduction in cancerous cells

Folates must be in the reduced form (FH$_4$) to be active

Folates are activated by dihydrofolate reductase (DHFR)

DHFR is inhibited by MTX (by binding irreversibly), causing an increase in the intracellular dihydrofolate pool (the inactive cofactor) and inhibition of both purine and thymidylate synthesis (TS)

MTX enters the cell through an energy-dependent and temperature-dependent process which is mediated by an intramembrane protein; this carrier mechanism is also used by naturally occurring reduced folates, including folinic acid (leucovorin), making this a competitive process

At high drug concentrations (>20 µM), MTX enters the cell by a second mechanism which is not shared by reduced folates; the process may be passive diffusion or a specific, saturable process, and provides a rationale for high-dose MTX

A small fraction of MTX is converted intracellularly to polyglutamates, which leads to a prolonged inhibition of DHFR

Local Anesthetic/Vasoconstrictor Precautions No information available to require special precautions

Effects on Dental Treatment Methotrexate commonly causes ulceration stomatitis, gingivitis, and pharyngitis associated with oral discomfort

Other Adverse Effects

>10%:
  Mucositis: Dose-dependent; appears in 3-7 days after therapy, resolving within 2 weeks
  Cardiovascular: Vasculitis
  Central nervous system (with I.T. administration only):
    Arachnoiditis: Acute reaction manifested as severe headache, nuchal rigidity, vomiting, and fever; may be alleviated by reducing the dose
    Subacute toxicity: 10% of patients treated with 12-15 mg/m^2 of I.T. MTX may develop this in the second or third week of therapy; consists of motor paralysis of extremities, cranial nerve palsy, seizures, or coma. This has also been seen in pediatric cases receiving very high-dose MTX (when enough MTX can get across into the CSF).
    Demyelinating encephalopathy: Seen months or years after receiving MTX; usually in association with cranial irradiation or other systemic chemotherapy
  Dermatologic: Reddening of skin
  Gastrointestinal: Ulcerative stomatitis, pharyngitis, glossitis, gingivitis, nausea, vomiting, diarrhea, anorexia, intestinal perforation
  Emetic potential:
    <100 mg: Moderately low (10% to 30%)
    ≥100 mg or <250 mg: Moderate (30% to 60%)
    ≥250 mg: Moderately high (60% to 90%)
  Hematologic: Leukopenia, thrombocytopenia
  Renal: Renal failure, azotemia, hyperuricemia, nephropathy

1% to 10%:
  Central nervous system: Dizziness, malaise, encephalopathy, seizures, fever, chills
  Dermatitis: Alopecia, rash, photosensitivity, depigmentation or hyperpigmentation of skin
  Endocrine & metabolic: Diabetes
  Hematologic: Hemorrhage
  Hepatic abnormalities: Cirrhosis and portal fibrosis have been associated with chronic MTX therapy; acute elevation of liver enzymes are common after high-dose MTX, and usually resolve within 10 days
  Myelosuppressive: This is the primary dose-limiting factor (along with mucositis) of MTX; occurs about 5-7 days after MTX therapy, and should resolve within 2 weeks
    WBC: Mild
    Platelets: Moderate
    Onset (days): 7
    Nadir (days): 10
    Recovery (days): 21

(Continued)

Methotrexate *(Continued)*

Ocular: Blurred vision

Neuromuscular & skeletal: Arthralgia

Pneumonitis: Associated with fever, cough, and interstitial pulmonary infiltrates; treatment is to withhold MTX during the acute reaction

Renal dysfunction: Manifested by an abrupt rise in serum creatinine and BUN and a fall in urine output; more common with high-dose MTX, and may be due to precipitation of the drug. The best treatment is prevention: Aggressively hydrate with 3 L/m^2/day starting 12 hours before therapy and continue for 24-36 hours; alkalinize the urine by adding 50 mEq of bicarbonate to each liter of fluid; keep urine flow over 100 mL/hour and urine pH >7.

Renal: Vasculitis, cystitis

Miscellaneous: Anaphylaxis, decreased resistance to infection

Drug Interactions

Decreased effect: Decreased phenytoin, 5-FU, nonsteroidal anti-inflammatory drugs (NSAIDs)

Corticosteroids: Reported to decrease uptake of MTX into leukemia cells. Administration of these drugs should be separated by 12 hours. Dexamethasone has been reported to not affect methotrexate influx into cells.

Increased toxicity:

Live virus vaccines cause vaccinia infections

Vincristine: Inhibits MTX efflux from the cell, leading to increased and prolonged MTX levels in the cell; the dose of VCR needed to produce this effect is not achieved clinically

Organic acids: Salicylates, sulfonamides, probenecid, and high doses of penicillins compete with MTX for transport and reduce renal tubular secretion. Salicylates and sulfonamides may also displace MTX from plasma proteins, increasing MTX levels.

Ara-C: Increased formation of the Ara-C nucleotide can occur when MTX precedes Ara-C, thus promoting the action of Ara-C

Cyclosporine: CSA and MTX interfere with each others renal elimination, which may result in increased toxicity

Drug Uptake

Absorption:

Oral: Rapid; well absorbed orally at low doses (<30 mg/m^2), incomplete absorption after large doses

I.M. injection: Completely absorbed

Serum half-life: 8-12 hours with high doses and 3-10 hours with low doses

Time to peak serum concentration:

Oral: 1-2 hours

Parenteral: 30-60 minutes

Pregnancy Risk Factor D

Methotrimeprazine Hydrochloride

(meth oh trye mep' ra zeen hye droe klor' ide)

Brand Names Levoprome®

Therapeutic Category Analgesic, Non-narcotic; Phenothiazine Derivative; Sedative

Synonyms Levomepromazine

Use Relief of moderate to severe pain in nonambulatory patients; for analgesia and sedation when respiratory depression is to be avoided, as in obstetrics; preanesthetic for producing sedation, somnolence and relief of apprehension and anxiety

Usual Dosage Adults: I.M.:

Sedation analgesia: 10-20 mg every 4-6 hours as needed

Preoperative medication: 2-20 mg, 45 minutes to 3 hours before surgery

Postoperative analgesia: 2.5-7.5 mg every 4-6 hours is suggested as necessary since residual effects of anesthetic may be present

Pre- and postoperative hypotension: I.M.: 5-10 mg

Mechanism of Action Methotrimeprazine is a phenothiazine with sites of action thought to be in the thalamus, hypothalamus, reticular and limbic systems, producing suppression of sensory impulses. This results with sedation, an elevated pain threshold, and induction of amnesia. The analgesic effect of methotrimeprazine is comparable to meperidine and morphine without the respiratory suppression. This agent also has antihistamine, anticholinergic, and antiepinephrine effects.

Local Anesthetic/Vasoconstrictor Precautions No information available to require special precautions

Effects on Dental Treatment Anticholinergic side effects can cause a reduction of saliva production or secretion contributes to discomfort and dental disease (ie, caries, oral candidiasis and periodontal disease); phenothiazines can cause extrapyramidal reactions which may appear as muscle twitching or increased motor activity of the face, neck or head

Other Adverse Effects
>10%:
Cardiovascular: Hypotension, orthostatic hypotension
Central nervous system: Pseudoparkinsonism, akathisia, dystonias, tardive dyskinesia (persistent)
Gastrointestinal: Constipation
Ocular: Pigmentary retinopathy
Respiratory: Nasal congestion
Miscellaneous: Decreased sweating
1% to 10%:
Central nervous system: Dizziness
Dermatologic: Increased sensitivity to sun, skin rash
Endocrine & metabolic: Changes in menstrual cycle, changes in libido, pain in breasts
Gastrointestinal: Weight gain, nausea, vomiting, stomach pain
Genitourinary: Difficulty in urination, ejaculatory disturbances
Neuromuscular & skeletal: Trembling of fingers
<1%:
Central nervous system: Neuroleptic malignant syndrome (NMS)
Dermatologic: Discoloration of skin (blue-gray)
Endocrine & metabolic: Galactorrhea
Genitourinary: Priapism
Hematologic: Agranulocytosis, leukopenia
Hepatic: Cholestatic jaundice, hepatotoxicity
Ocular: Cornea and lens changes, pigmentary retinopathy
Miscellaneous: Impairment of temperature regulation, lowering of seizures threshold

Drug Interactions Increased toxicity: Additive effects with other CNS-depressants

Drug Uptake
Peak effect: Within 20-40 minutes
Duration: 4 hours
Serum half-life, elimination: 20 hours
Time to peak serum concentration: Within 0.5-1.5 hours

Pregnancy Risk Factor C

Methoxsalen (meth ox′ a len)

Brand Names Oxsoralen® Topical; Oxsoralen-Ultra® Oral

Therapeutic Category Psoralen

Synonyms Methoxypsoralen; 8-Methoxypsoralen; 8-MOP

Use Symptomatic control of severe, recalcitrant, disabling psoriasis in conjunction with long wave ultraviolet radiation; induce repigmentation in vitiligo topical repigmenting agent in conjunction with controlled doses of ultraviolet A (UVA) or sunlight

Usual Dosage
Psoriasis: Adults: Oral: 10-70 mg 1½-2 hours before exposure to ultraviolet light, 2-3 times at least 48 hours apart; dosage is based upon patient's body weight and skin type

Vitiligo: Children >12 years and Adults:
Oral: 20 mg 2-4 hours before exposure to UVA light or sunlight; limit exposure to 15-40 minutes based on skin basic color and exposure
Topical: Apply lotion 1-2 hours before exposure to UVA light, no more than once weekly

Mechanism of Action Bonds covalently to pyrimidine bases in DNA, inhibits the synthesis of DNA, and suppresses cell division. The augmented sunburn reaction involves excitation of the methoxsalen molecule by radiation in the long-wave ultraviolet light (UVA), resulting in transference of energy to the methoxsalen molecule producing an excited state ("triplet electronic state"). The molecule, in this "triplet state", then reacts with cutaneous DNA.

Local Anesthetic/Vasoconstrictor Precautions No information available to require special precautions

Effects on Dental Treatment No effects or complications reported

Other Adverse Effects
>10%:
Dermatologic: Itching

(Continued)

Methoxsalen *(Continued)*

Gastrointestinal: Nausea
1% to 10%:
Cardiovascular: Severe edema, hypotension
Central nervous system: Nervousness, vertigo, depression
Dermatologic: Painful blistering, burning, and peeling of skin; pruritus, freckling, hypopigmentation, rash, cheilitis, erythema
Neuromuscular & skeletal: Loss of muscle coordination

Drug Uptake
Time to peak serum concentration: Oral: 2-4 hours

Pregnancy Risk Factor C

Comments Absorption is increased with food; peak levels occur in 30 minutes to 1 hour after ingestion; plasma half-life is approximately 2 hours

Methoxycinnamate and Oxybenzone

(meth ox′ ee sin′ a mate & ox i ben′ zone)

Brand Names PreSun® 29 [OTC]; Ti-Screen® [OTC]

Therapeutic Category Sunscreen

Synonyms Sunscreen, PABA-Free

Use Reduce the chance of premature aging of the skin and skin cancer from overexposure to the sun

Local Anesthetic/Vasoconstrictor Precautions No information available to require special precautions

Effects on Dental Treatment No effects or complications reported

Methoxypsoralen *see* Methoxsalen *on previous page*
8-Methoxypsoralen *see* Methoxsalen *on previous page*

Methscopolamine Bromide (meth skoe pol′ a meen broe′ mide)

Brand Names Pamine®

Therapeutic Category Anticholinergic Agent; Antispasmodic Agent, Gastrointestinal

Use Adjunctive therapy in the treatment of peptic ulcer

Usual Dosage Adults: Oral: 2.5 mg 30 minutes before meals or food and 2.5-5 mg at bedtime

Mechanism of Action Methscopolamine is a peripheral anticholinergic agent that does not cross the blood-brain barrier and provides a peripheral blockade of muscarinic receptors. This agent reduces the volume and the total acid content of gastric secretions, inhibits salivation, and reduces gastrointestinal motility.

Local Anesthetic/Vasoconstrictor Precautions No information available to require special precautions

Effects on Dental Treatment Anticholinergic side effects can cause a reduction of saliva production or secretion contributes to discomfort and dental disease (ie, caries, oral candidiasis and periodontal disease)

Other Adverse Effects
>10%:
Gastrointestinal: Constipation, dry mouth
Miscellaneous: Decreased sweating; dry skin, nose, or throat
1% to 10%: Difficulty in swallowing
<1%:
Cardiovascular: Tachycardia
Central nervous system: Confusion, drowsiness, nervousness, insomnia, headache, loss of memory, weakness, tiredness
Dermatologic: Rash
Gastrointestinal: Bloated feeling, nausea, vomiting
Genitourinary: Urinary retention
Ocular: Increased intraocular pressure, blurred vision

Drug Interactions No data reported

Pregnancy Risk Factor C

Methsuximide (meth sux′ i mide)

Brand Names Celontin®

Canadian/Mexican Brand Names Celontin® (Canada)

Therapeutic Category Anticonvulsant, Succinimide

Use Control of absence (petit mal) seizures; useful adjunct in refractory, partial complex (psychomotor) seizures

Usual Dosage Oral:
Children: Initial: 10-15 mg/kg/day in 3-4 divided doses; increase weekly up to maximum of 30 mg/kg/day

Adults: 300 mg/day for the first week; may increase by 300 mg/day at weekly intervals up to 1.2 g/day in 2-4 divided doses/day

Mechanism of Action Increases the seizure threshold and suppresses paroxysmal spike-and-wave pattern in absence seizures; depresses nerve transmission in the motor cortex

Local Anesthetic/Vasoconstrictor Precautions No information available to require special precautions

Effects on Dental Treatment No effects or complications reported

Other Adverse Effects

>10%:

Central nervous system: Ataxia, dizziness, drowsiness, headache
Dermatologic: Stevens-Johnson syndrome or SLE
Gastrointestinal: Anorexia, nausea, vomiting, weight loss
Miscellaneous: Hiccups

1% to 10%: Central nervous system: Aggressiveness, mental depression, nightmares, weakness, tiredness

<1%:

Central nervous system: Paranoid psychosis
Dermatologic: Urticaria, exfoliative dermatitis
Hematologic: Agranulocytosis, leukopenia, aplastic anemia, thrombocytopenia, pancytopenia

Drug Interactions No data reported

Drug Uptake

Serum half-life: 2-4 hours
Time to peak serum concentration: Oral: Within 1-3 hours

Pregnancy Risk Factor C

Methyclothiazide (meth i kloe thye′ a zide)

Related Information

Cardiovascular Diseases *on page 912*

Brand Names Aquatensen®; Enduron®

Therapeutic Category Diuretic, Thiazide Type

Use Management of mild to moderate hypertension; treatment of edema in congestive heart failure and nephrotic syndrome

Usual Dosage Oral:

Children: 0.05-0.2 mg/kg/day

Adults:
Edema: 2.5-10 mg/day
Hypertension: 2.5-5 mg/day

Mechanism of Action Inhibits sodium reabsorption in the distal tubules causing increased excretion of sodium and water, as well as, potassium and hydrogen ions

Local Anesthetic/Vasoconstrictor Precautions No information available to require special precautions

Effects on Dental Treatment No effects or complications reported

Other Adverse Effects

1% to 10%: Endocrine & metabolic: Hypokalemia

<1%:

Cardiovascular: Hypotension
Central nervous system: Drowsiness
Dermatologic: Photosensitivity, rash
Endocrine & metabolic: Fluid and electrolyte imbalances (hypocalcemia, hypomagnesemia, hyponatremia), hyperglycemia
Gastrointestinal: Nausea, vomiting, anorexia
Genitourinary: Uremia
Hematologic: Rarely blood dyscrasias, aplastic anemia, hemolytic anemia, leukopenia, agranulocytosis, thrombocytopenia
Hepatic: Hepatitis
Neuromuscular & skeletal: Paresthesia
Renal: Polyuria, prerenal azotemia

Drug Interactions Increased toxicity/levels of lithium

Drug Uptake

Onset of diuresis: Oral: 2 hours
Peak effect: 6 hours
Duration: ~1 day

Pregnancy Risk Factor D

Methyclothiazide and Cryptenamine Tannates
(meth i kloe thye' a zide & krip ten' a meen tan' ates)

Brand Names Diutensin®

Therapeutic Category Antihypertensive Agent, Combination

Synonyms Cryptenamine Tannates and Methyclothiazide

Use Management of hypertension

Local Anesthetic/Vasoconstrictor Precautions No information available to require special precautions

Effects on Dental Treatment No effects or complications reported

Methyclothiazide and Deserpidine
(meth i kloe thye' a zide & de ser' pi deen)

Brand Names Enduronyl®; Enduronyl® Forte

Therapeutic Category Antihypertensive Agent, Combination

Use Management of mild to moderately severe hypertension

Local Anesthetic/Vasoconstrictor Precautions No information available to require special precautions

Effects on Dental Treatment No effects or complications reported

Methyclothiazide and Pargyline
(meth i kloe thye' a zide & par' gi leen)

Brand Names Eutron®

Therapeutic Category Antihypertensive Agent, Combination

Synonyms Pargyline and Methyclothiazide

Use Management of hypertension

Local Anesthetic/Vasoconstrictor Precautions No information available to require special precautions

Effects on Dental Treatment No effects or complications reported

Methylbenzethonium Chloride
(meth il ben ze thoe' nee um klor' ide)

Brand Names Diaparene® [OTC]; Puri-Clens™ [OTC]; Sween® Cream [OTC]

Therapeutic Category Topical Skin Product

Use Diaper rash and ammonia dermatitis

Local Anesthetic/Vasoconstrictor Precautions No information available to require special precautions

Effects on Dental Treatment No effects or complications reported

Methylcellulose (meth il sel' yoo lose)

Brand Names Citrucel® [OTC]

Therapeutic Category Ophthalmic Agent, Miscellaneous

Use Adjunct in treatment of constipation

Local Anesthetic/Vasoconstrictor Precautions No information available to require special precautions

Effects on Dental Treatment No effects or complications reported

Comments Each dose contains sodium 3 mg, potassium 105 mg, and 60 calories from sucrose

Methyldopa (meth il doe' pa)

Related Information

Cardiovascular Diseases on page 912

Brand Names Aldomet®

Canadian/Mexican Brand Names Apo-Methyldopa® (Canada); Dopamet® (Canada); Medimet® (Canada); Novo-Medopa® (Canada); Nu-Medopa® (Canada)

Therapeutic Category Alpha-Adrenergic Blockers - Peripheral-Acting (Alpha$_1$-Blockers)

Synonyms Metildopa (Mexico)

Use Management of moderate to severe hypertension

Usual Dosage

Children:

Oral: Initial: 10 mg/kg/day in 2-4 divided doses; increase every 2 days as needed to maximum dose of 65 mg/kg/day; do not exceed 3 g/day

I.V.: 5-10 mg/kg/dose every 6-8 hours up to a total dose of 65 mg/kg/24 hours or 3 g/24 hours

Adults:

Oral: Initial: 250 mg 2-3 times/day; increase every 2 days as needed; usual dose 1-1.5 g/day in 2-4 divided doses; maximum dose: 3 g/day

I.V.: 250-1000 mg every 6-8 hours; maximum dose: 1 g every 6 hours

Mechanism of Action Stimulation of central alpha-adrenergic receptors by a false transmitter that results in a decreased sympathetic outflow to the heart, kidneys, and peripheral vasculature

Local Anesthetic/Vasoconstrictor Precautions No information available to require special precautions

Effects on Dental Treatment Anticholinergic side effects can cause a reduction of saliva production or secretion. This may result in discomfort and dental disease (ie, caries, oral candidiasis and periodontal disease)

Other Adverse Effects

>10%: Cardiovascular: Peripheral edema

1% to 10%:
Central nervous system: Drug fever, mental depression, anxiety, nightmares, drowsiness, headache
Gastrointestinal: Dry mouth

<1%:
Cardiovascular: Orthostatic hypotension, bradycardia (sinus)
Central nervous system: Fever, chills, sedation, vertigo, depression, memory lapse
Dermatologic: Rash
Endocrine & metabolic: Sodium retention, sexual dysfunction, gynecomastia
Gastrointestinal: Colitis, pancreatitis, diarrhea, nausea, vomiting
Genitourinary: Decreased libido
Hematologic: Thrombocytopenia, hemolytic anemia, positive Coombs' test, leukopenia, transient leukopenia or granulocytopenia
Hepatic: Cholestasis or hepatitis and heptocellular injury, increased liver enzymes, jaundice, cirrhosis
Neuromuscular & skeletal: Paresthesias, weakness
Respiratory: Troubled breathing
Miscellaneous: SLE-like syndrome, hyperprolactinemia, "black" tongue

Drug Interactions

Decreased effect: Iron supplements can interact and cause a significant **increase** in blood pressure
Increased toxicity: Lithium causes increased lithium toxicity; tolbutamide and levodopa effects/toxicity increased

Drug Uptake

Peak hypotensive effect: Oral, parenteral: Within 3-6 hours
Duration: 12-24 hours
Serum half-life: 75-80 minutes
End stage renal disease: 6-16 hours

Pregnancy Risk Factor B

Methyldopa and Chlorothiazide see Chlorothiazide and Methyldopa on page 188

Methyldopa and Hydrochlorothiazide
(meth il doe' pa & hye droe klor oh thye' a zide)

Brand Names Aldoril®

Therapeutic Category Antihypertensive Agent, Combination

Synonyms Hydrochlorothiazide and Methyldopa

Use Management of moderate to severe hypertension

Local Anesthetic/Vasoconstrictor Precautions No information available to require special precautions

Effects on Dental Treatment Anticholinergic side effects can cause a reduction of saliva production or secretion. This may result in discomfort and dental disease (ie, caries, oral candidiasis and periodontal disease)

Methylergonovine Maleate (meth il er goe noe' veen mal' ee ate)

Brand Names Methergine®

Therapeutic Category Ergot Alkaloid and Derivative

Synonyms Metilergometrina, Maleato De (Mexico)

Use Prevention and treatment of postpartum and postabortion hemorrhage caused by uterine atony or subinvolution

Usual Dosage Adults:

Oral: 0.2 mg 3-4 times/day for 2-7 days
I.M.: 0.2 mg after delivery of anterior shoulder, after delivery of placenta, or during puerperium; may be repeated as required at intervals of 2-4 hours
I.V.: Same dose as I.M., but should not be routinely administered I.V. because of possibility of inducing sudden hypertension and cerebrovascular accident

Mechanism of Action Similar smooth muscle actions as seen with ergotamine; however, it affects primarily uterine smooth muscles producing sustained contractions and thereby shortens the third stage of labor
(Continued)

Methylergonovine Maleate *(Continued)*

Local Anesthetic/Vasoconstrictor Precautions No information available to require special precautions

Effects on Dental Treatment No effects or complications reported

Other Adverse Effects

>10%:
  Cardiovascular: Hypertension
  Central nervous system: Headache, seizures
1% to 10%: Gastrointestinal: Nausea, vomiting
<1%:
  Cardiovascular: Temporary chest pain, palpitations
  Central nervous system: Hallucinations, dizziness
  Gastrointestinal: Diarrhea
  Local: Thrombophlebitis
  Neuromuscular & skeletal: Leg cramps
  Otic: Tinnitus
  Renal: Hematuria, water intoxication
  Respiratory: Dyspnea, nasal congestion
  Miscellaneous: Diaphoresis, foul taste

Drug Interactions No data reported

Drug Uptake

Onset of oxytocic effect:
  Oral: 5-10 minutes
  I.M.: 2-5 minutes
  I.V.: Immediately
Duration of action:
  Oral: ~3 hours
  I.M.: ~3 hours
  I.V.: 45 minutes
Absorption: Rapid
Serum half-life (biphasic):
  Initial: 1-5 minutes
  Terminal: 30 minutes to 2 hours
Time to peak serum concentration: Within 30 minutes to 3 hours

Pregnancy Risk Factor C

Methylmorphine (Canada) *see* Codeine *on page 227*

Methylone® *see* Methylprednisolone *on next page*

Methylphenidate Hydrochloride

(meth il fen′ i date hye droe klor′ ide)

Brand Names Ritalin®; Ritalin-SR®

Canadian/Mexican Brand Names PMS-Methylphenidate® (Canada)

Therapeutic Category Central Nervous System Stimulant, Nonamphetamine

Synonyms Metifenidato, Clorhidrato De (Mexico)

Use Treatment of attention deficit disorder and symptomatic management of narcolepsy; many **unlabeled uses**

Usual Dosage Oral: (Discontinue periodically to re-evaluate or if no improvement occurs within 1 month)

Children ≥6 years: Attention deficit disorder: Initial: 0.3 mg/kg/dose or 2.5-5 mg/dose given before breakfast and lunch; increase by 0.1 mg/kg/dose or by 5-10 mg/day at weekly intervals; usual dose: 0.5-1 mg/kg/day; maximum dose: 2 mg/kg/day or 60 mg/day

Adults:
  Narcolepsy: 10 mg 2-3 times/day, up to 60 mg/day
  Depression: Initial: 2.5 mg every morning before 9 AM; dosage may be increased by 2.5-5 mg every 2-3 days as tolerated to a maximum of 20 mg/day; may be divided (ie, 7 AM and 12 noon), but should not be given after noon; do not use sustained release product

Mechanism of Action Blocks the reuptake mechanism of dopaminergic neurons; appears to stimulate the cerebral cortex and subcortical structures similar to amphetamines

Local Anesthetic/Vasoconstrictor Precautions No information available to require special precautions

Effects on Dental Treatment Up to 10% of patients taking dextroamphetamines may present with hypertension. The use of local anesthetic without vasoconstrictor is recommended in these patients.

Other Adverse Effects

>10%:
  Cardiovascular: Tachycardia

Central nervous system: Nervousness, insomnia
Gastrointestinal: Anorexia
1% to 10%:
Central nervous system: Dizziness, drowsiness
Gastrointestinal: Stomach pain
Miscellaneous: Hypersensitivity reactions
<1%:
Cardiovascular: Hypertension, hypotension, palpitations, cardiac arrhythmias
Central nervous system: Movement disorders, precipitation of Tourette's syndrome, and toxic psychosis (rare), fever, headache, convulsions
Dermatologic: Rash
Gastrointestinal: Nausea, weight loss, vomiting
Endocrine & metabolic: Growth retardation
Hematologic: Thrombocytopenia, anemia, leukopenia
Ocular: Blurred vision

Drug Interactions
Decreased effect: Effects of guanethidine, bretylium may be antagonized by methylphenidate
Increased toxicity: May increase serum concentrations of tricyclic antidepressants, warfarin, phenytoin, phenobarbital, and primidone; MAO inhibitors may potentiate effects of methylphenidate

Drug Uptake
Immediate release tablet:
Duration: 3-6 hours
Sustained release tablet:
Peak effect: Within 4-7 hours
Duration: 8 hours
Absorption: Slow and incomplete from GI tract
Serum half-life: 2-4 hours

Pregnancy Risk Factor C

Methylprednisolone (meth ill pred niss' oh lone)
Related Information
Corticosteroid Equivalencies Comparison *on page 1017*
Corticosteroids, Topical Comparison *on page 1018*
Respiratory Diseases *on page 924*

Brand Names Adlone®; A-Methapred®; depMedalone®; Depoject®; Depo-Medrol®; Depopred®; Duralone®; Medralone®; Medrol®; Methylone®; Solu-Medrol®

Canadian/Mexican Brand Names Cryosolona® (Mexico)

Therapeutic Category Adrenal Corticosteroid; Anti-inflammatory Agent; Corticosteroid, Systemic; Corticosteroid, Topical (Low Potency)

Use
Dental: Treatment of a variety of oral diseases of allergic, inflammatory or autoimmune origin
Medical: Primarily as an anti-inflammatory or immunosuppressant agent in the treatment of a variety of diseases including those of hematologic, allergic, inflammatory, neoplastic, and autoimmune origin

Usual Dosage Only sodium succinate salt may be given I.V.. Methylprednisolone sodium succinate is highly soluble and has a rapid effect by I.M. and I.V. routes. Methylprednisolone acetate has a low solubility and has a sustained I.M. effect.

Children:
Anti-inflammatory or immunosuppressive: Oral, I.M., I.V. (sodium succinate): 0.12-1.7 mg/kg/day or 5-25 mg/m^2/day in divided doses every 6-12 hours
Topical: Apply sparingly 2-4 times/day
Adults:
Anti-inflammatory or immunosuppressive: Oral: 2-60 mg/day in 1-4 divided doses to start, followed by gradual reduction in dosage to the lowest possible level consistent with maintaining an adequate clinical response
I.M. (sodium succinate): 10-80 mg/day once daily
I.M. (acetate): 40-120 mg every 1-2 weeks
I.V. (sodium succinate): 10-40 mg over a period of several minutes and repeated I.V. or I.M. at intervals depending on clinical response; when high dosages are needed, give 30 mg/kg over a period of 10-20 minutes and may be repeated every 4-6 hours for 48 hours
Topical: Apply sparingly 2-4 times/day

Mechanism of Action Decreases inflammation by suppression of migration of polymorphonuclear leukocytes and reversal of increased capillary permeability
(Continued)

Methylprednisolone *(Continued)*

Local Anesthetic/Vasoconstrictor Precautions No information available to require special precautions

Effects on Dental Treatment No effects or complications reported

Other Adverse Effects >10%:

Central nervous system: Insomnia, nervousness

Gastrointestinal: Increased appetite, indigestion

Oral manifestations: No data reported

Contraindications Serious infections, except septic shock or tuberculous meningitis; known hypersensitivity to methylprednisolone; viral, fungal, or tubercular skin lesions; administration of live virus vaccines

Warnings/Precautions

Use with caution in patients with hyperthyroidism, cirrhosis, nonspecific ulcerative colitis, hypertension, osteoporosis, thromboembolic tendencies, CHF, convulsive disorders, myasthenia gravis, thrombophlebitis, peptic ulcer, diabetes

Acute adrenal insufficiency may occur with abrupt withdrawal after long-term therapy or with stress; young pediatric patients may be more susceptible to adrenal axis suppression from topical therapy

Because of the risk of adverse effects, systemic corticosteroids should be used cautiously in the elderly, in the smallest possible dose, and for the shortest possible time.

Drug Interactions Phenytoin, phenobarbital, rifampin increases clearance of methylprednisolone; potassium depleting diuretics enhance potassium depletion; skin test antigens, immunizations increase response and increase potential infections; methylprednisolone may increase circulating glucose levels → may need adjustments of insulin or oral hypoglycemics

Drug Uptake Methylprednisolone sodium succinate is highly soluble and has a rapid effect by I.M. and I.V. routes; methylprednisolone acetate has a low solubility and has a sustained I.M. effect

Time to obtain peak effect and the duration of these effects is dependent upon the route of administration. See table.

Route	Peak Effect	Duration
Oral	1-2 h	30-36 h
I.M.	4-8 d	1-4 wk
Intra-articular	1 wk	1-5 wk

Serum half-life: 3-3.5 hours

Pregnancy Risk Factor C

Breast-feeding Considerations No data reported

Dosage Forms

Injection, as sodium succinate: 40 mg (1 mL, 3 mL); 125 mg (2 mL, 5 mL); 500 mg (1 mL, 4 mL, 8 mL, 20 mL); 1,000 mg (1 mL, 8 mL, 50 mL); 2,000 mg (30.6 mL)

Injection, as acetate: 20 mg/mL (5 mL, 10 mL); 40 mg/mL (1 mL, 5 mL, 10 mL); 80 mg/mL (1 mL, 5 mL)

Ointment, topical, as acetate: 0.25% (30 g); 1% (30 g)

Tablet: 2 mg, 4 mg, 8 mg, 16 mg, 24 mg, 32 mg

Tablet, dose pack: 4 mg (21s)

Dietary Considerations Should be taken after meals or with food or milk; limit caffeine; need diet rich in pyridoxine, vitamin C, vitamin D, folate, calcium, phosphorus, and protein

Generic Available Yes

Methyltestosterone *(meth il tes tos' te rone)*

Brand Names Android®; Metandren®; Oreton® Methyl; Testred®; Virilon®

Therapeutic Category Androgen

Use

Male: Hypogonadism; delayed puberty; impotence and climacteric symptoms

Female: Palliative treatment of metastatic breast cancer; postpartum breast pain and/or engorgement

Usual Dosage Adults (buccal absorption produces twice the androgenic activity of oral tablets):

Male:

Oral: 10-40 mg/day

Buccal: 5-25 mg/day

Female:
    Breast pain/engorgement:
        Oral: 80 mg/day for 3-5 days
        Buccal: 40 mg/day for 3-5 days
    Breast cancer:
        Oral: 50-200 mg/day
        Buccal: 25-100 mg/day

Mechanism of Action Stimulates receptors in organs and tissues to promote growth and development of male sex organs and maintains secondary sex characteristics in androgen-deficient males

Local Anesthetic/Vasoconstrictor Precautions No information available to require special precautions

Effects on Dental Treatment No effects or complications reported

Other Adverse Effects
>10%:
    Male: Virilism, priapism
    Female: Virilism, menstrual problems (amenorrhea), breast soreness
    Dermatologic: Edema, acne
1% to 10%:
    Females: Hirsutism (increase in pubic hair growth)
    Men: Prostatic hypertrophy, prostatic carcinoma, impotence, testicular atrophy
    Gastrointestinal: GI irritation, nausea, vomiting
    Hepatic: Hepatic dysfunction
<1%:
    Endocrine & metabolic: Gynecomastia, amenorrhea, hypercalcemia
    Hematologic: Leukopenia, polycythemia
    Hepatic: Hepatic necrosis, cholestatic hepatitis
    Miscellaneous: Hypersensitivity reactions

Drug Interactions Decreased effect: Oral anticoagulant effect or insulin requirements may be increased

Drug Uptake
    Absorption: From GI tract and oral mucosa

Pregnancy Risk Factor X

Methysergide Maleate (meth i ser' jide mal' ee ate)

Brand Names Sansert®

Therapeutic Category Ergot Alkaloid and Derivative

Use Prophylaxis of vascular headache

Usual Dosage Adults: Oral: 4-8 mg/day with meals; if no improvement is noted after 3 weeks, drug is unlikely to be beneficial; must not be given continuously for longer than 6 months, and a drug-free interval of 3-4 weeks must follow each 6-month course

Mechanism of Action Ergotamine congener, however actions appear to differ; methysergide has minimal ergotamine-like oxytocic or vasoconstrictive properties, and has significantly greater serotonin-like properties

Local Anesthetic/Vasoconstrictor Precautions No information available to require special precautions

Effects on Dental Treatment No effects or complications reported

Other Adverse Effects
>10%:
    Cardiovascular: Postural hypotension, peripheral ischemia
    Central nervous system: Insomnia
    Gastrointestinal: Nausea, vomiting, abdominal pain, diarrhea
1% to 10%:
    Cardiovascular: Peripheral edema, tachycardia, bradycardia
    Dermatologic: Skin rash
    Gastrointestinal: Heartburn
<1%:
    Central nervous system: Insomnia, overstimulation, drowsiness, mild euphoria, lethargy, mental depression, vertigo, unsteadiness, confusion, hyperesthesia, rebound headache may occur if methysergide is discontinued abruptly
    Ocular: Visual disturbances
    Respiratory: Fibrosis

Drug Interactions No data reported

Drug Uptake
    Serum half-life, plasma elimination: ~10 hours

Pregnancy Risk Factor X

Meticorten® *see* Prednisone *on page 719*

Metifenidato, Clorhidrato De (Mexico) *see* Methylphenidate Hydrochloride *on page 568*

Metildopa (Mexico) *see* Methyldopa *on page 566*

Metilergometrina, Maleato De (Mexico) *see* Methylergonovine Maleate *on page 567*

Metimyd® *see* Sodium Sulfacetamide and Prednisolone Acetate *on page 794*

Metipranolol Hydrochloride (met i pran' oh lol hye droe klor' ide)
Brand Names OptiPranolol®
Therapeutic Category Antiglaucoma Agent; Beta-Adrenergic Blocker, Ophthalmic
Use Agent for lowering intraocular pressure in patients with chronic open-angle glaucoma
Usual Dosage Ophthalmic: Adults: Instill 1 drop in the affected eye(s) twice daily
Mechanism of Action Beta-adrenoceptor-blocking agent; lacks intrinsic sympathomimetic activity and membrane-stabilizing effects and possesses only slight local anesthetic activity; mechanism of action of metipranolol in reducing intraocular pressure appears to be via reduced production of aqueous humor. This effect may be related to a reduction in blood flow to the iris root-ciliary body. It remains unclear if the reduction in intraocular pressure observed with beta-blockers is actually secondary to beta-adrenoceptor blockade.
Local Anesthetic/Vasoconstrictor Precautions No information available to require special precautions
Effects on Dental Treatment No effects or complications reported
Other Adverse Effects
>10%: Ocular: Mild ocular stinging and discomfort, eye irritation
1% to 10%: Ocular: Blurred vision, browache
<1%:
Cardiovascular: Bradycardia, A-V block, congestive heart failure
Central nervous system: Asthenia
Ocular: Conjunctivitis, blepharitis, tearing, erythema, itching, keratitis, photophobia, decreased corneal sensitivity
Respiratory: Bronchospasm
Drug Interactions No data reported
Drug Uptake
Onset of action: ≤30 minutes
Maximum effects: ~2 hours
Duration of action: Intraocular pressure reduction has persisted for 24 hours following ocular instillation
Serum half-life, elimination: ~3 hours
Pregnancy Risk Factor C

Metoclopramida (Mexico) *see* Metoclopramide *on this page*

Metoclopramide (met oh kloe pra' mide)
Related Information
Endocrine Disorders & Pregnancy *on page 927*
Brand Names Clopra®; Maxolon®; Octamide®; Reglan®
Canadian/Mexican Brand Names Apo-Metoclop® (Canada); Maxeran® (Canada); Carnotprim Primperan® (Mexico); Carnotprim Primperan® Retard (Mexico); Meclomid® (Mexico); Plasil® (Mexico); Pramotil® (Mexico)
Therapeutic Category Antiemetic
Synonyms Metoclopramida (Mexico)
Use Symptomatic treatment of diabetic gastric stasis, gastroesophageal reflux; prevention of nausea associated with chemotherapy or postsurgery and facilitates intubation of the small intestine
Usual Dosage
Children:
Gastroesophageal reflux: Oral: 0.1-0.2 mg/kg/dose up to 4 times/day; efficacy of continuing metoclopramide beyond 12 weeks in reflux has not been determined; total daily dose should not exceed 0.5 mg/kg/day
Gastrointestinal hypomotility (gastroparesis): Oral, I.M., I.V.: 0.1 mg/kg/dose up to 4 times/day, not to exceed 0.5 mg/kg/day
Antiemetic (chemotherapy-induced emesis): I.V.: 1-2 mg/kg 30 minutes before chemotherapy and every 2-4 hours
Facilitate intubation: I.V.:
<6 years: 0.1 mg/kg
6-14 years: 2.5-5 mg

Adults:

Gastroesophageal reflux: Oral: 10-15 mg/dose up to 4 times/day 30 minutes before meals or food and at bedtime; single doses of 20 mg are occasionally needed for provoking situations; efficacy of continuing metoclopramide beyond 12 weeks in reflux has not been determined

Gastrointestinal hypomotility (gastroparesis):

Oral: 10 mg 30 minutes before each meal and at bedtime for 2-8 weeks

I.V. (for severe symptoms): 10 mg over 1-2 minutes; 10 days of I.V. therapy may be necessary for best response

Antiemetic (chemotherapy-induced emesis): I.V.: 1-2 mg/kg 30 minutes before chemotherapy and every 2-4 hours to every 4-6 hours (and usually given with diphenhydramine 25-50 mg I.V./oral)

Postoperative nausea and vomiting: I.M.: 10 mg near end of surgery; 20 mg doses may be used

Facilitate intubation: I.V.: 10 mg

Elderly:

Gastroesophageal reflux: Oral: 5 mg 4 times/day (30 minutes before meals and at bedtime); increase dose to 10 mg 4 times/day if no response at lower dose

Gastrointestinal hypomotility:

Oral: Initial: 5 mg 30 minutes before meals and at bedtime for 2-8 weeks; increase if necessary to 10 mg doses

I.V.: Initiate at 5 mg over 1-2 minutes; increase to 10 mg if necessary

Postoperative nausea and vomiting: I.M.: 5 mg near end of surgery; may repeat dose if necessary

Mechanism of Action Blocks dopamine receptors in chemoreceptor trigger zone of the CNS; enhances the response to acetylcholine of tissue in upper GI tract causing enhanced motility and accelerated gastric emptying without stimulating gastric, biliary, or pancreatic secretions

Local Anesthetic/Vasoconstrictor Precautions No information available to require special precautions

Effects on Dental Treatment No effects or complications reported

Other Adverse Effects

>10%:

Central nervous system: Weakness, restlessness, drowsiness

Gastrointestinal: Diarrhea

1% to 10%:

Central nervous system: Insomnia, depression

Dermatologic: Skin rash

Endocrine & metabolic: Breast tenderness, prolactin stimulation

Gastrointestinal: Nausea, dry mouth

<1%:

Cardiovascular: Tachycardia, hypertension or hypotension

Central nervous system: Extrapyramidal reactions•, tardive dyskinesia, fatigue, anxiety, agitation

Gastrointestinal: Constipation

Hematologic: Methemoglobinemia

•**Note:** A recent study suggests the incidence of extrapyramidal reactions due to metoclopramide may be as high as 34% and the incidence appears more often in the elderly

Drug Interactions

Decreased effect: Anticholinergic agents antagonize metoclopramide's actions

Increased toxicity: Opiate analgesics causes increased CNS depression

Drug Uptake

Onset of effect:

Oral: Within 0.5-1 hour

I.V.: Within 1-3 minutes

Duration of therapeutic effect: 1-2 hours, regardless of route administered

Serum half-life, normal renal function: 4-7 hours (may be dose-dependent)

Pregnancy Risk Factor B

Metolazone (me tole′ a zone)

Related Information

Cardiovascular Diseases on page 912

Brand Names Mykrox®; Zaroxolyn®

Therapeutic Category Diuretic, Thiazide Type

Use Management of mild to moderate hypertension; treatment of edema in congestive heart failure and nephrotic syndrome, impaired renal function

Usual Dosage Oral:

Children: 0.2-0.4 mg/kg/day divided every 12-24 hours

(Continued)

Metolazone *(Continued)*

Adults:
Edema: 5-20 mg/dose every 24 hours
Hypertension: 2.5-5 mg/dose every 24 hours
Hypertension (Mykrox®): 0.5 mg/day; if response is not adequate, increase dose to maximum of 1 mg/day

Not dialyzable (0% to 5%) via hemo- or peritoneal dialysis; supplemental dose is not necessary

Mechanism of Action Inhibits sodium reabsorption in the distal tubules causing increased excretion of sodium and water, as well as, potassium and hydrogen ions

Local Anesthetic/Vasoconstrictor Precautions No information available to require special precautions

Effects on Dental Treatment No effects or complications reported

Other Adverse Effects
1% to 10%: Endocrine & metabolic: Hypokalemia
<1%:
Cardiovascular: Hypotension
Central nervous system: Drowsiness
Dermatologic: Photosensitivity, rash
Endocrine & metabolic: Fluid and electrolyte imbalances (hypocalcemia, hypomagnesemia, hyponatremia), hyperglycemia
Gastrointestinal: Nausea, vomiting, anorexia
Genitourinary: Uremia
Hematologic: Rarely blood dyscrasias, aplastic anemia, hemolytic anemia, leukopenia, agranulocytosis, thrombocytopenia
Hepatic: Hepatitis
Neuromuscular & skeletal: Paresthesia
Renal: Prerenal azotemia, polyuria

Drug Interactions
Increased toxicity:
Concurrent administration with furosemide may cause excessive volume and electrolyte depletion
Increased digitalis glycosides toxicity
Increased lithium toxicity

Drug Uptake Same for all routes:
Onset of diuresis: Within 60 minutes
Duration: 12-24 hours
Absorption: Oral: Incomplete
Serum half-life: 6-20 hours, renal function dependent

Pregnancy Risk Factor D

Metoprolol *(me toe' proe lole tar' trate)*

Related Information
Cardiovascular Diseases *on page 912*

Brand Names Lopressor® [Tartrate]; Toprol XL® [Succinate]

Canadian/Mexican Brand Names Apo-Metoprolol® (Type L) (Canada); Betaloc® (Canada); Betaloc Durules® (Canada); Novo-Metoprolol® (Canada); Nu-Metop® (Canada); Kenaprol® (Mexico); Lopresor® (Mexico); Proken® M (Mexico); Prolaken® (Mexico); Ritmolol® (Mexico); Seloken® (Mexico); Selopres® (Mexico)

Therapeutic Category Beta-Adrenergic Blocker, Cardioselective

Use Treatment of hypertension and angina pectoris; prevention of myocardial infarction, atrial fibrillation, flutter, symptomatic treatment of hypertrophic suba-ortic stenosis

Unlabeled use: Treatment of ventricular arrhythmias, atrial ectopy, migraine prophylaxis, essential tremor, aggressive behavior

Usual Dosage
Children: Oral: 1-5 mg/kg/24 hours divided twice daily; allow 3 days between dose adjustments
Adults:
Oral: 100-450 mg/day in 2-3 divided doses, begin with 50 mg twice daily and increase doses at weekly intervals to desired effect
I.V.: 5 mg every 2 minutes for 3 doses in early treatment of myocardial infarction; thereafter give 50 mg orally every 6 hours 15 minutes after last I.V. dose and continue for 48 hours; then administer a maintenance dose of 100 mg twice daily
Elderly: Oral: Initial: 25 mg/day; usual range: 25-300 mg/day

Hemodialysis: Administer dose posthemodialysis or administer 50 mg supplemental dose supplemental dose is not necessary following peritoneal dialysis

Mechanism of Action Selective inhibitor of beta$_1$-adrenergic receptors; competitively blocks beta$_1$-receptors, with little or no effect on beta$_2$-receptors at doses <100 mg; does not exhibit any membrane stabilizing or intrinsic sympathomimetic activity

Local Anesthetic/Vasoconstrictor Precautions No information available to require special precautions

Effects on Dental Treatment Non-cardioselective beta-blockers (ie, propranolol, nadolol) enhance the pressor response to epinephrine, resulting in hypertension and bradycardia. This has not been reported for metoprolol, a cardioselective beta-blocker. Therefore, local anesthetic with vasoconstrictor can be safely used in patients medicated with metoprolol. Many nonsteroidal anti-inflammatory drugs such as ibuprofen and indomethacin can reduce the hypotensive effect of beta-blockers after 3 or more weeks of therapy with the NSAID. Short-term NSAID use (ie, 3 days) requires no special precautions in patients taking beta-blockers.

Other Adverse Effects

>10%: Central nervous system: Mental depression, tiredness, weakness, dizziness

1% to 10%:

Cardiovascular: Bradycardia, irregular heartbeat, reduced peripheral circulation

Gastrointestinal: Heartburn

Respiratory: Wheezing

<1%:

Cardiovascular: Chest pain, heart failure, Raynaud's phenomena

Central nervous system: Insomnia, nightmares, confusion, headache

Dermatologic: Rash, itching

Endocrine & metabolic: Decreased sexual activity

Gastrointestinal: Constipation, nausea, vomiting, stomach discomfort

Genitourinary: Impotence

Miscellaneous: Cold extremities

Drug Interactions

Decreased effect of beta-blockers:

Barbiturates (increased liver metabolism of beta-blockers to result in lower serum levels)

NSAIDs (attenuate the hypotensive therapeutic effects of beta-blockers)

Rifampin (increased liver metabolism of beta-blockers to result in lower serum levels)

Increased effects of beta-blockers:

Calcium channel blockers (increase serum levels of beta-blockers by unknown mechanism to enhance hypotension)

Beta-blockers increase the effects of:

Epinephrine (vasoconstrictor; initial hypertensive episode followed by bradycardia) only from non-cardioselective type beta-blockers

Phenylephrine (Neosynephrine®; enhanced pressor response)

Theophylline (inhibit theophylline metabolism causing increase in serum concentrations)

Drug Uptake

Peak antihypertensive effect: Oral: Within 1.5-4 hours

Duration: 10-20 hours

Absorption: 95%

Serum half-life: 3-4 hours

End stage renal disease: 2.5-4.5 hours

Pregnancy Risk Factor B

Selected Readings

Foster CA and Aston SJ, "Propranolol-Epinephrine Interaction: A Potential Disaster," *Plast Reconstr Surg*, 1983, 72(1):74-8.

Wong DG, Spence JD, Lamki L, et al, "Effect of Nonsteroidal Anti-Inflammatory Drugs on Control of Hypertension of Beta-Blockers and Diuretics," *Lancet*, 1986, 1(8488):997-1001.

Wynn RL, "Dental Nonsteroidal Anti-Inflammatory Drugs and Prostaglandin-Based Drug Interactions, Part Two," *Gen Dent*, 1992, 40(2):104, 106, 108.

Wynn RL, "Epinephrine Interactions With Beta-Blockers," *Gen Dent*, 1994, 42(1):16, 18.

Metotrexato (Mexico) *see* Methotrexate *on page 559*

Metreton® *see* Prednisolone *on page 718*

Metrodin® *see* Urofollitropin *on page 885*

MetroGel® *see* Metronidazole *on next page*

Metro I.V.® *see* Metronidazole *on next page*

Metronidazole (me troe ni′ da zole)

Related Information

Oral Bacterial Infections *on page 945*
Oral Nonviral Soft Tissue Ulcerations or Erosions *on page 955*

Brand Names Flagyl®; Helidac® Combination; MetroGel®; Metro I.V.®; Proto-stat®

Canadian/Mexican Brand Names Apo-Metronidazole® (Canada); Novo-Nidazol® (Canada); Ameblin® (Mexico); Flagenase® (Mexico); Milezzol® (Mexico); Otrozol® (Mexico); Vatrix-S® (Mexico); Vertisal® (Mexico)

Therapeutic Category Amebicide; Antibiotic, Anaerobic; Antibiotic, Topical; Antiprotozoal

Use

Dental: Treatment of oral soft tissue infections due to anaerobic bacteria including all anaerobic cocci, anaerobic gram-negative bacilli (*Bacteroides*), and gram-positive spore-forming bacilli (*Clostridium*). Useful as single agent or in combination with amoxicillin, Augmentin®, or ciprofloxacin in the treatment of periodontitis associated with the presence of *Actinobacillus actinomycetemcomitans*, (AA).

Medical: Treatment of susceptible anaerobic bacterial and protozoal infections in the following conditions: amebiasis, symptomatic and asymptomatic trichomoniasis; skin and skin structure infections; CNS infections; intra-abdominal infections; systemic anaerobic infections; topically for the treatment of acne rosacea; treatment of antibiotic-associated pseudomembranous colitis (AAPC); Helidac® in combination with an H_2 antagonist for the treatment active duodenal ulcer associated with *H. pylori* infection

Usual Dosage Adults: Oral:

Anaerobic infections: 500 mg every 6-8 hours, not to exceed 4 g/day
Treatment of periodontitis associated with AA:
Oral, singly: 200-400 mg 3 times/day for 7-10 days;
In combination: metronidazole plus Augmentin® 250 mg 3 times/day of each for 7 days; metronidazole 250 mg plus amoxicillin 375 mg each 3 times/day for 7 days; metronidazole plus ciprofloxacin 500 mg each twice daily for 8 days

Helidac®: Take metronidazole 250 mg tablet, bismuth subsalicylate 262.4 mg tablet x2, and tetracycline 500 mg capsule plus an H_2 antagonist four times daily at meals and bedtime for 14 days; chew and swallow the bismuth subsalicylate tablets, swallow the metronidazole tablet and tetracycline capsule with a full glass of water

Mechanism of Action Reduced to a product which interacts with DNA to cause a loss of helical DNA structure and strand breakage resulting in inhibition of protein synthesis and cell death in susceptible organisms

Local Anesthetic/Vasoconstrictor Precautions No information available to require special precautions

Effects on Dental Treatment No effects or complications reported

Other Adverse Effects

>10%:
Central nervous system: Dizziness, headache
Gastrointestinal: Nausea, diarrhea, loss of appetite, vomiting
<1%: Endocrine & metabolic: Disulfiram-type reaction with alcohol

Oral manifestations: <1%: Dry mouth, metallic taste

Contraindications Hypersensitivity to metronidazole or any component, 1st trimester of pregnancy

Warnings/Precautions Use with caution in patients with liver impairment, blood dyscrasias; history of seizures, congestive heart failure, or other sodium retaining states; reduce dosage in patients with severe liver impairment, CNS disease, and severe renal failure. Has been shown to be carcinogenic in rodents.

Drug Interactions Phenytoin, phenobarbital cause decreased metronidazole half-life; alcohol, disulfiram cause disulfiram-like reactions which includes flushing, headache, nausea, and in some patients, vomiting and chest and/or abdominal pain, therefore, absolutely contraindicated with alcohol; warfarin increases PT prolongation

Drug Uptake

Absorption: Oral: ~80%
Time to peak serum concentration: Within 1-2 hours
Serum half-life: 6-8 hours, increases with hepatic impairment
Influence of food: No effect on extent of absorption, but delays rate and decreases maximum concentration

Pregnancy Risk Factor B

Breast-feeding Considerations Not compatible; resume breast-feeding 12-24 hours after last dose

Dosage Forms

Gel, topical: 0.75% [7.5 mg/mL] (30 g)

Injection, ready to use: 5 mg/mL (100 mL)

Powder for injection, as hydrochloride: 500 mg

Tablet: 250 mg, 500 mg

Helidac® (One day supply): Contains metronidazole 250 mg tablet (#4), bismuth subsalicylate 262.4 mg tablet [Pepto-Bismol®] (#8), and tetracycline 500 mg capsule (#4)

Dietary Considerations May be taken with food because of gastric irritation, however, there is delayed absorption with food

Generic Available Yes

Selected Readings

Eisenberg L, Suchow R, Coles RS, et al, "The Effects of Metronidazole Administration on Clinical and Microbiologic Parameters of Periodontal Disease," *Clin Prev Dent*, 1991, 13(1):28-34.

Jenkins WM, MacFarlane TW, Gilmour WH, et al, "Systemic Metronidazole in the Treatment of Periodontitis," *J Clin Periodontol*, 1989, 16(7):433-50.

Loesche WJ, Giordano JR, Hujoel P, et al, "Metronidazole in Periodontitis: Reduced Need for Surgery," *J Clin Periodontol*, 1992, 19(2):103-12.

Loesche WJ, Schmidt E, Smith BA, et al, "Effects of Metronidazole on Periodontal Treatment Needs," *J Periodontol*, 1991, 62(4):247-57.

Soder PO, Frithiof L, Wikner S, et al, "The Effect of Systemic Metronidazole After Nonsurgical Treatment in Moderate and Advanced Periodontitis in Young Adults," *J Periodontol*, 1990, 61(5):281-8.

Mevacor® see Lovastatin *on page 516*

Mexiletina (Mexico) see Mexiletine *on this page*

Mexiletine (mex' i le teen)

Related Information

Cardiovascular Diseases *on page 912*

Brand Names Mexitil®

Therapeutic Category Antiarrhythmic Agent, Class I-B; Antiarrhythmic Agent (Supraventricular & Ventricular)

Synonyms Mexiletina (Mexico)

Use Management of serious ventricular arrhythmias; suppression of PVCs

Unlabeled use: Diabetic neuropathy

Usual Dosage Adults: Oral: Initial: 200 mg every 8 hours (may load with 400 mg if necessary); adjust dose every 2-3 days; usual dose: 200-300 mg every 8 hours; maximum dose: 1.2 g/day (some patients respond to every 12-hour dosing); patients with hepatic impairment or CHF may require dose reduction; when switching from another antiarrhythmic, initiate a 200 mg dose 6-12 hours after stopping former agents, 3-6 hours after stopping procainamide

Mechanism of Action Class IB antiarrhythmic, structurally related to lidocaine, which may cause increase in systemic vascular resistance and decrease in cardiac output; no significant negative inotropic effect; inhibits inward sodium current, decreases rate of rise of phase 0, increases effective refractory period/action potential duration ratio

Local Anesthetic/Vasoconstrictor Precautions No information available to require special precautions

Effects on Dental Treatment No effects or complications reported

Other Adverse Effects

>10%:

Central nervous system: Lightheadedness, dizziness, nervousness

Neuromuscular & skeletal: Trembling, unsteady gait

1% to 10%:

Cardiovascular: Chest pain, premature ventricular contractions

Central nervous system: Confusion, headache, numbness of fingers or toes, insomnia

Dermatologic: Rash

Gastrointestinal: Constipation or diarrhea

Hepatic: Increased LFTs

Neuromuscular & skeletal: Weakness

Ocular: Blurred vision

Otic: Tinnitus

Respiratory: Shortness of breath

<1%:

Hematologic: Leukopenia, agranulocytosis, thrombocytopenia, positive anti-nuclear antibody

Ocular: Diplopia

(Continued)

Mexiletine *(Continued)*

Drug Interactions
Decreased plasma levels: Phenobarbital, phenytoin, rifampin, and other hepatic enzyme inducers, cimetidine and drugs which make the urine acidic
Increased effect: Allopurinol
Increased toxicity/levels of caffeine and theophylline

Drug Uptake
Absorption: Elderly have a slightly slower rate of absorption but extent of absorption is the same as young adults
Serum half-life: Adults: 10-14 hours (average: 14.4 hours elderly, 12 hours in younger adults); increase in half-life with hepatic or heart failure
Time to peak: Peak levels attained in 2-3 hours

Pregnancy Risk Factor C

Mexitil® *see* Mexiletine *on previous page*
Mezlin® *see* Mezlocillin Sodium *on this page*

Mezlocillin Sodium *(mez loe sil' in sow' dee um)*

Brand Names Mezlin®
Therapeutic Category Antibiotic, Penicillin
Use Treatment of infections caused by susceptible gram-negative aerobic bacilli (*Klebsiella*, *Proteus*, *Escherichia coli*, *Enterobacter*, *Pseudomonas aeruginosa*, *Serratia*) involving the skin and skin structure, bone and joint, respiratory tract, urinary tract, gastrointestinal tract, as well as, septicemia

Usual Dosage I.M., I.V.:
Children: 200-300 mg/kg/day divided every 4-6 hours; maximum: 24 g/day
Adults:
Uncomplicated urinary tract infection: 1.5-2 g every 6 hours
Serious infections: 3-4 g every 4-6 hours

Mechanism of Action Interferes with bacterial cell wall synthesis during active multiplication causing cell death and resultant bactericidal activity against susceptible bacteria

Local Anesthetic/Vasoconstrictor Precautions No information available to require special precautions

Effects on Dental Treatment Prolonged use of penicillins may lead to development of oral candidiasis

Other Adverse Effects
1% to 10%: Gastrointestinal: Nausea, diarrhea
<1%:
Central nervous system: Fever, seizures, dizziness, headache
Dermatologic: Rash, exfoliative dermatitis
Endocrine & metabolic: Hypokalemia, hypernatremia
Gastrointestinal: Vomiting
Hematologic: Eosinophilia, leukopenia, neutropenia, thrombocytopenia, agranulocytosis, hemolytic anemia, prolonged bleeding time, positive Coombs' [direct]
Hepatic: Hepatotoxicity, elevated liver enzymes
Renal: Hematuria, elevated serum creatinine and BUN, interstitial nephritis
Miscellaneous: Serum sickness-like reactions

Drug Interactions Aminoglycosides (synergy), probenecid (decreased clearance), vecuronium (increased duration of neuromuscular blockade), heparin (increased risk of bleeding)

Drug Uptake
Absorption: I.M.: 63%
Serum half-life: Dose dependent:
Children 2-19 years: 0.9 hour
Adults: 50-70 minutes, increased in renal impairment
Time to peak serum concentration:
I.M.: 45-90 minutes after administration
I.V. infusion: Within 5 minutes

Pregnancy Risk Factor B

Miacalcin® *see* Calcitonin *on page 138*
Micatin® **[OTC]** *see* Miconazole *on this page*

Miconazole *(mi kon' a zole)*

Brand Names Micatin® [OTC]; Monistat™; Monistat-Derm™; Monistat i.v.™
Canadian/Mexican Brand Names Aloid® (Mexico); Daktarin® (Mexico); Dermifun® (Mexico); Fungiquim® (Mexico); Gyno-Daktarin® (Mexico); Gyno-Daktarin® V (Mexico); Neomicol® (Mexico)
Therapeutic Category Antifungal Agent, Topical; Antifungal Agent, Vaginal

Use

I.V.: Treatment of severe systemic fungal infections and fungal meningitis that are refractory to standard treatment

Topical: Treatment of vulvovaginal candidiasis and a variety of skin and mucous membrane fungal infections

Usual Dosage

Children:

I.V.: 20-40 mg/kg/day divided every 8 hours

Topical: Apply twice daily for up to 1 month

Adults:

Topical: Apply twice daily for up to 1 month

I.T.: 20 mg every 1-2 days

I.V.: Initial: 200 mg, then 1.2-3.6 g/day divided every 8 hours for up to 20 weeks

Bladder candidal infections: 200 mg diluted solution instilled in the bladder

Vaginal: Insert contents of 1 applicator of vaginal cream (100 mg) or 100 mg suppository at bedtime for 7 days, or 200 mg suppository at bedtime for 3 days

Not dialyzable (0% to 5%)

Mechanism of Action Inhibits biosynthesis of ergosterol, damaging the fungal cell wall membrane, which increases permeability causing leaking of nutrients

Local Anesthetic/Vasoconstrictor Precautions No information available to require special precautions

Effects on Dental Treatment No effects or complications reported

Other Adverse Effects

>10%:

Central nervous system: Fever, chills

Dermatologic: Skin rash, itching

Local: Pain at injection site

Gastrointestinal: Anorexia, diarrhea, nausea, vomiting

1% to 10%: Hematologic: Anemia, thrombocytopenia

<1%:

Cardiovascular: Flushing of face or skin

Central nervous system: Drowsiness

Drug Interactions Warfarin (increased anticoagulant effect), oral sulfonylureas, amphotericin B (decreased antifungal effect of both agents), phenytoin (levels may be increased)

Drug Uptake

Serum half-life, multiphasic:

Initial: 40 minutes

Secondary: 126 minutes

Terminal phase: 24 hours

Pregnancy Risk Factor C

Dosage Forms

Cream:

Topical, as nitrate: 2% [20 mg/g] (15 g, 30 g, 85 g)

Vaginal, as nitrate: 2% [20 mg/g] (45 g is equivalent to 7 doses)

Injection: 1% [10 mg/mL] (20 mL)

Lotion, as nitrate: 2% [20 mg/g] (30 mL, 60 mL)

Powder, topical: 2% [20 mg/g] (45 g, 90 g)

Spray, topical: 2% [20 mg/g] (105 mL)

Suppository, vaginal, as nitrate: 100 mg (7s); 200 mg (3s)

Generic Available No

MICRhoGAM™ *see* Rh$_o$(D) Immune Globulin *on page 767*

Microfibrillar Collagen Hemostat

(mi kro fi′ bri lar kol′ la jen hee′ moe stat)

Brand Names Avitene®

Therapeutic Category Hemostatic Agent

Use

Dental & Medical: Adjunct to hemostasis when control of bleeding by ligature is ineffective or impractical

Usual Dosage Apply dry directly to source of bleeding

Mechanism of Action Microfibrillar collagen hemostat (MCH) is an absorbable topical hemostatic agent prepared from purified bovine corium collagen and shredded into fibrils. Physically, microfibrillar collagen hemostat yields a large surface area. Chemically, it is collagen with hydrochloric acid noncovalently bound to some of the available amino groups in the collagen molecules. When in contact with a bleeding surface, microfibrillar collagen hemostat attracts platelets which adhere to its fibrils and undergo the release phenomenon. This

(Continued)

Microfibrillar Collagen Hemostat *(Continued)*

triggers aggregation of the platelets into thrombi in the interstices of the fibrous mass, initiating the formation of a physiologic platelet plug.

Local Anesthetic/Vasoconstrictor Precautions No information available to require special precautions

Effects on Dental Treatment No effects or complications reported

Other Adverse Effects 1% to 10%:
Local: Adhesion formation
Miscellaneous: Potentiation of infection, allergic reaction

Oral manifestations: No data reported

Contraindications Closure of skin incisions, contaminated wounds

Warnings/Precautions Fragments of MCH may pass through filters of blood scavenging systems, avoid reintroduction of blood from operative sites treated with MCH; after several minutes remove excess material

Drug Interactions No data reported

Drug Uptake Resorption: By animal tissue in 3 months

Pregnancy Risk Factor C

Breast-feeding Considerations No data reported

Dosage Forms
Fibrous: 1 g, 5 g
Nonwoven web: 70 mm x 70 mm x 1 mm; 70 mm x 35 mm x 1 mm

Dietary Considerations No data reported

Generic Available No

Micro-K® *see* Potassium Chloride *on page 708*

Micronase® *see* Glyburide *on page 401*

microNefrin® *see* Epinephrine, Racemic *on page 314*

Micronor® *see* Norethindrone *on page 627*

Microsulfon® *see* Sulfadiazine *on page 807*

Midamor® *see* Amiloride Hydrochloride *on page 45*

Midazolam Hydrochloride (mid′ aye zoe lam hye droe klor′ ide)

Brand Names Versed®

Canadian/Mexican Brand Names Dormicum® (Mexico)

Therapeutic Category Benzodiazepine; Hypnotic; Sedative

Use
Dental: Sedation component in I.V. conscious sedation in oral surgery patients
Medical: In medicine, preoperative sedation and provides conscious sedation prior to diagnostic or radiographic procedures

Usual Dosage
Children:
Preoperative sedation:
I.M.: 0.07-0.08 mg/kg 30-60 minutes presurgery
I.V.: 0.035 mg/kg/dose, repeat over several minutes as required to achieve the desired sedative effect up to a total dose of 0.1-0.2 mg/kg
Conscious sedation for procedures:
Oral, Intranasal: 0.2-0.4 mg/kg (maximum: 15 mg) 30-45 minutes before the procedure
I.V.: 0.05 mg/kg 3 minutes before procedure

Adults: Conscious sedation: I.V.: Initial: 0.5-2 mg slow I.V. over at least 2 minutes; slowly titrate to effect by repeating doses every 2-3 minutes if needed; usual total dose: 2.5-5 mg; use decreased doses in elderly

Healthy Adults <60 years: I.V.: Some patients respond to doses as low as 1 mg; no more than 2.5 mg should be administered over a period of 2 minutes. Additional doses of midazolam may be administered after a 2-minute waiting period and evaluation of sedation after each dose increment. A total dose >5 mg is generally not needed. If narcotics or other CNS depressants are administered concomitantly, the midazolam dose should be reduced by 30%.

Mechanism of Action Depresses all levels of the CNS, including the limbic and reticular formation, probably through the increased action of gamma-aminobutyric acid (GABA), which is a major inhibitory neurotransmitter in the brain

Local Anesthetic/Vasoconstrictor Precautions No information available to require special precautions

Effects on Dental Treatment No effects or complications reported

Other Adverse Effects
>10%: Hiccups
1% to 10%:
Central nervous system: Drowsiness, ataxia, amnesia, dizziness, sedation

Respiratory: Respiratory depression, apnea, laryngospasm, bronchospasm

Oral manifestations: No data reported

Contraindications Hypersensitivity to midazolam or any component (cross-sensitivity with other benzodiazepines may occur); uncontrolled pain; existing CNS depression; shock; narrow-angle glaucoma

Warnings/Precautions Use with caution in patients with congestive heart failure, renal impairment, pulmonary disease, hepatic dysfunction, the elderly, and those receiving concomitant narcotics; midazolam may cause respiratory depression/arrest; deaths and hypoxic encephalopathy have resulted when these were not promptly recognized and treated appropriately

Drug Interactions Theophylline may antagonize the sedative effects of midazolam; CNS depressants cause increased sedation and respiratory depression; doses of general anesthetic agents should be reduced when used in conjunction with midazolam; cimetidine may increase midazolam serum concentrations

Note: If narcotics or other CNS depressants are administered concomitantly, the midazolam dose should be reduced by 30%, if <65 years of age or by at least 50%, if >65 years of age.

Drug Uptake
Onset of action:
I.M.: Within 15-60 minutes
I.V.: Within 1-5 minutes
Serum half-life: 1-4 hours, increased with cirrhosis, CHF, obesity, elderly
Time to recovery: Usually within 2 hours, but may take up to 6 hours

Pregnancy Risk Factor D

Breast-feeding Considerations No data reported

Dosage Forms Injection: 1 mg/mL (2 mL, 5 mL, 10 mL); 5 mg/mL (1 mL, 2 mL, 5 mL, 10 mL)

Dietary Considerations No data reported

Generic Available No

Midol® 200 [OTC] *see* Ibuprofen *on page 447*

Midol® PM [OTC] *see* Acetaminophen and Diphenhydramine *on page 16*

Midrin® *see* Acetaminophen and Isometheptene Mucate *on page 16*

Miflex® *see* Chlorzoxazone *on page 200*

Milontin® *see* Phensuximide *on page 683*

Milrinone Lactate (mil′ ri none lak′ tate)

Brand Names Primacor®

Therapeutic Category Cardiovascular Agent, Other

Use Short-term I.V. therapy of congestive heart failure; used for calcium antagonist intoxication

Usual Dosage Adults: I.V.: Loading dose: 50 mcg/kg administered over 10 minutes followed by a maintenance dose titrated according to the hemodynamic and clinical response

Mechanism of Action Phosphodiesterase inhibitor resulting in vasodilation

Local Anesthetic/Vasoconstrictor Precautions No information available to require special precautions

Effects on Dental Treatment No effects or complications reported

Other Adverse Effects
>10%: Cardiovascular: Ventricular arrhythmias
1% to 10%:
Cardiovascular: Supraventricular arrhythmias, hypotension, angina, chest pain
Central nervous system: Headache
<1%:
Cardiovascular: Ventricular fibrillation
Endocrine & metabolic: Hypokalemia
Hematologic: Thrombocytopenia
Neuromuscular & skeletal: Tremor

Drug Interactions No data reported

Drug Uptake
Serum level: I.V.: Following a 125 mcg/kg dose, peak plasma concentrations of ~1000 ng/mL were observed at 2 minutes postinjection, decreasing to <100 ng/mL in 2 hours
Therapeutic effect: Oral: Following doses of 7.5-15 mg, peak hemodynamic effects occurred at 90 minutes
Serum half-life, elimination: I.V.: 136 minutes in patients with CHF; patients with severe CHF have a more prolonged half-life, with values ranging from 1.7-2.7 hours. Patients with CHF have a reduction in the systemic clearance
(Continued)

Milrinone Lactate (Continued)

of milrinone, resulting in a prolonged elimination half-life. Alternatively, one study reported that 1 month of therapy with milrinone did not change the pharmacokinetic parameters for patients with CHF despite improvement in cardiac function.

Pregnancy Risk Factor C

Miltown® *see* Meprobamate *on page 543*

Mini-Gamulin® Rh *see* Rh₀(D) Immune Globulin *on page 767*

Minipress® *see* Prazosin Hydrochloride *on page 717*

Minitran® *see* Nitroglycerin *on page 623*

Minizide® *see* Prazosin and Polythiazide *on page 717*

Minociclina (Mexico) *see* Minocycline Hydrochloride *on this page*

Minocin® *see* Minocycline Hydrochloride *on this page*

Minocin® IV *see* Minocycline Hydrochloride *on this page*

Minocycline Hydrochloride (mi noe sye' kleen hye droe klor' ide)

Brand Names Minocin®; Minocin® IV

Canadian/Mexican Brand Names Apo-Minocycline® (Canada); Syn-Minocycline® (Canada)

Therapeutic Category Antibiotic, Tetracycline Derivative

Synonyms Minociclina (Mexico)

Use

Dental: Treatment of periodontitis associated with presence of *Actinobacillus actinomycetemocomitams* (AA); as adjunctive therapy in recurrent aphthous ulcers

Medical: Treatment of susceptible bacterial infections of both gram-negative and gram-positive organisms; acne, meningococcal carrier state

Usual Dosage Infection: Oral, I.V.:

Children >8 years: Initial: 4 mg/kg followed by 2 mg/kg/dose every 12 hours

Adults: 200 mg stat, 100 mg every 12 hours not to exceed 400 mg/24 hours

Mechanism of Action Inhibits bacterial protein synthesis by binding with the 30S and possibly the 50S ribosomal subunit(s) of susceptible bacteria; cell wall synthesis is not affected

Local Anesthetic/Vasoconstrictor Precautions No information available to require special precautions

Effects on Dental Treatment Tetracycline's are not recommended for use during pregnancy or in children ≤8 years of age since they have been reported to cause enamel hypoplasia and permanent teeth discoloration. The use of tetracycline's should only be used in these patients if other agents are contraindicated or alternative antimicrobials will not eradicate the organism. Long-term use associated with oral candidiasis.

Other Adverse Effects

>10%: Miscellaneous: Discoloration of teeth in children

1% to 10%:

Dermatologic: Photosensitivity

Gastrointestinal: Nausea, diarrhea

Oral manifestations: Opportunistic "superinfection" with *Candida albicans*

Warnings/Precautions Use of tetracyclines during tooth development may cause permanent discoloration of the teeth and enamel, hypoplasia and retardation of skeletal development and bone growth with risk being the greatest for children <4 years of age and those receiving high doses; use with caution in patients with renal or hepatic impairment and in pregnancy; dosage modification required in patients with renal impairment; pseudotumor cerebri has been reported with tetracycline use; outdated drug can cause nephropathy.

Drug Interactions Decreased effect with antacids (aluminum, calcium, zinc, or magnesium), bismuth salts, barbiturates, carbamazepine, hydantoins; decreased effect of oral contraceptives; increased effect of warfarin

Drug Uptake Serum half-life: 15 hours

Pregnancy Risk Factor D

Breast-feeding Considerations No data reported

Dosage Forms

Capsule: 50 mg, 100 mg

Capsule (Dynacin®): 50 mg, 100 mg

Capsule, pellet-filled (Minocin®): 50 mg, 100 mg

Injection (Minocin® IV): 100 mg

Suspension, oral (Minocin®)50 mg/5 mL (60 mL)

Dietary Considerations No data reported

Generic Available Yes

Minodyl® *see Minoxidil on this page*

Minoxidil (mi nox' i dil)
Related Information
Cardiovascular Diseases *on page 912*
Brand Names Loniten®; Minodyl®; Rogaine®
Canadian/Mexican Brand Names Apo-Gain® (Canada); Gen-Minoxidil® (Canada); Regaine® (Mexico)
Therapeutic Category Vasodilator
Use Management of severe hypertension (usually in combination with a diuretic and beta-blocker); treatment of male pattern baldness (alopecia androgenetica)
Usual Dosage
Children <12 years: Hypertension: Oral: Initial: 0.1-0.2 mg/kg once daily; maximum: 5 mg/day; increase gradually every 3 days; usual dosage: 0.25-1 mg/kg/day in 1-2 divided doses; maximum: 50 mg/day
Children >12 years and Adults:
Hypertension: Oral: Initial: 5 mg once daily, increase gradually every 3 days; usual dose: 10-40 mg/day in 1-2 divided doses; maximum: 100 mg/day
Alopecia: Topical: Apply twice daily; 4 months of therapy may be necessary for hair growth
Elderly: Initial: 2.5 mg once daily; increase gradually

Supplemental dose is not necessary via hemo- or peritoneal dialysis
Mechanism of Action Produces vasodilation by directly relaxing arteriolar smooth muscle, with little effect on veins; effects may be mediated by cyclic AMP; stimulation of hair growth is secondary to vasodilation, increased cutaneous blood flow and stimulation of resting hair follicles
Local Anesthetic/Vasoconstrictor Precautions No information available to require special precautions
Effects on Dental Treatment No effects or complications reported
Other Adverse Effects
>10%:
Cardiovascular: EKG changes, tachycardia, congestive heart failure, edema
Dermatologic: Hypertrichosis (commonly occurs within 1-2 months of therapy)
1% to 10%: Endocrine & metabolic: Fluid and electrolyte imbalance
<1%:
Cardiovascular: Angina, pericardial effusion tamponade
Central nervous system: Dizziness
Endocrine & metabolic: Breast tenderness
Dermatologic: Rashes, headache, coarsening facial features, dermatologic reactions, Stevens-Johnson syndrome, sunburn
Gastrointestinal: Weight gain
Hematologic: Thrombocytopenia, leukopenia
Drug Interactions Increased toxicity:
Concurrent administration with guanethidine may cause profound orthostatic hypotensive effects
Additive hypotensive effects with other hypotensive agents or diuretics
Drug Uptake
Onset of hypotensive effect: Oral: Within 30 minutes
Peak effect: Within 2-8 hours
Duration: Up to 2-5 days
Serum half-life: Adults: 3.5-4.2 hours
Pregnancy Risk Factor C

Mintezol® *see Thiabendazole on page 836*
Minute-Gel® *see Fluoride on page 374*
Miochol® *see Acetylcholine Chloride on page 21*
Miostat® *see Carbachol on page 150*

Mirtazapine (mir taz' a peen)
Brand Names Remeron®
Therapeutic Category Antidepressant, Tetracyclic
Use Treatment of depression
Usual Dosage Adults: Oral: Starting dose is 15 mg/day, usually given in the evening
Local Anesthetic/Vasoconstrictor Precautions No information available to require special precautions
Effects on Dental Treatment Significant xerostomia occurs in up to 25% of patients
(Continued)

Mirtazapine *(Continued)*
Other Adverse Effects >10%:
Central nervous system: Drowsiness, insomnia
Gastrointestinal: Constipation, weight gain

Warnings/Precautions Use with caution in patients with cardiac conduction disturbances, history of hyperthyroid, renal, or hepatic dysfunction; safe use of tricyclic antidepressants in children <12 years of age has not been established; to avoid cholinergic crisis do not discontinue abruptly in patients receiving high doses chronically

Drug Interactions
Decreased effect: Barbiturates, phenytoin, carbamazepine
Increased toxicity: CNS depressants, MAO inhibitors (hyperpyretic crisis), anticholinergics, sympathomimetics, thyroid increases cardiotoxicity, phenothiazines (seizures), benzodiazepines

Pregnancy Risk Factor B
Generic Available No

Misoprostol *(mye soe prost' ole)*
Brand Names Cytotec®
Therapeutic Category Prostaglandin
Use Prevention of NSAID-induced gastric ulcers
Usual Dosage Adults: Oral: 200 mcg 4 times/day with food; if not tolerated, may decrease dose to 100 mcg 4 times/day with food or 200 mcg twice daily with food

Mechanism of Action Misoprostol is a synthetic prostaglandin E$_1$ analog that replaces the protective prostaglandins consumed with prostaglandin-inhibiting therapies eg, nonsteroidal anti-inflammatory drugs

Local Anesthetic/Vasoconstrictor Precautions No information available to require special precautions
Effects on Dental Treatment No effects or complications reported
Other Adverse Effects
>10%: Gastrointestinal: Diarrhea, abdominal pain
1% to 10%:
Central nervous system: Headache
Gastrointestinal: Constipation, flatulence
<1%:
Gastrointestinal: Nausea, vomiting
Genitourinary: Uterine stimulation, vaginal bleeding

Drug Interactions No data reported
Drug Uptake
Absorption: Oral: Rapid
Serum half-life (parent and metabolite combined): 1.5 hours
Time to peak serum concentration (active metabolite): Within 15-30 minutes

Pregnancy Risk Factor X

Mithracin® *see* Plicamycin *on page 700*

Mitomycin *(mye toe mye' sin)*
Brand Names Mutamycin®
Therapeutic Category Antineoplastic Agent, Antibiotic
Synonyms Mitomycin-C; MTC
Use Therapy of disseminated adenocarcinoma of stomach, colon, or pancreas in combination with other approved chemotherapeutic agents; bladder cancer, breast cancer

Usual Dosage Refer to individual protocols.
Children and Adults: I.V.:
Single agent therapy: 20 mg/m^2 every 6-8 weeks
Combination therapy: 10 mg/m^2 every 6-8 weeks
Bone marrow transplant:
40-50 mg/m^2
2-40 mg/m^2/day for 3 days
Total cumulative dose should not exceed 50 mg/m^2; see table.

Nadir After Prior Dose/mm^3		% of Prior Dose to Be Given
Leukocytes	Platelets	
4000	>100,000	100
3000-3999	75,000-99,999	100
2000-2999	25,000-74,999	70
2000	<25,000	50

Mechanism of Action Isolated from *Streptomyces caespitosus*; acts primarily as an alkylating agent and produces DNA cross-linking (primarily with guanine and cytosine pairs); cell-cycle nonspecific; inhibits DNA and RNA synthesis by alkylation and cross-linking the strands of DNA

Local Anesthetic/Vasoconstrictor Precautions No information available to require special precautions

Effects on Dental Treatment No effects or complications reported

Other Adverse Effects

>10%:

Gastrointestinal: **Emetic potential:** Moderately high (60% to 90%); **nausea and vomiting (mild to moderate) seen in almost 100% of patients**; usually begins 1-2 hours after treatment and persists for 3 hours to 4 days; other toxicities include stomatitis, hepatic toxicity, diarrhea, anorexia

Extravasation: May cause severe tissue irritation if infiltrated; can progress to cellulitis, ulceration, and sloughing of tissue

Myelosuppressive: Dose-related toxicity and may be cumulative; related to both total dose (incidence higher at doses >50 mg) and schedule

1% to 10%:

Central nervous system: Extremity tingling

Dermatologic: Discolored fingernails (violet), alopecia

Gastrointestinal: Mouth ulcers

Respiratory: Interstitial pneumonitis or pulmonary fibrosis have been noticed in 7% of patients, and it occurs independent of dosing. Manifested as dry cough and progressive dyspnea; usually is responsive to steroid therapy.

Renal: Elevation of creatinine seen in 2% of patients; hemolytic uremic syndrome observed in <10% of patients and is dose-dependent (doses >30 mg have higher risk)

<1%:

Cardiovascular: Cardiac failure (in patients treated with doses >30 mg)

Central nervous system: Malaise, fever

Dermatologic: Pruritus, rash

Hematologic: Bone marrow suppression (leukopenia, thrombocytopenia), microangiopathic hemolytic anemia

Local: Thrombophlebitis

Neuromuscular & skeletal: Paresthesia, weakness

Drug Uptake

Absorption: Fairly well from the GI tract

Serum half-life: 23-78 minutes

Terminal: 50 minutes

Pregnancy Risk Factor C

Mitomycin-C *see* Mitomycin *on previous page*

Mitotane (mye' toe tane)

Brand Names Lysodren®

Therapeutic Category Antiadrenal Agent; Antineoplastic Agent, Miscellaneous

Synonyms o,p'-DDD

Use Treatment of inoperable adrenal cortical carcinoma

Usual Dosage Oral:

Children: 0.1-0.5 mg/kg or 1-2 g/day in divided doses increasing gradually to a maximum of 5-7 g/day

Adults: Start at 1-6 g/day in divided doses, then increase incrementally to 8-10 g/day in 3-4 divided doses; dose is changed on basis of side effect with aim of giving as high a dose as tolerated; maximum daily dose: 18 g

Mechanism of Action Causes adrenal cortical atrophy; drug affects mitochondria in adrenal cortical cells and decreases production of cortisol; also alters the peripheral metabolism of steroids

Local Anesthetic/Vasoconstrictor Precautions No information available to require special precautions

Effects on Dental Treatment No effects or complications reported

Other Adverse Effects

>10%:

Central nervous system: Visual disturbances, double vision, vertigo, blurred vision, mental depression, dizziness; all are reversible with discontinuation of the drug and can occur in 15% to 26% of patients

Dermatologic: Rash (15%) which may subside without discontinuation of therapy, hyperpigmentation

Gastrointestinal: 75% to 80% will experience nausea, vomiting, and anorexia; diarrhea can occur in 20% of patients

(Continued)

Mitotane *(Continued)*

1% to 10%:
Cardiovascular: Orthostatic hypotension
Central nervous system: Fever
Endocrine & metabolic: Flushing of skin
Genitourinary: Hemorrhagic cystitis
Neuromuscular & skeletal: Myalgia

<1%:
Adrenal insufficiency: May develop and may require steroid replacement
Cardiovascular: Hypertension, flushing
Central nervous system: Lethargy, somnolence, mental depression, irritability, confusion, fatigue, headache, fever, hyperpyrexia
Dermatologic: Rash
Endocrine & metabolic: Hypercholesterolemia
Genitourinary: Albuminuria, hemorrhagic cystitis
Myelosuppressive:
  WBC: None
  Platelets: None
Neuromuscular & skeletal: Tremor, weakness
Ocular: Lens opacities, toxic retinopathy
Renal: Hypouricemia, hematuria
Respiratory: Shortness of breath, wheezing

Drug Uptake
Absorption: Oral: ~35% to 40%
Time to peak serum concentration: Within 3-5 hours
Serum half-life: 18-159 days

Pregnancy Risk Factor C

Comments Myelosuppressive effects:
WBC: None
Platelets: None

Mitoxantrone Hydrochloride

(mye toe zan' trone hye droe klor' ide)

Brand Names Novantrone®

Canadian/Mexican Brand Names Novantrone® (Mexico); Misostol (Mexico)

Therapeutic Category Antineoplastic Agent, Anthracycline; Antineoplastic Agent, Antibiotic

Synonyms DHAD

Use FDA approved for remission-induction therapy of acute nonlymphocytic leukemia (ANLL); mitoxantrone is also active against other various leukemias, lymphoma, and breast cancer, and moderately active against pediatric sarcoma

Usual Dosage
Refer to individual protocols. I.V. (may dilute in D_5W or NS):
ANLL leukemias:
  Children ≤2 years: 0.4 mg/kg/day once daily for 3-5 days
  Children >2 years and Adults: 12 mg/m²/day once daily for 3 days; acute leukemia in relapse: 8-12 mg/m²/day once daily for 4-5 days

Solid tumors:
  Children: 18-20 mg/m² every 3-4 weeks **OR** 5-8 mg/m² every week
  Adults: 12-14 mg/m² every 3-4 weeks **OR** 2-4 mg/m²/day for 5 days
  Maximum total dose: 80-120 mg/m² in patients with predisposing factor and <160 mg in patients with no predisposing factor

Mechanism of Action Analogue of the anthracyclines, but different in mechanism of action, cardiac toxicity, and potential for tissue necrosis; mitoxantrone does intercalate DNA; binds to nucleic acids and inhibits DNA and RNA synthesis by template disordering and steric obstruction; replication is decreased by binding to DNA topoisomerase II (enzyme responsible for DNA helix supercoiling); active throughout entire cell cycle; does not appear to produce free radicals

Local Anesthetic/Vasoconstrictor Precautions No information available to require special precautions

Effects on Dental Treatment No effects or complications reported

Other Adverse Effects
>10%:
Central nervous system: Headache
Dermatologic: Alopecia
Gastrointestinal: **Emetic potential:** Moderate (31% to 72%); nausea, vomiting, diarrhea, abdominal pain, mucositis, stomatitis, GI bleeding
Genitourinary: Discoloration of urine (blue-green)

Hepatic: Abnormal LFTs
Respiratory: Coughing, shortness of breath
1% to 10%:
Cardiac toxicity: Much reduced compared to doxorubicin and has been reported primarily in patients who have received prior anthracycline therapy, congestive heart failure, hypotension
Central nervous system: Seizures, fever
Dermatologic: Pruritus, skin desquamation
Hepatic: Transient elevation of liver enzymes, jaundice
Ocular: Conjunctivitis
Renal: Renal failure
<1%: Local: Pain or redness at injection site
Drug Uptake
Absorption: Oral: Poor
Serum half-life: Terminal: 37 hours; may be prolonged with liver impairment
Pregnancy Risk Factor D

Mitran® see Chlordiazepoxide on page 183

Mitrolan® Chewable Tablet [OTC] see Calcium Polycarbophil on page 146

MK594 see Losartan Potassium on page 515

M-KYA® [OTC] see Quinine Sulfate on page 760

MMR see Measles, Mumps, and Rubella Vaccines, Combined on page 528

M-M-R® II see Measles, Mumps, and Rubella Vaccines, Combined on page 528

Moban® see Molindone Hydrochloride on next page

Modane® [OTC] see Phenolphthalein on page 682

Modane® Bulk [OTC] see Psyllium on page 750

Modane® Plus [OTC] see Docusate and Phenolphthalein on page 295

Modane® Soft [OTC] see Docusate on page 295

Modicon™ see Ethinyl Estradiol and Norethindrone on page 339

Modical® [OTC] see Glucose Polymers on page 400

Moduretic® see Amiloride and Hydrochlorothiazide on page 45

Moexipril Hydrochloride (mo ex' i pril hye droe klor' ide)

Related Information
Cardiovascular Diseases on page 912

Brand Names Univasc®

Therapeutic Category Angiotensin-Converting Enzyme (ACE) Inhibitors

Use Treatment of hypertension, alone or in combination with thiazide diuretics

Usual Dosage Adults: Oral: Initial: 7.5 mg once daily (in patients **not** receiving diuretics), one hour prior to a meal **or** 3.75 mg once daily (when combined with thiazide diuretics); maintenance dose: 7.5-30 mg/day in 1 or 2 divided doses one hour before meals

Mechanism of Action Competitive inhibitor of angiotensin-converting enzyme (ACE); prevents conversion of angiotensin I to angiotensin II, a potent vasoconstrictor; results in lower levels of angiotensin II which causes an increase in plasma renin activity and a reduction in aldosterone secretion

Local Anesthetic/Vasoconstrictor Precautions No information available to require special precautions

Effects on Dental Treatment No effects or complications reported

Other Adverse Effects
1% to 10%:
Central nervous system: Headache, dizziness, fatigue
Dermatologic: Rash, pruritus, alopecia, flushing, rash
Endocrine & metabolic: Hyperkalemia
Gastrointestinal: Diarrhea
Genitourinary: Urinary frequency
Renal: Oliguria, reversible increases in creatinine or BUN
Respiratory: Nonproductive cough (6%), pharyngitis, upper respiratory infections, rhinitis
Miscellaneous: Flu-like symptoms
<1%:
Cardiovascular: Symptomatic hypotension, chest pain, angina, peripheral edema, myocardial infarction, palpitations, arrhythmias
Central nervous system: Sleep disturbances, anxiety, mood changes
Dermatologic: Angioedema, photosensitivity, pemphigus
Endocrine & metabolic: Hypercholesterolemia
Gastrointestinal: Abdominal pain, taste disturbance, constipation, vomiting, dry mouth, changes in appetite, pancreatitis, altered taste perception
Hematologic: Neutropenia
Hepatic: Elevated LFTs
(Continued)

Moexipril Hydrochloride *(Continued)*

Neuromuscular & skeletal: Myalgia, arthralgia
Renal: Proteinuria
Respiratory: Bronchospasm, dyspnea

Drug Uptake
Absorption: Food decreases bioavailability (AUC decreased by ~40%)
Serum half-life:
Moexipril: 1 hour
Moexiprilat: 2-10 hours
Time to peak: 1.5 hours

Pregnancy Risk Factor C (1st trimester); D (2nd and 3rd trimesters)

Moi-Stir® [OTC] *see* Saliva Substitute *on page 778*
Moisture® Ophthalmic Drops [OTC] *see* Artificial Tears *on page 75*

Molindone Hydrochloride (moe lin' done hye droe klor' ide)

Brand Names Moban®
Therapeutic Category Antipsychotic Agent
Use Management of psychotic disorder
Usual Dosage Oral:
Children:
3-5 years: 1-2.5 mg/day divided into 4 doses
5-12 years: 0.5-1 mg/kg/day in 4 divided doses

Adults: 50-75 mg/day increase at 3- to 4-day intervals up to 225 mg/day

Mechanism of Action Mechanism of action mimics that of chlorpromazine; however, it produces more extrapyramidal effects and less sedation than chlorpromazine

Local Anesthetic/Vasoconstrictor Precautions No information available to require special precautions

Effects on Dental Treatment Anticholinergic side effects can cause a reduction of saliva production or secretion. This may result in discomfort and dental disease (ie, caries, oral candidiasis and periodontal disease); molindone can cause extrapyramidal reactions which may appear as muscle twitching or increased motor activity of the face, neck or head

Other Adverse Effects
>10%:
Cardiovascular: Orthostatic hypotension
Central nervous system: Akathisia, extrapyramidal effects, persistent tardive dyskinesia
Gastrointestinal: Constipation, dry mouth
Ocular: Blurred vision
Miscellaneous: Decreased sweating
1% to 10%:
Central nervous system: Mental depression
Endocrine & metabolic: Change in menstrual periods, swelling of breasts
<1%:
Cardiovascular: Tachycardia, arrhythmias
Central nervous system: Sedation, drowsiness, restlessness, anxiety, seizures, neuroleptic malignant syndrome (NMS)
Dermatologic: Hyperpigmentation, pruritus, rash, photosensitivity
Endocrine & metabolic: Galactorrhea, gynecomastia
Gastrointestinal: Weight gain
Genitourinary: Urinary retention
Hematologic: Agranulocytosis (more often in women between fourth and tenth weeks of therapy), leukopenia (usually in patients with large doses for prolonged periods)
Ocular: Retinal pigmentation
Miscellaneous: Altered central temperature regulation

Drug Interactions Increased toxicity: CNS depressants, antihypertensives, anticonvulsants

Drug Uptake
Serum half-life: 1.5 hours
Time to peak serum concentration: Oral: Within 1.5 hours

Pregnancy Risk Factor C

Mol-Iron® [OTC] *see* Ferrous Sulfate *on page 360*
Molybdenum *see* Trace Metals *on page 857*
Molypen® *see* Trace Metals *on page 857*
Mometasona, Furoata De (Mexico) *see* Mometasone Furoate *on next page*

Mometasone Furoate (moe met' a sone fyoor' oh ate)
Brand Names Elocon®
Canadian/Mexican Brand Names Elocom® (Canada); Elomet® (Mexico)
Therapeutic Category Corticosteroid, Topical (Medium Potency)
Synonyms Mometasona, Furoata De (Mexico)
Use Relief of the inflammatory and pruritic manifestations of corticosteroid-responsive dermatoses (medium potency topical corticosteroid)
Usual Dosage Adults: Topical: Apply sparingly to area once daily, do not use occlusive dressings
Mechanism of Action May depress the formation, release, and activity of endogenous chemical mediators of inflammation (kinins, histamine, liposomal enzymes, prostaglandins). Leukocytes and macrophages may have to be present for the initiation of responses mediated by the above substances. Inhibits the margination and subsequent cell migration to the area of injury, and also reverses the dilatation and increased vessel permeability in the area resulting in decreased access of cells to the sites of injury.
Local Anesthetic/Vasoconstrictor Precautions No information available to require special precautions
Effects on Dental Treatment No effects or complications reported
Other Adverse Effects <1%:
Dermatologic: Acne, hypopigmentation, allergic dermatitis, maceration of the skin, skin atrophy, striae, miliaria
Endocrine & metabolic: HPA suppression, Cushing's syndrome, growth retardation
Local: Burning, itching, irritation, dryness, folliculitis, hypertrichosis
Miscellaneous: Secondary infection
Drug Interactions No data reported
Pregnancy Risk Factor C

MOM/Mineral Oil Emulsion see Magnesium Hydroxide and Mineral Oil Emulsion on page 523

Monistat™ see Miconazole on page 578

Monistat-Derm™ see Miconazole on page 578

Monistat i.v.™ see Miconazole on page 578

Monobenzone (mon oh ben' zone)
Brand Names Benoquin®
Therapeutic Category Topical Skin Product
Use Final depigmentation in extensive vitiligo
Local Anesthetic/Vasoconstrictor Precautions No information available to require special precautions
Effects on Dental Treatment No effects or complications reported
Other Adverse Effects 1% to 10%: Irritation, burning sensation, dermatitis

Monocid® see Cefonicid Sodium on page 166

Monoclate-P® see Antihemophilic Factor (Human) on page 68

Monoclonal Antibody see Muromonab-CD3 on page 594

Monoethanolamine (Canada) see Ethanolamine Oleate on page 333

Mono-Gesic® see Salsalate on page 779

Monoket® see Isosorbide Mononitrate on page 474

Mononine® see Factor IX Complex (Human) on page 350

Monopril® see Fosinopril on page 387

8-MOP see Methoxsalen on page 563

More Attenuated Enders Strain see Measles Virus Vaccine, Live on page 529

More-Dophilus® [OTC] see Lactobacillus acidophilus and Lactobacillus bulgaricus on page 488

Morfina (Mexico) see Morphine Sulfate on next page

Moricizine Hydrochloride (mor i' siz een hye droe klor' ide)
Related Information
Cardiovascular Diseases on page 912
Brand Names Ethmozine®
Therapeutic Category Antiarrhythmic Agent, Class I; Antiarrhythmic Agent (Supraventricular & Ventricular)
Use For treatment of ventricular tachycardia and life-threatening ventricular arrhythmias

Unlabeled use: PVCs, complete and nonsustained ventricular tachycardia
(Continued)

589

Moricizine Hydrochloride *(Continued)*

Usual Dosage Adults: Oral: 200-300 mg every 8 hours, adjust dosage at 150 mg/day at 3-day intervals. See table for dosage recommendations of transferring from other antiarrhythmic agents to Ethmozine®.

Moricizine

Transferred From	Start Ethmozine®
Encainide, propafenone, tocainide, or mexiletine	8-12 hours after last dose
Flecainide	12-24 hours after last dose
Procainamide	3-6 hours after last dose
Quinidine, disopyramide	6-12 hours after last dose

Mechanism of Action Class I antiarrhythmic agent; reduces the fast inward current carried by sodium ions, shortens Phase I and Phase II repolarization, resulting in decreased action potential duration and effective refractory period

Local Anesthetic/Vasoconstrictor Precautions No information available to require special precautions

Effects on Dental Treatment No effects or complications reported

Other Adverse Effects
>10%: Central nervous system: Dizziness
1% to 10%:
    Cardiovascular: Proarrhythmia, palpitations, cardiac death, EKG abnormalities, congestive heart failure
    Central nervous system: Headache, fatigue, insomnia
    Gastrointestinal: Nausea, diarrhea, ileus
    Genitourinary: Decreased libido
    Ocular: Blurred vision, periorbital edema
    Respiratory: Dyspnea
<1%:
    Cardiovascular: Ventricular tachycardia, cardiac chest pain, hypotension or hypertension, syncope, supraventricular arrhythmias, myocardial infarction
    Central nervous system: Anxiety, drug fever, confusion, loss of memory, vertigo, anorexia
    Dermatologic: Rash, dry skin
    Gastrointestinal: GI upset, vomiting, dyspepsia, flatulence, bitter taste
    Genitourinary: Urinary retention, urinary incontinence, impotence
    Neuromuscular & skeletal: Tremor
    Otic: Tinnitus
    Respiratory: Apnea
    Miscellaneous: Sweating

Drug Interactions
Decreased levels of theophylline (50%)
Increased levels with cimetidine (50%)

Drug Uptake
Serum half-life:
    Normal patients: 3-4 hours
    Cardiac disease patients: 6-13 hours

Pregnancy Risk Factor B

Morphine Sulfate *(mor' feen sul' fate)*

Related Information
Narcotic Agonist Charts *on page 1019*

Brand Names Astramorph™ PF Injection; Duramorph® Injection; Infumorph™ Injection; Kadian® Capsule; MS Contin® Oral; MSIR® Oral; MS/L®; MS/S®; OMS® Oral; Oramorph SR™ Oral; RMS® Rectal; Roxanol™ Oral; Roxanol Rescudose®; Roxanol SR™ Oral

Canadian/Mexican Brand Names Epimorph® (Canada); Morphine-HP® (Canada); MS-IR® (Canada); Statex® (Canada); MST-Continus® (Mexico)

Therapeutic Category Analgesic, Narcotic

Synonyms Morfina (Mexico)

Use Relief of moderate to severe acute and chronic pain; pain of myocardial infarction; relieves dyspnea of acute left ventricular failure and pulmonary edema; preanesthetic medication

Usual Dosage Doses should be titrated to appropriate effect; when changing routes of administration in chronically treated patients, please note that oral doses are approximately one-half as effective as parenteral dose

Children:

Oral: Tablet and solution (prompt release): 0.2-0.5 mg/kg/dose every 4-6 hours as needed; tablet (controlled release): 0.3-0.6 mg/kg/dose every 12 hours

I.M., I.V., S.C.: 0.1-0.2 mg/kg/dose every 2-4 hours as needed; usual maximum: 15 mg/dose; may initiate at 0.05 mg/kg/dose

I.V., S.C. continuous infusion: Sickle cell or cancer pain: 0.025-2 mg/kg/hour; postoperative pain: 0.01-0.04 mg/kg/hour

Sedation/analgesia for procedures: I.V.: 0.05-0.1 mg/kg 5 minutes before the procedure

Adolescents >12 years: Sedation/analgesia for procedures: I.V.: 3-4 mg and repeat in 5 minutes if necessary

Adults:

Oral: Prompt release: 10-30 mg every 4 hours as needed; controlled release: 15-30 mg every 8-12 hours

I.M., I.V., S.C.: 2.5-20 mg/dose every 2-6 hours as needed; usual: 10 mg/dose every 4 hours as needed

I.V., S.C. continuous infusion: 0.8-10 mg/hour; may increase depending on pain relief/adverse effects; usual range: up to 80 mg/hour

Epidural: Initial: 5 mg in lumbar region; if inadequate pain relief within 1 hour, give 1-2 mg, maximum dose: 10 mg/24 hours

Intrathecal ($1/10$ of epidural dose): 0.2-1 mg/dose; repeat doses **not** recommended

Rectal: 10-20 mg every 4 hours

Mechanism of Action Binds to opiate receptors in the CNS, causing inhibition of ascending pain pathways, altering the perception of and response to pain; produces generalized CNS depression

Local Anesthetic/Vasoconstrictor Precautions No information available to require special precautions

Effects on Dental Treatment Anticholinergic side effects can cause a reduction of saliva production or secretion contributes to discomfort and dental disease (ie, caries, oral candidiasis and periodontal disease)

Other Adverse Effects

Central nervous system: CNS depression, drowsiness, sedation, sweating, flushing, increased intracranial pressure

Endocrine & metabolic: Antidiuretic hormone release

Miscellaneous: Physical and psychological dependence

>10%:

Cardiovascular: Palpitations, hypotension, bradycardia

Central nervous system: Weakness, dizziness

Gastrointestinal: Nausea, vomiting, constipation, dry mouth

Local: Pain at injection site

Miscellaneous: Histamine release

1% to 10%:

Central nervous system: Restlessness, headache, false feeling of well being, confusion

Gastrointestinal: Anorexia, GI irritation, dry mouth, paralytic ileus

Genitourinary: Decreased urination

Neuromuscular & skeletal: Trembling

Ocular: Vision problems

Respiratory: Respiratory depression, shortness of breath

<1%:

Cardiovascular: Peripheral vasodilation

Central nervous system: Insomnia, mental depression, hallucinations, paradoxical CNS stimulation, increased intracranial pressure

Dermatologic: Pruritus

Neuromuscular & skeletal: Muscle rigidity

Ocular: Miosis

Miscellaneous: Biliary or urinary tract spasm

Drug Interactions

Decreased effect: Phenothiazines may antagonize the analgesic effect of morphine and other opiate agonists

Increased toxicity: CNS depressants, tricyclic antidepressants may potentiate the effects of morphine and other opiate agonists; dextroamphetamine may enhance the analgesic effect of morphine and other opiate agonists

Drug Uptake

Absorption: Oral: Variable

Serum half-life:

Adults: 2-4 hours

(Continued)

591

Morphine Sulfate *(Continued)*

Pregnancy Risk Factor B (D if used for prolonged periods or in high doses at term)

Morrhuate Sodium *(mor' yoo ate sow' dee um)*

Brand Names Scleromate™

Therapeutic Category Sclerosing Agent

Use Treatment of small, uncomplicated varicose veins of the lower extremities

Usual Dosage I.V.:

Children 1-18 years: Esophageal hemorrhage: 2, 3, or 4 mL of 5% repeated every 3-4 days until bleeding is controlled, then every 6 weeks until varices obliterated

Adults: 50-250 mg, repeated at 5- to 7-day intervals (50-100 mg for small veins, 150-250 mg for large veins)

Mechanism of Action Both varicose veins and esophageal varices are treated by the thrombotic action of morrhuate sodium. By causing inflammation of the vein's intima, a thrombus is formed. Occlusion secondary to the fibrous tissue and the thrombus results in the obliteration of the vein.

Local Anesthetic/Vasoconstrictor Precautions No information available to require special precautions

Effects on Dental Treatment No effects or complications reported

Other Adverse Effects

>10%:

Cardiovascular: Thrombosis, valvular incompetency

Dermatologic: Urticaria

Local: Burning at the site of injection, severe extravasation effects

<1%:

Cardiovascular: Vascular collapse

Central nervous system: Drowsiness, headache, dizziness

Gastrointestinal: Nausea, vomiting

Neuromuscular & skeletal: Weakness

Respiratory: Asthma

Miscellaneous: Anaphylaxis

Drug Interactions No data reported

Drug Uptake

Onset of action: ~5 minutes

Absorption: Most of the dose stays at the site of injection

Pregnancy Risk Factor C

Motofen® *see* Difenoxin and Atropine *on page 277*

Motrin® *see* Ibuprofen *on page 447*

Motrin® **IB [OTC]** *see* Ibuprofen *on page 447*

Motrin® **IB Sinus [OTC]** *see* Pseudoephedrine and Ibuprofen *on page 750*

MouthKote® **[OTC]** *see* Saliva Substitute *on page 778*

Mouth Pain, Cold Sore, Canker Sore Products *see page 1063*

Mouthwash, Antiseptic

Related Information

Oral Bacterial Infections *on page 945*

Oral Nonviral Soft Tissue Ulcerations or Erosions *on page 955*

Oral Rinse Products *on page 1067*

Brand Names Cool Mint Listerine® Antiseptic [OTC]; Fresh Burst Listerine® Antiseptic [OTC]; Listerine® Antiseptic [OTC]

Therapeutic Category Antimicrobial Mouth Rinse; Antiplaque Agent; Mouthwash

Use Help prevent and reduce plaque and gingivitis; bad breath

Usual Dosage Rinse full strength for 30 seconds with 20 mL (2/3 fluid ounce or 4 teaspoonfuls) morning and night

Local Anesthetic/Vasoconstrictor Precautions No information available to require special precautions

Effects on Dental Treatment No effects or complications reported

Other Adverse Effects Oral manifestations: No data reported

Contraindications Known hypersensitivity to any of its components

Dosage Forms Rinse: 250 mL, 500 mL, 1000 mL

Comments

Active ingredients:

Listerine® Antiseptic: Thymol 0.064%, eucalyptus 0.092%, methyl salicylate 0.060%, menthol 0.042%, alcohol 26.9%, water, benzoic acid, poloxamer 407, sodium benzoate, caramel

Fresh Burst Listerine® Antiseptic: Thymol 0.064%, eucalyptus 0.092%, methyl salicylate 0.060%, menthol 0.042%, alcohol 26.9%, water, benzoic acid, poloxamer 407, sodium benzoate, flavoring, sodium, saccharin, sodium citrate, citric acid, D&C yellow #10, FD&C green #3

Cool Mint Listerine® Antiseptic: Thymol 0.064%, eucalyptus 0.092%, methyl salicylate 0.060%, menthol 0.042%, alcohol 26.9%, water, benzoic acid, poloxamer 407, sodium benzoate, flavoring, sodium, saccharin, sodium citrate, citric acid, FD&C green #3

The following information is endorsed on the label of the Listerine® products by the Council on Scientific Affairs, American Dental Association: "Listerine Antiseptic has been shown to help prevent and reduce supragingival plaque accumulation and gingivitis when used in a conscientiously applied program of oral hygiene and regular professional care. Its effect on periodontitis has not been determined."

6-MP *see* Mercaptopurine *on page 544*

M-R-VAX® II *see* Measles and Rubella Vaccines, Combined *on page 527*

MS Contin® Oral *see* Morphine Sulfate *on page 590*

MSIR® Oral *see* Morphine Sulfate *on page 590*

MS/L® *see* Morphine Sulfate *on page 590*

MS/S® *see* Morphine Sulfate *on page 590*

MTC *see* Mitomycin *on page 584*

M.T.E.-4® *see* Trace Metals *on page 857*

M.T.E.-5® *see* Trace Metals *on page 857*

M.T.E.-6® *see* Trace Metals *on page 857*

Mucomyst® *see* Acetylcysteine *on page 21*

Mucoplex® [OTC] *see* Vitamin B Complex *on page 899*

Mucosil™ *see* Acetylcysteine *on page 21*

Multe-Pak-4® *see* Trace Metals *on page 857*

Multiple Sulfonamides *see* Sulfadiazine, Sulfamethazine, and Sulfamerazine *on page 808*

Multitest CMI® *see* Skin Test Antigens, Multiple *on page 790*

Multi Vit® Drops [OTC] *see* Vitamins, Multiple *on page 901*

Mumps, Measles and Rubella Vaccines, Combined *see* Measles, Mumps, and Rubella Vaccines, Combined *on page 528*

Mumpsvax® *see* Mumps Virus Vaccine, Live, Attenuated *on this page*

Mumps Virus Vaccine, Live, Attenuated

(mumpz vye' rus vak seen', live, a ten yoo' ate ed)

Brand Names Mumpsvax®

Therapeutic Category Vaccine, Live Virus

Use Immunization against mumps in children ≥12 months and adults

Usual Dosage 1 vial (5000 units) S.C. in outer aspect of the upper arm, no booster

Local Anesthetic/Vasoconstrictor Precautions No information available to require special precautions

Effects on Dental Treatment No effects or complications reported

Other Adverse Effects
>10%: Local: Burning or stinging at injection site
1% to 10%:
  Central nervous system: Fever ≤100°F
  Dermatologic: Rash
  Endocrine & metabolic: Parotitis
<1%:
  Central nervous system: Convulsions, confusion, severe or continuing headache, fever >103°F
  Genitourinary: Orchitis in postpubescent and adult males
  Hematologic: Thrombocytopenic purpura
  Miscellaneous: Anaphylactic reactions

Pregnancy Risk Factor X

Comments Federal law requires that the date of administration, the vaccine manufacturer, lot number of vaccine, and the administering person's name, title and address be entered into the patient's permanent medical record

Mupirocin (myoo peer' oh sin)

Brand Names Bactroban®

Canadian/Mexican Brand Names Mupiban® (Mexico)

Therapeutic Category Antibiotic, Topical

(Continued)

Mupirocin *(Continued)*

Use Topical treatment of impetigo due to *Staphylococcus aureus*, beta-hemo-lytic *Streptococcus*, and *S. pyogenes*

Usual Dosage Children and Adults: Topical: Apply small amount to affected area 2-5 times/day for 5-14 days

Mechanism of Action Binds to bacterial isoleucyl transfer-RNA synthetase resulting in the inhibition of protein and RNA synthesis

Local Anesthetic/Vasoconstrictor Precautions No information available to require special precautions

Effects on Dental Treatment No effects or complications reported

Other Adverse Effects 1% to 10%:
Dermatologic: Pruritus, rash, erythema, dry skin
Local: Burning, stinging, pain, tenderness, swelling

Drug Interactions No data reported

Drug Uptake
Absorption: Topical: Penetrates the outer layers of the skin; systemic absorption minimal through intact skin
Serum half-life: 17-36 minutes

Pregnancy Risk Factor B

Murine® Ear Drops [OTC] *see* Carbamide Peroxide *on page 152*
Murine® Plus [OTC] *see* Tetrahydrozoline Hydrochloride *on page 831*
Murine® Solution [OTC] *see* Artificial Tears *on page 75*
Murocel® Ophthalmic Solution [OTC] *see* Artificial Tears *on page 75*
Murocoll-2® Ophthalmic *see* Phenylephrine and Scopolamine *on page 685*

Muromonab-CD3 *(myoo roe moe' nab see dee three)*

Brand Names Orthoclone® OKT3
Canadian/Mexican Brand Names Orthoclone® OKT3 (Mexico)
Therapeutic Category Immunosuppressant Agent
Synonyms Monoclonal Antibody; OKT3

Use Treatment of acute allograft rejection in renal transplant patients; effective in reversing acute hepatic, cardiac, and bone marrow transplant rejection episodes resistant to conventional treatment

Usual Dosage I.V. **(refer to individual protocols)**:
Children <30 kg: 2.5 mg/day once daily for 7-14 days
Children >30 kg: 5 mg/day once daily for 7-14 days
or
Children <12 years: 0.1 mg/kg/day once daily for 10-14 days
Children ≥12 years and Adults: 5 mg/day once daily for 10-14 days

Removal by dialysis: Molecular size of OKT_3 is 150,000 daltons; not dialyzed by most standard dialyzers; however, may be dialyzed by high flux dialysis; OKT_3 will be removed by plasmapheresis; administer following dialysis treatments

Mechanism of Action Reverses graft rejection by binding to T-cells and interfering with their function

Local Anesthetic/Vasoconstrictor Precautions No information available to require special precautions

Effects on Dental Treatment No effects or complications reported

Other Adverse Effects
>10%:
Cardiovascular: Tachycardia
Central nervous system: Dizziness, faintness
Gastrointestinal: Diarrhea, nausea, vomiting
Neuromuscular & skeletal: Trembling
Respiratory: Shortness of breath
1% to 10%:
Central nervous system: Headache, stiff neck
Ocular: Photophobia
Respiratory: Pulmonary edema
<1%:
Cardiovascular: Hypertension, hypotension, chest pain, tightness in chest
Central nervous system: Aseptic meningitis, seizures, tiredness, confusion, coma, hallucinations, pyrexia
Dermatologic: Pruritus, rash
Neuromuscular & skeletal: Joint pain, tremor
Renal: Increased BUN/creatinine
Respiratory: Dyspnea, wheezing
Sensitivity reactions: Anaphylactic-type reactions
Miscellaneous: Flu-like symptoms (ie, fever, chills), infection

Drug Uptake
Absorption: I.V.: Immediate
Time to steady-state: Trough level: 3-14 days; pretreatment levels are restored within 7 days after treatment is terminated
Pregnancy Risk Factor C
Comments Recommend decreasing dose of prednisone to 0.5 mg/kg, azathioprine to 0.5 mg/kg (approximate 50% decrease in dose), and discontinuing cyclosporine while patient is receiving OKT$_3$

Muro's Opcon® *see* Naphazoline Hydrochloride *on page 605*

Mus-Lac® *see* Chlorzoxazone *on page 200*

Mutamycin® *see* Mitomycin *on page 584*

M.V.I.® *see* Vitamins, Multiple *on page 901*

M.V.I.®-12 *see* Vitamins, Multiple *on page 901*

M.V.I.® Concentrate *see* Vitamins, Multiple *on page 901*

M.V.I.® Pediatric *see* Vitamins, Multiple *on page 901*

Myambutol® *see* Ethambutol Hydrochloride *on page 332*

Mycelex® Troche *see* Clotrimazole *on page 223*

Mycifradin® Sulfate *see* Neomycin Sulfate *on page 611*

Mycobutin® *see* Rifabutin *on page 769*

Mycogen® II *see* Nystatin and Triamcinolone *on page 632*

Mycolog®-II *see* Nystatin and Triamcinolone *on page 632*

Myconel® *see* Nystatin and Triamcinolone *on page 632*

Mycophenolate Mofetil (mye koe fen' oh late moe' fe til)
Brand Names CellCept®
Therapeutic Category Immunosuppressant Agent
Use Immunosuppressant used with corticosteroids and cyclosporine to prevent organ rejection in patients receiving allogenic renal transplants
Usual Dosage Oral:
Children: Doses of 15-23 mg/kg given twice daily have been used, further studies are necessary
Adults: 1 g twice daily within 72 hours of transplant (although 3 g/day has been given in some clinical trials, there was decreased tolerability and no efficacy advantage)
Local Anesthetic/Vasoconstrictor Precautions No information available to require special precautions
Effects on Dental Treatment No effects or complications reported
Drug Uptake
Absorption: Mycophenolate mofetil is hydrolized to mycophenolic acid in the liver and gastrointestinal tract; food does not alter the extent of absorption, but the maximum concentration is decreased
Serum half-life: 18 hours
Serum concentrations: Correlation of toxicity or efficacy is still being developed, however, one study indicated that 12-hour AUCs of >40 mcg/mL/hour were correlated with efficacy and decreased episodes of rejection

Mycostatin® *see* Nystatin *on page 632*

Myco-Triacet® II *see* Nystatin and Triamcinolone *on page 632*

Mydfrin® Ophthalmic Solution *see* Phenylephrine Hydrochloride *on page 685*

Mydriacyl® Ophthalmic *see* Tropicamide *on page 881*

Mykrox® *see* Metolazone *on page 573*

Mylanta® [OTC] *see* Aluminum Hydroxide, Magnesium Hydroxide, and Simethicone *on page 41*

Mylanta® Gas [OTC] *see* Simethicone *on page 788*

Mylanta®-II [OTC] *see* Aluminum Hydroxide, Magnesium Hydroxide, and Simethicone *on page 41*

Myleran® *see* Busulfan *on page 131*

Mylicon® [OTC] *see* Simethicone *on page 788*

Mylosar® *see* Azacitidine *on page 88*

Myminic® Expectorant [OTC] *see* Guaifenesin and Phenylpropanolamine *on page 409*

Myochrysine® *see* Gold Sodium Thiomalate *on page 404*

Myoflex® [OTC] *see* Triethanolamine Salicylate *on page 868*

Myotonachol™ *see* Bethanechol Chloride *on page 112*

Myphetane DC® *see* Brompheniramine, Phenylpropanolamine, and Codeine *on page 125*

Myphetapp® [OTC] *see* Brompheniramine and Phenylpropanolamine *on page 123*

Mysoline® *see* Primidone *on page 723*
Mytelase® Caplets® *see* Ambenonium Chloride *on page 43*
Mytrex® *see* Nystatin and Triamcinolone *on page 632*
Mytussin® [OTC] *see* Guaifenesin *on page 407*
Mytussin® AC *see* Guaifenesin and Codeine *on page 408*
Mytussin® DAC *see* Guaifenesin, Pseudoephedrine, and Codeine *on page 410*
Mytussin® DM [OTC] *see* Guaifenesin and Dextromethorphan *on page 408*

Nabilone (na' bi lone)
Brand Names Cesamet®
Therapeutic Category Antiemetic
Use Treatment of nausea and vomiting associated with cancer chemotherapy
Usual Dosage Oral:
Children >4 years:
<18 kg: 0.5 mg twice daily
18-30 kg: 1 mg twice daily
>30 kg: 1 mg 3 times/day

Adults: 1-2 mg twice daily beginning 1-3 hours before chemotherapy is administered and continuing around-the-clock until 1 dose after chemotherapy is completed; maximum daily dose: 6 mg divided in 3 doses
Mechanism of Action Nabilone is a synthetic cannabinoid utilized as an antiemetic drug in the control of nausea and vomiting in patients receiving cancer chemotherapy; like delta-9-tetrahydrocannabinol (the active principal of marijuana), nabilone is a dibenzo(b,d)pyrans
Local Anesthetic/Vasoconstrictor Precautions No information available to require special precautions
Effects on Dental Treatment No effects or complications reported
Other Adverse Effects
>10%:
Central nervous system: Dizziness, drowsiness, vertigo, euphoria, clumsiness
Gastrointestinal: Dry mouth
1% to 10%:
Cardiovascular: Orthostatic hypotension
Central nervous system: Ataxia, depression
Ocular: Blurred vision
<1%:
Central nervous system: Changes of mood, confusion, hallucinations, headache
Gastrointestinal: Loss of appetite
Respiratory: Difficulty in breathing
Drug Interactions No data reported
Drug Uptake
Absorption: Rapid
Serum half-life: 35 hours
Pregnancy Risk Factor C

Nabumetone (na byoo' me tone)
Related Information
Nonsteroidal Anti-Inflammatory Agents, Comparative Dosages, and Pharmacokinetics *on page 1021*
Rheumatoid Arthritis, Osteoarthritis, and Joint Prostheses *on page 930*
Brand Names Relafen®
Therapeutic Category Nonsteroidal Anti-inflammatory Agent (NSAID), Oral
Use Management of osteoarthritis and rheumatoid arthritis

Unlabeled use: Sunburn, mild to moderate pain
Usual Dosage Adults: Oral: 1000 mg/day; an additional 500-1000 mg may be needed in some patients to obtain more symptomatic relief; may be administered once or twice daily
Mechanism of Action Nabumetone is a nonacidic, nonsteroidal anti-inflammatory drug that is rapidly metabolized after absorption to a major active metabolite, 6-methoxy-2-naphthylacetic acid. As found with previous nonsteroidal anti-inflammatory drugs, nabumetone's active metabolite inhibits the cyclo-oxygenase enzyme which is indirectly responsible for the production of inflammation and pain during arthritis by way of enhancing the production of endoperoxides and prostaglandins E_2 and I_2 (prostacyclin). The active metabolite of nabumetone is felt to be the compound primarily responsible for therapeutic effect. Comparatively, the parent drug is a poor inhibitor of prostaglandin synthesis.

Local Anesthetic/Vasoconstrictor Precautions No information available to require special precautions

Effects on Dental Treatment No effects or complications reported

Other Adverse Effects

>10%:

Central nervous system: Dizziness

Dermatologic: Skin rash

Gastrointestinal: Abdominal cramps, heartburn, indigestion, nausea

1% to 10%:

Cardiovascular: Fluid retention

Central nervous system: Headache, nervousness

Dermatologic: Itching

Gastrointestinal: Vomiting

Otic: Ringing in ears

<1%:

Cardiovascular: Congestive heart failure, hypertension, arrhythmia, tachycardia, hot flushes

Central nervous system: Epistaxis, confusion, hallucinations, aseptic meningitis, mental depression, drowsiness, insomnia

Dermatologic: Angioedema, hives, erythema multiforme, toxic epidermal necrolysis, Stevens-Johnson syndrome

Endocrine & metabolic: Polydipsia

Gastrointestinal: Gastritis, GI ulceration

Genitourinary: Cystitis

Hematologic: Agranulocytosis, anemia, hemolytic anemia, bone marrow depression, leukopenia, thrombocytopenia

Hepatic: Hepatitis

Neuromuscular & skeletal: Peripheral neuropathy

Ocular: Toxic amblyopia, blurred vision, conjunctivitis, dry eyes

Otic: Decreased hearing

Renal: Polyuria, acute renal failure

Respiratory: Allergic rhinitis, shortness of breath

Drug Interactions No data reported

Drug Uptake

Serum half-life, elimination: Major metabolite: 24 hours

Time to peak serum concentration: Metabolite: Oral: Within 3-6 hours

Pregnancy Risk Factor C

Nadolol (nay doe' lole)

Related Information

Cardiovascular Diseases *on page 912*

Brand Names Corgard®

Canadian/Mexican Brand Names Apo-Nadol® (Canada); Syn-Nadolol® (Canada)

Therapeutic Category Antianginal Agent; Beta-Adrenergic Blocker, Noncardioselective

Use Treatment of hypertension and angina pectoris; prevention of myocardial infarction; prophylaxis of migraine headaches

Usual Dosage Oral:

Children: No information regarding pediatric dosage is currently available in the literature

Adults: Initial: 40-80 mg/day, increase dosage gradually by 40-80 mg increments at 3- to 7-day intervals until optimum clinical response is obtained with profound slowing of heart rate; doses up to 160-240 mg/day in angina and 240-320 mg/day in hypertension may be necessary; doses as high as 640 mg/day have been used

Elderly: Initial: 20 mg/day; increase doses by 20 mg increments at 3- to 7-day intervals; usual dosage range: 20-240 mg/day

Mechanism of Action Competitively blocks response to beta$_1$- and beta$_2$-adrenergic stimulation; does not exhibit any membrane stabilizing or intrinsic sympathomimetic activity

Local Anesthetic/Vasoconstrictor Precautions Use with caution; epinephrine has interacted with nonselective beta-blockers to result in initial hypertensive episode followed by bradycardia

Effects on Dental Treatment Non-cardioselective beta-blockers (ie, propranolol, nadolol) enhance the pressor response to epinephrine, resulting in hypertension and bradycardia. Many nonsteroidal anti-inflammatory drugs such as ibuprofen and indomethacin can reduce the hypotensive effect of beta-blockers after 3 or more weeks of therapy with the NSAID. Short-term NSAID use (ie, 3 days) requires no special precautions in patients taking beta-blockers.

(Continued)

Nadolol *(Continued)*

Other Adverse Effects

>10%: Cardiovascular: Bradycardia

1% to 10%:

Cardiovascular: Reduced peripheral circulation

Central nervous system: Mental depression

Endocrine & metabolic: Decreased sexual ability

Gastrointestinal: Constipation

Neuromuscular & skeletal: Weakness

Respiratory: Breathing difficulty, wheezing

<1%:

Cardiovascular: Congestive heart failure, chest pain, orthostatic hypotension, Raynaud's syndrome, congestive heart failure, edema, Raynaud's phenomena

Central nervous system: Drowsiness, nightmares, vivid dreams, tingling of toes and fingers, insomnia, lethargy, dizziness, fatigue, confusion, headache

Dermatologic: Itching, rash

Gastrointestinal: Vomiting, stomach discomfort, diarrhea, nausea

Genitourinary: Impotence

Hematologic: Thrombocytopenia

Ocular: Dry eyes

Respiratory: Stuffy nose

Miscellaneous: Cold extremities

Drug Interactions

Decreased effect of beta-blockers:

Barbiturates (increased liver metabolism of beta-blockers to result in lower serum levels)

NSAIDs (attenuate the hypotensive therapeutic effects of beta-blockers)

Rifampin (increased liver metabolism of beta-blockers to result in lower serum levels)

Increased effects of beta-blockers:

Calcium channel blockers (increase serum levels of beta-blockers by unknown mechanism to enhance hypotension)

Beta-blockers increase the effects of:

Epinephrine (vasoconstrictor; initial hypertensive episode followed by bradycardia) only from non-cardioselective type beta-blockers

Phenylephrine (Neosynephrine®; enhanced pressor response)

Theophylline (inhibit theophylline metabolism causing increase in serum concentrations)

Drug Uptake

Duration of effect: 24 hours

Absorption: Oral: 30% to 40%

Time to peak serum concentration: Within 2-4 hours persisting for 17-24 hours

Serum half-life: Adults: 10-24 hours; increased half-life with decreased renal function

End stage renal disease: 45 hours

Pregnancy Risk Factor C

Nafarelin Acetate *(naf' a re lin as' e tate)*

Brand Names Synarel®

Therapeutic Category Hormone, Posterior Pituitary; Luteinizing Hormone-Releasing Hormone Analog

Use Treatment of endometriosis, including pain and reduction of lesions; treatment of central precocious puberty (gonadotropin-dependent precocious puberty) in children of both sexes

Usual Dosage

Endometriosis: Adults: Female: 1 spray (200 mcg) in 1 nostril each morning and the other nostril each evening starting on days 2-4 of menstrual cycle for 6 months

Central precocious puberty: Children: Males/Females: 2 sprays (400 mcg) into each nostril in the morning 2 sprays (400 mcg) into each nostril in the evening. If inadequate suppression, may increase dose to 3 sprays (600 mcg) into alternating nostrils 3 times/day.

Mechanism of Action Potent synthetic decapeptide analogue of gonadotropin-releasing hormone (GnRH; LHRH) which is approximately 200 times more potent than GnRH in terms of pituitary release of luteinizing hormone (LH) and follicle-stimulating hormone (FSH). Effects on the pituitary gland and sex hormones are dependent upon its length of administration. After acute administration, an initial stimulation of the release of LH and FSH from the pituitary is observed; an increase in androgens and estrogens subsequently follows. Continued administration of nafarelin, however, suppresses gonado-trope responsiveness to endogenous GnRH resulting in reduced secretion of LH and FSH and, secondarily, decreased ovarian and testicular steroid production.

Local Anesthetic/Vasoconstrictor Precautions No information available to require special precautions

Effects on Dental Treatment No effects or complications reported

Other Adverse Effects

>10%:
Central nervous system: Headache, emotional lability
Dermatologic: Acne
Endocrine & metabolic: Hot flashes, decreased libido, decreased breast size
Genitourinary: Vaginal dryness
Neuromuscular & skeletal: Myalgia
Respiratory: Nasal irritation

1% to 10%:
Cardiovascular: Edema
Central nervous system: Insomnia
Dermatologic: Urticaria, rash, pruritus
Respiratory: Shortness of breath, chest pain
Miscellaneous: Seborrhea

<1%:
Endocrine & metabolic: Increased libido
Gastrointestinal: weight loss

Drug Interactions No data reported

Drug Uptake
Absorption: Not absorbed from GI tract
Maximum serum concentration: 10-45 minutes

Pregnancy Risk Factor X

Nafazair® *see* Naphazoline Hydrochloride *on page 605*

Nafazolina, Clorhidrato De (Mexico) *see* Naphazoline Hydrochloride *on page 605*

Nafcil™ *see* Nafcillin Sodium *on this page*

Nafcillin Sodium (naf sil' in sow' dee um)

Brand Names Nafcil™; Nallpen®; Unipen®

Therapeutic Category Antibiotic, Penicillin

Use Treatment of susceptible bacterial infections such as osteomyelitis, septi-cemia, endocarditis, and CNS infections due to penicillinase-producing strains of *Staphylococcus*

Usual Dosage
Children: I.M., I.V.:
Mild to moderate infections: 50-100 mg/kg/day in divided doses every 6 hours
Severe infections: 100-200 mg/kg/day in divided doses every 4-6 hours
Maximum dose: 12 g/day
Adults:
I.M.: 500 mg every 4-6 hours
I.V.: 500-2000 mg every 4-6 hours

Mechanism of Action Interferes with bacterial cell wall synthesis during active multiplication, causing cell wall death and resultant bactericidal activity against susceptible bacteria

Local Anesthetic/Vasoconstrictor Precautions No information available to require special precautions

Effects on Dental Treatment Prolonged use of penicillins may lead to the development of oral candidiasis

Other Adverse Effects <1%:
Central nervous system: Fever, pain
Dermatologic: Skin rash
Gastrointestinal: Nausea, diarrhea
Hematologic: Neutropenia
Local: Thrombophlebitis; oxacillin (less likely to cause phlebitis) is often preferred in pediatric patients
Renal: Acute interstitial nephritis
Miscellaneous: Hypersensitivity reactions

Drug Interactions
Decreased effect: Chloramphenicol may decrease nafcillin levels; oral contra-ceptive may have a decreased effectiveness
Increased effect: Probenecid may increase nafcillin levels
Increased toxicity: Oral anticoagulants, heparin increase risk of bleeding
(Continued)

Nafcillin Sodium *(Continued)*

Drug Uptake
Absorption: Oral: Poor and erratic
Serum half-life:
  Adults: 0.5-1.5 hours, with normal hepatic function
  End stage renal disease: 1.2 hours
Time to peak serum concentration:
  Oral: Within 2 hours
  I.M.: Within 0.5-1 hour
Pregnancy Risk Factor B

Naftifine Hydrochloride (naf' ti feen hye droe klor' ide)
Brand Names Naftin®
Therapeutic Category Antifungal Agent, Topical
Use Topical treatment of tinea cruris (jock itch), tinea corporis (ring worm), and tinea pedis (athlete's foot)
Usual Dosage Adults: Topical: Apply cream once daily and gel twice daily (morning and evening) for up to 4 weeks
Mechanism of Action Synthetic, broad-spectrum antifungal agent in the allylamine class; appears to have both fungistatic and fungicidal activity. Exhibits antifungal activity by selectively inhibiting the enzyme squalene epoxidase in a dose-dependent manner which results in the primary sterol, ergosterol, within the fungal membrane not being synthesized.
Local Anesthetic/Vasoconstrictor Precautions No information available to require special precautions
Effects on Dental Treatment No effects or complications reported
Other Adverse Effects
>10%: Local: Burning, stinging
1% to 10%: Local: Dryness, erythema, itching, irritation
Drug Interactions No data reported
Drug Uptake
Absorption: Systemic, 6% for cream, ≤4% for gel
Serum half-life: 2-3 days
Pregnancy Risk Factor B

Naftin® *see* Naftifine Hydrochloride *on this page*

Nalbufina, Clorhidrato De (Mexico) *see* Nalbuphine Hydrochloride *on this page*

Nalbuphine Hydrochloride (nal' byoo feen hye droe klor' ide)
Related Information
Narcotic Agonist Charts *on page 1019*
Brand Names Nubain®
Therapeutic Category Analgesic, Narcotic
Synonyms Nalbufina, Clorhidrato De (Mexico)
Use Relief of moderate to severe pain; preoperative analgesia, postoperative and surgical anesthesia, and obstetrical analgesia during labor and delivery
Usual Dosage I.M., I.V., S.C.:
Children 10 months to 14 years: Premedication: 0.2 mg/kg; maximum: 20 mg/dose

Adults: 10 mg/70 kg every 3-6 hours; maximum single dose: 20 mg; maximum daily dose: 160 mg
Mechanism of Action Binds to opiate receptors in the CNS, causing inhibition of ascending pain pathways, altering the perception of and response to pain; produces generalized CNS depression
Local Anesthetic/Vasoconstrictor Precautions No information available to require special precautions
Effects on Dental Treatment Anticholinergic side effects can cause a reduction of saliva production or secretion contributes to discomfort and dental disease (ie, caries, oral candidiasis and periodontal disease)
Other Adverse Effects
>10%:
  Central nervous system: Drowsiness, CNS depression
  Miscellaneous: Histamine release, narcotic withdrawal
1% to 10%:
  Cardiovascular: Hypotension, flushing
  Central nervous system: Dry mouth, dizziness, headache, weakness
  Dermatologic: Urticaria, skin rash
  Gastrointestinal: Nausea, vomiting, anorexia
  Local: Pain at injection site

Respiratory: Pulmonary edema

<1%:

Cardiovascular: Hypertension, tachycardia

Central nervous system: Mental depression, hallucinations, confusion, paradoxical CNS stimulation, nervousness, restlessness, nightmares, insomnia

Gastrointestinal: GI irritation, ureteral spasm, biliary spasm

Genitourinary: Decreased urination, toxic megacolon

Ocular: Blurred vision

Respiratory: Shortness of breath, respiratory depression

Drug Interactions Increased toxicity: Barbiturate anesthetics cause increased CNS depression

Drug Uptake Serum half-life: 3.5-5 hours

Pregnancy Risk Factor B (D if used for prolonged periods or in high doses at term)

Naldecon® *see* Chlorpheniramine, Phenyltoloxamine, Phenylpropanolamine, and Phenylephrine *on page 194*

Naldecon® DX Adult Liquid [OTC] *see* Guaifenesin, Phenylpropanolamine, and Dextromethorphan *on page 410*

Naldecon-EX® Children's Syrup [OTC] *see* Guaifenesin and Phenylpropanolamine *on page 409*

Naldecon® Senior DX [OTC] *see* Guaifenesin and Dextromethorphan *on page 408*

Naldecon® Senior EX [OTC] *see* Guaifenesin *on page 407*

Naldelate® *see* Chlorpheniramine, Phenyltoloxamine, Phenylpropanolamine, and Phenylephrine *on page 194*

Nalfon® *see* Fenoprofen Calcium *on page 356*

Nalgest® *see* Chlorpheniramine, Phenyltoloxamine, Phenylpropanolamine, and Phenylephrine *on page 194*

Nalidixic Acid (nal i dix' ik as' id)

Brand Names NegGram®

Therapeutic Category Antibiotic, Quinolone

Synonyms Nalidixio Acido (Mexico)

Use Treatment of urinary tract infections

Usual Dosage Oral:

Children 3 months to 12 years: 55 mg/kg/day divided every 6 hours; suppressive therapy is 33 mg/kg/day divided every 6 hours

Adults: 1 g 4 times/day for 2 weeks; then suppressive therapy of 500 mg 4 times/day

Mechanism of Action Inhibits DNA polymerization in late stages of chromosomal replication

Local Anesthetic/Vasoconstrictor Precautions No information available to require special precautions

Effects on Dental Treatment No effects or complications reported

Other Adverse Effects

>10%: Central nervous system: Dizziness, drowsiness, headache

1% to 10%: Gastrointestinal: Nausea, vomiting

<1%:

Central nervous system: Increased intracranial pressure, malaise, vertigo, confusion, toxic psychosis, convulsions, fever, chills

Dermatologic: Rash, urticaria, photosensitivity reactions

Endocrine & metabolic: Metabolic acidosis

Hematologic: Leukopenia, thrombocytopenia

Hepatic: Hepatotoxicity

Ocular: Visual disturbances

Drug Interactions

Decreased effect with antacids

Increased effect of warfarin

Drug Uptake

Serum half-life: 6-7 hours; increases significantly with renal impairment

Time to peak serum concentration: Oral: Within 1-2 hours

Pregnancy Risk Factor B

Nalidixio Acido (Mexico) *see* Nalidixic Acid *on this page*

Nallpen® *see* Nafcillin Sodium *on page 599*

Nalmefene Hydrochloride (nal' me feen hye droe klor' ide)

Brand Names Revex®

Therapeutic Category Antidote, Narcotic Agonist

(Continued)

Nalmefene Hydrochloride *(Continued)*

Use Complete or partial of opioid drug effects; management of known or suspected opioid overdose

Usual Dosage

Reversal of postoperative opioid depression: Blue labeled product (100 mcg/mL): Titrate to reverse the undesired effects of opioids; initial dose for nonopioid dependent patients: 0.25 mcg/kg followed by 0.25 mcg/kg incremental doses at 2- to 5-minute intervals; after a total dose of >1 mcg/kg, further therapeutic response is unlikely

Management of known/suspected opioid overdose: Green labeled product (1000 mcg/mL): Initial dose: 0.5 mg/70 kg; may repeat with 1 mg/70 kg in 2-5 minutes; further increase beyond a total dose of 1.5 mg/70 kg will not likely result in improved response and may result in cardiovascular stress and precipitated withdrawal syndrome. (If opioid dependency is suspected, administer a challenge dose of 0.1 mg/70 kg; if no withdrawal symptoms are observed in 2 minutes, the recommended doses can be administered.)

Local Anesthetic/Vasoconstrictor Precautions No information available to require special precautions

Effects on Dental Treatment No effects or complications reported

Other Adverse Effects

>10%: Gastrointestinal: Nausea

1% to 10%:
Cardiovascular: Tachycardia, hypertension
Central nervous system: Postoperative pain, fever, dizziness
Gastrointestinal: Vomiting

<1%:
Cardiovascular: Hypotension, vasodilation, arrhythmia
Central nervous system: Headache, chills, nervousness, confusion
Gastrointestinal: Diarrhea dry mouth
Genitourinary: Urinary retention
Neuromuscular & skeletal: Tremor
Miscellaneous: Withdrawal syndrome

Drug Uptake

Onset of action: I.M., S.C.: 5-15 minutes
Serum half-life: 10.8 hours
Time to peak serum concentration: 2.3 hours

Comments Nalmefene is supplied in two concentrations 100 mcg/mL has a blue label, 1000 mcg/mL has a green label; proper steps should be used to prevent use of the incorrect dosage strength; duration of action of nalmefene is as long as most opioid analgesics; may cause acute withdrawal symptoms in individuals who have some degree of tolerance to and dependence on opioids

Naloxone Hydrochloride *(nal ox' one hye droe klor' ide)*

Related Information

Narcotic Agonist Charts *on page 1019*

Brand Names Narcan®

Therapeutic Category Narcotic Antagonist

Use

Dental: Reverses CNS and respiratory depressant effects of fentanyl and meperidine during I.V. conscious state
Medical: Reverses CNS and respiratory depression in suspected narcotic overdose; neonatal opiate depression; coma of unknown etiology

Usual Dosage Adults: Narcotic overdose: I.V.: 0.4-2 mg every 2-3 minutes as needed; may need to repeat doses every 20-60 minutes, if no response is observed after 10 mg, question the diagnosis. **Note:** Use 0.1-0.2 mg increments in patients who are opioid-dependent and in postoperative patients to avoid large cardiovascular changes.

Mechanism of Action Competes and displaces narcotics at narcotic receptor sites (mu, kappa, delta, and sigma subtypes)

Local Anesthetic/Vasoconstrictor Precautions No information available to require special precautions

Effects on Dental Treatment No effects or complications reported

Other Adverse Effects 1% to 10%:
Cardiovascular: Hypertension, hypotension, tachycardia, ventricular arrhythmias
Central nervous system: Insomnia, irritability, anxiety
Dermatologic: Rash
Gastrointestinal: Nausea, vomiting
Ocular: Blurred vision
Miscellaneous: Narcotic withdrawal, sweating

Oral manifestations: No data reported

Contraindications Hypersensitivity to naloxone or any component

Warnings/Precautions Use with caution in patients with cardiovascular disease; excessive dosages should be avoided after use of opiates in surgery, because naloxone may cause an increase in blood pressure and reversal of anesthesia; may precipitate withdrawal symptoms in patients addicted to opiates, including pain, hypertension, sweating, agitation, irritability, shrill cry, failure to feed

Drug Interactions Decreased effect of narcotic analgesics

Drug Uptake
Onset of effect: I.V.: Within 2 minutes
Time to peak serum concentration: 5-15 minutes
Duration of effect: 20-60 minutes; since shorter than that of most opioids, repeated doses are usually needed
Serum half-life: 1-1.5 hours

Pregnancy Risk Factor B

Breast-feeding Considerations No data reported

Dosage Forms Injection: 0.02 mg/mL (2 mL); 0.4 mg/mL (1 mL, 2 mL, 10 mL); 1 mg/mL (2 mL, 10 mL)

Dietary Considerations No data reported

Generic Available Yes

Comments Naloxone is an antagonist to all narcotic analgesics. Its use in dental practice is to reverse overdose effects of the two narcotic agents fentanyl and meperidine, used in the technique of I.V. conscious sedation.

Nalspan® *see* Chlorpheniramine, Phenyltoloxamine, Phenylpropanolamine, and Phenylephrine *on page 194*

Naltrexone Hydrochloride (nal trex' one hye droe klor' ide)

Brand Names Trexan™

Therapeutic Category Narcotic Antagonist

Use Adjunct to the maintenance of an opioid-free state in detoxified individual

Usual Dosage Do not give until patient is opioid-free for 7-10 days as required by urine analysis

Adults: Oral: 25 mg; if no withdrawal signs within 1 hour give another 25 mg; maintenance regimen is flexible, variable and individualized (50 mg/day to 100-150 mg 3 times/week)

Mechanism of Action Naltrexone is a cyclopropyl derivative of oxymorphone similar in structure to naloxone and nalorphine (a morphine derivative); it acts as a competitive antagonist at opioid receptor sites

Local Anesthetic/Vasoconstrictor Precautions No information available to require special precautions

Effects on Dental Treatment No effects or complications reported

Other Adverse Effects
>10%:
Central nervous system: Insomnia, nervousness, headache
Gastrointestinal: Abdominal cramping, nausea, vomiting
Neuromuscular & skeletal: Joint pain
1% to 10%:
Central nervous system: Dizziness, anorexia
Dermatologic: Skin rash
Endocrine & metabolic: Polydipsia
Respiratory: Sneezing
<1%:
Central nervous system: Insomnia, irritability, anxiety
Hematologic: Thrombocytopenia, agranulocytosis, hemolytic anemia
Ocular: Blurred vision
Miscellaneous: Narcotic withdrawal

Drug Interactions No data reported

Drug Uptake
Duration of action:
50 mg: 24 hours
100 mg: 48 hours
150 mg: 72 hours
Absorption: Oral: Almost completely
Serum half-life: 4 hours; 6-β-naltrexol: 13 hours
Time to peak serum concentration: Within 60 minutes

Pregnancy Risk Factor C

Nandrolone (nan' droe lone)

Brand Names Androlone®; Androlone®-D; Deca-Durabolin®; Durabolin®; Hybolin™ Decanoate; Hybolin™ Improved; Neo-Durabolic

Therapeutic Category Androgen

Use Control of metastatic breast cancer; management of anemia of renal insufficiency

Usual Dosage Deep I.M. (into gluteal muscle):

Children 2-13 years: (decanoate): 25-50 mg every 3-4 weeks

Adults:

Male:

Breast cancer (phenpropionate): 50-100 mg/week

Anemia of renal insufficiency (decanoate): 100-200 mg/week

Female: 50-100 mg/week

Breast cancer (phenproprionate): 50-100 mg/week

Anemia of renal insufficiency (decanoate): 50-100 mg/week

Mechanism of Action Promotes tissue-building processes, increases production of erythropoietin, causes protein anabolism; increases hemoglobin and red blood cell volume

Local Anesthetic/Vasoconstrictor Precautions No information available to require special precautions

Effects on Dental Treatment No effects or complications reported

Other Adverse Effects

Male:

Postpubertal:

>10%:

Dermatologic: Acne

Endocrine & metabolic: Bladder irritability, priapism, gynecomastia

1% to 10%:

Central nervous system: Insomnia

Endocrine & metabolic: Decreased libido, hepatic dysfunction, chills, prostatic hypertrophy (elderly)

Gastrointestinal: Nausea, diarrhea

Hematologic: Iron deficiency anemia, suppression of clotting factors

<1%:

Hepatic: Hepatic necrosis, hepatocellular carcinoma

Prepubertal:

>10%:

Dermatologic: Acne

Endocrine & metabolic: Virilism

1% to 10%:

Central nervous system: Chills, insomnia, factors

Dermatologic: Hyperpigmentation

Gastrointestinal: Diarrhea, nausea

Hematologic: Iron deficiency anemia, suppression of clotting

<1%: Hepatic: necrosis, hepatocellular carcinoma

Female:

>10%: Endocrine & metabolic: Virilism

1% to 10%:

Central nervous system: Chills, insomnia

Endocrine & metabolic: Hypercalcemia

Gastrointestinal: Nausea, diarrhea

Hematologic: Iron deficiency anemia, suppression of clotting factors

Hepatic: Hepatic dysfunction

<1%: Hepatic: Hepatic necrosis, hepatocellular carcinoma

Drug Interactions Increased toxicity: Oral anticoagulants, insulin, oral hypoglycemic agents, adrenal steroids, ACTH

Pregnancy Risk Factor X

Naphazoline and Antazoline (naf az' oh leen & an taz' oh leen)

Brand Names Albalon-A® Ophthalmic; Antazoline-V® Ophthalmic; Vasocon-A® [OTC] Ophthalmic

Therapeutic Category Ophthalmic Agent, Vasoconstrictor

Use Topical ocular congestion, irritation and itching

Local Anesthetic/Vasoconstrictor Precautions No information available to require special precautions

Effects on Dental Treatment No effects or complications reported

Other Adverse Effects 1% to 10%:

Cardiovascular: Systemic cardiovascular stimulation, hypertension

Central nervous system: Nervousness, dizziness, headache

Gastrointestinal: Nausea

Local: Transient stinging
Neuromuscular & skeletal: Weakness
Ocular: Mydriasis, intraocular pressure (increased), blurring of vision
Respiratory: Nasal mucosa irritation, dryness, rebound congestion
Miscellaneous: Sweating

Comments Discontinue drug and consult physician if ocular pain or visual changes occur, ocular redness or irritation, or condition worsens or persists for more than 72 hours

Naphazoline and Pheniramine (naf az' oh leen & fen nir' a meen)
Brand Names Naphcon-A® Ophthalmic [OTC]
Therapeutic Category Ophthalmic Agent, Vasoconstrictor
Synonyms Pheniramine and Naphazoline
Use Topical ocular vasoconstrictor
Local Anesthetic/Vasoconstrictor Precautions No information available to require special precautions
Effects on Dental Treatment No effects or complications reported
Other Adverse Effects 1% to 10%:
Cardiovascular: Systemic effects due to absorption (hypertension, cardiac irregularities, hyperglycemia)
Ocular: Pupillary dilation, increase in intraocular pressure

Naphazoline Hydrochloride (naf az' oh leen hye droe klor' ide)
Brand Names AK-Con®; Albalon® Liquifilm®; Allerest® Eye Drops [OTC]; Clear Eyes® [OTC]; Comfort® [OTC]; Degest® 2 [OTC]; Estivin® II [OTC]; I-Naphline®; Muro's Opcon®; Nafazair®; Naphcon Forte®; Naphcon® [OTC]; Opcon®; Privine®; VasoClear® [OTC]; Vasocon Regular®
Canadian/Mexican Brand Names Nazil® Ofteno (Mexico)
Therapeutic Category Adrenergic Agonist Agent, Ophthalmic; Decongestant, Nasal; Nasal Agent, Vasoconstrictor; Ophthalmic Agent, Vasoconstrictor
Synonyms Nafazolina, Clorhidrato De (Mexico)
Use Topical ocular vasoconstrictor; will temporarily relieve congestion, itching, and minor irritation, and to control hyperemia in patients with superficial corneal vascularity
Usual Dosage
Nasal:
Children:
<6 years: Intranasal: Not recommended (especially infants) due to CNS depression
6-12 years: 1 spray of 0.05% into each nostril every 6 hours if necessary; therapy should not exceed 3-5 days
Children >12 years and Adults: 0.05%, instill 1-2 drops or sprays every 6 hours if needed; therapy should not exceed 3-5 days

Ophthalmic:
Children <6 years: Not recommended for use due to CNS depression (especially in infants)
Children >6 years and Adults: Instill 1-2 drops into conjunctival sac of affected eye(s) every 3-4 hours; therapy generally should not exceed 3-4 days
Mechanism of Action Stimulates alpha-adrenergic receptors in the arterioles of the conjunctiva and the nasal mucosa to produce vasoconstriction
Local Anesthetic/Vasoconstrictor Precautions No information available to require special precautions
Effects on Dental Treatment No effects or complications reported
Other Adverse Effects 1% to 10%:
Cardiovascular: Systemic cardiovascular stimulation
Central nervous system: Dizziness, headache, nervousness
Gastrointestinal: Nausea
Local: Transient stinging, nasal mucosa irritation, dryness, sneezing, rebound congestion
Ocular: Mydriasis, increased intraocular pressure, blurring of vision
Drug Interactions Increased toxicity: Anesthetics (discontinue mydriatic prior to use of anesthetics that sensitize the myocardium to sympathomimetics, ie, cyclopropane, halothane), MAO inhibitors, tricyclic antidepressants causes hypertensive reactions
Drug Uptake
Onset of decongestant action: Topical: Within 10 minutes
Duration: 2-6 hours
Pregnancy Risk Factor C

Naphcon® [OTC] *see* Naphazoline Hydrochloride *on this page*

Naphcon-A® Ophthalmic [OTC] *see* Naphazoline and Pheniramine *on previous page*

Naphcon Forte® *see* Naphazoline Hydrochloride *on previous page*

Naprosyn® (Naproxen Base) *see* Naproxen *on this page*

Naproxen (na prox' en)
Related Information
Dental Drug Interactions: Update on Drug Combinations Requiring Special Considerations *on page 1022*

Nonsteroidal Anti-Inflammatory Agents, Comparative Dosages, and Pharmacokinetics *on page 1021*

Oral Pain *on page 940*

Rheumatoid Arthritis, Osteoarthritis, and Joint Prostheses *on page 930*

Temporomandibular Dysfunction (TMD) *on page 963*

Brand Names Aleve® (Naproxen Sodium) (OTC); Anaprox® (Naproxen Sodium); Naprosyn® (Naproxen Base)

Canadian/Mexican Brand Names Apo-Naproxen® (Canada); Naxen® (Canada); Novo-Naprox® (Canada); Nu-Naprox® (Canada); Atiquim® (Mexico); Atiflan® (Mexico); Dafloxen® (Mexico); Faraxen® (Mexico); Flanax® (Mexico); Flexen® (Mexico); Flogen® (Mexico); Fuxen® (Mexico); Naprodil® (Mexico); Naxen® (Mexico); Naxil® (Mexico); Pactens® (Mexico); Pronaxil® (Mexico); Supradol® (Mexico); Velsay® (Mexico)

Therapeutic Category Analgesic, Non-narcotic; Anti-inflammatory Agent; Nonsteroidal Anti-inflammatory Agent (NSAID)

Use
Dental: Management of pain and swelling

Medical: Management of inflammatory disease and rheumatoid disorders (including juvenile rheumatoid arthritis); acute gout; mild to moderate pain; dysmenorrhea; fever, migraine headache

Usual Dosage Adults: Oral:
Naproxen base: Initial: 500 mg, then 250 mg every 6-8 hours

Naproxen sodium: Initial: 550 mg, then 275 mg every 6-8 hours

Maximum daily dose: 1250 mg/day naproxen base and 1375 mg naproxen sodium

Mechanism of Action Inhibits prostaglandin synthesis by decreasing the activity of the enzyme, cyclo-oxygenase, which results in decreased formation of prostaglandin precursors

Local Anesthetic/Vasoconstrictor Precautions No information available to require special precautions

Effects on Dental Treatment Use with caution in patients taking anticoagulants

Other Adverse Effects >10%: Gastrointestinal: Nausea, heartburn, ulcers, indigestion

Oral manifestations: No data reported

Contraindications Hypersensitivity to naproxen, aspirin, or other nonsteroidal anti-inflammatory drugs (NSAIDs)

Warnings/Precautions Use with caution in patients with GI disease (bleeding or ulcers), cardiovascular disease (CHF, hypertension), renal or hepatic impairment, and patients receiving anticoagulants; perform ophthalmologic evaluation for those who develop eye complaints during therapy (blurred vision, diminished vision, changes in color vision, retinal changes); NSAIDs may mask signs/symptoms of infections; photosensitivity reported; elderly are at especially high-risk for adverse effects

Drug Interactions Decreased effect of furosemide; naproxen could displace other highly protein bound drugs, such as oral anticoagulants, hydantoins, salicylates, sulfonamides, and sulfonylureas; naproxen and warfarin may result in slight increase in free warfarin; naproxen and probenecid may result in increased plasma half-life of naproxen; naproxen and methotrexate may result in significantly increased and prolonged blood methotrexate concentration, which may be severe or fatal

Drug Uptake
Onset of effect: 1 hour

Duration of effect: Up to 7 hours

Time to peak serum concentration: Within 1-2 hours and persisting for up to 12 hours

Serum half-life: 12-15 hours

Pregnancy Risk Factor B (D if used in the 3rd trimester or near delivery)

Breast-feeding Considerations May be taken while breast-feeding

Dosage Forms
Suspension, oral: 125 mg/5 mL (480 mL)

Tablet, as sodium: 275 mg (250 mg base); 550 mg (500 mg base)
Tablet: 250 mg, 375 mg, 500 mg
Dietary Considerations May be taken with food, milk, or antacids to decrease GI adverse effects
Generic Available No
Comments The sodium salt of naproxen provides better effects because of better oral absorption; the sodium salt also provides a faster onset and a longer duration of action
Selected Readings
Brooks PM and Day RO, "Nonsteroidal Anti-inflammatory Drugs-Differences and Similarities," *N Engl J Med*, 1991, 324(24):1716-25.
Forbes JA, Keller CK, Smith JW, et al, "Analgesic Effect of Naproxen Sodium, Codeine, a Naproxen-Codeine Combination and Aspirin on the Postoperative Pain of Oral Surgery," *Pharmacotherapy*, 1986, 6(5):211-8.

Naqua® *see* Trichlormethiazide *on page 867*

Narcan® *see* Naloxone Hydrochloride *on page 602*

Narcotic Agonist Charts *see page 1019*

Nardil® *see* Phenelzine Sulfate *on page 679*

Naropin® *see* Ropivacaine Hydrochloride *on page 775*

Nasabid™ *see* Guaifenesin and Pseudoephedrine *on page 409*

Nasacort® *see* Triamcinolone *on page 862*

Nasahist B® *see* Brompheniramine Maleate *on page 124*

Nasalcrom® *see* Cromolyn Sodium *on page 235*

Nasalide® *see* Flunisolide *on page 372*

Natabec® **[OTC]** *see* Vitamins, Multiple *on page 901*

Natabec® **FA [OTC]** *see* Vitamins, Multiple *on page 901*

Natabec® **Rx** *see* Vitamins, Multiple *on page 901*

Natacyn® *see* Natamycin *on this page*

Natalins® **[OTC]** *see* Vitamins, Multiple *on page 901*

Natalins® **Rx** *see* Vitamins, Multiple *on page 901*

Natamycin (na ta mye' sin)
Brand Names Natacyn®
Therapeutic Category Antifungal Agent, Ophthalmic
Use Treatment of blepharitis, conjunctivitis, and keratitis caused by susceptible fungi (*Aspergillus, Candida*), *Cephalosporium, Curvularia, Fusarium, Penicillium, Microsporum, Epidermophyton, Blastomyces dermatitidis, Coccidioides immitis, Cryptococcus neoformans, Histoplasma capsulatum, Sporothrix schenckii, Trichomonas vaginalis*
Usual Dosage Adults: Ophthalmic: Instill 1 drop in conjunctival sac every 1-2 hours, after 3-4 days reduce to one drop 6-8 times/day; usual course of therapy is 2-3 weeks.
Mechanism of Action Increases cell membrane permeability in susceptible fungi
Local Anesthetic/Vasoconstrictor Precautions No information available to require special precautions
Effects on Dental Treatment No effects or complications reported
Other Adverse Effects <1%: Ocular: Blurred vision, photophobia, eye pain, eye irritation not present before therapy
Drug Interactions Increased toxicity: Topical corticosteroids (concomitant use contraindicated)
Drug Uptake
Absorption: Ophthalmic: <2% systemically absorbed
Pregnancy Risk Factor C

Nature's Tears® **Solution [OTC]** *see* Artificial Tears *on page 75*

Naturetin® *see* Bendroflumethiazide *on page 101*

Naus-A-Way® **[OTC]** *see* Phosphorated Carbohydrate Solution *on page 690*

Nausetrol® **[OTC]** *see* Phosphorated Carbohydrate Solution *on page 690*

Navane® *see* Thiothixene *on page 842*

Navelbine® *see* Vinorelbine Tartrate *on page 897*

N-B-P® **Ointment** *see* Bacitracin, Neomycin, and Polymyxin B *on page 94*

ND-Stat® *see* Brompheniramine Maleate *on page 124*

Nebcin® *see* Tobramycin *on page 849*

NebuPent™ *see* Pentamidine Isethionate *on page 670*

Nedocromil Sodium (ne doe kroe' mil sow' dee um)
Related Information
Respiratory Diseases *on page 924*
(Continued)

Nedocromil Sodium *(Continued)*

Brand Names Tilade® Inhalation Aerosol

Therapeutic Category Antiasthmatic; Antihistamine, Inhalation

Use Maintenance therapy in patients with mild to moderate bronchial asthma

Usual Dosage Children >12 years and Adults: Inhalation: 2 inhalations 4 times/day; may reduce dosage to 2-3 times/day once desired clinical response to initial dose is observed

Local Anesthetic/Vasoconstrictor Precautions No information available to require special precautions

Effects on Dental Treatment No effects or complications reported

Other Adverse Effects 1% to 10%:

Central nervous system: Dizziness, headache, chest pain, fatigue
Gastrointestinal: Nausea, vomiting, dry mouth, diarrhea, unpleasant taste
Respiratory: Coughing, pharyngitis, rhinitis, bronchitis, dyspnea, bronchospasm

Drug Uptake

Duration of therapeutic effect: 2 hours
Serum half-life: 1.5-2 hours

Comments Not a bronchodilator and, therefore, should not be used for reversal of acute bronchospasm; has no known therapeutic systemic activity when delivered by inhalation

N.E.E.® 1/35 *see* Ethinyl Estradiol and Norethindrone *on page 339*

Nefazodone *(nef ay' zoe done)*

Brand Names Serzone®

Therapeutic Category Antidepressant, Miscellaneous

Use Treatment of depression

Usual Dosage Oral: Adults: 200 mg/day, administered in two divided doses initially, with a range of 300-600 mg/day in two divided doses thereafter

Mechanism of Action Inhibits reuptake of serotonin and norepinephrine by the presynaptic neuronal membrane and desensitization of adenyl cyclase, down regulation of beta-adrenergic receptors, and down regulation of serotonin receptors

Local Anesthetic/Vasoconstrictor Precautions No information available to require special precautions

Effects on Dental Treatment Up to 10% of patients will have significant dry mouth which will disappear with cessation of drug therapy

Other Adverse Effects

>10%:

Central nervous system: Headache, drowsiness, insomnia, agitation, dizziness, confusion
Gastrointestinal: Dry mouth, nausea
Neuromuscular & skeletal: Tremor

1% to 10%:

Cardiovascular: Postural hypotension
Central nervous system: Asthenia
Gastrointestinal: Constipation, vomiting
Ocular: Blurred vision, amblyopia

<1%: Prolonged priapism, diarrhea

Drug Interactions

Decreased effect: Clonidine, methyldopa, diuretics, oral hypoglycemics, anticoagulants
Increased toxicity: Terfenadine and astemizole (increased concentrations have been associated with serious ventricular arrhythmias and death), fluoxetine, triazolam (reduce triazolam dose by 75%), alprazolam (reduce alprazolam dose by 50%), phenytoin, CNS depressants, MAO inhibitors (allow 14 days after MAO inhibitors are stopped or 7 days after nefazodone is stopped); digoxin serum levels may increase

Drug Uptake

Onset of action: Therapeutic effects take at least 2 weeks to appear
Serum half-life: 2-4 hours (parent compound), active metabolites persist longer
Time to peak serum concentration: 30 minutes, prolonged in presence of food

Pregnancy Risk Factor C

NegGram® *see* Nalidixic Acid *on page 601*

Nelova™ 0.5/35E *see* Ethinyl Estradiol and Norethindrone *on page 339*

Nelova™ 1/50M *see* Mestranol and Norethindrone *on page 547*

Nelova™ 10/11 *see* Ethinyl Estradiol and Norethindrone *on page 339*

Nembutal® *see* Pentobarbital *on page 672*

Neo-Calglucon® [OTC] *see* Calcium Glubionate *on page 142*
Neo-Cortef® Ophthalmic *see* Neomycin and Hydrocortisone *on this page*
Neo-Cortef® Topical *see* Neomycin and Hydrocortisone *on this page*
NeoDecadron® Ophthalmic *see* Neomycin and Dexamethasone *on this page*
NeoDecadron® Topical *see* Neomycin and Dexamethasone *on this page*
Neo-Dexameth® Ophthalmic *see* Neomycin and Dexamethasone *on this page*
Neo-Durabolic *see* Nandrolone *on page 604*
Neofed® [OTC] *see* Pseudoephedrine *on page 749*
Neo-fradin® *see* Neomycin Sulfate *on page 611*
Neoloid® [OTC] *see* Castor Oil *on page 161*
Neomixin® *see* Bacitracin, Neomycin, and Polymyxin B *on page 94*

Neomycin and Dexamethasone
(nee oh mye' sin & dex a meth' a sone)
Brand Names AK-Neo-Dex® Ophthalmic; NeoDecadron® Ophthalmic; NeoDecadron® Topical; Neo-Dexameth® Ophthalmic
Therapeutic Category Antibiotic, Ophthalmic; Corticosteroid, Ophthalmic
Synonyms Dexamethasone and Neomycin
Use Treatment of steroid responsive inflammatory conditions of the palpebral and bulbar conjunctiva, lid, cornea, and anterior segment of the globe
Local Anesthetic/Vasoconstrictor Precautions No information available to require special precautions
Effects on Dental Treatment No effects or complications reported
Other Adverse Effects <1%:
Local: Transient stinging, burning, or local irritation
Ocular: Intraocular pressure (increased), mydriasis, ptosis, epithelial punctate keratitis, and possible corneal or scleral malacia can occur

Neomycin and Hydrocortisone
(nee oh mye' sin & hye droe kor' ti sone)
Brand Names Neo-Cortef® Ophthalmic; Neo-Cortef® Topical
Therapeutic Category Antibiotic, Topical; Corticosteroid, Topical (Low Potency)
Use Treatment of susceptible topical bacterial infections with associated swelling
Local Anesthetic/Vasoconstrictor Precautions No information available to require special precautions
Effects on Dental Treatment No effects or complications reported

Neomycin and Polymyxin B (nee oh mye' sin & pol i mix' in bee)
Brand Names Neosporin® G.U. Irrigant; Neosporin® Cream [OTC]; Statrol®
Therapeutic Category Antibiotic, Topical; Antibiotic, Urinary Irrigation
Use Short-term as a continuous irrigant or rinse in the urinary bladder to prevent bacteriuria and gram-negative rod septicemia associated with the use of indwelling catheters; to help prevent infection in minor cuts, scrapes, and burns; treatment of superficial ocular infections involving the conjunctiva or cornea
Usual Dosage Children and Adults:
Bladder irrigation: **Not for injection**; add 1 mL irrigant to 1 liter isotonic saline solution and connect container to the inflow of lumen of 3-way catheter. Continuous irrigant or rinse in the urinary bladder for up to a maximum of 10 days with administration rate adjusted to patient's urine output; usually no more than 1 L of irrigant is used per day.
Ophthalmic:
Ointment: Instill 1/2" ribbon into the conjunctival sac every 3-4 hours for acute infections or 2-3 times/day for mild to moderate infections for 7-10 days
Solution: Instill 1-2 drops every 15-30 minutes for acute infections; 1-2 drops every 3-6 hours for mild-moderate infections.
Topical: Apply cream 1-4 times/day to affected area
Mechanism of Action Refer to individual monographs for Neomycin and Polymyxin
Local Anesthetic/Vasoconstrictor Precautions No information available to require special precautions
Effects on Dental Treatment No effects or complications reported
Other Adverse Effects 1% to 10%:
Dermatologic: Contact dermatitis, erythema, rash, urticaria
Genitourinary: Nephrotoxicity, bladder irritation
Local: Burning
Neuromuscular & skeletal: Neuromuscular blockade
(Continued)

Neomycin and Polymyxin B *(Continued)*
Otic: Ototoxicity
Drug Interactions No data reported
Drug Uptake Absorption: Topical: Not absorbed following application to intact skin; absorbed through denuded or abraded skin, peritoneum, wounds, or ulcers
Pregnancy Risk Factor C (D G.U. irrigant)

Neomycin, Polymyxin B, and Dexamethasone
(nee oh mye' sin, pol i mix' in bee, & dex a meth' a sone)
Brand Names AK-Trol®; Dexacidin®; Dexasporin®; Maxitrol®
Therapeutic Category Antibiotic, Ophthalmic
Use Steroid-responsive inflammatory ocular conditions in which a corticosteroid is indicated and where bacterial infection or a risk of bacterial infection exists
Usual Dosage Children and Adults: Ophthalmic:
Ointment: Place a small amount (~½") in the affected eye 3-4 times/day or apply at bedtime as an adjunct with drops
Solution: Instill 1-2 drops into affected eye(s) every 3-4 hours; in severe disease, drops may be used hourly and tapered to discontinuation
Mechanism of Action Refer to Individual Monographs for neomycin, polymyxin B, and dexamethasone
Local Anesthetic/Vasoconstrictor Precautions No information available to require special precautions
Effects on Dental Treatment No effects or complications reported
Other Adverse Effects 1% to 10%: Ocular: Cutaneous sensitization, pain, development of glaucoma, cataract, increased intraocular pressure, optic nerve damage, contact dermatitis, delayed wound healing
Drug Interactions No data reported
Pregnancy Risk Factor C

Neomycin, Polymyxin B, and Gramicidin
(nee oh mye' sin, pol i mix' in bee, & gram i sye' din)
Related Information
Antimicrobial Prophylaxis in Surgical Patients *on page 1042*
Brand Names AK-Spore® Ophthalmic Solution; Neosporin® Ophthalmic Solution; Ocutricin® Ophthalmic Solution
Canadian/Mexican Brand Names Neosporin® Oftalmico (Mexico)
Therapeutic Category Antibiotic, Ophthalmic
Use Treatment of superficial ocular infection, infection prophylaxis in minor skin abrasions
Usual Dosage Children and Adults: Ophthalmic: Instill 1-2 drops 4-6 times/day or more frequently as required for severe infections
Mechanism of Action Interferes with bacterial protein synthesis by binding to 30S ribosomal subunits; binds to phospholipids, alters permeability, and damages the bacterial cytoplasmic membrane permitting leakage of intracellular constituents
Local Anesthetic/Vasoconstrictor Precautions No information available to require special precautions
Effects on Dental Treatment No effects or complications reported
Other Adverse Effects 1% to 10%:
Local: Itching, reddening, failure to heal, edema
Ocular: Low grade conjunctivitis
Drug Interactions No data reported
Pregnancy Risk Factor C

Neomycin, Polymyxin B, and Hydrocortisone
(nee oh mye' sin, pol i mix' in bee, & hye droe kor' ti sone)
Brand Names AK-Spore H.C.® Ophthalmic Suspension; AK-Spore H.C.® Otic; AntibiOtic® Otic; Bacticort® Otic; Cortatrigen® Otic; Cortisporin® Ophthalmic Suspension; Cortisporin® Otic; Cortisporin® Topical Cream; Drotic® Otic; LazerSporin-C® Otic; Octicair® Otic; Ocutricin® HC Otic; Otocort® Otic; Otomycin-HPN® Otic; Otosporin® Otic; PediOtic® Otic
Therapeutic Category Antibiotic, Ophthalmic; Antibiotic, Otic; Antibiotic, Topical; Corticosteroid, Ophthalmic; Corticosteroid, Otic; Corticosteroid, Topical (Low Potency)
Use Steroid-responsive inflammatory condition for which a corticosteroid is indicated and where bacterial infection or a risk of bacterial infection exists
Usual Dosage Duration of use should be limited to 10 days unless otherwise directed by the physician

Otic solution is used **only** for swimmer's ear (infections of external auditory canal)

Otic:
Children: Instill 3 drops into affected ear 3-4 times/day
Adults: Instill 4 drops 3-4 times/day; otic suspension is the preferred otic preparation

Children and Adults:
Ophthalmic: Drops: Instill 1-2 drops 2-4 times/day, or more frequently as required for severe infections; in acute infections, instill 1-2 drops every 15-30 minutes gradually reducing the frequency of administration as the infection is controlled
Topical: Apply a thin layer 1-4 times/day

Mechanism of Action Refer to individual monographs for neomycin, Polymyxin B, and Hydrocortisone

Local Anesthetic/Vasoconstrictor Precautions No information available to require special precautions

Effects on Dental Treatment No effects or complications reported

Other Adverse Effects
>10%: Miscellaneous: Hypersensitivity
1% to 10%:
Local: Contact dermatitis, erythema, rash, urticaria, burning, itching, swelling, pain, stinging
Neuromuscular & skeletal: Neuromuscular blockade
Ocular: Elevation of intraocular pressure, glaucoma, cataracts, conjunctival erythema
Otic: Ototoxicity
Renal: Nephrotoxicity
Miscellaneous: Sensitization to neomycin, secondary infections, bladder irritation

Drug Interactions No data reported

Pregnancy Risk Factor C

Neomycin, Polymyxin B, and Prednisolone
(nee oh mye' sin, pol i mix' in bee, & pred niss' oh lone)

Brand Names Poly-Pred®

Therapeutic Category Antibiotic, Ophthalmic; Corticosteroid, Ophthalmic

Use Steroid-responsive inflammatory ocular condition in which bacterial infection or a risk of bacterial ocular infection exists

Usual Dosage Children and Adults: Ophthalmic: Instill 1-2 drops every 3-4 hours; acute infections may require every 30-minute instillation initially with frequency of administration reduced as the infection is brought under control. To treat the lids: Instill 1-2 drops every 3-4 hours, close the eye and rub the excess on the lids and lid margins.

Mechanism of Action Refer to individual monographs for Neomycin, Polymyxin B, and Prednisolone

Local Anesthetic/Vasoconstrictor Precautions No information available to require special precautions

Effects on Dental Treatment No effects or complications reported

Other Adverse Effects 1% to 10%:
Dermatologic: Cutaneous sensitization, skin rash, delayed wound healing
Ocular: Increased intraocular pressure, glaucoma, optic nerve damage, cataracts, conjunctival sensitization

Drug Interactions No data reported

Pregnancy Risk Factor C

Neomycin Sulfate (nee oh mye' sin sul' fate)

Related Information
Antimicrobial Prophylaxis in Surgical Patients *on page 1042*

Brand Names Mycifradin® Sulfate; Neo-fradin®; Neo-Tabs®

Therapeutic Category Ammonium Detoxicant; Antibiotic, Aminoglycoside; Antibiotic, Topical

Use Prepares GI tract for surgery; treat minor skin infections; treat diarrhea caused by *E. coli*; adjunct in the treatment of hepatic encephalopathy, as irrigant during surgery

Usual Dosage
Children: Oral:
Preoperative intestinal antisepsis: 90 mg/kg/day divided every 4 hours for 2 days; or 25 mg/kg at 1 PM, 2 PM, and 11 PM on the day preceding surgery as an adjunct to mechanical cleansing of the intestine and in combination with erythromycin base

(Continued)

Neomycin Sulfate *(Continued)*

Hepatic coma: 50-100 mg/kg/day in divided doses every 6-8 hours or 2.5-7 g/m²/day divided every 4-6 hours for 5-6 days not to exceed 12 g/day

Children and Adults: Topical: Apply ointment 1-4 times/day; topical solutions containing 0.1% to 1% neomycin have been used for irrigation

Adults: Oral:

Preoperative intestinal antisepsis: 1 g each hour for 4 doses then 1 g every 4 hours for 5 doses; or 1 g at 1 PM, 2 PM, and 11 PM on day preceding surgery as an adjunct to mechanical cleansing of the bowel and oral erythromycin; or 6 g/day divided every 4 hours for 2-3 days

Hepatic coma: 500-2000 mg every 6-8 hours or 4-12 g/day divided every 4-6 hours for 5-6 days

Chronic hepatic insufficiency: 4 g/day for an indefinite period

Dialyzable (50% to 100%)

Mechanism of Action Interferes with bacterial protein synthesis by binding to 30S ribosomal subunits

Local Anesthetic/Vasoconstrictor Precautions No information available to require special precautions

Effects on Dental Treatment No effects or complications reported

Other Adverse Effects

1% to 10%:

Dermatologic: Dermatitis, rash, urticaria, erythema

Local: Burning

Ocular: Contact conjunctivitis

<1%:

Gastrointestinal: Nausea, vomiting, diarrhea

Neuromuscular & skeletal: Neuromuscular blockade

Otic: Ototoxicity

Renal: Nephrotoxicity

Drug Interactions

Decreased effect: May decrease GI absorption of digoxin and methotrexate

Increased effect: Synergistic effects with penicillins

Increased toxicity:

Oral neomycin may potentiate the effects of oral anticoagulants

Increased adverse effects with other neurotoxic, ototoxic, or nephrotoxic drugs

Drug Uptake

Absorption: Oral, percutaneous: Poor (3%)

Serum half-life: 3 hours (age and renal function dependent)

Time to peak serum concentration:

Oral: 1-4 hours

I.M.: Within 2 hours

Pregnancy Risk Factor C

Neonatal Trace Metals *see* Trace Metals *on page 857*

Neopap® [OTC] *see* Acetaminophen *on page 14*

Neoquess® *see* Dicyclomine Hydrochloride *on page 273*

Neosar® *see* Cyclophosphamide *on page 240*

Neosporin® *see* Bacitracin, Neomycin, and Polymyxin B *on page 94*

Neosporin® Cream [OTC] *see* Neomycin and Polymyxin B *on page 609*

Neosporin® G.U. Irrigant *see* Neomycin and Polymyxin B *on page 609*

Neosporin® Ophthalmic Solution *see* Neomycin, Polymyxin B, and Gramicidin *on page 610*

Neo-Synephrine® 12 Hour Nasal Solution [OTC] *see* Oxymetazoline Hydrochloride *on page 649*

Neo-Synephrine® Nasal Solution [OTC] *see* Phenylephrine Hydrochloride *on page 685*

Neo-Synephrine® Ophthalmic Solution *see* Phenylephrine Hydrochloride *on page 685*

Neo-Tabs® *see* Neomycin Sulfate *on previous page*

Neothylline® *see* Dyphylline *on page 305*

Neotrace-4® *see* Trace Metals *on page 857*

Neotricin HC® Ophthalmic Ointment *see* Bacitracin, Neomycin, Polymyxin B, and Hydrocortisone *on page 95*

NeoVadrin® [OTC] *see* Vitamins, Multiple *on page 901*

NeoVadrin® B Complex [OTC] *see* Vitamin B Complex *on page 899*

Nephrocaps® [OTC] *see* Vitamin B Complex With Vitamin C and Folic Acid *on page 900*

Nephro-Fer™ [OTC] see Ferrous Fumarate on page 359
Nephron® see Epinephrine, Racemic on page 314
Nephrox Suspension [OTC] see Aluminum Hydroxide on page 39
Neptazane® see Methazolamide on page 554
Nervocaine® see Lidocaine Hydrochloride on page 502
Nesacaine® see Chloroprocaine Hydrochloride on page 185
Nesacaine®-MPF see Chloroprocaine Hydrochloride on page 185
Nestrex® see Pyridoxine Hydrochloride on page 753
Netilmicina Sulfato De (Mexico) see Netilmicin Sulfate on this page

Netilmicin Sulfate (ne til mye' sin sul' fate)

Brand Names Netromycin®
Canadian/Mexican Brand Names Netromicina® (Mexico)
Therapeutic Category Antibiotic, Aminoglycoside
Synonyms Netilmicina Sulfato De (Mexico)
Use Short-term treatment of serious or life-threatening infections including septicemia, peritonitis, intra-abdominal abscess, lower respiratory tract infections, urinary tract infections; skin, bone, and joint infections caused by sensitive *Pseudomonas aeruginosa*, *Escherichia coli*, *Proteus*, *Klebsiella*, *Serratia*, *Enterobacter*, *Citrobacter*, and *Staphylococcus*
Usual Dosage Individualization is critical because of the low therapeutic index. Use of ideal body weight (IBW) for determining the mg/kg/dose appears to be more accurate than dosing on the basis of total body weight (TBW). In morbid obesity, dosage requirement may best be estimated using a dosing weight of IBW + 0.4 (TBW - IBW). Peak and trough plasma drug levels should be determined, particularly in critically ill patients with serious infections or in disease states known to significantly alter aminoglycoside pharmacokinetics (eg, cystic fibrosis, burns, or major surgery).

Once daily dosing: Higher peak serum drug concentration to MIC ratios, demonstrated aminoglycoside postantibiotic effect, decreased renal cortex drug uptake, and improved cost-time efficiency are supportive reasons for the use of once daily dosing regimens for aminoglycosides. Current research indicates these regimens to be as effective for nonlife-threatening infections, with no higher incidence of nephrotoxicity, than those requiring multiple daily doses. Doses are determined by calculating the entire day's dose via usual multiple dose calculation techniques and administering this quantity as a single dose. Doses are then adjusted to maintain mean serum concentrations above the MIC(s) of the causative organism(s). (Example: 4.5-6.5 mg/kg as a single dose; expected Cp_{max}: 10-20 mcg/mL, and Cp_{min}: <1 mcg/mL). Further research is needed for universal recommendation in all patient populations and gram-negative disease; exceptions may include those with known high clearance (eg, children, patients with cystic fibrosis, or burns who may require shorter dosage intervals) and patients with renal function impairment for whom longer than conventional dosage intervals are usually required.

I.M., I.V.:
Children 6 weeks to 12 years: 1-2.5 mg/kg/dose every 8 hours
Children >12 years and Adults: 1.5-2 mg/kg/dose every 8-12 hours
Some clinicians suggest a daily dose of 4-7 mg/kg for all patients with normal renal function. This dose is at least as efficacious with similar, if not less, toxicity than conventional dosing.

Mechanism of Action Interferes with protein synthesis in bacterial cell by binding to ribosomal subunit
Local Anesthetic/Vasoconstrictor Precautions No information available to require special precautions
Effects on Dental Treatment No effects or complications reported
Other Adverse Effects
>10%:
Central nervous system: Neurotoxicity
Otic: Ototoxicity (auditory), ototoxicity (vestibular)
Renal: Decreased creatinine clearance, nephrotoxicity
1% to 10%:
Cardiovascular: Swelling
Dermatologic: Skin itching, redness, rash
<1%:
Central nervous system: Drowsiness, headache, pseudomotor cerebri
Dermatologic: Photosensitivity, erythema
Gastrointestinal: Anorexia, nausea, vomiting, weight loss, increased salivation, enterocolitis
(Continued)

Netilmicin Sulfate *(Continued)*

Hematologic: Granulocytopenia, agranulocytosis, thrombocytopenia
Local: Burning, stinging
Neuromuscular & skeletal: Weakness, tremors, muscle cramps
Respiratory: Difficulty in breathing
Drug Interactions Increased toxicity:
Penicillins, cephalosporins, amphotericin B, loop diuretics, vancomycin cause increased nephrotoxic potential
Neuromuscular blocking agents cause increased neuromuscular blockade
Drug Uptake
Absorption: I.M.: Well absorbed
Serum half-life: 2-3 hours (age and renal function dependent)
Time to peak serum concentration: I.M.: Within 0.5-1 hour
Pregnancy Risk Factor D

Netromycin® *see* Netilmicin Sulfate *on previous page*

Neucalm® *see* Hydroxyzine *on page 443*

Neupogen® Injection *see* Filgrastim *on page 362*

Neuramate® *see* Meprobamate *on page 543*

Neurontin® *see* Gabapentin *on page 392*

Neutra-Phos® *see* Potassium Phosphate and Sodium Phosphate *on page 713*

Neutra-Phos®-K *see* Potassium Phosphate *on page 711*

Neutrexin™ *see* Trimetrexate Glucuronate *on page 875*

Neutrogena® [OTC] *see* Benzoyl Peroxide *on page 104*

Neutrogena® T/Derm *see* Coal Tar *on page 225*

Nevirapine (ne vye' re peen)

Brand Names Viramune®
Therapeutic Category Antiviral Agent, Parenteral
Use In combination therapy with nucleoside antiretroviral agents in HIV-1 infected adults previously treated for whom current therapy is deemed inadequate
Usual Dosage Adults: Oral: 200 mg once daily for 2 weeks followed by 200 mg twice daily
Mechanism of Action Nevirapine is a non-nucleoside reverse transcriptase inhibitor specific for HIV-1; nevirapine does not require intracellular phosphorylation for antiviral activity
Local Anesthetic/Vasoconstrictor Precautions No information available to require special precautions
Effects on Dental Treatment No effects or complications reported
Other Adverse Effects >10%:
Central nervous system: Headache, somnolence, drug fever
Dermatologic: Rash
Gastrointestinal: Diarrhea, nausea
Hepatic: LFTs (elevated)
Contraindications Previous hypersensitivity to nevirapine
Drug Uptake
Absorption: Rapidly absorbed with peak levels occurring within 2 hours of administration
Serum half-life: 22-84 hours
Pregnancy Risk Factor C
Generic Available No
Comments All product information was not available at the time of this writing
Selected Readings
D'Aquila RT, Hughes MD, Johnson VA, et al, "Nevirapine, Zidovudine, and Didanosine Compared With Zidovudine and Didanosine in Patients With HIV-1 Infection," *Ann Intern Med*, 1996, 124:1019-30.
Hammer SM, Kessler HA, and Saag MS, "Issues in Combination Antiretroviral Therapy: A Review," *J Acquired Immune Deficiency Syndromes*, 1994, 7(Suppl 2):S24-37.

New Decongestant® *see* Chlorpheniramine, Phenyltoloxamine, Phenylpropanolamine, and Phenylephrine *on page 194*

N.G.T.® *see* Nystatin and Triamcinolone *on page 632*

Niac® [OTC] *see* Niacin *on this page*

Niacels™ [OTC] *see* Niacin *on this page*

Niacin (nye' a sin)

Related Information
Cardiovascular Diseases *on page 912*
Brand Names Niac® [OTC]; Niacels™ [OTC]; Nicobid® [OTC]; Nicolar® [OTC]; Nicotinex [OTC]; Slo-Niacin® [OTC]

Therapeutic Category Lipid Lowering Drugs; Vitamin, Water Soluble

Use Adjunctive treatment of hyperlipidemias; peripheral vascular disease and circulatory disorders; treatment of pellagra; dietary supplement

Usual Dosage Give I.M., I.V., or S.C. only if oral route is unavailable and use only for vitamin deficiencies (not for hyperlipidemia)

Children: Pellagra: Oral: 50-100 mg/dose 3 times/day
    Oral: Recommended daily allowances:
       0-0.5 years: 5 mg/day
       0.5-1 year: 6 mg/day
       1-3 years: 9 mg/day
       4-6 years: 12 mg/day
       7-10 years: 13 mg/day
    Males:
       11-14 years: 17 mg/day
       15-18 years: 20 mg/day
       19-24 years: 19 mg/day
    Females: 11-24 years: 15 mg/day

Adults: Oral:
    Recommended daily allowances:
    Males: 25-50 years: 19 mg/day; >51 years: 15 mg/day
    Females: 25-50 years: 15 mg/day; >51 years: 13 mg/day
    Hyperlipidemia: 1.5-6 g/day in 3 divided doses with or after meals
    Pellagra: 50-100 mg 3-4 times/day, maximum: 500 mg/day
    Niacin deficiency: 10-20 mg/day, maximum: 100 mg/day

Mechanism of Action Component of two coenzymes which is necessary for tissue respiration, lipid metabolism, and glycogenolysis; inhibits the synthesis of very low density lipoproteins

Local Anesthetic/Vasoconstrictor Precautions No information available to require special precautions

Effects on Dental Treatment No effects or complications reported

Other Adverse Effects

1% to 10%:
    Cardiovascular: Generalized flushing with sensation of warmth
    Central nervous system: Headache
    Gastrointestinal: Bloating, flatulence, nausea
    Hepatic: Abnormalities of hepatic function tests, jaundice
    Neuromuscular & skeletal: Tingling in extremities
    Miscellaneous: Increased sebaceous gland activity

<1%:
    Cardiovascular: Tachycardia, syncope, vasovagal attacks
    Central nervous system: Dizziness
    Dermatologic: Skin rash
    Hepatic: Chronic liver damage
    Ocular: Blurred vision
    Respiratory: Wheezing

Drug Interactions

Decreased effect of oral hypoglycemics; may inhibit uricosuric effects of sulfin-pyrazone and probenecid

Decreased toxicity (flush) with aspirin

Increased toxicity with lovastatin (myopathy) and possibly with other HMG-CoA reductase inhibitors; adrenergic blocking agents → additive vasodilating effect and postural hypotension

Drug Uptake

Peak serum concentrations: Oral: Within 45 minutes
Serum half-life: 45 minutes

Pregnancy Risk Factor A (C if used in doses greater than RDA suggested doses)

Niacinamide (nye a sin' a mide)

Therapeutic Category Vitamin, Water Soluble

Use Prophylaxis and treatment of pellagra

Usual Dosage Oral:

Children: Pellagra: 100-300 mg/day in divided doses

Adults: 50 mg 3-10 times/day
    Pellagra: 300-500 mg/day
    Recommended daily allowance: 13-19 mg/day

Mechanism of Action Used by the body as a source of niacin; is a component of two coenzymes which is necessary for tissue respiration, lipid metabolism, and glycogenolysis; inhibits the synthesis of very low density lipoproteins (Continued)

Niacinamide *(Continued)*

Local Anesthetic/Vasoconstrictor Precautions No information available to require special precautions

Effects on Dental Treatment No effects or complications reported

Other Adverse Effects

1% to 10%:

Gastrointestinal: Bloating, flatulence, nausea

Neuromuscular & skeletal: Tingling in extremities

Miscellaneous: Increased sebaceous gland activity

<1%:

Cardiovascular: Tachycardia

Dermatologic: Skin rash

Ocular: Blurred vision

Respiratory: Wheezing

Drug Interactions No data reported

Drug Uptake

Absorption: Rapid from GI tract

Serum half-life: 45 minutes

Time to peak serum concentration: 20-70 minutes

Pregnancy Risk Factor A (C if used in doses greater than RDA suggested doses)

Nicardipina (Mexico) *see* Nicardipine Hydrochloride *on this page*

Nicardipine Hydrochloride (nye kar' de peen hye droe klor' ide)

Related Information

Calcium Channel Blockers & Gingival Hyperplasia *on page 1010*

Cardiovascular Diseases *on page 912*

Brand Names Cardene®; Cardene® SR

Canadian/Mexican Brand Names Ridene® (Mexico)

Therapeutic Category Antianginal Agent; Calcium Channel Blocker

Synonyms Nicardipina (Mexico)

Use Chronic stable angina; management of essential hypertension, migraine prophylaxis

Unlabeled use: CHF

Usual Dosage Adults:

Oral: 40 mg 3 times/day (allow 3 days between dose increases)

Oral, sustained release: Initial: 30 mg twice daily, titrate up to 60 mg twice daily

I.V. (dilute to 0.1 mg/mL): Initial: 5 mg/hour increased by 2.5 mg/hour every 15 minutes to a maximum of 15 mg/hour

Mechanism of Action Inhibits calcium ion from entering the "slow channels" or select voltage-sensitive areas of vascular smooth muscle and myocardium during depolarization, producing a relaxation of coronary vascular smooth muscle and coronary vasodilation; increases myocardial oxygen delivery in patients with vasospastic angina

Local Anesthetic/Vasoconstrictor Precautions No information available to require special precautions

Effects on Dental Treatment Other drugs of this class can cause gingival hyperplasia (ie, nifedipine) but there have been no reports for nicardipine

Other Adverse Effects

1% to 10%:

Cardiovascular: Flushing, palpitations, tachycardia

Central nervous system: Headache, asthenia, dizziness, nausea, somnolence

Miscellaneous: Pedal edema

<1%:

Cardiovascular: Edema, tachycardia, syncope, abnormal EKG

Central nervous system: Insomnia, malaise, abnormal dreams

Dermatologic: Rash

Gastrointestinal: Vomiting, constipation, dyspepsia, dry mouth

Genitourinary: Nocturia

Neuromuscular & skeletal: Tremor

Drug Interactions

Increased toxicity/effect/levels:

Calcium channel blockers (CCB) and H_2-blockers cause increased bioavailability CCB

CCB and beta-blockers cause increased cardiac depressant effects on A-V conduction

H_2-blockers cause increased bioavailability of nicardipine

Severe hypotension has been reported during fentanyl anesthesia with concomitant use of beta-blockers and calcium channel blockers; even though such interactions have not been seen specifically with nicardipine, caution is suggested in using nicardipine with fentanyl

Drug Uptake
Absorption: Oral: Well absorbed, ~100%
Serum half-life: 2-4 hours
Time to peak: Peak serum levels occur within 20-120 minutes and an onset of hypotension occurs within 20 minutes

Pregnancy Risk Factor C

Niclocide® *see* Niclosamide *on this page*

Niclosamide (ni kloe' sa mide)
Brand Names Niclocide®
Therapeutic Category Anthelmintic
Use Treatment of intestinal beef and fish tapeworm infections and dwarf tapeworm infections
Usual Dosage Oral:
Beef and fish tapeworm:
Children:
11-34 kg: 1 g (2 tablets) as a single dose
>34 kg: 1.5 g (3 tablets) as a single dose
Adults: 2 g (4 tablets) in a single dose
May require a second course of treatment 7 days later

Dwarf tapeworm:
Children:
11-34 g: 1 g (2 tablets) chewed thoroughly in a single dose the first day, then 500 mg/day (1 tablet) for next 6 days
>34 g: 1.5 g (3 tablets) in a single dose the first day, then 1 g/day for 6 days
Adults: 2 g (4 tablets) in a single daily dose for 7 days
Mechanism of Action Inhibits the synthesis of ATP through inhibition of oxidative phosphorylation in the mitochondria of cestodes
Local Anesthetic/Vasoconstrictor Precautions No information available to require special precautions
Effects on Dental Treatment No effects or complications reported
Other Adverse Effects
1% to 10%:
Central nervous system: Drowsiness, dizziness, headache
Gastrointestinal: Nausea, vomiting, loss of appetite, diarrhea
<1%:
Cardiovascular: Palpitations
Central nervous system: Fever
Dermatologic: Rash, pruritus ani, alopecia
Gastrointestinal: Constipation
Neuromuscular & skeletal: Weakness, backache
Miscellaneous: Oral irritation, rectal bleeding, bad taste in mouth, sweating, edema in the arm
Drug Interactions No data reported
Drug Uptake
Absorption: Oral: Not significant
Pregnancy Risk Factor B

Nicobid® [OTC] *see* Niacin *on page 614*
Nicoderm® *see* Nicotine *on this page*
Nicolar® [OTC] *see* Niacin *on page 614*
Nicorette® *see* Nicotine *on this page*

Nicotine (nik oh teen')
Brand Names Habitrol™; Nicoderm®; Nicorette®; Nicotrol®; ProStep®
Canadian/Mexican Brand Names Nicorette® Plus (Canada); Nicolan® (Mexico); Nicotinell®-TTS (Mexico)
Therapeutic Category Smoking Deterrent
Use
Dental: Treatment aid to smoking cessation while participating in a behavioral modification program under dental or medical supervision
Medical: None
Usual Dosage
Gum: Chew 1 piece of gum when urge to smoke, up to 30 pieces/day; most patients require 10-12 pieces of gum/day
(Continued)

Nicotine *(Continued)*

Transdermal patch (patients should be advised to completely stop smoking upon initiation of therapy): Apply new patch every 24 hours to nonhairy, clean, dry skin on the upper body or upper outer arm; each patch should be applied to a different site

Initial starting dose: 21 mg/day for 4-8 weeks for most patients

First weaning dose: 14 mg/day for 2-4 weeks

Second weaning dose: 7 mg/day for 2-4 weeks

Initial starting dose for patients <100 pounds, smoke <10 cigarettes/day, have a history of cardiovascular disease: 14 mg/day for 4-8 weeks followed by 7 mg/day for 2-4 weeks

In patients who are receiving >600 mg/day of cimetidine: Decrease to the next lower patch size

Benefits of use of nicotine transdermal patches beyond 3 months have not been demonstrated

Mechanism of Action Nicotine is one of two naturally-occurring alkaloids which exhibit their primary effects via autonomic ganglia stimulation. The other alkaloid is lobeline which has many actions similar to those of nicotine but is less potent. Nicotine is a potent ganglionic and central nervous system stimulant, the actions of which are mediated via nicotine-specific receptors. Biphasic actions are observed depending upon the dose administered. The main effect of nicotine in small doses is stimulation of all autonomic ganglia; with larger doses, initial stimulation is followed by blockade of transmission. Biphasic effects are also evident in the adrenal medulla; discharge of catecholamines occurs with small doses, whereas prevention of catecholamines release is seen with higher doses as a response to splanchnic nerve stimulation. Stimulation of the central nervous system (CNS) is characterized by tremors and respiratory excitation. However, convulsions may occur with higher doses, along with respiratory failure secondary to both central paralysis and peripheral blockade to respiratory muscles.

Local Anesthetic/Vasoconstrictor Precautions No information available to require special precautions

Effects on Dental Treatment No effects or complications reported

Other Adverse Effects

Chewing gum:

>10%:

Cardiovascular: Tachycardia

Central nervous system: Headache (mild)

Gastrointestinal: Nausea, vomiting, indigestion, excessive salivation, belching, increased appetite

Neuromuscular & skeletal: Jaw muscle ache

Miscellaneous: Mouth or throat soreness, hiccups

1% to 10%:

Central nervous system: Insomnia, dizziness, nervousness

Endocrine & metabolic: Dysmenorrhea

Gastrointestinal: GI distress, eructation

Neuromuscular & skeletal: Muscle pain

Respiratory: Hoarseness

Miscellaneous: Hiccups

<1%:

Cardiovascular: Atrial fibrillation

Dermatologic: Erythema, itching, hypersensitivity reactions

Transdermal systems:

>10%:

Cardiovascular: Tachycardia

Central nervous system: Headache (mild)

Dermatologic: Pruritus, erythema

Gastrointestinal: Increased appetite

1% to 10%:

Central nervous system: Insomnia, nervousness

Endocrine & metabolic: Dysmenorrhea

Neuromuscular & skeletal: Muscle pain

<1%:

Cardiovascular: Atrial fibrillation

Dermatologic: Itching, hypersensitivity reactions

Oral manifestations: >10%: Chewing gum: Excessive salivation, mouth, or throat soreness

Contraindications Nonsmokers, patients with a history of hypersensitivity or allergy to nicotine or any components used in the transdermal system, pregnant or nursing women, patients who are smoking during the postmyocardial infarction period, patients with life-threatening arrhythmias, or severe or worsening angina pectoris, active temporomandibular joint disease (gum)

Warnings/Precautions Use with caution in oropharyngeal inflammation and in patients with history of esophagitis, peptic ulcer, coronary artery disease, vasospastic disease, angina, hypertension, hyperthyroidism, diabetes, and hepatic dysfunction; nicotine is known to be one of the most toxic of all poisons; while the gum is being used to help the patient overcome a health hazard, it also must be considered a hazardous drug vehicle

Drug Interactions

Smoking cessation may alter response to concomitant medications:

Decreased effect of caffeine, imipramine, oxazepam, pentazocine, propranolol, theophylline, glutethimide

Increased effect of furosemide, insulin, propoxyphene

Smoking and nicotine can increase circulating cortisol and catecholamines; therapy with adrenergic agonists or adrenergic blockers may need to be adjusted

Decrease dose of patch in patients taking lithium

Drug Uptake

Time to peak serum concentration:

Gum: 15-30 minutes

Transdermal: 8-9 hours

Duration of effect: Transdermal: 24 hours

Serum half-life:

Nicotine: 1-2 hours

Cotinine: 15-20 hours

Pregnancy Risk Factor D (transdermal)/X (chewing gum)

Breast-feeding Considerations No data reported

Dosage Forms

Patch, transdermal:

Habitrol™: 21 mg/day; 14 mg/day; 7 mg/day (30 systems/box)

Nicoderm®: 21 mg/day; 14 mg/day; 7 mg/day (14 systems/box)

ProStep®: 22 mg/day; 11 mg/day (7 systems/box)

Pieces, chewing gum, as polacrilex: 2 mg/square (96 pieces/box)

Dietary Considerations No data reported

Generic Available No

Comments At least 10 reported studies have documented the effectiveness of nicotine patches in smoking cessation. Approximately 45% of treated patients quit smoking after 6 weeks of patch therapy. Control patients given placebo patches accounted for about a 20% success rate. At 52 weeks, approximately 1/2 of the 45% 6-week successful patients continued to abstain. Control placebo patients accounted for an approximate 11% success rate after 52 weeks.

Selected Readings

Li Wan Po A, "Transdermal Nicotine in Smoking Cessation: A Meta-Analysis," *Eur J Clin Pharmacol*, 1993, 45(6):519-28.

Transdermal Nicotine Study Group, "Transdermal Nicotine for Smoking Cessation. Six-month Results from Two Multicenter Controlled Clinical Trials," *JAMA*, 1991, 266(22):3133-8.

Westman EC, Levin ED, and Rose JE, "The Nicotine Patch in Smoking Cessation," *Arch Intern Med*, 1993, 153(16):1917-23.

Wynn RL, "Nicotine Patches in Smoking Cessation," *AGD Impact*, 1994, 22:14.

Nicotinex [OTC] *see* Niacin *on page 614*

Nicotrol® *see* Nicotine *on page 617*

Nidryl® [OTC] *see* Diphenhydramine Hydrochloride *on page 288*

Nifedipine (nye fed' i peen)

Related Information

Calcium Channel Blockers & Gingival Hyperplasia *on page 1010*

Cardiovascular Diseases *on page 912*

Brand Names Adalat®; Adalat® CC; Procardia®; Procardia XL®

Canadian/Mexican Brand Names Adalat PA® (Canada); Apo-Nifed® (Canada); Gen-Nifedipine® (Canada); Novo-Nifedin® (Canada); Nu-Nifedin® (Canada); Adalat® Oros (Mexico); Adalat® Retard (Mexico); Corogal® (Mexico); Corotrend® (Mexico); Corotrend® Retard (Mexico); Nifedipres® (Mexico); Noviken-N® (Mexico)

Therapeutic Category Antianginal Agent; Calcium Channel Blocker

Synonyms Nifedipino (Mexico)

Use Angina, hypertrophic cardiomyopathy, hypertension (sustained release only), pulmonary hypertension

Usual Dosage Capsule may be punctured and drug solution administered sublingually to reduce blood pressure

(Continued)

Nifedipine *(Continued)*

Children: Oral, S.L.:
Hypertensive emergencies: 0.25-0.5 mg/kg/dose
Hypertrophic cardiomyopathy: 0.6-0.9 mg/kg/24 hours in 3-4 divided doses

Adults:
Initial: 10 mg 3 times/day as capsules or 30 mg once daily as sustained release
Usual dose: 10-30 mg 3 times/day as capsules or 30-60 mg once daily as sustained release
Maximum dose: 120-180 mg/day
Increase sustained release at 7- to 14-day intervals

Not removed by hemo- or peritoneal dialysis; supplemental dose is not necessary

Mechanism of Action Inhibits calcium ion from entering the "slow channels" or select voltage-sensitive areas of vascular smooth muscle and myocardium during depolarization, producing a relaxation of coronary vascular smooth muscle and coronary vasodilation; increases myocardial oxygen delivery in patients with vasospastic angina

Local Anesthetic/Vasoconstrictor Precautions No information available to require special precautions

Effects on Dental Treatment Nifedipine has the greatest incidence in causing gingival hyperplasia than any other calcium channel blocker. Effects from the use of nifedipine (30-100 mg/day) have appeared after 1-9 months. Discontinuance of the drug results in complete disappearance or marked regression of symptoms; symptoms will reappear upon remedication. Marked regression occurs after 1 week and complete disappearance of symptoms has occurred within 15 days. If a gingivectomy is performed and use of the drug is continued or resumed, hyperplasia usually will reoccur. The success of the gingivectomy usually requires that the medication be discontinued or that a switch to a noncalcium channel blocker be made. If for some reason, nifedipine cannot be discontinued, hyperplasia has not reoccurred after gingivectomy when extensive plaque control was performed. If nifedipine is changed to another class of cardiovascular agent, the gingival hyperplasia will probably regress and disappear. A switch to another calcium channel blocker probably may result in continued hyperplasia.

Other Adverse Effects

\>10%:
Cardiovascular: Flushing
Central nervous system: Dizziness, lightheadedness, giddiness, headache
Gastrointestinal: Nausea, heartburn
Neuromuscular & skeletal: Weakness
Miscellaneous: Heat sensation

1% to 10%:
Cardiovascular: Peripheral edema, palpitations, hypotension
Central nervous system: Nervousness, mood changes
Neuromuscular & skeletal: Muscle cramps, tremor
Respiratory: Dyspnea, cough, nasal congestion
Miscellaneous: Sore throat

<1%:
Cardiovascular: Tachycardia, syncope, peripheral edema
Central nervous system: Giddiness, fever, chills
Dermatologic: Dermatitis, urticaria, purpura
Gastrointestinal: Diarrhea, constipation, gingival hyperplasia
Hematologic: Thrombocytopenia, leukopenia, anemia
Neuromuscular & skeletal: Joint stiffness, arthritis with increased ANA
Ocular: Blurred vision, transient blindness
Respiratory: Shortness of breath
Miscellaneous: Sweating

Drug Interactions

Increased toxicity/effect/levels:
H_2-blockers cause increased bioavailability of nifedipine
Beta-blockers cause increased cardiac depressant effects on A-V conduction
Severe hypotension has been reported during fentanyl anesthesia with concomitant use of beta-blockers and calcium channel blockers; even though such interactions have not been seen specifically with nifedipine, caution is suggested in using nifedipine with fentanyl

Drug Uptake

Onset of action:
Oral: Within 20 minutes

S.L.: Within 1-5 minutes
Serum half-life:
Adults, normal: 2-5 hours
Adults with cirrhosis: 7 hours
Pregnancy Risk Factor C
Selected Readings
Lederman D, Lumerman H, Reuben S, et al, "Gingival Hyperplasia Associated With Nifedi-pine Therapy," *Oral Surg Oral Med Oral Pathol*, 1984, 57(6):620-2.

Lucas RM, Howell LP, and Wall BA, "Nifedipine-Induced Gingival Hyperplasia: A Histo-chemical and Ultrastructural Study," *J Periodontol*, 1985, 56(4):211-5.

Nishikawa SJ, Tada H, Hamasaki A, et al, "Nifedipine-Induced Gingival Hyperplasia: A Clinical and In Vitro Study," *J Periodontol*, 1991, 62(1):30-5.

Wynn RL, "Calcium Channel Blockers and Gingival Hyperplasia," *Gen Dent*, 1991, 39(4):240-3.

Wynn RL, "Update on Calcium Channel Blocker-Induced Gingival Hyperplasia," *Gen Dent*, 1995, 43:218-22.

Nifedipino (Mexico) *see* Nifedipine *on page 619*

Niferex® [OTC] *see* Polysaccharide-Iron Complex *on page 705*

Niferex®-PN *see* Vitamins, Multiple *on page 901*

Nilandron® *see* Nilutamide *on this page*

Niloric® *see* Ergoloid Mesylates *on page 318*

Nilstat® *see* Nystatin *on page 632*

Nilutamide (ni lu' ta mide)
Brand Names Nilandron®
Canadian/Mexican Brand Names Anandron® (Can)
Therapeutic Category Antineoplastic Agent, Miscellaneous
Use Use with orchiectomy for the treatment of metastatic prostate cancer
Usual Dosage Adults: Oral: 300 mg (6-50 mg tablets) once daily for 30 days, then 150 mg (3-50 mg tablets) once daily; starting on the same day or day after surgical castration
Local Anesthetic/Vasoconstrictor Precautions No information available to require special precautions
Effects on Dental Treatment No effects or complications reported

NIM *see* Bleomycin Sulfate *on page 117*

Nimodipina (Mexico) *see* Nimodipine *on this page*

Nimodipine (nye moe' di peen)
Related Information
Calcium Channel Blockers & Gingival Hyperplasia *on page 1010*
Cardiovascular Diseases *on page 912*
Brand Names Nimotop®
Therapeutic Category Calcium Channel Blocker
Synonyms Nimodipina (Mexico)
Use Improvement of neurological deficits due to spasm following subarachnoid hemorrhage from ruptured congenital intracranial aneurysms in patients who are in good neurological condition postictus
Usual Dosage Adults: Oral: 60 mg every 4 hours for 21 days, start therapy within 96 hours after subarachnoid hemorrhage

Not removed by hemo- or peritoneal dialysis; supplemental dose is not neces-sary
Mechanism of Action Nimodipine shares the pharmacology of other calcium channel blockers; animal studies indicate that nimodipine has a greater effect on cerebral arterials than other arterials; this increased specificity may be due to the drug's increased lipophilicity and cerebral distribution as compared to nifedipine; inhibits calcium ion from entering the "slow channels" or select voltage sensitive areas of vascular smooth muscle and myocardium during depolarization
Local Anesthetic/Vasoconstrictor Precautions No information available to require special precautions
Effects on Dental Treatment Other drugs of this class can cause gingival hyperplasia (ie, nifedipine) but there have been no reports for nimodipine
Other Adverse Effects
1% to 10%: Cardiovascular: Reductions in systemic blood pressure
<1%:
Cardiovascular: Edema, EKG abnormalities, tachycardia, bradycardia
Central nervous system: Headache, depression
Dermatologic: Rash, acne
Gastrointestinal: Diarrhea, nausea
Hematologic: Hemorrhage
(Continued)

Nimodipine (Continued)

Hepatic: Hepatitis
Neuromuscular & skeletal: Muscle cramps
Respiratory: Dyspnea

Drug Interactions
Increased toxicity/effect/levels:
H_2 blockers cause increased bioavailability of nimodipine
Beta-blockers cause increased cardiac depressant effects on A-V conduction
Severe hypotension has been reported during fentanyl anesthesia with concomitant use of beta-blockers and calcium channel blockers; even though such interactions have not been seen specifically with nimodipine, caution is suggested in using nimodipine with fentanyl

Drug Uptake
Serum half-life: 3 hours, increases with reduced renal function
Time to peak serum concentration: Oral: Within 1 hour

Pregnancy Risk Factor C

Nimotop® see Nimodipine on previous page
Nipent™ Injection see Pentostatin on page 674
Nipride® see Nitroprusside Sodium on page 625

Nisoldipine (nye' sole di peen)

Related Information
Cardiovascular Diseases on page 912

Brand Names Sular™

Therapeutic Category Calcium Channel Blocker

Use Management of hypertension, may be used alone or in combination with other antihypertensive agents

Usual Dosage Adults: Oral: Initial: 20 mg once daily, then increase by 10 mg per week (or longer intervals) to attain adequate control of blood pressure; doses >60 mg once daily are not recommended

Local Anesthetic/Vasoconstrictor Precautions No information available to require special precautions

Effects on Dental Treatment No effects or complications reported

Warnings/Precautions Increased angina and/or myocardial infarction in patients with coronary artery disease

Dosage Forms Tablet, extended release: 10 mg, 20 mg, 30 mg, 40 mg

Nitro-Bid® see Nitroglycerin on next page
Nitrocine® see Nitroglycerin on next page
Nitrodisc® see Nitroglycerin on next page
Nitro-Dur® see Nitroglycerin on next page

Nitrofurantoin (nye troe fyoor an' toyn)

Brand Names Furadantin®; Furalan®; Furan®; Furanite®; Macrobid®; Macrodantin®

Canadian/Mexican Brand Names Apo-Nitrofurantoin® (Canada); Nephronex® (Canada); Novo-Furan® (Canada); Furadantina® (Mexico); Macrodantina® (Mexico)

Therapeutic Category Antibiotic, Miscellaneous

Synonyms Nitrofurantoina (Mexico)

Use Prevention and treatment of urinary tract infections caused by susceptible gram-negative and some gram-positive organisms; *Pseudomonas*, *Serratia*, and most species of *Proteus* are generally resistant to nitrofurantoin

Usual Dosage Oral:
Children >1 month: 5-7 mg/kg/day in divided doses every 6 hours; maximum: 400 mg/day
Chronic therapy: 1-2 mg/kg/day in divided doses every 24 hours; maximum dose: 400 mg/day
Adults: 50-100 mg/dose every 6 hours (not to exceed 400 mg/24 hours)
Prophylaxis: 50-100 mg/dose at at bedtime

Mechanism of Action Inhibits several bacterial enzyme systems including acetyl coenzyme A interfering with metabolism and possibly cell wall synthesis

Local Anesthetic/Vasoconstrictor Precautions No information available to require special precautions

Effects on Dental Treatment No effects or complications reported

Other Adverse Effects
>10%:
Cardiovascular: Chest pains

Central nervous system: Chills, fever
Gastrointestinal: Stomach upset, diarrhea, loss of appetite, vomiting
Respiratory: Cough, difficult breathing
1% to 10%:
Central nervous system: Tiredness, drowsiness, headache, dizziness, numbness
Gastrointestinal: Sore throat
Neuromuscular & skeletal: Weakness, tingling
<1%:
Dermatologic: Skin rash, itching
Hematologic: Hemolytic anemia
Hepatic: Hepatitis
Neuromuscular & skeletal: Arthralgia
Drug Interactions
Decreased effect: Antacids (decreases absorption of nitrofurantoin)
Increased toxicity: Probenecid (decreases renal excretion of nitrofurantoin)
Drug Uptake
Absorption: Well absorbed from GI tract; the macrocrystalline form is absorbed more slowly due to slower dissolution, but causes less GI distress
Serum half-life: 20-60 minutes; prolonged with renal impairment
Pregnancy Risk Factor B

Nitrofurantoina (Mexico) *see* Nitrofurantoin *on previous page*
Nitrofurazona (Mexico) *see* Nitrofurazone *on this page*

Nitrofurazone (nye troe fyoor' a zone)
Brand Names Furacin®
Therapeutic Category Antibacterial, Topical
Synonyms Nitrofurazona (Mexico)
Use Antibacterial agent in second and third degree burns and skin grafting
Usual Dosage Children and Adults: Topical: Apply once daily or every few days to lesion or place on gauze
Mechanism of Action A broad antibacterial spectrum; it acts by inhibiting bacterial enzymes involved in carbohydrate metabolism; effective against a wide range of gram-negative and gram-positive organisms; bactericidal against most bacteria commonly causing surface infections including *Staphylococcus aureus*, *Streptococcus*, *Escherichia coli*, *Enterobacter cloacae*, *Clostridium perfringens*, *Aerobacter aerogenes*, and *Proteus* sp; not particularly active against most *Pseudomonas aeruginosa* strains and does not inhibit viruses or fungi. Topical preparations of nitrofurazone are readily soluble in blood, pus, and serum and are nonmacerating.
Local Anesthetic/Vasoconstrictor Precautions No information available to require special precautions
Effects on Dental Treatment No effects or complications reported
Other Adverse Effects Women should inform their physicians if signs or symptoms of any of the following occur thromboembolic or thrombotic disorders including sudden severe headache or vomiting, disturbance of vision or speech, loss of vision, numbness or weakness in an extremity, sharp or crushing chest pain, calf pain, shortness of breath, severe abdominal pain or mass, mental depression or unusual bleeding

Women should discontinue taking the medication if they suspect they are pregnant or become pregnant. Notify physician if area under dermal patch becomes irritated or a rash develops.
Drug Interactions Decreased effect: Sutilains decrease activity of nitrofurazone
Pregnancy Risk Factor C

Nitrogard® *see* Nitroglycerin *on this page*
Nitroglicerina (Mexico) *see* Nitroglycerin *on this page*

Nitroglycerin (nye troe gli' ser in)
Related Information
Cardiovascular Diseases *on page 912*
Brand Names Deponit®; Minitran®; Nitro-Bid®; Nitrocine®; Nitrodisc®; Nitro-Dur®; Nitrogard®; Nitroglyn®; Nitrol®; Nitrolingual®; Nitrong®; Nitrostat®; Transdermal-NTG®; Transderm-Nitro®; Tridil®
Canadian/Mexican Brand Names Cardinit® (Mexico); Nitradisc® (Mexico); Nitroderm-TTS® (Mexico)
Therapeutic Category Antianginal Agent; Nitrate; Vasodilator, Coronary
Synonyms Nitroglicerina (Mexico)
(Continued)

Nitroglycerin *(Continued)*

Use Treatment of angina pectoris; I.V. for congestive heart failure (especially when associated with acute myocardial infarction); pulmonary hypertension; hypertensive emergencies occurring perioperatively (especially during cardiovascular surgery)

Usual Dosage Note: Hemodynamic and antianginal tolerance often develop within 24-48 hours of continuous nitrate administration

Children: Pulmonary hypertension: Continuous infusion: Start 0.25-0.5 mcg/kg/minute and titrate by 1 mcg/kg/minute at 20- to 60-minute intervals to desired effect; usual dose: 1-3 mcg/kg/minute; maximum: 5 mcg/kg/minute

Adults:

Buccal: Initial: 1 mg every 3-5 hours while awake (3 times/day); titrate dosage upward if angina occurs with tablet in place

Oral: 2.5-9 mg 2-4 times/day (up to 26 mg 4 times/day)

I.V.: 5 mcg/minute, increase by 5 mcg/minute every 3-5 minutes to 20 mcg/minute; if no response at 20 mcg/minute increase by 10 mcg/minute every 3-5 minutes, up to 200 mcg/minute

Ointment: 1" to 2" every 8 hours up to 4" to 5" every 4 hours

Patch, transdermal: 0.2-0.4 mg/hour initially and titrate to doses of 0.4-0.8 mg/hour; tolerance is minimized by using a patch-on period of 12-14 hours and patch-off period of 10-12 hours

Sublingual: 0.2-0.6 mg every 5 minutes for maximum of 3 doses in 15 minutes; may also use prophylactically 5-10 minutes prior to activities which may provoke an attack

Translingual: 1-2 sprays into mouth under tongue every 3-5 minutes for maximum of 3 doses in 15 minutes, may also be used 5-10 minutes prior to activities which may provoke an attack prophylactically

May need to use nitrate-free interval (10-12 hours/day) to avoid tolerance development; tolerance may possibly be reversed with acetylcysteine; gradually decrease dose in patients receiving NTG for prolonged period to avoid withdrawal reaction

Mechanism of Action Reduces cardiac oxygen demand by decreasing left ventricular pressure and systemic vascular resistance; dilates coronary arteries and improves collateral flow to ischemic regions

Local Anesthetic/Vasoconstrictor Precautions No information available to require special precautions

Effects on Dental Treatment No effects or complications reported

Other Adverse Effects

>10%:

Cardiovascular: Postural hypotension

Central nervous system: Headache, flushing, lightheadedness, dizziness

Neuromuscular & skeletal: Weakness

1% to 10%: Dermatologic: Drug rash, exfoliative dermatitis

<1%:

Cardiovascular: Reflex tachycardia, bradycardia, coronary vascular insufficiency, arrhythmias

Dermatologic: Allergic contact dermatitis, exfoliative dermatitis

Gastrointestinal: Nausea, vomiting

Hematologic: Methemoglobinemia (overdose)

Miscellaneous: Perspiration, collapse, alcohol intoxication

Drug Interactions

Decreased effect: I.V. nitroglycerin may antagonize the anticoagulant effect of heparin, monitor closely; may need to decrease heparin dosage when nitroglycerin is discontinued

Increased toxicity: Alcohol, beta-blockers, calcium channel blockers may enhance nitroglycerin's hypotensive effect

Drug Uptake

Onset and duration of action is dependent upon dosage form administered

Serum half-life: 1-4 minutes

Pregnancy Risk Factor C

Nitroglyn® *see* Nitroglycerin *on previous page*

Nitrol® *see* Nitroglycerin *on previous page*

Nitrolingual® *see* Nitroglycerin *on previous page*

Nitrong® *see* Nitroglycerin *on previous page*

Nitropress® *see* Nitroprusside Sodium *on next page*

Nitroprusside Sodium (nye troe pruss' ide sow' dee um)

Brand Names Nipride®; Nitropress®

Therapeutic Category Vasodilator

Use Management of hypertensive crises; congestive heart failure; used for controlled hypotension to reduce bleeding during surgery

Usual Dosage Administration requires the use of an infusion pump. Average dose: 5 mcg/kg/minute

Children: Pulmonary hypertension: I.V.: Initial: 1 mcg/kg/minute by continuous I.V. infusion; increase in increments of 1 mcg/kg/minute at intervals of 20-60 minutes; titrating to the desired response; usual dose: 3 mcg/kg/minute, rarely need >4 mcg/kg/minute; maximum: 5 mcg/kg/minute.

Adults: I.V.: Initial: 0.3-0.5 mcg/kg/minute; increase in increments of 0.5 mcg/kg/minute, titrating to the desired hemodynamic effect or the appearance of headache or nausea; usual dose: 3 mcg/kg/minute; rarely need >4 mcg/kg/minute; maximum: 10 mcg/kg/minute. When >500 mcg/kg is administered by prolonged infusion of faster than 2 mcg/kg/minute, cyanide is generated faster than an unaided patient can handle.

Mechanism of Action Causes peripheral vasodilation by direct action on venous and arteriolar smooth muscle, thus reducing peripheral resistance; will increase cardiac output by decreasing afterload; reduces aortal and left ventricular impedance

Local Anesthetic/Vasoconstrictor Precautions No information available to require special precautions

Effects on Dental Treatment No effects or complications reported

Other Adverse Effects 1% to 10%:

Cardiovascular: Excessive hypotensive response, palpitations
Central nervous system: Disorientation, psychosis, headache, restlessness
Endocrine & metabolic: Thyroid suppression
Gastrointestinal: Nausea, vomiting
Hematologic: Thiocyanate toxicity
Neuromuscular & skeletal: Weakness, muscle spasm
Otic: Tinnitus
Respiratory: Hypoxia
Miscellaneous: Sweating, substernal distress

Drug Interactions No data reported

Drug Uptake

Onset of hypotensive effect: <2 minutes
Duration: Within 1-10 minutes following discontinuation of therapy, effects cease
Serum half-life:
Parent drug: <10 minutes
Thiocyanate: 2.7-7 days

Pregnancy Risk Factor C

Nitrostat® *see* Nitroglycerin *on page 623*

Nitrous Oxide (nye' trus ok' side)

Related Information

Patients Requiring Sedation *on page 965*

Therapeutic Category Decongestant, Ophthalmic

Use

Dental: To induce sedation and analgesia in anxious dental patients
Medical: A principal adjunct to inhalation and intravenous general anesthesia in medical patients undergoing surgery; prehospital relief of pain of differing etiologies (ie, burns, fractures, back injury, abrasions, lacerations)

Usual Dosage Children and Adults: For sedation and analgesia: Concentrations of 25% to 50% nitrous oxide with oxygen inhaled through the nose via a nasal mask

Mechanism of Action General CNS depressant action; may act similarly as inhalant general anesthetics by mildly stabilizing axonal membranes to partially inhibit action potentials leading to sedation; may partially act on opiate receptor systems to cause mild analgesia

Local Anesthetic/Vasoconstrictor Precautions No information available to require special precautions

Effects on Dental Treatment No effects or complications reported

Other Adverse Effects

An increased risk of renal and hepatic diseases and peripheral neuropathy similar to that of vitamin B_{12} deficiency have been reported in dental personnel who work in areas where nitrous oxide is used

(Continued)

Nitrous Oxide (Continued)

Methionine synthase, a vitamin B$_{12}$ dependent enzyme, is inactivated following very prolonged administration of nitrous oxide, and the subsequent interference with DNA synthesis prevents production of both leukocytes and red blood cells by bone marrow. These effects do not occur within the time frame of clinical sedation

Female dental personnel who were exposed to unscavenged nitrous oxide for more than 5 hours/week were significantly less fertile than women who were not exposed, or who were exposed to lower levels of scavenged or unscavenged nitrous oxide. Fertility was measured by the number of menstrual cycles, without use of contraception, required to become pregnant. Women who were exposed to nitrous oxide for more than 5 hours/week were only 41% as likely as unexposed women to conceive during each monthly cycle.

Oral manifestations: No data reported

Contraindications Nitrous oxide should not be administered without oxygen. Nitrous oxide should not be given to patients after a full meal

Warnings/Precautions Nausea and vomiting occurs postoperatively in ~15% of patients. Prolonged use may produce bone marrow suppression and/or neurologic dysfunction. Oxygen should be briefly administered during emergence from prolonged anesthesia with nitrous oxide to prevent diffusion hypoxia. Patients with vitamin B$_{12}$ deficiency (pernicious anemia) and those with other nutritional deficiencies (alcoholics) are at increased risk of developing neurologic disease and bone marrow suppression with exposure to nitrous oxide. May be addictive

Drug Interactions No data reported

Drug Uptake Nitrous oxide is rapidly absorbed via inhalation. The blood/gas partition coefficient is 0.5. The gas is rapidly eliminated via the lungs, with minimal amounts eliminated through the skin.

Onset time: Inhalation: 5-10 minutes

Pregnancy Risk Factor No data reported

Breast-feeding Considerations No data reported

Dosage Forms Supplied in blue cylinders

Dietary Considerations No data reported

Comments Results of a mail survey of more than 30,000 dentists and 30,000 chairside assistants, who were exposed to trace anesthetics in dental operatories were published in 1980 (Cohen et al, 1980). This study suggested that long-term exposure to nitrous oxide and to nitrous oxide/halogenated anesthetics was associated with an increase in general health problems and reproductive difficulties in these dental personnel. Schuyt et al (1986) observed that 4 female dental personnel who were exposed to inhalation sedation with 35% nitrous oxide reported 6 spontaneous abortions among 7 pregnancies over 17 months

Selected Readings

Baird PA, "Occupational Exposure to Nitrous Oxide - Not a Laughing Matter," *N Engl J Med*, 1992, 327(14):1026-7.

Cohen EN, Gift HC, Brown BW, et al, "Occupational Disease in Dentistry and Chronic Exposure to Trace Anesthetic Gases," *J Am Dent Assoc*, 1980, 101(1):21-31.

Rowland AS, Baird DD, Weinberg CR, et al, "Reduced Fertility Among Women Employed as Female Dental Assistants Exposed to High Levels of Nitrous Oxide," *N Engl J Med*, 1992, 327(14):993-7.

Schuyt HC, Brakel K, Oostendorp SG, et al, "Abortions Among Dental Personnel Exposed to Nitrous Oxide," *Anaesthesia*, 1986, 41(1):82-3.

Wynn RL, "Nitrous Oxide and Fertility, Part I," *Gen Dent*, 1993, 41(2):122-3.

Wynn RL, "Nitrous Oxide and Fertility, Part II," *Gen Dent*, 1993, 41(3):212, 214.

Nix™ [OTC] see Permethrin on page 676

Nizatidina (Mexico) see Nizatidine on this page

Nizatidine (ni za' ti deen)

Brand Names Axid®

Therapeutic Category Histamine-2 Antagonist

Synonyms Nizatidina (Mexico)

Use Treatment and maintenance of duodenal ulcer; treatment of gastroesophageal reflux disease (GERD)

Usual Dosage Adults: Active duodenal ulcer: Oral:

Treatment: 300 mg at bedtime or 150 mg twice daily

Maintenance: 150 mg/day

Mechanism of Action Nizatidine is an H$_2$-receptor antagonist. In healthy volunteers, nizatidine has been effective in suppressing gastric acid secretion induced by pentagastrin infusion or food. Nizatidine reduces gastric acid secretion by 29.4% to 78.4%. This compares with a 60.3% reduction by cimetidine.

Nizatidine 100 mg is reported to provide equivalent acid suppression as cimetidine 300 mg.

Local Anesthetic/Vasoconstrictor Precautions No information available to require special precautions

Effects on Dental Treatment No effects or complications reported

Other Adverse Effects

1% to 10%:

Central nervous system: Dizziness, headache

Gastrointestinal: Constipation, diarrhea

<1%:

Cardiovascular: Bradycardia, tachycardia, palpitations, hypertension

Central nervous system: Fever, dizziness, weakness, fatigue, seizures, insomnia, drowsiness

Dermatologic: Acne, pruritus, urticaria, dry skin

Gastrointestinal: Abdominal discomfort, flatulence, belching, anorexia

Hematologic: Agranulocytosis, neutropenia, thrombocytopenia

Hepatic: Increases in AST, ALT

Neuromuscular & skeletal: Paresthesia

Renal: Increases in BUN, creatinine; proteinuria

Respiratory: Bronchospasm

Miscellaneous: Allergic reaction

Drug Interactions No data reported

Pregnancy Risk Factor C

Nizoral® see Ketoconazole on page 481

N-Methylhydrazine see Procarbazine Hydrochloride on page 727

Noctec® see Chloral Hydrate on page 180

Nolahist® [OTC] see Phenindamine Tartrate on page 680

Nolamine® see Chlorpheniramine, Phenindamine, and Phenylpropanolamine on page 192

Nolex® LA see Guaifenesin and Phenylpropanolamine on page 409

Nolvadex® see Tamoxifen Citrate on page 818

Nonoxynol 9 (non oks' i nole nine)

Brand Names Because® [OTC]; Delfen® [OTC]; Emko® [OTC]; Encare® [OTC]; Gynol II® [OTC]; Intercept™ [OTC]; Koromex® [OTC]; Ramses® [OTC]; Semicid® [OTC]; Shur-Seal® [OTC]

Therapeutic Category Spermicide

Use Spermatocide in contraception

Local Anesthetic/Vasoconstrictor Precautions No information available to require special precautions

Effects on Dental Treatment No effects or complications reported

Nonsteroidal Anti-Inflammatory Agents, Comparative Dosages, and Pharmacokinetics see page 1021

Nonviral Infectious Diseases see page 932

Norcet® [5/500] see Hydrocodone and Acetaminophen on page 431

Nordette® see Ethinyl Estradiol and Levonorgestrel on page 337

Nordryl® see Diphenhydramine Hydrochloride on page 288

Norethin™ 1/35E see Ethinyl Estradiol and Norethindrone on page 339

Norethin™ 1/50M see Mestranol and Norethindrone on page 547

Norethindrone (nor eth in' drone)

Related Information

Endocrine Disorders & Pregnancy on page 927

Brand Names Aygestin®; Micronor®; Norlutate®; Norlutin®; Nor-Q.D.®

Canadian/Mexican Brand Names Syngestal® (Mexico)

Therapeutic Category Contraceptive, Oral; Contraceptive, Progestin Only; Progestin Derivative

Synonyms Noretindrona (Mexico)

Use Treatment of amenorrhea; abnormal uterine bleeding; endometriosis, oral contraceptive; **higher rate of failure with progestin only contraceptives**

Mechanism of Action Inhibits secretion of pituitary gonadotropin (LH) which prevents follicular maturation and ovulation

Local Anesthetic/Vasoconstrictor Precautions No information available to require special precautions

Effects on Dental Treatment Caution is not required in prescribing antibiotics to female dental patients taking progestin only contraceptives since there is no interaction with the progesterone ingredient

(Continued)

Norethindrone *(Continued)*

Other Adverse Effects

>10%:

Cardiovascular: Edema

Central nervous system: Weakness

Endocrine & metabolic: Breakthrough bleeding, spotting, changes in menstrual flow, amenorrhea

Gastrointestinal: Anorexia

1% to 10%:

Cardiovascular: Embolism, central thrombosis

Central nervous system: Mental depression, fever, insomnia

Dermatologic: Melasma or chloasma, allergic rash with or without pruritus

Endocrine & metabolic: Changes in cervical erosion and secretions, weight gain or loss, increased breast tenderness

Hepatic: Cholestatic jaundice

Local: Thrombophlebitis

Drug Interactions Decreased effect: Aminoglutethimide may decrease effects by increasing hepatic metabolism

Pregnancy Risk Factor X

Noretindrona (Mexico) *see* Norethindrone *on previous page*

Norflex™ *see* Orphenadrine Citrate *on page 640*

Norfloxacin *(nor flox' a sin)*

Brand Names Chibroxin™; Noroxin®

Canadian/Mexican Brand Names Floxacin® (Mexico); Oranor® (Mexico)

Therapeutic Category Antibiotic, Quinolone

Synonyms Norfloxacina (Mexico)

Use Complicated and uncomplicated urinary tract infections caused by susceptible gram-negative and gram-positive bacteria; ophthalmic solution for conjunctivitis

Usual Dosage

Ophthalmic: Children >1 year and Adults: Instill 1-2 drops in affected eye(s) 4 times/day for up to 7 days

Oral: Adults:

Urinary tract infections: 400 mg twice daily for 3-21 days depending on severity of infection or organism sensitivity; maximum: 800 mg/day

Uncomplicated gonorrhea: 800 mg as a single dose (CDC recommends as an alternative regimen to ciprofloxacin or ofloxacin)

Prostatitis: 400 mg every 12 hours for 4 weeks

Mechanism of Action Norfloxacin is a DNA gyrase inhibitor. DNA gyrase is an essential bacterial enzyme that maintains the superhelical structure of DNA. DNA gyrase is required for DNA replication and transcription, DNA repair, recombination, and transposition; bactericidal

Local Anesthetic/Vasoconstrictor Precautions No information available to require special precautions

Effects on Dental Treatment No effects or complications reported

Other Adverse Effects

1% to 10%:

Central nervous system: Headache, dizziness, fatigue

Gastrointestinal: Nausea

<1%:

Central nervous system: Somnolence, depression, insomnia, fever, asthenia

Dermatologic: Pruritus, hyperhidrosis, erythema, rash

Gastrointestinal: Abdominal pain, dyspepsia, constipation, flatulence, heartburn, dry mouth, diarrhea, vomiting, loose stools, anorexia, bitter taste, GI bleeding

Hepatic: Increased liver enzymes

Neuromuscular & skeletal: Back pain

Renal: Increased serum creatinine and BUN, acute renal failure

Drug Interactions

Decreased effect: Decreased absorption with antacids containing aluminum, magnesium, and/or calcium (by up to 98% if given at the same time)

Increased toxicity/serum levels: Quinolones cause increased levels of caffeine, warfarin, cyclosporine, and theophylline; azlocillin, cimetidine, probenecid increase quinolone levels

Drug Uptake

Absorption: Oral: Rapid, up to 40%

Serum half-life: 4.8 hours (can be higher with reduced glomerular filtration rates)

Time to peak serum concentration: Within 1-2 hours

Pregnancy Risk Factor C

Norfloxacina (Mexico) *see* Norfloxacin *on previous page*

Norgesic® *see* Orphenadrine, Aspirin, and Caffeine *on page 640*

Norgesic® Forte *see* Orphenadrine, Aspirin, and Caffeine *on page 640*

Norgestimate and Ethinyl Estradiol *see* Ethinyl Estradiol and Norgestimate *on page 340*

Norgestrel (nor jes' trel)
Related Information
Endocrine Disorders & Pregnancy *on page 927*
Brand Names Ovrette®
Therapeutic Category Contraceptive, Oral; Progestin Derivative
Use Prevention of pregnancy; **progestin only products have higher risk of failure in contraceptive use**
Usual Dosage Administer daily, starting the first day of menstruation, take one tablet at the same time each day, every day of the year. If one dose is missed, take as soon as remembered, then next tablet at regular time; if two doses are missed, take one tablet and discard the other, then take daily at usual time; if three doses are missed, use an additional form of birth control until menses or pregnancy is ruled out
Mechanism of Action Inhibits secretion of pituitary gonadotropin (LH) which prevents follicular maturation and ovulation
Local Anesthetic/Vasoconstrictor Precautions No information available to require special precautions
Effects on Dental Treatment Caution is not required in prescribing antibiotics to female dental patients taking progestin only contraceptives since there is no interaction with the progesterone ingredient
Other Adverse Effects
>10%:
Cardiovascular: Edema
Central nervous system: Weakness
Endocrine & metabolic: Breakthrough bleeding, spotting, changes in menstrual flow, amenorrhea
Gastrointestinal: Anorexia
1% to 10%:
Cardiovascular: Embolism, central thrombosis
Central nervous system: Mental depression, fever, insomnia
Dermatologic: Melasma or chloasma, allergic rash with or without pruritus
Endocrine & metabolic: Changes in cervical erosion and secretions, weight gain or loss, increased breast tenderness
Hepatic: Cholestatic jaundice
Local: Thrombophlebitis
Drug Interactions Decreased effect: Aminoglutethimide may decrease effects by increasing hepatic metabolism
Pregnancy Risk Factor X

Norinyl® 1+35 *see* Ethinyl Estradiol and Norethindrone *on page 339*

Norinyl® 1+50 *see* Mestranol and Norethindrone *on page 547*

Norisodrine® *see* Isoproterenol *on page 472*

Norlutate® *see* Norethindrone *on page 627*

Norlutin® *see* Norethindrone *on page 627*

Normodyne® *see* Labetalol Hydrochloride *on page 486*

Noroxin® *see* Norfloxacin *on previous page*

Norpace® *see* Disopyramide Phosphate *on page 292*

Norpanth® *see* Propantheline Bromide *on page 736*

Norplant® *see* Levonorgestrel *on page 497*

Norpramin® *see* Desipramine Hydrochloride *on page 257*

Nor-Q.D.® *see* Norethindrone *on page 627*

Nortriptilina Clorhidrato De (Mexico) *see* Nortriptyline Hydrochloride *on this page*

Nortriptyline Hydrochloride (nor trip' ti leen hye droe klor' ide)
Brand Names Aventyl® Hydrochloride; Pamelor®
Therapeutic Category Antidepressant, Tricyclic
Synonyms Nortriptilina Clorhidrato De (Mexico)
Use Treatment of various forms of depression, often in conjunction with psychotherapy. Maximum antidepressant effect may not be seen for 2 or more weeks after initiation of therapy; has also demonstrated effectiveness for chronic pain. (Continued)

Nortriptyline Hydrochloride *(Continued)*

Usual Dosage Oral:
   Nocturnal enuresis:
      Children:
         6-7 years (20-25 kg): 10 mg/day
         8-11 years (25-35 kg): 10-20 mg/day
         >11 years (35-54 kg): 25-35 mg/day
   Depression:
      Adolescents: 30-50 mg/day in divided doses
      Adults: 25 mg 3-4 times/day up to 150 mg/day
      Elderly:
         Initial: 10-25 mg at bedtime
         Dosage can be increased by 25 mg every 3 days for inpatients and weekly
            for outpatients if tolerated
         Usual maintenance dose: 75 mg as a single bedtime dose, however, lower
            or higher doses may be required to stay within the therapeutic window

Mechanism of Action Traditionally believed to increase the synaptic concentration of serotonin and/or norepinephrine in the central nervous system by inhibition of their reuptake by the presynaptic neuronal membrane. However, additional receptor effects have been found including desensitization of adenyl cyclase, down regulation of beta-adrenergic receptors, and down regulation of serotonin receptors.

Local Anesthetic/Vasoconstrictor Precautions Use with caution; epinephrine, norepinephrine and levonordefrin have been shown to have an increased pressor response in combination with TCAs

Effects on Dental Treatment Long-term treatment with TCAs such as amoxapine increases the risk of caries by reducing salivation and salivary buffer capacity

Other Adverse Effects
   Neuromuscular & skeletal: Tremor

   >10%:
      Central nervous system: Dizziness, drowsiness, headache, weakness
      Gastrointestinal: Dry mouth, constipation, increased appetite, nausea, unpleasant taste, weight gain
   1% to 10%:
      Anticholinergic: Dry mouth, blurred vision, constipation, urinary retention, increased intraocular pressure
      Cardiovascular: Postural hypotension, arrhythmias, tachycardia, sudden death
      Central nervous system: Confusion, delirium, hallucinations, nervousness, restlessness, parkinsonian syndrome, excessive sweating, insomnia
      Gastrointestinal: Diarrhea, heartburn
      Genitourinary: Difficult urination, sexual dysfunction
      Ocular: Blurred vision, eye pain
      Neuromuscular & skeletal: Fine muscle tremors
   <1%:
      Central nervous system: Anxiety, seizures
      Dermatologic: Alopecia, photosensitivity
      Endocrine & metabolic: Breast enlargement, galactorrhea, SIADH
      Genitourinary: Testicular swelling
      Hematologic: Leukopenia, rarely agranulocytosis, eosinophilia
      Hepatic: Increased liver enzymes, cholestatic jaundice
      Ocular: Increased intraocular pressure
      Otic: Tinnitus
      Miscellaneous: Allergic reactions, trouble with gums, decreased lower esophageal sphincter tone may cause GE reflux

Drug Interactions Blocks the uptake of guanethidine and thus prevents the hypotensive effect of guanethidine; may be additive with or may potentiate the action of other CNS depressants such as sedatives or hypnotics; potentiates the pressor and cardiac effects of sympathomimetic agents such as isoproterenol, epinephrine, etc; with MAO inhibitors, hyperpyrexia, hypertension, tachycardia, confusion, seizures, and death have been reported; anticholinergic effect seen with other anticholinergic agents; cimetidine reduces the metabolism of nortriptyline; may increase the prothrombin time in patients stabilized on warfarin

Drug Uptake
   Onset of action: 1-3 weeks before therapeutic effects are seen
   Serum half-life: 28-31 hours
   Time to peak serum concentration: Oral: Within 7-8.5 hours

Pregnancy Risk Factor D

ALPHABETICAL LISTING OF DRUGS

Selected Readings

Boakes AJ, Laurence DR, Teoh PC, et al, "Interactions Between Sympathomimetic Amines and Antidepressant Agents in Man," *Br Med J*, 1973, 1(849):311-5.

Jastak JT and Yagiela JA, "Vasoconstrictors and Local Anesthesia: A Review and Rationale for Use," *J Am Dent Assoc*, 1983, 107(4):623-30.

Larochelle P, Hamet P, and Enjalbert M, "Responses to Tyramine and Norepinephrine After Imipramine and Trazodone," *Clin Pharmacol Ther*, 1979, 26(1):24-30.

Mitchell JR, "Guanethidine and Related Agents. III Antagonism by Drugs Which Inhibit the Norepinephrine Pump in Man," *J Clin Invest*, 1970, 49(8):1596-604.

Rundegren J, van Dijken J, Mörnstad H, et al, "Oral Conditions in Patients Receiving Long-Term Treatment With Cyclic Antidepressant Drugs," *Swed Dent J*, 1985, 9(2):55-64.

Svedmyr N, "The Influence of a Tricyclic Antidepressive Agent (Protriptyline) on Some of the Circulatory Effects of Noradrenaline and Adrenalin in Man," *Life Sci*, 1968, 7(1):77-84.

Norvasc® see Amlodipine on page 53

Norvir® see Ritonavir on page 773

Nōstrilla® see Oxymetazoline Hydrochloride on page 649

Nōstrilla® Long Acting Nasal Solution [OTC] see Oxymetazoline Hydrochloride on page 649

Nostril® Nasal Solution [OTC] see Phenylephrine Hydrochloride on page 685

Novacet® Topical see Sulfur and Sodium Sulfacetamide on page 813

Novafed® see Pseudoephedrine on page 749

Novahistine® DH see Chlorpheniramine, Pseudoephedrine, and Codeine on page 195

Novahistine® Elixir [OTC] see Chlorpheniramine and Phenylephrine on page 190

Novahistine® Expectorant see Guaifenesin, Pseudoephedrine, and Codeine on page 410

Novantrone® see Mitoxantrone Hydrochloride on page 586

Novocain® see Procaine Hydrochloride on page 727

Novolin® 70/30 see Insulin Preparations on page 459

Novolin® L see Insulin Preparations on page 459

Novolin® N see Insulin Preparations on page 459

Novolin® R see Insulin Preparations on page 459

NP-27® [OTC] see Tolnaftate on page 855

NPH Iletin® I see Insulin Preparations on page 459

NPH Insulin see Insulin Preparations on page 459

NPH-N see Insulin Preparations on page 459

NSC-102816 see Azacitidine on page 88

NTZ® Nasal Solution [OTC] see Oxymetazoline Hydrochloride on page 649

Nubain® see Nalbuphine Hydrochloride on page 600

Nucofed® see Guaifenesin, Pseudoephedrine, and Codeine on page 410

Nucofed® Pediatric Expectorant see Guaifenesin, Pseudoephedrine, and Codeine on page 410

Nucotuss® see Guaifenesin, Pseudoephedrine, and Codeine on page 410

Nu-Iron® [OTC] see Polysaccharide-Iron Complex on page 705

Nullo® [OTC] see Chlorophyll on page 185

NuLYTELY® see Polyethylene Glycol-Electrolyte Solution on page 703

Numorphan® see Oxymorphone Hydrochloride on page 651

Numzitdent® [OTC] see Benzocaine on page 102

Numzit Teething® [OTC] see Benzocaine on page 102

Nupercainal® [OTC] see Dibucaine on page 270

Nuprin® [OTC] see Ibuprofen on page 447

Nu-Tears® II Solution [OTC] see Artificial Tears on page 75

Nu-Tears® Solution [OTC] see Artificial Tears on page 75

Nutraplus® [OTC] see Urea on page 884

Nutropin® see Human Growth Hormone on page 426

Nydrazid® see Isoniazid on page 471

Nylidrin Hydrochloride (nye' li drin)

Brand Names Arlidin®

Canadian/Mexican Brand Names PMS-Nylidrin® (Canada)

Therapeutic Category Vasodilator, Peripheral

Use Considered "possibly effective" for increasing blood supply to treat peripheral disease (arteriosclerosis obliterans, diabetic vascular disease, nocturnal leg cramps, Raynaud's disease, frost bite, ischemic ulcer, thrombophlebitis) and circulatory disturbances of the inner ear (cochlear ischemia, macular or ampullar ischemia, etc)

Mechanism of Action Nylidrin is a peripheral vasodilator; this results from direct relaxation of vascular smooth muscle and beta agonist action. Nylidrin (Continued)

Nylidrin Hydrochloride *(Continued)*

does not appear to affect cutaneous blood flow; it reportedly increases heart rate and cardiac output; cutaneous blood flow is not enhanced to any appreciable extent.

Local Anesthetic/Vasoconstrictor Precautions No information available to require special precautions

Effects on Dental Treatment No effects or complications reported

Other Adverse Effects

1% to 10%:
Central nervous system: Nervousness
Neuromuscular & skeletal: Trembling
<1%:
Cardiovascular: Palpitations, postural hypotension
Central nervous system: Dizziness
Gastrointestinal: Nausea, vomiting
Neuromuscular & skeletal: Weakness

Drug Interactions No data reported

Pregnancy Risk Factor C

Nystatin (nye stat' in)

Related Information

Oral Fungal Infections *on page 948*
Patients Undergoing Cancer Therapy *on page 967*

Brand Names Mycostatin®; Nilstat®

Canadian/Mexican Brand Names Mestatin® (Canada); Nadostine® (Canada); Nyaderm® PMS-Nystatin® (Canada); Micostatin® (Mexico); Nistaquim® (Mexico)

Therapeutic Category Antifungal Agent, Oral Nonabsorbed; Antifungal Agent, Topical; Antifungal Agent, Vaginal

Use

Dental: Treatment of susceptible cutaneous, mucocutaneous, and oral cavity fungal infections normally caused by the *Candida* species
Medical: None

Usual Dosage Oral candidiasis: Suspension (swish and swallow orally):
Children and Adults: 400,000-600,000 units 4 times/day; troche: 200,000-400,000 units 4-5 times/day
Adults: 400,000-600,000 units 4 times/day; pastilles: 200,000-400,000 units 4-5 times/day

Mechanism of Action Binds to sterols in fungal cell membrane, changing the cell wall permeability allowing for leakage of cellular contents

Local Anesthetic/Vasoconstrictor Precautions No information available to require special precautions

Effects on Dental Treatment No effects or complications reported

Other Adverse Effects

1% to 10%: Gastrointestinal: Nausea, vomiting, diarrhea, abdominal pain
<1%:
Miscellaneous: Hypersensitivity reactions
Dermatologic: Contact dermatitis, Stevens-Johnson syndrome

Oral manifestations: No data reported

Contraindications Hypersensitivity to nystatin or any component

Drug Interactions No data reported

Drug Uptake

Absorption: Not absorbed through mucous membranes or intact skin; poorly absorbed from GI tract
Onset of symptomatic relief from candidiasis: Within 24-72 hours

Pregnancy Risk Factor B/C (oral)

Breast-feeding Considerations Compatible (not absorbed orally)

Dosage Forms

Powder, for preparation of oral suspension: 50 million units, 1 billion units, 2 billion units, 5 billion units
Suspension, oral: 100,000 units/mL (5 mL, 60 mL, 480 mL)
Tablet: Oral: 500,000 units
Troche: 200,000 units

Dietary Considerations No data reported

Generic Available Yes

Nystatin and Triamcinolone (nye stat' in & trye am sin' oh lone)

Related Information

Oral Fungal Infections *on page 948*

Brand Names Dermacomb®; Mycogen® II; Mycolog®-II; Myconel®; Myco-Triacet® II; Mytrex®; N.G.T.®; Tri-Statin® II

Therapeutic Category Antifungal Agent, Topical; Corticosteroid, Topical (Medium Potency)

Use Treatment of cutaneous candidiasis

Usual Dosage Children and Adults: Topical: Apply sparingly 2-4 times/day

Mechanism of Action Nystatin is an antifungal agent that binds to sterols in fungal cell membrane, changing the cell wall permeability allowing for leakage of cellular contents. Triamcinolone is a synthetic corticosteroid; it decreases inflammation by suppression of migration of polymorphonuclear leukocytes and reversal of increased capillary permeability. It suppresses the immune system reducing activity and volume of the lymphatic system. It suppresses adrenal function at high doses.

Local Anesthetic/Vasoconstrictor Precautions No information available to require special precautions

Effects on Dental Treatment No effects or complications reported

Other Adverse Effects 1% to 10%:
Dermatologic: Dryness, folliculitis, hypertrichosis, acne, hypopigmentation, allergic dermatitis, maceration of the skin, skin atrophy
Local: Burning, itching, irritation
Miscellaneous: Increased incidence of secondary infection

Contraindications Known hypersensitivity to nystatin or triamcinolone

Warnings/Precautions Avoid use of occlusive dressings; limit therapy to least amount necessary for effective therapy, pediatric patients may be more susceptible to HPA axis suppression due to larger BSA to weight ratio

Drug Interactions No data reported

Pregnancy Risk Factor C

Breast-feeding Considerations
Nystatin: Compatible
Triamcinolone: No data reported

Dosage Forms
Cream: Nystatin 100,000 units and triamcinolone acetonide 0.1% (1.5 g, 15 g, 30 g, 60 g, 120 g)
Ointment, topical: Nystatin 100,000 units and triamcinolone acetonide 0.1% (15 g, 30 g, 60 g, 120 g)

Dietary Considerations No data reported

Generic Available Yes

Nytol® [OTC] see Diphenhydramine Hydrochloride on page 288

Occucoat™ see Hydroxypropyl Methylcellulose on page 442

Occupational Exposure to Bloodborne Pathogens (Universal Precautions) see page 1030

OCL® see Polyethylene Glycol-Electrolyte Solution on page 703

Octamide® see Metoclopramide on page 572

Octicair® Otic see Neomycin, Polymyxin B, and Hydrocortisone on page 610

Octocaine® see Lidocaine Hydrochloride on page 502

Octocaine® 50 see Lidocaine and Epinephrine on page 499

Octocaine® 100 see Lidocaine and Epinephrine on page 499

Octreotide Acetate (ok tree' oh tide as' e tate)

Brand Names Sandostatin®

Canadian/Mexican Brand Names Sandostatina® (Mexico)

Therapeutic Category Antisecretory Agent; Somatostatin Analog

Use Control of symptoms in patients with metastatic carcinoid, vasoactive intestinal peptide-secreting tumors (VIPomas), and secretory diarrhea

Usual Dosage Adults: S.C.: Initial: 50 mcg 1-2 times/day and titrate dose based on patient tolerance and response
Carcinoid: 100-600 mcg/day in 2-4 divided doses
VIPomas: 200-300 mcg/day in 2-4 divided doses
Diarrhea: Initial: I.V.: 50-100 mcg every 8 hours; increase by 100 mcg/dose at 48-hour intervals; maximum dose: 500 mcg every 8 hours
Esophageal varices bleeding: I.V. bolus: 25-50 mcg followed by continuous I.V. infusion of 25-50 mcg/hour

Mechanism of Action Mimics natural somatostatin by inhibiting serotonin release, and the secretion of gastrin, VIP, insulin, glucagon, secretin, motilin, and pancreatic polypeptide

Local Anesthetic/Vasoconstrictor Precautions No information available to require special precautions

Effects on Dental Treatment No effects or complications reported
(Continued)

Octreotide Acetate *(Continued)*

Other Adverse Effects
1% to 10%:
  Cardiovascular: Flushing, edema
  Central nervous system: Headache, dizziness, fatigue
  Endocrine & metabolic: Hyperglycemia, hypoglycemia
  Gastrointestinal: Nausea, diarrhea, abdominal pain, vomiting
  Local: Pain at injection site
  Neuromuscular & skeletal: Weakness
  Miscellaneous: Fat malabsorption
<1%:
  Cardiovascular: Chest pain
  Central nervous system: Anxiety, fever
  Dermatologic: Erythema, hair loss, rash
  Endocrine & metabolic: Galactorrhea
  Gastrointestinal: Constipation, flatulence, throat discomfort
  Hepatic: Hepatitis
  Respiratory: Shortness of breath, rhinorrhea
  Ocular: Burning eyes
  Neuromuscular & skeletal: Leg cramps, Bell's palsy

Drug Uptake
Duration of action: 6-12 hours
Absorption:
  Oral: Absorbed but still under study
  S.C.: Rapid
Serum half-life: 60-110 minutes

Pregnancy Risk Factor B

Comments Doses of 1-10 mcg/kg every 12 hours have been used in children beginning at the low end of the range and increasing by 0.3 mcg/kg/dose at 3-day intervals; suppression of growth hormone (animal data) is of concern when used as long-term therapy

Ocu-Carpine® *see* Pilocarpine *on page 691*

OcuCoat® Ophthalmic Solution [OTC] *see* Artificial Tears *on page 75*

OcuCoat® PF Ophthalmic Solution [OTC] *see* Artificial Tears *on page 75*

Ocu-Drop® [OTC] *see* Tetrahydrozoline Hydrochloride *on page 831*

Ocuflox™ *see* Ofloxacin *on this page*

Ocupress® *see* Carteolol Hydrochloride *on page 158*

Ocusert® Pilo *see* Pilocarpine *on page 691*

Ocusert Pilo-20® *see* Pilocarpine *on page 691*

Ocusert Pilo-40® *see* Pilocarpine *on page 691*

Ocutricin® *see* Bacitracin, Neomycin, and Polymyxin B *on page 94*

Ocutricin® HC Otic *see* Neomycin, Polymyxin B, and Hydrocortisone *on page 610*

Ocutricin® Ophthalmic Solution *see* Neomycin, Polymyxin B, and Gramicidin *on page 610*

Ofloxacin *(oh floks' a sin)*

Related Information
Nonviral Infectious Diseases *on page 932*

Brand Names Floxin®; Ocuflox™

Canadian/Mexican Brand Names Bactocin® (Mexico); Floxil® (Mexico); Floxstat® (Mexico)

Therapeutic Category Antibiotic, Quinolone

Synonyms Ofloxacina (Mexico)

Use Quinolone antibiotic for skin and skin structure, lower respiratory and urinary tract infections, and sexually transmitted diseases, bacterial conjunctivitis caused by susceptible organisms

Usual Dosage
Children >1 year and Adults: Ophthalmic: Instill 1-2 drops in affected eye(s) every 2-4 hours for the first 2 days, then use 4 times/day for an additional 5 days

Adults: Oral, I.V.: 200-400 mg every 12 hours for 7-10 days for most infections or for 6 weeks for prostatitis

Mechanism of Action Ofloxacin, a fluorinated quinolone, is a pyridine carboxylic acid derivative which exerts a broad spectrum bactericidal effect. It inhibits DNA gyrase, an essential bacterial enzyme that maintains the superhelical structure of DNA. DNA gyrase is required for DNA replication and transcription, DNA repair, recombination, and transposition within the bacteria.

Local Anesthetic/Vasoconstrictor Precautions No information available to require special precautions

Effects on Dental Treatment No effects or complications reported

Other Adverse Effects

>10%: Gastrointestinal: Nausea

1% to 10%:

Cardiovascular: Chest pain

Central nervous system: Headache, insomnia, dizziness, fatigue, somnolence, sleep disorders, nervousness, pyrexia

Dermatologic: External genital pruritus in women, rash, pruritus

Gastrointestinal: Diarrhea, vomiting, GI distress, pain and cramps, abdominal cramps, flatulence, dysgeusia, dry mouth, decreased appetite

Genitourinary: Vaginitis

Neuromuscular & skeletal: Trunk pain

Ocular: Superinfection (ophthalmic), photophobia, lacrimation, dry eyes, stinging, visual disturbances

<1%:

Cardiovascular: Syncope, edema, hypertension, palpitations, vasodilation

Central nervous system: Anxiety, cognitive change, depression, dream abnormality, euphoria, hallucinations, vertigo, asthenia, chills, malaise, extremity pain

Gastrointestinal: Thirst, weight loss

Neuromuscular & skeletal: Paresthesia

Ocular: Photophobia

Otic: Decreased hearing acuity, tinnitus

Respiratory: Cough

Drug Interactions

Decreased effect: decreased absorption with antacids containing aluminum, magnesium, and/or calcium (by up to 98% if given at the same time)

Increased toxicity/serum levels: Quinolones cause increased caffeine, warfarin, cyclosporine, and theophylline levels; azlocillin, cimetidine, probenecid increase quinolone levels

Drug Uptake

Absorption: Well absorbed; administration with food causes only minor alterations in absorption

Serum half-life, elimination 5-7.5 hours

Pregnancy Risk Factor C

Ofloxacina (Mexico) see Ofloxacin on previous page

Ogen® see Estropipate on page 330

OKT3 see Muromonab-CD3 on page 594

Olanzapine (oh lan' za peen)

Brand Names Zyprexa®

Therapeutic Category Antipsychotic Agent

Use Treatment of manifestations of psychotic disorders

Usual Dosage Adults: Oral: Usual starting dose: 5-10 mg/day, given in a once-a-day dosing schedule; up to a maximum of 20 mg/day

Local Anesthetic/Vasoconstrictor Precautions No information available to require special precautions

Effects on Dental Treatment No effects or complications reported

Pregnancy Risk Factor C

Comments Olanzapine (Zyprexa®) is chemically similar to clozapine (Clozaril®), but without as many side effects. Also, olanzapine (Zyprexa®) does not produce side effects such as Parkinson's disease-like tremors which are associated with other antipsychotics such as haloperidol.

Olsalazine Sodium (ole sal' a zeen sow' dee um)

Brand Names Dipentum®

Therapeutic Category 5-Aminosalicylic Acid Derivative; Anti-inflammatory Agent

Use Maintenance of remission of ulcerative colitis in patients intolerant to sulfasalazine

Usual Dosage Adults: Oral: 1 g/day in 2 divided doses

Mechanism of Action The mechanism of action appears to be topical rather than systemic

Local Anesthetic/Vasoconstrictor Precautions No information available to require special precautions

Effects on Dental Treatment No effects or complications reported

Other Adverse Effects

>10%: Gastrointestinal: Diarrhea, cramps, abdominal pain

(Continued)

Olsalazine Sodium *(Continued)*

1% to 10%:
Central nervous system: Headache, fatigue, depression
Dermatologic: Rash, itching
Gastrointestinal: Nausea, dyspepsia, bloating, anorexia
Neuromuscular & skeletal: Arthralgia
<1%:
Central nervous system: Fever
Gastrointestinal: Bloody diarrhea
Hematologic: Blood dyscrasias
Hepatic: Hepatitis
Drug Interactions No data reported
Drug Uptake
Absorption: <3%; very little intact olsalazine is systemically absorbed
Serum half-life, elimination: 56 minutes or 55 hours depending on the analysis used
Pregnancy Risk Factor C

Omeprazole (oh me′ pray zol)
Brand Names Prilosec™
Canadian/Mexican Brand Names Losec® (Canada); Inhibitron® (Mexico); Ozoken® (Mexico); Prazidec® (Mexico); Ulsen® (Mexico)
Therapeutic Category Gastric Acid Secretion Inhibitor
Synonyms Omeprazol (Mexico)
Use Short-term (4-8 weeks) treatment of severe erosive esophagitis (grade 2 or above), diagnosed by endoscopy and short-term treatment of symptomatic gastroesophageal reflux disease (GERD) poorly responsive to customary medical treatment; pathological hypersecretory conditions; peptic ulcer disease

Unlabeled use: Gastric ulcer therapy and healing NSAID-induced ulcers
Usual Dosage Adults: Oral:
Active duodenal ulcer: 20 mg/day for 4-8 weeks

GERD or severe erosive esophagitis: 20 mg/day for 4-8 weeks

Pathological hypersecretory conditions: 60 mg once daily to start; doses up to 120 mg 3 times/day have been administered; administer daily doses >80 mg in divided doses

Helicobacter pylori: Combination therapy with bismuth subsalicylate, tetracycline, clarithromycin, and H_2 antagonist; or clarithromycin and omeprazole. Adult dose: Oral: 20 mg twice daily

Gastric ulcers: 40 mg/day for 4-8 weeks
Mechanism of Action Suppresses gastric acid secretion by inhibiting the parietal cell H+/K+ ATP pump
Local Anesthetic/Vasoconstrictor Precautions No information available to require special precautions
Effects on Dental Treatment No effects or complications reported
Other Adverse Effects
1% to 10%:
Cardiovascular: Angina, tachycardia, bradycardia, edema
Central nervous system: Headache (7%), dizziness, asthenia
Dermatologic: Rash, urticaria, pruritus, dry skin
Gastrointestinal: Diarrhea, nausea, abdominal pain, vomiting, constipation, anorexia, irritable colon, fecal discoloration, esophageal candidiasis, dry mouth, taste alterations
Genitourinary: Testicular pain, urinary tract infection, urinary frequency
Neuromuscular & skeletal: Back pain, asthenia occurred in more frequently than 1% of patients, muscle cramps, myalgia, joint pain, leg pain
Renal: Pyuria, proteinuria, hematuria, glycosuria
Respiratory: Cough
<1%:
Cardiovascular: Chest pain
Central nervous system: Fever, fatigue, malaise, apathy, somnolence, nervousness, anxiety, pain
Gastrointestinal: Abdominal swelling
Drug Interactions
Cytochrome P-450 1A2 enzyme inducer and cytochrome P-450 IIC enzyme inhibitor
Decreased effect: Decreased ketoconazole; decreased itraconazole because of reduced absorption from gastrointestinal tract

Increased toxicity: Diazepam causes increased half-life; increased digoxin, increased phenytoin, increased warfarin

Drug Uptake
Onset of antisecretory action: Oral: Within 1 hour
Duration: 72 hours
Serum half-life: 30-90 minutes

Pregnancy Risk Factor C

Omeprazol (Mexico) *see* Omeprazole *on previous page*

OmniHIB® *see Haemophilus* b Conjugate Vaccine *on page 414*

Omnipen® *see* Ampicillin *on page 62*

OMS® Oral *see* Morphine Sulfate *on page 590*

Oncaspar® *see* Pegaspargase *on page 662*

Oncovin® Injection *see* Vincristine Sulfate *on page 896*

Ondansetron (on dan' se tron)
Brand Names Zofran®

Therapeutic Category Antiemetic

Use May be prescribed for patients who are refractory to or have severe adverse reactions to standard antiemetic therapy. Ondansetron may be prescribed for young patients (ie, <45 years of age who are more likely to develop extrapyramidal reactions to high-dose metoclopramide) who are to receive highly emetogenic chemotherapeutic agents as listed:

Agents with high emetogenic potential (>90%) (dose/m^2):
Carmustine ≥200 mg
Cisplatin ≥75 mg
Cyclophosphamide ≥1000 mg
Cytarabine ≥1000 mg
Dacarbazine ≥500 mg
Ifosfamide ≥1000 mg
Lomustine ≥60 mg
Mechlorethamine
Pentostatin
Streptozocin

or two agents classified as having high or moderately high emetogenic potential as listed:

Agents with moderately high emetogenic potential (60% to 90%) (dose/m^2):
Carmustine <200 mg
Cisplatin <75 mg
Cyclophosphamide 1000 mg
Cytarabine 250-1000 mg
Dacarbazine <500 mg
Doxorubicin ≥75 mg
Ifosfamide
Lomustine <60 mg
Methotrexate ≥250 mg
Mitomycin
Mitoxantrone
Procarbazine

Ondansetron should not be prescribed for chemotherapeutic agents with a low emetogenic potential (eg, bleomycin, busulfan, cyclophosphamide <1000 mg, etoposide, 5-fluorouracil, vinblastine, vincristine)

Usual Dosage
Oral:
Children 4-11 years: 4 mg 30 minutes before chemotherapy; repeat 4 and 8 hours after initial dose
Children >11 years and Adults: 8 mg 30 minutes before chemotherapy; repeat 4 and 8 hours after initial dose or every 8 hours for a maximum of 48 hours

I.V.: Administer either three 0.15 mg/kg doses or a single 32 mg dose; with the 3-dose regimen, the initial dose is given 30 minutes prior to chemotherapy with subsequent doses administered 4 and 8 hours after the first dose. With the single-dose regimen 32 mg is infused over 15 minutes beginning 30 minutes before the start of emetogenic chemotherapy. Dosage should be calculated based on weight:
Children: Pediatric dosing should follow the manufacturer's guidelines for 0.15 mg/kg/dose administered 30 minutes prior to chemotherapy, 4 and 8 hours after the first dose. While not as yet FDA-approved, literature
(Continued)

Ondansetron *(Continued)*

supports the day's total dose administered as a single dose 30 minutes prior to chemotherapy.

Adults:

>80 kg: 12 mg IVPB

45-80 kg: 8 mg IVPB

<45 kg: 0.15 mg/kg/dose IVPB

Mechanism of Action Selective 5-HT$_3$ receptor antagonist, blocking serotonin, both peripherally on vagal nerve terminals and centrally in the chemoreceptor trigger zone

Local Anesthetic/Vasoconstrictor Precautions No information available to require special precautions

Effects on Dental Treatment No effects or complications reported

Other Adverse Effects

>10%:

Central nervous system: Headache, fever

Gastrointestinal: Constipation, diarrhea

1% to 10%:

Central nervous system: Dizziness, weakness

Gastrointestinal: Abdominal cramps, dry mouth

<1%:

Cardiovascular: Tachycardia

Central nervous system: Lightheadedness, seizures

Dermatologic: Rash

Endocrine & metabolic: Hypokalemia

Hepatic: Transient elevations in serum levels of aminotransferases and bilirubin

Respiratory: Bronchospasm, shortness of breath, wheezing

Drug Interactions

Decreased effect: Metabolized by the hepatic cytochrome P-450 enzymes; therefore, the drug's clearance and half-life may be changed with concomitant use of cytochrome P-450 inducers (eg, barbiturates, carbamazepine, rifampin, phenytoin, and phenylbutazone)

Increased toxicity: Inhibitors (eg, cimetidine, allopurinol, and disulfiram)

Drug Uptake

Serum half-life:

Children <15 years: 2-3 hours

Adults: 4 hours

Pregnancy Risk Factor B

Ony-Clear® Nail *see* Triacetin *on page 862*

OP-CCK *see* Sincalide *on page 789*

Opcon® *see* Naphazoline Hydrochloride *on page 605*

o,p′-DDD *see* Mitotane *on page 585*

Ophthacet® *see* Sodium Sulfacetamide *on page 793*

Ophthaine® *see* Proparacaine Hydrochloride *on page 737*

Ophthalgan® Ophthalmic *see* Glycerin *on page 402*

Ophthetic® *see* Proparacaine Hydrochloride *on page 737*

Ophthochlor® *see* Chloramphenicol *on page 182*

Ophthocort® Ophthalmic *see* Chloramphenicol, Polymyxin B, and Hydrocortisone *on page 183*

Opium Alkaloids *(oh′ pee um al′ ka loyds)*

Brand Names Pantopon®

Therapeutic Category Analgesic, Narcotic

Use For relief of severe pain

Local Anesthetic/Vasoconstrictor Precautions No information available to require special precautions

Effects on Dental Treatment 1% to 10% of patients will experience significant dry mouth

Other Adverse Effects

>10%:

Neuromuscular & skeletal: Weakness

Central nervous system: Tiredness, drowsiness, dizziness

Gastrointestinal: Nausea, vomiting

Cardiovascular: Hypotension

1% to 10%:

Central nervous system: Nervousness, headache, confusion restlessness, malaise

   Gastrointestinal: Anorexia, stomach cramps, dry mouth, constipation, biliary
     tract spasm
   Genitourinary: Ureteral spasms, decreased urination
   Local: Pain at injection site
   Respiratory: Troubled breathing, shortness of breath
  <1%:
   Central nervous system: Mental depression, paradoxical CNS stimulation,
     hallucinations
   Dermatologic: Skin rash, hives
   Gastrointestinal: Paralytic ileus
   Ocular: Intracranial pressure (increased)
   Miscellaneous: Histamine release, physical and psychological dependence
Comments Abrupt discontinuation after sustained use (generally >10 days)
may cause withdrawal symptoms

Opium Tincture (oh' pee um tingk' chur)
Therapeutic Category Analgesic, Narcotic; Antidiarrheal
Use Treatment of diarrhea or relief of pain
Usual Dosage Oral:
  Children:
   Diarrhea: 0.005-0.01 mL/kg/dose every 3-4 hours for a maximum of 6 doses/
     24 hours
   Analgesia: 0.01-0.02 mL/kg/dose every 3-4 hours
  Adults:
   Diarrhea: 0.3-1 mL/dose every 2-6 hours to maximum of 6 mL/24 hours
   Analgesia: 0.6-1.5 mL/dose every 3-4 hours
Mechanism of Action Contains many narcotic alkaloids including morphine;
its mechanism for gastric motility inhibition is primarily due to this morphine
content; it results in a decrease in digestive secretions, an increase in GI
muscle tone, and therefore a reduction in GI propulsion
Local Anesthetic/Vasoconstrictor Precautions No information available to
require special precautions
Effects on Dental Treatment No effects or complications reported
Other Adverse Effects
  >10%:
   Cardiovascular: Palpitations, hypotension, bradycardia
   Central nervous system: Weakness, drowsiness, dizziness
  1% to 10%:
   Central nervous system: Restlessness, headache, malaise
   Genitourinary: Decreased urination
   Miscellaneous: Histamine release
  <1%:
   Cardiovascular: Peripheral vasodilation
   Central nervous system: CNS depression, increased intracranial pressure,
     insomnia, mental depression
   Gastrointestinal: Nausea, vomiting, constipation, anorexia, stomach cramps
   Ocular: Miosis
   Respiratory: Respiratory depression
   Miscellaneous: Physical and psychological dependence, biliary or urinary
     tract spasm
Drug Interactions
  Decreased effect: Phenothiazines may antagonize the analgesic effect of
   opiate agonists
  Increased toxicity: CNS depressants, MAO inhibitors, tricyclic antidepressants
   may potentiate the effects of opiate agonists; dextroamphetamine may
   enhance the analgesic effect of opiate agonists
Drug Uptake
  Duration of effect: 4-5 hours
  Absorption: Variable from GI tract
Pregnancy Risk Factor B (D if used for prolonged periods or in high doses at
term)

Optigene® [OTC] *see* Tetrahydrozoline Hydrochloride *on page 831*
Optimine® *see* Azatadine Maleate *on page 89*
Optimoist® [OTC] *see* Saliva Substitute *on page 778*
OptiPranolol® *see* Metipranolol Hydrochloride *on page 572*
Optised® **Ophthalmic** [OTC] *see* Phenylephrine and Zinc Sulfate *on page 685*
OPV *see* Poliovirus Vaccine, Live, Trivalent, Oral *on page 702*
Orabase®-**B** [OTC] *see* Benzocaine *on page 102*
Orabase® **HCA** *see* Hydrocortisone *on page 436*

Orabase®-O [OTC] *see* Benzocaine *on page 102*

Orabase® Plain [OTC] *see* Gelatin, Pectin, and Methylcellulose *on page 395*

Orabase® With Benzocaine [OTC] *see* Benzocaine, Gelatin, Pectin, and Sodium Carboxymethylcellulose *on page 103*

Orajel® Brace-Aid Oral Anesthetic [OTC] *see* Benzocaine *on page 102*

Orajel® Brace-Aid Rinse [OTC] *see* Carbamide Peroxide *on page 152*

Orajel® Maximum Strength [OTC] *see* Benzocaine *on page 102*

Orajel® Mouth-Aid [OTC] *see* Benzocaine *on page 102*

Oral Bacterial Infections *see page 945*

Oral Fungal Infections *see page 948*

Oral Nonviral Soft Tissue Ulcerations or Erosions *see page 955*

Oral Pain *see page 940*

Oral Rinse Products *see page 1067*

Oral Viral Infections *see page 951*

Oraminic® II *see* Brompheniramine Maleate *on page 124*

Oramorph SR™ Oral *see* Morphine Sulfate *on page 590*

Orap™ *see* Pimozide *on page 694*

Orasept® [OTC] *see* Benzocaine *on page 102*

Orasol® [OTC] *see* Benzocaine *on page 102*

Orasone® *see* Prednisone *on page 719*

Oratect® [OTC] *see* Benzocaine *on page 102*

Orazinc® [OTC] *see* Zinc Supplements *on page 909*

Ordrine AT® Extended Release Capsule *see* Caramiphen and Phenylpropanolamine *on page 150*

Oretic® *see* Hydrochlorothiazide *on page 430*

Oreton® Methyl *see* Methyltestosterone *on page 570*

Orexin® [OTC] *see* Vitamin B Complex *on page 899*

Orfenadrina (Mexico) *see* Orphenadrine Citrate *on this page*

Organidin® *see* Iodinated Glycerol *on page 465*

Orimune® *see* Poliovirus Vaccine, Live, Trivalent, Oral *on page 702*

Orinase® *see* Tolbutamide *on page 853*

ORLAAM® *see* Levomethadyl Acetate Hydrochloride *on page 496*

Ormazine *see* Chlorpromazine Hydrochloride *on page 195*

Ornade® Spansule® *see* Chlorpheniramine and Phenylpropanolamine *on page 190*

Orphenadrine, Aspirin, and Caffeine
(or fen' a dreen, as' pir in, & kaf' een)

Brand Names Norgesic® Forte; Norgesic®

Therapeutic Category Analgesic, Non-narcotic; Muscle Relaxant; Skeletal Muscle Relaxant

Use Relief of discomfort associated with skeletal muscular conditions

Local Anesthetic/Vasoconstrictor Precautions No information available to require special precautions

Effects on Dental Treatment The peripheral anticholinergic effects of orphenadrine may decrease or inhibit salivary flow; normal salivation will return with cessation of drug therapy

Orphenadrine Citrate (or fen' a dreen sit' rate)

Related Information
Temporomandibular Dysfunction (TMD) *on page 963*

Brand Names Norflex™

Therapeutic Category Muscle Relaxant; Skeletal Muscle Relaxant

Synonyms Orfenadrina (Mexico)

Use Treatment of muscle spasm associated with acute painful musculoskeletal conditions; supportive therapy in tetanus

Usual Dosage Adults:
Oral: 100 mg twice daily
I.M., I.V.: 60 mg every 12 hours

Mechanism of Action Indirect skeletal muscle relaxant thought to work by central atropine-like effects; has some euphorgenic and analgesic properties

Local Anesthetic/Vasoconstrictor Precautions No information available to require special precautions

Effects on Dental Treatment The peripheral anticholinergic effects of orphenadrine may decrease or inhibit salivary flow; normal salivation will return with cessation of drug therapy

Other Adverse Effects
>10%:
Central nervous system: Drowsiness, dizziness
Ocular: Blurred vision
1% to 10%:
Cardiovascular: Flushing of face, tachycardia
Central nervous system: Weakness, fainting
Dermatologic: Skin rash
Gastrointestinal: Nausea, vomiting, constipation
Genitourinary: Decreased urination
Ocular: Nystagmus, increased intraocular pressure
Respiratory: Nasal congestion
<1%:
Central nervous system: Hallucinations
Hematologic: Aplastic anemia
Drug Interactions No data reported
Drug Uptake
Duration: 4-6 hours
Serum half-life: 14-16 hours
Pregnancy Risk Factor C

Ortho-Cept® see Ethinyl Estradiol and Desogestrel *on page 335*
Orthoclone® OKT3 see Muromonab-CD3 *on page 594*
Ortho-Cyclen® see Ethinyl Estradiol and Norgestimate *on page 340*
Ortho® Dienestrol see Dienestrol *on page 275*
Ortho-Est® see Estropipate *on page 330*
Ortho-Novum™ 1/35 see Ethinyl Estradiol and Norethindrone *on page 339*
Ortho-Novum™ 1/50 see Mestranol and Norethindrone *on page 547*
Ortho-Novum™ 7/7/7 see Ethinyl Estradiol and Norethindrone *on page 339*
Ortho-Novum™ 10/11 see Ethinyl Estradiol and Norethindrone *on page 339*
Ortho Tri-Cyclen® see Ethinyl Estradiol and Norgestimate *on page 340*
Or-Tyl® see Dicyclomine Hydrochloride *on page 273*
Orudis® see Ketoprofen *on page 483*
Orudis KT® [OTC] see Ketoprofen *on page 483*
Oruvail® see Ketoprofen *on page 483*
Os-Cal® 250 [OTC] see Calcium Carbonate *on page 140*
Os-Cal® 500 [OTC] see Calcium Carbonate *on page 140*
Osmoglyn® Ophthalmic see Glycerin *on page 402*
Otic Domeboro® see Aluminum Acetate and Acetic Acid *on page 39*
Otobiotic® Otic see Polymyxin B and Hydrocortisone *on page 704*
Otocalm® Ear see Antipyrine and Benzocaine *on page 70*
Otocort® Otic see Neomycin, Polymyxin B, and Hydrocortisone *on page 610*
Otomycin-HPN® Otic see Neomycin, Polymyxin B, and Hydrocortisone *on page 610*
Otosporin® Otic see Neomycin, Polymyxin B, and Hydrocortisone *on page 610*
Otrivin® [OTC] see Xylometazoline Hydrochloride *on page 905*
Ovcon® 35 see Ethinyl Estradiol and Norethindrone *on page 339*
Ovcon® 50 see Ethinyl Estradiol and Norethindrone *on page 339*
Ovral® see Ethinyl Estradiol and Norgestrel *on page 341*
Ovrette® see Norgestrel *on page 629*

Oxacillin Sodium (ox a sil' in sow' dee um)
Brand Names Bactocill®; Prostaphlin®
Therapeutic Category Antibiotic, Penicillin
Use Treatment of susceptible bacterial infections such as osteomyelitis, septicemia, endocarditis, and CNS infections due to penicillinase-producing strains of *Staphylococcus*
Usual Dosage
Children:
Oral: 50-100 mg/kg/day divided every 6 hours
I.M., I.V.: 150-200 mg/kg/day in divided doses every 6 hours; maximum dose: 12 g/day

Adults:
Oral: 500-1000 mg every 4-6 hours for at least 5 days
I.M., I.V.: 250 mg to 2 g/dose every 4-6 hours
Mechanism of Action Inhibits bacterial cell wall synthesis by binding to one or more of the penicillin binding proteins (PBPs); which in turn inhibits the final transpeptidation step of peptidoglycan synthesis in bacterial cell walls, thus
(Continued)

Oxacillin Sodium *(Continued)*

inhibiting cell wall biosynthesis. Bacteria eventually lyse due to ongoing activity of cell wall autolytic enzymes (autolysins and murein hydrolases) while cell wall assembly is arrested.

Local Anesthetic/Vasoconstrictor Precautions No information available to require special precautions

Effects on Dental Treatment Prolonged use of penicillins may lead to development of oral candidiasis

Other Adverse Effects

1% to 10%: Gastrointestinal: Nausea, diarrhea

<1%:

Central nervous system: Fever

Dermatologic: Rash

Gastrointestinal: Vomiting

Hematologic: Eosinophilia, leukopenia, neutropenia, thrombocytopenia, agranulocytosis

Hepatic: Hepatotoxicity, elevated AST

Renal: Hematuria, acute interstitial nephritis

Miscellaneous: Serum sickness-like reactions

Drug Interactions

Decreased effect: Efficacy of oral contraceptives may be reduced

Increased effect: Disulfiram, probenecid causes increased penicillin levels

Drug Uptake

Absorption: Oral: 35% to 67%

Serum half-life:

Children 1 week to 2 years: 0.9-1.8 hours

Adults: 23-60 minutes (prolonged with reduced renal function and in neonates)

Time to peak serum concentration:

Oral: Within 2 hours

I.M.: Within 30-60 minutes

Pregnancy Risk Factor B

Oxamniquine (ox am' ni kwin)

Brand Names Vansil™

Therapeutic Category Anthelmintic

Use Treat all stages of *Schistosoma mansoni* infection

Local Anesthetic/Vasoconstrictor Precautions No information available to require special precautions

Effects on Dental Treatment No effects or complications reported

Other Adverse Effects

>10%: Central nervous system: Dizziness, drowsiness, headache

<10%:

Central nervous system: Insomnia, malaise, hallucinations, behavior changes

Dermatologic: Rash, urticaria, pruritus

Gastrointestinal: GI effects

Genitourinary: Urine discoloration (orange/red)

Hepatic: LFTs (elevated)

Renal: Proteinuria

Comments Strains other than from the western hemisphere may require higher doses

Oxandrine® *see* Oxandrolone *on this page*

Oxandrolone (ox an' droe lone)

Brand Names Oxandrine®

Therapeutic Category Androgen

Use Treatment of catabolic or tissue-depleting processes

Local Anesthetic/Vasoconstrictor Precautions No information available to require special precautions

Effects on Dental Treatment No effects or complications reported

Other Adverse Effects

Male:

Postpubertal:

>10%: Bladder irritability, priapism, gynecomastia, acne

1% to 10%: Decreased libido, hepatic dysfunction, chills, nausea, diarrhea, insomnia, iron deficiency anemia, suppression of clotting factors, prostatic hypertrophy (geriatric)

<1%: Hepatic necrosis, hepatocellular carcinoma

Prepubertal: Virilism

>10%: Acne, virilism

1% to 10%: Hyperpigmentation, chills, diarrhea, nausea, insomnia, iron deficiency anemia, suppression of clotting factors

<1%: Hepatic necrosis, hepatocellular carcinoma

Female:

>10%: Virilism

1% to 10%: Hypercalcemia, hepatic dysfunction, nausea, chills, diarrhea, insomnia, iron deficiency anemia, suppression of clotting factors

<1%: Hepatic necrosis, hepatocellular carcinoma

Comments This medication is currently on the market as an Orphan Drug. It is distributed by Gynex Pharmaceuticals, Inc. to physicians who document their expertise in endocrinology and agree to participate in a study to gather data for the FDA.

Oxaprozin (ox a proe' zin)

Related Information

Rheumatoid Arthritis, Osteoarthritis, and Joint Prostheses *on page 930*

Brand Names Daypro™

Therapeutic Category Nonsteroidal Anti-inflammatory Agent (NSAID), Oral

Use Acute and long-term use in the management of signs and symptoms of osteoarthritis and rheumatoid arthritis

Usual Dosage Adults: Oral (individualize dosage to lowest effective dose to minimize adverse effects):

Osteoarthritis: 600-1200 mg once daily

Rheumatoid arthritis: 1200 mg once daily

Maximum dose: 1800 mg/day or 26 mg/kg (whichever is lower) in divided doses

Mechanism of Action Inhibits prostaglandin synthesis by decreasing the activity of the enzyme, cyclo-oxygenase, which results in decreased formation of prostaglandin precursors

Local Anesthetic/Vasoconstrictor Precautions No information available to require special precautions

Effects on Dental Treatment No effects or complications reported

Other Adverse Effects

>10%:

Central nervous system: Dizziness

Dermatologic: Skin rash

Gastrointestinal: Abdominal cramps, heartburn, indigestion, nausea

1% to 10%:

Cardiovascular: Angina pectoris, arrhythmia

Central nervous system: Dizziness, nervousness

Dermatologic: Skin rash, itching

Gastrointestinal: GI ulceration, vomiting

Genitourinary: Vaginal bleeding

Otic: Tinnitus

<1%:

Cardiovascular: Chest pain, congestive heart failure, hypertension, tachycardia

Central nervous system: Convulsions, forgetfulness, mental depression, drowsiness, nervousness, insomnia, weakness

Dermatologic: Hives, exfoliative dermatitis, erythema multiforme, Stevens-Johnson syndrome, angioedema

Gastrointestinal: Stomatitis

Genitourinary: Cystitis

Hematologic: Agranulocytosis, anemia, pancytopenia, leukopenia, thrombocytopenia

Hepatic: Hepatitis

Neuromuscular & skeletal: Peripheral neuropathy, trembling

Ocular: Blurred vision, change in vision

Otic: Decreased hearing

Renal: Interstitial nephritis, nephrotic syndrome, renal impairment

Respiratory: Shortness of breath, wheezing, laryngeal edema

Miscellaneous: Epistaxis, anaphylaxis, increased sweating

Drug Interactions Oxaprozin, like other NSAIDs, may cause increased toxicity of aspirin, oral anticoagulants, diuretics

Drug Uptake

Absorption: Almost completely

Serum half-life: 40-50 hours

Time to peak: 2-4 hours

Pregnancy Risk Factor C

Oxazepam (ox a′ ze pam)

Related Information
Patients Requiring Sedation *on page 965*

Brand Names Serax®

Canadian/Mexican Brand Names Apo-Oxazepam® (Canada); Novo-Oxazepam® (Canada); Oxpam® (Canada); PMS-Oxazepam® (Canada); Zapex® (Canada)

Therapeutic Category Benzodiazepine

Use Treatment of anxiety and management of alcohol withdrawal; may also be used as an anticonvulsant in management of simple partial seizures

Usual Dosage Oral:
Children: 1 mg/kg/day has been administered

Adults:
Anxiety: 10-30 mg 3-4 times/day
Alcohol withdrawal: 15-30 mg 3-4 times/day
Hypnotic: 15-30 mg
Not dialyzable (0% to 5%)

Mechanism of Action Benzodiazepine anxiolytic sedative that produces CNS depression at the subcortical level, except at high doses, whereby it works at the cortical level

Local Anesthetic/Vasoconstrictor Precautions No information available to require special precautions

Effects on Dental Treatment Over 10% of patients will experience dry mouth which disappears with cessation of drug therapy

Other Adverse Effects
>10%:
Cardiovascular: Tachycardia, chest pain
Central nervous system: Drowsiness, fatigue, impaired coordination, light-headedness, memory impairment, insomnia, anxiety, depression, headache
Dermatologic: Rash increased or decreased appetite
Endocrine & metabolic: Decreased libido
Gastrointestinal: Dry mouth, constipation, diarrhea, decreased salivation, nausea, vomiting
Neuromuscular & skeletal: Dysarthria
Ocular: Blurred vision
Miscellaneous: Sweating
1% to 10%:
Cardiovascular: Syncope, hypotension
Central nervous system: Confusion, nervousness, dizziness, akathisia
Dermatologic: Dermatitis
Gastrointestinal: Increased salivation, weight gain or loss
Neuromuscular & skeletal: Rigidity, tremor, muscle cramps
Ocular: Blurred vision
Otic: Tinnitus
Respiratory: Nasal congestion, hyperventilation
<1%:
Central nervous system: Reflex slowing
Endocrine & metabolic: Menstrual irregularities
Hematologic: Blood dyscrasias
Miscellaneous: Drug dependence

Drug Interactions Increased toxicity (CNS depression): Alcohol, tricyclic antidepressants, sedative-hypnotics, MAO inhibitors

Drug Uptake
Absorption: Oral: Almost completely
Serum half-life: 2.8-5.7 hours
Time to peak serum concentration: Within 2-4 hours

Pregnancy Risk Factor D

Oxiconazole Nitrate (ox i kon′ a zole nye′ trate)

Brand Names Oxistat®

Canadian/Mexican Brand Names Myfungar® (Mexico)

Therapeutic Category Antifungal Agent, Topical

Synonyms Oxiconazol, Nitrato De (Mexico)

Use Treatment of tinea pedis (athlete's foot), tinea cruris (jock itch), and tinea corporis (ring worm)

Usual Dosage Children and Adults: Topical: Apply once to twice daily to affected areas for 2 weeks (tinea corporis/tinea cruris) to 1 month (tinea pedis)

Mechanism of Action Inhibition of ergosterol synthesis. Effective for treatment of tinea pedis, tinea cruris, and tinea corporis. Active against *Trichophyton*

rubrum, *Trichophyton mentagrophytes*, *Trichophyton violaceum*, *Microsporum canis*, *Microsporum audouini*, *Microsporum gypseum*, *Epidermophyton floccosum*, *Candida albicans*, and *Malassezia furfur*.

Local Anesthetic/Vasoconstrictor Precautions No information available to require special precautions

Effects on Dental Treatment No effects or complications reported

Other Adverse Effects 1% to 10%: Local: Itching, transient burning, local irritation, stinging, erythema, dryness

Drug Interactions No data reported

Drug Uptake
Absorption: In each layer of the dermis; very little is absorbed systemically after one topical dose

Pregnancy Risk Factor B

Oxiconazol, Nitrato De (Mexico) *see* Oxiconazole Nitrate *on previous page*

Oxistat® *see* Oxiconazole Nitrate *on previous page*

Oxitetraciclina (Mexico) *see* Oxytetracycline Hydrochloride *on page 653*

Oxitocina (Mexico) *see* Oxytocin *on page 654*

Oxsoralen® Topical *see* Methoxsalen *on page 563*

Oxsoralen-Ultra® Oral *see* Methoxsalen *on page 563*

Oxtriphylline (ox trye′ fi lin)

Related Information
Respiratory Diseases *on page 924*

Brand Names Choledyl®

Therapeutic Category Antiasthmatic; Bronchodilator; Theophylline Derivative

Synonyms Choline Theophyllinate

Use Bronchodilator in symptomatic treatment of asthma and reversible bronchospasm

Local Anesthetic/Vasoconstrictor Precautions No information available to require special precautions

Effects on Dental Treatment Do not prescribe any erythromycin product to patients taking theophylline products. Erythromycin will delay the normal metabolic inactivation of theophyllines leading to increased blood levels; this has resulted in nausea, vomiting and CNS restlessness

Other Adverse Effects Uncommon with theophylline levels <20 mcg/mL
1% to 10%:
Cardiovascular: Tachycardia
Central nervous system: Nervousness, restlessness
Gastrointestinal: Nausea, vomiting
<1%:
Central nervous system: Insomnia, irritability, seizures
Dermatologic: Skin rash
Gastrointestinal: Gastric irritation
Neuromuscular & skeletal: Tremor
Miscellaneous: Allergic reactions

Comments Oxtriphylline is 64% theophylline

Oxy-5® [OTC] *see* Benzoyl Peroxide *on page 104*

Oxy-10® [OTC] *see* Benzoyl Peroxide *on page 104*

Oxybutynin Chloride (ox i byoo′ ti nin klor′ ide)

Brand Names Ditropan®

Therapeutic Category Antispasmodic Agent, Urinary

Use Antispasmodic for neurogenic bladder (urgency, frequency, urge incontinence) and uninhibited bladder

Usual Dosage Oral:
Children:
1-5 years: 0.2 mg/kg/dose 2-4 times/day
>5 years: 5 mg twice daily, up to 5 mg 4 times/day maximum
Adults: 5 mg 2-3 times/day up to 5 mg 4 times/day maximum
Elderly: 2.5-5 mg twice daily; increase by 2.5 mg increments every 1-2 days

Note: Should be discontinued periodically to determine whether the patient can manage without the drug and to minimize resistance to the drug

Mechanism of Action Direct antispasmodic effect on smooth muscle, also inhibits the action of acetylcholine on smooth muscle (exhibits $\frac{1}{5}$ the anticholinergic activity of atropine, but is 4-10 times the antispasmodic activity); does not block effects at skeletal muscle or at autonomic ganglia; increases bladder capacity, decreases uninhibited contractions, and delays desire to void; therefore, decreases urgency and frequency
(Continued)

Oxybutynin Chloride *(Continued)*

Local Anesthetic/Vasoconstrictor Precautions No information available to require special precautions

Effects on Dental Treatment Prolonged use of oxybutynin may decrease or inhibit salivary flow; normal salivation returns with cessation of drug therapy

Other Adverse Effects

>10%:
  Cardiovascular: Decreased sweating
  Central nervous system: Drowsiness
  Gastrointestinal: Dry mouth, constipation

1% to 10%:
  Cardiovascular: Tachycardia, palpitations
  Central nervous system: Drowsiness, weakness, dizziness, insomnia, fever, headache
  Dermatologic: Rash
  Endocrine & metabolic: Hot flushes, decreased flow of breast milk
  Gastrointestinal: Nausea, vomiting
  Genitourinary: Urinary hesitancy or retention, decreased sexual ability
  Ocular: Blurred vision, mydriatic effect

<1%:
  Ophthalmic: Increased intraocular pressure
  Miscellaneous: Allergic reaction

Drug Interactions

Increased toxicity:
  Additive sedation with CNS depressants and alcohol
  Additive anticholinergic effects with antihistamines and anticholinergic agents

Drug Uptake

Onset of effect: Oral: 30-60 minutes
Peak effect: 3-6 hours
Duration: 6-10 hours
Absorption: Oral: Rapid and well absorbed
Serum half-life: 1-2.3 hours
Time to peak serum concentration: Within 60 minutes

Pregnancy Risk Factor B

Oxycel® *see* Cellulose, Oxidized *on page 174*

Oxychlorosene Sodium (ox i klor′ oh seen sow′ dee um)

Brand Names Clorpactin® WCS-90

Therapeutic Category Antibiotic, Topical

Use Treating localized infections

Local Anesthetic/Vasoconstrictor Precautions No information available to require special precautions

Effects on Dental Treatment No effects or complications reported

Comments Product is available as powder which must be diluted with sterile water or isotonic saline

Oxycodone and Acetaminophen
(ox i koe′ done & a seet a min′ oh fen)

Related Information

Dental Drug Interactions: Update on Drug Combinations Requiring Special Considerations *on page 1022*
Narcotic Agonist Charts *on page 1019*
Oral Pain *on page 940*

Brand Names Percocet®; Roxicet®; Tylox®

Canadian/Mexican Brand Names Endocet® (Canada); Oxycocet® (Canada); Percocet-Demi® (Canada)

Therapeutic Category Analgesic, Narcotic

Use

Dental: Treatment of postoperative pain
Medical: Relief of pain

Usual Dosage Oral:

Children: Not recommended in pediatric dental patients
Adults: 1-2 tablets every 4-6 hours as needed for pain; maximum dose: 12 tablets/day

Mechanism of Action

Oxycodone, as with other narcotic (opiate) analgesics, blocks pain perception in the cerebral cortex by binding to specific receptor molecules (opiate receptors) within the neuronal membranes of synapses. This binding results in a decreased synaptic chemical transmission throughout the CNS thus inhibiting the flow of pain sensations into the higher centers. Mu and kappa are the two subtypes of the opiate receptor which oxycodone binds to to cause analgesia.

Acetaminophen inhibits the synthesis of prostaglandins in the CNS and peripherally blocks pain impulse generation; produces antipyresis from inhibition of hypothalamic heat-regulating center

Local Anesthetic/Vasoconstrictor Precautions No information available to require special precautions

Effects on Dental Treatment No effects or complications reported

Other Adverse Effects
>10%:
Central nervous system: Drowsiness, dizziness, sedation
Gastrointestinal: Nausea
1% to 10%: Gastrointestinal: Constipation

Oral manifestations: 1% to 10%: Dry mouth

Contraindications Patients with known G-6-PD deficiency; hypersensitivity to acetaminophen; hypersensitivity to oxycodone

Warnings/Precautions Use with caution in patients with hypersensitivity reactions to other phenanthrene derivative opioid agonists (morphine, codeine, hydrocodone, hydromorphone, levorphanol, oxymorphone); respiratory diseases including asthma, emphysema, COPD, or severe liver or renal insufficiency; some preparations contain sulfites which may cause allergic reactions; may be habit-forming

Enhanced analgesia has been seen in elderly patients on therapeutic doses of narcotics; duration of action may be increased in the elderly; the elderly may be particularly susceptible to the CNS depressant and constipating effects of narcotics

Drug Interactions The use of MAO inhibitors or tricyclic antidepressants with oxycodone may **increase** the effect of either the antidepressant or oxycodone; concurrent use of oxycodone with anticholinergics may cause paralytic ileus; patients taking other narcotic agents, antipsychotics, antianxiety agents or other CNS depressants (including alcohol) with oxycodone may experience an additive CNS depression

Drug Uptake
Onset of effect: Narcotic analgesia: 0.5-1 hour
Duration of effect: 4-6 hours
Serum half-life: Oxycodone: 2-3 hours

Pregnancy Risk Factor C

Breast-feeding Considerations
Oxycodone: No data reported
Acetaminophen: May be taken while breast-feeding

Dosage Forms
Capsule (Tylox®): Oxycodone hydrochloride 5 mg and acetaminophen 500 mg
Solution, oral (Roxicet®): Oxycodone hydrochloride 5 mg and acetaminophen 325 mg per 5 mL (5 mL, 500 mL)
Tablet (Percocet®): Oxycodone hydrochloride 5 mg and acetaminophen 325 mg

Dietary Considerations No data reported

Generic Available Yes

Comments Oxycodone, as with other narcotic analgesics, is recommended only for limited acute dosing (ie, 3 days or less). The most common adverse effect is nausea, followed by sedation and constipation. Oxycodone has an addictive liability, especially when given long term. The acetaminophen component requires use with caution in patients with alcoholic liver disease.

Selected Readings
Cooper SA, Precheur H, Rauch D, et al, "Evaluation of Oxycodone and Acetaminophen in Treatment of Postoperative Pain," *Oral Surg Oral Med Oral Pathol*, 1980, 50(6):496-501.
Dionne RA, "New Approaches to Preventing and Treating Postoperative Pain," *J Am Dent Assoc*, 1992, 123(6):26-34.
Gobetti JP, "Controlling Dental Pain," *J Am Dent Assoc*, 1992, 123(6):47-52.

Oxycodone and Aspirin (ox i koe' done & as' pir in)

Related Information
Dental Drug Interactions: Update on Drug Combinations Requiring Special Considerations *on page 1022*
Narcotic Agonist Charts *on page 1019*
Oral Pain *on page 940*

Brand Names Codoxy®; Percodan®; Percodan®-Demi; Roxiprin®

Canadian/Mexican Brand Names Endodan® (Canada); Oxcodan® (Canada)

Therapeutic Category Analgesic, Narcotic

(Continued)

Oxycodone and Aspirin *(Continued)*

Use
Dental: Treatment of postoperative pain
Medical: Relief of pain

Usual Dosage Oral:
Children: Not recommended in pediatric dental patients
Adults: Percodan®: 1 tablet every 6 hours as needed for pain or Percodan®-Demi: 1-2 tablets every 6 hours as needed for pain

Mechanism of Action
Oxycodone, as with other narcotic (opiate) analgesics, blocks pain perception in the cerebral cortex by binding to specific receptor molecules (opiate receptors) within the neuronal membranes of synapses. This binding results in a decreased synaptic chemical transmission throughout the CNS thus inhibiting the flow of pain sensations into the higher centers. Mu and kappa are the two subtypes of the opiate receptor which oxycodone binds to to cause analgesia.

Aspirin inhibits prostaglandin synthesis by decreasing the activity of the enzyme, cyclo-oxygenase, which results in decreased formation of prostaglandin precursors, acts on the hypothalamic heat-regulating center to reduce fever, blocks thromboxane synthetase action which prevents formation of the platelet-aggregating substance thromboxane A_2

Local Anesthetic/Vasoconstrictor Precautions
No information available to require special precautions

Effects on Dental Treatment
Use with caution in patients with platelet and bleeding disorders, renal dysfunction, erosive gastritis, or peptic ulcer disease, previous nonreaction does not guarantee future safe taking of medication; do not use aspirin in children <16 years of age for chickenpox or flu symptoms due to the association with Reye's syndrome

Avoid aspirin if possible, for 1 week prior to surgery because of the possibility of postoperative bleeding; use with caution in impaired hepatic function

Elderly are a high-risk population for adverse effects from nonsteroidal anti-inflammatory agents. As much as 60% of elderly with GI complications to NSAIDs can develop peptic ulceration and/or hemorrhage asymptomatically. Also, concomitant disease and drug use contribute to the risk for GI adverse effects. Use lowest effective dose for shortest period possible. Consider renal function decline with age. Use with caution in patients with history of asthma

Other Adverse Effects
>10%:
  Central nervous system: Drowsiness, dizziness, sedation
  Gastrointestinal: Nausea, heartburn, stomach pains, dyspepsia
1% to 10%: Gastrointestinal: Constipation

Oral manifestations: 1% to 10%: Dry mouth

Contraindications
Known hypersensitivity to oxycodone or aspirin; severe respiratory depression

Warnings/Precautions
Use with caution in patients with hypersensitivity to other phenanthrene derivative opioid agonists (morphine, codeine, hydrocodone, hydromorphone, oxymorphone, levorphanol); children and teenagers should not be given aspirin products if chickenpox or flu symptoms are present; aspirin use has been associated with Reye's syndrome; severe liver or renal insufficiency, pre-existing CNS and depression

Enhanced analgesia has been seen in elderly patients on therapeutic doses of narcotics; duration of action may be increased in the elderly; the elderly may be particularly susceptible to the CNS depressant and constipating effects of narcotics

Drug Interactions
The use of MAO inhibitors or tricyclic antidepressants with oxycodone may **increase** effect of either the antidepressant or oxycodone; concurrent use of oxycodone with anticholinergics may cause paralytic ileus; patients taking other narcotic agents, antipsychotics, antianxiety agents or other CNS depressants (including alcohol) with oxycodone and aspirin may experience an additive CNS depression; aspirin interacts with warfarin to cause bleeding

Drug Uptake
Onset of effect: Narcotic analgesia: 0.5-1 hour
Duration of effect 4-6 hours
Serum half-life: Oxycodone: 2-3 hours

Pregnancy Risk Factor D

Breast-feeding Considerations
Aspirin: Caution is suggested due to potential adverse effects in nursing infants

Oxycodone: No data reported

Dosage Forms Tablet:

Percodan®: Oxycodone hydrochloride 4.5 mg, oxycodone terephthalate 0.38 mg, and aspirin 325 mg

Percodan®-Demi: Oxycodone hydrochloride 2.25 mg, oxycodone terephthalate 0.19 mg, and aspirin 325 mg

Dietary Considerations May be taken with food or water

Generic Available Yes

Comments Oxycodone, as with other narcotic analgesics, is recommended only for limited acute dosing (ie, 3 days or less). The most common adverse effect is nausea, followed by sedation and constipation. Oxycodone has an addictive liability, especially when given long term. The oxycodone with aspirin could have anticoagulant effects and could possibly affect bleeding times.

Selected Readings

Dionne RA, "New Approaches to Preventing and Treating Postoperative Pain," *J Am Dent Assoc*, 1992, 123(6):26-34.

Gobetti JP, "Controlling Dental Pain," *J Am Dent Assoc*, 1992, 123(6):47-52.

Oxydess® II see Dextroamphetamine Sulfate *on page 265*

Oxygen (ok' si jen)

Therapeutic Category Decongestant, Ophthalmic

Use

Dental: Administered as a supplement with nitrous oxide to ensure adequate ventilation during sedation; a resuscitative agent for medical emergencies in dental office

Medical: To treat various clinical disorders, both respiratory and nonrespiratory; relief of arterial hypoxia and secondary complications; treatment of pulmonary hypertension, polycythemia secondary to hypoxemia, chronic disease states complicated by anemia, cancer, migraine headaches, coronary artery disease, seizure disorders, sickle-cell crisis and sleep apnea

Usual Dosage Children and Adults: Average rate of 2 L/minute

Mechanism of Action Increased oxygen in tidal volume and oxygenation of tissues at molecular level

Local Anesthetic/Vasoconstrictor Precautions No information available to require special precautions

Effects on Dental Treatment No effects or complications reported

Other Adverse Effects No data reported

Oral manifestations: No data reported

Contraindications No data reported

Warnings/Precautions Oxygen-induced hypoventilation is the greatest potential hazard of oxygen therapy. In patients with severe chronic obstructive pulmonary disease (COPD), the respiratory drive results from hypoxic stimulation of the carotid chemoreceptors. If this hypoxic drive is diminished by excessive oxygen therapy, hypoventilation may occur and further carbon dioxide retention with possible cessation of ventilation could result.

Drug Interactions No data reported

Pregnancy Risk Factor No data reported

Breast-feeding Considerations No data reported

Dosage Forms Liquid system with large reservoir holding 75-100 lb of liquid oxygen; compressed gas system consisting of high-pressure tank; tank sizes are "H" (6900 L of oxygen), "E" (622 L of oxygen) and "D" (356 L of oxygen)

Dietary Considerations No data reported

Oxymetazoline Hydrochloride

(ox i met az' oh leen hye droe klor' ide)

Related Information

Oral Bacterial Infections *on page 945*

Brand Names Afrin® Nasal Solution [OTC]; Allerest® 12 Hour Nasal Solution [OTC]; Chlorphed®-LA Nasal Solution [OTC]; Dristan® Long Lasting Nasal Solution [OTC]; Duration® Nasal Solution [OTC]; Neo-Synephrine® 12 Hour Nasal Solution [OTC]; Nōstrilla®; Nōstrilla® Long Acting Nasal Solution [OTC]; NTZ® Nasal Solution [OTC]; Sinarest® 12 Hour Nasal Solution; Vicks® Sinex® Long-Acting Nasal Solution [OTC]; 4-Way® Long Acting Nasal Solution [OTC]

Canadian/Mexican Brand Names Drixoral® Nasal (Canada)

Therapeutic Category Adrenergic Agonist Agent; Decongestant, Nasal; Nasal Agent, Vasoconstrictor

Use

Dental: Symptomatic relief of nasal mucosal congestion

(Continued)

Oxymetazoline Hydrochloride *(Continued)*

Medical:
  Adjunctive therapy of middle ear infections, associated with acute or chronic rhinitis, the common cold, sinusitis, hay fever, or other allergies
  Ophthalmic: Relief of redness of eye due to minor eye irritations
Usual Dosage Intranasal (therapy should not exceed 3-5 days):
  Children 2-5 years: 0.025% solution: Instill 2-3 drops in each nostril twice daily
  Children ≥6 years and Adults: 0.05% solution: Instill 2-3 drops or 2-3 sprays into each nostril twice daily
Mechanism of Action Stimulates alpha-adrenergic receptors in the arterioles of the nasal mucosa to produce vasoconstriction
Local Anesthetic/Vasoconstrictor Precautions No information available to require special precautions
Effects on Dental Treatment No effects or complications reported
Other Adverse Effects
  >10%:
    Local: Transient burning, stinging
    Respiratory: Dryness of the nasal mucosa, sneezing
  1% to 10%: Cardiovascular: Rebound congestion with prolonged use, hypertension, palpitations

  Oral manifestations: No data reported
Contraindications Hypersensitivity to oxymetazoline or any component
Warnings/Precautions Rebound congestion may occur with extended use (>3 days); use with caution in the presence of hypertension, diabetes, hyperthyroidism, heart disease, coronary artery disease, cerebral arteriosclerosis, or long-standing bronchial asthma
Drug Interactions Increased toxicity with MAO inhibitors
Drug Uptake
  Onset of effect: Intranasal: Within 5-10 minutes
  Duration: 5-6 hours
Pregnancy Risk Factor C
Breast-feeding Considerations No data reported
Dosage Forms Solution, nasal:
  Drops: 0.05% drops (15 mL, 20 mL)
  Drops, pediatric: 0.025% (20 mL)
  Spray: 0.05% (15 mL, 30 mL)
Dietary Considerations No data reported
Generic Available Yes

Oxymetholone *(ox i meth' oh lone)*

Brand Names Anadrol®
Canadian/Mexican Brand Names Anapolon® (Canada)
Therapeutic Category Anabolic Steroid
Use Anemias caused by the administration of myelotoxic drugs
Usual Dosage Adults: Erythropoietic effects: Oral: 1-5 mg/kg/day in 1 daily dose; maximum: 100 mg/day; give for a minimum trial of 3-6 months because response may be delayed
Mechanism of Action Stimulates receptors in organs and tissues to promote growth and development of male sex organs and maintains secondary sex characteristics in androgen-deficient males
Local Anesthetic/Vasoconstrictor Precautions No information available to require special precautions
Effects on Dental Treatment No effects or complications reported
Other Adverse Effects
  Male:
  Postpubertal:
    >10%:
      Dermatologic: Acne
      Endocrine & metabolic: Gynecomastia
      Genitourinary: Bladder irritability, priapism
    1% to 10%:
      Central nervous system: Insomnia, chills
      Endocrine & metabolic: Decreased libido
      Gastrointestinal: Nausea, diarrhea
      Genitourinary: Prostatic hypertrophy (elderly)
      Hematologic: Iron deficiency anemia, suppression of clotting factors
    Hepatic: Hepatic dysfunction
    <1%:
      Hepatic: Hepatic necrosis, hepatocellular carcinoma

Prepubertal:
>10%:
Dermatologic: Acne
Endocrine & metabolic: Virilism
1% to 10%:
Central nervous system: Chills, insomnia
Dermatologic: Hyperpigmentation
Gastrointestinal: Diarrhea, nausea
Hematologic: Iron deficiency anemia, suppression of clotting factors
<1%: Hepatic: Hepatic necrosis, hepatocellular carcinoma

Female:
>10%: Endocrine & metabolic: Virilism
1% to 10%:
Central nervous system: Chills, insomnia
Endocrine & metabolic: Hypercalcemia
Gastrointestinal: Nausea, diarrhea
Hematologic: Iron deficiency anemia, suppression of clotting factors
Hepatic: Hepatic dysfunction
<1%: Hepatic: Hepatic necrosis, hepatocellular carcinoma
Drug Interactions Increased toxicity: Increased oral anticoagulants, insulin requirements may be decreased
Drug Uptake
Serum half-life: 9 hours
Pregnancy Risk Factor X

Oxymorphone Hydrochloride (ox i mor' fone hye droe klor' ide)
Related Information
Narcotic Agonist Charts *on page 1019*
Brand Names Numorphan®
Therapeutic Category Analgesic, Narcotic
Use Management of moderate to severe pain and preoperatively as a sedative and a supplement to anesthesia
Usual Dosage Adults:
I.M., S.C.: 0.5 mg initially, 1-1.5 mg every 4-6 hours as needed
I.V.: 0.5 mg initially
Rectal: 5 mg every 4-6 hours
Mechanism of Action Oxymorphone hydrochloride (Numorphan®) is a potent narcotic analgesic with uses similar to those of morphine. The drug is a semisynthetic derivative of morphine (phenanthrene derivative) and is closely related to hydromorphone chemically (Dilaudid®).
Local Anesthetic/Vasoconstrictor Precautions No information available to require special precautions
Effects on Dental Treatment Anticholinergic side effects can cause a reduction of saliva production or secretion contributes to discomfort and dental disease (ie, caries, oral candidiasis and periodontal disease)
Other Adverse Effects
>10%:
Cardiovascular: Hypotension
Central nervous system: Weakness, tiredness, drowsiness, dizziness
Gastrointestinal: Nausea, vomiting, constipation
Miscellaneous: Histamine release
1% to 10%:
Central nervous system: Nervousness, headache, restlessness, malaise, confusion
Gastrointestinal: Anorexia, stomach cramps, dry mouth, biliary spasm
Genitourinary: Decreased urination, ureteral spasms
Local: Pain at injection site
Respiratory: Troubled breathing, shortness of breath
<1%:
Central nervous system: Mental depression, hallucinations, paradoxical CNS stimulation, increased intracranial pressure
Dermatologic: Skin rash, hives
Gastrointestinal: Paralytic ileus
Miscellaneous: Histamine release, physical and psychological dependence
Drug Interactions
Decreased effect with phenothiazines
Increased effect/toxicity with CNS depressants, TCAs, dextroamphetamine
Drug Uptake
Onset of analgesia:
I.V., I.M., S.C.: Within 5-10 minutes
(Continued)

Oxymorphone Hydrochloride *(Continued)*

Rectal: Within 15-30 minutes
Duration of analgesia: Parenteral, rectal: 3-4 hours
Pregnancy Risk Factor B (D if used for prolonged periods or in high doses at term)

Oxyphenbutazone (ox i fen byoo' ta zone)

Therapeutic Category Analgesic, Non-narcotic; Nonsteroidal Anti-inflammatory Agent (NSAID), Oral
Use Management of inflammatory disorders, as an analgesic in the treatment of mild to moderate pain and as an antipyretic; I.V. form used as an alternate to surgery in management of patent ductus arteriosus in premature neonates; acute gouty arthritis
Local Anesthetic/Vasoconstrictor Precautions No information available to require special precautions
Effects on Dental Treatment No effects or complications reported
Other Adverse Effects
>10%:
Central nervous system: Dizziness
Dermatologic: Skin rash
Gastrointestinal: Abdominal cramps, heartburn, indigestion, nausea
1% to 10%:
Central nervous system: Headache, nervousness
Dermatologic: Itching
Endocrine & metabolic: Fluid retention
Gastrointestinal: Vomiting
Otic: Ringing in ears
<1%:
Cardiovascular: Congestive heart failure, hypertension, arrhythmia, tachycardia
Central nervous system: Confusion, hallucinations, aseptic meningitis, mental depression, drowsiness, insomnia
Dermatologic: Hives, erythema multiforme, toxic epidermal necrolysis, Stevens-Johnson syndrome, angioedema
Endocrine & metabolic: Polydipsia, hot flashes
Gastrointestinal: Gastritis, GI ulceration
Genitourinary: Cystitis
Hematologic: Agranulocytosis, anemia, hemolytic anemia, bone marrow depression, leukopenia, thrombocytopenia
Hepatic: Hepatitis
Neuromuscular & skeletal: Neuropathy (peripheral)
Ocular: Toxic amblyopia, blurred vision, conjunctivitis, dry eyes
Otic: Decreased hearing
Renal: Polyuria, acute renal failure
Respiratory: Allergic rhinitis, shortness of breath, epistaxis

Oxyphencyclimine Hydrochloride
(ox i fen sye' kli meen hye droe klor' ide)
Brand Names Daricon®
Therapeutic Category Anticholinergic Agent; Antispasmodic Agent, Gastrointestinal
Use Adjunctive treatment of peptic ulcer
Local Anesthetic/Vasoconstrictor Precautions No information available to require special precautions
Effects on Dental Treatment >10%: Dry mouth
Other Adverse Effects
>10%:
Dermatologic: Dry skin
Gastrointestinal: Constipation, dry mouth and throat
Respiratory: Dry nose
Miscellaneous: Decreased sweating
1% to 10%:
Ocular: Sensitivity to light
Respiratory: Difficulty in swallowing
<1%:
Cardiovascular: Tachycardia
Central nervous system: Confusion, headache, loss of memory, tiredness, drowsiness, nervousness, insomnia
Dermatologic: Rash
Gastrointestinal: Bloated feeling, nausea, vomiting

Genitourinary: Urinary retention
Neuromuscular & skeletal: Weakness
Ocular: Intraocular pressure (increased), blurred vision

Oxytetracycline and Hydrocortisone
(ox i tet ra sye' kleen & hye droe kor' ti sone)

Brand Names Terra-Cortril® Ophthalmic Suspension

Therapeutic Category Antibiotic, Ophthalmic

Use Treatment of susceptible ophthalmic bacterial infections with associated swelling

Local Anesthetic/Vasoconstrictor Precautions No information available to require special precautions

Effects on Dental Treatment No effects or complications reported

Oxytetracycline and Polymyxin B
(ox i tet ra sye' kleen & pol i mix' in bee)

Brand Names Terak® Ophthalmic Ointment; Terramycin® Ophthalmic Ointment; Terramycin® w/Polymyxin B Ophthalmic Ointment

Therapeutic Category Antibiotic, Ophthalmic

Synonyms Polymyxin B and Oxytetracycline

Use Treatment of superficial ocular infections involving the conjunctiva and/or cornea

Local Anesthetic/Vasoconstrictor Precautions No information available to require special precautions

Effects on Dental Treatment No effects or complications reported

Oxytetracycline Hydrochloride
(ox i tet ra sye' kleen hye droe klor' ide)

Brand Names Terramycin® IV; Uri-Tet®

Canadian/Mexican Brand Names Oxitraklin® (Mexico); Terramicina® (Mexico)

Therapeutic Category Antibiotic, Tetracycline Derivative

Synonyms Oxitetraciclina (Mexico)

Use Treatment of susceptible bacterial infections; both gram-positive and gram-negative, as well as, *Rickettsia* and *Mycoplasma* organisms

Usual Dosage
Oral:
Children: 40-50 mg/kg/day in divided doses every 6 hours (maximum: 2 g/24 hours)
Adults: 250-500 mg/dose every 6 hours

I.M.:
Children >8 years: 15-25 mg/kg/day (maximum: 250 mg/dose) in divided doses every 8-12 hours
Adults: 250-500 mg every 24 hours or 300 mg/day divided every 8-12 hours

Mechanism of Action Inhibits bacterial protein synthesis by binding with the 30S and possibly the 50S ribosomal subunit(s) of susceptible bacteria, cell wall synthesis is not affected

Local Anesthetic/Vasoconstrictor Precautions No information available to require special precautions

Effects on Dental Treatment Tetracycline's are not recommended for use during pregnancy or in children ≤8 years of age since they have been reported to cause enamel hypoplasia and permanent teeth discoloration. The use of tetracycline's should only be used in these patients if other agents are contraindicated or alternative antimicrobials will not eradicate the organism. Long-term use associated with oral candidiasis.

Other Adverse Effects
>10%: Miscellaneous: Discoloration of teeth and enamel hypoplasia (infants)
1% to 10%:
Dermatologic: Photosensitivity
Gastrointestinal: Nausea, diarrhea
<1%:
Cardiovascular: Pericarditis
Central nervous system: Increased intracranial pressure, bulging fontanels in infants, pseudotumor cerebri
Dermatologic: Pruritus, exfoliative dermatitis, dermatologic effects
Endocrine & metabolic: Diabetes insipidus syndrome
Gastrointestinal: Vomiting, esophagitis, anorexia, abdominal cramps, antibiotic-associated pseudomembranous colitis, staphylococcal enterocolitis
Hepatic: Hepatotoxicity
Local: Thrombophlebitis
(Continued)

Oxytetracycline Hydrochloride *(Continued)*

Neuromuscular & skeletal: Paresthesia
Renal: Renal damage, acute renal failure, azotemia
Miscellaneous: Superinfections, anaphylaxis, pigmentation of nails, hypersensitivity reactions, candidal superinfection

Drug Interactions

Decreased effect with antacids containing aluminum, calcium or magnesium
Iron and bismuth subsalicylate may decrease oxytetracycline bioavailability
Barbiturates, phenytoin, and carbamazepine decrease oxytetracycline's half-life
Increased effect of warfarin

Drug Uptake

Absorption:
Oral: Adequate (~75%)
I.M.: Poor
Serum half-life: 8.5-9.6 hours (increases with renal impairment)
Time to peak serum concentration: Within 2-4 hours

Pregnancy Risk Factor D

Dosage Forms

Capsule: 250 mg
Injection, with lidocaine 2%: 5% [50 mg/mL] (2 mL, 10 mL); 12.5% [125 mg/mL] (2 mL)

Generic Available Yes

Oxytocin *(ox i toe' sin)*

Brand Names Pitocin®; Syntocinon®

Canadian/Mexican Brand Names Toesen® (Canada); Oxitopisa® (Mexico); Syntocinon® (Mexico); Xitocin® (Mexico)

Therapeutic Category Oxytocic Agent

Synonyms Oxitocina (Mexico)

Use Induces labor at term; controls postpartum bleeding; nasal preparation used to promote milk letdown in lactating females

Usual Dosage I.V. administration requires the use of an infusion pump

Adults:
Induction of labor: I.V.: 0.001-0.002 units/minute; increase by 0.001-0.002 units every 15-30 minutes until contraction pattern has been established; maximum dose should not exceed 20 milliunits/minute
Postpartum bleeding:
I.M.: Total dose of 10 units after delivery
I.V.: 10-40 units by I.V. infusion in 1000 mL of intravenous fluid at a rate sufficient to control uterine atony
Promotion of milk letdown: Intranasal: 1 spray or 3 drops in one or both nostrils 2-3 minutes before breast-feeding

Mechanism of Action Produces the rhythmic uterine contractions characteristic to delivery and stimulates breast milk flow during nursing

Local Anesthetic/Vasoconstrictor Precautions No information available to require special precautions

Effects on Dental Treatment No effects or complications reported

Other Adverse Effects

Fetal: <1%:
Cardiovascular: Bradycardia, arrhythmias, intracranial hemorrhage
Central nervous system: Brain damage
Hepatic: Neonatal jaundice
Respiratory: Hypoxia
Miscellaneous: Death
Maternal: <1%:
Cardiovascular: Cardiac arrhythmias, premature ventricular contractions, hypotension, tachycardia, arrhythmias
Central nervous system: Seizures, coma
Gastrointestinal: Nausea, vomiting
Hematologic: Postpartum hemorrhage, fatal afibrinogenemia, increased blood loss, pelvic hematoma
Miscellaneous: Death, increased uterine motility, anaphylactic reactions, SIADH with hyponatremia

Drug Interactions No data reported

Drug Uptake

Onset of uterine contractions: I.V.: Within 1 minute
Duration: <30 minutes
Serum half-life: 1-5 minutes

Pregnancy Risk Factor X

P-071 *see* Cetirizine Hydrochloride *on page 179*

Paclitaxel (pak' li tax el)
Brand Names Taxol®
Therapeutic Category Antineoplastic Agent, Antimicrotubular
Use Treatment of metastatic carcinoma of the ovary after failure of first-line or subsequent chemotherapy; treatment of metastatic breast cancer
Usual Dosage Corticosteroids (dexamethasone), H$_1$ antagonists (diphenhydramine), and H$_2$ antagonists (cimetidine or ranitidine), should be administered prior to paclitaxel administration to minimize potential for anaphylaxis
Adults: I.V. infusion: **Refer to individual protocol**
Ovarian carcinoma: 135-175 mg/m^2 over 1-24 hours administered every 3 weeks
Metastatic breast cancer: Treatment is still undergoing investigation; most protocols have used doses of 175-250 mg/m^2 over 1-24 hours every 3 weeks

Local Anesthetic/Vasoconstrictor Precautions No information available to require special precautions
Effects on Dental Treatment No effects or complications reported
Other Adverse Effects
>10%:
Bone marrow suppression: Major dose-limiting (ie, more severe at doses of 200-250 mg/m^2) toxicity
Dermatologic: Alopecia has been observed in almost all patients; loss of scalp hair occurs suddenly between day 14 and 21 and is reversible. Some patients experience a loss of all body hair. Local venous effects include erythema, tenderness, and discomfort during infusion and areas of extravasation include erythema, swelling, and induration. Necrotic changes and ulcers have not been reported even after extravasation of large volumes of infusate.
Hypersensitivity: Based on observations during early clinical trials, reactions were principally nonimmunologically mediated by the direct release of histamine or other vasoactive substances from mast cells and basophils
Neurotoxicity: Typically cumulative, with symptoms progressing after each treatment at both high and low doses. Patients with pre-existing neuropathies due to previous chemotherapy or coexisting medical illness (diabetes mellitus, alcoholism) appear to be predisposed to neurotoxicity. Neurotoxic effects such as sensory neuropathy, motor neuropathy, autonomic neuropathy, myopathy or myopathic effects, and central nervous system toxicity have been reported. Sensory neuropathy occurs invariably when the paclitaxel dose approaches 250 mg/m^2. Symptoms include numbness, tingling, and/or burning pain in the distal lower extremities, toes and/or fingers and begin as early as 24-72 hours after treatment with high single doses. Motor neuropathy occurs primarily at relatively high doses (250-275 mg/m^2) and in those patients with diabetes mellitus who may be more predisposed to toxic neuropathies. Myopathy effects are commonly observed after treatment with moderate to high doses (ie, >200 mg/m^2) administered over 6-24 hours. These symptoms generally occur 2-3 days after treatment and resolve within 5-6 days.
Miscellaneous: Hypersensitivity reactions, myalgia, abnormal liver function tests
1% to 10%:
Cardiovascular: Bradycardia, severe cardiovascular events
Gastrointestinal: Nausea and vomiting are not severe at any dose level
Irritant chemotherapy
Drug Interactions Increased toxicity:
In phase I trials, myelosuppression was more profound when given after cisplatin than with alternative sequence; pharmacokinetic data demonstrates a decrease in clearance of -33% when administered following cisplatin
Possibility of an inhibition of metabolism in patients treated with ketoconazole
Drug Uptake Administered by I.V. infusion and exhibits a biphasic decline in plasma concentrations
Serum half-life, mean, terminal: 5.3-17.4 hours after 1- and 6-hour infusions at dosing levels of 15-275 mg/m^2
Pregnancy Risk Factor D

PALS® [OTC] *see* Chlorophyll *on page 185*
Pamelor® *see* Nortriptyline Hydrochloride *on page 629*

Pamidronate Disodium (pa mi droe' nate dye sow' dee um)
Brand Names Aredia™
Therapeutic Category Antidote, Hypercalcemia; Biphosphonate Derivative
(Continued)

Pamidronate Disodium *(Continued)*

Use FDA-approved: Treatment of hypercalcemia associated with malignancy; treatment of osteolytic bone lesions associated with multiple myeloma; treatment of osteolytic bone metastases of breast cancer; moderate to severe Paget's disease of bone

Usual Dosage Drug must be diluted properly before administration and infused slowly (over at least 1 hour)

Adults: I.V.:

Moderate cancer-related hypercalcemia (corrected serum calcium: 12-13 mg/dL): 60-90 mg given as a slow infusion over 2-24 hours

Severe cancer-related hypercalcemia (corrected serum calcium: >13.5 mg/dL): 90 mg as a slow infusion over 2-24 hours

A period of 7 days should elapse before the use of second course; repeat infusions every 2-3 weeks have been suggested, however, could be administered every 2-3 months according to the degree and of severity of hypercalcemia and/or the type of malignancy

Osteolytic bone lesions with multiple myeloma: 90 mg in 500 mL D_5W, 0.45% NaCl or 0.9% NaCl administered over 4 hours on a monthly basis

Paget's disease: 30 mg in 500 mL 0.45% NaCl, 0.9% NaCl or D_5W administered over 4 hours for 3 consecutive days

Mechanism of Action A biphosphonate which inhibits bone resorption via actions on osteoclasts or on osteoclast precursors. Does not appear to produce any significant effects on renal tubular calcium handling and is poorly absorbed following oral administration (high oral doses have been reported effective); therefore, I.V. therapy is preferred.

Local Anesthetic/Vasoconstrictor Precautions No information available to require special precautions

Effects on Dental Treatment No effects or complications reported

Other Adverse Effects

1% to 10%:

Central nervous system: Malaise, fever, convulsions

Endocrine & metabolic: Hypomagnesemia, hypocalcemia, hypokalemia, hypophosphatemia, fluid overload

Gastrointestinal: GI symptoms, nausea, diarrhea, constipation, anorexia

Hepatic: Abnormal hepatic function

Neuromuscular & skeletal: Bone pain

Respiratory: Dyspnea

<1%:

Dermatologic: Skin rash, angioedema

Hematologic: Leukopenia, occult blood in stools

Neuromuscular & skeletal: Increased risk of fractures

Renal: Nephrotoxicity

Miscellaneous: Pain, hypersensitivity reactions, altered taste

Drug Interactions No data reported

Drug Uptake

Onset of effect: 24-48 hours

Maximum effect: 5-7 days

Absorption: Poorly from the GI tract; pharmacokinetic studies are lacking

Serum half-life, unmetabolized: 2.5 hours

Pregnancy Risk Factor C

Pamine® *see* Methscopolamine Bromide *on page 564*

p-Aminoclonidine *see* Apraclonidine Hydrochloride *on page 72*

Pamprin IB® [OTC] *see* Ibuprofen *on page 447*

Panadol® [OTC] *see* Acetaminophen *on page 14*

Pancrease® *see* Pancrelipase *on next page*

Pancrease® MT 4 *see* Pancrelipase *on next page*

Pancrease® MT 10 *see* Pancrelipase *on next page*

Pancrease® MT 16 *see* Pancrelipase *on next page*

Pancreatin *(pan' kree a tin)*

Brand Names Creon®; Digepepsin®; Donnazyme®; Hi-Vegi-Lip®

Therapeutic Category Pancreatic Enzyme

Use Replacement therapy in symptomatic treatment of malabsorption syndrome caused by pancreatic insufficiency

Local Anesthetic/Vasoconstrictor Precautions No information available to require special precautions

Effects on Dental Treatment No effects or complications reported

Other Adverse Effects

1% to 10%: High Doses:

Endocrine & metabolic: Hyperuricemia

Gastrointestinal: Nausea, cramps, constipation, diarrhea

Ocular: Lacrimation

Respiratory: Sneezing

Miscellaneous: Hyperuricosuria

<1%:

Dermatologic: Rash

Gastrointestinal: Irritation of the mouth

Respiratory: Shortness of breath, bronchospasm

Comments On a weight basis, pancreatin has $1/12$ the lipolytic activity of pancrelipase

Pancrelipase (pan kre li' pase)

Brand Names Cotazym®; Cotazym-S®; Creon® 10; Creon® 20; Ilozyme®; Ku-Zyme® HP; Pancrease®; Pancrease® MT 4; Pancrease® MT 10; Pancrease® MT 16; Protilase®; Ultrase® MT12; Ultrase® MT20; Ultrase® MT24; Viokase®; Zymase®

Therapeutic Category Pancreatic Enzyme

Synonyms Lipancreatin

Use Replacement therapy in symptomatic treatment of malabsorption syndrome caused by pancreatic insufficiency

Usual Dosage Oral:

Powder: Actual dose depends on the digestive requirements of the patient

Children <1 year: Start with $1/8$ teaspoonful with feedings

Adults: 0.7 g with meals

Enteric coated microspheres and microtablets: The following dosage recommendations are only an approximation for initial dosages. The actual dosage will depend on the digestive requirements of the individual patient.

Children:

<1 year: 2000 units of lipase with meals

1-6 years: 4000-8000 units of lipase with meals and 4000 units with snacks

7-12 years: 4000-12,000 units of lipase with meals and snacks

Adults: 4000-16,000 units of lipase with meals and with snacks or 1-3 tablets/capsules before or with meals and snacks; in severe deficiencies, dose may be increased to 8 tablets/capsules

Occluded feeding tubes: One tablet of Viokase® crushed with one 325 mg tablet of sodium bicarbonate (to activate the Viokase®) in 5 mL of water can be instilled into the nasogastric tube and clamped for 5 minutes; then, flushed with 50 mL of tap water

Mechanism of Action Replaces endogenous pancreatic enzymes to assist in digestion of protein, starch and fats

Local Anesthetic/Vasoconstrictor Precautions No information available to require special precautions

Effects on Dental Treatment No effects or complications reported

Other Adverse Effects

1% to 10%: High doses:

Endocrine & metabolic: Hyperuricemia

Gastrointestinal: Nausea, cramps, constipation, diarrhea

Ocular: Lacrimation

Respiratory: Sneezing

Miscellaneous: Hyperuricosuria

<1%:

Dermatologic: Rash

Gastrointestinal: Irritation of the mouth

Respiratory: Shortness of breath, bronchospasm

Drug Uptake

Absorption: Not absorbed, acts locally in GI tract

Pregnancy Risk Factor C

Comments Concomitant administration of conventional pancreatin enzymes with an H_2-receptor antagonist has been used to decrease the inactivation of enzyme activity

Panhematin® see Hemin on page 419

PanOxyl® [OTC] see Benzoyl Peroxide on page 104

PanOxyl®-AQ see Benzoyl Peroxide on page 104

Panscol® see Salicylic Acid on page 777

Panthoderm® [OTC] see Dexpanthenol on page 263

Pantopon® see Opium Alkaloids on page 638

Pantothenic Acid (pan toe then' ik as' id)
Therapeutic Category Vitamin, Water Soluble
Synonyms Calcium Pantothenate; Vitamin B_5
Use Pantothenic acid deficiency
Local Anesthetic/Vasoconstrictor Precautions No information available to require special precautions
Effects on Dental Treatment No effects or complications reported

Papaverine Hydrochloride (pa pav' er een hye droe klor' ide)
Brand Names Cerespan®; Genabid®; Pavabid®; Pavagen®; Pavased®; Pavaspan®; Pavasull®; Pavatab®; Pavatine®; Pavatym®; Paverolan®
Therapeutic Category Vasodilator
Use
Oral: Relief of peripheral and cerebral ischemia associated with arterial spasm; smooth muscle relaxant
Parenteral: Various vascular spasms associated with muscle spasms as in myocardial infarction, angina, peripheral and pulmonary embolism, peripheral vascular disease, angiospastic states, and visceral spasm (ureteral, biliary, and GI colic); testing for impotence
Usual Dosage
Children: I.M., I.V.: 1.5 mg/kg 4 times/day
Adults:
Oral: 100-300 mg 3-5 times/day
Oral, sustained release: 150-300 mg every 12 hours
I.M., I.V.: 30-120 mg every 3 hours as needed; for cardiac extrasystoles, give 2 doses 10 minutes apart I.V. or I.M.
Mechanism of Action Smooth muscle spasmolytic producing a generalized smooth muscle relaxation including: vasodilatation, gastrointestinal sphincter relaxation, bronchiolar muscle relaxation, and potentially a depressed myocardium (with large doses); muscle relaxation may occur due to inhibition or cyclic nucleotide phosphodiesterase, increasing cyclic AMP; muscle relaxation is unrelated to nerve innervation; papaverine increases cerebral blood flow in normal subjects; oxygen uptake is unaltered
Local Anesthetic/Vasoconstrictor Precautions No information available to require special precautions
Effects on Dental Treatment No effects or complications reported
Other Adverse Effects <1%:
Cardiovascular: Flushing of the face, tachycardias, hypotension, arrhythmias with rapid I.V. use
Central nervous system: Depression, dizziness, vertigo, drowsiness, sedation, lethargy, headache
Dermatologic: Pruritus
Gastrointestinal: Dry mouth, nausea, constipation
Hepatic: Hepatic hypersensitivity
Local: Thrombosis at the I.V. administration site
Respiratory: Apnea with rapid I.V. use
Miscellaneous: Sweating
Drug Interactions
Decreased effect: Papaverine decreases the effects of levodopa
Increased toxicity: Additive effects with CNS depressants or morphine
Drug Uptake
Onset of action: Oral: Rapid
Serum half-life: 0.5-1.5 hours
Pregnancy Risk Factor C

Para-Aminosalicylate Sodium
(pair' a-a mee' noe sa lis' i late sow' dee um)
Related Information
Nonviral Infectious Diseases *on page 932*
Therapeutic Category Analgesic, Non-narcotic; Salicylate
Synonyms PAS
Use Adjunctive treatment of tuberculosis
Local Anesthetic/Vasoconstrictor Precautions No information available to require special precautions
Effects on Dental Treatment No effects or complications reported
Other Adverse Effects 1% to 10%:
Endocrine & metabolic: Hypokalemia
Gastrointestinal: Nausea, vomiting, diarrhea
Hepatic: Hepatitis, jaundice
Miscellaneous: Allergy reactions

Comments Capsules contain bentonite which may decrease absorption of concomitantly ingested drugs

Paracetamol (Mexico) *see* Acetaminophen *on page 14*

Parachlorometaxylenol (pair' a klor oh met a zye' le nol)
Brand Names Metasep® [OTC]
Therapeutic Category Antiseborrheic Agent, Topical
Synonyms PCMX
Use Aid in relief of dandruff and associated conditions
Local Anesthetic/Vasoconstrictor Precautions No information available to require special precautions
Effects on Dental Treatment No effects or complications reported

Paraflex® *see* Chlorzoxazone *on page 200*
Parafon Forte™ DSC *see* Chlorzoxazone *on page 200*

Paramethasone Acetate (par a meth' a sone as' e tate)
Brand Names Haldrone®; Stemex®
Therapeutic Category Adrenal Corticosteroid
Use Treatment of variety of diseases including those of hematologic, allergic, inflammatory, neoplastic, and autoimmune in origin
Local Anesthetic/Vasoconstrictor Precautions No information available to require special precautions
Effects on Dental Treatment No effects or complications reported
Comments Likely to inhibit maturation and growth in adolescents; at high doses (>15 mg/d) increased urinary excretion of nitrogen and calcium will occur

Paraplatin® *see* Carboplatin *on page 155*
Par Decon® *see* Chlorpheniramine, Phenyltoloxamine, Phenylpropanolamine, and Phenylephrine *on page 194*
Paredrine® *see* Hydroxyamphetamine Hydrobromide *on page 440*

Paregoric (par e gor' ik)
Therapeutic Category Analgesic, Narcotic; Antidiarrheal
Use Treatment of diarrhea or relief of pain; neonatal opiate withdrawal
Usual Dosage Oral:
  Neonatal opiate withdrawal: Instill 3-6 drops every 3-6 hours as needed, or initially 0.2 mL every 3 hours; increase dosage by approximately 0.05 mL every 3 hours until withdrawal symptoms are controlled; it is rare to exceed 0.7 mL/dose. Stabilize withdrawal symptoms for 3-5 days, then gradually decrease dosage over a 2- to 4-week period.
  Children: 0.25-0.5 mL/kg 1-4 times/day
  Adults: 5-10 mL 1-4 times/day
Mechanism of Action Increases smooth muscle tone in GI tract, decreases motility and peristalsis, diminishes digestive secretions
Local Anesthetic/Vasoconstrictor Precautions No information available to require special precautions
Effects on Dental Treatment No effects or complications reported
Other Adverse Effects
  >10%:
    Cardiovascular: Hypotension
    Central nervous system: Weakness, drowsiness, dizziness
    Gastrointestinal: Constipation
  1% to 10%:
    Central nervous system: Restlessness, headache, malaise
    Genitourinary: Ureteral spasms, decreased urination
    Miscellaneous: Histamine release
  <1%:
    Cardiovascular: Peripheral vasodilation
    Central nervous system: Insomnia, CNS depression, mental depression, increased intracranial pressure
    Gastrointestinal: Anorexia, stomach cramps, nausea, vomiting
    Ocular: Miosis
    Respiratory: Respiratory depression
    Miscellaneous: Biliary or urinary tract spasm, physical and psychological dependence
Drug Interactions Increased effect/toxicity with CNS depressants (eg, alcohol, narcotics, benzodiazepines, TCAs, MAO inhibitors, phenothiazine)
Pregnancy Risk Factor B (D when used long-term or in high doses)

Paremyd® Ophthalmic *see* Hydroxyamphetamine and Tropicamide *on page 440*

Parepectolin® *see* Kaolin and Pectin With Opium *on page 480*

Pargen Fortified® *see* Chlorzoxazone *on page 200*

Par Glycerol® *see* Iodinated Glycerol *on page 465*

Pargyline and Methyclothiazide *see* Methyclothiazide and Pargyline *on page 566*

Parhist SR® *see* Chlorpheniramine and Phenylpropanolamine *on page 190*

Parlodel® *see* Bromocriptine Mesylate *on page 121*

Parnate® *see* Tranylcypromine Sulfate *on page 860*

Paromomycin Sulfate (par oh moe mye' sin sul' fate)
Brand Names Humatin®
Therapeutic Category Amebicide
Use Treatment of acute and chronic intestinal amebiasis due to susceptible *Entamoeba histolytica* (not effective in the treatment of extraintestinal amebiasis); tapeworm infestations; adjunctive management of hepatic coma; treatment of cryptosporidial diarrhea
Usual Dosage Oral:
  Intestinal amebiasis: Children and Adults: 25-35 mg/kg/day in 3 divided doses for 5-10 days
  Dientamoeba fragilis: Children and Adults: 25-30 mg/kg/day in 3 divided doses for 7 days
  Cryptosporidium: Adults with AIDS: 1.5-2.25 g/day in 3-6 divided doses for 10-14 days (occasionally courses of up to 4-8 weeks may be needed)
  Tapeworm (fish, dog, bovine, porcine):
    Children: 11 mg/kg every 15 minutes for 4 doses
    Adults: 1 g every 15 minutes for 4 doses
  Hepatic coma: Adults: 4 g/day in 2-4 divided doses for 5-6 days
  Dwarf tapeworm: Children and Adults: 45 mg/kg/dose every day for 5-7 days
Mechanism of Action Acts directly on ameba; has antibacterial activity against normal and pathogenic organisms in the GI tract; interferes with bacterial protein synthesis by binding to 30S ribosomal subunits
Local Anesthetic/Vasoconstrictor Precautions No information available to require special precautions
Effects on Dental Treatment No effects or complications reported
Other Adverse Effects
  1% to 10%: Gastrointestinal: Diarrhea, abdominal cramps, nausea, vomiting, heartburn
  <1%:
    Central nervous system: Headache, vertigo
    Dermatologic: Rash, pruritus, exanthema
    Gastrointestinal: Steatorrhea, secondary enterocolitis
    Hematologic: Eosinophilia
    Otic: Ototoxicity
Drug Uptake
  Absorption: Not absorbed via oral route
Pregnancy Risk Factor C

Paroxetina (Mexico) *see* Paroxetine *on this page*

Paroxetine (pa rox' e teen)
Related Information
  Vasoconstrictor Interactions With Antidepressants *on page 1108*
Brand Names Paxil™
Therapeutic Category Antidepressant, Selective Serotonin Reuptake Inhibitor
Synonyms Paroxetina (Mexico)
Use Treatment of depression; presently being investigated for obsessive-compulsive disorder
Usual Dosage Adults: Oral:
  Depression: 20 mg once daily (maximum: 60 mg/day), preferably in the morning; in elderly, debilitated, or patients with hepatic or renal impairment, start with 10 mg/day (maximum: 40 mg/day); adjust doses at 7-day intervals
  Panic disorder and obsessive compulsive disorder: Recommended average daily dose: 40 mg, this dosage should be given after an adequate trial on 20 mg/day and then titrating upward
Mechanism of Action Paroxetine is a selective serotonin reuptake inhibitor, chemically unrelated to tricyclic, tetracyclic, or other antidepressants; presumably, the inhibition of serotonin reuptake from brain synapse stimulated serotonin activity in the brain
Local Anesthetic/Vasoconstrictor Precautions Although caution should be used in patients taking tricyclic antidepressants, no interactions have been

reported with vasoconstrictor and paroxetine, a nontricyclic antidepressant which acts to increase serotonin

Effects on Dental Treatment Prolonged use of paroxetine may decrease or inhibit salivary flow; normal salivary flow will resume with cessation of drug therapy

Other Adverse Effects
>10%:
Central nervous system: Headache, asthenia, somnolence, dizziness, insomnia,
Gastrointestinal: Nausea, dry mouth, constipation, diarrhea
Genitourinary: Ejaculatory disturbances
Miscellaneous: Sweating
1% to 10%:
Cardiovascular: Palpitations, vasodilation, postural hypotension
Central nervous system: Nervousness, anxiety
Endocrine & metabolic: Decreased libido
Gastrointestinal: Anorexia, flatulence, vomiting
Neuromuscular & skeletal: Tremor, paresthesia
<1%:
Cardiovascular: Bradycardia, hypotension
Central nervous system: Migraine, akinesia
Dermatologic: Alopecia
Endocrine & metabolic: Amenorrhea
Gastrointestinal: Gastritis
Hematologic: Anemia, leukopenia
Neuromuscular & skeletal: Arthritis
Otic: Ear pain
Ocular: Eye pain
Respiratory: Asthma
Miscellaneous: Bruxism, thirst

Drug Interactions
Decreased effect of paroxetine when taken with phenobarbital, phenytoin
Increased toxicity: Alcohol, cimetidine, MAO inhibitors (hyperpyrexic crisis); increased effect/toxicity of tricyclic antidepressants, fluoxetine, sertraline, phenothiazines, class 1C antiarrhythmics, warfarin

Drug Uptake Serum half-life: 21 hours
Pregnancy Risk Factor B

Parsidol® see Ethopropazine Hydrochloride on page 343
Partuss® LA see Guaifenesin and Phenylpropanolamine on page 409
PAS see Para-Aminosalicylate Sodium on page 658
Pathilon® see Tridihexethyl Chloride on page 868
Pathocil® see Dicloxacillin Sodium on page 273
Patients Requiring Sedation see page 965
Patients Undergoing Cancer Therapy see page 967
Pavabid® see Papaverine Hydrochloride on page 658
Pavagen® see Papaverine Hydrochloride on page 658
Pavased® see Papaverine Hydrochloride on page 658
Pavaspan® see Papaverine Hydrochloride on page 658
Pavasull® see Papaverine Hydrochloride on page 658
Pavatab® see Papaverine Hydrochloride on page 658
Pavatine® see Papaverine Hydrochloride on page 658
Pavatym® see Papaverine Hydrochloride on page 658
Paverolan® see Papaverine Hydrochloride on page 658
Paxil™ see Paroxetine on previous page
Paxipam® see Halazepam on page 415
PBZ® see Tripelennamine on page 877
PBZ-SR® see Tripelennamine on page 877
PCE® see Erythromycin on page 321
PCMX see Parachlorometaxylenol on page 659
Pectin and Kaolin see Kaolin and Pectin on page 480
Pedameth® see Methionine on page 557
PediaCare® Oral see Pseudoephedrine on page 749
Pediacof® see Chlorpheniramine, Phenylephrine, and Codeine on page 192
Pediaflor® see Fluoride on page 374
Pediapred® see Prednisolone on page 718
PediaProfen™ see Ibuprofen on page 447
Pediazole® see Erythromycin and Sulfisoxazole on page 323

Pedi-Boro® [OTC] see Aluminum Sulfate and Calcium Acetate on page 41

Pedi-Cort V® Topical see Clioquinol and Hydrocortisone on page 216

Pedi-Dri Topical see Undecylenic Acid and Derivatives on page 884

PediOtic® Otic see Neomycin, Polymyxin B, and Hydrocortisone on page 610

Pedi-Pro Topical [OTC] see Undecylenic Acid and Derivatives on page 884

Pedituss® see Chlorpheniramine, Phenylephrine, and Codeine on page 192

Pedte-Pak-5® see Trace Metals on page 857

Pedtrace-4® see Trace Metals on page 857

PedvaxHIB™ see Haemophilus b Conjugate Vaccine on page 414

Pegademase Bovine (peg a' de mase boe' vine)

Brand Names Adagen™

Therapeutic Category Enzyme, Replacement Therapy

Use Enzyme replacement therapy for adenosine deaminase (ADA) deficiency in patients with severe combined immunodeficiency disease (SCID) who can not benefit from bone marrow transplant

Usual Dosage Children: I.M.: Dose given every 7 days, 10 units/kg the first dose, 15 units/kg the second dose, and 20 units/kg the third dose; maintenance dose: 20 units/kg/week is recommended depending on patient's ADA level; maximum single dose: 30 units/kg

Mechanism of Action Adenosine deaminase is an enzyme that catalyzes the deamination of both adenosine and deoxyadenosine. Hereditary lack of adenosine deaminase activity results in severe combined immunodeficiency disease, a fatal disorder of infancy characterized by profound defects of both cellular and humoral immunity. It is estimated that 25% of patients with the autosomal recessive form of severe combined immunodeficiency lack adenosine deaminase.

Local Anesthetic/Vasoconstrictor Precautions No information available to require special precautions

Effects on Dental Treatment No effects or complications reported

Other Adverse Effects <1%:
Central nervous system: Headache
Local: Pain at injection site

Drug Uptake
Plasma adenosine deaminase activity generally normalizes after 2-3 weeks of weekly I.M. injections
Absorption: Rapid
Serum half-life: 48-72 hours

Pregnancy Risk Factor C

Peganone® see Ethotoin on page 344

Pegaspargase (peg as' par jase)

Brand Names Oncaspar®

Therapeutic Category Antineoplastic Agent, Miscellaneous

Synonyms PEG-L-asparaginase

Use Induction treatment of acute lymphoblastic leukemia in combination with other chemotherapeutic agents in patients who have developed hypersensitivity to native forms of asparaginase derived from E. coli and/or Erwinia chrysanthemia, treatment of lymphoma

Usual Dosage
Dose must be individualized based upon clinical response and tolerance of the patient (refer to individual protocols)
I.M. administration is **preferred** over I.V. administration; I.M. administration may decrease the incidence of hepatotoxicity, coagulopathy, and GI and renal disorders

Children: I.M., I.V.:
Body surface area ≤0.6 m^2: 82.5 units/kg every 14 days
Body surface area ≥0.6 m^2: 2500 units/m^2 every 14 days
Adults: I.M., I.V.: 2,500 units/m^2 every 14 days

Mechanism of Action
Pegaspargase is a modified version of the enzyme asparaginase. The asparaginase used in the manufacture of pegaspargase is derived from Escherichia coli.
Some malignant cells (ie, lymphoblastic leukemia cells and those of lymphocyte derivation) must acquire the amino acid asparagine from surrounding fluid such as blood, whereas normal cells can synthesize their own asparagine. asparaginase is an enzyme that deaminates asparagine to aspartic acid and ammonia in the plasma and extracellular fluid and therefore deprives tumor cells of the amino acid for protein synthesis.

Local Anesthetic/Vasoconstrictor Precautions No information available to require special precautions

Effects on Dental Treatment No effects or complications reported

Other Adverse Effects

Overall, the adult patients had a somewhat higher incidence of asparaginase toxicities, except for hypersensitivity reactions, than the pediatric patients

>10%:

Hypersensitivity: Acute or delayed, acute anaphylaxis, bronchospasm, dyspnea, urticaria, arthralgia, erythema, induration, edema, pain, tenderness, hives, swelling lip

Pancreatic: Pancreatitis, (sometimes fulminant and fatal); increased serum amylase and lipase

Hepatic: Elevations of AST, ALT and bilirubin (direct and indirect); jaundice, ascites and hypoalbuminemia, fatty changes in the liver; liver failure

>5%:

Allergic reactions: rash, erythema, edema, pain, fever, chills, urticaria, dyspnea or bronchospasm

Emetic potential: Mild (>5%)

Miscellaneous: ALT increase, fever, malaise

1% to 5%:

Cardiovascular: Hypotension, tachycardia, thrombosis

Central nervous system: Chills

Dermatologic: Lip edema, rash, urticaria

Gastrointestinal: Abdominal pain

Hematologic: Decreased anticoagulant effect, disseminated intravascular coagulation, decreased fibrinogen, hemolytic anemia, leukopenia, pancytopenia, thrombocytopenia, increased thromboplastin

Local: Injection site hypersensitivity

Myelosuppressive effects:

WBC: Mild

Platelets: Mild

Onset (days): 7

Nadir (days): 14

Recovery (days): 21

Respiratory: Dyspnea

Drug Uptake

Serum half-life: 5.73 days

Pregnancy Risk Factor C

PEG-L-asparaginase see Pegaspargase on previous page

Pemoline (pem' oh leen)

Brand Names Cylert®

Therapeutic Category Central Nervous System Stimulant, Nonamphetamine

Use Treatment of attention deficit disorder with hyperactivity (ADDH); narcolepsy

Usual Dosage Children ≥6 years: Oral: Initial: 37.5 mg given once daily in the morning, increase by 18.75 mg/day at weekly intervals; usual effective dose range: 56.25-75 mg/day; maximum: 112.5 mg/day; dosage range: 0.5-3 mg/kg/24 hours; significant benefit may not be evident until third or fourth week of administration

Mechanism of Action Blocks the reuptake mechanism of dopaminergic neurons, appears to act at the cerebral cortex and subcortical structures; CNS and respiratory stimulant with weak sympathomimetic effects; actions may be mediated via increase in CNS dopamine

Local Anesthetic/Vasoconstrictor Precautions Pemoline has minimal sympathomimetic effects; there are no precautions in using vasoconstrictors

Effects on Dental Treatment No effects or complications reported

Other Adverse Effects

>10%:

Central nervous system: Insomnia

Gastrointestinal: Anorexia, weight loss

1% to 10%:

Central nervous system: Dizziness, drowsiness, mental depression

Dermatologic: Skin rash

Gastrointestinal: Stomach pain, nausea

<1%:

Central nervous system: Seizures, precipitation of Tourette's syndrome, hallucination, headache, movement disorders

Dermatologic: Skin rashes

Endocrine & metabolic: Growth reaction

Gastrointestinal: Diarrhea

(Continued)

663

Pemoline *(Continued)*

Hepatic: Increased liver enzymes (usually reversible upon discontinuation), hepatitis, jaundice

Drug Interactions Decreased effect of insulin

Drug Uptake
Duration: 8 hours
Serum half-life:
Children: 7-8.6 hours
Adults: 12 hours
Time to peak serum concentration: Oral: Within 2-4 hours

Pregnancy Risk Factor B

Penamp® *see Ampicillin on page 62*

Penbutolol Sulfate *(pen byoo' toe lole sul' fate)*

Related Information
Cardiovascular Diseases *on page 912*

Brand Names Levatol®

Therapeutic Category Beta-Adrenergic Blocker, Noncardioselective

Use Treatment of mild to moderate arterial hypertension

Mechanism of Action Blocks both beta$_1$- and beta$_2$-receptors and has mild intrinsic sympathomimetic activity; has negative inotropic and chronotropic effects and can significantly slow A-V nodal conduction

Local Anesthetic/Vasoconstrictor Precautions No information available to require special precautions

Effects on Dental Treatment No effects or complications reported

Other Adverse Effects
1% to 10%:
Cardiovascular: Congestive heart failure, irregular heart beat
Central nervous system: Mental depression, headache, dizziness
Neuromuscular & skeletal: Back pain, joint pain
<1%:
Cardiovascular: Bradycardia, chest pain, mesenteric arterial thrombosis, A-V block, persistent bradycardia, hypotension, chest pain, edema, Raynaud's phenomena
Central nervous system: Fatigue, insomnia, lethargy, impotence, nightmares, depression, confusion
Dermatologic: Purpura
Endocrine & metabolic: Hyperglycemia
Gastrointestinal: Ischemic colitis, constipation, nausea, diarrhea
Hematologic: Thrombocytopenia
Respiratory: Bronchospasm
Miscellaneous: Cold extremities

Penciclovir

Related Information
Oral Viral Infections *on page 951*

Brand Names Denavir®

Therapeutic Category Antiviral Agent, Topical

Use Antiviral cream for the treatment of recurrent herpes labialis (cold sores) in adults

Usual Dosage Apply cream at the first sign or symptom of cold sore (eg, tingling, swelling); apply every 2 hours during waking hours for 4 days

Mechanism of Action In cells infected with HSV-1 or HSV-2, viral thymidine kinase phosphorylates penciclovir to a monophosphate form which, in turn, is converted to penciclovir triphosphate by cellular kinases. Penciclovir triphosphate inhibits HSV polymerase competitively with deoxyguanosine triphosphate. Consequently, herpes viral DNA synthesis and, therefore, replication are selectively inhibited

Local Anesthetic/Vasoconstrictor Precautions No information available to require special precautions

Effects on Dental Treatment No effects or complications reported

Other Adverse Effects 1% to 10%:
Central nervous system: Headache
Local: Application site reaction

Oral manifestations: No data reported

Contraindications Patients with known hypersensitivity to the product or any of its components

Warnings/Precautions Penciclovir should only be used on herpes labialis on the lips and face; because no data are available, application to mucous membranes is not recommended. Avoid application in or near eyes since it may cause irritation. The effect of penciclovir has not been established in immunocompromised patients.

Drug Interactions No data reported

Drug Uptake Measurable penciclovir concentrations were not detected in plasma or urine of health male volunteers following single or repeat application of the 1% cream at a dose of 180 mg penciclovir daily (approximately 67 times the usual clinical dose)

Pregnancy Risk Factor B

Dosage Forms Cream: 10 mg/g (1%) (2 g tubes)

Generic Available No

Penetrex™ *see* Enoxacin *on page 310*

Penicilina G Procainica (Mexico) *see* Penicillin G Procaine *on page 667*

Penicillin G Benzathine and Procaine Combined
(pen i sil' in jee benz' a theen & proe' kane kom' bined)

Brand Names Bicillin® C-R 900/300 Injection; Bicillin® C-R Injection

Therapeutic Category Antibiotic, Penicillin

Synonyms Penicillin G Procaine and Benzathine Combined

Use Active against most gram-positive organisms, mostly streptococcal and pneumococcal

Local Anesthetic/Vasoconstrictor Precautions No information available to require special precautions

Effects on Dental Treatment No effects or complications reported

Other Adverse Effects 1% to 10%:

Central nervous system: Jarisch-Herxheimer reaction, CNS toxicity (convulsions, confusion, drowsiness, myoclonus)

Hematologic: Positive Coombs' reaction, hemolytic anemia

Renal: Interstitial nephritis

Miscellaneous: Hypersensitivity reactions

Penicillin G Benzathine, Parenteral
(pen i sil' in gee benz' a theen, pa ren' ter al)

Related Information

Dental Drug Interactions: Update on Drug Combinations Requiring Special Considerations *on page 1022*

Nonviral Infectious Diseases *on page 932*

Brand Names Bicillin® L-A; Permapen®

Canadian/Mexican Brand Names Megacillin® Susp (Canada); Benzetacil® (Mexico); Benzilfan® (Mexico)

Therapeutic Category Antibiotic, Penicillin

Use Active against some gram-positive organisms, few gram-negative organisms such as *Neisseria gonorrhoeae*, and some anaerobes and spirochetes; used only for the treatment of mild to moderately severe infections caused by organisms susceptible to low concentrations of penicillin G or for prophylaxis of infections caused by these organisms; used when patient cannot be kept in a hospital environment and neurosyphilis has been ruled out

The CDC and AAP do not currently recommend the use of penicillin G benzathine to treat congenital syphilis or neurosyphilis due to reported treatment failures and lack of published clinical data on its efficacy

Usual Dosage I.M.: Give undiluted injection; higher doses result in more sustained rather than higher levels. Use a penicillin G benzathine-penicillin G procaine combination to achieve early peak levels in acute infections.

Children:

Group A streptococcal upper respiratory infection: 25,000-50,000 units/kg as a single dose; maximum: 1.2 million units

Prophylaxis of recurrent rheumatic fever: 25,000-50,000 units/kg every 3-4 weeks; maximum: 1.2 million units/dose

Early syphilis: 50,000 units/kg as a single injection; maximum: 2.4 million units

Syphilis of more than 1-year duration: 50,000 units/kg every week for 3 doses; maximum: 2.4 million units/dose

Adults:

Group A streptococcal upper respiratory infection: 1.2 million units as a single dose

Prophylaxis of recurrent rheumatic fever: 1.2 million units every 3-4 weeks or 600,000 units twice monthly

Early syphilis: 2.4 million units as a single dose in 2 injection sites

Syphilis of more than 1-year duration: 2.4 million units in 2 injection sites once weekly for 3 doses

(Continued)

Penicillin G Benzathine, Parenteral *(Continued)*

Not indicated as single drug therapy for neurosyphilis, but may be given 1 time/week for 3 weeks following I.V. treatment (refer to Penicillin G monograph for dosing)

Mechanism of Action Interferes with bacterial cell wall synthesis during active multiplication, causing cell wall death and resultant bactericidal activity against susceptible bacteria

Local Anesthetic/Vasoconstrictor Precautions No information available to require special precautions

Effects on Dental Treatment No effects or complications reported

Other Adverse Effects

1% to 10%: Local: Local pain

<1%:

Central nervous system: Convulsions, confusion, drowsiness, fever

Dermatologic: Rash

Endocrine & metabolic: Electrolyte imbalance

Hematologic: Hemolytic anemia, positive Coombs' reaction

Local: Thrombophlebitis

Neuromuscular & skeletal: Myoclonus

Renal: Acute interstitial nephritis

Miscellaneous: Jarisch-Herxheimer reaction, hypersensitivity reactions, anaphylaxis

Drug Interactions

Decreased effect: Tetracyclines cause decreased penicillin effectiveness

Increased effect:

Probenecid causes increased penicillin levels

Drug Uptake

Absorption: I.M.: Slow

Time to peak serum concentration: Within 12-24 hours; serum levels are usually detectable for 1-4 weeks depending on the dose; larger doses result in more sustained levels rather than higher levels

Pregnancy Risk Factor B

Penicillin G, Parenteral, Aqueous

(pen i sil' in jee, pa ren' ter al, aye' kwee us)

Related Information

Antimicrobial Prophylaxis in Surgical Patients *on page 1042*

Dental Drug Interactions: Update on Drug Combinations Requiring Special Considerations *on page 1022*

Nonviral Infectious Diseases *on page 932*

Brand Names Pfizerpen®

Canadian/Mexican Brand Names Benzanil® (Mexico); Lentopenil® (Mexico)

Therapeutic Category Antibiotic, Penicillin

Use Active against some gram-positive organisms, generally not *Staphylococcus aureus*; some gram-negative such as *Neisseria gonorrhoeae*, and some anaerobes and spirochetes; although ceftriaxone is now the drug of choice for Lyme disease and gonorrhea

Usual Dosage I.M., I.V.:

Children (sodium salt is preferred in children): 100,000-250,000 units/kg/day in divided doses every 4 hours; maximum: 4.8 million units/24 hours

Severe infections: Up to 400,000 units/kg/day in divided doses every 4 hours; maximum dose: 24 million units/day

Adults: 2-24 million units/day in divided doses every 4 hours

Congenital syphilis:

Disseminated gonococcal infections or gonococcus ophthalmia (if organism proven sensitive): 100,000 units/kg/day in 2 equal doses (4 equal doses/day for infants >1 week)

Gonococcal meningitis: 150,000 units/kg in 2 equal doses (4 doses/day for infants >1 week)

Mechanism of Action Interferes with bacterial cell wall synthesis during active multiplication, causing cell wall death and resultant bactericidal activity against susceptible bacteria

Local Anesthetic/Vasoconstrictor Precautions No information available to require special precautions

Effects on Dental Treatment No effects or complications reported

Other Adverse Effects <1%:

Central nervous system: Convulsions, confusion, drowsiness, fever

Dermatologic: Rash

Endocrine & metabolic: Electrolyte imbalance

Hematologic: Hemolytic anemia, positive Coombs' reaction
Local: Thrombophlebitis
Neuromuscular & skeletal: Myoclonus
Renal: Acute interstitial nephritis
Miscellaneous: Jarisch-Herxheimer reaction, hypersensitivity reactions, anaphylaxis

Drug Interactions
Decreased effect: Tetracyclines cause decreased penicillin effectiveness
Increased effect: Probenecid causes increased penicillin levels

Drug Uptake
Time to peak serum concentration:
I.M.: Within 30 minutes
I.V. Within 1 hour
Serum half-life:
Children and adults with normal renal function: 20-50 minutes
End stage renal disease: 3.3-5.1 hours

Pregnancy Risk Factor B

Penicillin G Potassium, Oral (pen i sil′ in gee poe tass′ y um)
Related Information
Dental Drug Interactions: Update on Drug Combinations Requiring Special Considerations *on page 1022*

Therapeutic Category Antibiotic, Penicillin

Use Treatment of susceptible bacterial infections including most gram-positive organisms (except *Staphylococcus aureus*), some gram-negative organisms such as *Neisseria gonorrhoeae*, and some anaerobes and spirochetes

Usual Dosage Oral:
Children: 25-50 mg/kg/day or 40,000-80,000 units/kg/day divided every 6-8 hours hours
Adults: 125-500 mg every 6-8 hours

Mechanism of Action Inhibits bacterial cell wall synthesis by binding to one or more of the penicillin binding proteins (PBPs); which in turn inhibits the final transpeptidation step of peptidoglycan synthesis in bacterial cell walls, thus inhibiting cell wall biosynthesis. Bacteria eventually lyse due to ongoing activity of cell wall autolytic enzymes (autolysins and murein hydrolases) while cell wall assembly is arrested.

Local Anesthetic/Vasoconstrictor Precautions No information available to require special precautions

Effects on Dental Treatment Prolonged use of penicillins may lead to development of oral candidiasis

Other Adverse Effects <1%:
Central nervous system: Convulsions, confusion, drowsiness, fever
Dermatologic: Rash
Endocrine & metabolic: Electrolyte imbalance
Hematologic: Hemolytic anemia, positive Coombs' reaction
Neuromuscular & skeletal: Myoclonus
Renal: Acute interstitial nephritis
Miscellaneous: Jarisch-Herxheimer reaction, hypersensitivity reactions, anaphylaxis

Drug Interactions
Decreased effect: Tetracyclines causes decreased penicillin effectiveness
Increased effect:
Probenecid causes increased penicillin levels

Drug Uptake
Absorption: Oral: <30%; acid labile
Time to peak serum concentration: Oral: Within 0.5-1 hour

Pregnancy Risk Factor B

Dosage Forms
Powder for oral solution, as potassium: 400,000 units/5 mL (100 mL, 200 mL); 400,000 units = 250 mg
Tablet, as potassium: 200,000 units, 250,000 units, 400,000 units, 500,000 units, 800,000 units; 400,000 units = 250 mg

Generic Available Yes

Penicillin G Procaine (pen i sil′ in jee proe′ kane)
Related Information
Dental Drug Interactions: Update on Drug Combinations Requiring Special Considerations *on page 1022*

Brand Names Crysticillin® A.S.; Pfizerpen®-AS; Wycillin®

Canadian/Mexican Brand Names Ayercillin® (Canada); Penicil® (Mexico); Penipot® (Mexico); Penprocilina® (Mexico)
(Continued)

Penicillin G Procaine *(Continued)*

Therapeutic Category Antibiotic, Penicillin

Synonyms Penicilina G Procainica (Mexico)

Use Moderately severe infections due to *Neisseria gonorrhoeae, Treponema pallidum* and other penicillin G-sensitive microorganisms that are susceptible to low but prolonged serum penicillin concentrations

Usual Dosage I.M.:

Children: 25,000-50,000 units/kg/day in divided doses 1-2 times/day; not to exceed 4.8 million units/24 hours

Gonorrhea: 100,000 units/kg (maximum 4.8 million units) one time (in 2 injection sites) along with probenecid 25 mg/kg (maximum: 1 g orally) 30 minutes prior to procaine penicillin

Congenital syphilis: 50,000 units/kg/day for 10-14 days

Adults: 0.6-4.8 million units/day in divided doses every 12-24 hours

Uncomplicated gonorrhea: 1 g probenecid orally, then 4.8 million units procaine penicillin divided into 2 injection sites 30 minutes later

Endocarditis caused by susceptible viridans *Streptococcus* (when used in conjunction with an aminoglycoside): 1.2 million units every 6 hours for 2-4 weeks

Neurosyphilis: I.M.: 2-4 million units/day with 500 mg probenecid by mouth 4 times/day for 10-14 days; **penicillin G aqueous I.V. is the preferred agent**

Moderately dialyzable (20% to 50%)

Mechanism of Action Inhibits bacterial cell wall synthesis by binding to one or more of the penicillin binding proteins (PBPs); which in turn inhibits the final transpeptidation step of peptidoglycan synthesis in bacterial cell walls, thus inhibiting cell wall biosynthesis. Bacteria eventually lyse due to ongoing activity of cell wall autolytic enzymes (autolysins and murein hydrolases) while cell wall assembly is arrested.

Local Anesthetic/Vasoconstrictor Precautions No information available to require special precautions

Effects on Dental Treatment No effects or complications reported

Other Adverse Effects

>10%: Local: Pain at injection site

<1%:

Cardiovascular: Myocardial depression, vasodilation, conduction disturbances

Central nervous system: CNS stimulation, seizures, confusion, drowsiness, Jarisch-Herxheimer reaction

Hematologic: Hemolytic anemia, positive Coombs' reaction

Local: Sterile abscess at injection site

Neuromuscular & skeletal: Myoclonus

Renal: Interstitial nephritis

Miscellaneous: Pseudoanaphylactic reactions, hypersensitivity reactions

Drug Interactions

Decreased effect: Tetracyclines cause decreased penicillin effectiveness

Increased effect: Probenecid causes increased penicillin levels

Drug Uptake

Absorption: I.M.: Slowly absorbed

Time to peak serum concentration: Within 1-4 hours; can persist within the therapeutic range for 15-24 hours

Pregnancy Risk Factor B

Penicillin G Procaine and Benzathine Combined *see* Penicillin G Benzathine and Procaine Combined *on page 665*

Penicillin V Potassium *(pen i sil' in vee poe tass' y um)*

Related Information

Dental Drug Interactions: Update on Drug Combinations Requiring Special Considerations *on page 1022*
Oral Bacterial Infections *on page 945*
Oral Viral Infections *on page 951*

Brand Names Beepen-VK®; Betapen®-VK; Ledercillin® VK; Pen.Vee® K; Robicillin® VK; V-Cillin K®; Veetids®

Canadian/Mexican Brand Names Apo-Pen® VK (Canada); Nadopen-V® (Canada); Novo-Pen-VK® (Canada); Nu-Pen-VK® (Canada); PVF® K (Canada); Anapenil® (Mexico); Pen-Vi-K® (Mexico)

Therapeutic Category Antibiotic, Penicillin

Use

Dental: Antibiotic of first choice in treating common orofacial infections caused by aerobic gram-positive cocci and anaerobes. These orofacial infections include cellulitis, periapical abscess, periodontal abscess, acute suppurative pulpitis, oronasal fistula, pericoronitis, osteitis, osteomyelitis, postsurgical and post-traumatic infection. It is no longer recommended for dental procedure prophylaxis.

Medical: Treatment of moderate to severe susceptible bacterial infections involving the respiratory tract, otitis media, sinusitis, skin, and and urinary tract

Usual Dosage

Children <12 years: Daily dose: 25-50 mg/kg in divided doses every 6-8 hours for 7 days; maximum daily dose: 3 g

Children >12 years and Adults: 250-500 mg every 6 hours for at least 7 days

Mechanism of Action Inhibits bacterial cell wall synthesis by binding to one or more of the penicillin binding proteins (PBPs); which in turn inhibits the final transpeptidation step of peptidoglycan synthesis in bacterial cell walls, thus inhibiting cell wall biosynthesis. Bacteria eventually lyse due to ongoing activity of cell wall autolytic enzymes (autolysins and murein hydrolases) while cell wall assembly is arrested.

Local Anesthetic/Vasoconstrictor Precautions No information available to require special precautions

Effects on Dental Treatment Prolonged use of penicillins may lead to development of oral candidiasis

Other Adverse Effects

>10%: Gastrointestinal: Mild diarrhea, vomiting, nausea, oral candidiasis

1% to 10%: Miscellaneous: Hypersensitivity reactions

Oral manifestations: Oral candidiasis

Contraindications Known hypersensitivity to penicillin or any component

Warnings/Precautions Use with caution in patients with severe renal impairment (modify dosage), history of seizures, or hypersensitivity to cephalosporins

Drug Interactions Tetracyclines may decrease penicillin effectiveness; probenecid may increase penicillin levels; aminoglycosides cause synergistic efficacy

Drug Uptake

Absorption: Oral: 60% to 73% from GI tract

Time to peak serum concentration: Oral: Within 0.5-1 hour

Serum half-life: 0.5 hours

Pregnancy Risk Factor B

Breast-feeding Considerations No data reported; however, other penicillins may be taken while breast-feeding

Dosage Forms

Powder for oral solution: 125 mg/5 mL (3 mL, 100 mL, 150 mL, 200 mL); 250 mg/5 mL (100 mL, 150 mL, 200 mL)

Tablet: 125 mg, 250 mg, 500 mg

Dietary Considerations Peak concentration may be delayed with food; may be taken with water on an empty stomach 1 hour before or 2 hours after meals or may be taken with food

Generic Available Yes

Selected Readings

Wynn RL and Bergman SA, "Antibiotics and Their Use in the Treatment of Orofacial Infections," *Gen Dent*, 1994, 42(Pt 1):398-402 and 42(Pt 2):498-502.

Pentaerythritol Tetranitrate (pen ta er ith' ri tole te tra nye' trate)

Related Information

Cardiovascular Diseases *on page 912*

Brand Names Duotrate®; Peritrate®; Peritrate® SA

Therapeutic Category Antianginal Agent; Nitrate; Vasodilator, Coronary

Use Possibly effective for the prophylactic long-term management of angina pectoris. **Note:** Not indicated to abort acute anginal episodes

Usual Dosage Adults: Oral: 10-20 mg 4 times/day up to 40 mg 4 times/day before or after meals and at bedtime; sustained release preparation 80 mg twice daily; use lowest recommended doses in elderly initially; titrations up to 240 mg/day are tolerated, however, headache may occur with increasing doses (reduce dose for a few days; if headache returns or is persistent, an analgesic can be used to treat symptoms)

Mechanism of Action Stimulation of intracellular cyclic-GMP results in vascular smooth muscle relaxation of both arterial and venous vasculature. Increased venous pooling decreases left ventricular pressure (preload) and (Continued)

Pentaerythritol Tetranitrate *(Continued)*

arterial dilatation decreases arterial resistance (afterload). Therefore, this reduces cardiac oxygen demand by decreasing left ventricular pressure and systemic vascular resistance by dilating arteries. Additionally, coronary artery dilation improves collateral flow to ischemic regions; esophageal smooth muscle is relaxed via the same mechanism.

Local Anesthetic/Vasoconstrictor Precautions No information available to require special precautions

Effects on Dental Treatment No effects or complications reported

Other Adverse Effects

>10%:
  Cardiovascular: Flushing, postural hypotension
  Central nervous system: Headache, lightheadedness, dizziness
  Neuromuscular & skeletal: Weakness
1% to 10%: Dermatologic: Drug rash, exfoliative dermatitis
<1%:
  Gastrointestinal: Nausea, vomiting
  Hematologic: Methemoglobinemia (overdose)

Drug Interactions No data reported

Drug Uptake
  Onset of hemodynamic effect: Oral: Within 20-60 minutes
  Duration: 4-5 hours, or up to 12 hours with the sustained release formulations
  Serum half-life: 10 minutes

Pregnancy Risk Factor C

Pentagastrin *(pen ta gas' trin)*

Brand Names Peptavlon®

Therapeutic Category Diagnostic Agent, Gastric Acid Secretory Function

Use Evaluate gastric acid secretory function in pernicious anemia, gastric carcinoma; in suspected duodenal ulcer or Zollinger-Ellison tumor

Usual Dosage Adults:
  I.M., S.C.: 6 mcg/kg
  I.V. infusion: 0.1-12 mcg/kg/hour in 0.9% sodium chloride

Mechanism of Action Excites the oxyntic cells of the stomach to secrete to their maximum capacity similar to the naturally occurring hormone, gastrin

Local Anesthetic/Vasoconstrictor Precautions No information available to require special precautions

Effects on Dental Treatment No effects or complications reported

Other Adverse Effects
  >10%: Gastrointestinal: Abdominal pain, desire to defecate, nausea, vomiting
  1% to 10%:
    Cardiovascular: Flushing, tachycardia, palpitations, hypotension
    Central nervous system: Dizziness, faintness, headache
    Respiratory: Shortness of breath
  <1%: Miscellaneous: Allergic reactions

Drug Uptake
  Absorption: I.M., S.C.: Well absorbed
  Serum half-life: 1 minute

Pregnancy Risk Factor C

Pentam-300® *see* Pentamidine Isethionate *on this page*

Pentamidina (Mexico) *see* Pentamidine Isethionate *on this page*

Pentamidine Isethionate *(pen tam' i deen eye seth eye' oh nate)*

Brand Names NebuPent™; Pentam-300®

Canadian/Mexican Brand Names Pentacarinat® (Mexico)

Therapeutic Category Antibiotic, Miscellaneous

Synonyms Pentamidina (Mexico)

Use Treatment and prevention of pneumonia caused by *Pneumocystis carinii*; treatment of trypanosomiasis

Usual Dosage
  Children:
    Treatment: I.M., I.V. (I.V. preferred): 4 mg/kg/day once daily for 10-14 days
    Prevention:
      I.M., I.V.: 4 mg/kg monthly or every 2 weeks
      Inhalation (aerosolized pentamidine in children ≥5 years): 300 mg/dose given every 3-4 weeks via Respirgard® II inhaler (8 mg/kg dose has also been used in children <5 years)
    Treatment of trypanosomiasis: I.V.: 4 mg/kg/day once daily for 10 days

Adults:
Treatment: I.M., I.V. (I.V. preferred): 4 mg/kg/day once daily for 14 days
Prevention: Inhalation: 300 mg every 4 weeks via Respirgard® II nebulizer

Not removed by hemo or peritoneal dialysis or continuous arterio-venous or veno-venous hemofiltration (CAVH/CAVHD); supplemental dosage is not necessary

Mechanism of Action Interferes with RNA/DNA, phospholipids and protein synthesis, through inhibition of oxidative phosphorylation and/or interference with incorporation of nucleotides and nucleic acids into RNA and DNA, in protozoa

Local Anesthetic/Vasoconstrictor Precautions No information available to require special precautions

Effects on Dental Treatment No effects or complications reported

Other Adverse Effects
>10%:
Cardiovascular: Chest pain
Dermatologic: Skin rash
Endocrine & metabolic: Hyperkalemia
Local: Local reactions at injection site
Respiratory: Wheezing, dyspnea, coughing, pharyngitis
1% to 10%: Gastrointestinal: Bitter or metallic taste
<1%:
Cardiovascular: Hypotension, tachycardia
Central nervous system: Dizziness, fever, fatigue, Jarisch-Herxheimer-like reaction
Endocrine & metabolic: Hyperglycemia or hypoglycemia, hypocalcemia
Gastrointestinal: Pancreatitis, vomiting
Hematologic: Megaloblastic anemia, granulocytopenia, leukopenia, thrombocytopenia
Renal: Renal insufficiency
Respiratory: Extrapulmonary pneumocystosis, irritation of the airway
Miscellaneous: Pneumothorax, mild renal or hepatic injury

Drug Interactions No data reported

Drug Uptake
Absorption: I.M.: Well absorbed
Serum half-life, terminal: 6.4-9.4 hours; may be prolonged in patients with severe renal impairment

Pregnancy Risk Factor C

Pentasa® *see* Mesalamine *on page 546*

Pentaspan® *see* Pentastarch *on this page*

Pentastarch (pen' ta starch)
Brand Names Pentaspan®
Therapeutic Category Blood Modifiers
Use Adjunct in leukapheresis to improve the harvesting and increase the yield of leukocytes by centrifugal means
Local Anesthetic/Vasoconstrictor Precautions No information available to require special precautions
Effects on Dental Treatment No effects or complications reported

Pentazocine (pen taz' oh seen)
Related Information
Narcotic Agonist Charts *on page 1019*
Brand Names Talwin®; Talwin® NX
Therapeutic Category Analgesic, Narcotic
Use Relief of moderate to severe pain; has also been used as a sedative prior to surgery and as a supplement to surgical anesthesia
Usual Dosage
Children: I.M., S.C.:
5-8 years: 15 mg
8-14 years: 30 mg

Children >12 years and Adults: Oral: 50 mg every 3-4 hours; may increase to 100 mg/dose if needed, but should not exceed 600 mg/day
Adults:
I.M., S.C.: 30-60 mg every 3-4 hours, not to exceed total daily dose of 360 mg
I.V.: 30 mg every 3-4 hours
(Continued)

Pentazocine *(Continued)*

Mechanism of Action Binds to opiate receptors in the CNS, causing inhibition of ascending pain pathways, altering the perception of and response to pain; produces generalized CNS depression; partial agonist-antagonist

Local Anesthetic/Vasoconstrictor Precautions No information available to require special precautions

Effects on Dental Treatment No effects or complications reported

Other Adverse Effects

>10%:
Central nervous system: Euphoria, weakness, drowsiness
Gastrointestinal: Nausea, vomiting

1% to 10%:
Cardiovascular: Hypotension
Central nervous system: Malaise, headache, restlessness, nightmares
Dermatologic: Skin rash
Gastrointestinal: Dry mouth
Genitourinary: Ureteral spasm
Ocular: Blurred vision
Respiratory: Troubled breathing

<1%:
Cardiovascular: Palpitations, bradycardia, peripheral vasodilation
Central nervous system: Insomnia, CNS depression, sedation, hallucinations, confusion, disorientation, seizures may occur in seizure-prone patients, increased intracranial pressure
Dermatologic: Pruritus
Endocrine & metabolic: Antidiuretic hormone release
Gastrointestinal: GI irritation, constipation
Local: Tissue damage and irritation with I.M./S.C. use
Ocular: Miosis
Miscellaneous: Biliary or urinary tract spasm, histamine release physical and psychological dependence

Drug Interactions May potentiate or reduce analgesic effect of opiate agonist, (eg, morphine) depending on patients tolerance to opiates can precipitate withdrawal in narcotic addicts

Increased effect/toxicity with tripelennamine (can be lethal), CNS depressants (phenothiazines, tranquilizers, anxiolytics, sedatives, hypnotics, or alcohol)

Drug Uptake
Onset of action:
Oral, I.M., S.C.: Within 15-30 minutes
I.V.: Within 2-3 minutes
Duration:
Oral: 4-5 hours
Parenteral: 2-3 hours
Serum half-life: 2-3 hours; increased with decreased hepatic function

Pregnancy Risk Factor B (D if used for prolonged periods or in high doses at term)

Dosage Forms
Injection, as lactate: 30 mg/mL (1 mL, 1.5 mL, 2 mL, 10 mL)
Tablet: Pentazocine hydrochloride 50 mg and naloxone hydrochloride 0.5 mg

Generic Available No

Pentazocine Compound *(pen taz' oh seen kom' pownd)*

Brand Names Talacen®; Talwin® Compound

Therapeutic Category Analgesic, Narcotic

Use Relief of moderate to severe pain; has also been used as a sedative prior to surgery and as a supplement to surgical anesthesia

Local Anesthetic/Vasoconstrictor Precautions No information available to require special precautions

Effects on Dental Treatment No effects or complications reported

Comments Abrupt discontinuation after sustained use (generally >10 days) may cause withdrawal symptoms

Pentobarbital *(pen toe bar' bi tal)*

Brand Names Nembutal®

Therapeutic Category Barbiturate; Sedative

Use Short-term treatment of insomnia; preoperative sedation; high-dose barbiturate coma for treatment of increased intracranial pressure or status epilepticus unresponsive to other therapy

Usual Dosage

Children:

Sedative: Oral: 2-6 mg/kg/day divided in 3 doses; maximum: 100 mg/day

Hypnotic: I.M.: 2-6 mg/kg; maximum: 100 mg/dose

Rectal:

2 months to 1 year (10-20 lb): 30 mg

1-4 years (20-40 lb): 30-60 mg

5-12 years (40-80 lb): 60 mg

12-14 years (80-110 lb): 60-120 mg

or

<4 years: 3-6 mg/kg/dose

>4 years: 1.5-3 mg/kg/dose

Preoperative/preprocedure sedation: ≥6 months:

Oral, I.M., rectal: 2-6 mg/kg; maximum: 100 mg/dose

I.V.: 1-3 mg/kg to a maximum of 100 mg until asleep

Children 5-12 years: Conscious sedation prior to a procedure: I.V.: 2 mg/kg 5-10 minutes before procedures, may repeat one time

Adolescents: Conscious sedation: Oral, I.V.: 100 mg prior to a procedure

Adults:

Hypnotic:

Oral: 100-200 mg at bedtime or 20 mg 3-4 times/day for daytime sedation

I.M.: 150-200 mg

I.V.: Initial: 100 mg, may repeat every 1-3 minutes up to 200-500 mg total dose

Rectal: 120-200 mg at bedtime

Preoperative sedation: I.M.: 150-200 mg

Children and Adults: Barbiturate coma in head injury patients: I.V.: Loading dose: 5-10 mg/kg given slowly over 1-2 hours; monitor blood pressure and respiratory rate; Maintenance infusion: Initial: 1 mg/kg/hour; may increase to 2-3 mg/kg/hour; maintain burst suppression on EEG

Mechanism of Action Short-acting barbiturate with sedative, hypnotic, and anticonvulsant properties

Local Anesthetic/Vasoconstrictor Precautions No information available to require special precautions

Effects on Dental Treatment No effects or complications reported

Other Adverse Effects

Genitourinary: Oliguria

>10%:

Cardiovascular: Cardiac arrhythmias, bradycardia, hypotension, arterial spasm, and gangrene with inadvertent intra-arterial injection

Central nervous system: Drowsiness, lethargy, CNS excitation or depression, impaired judgment, "hangover" effect

Local: Pain at injection site, thrombophlebitis with I.V. use

1% to 10%:

Central nervous system: Confusion, mental depression, unusual excitement, nervousness, faint feeling, headache, insomnia, nightmares

Gastrointestinal: Nausea, vomiting, constipation

<1%:

Cardiovascular: Thrombophlebitis, hypotension

Central nervous system: Hallucinations

Dermatologic: Rash, exfoliative dermatitis, Stevens-Johnson syndrome

Endocrine & metabolic: Hypothermia

Hematologic: Agranulocytosis, thrombocytopenia, megaloblastic anemia

Respiratory: Laryngospasm, respiratory depression, apnea (especially with rapid I.V. use)

Drug Interactions

Decreased effect: Decreased chloramphenicol; decreased doxycycline effects

Increased toxicity: Increased CNS depressants, cimetidine; causes increase effect of pentobarbital

Drug Uptake

Onset of action:

Oral, rectal: 15-60 minutes

I.M.: Within 10-15 minutes

I.V.: Within 1 minute

Duration:

Oral, rectal: 1-4 hours

I.V.: 15 minutes

Serum half-life, terminal:

Children: 25 hours

Adults, normal: 22 hours; range: 35-50 hours

Pregnancy Risk Factor D

(Continued)

Pentolair® *see* Cyclopentolate Hydrochloride *on page 240*

Pentosan Polysulfate Sodium
Brand Names Elmiron®
Therapeutic Category Analgesic, Urinary
Use Bladder pain relief or discomfort associated with interstitial cystitis
Usual Dosage Adults: Oral: 100 mg 3 times/day
Local Anesthetic/Vasoconstrictor Precautions No information available to require special precautions
Effects on Dental Treatment No effects or complications reported
Pregnancy Risk Factor B

Pentostatin (pen' toe stat in)
Brand Names Nipent™ Injection
Therapeutic Category Antineoplastic Agent, Antimetabolite; Antineoplastic Agent, Nonirritant
Synonyms DCF; Deoxycoformycin; 2'-deoxycoformycin
Use Treatment of adult patients with alpha-interferon-refractory hairy cell leukemia; significant antitumor activity in various lymphoid neoplasms has been demonstrated; pentostatin also is known as 2'-deoxycoformycin; it is a purine analogue capable of inhibiting adenosine deaminase
Usual Dosage Refractory hairy cell leukemia: Adults (refer to individual protocols): 4 mg/m^2 every other week; I.V. bolus over ≥3-5 minutes in D_5W or NS at concentrations ≥2 mg/mL
Mechanism of Action An antimetabolite inhibiting adenosine deaminase (ADA), prevents ADA from controlling intracellular adenosine levels through the irreversible deamination of adenosine and deoxyadenosine. ADA is found to exhibit the highest activity in lymphoid tissue. Patients receiving pentostatin accumulate deoxyadenosine (dAdo) and deoxyadenosine 5'-triphosphate (dATP); accumulation of dATP results in cell death, probably through inhibiting DNA or RNA synthesis. Following a single dose, pentostatin has the ability to inhibit ADA for periods exceeding 1 week.
Local Anesthetic/Vasoconstrictor Precautions No information available to require special precautions
Effects on Dental Treatment No effects or complications reported
Other Adverse Effects
>10%:
  Central nervous system: Headache, neurologic disorder, fever, fatigue, chills, pain
  Dermatologic: Rash
  Gastrointestinal: Vomiting, nausea, anorexia, diarrhea
  Hematologic: Leukopenia, anemia, thrombocytopenia
  Hepatic: Hepatic disorder, liver function tests (abnormal)
  Neuromuscular & skeletal: Myalgia
  Respiratory: Coughing
  Miscellaneous: Allergic reaction
1% to 10%:
  Cardiovascular: Chest pain, arrhythmia, peripheral edema
  Central nervous system: Anxiety, confusion, depression, dizziness, insomnia, lethargy, coma, seizures, asthenia, malaise
  Dermatologic: Dry skin, eczema, pruritus
  Gastrointestinal: Constipation, flatulence, stomatitis, weight loss
  Genitourinary: Dysuria
  Hematologic: Myelosuppression
  Hepatic: Liver dysfunction
  Local: Thrombophlebitis
  Neuromuscular & skeletal: Arthralgia, paresthesia, back pain
  Ocular: Abnormal vision, eye pain, keratoconjunctivitis
  Otic: Ear pain
  Renal: Renal failure, hematuria
  Respiratory: Bronchitis, dyspnea, lung edema, pneumonia
  Miscellaneous: Death, opportunistic infections, sweating
Drug Uptake
  Serum half-life, terminal: 5-15 hours
Pregnancy Risk Factor D

Pentothal® Sodium *see* Thiopental Sodium *on page 839*
Pentoxifilina (Mexico) *see* Pentoxifylline *on next page*

Pentoxifylline (pen tox i' fi leen)
Brand Names Trental®
Canadian/Mexican Brand Names Peridane® (Mexico)
Therapeutic Category Blood Viscosity Reducer Agent
Synonyms Pentoxifilina (Mexico)
Use Symptomatic management of peripheral vascular disease, mainly intermittent claudication

Unapproved use: AIDS patients with increased TNF, CVA, cerebrovascular diseases, diabetic atherosclerosis, diabetic neuropathy, gangrene, hemodialysis shunt thrombosis, vascular impotence, cerebral malaria, septic shock, sickle cell syndromes, and vasculitis

Usual Dosage Adults: Oral: 400 mg 3 times/day with meals; may reduce to 400 mg twice daily if GI or CNS side effects occur
Mechanism of Action Mechanism of action remains unclear; is thought to reduce blood viscosity and improve blood flow by altering the rheology of red blood cells
Local Anesthetic/Vasoconstrictor Precautions No information available to require special precautions
Effects on Dental Treatment No effects or complications reported
Other Adverse Effects
1% to 10%:
Central nervous system: Dizziness, headache
Gastrointestinal: Dyspepsia, nausea, vomiting
<1%:
Cardiovascular: Mild hypotension, angina
Central nervous system: Agitation
Ocular: Blurred vision
Otic: Earache
Drug Interactions Increased effect/toxic potential with cimetidine (increased levels) and other H_2 antagonists, warfarin; increased effect of antihypertensives
Drug Uptake
Absorption: Oral: Well absorbed
Serum half-life:
Parent drug: 24-48 minutes
Metabolites: 60-96 minutes
Time to peak serum concentration: Within 2-4 hours
Pregnancy Risk Factor C

Pentrax® [OTC] *see* Coal Tar *on page 225*

Pen.Vee® K *see* Penicillin V Potassium *on page 668*

Pepcid® [OTC] *see* Famotidine *on page 352*

Peptavlon® *see* Pentagastrin *on page 670*

Pepto-Bismol® (subsalicylate) [OTC] *see* Bismuth *on page 114*

Pepto® Diarrhea Control [OTC *see* Loperamide Hydrochloride *on page 511*

Percocet® *see* Oxycodone and Acetaminophen *on page 646*

Percodan® *see* Oxycodone and Aspirin *on page 647*

Percodan®-Demi *see* Oxycodone and Aspirin *on page 647*

Percogesic® [OTC] *see* Acetaminophen and Phenyltoloxamine *on page 17*

Perdiem® Plain [OTC] *see* Psyllium *on page 750*

Perfectoderm® [OTC] *see* Benzoyl Peroxide *on page 104*

Perfenacina (Mexico) *see* Perphenazine *on page 677*

Pergolida, Mesilato De (Mexico) *see* Pergolide Mesylate *on this page*

Pergolide Mesylate (per' go lide mes' i late)
Brand Names Permax®
Therapeutic Category Anti-Parkinson's Agent; Ergot Alkaloid and Derivative
Synonyms Pergolida, Mesilato De (Mexico)
Use Adjunctive treatment to levodopa/carbidopa in the management of Parkinson's Disease
Usual Dosage When adding pergolide to levodopa/carbidopa, the dose of the latter can usually and should be decreased. Patients no longer responsive to bromocriptine may benefit by being switched to pergolide.

Adults: Oral: Start with 0.05 mg/day for 2 days, then increase dosage by 0.1 or 0.15 mg/day every 3 days over next 12 days, increase dose by 0.25 mg/day every 3 days until optimal therapeutic dose is achieved, up to 5 mg/day maximum; usual dosage range: 2-3 mg/day in 3 divided doses
(Continued)

Pergolide Mesylate *(Continued)*

Mechanism of Action Pergolide is a semisynthetic ergot alkaloid similar to bromocriptine but stated to be more potent and longer acting; it is a centrally-active dopamine agonist stimulating both D_1 and D_2 receptors

Local Anesthetic/Vasoconstrictor Precautions No information available to require special precautions

Effects on Dental Treatment Pergolide may decrease or inhibit salivary flow; normal salivary flow will resume with cessation of drug therapy; prolonged salivary reduction could enhance development of periodontal disease, oral candidiasis and discomfort

Other Adverse Effects
>10%:
Central nervous system: Dizziness, somnolence, insomnia, confusion, hallucinations, anxiety
Gastrointestinal: Nausea, constipation
Neuromuscular & skeletal: Dyskinesias, dystonia
Respiratory: Rhinitis
1% to 10%:
Cardiovascular: Myocardial infarction, postural hypotension, syncope, arrhythmias, peripheral edema, vasodilation, palpitations, chest pain, dyspnea
Central nervous system: Insomnia, abnormal vision, asthenia, chills
Gastrointestinal: Diarrhea, abdominal pain, vomiting, dry mouth, anorexia, weight gain
Miscellaneous: Flu syndrome

Drug Interactions Decreased effect: Dopamine antagonists, metoclopramide

Drug Uptake
Absorption: Oral: Well absorbed

Pregnancy Risk Factor B

Pergonal® *see* Menotropins *on page 538*
Periactin® *see* Cyproheptadine Hydrochloride *on page 244*
Peri-Colace® [OTC] *see* Docusate and Casanthranol *on page 295*
Peridex® *see* Chlorhexidine Gluconate *on page 184*

Perindopril Erbumine *(per in' doe pril er byoo' meen)*

Brand Names Aceon®
Therapeutic Category Antihypertensive
Use Treatment of hypertension
Usual Dosage Adults: Oral:
Congestive heart failure: 4 mg once daily
Hypertension: Initial: 4 mg/day but may be titrated to response; usual range: 4-8 mg/day, maximum: 16 mg/day
Mechanism of Action Competitive inhibitor of angiotensin-converting enzyme (ACE); prevents conversion of angiotensin I to angiotensin II, a potent vasoconstrictor; results in lower levels of angiotensin II which, in turn, causes an increase in plasma renin activity and a reduction in aldosterone secretion
Local Anesthetic/Vasoconstrictor Precautions No information available to require special precautions
Effects on Dental Treatment No effects or complications reported
Drug Uptake
Serum half-life:
Parent drug: 1.5-3 hours
Time to peak: Occurs in 1 and 3-4 hours for perindopril and perindoprilat, respectively after chronic therapy; (maximum perindoprilat serum levels are 2-3 times higher and T_{max} is shorter following chronic therapy); in CHF, the peak of perindoprilat is prolonged to 6 hours
Pregnancy Risk Factor D (especially during 2nd and 3rd trimester)

PerioGard® *see* Chlorhexidine Gluconate *on page 184*
Peritrate® *see* Pentaerythritol Tetranitrate *on page 669*
Peritrate® SA *see* Pentaerythritol Tetranitrate *on page 669*
Permapen® *see* Penicillin G Benzathine, Parenteral *on page 665*
Permax® *see* Pergolide Mesylate *on previous page*

Permethrin *(per meth' rin)*

Brand Names Elimite™; Nix™ [OTC]
Therapeutic Category Antiparasitic Agent, Topical; Scabicidal Agent
Use Single application treatment of infestation with *Pediculus humanus capitis* (head louse) and its nits or *Sarcoptes scabiei* (scabies)

Usual Dosage Topical: Children >2 months and Adults:

Head lice: After hair has been washed with shampoo, rinsed with water, and towel dried, apply a sufficient volume of topical liquid to saturate the hair and scalp. Leave on hair for 10 minutes before rinsing off with water; remove remaining nits; may repeat in 1 week if lice or nits still present.

Scabies: Apply cream from head to toe; leave on for 8-14 hours before washing off with water; for infants, also apply on the hairline, neck, scalp, temple, and forehead; may reapply in 1 week if live mites appear

Permethrin 5% cream was shown to be safe and effective when applied to an infant <1 month of age with neonatal scabies; time of application was limited to 6 hours before rinsing with soap and water

Mechanism of Action Inhibits sodium ion influx through nerve cell membrane channels in parasites resulting in delayed repolarization and thus paralysis and death of the pest

Local Anesthetic/Vasoconstrictor Precautions No information available to require special precautions

Effects on Dental Treatment No effects or complications reported

Other Adverse Effects 1% to 10%:

Dermatologic: Pruritus, erythema, rash of the scalp, numbness or scalp discomfort

Local: Burning, stinging, tingling, numbness or scalp discomfort, edema

Drug Interactions No data reported

Drug Uptake

Absorption: Topical: Minimal (<2%)

Pregnancy Risk Factor B

Permitil® see Fluphenazine on page 379

Pernox® [OTC] see Sulfur and Salicylic Acid on page 813

Perphenazine (per fen' a zeen)

Brand Names Trilafon®

Canadian/Mexican Brand Names Apo-Perphenazine® (Canada); PMS-Perphenazine® (Canada); Leptopsique® (Mexico)

Therapeutic Category Antiemetic; Antipsychotic Agent; Phenothiazine Derivative

Synonyms Perfenacina (Mexico)

Use Management of manifestations of psychotic disorders, depressive neurosis, alcohol withdrawal, nausea and vomiting, nonpsychotic symptoms associated with dementia in elderly, Tourette's syndrome, Huntington's chorea, spasmodic torticollis and Reye's syndrome

Usual Dosage

Children:

Psychoses: Oral:

1-6 years: 4-6 mg/day in divided doses

6-12 years: 6 mg/day in divided doses

>12 years: 4-16 mg 2-4 times/day

I.M.: 5 mg every 6 hours

Nausea/vomiting: I.M.: 5 mg every 6 hours

Adults:

Psychoses:

Oral: 4-16 mg 2-4 times/day not to exceed 64 mg/day

I.M.: 5 mg every 6 hours up to 15 mg/day in ambulatory patients and 30 mg/day in hospitalized patients

Nausea/vomiting:

Oral: 8-16 mg/day in divided doses up to 24 mg/day

I.M.: 5-10 mg every 6 hours as necessary up to 15 mg/day in ambulatory patients and 30 mg/day in hospitalized patients

I.V. (severe): 1 mg at 1- to 2-minute intervals up to a total of 5 mg

Not dialyzable (0% to 5%)

Mechanism of Action Blocks postsynaptic mesolimbic dopaminergic receptors in the brain; exhibits a strong alpha-adrenergic blocking effect and depresses the release of hypothalamic and hypophyseal hormones

Local Anesthetic/Vasoconstrictor Precautions No information available to require special precautions

Effects on Dental Treatment Significant hypotension may occur, especially when the drug is administered parenterally; orthostatic hypotension is due to alpha-receptor blockade, the elderly are at greater risk for orthostatic hypotension

(Continued)

677

Perphenazine *(Continued)*

Tardive dyskinesia: Prevalence rate may be 40% in elderly; development of the syndrome and the irreversible nature are proportional to duration and total cumulative dose over time

Extrapyramidal reactions are more common in elderly with up to 50% developing these reactions after 60 years of age; drug-induced **Parkinson's syndrome** occurs often; **Akathisia** is the most common extrapyramidal reaction in elderly

Increased confusion, memory loss, psychotic behavior, and agitation frequently occur as a consequence of anticholinergic effects

Antipsychotic associated sedation in nonpsychotic patients is extremely unpleasant due to feelings of depersonalization, derealization, and dysphoria

Other Adverse Effects

>10%:
  Cardiovascular: Hypotension, orthostatic hypotension
  Central nervous system: Pseudoparkinsonism, akathisia, dystonias, tardive dyskinesia (persistent), dizziness
  Gastrointestinal: Constipation
  Ocular: Pigmentary retinopathy
  Respiratory: Nasal congestion
  Miscellaneous: Decreased sweating

1% to 10%:
  Central nervous system: Dizziness
  Dermatologic: Increased sensitivity to sun, skin rash
  Endocrine & metabolic: Changes in menstrual cycle, changes in libido, pain in breasts
  Gastrointestinal: Weight gain, vomiting, stomach pain, nausea
  Genitourinary: Difficulty in urination, ejaculatory disturbances
  Neuromuscular & skeletal: Trembling of fingers

<1%:
  Central nervous system: Neuroleptic malignant syndrome (NMS)
  Dermatologic: Discoloration of skin (blue-gray), pigmentary retinopathy
  Endocrine & metabolic: Galactorrhea
  Genitourinary: Priapism
  Hematologic: Agranulocytosis, leukopenia
  Hepatic: Cholestatic jaundice, hepatotoxicity
  Ocular: Cornea and lens changes
  Miscellaneous: Impairment of temperature regulation, lowering of seizures threshold

Drug Interactions Increased toxicity: Additive effects with other CNS depressants

Drug Uptake
  Absorption: Oral: Well absorbed
  Serum half-life: 9 hours
  Time to peak serum concentration: Within 4-8 hours

Pregnancy Risk Factor C

Perphenazine and Amitriptyline *see* Amitriptyline and Perphenazine *on page 50*

Persa-Gel® *see* Benzoyl Peroxide *on page 104*

Persantine® *see* Dipyridamole *on page 290*

Pertofrane® *see* Desipramine Hydrochloride *on page 257*

Pertussin® CS [OTC] *see* Dextromethorphan *on page 266*

Pertussin® ES [OTC] *see* Dextromethorphan *on page 266*

Pethidine Hydrochloride (Canada) *see* Meperidine Hydrochloride *on page 539*

Pfizerpen® *see* Penicillin G, Parenteral, Aqueous *on page 666*

Pfizerpen®-AS *see* Penicillin G Procaine *on page 667*

PGE₁ *see* Alprostadil *on page 35*

Pharmaflur® *see* Fluoride *on page 374*

Phazyme® [OTC] *see* Simethicone *on page 788*

Phenameth® DM *see* Promethazine With Dextromethorphan *on page 735*

Phenaphen® With Codeine *see* Acetaminophen and Codeine *on page 15*

Phenazine® *see* Promethazine Hydrochloride *on page 733*

Phenazodine® *see* Phenazopyridine Hydrochloride *on next page*

Phenazopyridine Hydrochloride
(fen az oh peer' i deen hye droe klor' ide)

Brand Names Azo-Standard®; Baridium®; Eridium®; Geridium®; Phenazodine®; Pyridiate®; Pyridium®; Urodine®; Urogesic®

Canadian/Mexican Brand Names Phenazo® (Canada); Pyronium® (Canada); Vito Reins® (Canada); Azo Wintomylon® (Mexico); Madel® (Mexico); Urovalidin® (Mexico)

Therapeutic Category Analgesic, Urinary; Local Anesthetic, Urinary

Synonyms Fenazopiridina (Mexico)

Use Symptomatic relief of urinary burning, itching, frequency and urgency in association with urinary tract infection or following urologic procedures

Usual Dosage Oral:

Children: 12 mg/kg/day in 3 divided doses administered after meals for 2 days

Adults: 100-200 mg 3 times/day after meals for 2 days when used concomitantly with an antibacterial agent

Mechanism of Action An azo dye which exerts local anesthetic or analgesic action on urinary tract mucosa through an unknown mechanism

Local Anesthetic/Vasoconstrictor Precautions No information available to require special precautions

Effects on Dental Treatment No effects or complications reported

Other Adverse Effects

1% to 10%:
Central nervous system: Headache, dizziness
Gastrointestinal: Stomach cramps

<1%:
Central nervous system: Vertigo
Dermatologic: Skin pigmentation, rash
Hematologic: Methemoglobinemia, hemolytic anemia
Hepatic: Hepatitis
Renal: Acute renal failure

Drug Interactions No data reported

Pregnancy Risk Factor B

Phencen® *see* Promethazine Hydrochloride *on page 733*

Phen DH® w/Codeine *see* Chlorpheniramine, Pseudoephedrine, and Codeine *on page 195*

Phenelzine Sulfate (fen' el zeen sul' fate)
Brand Names Nardil®

Therapeutic Category Antidepressant, Monoamine Oxidase Inhibitor

Use Symptomatic treatment of atypical, nonendogenous or neurotic depression

The MAO inhibitors are usually reserved for patients who do not tolerate or respond to the traditional "cyclic" or "second generation" antidepressants. The brain activity of monoamine oxidase increases with age and even more so in patients with Alzheimer's disease. Therefore, the MAO inhibitors may have an increased role in patients with Alzheimer's disease who are depressed. Phenelzine is less stimulating than tranylcypromine.

Usual Dosage Oral:

Adults: 15 mg 3 times/day; may increase to 60-90 mg/day during early phase of treatment, then reduce to dose for maintenance therapy slowly after maximum benefit is obtained; takes 2-4 weeks for a significant response to occur

Elderly: Initial: 7.5 mg/day; increase by 7.5-15 mg/day every 3-4 days as tolerated; usual therapeutic dose: 15-60 mg/day in 3-4 divided doses

Mechanism of Action Thought to act by increasing endogenous concentrations of epinephrine, norepinephrine, dopamine and serotonin through inhibition of the enzyme (monoamine oxidase) responsible for the breakdown of these neurotransmitters

Local Anesthetic/Vasoconstrictor Precautions Attempts should be made to avoid use of vasoconstrictor due to possibility of hypertensive episodes with monoamine oxidase inhibitors

Effects on Dental Treatment Orthostatic hypotension in >10% of patients; meperidine should be avoided as an analgesic due to toxic reactions with MAO inhibitors

Other Adverse Effects

>10%:
Cardiovascular: Orthostatic hypotension
Central nervous system: Drowsiness, weakness
Endocrine & metabolic: Decreased sexual ability
Neuromuscular & skeletal: Trembling

(Continued)

679

Phenelzine Sulfate *(Continued)*

Ocular: Blurred vision

1% to 10%:

Cardiovascular; Tachycardia, peripheral edema

Central nervous system: Nervousness, chills

Gastrointestinal: Diarrhea, anorexia, dry mouth, constipation

<1%:

Central nervous system: Parkinsonism syndrome

Hematologic: Leukopenia

Hepatic: Hepatitis

Drug Interactions

Decreased effect of antihypertensives

Increased toxicity with disulfiram (possible seizures), fluoxetine (and other serotonin active agents), tricyclic antidepressants (cardiovascular instability), meperidine (cardiovascular instability), phenothiazines (hyperpyretic crisis), levodopa, sympathomimetics (hypertensive crisis), barbiturates, rauwolfia alkaloids (eg, reserpine), dextroamphetamine (psychoses), foods containing tyramine

Drug Uptake

Onset of action: Within 2-4 weeks

Absorption: Oral: Well absorbed

Duration: May continue to have a therapeutic effect and interactions 2 weeks after discontinuing therapy

Pregnancy Risk Factor C

Phenerbel-S® *see* Belladonna, Phenobarbital, and Ergotamine Tartrate *on page 99*

Phenergan® *see* Promethazine Hydrochloride *on page 733*

Phenergan® VC Syrup *see* Promethazine and Phenylephrine *on page 733*

Phenergan® VC With Codeine *see* Promethazine, Phenylephrine, and Codeine *on page 734*

Phenergan® With Codeine *see* Promethazine and Codeine *on page 733*

Phenergan® With Dextromethorphan *see* Promethazine With Dextromethorphan *on page 735*

Phenetron® *see* Chlorpheniramine Maleate *on page 191*

Phenhist® Expectorant *see* Guaifenesin, Pseudoephedrine, and Codeine *on page 410*

Phenindamine Tartrate *(fen in' dah meen tar' trate)*

Brand Names Nolahist® [OTC]

Therapeutic Category Decongestant, Nasal

Use Treatment of perennial and seasonal allergic rhinitis and chronic urticaria

Local Anesthetic/Vasoconstrictor Precautions No information available to require special precautions

Effects on Dental Treatment No effects or complications reported

Pheniramine and Naphazoline *see* Naphazoline and Pheniramine *on page 605*

Pheniramine, Phenylpropanolamine, and Pyrilamine

(fen eer' a meen, fen il proe pa nole' a meen, & peer il' a meen)

Brand Names Triaminic® Oral Infant Drops

Therapeutic Category Antihistamine/Decongestant Combination

Use Symptomatic relief of nasal congestion and postnasal drip as well as allergic rhinitis

Local Anesthetic/Vasoconstrictor Precautions No information available to require special precautions

Effects on Dental Treatment No effects or complications reported

Phenobarbital *(fee noe bar' bi tal)*

Brand Names Barbita®; Luminal®; Solfoton®

Canadian/Mexican Brand Names Barbilixir® (Canada); Alepsal® (Mexico)

Therapeutic Category Anticonvulsant, Barbiturate; Barbiturate; Hypnotic; Sedative

Synonyms Fenobarbital (Mexico)

Use Management of generalized tonic-clonic (grand mal) and partial seizures; neonatal seizures; febrile seizures in children; sedation; may also be used for prevention and treatment of neonatal hyperbilirubinemia and lowering of bilirubin in chronic cholestasis

Usual Dosage
Children:
Sedation: Oral: 2 mg/kg 3 times/day
Hypnotic: I.M., I.V., S.C.: 3-5 mg/kg at bedtime
Preoperative sedation: Oral, I.M., I.V.: 1-3 mg/kg 1-1.5 hours before procedure

Anticonvulsant: Status epilepticus: **Loading dose:** I.V.:
Children: 10-20 mg/kg in a single or divided dose; in select patients may give additional 5 mg/kg/dose every 15-30 minutes until seizure is controlled or a total dose of 40 mg/kg is reached
Adults: 300-800 mg initially followed by 120-240 mg/dose at 20-minute intervals until seizures are controlled or a total dose of 1-2 g

Anticonvulsant maintenance dose: Oral, I.V.:
Children:
1-5 years: 6-8 mg/kg/day in 1-2 divided doses
5-12 years: 4-6 mg/kg/day in 1-2 divided doses
Children >12 years and Adults: 1-3 mg/kg/day in divided doses or 50-100 mg 2-3 times/day

Adults:
Sedation: Oral, I.M.: 30-120 mg/day in 2-3 divided doses
Hypnotic: Oral, I.M., I.V., S.C.: 100-320 mg at bedtime
Preoperative sedation: I.M.: 100-200 mg 1-1.5 hours before procedure

Mechanism of Action Interferes with transmission of impulses from the thalamus to the cortex of the brain resulting in an imbalance in central inhibitory and facilitatory mechanisms

Local Anesthetic/Vasoconstrictor Precautions No information available to require special precautions

Effects on Dental Treatment No effects or complications reported

Other Adverse Effects
>10%:
Cardiovascular: Hypotension, cardiac arrhythmias, bradycardia, arterial spasm, and gangrene with inadvertent intra-arterial injection
Central nervous system: Dizziness, lightheadedness, "hangover" effect, drowsiness, lethargy, CNS excitation or depression, impaired judgment
Local: Pain at injection site, thrombophlebitis with I.V. use
1% to 10%:
Central nervous system: Confusion, mental depression, unusual excitement, nervousness, faint feeling, headache, insomnia, nightmares
Gastrointestinal: Nausea, vomiting, constipation
<1%:
Cardiovascular: Hypotension
Central nervous system: Hallucinations
Dermatologic: Exfoliative dermatitis, Stevens-Johnson syndrome, rash
Hematologic: Agranulocytosis, megaloblastic anemia, thrombocytopenia
Respiratory: Laryngospasm, respiratory depression, apnea (especially with rapid I.V. use)
Miscellaneous: Hypothermia

Drug Interactions
Decreased effect: Phenobarbital appears to increase the metabolism of the following drugs to cause a decrease in their actions: Phenothiazines, haloperidol, quinidine, cyclosporine, tricyclic antidepressants, corticosteroids, theophylline, ethosuximide, warfarin, oral contraceptives, chloramphenicol, griseofulvin, doxycycline, beta-blockers
Increased toxicity: Phenobarbital enhances the sedative effects of propoxyphene, benzodiazepines, CNS depressants, valproic acid, methylphenidate, chloramphenicol

Drug Uptake
Oral:
Onset of hypnosis: Within 20-60 minutes
Duration: 6-10 hours
I.V.:
Onset of action: Within 5 minutes
Duration: 4-10 hours
Absorption: Oral: 70% to 90%
Serum half-life:
Children: 37-73 hours
Adults: 53-140 hours
Time to peak serum concentration: Oral: Within 1-6 hours

Pregnancy Risk Factor D

Phenol (fee' nole)
Related Information
Mouth Pain, Cold Sore, Canker Sore Products *on page 1063*
Brand Names Baker's P&S Topical [OTC]; Cēpastat® [OTC]; Chloraseptic® Oral [OTC]
Therapeutic Category Pharmaceutical Aid
Synonyms Carbolic Acid
Use Relief of sore throat pain, mouth, gum, and throat irritations
Local Anesthetic/Vasoconstrictor Precautions No information available to require special precautions
Effects on Dental Treatment No effects or complications reported
Other Adverse Effects In overdose situation:
1% to 10%:
Cardiovascular: Hypotension, cardiovascular collapse, tachycardia, atrial and ventricular arrhythmias, edema
Central nervous system: slurred speech, CNS depression, agitation, confusion, seizures, coma
Dermatologic: White, red, or brown skin discoloration
Gastrointestinal: Nausea, vomiting, oral burns GI ulceration, GI bleeding
Genitourinary: Urine discoloration (green)
Hematologic: Hemorrhage
Local: Irritation, burns
Respiratory: Bronchospasm/wheezing, coughing, dyspnea, pneumonia, nephritis, pulmonary

When used for spinal neurolysis/motor point blocks: 1% to 10%:
Central nervous system: Dysrhythmias, headache, hyperesthesia, dysesthesia
Gastrointestinal: Bowel incontinence
Genitourinary: Urinary incontinence
Local: Tissue necrosis, pain at injection site
Neuromuscular & skeletal: Motor weakness, nerve damage
Respiratory: Pleural irritation
Comments Cepastat® contains 8 calories/lozenge (2 g sorbitol)

Phenolax® [OTC] *see* Phenolphthalein *on this page*

Phenolphthalein (fee nole thay' leen)
Brand Names Alophen Pills® [OTC]; Espotabs® [OTC]; Evac-U-Gen® [OTC]; Evac-U-Lax® [OTC]; Ex-Lax® [OTC]; Feen-a-Mint® [OTC]; Lax-Pills® [OTC]; Medilax® [OTC]; Modane® [OTC]; Phenolax® [OTC]; Prulet® [OTC]
Therapeutic Category Laxative, Stimulant
Synonyms Phenolphthalein, White; Phenolphthalein, Yellow
Use Stimulant laxative
Local Anesthetic/Vasoconstrictor Precautions No information available to require special precautions
Effects on Dental Treatment No effects or complications reported
Other Adverse Effects 1% to 10%:
Dermatologic: Rash
Endocrine & metabolic: Electrolyte imbalance
Gastrointestinal: Irritation and sensation of burning on rectal mucosa and proctitis, abdominal cramps, nausea, vomiting
Comments Yellow is 2-3 times more potent than white

Phenolphthalein, White *see* Phenolphthalein *on this page*
Phenolphthalein, Yellow *see* Phenolphthalein *on this page*

Phenoxybenzamine Hydrochloride
(fen ox ee ben' za meen hye droe klor' ide)
Brand Names Dibenzyline®
Therapeutic Category Alpha-Adrenergic Blocking Agent, Oral; Antihypertensive; Vasodilator, Coronary
Use Symptomatic management of pheochromocytoma; treatment of hypertensive crisis caused by sympathomimetic amines

Unlabeled use: Micturition problems associated with neurogenic bladder, functional outlet obstruction, and partial prostate obstruction
Usual Dosage Oral:
Children: Initial: 0.2 mg/kg (maximum: 10 mg) once daily, increase by 0.2 mg/kg increments; usual maintenance dose: 0.4-1.2 mg/kg/day every 6-8 hours, higher doses may be necessary

Adults: Initial: 10 mg twice daily, increase by 10 mg every other day until optimum dose is achieved; usual range: 20-40 mg 2-3 times/day

Mechanism of Action Produces long-lasting noncompetitive alpha-adrenergic blockade of postganglionic synapses in exocrine glands and smooth muscle; relaxes urethra and increases opening of the bladder

Local Anesthetic/Vasoconstrictor Precautions No information available to require special precautions

Effects on Dental Treatment No effects or complications reported

Other Adverse Effects
>10%:
Cardiovascular: Postural hypotension, tachycardia, syncope
Ocular: Miosis
Respiratory: Nasal congestion
1% to 10%:
Central nervous system: Lethargy, weakness, headache, confusion, tiredness, shock
Gastrointestinal: Vomiting, nausea, diarrhea, dry mouth
Genitourinary: Inhibition of ejaculation

Drug Interactions
Decreased effect: Alpha agonists
Increased toxicity: Beta-blockers (hypotension, tachycardia)

Drug Uptake
Onset of action: Oral: Within 2 hours
Duration: Can continue for 4 or more days
Serum half-life: 24 hours

Pregnancy Risk Factor C

Phensuximide (fen sux' i mide)

Brand Names Milontin®

Therapeutic Category Anticonvulsant, Succinimide

Use Control of absence (petit mal) seizures

Local Anesthetic/Vasoconstrictor Precautions No information available to require special precautions

Effects on Dental Treatment No effects or complications reported

Other Adverse Effects
>10%:
Central nervous system: Ataxia, dizziness, drowsiness, headache
Dermatologic: Stevens-Johnson syndrome
Gastrointestinal: Anorexia, nausea, vomiting, weight loss
Miscellaneous: Systemic lupus erythematosus (SLE), hiccups
1% to 10%:
Central nervous system: Mental depression, nightmares, tiredness
Neuromuscular & skeletal: Weakness
Miscellaneous: Aggressiveness
<1%:
Central nervous system: Paranoid psychosis
Dermatologic: Urticaria, exfoliative dermatitis
Hematologic: Agranulocytosis, leukopenia, aplastic anemia, thrombocytopenia, pancytopenia

Phentermine Hydrochloride (fen' ter meen hye droe klor' ide)

Brand Names Adipex-P®; Fastin®; Ionamin®

Canadian/Mexican Brand Names Diminex® (Mexico)

Therapeutic Category Anorexiant

Synonyms Fentermina (Mexico)

Use Short-term adjunct in exogenous obesity

Usual Dosage Oral:
Children 3-15 years: 5-15 mg/day for 4 weeks

Adults: 8 mg 3 times/day 30 minutes before meals or food or 15-37.5 mg/day before breakfast or 10-14 hours before retiring

Mechanism of Action Phentermine is structurally similar to dextroamphetamine and is comparable to dextroamphetamine as an appetite suppressant, but is generally associated with a lower incidence and severity of CNS side effects. Phentermine, like other anorexiants, stimulates the hypothalamus to result in decreased appetite; anorexiant effects are most likely mediated via norepinephrine and dopamine metabolism. However, other CNS effects or metabolic effects may be involved.

(Continued)

683

Phentermine Hydrochloride *(Continued)*

Local Anesthetic/Vasoconstrictor Precautions Use vasoconstriction with caution in patients taking phentermine. Amphetamines enhance the sympatho-mimetic response of epinephrine and norepinephrine leading to potential hypertension and cardiotoxicity.

Effects on Dental Treatment Up to 10% of patients may present with hypertension. The use of local anesthetic without vasoconstrictor is recommended in these patients.

Other Adverse Effects
>10%:
  Cardiovascular: Hypertension
  Central nervous system: Euphoria, nervousness, insomnia
1% to 10%:
  Central nervous system: Confusion, mental depression, restlessness
  Gastrointestinal: Nausea, vomiting, constipation
  Endocrine & metabolic: Changes in libido
  Hematologic: Blood dyscrasias
  Neuromuscular & skeletal: Tremor
  Ocular: Blurred vision
<1%:
  Cardiovascular: Tachycardia, arrhythmias
  Central nervous system: Insomnia, restlessness, nervousness, depression, headache
  Dermatologic: Alopecia
  Gastrointestinal: Nausea, vomiting, diarrhea, abdominal cramps
  Neuromuscular & skeletal: Myalgia, tremor
  Renal: Dysuria, polyuria
  Respiratory: Dyspnea
  Miscellaneous: Increased sweating

Drug Interactions
  Adrenergic blockers are inhibited by amphetamines
  Amphetamines enhance the activity of tricyclic or sympathomimetic agents
  MAO inhibitors slow the metabolism of amphetamines
  Amphetamines will counteract the sedative effects of antihistamines
  Amphetamines potentiate the analgesic effects of meperidine

Drug Uptake
  Absorption: Well absorbed; resin absorbed slower and produces more prolonged clinical effects
  Serum half-life: 20 hours

Pregnancy Risk Factor C

Phentolamine Mesylate *(fen tole' a meen mes' i late)*

Brand Names Regitine®

Canadian/Mexican Brand Names Rogitine® (Canada)

Therapeutic Category Alpha-Adrenergic Blocking Agent, Parenteral; Alpha-Adrenergic Inhibitors, Central; Antidote, Extravasation; Antihypertensive; Diagnostic Agent, Pheochromocytoma; Vasodilator, Coronary

Use Diagnosis of pheochromocytoma and treatment of hypertension associated with pheochromocytoma or other caused by excess sympathomimetic amines; as treatment of dermal necrosis after extravasation of drugs with alpha-adrenergic effects (norepinephrine, dopamine, epinephrine, dobutamine)

Usual Dosage
Treatment of alpha-adrenergic drug extravasation: S.C.:
  Children: 0.1-0.2 mg/kg diluted in 10 mL 0.9% sodium chloride infiltrated into area of extravasation within 12 hours
  Adults: Infiltrate area with small amount of solution made by diluting 5-10 mg in 10 mL 0.9% sodium chloride within 12 hours of extravasation
  If dose is effective, normal skin color should return to the blanched area within 1 hour

Diagnosis of pheochromocytoma: I.M., I.V.:
  Children: 0.05-0.1 mg/kg/dose, maximum single dose: 5 mg
  Adults: 5 mg

Surgery for pheochromocytoma: Hypertension: I.M., I.V.:
  Children: 0.05-0.1 mg/kg/dose given 1-2 hours before procedure; repeat as needed every 2-4 hours until hypertension is controlled; maximum single dose: 5 mg
  Adults: 5 mg given 1-2 hours before procedure and repeated as needed every 2-4 hours

Hypertensive crisis: Adults: 5-20 mg

Mechanism of Action Competitively blocks alpha-adrenergic receptors to produce brief antagonism of circulating epinephrine and norepinephrine to reduce hypertension caused by alpha effects of these catecholamines; also has a positive inotropic and chronotropic effect on the heart

Local Anesthetic/Vasoconstrictor Precautions No information available to require special precautions

Effects on Dental Treatment No effects or complications reported

Other Adverse Effects
>10%:
  Cardiovascular: Hypotension, tachycardia, arrhythmias, nasal congestion, reflex tachycardia, anginal pain, orthostatic hypotension
  Gastrointestinal: Nausea, vomiting, diarrhea, exacerbation of peptic ulcer, abdominal pain
1% to 10%:
  Cardiovascular: Flushing of face
  Central nervous system: Weakness, dizziness, fainting
  Respiratory: Nasal stuffiness
<1%:
  Cardiovascular: Myocardial infarction
  Central nervous system: Severe headache
  Miscellaneous: Exacerbation of peptic ulcer

Drug Interactions
Decreased effect: Epinephrine, ephedrine
Increased toxicity: Ethanol (disulfiram reaction)

Drug Uptake
Onset of action:
  I.M.: Within 15-20 minutes
  I.V.: Immediate
Duration:
  I.M.: 30-45 minutes
  I.V.: 15-30 minutes
Serum half-life: 19 minutes

Pregnancy Risk Factor C

Phenylalanine Mustard *see* Melphalan *on page 536*

Phenylephrine and Chlorpheniramine *see* Chlorpheniramine and Phenylephrine *on page 190*

Phenylephrine and Scopolamine
(fen il ef' rin & skoe pol' a meen)
Brand Names Murocoll-2® Ophthalmic
Therapeutic Category Ophthalmic Agent, Mydriatic
Synonyms Scopolamine and Phenylephrine
Use Mydriasis, cycloplegia, and to break posterior synechiae in iritis
Local Anesthetic/Vasoconstrictor Precautions Use with caution since phenylephrine is a sympathomimetic amine which could interact with epinephrine to cause a pressor response
Effects on Dental Treatment This form of phenylephrine will have no effect on dental treatment when given as eye drops

Phenylephrine and Zinc Sulfate (fen il ef' rin & zingk sul' fate)
Brand Names Optised® Ophthalmic [OTC]; Phenylzin® Ophthalmic [OTC]; Zincfrin® Ophthalmic [OTC]
Therapeutic Category Ophthalmic Agent, Miscellaneous
Use Soothe, moisturize, and remove redness due to minor eye irritation
Local Anesthetic/Vasoconstrictor Precautions No information available to require special precautions
Effects on Dental Treatment No effects or complications reported

Phenylephrine Hydrochloride (fen il ef' rin hye droe klor' ide)
Related Information
Dentin Hypersensitivity; High Caries Index; Xerostomia *on page 959*
Brand Names AK-Dilate® Ophthalmic Solution; AK-Nefrin® Ophthalmic Solution; Alconefrin® Nasal Solution [OTC]; Doktors® Nasal Solution [OTC]; I-Phrine® Ophthalmic Solution; Isopto® Frin Ophthalmic Solution; Mydfrin® Ophthalmic Solution; Neo-Synephrine® Nasal Solution [OTC]; Neo-Synephrine® Ophthalmic Solution; Nostril® Nasal Solution [OTC]; Prefrin™ Ophthalmic Solution; Relief® Ophthalmic Solution; Rhinall® Nasal Solution [OTC]; Sinarest® Nasal Solution [OTC]; St. Joseph® Measured Dose Nasal Solution [OTC]; Vicks® Sinex® Nasal Solution [OTC]
Canadian/Mexican Brand Names Dionephrine® (Canada)
(Continued)

Phenylephrine Hydrochloride *(Continued)*

Therapeutic Category Adrenergic Agonist Agent; Adrenergic Agonist Agent, Ophthalmic; Antiglaucoma Agent; Nasal Agent, Vasoconstrictor; Ophthalmic Agent, Mydriatic

Synonyms Fenilefrina (Mexico)

Use Treatment of hypotension, vascular failure in shock; as a vasoconstrictor in regional analgesia; symptomatic relief of nasal and nasopharyngeal mucosal congestion; as a mydriatic in ophthalmic procedures and treatment of wide-angle glaucoma; supraventricular tachycardia

Usual Dosage
Ophthalmic procedures:
Children and Adults: Instill 1 drop of 2.5% or 10% solution, may repeat in 10-60 minutes as needed
Nasal decongestant: (therapy should not exceed 5 continuous days)
Children:
2-6 years: Instill 1 drop every 2-4 hours of 0.125% solution as needed
6-12 years: Instill 1-2 sprays or instill 1-2 drops every 4 hours of 0.25% solution as needed
Children >12 years and Adults: Instill 1-2 sprays or instill 1-2 drops every 4 hours of 0.25% to 0.5% solution as needed; 1% solution may be used in adult in cases of extreme nasal congestion; do not use nasal solutions more than 3 days
Hypotension/shock:
Children:
I.M., S.C.: 0.1 mg/kg/dose every 1-2 hours as needed (maximum: 5 mg)
I.V. bolus: 5-20 mcg/kg/dose every 10-15 minutes as needed
I.V. infusion: 0.1-0.5 mcg/kg/minute
Adults:
I.M., S.C.: 2-5 mg/dose every 1-2 hours as needed (initial dose should not exceed 5 mg)
I.V. bolus: 0.1-0.5 mg/dose every 10-15 minutes as needed (initial dose should not exceed 0.5 mg)
I.V. infusion: 10 mg in 250 mL D_5W or NS (1:25,000 dilution) (40 mcg/mL); start at 100-180 mcg/minute (2-5 mL/minute; 50-90 drops/minute) initially; when blood pressure is stabilized, maintenance rate: 40-60 mcg/minute (20-30 drops/minute)
Paroxysmal supraventricular tachycardia: I.V.:
Children: 5-10 mcg/kg/dose over 20-30 seconds
Adults: 0.25-0.5 mg/dose over 20-30 seconds

Mechanism of Action Potent, direct-acting alpha-adrenergic stimulator with weak beta-adrenergic activity; causes vasoconstriction of the arterioles of the nasal mucosa and conjunctiva; activates the dilator muscle of the pupil to cause contraction; produces vasoconstriction of arterioles in the body; produces systemic arterial vasoconstriction

Local Anesthetic/Vasoconstrictor Precautions Use with caution since phenylephrine is a sympathomimetic amine which could interact with epinephrine to cause a pressor response

Effects on Dental Treatment Up to 10% of patients could experience tachycardia, palpitations, and dry mouth; use vasoconstrictor with caution

Other Adverse Effects
Nasal:
>10%: Respiratory: Burning, rebound congestion, sneezing
1% to 10%: Respiratory: Stinging, dryness

Ophthalmic:
>10%: Ocular: Transient stinging
1% to 10%:
Central nervous system: Headache, browache
Ocular: Blurred vision, photophobia, lacrimation

Systemic:
>10%: Neuromuscular & skeletal: Tremor
1% to 10%:
Cardiovascular: Peripheral vasoconstriction hypertension, angina, reflex bradycardia, arrhythmias
Central nervous system: Restlessness, excitability

Drug Interactions
Decreased effect of phenylephrine with alpha- and beta-adrenergic blocking agents
Increased effect of phenylephrine with oxytocic drugs
Increased toxicity: With sympathomimetics, tachycardia or arrhythmias may occur; with MAO inhibitors, actions may be potentiated

Drug Uptake
Onset of effect:
I.M., S.C.: Within 10-15 minutes
I.V.: Immediate
Duration:
I.M.: 30 minutes to 2 hours
I.V.: 15-30 minutes
S.C.: 1 hour
Serum half-life: 2.5 hours
Pregnancy Risk Factor C

Phenylfenesin® L.A. *see* Guaifenesin and Phenylpropanolamine *on page 409*

Phenylpropanolamine and Brompheniramine *see* Brompheniramine and Phenylpropanolamine *on page 123*

Phenylpropanolamine and Caramiphen *see* Caramiphen and Phenylpropanolamine *on page 150*

Phenylpropanolamine and Chlorpheniramine *see* Chlorpheniramine and Phenylpropanolamine *on page 190*

Phenylpropanolamine and Guaifenesin *see* Guaifenesin and Phenylpropanolamine *on page 409*

Phenylpropanolamine and Hydrocodone *see* Hydrocodone and Phenylpropanolamine *on page 435*

Phenylpropanolamine Hydrochloride
(fen il proe pa nole' a meen hye droe klor' ide)
Brand Names Acutrim® Precision Release® [OTC]; Control® [OTC]; Dex-A-Diet® [OTC]; Dexatrim® [OTC]; Maigret-50; Prolamine® [OTC]; Propadrine; Propagest® [OTC]; Rhindecon®; Stay Trim® Diet Gum [OTC]; Westrim® LA [OTC]
Therapeutic Category Adrenergic Agonist Agent; Anorexiant; Decongestant; Nasal Agent, Vasoconstrictor
Synonyms Fenilpropanolamina (Mexico)
Use Anorexiant; nasal decongestant
Usual Dosage Oral:
Children: Decongestant:
2-6 years: 6.25 mg every 4 hours
6-12 years: 12.5 mg every 4 hours not to exceed 75 mg/day

Adults:
Decongestant: 25 mg every 4 hours or 50 mg every 8 hours, not to exceed 150 mg/day
Anorexic: 25 mg 3 times/day 30 minutes before meals or 75 mg (timed release) once daily in the morning
Precision release: 75 mg after breakfast
Mechanism of Action Releases tissue stores of epinephrine and thereby produces an alpha- and beta-adrenergic stimulation; this causes vasoconstriction and nasal mucosa blanching; also appears to depress central appetite centers
Local Anesthetic/Vasoconstrictor Precautions Use with caution since phenylpropanolamine is a sympathomimetic amine which could interact with epinephrine to cause a pressor response
Effects on Dental Treatment Up to 10% of patients could experience tachycardia, palpitations, and dry mouth; use vasoconstrictor with caution
Other Adverse Effects
>10%: Cardiovascular: Hypertension, palpitations
1% to 10%:
Central nervous system: Insomnia, restlessness, dizziness
Gastrointestinal: Dry mouth, nausea
<1%:
Cardiovascular: Tightness in chest, bradycardia, arrhythmias angina
Central nervous system: Severe headache, anxiety, nervousness, restlessness
Genitourinary: Difficult urination
Drug Interactions
Decreased effect of antihypertensives
Increased effect/toxicity with MAO inhibitors (hypertensive crisis), beta-blockers (increased pressor effects)
Drug Uptake
Absorption: Oral: Well absorbed
Serum half-life: 4.6-6.6 hours
Pregnancy Risk Factor C

Phenyltoloxamine, Phenylpropanolamine, and Acetaminophen

(fen il tol ox a meen, fen il proe pa nole' a meen, & a seet a min' oh fen)

Brand Names Sinubid®

Therapeutic Category Analgesic, Non-narcotic; Antihistamine/Decongestant Combination

Use Intermittent symptomatic treatment of nasal congestion in sinus or other frontal headache; allergic rhinitis, vasomotor rhinitis, coryza; facial pain and pressure of acute and chronic sinusitis

Local Anesthetic/Vasoconstrictor Precautions Use with caution since phenylpropanolamine is a sympathomimetic amine which could interact with epinephrine to cause a pressor response

Effects on Dental Treatment

Acetaminophen: No effects or complications reported

Phenylpropanolamine: Up to 10% of patients could experience tachycardia, palpitations, and dry mouth; use vasoconstrictor with caution

Selected Readings

Barker JD Jr, de Carle DJ, and Anuras S, "Chronic Excessive Acetaminophen Use in Liver Damage," *Ann Intern Med*, 1977, 87(3):299-301.

Dionne RA, Campbell RA, Cooper SA, et al, "Suppression of Postoperative Pain by Preoperative Administration of Ibuprofen in Comparison to Placebo, Acetaminophen, and Acetaminophen Plus Codeine," *J Clin Pharmacol*, 1983, 23(1):37-43.

Licht H, Seeff LB, and Zimmerman HJ, "Apparent Potentiation of Acetaminophen Hepatotoxicity by Alcohol," *Ann Intern Med*, 1980, 92(4):511.

Phenylzin® Ophthalmic [OTC] *see* Phenylephrine and Zinc Sulfate *on page 685*

Phenytoin (fen' i toyn)

Related Information

Cardiovascular Diseases *on page 912*

Brand Names Dilantin®; Diphenylan Sodium®

Canadian/Mexican Brand Names Tremytoine® (Canada)

Therapeutic Category Antiarrhythmic Agent, Class I-B; Antiarrhythmic Agent (Supraventricular & Ventricular); Anticonvulsant, Hydantoin

Use Management of generalized tonic-clonic (grand mal), simple partial and complex partial seizures; prevention of seizures following head trauma/neurosurgery; ventricular arrhythmias, including those associated with digitalis intoxication, prolonged Q-T interval and surgical repair of congenital heart diseases in children; also used for epidermolysis bullosa

Usual Dosage

Status epilepticus: I.V.:

Children: Loading dose: 15-20 mg/kg in a single or divided dose; maintenance dose: Initial: 5 mg/kg/day in 2 divided doses, usual doses:

6 months to 3 years: 8-10 mg/kg/day

4-6 years: 7.5-9 mg/kg/day

7-9 years: 7-8 mg/kg/day

10-16 years: 6-7 mg/kg/day, some patients may require every 8 hours dosing

Adults: Loading dose: 15-20 mg/kg in a single or divided dose, followed by 100-150 mg/dose at 30-minute intervals up to a maximum of 1500 mg/24 hours; maintenance dose: 300 mg/day or 5-6 mg/kg/day in 3 divided doses or 1-2 divided doses using extended release

Anticonvulsant: Children and Adults: Oral:

Loading dose: 15-20 mg/kg; based on phenytoin serum concentrations and recent dosing history; administer oral loading dose in 3 divided doses given every 2-4 hours to decrease GI adverse effects and to ensure complete oral absorption; maintenance dose: same as I.V.

Mechanism of Action Stabilizes neuronal membranes and decreases seizure activity by increasing efflux or decreasing influx of sodium ions across cell membranes in the motor cortex during generation of nerve impulses; prolongs effective refractory period and suppresses ventricular pacemaker automaticity, shortens action potential in the heart

Local Anesthetic/Vasoconstrictor Precautions No information available to require special precautions

Effects on Dental Treatment Gingival hyperplasia is a common problem observed during the first 6 months of phenytoin therapy appearing as gingivitis or gum inflammation. To minimize severity and growth rate of gingival tissue begin a program of professional cleaning and patient plaque control within 10 days of starting anticonvulsant therapy.

Other Adverse Effects
>10%:
Central nervous system: Psychiatric changes, slurred speech, dizziness, drowsiness
Gastrointestinal: Constipation, nausea, vomiting, gingival hyperplasia
Neuromuscular & skeletal: Trembling
1% to 10%:
Central nervous system: Drowsiness, headache, insomnia
Dermatologic: Skin rash
Gastrointestinal: Anorexia, weight loss
Hematologic: Leukopenia, increase in serum creatinine
Hepatic: Hepatitis
<1%:
Cardiovascular: Hypotension, bradycardia, cardiac arrhythmias, cardiovascular collapse
Central nervous system: Confusion, fever, ataxia
Local: Thrombophlebitis
Neuromuscular & skeletal: Peripheral neuropathy, paresthesia
Ocular: Diplopia, nystagmus, blurred vision
Rarely seen effects: SLE-like syndrome, lymphadenopathy, hepatitis, Stevens-Johnson syndrome, blood dyscrasias, dyskinesias, pseudolymphoma, lymphoma
Miscellaneous: Venous irritation and pain

Drug Interactions Phenytoin is an inducer of cytochrome P-450 IIIA enzymes and is associated with many drug interactions

Decreased effect: Rifampin, cisplatin, vinblastine, bleomycin, folic acid, continuous NG feedings
Increased toxicity: Amiodarone decreases metabolism of phenytoin; disulfiram decreases metabolism of phenytoin; fluconazole, itraconazole decreases phenytoin serum concentrations; isoniazid may increase phenytoin serum concentrations
Increased effect/toxicity of valproic acid, ethosuximide, primidone, warfarin, oral contraceptives, corticosteroids, cyclosporine, theophylline, chloramphenicol, rifampin, doxycycline, quinidine, mexiletine, disopyramide, dopamine, nondepolarizing skeletal muscle relaxants

Drug Uptake
Absorption: Oral: Slow
Time to peak serum concentration (dependent upon formulation administered): Oral:
Extended-release capsule: Within 4-12 hours
Immediate release preparation: Within 2-3 hours
Pregnancy Risk Factor D

Phenytoin With Phenobarbital (fen' i toyn with fee noe bar' bi tal)
Brand Names Dilantin® With Phenobarbital
Therapeutic Category Anticonvulsant, Barbiturate; Anticonvulsant, Hydantoin
Use Management of generalized tonic-clonic (grand mal), simple partial and complex partial seizures
Local Anesthetic/Vasoconstrictor Precautions No information available to require special precautions
Effects on Dental Treatment Gingival hyperplasia is a common problem observed during the first 6 months of phenytoin therapy appearing as gingivitis or gum inflammation. To minimize severity and growth rate of gingival tissue begin a program of professional cleaning and patient plaque control within 10 days of starting anticonvulsant therapy.

Pherazine® w/DM see Promethazine With Dextromethorphan on page 735
Pherazine® With Codeine see Promethazine and Codeine on page 733
Phicon® [OTC] see Pramoxine Hydrochloride on page 714
Phillips'® LaxCaps® [OTC] see Docusate and Phenolphthalein on page 295
Phillips'® Milk of Magnesia [OTC] see Magnesium Hydroxide on page 522
pHisoHex® see Hexachlorophene on page 424
pHiso® Scrub see Hexachlorophene on page 424
Phos-Ex® see Calcium Acetate on page 139
Phos-Flur® see Fluoride on page 374
PhosLo® see Calcium Acetate on page 139
Phospholine Iodide® see Echothiophate Iodide on page 305

Phosphorated Carbohydrate Solution
(fos' for ate ed kar boe hye' drate soe loo' shun)
Brand Names Emecheck® [OTC]; Emetrol® [OTC]; Naus-A-Way® [OTC]; Nausetrol® [OTC]
Therapeutic Category Antiemetic
Synonyms Dextrose, Levulose and Phosphoric Acid; Levulose, Dextrose and Phosphoric Acid; Phosphoric Acid, Levulose and Dextrose
Use Relief of nausea associated with upset stomach that occurs with intestinal flu, pregnancy, food indiscretions, and emotional upsets
Local Anesthetic/Vasoconstrictor Precautions No information available to require special precautions
Effects on Dental Treatment No effects or complications reported
Other Adverse Effects 1% to 10%: Abdominal pain, diarrhea

Phosphoric Acid, Levulose and Dextrose *see* Phosphorated Carbohydrate Solution *on this page*

Phrenilin® *see* Butalbital Compound *on page 133*

Phrenilin® Forte® *see* Butalbital Compound *on page 133*

Phyllocontin® *see* Theophylline/Aminophylline *on page 832*

Phylloquinone (Canada) *see* Phytonadione *on this page*

Physostigmine (fye zoe stig' meen)
Brand Names Antilirium®; Isopto® Eserine®
Therapeutic Category Antidote, Anticholinergic Agent; Antiglaucoma Agent; Cholinergic Agent; Cholinergic Agent, Ophthalmic
Use Reverse toxic CNS effects caused by anticholinergic drugs; used as miotic in treatment of glaucoma
Usual Dosage
Children: Anticholinergic drug overdose: Reserve for life-threatening situations only: I.V.: 0.01-0.03 mg/kg/dose, (maximum: 0.5 mg/minute); may repeat after 5-10 minutes to a maximum total dose of 2 mg or until response occurs or adverse cholinergic effects occur
Adults: Anticholinergic drug overdose:
 I.M., I.V., S.C.: 0.5-2 mg to start, repeat every 20 minutes until response occurs or adverse effect occurs
 Repeat 1-4 mg every 30-60 minutes as life-threatening signs (arrhythmias, seizures, deep coma) recur; maximum I.V. rate: 1 mg/minute
Ophthalmic:
 Ointment: Instill a small quantity to lower fornix up to 3 times/day
 Solution: Instill 1-2 drops into eye(s) up to 4 times/day
Mechanism of Action Inhibits destruction of acetylcholine by acetylcholinesterase which facilitates transmission of impulses across myoneural junction and prolongs the central and peripheral effects of acetylcholine
Local Anesthetic/Vasoconstrictor Precautions No information available to require special precautions
Effects on Dental Treatment No effects or complications reported
Other Adverse Effects Ophthalmic:
>10%:
 Ocular: Lacrimation, marked miosis, blurred vision, eye pain
 Miscellaneous: Sweating
1% to 10%:
 Central nervous system: Headache, browache
 Dermatologic: Burning, redness
Drug Interactions No data reported with ophthalmic use
Drug Uptake
Onset of action:
 Ophthalmic instillation: Within 2 minutes
 Parenteral: Within 5 minutes
Absorption: I.M., ophthalmic, S.C.: Readily absorbed
Serum half-life: 15-40 minutes
Pregnancy Risk Factor C

Phytomenadione (Canada) *see* Phytonadione *on this page*

Phytonadione (fye toe na dye' one)
Brand Names AquaMEPHYTON®; Konakion®; Mephyton®
Therapeutic Category Vitamin, Fat Soluble
Synonyms Phylloquinone (Canada); Phytomenadione (Canada)
Use Prevention and treatment of hypoprothrombinemia caused by drug-induced or anticoagulant-induced vitamin K deficiency, hemorrhagic disease of the newborn; phytonadione is more effective and is preferred to other vitamin K

preparations in the presence of impending hemorrhage; oral absorption depends on the presence of bile salts

Usual Dosage I.V. route should be restricted for emergency use only

Minimum daily requirement: Not well established

Adults: 0.03 mcg/kg/day

Hemorrhagic disease of the newborn:

Prophylaxis: I.M., S.C.: 0.5-1 mg within 1 hour of birth

Treatment: I.M., S.C.: 1-2 mg/dose/day

Oral anticoagulant overdose:

Children and Adults: Oral, I.M., I.V., S.C.: 2.5-10 mg/dose; rarely up to 25-50 mg has been used; may repeat in 6-8 hours if given by I.M., I.V., S.C. route; may repeat 12-48 hours after oral route

Vitamin K deficiency: Due to drugs, malabsorption or decreased synthesis of vitamin K

Children:

Oral: 2.5-5 mg/24 hours

I.M., I.V.: 1-2 mg/dose as a single dose

Adults:

Oral: 5-25 mg/24 hours

I.M., I.V.: 10 mg

Mechanism of Action Promotes liver synthesis of clotting factors (II, VII, IX, X); however, the exact mechanism as to this stimulation is unknown. Menadiol is a water soluble form of vitamin K; phytonadione has a more rapid and prolonged effect than menadione; menadiol sodium diphosphate (K_4) is half as potent as menadione (K_3).

Local Anesthetic/Vasoconstrictor Precautions No information available to require special precautions

Effects on Dental Treatment No effects or complications reported

Other Adverse Effects <1%:

Cardiovascular: Transient flushing reaction, rarely hypotension, cyanosis

Central nervous system: Rarely dizziness

Gastrointestinal: Dysgeusia, GI upset (oral)

Hematologic: Hemolysis in neonates and in patients with G-6-PD deficiency

Local: Tenderness at injection site

Respiratory: Dyspnea

Miscellaneous: Sweating, anaphylaxis, hypersensitivity reactions, pain

Drug Interactions Warfarin sodium, dicumarol, and anisindione effects antagonized by phytonadione

Drug Uptake

Onset of increased coagulation factors:

Oral: Within 6-12 hours

Parenteral: Within 1-2 hours; patient may become normal after 12-14 hours

Absorption: Oral: Absorbed from the intestines in the presence of bile

Pregnancy Risk Factor C (X if used in third trimester or near term)

Pilagan® *see* Pilocarpine *on this page*

Pilocar® *see* Pilocarpine *on this page*

Pilocarpine (pye loe kar' peen)

Related Information

Dentin Hypersensitivity; High Caries Index; Xerostomia *on page 959*

Patients Undergoing Cancer Therapy *on page 967*

Brand Names Adsorbocarpine®; Akarpine®; Isopto® Carpine®; Ocu-Carpine®; Ocusert® Pilo; Ocusert Pilo-20®; Ocusert Pilo-40®; Pilagan®; Pilocar®; Pilopine HS®; Piloptic®; Pilostat®

Canadian/Mexican Brand Names Minims® Pilocarpine (Canada)

Therapeutic Category Antiglaucoma Agent; Cholinergic Agent, Ophthalmic; Ophthalmic Agent, Miotic

Use Management of chronic simple glaucoma, chronic and acute angle-closure glaucoma; counter effects of cycloplegics

Usual Dosage Adults:

Ophthalmic:

Nitrate solution: Shake well before using; instill 1-2 drops 2-4 times/day

Hydrochloride solution:

Instill 1-2 drops up to 6 times/day; adjust the concentration and frequency as required to control elevated intraocular pressure

To counteract the mydriatic effects of sympathomimetic agents: Instill 1 drop of a 1% solution in the affected eye

Gel: Instill 0.5" ribbon into lower conjunctival sac once daily at bedtime

(Continued)

Pilocarpine *(Continued)*

Ocular systems: Systems are labeled in terms of mean rate of release of pilocarpine over 7 days; begin with 20 mcg/hour at night and adjust based on response

Oral: 5 mg 3 times/day, titration up to 10 mg 3 times/day may be considered for patients who have not responded adequately

Mechanism of Action Directly stimulates cholinergic receptors in the eye causing miosis (by contraction of the iris sphincter), loss of accommodation (by constriction of ciliary muscle), and lowering of intraocular pressure (with decreased resistance to aqueous humor outflow)

Local Anesthetic/Vasoconstrictor Precautions No information available to require special precautions

Effects on Dental Treatment No effects or complications reported

Other Adverse Effects

>10%: Ocular: Blurred vision, miosis

1% to 10%:

Central nervous system: Headache

Genitourinary: Frequent urination

Local: Stinging, burning, lacrimation

Ocular: Ciliary spasm, retinal detachment, browache, photophobia, acute iritis, conjunctival and ciliary congestion early in therapy

Miscellaneous: Hypersensitivity reactions

<1%:

Cardiovascular: Hypertension, tachycardia

Gastrointestinal: Nausea, vomiting, diarrhea, salivation

Miscellaneous: Sweating

Drug Interactions Concurrent use with beta-blockers may cause conduction disturbances; pilocarpine may antagonize the effects of anticholinergic drugs

Drug Uptake

Ophthalmic instillation:

Miosis:

Onset of effect: Within 10-30 minutes

Duration: 4-8 hours

Intraocular pressure reduction:

Onset of effect: 1 hour required

Duration: 4-12 hours

Ocusert® Pilo application:

Miosis: Onset of effect: 1.5-2 hours

Reduced intraocular pressure:

Onset: Within 1.5-2 hours; miosis within 10-30 minutes

Duration: ~1 week

Pregnancy Risk Factor C

Dosage Forms See table.

Pilocarpine

Dosage Form	Strength %	1 mL	2 mL	15 mL	30 mL	3.5 g
Gel	4					x
Solution as hydrochloride	0.25			x		
	0.5			x	x	
	1	x	x	x	x	
	2	x	x	x	x	
	3			x	x	
	4	x	x	x	x	
	6			x	x	
	8		x			
	10			x		
Solution as nitrate	1			x		
	2			x		
	4			x		
Ocusert® Pilo-20: Releases 20 mcg/hour for 1 week						
Ocusert® Pilo-40: Releases 40 mcg/hour for 1 week						

Generic Available Yes: Solution

Pilocarpine and Epinephrine (pye loe kar' peen & ep i nef' rin)
Brand Names E-Pilo-x® Ophthalmic; P$_x$E$_x$® Ophthalmic
Therapeutic Category Antiglaucoma Agent; Ophthalmic Agent, Miotic
Use Treatment of glaucoma; counter effect of cycloplegics
Local Anesthetic/Vasoconstrictor Precautions No information available to require special precautions
Effects on Dental Treatment No effects or complications reported
Other Adverse Effects 1% to 10%:
Cardiovascular: Tachycardia, hypertension
Central nervous system: Headache
Ocular: Miosis, ciliary spasm, blurred vision, retinal detachment, stinging, lacrimation, itching, vitreous hemorrhages, photophobia, acute iritis
Miscellaneous: Hypersensitivity reactions, salivation

Pilocarpine (Dental) (pye loe kar' peen)
Brand Names Salagen®
Therapeutic Category Cholinergic Agent
Use
Dental: Treatment of xerostomia caused by radiation therapy in patients with head and neck cancer
Medical: No data reported
Usual Dosage Adults: 1-2 tablets 3-4 times/day not to exceed 30 mg/day; patients should be treated for a minimum of 90 days for optimum effects
Mechanism of Action Pilocarpine stimulates the muscarinic-type acetylcholine receptors in the salivary glands within the parasympathetic division of the autonomic nervous system to cause an increase in serous-type saliva
Local Anesthetic/Vasoconstrictor Precautions No information available to require special precautions
Effects on Dental Treatment Salivation - therapeutic effect
Other Adverse Effects
>10%: Miscellaneous: Sweating
1% to 10%:
Central nervous system: Chills, headache, dizziness
Gastrointestinal: Nausea
Genitourinary: Urinary frequency
Ocular: Lacrimation
Respiratory: Rhinitis, pharyngitis

Oral manifestations: Salivation (therapeutic effect)
Contraindications In patients with uncontrolled asthma, known hypersensitivity to pilocarpine and when miosis is undesirable (eg, narrow-angle glaucoma)
Warnings/Precautions In patients with chronic obstructive pulmonary disease, pilocarpine may stimulate the mucous cells of the respiratory tract and may increase airway resistance. Patients with cardiovascular disease may be unable to compensate for changes in heart rhythm that could be induced by pilocarpine.
Drug Interactions Concurrent use with anticholinergics may cause antagonism of pilocarpine's cholinergic effect; medications with cholinergic actions may result in additive cholinergic effects; beta-adrenergic receptor blocking drugs when used with pilocarpine may increase the possibility of myocardial conduction disturbances
Drug Uptake
Onset of action after single dose: 20 minutes
Time to peak serum concentration: 1.25 hours
Duration: 3-5 hours
Serum half-life: 0.76 hours
Pregnancy Risk Factor C
Breast-feeding Considerations May be taken while breast-feeding
Dosage Forms Tablet: 5 mg
Dietary Considerations No data reported
Generic Available No
Comments Pilocarpine may have potential as a salivary stimulant in individuals suffering from xerostomia induced by antidepressants and other medications. At the present time however, the FDA has not approved pilocarpine for use in drug-induced xerostomia. Clinical studies are needed to evaluate pilocarpine for this type of indication. In an attempt to discern the efficacy of pilocarpine as a salivary stimulant in patients suffering from Sjögren's syndrome (SS), Rhodus and Schuh studied 9 patients with SS given daily doses of pilocarpine over a 6-week period. A dose of 5 mg daily produced a significant overall
(Continued)

Pilocarpine (Dental) *(Continued)*

increase in both whole unstimulated salivary flow and parotid stimulated salivary flow. These results support the use of pilocarpine to increase salivary flow in patients with SS.

Selected Readings

Fox PC, Atkinson JC, Macynski AA, et al, " Pilocarpine Treatment of Salivary Gland Hypofunction and Dry Mouth (Xerostomia)," *Arch Intern Med*, 1991, 151:1149-52.

Greenspan D and Daniels TE, "The Use of Pilocarpine in Postradiation Xerostomia," *J Dent Res*, 1979, 58:420.

Johnson JT, Ferretti GA, Nethery WJ, et al, "Oral Pilocarpine for Post-Irradiation Xerostomia in Patients With Head and Neck Cancer," *N Engl J Med*, 1993, 329:390-5.

Rhodus NL and Schuh MJ, "Effects of Pilocarpine on Salivary Flow in Patients With Sjögren's Syndrome," *Oral Surg Oral Med Oral Pathol*, 1991, 72:545-9.

Schuller DE, Stevens P, Clausen KP, et al, "Treatment of Radiation Side Effects With Pilocarpine," *J Surg Oncol*, 1989, 42(4):272-6.

Valdez III, Wolf A, Atkinson JC, et al, "Use of Pilocarpine During Head and Neck Radiation Therapy to Reduce Xerostomia Salivary Dysfunction," *Cancer*, 1993, 71:1848-51.

Pilopine HS® *see Pilocarpine on page 691*

Piloptic® *see Pilocarpine on page 691*

Pilostat® *see Pilocarpine on page 691*

Pima® *see Potassium Iodide on page 711*

Pimozide *(pi' moe zide)*

Brand Names Orap™

Therapeutic Category Neuroleptic Agent

Use Suppression of severe motor and phonic tics in patients with Tourette's disorder

Usual Dosage Children >12 years and Adults: Oral: Initial: 1-2 mg/day, then increase dosage as needed every other day; range is usually 7-16 mg/day, maximum dose: 20 mg/day or 0.3 mg/kg/day should not be exceeded

Mechanism of Action A potent centrally acting dopamine receptor antagonist resulting in its characteristic neuroleptic effects

Local Anesthetic/Vasoconstrictor Precautions No information available to require special precautions

Effects on Dental Treatment No effects or complications reported

Other Adverse Effects

>10%:
  Cardiovascular: Tachycardia, orthostatic hypotension
  Central nervous system: Akathisia, akinesia, extrapyramidal effects
  Dermatologic: Skin rash
  Endocrine & metabolic: Swelling of breasts
  Gastrointestinal: Constipation, drowsiness, dry mouth

1% to 10%:
  Cardiovascular: Swelling of face
  Central nervous system: Tardive dyskinesia, mental depression
  Gastrointestinal: Diarrhea, anorexia

<1%:
  Central nervous system: Neuroleptic malignant syndrome (NMS)
  Hematologic: Blood dyscrasias
  Hepatic: Jaundice

Contraindications Simple tics other than Tourette's, history of cardiac dysrhythmias, known hypersensitivity to pimozide; use in patients receiving macrolide antibiotics such as clarithromycin, erythromycin, azithromycin, and dirithromycin

Drug Interactions Increased effect/toxicity of alfentanil, CNS depressants, guanabenz (increased sedation), MAO inhibitors

Drug Uptake
  Absorption: Oral: 50%
  Serum half-life: 50 hours
  Time to peak serum concentration: Within 6-8 hours

Pregnancy Risk Factor C

Selected Readings

"Pimozide (Orap) Contraindicated With Clarithromycin (Biaxin) and Other Macrolide Antibiotics," *FDA Medical Bulletin*, October 1996, 3.

Pindolol *(pin' doe lole)*

Related Information

Cardiovascular Diseases *on page 912*

Brand Names Visken®

Canadian/Mexican Brand Names Apo-Pindol® (Canada); Gen-Pindolol® (Canada); Novo-Pindol® (Canada); Nu-Pindol® (Canada); Syn-Pindol® (Canada)

Therapeutic Category Beta-Adrenergic Blocker, Noncardioselective
Use Management of hypertension

Unlabeled use: Ventricular arrhythmias/tachycardia, antipsychotic-induced akathisia, situational anxiety; aggressive behavior associated with dementia

Usual Dosage
Adults: Initial: 5 mg twice daily, increase as necessary by 10 mg/day every 3-4 weeks; maximum daily dose: 60 mg
Elderly: Initial: 5 mg once daily, increase as necessary by 5 mg/day every 3-4 weeks

Mechanism of Action Blocks both $beta_1$- and $beta_2$-receptors and has mild intrinsic sympathomimetic activity; pindolol has negative inotropic and chronotropic effects and can significantly slow A-V nodal conduction

Local Anesthetic/Vasoconstrictor Precautions Use with caution; epinephrine has interacted with nonselective beta-blockers to result in initial hypertensive episode followed by bradycardia

Effects on Dental Treatment Non-cardioselective beta-blockers (ie, propranolol, nadolol, pindolol) enhance the pressor response to epinephrine, resulting in hypertension and bradycardia. Many nonsteroidal anti-inflammatory drugs such as ibuprofen and indomethacin can reduce the hypotensive effect of beta-blockers after 3 or more weeks of therapy with the NSAID. Short-term NSAID use (ie, 3 days) requires no special precautions in patients taking beta-blockers.

Other Adverse Effects
>10%:
Central nervous system: Anxiety, dizziness, insomnia, weakness, tiredness
Endocrine & metabolic: Decreased sexual ability
Neuromuscular & skeletal: Joint pain
Miscellaneous: Back pain
1% to 10%:
Cardiovascular: Congestive heart failure, irregular heartbeat, reduced peripheral circulation,
Central nervous system: Hallucinations, nightmares, vivid dreams, numbness of extremities
Dermatologic: Skin rash, itching
Gastrointestinal: Diarrhea, nausea, vomiting, stomach discomfort
Respiratory: Breathing difficulty
<1%:
Cardiovascular: Bradycardia, chest pain
Central nervous system: Confusion, mental depression
Hematologic: Thrombocytopenia
Ocular: Dry eyes

Drug Interactions
Decreased effect of beta-blockers:
Barbiturates (increased liver metabolism of beta-blockers to result in lower serum levels)
NSAIDs (attenuate the hypotensive therapeutic effects of beta-blockers)
Rifampin (increased liver metabolism of beta-blockers to result in lower serum levels)
Increased effects of beta-blockers:
Calcium channel blockers (increase serum levels of beta-blockers by unknown mechanism to enhance hypotension)
Beta-Blockers increase the effects of:
Epinephrine (vasoconstrictor; initial hypertensive episode followed by bradycardia) only from non-cardioselective type beta-blockers

Drug Uptake
Absorption: Oral: Rapid, 50% to 95%
Serum half-life: 2.5-4 hours; increased with renal insufficiency, age, and cirrhosis
Time to peak serum concentration: Within 1-2 hours

Pregnancy Risk Factor B

Selected Readings
Foster CA and Aston SJ, "Propranolol-Epinephrine Interaction: A Potential Disaster," *Plast Reconstr Surg*, 1983, 72(1):74-8.
Wong DG, Spence JD, Lamki L, et al, "Effect of Nonsteroidal Anti-Inflammatory Drugs on Control of Hypertension of Beta-Blockers and Diuretics," *Lancet*, 1986, 1(8488):997-1001.
Wynn RL, "Dental Nonsteroidal Anti-Inflammatory Drugs and Prostaglandin-Based Drug Interactions, Part Two," *Gen Dent*, 1992, 40(2):104, 106, 108.
Wynn RL, "Epinephrine Interactions With Beta-Blockers," *Gen Dent*, 1994, 42(1):16, 18.

Pink Bismuth® (subsalicylate) [OTC] *see* Bismuth *on page 114*
Pin-Rid® [OTC] *see* Pyrantel Pamoate *on page 751*

Pin-X® [OTC] *see* Pyrantel Pamoate *on page 751*
Piperacilina (Mexico) *see* Piperacillin Sodium *on this page*

Piperacillin Sodium (pi per' a sil in sow' dee um)
Brand Names Pipracil®
Therapeutic Category Antibiotic, Penicillin
Synonyms Piperacilina (Mexico)
Use Treatment of susceptible infections such as septicemia, acute and chronic respiratory tract infections, skin and soft tissue infections, and urinary tract infections due to susceptible strains of *Pseudomonas*, *Proteus*, and *Escherichia coli* and *Enterobacter*, normally used with other antibiotics (ie, aminoglycosides)
Usual Dosage
Children: I.M., I.V.: 200-300 mg/kg/day in divided doses every 4-6 hours; maximum dose: 24 g/day
Higher doses have been used in cystic fibrosis: 350-500 mg/kg/day in divided doses every 4 hours

Adults:
I.M.: 2-3 g/dose every 6-12 hours; maximum: 24 g/24 hours
I.V.: 3-4 g/dose every 4-6 hours; maximum: 24 g/24 hours
Mechanism of Action Inhibits bacterial cell wall synthesis by binding to one or more of the penicillin binding proteins (PBPs); which in turn inhibits the final transpeptidation step of peptidoglycan synthesis in bacterial cell walls, thus inhibiting cell wall biosynthesis. Bacteria eventually lyse due to ongoing activity of cell wall autolytic enzymes (autolysins and murein hydrolases) while cell wall assembly is arrested.
Local Anesthetic/Vasoconstrictor Precautions No information available to require special precautions
Effects on Dental Treatment Prolonged use of penicillins may lead to development of oral candidiasis
Other Adverse Effects <1%:
Central nervous system: Convulsions, confusion, drowsiness, fever, Jarisch-Herxheimer reaction
Dermatologic: Rash
Endocrine & metabolic: Electrolyte imbalance
Hematologic: Hemolytic anemia, positive Coombs' reaction, abnormal platelet aggregation and prolonged prothrombin time (high doses)
Local: Thrombophlebitis
Neuromuscular: Myoclonus
Renal: Acute interstitial nephritis
Miscellaneous: Hypersensitivity reactions, anaphylaxis
Drug Interactions
Decreased effect: Tetracyclines cause decreased penicillin effectiveness
Increased effect: Probenecid causes increased penicillin levels
Drug Uptake
Absorption: I.M.: 70% to 80%
Serum half-life: Dose-dependent; prolonged with moderately severe renal or hepatic impairment:
Adults: 36-80 minutes
Time to peak serum concentration: I.M.: Within 30-50 minutes
Pregnancy Risk Factor B

Piperacillin Sodium and Tazobactam Sodium
(pi per' a sil in sow' dee um & ta zoe bak' tam sow' dee um)
Brand Names Zosyn™
Therapeutic Category Antibiotic, Penicillin
Use
Treatment of infections of lower respiratory tract, urinary tract, skin and skin structures, gynecologic, bone and joint infections, and septicemia caused by susceptible organisms. Tazobactam expands activity of piperacillin to include beta-lactamase producing strains of *S. aureus*, *H. influenzae*, *Enterobacteriaceae*, *Pseudomonas*, *Klebsiella*, *Citrobacter*, *Serratia*, *Bacteroides*, and other gram-negative anaerobes.
Application to nosocomial infections may be limited by restricted activity against gram-negative organisms producing class I beta-lactamases and inactivity against methicillin-resistant *Staphylococcus aureus*
Usual Dosage
Children <12 years: Not recommended due to lack of data

Children >12 years and Adults:
  Severe infections: I.V.: Piperacillin/tazobactam 4/0.5 g every 8 hours or 3/
    0.375 g every 6 hours
  Moderate infections: I.M.: Piperacillin/tazobactam 2/0.25 g every 6-1 hours;
    treatment should be continued for ≥7-10 days depending on severity of
    disease

Mechanism of Action Piperacillin interferes with bacterial cell wall synthesis
during active multiplication, causing cell wall death and resultant bactericidal
activity against susceptible bacteria; tazobactam prevents degradation of
piperacillin by binding to the active side on beta-lactamase; tazobactam
inhibits many beta-lactamases, including staphylococcal penicillinase and
Richmond and Sykes types II, III, IV, and V, including extended spectrum
enzymes; it has only limited activity against class I beta-lactamases other than
class Ic types

Local Anesthetic/Vasoconstrictor Precautions No information available to
require special precautions

Effects on Dental Treatment Prolonged use of penicillins may lead to development of oral candidiasis

Other Adverse Effects
  >10%: Gastrointestinal: Diarrhea
  1% to 10%:
    Central nervous system: Insomnia, headache
    Dermatologic: Rash, pruritus
    Gastrointestinal: Constipation, nausea, vomiting, dyspepsia
    Hematologic: Leukopenia
    Miscellaneous: Serum sickness-like reaction
  <1%:
    Cardiovascular: Hypertension, hypotension, edema
    Central nervous system: Dizziness, agitation, confusion
    Gastrointestinal: Pseudomembranous colitis
    Respiratory: Bronchospasm
  Several laboratory abnormalities have rarely been associated with piperacillin/
    tazobactam including reversible eosinophilia, and neutropenia (associated
    most often with prolonged therapy), positive direct Coombs' test, prolonged
    PT and PTT, transient elevations of LFT, increases in creatinine

Drug Interactions
  Decreased effect: Tetracyclines cause decreased penicillin effectiveness
  Increased effect: Probenecid causes increased penicillin levels

Drug Uptake Both AUC and peak concentrations are dose proportional
  Serum half-life:
    Piperacillin: 1 hour
    Metabolite: 1-1.5 hours
    Tazobactam: 0.7-0.9 hour

Pregnancy Risk Factor B

Piperazine Citrate (pi′ per a zeen sit′ rate)
Brand Names Vermizine®
Therapeutic Category Anthelmintic
Use Treatment of pinworm and roundworm infections (used as an alternative to
first-line agents, mebendazole, or pyrantel pamoate)
Usual Dosage Oral:
  Pinworms: Children and Adults: 65 mg/kg/day (not to exceed 2.5 g/day) as a
    single daily dose for 7 days; in severe infections, repeat course after a 1-
    week interval

  Roundworms:
    Children: 75 mg/kg/day as a single daily dose for 2 days; maximum: 3.5 g/
      day
    Adults: 3.5 g/day for 2 days (in severe infections, repeat course, after a 1-
      week interval)
Mechanism of Action Causes muscle paralysis of the roundworm by blocking
the effects of acetylcholine at the neuromuscular junction
Local Anesthetic/Vasoconstrictor Precautions No information available to
require special precautions
Effects on Dental Treatment No effects or complications reported
Other Adverse Effects <1%:
  Central nervous system: Dizziness, weakness, seizures, EEG changes, head-
    ache, vertigo
  Gastrointestinal: Nausea, vomiting, diarrhea
  Hematologic: Hemolytic anemia
  Ocular: Visual impairment
  (Continued)

Piperazine Citrate *(Continued)*

Respiratory: Bronchospasms
Miscellaneous: Hypersensitivity reactions
Drug Interactions None reported
Drug Uptake
Absorption: Well absorbed from GI tract
Time to peak serum concentration: 1 hour
Pregnancy Risk Factor B

Pipobroman (pi poe broe' man)

Brand Names Vercyte®
Therapeutic Category Antineoplastic Agent, Alkylating Agent
Use Treat polycythemia vera; chronic myelocytic leukemia
Usual Dosage Children >15 years and Adults: Oral:
Polycythemia: 1 mg/kg/day for 30 days; may increase to 1.5-3 mg/kg until hematocrit reduced to 50% to 55%; maintenance: 0.1-0.2 mg/kg/day
Myelocytic leukemia: 1.5-2.5 mg/kg/day until WBC drops to 10,000/mm^3 then start maintenance 7-175 mg/day; stop if WBC falls to <3000/mm^3 or platelets fall to <150,000/mm^3
Mechanism of Action An alkylating agent considered to be cell-cycle nonspecific and capable of killing tumor cells in any phase of the cell cycle. Alkylating agents form covalent cross-links with DNA thereby resulting in cytotoxic, mutagenic, and carcinogenic effects. The end result of the alkylation process results in the misreading of the DNA code and the inhibition of DNA, RNA, and protein synthesis in rapidly proliferating tumor cells.
Local Anesthetic/Vasoconstrictor Precautions No information available to require special precautions
Effects on Dental Treatment No effects or complications reported
Other Adverse Effects 1% to 10%:
Dermatologic: Rash
Gastrointestinal: Vomiting, diarrhea, nausea, abdominal cramps
Hematologic: Leukopenia, thrombocytopenia, anemia
Pregnancy Risk Factor D

Pipracil® *see Piperacillin Sodium on page 696*
Pirazinamida (Mexico) *see Pyrazinamide on page 752*

Pirbuterol Acetate (peer byoo' ter ole as' e tate)

Related Information
Respiratory Diseases *on page 924*
Brand Names Maxair™
Therapeutic Category Antiasthmatic; Beta-2-Adrenergic Agonist Agent; Bronchodilator
Use Prevention and treatment of reversible bronchospasm including asthma
Usual Dosage Children >12 years and Adults: 2 inhalations every 4-6 hours for prevention; two inhalations at an interval of at least 1-3 minutes, followed by a third inhalation in treatment of bronchospasm, not to exceed 12 inhalations/day
Mechanism of Action Pirbuterol is a beta$_2$-adrenergic agonist with a similar structure to albuterol, specifically a pyridine ring has been substituted for the benzene ring in albuterol. The increased beta$_2$ selectivity of pirbuterol results from the substitution of a tertiary butyl group on the nitrogen of the side chain, which subsequently imparts resistance of pirbuterol to degradation by monoamine oxidase and provides a lengthened duration of action in comparison to the less selective previous beta-agonist agents.
Local Anesthetic/Vasoconstrictor Precautions No information available to require special precautions
Effects on Dental Treatment No effects or complications reported
Other Adverse Effects
>10%:
Central nervous system: Nervousness, restlessness
Neuromuscular & skeletal: Trembling
1% to 10%:
Central nervous system: Headache, dizziness
Gastrointestinal: Taste changes, vomiting, nausea
<1%:
Cardiovascular: Hypertension, arrhythmias, chest pain
Central nervous system: Weakness, insomnia, numbness in hands
Dermatologic: Bruising
Gastrointestinal: Anorexia
Respiratory: Paradoxical bronchospasm

Drug Interactions Increased toxicity: Cardiovascular effects are potentiated in patients also receiving MAO inhibitors, tricyclic antidepressants, sympathomimetic agents (eg, amphetamine, dopamine, dobutamine), inhaled anesthetics (eg, enflurane)

Drug Uptake
Peak therapeutic effect:
Oral: 2-3 hours with peak serum concentration of 6.2-9.8 mcg/L
Inhalation: 0.5-1 hour
Serum half-life: 2-3 hours

Pregnancy Risk Factor C

Piridoxina (Mexico) *see* Pyridoxine Hydrochloride *on page 753*
Pirimetamina (Mexico) *see* Pyrimethamine *on page 754*

Piroxicam (peer ox' i kam)
Related Information
Nonsteroidal Anti-Inflammatory Agents, Comparative Dosages, and Pharmacokinetics *on page 1021*
Rheumatoid Arthritis, Osteoarthritis, and Joint Prostheses *on page 930*
Brand Names Feldene®
Canadian/Mexican Brand Names Apo-Piroxicam® (Canada); Novo-Piroxicam® (Canada); Nu-Pirox® (Canada); Pro-Piroxicam® (Canada); Artyflam® (Mexico); Citoken® (Mexico); Facicam® (Mexico); Flogosan® (Mexico); Oxicanol® (Mexico); Rogal® (Mexico); Piroxan® (Mexico); Piroxen® (Mexico)
Therapeutic Category Analgesic, Non-narcotic; Anti-inflammatory Agent; Nonsteroidal Anti-inflammatory Agent (NSAID), Oral
Use Management of inflammatory disorders; symptomatic treatment of acute and chronic rheumatoid arthritis, osteoarthritis, and ankylosing spondylitis; also used to treat sunburn
Usual Dosage Oral:
Children: 0.2-0.3 mg/kg/day once daily; maximum dose: 15 mg/day

Adults: 10-20 mg/day once daily; although associated with increase in GI adverse effects, doses >20 mg/day have been used (ie, 30-40 mg/day)
Mechanism of Action Inhibits prostaglandin synthesis, acts on the hypothalamus heat-regulating center to reduce fever, blocks prostaglandin synthetase action which prevents formation of the platelet-aggregating substance thromboxane A_2; decreases pain receptor sensitivity. Other proposed mechanisms of action for salicylate anti-inflammatory action are lysosomal stabilization, kinin and leukotriene production, alteration of chemotactic factors, and inhibition of neutrophil activation. This latter mechanism may be the most significant pharmacologic action to reduce inflammation.

Local Anesthetic/Vasoconstrictor Precautions No information available to require special precautions
Effects on Dental Treatment No effects or complications reported
Other Adverse Effects
>10%:
Central nervous system: Dizziness
Dermatologic: Skin rash
Gastrointestinal: Abdominal cramps, heartburn, indigestion, nausea
1% to 10%:
Cardiovascular: Fluid retention
Central nervous system: Headache, nervousness
Dermatologic: Itching
Gastrointestinal: Vomiting
Otic: Ringing in ears
<1%:
Cardiovascular; Congestive heart failure, hypertension, arrhythmias, tachycardia, hot flushes
Central nervous system: Epistaxis, confusion, hallucinations, aseptic meningitis, mental depression, drowsiness, insomnia
Dermatologic: Hives, erythema multiforme, toxic epidermal necrolysis, Stevens-Johnson syndrome, angioedema
Endocrine & metabolic: Polydipsia
Gastrointestinal: Gastritis, GI ulceration
Genitourinary: Cystitis
Hematologic: Agranulocytosis, anemia, hemolytic anemia, bone marrow depression, leukopenia, thrombocytopenia
Hepatic: Hepatitis
Neuromuscular & skeletal: Peripheral neuropathy
Ocular: Toxic amblyopia, blurred vision, conjunctivitis, dry eyes
Otic: Decreased hearing
(Continued)

Piroxicam *(Continued)*

Renal: Polyuria, acute renal failure
Respiratory: Allergic rhinitis, shortness of breath

Drug Interactions
Decreased effect of diuretics, beta-blockers; decreased effect with aspirin, antacids, cholestyramine
Increased effect/toxicity of lithium, warfarin, methotrexate (controversial)

Drug Uptake
Onset of analgesia: Oral: Within 1 hour
Serum half-life: 45-50 hours

Pregnancy Risk Factor B (D if used in the 3rd trimester)

Pitocin® *see* Oxytocin *on page 654*

Pitressin® *see* Vasopressin *on page 891*

Pix Carbonis *see* Coal Tar *on page 225*

Placidyl® *see* Ethchlorvynol *on page 334*

Plaquenil® *see* Hydroxychloroquine Sulfate *on page 440*

Platinol® *see* Cisplatin *on page 210*

Platinol®-AQ *see* Cisplatin *on page 210*

Plendil® *see* Felodipine *on page 354*

Plicamycin *(plye kay mye' sin)*

Brand Names Mithracin®

Therapeutic Category Antidote, Hypercalcemia; Antineoplastic Agent, Antibiotic

Use Malignant testicular tumors, in the treatment of hypercalcemia and hypercalciuria of malignancy not responsive to conventional treatment; Paget's disease

Usual Dosage Refer to individual protocols. Dose should be diluted in 1 L of D_5W or NS and administered over 4-6 hours

Dosage should be based on the patient's body weight. If a patient has abnormal fluid retention (ie, edema, hydrothorax or ascites), the patient's ideal weight rather than actual body weight should be used to calculate the dose.

Adults: I.V.:
Testicular cancer: 25-30 mcg/kg/day for 8-10 days
Blastic chronic granulocytic leukemia: 25 mcg/kg over 2-4 hours every other day for 3 weeks
Paget's disease: 15 mcg/kg/day once daily for 10 days
Hypercalcemia:
25 mcg/kg single dose which may be repeated in 48 hours if no response occurs
or 25 mcg/kg for 3-4 days
or 25-50 mcg/kg every other day for 3-8 doses

Mechanism of Action Potent osteoclast inhibitor; may inhibit parathyroid hormone effect on osteoclasts; inhibits bone resorption; forms a complex with DNA in the presence of magnesium or other divalent cations inhibiting DNA-directed RNA synthesis

Local Anesthetic/Vasoconstrictor Precautions No information available to require special precautions

Effects on Dental Treatment No effects or complications reported

Other Adverse Effects
>10%: Gastrointestinal: Nausea and vomiting occur in almost 100% of patients within the first 6 hours after treatment; incidence increases with rapid injection; stomatitis has also occurred; anorexia, diarrhea
1% to 10%:
Central nervous system: Headache, fever, mental depression, drowsiness, weakness
Myelosuppression: Mild leukopenia and thrombocytopenia
Clotting disorders: May also depress hepatic synthesis of clotting factors, leading to a form of coagulopathy; petechiae, increased prothrombin time, epistaxis, and thrombocytopenia may be seen and may require discontinuation of the drug
Endocrine & metabolic: Hypocalcemia
Extravasation: Is an irritant; may produce local tissue irritation or cellulitis if infiltrated; if extravasation occurs, follow hospital procedure, discontinue I.V., and apply ice for 24 hours
Irritant chemotherapy
Hepatic: Elevation in liver enzymes, hepatotoxicity
Renal: Nephrotoxicity, azotemia

Miscellaneous: Facial flushing, hemorrhagic diathesis
Drug Interactions Increased toxicity: Calcitonin, etidronate, glucagon, causes additive hypoglycemic effects
Drug Uptake
Decreasing calcium levels:
Onset of action: Within 24 hours
Peak effect: 48-72 hours
Duration: 5-15 days
Serum half-life, plasma: 1 hour
Pregnancy Risk Factor D

Podocon-25® *see* Podophyllum Resin *on this page*

Podofilox (po do fil' ox)
Brand Names Condylox®
Therapeutic Category Keratolytic Agent
Use Treatment of external genital warts
Local Anesthetic/Vasoconstrictor Precautions No information available to require special precautions
Effects on Dental Treatment No effects or complications reported

Podofin® *see* Podophyllum Resin *on this page*

Podophyllin and Salicylic Acid (po dof' fil um & sal i sil' ik as' id)
Brand Names Verrex-C&M®
Therapeutic Category Keratolytic Agent
Synonyms Salicylic Acid and Podophyllin
Use Topical treatment of benign growths including external genital and perianal warts, papillomas, fibroids
Local Anesthetic/Vasoconstrictor Precautions No information available to require special precautions
Effects on Dental Treatment No effects or complications reported

Podophyllum Resin (po dof' fil um rez' in)
Brand Names Podocon-25®; Podofin®
Canadian/Mexican Brand Names Podofilm® (Canada)
Therapeutic Category Keratolytic Agent
Use Topical treatment of benign growths including external genital and perianal warts, papillomas, fibroids; compound benzoin tincture generally is used as the medium for topical application
Usual Dosage Topical:
Children and Adults: 10% to 25% solution in compound benzoin tincture; apply drug to dry surface, use 1 drop at a time allowing drying between drops until area is covered; total volume should be limited to <0.5 mL per treatment session

Condylomata acuminatum: 25% solution is applied daily; use a 10% solution when applied to or near mucous membranes

Verrucae: 25% solution is applied 3-5 times/day directly to the wart
Mechanism of Action Directly affects epithelial cell metabolism by arresting mitosis through binding to a protein subunit of spindle microtubules (tubulin)
Local Anesthetic/Vasoconstrictor Precautions No information available to require special precautions
Effects on Dental Treatment No effects or complications reported
Other Adverse Effects Local: Pain, swelling
1% to 10%:
Dermatologic: Pruritus
Gastrointestinal: Nausea, vomiting, abdominal pain, diarrhea
<1%:
Central nervous system: Confusion, lethargy, hallucinations
Genitourinary: Renal failure
Hematologic: Leukopenia, thrombocytopenia
Hepatic: Hepatotoxicity
Neuromuscular & skeletal: Peripheral neuropathy
Drug Interactions No data reported
Pregnancy Risk Factor X

Point-Two® *see* Fluoride *on page 374*
Poison Information Centers *see page 1086*
Poladex® *see* Dexchlorpheniramine Maleate *on page 261*
Polaramine® *see* Dexchlorpheniramine Maleate *on page 261*
Polargen® *see* Dexchlorpheniramine Maleate *on page 261*

Poliovirus Vaccine, Inactivated
(poe′ lee oh vye′ rus vak seen′ in ak ti vay′ ted)
Brand Names IPOL™
Therapeutic Category Vaccine, Live Virus and Inactivated Virus
Synonyms Enhanced-potency Inactivated Poliovirus Vaccine; IPV; Salk Vaccine
Use Although a protective immune response to E-IPV cannot be assured in the immunocompromised individual, E-IPV is recommended because the vaccine is safe and some protection may result from its administration.
Usual Dosage Subcutaneous: **Enhanced-potency inactivated poliovirus vaccine (E-IPV) is preferred for primary vaccination of adults**, two doses S.C. 4-8 weeks apart, a third dose 6-12 months after the second. For adults with a completed primary series and for whom a booster is indicated, either OPV or E-IPV can be given. If immediate protection is needed, either OPV or E-IPV is recommended.
Local Anesthetic/Vasoconstrictor Precautions No information available to require special precautions
Effects on Dental Treatment No effects or complications reported
Other Adverse Effects All serious adverse reactions must be reported to the FDA
1% to 10%:
  Dermatologic: Skin rash
  Central nervous system: Fever >101.3°F
  Local: Tenderness or pain at injection site
<1%:
  Central nervous system: Tiredness, weakness, fussiness, sleepiness, crying, Guillain-Barré
  Dermatologic: Reddening of skin, erythema
  Gastrointestinal: Decreased appetite
  Respiratory: Difficulty in breathing
Drug Interactions Decreased effect with immunosuppressive agents, immune globulin, other live vaccines within 1 month; may temporarily suppress tuberculin skin test sensitivity (4-6 weeks)
Pregnancy Risk Factor C

Poliovirus Vaccine, Live, Trivalent, Oral
(poe′ lee oh vye′ rus vak seen′, live, try vay′ lent, or′ al)
Brand Names Orimune®
Therapeutic Category Vaccine, Live Virus
Synonyms OPV; Sabin Vaccine; TOPV
Use Poliovirus immunization
Local Anesthetic/Vasoconstrictor Precautions No information available to require special precautions
Effects on Dental Treatment No effects or complications reported
Other Adverse Effects All serious adverse reactions must be reported to the Vaccine Adverse Event Reporting System (1-800-822-7967)
Comments
Oral vaccine: Live, attenuated vaccine
Federal law requires that the date of administration, the vaccine manufacturer, lot number of vaccine, and the administering person's name, title and address be entered into the patient's permanent medical record; live virus vaccine

Polocaine® 2% *see* Mepivacaine With Levonordefrin *on page 542*
Polocaine® 3% *see* Mepivacaine Dental Anesthetic *on page 541*
Polycillin® *see* Ampicillin *on page 62*
Polycillin-PRB® *see* Ampicillin and Probenecid *on page 63*
Polycitra®-K *see* Potassium Citrate and Citric Acid *on page 710*
Polycose® [OTC] *see* Glucose Polymers *on page 400*

Polyestradiol Phosphate (pol i es tra dye′ ole fos′ fate)
Brand Names Estradurin®
Therapeutic Category Estrogen Derivative
Use Palliative treatment of advanced, inoperable carcinoma of the prostate
Usual Dosage Adults: Deep I.M.: 40 mg every 2-4 weeks or less frequently; maximum dose: 80 mg
Mechanism of Action Estrogens exert their primary effects on the interphase DNA-protein complex (chromatin) by binding to a receptor (usually located in the cytoplasm of a target cell) and initiating translocation of the hormone-receptor complex to the nucleus

Local Anesthetic/Vasoconstrictor Precautions No information available to require special precautions

Effects on Dental Treatment No effects or complications reported

Other Adverse Effects

>10%:
  Cardiovascular: Peripheral edema
  Endocrine & metabolic: Enlargement of breasts (female and male), breast tenderness
  Gastrointestinal: Nausea, anorexia, bloating

1% to 10%:
  Central nervous system: Headache
  Endocrine & metabolic: Increased libido (female), decrease libido (male)
  Gastrointestinal: Vomiting, diarrhea

<1%:
  Cardiovascular: Hypertension, thromboembolism, stroke, myocardial infarction, edema
  Central nervous system: Depression, dizziness, anxiety
  Dermatologic: Chloasma, melasma, rash
  Endocrine: Breast tumors, amenorrhea, alterations in frequency and flow of menses, decreased glucose tolerance, increased triglycerides and LDL
  Gastrointestinal: Nausea, GI distress
  Hepatic: Cholestatic jaundice
  Miscellaneous: Intolerance to contact lenses, increased susceptibility to *Candida* infection

Drug Interactions No data reported

Drug Uptake
90% of injected dose leaves blood stream within 24 hours
Passive storage in reticuloendothelial system
Increasing the dose prolongs duration of action

Pregnancy Risk Factor X

Polyethylene Glycol-Electrolyte Solution

(pol i eth' i leen gly' kol ee lek' troe lite soe loo' shun)

Brand Names Co-Lav®; Colovage®; CoLyte®; Go-Evac®; GoLYTELY®; NuLYTELY®; OCL®

Therapeutic Category Laxative, Bowel Evacuant

Synonyms Electrolyte Lavage Solution

Use For bowel cleansing prior to GI examination

Usual Dosage The recommended dose for adults is 4 L of solution prior to gastrointestinal examination, as ingestion of this dose produces a satisfactory preparation in >95% of patients. Ideally the patient should fast for approximately 3-4 hours prior to administration, but in no case should solid food be given for at least 2 hours before the solution is given. The solution is usually administered orally, but may be given via nasogastric tube to patients who are unwilling or unable to drink the solution.

Children: Oral: 25-40 mL/kg/hour for 4-10 hours

Adults:
  Oral: At a rate of 240 mL (8 oz) every 10 minutes, until 4 liters are consumed or the rectal effluent is clear; rapid drinking of each portion is preferred to drinking small amounts continuously
  Nasogastric tube: At a rate of 20-30 mL/minute (1.2-1.8 L/hour); the first bowel movement should occur approximately 1 hour after the start of administration

Mechanism of Action Induces catharsis by strong electrolyte and osmotic effects

Local Anesthetic/Vasoconstrictor Precautions No information available to require special precautions

Effects on Dental Treatment No effects or complications reported

Other Adverse Effects GI side effect may be reduced by premedication with single doses of simethicone and metoclopramide, given 30 minutes to 1 hour prior to beginning prep

>10%: Gastrointestinal: Nausea, abdominal fullness, bloating
1% to 10%: Gastrointestinal: Abdominal cramps, vomiting, anal irritation
<1%: Dermatologic: Skin rash

Drug Uptake Onset of effect: Oral: Within 1-2 hours

Pregnancy Risk Factor C

Comments Do not add flavorings as additional ingredients before use

Polyflex® see Chlorzoxazone *on page 200*
Polygam® see Immune Globulin, Intravenous *on page 454*

Polygam® S/D see Immune Globulin, Intravenous on page 454

Poly-Histine CS® see Brompheniramine, Phenylpropanolamine, and Codeine on page 125

Polymox® see Amoxicillin Trihydrate on page 58

Polymyxin B and Hydrocortisone
(pol i mix' in bee & hye droe kor' ti sone)

Brand Names Otobiotic® Otic; Pyocidin-Otic®

Therapeutic Category Antibacterial, Otic; Corticosteroid, Otic

Use Treatment of superficial bacterial infections of external ear canal

Local Anesthetic/Vasoconstrictor Precautions No information available to require special precautions

Effects on Dental Treatment No effects or complications reported

Polymyxin B and Oxytetracycline see Oxytetracycline and Polymyxin B on page 653

Polymyxin B and Trimethoprim see Trimethoprim and Polymyxin B on page 874

Polymyxin B Sulfate (pol i mix' in bee sul' fate)

Brand Names Aerosporin®

Therapeutic Category Antibiotic, Ophthalmic; Antibiotic, Topical

Use

Topical: Wound irrigation and bladder irrigation against *Pseudomonas aeruginosa*; used occasionally for gut decontamination

Parenteral use of polymyxin B has mainly been replaced by less toxic antibiotics; it is reserved for life-threatening infections caused by organisms resistant to the preferred drugs

Usual Dosage

Otic: 1-2 drops, 3-4 times/day; should be used sparingly to avoid accumulation of excess debris

Children ≥2 years and Adults:

I.M.: 25,000-30,000 units/kg/day divided every 4-6 hours

I.V.: 15,000-25,000 units/kg/day divided every 12 hours or by continuous infusion

Intrathecal: 50,000 units/day for 3-4 days, then every other day for at least 2 weeks

Total daily dose should not exceed 2,000,000 units/day

Bladder irrigation: Continuous irrigant or rinse in the urinary bladder for up to 10 days using 20 mg (equal to 200,000 units) added to 1 L of normal saline; usually no more than 1 L of irrigant is used per day unless urine flow rate is high; administration rate is adjusted to patient's urine output

Topical irrigation or topical solution: 500,000 units/L of normal saline; topical irrigation should not exceed 2 million units/day in adults

Gut sterilization: Oral: 15,000-25,000 units/kg/day in divided doses every 6 hours

Clostridium difficile enteritis: Oral: 25,000 units every 6 hours for 10 days

Ophthalmic: A concentration of 0.1% to 0.25% is administered as 1-3 drops every hour, then increasing the interval as response indicates to 1-2 drops 4-6 times/day

Mechanism of Action Binds to phospholipids, alters permeability, and damages the bacterial cytoplasmic membrane permitting leakage of intracellular constituents

Local Anesthetic/Vasoconstrictor Precautions No information available to require special precautions

Effects on Dental Treatment No effects or complications reported

Other Adverse Effects <1%:

Cardiovascular: Facial flushing

Central nervous system: Neurotoxicity (irritability, weakness, drowsiness, ataxia, perioral paresthesia, numbness of the extremities, and blurring of vision)

Dermatologic: Urticarial rash

Endocrine & metabolic: Hypocalcemia, hyponatremia, hypokalemia, hypochloremia

Neuromuscular & skeletal: Neuromuscular blockade

Renal: Nephrotoxicity

Respiratory: Respiratory arrest

Miscellaneous: Drug fever, anaphylactoid reaction, meningeal irritation with intrathecal administration

Drug Interactions Increased/prolonged effect of neuromuscular blocking agents

Drug Uptake
Absorption: Well absorbed from the peritoneum; minimal absorption from the GI tract (except in neonates) from mucous membranes or intact skin
Serum half-life: 4.5-6 hours, increased with reduced renal function
Time to peak serum concentration: I.M.: Within 2 hours
Pregnancy Risk Factor B

Polymyxin E see Colistin Sulfate on page 231

Poly-Pred® see Neomycin, Polymyxin B, and Prednisolone on page 611

Polysaccharide-Iron Complex
(pol i sak' a ride-eye' ern kom' pleks)
Brand Names Hytinic® [OTC]; Niferex® [OTC]; Nu-Iron® [OTC]
Therapeutic Category Iron Salt
Use Prevention and treatment of iron deficiency anemias
Local Anesthetic/Vasoconstrictor Precautions No information available to require special precautions
Effects on Dental Treatment No effects or complications reported
Other Adverse Effects
>10%: Gastrointestinal: Stomach cramping, constipation, nausea, vomiting, dark stools, GI irritation, epigastric pain, nausea
1% to 10%:
Gastrointestinal: Heartburn, diarrhea
Genitourinary: Discolored urine
Miscellaneous: Staining of teeth
<1%: Dermatologic: Contact irritation
Comments 100% elemental iron

Polysporin® see Bacitracin and Polymyxin B on page 94

Polytar® [OTC] see Coal Tar on page 225

Polythiazide (pol i thye' a zide)
Related Information
Cardiovascular Diseases on page 912
Brand Names Renese®
Therapeutic Category Diuretic, Thiazide Type
Use Adjunctive therapy in treatment of edema and hypertension
Usual Dosage Adults: Oral: 1-4 mg/day
Mechanism of Action The diuretic mechanism of action of the thiazides is primarily inhibition of sodium, chloride, and water reabsorption in the renal distal tubules, thereby producing diuresis with a resultant reduction in plasma volume. The antihypertensive mechanism of action of the thiazides is unknown. It is known that doses of thiazides produce greater reductions in blood pressure than equivalent diuretic doses of loop diuretics (eg, furosemide). There has been speculation that the thiazides may have some influence on vascular tone mediated through sodium depletion, but this remains to be proven.
Local Anesthetic/Vasoconstrictor Precautions No information available to require special precautions
Effects on Dental Treatment No effects or complications reported
Other Adverse Effects
1% to 10%: Endocrine & metabolic: Hypokalemia
<1%:
Cardiovascular: Hypotension
Central nervous system: Drowsiness
Dermatologic: Photosensitivity, rash
Endocrine & metabolic: Fluid and electrolyte imbalances (hypocalcemia, hypomagnesemia, hyponatremia), hyperglycemia
Gastrointestinal: Nausea, vomiting, anorexia
Genitourinary: Uremia
Hematologic: Rarely blood dyscrasias
Hepatic: Hepatitis
Renal: Prerenal azotemia, polyuria
Drug interactions Increased toxicity/levels of lithium
Drug Uptake
Onset of diuretic effect: Within ~2 hours
Duration: 24-48 hours
Pregnancy Risk Factor D

Polytrim® Ophthalmic see Trimethoprim and Polymyxin B on page 874

Poly-Vi-Flor® see Vitamins, Multiple on page 901

Polyvinyl Alcohol see Artificial Tears on page 75

Poly-Vi-Sol® [OTC] *see* Vitamins, Multiple *on page 901*

Pondimin® *see* Fenfluramine Hydrochloride *on page 355*

Ponstel® *see* Mefenamic Acid *on page 534*

Pontocaine® *see* Tetracaine Hydrochloride *on page 828*

Pontocaine® **With Dextrose Injection** *see* Tetracaine With Dextrose *on page 829*

Porcelana® [OTC] *see* Hydroquinone *on page 439*

Pork NPH Iletin® II *see* Insulin Preparations *on page 459*

Pork Regular Iletin® II *see* Insulin Preparations *on page 459*

Posture® [OTC] *see* Calcium Phosphate, Tribasic *on page 145*

Potasalan® *see* Potassium Chloride *on page 708*

Potassium Acetate (poe tass' ee um as' e tate)

Therapeutic Category Electrolyte Supplement, Parenteral; Potassium Salt

Use Potassium deficiency; to avoid chloride when high concentration of potassium is needed, source of bicarbonate

Usual Dosage I.V. doses should be incorporated into the patient's maintenance I.V. fluids, intermittent I.V. potassium administration should be reserved for severe depletion situations and requires EKG monitoring; doses listed as mEq of potassium

Treatment of hypokalemia: I.V.:
Children: 2-5 mEq/kg/day
Adults: 40-100 mEq/day
I.V. intermittent infusion (must be diluted prior to administration):
Children: 0.5-1 mEq/kg/dose (maximum: 30 mEq) to infuse at 0.3-0.5 mEq/kg/hour (maximum: 1 mEq/kg/hour)
Adults: 10-20 mEq/dose (maximum: 40 mEq/dose) to infuse over 2-3 hours (maximum: 40 mEq over 1 hour)

Mechanism of Action Potassium is the major cation of intracellular fluid and is essential for the conduction of nerve impulses in heart, brain, and skeletal muscle; contraction of cardiac, skeletal and smooth muscles; maintenance of normal renal function, acid-base balance, carbohydrate metabolism, and gastric secretion

Local Anesthetic/Vasoconstrictor Precautions No information available to require special precautions

Effects on Dental Treatment No effects or complications reported

Other Adverse Effects
>10%: Gastrointestinal: Diarrhea, nausea, stomach pain, flatulence, vomiting (oral)
1% to 10%:
Cardiovascular: Bradycardia
Endocrine & metabolic: Hyperkalemia
Respiratory: Difficult breathing, weakness
Local: Local tissue necrosis with extravasation
<1%:
Cardiovascular: Chest pain
Central nervous system: Mental confusion
Endocrine & metabolic: Alkalosis
Gastrointestinal: Abdominal pain
Local: Phlebitis
Neuromuscular & skeletal: Paresthesias, paralysis
Miscellaneous: Throat pain

Drug Interactions Increased effect/levels with potassium-sparing diuretics, salt substitutes, ACE inhibitors

Drug Uptake
Absorption: Absorbed well from upper GI tract

Pregnancy Risk Factor C

Potassium Acetate, Potassium Bicarbonate, and Potassium Citrate

(poe tass' ee um as' e tate, poe tass' ee um bye kar' bun ate, & poe tass' ee um sit' rate)

Brand Names Tri-K®; Trikates®

Therapeutic Category Electrolyte Supplement, Oral; Potassium Salt

Use Treatment or prevention of hypokalemia

Local Anesthetic/Vasoconstrictor Precautions No information available to require special precautions

Effects on Dental Treatment No effects or complications reported

Potassium Acid Phosphate (poe tass' ee um as' id fos' fate)

Brand Names K-Phos® Original

Therapeutic Category Electrolyte Supplement, Oral; Potassium Salt; Urinary Acidifying Agent

Use Acidifies urine and lowers urinary calcium concentration; reduces odor and rash caused by ammoniacal urine; increases the antibacterial activity of methenamine

Usual Dosage Adults: Oral: 1000 mg dissolved in 6-8 oz of water 4 times/day with meals and at bedtime; for best results, soak tablets in water for 2-5 minutes, then stir and swallow

Mechanism of Action The principal intracellular cation; involved in transmission of nerve impulses, muscle contractions, enzyme activity, and glucose utilization

Local Anesthetic/Vasoconstrictor Precautions No information available to require special precautions

Effects on Dental Treatment No effects or complications reported

Other Adverse Effects

>10%: Gastrointestinal: Diarrhea, nausea, stomach pain, flatulence, vomiting

1% to 10%:

Cardiovascular: Bradycardia

Central nervous system: Weakness

Endocrine & metabolic: Hyperkalemia

Local: Local tissue necrosis with extravasation

Respiratory: Difficult breathing

<1%:

Cardiovascular: Chest pain, irregular heartbeat, edema

Central nervous system: Mental confusion, tetany, pain/weakness of extremities

Endocrine & metabolic: Hyperphosphatemia, hypocalcemia, alkalosis

Gastrointestinal: Abdominal pain, weight gain

Genitourinary: Decreased urine output

Local: Phlebitis

Neuromuscular & skeletal: Paresthesias, paralysis, bone/joint pain

Respiratory: Shortness of breath

Miscellaneous: Thirst, throat pain

Drug Interactions

Increased effect/levels with potassium-sparing diuretics, salt substitutes, salicylates, ACE inhibitors

Drug Uptake

Absorption: Absorbed well from upper GI tract

Pregnancy Risk Factor C

Potassium Bicarbonate (poe tass' ee um bye kar' bun ate)

Brand Names K+ Care® Effervescent; K-Electrolyte® Effervescent; K-Gen® Effervescent; K-Lyte® Effervescent

Therapeutic Category Electrolyte Supplement, Oral; Potassium Salt

Use Potassium deficiency, hypokalemia

Local Anesthetic/Vasoconstrictor Precautions No information available to require special precautions

Effects on Dental Treatment No effects or complications reported

Potassium Bicarbonate and Potassium Chloride, Effervescent

(poe tass' ee um bye kar' bun ate, & poe tass' ee um klor' ide ef er ves' ent)

Brand Names Klorvess® Effervescent; K-Lyte/CL®

Therapeutic Category Electrolyte Supplement, Oral; Potassium Salt

Use Treatment or prevention of hypokalemia

Local Anesthetic/Vasoconstrictor Precautions No information available to require special precautions

Effects on Dental Treatment No effects or complications reported

Potassium Bicarbonate and Potassium Citrate, Effervescent

(poe tass' ee um bye kar' bun ate & poe tass' ee um sit' rate ef er ves' ent)

Brand Names Effer-K™; Klor-Con®/EF; K-Lyte®; K-Vescent®

Therapeutic Category Electrolyte Supplement, Oral; Potassium Salt

Use Treatment or prevention of hypokalemia

(Continued)

Potassium Bicarbonate and Potassium Citrate, Effervescent *(Continued)*

Usual Dosage Oral:

Children: 1-4 mEq/kg/24 hours in divided doses as required to maintain normal serum potassium

Adults:
Prevention: 16-24 mEq/day in 2-4 divided doses
Treatment: 40-100 mEq/day in 2-4 divided doses

Mechanism of Action Needed for the conduction of nerve impulses in heart, brain, and skeletal muscle; contraction of cardiac, skeletal and smooth muscles; maintenance of normal renal function

Local Anesthetic/Vasoconstrictor Precautions No information available to require special precautions

Effects on Dental Treatment No effects or complications reported

Other Adverse Effects

>10%: Gastrointestinal: Diarrhea, nausea, stomach pain, flatulence, vomiting

1% to 10%:
Cardiovascular: Bradycardia
Central nervous system: Weakness
Endocrine & metabolic: Hyperkalemia
Local: Local tissue necrosis with extravasation
Respiratory: Difficult breathing

<1%:
Cardiovascular: Chest pain
Central nervous system: Mental confusion
Endocrine & metabolic: Alkalosis
Gastrointestinal: Abdominal pain
Local: Phlebitis
Neuromuscular & skeletal: Paresthesias, paralysis
Miscellaneous: Throat pain

Drug Interactions Increased effect/levels with potassium-sparing diuretics, salt substitutes, ACE inhibitors

Drug Uptake

Absorption: Absorbed well from upper GI tract

Pregnancy Risk Factor C

Potassium Bicarbonate, Potassium Chloride, and Potassium Citrate

(poe tass' ee um bye kar' bun ate, poe tass' ee um klor' ide & poe tass' ee um sit' rate)

Brand Names Kaochlor-Eff®

Therapeutic Category Electrolyte Supplement, Oral; Potassium Salt

Use Treatment or prevention of hypokalemia

Local Anesthetic/Vasoconstrictor Precautions No information available to require special precautions

Effects on Dental Treatment No effects or complications reported

Potassium Chloride (poe tass' ee um klor' ide)

Brand Names Cena-K®; Gen-K®; K+8®; Kaochlor® S-F; Kaon-CL®; Kato®; K-Dur®; K-Lor™; Klor-con®; Klorvess®; Klotrix®; K-Tab®; Micro-K®; Potasalan®; Rum-K®; Slow-K®

Canadian/Mexican Brand Names Celek® 20 (Mexico); Clor-K-Zaf® (Mexico); Cloruro® De Potasio (Mexico); Kaliolite® (Mexico)

Therapeutic Category Electrolyte Supplement, Oral; Electrolyte Supplement, Parenteral; Potassium Salt

Use Treatment or prevention of hypokalemia

Usual Dosage I.V. doses should be incorporated into the patient's maintenance I.V. fluids; intermittent I.V. potassium administration should be reserved for severe depletion situations in patients undergoing EKG monitoring.

Normal daily requirements: Oral, I.V.:
Children: 2-3 mEq/kg/day
Adults: 40-80 mEq/day

Prevention during diuretic therapy: Oral:
Children: 1-2 mEq/kg/day in 1-2 divided doses
Adults: 20-40 mEq/day in 1-2 divided doses

Treatment of hypokalemia: Children:

Oral: 1-2 mEq/kg initially, then as needed based on frequently obtained lab values. If deficits are severe or ongoing losses are great, I.V. route should be considered.

I.V.: 1 mEq/kg over 1-2 hours initially, then repeated as needed based on frequently obtained lab values; severe depletion or ongoing losses may require >200% of normal limit needs

I.V. intermittent infusion: Dose should not exceed 1 mEq/kg/hour, or 40 mEq/ hour; if it exceeds 0.5 mEq/kg/hour, physician should be at bedside and patient should have continuous EKG monitoring

Treatment of hypokalemia: Adults:

I.V. intermittent infusion: 10-20 mEq/hour, not to exceed 40 mEq/hour and 150 mEq/day. See table.

Potassium Dosage/Rate of Infusion Guidelines

Serum Potassium⁺	Maximum Infusion Rate	Maximum Concentration	Maximum 24-Hour Dose
>2.5 mEq/L	10 mEq/h	40 mEq/L	200 mEq
<2.5 mEq/L	40 mEq/h	80 mEq/L	400 mEq

Potassium >2.5 mEq/L:

Oral: 60-80 mEq/day plus additional amounts if needed

I.V.: 10 mEq over 1 hour with additional doses if needed

Potassium <2.5 mEq/L:

Oral: Up to 40-60 mEq initial dose, followed by further doses based on lab values; deficits at a plasma level of 2 mEq/L may be as high as 400-800 mEq of potassium

I.V.: Up to 40 mEq over 1 hour, with doses based on frequent lab monitoring; deficits at a plasma level of 2 mEq/L may be as high as 400-800 mEq of potassium

Mechanism of Action Potassium is the major cation of intracellular fluid and is essential for the conduction of nerve impulses in heart, brain, and skeletal muscle; contraction of cardiac, skeletal and smooth muscles; maintenance of normal renal function, acid-base balance, carbohydrate metabolism, and gastric secretion

Local Anesthetic/Vasoconstrictor Precautions No information available to require special precautions

Effects on Dental Treatment No effects or complications reported

Other Adverse Effects

>10%: Gastrointestinal: Diarrhea, nausea, stomach pain, flatulence, vomiting (oral)

1% to 10%:

Cardiovascular: Bradycardia

Central nervous system: Weakness

Endocrine & metabolic: Hyperkalemia

Local: Local tissue necrosis with extravasation, pain at the site of injection

Respiratory: Difficult breathing

<1%:

Cardiovascular: Chest pain, arrhythmias, heart block, hypotension

Central nervous system: Mental confusion

Endocrine & metabolic: Alkalosis

Gastrointestinal: Abdominal pain

Local: Phlebitis

Neuromuscular & skeletal: Paresthesias, paralysis

Miscellaneous: Throat pain

Drug Interactions No data reported

Drug Uptake

Absorption: Absorbed well from upper GI tract

Pregnancy Risk Factor A

Potassium Chloride and Potassium Gluconate

(poe tass′ ee um klor′ ide & poe tass′ ee um gloo′ coe nate)

Brand Names Kolyum®

Therapeutic Category Electrolyte Supplement, Oral; Potassium Salt

Use Treatment or prevention of hypokalemia

Local Anesthetic/Vasoconstrictor Precautions No information available to require special precautions

Effects on Dental Treatment No effects or complications reported

Potassium Citrate (poe tass' ee um sit' rate)

Brand Names Urocit®-K

Therapeutic Category Alkalinizing Agent, Oral

Use Prevention of uric acid nephrolithiasis; prevention of calcium renal stones in patients with hypocitraturia; urinary alkalinizer when sodium citrate is contraindicated

Local Anesthetic/Vasoconstrictor Precautions No information available to require special precautions

Effects on Dental Treatment No effects or complications reported

Comments Parenteral K_3PO_4 contains 3 mmol of phosphorous/mL and 4.4 mEq of potassium/mL. If ordering by phosphorous content, use mmol instead of mEq since the mEq value for phosphorous varies with the pH of the solution due to valence changes of the phosphorus ion. (1 mmol of phosphorous = 31 mg)

Potassium Citrate and Citric Acid

(poe tass' ee um sit' rate & si' trik as' id)

Brand Names Polycitra®-K

Therapeutic Category Electrolyte Supplement, Oral; Potassium Salt

Use Treatment of metabolic acidosis; alkalinizing agent in conditions where long-term maintenance of an alkaline urine is desirable

Local Anesthetic/Vasoconstrictor Precautions No information available to require special precautions

Effects on Dental Treatment No effects or complications reported

Comments Potassium citrate 3.4 mmol/5 mL and citric acid 1.6 mmol/5 mL = total of 5.0 mmol/5 mL citrate content

Potassium Citrate and Potassium Gluconate

(poe tass' ee um sit' rate & poe tass' ee um gloo' coe nate)

Brand Names Twin-K®

Therapeutic Category Electrolyte Supplement, Oral; Potassium Salt

Use Treatment or prevention of hypokalemia

Local Anesthetic/Vasoconstrictor Precautions No information available to require special precautions

Effects on Dental Treatment No effects or complications reported

Potassium Gluconate (poe tass' ee um gloo' coe nate)

Brand Names Kaon®; Kaylixir®; K-G® Elixir

Therapeutic Category Electrolyte Supplement, Oral; Potassium Salt

Use Treatment or prevention of hypokalemia

Usual Dosage Oral (doses listed as mEq of potassium):

Normal daily requirement:
  Children: 2-3 mEq/kg/day
  Adults: 40-80 mEq/day

Prevention of hypokalemia during diuretic therapy:
  Children: 1-2 mEq/kg/day in 1-2 divided doses
  Adults: 20-40 mEq/kg/day in 1-2 divided doses

Treatment of hypokalemia:
  Children: 2-5 mEq/kg/day in 2-4 divided doses
  Adults: 40-100 mEq/day in 2-4 divided doses

Mechanism of Action Potassium is the major cation of intracellular fluid and is essential for the conduction of nerve impulses in heart, brain, and skeletal muscle; contraction of cardiac, skeletal and smooth muscles; maintenance of normal renal function, acid-base balance, carbohydrate metabolism, and gastric secretion

Local Anesthetic/Vasoconstrictor Precautions No information available to require special precautions

Effects on Dental Treatment No effects or complications reported

Other Adverse Effects

>10%: Gastrointestinal: Diarrhea, nausea, stomach pain, flatulence, vomiting (oral)

1% to 10%:
  Cardiovascular: Bradycardia
  Endocrine & metabolic: Hyperkalemia
  Neuromuscular & skeletal: Weakness
  Respiratory: Difficult breathing

<1%:
  Cardiovascular: Chest pain
  Central nervous system: Mental confusion
  Endocrine & metabolic: Alkalosis

Local: Phlebitis
Neuromuscular & skeletal: Paresthesias, paralysis
Miscellaneous: Throat pain
Drug Interactions
Increased effect/levels with potassium-sparing diuretics, salt substitutes, ACE inhibitors
Increased effect of digitalis
Drug Uptake
Absorption: Absorbed well from upper GI tract
Pregnancy Risk Factor A

Potassium Iodide (poe tass' ee um eye' oh dide)
Related Information
Endocrine Disorders & Pregnancy *on page 927*
Brand Names Iosat®; Pima®; Potassium Iodide Enseals®; SSKI®; Thyro-Block®
Therapeutic Category Antithyroid Agent; Expectorant
Use Facilitate bronchial drainage and cough; reduce thyroid vascularity prior to thyroidectomy and management of thyrotoxic crisis; block thyroidal uptake of radioactive isotopes of iodine in a radiation emergency
Usual Dosage Oral:
Adults: RDA: 130 mcg

Expectorant:
Children: 60-250 mg every 6-8 hours; maximum single dose: 500 mg
Adults: 300-650 mg 2-3 times/day
Preoperative thyroidectomy: Children and Adults: 50-250 mg (1-5 drops SSKI®) 3 times/day **or** 0.1-0.3 mL (3-5 drops) of strong iodine (Lugol's solution) 3 times/day; give for 10 days before surgery
Thyrotoxic crisis:
Children and Adults: 300-500 mg (6-10 drops SSKI®) 3 times/day or 1 mL strong iodine (Lugol's solution) 3 times/day
Graves' disease in neonates: 1 drop of strong iodine (Lugol's solution) 3 times/day
Sporotrichosis:
Initial:
Preschool: 50 mg/dose 3 times/day
Children: 250 mg/dose 3 times/day
Adults: 500 mg/dose 3 times/day
Oral increase 50 mg/dose daily
Maximum dose:
Preschool: 500 mg/dose 3 times/day
Children and Adults: 1-2 g/dose 3 times/day
Continue treatment for 4-6 weeks after lesions have completely healed
Mechanism of Action Reduces viscosity of mucus by increasing respiratory tract secretions; inhibits secretion of thyroid hormone, fosters colloid accumulation in thyroid follicles
Local Anesthetic/Vasoconstrictor Precautions No information available to require special precautions
Effects on Dental Treatment No effects or complications reported
Other Adverse Effects 1% to 10%:
Central nervous system: Fever, headache
Dermatologic: Urticaria, acne, angioedema
Endocrine & metabolic: Goiter with hypothyroidism
Gastrointestinal: Metallic taste, GI upset
Hematologic: Cutaneous and mucosal hemorrhage, eosinophilia
Neuromuscular & skeletal: Arthralgia
Respiratory: Rhinitis
Miscellaneous: Lymph node enlargement, soreness of teeth and gums
Drug Interactions Increased toxicity: Lithium causes additive hypothyroid effects
Drug Uptake
Onset of action: 24-48 hours
Peak effect: 10-15 days after continuous therapy
Pregnancy Risk Factor D

Potassium Iodide Enseals® *see* Potassium Iodide *on this page*

Potassium Phosphate (poe tass' ee um fos' fate)
Brand Names Neutra-Phos®-K
Therapeutic Category Electrolyte Supplement, Parenteral; Phosphate Salt; Potassium Salt
Use Treatment and prevention of hypophosphatemia or hypokalemia
(Continued)

Potassium Phosphate *(Continued)*

Usual Dosage I.V. doses should be incorporated into the patient's maintenance I.V. fluids; intermittent I.V. infusion should be reserved for severe depletion situations in patients undergoing continuous EKG monitoring. It is difficult to determine total body phosphorus deficit; the following dosages are empiric guidelines:

Normal requirements elemental phosphorus: Oral:
0-6 months: 240 mg
6-12 months: 360 mg
1-10 years: 800 mg
>10 years: 1200 mg
Pregnancy lactation: Additional 400 mg/day

Adults RDA: 800 mg

Treatment: It is difficult to provide concrete guidelines for the treatment of severe hypophosphatemia because the extent of total body deficits and response to therapy are difficult to predict. Aggressive doses of phosphate may result in a transient serum elevation followed by redistribution into intracellular compartments or bone tissue. It is recommended that repletion of severe hypophosphatemia (<1 mg/dL in adults) be done I.V. because large doses of oral phosphate may cause diarrhea and intestinal absorption may be unreliable

Pediatric I.V. phosphate repletion: Children: 0.25-0.5 mmol/kg **administer over 4-6 hours and repeat if symptomatic hypophosphatemia persists**; to assess the need for further phosphate administration, obtain serum inorganic phosphate after administration of the first dose and base further doses on serum levels and clinical status

Adult I.V. phosphate repletion:
Initial dose: 0.08 mmol/kg if recent uncomplicated hypophosphatemia
Initial dose: 0.16 mmol/kg if prolonged hypophosphatemia with presumed total body deficits; increase dose by 25% to 50% if patient symptomatic with severe hypophosphatemia
Do not exceed 0.24 mmol/kg/day; administer over 6 hours by I.V. infusion

With orders for I.V. phosphate, there is considerable confusion associated with the use of millimoles (mmol) versus milliequivalents (mEq) to express the phosphate requirement. Because inorganic phosphate exists as monobasic and dibasic anions, with the mixture of valences dependent on pH, ordering by mEq amounts is unreliable and may lead to large dosing errors. In addition, I.V. phosphate is available in the sodium and potassium salt; therefore, the content of these cations must be considered when ordering phosphate. The most reliable method of ordering I.V. phosphate is by millimoles, then specifying the potassium or sodium salt. For example, an order for 15 mmol of phosphate as potassium phosphate in one liter of normal saline would also provide 22 mEq of potassium.

Phosphate maintenance electrolyte requirement in parenteral nutrition: 2 mmol/kg/24 hours or 35 mmol/kcal/24 hours; maximum: 15-30 mmol/24 hours

Maintenance:
I.V. solutions:
Children: 0.5-1.5 mmol/kg/24 hours I.V. or 2-3 mmol/kg/24 hours orally in divided doses
Adults: 15-30 mmol/24 hours I.V. or 50-150 mmol/24 hours orally in divided doses
Oral:
Children <4 years: 1 capsule (250 mg phosphorus/8 mmol) 4 times/day; dilute as instructed
Children >4 years and Adults: 1-2 capsules (250-500 mg phosphorus/8-16 mmol) 4 times/day; dilute as instructed

Fleet® Phospho®-Soda: Laxative: Oral: Single dose
Children: 5-15 mL
Adults: 20-30 mL mixed with 120 mL cold water

Local Anesthetic/Vasoconstrictor Precautions No information available to require special precautions
Effects on Dental Treatment No effects or complications reported
Other Adverse Effects
>10%: Gastrointestinal: Diarrhea, nausea, stomach pain, flatulence, vomiting
1% to 10%:
Cardiovascular: Bradycardia

Endocrine & metabolic: Hyperkalemia
Neuromuscular & skeletal: Weakness
Respiratory: Difficult breathing
<1%:
Cardiovascular: Chest pain
Central nervous system: Mental confusion
Endocrine & metabolic: Alkalosis
Gastrointestinal: Abdominal pain
Local: Phlebitis
Neuromuscular & skeletal: Paresthesias, paralysis
Renal: Acute renal failure
Miscellaneous: Throat pain

Drug Interactions
Decreased effect/levels with aluminum and magnesium-containing antacids or sucralfate which can act as phosphate binders
Increased effect/levels with potassium-sparing diuretics, salt substitutes, or ACE-inhibitors
Increased effect of digitalis

Pregnancy Risk Factor C

Potassium Phosphate and Sodium Phosphate
(poe tass' ee um fos' fate & sow' dee um fos' fate)
Brand Names K-Phos® Neutral; Neutra-Phos®; Uro-KP-Neutral®
Therapeutic Category Electrolyte Supplement, Oral; Phosphate Salt; Potassium Salt
Use Treatment of conditions associated with excessive renal phosphate loss or inadequate GI absorption of phosphate; to acidify the urine to lower calcium concentrations; to increase the antibacterial activity of methenamine; reduce odor and rash caused by ammonia in urine
Usual Dosage All dosage forms to be mixed in 6-8 oz of water prior to administration
Children: 2-3 mmol phosphate/kg/24 hours given 4 times/day **or** 1 capsule 4 times/day
Adults: 1-2 capsules (250-500 mg phosphorus/8-16 mmol) 4 times/day after meals and at bedtime
Local Anesthetic/Vasoconstrictor Precautions No information available to require special precautions
Effects on Dental Treatment No effects or complications reported
Other Adverse Effects
>10%: Gastrointestinal: Diarrhea, nausea, stomach pain, flatulence, vomiting
1% to 10%:
Cardiovascular: Bradycardia
Endocrine & metabolic: Hyperkalemia
Neuromuscular & skeletal: Weakness
Respiratory: Difficult breathing
<1%:
Cardiovascular: Irregular heartbeat, shortness of breath, chest pain, edema
Central nervous system: Mental confusion, tetany
Endocrine & metabolic: Alkalosis
Genitourinary: Decreased urine output
Local: Phlebitis
Neuromuscular & skeletal: Paresthesias, paralysis, pain/weakness of extremities, bone/joint pain
Renal: Acute renal failure
Miscellaneous: Thirst, throat pain, weight gain
Drug Interactions
Decreased effect/levels with aluminum and magnesium-containing antacids or sucralfate which can act as phosphate binders
Increased effect/levels with potassium-sparing diuretics or ACE-inhibitors
Increased effect/levels of digitalis, salicylates
Pregnancy Risk Factor C

Povidone-Iodine (poe' vi done eye' oh dine)
Related Information
Patients Undergoing Cancer Therapy *on page 967*
Brand Names Betadine® [OTC]; Efodine® [OTC]; Iodex® Regular; Isodine® [OTC]
Therapeutic Category Antibacterial, Topical
Use External antiseptic with broad microbicidal spectrum against bacteria, fungi, viruses, protozoa, and yeasts
(Continued)

Povidone-Iodine (Continued)

Usual Dosage
Shampoo: Apply 2 tsp to hair and scalp, lather and rinse; repeat application 2 times/week until improvement is noted, then shampoo weekly
Topical: Apply as needed for treatment and prevention of susceptible microbial infections

Mechanism of Action Povidone-iodine is known to be a powerful broad spectrum germicidal agent effective against a wide range of bacteria, viruses, fungi, protozoa, and spores.

Local Anesthetic/Vasoconstrictor Precautions No information available to require special precautions

Effects on Dental Treatment No effects or complications reported

Other Adverse Effects
1% to 10%:
Dermatologic: Rash, pruritus
Local: Local edema
<1%:
Endocrine & metabolic: Metabolic acidosis
Local: Systemic absorption in extensive burns causing ioderma
Renal: Renal impairment

Drug Interactions No data reported

Drug Uptake Absorption: In normal individuals, topical application results in very little systemic absorption; with vaginal administration, however, absorption is rapid and serum concentrations of total iodine and inorganic iodide are increased significantly

Pregnancy Risk Factor D

PPD see Tuberculin Purified Protein Derivative on page 882

Pramet® FA see Vitamins, Multiple on page 901

Pramilet® FA see Vitamins, Multiple on page 901

Pramosone® see Pramoxine and Hydrocortisone on this page

Pramoxine and Hydrocortisone
(pra mox' een & hye droe kor' ti sone)

Brand Names Enzone®; Pramosone®; Proctofoam®-HC; Zone-A Forte®

Therapeutic Category Anti-inflammatory Agent; Corticosteroid, Topical (Low Potency); Local Anesthetic, Topical

Synonyms Hydrocortisone and Pramoxine

Use Treatment of severe anorectal or perianal swelling

Local Anesthetic/Vasoconstrictor Precautions No information available to require special precautions

Effects on Dental Treatment No effects or complications reported

Pramoxine Hydrochloride (pra mox' een hye droe klor' ide)

Brand Names Itch-X® [OTC]; Phicon® [OTC]; Prax® [OTC]; Proctofoam® [OTC]; Tronolane® [OTC]; Tronothane® [OTC]

Therapeutic Category Local Anesthetic, Topical

Use Temporary relief of pain and itching associated with anogenital pruritus or irritation; dermatosis, minor burns, or hemorrhoids

Usual Dosage Adults: Topical: Apply as directed, usually every 3-4 hours to affected area (maximum adult dose: 200 mg)

Mechanism of Action Pramoxine, like other anesthetics, decreases the neuronal membrane's permeability to sodium ions; both initiation and conduction of nerve impulses are blocked, thus depolarization of the neuron is inhibited

Local Anesthetic/Vasoconstrictor Precautions No information available to require special precautions

Effects on Dental Treatment No effects or complications reported

Other Adverse Effects
1% to 10%:
Dermatologic: Angioedema
Local: Contact dermatitis, burning, stinging
<1%:
Cardiovascular: Edema
Dermatologic: Tenderness, urticaria
Genitourinary: Urethritis
Hematologic: Methemoglobinemia in infants

Drug Interactions No data reported

Drug Uptake
Onset of therapeutic effect: Within 2-5 minutes

Peak effect: 3-5 minutes
Duration: May last for several days
Pregnancy Risk Factor C

Pravachol® *see* Pravastatin Sodium *on this page*

Pravastatin Sodium (pra′ va stat in sow′ dee um)
Related Information
Cardiovascular Diseases *on page 912*
Brand Names Pravachol®
Therapeutic Category HMG-CoA Reductase Inhibitor; Lipid Lowering Drugs
Use Adjunct to diet for the reduction of elevated total and LDL-cholesterol levels in patients with hypercholesterolemia (Type IIa, IIb, and IIc); used in hypercholesterolemic patients without clinically evident heart disease to reduce the risk of myocardial infarction, to reduce the risk for revascularization, and reduce the risk of death due to cardiovascular causes with no increase in death from non-cardiovascular diseases
Usual Dosage Adults: Oral: 10-20 mg once daily at bedtime, may increase to 40 mg/day at bedtime
Mechanism of Action Pravastatin is a competitive inhibitor of 3-hydroxy-3-methylglutaryl coenzyme A (HMG-CoA) reductase, which is the rate-limiting enzyme involved in *de novo* cholesterol synthesis.
Local Anesthetic/Vasoconstrictor Precautions No information available to require special precautions
Effects on Dental Treatment No effects of complications reported
Other Adverse Effects
1% to 10%:
Central nervous system: Headache, dizziness
Dermatologic: Rash
Gastrointestinal: flatulence, abdominal cramps, diarrhea, constipation, nausea, dyspepsia, heartburn
Neuromuscular & skeletal: Myalgia
Miscellaneous: Elevated creatine phosphokinase (CPK)
<1%:
Gastrointestinal: Dysgeusia
Ocular: Lenticular opacities, blurred vision
Drug Interactions
Increased effect with cholestyramine
Increased effect/toxicity of oral anticoagulants
Increased toxicity with gemfibrozil, clofibrate
Concurrent use of erythromycin and HMG-CoA reductase inhibitors may result in rhabdomyolysis
Drug Uptake
Absorption: Poor
Serum half-life, elimination: ~2-3 hours
Time to peak serum concentration: 1-1.5 hours
Pregnancy Risk Factor X

Prax® [OTC] *see* Pramoxine Hydrochloride *on previous page*

Prazepam (pra′ ze pam)
Brand Names Centrax®
Therapeutic Category Antianxiety Agent; Anticonvulsant, Benzodiazepine; Benzodiazepine; Tranquilizer, Minor
Use Treatment of anxiety and management of alcohol withdrawal; may also be used as an anticonvulsant in management of simple partial seizures
Usual Dosage Adults: Oral: 30 mg/day in divided doses, may increase gradually to a maximum of 60 mg/day
Mechanism of Action Benzodiazepine anxiolytic sedative that produces CNS depression at the subcortical level, except at high doses, whereby it works at the cortical level
Local Anesthetic/Vasoconstrictor Precautions No information available to require special precautions
Effects on Dental Treatment Over 10% of patients will experience dry mouth which disappears with cessation of drug therapy
Other Adverse Effects
>10%:
Cardiovascular Tachycardia, chest pain
Central nervous system: Drowsiness, fatigue, impaired coordination, light-headedness, memory impairment, insomnia, anxiety, depression, headache
(Continued)

Prazepam *(Continued)*

Dermatologic: Rash
Endocrine & metabolic: Decreased libido
Gastrointestinal: Dry mouth, constipation, diarrhea, decreased salivation, nausea, vomiting, increased or decreased appetite
Neuromuscular & skeletal: Dysarthria
Ocular: Blurred vision
Miscellaneous: Sweating

1% to 10%:
Cardiovascular: Syncope, hypotension
Central nervous system: Confusion, nervousness, dizziness, akathisia
Dermatologic: Dermatitis
Gastrointestinal: Weight gain or loss, increased salivation
Ocular: Blurred vision
Otic: Tinnitus
Neuromuscular & skeletal: Muscle cramps, rigidity, tremor
Respiratory: Hyperventilation, nasal congestion

<1%:
Central nervous system: Reflex slowing
Endocrine & metabolic: Menstrual irregularities
Hematologic: Blood dyscrasias
Miscellaneous: Drug dependence

Drug Interactions Increased toxicity (CNS depression): Oral anticoagulants, alcohol, tricyclic antidepressants, sedative-hypnotics, MAO inhibitors

Drug Uptake
Duration: 48 hours
Serum half-life:
Parent drug: 78 minutes
Desmethyldiazepam: 30-100 hours

Pregnancy Risk Factor D

Praziquantel (pray zi kwon' tel)

Brand Names Biltricide®
Canadian/Mexican Brand Names Cisticid® (Mexico); Tecprazin (Mexico)
Therapeutic Category Anthelmintic
Use Treatment of all stages of schistosomiasis caused by *Schistosoma* species pathogenic to humans; also active in the treatment of clonorchiasis, opisthorchiasis, cysticercosis, and many intestinal tapeworm infections and trematode
Usual Dosage Children >4 years and Adults: Oral:
Schistosomiasis: 20 mg/kg/dose 2-3 times/day for 1 day at 4- to 6-hour intervals
Flukes: 25 mg/kg/dose every 8 hours for 1-2 days
Cysticercosis: 50 mg/kg/day divided every 8 hours for 14 days
Tapeworms: 10-20 mg/kg as a single dose (25 mg/kg for *Hymenolepis nana*)
Mechanism of Action Increases the cell permeability to calcium in schistosomes, causing strong contractions and paralysis of worm musculature leading to detachment of suckers from the blood vessel walls and to dislodgment
Local Anesthetic/Vasoconstrictor Precautions No information available to require special precautions
Effects on Dental Treatment No effects or complications reported
Other Adverse Effects
1% to 10%:
Central nervous system: Dizziness, drowsiness, headache, malaise
Gastrointestinal: Abdominal pain, loss of appetite, nausea, vomiting
Miscellaneous: Sweating
<1%:
Central nervous system: Fever
Dermatologic: Skin rash, hives, itching
Gastrointestinal: Diarrhea
Miscellaneous: CSF reaction syndrome in patients being treated for neurocysticercosis
Drug Uptake
Absorption: Oral: ~80%; CSF concentration is 14% to 20% of plasma concentration
Serum half-life:
Parent drug: 0.8-1.5 hours
Metabolites: 4.5 hours
Time to peak serum concentration: Within 1-3 hours
Pregnancy Risk Factor B

Prazosin and Polythiazide (pra' zoe sin & pol i thye' a zide)
Brand Names Minizide®
Therapeutic Category Antihypertensive Agent, Combination
Use Management of mild to moderate hypertension
Local Anesthetic/Vasoconstrictor Precautions No information available to require special precautions
Effects on Dental Treatment No effects or complications reported

Prazosin Hydrochloride (pra' zoe sin hye droe klor' ide)
Related Information
Cardiovascular Diseases *on page 912*
Brand Names Minipress®
Canadian/Mexican Brand Names Apo-Prazo® (Canada); Novo-Prazin® (Canada); Nu-Prazo® (Canada)
Therapeutic Category Alpha-Adrenergic Blockers - Peripheral-Acting (Alpha$_1$-Blockers); Antihypertensive; Vasodilator, Coronary
Use Treatment of hypertension, severe congestive heart failure (in conjunction with diuretics and cardiac glycosides); reduce mortality in stable postmyocardial patients with left ventricular dysfunction (ejection fraction ≤40%)
Unlabeled use: Symptoms of benign prostatic hypertrophy
Usual Dosage Oral:
Children: Initial: 5 mcg/kg/dose (to assess hypotensive effects); usual dosing interval: every 6 hours; increase dosage gradually up to maximum of 25 mcg/kg/dose every 6 hours
Adults: Initial: 1 mg/dose 2-3 times/day; usual maintenance dose: 3-15 mg/day in divided doses 2-4 times/day; maximum daily dose: 20 mg
Mechanism of Action Competitively inhibits postsynaptic alpha-adrenergic receptors which results in vasodilation of veins and arterioles and a decrease in total peripheral resistance and blood pressure
Local Anesthetic/Vasoconstrictor Precautions No information available to require special precautions
Effects on Dental Treatment Significant orthostatic hypotension a possibility; monitor patient when getting out of dental chair; significant dry mouth in up to 10% of patients
Other Adverse Effects
>10%:
Cardiovascular: Orthostatic hypotension
Central nervous system: Dizziness, lightheadedness, drowsiness, headache, malaise
1% to 10%:
Cardiovascular: Edema, palpitations
Central nervous system: Fatigue, nervousness
Gastrointestinal: Dry mouth
Genitourinary: Urinary incontinence
<1%:
Cardiovascular: Angina
Central nervous system: Nightmares, hypothermia
Dermatologic: Rash
Endocrine & metabolic: Sexual dysfunction
Gastrointestinal: Nausea
Genitourinary: Priapism, urinary frequency
Respiratory: Dyspnea, nasal congestion
Drug Interactions
Decreased effect (antihypertensive) with NSAIDs
Increased effect (hypotensive) with diuretics and antihypertensive medications (especially beta-blockers)
Drug Uptake
Onset of hypotensive effect: Within 2 hours
Maximum decrease: 2-4 hours
Duration: 10-24 hours
Serum half-life: 2-4 hours; increased with congestive heart failure
Pregnancy Risk Factor C

Precose® *see* Acarbose *on page 12*
Predair® *see* Prednisolone *on next page*
Predaject® *see* Prednisolone *on next page*
Predalone T.B.A.® *see* Prednisolone *on next page*
Predcor® *see* Prednisolone *on next page*
Predcor-TBA® *see* Prednisolone *on next page*
Pred Forte® *see* Prednisolone *on next page*

Pred-G® Ophthalmic *see* Prednisolone and Gentamicin *on next page*
Pred Mild® *see* Prednisolone *on this page*

Prednicarbate (pred' ni kar bate)
Brand Names Dermatop®
Therapeutic Category Corticosteroid, Topical (Medium Potency)
Use Relief of the inflammatory and pruritic manifestations of corticosteroid-responsive dermatoses (medium potency topical corticosteroid)
Usual Dosage Adults: Topical: Apply a thin film to affected area twice daily
Mechanism of Action Topical corticosteroids have anti-inflammatory, antipruritic, vasoconstrictive, and antiproliferative actions
Local Anesthetic/Vasoconstrictor Precautions No information available to require special precautions
Effects on Dental Treatment No effects or complications reported
Other Adverse Effects <10%:
  Dermatologic: Acne, hypopigmentation, allergic dermatitis, maceration of the skin, skin atrophy
  Endocrine & metabolic: HPA suppression, Cushing's syndrome, growth retardation
  Local: Burning, itching, irritation, dryness, folliculitis, hypertrichosis
  Miscellaneous: Secondary infection
Drug Interactions No data reported
Pregnancy Risk Factor C

Prednicen-M® *see* Prednisone *on next page*

Prednisolone (pred niss' oh lone)
Related Information
  Corticosteroid Equivalencies Comparison *on page 1017*
  Corticosteroids, Topical Comparison *on page 1018*
  Respiratory Diseases *on page 924*
Brand Names AK-Pred®; Articulose-50®; Delta-Cortef®; Econopred®; Econopred® Plus; Hydeltrasol®; Hydeltra-T.B.A.®; Inflamase®; Inflamase® Mild; Key-Pred®; Key-Pred-SP®; Metreton®; Pediapred®; Predair®; Predaject®; Predalone T.B.A.®; Predcor®; Predcor-TBA®; Pred Forte®; Pred Mild®; Prelone®
Canadian/Mexican Brand Names Novo-Prednisolone® (Canada); Fisopred® (Mexico); Sophipren® Ofteno (Mexico)
Therapeutic Category Adrenal Corticosteroid; Anti-inflammatory Agent; Corticosteroid, Ophthalmic; Corticosteroid, Systemic
Use
  Dental: Treatment of a variety of oral diseases of allergic, inflammatory or autoimmune origin
  Medical: Treatment of palpebral and bulbar conjunctivitis; corneal injury from chemical, radiation, thermal burns, or foreign body penetration; endocrine disorders, rheumatic disorders, collagen diseases, dermatologic diseases, allergic states, ophthalmic diseases, respiratory diseases, hematologic disorders, neoplastic diseases, edematous states, and gastrointestinal diseases; useful in patients with inability to activate prednisone (liver disease)
Usual Dosage Dose depends upon condition being treated and response of patient; dosage for infants and children should be based on severity of the disease and response of the patient rather than on strict adherence to dosage indicated by age, weight, or body surface area. Consider alternate day therapy for long-term therapy. Discontinuation of long-term therapy requires gradual withdrawal by tapering the dose.

  Children: Anti-inflammatory or immunosuppressive dose: Oral, I.V., I.M. (sodium phosphate salt): 0.1-2 mg/kg/day in divided doses 1-4 times/day
  Adults: Oral, I.V., I.M. (sodium phosphate salt): 5-60 mg/day
  Elderly: Use lowest effective adult dose
Mechanism of Action Decreases inflammation by suppression of migration of polymorphonuclear leukocytes and reversal of increased capillary permeability; suppresses the immune system by reducing activity and volume of the lymphatic system
Local Anesthetic/Vasoconstrictor Precautions No information available to require special precautions
Effects on Dental Treatment No effects or complications reported
Other Adverse Effects >10%:
  Central nervous system: Insomnia, nervousness
  Gastrointestinal: Increased appetite, indigestion

  Oral manifestations: No data reported

Contraindications Acute superficial herpes simplex keratitis; systemic fungal infections; varicella; hypersensitivity to prednisolone or any component

Warnings/Precautions Use with caution in patients with hyperthyroidism, cirrhosis, nonspecific ulcerative colitis, hypertension, osteoporosis, thrombo-embolic tendencies, CHF, convulsive disorders, myasthenia gravis, thrombo-phlebitis, peptic ulcer, diabetes; acute adrenal insufficiency may occur with abrupt withdrawal after long-term therapy or with stress; young pediatric patients may be more susceptible to adrenal axis suppression from topical therapy. Because of the risk of adverse effects, systemic corticosteroids should be used cautiously in the elderly, in the smallest possible dose, and for the shortest possible time.

Drug Interactions Decreased effect with barbiturates, phenytoin, rifampin; decreased effect of salicylates, vaccines, toxoids

Drug Uptake
Absorption: Rapid and nearly complete
Serum half-life: 3.6 hours; biological: 18-36 hours

Pregnancy Risk Factor C

Breast-feeding Considerations May be taken while breast-feeding

Dosage Forms
Injection, as acetate (for I.M., intralesional, intra-articular, or soft tissue administration only): 25 mg/mL (10 mL, 30 mL); 50 mg/mL (30 mL)
Injection, as sodium phosphate (for I.M., I.V., intra-articular, intralesional, or soft tissue administration): 20 mg/mL (2 mL, 5 mL, 10 mL)
Injection, as tebutate (for intra-articular, intralesional, soft tissue administration only): 20 mg/mL (1 mL, 5 mL, 10 mL)
Liquid, oral, as sodium phosphate: 5 mg/5 mL (120 mL)
Solution, ophthalmic, as sodium phosphate: 0.125% (5 mL, 10 mL, 15 mL); 1% (5 mL, 10 mL, 15 mL)
Syrup: 15 mg/5 mL (240 mL)
Tablet: 5 mg

Dietary Considerations Should be taken after meals or with food or milk to decrease GI effects; limit caffeine; increase dietary intake of pyridoxine, vitamin C, vitamin D, folate, calcium, and phosphorus

Generic Available Yes

Prednisolone and Gentamicin
(pred nis' oh lone & jen ta mye' sin)
Brand Names Pred-G® Ophthalmic
Therapeutic Category Antibiotic, Ophthalmic; Corticosteroid, Ophthalmic
Synonyms Gentamicin and Prednisolone
Use Treatment of steroid responsive inflammatory conditions and superficial ocular infections due to strains of microorganisms susceptible to gentamicin such as *Staphylococcus*, *E. coli*, *H. influenzae*, *Klebsiella*, *Neisseria*, *Pseudomonas*, *Proteus*, and *Serratia* species
Local Anesthetic/Vasoconstrictor Precautions No information available to require special precautions
Effects on Dental Treatment No effects or complications reported
Other Adverse Effects 1% to 10%:
Dermatologic: Delayed wound healing
Local: Burning, stinging
Ocular: Intraocular pressure (increased), glaucoma, superficial punctate keratitis, infrequent optic nerve damage, posterior subcapsular cataract formation
Miscellaneous: Development of secondary infection, allergic sensitization

Prednisone (pred' ni sone)
Related Information
Corticosteroid Equivalencies Comparison *on page 1017*
Oral Nonviral Soft Tissue Ulcerations or Erosions *on page 955*
Respiratory Diseases *on page 924*
Rheumatoid Arthritis, Osteoarthritis, and Joint Prostheses *on page 930*
Brand Names Deltasone®; Liquid Pred®; Meticorten®; Orasone®; Prednicen-M®; Sterapred®
Canadian/Mexican Brand Names Apo-Prednisone® (Canada); Jaa-Prednisone® (Canada); Novo-Prednisone® (Canada); Wimpred® (Canada)
Therapeutic Category Adrenal Corticosteroid; Anti-inflammatory Agent; Corticosteroid, Systemic
Use
Dental: Treatment of a variety of oral diseases of allergic, inflammatory or autoimmune origin
Medical: Treatment of a variety of diseases including adrenocortical insufficiency, hypercalcemia, rheumatic and collagen disorders; dermatologic,
(Continued)

719

Prednisone *(Continued)*

ocular, respiratory, gastrointestinal, and neoplastic diseases; organ transplantation; not available in injectable form, prednisolone must be used

Usual Dosage Dose depends upon condition being treated and response of patient; dosage for infants and children should be based on severity of the disease and response of the patient rather than on strict adherence to dosage indicated by age, weight, or body surface area. Consider alternate day therapy for long-term therapy. Discontinuation of long-term therapy requires gradual withdrawal by tapering the dose.

Children: Oral: Anti-inflammatory or immunosuppressive dose: 0.05-2 mg/kg/day divided 1-4 times/day

Adults: 5-60 mg/day in divided doses 1-4 times/day

Elderly: Use the lowest effective dose

Mechanism of Action Decreases inflammation by suppression of migration of polymorphonuclear leukocytes and reversal of increased capillary permeability; suppresses the immune system by reducing activity and volume of the lymphatic system; suppresses adrenal function at high doses

Local Anesthetic/Vasoconstrictor Precautions No information available to require special precautions

Effects on Dental Treatment No effects or complications reported

Other Adverse Effects >10%:

Central nervous system: Insomnia, nervousness

Gastrointestinal: Increased appetite, indigestion

Oral manifestations: No data reported

Contraindications Serious infections, except septic shock or tuberculous meningitis; systemic fungal infections; hypersensitivity to prednisone or any component; varicella

Warnings/Precautions Use with caution in patients with hypothyroidism, cirrhosis, hypertension, congestive heart failure, ulcerative colitis, thromboembolic disorders, and patients with an increased risk for peptic ulcer disease; may retard bone growth; gradually taper dose to withdraw therapy. Because of the risk of adverse effects, systemic corticosteroids should be used cautiously in the elderly, in the smallest possible dose, and for the shortest possible time.

Drug Interactions Decreased effect with barbiturates, phenytoin, rifampin; decreased effect of salicylates, vaccines, toxoids

Drug Uptake Prednisone is inactive and must be metabolized to prednisolone which may be impaired in patients with impaired liver function

Absorption: Rapid and nearly complete

Serum half-life: Normal renal function: 2.5-3.5 hours

Pregnancy Risk Factor B

Breast-feeding Considerations May be taken while breast-feeding

Dosage Forms

Solution, oral: Concentrate (30% alcohol): 5 mg/mL (30 mL); Nonconcentrate (5% alcohol): 5 mg/5 mL (5 mL, 500 mL)

Syrup: 5 mg/5 mL (120 mL, 240 mL)

Tablet: 1 mg, 2.5 mg, 5 mg, 10 mg, 20 mg, 50 mg

Dietary Considerations Should be taken after meals or with food or milk; limit caffeine; increase dietary intake of pyridoxine, vitamin C, vitamin D, folate, calcium, and phosphorus

Generic Available Yes

Predominant Cultivable Microorganisms From Various Sites of the Oral Cavity *see page 1045*

Prefrin™ Ophthalmic Solution *see Phenylephrine Hydrochloride on page 685*

Pregnyl® *see Chorionic Gonadotropin on page 203*

Prelone® *see Prednisolone on page 718*

Premarin® *see Estrogens, Conjugated on page 327*

Premarin® With Methyltestosterone Oral *see Estrogens With Methyltestosterone on page 329*

Premphase™ *see Estrogens and Medroxyprogesterone on page 327*

Prempro™ *see Estrogens and Medroxyprogesterone on page 327*

Prenavite® [OTC] *see Vitamins, Multiple on page 901*

Pre-Par® *see Ritodrine Hydrochloride on page 773*

Pre-Pen® *see Benzylpenicilloyl-polylysine on page 107*

Prescription Writing *see page 1100*

PreSun® 29 [OTC] *see Methoxycinnamate and Oxybenzone on page 564*

Prevacid® *see Lansoprazole on page 490*

PreviDent® *see Fluoride on page 374*

Prilocaine (pril' oh kane)

Related Information

Oral Pain *on page 940*

Brand Names Citanest Plain 4% Injection

Therapeutic Category Dental/Local Anesthetics; Local Anesthetic, Injectable

Use Dental: Amide-type anesthetic used for local infiltration anesthesia; injection near nerve trunks to produce nerve block

Usual Dosage The lowest dose needed to provide effective anesthesia should be administered; maximum recommended dose for normal healthy adults is not more than 600 mg prilocaine hydrochloride

Mechanism of Action Local anesthetics bind selectively to the intracellular surface of sodium channels to block influx of sodium into the axon. As a result, depolarization necessary for action potential propagation and subsequent nerve function is prevented. The block at the sodium channel is reversible. When drug diffuses away from the axon, sodium channel function is restored and nerve propagation returns.

Local Anesthetic/Vasoconstrictor Precautions No information available to require special precautions

Effects on Dental Treatment No effects or complications reported

Other Adverse Effects Degree of adverse effects in the central nervous system and cardiovascular system are directly related to the blood levels of local anesthetic. The effects below are more likely to occur after systemic administration rather than infiltration.

Cardiovascular: Myocardial effects include a decrease in contraction force as well as a decrease in electrical excitability and myocardial conduction rate resulting in bradycardia and reduction in cardiac output.

Central nervous system: High blood levels result in anxiety, restlessness, disorientation, confusion, dizziness, tremors and seizures. This is followed by depression of CNS resulting in drowsiness, unconsciousness and possible respiratory arrest. Nausea and vomiting may also occur. In some cases, symptoms of CNS stimulation may be absent and the primary CNS effects are drowsiness and unconsciousness.

Hypersensitivity reactions: May be manifest as dermatologic reactions and edema at injection site. Asthmatic syndromes have occurred.

Psychogenic reactions: It is common to misinterpret psychogenic responses to local anesthetic injection as an allergic reaction. Intraoral injections are perceived by many patients as a stressful procedure in dentistry. Common symptoms to this stress are sweating, palpitations, hyperventilation, generalized pallor and a fainting feeling

Oral manifestations: No data reported

Contraindications Hypersensitivity to local anesthetics of the amide type

Warnings/Precautions Aspirate the syringe after tissue penetration and before injection to minimize chance of direct vascular injection

Drug Interactions No data reported

Drug Uptake

Infiltration

Onset: ~2 minutes

Duration: Complete anesthesia for procedures lasting 20 minutes

Inferior alveolar nerve block

Onset: ~3 minutes

Duration: ~2.5 hours

Pregnancy Risk Factor No data reported

Breast-feeding Considerations Usual infiltration doses of prilocaine given to nursing mothers has not been shown to affect the health of the nursing infant

Dosage Forms Prilocaine hydrochloride 4%, 1.8 mL cartridges, containers of 100

Dietary Considerations No data reported

Selected Readings

Jastak JT and Yagiela JA, "Vasoconstrictors and Local Anesthesia: A Review and Rationale for Use," *J Am Dent Assoc*, 1983, 107(4):623-30.

MacKenzie TA and Young ER, "Local Anesthetic Update," *Anesth Prog*, 1993, 40(2):29-34.

Wynn RL, "Epinephrine Interactions With Beta-Blockers," *Gen Dent*, 1994, 42(1):16, 18.

Yagiela JA, "Local Anesthetics," *Anesth Prog*, 1991, 38(4-5):128-41.

Prilocaine With Epinephrine (pril' oh kane with ep i nef' rin)

Related Information

Oral Pain *on page 940*

Brand Names Citanest Forte® with Epinephrine

Canadian/Mexican Brand Names Citanest® Forte (Canada); Citanest® Octapresin (Mexico)

(Continued)

Prilocaine With Epinephrine *(Continued)*

Therapeutic Category Dental/Local Anesthetics; Local Anesthetic, Injectable

Use Dental: Amide-type anesthetic used for local infiltration anesthesia; injection near nerve trunks to produce nerve block

Usual Dosage The lowest dose needed to provide effective anesthesia should be administered; the maximum recommended dose for normal healthy adults is not more than 600 mg prilocaine

Mechanism of Action Local anesthetics bind selectively to the intracellular surface of sodium channels to block influx of sodium into the axon. As a result, depolarization necessary for action potential propagation and subsequent nerve function is prevented. The block at the sodium channel is reversible. When drug diffuses away from the axon, sodium channel function is restored and nerve propagation returns.

Epinephrine prolongs the duration of the anesthetic actions of prilocaine by causing vasoconstriction (alpha adrenergic receptor agonist) of the vasculature surrounding the nerve axons. This prevents the diffusion of prilocaine away from the nerves resulting in a longer retention in the axon.

Local Anesthetic/Vasoconstrictor Precautions No information available to require special precautions

Effects on Dental Treatment No effects or complications reported

Other Adverse Effects Degree of adverse effects in the CNS and cardiovascular system are directly related to the blood levels of prilocaine. The effects below are more likely to occur after systemic administration rather than infiltration.

Cardiovascular: Myocardial effects include a decrease in contraction force as well as a decrease in electrical excitability and myocardial conduction rate resulting in bradycardia and reduction in cardiac output.

Central nervous system: High blood levels result in anxiety, restlessness, disorientation, confusion, dizziness, tremors and seizures. This is followed by depression of CNS resulting in drowsiness, unconsciousness and possible respiratory arrest. Nausea and vomiting may also occur. In some cases, symptoms of CNS stimulation may be absent and the primary CNS effects are drowsiness and unconsciousness.

Hypersensitivity reactions: Extremely rare, but may be manifest as dermatologic reactions and edema at injection site. Asthmatic syndromes have occurred. Patients may exhibit hypersensitivity to bisulfites contained in local anesthetic solution to prevent oxidation of epinephrine. In general, patients reacting to bisulfites have a history of asthma and their airways are hyperreactive to asthmatic syndrome.

Psychogenic reactions: It is common to misinterpret psychogenic responses to local anesthetic injection as an allergic reaction. Intraoral injections are perceived by many patients as a stressful procedure in dentistry. Common symptoms to this stress are sweating, palpitations, hyperventilation, generalized pallor, and a fainting feeling.

Oral manifestations: No data reported

Contraindications Hypersensitivity to local anesthetics of the amide-type

Warnings/Precautions Should be avoided in patients with uncontrolled hyperthyroidism. Should be used in minimal amounts in patients with significant cardiovascular problems (because of epinephrine component). Aspirate the syringe after tissue penetration and before injection to minimize chance of direct vascular injection

Drug Interactions Due to epinephrine component, use with tricyclic antidepressants or MAO inhibitors could result in increased pressor response; use with nonselective beta-blockers (ie, propranolol) could result in serious hypertension and reflex bradycardia

Drug Uptake
Onset of action:
Infiltration <2 minutes
Inferior alveolar nerve block: <3 minutes
Duration:
Infiltration 2.25 hours
Inferior alveolar nerve block: 3 hours

Pregnancy Risk Factor C

Breast-feeding Considerations Usual infiltration doses of prilocaine with epinephrine given to nursing mothers has not been shown to affect the health of the nursing infant

Dosage Forms Injection: Prilocaine hydrochloride 4% with epinephrine 1:200,000 (1.8 mL cartridges, in boxes of 100)

Dietary Considerations No data reported

Selected Readings

Jastak JT and Yagiela JA, "Vasoconstrictors and Local Anesthesia: A Review and Rationale for Use," *J Am Dent Assoc*, 1983, 107(4):623-30.

MacKenzie TA and Young ER, "Local Anesthetic Update," *Anesth Prog*, 1993, 40(2):29-34.

Wynn RL, "Epinephrine Interactions With Beta-Blockers," *Gen Dent*, 1994, 42(1):16, 18.

Yagiela JA, "Local Anesthetics," *Anesth Prog*, 1991, 38(4-5):128-41.

Prilosec™ *see* Omeprazole *on page 636*

Primacor® *see* Milrinone Lactate *on page 581*

Primaquine Phosphate (prim′ a kween fos′ fate)

Therapeutic Category Antimalarial Agent

Use Provides radical cure of *P. vivax* or *P. ovale* malaria after a clinical attack has been confirmed by blood smear or serologic titer and postexposure prophylaxis

Usual Dosage Oral:
Children: 0.3 mg base/kg/day once daily for 14 days (not to exceed 15 mg/day) or 0.9 mg base/kg once weekly for 8 weeks not to exceed 45 mg base/week
Adults: 15 mg/day (base) once daily for 14 days or 45 mg base once weekly for 8 weeks

Mechanism of Action Eliminates the primary tissue exoerythrocytic forms of *P. falciparum*; disrupts mitochondria and binds to DNA

Local Anesthetic/Vasoconstrictor Precautions No information available to require special precautions

Effects on Dental Treatment No effects or complications reported

Other Adverse Effects
>10%:
Gastrointestinal: Abdominal pain, nausea, vomiting
Hematologic: Hemolytic anemia
1% to 10%: Hematologic: Methemoglobinemia
<1%:
Cardiovascular: Arrhythmias
Central nervous system: Headache
Dermatologic: Pruritus
Hematologic: Leukopenia, agranulocytosis, leukocytosis
Miscellaneous: Interference with visual accommodation

Drug Interactions Increased toxicity/levels with quinacrine

Drug Uptake
Absorption: Oral: Well absorbed
Serum half-life: 3.7-9.6 hours
Time to peak serum concentration: Within 1-2 hours

Pregnancy Risk Factor C

Primaxin® *see* Imipenem/Cilastatin *on page 451*

Primidone (pri′ mi done)

Brand Names Mysoline®

Canadian/Mexican Brand Names Apo-Primidone® (Canada); Sertan® (Canada)

Therapeutic Category Anticonvulsant, Barbiturate

Use Management of grand mal, complex partial, and focal seizures

Unlabeled use: Benign familial tremor (essential tremor)

Usual Dosage Oral:
Children <8 years: Initial: 50-125 mg/day given at bedtime; increase by 50-125 mg/day increments every 3-7 days; usual dose: 10-25 mg/kg/day in divided doses 3-4 times/day
Children >8 years and Adults: Initial: 125-250 mg/day at bedtime; increase by 125-250 mg/day every 3-7 days; usual dose: 750-1500 mg/day in divided doses 3-4 times/day with maximum dosage of 2 g/day

Mechanism of Action Decreases neuron excitability, raises seizure threshold similar to phenobarbital; primidone has two active metabolites, phenobarbital and phenylethylmalonamide (PEMA); PEMA may enhance the activity of phenobarbital

Local Anesthetic/Vasoconstrictor Precautions No information available to require special precautions

Effects on Dental Treatment No effects or complications reported

Other Adverse Effects
>10%: Central nervous system: Drowsiness, vertigo, ataxia, lethargy, behavior change, sedation, headache
1% to 10%:
Gastrointestinal: Nausea, vomiting, anorexia
Genitourinary: Impotence
(Continued)

Primidone *(Continued)*

<1%:
  Central nervous system: Behavior change
  Dermatologic: Rash
  Hematologic: Leukopenia, malignant lymphoma-like syndrome, megalo-
    blastic anemia
  Hepatic: Systemic lupus-like syndrome
  Ocular: Diplopia, nystagmus

Drug Interactions

Decreased effect: Primidone may decrease serum concentrations of ethosuximide, valproic acid, griseofulvin; phenytoin may decrease primidone serum
  concentrations

Increased toxicity: Methylphenidate may increase primidone serum concentrations; valproic acid may increase phenobarbital concentrations derived from
  primidone

Drug Uptake

Serum half-life (age dependent):
  Primidone: 10-12 hours
  PEMA: 16 hours
  Phenobarbital: 52-118 hours
Time to peak serum concentration: Oral: Within 4 hours

Pregnancy Risk Factor D

Principen® *see* Ampicillin *on page 62*

Prinivil® *see* Lisinopril *on page 506*

Prinzide® *see* Lisinopril and Hydrochlorothiazide *on page 507*

Priscoline® *see* Tolazoline Hydrochloride *on page 852*

Privine® *see* Naphazoline Hydrochloride *on page 605*

Proampacin® *see* Ampicillin and Probenecid *on page 63*

Proaqua® *see* Benzthiazide *on page 105*

Probalan® *see* Probenecid *on this page*

Pro-Banthine® *see* Propantheline Bromide *on page 736*

Proben-C® *see* Colchicine and Probenecid *on page 229*

Probenecid *(proe ben' e sid)*

Related Information

Dental Drug Interactions: Update on Drug Combinations Requiring Special
  Considerations *on page 1022*

Brand Names Benemid®; Probalan®

Canadian/Mexican Brand Names Benuryl® (Canada); Benecid®
Probenecida Valdecasas (Mexico)

Therapeutic Category Adjuvant Therapy, Penicillin Level Prolongation; Uric
Acid Lowering Agent

Use Prevention of gouty arthritis; hyperuricemia; prolongation of beta-lactam
effect (ie, serum levels)

Usual Dosage Oral:
Children:
  <2 years: Not recommended
  2-14 years: Prolong penicillin serum levels: 25 mg/kg starting dose, then 40
    mg/kg/day given 4 times/day
  Gonorrhea: <45 kg: 25 mg/kg x 1 (maximum: 1 g/dose) 30 minutes before
    penicillin, ampicillin or amoxicillin
Adults:
  Hyperuricemia with gout: 250 mg twice daily for one week; increase to 250-
    500 mg/day; may increase by 500 mg/month, if needed, to maximum of 2-3
    g/day (dosages may be increased by 500 mg every 6 months if serum
    urate concentrations are controlled)
  Prolong penicillin serum levels: 500 mg 4 times/day
  Gonorrhea: 1 g 30 minutes before penicillin, ampicillin or amoxicillin

Mechanism of Action Competitively inhibits the reabsorption of uric acid at
the proximal convoluted tubule, thereby promoting its excretion and reducing
serum uric acid levels; increases plasma levels of weak organic acids (penicillins, cephalosporins, or other beta-lactam antibiotics) by competitively inhibiting their renal tubular secretion

Local Anesthetic/Vasoconstrictor Precautions No information available to
require special precautions

Effects on Dental Treatment No effects or complications reported

Other Adverse Effects
>10%:
  Central nervous system: Headache

Gastrointestinal: Anorexia, nausea, vomiting
Neuromuscular & skeletal: Gouty arthritis (acute)
1% to 10%:
Central nervous system: Dizziness
Cardiovascular: Flushing of face
Dermatologic: Skin rash, itching
Genitourinary: Painful urination
Renal: Renal calculi
Miscellaneous: Sore gums
<1%:
Hematologic: Leukopenia, hemolytic anemia, aplastic anemia
Hepatic: Hepatic necrosis
Renal: Urate nephropathy, nephrotic syndrome
Miscellaneous: Anaphylaxis
Drug Interactions
Decreased effect:
Salicylates (high dose) cause decreased uricosuria
Decreased urinary levels of nitrofurantoin cause decreased efficacy
Increased toxicity:
Increased methotrexate toxic potential
Increased penicillin and cephalosporin (beta-lactam) serum levels
Increased toxicity of acyclovir, thiopental, benzodiazepines, dapsone, sulfonylureas, zidovudine
Drug Uptake
Onset of action: Effect on penicillin levels reached in about 2 hours
Absorption: Rapid and complete from GI tract
Serum half-life: Normal renal function: 6-12 hours and is dose dependent
Time to peak serum concentration: 2-4 hours
Pregnancy Risk Factor B

Probenecid and Colchicine *see* Colchicine and Probenecid *on page 229*

Probucol (proe' byoo kole)
Related Information
Cardiovascular Diseases *on page 912*
Brand Names Lorelco®
Canadian/Mexican Brand Names Lesterol® (Mexico)
Therapeutic Category Lipid Lowering Drugs
Use Adjunct to dietary therapy to decrease elevated serum total and LDL cholesterol concentrations in primary hypercholesterolemia
Mechanism of Action Increases the fecal loss of bile acid-bound low density lipoprotein cholesterol, decreases the synthesis of cholesterol and inhibits enteral cholesterol absorption
Local Anesthetic/Vasoconstrictor Precautions No information available to require special precautions
Effects on Dental Treatment No effects or complications reported
Other Adverse Effects
>10%:
Cardiovascular: Q-T prolongation, serious arrhythmias
Gastrointestinal: Bloating, diarrhea, stomach pain, nausea, vomiting
1% to 10%: Central nervous system: Dizziness, headache, numbness of extremities
<1%:
Cardiovascular: Tachycardia
Hematologic: Anemia, Thrombocytopenia
Drug Interactions Increased toxicity: Drugs that prolong the Q-T interval (eg, tricyclic antidepressants, some antiarrhythmic agents, phenothiazines) or with drugs that affect the atrial rate (eg, beta-adrenergic blocking agents) or that can cause A-V block (eg, digoxin)
Pregnancy Risk Factor B

Procainamide Hydrochloride
(proe kane a' mide hye droe klor' ide)
Related Information
Cardiovascular Diseases *on page 912*
Brand Names Procan® SR; Promine®; Pronestyl®; Rhythmin®
Canadian/Mexican Brand Names Apo-Procainamide® (Canada)
Therapeutic Category Antiarrhythmic Agent, Class I-A; Antiarrhythmic Agent (Supraventricular & Ventricular)
Use Treatment of ventricular tachycardia, premature ventricular contractions, paroxysmal atrial tachycardia, and atrial fibrillation; to prevent recurrence of
(Continued)

Procainamide Hydrochloride *(Continued)*

ventricular tachycardia, paroxysmal supraventricular tachycardia, atrial fibrillation or flutter

Usual Dosage Must be titrated to patient's response

Children:

Oral: 15-50 mg/kg/24 hours divided every 3-6 hours; maximum: 4 g/24 hours

I.M.: 20-30 mg/kg/24 hours divided every 4-6 hours in divided doses; maximum: 4 g/24 hours

I.V. (infusion requires use of an infusion pump):

Load: 3-6 mg/kg/dose over 5 minutes not to exceed 100 mg/dose; may repeat every 5-10 minutes to maximum of 15 mg/kg/load

Maintenance as continuous I.V. infusion: 20-80 mcg/kg/minute; maximum: 2 g/24 hours

Adults:

Oral: 250-500 mg/dose every 3-6 hours or 500 mg to 1 g every 6 hours sustained release; usual dose: 50 mg/kg/24 hours; maximum: 4 g/24 hours

I.M.: 0.5-1 g every 4-8 hours until oral therapy is possible

I.V. (infusion requires use of an infusion pump): Loading dose: 15-18 mg/kg administered as slow infusion over 25-30 minutes or 100-200 mg/dose repeated every 5 minutes as needed to a total dose of 1 g; maintenance dose: 1-6 mg/minute by continuous infusion

Infusion rate: 2 g/250 mL D_5W/NS (I.V. infusion requires use of an infusion pump):

1 mg/minute: 7 mL/hour

2 mg/minute: 15 mL/hour

3 mg/minute: 21 mL/hour

4 mg/minute: 30 mL/hour

5 mg/minute: 38 mL/hour

6 mg/minute: 45 mL/hour

Refractory ventricular fibrillation: 30 mg/minute, up to a total of 17 mg/kg; I.V. maintenance infusion: 1-4 mg/minute; monitor levels and do not exceed 3 mg/minute for >24 hours in adults with renal failure

ACLS guidelines: I.V.: Infuse 20 mg/minute until arrhythmia is controlled, hypotension occurs, QRS complex widens by 50% of its original width, or total of 17 mg/kg is given

Mechanism of Action Decreases myocardial excitability and conduction velocity and may depress myocardial contractility, by increasing the electrical stimulation threshold of ventricle, HIS-Purkinje system and through direct cardiac effects

Local Anesthetic/Vasoconstrictor Precautions No information available to require special precautions

Effects on Dental Treatment No effects or complications reported

Other Adverse Effects

>10%: Miscellaneous: SLE-like syndrome

1% to 10%:

Cardiovascular: Tachycardia, arrhythmias, A-V block, Q-T prolongation, widening QRS complex

Central nervous system: Dizziness, lightheadedness

Gastrointestinal: Diarrhea

<1%:

Cardiovascular: Hypotension

Central nervous system: Confusion, hallucinations, mental depression, confusion, disorientation, fever

Dermatologic: Rash

Gastrointestinal: Nausea, vomiting, GI complaints

Hematologic: Hemolytic anemia, agranulocytosis, neutropenia, thrombocytopenia, positive Coombs' test

Neuromuscular & skeletal: Arthralgia, myalgia

Respiratory: Pleural effusion

Miscellaneous: Drug fever

Drug Interactions

Increased plasma/NAPA concentrations with cimetidine, ranitidine, beta-blockers, and amiodarone

Increased effect of skeletal muscle relaxants, quinidine and lidocaine and neuromuscular blockers (succinylcholine)

Increased NAPA levels/toxicity with trimethoprim

Drug Uptake

Onset of action: I.M. 10-30 minutes

Serum half-life:
Procainamide: (Dependent upon hepatic acetylator, phenotype, cardiac function, and renal function):
Adults: 2.5-4.7 hours
Anephric: 11 hours
NAPA: (Dependent upon renal function):
Children: 6 hours
Adults: 6-8 hours
Anephric: 42 hours
Time to peak serum concentration:
Capsule: Within 45 minutes to 2.5 hours
I.M.: 15-60 minutes
Pregnancy Risk Factor C

Procaine Hydrochloride (proe' kane hye droe klor' ide)
Related Information
Oral Pain on page 940
Brand Names Novocain®
Therapeutic Category Dental/Local Anesthetics; Local Anesthetic, Injectable
Use Produces spinal anesthesia and epidural and peripheral nerve block by injection and infiltration methods
Usual Dosage Dose varies with procedure, desired depth, and duration of anesthesia, desired muscle relaxation, vascularity of tissues, physical condition, and age of patient
Mechanism of Action Blocks both the initiation and conduction of nerve impulses by decreasing the neuronal membrane's permeability to sodium ions, which results in inhibition of depolarization with resultant blockade of conduction
Local Anesthetic/Vasoconstrictor Precautions No information available to require special precautions
Effects on Dental Treatment This is no longer a useful anesthetic in dentistry because of high incidence of allergic reactions
Other Adverse Effects
1% to 10%: Local: Burning sensation at site of injection, pain, tissue irritation
<1%:
Central nervous system: Aseptic meningitis resulting in paralysis can occur, CNS stimulation followed by CNS depression, chills
Dermatologic: Skin discoloration
Gastrointestinal: Nausea, vomiting
Ocular: Miosis
Otic: Tinnitus
Miscellaneous: Anaphylactoid reaction
Drug Interactions
Decreased effect of sulfonamides with the PABA metabolite of procaine, chloroprocaine, and tetracaine
Decreased/increased effect of vasopressors, ergot alkaloids, and MAO inhibitors on blood pressure when using anesthetic solutions with a vasoconstrictor
Drug Uptake
Onset of effect: Injection: Within 2-5 minutes
Duration: 0.5-1.5 hours (dependent upon patient, type of block, concentration, and method of anesthesia)
Serum half-life: 7.7 minutes
Pregnancy Risk Factor C
Dosage Forms Injection: 1% [10 mg/mL] (2 mL, 6 mL, 30 mL, 100 mL); 2% [20 mg/mL] (30 mL, 100 mL); 10% (2 mL)
Generic Available Yes

Pro-Cal-Sof® [OTC] see Docusate on page 295

Procan® SR see Procainamide Hydrochloride on page 725

Procarbazine Hydrochloride (proe kar' ba zeen hye droe klor' ide)
Brand Names Matulane®
Canadian/Mexican Brand Names Natulan® (Mexico)
Therapeutic Category Antineoplastic Agent, Miscellaneous
Synonyms Benzmethyzin; N-Methylhydrazine
Use Treatment of Hodgkin's disease, non-Hodgkin's lymphoma, brain tumor, bronchogenic carcinoma
Usual Dosage Refer to individual protocols
(Continued)

Procarbazine Hydrochloride *(Continued)*

Oral (dose based on patients ideal weight if the patients has abnormal fluid retention):

Children:

BMT aplastic anemia conditioning regimen: 12.5 mg/kg/dose every other day for 4 doses

Hodgkin's disease: MOPP/IC-MOPP regimens: 100 mg/m^2/day for 14 days and repeated every 4 weeks

Neuroblastoma and medulloblastoma: Doses as high as 100-200 mg/m^2/day once daily have been used

Adults: Initial: 2-4 mg/kg/day in single or divided doses for 7 days then increase dose to 4-6 mg/kg/day until response is obtained or leukocyte count decreased <4000/mm^3 or the platelet count decreased <100,000/mm^3; maintenance: 1-2 mg/kg/day

In MOPP, 100 mg/m^2/day on days 1-14 of a 28-day cycle

Mechanism of Action Mechanism of action is not clear, methylating of nucleic acids; inhibits DNA, RNA, and protein synthesis; may damage DNA directly and suppresses mitosis; metabolic activation required by host

Local Anesthetic/Vasoconstrictor Precautions No information available to require special precautions

Effects on Dental Treatment No effects or complications reported

Other Adverse Effects

>10%:

Central nervous system: Paresthesia, neuropathies, mental depression, manic reactions, hallucinations, dizziness, headache, nervousness, insomnia, nightmares, nystagmus, ataxia, disorientation, foot drop, decreased reflexes, tremors, confusion, and seizures

Endocrine & metabolic: Amenorrhea

Gastrointestinal: Severe nausea and vomiting occur frequently and may be dose-limiting; anorexia, abdominal pain, stomatitis, dysphagia, diarrhea, and constipation; use a nonphenothiazine antiemetic, when possible

Emetic potential: Moderately high (60% to 90%)

Hematologic: May be dose-limiting toxicity; procarbazine should be discontinued if leukocyte count is <4000/mm^3 or platelet count <100,000/mm^3

Respiratory: Pleural effusion, cough

1% to 10%:

Central nervous system: Headache, mental depression

Dermatologic: Alopecia, hyperpigmentation

Gastrointestinal: Diarrhea, stomatitis, constipation, anorexia

Hepatic: Hepatotoxicity

Neuromuscular & skeletal: Neuropathy (peripheral)

<1%:

Cardiovascular: Hypotension (orthostatic), hypertensive crisis

Central nervous system: Nervousness, irritability

Dermatologic: Dermatitis, hypersensitivity rash

Neuromuscular & skeletal: Arthralgia, myalgia

Ocular: Nystagmus, diplopia, photophobia

Miscellaneous: Flu-like syndrome

Miscellaneous: Pneumonitis, secondary malignancy, pruritus, allergic reactions, jaundice, hoarseness, somnolence, disulfiram-like reaction of alcohol, cessation of menses

Drug Uptake

Absorption: Oral: Rapid and complete

Serum half-life: 1 hour

Pregnancy Risk Factor D

Procardia® *see* Nifedipine *on page 619*

Procardia XL® *see* Nifedipine *on page 619*

Prochlorperazine *(proe klor per' a zeen)*

Brand Names Compazine®

Canadian/Mexican Brand Names Nu-Prochlor® (Canada); PMS-Prochlorperazine® (Canada); Prorazin® (Canada)

Therapeutic Category Antiemetic; Antipsychotic Agent; Phenothiazine Derivative

Use Management of nausea and vomiting; acute and chronic psychosis

Usual Dosage

Antiemetic: Children:

Oral, rectal:

>10 kg: 0.4 mg/kg/24 hours in 3-4 divided doses; **or**

9-14 kg: 2.5 mg every 12-24 hours as needed; maximum: 7.5 mg/day
14-18 kg: 2.5 mg every 8-12 hours as needed; maximum: 10 mg/day
18-39 kg: 2.5 mg every 8 hours or 5 mg every 12 hours as needed; maximum: 15 mg/day
I.M.: 0.1-0.15 mg/kg/dose; usual: 0.13 mg/kg/dose; change to oral as soon as possible
I.V.: Not recommended in children <10 kg or <2 years

Antiemetic: Adults:
Oral: 5-10 mg 3-4 times/day; usual maximum: 40 mg/day
I.M.: 5-10 mg every 3-4 hours; usual maximum: 40 mg/day
I.V.: 2.5-10 mg; maximum 10 mg/dose or 40 mg/day; may repeat dose every 3-4 hours as needed
Rectal: 25 mg twice daily

Antipsychotic:
Children 2-12 years:
Oral, rectal: 2.5 mg 2-3 times/day; increase dosage as needed to maximum daily dose of 20 mg for 2-5 years and 25 mg for 6-12 years
I.M.: 0.13 mg/kg/dose; change to oral as soon as possible
Adults:
Oral: 5-10 mg 3-4 times/day; doses up to 150 mg/day may be required in some patients for treatment of severe disturbances
I.M.: 10-20 mg every 4-6 hours may be required in some patients for treatment of severe disturbances; change to oral as soon as possible

Dementia behavior (nonpsychotic): Elderly: Initial: 2.5-5 mg 1-2 times/day; increase dose at 4- to 7-day intervals by 2.5-5 mg/day; increase dosing intervals (twice daily, 3 times/day, etc) as necessary to control response or side effects; maximum daily dose should probably not exceed 75 mg in elderly; gradual increases (titration) may prevent some side effects or decrease their severity

Not dialyzable (0% to 5%)

Mechanism of Action Blocks postsynaptic mesolimbic dopaminergic D_1 and D_2 receptors in the brain, including the medullary chemoreceptor trigger zone; exhibits a strong alpha-adrenergic and anticholinergic blocking effect and depresses the release of hypothalamic and hypophyseal hormones; believed to depress the reticular activating system, thus affecting basal metabolism, body temperature, wakefulness, vasomotor tone and emesis

Local Anesthetic/Vasoconstrictor Precautions No information available to require special precautions

Effects on Dental Treatment Significant hypotension may occur especially when the drug is administered parenterally; orthostatic hypotension is due to alpha-receptor blockade, the elderly are at greater risk for orthostatic hypotension

Tardive dyskinesia: Prevalence rate may be 40% in elderly; development of the syndrome and the irreversible nature are proportional to duration and total cumulative dose over time

Extrapyramidal reactions are more common in elderly with up to 50% developing these reactions after 60 years of age; drug-induced **Parkinson's syndrome** occurs often; **Akathisia** is the most common extrapyramidal reaction in elderly

Increased confusion, memory loss, psychotic behavior, and agitation frequently occur as a consequence of anticholinergic effects

Antipsychotic associated sedation in nonpsychotic patients is extremely unpleasant due to feelings of depersonalization, derealization, and dysphoria

Other Adverse Effects Incidence of extrapyramidal reactions are higher with prochlorperazine than chlorpromazine
Central nervous system: Sedation, drowsiness, restlessness, anxiety, extrapyramidal reactions, parkinsonian signs and symptoms, seizures, altered central temperature regulation
Endocrine & metabolic: Amenorrhea, galactorrhea, gynecomastia
Gastrointestinal: Weight gain, GI upset
Miscellaneous: Photosensitivity, hyperpigmentation, pruritus, rash, anaphylactoid reactions

>10%:
Cardiovascular: Hypotension (especially with I.V. use), orthostatic hypotension, tachycardia, arrhythmias
Central nervous system: Pseudoparkinsonism, akathisia, tardive dyskinesia (persistent), decreased sweating, dizziness
Gastrointestinal: Dry mouth, constipation
(Continued)

Prochlorperazine *(Continued)*

    Genitourinary: Urinary retention
    Neuromuscular & skeletal: Dystonias
    Ocular: Pigmentary retinopathy, blurred vision
    Respiratory: Nasal congestion
1% to 10%:
    Central nervous system: Dizziness, trembling of fingers
    Dermatologic: Increased sensitivity to sun, skin rash
    Endocrine & metabolic: Changes in menstrual cycle pain in breasts, changes in libido
    Gastrointestinal: Weight gain, nausea, vomiting, stomach pain
    Genitourinary: Difficulty in urination, ejaculatory disturbances
<1%:
    Central nervous system: Neuroleptic malignant syndrome (NMS)
    Dermatologic: Discoloration of skin (blue-gray)
    Endocrine & metabolic: Galactorrhea
    Genitourinary: Priapism
    Hematologic: Agranulocytosis, leukopenia, thrombocytopenia
    Hepatic: Cholestatic jaundice, hepatotoxicity
    Ocular: Cornea and lens changes, pigmentary retinopathy
    Miscellaneous: Impairment of temperature regulation lowering of seizures threshold

Drug Interactions Increased toxicity: Additive effects with other CNS depressants

Drug Uptake
    Onset of effect:
        Oral: Within 30-40 minutes
        I.M.: Within 10-20 minutes
        Rectal: Within 60 minutes
    Duration: Persists longest with I.M. and oral extended-release doses (12 hours); shortest following rectal and immediate release oral administration (3-4 hours)
    Serum half-life: 23 hours

Pregnancy Risk Factor C

Procrit® *see* Epoetin Alfa *on page 315*

Proctofoam® [OTC] *see* Pramoxine Hydrochloride *on page 714*

Proctofoam®-HC *see* Pramoxine and Hydrocortisone *on page 714*

Procyclidine Hydrochloride (proe sye′ kli deen hye droe klor′ ide)

Brand Names Kemadrin®
Canadian/Mexican Brand Names PMS-Procyclidine® (Canada); Procyclid® (Canada)
Therapeutic Category Anticholinergic Agent; Anti-Parkinson's Agent
Use Relieves symptoms of parkinsonian syndrome and drug-induced extrapyramidal symptoms
Usual Dosage Adults: Oral: 2.5 mg 3 times/day after meals; if tolerated, gradually increase dose, maximum of 20 mg/day if necessary
Mechanism of Action Thought to act by blocking excess acetylcholine at cerebral synapses; many of its effects are due to its pharmacologic similarities with atropine
Local Anesthetic/Vasoconstrictor Precautions No information available to require special precautions
Effects on Dental Treatment Prolonged use of antidyskinetics may decrease or inhibit salivary flow and could contribute to development of periodontal disease, oral candidiasis or discomfort
Other Adverse Effects
    >10%:
        Gastrointestinal: Constipation, dry mouth
        Miscellaneous: Decreased sweating; dry nose, throat, or skin
    1% to 10%: Decreased flow of breast milk, difficulty in swallowing, increased sensitivity to light
    <1%:
        Cardiovascular: Orthostatic hypotension, ventricular fibrillation, tachycardia, palpitations
        Central nervous system: Confusion, drowsiness, headache, loss of memory, weakness, tiredness, ataxia
        Dermatologic: Skin rash
        Gastrointestinal: Bloated feeling, nausea, vomiting
        Genitourinary: Difficult urination
        Ocular: Increased intraocular pain, blurred vision

Drug Interactions
Decreased effect of psychotropics
Increased toxicity with phenothiazines, meperidine, TCAs

Drug Uptake
Onset of effect: Oral: Within 30-40 minutes
Duration: 4-6 hours

Pregnancy Risk Factor C

Profasi® HP *see* Chorionic Gonadotropin *on page 203*

Profenal® *see* Suprofen *on page 815*

Profen II® *see* Guaifenesin and Phenylpropanolamine *on page 409*

Profen LA® *see* Guaifenesin and Phenylpropanolamine *on page 409*

Profilate® OSD *see* Antihemophilic Factor (Human) *on page 68*

Profilnine® Heat-Treated *see* Factor IX Complex (Human) *on page 350*

Progestaject® *see* Progesterone *on this page*

Progesterona (Mexico) *see* Progesterone *on this page*

Progesterone (proe jes' ter one)

Brand Names Gesterol®; Progestaject®
Canadian/Mexican Brand Names PMS-Progesterone® (Canada); Progesterone Oil (Canada); Utrogestan® (Mexico)
Therapeutic Category Progestin Derivative
Synonyms Progesterona (Mexico)
Use Endometrial carcinoma or renal carcinoma as well as secondary amenorrhea or abnormal uterine bleeding due to hormonal imbalance
Usual Dosage Adults: Female: Insert a single system into the uterine cavity; contraceptive effectiveness is retained for 1 year and system must be replaced 1 year after insertion
Mechanism of Action Natural steroid hormone that induces secretory changes in the endometrium, promotes mammary gland development, relaxes uterine smooth muscle, blocks follicular maturation and ovulation, and maintains pregnancy
Local Anesthetic/Vasoconstrictor Precautions No information available to require special precautions
Effects on Dental Treatment Progestins may predispose the patient to gingival bleeding
Other Adverse Effects
>10%:
  Cardiovascular: Edema
  Central nervous system: Weakness
  Endocrine & metabolic: Breakthrough bleeding, spotting, changes in menstrual flow, amenorrhea
  Gastrointestinal: Anorexia
  Local: Pain at injection site
1% to 10%:
  Cardiovascular: Embolism, central thrombosis
  Central nervous system: Mental depression, fever, insomnia
  Dermatologic: Melasma or chloasma, allergic rash with or without pruritus
  Endocrine: Changes in cervical erosion and secretions, weight gain or loss, increased breast tenderness
  Hepatic: Cholestatic jaundice
  Local: Thrombophlebitis
Drug Interactions Decreased effect: Aminoglutethimide may decrease effect by increasing hepatic metabolism
Drug Uptake
Duration of action: 24 hours
Serum half-life: 5 minutes
Pregnancy Risk Factor X

Proglycem® *see* Diazoxide *on page 269*

Prograf® *see* Tacrolimus *on page 817*

ProHIBiT® *see* Haemophilus b Conjugate Vaccine *on page 414*

Prolamine® [OTC] *see* Phenylpropanolamine Hydrochloride *on page 687*

Prolastin® Injection *see* Alpha₁-Proteinase Inhibitor, Human *on page 34*

Proleukin® *see* Aldesleukin *on page 29*

Prolixin® *see* Fluphenazine *on page 379*

Prolixin Decanoate® *see* Fluphenazine *on page 379*

Prolixin Enanthate® *see* Fluphenazine *on page 379*

Proloprim® *see* Trimethoprim *on page 874*

Promazine Hydrochloride (proe′ ma zeen hye droe klor′ ide)

Brand Names Sparine®

Therapeutic Category Antipsychotic Agent; Phenothiazine Derivative

Use Management of manifestations of psychotic disorders; depressive neurosis; alcohol withdrawal; nausea and vomiting; nonpsychotic symptoms associated with dementia in elderly, Tourette's syndrome; Huntington's chorea; spasmodic torticollis and Reye's syndrome

Usual Dosage Oral, I.M.:

Children >12 years: Antipsychotic: 10-25 mg every 4-6 hours

Adults:
Psychosis: 10-200 mg every 4-6 hours not to exceed 1000 mg/day
Antiemetic: 25-50 mg every 4-6 hours as needed

Not dialyzable (0% to 5%)

Mechanism of Action Blocks postsynaptic mesolimbic dopaminergic D_1 and D_2 receptors in the brain; exhibits a strong alpha-adrenergic blocking and anticholinergic effect, depresses the release of hypothalamic and hypophyseal hormones; believed to depress the reticular activating system thus affecting basal metabolism, body temperature, wakefulness, vasomotor tone, and emesis

Local Anesthetic/Vasoconstrictor Precautions No information available to require special precautions

Effects on Dental Treatment Significant hypotension may occur, especially when the drug is administered parenterally; orthostatic hypotension is due to alpha-receptor blockade, the elderly are at greater risk for orthostatic hypotension

Tardive dyskinesia: Prevalence rate may be 40% in elderly; development of the syndrome and the irreversible nature are proportional to duration and total cumulative dose over time

Extrapyramidal reactions are more common in elderly with up to 50% developing these reactions after 60 years of age; drug-induced **Parkinson's syndrome** occurs often; **Akathisia** is the most common extrapyramidal reaction in elderly

Increased confusion, memory loss, psychotic behavior, and agitation frequently occur as a consequence of anticholinergic effects

Antipsychotic associated sedation in nonpsychotic patients is extremely unpleasant due to feelings of depersonalization, derealization, and dysphoria

Other Adverse Effects

>10%:
Cardiovascular: Hypotension, orthostatic hypotension
Central nervous system: Pseudoparkinsonism, akathisia, dystonias, tardive dyskinesia (persistent), dizziness
Gastrointestinal: Constipation
Ocular: Pigmentary retinopathy
Respiratory: Nasal congestion
Miscellaneous: Decreased sweating

1% to 10%:
Central nervous system: Dizziness
Dermatologic: Increased sensitivity to sun, skin rash
Endocrine & metabolic: Changes in menstrual cycle, changes in libido, pain in breasts
Gastrointestinal: Weight gain, nausea, vomiting, stomach pain
Genitourinary: Difficulty in urination, ejaculatory disturbances
Neuromuscular & skeletal: Trembling of fingers

<1%:
Central nervous system: Neuroleptic malignant syndrome (NMS)
Dermatologic: Discoloration of skin (blue-gray), pigmentary retinopathy
Endocrine & metabolic: Galactorrhea
Genitourinary: Priapism
Hematologic: Agranulocytosis, leukopenia
Hepatic: Cholestatic jaundice, hepatotoxicity
Ocular: Cornea and lens changes
Miscellaneous: Impairment of temperature regulation, lowering of seizures threshold

Drug Interactions Increased toxicity: Additive effects with other CNS depressants

Drug Uptake The specific pharmacokinetics of promazine are poorly established but probably resemble those of other phenothiazines.

Serum half-life: Most phenothiazines have long half-lives in the range of 24 hours or more

Pregnancy Risk Factor C

Prometa® *see* Metaproterenol Sulfate *on page 550*

Prometh® *see* Promethazine Hydrochloride *on this page*

Promethazine and Codeine (proe meth' a zeen & koe' deen)

Brand Names Phenergan® With Codeine; Pherazine® With Codeine; Prothazine-DC®

Therapeutic Category Antihistamine; Antitussive; Cough Preparation

Use Temporary relief of coughs and upper respiratory symptoms associated with allergy or the common cold

Local Anesthetic/Vasoconstrictor Precautions No information available to require special precautions

Effects on Dental Treatment Although promethazine is a phenothiazine derivative, extrapyramidal reactions or tardive dyskinesias are not seen with the use of this drug.

Promethazine and Phenylephrine
(proe meth' a zeen & fen il ef' rin)

Brand Names Phenergan® VC Syrup; Promethazine VC Plain Syrup; Promethazine VC Syrup; Prometh VC Plain Liquid

Therapeutic Category Antihistamine/Decongestant Combination

Use Temporary relief of upper respiratory symptoms associated with allergy or the common cold

Local Anesthetic/Vasoconstrictor Precautions

Phenylephrine: Use with caution since phenylephrine is a sympathomimetic amine which could interact with epinephrine to cause a pressor response

Promethazine: No information available to require special precautions

Effects on Dental Treatment

Phenylephrine: Up to 10% of patients could experience tachycardia, palpitations, and dry mouth; use vasoconstrictor with caution

Although promethazine is a phenothiazine derivative, extrapyramidal reactions or tardive dyskinesias are not seen with the use of this drug.

Promethazine Hydrochloride
(proe meth' a zeen hye droe klor' ide)

Brand Names Anergan®; Phenazine®; Phencen®; Phenergan®; Prometh®; Prorex®; V-Gan®

Therapeutic Category Antiemetic; Antihistamine; Phenothiazine Derivative; Sedative

Use Symptomatic treatment of various allergic conditions, antiemetic, motion sickness, and as a sedative

Usual Dosage

Children:

Antihistamine: Oral, rectal: 0.1 mg/kg/dose every 6 hours during the day and 0.5 mg/kg/dose at bedtime as needed

Antiemetic: Oral, I.M., I.V., rectal: 0.25-1 mg/kg 4-6 times/day as needed

Motion sickness: Oral, rectal: 0.5 mg/kg/dose 30 minutes to 1 hour before departure, then every 12 hours as needed

Sedation: Oral, I.M., I.V., rectal: 0.5-1 mg/kg/dose every 6 hours as needed

Adults:

Antihistamine (including allergic reactions to blood or plasma):

Oral, rectal: 12.5 mg 3 times/day and 25 mg at bedtime

I.M., I.V.: 25 mg, may repeat in 2 hours when necessary; switch to oral route as soon as feasible

Antiemetic: Oral, I.M., I.V., rectal: 12.5-25 mg every 4 hours as needed

Motion sickness: Oral, rectal: 25 mg 30-60 minutes before departure, then every 12 hours as needed

Sedation: Oral, I.M., I.V., rectal: 25-50 mg/dose

Not dialyzable (0% to 5%)

Mechanism of Action Blocks postsynaptic mesolimbic dopaminergic receptors in the brain; exhibits a strong alpha-adrenergic blocking effect and depresses the release of hypothalamic and hypophyseal hormones; competes with histamine for the H_1-receptor; reduces stimuli to the brainstem reticular system

Local Anesthetic/Vasoconstrictor Precautions No information available to require special precautions

(Continued)

Promethazine Hydrochloride *(Continued)*

Effects on Dental Treatment Significant hypotension may occur, especially when the drug is administered parenterally; orthostatic hypotension is due to alpha-receptor blockade, the elderly are at greater risk for orthostatic hypotension

Tardive dyskinesia: Prevalence rate may be 40% in elderly; development of the syndrome and the irreversible nature are proportional to duration and total cumulative dose over time

Extrapyramidal reactions are more common in elderly with up to 50% developing these reactions after 60 years of age; drug-induced **Parkinson's syndrome** occurs often; **akathisia** is the most common extrapyramidal reaction in elderly

Increased confusion, memory loss, psychotic behavior, and agitation frequently occur as a consequence of anticholinergic effects

Antipsychotic associated sedation in nonpsychotic patients is extremely unpleasant due to feelings of depersonalization, derealization, and dysphoria

Other Adverse Effects
Hematologic: Thrombocytopenia
Hepatic: Jaundice

>10%:
Central nervous system: Slight to moderate drowsiness
Respiratory: Thickening of bronchial secretions
1% to 10%:
Central nervous system: Headache, fatigue, nervousness, dizziness
Gastrointestinal: Dry mouth, abdominal pain, nausea, diarrhea, appetite increase, weight increase
Neuromuscular & skeletal: Arthralgia
Respiratory: Pharyngitis
<1%:
Cardiovascular: Tachycardia, bradycardia, palpitations, hypotension
Central nervous system: Sedation (pronounced), confusion, excitation, extrapyramidal reactions with high doses, dystonia, faintness with I.V. administration, depression, dizziness, insomnia, sedation (pronounced)
Dermatologic: Photosensitivity, allergic reactions, rash, angioedema
Genitourinary: Urinary retention
Hepatic: Hepatitis
Neuromuscular & skeletal: Tremor, paresthesia, myalgia
Ocular: Blurred vision
Respiratory: Irregular respiration, bronchospasm
Miscellaneous: Epistaxis

Drug Interactions Increased toxicity: Additive effects with other CNS depressants

Drug Uptake
Onset of effect: I.V.: Within 20 minutes (3-5 minutes with I.V. injection)
Duration: 2-6 hours

Pregnancy Risk Factor C

Promethazine, Phenylephrine, and Codeine
(proe meth' a zeen, fen il ef' rin, & koe' deen)

Brand Names Mallergan-VC® With Codeine; Phenergan® VC With Codeine

Therapeutic Category Antihistamine/Decongestant Combination; Antitussive; Cough Preparation

Use Temporary relief of coughs and upper respiratory symptoms including nasal congestion

Local Anesthetic/Vasoconstrictor Precautions
Phenylephrine: Use with caution since phenylephrine is a sympathomimetic amine which could interact with epinephrine to cause a pressor response
Promethazine: No information available to require special precautions

Effects on Dental Treatment
Phenylephrine: Up to 10% of patients could experience tachycardia, palpitations, and dry mouth; use vasoconstrictor with caution
Although promethazine is a phenothiazine derivative, extrapyramidal reactions or tardive dyskinesias are not seen with the use of this drug.

Promethazine VC Plain Syrup *see* Promethazine and Phenylephrine *on previous page*

Promethazine VC Syrup *see* Promethazine and Phenylephrine *on previous page*

Promethazine With Dextromethorphan
(proe meth′ a zeen with deks troe meth or′ fan)

Brand Names Phenameth® DM; Phenergan® With Dextromethorphan; Pherazine® w/DM

Therapeutic Category Antitussive; Cough Preparation

Use Temporary relief of coughs and upper respiratory symptoms associated with allergy or the common cold

Local Anesthetic/Vasoconstrictor Precautions No information available to require special precautions

Effects on Dental Treatment Although promethazine is a phenothiazine derivative, extrapyramidal reactions or tardive dyskinesias are not seen with the use of this drug.

Prometh VC Plain Liquid see Promethazine and Phenylephrine on page 733

Promine® see Procainamide Hydrochloride on page 725

Promit® see Dextran 1 on page 264

Pronestyl® see Procainamide Hydrochloride on page 725

Propacet® see Propoxyphene and Acetaminophen on page 741

Propadrine see Phenylpropanolamine Hydrochloride on page 687

Propafenona, Clorhidrato De (Mexico) see Propafenone Hydrochloride on this page

Propafenone Hydrochloride (proe pa feen′ one hye droe klor′ ide)
Related Information
Cardiovascular Diseases on page 912

Brand Names Rythmol®

Canadian/Mexican Brand Names Norfenon® (Mexico)

Therapeutic Category Antiarrhythmic Agent, Class I-C; Antiarrhythmic Agent (Supraventricular & Ventricular)

Synonyms Propafenona, Clorhidrato De (Mexico)

Use Life-threatening ventricular arrhythmias

Unlabeled use: Supraventricular tachycardias, including those patients with Wolff-Parkinson-White syndrome

Usual Dosage Adults: Oral: 150 mg every 8 hours, increase at 3- to 4-day intervals up to 300 mg every 8 hours. **Note:** Patients who exhibit significant widening of QRS complex or second or third degree A-V block may need dose reduction.

Mechanism of Action Propafenone is a 1C antiarrhythmic agent which possesses local anesthetic properties, blocks the fast inward sodium current, and slows the rate of increase of the action potential. prolongs conduction and refractoriness in all areas of the myocardium, with a slightly more pronounced effect on intraventricular conduction; it prolongs effective refractory period, reduces spontaneous automaticity and exhibits some beta-blockade activity.

Local Anesthetic/Vasoconstrictor Precautions No information available to require special precautions

Effects on Dental Treatment Over 10% of patients will experience significant dry mouth; normal salivary flow will resume with cessation of drug therapy

Other Adverse Effects
>10%:
Central nervous system: Dizziness, drowsiness
Gastrointestinal: Dry mouth
1% to 10%:
Cardiovascular: A-V block (first and second degree), cardiac conduction disturbances, palpitations, congestive heart failure, angina, bradycardia
Central nervous system: Dizziness, headache, anxiety, loss of balance
Gastrointestinal: Altered taste, constipation, nausea, vomiting, abdominal pain, dyspepsia, anorexia, flatulence, diarrhea
Ocular: Blurred vision
Respiratory: Dyspnea
<1%:
Cardiovascular: New or worsened arrhythmias (proarrhythmic effect), bundle branch block
Central nervous system: Abnormal speech, vision, or dreams, numbness
Hematologic: Leukopenia, thrombocytopenia, agranulocytosis
Neuromuscular & skeletal: Paresthesias

Drug Interactions
Decreased levels with rifampin
Increased levels with cimetidine, quinidine, and beta-blockers
(Continued)

Propafenone Hydrochloride *(Continued)*

Increased effect/levels of warfarin, beta-blockers metabolized by the liver, local anesthetics, cyclosporine, and digoxin (**Note:** Reduce dose of digoxin by 25%)

Drug Uptake

Absorption: Well absorbed

Serum half-life after a single dose (100-300 mg): 2-8 hours; half-life after chronic dosing ranges from 10-32 hours

Time to peak: Peak levels occur in 2 hours with a 150 mg dose and 3 hours after a 300 mg dose; this agent exhibits nonlinear pharmacokinetics; when dose is increased from 300 mg to 900 mg/day, serum concentrations increase tenfold; this nonlinearity is thought to be due to saturable first-pass hepatic enzyme metabolism

Pregnancy Risk Factor C

Propagest® [OTC] *see* Phenylpropanolamine Hydrochloride *on page 687*

Propantheline Bromide *(proe pan' the leen broe' mide)*

Brand Names Norpanth®; Pro-Banthine®

Therapeutic Category Anticholinergic Agent; Antispasmodic Agent, Gastrointestinal

Use

Dental: Induce dry field (xerostomia) in oral cavity

Medical: Adjunctive treatment of peptic ulcer, irritable bowel syndrome, pancreatitis, ureteral and urinary bladder spasm; reduce duodenal motility during diagnostic radiologic procedures

Usual Dosage Adults: 15-30 mg as a single dose to induce xerostomia 1 hour before procedure

Mechanism of Action Competitively blocks the action of acetylcholine at postganglionic parasympathetic receptor sites

Local Anesthetic/Vasoconstrictor Precautions No information available to require special precautions

Effects on Dental Treatment Significant xerostomia in >10% of patients

Other Adverse Effects

>10%:

Gastrointestinal: Constipation

Miscellaneous: Decreased sweating

1% to 10%: Respiratory: Difficulty in swallowing

Oral manifestations: Dry mouth (therapeutic effect)

Contraindications Narrow-angle glaucoma, known hypersensitivity to propantheline; ulcerative colitis; toxic megacolon; obstructive disease of the GI or urinary tract

Warnings/Precautions Use with caution in patients with hyperthyroidism, hepatic, cardiac, or renal disease, hypertension, GI infections, or other endocrine diseases

Drug Interactions Decreased effect with antacids (decreases absorption); decreased effect of sustained release dosage forms (decreases absorption); increased effect/toxicity with anticholinergics, disopyramide, narcotic analgesics, bretylium, type I antiarrhythmics, antihistamines, phenothiazines, TCAs, corticosteroids (increases intraocular pressure), CNS depressants (sedation), adenosine, amiodarone, beta-blockers, amoxapine

Drug Uptake

Onset of effect: Oral: Within 30-45 minutes

Duration: 4-6 hours

Serum half-life: 1.6 hours (average)

Pregnancy Risk Factor C

Breast-feeding Considerations No data reported; however, atropine may be taken while breast-feeding

Dosage Forms Tablet: 7.5 mg, 15 mg

Dietary Considerations Should be taken 30 minutes before meals so that the drug's peak effect occurs at the proper time

Generic Available Yes: 15 mg tablet

Proparacaine and Fluorescein *(proe par' a kane & flure' e seen)*

Brand Names Fluoracaine®; I-Parescein®

Therapeutic Category Diagnostic Agent, Ophthalmic Dye; Local Anesthetic, Ophthalmic

Use Anesthesia for tonometry, gonioscopy; suture removal from cornea; removal of corneal foreign body; cataract extraction, glaucoma surgery

Usual Dosage
Ophthalmic surgery: Children and Adults: Instill 1 drop in each eye every 5-10 minutes for 5-7 doses
Tonometry, gonioscopy, suture removal: Adults: Instill 1-2 drops in each eye just prior to procedure
Mechanism of Action Prevents initiation and transmission of impulse at the nerve cell membrane by decreasing ion permeability through stabilizing
Local Anesthetic/Vasoconstrictor Precautions No information available to require special precautions
Effects on Dental Treatment No effects or complications reported
Other Adverse Effects
1% to 10%: Local: Burning, stinging of eye
<1%: Local: Allergic contact dermatitis, irritation, sensitization, keratitis, iritis, erosion of the corneal epithelium, conjunctival congestion and hemorrhage, corneal opacification
Drug Interactions No data reported
Drug Uptake
Onset of action: Within 20 seconds of instillation
Duration: 15-20 minutes
Pregnancy Risk Factor C

Proparacaine Hydrochloride (proe par' a kane hye droe klor' ide)
Brand Names AK-Taine®; Alcaine®; I-Paracaine®; Ophthaine®; Ophthetic®
Therapeutic Category Local Anesthetic, Ophthalmic
Use Anesthesia for tonometry, gonioscopy; suture removal from cornea; removal of corneal foreign body; cataract extraction, glaucoma surgery; short operative procedure involving the cornea and conjunctiva
Usual Dosage Children and Adults:
Ophthalmic surgery: Instill 1 drop of 0.5% solution in eye every 5-10 minutes for 5-7 doses
Tonometry, gonioscopy, suture removal: Instill 1-2 drops of 0.5% solution in eye just prior to procedure
Mechanism of Action Prevents initiation and transmission of impulse at the nerve cell membrane by decreasing ion permeability through stabilizing
Local Anesthetic/Vasoconstrictor Precautions No information available to require special precautions
Effects on Dental Treatment No effects or complications reported
Other Adverse Effects
1% to 10%: Local: Burning, stinging, redness
<1%:
Cardiovascular: Arrhythmias
Central nervous system: CNS depression
Dermatologic: Allergic contact dermatitis, irritation, sensitization
Ocular: Lacrimation, keratitis, iritis, erosion of the corneal epithelium, conjunctival congestion and hemorrhage, corneal opacification, blurred vision
Miscellaneous: Increased sweating
Drug Interactions Increased effect of phenylephrine, tropicamide
Drug Uptake
Onset of action: Within 20 seconds of instillation
Duration: 15-20 minutes
Pregnancy Risk Factor C
Dosage Forms Ophthalmic, solution: 0.5% (2 mL, 15 mL)
Generic Available Yes

Propine® see Dipivefrin on page 290

Propiomazine Hydrochloride
(proe pee oh' ma zeen hye droe klor' ide)
Brand Names Largon® Injection
Therapeutic Category Antianxiety Agent; Antiemetic; Phenothiazine Derivative; Sedative; Tranquilizer, Minor
Use Relief of restlessness, nausea and apprehension before and during surgery or during labor
Local Anesthetic/Vasoconstrictor Precautions No information available to require special precautions
Effects on Dental Treatment No effects or complications reported
Other Adverse Effects
>10%:
Central nervous system: Dizziness, drowsiness
Gastrointestinal: Dry mouth
(Continued)

Propiomazine Hydrochloride *(Continued)*

1% to 10%:
Cardiovascular: Tachycardia
Central nervous system: Confusion
Dermatologic: Skin rash
Gastrointestinal: Diarrhea, stomach pain
Respiratory: Shortness of breath
<1%: Central nervous system: Neuroleptic malignant syndrome

Comments Do not use injection if cloudy or contains a precipitate

Proplex® T *see Factor IX Complex (Human) on page 350*

Propofol *(proe' po fole)*

Brand Names Diprivan® Injection
Therapeutic Category General Anesthetic, Intravenous
Use Induction or maintenance of anesthesia; sedation

Not recommended for use in children <3 years of age; not recommended for sedation of PICU patients, especially at high doses or for prolonged periods of time; metabolic acidosis with fatal cardiac failure has occurred in several children (4 weeks to 11 years of age) who received propofol infusions at average rates of infusion of 4.5-10 mg/kg/hour for 66-115 hours (maximum rates of infusion 6.2-11.5 mg/kg/hour); see Parke, 1992; Strickland, 1995; and Bray, 1995

Usual Dosage Dosage must be individualized based on total body weight and titrated to the desired clinical effect; however, as a general guideline:

No pediatric dose has been established; however, induction for children 1-12 years 2-2.8 mg/kg has been used

Induction: I.V.:
Adults ≤55 years, and/or ASA I or II patients: 2-2.5 mg/kg of body weight (approximately 40 mg every 10 seconds until onset of induction)
Elderly, debilitated, hypovolemic, and/or ASA III or IV patients: 1-1.5 mg/kg of body weight (approximately 20 mg every 10 seconds until onset of induction)

Maintenance: I.V. infusion:
Adults ≤55 years, and/or ASA I or II patients: 0.1-0.2 mg/kg of body weight/minute (6-12 mg/kg of body weight/hour)
Elderly, debilitated, hypovolemic, and/or ASA III or IV patients: 0.05-0.1 mg/kg of body weight/minute (3-6 mg/kg of body weight/hour)

I.V. intermittent: 25-50 mg increments, as needed

ICU sedation: Rapid bolus injection should be avoided. Bolus injection can result in hypotension, oxyhemoglobin desaturation, apnea, airway obstruction, and oxygen desaturation. The preferred route of administration is slow infusion. Doses are based on individual need and titrated to response. Recommended starting dose: 1-3 mg/kg/hour
Adjustments in dose can occur at 3- to 5-minute intervals. An 80% reduction in dose should be considered in elderly, debilitated, and ASA II or IV patients. Once sedation is established, the dose should be decreased for the maintenance infusion period and adjusted to response. The dose required for maintenance is 1.5-4.5 mg/kg/hour or 25-75 mcg/kg/minute. An alternative, but less preferred method of administration is intermittent slow I.V. bolus injection of 10-20 mg, administered over 3-5 minutes.

Mechanism of Action Propofol is a hindered phenolic compound with intravenous general anesthetic properties. The drug is unrelated to any of the currently used barbiturate, opioid, benzodiazepine, arylcyclohexylamine, or imidazole intravenous anesthetic agents.

Local Anesthetic/Vasoconstrictor Precautions No information available to require special precautions
Effects on Dental Treatment No effects or complications reported
Other Adverse Effects
>10%: Gastrointestinal: Nausea
1% to 10%:
Cardiovascular: Hypotension, bradycardia, apnea, flushing
Central nervous system: Fever
Gastrointestinal: Vomiting, abdominal cramping
Respiratory: Cough
<1%:
Cardiovascular: Chest pain, tachycardia, syncope
Central nervous system: Agitation, somnolence, confusion
Dermatologic: Pruritus

    Gastrointestinal: Dry mouth, diarrhea
    Neuromuscular & skeletal: Tremor, twitching
    Otic: Ear pain
    Respiratory: Bronchospasm, dyspnea

Drug Uptake
    Onset of anesthesia: Within 9-51 seconds (average 30 seconds) after bolus infusion (dose dependent)
    Duration: 3-10 minutes depending on the dose and the rate of administration
    Serum half-life, elimination (biphasic):
        Initial: 40 minutes
        Terminal: 1-3 days

Pregnancy Risk Factor B

Comments Formulated into an emulsion containing 10% w/v soybean oil, 1.2% w/v purified egg phosphatide, and 2.25% w/v glycerol; this emulsion vehicle is chemically similar to 10% Intralipid®

Propoxycaine and Procaine (proe pox' i kane & proe' kane)

Related Information
    Oral Pain *on page 940*

Brand Names Ravocaine® and Novocain® with Levophed®; Ravocaine® and Novocain® with Neo-Cobefrin®

Therapeutic Category Dental/Local Anesthetics; Local Anesthetic, Injectable

Use Dental: Ester-type anesthetic used for local infiltration anesthesia; injection near nerve trunks to produce nerve block

Usual Dosage The lowest dose needed to provide effective anesthesia should be administered. The 1.8 mL cartridge contains 43.2 mg of the anesthetics (7.2 mg propoxycaine hydrochloride and 36 mg procaine hydrochloride).
    Children: Based on a dose of 3 mg/lb body weight, maximum: 5 cartridges are usually adequate for any procedure
    Adults: 5 cartridges (216 mg of total anesthetics) are usually adequate to affect anesthesia of the entire oral cavity. A dose of 3 mg/lb body weight may be administered for one procedure

Mechanism of Action Local anesthetics bind selectively to the intracellular surface of sodium channels to block influx of sodium into the axon. As a result, depolarization necessary for action potential propagation and subsequent nerve function is prevented. The block at the sodium channel is reversible. When drug diffuses away from the axon, sodium channel function is restored and nerve propagation is subsequently restored.

Norepinephrine (Levophed®) and levonordefrin (Neocobefrin®) prolong the duration of the anesthetic actions of propoxycaine and procaine by causing vasoconstriction (alpha adrenergic receptor agonist) of the vasculature surrounding the nerve axons. This prevents the diffusion of local anesthetic away from the nerves resulting in a longer retention in the axon.

Local Anesthetic/Vasoconstrictor Precautions No information available to require special precautions

Effects on Dental Treatment No effects or complications reported

Other Adverse Effects Degree of adverse effects in the CNS and cardiovascular system are directly related to the blood levels of local anesthetic. The effects below are more likely to occur after systemic administration rather than infiltration.

    Cardiovascular: Myocardial effects include a decrease in contraction force as well as a decrease in electrical excitability and myocardial conduction rate resulting in bradycardia and reduction in cardiac output.
    Central nervous system: High blood levels result in anxiety, restlessness, disorientation, confusion, dizziness, tremors and seizures. This is followed by depression of CNS resulting in drowsiness, unconsciousness and possible respiratory arrest. Nausea and vomiting may also occur. In some cases, symptoms of CNS stimulation may be absent and the primary CNS effects are drowsiness and unconsciousness
    Hypersensitivity reactions: May be manifest as dermatologic reactions and edema at injection site. Asthmatic syndromes have occurred. Patients may exhibit hypersensitivity to bisulfites contained in local anesthetic solution to prevent oxidation of norepinephrine or levonordefrin. In general, patients reacting to bisulfites have a history of asthma and their airways are hyperreactive to asthmatic syndrome
    Psychogenic reactions: It is common to misinterpret psychogenic responses to local anesthetic injection as an allergic reaction. Intraoral injections are perceived by many patients as a stressful procedure in dentistry. Common symptoms to this stress are sweating, palpitations, hyperventilation, generalized pallor, and a fainting feeling

(Continued)

Propoxycaine and Procaine *(Continued)*

Oral manifestations: No data reported

Contraindications Hypersensitivity to local anesthetics of the ester type

Warnings/Precautions Should be avoided in patients with uncontrolled hyperthyroidism. Should be used in minimal amounts in patients with significant cardiovascular problems (because of norepinephrine or levonordefrin component). Aspirate the syringe after tissue penetration and before injection to minimize chance of direct vascular injection

Drug Interactions Due to norepinephrine or levonordefrin component, use with tricyclic antidepressants or MAO inhibitors could result in increased pressor response

Drug Uptake
Onset of action: 2-5 minutes
Duration 2-3 hours

Pregnancy Risk Factor No data reported

Breast-feeding Considerations No data reported

Dosage Forms Injection:
Ravocaine® and Novocain® with Levophed®: Propoxycaine hydrochloride 7.2 mg and procaine 36 mg with norepinephrine 0.12 mg/1.8 mL dental cartridge
Ravocaine® and Novocain® with Neo-Cobefrin®: Propoxycaine hydrochloride 7.2 mg and procaine 36 mg with levonordefrin 0.09 mg/1.8 mL dental cartridge

Dietary Considerations No data reported

Selected Readings
Jastak JT and Yagiela JA, "Vasoconstrictors and Local Anesthesia: A Review and Rationale for Use," *J Am Dent Assoc*, 1983, 107(4):623-30.
MacKenzie TA and Young ER, "Local Anesthetic Update," *Anesth Prog*, 1993, 40(2):29-34.
Wynn RL, "Epinephrine Interactions With Beta-Blockers," *Gen Dent*, 1994, 42(1):16, 18.
Yagiela JA, "Local Anesthetics," *Anesth Prog*, 1991, 38(4-5):128-41.

Propoxyphene *(proe pox' i feen)*

Related Information
Narcotic Agonist Charts *on page 1019*

Brand Names Darvon®; Darvon-N®; Dolene®

Canadian/Mexican Brand Names Novo-Propoxyn® (Canada)

Therapeutic Category Analgesic, Narcotic

Use Management of mild to moderate pain

Usual Dosage Oral:
Children: Doses for children are not well established; doses of the hydrochloride of 2-3 mg/kg/d divided every 6 hours have been used
Adults:
Hydrochloride: 65 mg every 3-4 hours as needed for pain; maximum: 390 mg/day
Napsylate: 100 mg every 4 hours as needed for pain; maximum: 600 mg/day

Mechanism of Action Binds to opiate receptors in the CNS, causing inhibition of ascending pain pathways, altering the perception of and response to pain; produces generalized CNS depression

Local Anesthetic/Vasoconstrictor Precautions No information available to require special precautions

Effects on Dental Treatment No effects or complications reported

Other Adverse Effects Hepatic: Increased liver enzymes
>10%:
Cardiovascular: Hypotension
Central nervous system: Dizziness, lightheadedness, weakness, sedation, paradoxical excitement and insomnia, tiredness, drowsiness
Gastrointestinal: GI upset, nausea, vomiting, constipation
Miscellaneous: Histamine release
1% to 10%:
Central nervous system: Nervousness, headache, restlessness, malaise, confusion
Gastrointestinal: Anorexia, stomach cramps, dry mouth, biliary spasm
Genitourinary: Decreased urination, ureteral spasms
Local: Pain at injection site
Respiratory: Troubled breathing, shortness of breath
<1%:
Central nervous system: Mental depression hallucinations, paradoxical CNS stimulation, increased intracranial pressure
Dermatologic: Rash, hives
Gastrointestinal: Paralytic ileus
Miscellaneous: Psychologic and physical dependence with prolonged use, histamine release

Drug Interactions

Decreased effect with charcoal, cigarette smoking

Increased toxicity: CNS depressants may potentiate pharmacologic effects; propoxyphene may inhibit the metabolism and increase the serum concentrations of carbamazepine, phenobarbital, MAO inhibitors, tricyclic antidepressants, and warfarin

Drug Uptake

Onset of effect: Oral: Within 0.5-1 hour

Duration: 4-6 hours

Serum half-life: Adults:

Parent drug: 8-24 hours (mean: ~15 hours)

Norpropoxyphene: 34 hours

Pregnancy Risk Factor C (D if used for prolonged periods)

Dosage Forms

Capsule, as hydrochloride: 32 mg, 65 mg

Suspension, oral, as napsylate: 50 mg/5 mL (480 mL)

Tablet, as napsylate: 100 mg

Dietary Considerations Should be taken with glass of water on empty stomach

Generic Available Yes: Capsule

Propoxyphene and Acetaminophen

(proe pox′ i feen & a seet a min′ oh fen)

Brand Names Darvocet-N®; Darvocet-N® 100; E-Lor®; Genagesic®; Propacet®; Wygesic®

Therapeutic Category Analgesic, Narcotic

Use

Dental: Management of postoperative pain

Medical: Relief of pain

Usual Dosage

Children: Not recommended in pediatric dental patients

Adults:

Darvocet-N®: 1-2 tablets every 4 hours as needed; maximum: 600 mg propoxyphene napsylate/day

Darvocet-N® 100: 1 tablet every 4 hours as needed; maximum: 600 mg propoxyphene napsylate/day

Mechanism of Action

Propoxyphene is a weak narcotic analgesic which acts through binding to opiate receptors to inhibit ascending pain pathways

Propoxyphene, as with other narcotic (opiate) analgesics, blocks pain perception in the cerebral cortex by binding to specific receptor molecules (opiate receptors) within the neuronal membranes of synapses. This binding results in a decreased synaptic chemical transmission throughout the CNS thus inhibiting the flow of pain sensations into the higher centers. Mu and kappa are the two subtypes of the opiate receptor which propoxyphene binds to to cause analgesia.

Acetaminophen inhibits the synthesis of prostaglandins in the CNS and peripherally blocks pain impulse generation; produces antipyresis from inhibition of hypothalamic heat-regulating center

Local Anesthetic/Vasoconstrictor Precautions No information available to require special precautions

Effects on Dental Treatment No effects or complications reported

Other Adverse Effects 1% to 10%:

Central nervous system: Dizziness, lightheadedness, headache, sedation

Gastrointestinal: Nausea, vomiting

Neuromuscular & skeletal: Weakness

Miscellaneous: Psychologic and physical dependence

Oral manifestations: No data reported

Contraindications Hypersensitivity to propoxyphene, acetaminophen, or any component; patients with known G-6-PD deficiency

Warnings/Precautions When given in excessive doses, either alone or in combination with other CNS depressants, propoxyphene is a major cause of drug-related deaths; do not exceed recommended dosage; give with caution in patients dependent on opiates, substitution may result in acute opiate withdrawal symptoms

Drug Interactions Decreased effect with charcoal, cigarette smoking; increased toxicity with cimetidine, CNS depressants; increased toxicity/effect of carbamazepine, phenobarbital, TCAs, MAO inhibitors, benzodiazepines

Drug Uptake

Onset of action: 15-60 minutes

(Continued)

Propoxyphene and Acetaminophen *(Continued)*

Time to peak serum concentration: 2-2.5 hours

Duration: 4-6 hours

Serum half-life:

Propoxyphene: 6-12 hours

Norpropoxyphene: 30-36 hours

Pregnancy Risk Factor C

Breast-feeding Considerations Both propoxyphene and acetaminophen may be taken while breast-feeding

Dosage Forms Tablet:

Darvocet-N®: Propoxyphene napsylate 50 mg and acetaminophen 325 mg

Darvocet-N® 100: Propoxyphene napsylate 100 mg and acetaminophen 650 mg

E-Lor®, Genagesic®, Wygesic®: Propoxyphene hydrochloride 65 mg and acetaminophen 650 mg

Dietary Considerations Should be taken with water on an empty stomach

Generic Available Yes

Comments Propoxyphene is a narcotic analgesic and shares many properties including addiction liability. The acetaminophen component requires use with caution in patients with alcoholic liver disease.

Selected Readings

Miller RR, Feingold A, and Paxinos J, "Propoxyphene Hydrochloride: A Critical Review," *JAMA*, 1970, 213(6):996-1006.

Propoxyphene and Aspirin (proe pox' i feen & as' pir in)

Related Information

Narcotic Agonist Charts *on page 1019*

Brand Names Bexophene®; Darvon® Compound-65 Pulvules®; Darvon®-N With ASA

Canadian/Mexican Brand Names Darvon-N® with ASA (Canada); Novo-Propoxyn Compound (contains caffeine) (Canada); Darvon-N® Compound (contains caffeine) (Canada)

Therapeutic Category Analgesic, Narcotic

Use

Dental: Management of postoperative pain

Medical: Relief of pain

Usual Dosage Oral:

Children: Not recommended

Adults: 1-2 capsules every 4 hours as needed

Mechanism of Action

Propoxyphene is a weak narcotic analgesic which acts through binding to opiate receptors to inhibit ascending pain pathways

Propoxyphene, as with other narcotic (opiate) analgesics, blocks pain perception in the cerebral cortex by binding to specific receptor molecules (opiate receptors) within the neuronal membranes of synapses. This binding results in a decreased synaptic chemical transmission throughout the CNS thus inhibiting the flow of pain sensations into the higher centers. Mu and kappa are the two subtypes of the opiate receptor which propoxyphene binds to to cause analgesia.

Aspirin inhibits prostaglandin synthesis by decreasing the activity of the enzyme, cyclo-oxygenase, which results in decreased formation of prostaglandin precursors, acts on the hypothalamic heat-regulating center to reduce fever, blocks thromboxane synthetase action which prevents formation of the platelet-aggregating substance thromboxane A_2

Local Anesthetic/Vasoconstrictor Precautions No effects or complications reported

Effects on Dental Treatment Use with caution in patients with platelet and bleeding disorders, renal dysfunction, erosive gastritis, or peptic ulcer disease, previous nonreaction does not guarantee future safe taking of medication; do not use aspirin in children <16 years of age for chickenpox or flu symptoms due to the association with Reye's syndrome

Avoid aspirin if possible, for 1 week prior to surgery because of the possibility of postoperative bleeding; use with caution in impaired hepatic function

Elderly are a high-risk population for adverse effects from nonsteroidal anti-inflammatory agents. As much as 60% of elderly with GI complications to NSAIDs can develop peptic ulceration and/or hemorrhage asymptomatically. Also, concomitant disease and drug use contribute to the risk for GI adverse effects. Use lowest effective dose for shortest period possible. Consider renal function decline with age. Use with caution in patients with history of asthma

Other Adverse Effects 1% to 10%:
Central nervous system: Dizziness, lightheadedness, headache, sedation
Gastrointestinal: Nausea, vomiting
Neuromuscular & skeletal: Weakness
Miscellaneous: Psychologic and physical dependence

Oral manifestations: No data reported

Contraindications Hypersensitivity to propoxyphene, aspirin or any component

Warnings/Precautions When given in excessive doses, either alone or in combination with other CNS depressants, propoxyphene is a major cause of drug-related deaths; do not exceed recommended dosage; because of aspirin component, children and teenagers should not use for chickenpox or flu symptoms before a physician is consulted about Reye's syndrome

Drug Interactions Decreased effect with charcoal, cigarette smoking; increased toxicity with cimetidine, CNS depressants; increased toxicity/effect of carbamazepine, phenobarbital, TCAs, warfarin, MAO inhibitors, benzodiazepines, warfarin (bleeding); see Aspirin

Drug Uptake
Onset of action: 15-60 minutes
Time to peak serum concentration: 2-2.5 hours
Duration: 4-6 hours
Serum half-life:
Propoxyphene: 6-12 hours
Norpropoxyphene: 30-36 hours

Pregnancy Risk Factor D

Breast-feeding Considerations
Propoxyphene: May be taken while breast-feeding
Aspirin: Use cautiously due to potential adverse effects in nursing infants

Dosage Forms
Capsule: Propoxyphene hydrochloride 65 mg and aspirin 389 mg with caffeine 32.4 mg
Tablet (Darvon-N® with A.S.A.): Propoxyphene napsylate 100 mg and aspirin 325 mg

Dietary Considerations No data reported

Generic Available Yes

Comments Propoxyphene is a narcotic analgesic and shares many properties including addiction liability. The aspirin component could have anticoagulant effects and could possibly affect bleeding times.

Selected Readings
Miller RR, Feingold A, and Paxinos J, "Propoxyphene Hydrochloride: A Critical Review," *JAMA*, 1970, 213(6):996-1006.

Propranolol and Hydrochlorothiazide
(proe pran' oh lole & hye droe klor oh thye' a zide)
Brand Names Inderide®
Therapeutic Category Antihypertensive Agent, Combination
Use Management of hypertension
Local Anesthetic/Vasoconstrictor Precautions Use with caution; epinephrine has interacted with nonselective beta-blockers to result in initial hypertensive episode followed by bradycardia
Effects on Dental Treatment Non-cardioselective beta-blockers (ie, propranolol, nadolol) enhance the pressor response to epinephrine, resulting in hypertension and bradycardia. Many nonsteroidal anti-inflammatory drugs such as ibuprofen and indomethacin can reduce the hypotensive effect of beta-blockers after 3 or more weeks of therapy with the NSAID. Short-term NSAID use (ie, 3 days) requires no special precautions in patients taking beta-blockers.

Propranolol Hydrochloride (proe pran' oh lole hye droe klor' ide)
Related Information
Cardiovascular Diseases *on page 912*
Endocrine Disorders & Pregnancy *on page 927*
Brand Names Betachron E-R®; Inderal®; Inderal® LA
Canadian/Mexican Brand Names Apo-Propranolol® (Canada); Detensol® (Canada); Nu-Propranolol® (Canada); PMS-Propranolol® (Mexico); Inderalici® (Mexico)
Therapeutic Category Antianginal Agent; Antiarrhythmic Agent, Class I-B; Antiarrhythmic Agent, Class II; Antiarrhythmic Agent (Supraventricular & Ventricular); Beta-Adrenergic Blocker, Noncardioselective
(Continued)

Propranolol Hydrochloride (Continued)

Use Management of hypertension, angina pectoris, pheochromocytoma, essential tremor, tetralogy of Fallot cyanotic spells, and arrhythmias (such as atrial fibrillation and flutter, A-V nodal re-entrant tachycardias, and catecholamine-induced arrhythmias); prevention of myocardial infarction, migraine headache; symptomatic treatment of hypertrophic subaortic stenosis

Unlabeled use: Tremor due to Parkinson's disease, alcohol withdrawal, aggressive behavior, antipsychotic-induced akathisia, esophageal varices bleeding, anxiety, schizophrenia, acute panic, and gastric bleeding in portal hypertension

Usual Dosage

Tachyarrhythmias:

Oral:

Children: Initial: 0.5-1 mg/kg/day in divided doses every 6-8 hours; titrate dosage upward every 3-7 days; usual dose: 2-4 mg/kg/day; higher doses may be needed; do not exceed 16 mg/kg/day or 60 mg/day

Adults: 10-30 mg/dose every 6-8 hours

Elderly: Initial: 10 mg twice daily; increase dosage every 3-7 days; usual dosage range: 10-320 mg given in 2 divided doses

I.V.:

Children: 0.01-0.1 mg/kg slow IVP over 10 minutes; maximum dose: 1 mg

Adults: 1 mg/dose slow IVP; repeat every 5 minutes up to a total of 5 mg

Hypertension: Oral:

Children: Initial: 0.5-1 mg/kg/day in divided doses every 6-12 hours; increase gradually every 3-7 days; maximum: 2 mg/kg/24 hours

Adults: Initial: 40 mg twice daily; increase dosage every 3-7 days; usual dose: ≤320 mg divided in 2-3 doses/day; maximum daily dose: 640 mg

Migraine headache prophylaxis: Oral:

Children: 0.6-1.5 mg/kg/day **or**

≤35 kg: 10-20 mg 3 times/day

>35 kg: 20-40 mg 3 times/day

Adults: Initial: 80 mg/day divided every 6-8 hours; increase by 20-40 mg/dose every 3-4 weeks to a maximum of 160-240 mg/day given in divided doses every 6-8 hours; if satisfactory response not achieved within 6 weeks of starting therapy, drug should be withdrawn gradually over several weeks

Tetralogy spells: Children:

Oral: 1-2 mg/kg/day every 6 hours as needed, may increase by 1 mg/kg/day to a maximum of 5 mg/kg/day, or if refractory may increase slowly to a maximum of 10-15 mg/kg/day

I.V.: 0.15-0.25 mg/kg/dose slow IVP; may repeat in 15 minutes

Thyrotoxicosis:

Adolescents and Adults: Oral: 10-40 mg/dose every 6 hours

Adults: I.V.: 1-3 mg/dose slow IVP as a single dose

Adults: Oral:

Angina: 80-320 mg/day in doses divided 2-4 times/day

Pheochromocytoma: 30-60 mg/day in divided doses

Myocardial infarction prophylaxis: 180-240 mg/day in 3-4 divided doses

Hypertrophic subaortic stenosis: 20-40 mg 3-4 times/day

Essential tremor: 40 mg twice daily initially; maintenance doses: usually 120-320 mg/day

Mechanism of Action Nonselective beta-adrenergic blocker (class II antiarrhythmic); competitively blocks response to beta$_1$- and beta$_2$-adrenergic stimulation which results in decreases in heart rate, myocardial contractility, blood pressure, and myocardial oxygen demand

Local Anesthetic/Vasoconstrictor Precautions Use with caution; epinephrine has interacted with nonselective beta-blockers to result in initial hypertensive episode followed by bradycardia

Effects on Dental Treatment Non-cardioselective beta-blockers (ie, propranolol, nadolol) enhance the pressor response to epinephrine, resulting in hypertension and bradycardia. Many nonsteroidal anti-inflammatory drugs such as ibuprofen and indomethacin can reduce the hypotensive effect of beta-blockers after 3 or more weeks of therapy with the NSAID. Short-term NSAID use (ie, 3 days) requires no special precautions in patients taking beta-blockers.

Other Adverse Effects

>10%:

Cardiovascular: Bradycardia

Central nervous system: Mental depression

Endocrine & metabolic: Decreased sexual ability

1% to 10%:

Cardiovascular: Congestive heart failure, reduced peripheral circulation

Central nervous system: Confusion, hallucinations, dizziness, insomnia, weakness, tiredness

Dermatologic: Skin rash

Gastrointestinal: Diarrhea, nausea, vomiting, stomach discomfort

Respiratory: Wheezing

<1%:

Cardiovascular: Chest pain, hypotension, impaired myocardial contractility, worsening of A-V conduction disturbances

Central nervous system: Nightmares, vivid dreams, lethargy

Dermatologic: Red, scaling, or crusted skin

Endocrine & metabolic: Hypoglycemia, hyperglycemia

Gastrointestinal: GI distress

Hematologic: Leukopenia, thrombocytopenia, agranulocytosis

Respiratory: Bronchospasm

Miscellaneous: Cold extremities

Drug Interactions

Decreased effect of beta-blockers with aluminum salts, barbiturates, calcium salts, cholestyramine, colestipol, NSAIDs, penicillins (ampicillin), rifampin, salicylates and sulfinpyrazone due to decreased bioavailability and plasma levels

Increased effect/toxicity of beta-blockers with calcium blockers (diltiazem, felodipine, nicardipine), contraceptives, flecainide, haloperidol (propranolol, hypotensive effects), H_2 antagonists (metoprolol, propranolol only by cimetidine, possibly ranitidine), hydralazine (metoprolol, propranolol), loop diuretics (propranolol, not atenolol), MAO inhibitors (metoprolol, nadolol, bradycardia), phenothiazines (propranolol), propafenone (metoprolol, propranolol), quinidine (in extensive metabolizers), ciprofloxacin, thyroid hormones (metoprolol, propranolol, when hypothyroid patient is converted to euthyroid state)

Beta-blockers may increase the effect/toxicity• of flecainide, haloperidol (hypotensive effects), hydralazine, phenothiazines, acetaminophen, anticoagulants (propranolol, warfarin), benzodiazepines (not atenolol), clonidine (hypertensive crisis after or during withdrawal of either agent), epinephrine (initial hypertensive episode followed by bradycardia), nifedipine and verapamil lidocaine, ergots (peripheral ischemia), prazosin (postural hypotension)

Beta-blockers may decrease the effect of sulfonylureas

Beta-blockers may also affect the action or levels of ethanol, disopyramide, nondepolarizing muscle relaxants and theophylline although the effects are difficult to predict

Drug Uptake

Onset of beta blockade: Oral: Within 1-2 hours

Duration: ~6 hours

Serum half-life:

Children: 3.9-6.4 hours

Adults: 4-6 hours

Pregnancy Risk Factor C

Selected Readings

Foster CA and Aston SJ, "Propranolol-Epinephrine Interaction: A Potential Disaster," *Plast Reconstr Surg*, 1983, 72(1):74-8.

Wong DG, Spence JD, Lamki L, et al, "Effect of Nonsteroidal Anti-Inflammatory Drugs on Control of Hypertension of Beta-Blockers and Diuretics," *Lancet*, 1986, 1(8488):997-1001.

Wynn RL, "Dental Nonsteroidal Anti-Inflammatory Drugs and Prostaglandin-Based Drug Interactions, Part Two," *Gen Dent*, 1992, 40(2):104, 106, 108.

Wynn RL, "Epinephrine Interactions With Beta-Blockers," *Gen Dent*, 1994, 42(1):16, 18.

Propulsid® see Cisapride *on page 209*

Propylene Glycol and Salicylic Acid see Salicylic Acid and Propylene Glycol *on page 778*

Propylhexedrine (proe pil hex' e dreen)

Brand Names Benzedrex® [OTC]

Therapeutic Category Decongestant

Use Topical nasal decongestant

Local Anesthetic/Vasoconstrictor Precautions No information available to require special precautions

Effects on Dental Treatment No effects or complications reported

Comments Drug has been extracted from inhaler and injected I.V. as an amphetamine substitute

Propylthiouracil (proe pil thye oh yoor' a sil)

Related Information
Endocrine Disorders & Pregnancy *on page 927*

Canadian/Mexican Brand Names Propyl-Thyracil® (Canada)

Therapeutic Category Antithyroid Agent

Use Palliative treatment of hyperthyroidism as an adjunct to ameliorate hyperthyroidism in preparation for surgical treatment or radioactive iodine therapy and in the management of thyrotoxic crisis. The use of antithyroid thioamides is as effective in elderly as they are in younger adults; however, the expense, potential adverse effects, and inconvenience (compliance, monitoring) make them undesirable. The use of radioiodine, due to ease of administration and less concern for long-term side effects and reproduction problems, makes it a more appropriate therapy.

Usual Dosage Oral: Administer in 3 equally divided doses at approximately 8-hour intervals. Adjust dosage to maintain T_3, T_4, and TSH levels in normal range; elevated T_3 may be sole indicator of inadequate treatment. Elevated TSH indicates excessive antithyroid treatment.

Children: Initial: 5-7 mg/kg/day in divided doses every 8 hours **or**
6-10 years: 50-150 mg/day
>10 years: 150-300 mg/day
Maintenance: $1/3$ to $2/3$ of the initial dose in divided doses every 8-12 hours. This usually begins after 2 months on an effective initial dose.

Adults: Initial: 300-450 mg/day in divided doses every 8 hours (severe hyperthyroidism may require 600-1200 mg/day); maintenance: 100-150 mg/day in divided doses every 8-12 hours

Elderly: Use lower dose recommendations; initial dose: 150-300 mg/day

Mechanism of Action Inhibits the synthesis of thyroid hormones by blocking the oxidation of iodine in the thyroid gland; blocks synthesis of thyroxine and triiodothyronine

Local Anesthetic/Vasoconstrictor Precautions No information available to require special precautions

Effects on Dental Treatment No effects or complications reported

Other Adverse Effects
>10%:
Central nervous system: Fever
Dermatologic: Skin rash
Hematologic: Leukopenia
1% to 10%:
Central nervous system: Dizziness
Gastrointestinal: Nausea, vomiting, loss of taste, stomach pain
Hematologic: Agranulocytosis
Miscellaneous: SLE-like syndrome
<1%:
Cardiovascular: Edema, cutaneous vasculitis
Central nervous system: Drowsiness, neuritis, vertigo, headache
Dermatologic: Rash, urticaria, pruritus, exfoliative dermatitis, hair loss
Gastrointestinal: Constipation, weight gain
Hematologic: Agranulocytosis, thrombocytopenia, bleeding, aplastic anemia
Hepatic: Cholestatic jaundice, hepatitis
Neuromuscular & skeletal: Arthralgia, paresthesia
Renal: Nephritis
Miscellaneous: Swollen salivary glands, goiter

Drug Interactions Increased effect: Increased anticoagulant activity

Drug Uptake
Onset of action: For significant therapeutic effects 24-36 hours are required
Peak effect: Remissions of hyperthyroidism do not usually occur before 4 months of continued therapy
Serum half-life: 1.5-5 hours
End stage renal disease: 8.5 hours
Time to peak serum concentration: Oral: Within 1 hour; persists for 2-3 hours

Pregnancy Risk Factor D

Prorex® *see* Promethazine Hydrochloride *on page 733*

Proscar® *see* Finasteride *on page 363*

Pro-Sof® [OTC] *see* Docusate *on page 295*

Pro-Sof® Plus [OTC] *see* Docusate and Casanthranol *on page 295*

ProSom™ *see* Estazolam *on page 324*

Prostaglandin E₁ *see* Alprostadil *on page 35*

Prostaphlin® *see* Oxacillin Sodium *on page 641*

ProStep® *see* Nicotine *on page 617*

Prostin VR Pediatric® Injection *see* Alprostadil *on page 35*

Protamine Sulfate (proe' ta meen sul' fate)
Therapeutic Category Antidote, Heparin
Use Treatment of heparin overdosage; neutralize heparin during surgery or dialysis procedures
Usual Dosage Protamine dosage is determined by the dosage of heparin; 1 mg of protamine neutralizes 90 USP units of heparin (lung) and 115 USP units of heparin (intestinal); maximum dose: 50 mg

In the situation of heparin overdosage, since blood heparin concentrations decrease rapidly **after** administration, adjust the protamine dosage depending upon the duration of time since heparin administration as follows:

Time Elapsed	Dose of Protamine (mg) to Neutralize 100 units of Heparin
Immediate	1-1.5
30-60 min	0.5-0.75
>2 h	0.25-0.375

If heparin administered by deep S.C. injection, use 1-1.5 mg protamine per 100 units heparin; this may be done by a portion of the dose (eg, 25-50 mg) given slowly I.V. followed by the remaining portion as a continuous infusion over 8-16 hours (the expected absorption time of the S.C. heparin dose)
Mechanism of Action Combines with strongly acidic heparin to form a stable complex (salt) neutralizing the anticoagulant activity of both drugs
Local Anesthetic/Vasoconstrictor Precautions No information available to require special precautions
Effects on Dental Treatment No effects or complications reported
Other Adverse Effects
>10%:
　Cardiovascular: Sudden fall in blood pressure, bradycardia
　Respiratory: Dyspnea
1% to 10%: Hematologic: Hemorrhage
<1%:
　Cardiovascular: Flushing, pulmonary hypertension
　Central nervous system: Lassitude
　Gastrointestinal: Nausea, vomiting
　Miscellaneous: Hypersensitivity reactions
Drug Uptake Onset of effect: I.V. injection: Heparin neutralization occurs within 5 minutes
Pregnancy Risk Factor C
Comments Heparin rebound associated with anticoagulation and bleeding has been reported to occur occasionally; symptoms typically occur 8-9 hours after protamine administration, but may occur as long as 18 hours later

Prothazine-DC® *see* Promethazine and Codeine *on page 733*
Protilase® *see* Pancrelipase *on page 657*

Protirelin (proe tye' re lin)
Brand Names Relefact® TRH Injection; Thypinone® Injection
Therapeutic Category Diagnostic Agent, Thyroid Function
Synonyms Lopremone; Thyrotropin Releasing Hormone; TRH
Use Adjunct in the diagnostic assessment of thyroid function, and an adjunct to other diagnostic procedures in assessment of patients with pituitary or hypothalamic dysfunction; also causes release of prolactin from the pituitary and is used to detect defective control of prolactin secretion.
Usual Dosage I.V.:
　Children <6 years: Experience limited, but doses of 7 mcg/kg have been administered
　Children 6-16 years: 7 mcg/kg to a maximum dose of 500 mcg
　Adults: 500 mcg (range 200-500 mcg)
Mechanism of Action Increase release of thyroid stimulating hormone from the anterior pituitary
Local Anesthetic/Vasoconstrictor Precautions No information available to require special precautions
Effects on Dental Treatment No effects or complications reported
Other Adverse Effects
>10%:
　Cardiovascular: Flushing of face
　Central nervous system: Headache, lightheadedness
(Continued)

Protirelin (Continued)

    Gastrointestinal: Nausea, dry mouth
    Genitourinary: Urge to urinate
1% to 10%:
    Central nervous system: Anxiety
    Endocrine & metabolic: Breast enlargement and leaking in lactating women
    Gastrointestinal: Bad taste in mouth, abdominal discomfort
    Neuromuscular & skeletal: Tingling
    Miscellaneous: Sweating
<1%:
    Cardiovascular: Severe hypotension
    Ocular: Temporary loss of vision

Drug Uptake
    Peak TSH levels: 20-30 minutes
    Duration: TSH returns to baseline after ~3 hours
    Serum half-life, mean plasma: 5 minutes

Pregnancy Risk Factor C

Protostat® see Metronidazole on page 576

Protriptyline Hydrochloride (proe trip' ti leen hye droe klor' ide)

Brand Names Vivactil®
Canadian/Mexican Brand Names Triptil® (Canada)
Therapeutic Category Antidepressant, Tricyclic
Use Treatment of various forms of depression, often in conjunction with psycho-therapy
Usual Dosage Oral:
    Adolescents: 15-20 mg/day
    Adults: 15-60 mg in 3-4 divided doses
    Elderly: 15-20 mg/day
Mechanism of Action Increases the synaptic concentration of serotonin and/or norepinephrine in the central nervous system by inhibition of their reuptake by the presynaptic neuronal membrane
Local Anesthetic/Vasoconstrictor Precautions No information available to require special precautions
Effects on Dental Treatment Long-term treatment with TCAs such as amoxa-pine increases the risk of caries by reducing salivation and salivary buffer capacity
Other Adverse Effects
>10%:
    Central nervous system: Dizziness, drowsiness, headache, weakness
    Gastrointestinal: Dry mouth, constipation, unpleasant taste, weight gain, increased appetite, nausea
1% to 10%:
    Cardiovascular: Arrhythmias, hypotension
    Central nervous system: Confusion, delirium, hallucinations, nervousness, restlessness, parkinsonian syndrome
    Gastrointestinal: Diarrhea, heartburn
    Genitourinary: Difficult urination, insomnia
    Neuromuscular & skeletal: Fine muscle tremors, sexual function impairment
    Ocular: Blurred vision, eye pain
    Miscellaneous: Excessive sweating
<1%:
    Central nervous system: Anxiety, seizures
    Dermatologic: Alopecia, photosensitivity
    Endocrine & metabolic: Breast enlargement, galactorrhea, SIADH
    Genitourinary: Testicular swelling
    Hematologic: Agranulocytosis, leukopenia, eosinophilia
    Hepatic: Cholestatic jaundice, increased liver enzymes
    Ocular: Increased intraocular pressure
    Otic: Tinnitus
    Miscellaneous: Trouble with gums, decreased lower esophageal sphincter tone may cause GE reflux, allergic reactions
Drug Interactions
    Decreased effect: Phenobarbital may increase the metabolism of protriptyline; protriptyline blocks the uptake of guanethidine and thus prevents the hypo-tensive effect of guanethidine
    Increased toxicity: Clonidine causes hypertensive crisis; protriptyline may be additive with or may potentiate the action of other CNS depressants such as sedatives or hypnotics; with MAO inhibitors, hyperpyrexia, hypertension, tachycardia, confusion, and seizures; protriptyline may increase the

prothrombin time in patients stabilized on warfarin; protriptyline potentiates the pressor and cardiac effects of sympathomimetic agents such as isoproterenol, epinephrine, etc; cimetidine and methylphenidate may decrease the metabolism of protriptyline

Additive anticholinergic effects seen with other anticholinergic agents

Drug Uptake

Maximum antidepressant effect: 2 weeks of continuous therapy is commonly required

Serum half-life: 54-92 hours, averaging 74 hours

Time to peak serum concentration: Oral: Within 24-30 hours

Pregnancy Risk Factor C

Selected Readings

Boakes AJ, Laurence DR, Teoh PC, et al, "Interactions Between Sympathomimetic Amines and Antidepressant Agents in Man," *Br Med J*, 1973, 1(849):311-5.

Jastak JT and Yagiela JA, "Vasoconstrictors and Local Anesthesia: A Review and Rationale for Use," *J Am Dent Assoc*, 1983, 107(4):623-30.

Larochelle P, Hamet P, and Enjalbert M, "Responses to Tyramine and Norepinephrine After Imipramine and Trazodone," *Clin Pharmacol Ther*, 1979, 26(1):24-30.

Mitchell JR, "Guanethidine and Related Agents. III Antagonism by Drugs Which Inhibit the Norepinephrine Pump in Man," *J Clin Invest*, 1970, 49(8):1596-604.

Rundegren J, van Dijken J, Mörnstad H, et al, "Oral Conditions in Patients Receiving Long-Term Treatment With Cyclic Antidepressant Drugs," *Swed Dent J*, 1985, 9(2):55-64.

Svedmyr N, "The Influence of a Tricyclic Antidepressive Agent (Protriptyline) on Some of the Circulatory Effects of Noradrenaline and Adrenalin in Man," *Life Sci*, 1968, 7(1):77-84.

Protropin® *see* Human Growth Hormone *on page 426*

Provatene® [OTC] *see* Beta-Carotene *on page 109*

Proventil® *see* Albuterol *on page 27*

Provera® *see* Medroxyprogesterone Acetate *on page 533*

Proxigel® [OTC] *see* Carbamide Peroxide *on page 152*

Prozac® *see* Fluoxetine Hydrochloride *on page 377*

PRP-D *see* Haemophilus b Conjugate Vaccine *on page 414*

Prulet® [OTC] *see* Phenolphthalein *on page 682*

P&S® [OTC] *see* Salicylic Acid *on page 777*

Pseudo-Car® DM *see* Carbinoxamine, Pseudoephedrine, and Dextromethorphan *on page 155*

Pseudoefedrina (Mexico) *see* Pseudoephedrine *on this page*

Pseudoephedrine (soo doe e fed' rin)

Brand Names Afrinol® [OTC]; Cenafed® [OTC]; Decofed® Syrup [OTC]; Drixoral® Non-Drowsy [OTC]; Efidac/24® [OTC]; Neofed® [OTC]; Novafed®; PediaCare® Oral; Sudafed® [OTC]; Sudafed® 12 Hour [OTC]; Sufedrin® [OTC]

Canadian/Mexican Brand Names Balminil® Decongestant (Canada); Eltor® (Canada); PMS-Pseudoephedrine® (Canada); Robidrine® (Canada)

Therapeutic Category Adrenergic Agonist Agent; Decongestant

Synonyms Pseudoefedrina (Mexico)

Use Temporary symptomatic relief of nasal congestion due to common cold, upper respiratory allergies, and sinusitis; also promotes nasal or sinus drainage

Usual Dosage Oral:

Children:

<2 years: 4 mg/kg/day in divided doses every 6 hours

2-5 years: 15 mg every 6 hours; maximum: 60 mg/24 hours

6-12 years: 30 mg every 6 hours; maximum: 120 mg/24 hours

Adults: 30-60 mg every 4-6 hours, sustained release: 120 mg every 12 hours; maximum: 240 mg/24 hours

Mechanism of Action Directly stimulates alpha-adrenergic receptors of respiratory mucosa causing vasoconstriction; directly stimulates beta-adrenergic receptors causing bronchial relaxation, increased heart rate and contractility

Local Anesthetic/Vasoconstrictor Precautions Use with caution since pseudoephedrine is a sympathomimetic amine which could interact with epinephrine to cause a pressor response

Effects on Dental Treatment Up to 10% of patients could experience tachycardia, palpitations, and dry mouth; use vasoconstrictor with caution

Other Adverse Effects

>10%:

Cardiovascular: Tachycardia, palpitations, arrhythmias

Central nervous system: Nervousness, transient stimulation, insomnia, excitability, dizziness, drowsiness, headache

Neuromuscular & skeletal: Tremor

1% to 10%:

Central nervous system: Dizziness, headache, diaphoresis, weakness

(Continued)

Pseudoephedrine *(Continued)*

Gastrointestinal: Dry mouth

<1%:

Central nervous system: Convulsions, hallucinations

Gastrointestinal: Nausea, vomiting

Genitourinary: Difficult urination

Respiratory: Shortness of breath, troubled breathing

Drug Interactions Increased toxicity with MAO inhibitors (hypertensive crisis) sympathomimetics, CNS depressants, alcohol (sedation)

Drug Uptake

Onset of decongestant effect: Oral: 15-30 minutes

Duration: 4-6 hours (up to 12 hours with extended release formulation administration)

Serum half-life: 9-16 hours

Pregnancy Risk Factor C

Pseudoephedrine and Azatadine *see* Azatadine and Pseudoephedrine *on page 89*

Pseudoephedrine and Chlorpheniramine *see* Chlorpheniramine and Pseudoephedrine *on page 191*

Pseudoephedrine and Dexbrompheniramine *see* Dexbrompheniramine and Pseudoephedrine *on page 261*

Pseudoephedrine and Dextromethorphan

(soo doe e fed' rin & deks troe meth or' fan)

Brand Names Drixoral® Cough & Congestion Liquid Caps [OTC]; Vicks® 44D Cough & Head Congestion; Vicks® 44 Non-Drowsy Cold & Cough Liqui-Caps [OTC]

Therapeutic Category Adrenergic Agonist Agent; Antitussive; Decongestant

Use Temporary symptomatic relief of nasal congestion due to common cold, upper respiratory allergies, and sinusitis; also promotes nasal or sinus drainage; symptomatic relief of coughs caused by minor viral upper respiratory tract infections or inhaled irritants; most effective for a chronic nonproductive cough

Local Anesthetic/Vasoconstrictor Precautions Use with caution since pseudoephedrine is a sympathomimetic amine which could interact with epinephrine to cause a pressor response

Effects on Dental Treatment Up to 10% of patients could experience tachycardia, palpitations, and dry mouth; use vasoconstrictor with caution

Pseudoephedrine and Guaifenesin *see* Guaifenesin and Pseudoephedrine *on page 409*

Pseudoephedrine and Ibuprofen

(soo doe e fed' rin & eye byoo proe' fen)

Brand Names Advil® Cold & Sinus Caplets [OTC]; Dimetapp® Sinus Caplets [OTC]; Dristan® Sinus Caplets [OTC]; Motrin® IB Sinus [OTC]; Sine-Aid® IB [OTC]

Therapeutic Category Adrenergic Agonist Agent; Analgesic, Non-narcotic; Decongestant

Use Temporary symptomatic relief of nasal congestion due to common cold, upper respiratory allergies, and sinusitis; also promotes nasal or sinus drainage; sinus headaches and pains

Local Anesthetic/Vasoconstrictor Precautions Use with caution since pseudoephedrine is a sympathomimetic amine which could interact with epinephrine to cause a pressor response

Effects on Dental Treatment Up to 10% of patients could experience tachycardia, palpitations, and dry mouth; use vasoconstrictor with caution

Pseudo-Gest Plus® Tablet [OTC] *see* Chlorpheniramine and Pseudoephedrine *on page 191*

Psorcon™ *see* Diflorasone Diacetate *on page 278*

psoriGel® [OTC] *see* Coal Tar *on page 225*

Psyllium (sil' i yum)

Brand Names Effer-Syllium® [OTC]; Fiberall® [OTC]; Hydrocil® [OTC]; Konsyl® [OTC]; Konsyl-D® [OTC]; Metamucil® [OTC]; Metamucil® Instant Mix [OTC]; Modane® Bulk [OTC]; Perdiem® Plain [OTC]; Reguloid® [OTC]; Serutan® [OTC]; Siblin® [OTC]; Syllact® [OTC]; V-Lax® [OTC]

Canadian/Mexican Brand Names Fibrepur® (Canada); Novo-Mucilax® (Canada); Prodiem® Plain (Canada)

Therapeutic Category Laxative, Bulk-Producing

Use Treatment of chronic atonic or spastic constipation and in constipation associated with rectal disorders; management of irritable bowel syndrome

Usual Dosage Oral (administer at least 3 hours before or after drugs):

Children 6-11 years: (Approximately ½ adult dosage) ½ to 1 rounded teaspoonful in 4 oz glass of liquid 1-3 times/day

Adults: 1-2 rounded teaspoonfuls or 1-2 packets or 1-2 wafers in 8 oz glass of liquid 1-3 times/day

Mechanism of Action Adsorbs water in the intestine to form a viscous liquid which promotes peristalsis and reduces transit time

Local Anesthetic/Vasoconstrictor Precautions No information available to require special precautions

Effects on Dental Treatment No effects or complications reported

Other Adverse Effects 1% to 10%:

Gastrointestinal: Esophageal or bowel obstruction, diarrhea, constipation, abdominal cramps

Respiratory: Bronchospasm, anaphylaxis upon inhalation in susceptible individuals, rhinoconjunctivitis

Drug Interactions Decreased effect of warfarin, digitalis, potassium-sparing diuretics, salicylates, tetracyclines, nitrofurantoin

Drug Uptake

Onset of action: 12-24 hour, but full effect may take 2-3 days

Absorption: Oral: Generally not absorbed following administration, small amounts of grain extracts present in the preparation have been reportedly absorbed following colonic hydrolysis

Pregnancy Risk Factor C

P.T.E.-4® *see* Trace Metals *on page 857*

P.T.E.-5® *see* Trace Metals *on page 857*

Pulmozyme® *see* Dornase Alfa *on page 296*

Puralube® Tears Solution [OTC] *see* Artificial Tears *on page 75*

Purge® [OTC] *see* Castor Oil *on page 161*

Puri-Clens™ [OTC] *see* Methylbenzethonium Chloride *on page 566*

Purinethol® *see* Mercaptopurine *on page 544*

P-V-Tussin® *see* Hydrocodone, Phenylephrine, Pyrilamine, Phenindamine, Chlorpheniramine, and Ammonium Chloride *on page 435*

P$_x$E$_x$® Ophthalmic *see* Pilocarpine and Epinephrine *on page 693*

Pyocidin-Otic® *see* Polymyxin B and Hydrocortisone *on page 704*

Pyonto® [OTC] *see* Pyrethrins *on page 753*

Pyrantel Pamoate (pi ran' tel pam' oh ate)

Brand Names Antiminth® [OTC]; Pin-Rid® [OTC]; Pin-X® [OTC]; Reese's® Pinworm Medicine [OTC]

Canadian/Mexican Brand Names Combantrin® (Mexico)

Therapeutic Category Anthelmintic

Use Roundworm (*Ascaris lumbricoides*), pinworm (*Enterobius vermicularis*), and hookworm (*Ancylostoma duodenale* and *Necator americanus*) infestations, and trichostrongyliasis

Usual Dosage Children and Adults (purgation is not required prior to use): Oral: Roundworm, pinworm, or trichostrongyliasis: 11 mg/kg administered as a single dose; maximum dose: 1 g. (**Note:** For pinworm infection, dosage should be repeated in 2 weeks and all family members should be treated).

Hookworm: 11 mg/kg administered once daily for 3 days

Mechanism of Action Causes the release of acetylcholine and inhibits cholinesterase; acts as a depolarizing neuromuscular blocker, paralyzing the helminths

Local Anesthetic/Vasoconstrictor Precautions No information available to require special precautions

Effects on Dental Treatment No effects or complications reported

Other Adverse Effects

1% to 10%: Gastrointestinal: Anorexia, nausea, vomiting, abdominal cramps, diarrhea

<1%:

Central nervous system: Dizziness, drowsiness, insomnia, headache

Dermatologic: Rash

Gastrointestinal: Tenesmus

Hepatic: Liver enzymes (elevated)

Neuromuscular & skeletal: Weakness

Drug Uptake

Absorption: Oral: Poor

Time to peak serum concentration: Within 1-3 hours

(Continued)

Pyrantel Pamoate *(Continued)*

Pregnancy Risk Factor C

Comments Purgation is not required prior to use

Pyrazinamide *(peer a zin' a mide)*

Related Information

Nonviral Infectious Diseases *on page 932*

Canadian/Mexican Brand Names PMS-Pyrazinamide® (Canada); Tebrazid® (Canada); Braccopril® (Mexico)

Therapeutic Category Antitubercular Agent

Synonyms Pirazinamida (Mexico)

Use Adjunctive treatment of tuberculosis in combination with other anti-tuberculosis agents

Usual Dosage Oral (calculate dose on ideal body weight rather than total body weight): **Note:** A four-drug regimen (isoniazid, rifampin, pyrazinamide, and either streptomycin or ethambutol) is preferred for the initial, empiric treatment of TB. When the drug susceptibility results are available, the regimen should be altered as appropriate.

Patients with TB and without HIV infection:

OPTION 1:

Isoniazid resistance rate <4%: Administer daily isoniazid, rifampin, and pyrazinamide for 8 weeks followed by isoniazid and rifampin daily or directly observed therapy (DOT) 2-3 times/week for 16 weeks

If isoniazid resistance rate is not documented, ethambutol or streptomycin should also be administered until susceptibility to isoniazid or rifampin is demonstrated. Continue treatment for at least 6 months or 3 months beyond culture conversion.

OPTION 2: Administer daily isoniazid, rifampin, pyrazinamide, and either streptomycin or ethambutol for 2 weeks followed by DOT 2 times/week administration of the same drugs for 6 weeks, and subsequently, with isoniazid and rifampin DOT 2 times/week administration for 16 weeks

OPTION 3: Administer isoniazid, rifampin, pyrazinamide, and either etham-butol or streptomycin by DOT 3 times/week for 6 months

Patients with TB and with HIV infection:

Administer any of the above OPTIONS 1, 2 or 3, however, treatment should be continued for a total of 9 months and at least 6 months beyond culture conversion

Note: Some experts recommend that the duration of therapy should be extended to 9 months for patients with disseminated disease, miliary disease, disease involving the bones or joints, or tuberculosis lymphade-nitis

Children and Adults:

Daily therapy: 15-30 mg/kg/day (maximum: 2 g/day)

Directly observed therapy (DOT): Twice weekly: 50-70 mg/kg (maximum: 4 g)

DOT: 3 times/week: 50-70 mg/kg (maximum: 3 g)

Elderly: Start with a lower daily dose (15 mg/kg) and increase as tolerated

Mechanism of Action Converted to pyrazinoic acid in susceptible strains of *Mycobacterium* which lowers the pH of the environment

Local Anesthetic/Vasoconstrictor Precautions No information available to require special precautions

Effects on Dental Treatment No effects or complications reported

Other Adverse Effects

1% to 10%:

Central nervous system: Malaise

Gastrointestinal: Nausea, vomiting, anorexia

Neuromuscular & skeletal: Arthralgia, myalgia

<1%:

Central nervous system: Fever

Dermatologic: Skin rash, itching, acne, photosensitivity

Hematologic: Porphyria, thrombocytopenia

Hepatic: Hepatotoxicity

Neuromuscular & skeletal: Gout

Renal: Dysuria, interstitial nephritis

Drug Interactions No data reported

Drug Uptake Bacteriostatic or bactericidal depending on the drug's concentration at the site of infection

Absorption: Oral: Well absorbed

Serum half-life: 9-10 hours, increased with reduced renal or hepatic function

End stage renal disease: 9 hours
Time to peak serum concentration: Within 2 hours
Pregnancy Risk Factor C

Pyrethrins (pye re′ thrins)
Brand Names A-200™ Pyrinate [OTC]; Barc™ [OTC]; Blue® [OTC]; Control-L™ [OTC]; End Lice® [OTC]; Pyonto® [OTC]; Pyrinyl II® [OTC]; RID® [OTC]; Tisit® [OTC]
Canadian/Mexican Brand Names Lice-Enz® (Canada)
Therapeutic Category Antiparasitic Agent, Topical; Pediculocide
Use Treatment of *Pediculus humanus* infestations (head lice, body lice, pubic lice and their eggs)
Usual Dosage Application of pyrethrins: Topical:
Apply enough solution to completely wet infested area, including hair
Allow to remain on area for 10 minutes
Wash and rinse with large amounts of warm water
Use fine-toothed comb to remove lice and eggs from hair
Shampoo hair to restore body and luster
Treatment may be repeated if necessary once in a 24-hour period
Repeat treatment in 7-10 days to kill newly hatched lice
Mechanism of Action Pyrethrins are derived from flowers that belong to the chrysanthemum family. The mechanism of action on the neuronal membranes of lice is similar to that of DDT. Piperonyl butoxide is usually added to pyrethrin to enhance the product's activity by decreasing the metabolism of pyrethrins in arthropods.
Local Anesthetic/Vasoconstrictor Precautions No information available to require special precautions
Effects on Dental Treatment No effects or complications reported
Other Adverse Effects 1% to 10%: Local: Pruritus, burning, stinging, irritation with repeat use
Drug Interactions No data reported
Drug Uptake
Onset of action: ~30 minutes
Absorption: Topical into the system is minimal
Pregnancy Risk Factor C

Pyridiate® *see* Phenazopyridine Hydrochloride *on page 679*
Pyridium® *see* Phenazopyridine Hydrochloride *on page 679*

Pyridoxine Hydrochloride (peer i dox′ een hye droe klor′ ide)
Brand Names Beesix®; Nestrex®
Canadian/Mexican Brand Names Benadon® (Mexico)
Therapeutic Category Antidote, Cycloserine Toxicity; Antidote, Hydralazine Toxicity; Antidote, Isoniazid Toxicity; Vitamin, Water Soluble
Synonyms Piridoxina (Mexico)
Use Prevents and treats vitamin B_6 deficiency, pyridoxine-dependent seizures in infants, adjunct to treatment of acute toxicity from isoniazid, cycloserine, or hydralazine overdose
Usual Dosage
Recommended daily allowance (RDA):
Children:
1-3 years: 0.9 mg
4-6 years: 1.3 mg
7-10 years: 1.6 mg
Adults:
Male: 1.7-2.0 mg
Female: 1.4-1.6 mg
Dietary deficiency: Oral:
Children: 5-25 mg/24 hours for 3 weeks, then 1.5-2.5 mg/day in multiple vitamin product
Adults: 10-20 mg/day for 3 weeks
Drug-induced neuritis (eg, isoniazid, hydralazine, penicillamine, cycloserine): Oral:
Children:
Treatment: 10-50 mg/24 hours
Prophylaxis: 1-2 mg/kg/24 hours
Adults:
Treatment: 100-200 mg/24 hours
Prophylaxis: 25-100 mg/24 hours
Treatment of seizures and/or coma from acute isoniazid toxicity, a dose of pyridoxine hydrochloride equal to the amount of INH ingested can be given
(Continued)

753

Pyridoxine Hydrochloride *(Continued)*

I.M./I.V. in divided doses together with other anticonvulsants; if the amount INH ingested is not known, administer 5 g I.V. pyridoxine

Treatment of acute hydralazine toxicity, a pyridoxine dose of 25 mg/kg in divided doses I.M./I.V. has been used

Mechanism of Action Precursor to pyridoxal, which functions in the metabolism of proteins, carbohydrates, and fats; pyridoxal also aids in the release of liver and muscle-stored glycogen and in the synthesis of GABA (within the central nervous system) and heme

Local Anesthetic/Vasoconstrictor Precautions No information available to require special precautions

Effects on Dental Treatment No effects or complications reported

Other Adverse Effects <1%:

Central nervous system: Sensory neuropathy, seizures have occurred following I.V. administration of very large doses, headache

Gastrointestinal: Nausea

Endocrine & metabolic: Decreased serum folic acid secretions

Neuromuscular & skeletal: Paresthesia

Miscellaneous: Allergic reactions have been reported, increased AST

Drug Interactions Decreased serum levels of levodopa, phenobarbital, and phenytoin

Drug Uptake

Absorption: Enteral, parenteral: Well absorbed from GI tract

Serum half-life: 15-20 days

Pregnancy Risk Factor A (C if dose exceeds RDA recommendation)

Pyrimethamine (peer i meth' a meen)

Brand Names Daraprim®

Canadian/Mexican Brand Names Daraprim® (Mexico)

Therapeutic Category Antimalarial Agent

Synonyms Pirimetamina (Mexico)

Use Prophylaxis of malaria due to susceptible strains of plasmodia; used in conjunction with quinine and sulfadiazine for the treatment of uncomplicated attacks of chloroquine-resistant *P. falciparum* malaria; used in conjunction with fast-acting schizonticide to initiate transmission control and suppression cure; synergistic combination with sulfonamide in treatment of toxoplasmosis

Usual Dosage

Malaria chemoprophylaxis (for areas where chloroquine-resistant *P. falciparum* exists): Begin prophylaxis 2 weeks before entering endemic area:

Children: 0.5 mg/kg once weekly; not to exceed 25 mg/dose

or

Children:

<4 years: 6.25 mg once weekly

4-10 years: 12.5 mg once weekly

Children >10 years and Adults: 25 mg once weekly

Dosage should be continued for all age groups for at least 6-10 weeks after leaving endemic areas

Chloroquine-resistant *P. falciparum* malaria (when used in conjunction with quinine and sulfadiazine):

Children:

<10 kg: 6.25 mg/day once daily for 3 days

10-20 kg: 12.5 mg/day once daily for 3 days

20-40 kg: 25 mg/day once daily for 3 days

Adults: 25 mg twice daily for 3 days

Toxoplasmosis:

Infants for congenital toxoplasmosis: Oral: 1 mg/kg once daily for 6 months with sulfadiazine then every other month with sulfa, alternating with spiramycin.

Children: Loading dose: 2 mg/kg/day divided into 2 equal daily doses for 1-3 days (maximum: 100 mg/day) followed by 1 mg/kg/day divided into 2 doses for 4 weeks; maximum: 25 mg/day

With sulfadiazine or trisulfapyrimidines: 2 mg/kg/day divided every 12 hours for 3 days followed by 1 mg/kg/day once daily or divided twice daily for 4 weeks given with trisulfapyrimidines or sulfadiazine

Adults: 50-75 mg/day together with 1-4 g of a sulfonamide for 1-3 weeks depending on patient's tolerance and response, then reduce dose by 50% and continue for 4-5 weeks **or** 25-50 mg/day for 3-4 weeks

Mechanism of Action Inhibits parasitic dihydrofolate reductase, resulting in inhibition of vital tetrahydrofolic acid synthesis

Local Anesthetic/Vasoconstrictor Precautions No information available to require special precautions

Effects on Dental Treatment No effects or complications reported

Other Adverse Effects

1% to 10%:

Gastrointestinal: Anorexia, abdominal cramps, vomiting

Hematologic: Megaloblastic anemia, leukopenia, thrombocytopenia, agranulocytosis

<1%:

Central nervous system: Insomnia, lightheadedness, fever, malaise, seizures, depression

Dermatologic: Skin rash, dermatitis, abnormal skin pigmentation

Gastrointestinal: Diarrhea, dry mouth, atrophic glossitis

Hematologic: Pulmonary eosinophilia

Drug Interactions

Decreased effect: Pyrimethamine effectiveness decreased by acid

Increased effect: Sulfonamides (synergy), methotrexate, TMP/SMX

Drug Uptake

Absorption: Oral: Well absorbed

Serum half-life: 80-95 hours

Pregnancy Risk Factor C

Pyrinyl II® [OTC] *see* Pyrethrins *on page 753*

Pyrithione Zinc (peer i thye′ one zink)

Brand Names DHS Zinc® [OTC]; Head & Shoulders® [OTC]; Sebulon® [OTC]; Theraplex Z® [OTC]; Zincon® Shampoo [OTC]; ZNP® Bar [OTC]

Therapeutic Category Antiseborrheic Agent, Topical

Use Relieves the itching, irritation and scalp flaking associated with dandruff and/or seborrheal dermatitis of the scalp

Local Anesthetic/Vasoconstrictor Precautions No information available to require special precautions

Effects on Dental Treatment No effects or complications reported

Quadra-Hist® *see* Chlorpheniramine, Phenyltoloxamine, Phenylpropanolamine, and Phenylephrine *on page 194*

Quazepam (kway′ ze pam)

Brand Names Doral®

Therapeutic Category Benzodiazepine; Hypnotic; Sedative

Use Treatment of insomnia; more likely than triazolam to cause daytime sedation and fatigue; is classified as a long-acting benzodiazepine hypnotic (like flurazepam - Dalmane®), this long duration of action may prevent withdrawal symptoms when therapy is discontinued

Usual Dosage Adults: Oral: Initial: 15 mg at bedtime, in some patients the dose may be reduced to 7.5 mg after a few nights

Mechanism of Action Depresses all levels of the CNS, including the limbic and reticular formation, probably through the increased action of gamma-aminobutyric acid (GABA), which is a major inhibitory neurotransmitter in the brain

Local Anesthetic/Vasoconstrictor Precautions No information available to require special precautions

Effects on Dental Treatment Over 10% of patients will experience dry mouth which disappears with cessation of drug therapy

Other Adverse Effects

>10%:

Cardiovascular: Tachycardia, chest pain

Central nervous system: Drowsiness, fatigue, impaired coordination, lightheadedness, memory impairment, insomnia, anxiety, depression, headache

Dermatologic: Rash

Endocrine & metabolic: Decreased libido

Gastrointestinal: Dry mouth, constipation, diarrhea, decreased salivation, nausea, vomiting, increased or decreased appetite

Neuromuscular & skeletal: Dysarthria

Ocular: Blurred vision

Miscellaneous: Sweating

1% to 10%:

Cardiovascular: Syncope, hypotension

Central nervous system: Confusion, nervousness, dizziness, akathisia

Dermatologic: Dermatitis

Gastrointestinal: Increased salivation, weight gain or loss

(Continued)

Quazepam *(Continued)*

    Neuromuscular & skeletal: Rigidity, tremor, muscle cramps
    Otic: Tinnitus
    Respiratory: Nasal congestion, hyperventilation
  <1%:
    Central nervous system: Reflex slowing
    Endocrine & metabolic: Menstrual irregularities
    Hematologic: Blood dyscrasias
    Miscellaneous: Drug dependence

Drug Interactions Increased effect/toxicity with CNS depressants (narcotics, alcohol, MAO inhibitors, TCAs, anesthetics, barbiturates, phenothiazines)

Drug Uptake
  Absorption: Oral: Rapid
  Serum half-life:
    Parent drug: 25-41 hours
    Active metabolite: 40-114 hours

Pregnancy Risk Factor X

Questran® *see* Cholestyramine Resin *on page 201*

Questran® Light *see* Cholestyramine Resin *on page 201*

Quibron® *see* Theophylline and Guaifenesin *on page 836*

Quibron®-T *see* Theophylline/Aminophylline *on page 832*

Quibron®-T/SR *see* Theophylline/Aminophylline *on page 832*

Quiess® *see* Hydroxyzine *on page 443*

Quinaglute® Dura-Tabs® *see* Quinidine *on page 759*

Quinalan® *see* Quinidine *on page 759*

Quinamm® *see* Quinine Sulfate *on page 760*

Quinapril Hydrochloride (kwin′ a pril hye droe klor′ ide)

Related Information
  Cardiovascular Diseases *on page 912*

Brand Names Accupril®

Canadian/Mexican Brand Names Acupril® (Mexico)

Therapeutic Category Angiotensin-Converting Enzyme (ACE) Inhibitors

Synonyms Quinaprilo, Clorhidrato De (Mexico)

Use Management of hypertension and treatment of congestive heart failure; increase circulation in Raynaud's phenomenon; idiopathic edema

  Unlabeled use: Hypertensive crisis, diabetic nephropathy, rheumatoid arthritis, diagnosis of anatomic renal artery stenosis, hypertension secondary to scleroderma renal crisis, diagnosis of aldosteronism, idiopathic edema, Bartter's syndrome, postmyocardial infarction for prevention of ventricular failure

Usual Dosage
  Adults: Oral: Initial: 10 mg once daily, adjust according to blood pressure response at peak and trough blood levels; in general, the normal dosage range is 20-80 mg/day
  Elderly: Initial: 2.5-5 mg/day; increase dosage at increments of 2.5-5 mg at 1- to 2-week intervals

Mechanism of Action Competitive inhibitor of angiotensin-converting enzyme (ACE); prevents conversion of angiotensin I to angiotensin II, a potent vasoconstrictor; results in lower levels of angiotensin II which causes an increase in plasma renin activity and a reduction in aldosterone secretion; a CNS mechanism may also be involved in hypotensive effect as angiotensin II increases adrenergic outflow from CNS; vasoactive kallikreins may be decreased in conversion to active hormones by ACE inhibitors, thus reducing blood pressure

Local Anesthetic/Vasoconstrictor Precautions No information available to require special precautions

Effects on Dental Treatment No effects or complications reported

Other Adverse Effects
  1% to 10%:
    Cardiovascular: Hypotension
    Central nervous system: Dizziness, headache, fatigue
    Gastrointestinal: Diarrhea
    Renal: Increased BUN and serum creatinine
    Respiratory: Upper respiratory symptoms, cough

<1%:
>
> Cardiovascular: Chest discomfort, flushing, myocardial infarction, angina pectoris, orthostatic hypotension, rhythm disturbances, tachycardia, peripheral edema, vasculitis, palpitations, syncope
>
> Central nervous system: Fever, malaise, depression, somnolence, insomnia
>
> Dermatologic: Urticaria, pruritus, angioedema
>
> Endocrine & metabolic: Gout
>
> Gastrointestinal: Pancreatitis, abdominal pain, anorexia, constipation, flatulence, dry mouth
>
> Hematologic: Neutropenia, bone marrow depression
>
> Hepatic: Hepatitis
>
> Neuromuscular & skeletal: Joint pain, shoulder pain
>
> Ocular: Blurred vision
>
> Respiratory: Bronchitis, sinusitis, pharyngeal pain
>
> Miscellaneous: Diaphoresis

Drug Interactions See table.

Drug-Drug Interactions With ACEIs

Precipitant Drug	Drug (Category) and Effect	Description
Antacids	ACE Inhibitors: decreased	Decreased bioavailability of ACEIs. May be more likely with captopril. Separate administration times by 1-2 hours.
NSAIDs (indomethacin)	ACEIs: decreased	Reduced hypotensive effects of ACEIs. More prominent in low renin or volume dependent hypertensive patients.
Phenothiazines	ACEIs: increased	Pharmacologic effects of ACEIs may be increased.
ACEIs	Allopurinol: increased	Higher risk of hypersensitivity reaction possible when given concurrently. Three case reports of Stevens-Johnson syndrome with captopril.
ACEIs	Digoxin: increased	Increased plasma digoxin levels.
ACEIs	Lithium: increased	Increased serum lithium levels and symptoms of toxicity may occur.
ACEIs	Potassium preps/ potassium sparing diuretics increased	Coadministration may result in elevated potassium levels.

Drug Uptake

Serum half-life, elimination:

Quinapril: 0.8 hours

Quinaprilat: 2 hours

Time to peak serum concentration:

Quinapril: 1 hour

Quinaprilat: ~2 hours

Pregnancy Risk Factor D

Quinaprilo, Clorhidrato De (Mexico) *see* Quinapril Hydrochloride *on previous page*

Quinestrol (kwin ess' trole)

Related Information

Endocrine Disorders & Pregnancy *on page 927*

Brand Names Estrovis®

Therapeutic Category Estrogen Derivative

Use Atrophic vaginitis; hypogonadism; primary ovarian failure; vasomotor symptoms of menopause; prostatic carcinoma; osteoporosis prophylactic

Usual Dosage Adults: Female: Oral: 100 mcg once daily for 7 days; followed by 100 mcg/week beginning 2 weeks after inception of treatment; may increase to 200 mcg/week if necessary

Mechanism of Action Increases the synthesis of DNA, RNA, and various proteins in target tissues; reduces the release of gonadotropin-releasing hormone from the hypothalamus; reduces FSH and LH release from the pituitary

Local Anesthetic/Vasoconstrictor Precautions No information available to require special precautions

Effects on Dental Treatment No effects or complications reported

(Continued)

757

Quinestrol *(Continued)*

Other Adverse Effects

>10%:

Cardiovascular: Peripheral edema

Endocrine & metabolic: Enlargement of breasts (female and male), breast tenderness

Gastrointestinal: Nausea, anorexia, bloating

1% to 10%:

Central nervous system: Headache

Endocrine & metabolic: Increased libido (female), decreased libido (male)

Gastrointestinal: Vomiting, diarrhea

<1%:

Cardiovascular: Hypertension, thromboembolism, stroke, myocardial infarction, edema

Central nervous system: Depression, dizziness, anxiety

Dermatologic: Chloasma, melasma, rash

Endocrine: Breast tumors, amenorrhea, alterations in frequency and flow of menses, decreased glucose tolerance, increased triglycerides and LDL

Gastrointestinal: Nausea, GI distress

Hepatic: Cholestatic jaundice

Miscellaneous: Intolerance to contact lenses, increased susceptibility to *Candida* infection

Drug Interactions No significant interactions reported

Drug Uptake

Onset of therapeutic effect: Commonly within 3 days of treatment

Duration: Can persist for as long as 4 months

Serum half-life: 120 hours

Pregnancy Risk Factor X

Quinethazone (kwin eth' a zone)

Related Information

Cardiovascular Diseases *on page 912*

Brand Names Hydromox®

Therapeutic Category Diuretic, Thiazide Type

Use Adjunctive therapy in treatment of edema and hypertension

Usual Dosage Adults: Oral: 50-100 mg once daily up to a maximum of 200 mg/day

Mechanism of Action Quinethazone is a quinazoline derivative which increases the renal excretion of sodium and chloride and an accompanying volume of water due to inhibition of the tubular mechanism of electrolyte reabsorption.

Local Anesthetic/Vasoconstrictor Precautions No information available to require special precautions

Effects on Dental Treatment No effects or complications reported

Other Adverse Effects

1% to 10%: Endocrine & metabolic: Hypokalemia

<1%:

Cardiovascular: Hypotension

Central nervous system: Drowsiness

Dermatologic: Photosensitivity, rash

Endocrine & metabolic: Fluid and electrolyte imbalances (hypocalcemia, hypomagnesemia, hyponatremia), hyperglycemia

Gastrointestinal: Nausea, vomiting, anorexia

Genitourinary: Uremia

Hematologic: Aplastic anemia, hemolytic anemia, leukopenia, agranulocytosis, thrombocytopenia

Hepatic: Hepatitis

Renal: Prerenal azotemia, polyuria

Drug Interactions

Decreased effect of oral hypoglycemics; decreased absorption with cholestyramine and colestipol

Increased effect with furosemide and other loop diuretics

Increased toxicity/levels of lithium

Drug Uptake

Onset of action: 2 hours

Duration: 18-24 hours

Pregnancy Risk Factor D

Quinidex® Extentabs® *see* Quinidine *on next page*

Quinidina (Mexico) *see* Quinidine *on next page*

Quinidine (kwin' i deen)

Related Information
Cardiovascular Diseases *on page 912*

Brand Names Cardioquin®; Quinaglute® Dura-Tabs®; Quinalan®; Quinidex® Extentabs®; Quinora®

Canadian/Mexican Brand Names Quini Durules® (Mexico)

Therapeutic Category Antiarrhythmic Agent, Class I-A; Antiarrhythmic Agent (Supraventricular & Ventricular)

Synonyms Quinidina (Mexico)

Use Prophylaxis after cardioversion of atrial fibrillation and/or flutter to maintain normal sinus rhythm; also used to prevent reoccurrence of paroxysmal supraventricular tachycardia, paroxysmal A-V junctional rhythm, paroxysmal ventricular tachycardia, paroxysmal atrial fibrillation, and atrial or ventricular premature contractions; also has activity against *Plasmodium falciparum* malaria

Usual Dosage Dosage expressed in terms of the salt: 267 mg of quinidine gluconate = 200 mg of quinidine sulfate

Children: Test dose for idiosyncratic reaction (sulfate, oral or gluconate, I.M.): 2 mg/kg or 60 mg/m^2

Oral (quinidine sulfate): 15-60 mg/kg/day in 4-5 divided doses or 6 mg/kg every 4-6 hours; usual 30 mg/kg/day or 900 mg/m^2/day given in 5 daily doses

I.V. **not** recommended (quinidine gluconate): 2-10 mg/kg/dose given at a rate ≤10 mg/minute every 3-6 hours as needed

Adults: Test dose: Oral, I.M.: 200 mg administered several hours before full dosage (to determine possibility of idiosyncratic reaction)

Oral:

Sulfate: 100-600 mg/dose every 4-6 hours; begin at 200 mg/dose and titrate to desired effect (maximum daily dose: 3-4 g)

Gluconate: 324-972 mg every 8-12 hours

I.M.: 400 mg/dose every 4-6 hours

I.V.: 200-400 mg/dose diluted and given at a rate ≤10 mg/minute

Mechanism of Action Class 1A antiarrhythmic agent; depresses phase O of the action potential; decreases myocardial excitability and conduction velocity, and myocardial contractility by decreasing sodium influx during depolarization and potassium efflux in repolarization; also reduces calcium transport across cell membrane

Local Anesthetic/Vasoconstrictor Precautions No information available to require special precautions

Effects on Dental Treatment When taken over a long period of time, the anticholinergic side effects from quinidine can cause a reduction of saliva production or secretion contributing to discomfort and dental disease (ie, caries, oral candidiasis and periodontal disease)

Other Adverse Effects

>10%: Gastrointestinal: Bitter taste, diarrhea, anorexia, nausea, vomiting, stomach cramping

1% to 10%:

Cardiovascular: Hypotension, syncope

Central nervous system: Lightheadedness, severe headache

Dermatologic: Skin rash

Ocular: Blurred vision

Otic: Tinnitus

Respiratory: Wheezing

<1%:

Cardiovascular: Tachycardia, heart block, ventricular fibrillation, vascular collapse

Central nervous system: Confusion, delirium, fever

Dermatologic: Angioedema

Gastrointestinal: Vertigo

Hematologic: Anemia, thrombocytopenic purpura, blood dyscrasias

Otic: Impaired hearing

Respiratory: Respiratory depression

Drug Interactions

Decreased effect: Phenobarbital, phenytoin, and rifampin may decrease quinidine serum concentrations

Increased toxicity:

Verapamil, amiodarone, alkalinizing agents, and cimetidine may increase quinidine serum concentrations

Quinidine may increase plasma concentration of digoxin, digoxin dosage may need to be reduced (by one-half) when quinidine is initiated

(Continued)

759

Quinidine *(Continued)*

Beta-blockers + quinidine may cause enhanced bradycardia
Quinidine may enhance coumarin anticoagulants

Drug Uptake
Serum half-life:
Children: 2.5-6.7 hours
Adults: 6-8 hours; increased half-life with elderly, cirrhosis, and congestive heart failure

Pregnancy Risk Factor C

Quinine Sulfate (kwye′ nine sul′ fate)

Brand Names Formula Q® [OTC]; Legatrin® [OTC]; M-KYA® [OTC]; Quinamm®; Quiphile®; Q-vel®

Therapeutic Category Antimalarial Agent; Muscle Relaxant; Skeletal Muscle Relaxant

Use Suppression or treatment of chloroquine-resistant *P. falciparum* malaria; treatment of *Babesia microti* infection; prevention and treatment of nocturnal recumbency leg muscle cramps

Usual Dosage Oral:
Children:
Treatment of chloroquine-resistant malaria: 25 mg/kg/day in divided doses every 8 hours for 3-7 days in conjunction with another agent
Babesiosis: 25 mg/kg/day, (up to a maximum of 650 mg/dose) divided every 8 hours for 7 days
Adults:
Treatment of chloroquine-resistant malaria: 650 mg every 8 hours for 3-7 days in conjunction with another agent
Suppression of malaria: 325 mg twice daily and continued for 6 weeks after exposure
Babesiosis: 650 mg every 6-8 hours for 7 days
Leg cramps: 200-300 mg at bedtime

Mechanism of Action Depresses oxygen uptake and carbohydrate metabolism; intercalates into DNA, disrupting the parasite's replication and transcription; affects calcium distribution within muscle fibers and decreases the excitability of the motor end-plate region; cardiovascular effects similar to quinidine

Local Anesthetic/Vasoconstrictor Precautions No information available to require special precautions

Effects on Dental Treatment No effects or complications reported

Other Adverse Effects
>10%:
Central nervous system: Severe headache
Gastrointestinal: Nausea, vomiting, diarrhea
Ocular: Blurred vision
Otic: Tinnitus
<1%:
Cardiovascular: Flushing of the skin, anginal symptoms
Central nervous system: Fever
Dermatologic: Rash, pruritus
Endocrine & metabolic: Hypoglycemia
Gastrointestinal: Epigastric pain
Hematologic: Hemolysis, thrombocytopenia
Hepatic: Hepatitis
Ocular: Nightblindness, diplopia, optic atrophy
Otic: Impaired hearing
Miscellaneous: Hypersensitivity reactions

Drug Interactions
Decreased effect: Phenobarbital, phenytoin, and rifampin may decrease quinine serum concentrations
Increased toxicity:
Verapamil, amiodarone, alkalizing agents, and cimetidine may increase quinidine serum concentrations
Quinidine may increase plasma concentration of digoxin, digoxin dosage may need to be reduced (by one-half) when quinidine is initiated
Beta-blockers + quinidine may cause enhanced bradycardia
Quinidine may enhance coumarin anticoagulants

Drug Uptake
Absorption: Oral: Readily absorbed mainly from the upper small intestine
Serum half-life:
Children: 6-12 hours

Adults: 8-14 hours
Time to peak serum concentration: Within 1-3 hours
Pregnancy Risk Factor D

Quinora® see Quinidine on page 759

Quinsana® **Plus Topical [OTC]** see Undecylenic Acid and Derivatives on page 884

Quiphile® see Quinine Sulfate on previous page

Q-vel® see Quinine Sulfate on previous page

Rabies Immune Globulin, Human
(ray' beez i' myun glob' yoo lin hyu' min)
Related Information
Animal and Human Bites Guidelines on page 976
Brand Names Hyperab®; Imogam®
Therapeutic Category Immune Globulin
Use Part of postexposure prophylaxis of persons with rabies exposure who lack a history or pre-exposure or postexposure prophylaxis with rabies vaccine or a recently documented neutralizing antibody response to previous rabies vaccination; although it is preferable to give RIG with the first dose of vaccine, it can be given up to 8 days after vaccination
Usual Dosage Children and Adults: I.M.: 20 units/kg in a single dose (RIG should always be administered in conjunction with rabies vaccine (HDCV)); infiltrate $1/2$ of the dose locally around the wound; give the remainder I.M.
Mechanism of Action Rabies immune globulin is a solution of globulins dried from the plasma or serum of selected adult human donors who have been immunized with rabies vaccine and have developed high titers of rabies antibody. It generally contains 10% to 18% of protein of which not less than 80% is monomeric immunoglobulin G.
Local Anesthetic/Vasoconstrictor Precautions No information available to require special precautions
Effects on Dental Treatment No effects or complications reported
Other Adverse Effects
1% to 10%:
Central nervous system: Fever (mild)
Local: Soreness at injection site
<1%:
Dermatologic: Urticaria, angioedema
Neuromuscular & skeletal: Stiffness, soreness of muscles
Miscellaneous: Anaphylactic shock
Drug Interactions
Decreased effect: Live vaccines, corticosteroids, immunosuppressive agents; should not be administered within 3 months
Pregnancy Risk Factor C

Rabies Virus Vaccine (ray' beez vye' rus vak' seen)
Related Information
Animal and Human Bites Guidelines on page 976
Brand Names Imovax® Rabies I.D. Vaccine; Imovax® Rabies Vaccine
Therapeutic Category Vaccine, Inactivated Virus
Use Veterinarians, animal handlers, certain laboratory workers, and persons living in or visiting countries for longer than 1 month where rabies is a constant threat.

Complete pre-exposure prophylaxis does not eliminate the need for additional therapy with rabies vaccine after a rabies exposure. The Food and Drug Administration has not approved the I.D. use of rabies vaccine for postexposure prophylaxis. Recommendations for I.D. use of HDCV are currently being discussed. The decision for postexposure rabies vaccination depends on the species of biting animal, the circumstances of biting incident, and the type of exposure (bite, saliva contamination of wound, and so on). The type of and schedule for postexposure prophylaxis depends upon the person's previous rabies vaccination status or the result of a previous or current serologic test for rabies antibody. For postexposure prophylaxis, rabies vaccine should always be administered I.M., **not** I.D.
Usual Dosage
Pre-exposure prophylaxis: Two 1 mL doses I.M. 1 week apart, third dose 3 weeks after second. If exposure continues, booster doses can be given every 2 years, or an antibody titer determined and a booster dose given if the titer is inadequate.
Postexposure prophylaxis: All postexposure treatment should begin with immediate cleansing of the wound with soap and water
(Continued)

Rabies Virus Vaccine *(Continued)*

Persons not previously immunized as above: Rabies immune globulin 20 units/ kg body weight, half infiltrated at bite site if possible, remainder I.M.; and 5 doses of rabies vaccine, 1 mL I.M., one each on days 0, 3, 7, 14, 28

Persons who have previously received postexposure prophylaxis with rabies vaccine, received a recommended I.M. pre-exposure series of rabies vaccine or have a previously documented rabies antibody titer considered adequate: Two doses of rabies vaccine, 1 mL I.M., one each on days 0 and 3

Mechanism of Action Rabies vaccine is an inactivated virus vaccine which promotes immunity by inducing an active immune response. The production of specific antibodies requires about 7-10 days to develop. Rabies immune globulin or antirabies serum, equine (ARS) is given in conjunction with rabies vaccine to provide immune protection until an antibody response can occur.

Local Anesthetic/Vasoconstrictor Precautions No information available to require special precautions

Effects on Dental Treatment No effects or complications reported

Other Adverse Effects >10%:

Central nervous system: Dizziness, malaise, encephalomyelitis, transverse myelitis, fever

Dermatologic: Itching, pain, local discomfort, swelling, erythema

Gastrointestinal: Nausea, headache, abdominal pain

Neuromuscular & skeletal: Neuroparalytic reactions, muscle aches

Drug Interactions Decreased effect with immunosuppressive agents, corticosteroids, antimalarial drugs (ie, chloroquine); persons on these drugs should receive RIG (3 doses/1 mL each) by the I.M. route

Drug Uptake

Onset of effect: I.M.: Rabies antibody appears in the serum within 7-10 days

Peak effect: Within 30-60 days and persists for at least 1 year

Pregnancy Risk Factor C

Racet® Topical *see* Clioquinol and Hydrocortisone *on page 216*

Ramipril (ra mi′ pril)

Related Information

Cardiovascular Diseases *on page 912*

Brand Names Altace™

Canadian/Mexican Brand Names Ramace® (Mexico); Tritace® (Mexico)

Therapeutic Category Angiotensin-Converting Enzyme (ACE) Inhibitors

Use Treatment of hypertension, alone or in combination with thiazide diuretics

Unlabeled use: Congestive heart failure

Usual Dosage Adults: Oral: 2.5-5 mg once daily, maximum: 20 mg/day

Mechanism of Action Ramipril is an angiotensin-converting enzyme (ACE) inhibitor which prevents the formation of angiotensin II from angiotensin I and exhibits pharmacologic effects that are similar to captopril. Ramipril must undergo enzymatic saponification by esterases in the liver to its biologically active metabolite, ramiprilat. The pharmacodynamic effects of ramipril result from the high-affinity, competitive, reversible binding of ramiprilat to angiotensin-converting enzyme thus preventing the formation of the potent vasoconstrictor angiotensin II. This isomerized enzyme-inhibitor complex has a slow rate of dissociation, which results in high potency and a long duration of action; a CNS mechanism may also be involved in the hypotensive effect as angiotensin II increases adrenergic outflow from CNS; vasoactive kallikreins may be decreased in conversion to active hormones by ACE inhibitors, thus reducing blood pressure

Local Anesthetic/Vasoconstrictor Precautions No information available to require special precautions

Effects on Dental Treatment No effects or complications reported

Other Adverse Effects

1% to 10%:

Cardiovascular: Tachycardia, chest pain, palpitations,

Central nervous system: Insomnia, headache, dizziness, fatigue, malaise

Dermatologic: Rash, pruritus, alopecia

Gastrointestinal: Dysgeusia, abdominal pain, vomiting, nausea, diarrhea, anorexia, constipation, loss of taste perception

Neuromuscular & skeletal: Paresthesia

Renal: Oliguria

Respiratory: Transient cough

<1%:

Cardiovascular: Hypotension

Dermatologic: Angioedema

Endocrine & metabolic: Hyperkalemia
Hematologic: Neutropenia, agranulocytosis
Renal: Proteinuria; increased BUN, serum creatinine
Drug Interactions See table.

Drug-Drug Interactions With ACEIs

Precipitant Drug	Drug (Category) and Effect	Description
Antacids	ACE Inhibitors: decreased	Decreased bioavailability of ACEIs. May be more likely with captopril. Separate administration times by 1-2 hours.
NSAIDs (indomethacin)	ACEIs: decreased	Reduced hypotensive effects of ACEIs. More prominent in low renin or volume dependent hypertensive patients.
Phenothiazines	ACEIs: increased	Pharmacologic effects of ACEIs may be increased.
ACEIs	Allopurinol: increased	Higher risk of hypersensitivity reaction possible when given concurrently. Three case reports of Stevens-Johnson syndrome with captopril.
ACEIs	Digoxin: increased	Increased plasma digoxin levels.
ACEIs	Lithium: increased	Increased serum lithium levels and symptoms of toxicity may occur.
ACEIs	Potassium preps/ potassium sparing diuretics increased	Coadministration may result in elevated potassium levels.

Drug Uptake
Absorption: Well absorbed from GI tract (50% to 60%)
Serum half-life: Ramiprilat: >50 hours
Time to peak serum concentration: ~1 hour
Pregnancy Risk Factor D

Ramses® [OTC] *see* Nonoxynol 9 *on page 627*
Ranitidina (Mexico) *see* Ranitidine Hydrochloride *on this page*

Ranitidine Bismuth Citrate (ra ni' ti deen biz' muth cit' rate)
Brand Names Tritec®
Therapeutic Category Histamine-2 Antagonist; *H. pylori* Agent
Use Used in combination with clarithromycin for the treatment of active duodenal ulcer associated with *H. pylori* infection; not to be used alone for the treatment of active duodenal ulcer
Usual Dosage Adults: Oral: 400 mg twice daily for 4 weeks with clarithromycin 500 mg 3 times/day for first 2 weeks
Local Anesthetic/Vasoconstrictor Precautions No information available to require special precautions
Effects on Dental Treatment No effects or complications reported
Warnings/Precautions Use in children has not been established
Pregnancy Risk Factor C

Ranitidine Hydrochloride (ra ni' ti deen hye droe klor' ide)
Related Information
Dental Drug Interactions: Update on Drug Combinations Requiring Special Considerations *on page 1022*
Brand Names Zantac®
Canadian/Mexican Brand Names Apo-Ranitidine® (Canada); Novo-Ranidine® (Canada); Nu-Ranit® (Canada); Acloral® (Mexico); Alter-H₂® (Mexico); Anistal® (Mexico); Azantac® (Mexico); Cauteridol® (Mexico); Credaxol® (Mexico); Galidrin® (Mexico); Gastrec® (Mexico); Microtid® (Mexico); Neugal® (Mexico); Ranifur® (Mexico); Ranisen® (Mexico)
Therapeutic Category Histamine-2 Antagonist
Synonyms Ranitidina (Mexico)
Use Short-term treatment of active duodenal ulcers and benign gastric ulcers; long-term prophylaxis of duodenal ulcer and gastric hypersecretory states, gastroesophageal reflux, recurrent postoperative ulcer, upper GI bleeding, prevention of acid-aspiration pneumonitis during surgery, and prevention of stress-induced ulcers; causes fewer interactions than cimetidine
Usual Dosage Giving oral dose at 6 PM may be better than 10 PM bedtime, the highest acid production usually starts at approximately 7 PM, thus giving at 6 PM controls acid secretion better
(Continued)

763

Ranitidine Hydrochloride *(Continued)*

Children:
  Oral: 1.25-2.5 mg/kg/dose every 12 hours; maximum: 300 mg/day
  I.M., I.V.: 0.75-1.5 mg/kg/dose every 6-8 hours, maximum daily dose: 400 mg
  Continuous infusion: 0.1-0.25 mg/kg/hour (preferred for stress ulcer prophylaxis in patients with concurrent maintenance I.V.s or TPNs)

Adults:
  Short-term treatment of ulceration: 150 mg/dose twice daily or 300 mg at bedtime
  Prophylaxis of recurrent duodenal ulcer: Oral: 150 mg at bedtime
  Gastric hypersecretory conditions:
    Oral: 150 mg twice daily, up to 6 g/day
    I.M., I.V.: 50 mg/dose every 6-8 hours (dose not to exceed 400 mg/day)
    I.V.: 50 mg/dose IVPB every 6-8 hours (dose not to exceed 400 mg/day)
  or
    Continuous I.V. infusion: Initial: 50 mg IVPB, followed by 6.25 mg/hour titrated to gastric pH >4.0 for prophylaxis or >7.0 for treatment; **continuous I.V. infusion is preferred in patients with active bleeding**
  Gastric hypersecretory conditions: Doses up to 2.5 mg/kg/hour (220 mg/hour) have been used

Mechanism of Action Competitive inhibition of histamine at H_2-receptors of the gastric parietal cells, which inhibits gastric acid secretion, gastric volume and hydrogen ion concentration reduced

Local Anesthetic/Vasoconstrictor Precautions No information available to require special precautions

Effects on Dental Treatment No effects or complications reported

Other Adverse Effects
  Endocrine & metabolic: Gynecomastia
  Hepatic: Hepatitis
  Neuromuscular & skeletal: Arthralgias

1% to 10%:
  Central nervous system: Dizziness, sedation, malaise, headache, drowsiness
  Dermatologic: Rash
  Gastrointestinal: Constipation, nausea, vomiting, diarrhea
<1%:
  Cardiovascular: Bradycardia, tachycardia
  Central nervous system: Fever, confusion
  Hematologic: Thrombocytopenia, neutropenia, agranulocytosis
  Respiratory: Bronchospasm

Drug Interactions
  Decreased effect: Variable effects on warfarin; antacids may decrease absorption of ranitidine; ketoconazole and itraconazole absorptions are decreased
  May produce altered serum levels of procainamide and ferrous sulfate
  Decreased effect of nondepolarizing muscle relaxants, cefpodoxime, cyanocobalamin (decreased absorption), diazepam, oxaprozin
  Decreased toxicity of atropine
  Increased toxicity of cyclosporine (increased serum creatinine), gentamicin (neuromuscular blockade), glipizide, glyburide, midazolam (increased concentrations), metoprolol, pentoxifylline, phenytoin, quinidine

Drug Uptake
  Absorption: Oral: 50% to 60%
  Serum half-life:
    Children 3.5-16 years: 1.8-2 hours
    Adults: 2-2.5 hours
    End stage renal disease: 6-9 hours
  Time to peak serum concentration: Oral: Within 1-3 hours and persisting for 8 hours

Pregnancy Risk Factor B

Raudixin® *see* Rauwolfia Serpentina *on this page*
Rauverid® *see* Rauwolfia Serpentina *on this page*

Rauwolfia Serpentina (rah wool′ fee a ser pen teen′ ah)
  Brand Names Raudixin®; Rauverid®; Wolfina®
  Therapeutic Category Antihypertensive; Rauwolfia Alkaloid
  Synonyms Whole Root Rauwolfia
  Use Mild essential hypertension; relief of agitated psychotic states

Local Anesthetic/Vasoconstrictor Precautions No information available to require special precautions

Effects on Dental Treatment No effects or complications reported

Ravocaine® and Novocain® with Levophed® *see* Propoxycaine and Procaine *on page 739*

Ravocaine® and Novocain® with Neo-Cobefrin® *see* Propoxycaine and Procaine *on page 739*

Rea-Lo® [OTC] *see* Urea *on page 884*

Recombinate® *see* Antihemophilic Factor (Recombinant) *on page 70*

Recombivax HB® *see* Hepatitis B Vaccine *on page 422*

Redisol® *see* Cyanocobalamin *on page 237*

Redux® *see* Dexfenfluramine Hydrochloride *on page 262*

Reese's® Pinworm Medicine [OTC] *see* Pyrantel Pamoate *on page 751*

Reference Values for Adults *see page 1046*

Refresh® Ophthalmic Solution [OTC] *see* Artificial Tears *on page 75*

Refresh® Plus Ophthalmic Solution [OTC] *see* Artificial Tears *on page 75*

Regitine® *see* Phentolamine Mesylate *on page 684*

Reglan® *see* Metoclopramide *on page 572*

Regulace® [OTC] *see* Docusate and Casanthranol *on page 295*

Regular (Concentrated) Iletin® II U-500 *see* Insulin Preparations *on page 459*

Regular Iletin® I *see* Insulin Preparations *on page 459*

Regular Insulin *see* Insulin Preparations *on page 459*

Regular Purified Pork Insulin *see* Insulin Preparations *on page 459*

Regulax SS® [OTC] *see* Docusate *on page 295*

Reguloid® [OTC] *see* Psyllium *on page 750*

Regutol® [OTC] *see* Docusate *on page 295*

Rela® *see* Carisoprodol *on page 157*

Relafen® *see* Nabumetone *on page 596*

Relaxadon® *see* Hyoscyamine, Atropine, Scopolamine, and Phenobarbital *on page 444*

Relefact® TRH Injection *see* Protirelin *on page 747*

Relief® Ophthalmic Solution *see* Phenylephrine Hydrochloride *on page 685*

Remeron® *see* Mirtazapine *on page 583*

Remifentanil (rem i fen' ta nil)

Brand Names Ultiva®

Therapeutic Category Analgesic, Narcotic; General Anesthetic, Intravenous

Use General anesthesia

Usual Dosage Adults: I.V.: Dose is individualized

Local Anesthetic/Vasoconstrictor Precautions No information available to require special precautions

Effects on Dental Treatment No effects or complications reported

Renacidin® *see* Citric Acid Bladder Mixture *on page 211*

Renese® *see* Polythiazide *on page 705*

Renoquid® *see* Sulfacytine *on page 807*

Renormax® *see* Spirapril *on page 798*

Rentamine® *see* Chlorpheniramine, Ephedrine, Phenylephrine, and Carbetapentane *on page 191*

ReoPro™ *see* Abciximab *on page 12*

Repan® *see* Butalbital Compound *on page 133*

Reposans-10® *see* Chlordiazepoxide *on page 183*

Resaid® *see* Chlorpheniramine and Phenylpropanolamine *on page 190*

Rescaps-D® S.R. Capsule *see* Caramiphen and Phenylpropanolamine *on page 150*

Rescon Liquid [OTC] *see* Chlorpheniramine and Phenylpropanolamine *on page 190*

Reserpina (Mexico) *see* Reserpine *on this page*

Reserpine (re ser' peen)

Related Information

Cardiovascular Diseases *on page 912*

Brand Names Serpalan®; Serpasil®

Canadian/Mexican Brand Names Novo-Reserpine® (Canada)

Therapeutic Category Alpha-Adrenergic Blockers - Peripheral-Acting (Alpha$_1$-Blockers)

(Continued)

Reserpine *(Continued)*

Synonyms Reserpina (Mexico)

Use Management of mild to moderate hypertension

Unlabeled use: Management of tardive dyskinesia

Usual Dosage Oral (full antihypertensive effects may take as long as 3 weeks):

Children: 0.01-0.02 mg/kg/24 hours divided every 12 hours; maximum dose: 0.25 mg/day

Adults: 0.1-0.25 mg/day in 1-2 doses; initial: 0.5 mg/day for 1-2 weeks; maintenance: reduce to 0.1-0.25 mg/day

Elderly: Initial: 0.05 mg once daily, increasing by 0.05 mg every week as necessary

Mechanism of Action Reduces blood pressure via depletion of sympathetic biogenic amines (norepinephrine and dopamine); this also commonly results in sedative effects

Local Anesthetic/Vasoconstrictor Precautions No information available to require special precautions

Effects on Dental Treatment No effects or complications reported

Other Adverse Effects

>10%:

Central nervous system: Dizziness

Gastrointestinal: Anorexia, diarrhea, dry mouth, nausea, vomiting

Respiratory: Nasal congestion

1% to 10%:

Cardiovascular: Peripheral edema, arrhythmias, bradycardia, chest pain

Central nervous system: Headache

Genitourinary: Impotence

Miscellaneous: Black stools, bloody vomit

<1%:

Cardiovascular: Hypotension

Central nervous system: Drowsiness, fatigue, mental depression, parkinsonism

Dermatologic: Skin rash

Gastrointestinal: Increased gastric acid secretion

Genitourinary: Urination difficulty

Neuromuscular & skeletal: Trembling of hands/fingers

Miscellaneous: Sodium and water retention

Drug Interactions

Decreased effect of indirect-acting sympathomimetics

Increased effect/toxicity of MAO inhibitors, direct-acting sympathomimetics, and tricyclic antidepressants

Drug Uptake

Onset of antihypertensive effect: Within 3-6 days

Duration: 2-6 weeks

Absorption: Oral: ~40%

Serum half-life: 50-100 hours

Pregnancy Risk Factor C

Reserpine and Chlorothiazide see Chlorothiazide and Reserpine *on page 189*

Reserpine and Hydrochlorothiazide see Hydrochlorothiazide and Reserpine *on page 431*

Respa-1st® see Guaifenesin and Pseudoephedrine *on page 409*

Respaire®-60 SR see Guaifenesin and Pseudoephedrine *on page 409*

Respaire®-120 SR see Guaifenesin and Pseudoephedrine *on page 409*

Respbid® see Theophylline/Aminophylline *on page 832*

Respinol-G® see Guaifenesin, Phenylpropanolamine, and Phenylephrine *on page 410*

Respiratory Diseases see page 924

Resporal [OTC] see Dexbrompheniramine and Pseudoephedrine *on page 261*

Restoril® see Temazepam *on page 819*

Retin-A™ see Tretinoin *on page 862*

Retrovir® see Zidovudine *on page 907*

Revex® see Nalmefene Hydrochloride *on page 601*

Rēv-Eyes™ see Dapiprazole Hydrochloride *on page 251*

R-Gen® see Iodinated Glycerol *on page 465*

R-Gene® see Arginine Hydrochloride *on page 73*

rGM-CSF see Sargramostim *on page 780*

Rheaban® [OTC] see Attapulgite *on page 86*

Rheomacrodex® see Dextran *on page 263*

Rhesonativ® see Rh₀(D) Immune Globulin *on this page*

Rheumatoid Arthritis, Osteoarthritis, and Joint Prostheses *see page 930*

Rheumatrex® *see Methotrexate on page 559*

Rhinall® Nasal Solution [OTC] *see Phenylephrine Hydrochloride on page 685*

Rhinatate® Tablet *see Chlorpheniramine, Pyrilamine, and Phenylephrine on page 195*

Rhindecon® *see Phenylpropanolamine Hydrochloride on page 687*

Rhinocort™ *see Budesonide on page 126*

Rhinosyn-DMX® [OTC] *see Guaifenesin and Dextromethorphan on page 408*

Rhinosyn® Liquid [OTC] *see Chlorpheniramine and Pseudoephedrine on page 191*

Rhinosyn-PD® Liquid [OTC] *see Chlorpheniramine and Pseudoephedrine on page 191*

Rh₀(D) Immune Globulin (ar aych oh (dee) i myun′ glob′ yoo lin)

Brand Names HypRho®-D; HypRho®-D Mini-Dose; MICRhoGAM™; Mini-Gamulin® Rh; Rhesonativ®; RhoGAM™

Canadian/Mexican Brand Names Anti-Rho(D)® (Mexico); Probi-Rho(D) (Mexico)

Therapeutic Category Immune Globulin

Use Prevent isoimmunization in Rh-negative individuals exposed to Rh-positive blood during delivery of an Rh-positive infant, as a result of an abortion, following amniocentesis or abdominal trauma, or following a transfusion accident; to prevent hemolytic disease of the newborn if there is a subsequent pregnancy with an Rh-positive fetus

Usual Dosage Adults (administered I.M. to mothers **not** to infant) I.M.:
Obstetrical usage: 1 vial (300 mcg) prevents maternal sensitization if fetal packed red blood cell volume that has entered the circulation is <15 mL; if it is more, give additional vials. The number of vials = RBC volume of the calculated fetomaternal hemorrhage divided by 15 mL

Postpartum prophylaxis: 300 mcg within 72 hours of delivery

Antepartum prophylaxis: 300 mcg at approximately 26-28 weeks gestation; followed by 300 mcg within 72 hours of delivery if infant is Rh-positive

Following miscarriage, abortion, or termination of ectopic pregnancy at up to 13 weeks of gestation: 50 mcg ideally within 3 hours, but may be given up to 72 hours after; if pregnancy has been terminated at 13 or more weeks of gestation, administer 300 mcg

Mechanism of Action Suppresses the immune response and antibody formation of Rh-negative individuals to Rh-positive red blood cells

Local Anesthetic/Vasoconstrictor Precautions No information available to require special precautions

Effects on Dental Treatment No effects or complications reported

Other Adverse Effects <1%:
Central nervous system: Lethargy, temperature elevation
Gastrointestinal: Splenomegaly
Hepatic: Bilirubin (elevated)
Local: Pain at the injection site
Neuromuscular & skeletal: Myalgia

Drug Uptake
Serum half-life: 23-26 days

Pregnancy Risk Factor C

Comments Administered I.M. to mothers **not** to infant; will prevent hemolytic disease of newborn in subsequent pregnancy

RhoGAM™ see Rh₀(D) Immune Globulin *on this page*

***r*HuEPO-α** *see Epoetin Alfa on page 315*

Rhythmin® *see Procainamide Hydrochloride on page 725*

Ribavirin (rye ba vye′ rin)

Brand Names Virazole® Aerosol

Canadian/Mexican Brand Names Vilona® (Mexico); Virazide® (Mexico); Vilona Pediatrica® (Mexico)

Therapeutic Category Antiviral Agent, Inhalation Therapy

Synonyms RTCA; Tribavirin

Use Treatment of patients with respiratory syncytial virus (RSV) infections; specially indicated for treatment of severe lower respiratory tract RSV infections in patients with an underlying compromising condition (prematurity, bronchopulmonary dysplasia and other chronic lung conditions, congenital heart (Continued)

Ribavirin *(Continued)*

disease, immunodeficiency, immunosuppression), and recent transplant recipients; may also be used in other viral infections including influenza A and B and adenovirus

Usual Dosage Children and Adults:

Aerosol inhalation: Use with Viratek® small particle aerosol generator (SPAG-2) at a concentration of 20 mg/mL (6 g reconstituted with 300 mL of sterile water without preservatives)

Aerosol only: 12-18 hours/day for 3 days, up to 7 days in length

Mechanism of Action Inhibits replication of RNA and DNA viruses; inhibits influenza virus RNA polymerase activity and inhibits the initiation and elongation of RNA fragments resulting in inhibition of viral protein synthesis

Local Anesthetic/Vasoconstrictor Precautions No information available to require special precautions

Effects on Dental Treatment No effects or complications reported

Other Adverse Effects

1% to 10%:

Central nervous system: Fatigue, headache, insomnia

Gastrointestinal: Nausea, anorexia

Hematologic: Anemia

<1%:

Cardiovascular: Hypotension, cardiac arrest, digitalis toxicity

Dermatologic: Rash, skin irritation

Ocular: Conjunctivitis

Respiratory: Mild bronchospasm, worsening of respiratory function, apnea, accumulation of fluid in ventilator tubing

Drug Uptake

Absorption: Absorbed systemically from the respiratory tract following nasal and oral inhalation; absorption is dependent upon respiratory factors and method of drug delivery; maximal absorption occurs with the use of the aerosol generator via an endotracheal tube; highest concentrations are found in the respiratory tract and erythrocytes

Serum half-life, plasma:

Children: 6.5-11 hours

Adults: 24 hours, much longer in the erythrocyte (16-40 days), which can be used as a marker for intracellular metabolism

Time to peak serum concentration: Inhalation: Within 60-90 minutes

Pregnancy Risk Factor X

Comments RSV season is usually December to April; viral shedding period for RSV is usually 3-8 days

Riboflavin (rye' boe flay vin)

Brand Names Riobin®

Therapeutic Category Vitamin, Water Soluble

Synonyms Riboflavina (Mexico)

Use Dental and Medical: Prevent riboflavin deficiency and treat ariboflavinosis

Usual Dosage Oral:

Riboflavin deficiency:

Children: 2.5-10 mg/day in divided doses

Adults: 5-30 mg/day in divided doses

Recommended daily allowance:

Children: 0.4-1.8 mg

Adults: 1.2-1.7 mg

Mechanism of Action Component of flavoprotein enzymes that work together, which are necessary for normal tissue respiration; also needed for activation of pyridoxine and conversion of tryptophan to niacin

Local Anesthetic/Vasoconstrictor Precautions No information available to require special precautions

Effects on Dental Treatment No effects or complications reported

Warnings/Precautions Riboflavin deficiency often occurs in the presence of other B vitamin deficiencies

Drug Interactions Decreased absorption with probenecid

Drug Uptake

Absorption: Readily via GI tract, however, food increases extent of GI absorption; GI absorption is decreased in patients with hepatitis, cirrhosis, or biliary obstruction

Serum half-life, biologic: 66-84 minutes

Pregnancy Risk Factor A (C if dose exceeds RDA recommendation)

Dosage Forms Tablet: 25 mg, 50 mg, 100 mg

Generic Available Yes

Riboflavina (Mexico) *see Riboflavin on previous page*
RID® [OTC] *see Pyrethrins on page 753*
Ridaura® *see Auranofin on page 87*

Rifabutin (rif a bu′ tin)
Related Information
Nonviral Infectious Diseases *on page 932*
Systemic Viral Diseases *on page 934*
Brand Names Mycobutin®
Therapeutic Category Antibiotic, Miscellaneous; Antitubercular Agent
Use Adjunctive therapy for the prevention of disseminated *Mycobacterium avium* complex (MAC) in patients with advanced HIV infection
Usual Dosage Oral:
Children: Efficacy and safety of rifabutin have not been established in children; a limited number of HIV-positive children with MAC have been given rifabutin for MAC prophylaxis; doses of 5 mg/kg/day have been useful
Adults: 300 mg once daily; for patients who experience gastrointestinal upset, rifabutin can be administered 150 mg twice daily with food
Mechanism of Action Inhibits DNA-dependent RNA polymerase at the beta subunit which prevents chain initiation
Local Anesthetic/Vasoconstrictor Precautions No information available to require special precautions
Effects on Dental Treatment No effects or complications reported
Other Adverse Effects
>10%:
Dermatologic: Rash
Hematologic: Neutropenia, leukopenia
Miscellaneous: Discolored urine
1% to 10%:
Central nervous system: Headache
Gastrointestinal: Vomiting, nausea, abdominal pain, diarrhea, anorexia, flatulence, eructation
Hematologic: Anemia, thrombocytopenia
Neuromuscular & skeletal: Myalgia
<1%:
Cardiovascular: Chest pain
Central nervous system: Fever, insomnia
Gastrointestinal: Dyspepsia, flatulence, nausea, vomiting, taste perversion
Drug Interactions Decreased plasma concentration (due to induction of liver enzymes) of verapamil, methadone, digoxin, cyclosporine, corticosteroids, oral anticoagulants, theophylline, barbiturates, chloramphenicol, ketoconazole, oral contraceptives, quinidine, halothane
Drug Uptake
Absorption: Oral: Readily absorbed 53%
Serum half life, terminal: 45 hours (range: 16-69 hours)
Peak serum level: Within 2-4 hours
Pregnancy Risk Factor B

Rifadin® *see Rifampin on this page*
Rifamate® *see Rifampin and Isoniazid on page 771*
Rifampicina (Mexico) *see Rifampin on this page*

Rifampin (rif′ am pin)
Related Information
Nonviral Infectious Diseases *on page 932*
Brand Names Rifadin®; Rimactane®
Canadian/Mexican Brand Names Rifadin® (Canada); Rimactane® (Canada); Rofact® (Canada)
Therapeutic Category Antibiotic, Miscellaneous; Antitubercular Agent
Synonyms Rifampicina (Mexico)
Use Management of active tuberculosis; eliminate meningococci from asymptomatic carriers; prophylaxis of *Haemophilus influenzae* type B infection; used in combination with other anti-infectives in the treatment of staphylococcal infections
Usual Dosage I.V. infusion dose is the same as for the oral route
Tuberculosis therapy: Oral:
Note: A four-drug regimen (isoniazid, rifampin, pyrazinamide, and either streptomycin or ethambutol) is preferred for the initial, empiric treatment of TB. When the drug susceptibility results are available, the regimen should be altered as appropriate.
(Continued)

Rifampin *(Continued)*

Patients with TB and without HIV infection:
OPTION 1:
Isoniazid resistance rate <4%: Administer daily isoniazid, rifampin, and pyrazinamide for 8 weeks followed by isoniazid and rifampin daily or directly observed therapy (DOT) 2-3 times/week for 16 weeks

If isoniazid resistance rate is not documented, ethambutol or streptomycin should also be administered until susceptibility to isoniazid or rifampin is demonstrated. Continue treatment for at least 6 months or 3 months beyond culture conversion.

OPTION 2: Administer daily isoniazid, rifampin, pyrazinamide, and either streptomycin or ethambutol for 2 weeks followed by DOT 2 times/week administration of the same drugs for 6 weeks, and subsequently, with isoniazid and rifampin DOT 2 times/week administration for 16 weeks

OPTION 3: Administer isoniazid, rifampin, pyrazinamide, and either ethambutol or streptomycin by DOT 3 times/week for 6 months

Patients with TB and with HIV infection:
Administer any of the above OPTIONS 1, 2 or 3, however, treatment should be continued for a total of 9 months and at least 6 months beyond culture conversion

Note: Some experts recommend that the duration of therapy should be extended to 9 months for patients with disseminated disease, miliary disease, disease involving the bones or joints, or tuberculosis lymphadenitis

Children <12 years of age: Oral:
Daily therapy: 10-20 mg/kg/day in divided doses every 12-24 hours (maximum: 600 mg/day)
Directly observed therapy (DOT): Twice weekly: 10-20 mg/kg (maximum: 600 mg)
DOT: 3 times/week: 10-20 mg/kg (maximum: 600 mg)

Adults: Oral:
Daily therapy: 10 mg/kg/day (maximum: 600 mg/day)
Directly observed therapy (DOT): Twice weekly: 10 mg/kg (maximum: 600 mg)
DOT: 3 times/week: 10 mg/kg (maximum: 600 mg)

H. influenzae prophylaxis: Oral:
Children: 20 mg/kg/day every 24 hours for 4 days, not to exceed 600 mg/dose
Adults: 600 mg every 24 hours for 4 days

Meningococcal prophylaxis: Oral:
<1 month: 10 mg/kg/day in divided doses every 12 hours for 2 days
Children: 20 mg/kg/day in divided doses every 12 hours for 2 days
Adults: 600 mg every 12 hours for 2 days

Nasal carriers of *Staphylococcus aureus*: Oral:
Children: 15 mg/kg/day divided every 12 hours for 5-10 days in combination with other antibiotics
Adults: 600 mg/day for 5-10 days in combination with other antibiotics

Synergy for *Staphylococcus aureus* infections: Oral: Adults: 300-600 mg twice daily with other antibiotics

Mechanism of Action Inhibits bacterial RNA synthesis by binding to the beta subunit of DNA-dependent RNA polymerase, blocking RNA transcription

Local Anesthetic/Vasoconstrictor Precautions No information available to require special precautions

Effects on Dental Treatment No effects or complications reported

Other Adverse Effects
1% to 10%:
Gastrointestinal: Diarrhea, stomach cramps
Miscellaneous: Discoloration of urine, feces, saliva, sputum, sweat, and tears (reddish orange); fungal overgrowth
<1%:
Central nervous system: Drowsiness, fatigue, ataxia, confusion, fever, headache
Dermatologic: Rash, pruritus
Gastrointestinal: Nausea, vomiting, stomatitis
Hematologic: Eosinophilia, blood dyscrasias (leukopenia, thrombocytopenia)
Hepatic: Hepatitis
Local: Irritation at the I.V. site
Renal: Renal failure

Miscellaneous: Flu-like syndrome

Drug Interactions Inducer of both Cytochrome P-450 3A and cytochrome P-450 2D6

Decreased effect: Rifampin induces liver enzymes which may decrease the plasma concentration of verapamil, methadone, digoxin, cyclosporine, corticosteroids, oral anticoagulants, theophylline, barbiturates, chloramphenicol, ketoconazole, oral contraceptives, quinidine, halothane, ketoconazole

Drug Uptake

Absorption: Oral: Well absorbed

Time to peak serum concentration: Oral: 2-4 hours and persisting for up to 24 hours; food may delay or slightly reduce

Serum half-life: 3-4 hours, prolonged with hepatic impairment

Pregnancy Risk Factor C

Rifampin and Isoniazid (rif' am pin & eye soe nye' a zid)

Brand Names Rifamate®

Therapeutic Category Antibiotic, Miscellaneous; Antitubercular Agent

Use Management of active tuberculosis; see individual monographs for additional information

Local Anesthetic/Vasoconstrictor Precautions No information available to require special precautions

Effects on Dental Treatment No effects or complications reported

Rifampin, Isoniazid, and Pyrazinamide

(rif' am pin , eye soe nye' a zid, & peer a zin' a mide)

Brand Names Rifater®

Therapeutic Category Antibiotic, Miscellaneous; Antitubercular Agent

Use Management of active tuberculosis

Local Anesthetic/Vasoconstrictor Precautions No information available to require special precautions

Effects on Dental Treatment No effects or complications reported

Rifater® see Rifampin, Isoniazid, and Pyrazinamide on this page

Rilutek® see Riluzole on this page

Riluzole (ril' yoo zole)

Brand Names Rilutek®

Therapeutic Category Amyotrophic Lateral Sclerosis (ALS) Agent

Use Treatment of amyotrophic lateral sclerosis (ALS), also know as Lou Gehrig's disease

Usual Dosage Adults: Oral: 50 mg every 12 hours; no increased benefit can be expected from higher daily doses, but adverse events are increased

Local Anesthetic/Vasoconstrictor Precautions No information available to require special precautions

Effects on Dental Treatment No effects or complications reported

Drug Uptake

Absorption: Well absorbed (90%); a high fat meal decreases absorption of riluzole (decreasing AUC by 20% and peak blood levels by 45%)

Rimactane® see Rifampin on page 769

Rimantadine Hydrochloride (ri man' ta deen hye droe klor' ide)

Related Information

Systemic Viral Diseases on page 934

Brand Names Flumadine®

Therapeutic Category Antiviral Agent, Oral

Use Prophylaxis (adults and children >1 year) and treatment (adults) of influenza A viral infection

Usual Dosage Oral:

Prophylaxis:

Children <10 years: 5 mg/kg give once daily; maximum: 150 mg

Children >10 years and Adults: 100 mg twice daily; decrease to 100 mg/day in elderly or in patients with severe hepatic or renal impairment (Cl_{cr} ≤10 mL/minute)

Treatment: Adults: 100 mg twice daily; decrease to 100 mg/day in elderly or in patients with severe hepatic or renal impairment (Cl_{cr} ≤10 mL/minute)

Mechanism of Action Exerts its inhibitory effect on three antigenic subtypes of influenza A virus (H1N1, H2N2, H3N2) early in the viral replicative cycle, possibly inhibiting the uncoating process; it has no activity against influenza B virus and is 2- to 8-fold more active than amantadine

(Continued)

Rimantadine Hydrochloride *(Continued)*

Local Anesthetic/Vasoconstrictor Precautions No information available to require special precautions

Effects on Dental Treatment No effects or complications reported

Other Adverse Effects 1% to 10%:

Cardiovascular: Orthostatic hypotension, edema

Central nervous system: Dizziness, confusion, headache, insomnia, difficulty in concentrating, anxiety, restlessness, irritability, hallucinations; incidence of CNS side effects may be less than that associated with amantadine

Gastrointestinal: Nausea, vomiting, dry mouth, abdominal pain, anorexia

Genitourinary: Urinary retention

Drug Interactions

Acetaminophen: Reduction in AUC and peak concentration of rimantadine

Aspirin: Peak plasma and AUC concentrations of rimantadine are reduced

Cimetidine: Rimantadine clearance is decreased (~16%)

Drug Uptake

Absorption: Tablet and syrup formulations are equally absorbed; T_{max}: 6 hours

Serum half-life: 25.4 hours (increased in elderly)

Pregnancy Risk Factor C

Rimexolone (ri mex' oh lone)

Brand Names Vexol® Ophthalmic Suspension

Therapeutic Category Anti-inflammatory Agent, Ophthalmic; Corticosteroid, Ophthalmic

Use Treatment of swelling after ocular surgery and the treatment of anterior uveitis

Local Anesthetic/Vasoconstrictor Precautions No information available to require special precautions

Effects on Dental Treatment No effects or complications reported

Riobin® *see* Riboflavin *on page 768*

Riopan® [OTC] *see* Magaldrate *on page 520*

Riopan Plus® [OTC] *see* Magaldrate and Simethicone *on page 521*

Risperdal® *see* Risperidone *on this page*

Risperidona (Mexico) *see* Risperidone *on this page*

Risperidone (ris per' i done)

Brand Names Risperdal®

Therapeutic Category Antipsychotic Agent

Synonyms Risperidona (Mexico)

Use Management of psychotic disorders (eg, schizophrenia); nonpsychotic symptoms associated with dementia in elderly

Usual Dosage

Recommended starting dose: 1 mg twice daily; slowly increase to the optimum range of 4-8 mg/day; daily dosages >10 mg does not appear to confer any additional benefit, and the incidence of extrapyramidal reactions is higher than with lower doses

Mechanism of Action Risperidone is a benzisoxazole derivative, mixed serotonin-dopamine antagonist; binds to 5-HT$_2$ receptors in the CNS and in the periphery with a very high affinity; binds to dopamine-D$_2$ receptors with less affinity. The binding affinity to the dopamine-D$_2$ receptor is 20 times lower than the 5-HT$_2$ affinity. The addition of serotonin antagonism to dopamine antagonism (classic neuroleptic mechanism) is thought to improve negative symptoms of psychoses and reduce the incidence of extrapyramidal side effects.

Local Anesthetic/Vasoconstrictor Precautions No information available to require special precautions

Effects on Dental Treatment Up to 10% of dental patients will experience significant dry mouth and orthostatic hypotension. These effects disappear with cessation of drug therapy.

Other Adverse Effects

1% to 10%:

Cardiovascular: Hypotension (especially orthostatic), tachycardia, arrhythmias, abnormal T waves with prolonged ventricular repolarization; EKG changes, syncope

Central nervous system: Sedation (occurs at daily doses ≥20 mg/day), headache, dizziness, restlessness, anxiety, extrapyramidal reactions, dystonic reactions, pseudoparkinson signs and symptoms, tardive dyskinesia, neuroleptic malignant syndrome, altered central temperature regulation

Dermatologic: Photosensitivity (rare)

Endocrine & metabolic: Amenorrhea, galactorrhea, gynecomastia

Gastrointestinal: Constipation, adynamic ileus, GI upset, dry mouth (problem for denture user), nausea and anorexia, weight gain

Genitourinary: Urinary retention, overflow incontinence, priapism, sexual dysfunction (up to 60%)

Hematologic: Agranulocytosis, leukopenia (usually in patients with large doses for prolonged periods)

Hepatic: Cholestatic jaundice

Ocular: Blurred vision, retinal pigmentation, decreased visual acuity (may be irreversible)

<1%: Seizures

Drug Interactions
May antagonize effects of levodopa; carbamazepine decreases risperidone serum concentrations; clozapine decreases clearance of risperidone

Drug Uptake
Absorption: Oral: Rapid
Serum half-life: 24 hours (risperidone and its active metabolite)
Time to peak: Peak plasma concentrations within 1 hour

Pregnancy Risk Factor C

Ritalin® *see* Methylphenidate Hydrochloride *on page 568*

Ritalin-SR® *see* Methylphenidate Hydrochloride *on page 568*

Ritodrine Hydrochloride (ri′ toe dreen hye droe klor′ ide)

Brand Names Pre-Par®; Yutopar®

Therapeutic Category Adrenergic Agonist Agent; Beta-2-Adrenergic Agonist Agent

Use Inhibits uterine contraction in preterm labor

Usual Dosage Adults:

I.V.: 50-100 mcg/minute; increase by 50 mcg/minute every 10 minutes; continue for 12 hours after contractions have stopped

Oral: Start 30 minutes before stopping I.V. infusion; 10 mg every 2 hours for 24 hours, then 10-20 mg every 4-6 hours up to 120 mg/day

Hemodialysis effects: Removed by hemodialysis

Mechanism of Action Tocolysis due to its uterine beta$_2$-adrenergic receptor stimulating effects; this agent's beta$_2$ effects can also cause bronchial relaxation and vascular smooth muscle stimulation

Local Anesthetic/Vasoconstrictor Precautions No information available to require special precautions

Effects on Dental Treatment No effects or complications reported

Other Adverse Effects

>10%:

Cardiovascular: Increases in maternal and fetal heart rates and maternal hypertension, palpitations

Endocrine & metabolic: Temporary hyperglycemia

Gastrointestinal: Nausea, vomiting

Neuromuscular & skeletal: Tremor

1% to 10%:

Cardiovascular: Chest pain

Central nervous system: Nervousness, anxiety, restlessness

<1%:

Hepatic: Impaired liver function

Miscellaneous: Anaphylactic shock, ketoacidosis

Drug Interactions
Decreased effect with beta-blockers

Increased effect/toxicity with meperidine, sympathomimetics, diazoxide, magnesium, betamethasone (pulmonary edema), potassium-depleting diuretics, general anesthetics

Drug Uptake
Absorption: Oral: Rapid
Serum half-life: 15 hours
Time to peak serum concentration: Within 0.5-1 hour

Pregnancy Risk Factor B

Ritonavir (rye ton′ a veer)

Related Information
Systemic Viral Diseases *on page 934*

Brand Names Norvir®

Therapeutic Category Antiviral Agent, Oral; Protease Inhibitor

Use Treatment of HIV, especially advanced cases; usually is used as part of triple or double therapy with other nucleoside and protease inhibitors

Usual Dosage Adults: Oral: 600 mg twice daily with meals

(Continued)

Ritonavir *(Continued)*

Dosing adjustment in renal impairment: None necessary
Dosing adjustment in hepatic impairment: Not determined; caution advised with severe impairment

Mechanism of Action As a protease inhibitor, ritonavir prevents cleavage of protein precursors essential for HIV infection of new cells and viral replication. Saquinavir- and zidovudine-resistant HIV isolates are generally susceptible to ritonavir. Used in combination therapy, resistance to ritonavir develops slowly; strains resistant to ritonavir are cross-resistant to indinavir and saquinavir.

Local Anesthetic/Vasoconstrictor Precautions No information available to require special precautions

Effects on Dental Treatment No effects or complications reported

Other Adverse Effects
1% to 10%:
Central nervous system: Asthenia
Gastrointestinal: Nausea, vomiting, diarrhea, altered taste
Neuromuscular & skeletal: Circumoral and peripheral paresthesias
<1%:
Central nervous system: Headache, confusion
Endocrine & metabolic: Elevated triglycerides, cholesterol
Hepatic: Elevated LFTs

Contraindications Hypersensitivity to ritonavir or any of its components; avoid use with astemizole, terfenadine, and rifabutin

Warnings/Precautions Use caution in patients with hepatic insufficiency; safety and efficacy have not been established in children <16 years of age; use caution with benzodiazepines, antiarrhythmics (flecainide, encainide, bepridil, amiodarone, quinidine) and certain analgesics (meperidine, piroxicam, propoxyphene)

Drug Interactions
Decreased effect: Concurrent use of rifampin, rifabutin, dexamethasone, and many anticonvulsants lowers serum concentration of ritonavir
Increased toxicity: Ketoconazole increases ritonavir's plasma levels; ritonavir may decrease metabolism of terfenadine and astemizole and result in rare but serious cardiac arrhythmias; enhanced cardiac effects when administered with flecainide, encainide, quinidine, amiodarone, bepridil. Increased toxic effects also possible with coadministration with cisapride and benzodiazepines.

Drug Uptake
Absorption: Well absorbed; T_{max}: 2-4 hours
Half-life: 3-5 hours

Pregnancy Risk Factor B

Dosage Forms
Capsule: 100 mg
Solution: 80 mg/mL

RMS® Rectal *see* Morphine Sulfate *on page 590*

Robafen® AC *see* Guaifenesin and Codeine *on page 408*

Robafen® CF [OTC] *see* Guaifenesin, Phenylpropanolamine, and Dextromethorphan *on page 410*

Robafen DM® [OTC] *see* Guaifenesin and Dextromethorphan *on page 408*

Robaxin® *see* Methocarbamol *on page 557*

Robaxisal® *see* Methocarbamol and Aspirin *on page 558*

Robicillin® VK *see* Penicillin V Potassium *on page 668*

Robinul® *see* Glycopyrrolate *on page 403*

Robinul® Forte *see* Glycopyrrolate *on page 403*

Robitussin® [OTC] *see* Guaifenesin *on page 407*

Robitussin® A-C *see* Guaifenesin and Codeine *on page 408*

Robitussin-CF® [OTC] *see* Guaifenesin, Phenylpropanolamine, and Dextromethorphan *on page 410*

Robitussin® Cough Calmers [OTC] *see* Dextromethorphan *on page 266*

Robitussin®-DAC *see* Guaifenesin, Pseudoephedrine, and Codeine *on page 410*

Robitussin®-DM [OTC] *see* Guaifenesin and Dextromethorphan *on page 408*

Robitussin-PE® [OTC] *see* Guaifenesin and Pseudoephedrine *on page 409*

Robitussin® Pediatric [OTC] *see* Dextromethorphan *on page 266*

Robitussin® Severe Congestion Liqui-Gels [OTC] *see* Guaifenesin and Pseudoephedrine *on page 409*

Robomol® *see* Methocarbamol *on page 557*

Rocaltrol® *see* Calcitriol *on page 139*

Rocephin® *see* Ceftriaxone Sodium *on page 172*

Rocky Mountain Spotted Fever Vaccine
(rok′ ee moun′ ten spot′ ted fee′ ver vak seen′)
Therapeutic Category Vaccine, Live Bacteria
Local Anesthetic/Vasoconstrictor Precautions No information available to require special precautions
Effects on Dental Treatment No effects or complications reported

Roferon-A® *see* Interferon Alfa-2a *on page 461*

Rogaine® *see* Minoxidil *on page 583*

Rolaids® Calcium Rich [OTC] *see* Calcium Carbonate *on page 140*

Rolatuss® Plain Liquid *see* Chlorpheniramine and Phenylephrine *on page 190*

Romazicon™ *see* Flumazenil *on page 370*

Rondamine®-DM Drops *see* Carbinoxamine, Pseudoephedrine, and Dextromethorphan *on page 155*

Rondec®-DM *see* Carbinoxamine, Pseudoephedrine, and Dextromethorphan *on page 155*

Rondec® Drops *see* Carbinoxamine and Pseudoephedrine *on page 154*

Rondec® Filmtab® *see* Carbinoxamine and Pseudoephedrine *on page 154*

Rondec® Syrup *see* Carbinoxamine and Pseudoephedrine *on page 154*

Rondec-TR® *see* Carbinoxamine and Pseudoephedrine *on page 154*

Ropivacaine Hydrochloride (roe piv′ a kane hye droe klor′ ide)
Related Information
  Oral Pain *on page 940*
Brand Names Naropin®
Therapeutic Category Local Anesthetic, Injectable
Use Production of local or regional anesthesia for surgery, postoperative pain management and obstetrical procedures by infiltration anesthesia and nerve block anesthesia
Usual Dosage Analgesia in postoperative pain management: With infiltration of 100-200 mg, the time to first request for an analgesia was 2-6 hours
Mechanism of Action Local anesthetics bind selectively to the intracellular surface of sodium channels to block influx of sodium into the axon. As a result, depolarization necessary for action potential propagation and subsequent nerve function is prevented. The block at the sodium channel is reversible. When drug diffuses away from the axon, sodium channel function is restored and nerve propagation returns.
Local Anesthetic/Vasoconstrictor Precautions No information available to require special precautions
Effects on Dental Treatment No effects or complications reported
Generic Available No
Comments Not available with vasoconstrictor (epinephrine) and not available in dental (1-8 mL) carpules

Rowasa® *see* Mesalamine *on page 546*

Roxanol™ Oral *see* Morphine Sulfate *on page 590*

Roxanol Rescudose® *see* Morphine Sulfate *on page 590*

Roxanol SR™ Oral *see* Morphine Sulfate *on page 590*

Roxicet® *see* Oxycodone and Acetaminophen *on page 646*

Roxiprin® *see* Oxycodone and Aspirin *on page 647*

R-Tannamine® Tablet *see* Chlorpheniramine, Pyrilamine, and Phenylephrine *on page 195*

R-Tannate® Tablet *see* Chlorpheniramine, Pyrilamine, and Phenylephrine *on page 195*

RTCA *see* Ribavirin *on page 767*

Rubella and Measles Vaccines, Combined *see* Measles and Rubella Vaccines, Combined *on page 527*

Rubella and Mumps Vaccines, Combined
(rue bel′ a & mumpz vak seens′ kom bined′)
Brand Names Biavax® II
Therapeutic Category Vaccine, Live Virus
Use Promote active immunity to rubella and mumps by inducing production of antibodies
Usual Dosage Children >12 months and Adults: 1 vial in outer aspect of the upper arm; children vaccinated before 12 months of age should be revaccinated
(Continued)

Rubella and Mumps Vaccines, Combined *(Continued)*

Local Anesthetic/Vasoconstrictor Precautions No information available to require special precautions

Effects on Dental Treatment No effects or complications reported

Other Adverse Effects 1% to 10%:
Central nervous system: Febrile seizures, fever
Local: Burning, stinging
Neuromuscular & skeletal: Soreness
Miscellaneous: Allergic reactions

Pregnancy Risk Factor X

Comments Federal law requires that the date of administration, the vaccine manufacturer, lot number of vaccine, and the administering person's name, title and address be entered into the patient's permanent medical record

Rubella, Measles and Mumps Vaccines, Combined *see* Measles, Mumps, and Rubella Vaccines, Combined *on page 528*

Rubella Virus Vaccine, Live *(rue bel′ a vye′ rus vak seen′ live)*

Brand Names Meruvax® II

Canadian/Mexican Brand Names Rimevax (Mexico)

Therapeutic Category Vaccine, Live Virus

Synonyms German Measles Vaccine

Use Provide vaccine-induced immunity to rubella

Usual Dosage Children ≥12 months and Adults: S.C.: 0.5 mL in outer aspect of upper arm; children vaccinated before 12 months of age should be revaccinated

Mechanism of Action Rubella vaccine is a live attenuated vaccine that contains the Wistar Institute RA 27/3 strain, which is adapted to and propagated in human diploid cell culture. It is the only strain of rubella vaccine marketed in the U.S. Antibody titers after immunization last 6 years without significant decline; 90% of those vaccinated have protection for at least 15 years.

Local Anesthetic/Vasoconstrictor Precautions No information available to require special precautions

Effects on Dental Treatment No effects or complications reported

Other Adverse Effects
>10%:
Dermatologic: Tenderness and erythema, urticaria, rash
Neuromuscular & skeletal: Arthralgias
1% to 10%:
Central nervous system: Malaise, fever, headache
Gastrointestinal: Sore throat
Miscellaneous: Lymphadenopathy
<1%:
Ocular: Optic neuritis
Miscellaneous: Hypersensitivity, allergic reactions to the vaccine

Drug Uptake
Onset of effect: Antibodies to the vaccine are detectable within 2-4 weeks following immunization
Duration: Protection against both clinical rubella and asymptomatic viremia is probably life-long. Vaccine-induced antibody levels have been shown to persist for at least 10 years without substantial decline. If the present pattern continues, it will provide a basis for the expectation that immunity following vaccination will be permanent. However, continued surveillance will be required to demonstrate this point.

Pregnancy Risk Factor X

Comments Federal law requires that the date of administration, the vaccine manufacturer, lot number of vaccine, and the administering person's name, title and address be entered into the patient's permanent record

Rubeola Vaccine *see* Measles Virus Vaccine, Live *on page 529*

Rubex® *see* Doxorubicin Hydrochloride *on page 299*

Rubidomycin Hydrochloride *see* Daunorubicin Hydrochloride *on page 252*

Rubramin-PC® *see* Cyanocobalamin *on page 237*

Rufen® *see* Ibuprofen *on page 447*

Rum-K® *see* Potassium Chloride *on page 708*

Ru-Tuss® DE *see* Guaifenesin and Pseudoephedrine *on page 409*

Ru-Tuss® Liquid *see* Chlorpheniramine and Phenylephrine *on page 190*

Ru-Vert-M® *see* Meclizine Hydrochloride *on page 530*

Rymed® *see* Guaifenesin and Pseudoephedrine *on page 409*

Rymed-TR® *see* Guaifenesin and Phenylpropanolamine *on page 409*

Ryna-C® Liquid *see* Chlorpheniramine, Pseudoephedrine, and Codeine *on page 195*

Ryna-CX® *see* Guaifenesin, Pseudoephedrine, and Codeine *on page 410*

Ryna® Liquid [OTC] *see* Chlorpheniramine and Pseudoephedrine *on page 191*

Rynatan® Pediatric Suspension *see* Chlorpheniramine, Pyrilamine, and Phenylephrine *on page 195*

Rynatan® Tablet *see* Chlorpheniramine, Pyrilamine, and Phenylephrine *on page 195*

Rynatuss® Pediatric Suspension *see* Chlorpheniramine, Ephedrine, Phenylephrine, and Carbetapentane *on page 191*

Rythmol® *see* Propafenone Hydrochloride *on page 735*

S-2® *see* Epinephrine, Racemic *on page 314*

S5614 *see* Dexfenfluramine Hydrochloride *on page 262*

Sabin Vaccine *see* Poliovirus Vaccine, Live, Trivalent, Oral *on page 702*

Safe Tussin 30 Liquid® [OTC] *see* Guaifenesin and Dextromethorphan *on page 408*

Safe Writing Practices *see page 1103*

SalAc® [OTC] *see* Salicylic Acid *on this page*

Salacid® *see* Salicylic Acid *on this page*

Salagen® *see* Pilocarpine (Dental) *on page 693*

Salbutamol (Mexico) *see* Albuterol *on page 27*

Saleto-200® [OTC] *see* Ibuprofen *on page 447*

Saleto-400® *see* Ibuprofen *on page 447*

Salflex® *see* Salsalate *on page 779*

Salgesic® *see* Salsalate *on page 779*

Salicilico, Acido (Mexico) *see* Salicylic Acid *on this page*

Salicylic Acid (sal i sil' ik as' id)

Brand Names ClearAway®; Compound W® [OTC]; Hydrisalic™; Ionil® [OTC]; Keralyt®; Panscol®; P&S® [OTC]; SalAc® [OTC]; Salacid®; Saligel™; Trans-Ver-Sal®

Canadian/Mexican Brand Names Acnex® (Canada); Acnomel® (Canada); Trans-Planta® (Canada); Trans-Ver-Sal® (Canada)

Therapeutic Category Keratolytic Agent

Synonyms Salicilico, Acido (Mexico)

Use Topically for its keratolytic effect in controlling seborrheic dermatitis or psoriasis of body and scalp, dandruff, and other scaling dermatoses; also used to remove warts, corns, and calluses

Usual Dosage

Lotion, cream, gel: Apply a thin layer to affected area once or twice daily

Plaster: Cut to size that covers the corn or callus, apply and leave in place for 48 hours; do not exceed 5 applications over a 14-day period

Solution: Apply a thin layer directly to wart using brush applicator once daily as directed for 1 week or until wart is removed

Mechanism of Action Produces desquamation of hyperkeratotic epithelium via dissolution of the intercellular cement which causes the cornified tissue to swell, soften, macerate, and desquamate. Salicylic acid is keratolytic at concentrations of 3% to 6%; it becomes destructive to tissue at concentrations >6%. Concentrations of 6% to 60% are used to remove corns and warts and in the treatment of psoriasis and other hyperkeratotic disorders.

Local Anesthetic/Vasoconstrictor Precautions No information available to require special precautions

Effects on Dental Treatment No effects or complications reported

Other Adverse Effects

>10%: Local: Burning and irritation at site of exposure on normal tissue

1% to 10%:

Central nervous system: Dizziness, mental confusion, headache

Otic: Tinnitus

Respiratory: Hyperventilation

Drug Interactions No data reported

Drug Uptake

Absorption: Absorbed percutaneously, but systemic toxicity is unlikely with normal use

Time to peak serum concentration: Topical: Within 5 hours of application with occlusion

Pregnancy Risk Factor C

Salicylic Acid and Benzoic Acid *see* Benzoic Acid and Salicylic Acid *on page 104*

Salicylic Acid and Lactic Acid (sal i sil' ik as' id & lak' tik as' id)
Brand Names Duofilm® Solution
Therapeutic Category Keratolytic Agent
Synonyms Lactic Acid and Salicylic Acid
Use Treatment of benign epithelial tumors such as warts
Local Anesthetic/Vasoconstrictor Precautions No information available to require special precautions
Effects on Dental Treatment No effects or complications reported
Comments Protect normal skin tissue with a ring of petrolatum surrounding the affected area; prior to application, soak affected area in hot water for at least 5 minutes; dry thoroughly with a clean towel

Salicylic Acid and Podophyllin *see* Podophyllin and Salicylic Acid *on page 701*

Salicylic Acid and Propylene Glycol
(sal i sil' ik as' id & proe' pi leen glye' cole)
Brand Names Keralyt® Gel
Therapeutic Category Keratolytic Agent
Synonyms Propylene Glycol and Salicylic Acid
Use Removal of excessive keratin in hyperkeratotic skin disorders, including various ichthyosis, keratosis palmaris and plantaris and psoriasis; may be used to remove excessive keratin in dorsal and plantar hyperkeratotic lesions
Local Anesthetic/Vasoconstrictor Precautions No information available to require special precautions
Effects on Dental Treatment No effects or complications reported

Salicylic Acid and Sulfur *see* Sulfur and Salicylic Acid *on page 813*
Saligel™ *see* Salicylic Acid *on previous page*
Salivart® [OTC] *see* Saliva Substitute *on this page*

Saliva Substitute (sa lye' va sub' stee tute)
Related Information
Artificial Saliva Products *on page 1050*
Patients Undergoing Cancer Therapy *on page 967*
Brand Names Glandosane® Spray [OTC]; Moi-Stir® [OTC]; MouthKote® [OTC]; Optimoist® [OTC]; Salivart® [OTC]; Xero-Lube® [OTC]
Therapeutic Category Gastrointestinal Agent, Miscellaneous; Saliva Substitute
Use Relief of dry mouth and throat in xerostomia
Usual Dosage Use as needed
Local Anesthetic/Vasoconstrictor Precautions No information available to require special precautions
Effects on Dental Treatment No effects or complications reported
Dosage Forms
Solution: 50 mL, 60 mL, 75 mL, 120 mL, 180 mL
Swabstix: 300s
Generic Available No

Salk Vaccine *see* Poliovirus Vaccine, Inactivated *on page 702*
Salmeterol, Hidroxinaftoato De (Mexico) *see* Salmeterol Xinafoate *on this page*

Salmeterol Xinafoate (sal me' te role zee na' foe ate)
Related Information
Respiratory Diseases *on page 924*
Brand Names Serevent®
Canadian/Mexican Brand Names Zantirel® (Mexico)
Therapeutic Category Adrenergic Agonist Agent; Antiasthmatic; Beta-2-Adrenergic Agonist Agent; Bronchodilator
Synonyms Salmeterol, Hidroxinaftoato De (Mexico)
Use Maintenance treatment of asthma and in prevention of bronchospasm in patients >12 years of age with reversible obstructive airway disease, including patients with symptoms of nocturnal asthma, who require regular treatment with inhaled, short-acting beta$_2$ agonists; prevention of exercise-induced bronchospasm
Usual Dosage
Inhalation: 42 mcg (2 puffs) twice daily (12 hours apart) for maintenance and prevention of symptoms of asthma

Prevention of exercise-induced asthma: 42 mcg (2 puffs) 30-60 minutes prior to exercise; additional doses should not be used for 12 hours

Mechanism of Action Relaxes bronchial smooth muscle by selective action on beta$_2$-receptors with little effect on heart rate; because salmeterol acts locally in the lung, therapeutic effect is not predicted by plasma levels

Local Anesthetic/Vasoconstrictor Precautions No information available to require special precautions

Effects on Dental Treatment No effects or complications reported

Other Adverse Effects

>10%:
 Central nervous system: Headache
 Respiratory: Pharyngitis

1% to 10%:
 Cardiovascular: Tachycardia, palpitations, elevation or depression of blood pressure, cardiac arrhythmias
 Central nervous system: Nervousness, CNS stimulation, hyperactivity, insomnia, malaise, dizziness
 Gastrointestinal: GI upset, diarrhea, nausea
 Neuromuscular & skeletal: Tremors (may be more common in the elderly), myalgias, back pain, joint pain
 Respiratory: Upper respiratory infection, cough, bronchitis

<1%: Miscellaneous: Immediate hypersensitivity reactions (rash, urticaria, bronchospasm)

Drug Interactions Vascular-system effects of salmeterol may be potentiated by MAO inhibitors and tricyclic antidepressants

Drug Uptake
 Onset of action: 5-20 minutes (average 10 minutes)
 Duration: 12 hours
 Serum half-life: 3-4 hours

Pregnancy Risk Factor C

Salsalate (sal' sa late)

Related Information
 Rheumatoid Arthritis, Osteoarthritis, and Joint Prostheses *on page 930*

Brand Names Argesic®-SA; Artha-G®; Disalcid®; Mono-Gesic®; Salflex®; Salgesic®; Salsitab®

Therapeutic Category Analgesic, Non-narcotic; Anti-inflammatory Agent; Antipyretic; Nonsteroidal Anti-inflammatory Agent (NSAID), Oral; Salicylate

Use Treatment of minor pain or fever; arthritis

Usual Dosage Adults: Oral: 3 g/day in 2-3 divided doses

 Dosing comments in renal impairment: In patients with end stage renal disease undergoing hemodialysis: 750 mg twice daily with an additional 500 mg after dialysis

Mechanism of Action Inhibits prostaglandin synthesis, acts on the hypothalamus heat-regulating center to reduce fever, blocks prostaglandin synthetase action which prevents formation of the platelet-aggregating substance thromboxane A$_2$

Local Anesthetic/Vasoconstrictor Precautions No information available to require special precautions

Effects on Dental Treatment No effects or complications reported

Other Adverse Effects

>10%: Gastrointestinal: Nausea, heartburn, stomach pains, dyspepsia, epigastric discomfort

1% to 10%:
 Central nervous system: Weakness, tiredness
 Dermatologic: Skin rash
 Gastrointestinal: Gastrointestinal ulceration
 Hematologic: Hemolytic anemia
 Respiratory: Troubled breathing
 Miscellaneous: Anaphylactic shock

<1%:
 Central nervous system: Insomnia, nervousness, jitters
 Hematologic: Leukopenia, thrombocytopenia, iron deficiency anemia, does not appear to inhibit platelet aggregation, occult bleeding
 Hepatic: Hepatotoxicity
 Renal: Impaired renal function
 Respiratory: Bronchospasm

Drug Interactions
 Decreased effect with urinary alkalinizers, antacids, corticosteroids; decreased effect of uricosurics, spironolactone
 Increased effect/toxicity of oral anticoagulants, hypoglycemics, methotrexate
 (Continued)

Salsalate *(Continued)*

Drug Uptake
Onset of action: Therapeutic effects occur within 3-4 days of continuous dosing
Absorption: Oral: Completely from the small intestine
Serum half-life: 7-8 hours

Pregnancy Risk Factor C

Salsitab® *see* Salsalate *on previous page*

Sal-Tropine® *see* Atropine Sulfate *on page 85*

Saluron® *see* Hydroflumethiazide *on page 437*

Salutensin® *see* Hydroflumethiazide and Reserpine *on page 438*

Salutensin-Demi® *see* Hydroflumethiazide and Reserpine *on page 438*

Sandimmune® *see* Cyclosporine *on page 243*

Sandoglobulin® *see* Immune Globulin, Intravenous *on page 454*

Sandostatin® *see* Octreotide Acetate *on page 633*

Sani-Supp® Suppository [OTC] *see* Glycerin *on page 402*

Sanorex® *see* Mazindol *on page 527*

Sansert® *see* Methysergide Maleate *on page 571*

Santyl® *see* Collagenase *on page 232*

Saquinavir Mesylate *(sa kwin' a veer mes' i late)*

Related Information
Systemic Viral Diseases *on page 934*

Brand Names Invirase®

Therapeutic Category Antiviral Agent, Oral

Use Treatment of advanced HIV infection, used in combination with older nucleoside analog medications

Usual Dosage Oral: 600 mg 3 times/day within 2 hours after a full meal; use in combination with a nucleoside analog (AZT or ddC)

Local Anesthetic/Vasoconstrictor Precautions No information available to require special precautions

Effects on Dental Treatment No effects or complications reported

Drug Uptake
Absorption: Incomplete; food, especially high fat diets, may increase the absorption and oral bioavailability of saquinavir by five-fold

Sargramostim *(sar gram' oh stim)*

Brand Names Leukine™

Canadian/Mexican Brand Names Leucomax® (Mexico)

Therapeutic Category Colony Stimulating Factor

Synonyms GM-CSF; Granulocyte-Macrophage Colony Stimulating Factor; rGM-CSF

Use Myeloid reconstitution after autologous bone marrow transplantation; to accelerate myeloid recovery in patients with non-Hodgkin's lymphoma, Hodgkin's lymphoma, and acute lymphoblastic leukemia undergoing autologous BMT; following induction chemotherapy in patients with acute myelogenous leukemia to shorten time to neutrophil recovery

Usual Dosage All orders should be scheduled between 8 AM and 10 AM daily
Children and Adults: I.V. infusion over ≥2 hours or S.C.
Bone marrow transplantation failure or engraftment delay: I.V.: 250 mcg/m^2/day for 14 days. The dose can be repeated after 7 days off therapy if engraftment has not occurred. If engraftment still has not occurred, a third course of 500 mcg/m^2/day for 14 days may be tried after another 7 days off therapy. If there is still no engraftment, it is unlikely that further dose escalation be beneficial.
Myeloid reconstitution after autologous bone marrow transplant: I.V.: 250 mcg/m^2/day to begin 2-4 hours after the marrow infusion on day 0 of autologous bone marrow transplant or ≥24 hours after chemotherapy or 12 hours after last dose of radiotherapy. If significant adverse effects or "first dose" reaction is seen at this dose, discontinue the drug until toxicity resolves, then restart at a reduced dose of 125 mcg/m^2/day.
Length of therapy: Bone marrow transplant patients: GM-CSF should be administered daily for up to 30 days or until the ANC has reached 1000/mm^3 for 3 consecutive days following the expected chemotherapy-induced neutrophil-nadir
Cancer chemotherapy recovery: I.V.: 3-15 mcg/kg/day for 14-21 days; maximum daily dose is 15 mcg/kg/day due to dose-related adverse effects; **discontinue therapy** if the ANC count is >20,000/mm^3

Excessive blood counts return to normal or baseline levels within 3-7 days following cessation of therapy

Mechanism of Action Stimulates proliferation, differentiation and functional activity of neutrophils, eosinophils, monocytes, and macrophages; see table.

Proliferation/Differentiation	G-CSF (Filgrastim)	GM-CSF (Sargramostim)
Neutrophils	Yes	Yes
Eosinophils	No	Yes
Macrophages	No	Yes
Neutrophil migration	Enhanced	Inhibited

Local Anesthetic/Vasoconstrictor Precautions No information available to require special precautions

Effects on Dental Treatment No effects or complications reported

Other Adverse Effects

>10%:
Cardiovascular: Tachycardia
Central nervous system: Neutropenic fever, fever
Dermatologic: Alopecia
Gastrointestinal: Nausea, vomiting, diarrhea, mucositis
Hematologic: Thrombocytopenia
Neuromuscular & skeletal: Skeletal pain

1% to 10%:
Cardiovascular: Chest pain, peripheral edema
Central nervous system: Headache
Dermatologic: Skin rash
Endocrine & metabolic: Fluid retention
Gastrointestinal: Anorexia, stomatitis, sore throat, constipation
Hematologic: Leukocytosis, capillary leak syndrome
Neuromuscular & skeletal: Weakness
Local: Pain at injection site
Respiratory: Dyspnea, cough

<1%:
Cardiovascular: Transient supraventricular arrhythmia, pericarditis
Local: Thrombophlebitis
Miscellaneous: Anaphylactic reaction

Drug Uptake
Onset of action: Increase in WBC in 7-14 days
Duration: WBC will return to baseline within 1 week after discontinuing drug
Serum half-life: 2 hours
Time to peak serum concentration: S.C.: Within 1-2 hours

Pregnancy Risk Factor C

Comments Has been demonstrated to accelerate myeloid engraftment in autologous bone marrow transplant, decrease median duration of antibiotic administration, reduce the median duration of infectious episodes, and shorten the median duration of hospitalization, no difference in relapse rate or survival or disease response has been found in placebo-controlled trials. Safety and efficacy of GM-CSF given simultaneously with cytotoxic chemotherapy have not been established. Concurrent treatment may increase myelosuppression. Precaution should be exercised in the usage of GM-CSF in any malignancy with myeloid characteristics. GM-CSF can potentially act as a growth factor for any tumor type, particularly myeloid malignancies. Tumors of nonhematopoietic origin may have surface receptors for GM-CSF.

Sarna [OTC] see Camphor, Menthol, and Phenol on page 146

Sastid® Plain Therapeutic Shampoo and Acne Wash [OTC] see Sulfur and Salicylic Acid on page 813

Scabene® see Lindane on page 504

Scleromate™ see Morrhuate Sodium on page 592

Scopolamine (skoe pol′ a meen)

Brand Names Isopto® Hyoscine; Transderm Scop®

Therapeutic Category Anticholinergic Agent; Anticholinergic Agent, Ophthalmic; Anticholinergic Agent, Transdermal; Ophthalmic Agent, Mydriatic

Use Preoperative medication to produce amnesia and decrease salivation and respiratory secretions to produce cycloplegia and mydriasis; treatment of iridocyclitis, prevention of nausea and vomiting by motion; produces more CNS depression, mydriasis, and cycloplegia but less effective in preventing reflex bradycardia and effecting the intestines than atropine

(Continued)

Scopolamine *(Continued)*

Usual Dosage
Preoperatively:
Children: I.M., S.C.: 6 mcg/kg/dose (maximum: 0.3 mg/dose) or 0.2 mg/m^2 may be repeated every 6-8 hours **or** alternatively:
4-7 months: 0.1 mg
7 months to 3 years: 0.15 mg
3-8 years: 0.2 mg
8-12 years: 0.3 mg
Adults: I.M., I.V., S.C.: 0.3-0.65 mg; may be repeated every 4-6 hours

Motion sickness: Transdermal: Children >12 years and Adults: Apply 1 disc behind the ear at least 4 hours prior to exposure and every 3 days as needed; effective if applied as soon as 2-3 hours before anticipated need, best if 12 hours before

Ophthalmic:
Refraction:
Children: Instill 1 drop of 0.25% to eye(s) twice daily for 2 days before procedure
Adults: Instill 1-2 drops of 0.25% to eye(s) 1 hour before procedure
Iridocyclitis:
Children: Instill 1 drop of 0.25% to eye(s) up to 3 times/day
Adults: Instill 1-2 drops of 0.25% to eye(s) up to 4 times/day

Mechanism of Action Blocks the action of acetylcholine at parasympathetic sites in smooth muscle, secretory glands and the CNS; increases cardiac output, dries secretions, antagonizes histamine and serotonin

Local Anesthetic/Vasoconstrictor Precautions No information available to require special precautions

Effects on Dental Treatment Over 10% of patients medicated with scopolamine patch (Transderm Scop) will experience significant dry mouth. This will disappear with cessation of drug therapy.

Other Adverse Effects
Ophthalmic:
>10%: Ocular: Blurred vision, photophobia
1% to 10%:
Ocular: Local irritation, increased intraocular pressure
Respiratory: Congestion
<1%:
Cardiovascular: Vascular congestion, edema
Central nervous system: Drowsiness
Dermatologic: Eczematoid dermatitis
Ocular: Follicular conjunctivitis
Miscellaneous: Exudate
Systemic:
>10%:
Gastrointestinal: Constipation, dry mouth
Local: Irritation at injection site
Miscellaneous: Decreased sweating, dry nose, throat, or skin
1% to 10%: Decreased flow of breast milk, difficulty in swallowing, increased sensitivity to light
<1%:
Cardiovascular: Orthostatic hypotension
Central nervous system: Confusion, drowsiness, headache, loss of memory, ataxia, weakness, tiredness
Dermatologic: Skin rash
Gastrointestinal: Bloated feeling, nausea, vomiting
Genitourinary: Difficult urination
Ocular: Increased intraocular pain, blurred vision, ventricular fibrillation, tachycardia, palpitations
Note: Systemic adverse effects have been reported following ophthalmic administration

Drug Interactions
Decreased effect of acetaminophen, levodopa, ketoconazole, digoxin, riboflavin, potassium chloride in wax matrix preparations
Increased toxicity: Additive adverse effects with other anticholinergic agents; GI absorption of the following drugs may be affected: acetaminophen, levodopa, ketoconazole, digoxin, riboflavin, potassium chloride wax-matrix preparations

Drug Uptake
Onset of effect:
Oral, I.M.: 0.5-1 hour

I.V.: 10 minutes
Duration of effect:
  Oral, I.M.: 4-6 hours
  I.V.: 2 hours
Absorption: Well absorbed by all routes of administration
Pregnancy Risk Factor C

Scopolamine and Phenylephrine see Phenylephrine and Scopolamine on page 685

Scot-Tussin® [OTC] see Guaifenesin on page 407

Scot-Tussin® DM Cough Chasers [OTC] see Dextromethorphan on page 266

Sebaquin® [OTC] see Iodoquinol on page 466

Sebizon® see Sodium Sulfacetamide on page 793

Sebulex® [OTC] see Sulfur and Salicylic Acid on page 813

Sebulon® [OTC] see Pyrithione Zinc on page 755

Secobarbital and Amobarbital see Amobarbital and Secobarbital on page 55

Secobarbital Sodium (see koe bar' bi tal sow' dee um)
Brand Names Seconal™
Canadian/Mexican Brand Names Novo-Secobarb® (Canada)
Therapeutic Category Barbiturate; Hypnotic; Sedative
Use Short-term treatment of insomnia and as preanesthetic agent
Usual Dosage Hypnotic:
  Children: I.M.: 3-5 mg/kg/dose; maximum: 100 mg/dose

  Adults:
    I.M.: 100-200 mg/dose
    I.V.: 50-250 mg/dose

  Slightly dialyzable (5% to 20%)
Mechanism of Action Interferes with transmission of impulses from the thalamus to the cortex of the brain resulting in an imbalance in central inhibitory and facilitatory mechanisms
Local Anesthetic/Vasoconstrictor Precautions No information available to require special precautions
Effects on Dental Treatment No effects or complications reported
Other Adverse Effects
  >10%:
    Central nervous system: Dizziness, lightheadedness, drowsiness, "hang-over" effect
    Local: Pain at injection site
  1% to 10%:
    Central nervous system: Confusion, mental depression, unusual excitement, nervousness, faint feeling, headache, insomnia, nightmares
    Gastrointestinal: Constipation, nausea, vomiting
  <1%:
    Cardiovascular: Hypotension
    Central nervous system: Hallucinations
    Dermatologic: Skin rash, exfoliative dermatitis, Stevens-Johnson syndrome
    Hematologic: Megaloblastic anemia, thrombocytopenia, agranulocytosis
    Local: Thrombophlebitis
    Respiratory: Respiratory depression
Drug Interactions
  Decreased effect of betamethasone and other corticosteroids, TCAs, chloramphenicol, estrogens, cyclophosphamide, oral anticoagulants, doxycycline, theophylline
  Increased effect/toxicity with CNS depressants, chloramphenicol, chlorpropamide
Drug Uptake
  Onset of hypnosis:
    Oral: Within 1-3 minutes
    I.V. injection: Within 15-30 minutes
  Duration: ~15 minutes
  Absorption: Oral: Well absorbed (90%)
  Serum half-life: 25 hours
  Time to peak serum concentration: Within 2-4 hours
Pregnancy Risk Factor D

Seconal™ see Secobarbital Sodium on this page
Secran® see Vitamins, Multiple on page 901

Secretin (see' kre tin)
Brand Names Secretin-Ferring Injection
Therapeutic Category Diagnostic Agent, Pancreatic Exocrine Insufficiency; Diagnostic Agent, Zollinger-Ellison Syndrome and Pancreatic Exocrine Disease
Use Diagnosis of Zollinger-Ellison syndrome, chronic pancreatic dysfunction, and some hepatobiliary diseases such as obstructive jaundice resulting from cancer or stones in the biliary tract
Usual Dosage Potency of secretin is expressed in terms of clinical units (CU).
I.V.:
Pancreatic function: 1 CU/kg slow I.V. injection over 1 minute
Zollinger-Ellison: 2 CU/kg slow I.V. injection over 1 minute
Mechanism of Action Hormone normally secreted by duodenal mucosa and upper jejunal mucosa which increases the volume and bicarbonate content of pancreatic juice; stimulates the flow of hepatic bile with a high bicarbonate concentration, stimulates gastrin release in patients with Zollinger-Ellison syndrome
Local Anesthetic/Vasoconstrictor Precautions No information available to require special precautions
Effects on Dental Treatment No effects or complications reported
Other Adverse Effects <1%:
Cardiovascular: Venous spasm
Central nervous system: Fainting
Miscellaneous: Hypersensitivity reactions
Drug Uptake
Inactivated by proteolytic enzymes if administered orally
Peak output of pancreatic secretions: Within 30 minutes
Duration of action: At least 2 hours
Comments Potency of secretin is expressed in terms of clinical units

Secretin-Ferring Injection see Secretin on this page
Sectral® see Acebutolol Hydrochloride on page 12
Sedapap-10® see Butalbital Compound on page 133
Seldane® see Terfenadine on page 823
Seldane-D® see Terfenadine and Pseudoephedrine on page 824

Selegiline Hydrochloride (seh ledge' ah leen hye droe klor' ide)
Brand Names Eldepryl®
Canadian/Mexican Brand Names Novo-Selegiline® (Canada)
Therapeutic Category Anti-Parkinson's Agent
Use Adjunct in the management of parkinsonian patients in which levodopa/carbidopa therapy is deteriorating
Unlabeled use: Early Parkinson's disease
Investigational use: Alzheimer's disease
Selegiline is also being studied in Alzheimer's disease. Small studies have shown some improvement in behavioral and cognitive performance in patients, however, further study is needed.
Usual Dosage Oral:
Adults: 5 mg twice daily with breakfast and lunch or 10 mg in the morning
Elderly: Initial: 5 mg in the morning, may increase to a total of 10 mg/day
Mechanism of Action Potent monoamine oxidase (MAO) type-B inhibitor; MAO-B plays a major role in the metabolism of dopamine; selegiline may also increase dopaminergic activity by interfering with dopamine reuptake at the synapse
Local Anesthetic/Vasoconstrictor Precautions Selegiline in doses of 10 mg a day or less does not inhibit type-A MAO. Therefore, there are no precautions with the use of vasoconstrictors.
Effects on Dental Treatment Anticholinergic side effects can cause a reduction of saliva production or secretion contributing to discomfort and dental disease (ie, caries, oral candidiasis and periodontal disease)
Other Adverse Effects
>10%:
Central nervous system: Mood changes, dyskinesias, dizziness
Gastrointestinal: Nausea, vomiting, dry mouth, abdominal pain
1% to 10%:
Cardiovascular: Orthostatic hypotension, arrhythmias, hypertension
Central nervous system: Hallucinations, confusion, depression, insomnia, agitation, loss of balance
Neuromuscular & skeletal: Increased involuntary movements, bradykinesia, muscle twitches

Miscellaneous: Bruxism

Drug Interactions Meperidine in combination with selegiline has caused agitation and delirium; it may be prudent to avoid other opioids as well

Drug Uptake
Onset of therapeutic effects: Within 1 hour
Duration: 24-72 hours
Serum half-life: 9 minutes

Pregnancy Risk Factor C

Selenium *see* Trace Metals *on page 857*

Selenium Sulfide (se lee' nee um sul' fide)
Brand Names Exsel®; Selsun®; Selsun Blue® [OTC]; Selsun Gold® for Women [OTC]

Canadian/Mexican Brand Names Versel® (Canada)

Therapeutic Category Shampoos

Use Treatment of itching and flaking of the scalp associated with dandruff, to control scalp seborrheic dermatitis; treatment of tinea versicolor

Usual Dosage I.V. in TPN solutions:
Children: 3 mcg/kg/day
Adults:
Metabolically stable: 20-40 mcg/day
Deficiency from prolonged TPN support: 100 mcg/day for 24 and 21 days

Mechanism of Action May block the enzymes involved in growth of epithelial tissue

Local Anesthetic/Vasoconstrictor Precautions No information available to require special precautions

Effects on Dental Treatment No effects or complications reported

Other Adverse Effects
>10%: Dermatologic: Unusual dryness or oiliness of scalp
1% to 10%:
Central nervous system: Lethargy
Dermatologic: Hair loss or discoloration
Gastrointestinal: Vomiting following long-term use on damaged skin, abdominal pain, garlic breath
Local: Irritation
Neuromuscular & skeletal: Tremors
Miscellaneous: Perspiration

Drug Interactions No data reported

Drug Uptake
Absorption: Topical: Not absorbed through intact skin, but can be absorbed through damaged skin

Pregnancy Risk Factor C

Sele-Pak® *see* Trace Metals *on page 857*

Selepen® *see* Trace Metals *on page 857*

Selestoject® *see* Betamethasone *on page 109*

Selsun® *see* Selenium Sulfide *on this page*

Selsun Blue® [OTC] *see* Selenium Sulfide *on this page*

Selsun Gold® for Women [OTC] *see* Selenium Sulfide *on this page*

Semicid® [OTC] *see* Nonoxynol 9 *on page 627*

Semprex-D® *see* Acrivastine and Pseudoephedrine *on page 22*

Senna (sen' na)
Brand Names Black Draught® [OTC]; Senna-Gen® [OTC]; Senokot® [OTC]; Senolax® [OTC]; X-Prep® Liquid [OTC]

Therapeutic Category Laxative, Stimulant

Use Short-term treatment of constipation; evacuate the colon for bowel or rectal examinations

Local Anesthetic/Vasoconstrictor Precautions No information available to require special precautions

Effects on Dental Treatment No effects or complications reported

Other Adverse Effects 1% to 10%: Gastrointestinal: Nausea, vomiting, diarrhea, abdominal cramps

Comments Some patients will experience considerable griping

Senna-Gen® [OTC] *see* Senna *on this page*

Senokot® [OTC] *see* Senna *on this page*

Senolax® [OTC] *see* Senna *on this page*

Sensorcaine® *see* Bupivacaine Hydrochloride *on page 127*

Sensorcaine®-MPF *see* Bupivacaine Hydrochloride *on page 127*

Septa® *see* Bacitracin, Neomycin, and Polymyxin B *on page 94*

Septisol® *see* Hexachlorophene *on page 424*

Septra® *see* Trimethoprim and Sulfamethoxazole *on page 874*

Septra® DS *see* Trimethoprim and Sulfamethoxazole *on page 874*

Ser-A-Gen® *see* Hydralazine, Hydrochlorothiazide, and Reserpine *on page 429*

Ser-Ap-Es® *see* Hydralazine, Hydrochlorothiazide, and Reserpine *on page 429*

Serathide® *see* Hydralazine, Hydrochlorothiazide, and Reserpine *on page 429*

Serax® *see* Oxazepam *on page 644*

Serentil® *see* Mesoridazine Besylate *on page 547*

Serevent® *see* Salmeterol Xinafoate *on page 778*

Sermorelin Acetate (ser moe rel' in as' e tate)
Brand Names Geref® Injection

Therapeutic Category Diagnostic Agent, Pituitary Function

Use Evaluate ability of the somatotroph of the pituitary gland to secrete growth hormone

Local Anesthetic/Vasoconstrictor Precautions No information available to require special precautions

Effects on Dental Treatment No effects or complications reported

Other Adverse Effects 1% to 10%:
Cardiovascular: Transient flushing of the face, tightness in the chest
Central nervous system: Headache
Gastrointestinal: Nausea, vomiting
Local: Pain, redness, and/or swelling at the injection site

Seromycin® Pulvules® *see* Cycloserine *on page 242*

Serophene® *see* Clomiphene Citrate *on page 218*

Serpalan® *see* Reserpine *on page 765*

Serpasil® *see* Reserpine *on page 765*

Sertraline Hydrochloride (ser' tra leen hye droe klor' ide)
Related Information
Vasoconstrictor Interactions With Antidepressants *on page 1108*

Brand Names Zoloft™

Therapeutic Category Antidepressant, Selective Serotonin Reuptake Inhibitor

Use Treatment of major depression; also being studied for use in obesity and obsessive-compulsive disorder

Usual Dosage Oral:
Adults: Start with 50 mg/day in the morning and increase by 50 mg/day increments every 2-3 days if tolerated to 100 mg/day; additional increases may be necessary; maximum dose: 200 mg/day. If somnolence is noted, give at bedtime.

Elderly: Start treatment with 25 mg/day in the morning and increase by 25 mg/day increments every 2-3 days if tolerated to 75-100 mg/day; additional increases may be necessary; maximum dose: 200 mg/day

Hemodialysis effects: Not removed by hemodialysis

Mechanism of Action Antidepressant with selective inhibitory effects on presynaptic serotonin (5-HT) reuptake

Local Anesthetic/Vasoconstrictor Precautions Although caution should be used in patients taking tricyclic antidepressants, no interactions have been reported with vasoconstrictor and sertraline, a nontricyclic antidepressant which acts to increase serotonin

Effects on Dental Treatment No effects or complications reported

Other Adverse Effects
1% to 10%: In clinical trials, dizziness and nausea were two most frequent side effects that led to discontinuation of therapy
Cardiovascular: Palpitations
Central nervous system: Insomnia, agitation, dizziness, headache, somnolence, nervousness, fatigue
Dermatologic: Dermatological reactions, sweating
Gastrointestinal: Dry mouth, diarrhea or loose stools, nausea, constipation
Genitourinary: Sexual dysfunction in men, micturition disorders
Neuromuscular & skeletal: Pain, tremors
Ocular: Visual difficulty
Otic: Tinnitus

Drug Interactions
All serotonin reuptake inhibitors are capable of inhibiting cytochrome P-450 IID6 isoenzyme enzyme system.

Increased/decreased effect of lithium (both increases and decreases level has been reported)

Increased toxicity of diazepam, trazodone via decreased clearance; increased toxicity with MAO inhibitors (hyperpyrexia, tremors, seizures, delirium, coma)

Displace protein bound drugs

Drug Uptake
Absorption: Slow
Serum half-life:
Parent: 24 hours
Metabolites: 66 hours

Pregnancy Risk Factor B

Serutan® [OTC] *see* Psyllium *on page 750*

Serzone® *see* Nefazodone *on page 608*

Shur-Seal® [OTC] *see* Nonoxynol 9 *on page 627*

Siblin® [OTC] *see* Psyllium *on page 750*

Silace-C® [OTC] *see* Docusate and Casanthranol *on page 295*

Silain® [OTC] *see* Simethicone *on next page*

Silaminic® Cold Syrup [OTC] *see* Chlorpheniramine and Phenylpropanolamine *on page 190*

Silaminic® Expectorant [OTC] *see* Guaifenesin and Phenylpropanolamine *on page 409*

Sildicon-E® [OTC] *see* Guaifenesin and Phenylpropanolamine *on page 409*

Siltussin-CF® [OTC] *see* Guaifenesin, Phenylpropanolamine, and Dextromethorphan *on page 410*

Silvadene® *see* Silver Sulfadiazine *on next page*

Silver Nitrate (sil′ ver nye′ trate)

Therapeutic Category Ophthalmic Agent, Miscellaneous; Topical Skin Product

Synonyms AgNO₃

Use Prevention of gonococcal ophthalmia neonatorum; cauterization of wounds and sluggish ulcers, removal of granulation tissue and warts

Usual Dosage
Children and Adults:
Ointment: Apply in an apertured pad on affected area or lesion for approximately 5 days
Sticks: Apply to mucous membranes and other moist skin surfaces only on area to be treated 2-3 times/week for 2-3 weeks
Topical solution: Apply a cotton applicator dipped in solution on the affected area 2-3 times/week for 2-3 weeks

Mechanism of Action Free silver ions precipitate bacterial proteins by combining with chloride in tissue forming silver chloride; coagulates cellular protein to form an eschar; silver ions or salts or colloidal silver preparations can inhibit the growth of both gram-positive and gram-negative bacteria. This germicidal action is attributed to the precipitation of bacterial proteins by liberated silver ions. Silver nitrate coagulates cellular protein to form an eschar, and this mode of action is the postulated mechanism for control of benign hematuria, rhinitis, and recurrent pneumothorax.

Local Anesthetic/Vasoconstrictor Precautions No information available to require special precautions

Effects on Dental Treatment No effects or complications reported

Other Adverse Effects
>10%:
Local: Burning and skin irritation
Ocular: Chemical conjunctivitis
1% to 10%:
Dermatologic: Staining of the skin
Hematologic: Methemoglobinemia
Ocular: Cauterization of the cornea, blindness

Drug Uptake
Absorption: Because silver ions readily combine with protein, there is minimal GI and cutaneous absorption of the 0.5% and 1% preparations

Pregnancy Risk Factor C

Comments Applicators are **not** for ophthalmic use

Silver Protein, Mild (sil′ ver pro′ teen mild)

Brand Names Argyrol® S.S. 20%

Therapeutic Category Antibiotic, Topical

(Continued)

Silver Protein, Mild *(Continued)*

Use Stain and coagulate mucus in eye surgery which is then removed by irrigation; eye infections

Local Anesthetic/Vasoconstrictor Precautions No information available to require special precautions

Effects on Dental Treatment No effects or complications reported

Silver Sulfadiazine *(sil' ver sul fa dye' a zeen)*

Brand Names Silvadene®; SSD™; SSD-AF™; Thermazene™

Canadian/Mexican Brand Names Dermazin® (Canada); Flamazine® (Canada)

Therapeutic Category Antibacterial, Topical

Use Prevention and treatment of infection in second and third degree burns

Usual Dosage Children and Adults: Topical: Apply once or twice daily with a sterile-gloved hand; apply to a thickness of $1/16$"; burned area should be covered with cream at all times

Mechanism of Action Acts upon the bacterial cell wall and cell membrane. Bactericidal for many gram-negative and gram-positive bacteria and is effective against yeast. Active against *Pseudomonas aeruginosa, Pseudomonas maltophilia, Enterobacteriae* species, *Klebsiella* species, *Serratia* species, *Escherichia coli, Proteus mirabilis, Morganella morganii, Providencia rettgeri, Proteus vulgaris, Providencia* species, *Citrobacter* species, *Acinetobacter calcoaceticus, Staphylococcus aureus, Staphylococcus epidermidis, Enterococcus* species, *Candida albicans, Corynebacterium diphtheriae,* and *Clostridium perfringens*

Local Anesthetic/Vasoconstrictor Precautions No information available to require special precautions

Effects on Dental Treatment No effects or complications reported

Other Adverse Effects
>10%: Local: Pain, burning
1% to 10%:
Dermatologic: Itching, rash, erythema multiforme, skin discoloration
Genitourinary: Interstitial nephritis
Hematologic: Hemolytic anemia, leukopenia, agranulocytosis, aplastic anemia
Hepatic: Hepatitis
Sensitivity reactions: Allergic reactions may be related to sulfa component
<1%: Ocular: Photosensitivity

Drug Interactions Decreased effect: Topical proteolytic enzymes are inactivated

Drug Uptake
Absorption: Significant percutaneous absorption of sulfadiazine can occur especially when applied to extensive burns
Serum half-life: 10 hours and is prolonged in patients with renal insufficiency
Time to peak serum concentration: Within 3-11 days of continuous therapy

Pregnancy Risk Factor C

Simethicone *(sye meth' i kone)*

Brand Names Flatulex® [OTC]; Gas Relief® [OTC]; Gas-X® [OTC]; Mylanta® Gas [OTC]; Mylicon® [OTC]; Phazyme® [OTC]; Silain® [OTC]

Canadian/Mexican Brand Names Ovol® (Canada)

Therapeutic Category Antiflatulent

Use Relieves flatulence and functional gastric bloating, and postoperative gas pains

Usual Dosage Oral:
Children <12 years: 40 mg 4 times/day
Children >12 years and Adults: 40-120 mg after meals and at bedtime as needed, not to exceed 500 mg/day

Mechanism of Action Decreases the surface tension of gas bubbles thereby disperses and prevents gas pockets in the GI system

Local Anesthetic/Vasoconstrictor Precautions No information available to require special precautions

Effects on Dental Treatment No effects or complications reported

Other Adverse Effects No data reported

Drug Interactions No data reported

Pregnancy Risk Factor C

Simethicone and Calcium Carbonate *see* Calcium Carbonate and Simethicone *on page 141*

Simethicone and Magaldrate *see* Magaldrate and Simethicone *on page 521*

Simron® [OTC] *see* Ferrous Gluconate *on page 360*

Simvastatin (sim' va stat in)
Related Information
Cardiovascular Diseases *on page 912*
Brand Names Zocor™
Therapeutic Category HMG-CoA Reductase Inhibitor; Lipid Lowering Drugs
Use Adjunct to dietary therapy to decrease elevated serum total and LDL cholesterol concentrations in primary hypercholesterolemia
Usual Dosage Adults: Oral: Start with 5-10 mg/day as a single bedtime dose; if LDL is ≤90 mg/dL start with 5 mg; if LDL >100 mg/dL, start with 10 mg/day; increase every 4 weeks as needed; maximum dose: 40 mg/day
Mechanism of Action Simvastatin is a methylated derivative of lovastatin that acts by competitively inhibiting 3 hydroxy 3 methylglutaryl coenzyme A reductase (HMB CoA reductase), the enzyme that catalyzes the rate-limiting step in cholesterol biosynthesis
Local Anesthetic/Vasoconstrictor Precautions No information available to require special precautions
Effects on Dental Treatment No effects or complications reported
Other Adverse Effects
1% to 10%:
Central nervous system: Headache, dizziness
Dermatologic: Rash
Gastrointestinal: Flatulence, abdominal cramps, diarrhea, constipation, nausea, dyspepsia, heartburn
Neuromuscular & skeletal: Myalgia
Renal: Elevated creatine phosphokinase (CPK)
<1%:
Central nervous system: Dizziness
Gastrointestinal: Dysgeusia
Ocular: Lenticular opacities, blurred vision
Drug Interactions
Increased effect of warfarin, erythromycin, niacin
Increased toxicity of cyclosporin, gemfibrozil
Concurrent use of erythromycin and HMG-CoA reductase inhibitors may result in rhabdomyolysis
Drug Uptake
Absorption: Oral: Although 85% is absorbed following administration, <5% reaches the general circulation due to an extensive first-pass effect
Time to peak concentrations: 1.3-2.4 hours
Pregnancy Risk Factor X

Sinarest® 12 Hour Nasal Solution *see* Oxymetazoline Hydrochloride *on page 649*

Sinarest® Nasal Solution [OTC] *see* Phenylephrine Hydrochloride *on page 685*

Sincalide (sin' ka lide)
Brand Names Kinevac®
Therapeutic Category Diagnostic Agent, Gallbladder Function
Synonyms C8-CCK; OP-CCK
Use Postevacuation cholecystography; gallbladder bile sampling; stimulate pancreatic secretion for analysis
Usual Dosage Adults: I.V.:
Contraction of gallbladder: 0.02 mcg/kg over 30 seconds to 1 minute, may repeat in 15 minutes a 0.04 mcg/kg dose
Pancreatic function: 0.02 mcg/kg over 30 minutes administered after secretin
Mechanism of Action Stimulates contraction of the gallbladder and simultaneous relaxation of the sphincter of Oddi, inhibits gastric emptying, and increases intestinal motility. Graded doses have been shown to produce graded decreases in small intestinal transit time, thought to be mediated by acetylcholine.
Local Anesthetic/Vasoconstrictor Precautions No information available to require special precautions
Effects on Dental Treatment No effects or complications reported
Other Adverse Effects 1% to 10%:
Cardiovascular: Flushing
Central nervous system: Dizziness
Gastrointestinal: Nausea, abdominal pain, urge to defecate
Drug Uptake
Onset of action: Contraction of the gallbladder occurs within 5-15 minutes
(Continued)

789

Sincalide *(Continued)*

Duration: ~1 hour

Pregnancy Risk Factor B

Comments Preparation of solution: To reconstitute, add 5 mL sterile water for injection to the vial; the solution may be kept at room temperature; use within 24 hours after reconstitution; delivers 1 mcg/mL

Sine-Aid® IB [OTC] *see* Pseudoephedrine and Ibuprofen *on page 750*

Sinemet® *see* Levodopa and Carbidopa *on page 495*

Sinequan® *see* Doxepin Hydrochloride *on page 298*

Sinubid® *see* Phenyltoloxamine, Phenylpropanolamine, and Acetaminophen *on page 688*

Sinufed® Timecelles® *see* Guaifenesin and Pseudoephedrine *on page 409*

Sinumist®-SR Capsulets® *see* Guaifenesin *on page 407*

Sinusol-B® *see* Brompheniramine Maleate *on page 124*

Sinutab® Tablets [OTC] *see* Acetaminophen, Chlorpheniramine, and Pseudoephedrine *on page 17*

SK and F 104864 *see* Topotecan Hydrochloride *on page 855*

Skelaxin® *see* Metaxalone *on page 551*

Skelex® *see* Chlorzoxazone *on page 200*

SKF 104864 *see* Topotecan Hydrochloride *on page 855*

SKF 104864-A *see* Topotecan Hydrochloride *on page 855*

Skin Test Antigens, Multiple *(skin test an' tee gens mul' ti pul)*

Brand Names Multitest CMI®

Therapeutic Category Diagnostic Agent, Skin Test

Use Detection of nonresponsiveness to antigens by means of delayed hypersensitivity skin testing

Usual Dosage Select only test sites that permit sufficient surface area and subcutaneous tissue to allow adequate penetration of all eight points, avoid hairy areas

Press loaded unit into the skin with sufficient pressure to puncture the skin and allow adequate penetration of all points, maintain firm contact for at least 5 seconds, during application the device should not be "rocked" back and forth and side to side without removing any of the test heads from the skin sites

If adequate pressure is applied it will be possible to observe:

1. The puncture marks of the nine tines on each of the eight test heads
2. An imprint of the circular platform surrounding each test head
3. Residual antigen and glycerin at each of the eight sites

If any of the above three criteria are not fully followed, the test results may not be reliable

Reading should be done in good light, read the test sites at both 24 and 48 hours, the largest reaction recorded from the two readings at each test site should be used; if two readings are not possible, a single 48 hour is recommended

A positive reaction from any of the seven delayed hypersensitivity skin test antigens is **induration ≥2 mm** providing there is no induration at the negative control site; the size of the induration reactions with this test may be smaller than those obtained with other intradermal procedures

Local Anesthetic/Vasoconstrictor Precautions No information available to require special precautions

Effects on Dental Treatment No effects or complications reported

Other Adverse Effects 1% to 10%: Local: Irritation

Pregnancy Risk Factor C

Comments Contains disposable plastic applicator consisting of eight sterile test heads preloaded with the following seven delayed hypersensitivity skin test antigens and glycerin negative control for percutaneous administration

Test Head No. 1 = Tetanus toxoid antigen
Test Head No. 2 = Diphtheria toxoid antigen
Test Head No. 3 = *Streptococcus* antigen
Test Head No. 4 = Tuberculin, old
Test Head No. 5 = Glycerin negative control
Test Head No. 6 = *Candida* antigen
Test Head No. 7 = *Trichophyton* antigen
Test Head No. 8 = *Proteus* antigen

Slo-bid™ *see* Theophylline/Aminophylline *on page 832*

Slo-Niacin® [OTC] *see* Niacin *on page 614*

Slo-Phyllin® *see* Theophylline/Aminophylline *on page 832*

Slo-Phyllin® GG *see* Theophylline and Guaifenesin *on page 836*

Slow FE® [OTC] *see* Ferrous Sulfate *on page 360*

Slow-K® *see* Potassium Chloride *on page 708*

Slow-Mag® [OTC] *see* Magnesium Chloride *on page 521*

SMZ-TMP *see* Trimethoprim and Sulfamethoxazole *on page 874*

Snaplets-EX® [OTC] *see* Guaifenesin and Phenylpropanolamine *on page 409*

Sodium Ascorbate (sow' dee um a skor' bate)

Brand Names Cenolate®

Therapeutic Category Urinary Acidifying Agent; Vitamin, Water Soluble

Use Dental and Medical: Prevention and treatment of scurvy and to acidify urine

Usual Dosage Oral, I.V.:

Children:

Scurvy: 100-300 mg/day in divided doses for at least 2 weeks

Urinary acidification: 500 mg every 6-8 hours

Dietary supplement: 35-45 mg/day

Adults:

Scurvy: 100-250 mg 1-2 times/day for at least 2 weeks

Urinary acidification: 4-12 g/day in divided doses

Dietary supplement: 50-60 mg/day

Prevention and treatment of cold: 1-3 g/day

Local Anesthetic/Vasoconstrictor Precautions No information available to require special precautions

Effects on Dental Treatment No effects or complications reported

Other Adverse Effects 1% to 10%:

Cardiovascular: Hypotension with rapid I.V. administration

Gastrointestinal: Diarrhea

Local: Soreness at injection site

Miscellaneous: Precipitation of cystine, oxalate or urate renal stones

Contraindications Large doses during pregnancy

Warnings/Precautions Use with caution in diabetics, patients with renal calculi, and those on sodium-restricted diets

Drug Interactions No data reported

Drug Uptake

Therapeutic serum levels: 0.4-1.5 mg/dL

Time to peak serum concentration: Oral: Within 2-3 hours

Pregnancy Risk Factor C

Breast-feeding Considerations No data reported

Dosage Forms

Crystals: 1020 mg per ¼ teaspoonful [ascorbic acid 900 mg]

Injection: 250 mg/mL [ascorbic acid 222 mg/mL] (30 mL); 562.5 mg/mL [ascorbic acid 500 mg/mL] (1 mL, 2 mL)

Tablet: 585 mg [ascorbic acid 500 mg]

Generic Available Yes

Sodium Benzoate and Caffeine *see* Caffeine and Sodium Benzoate *on page 136*

Sodium Cellulose Phosphate *see* Cellulose Sodium Phosphate *on page 175*

Sodium Cromoglycate (Canada) *see* Cromolyn Sodium *on page 235*

Sodium Fluoride *see* Fluoride *on page 374*

Sodium Hyaluronate (sow' dee um hye al yoor on' nate)

Brand Names Amvisc®; Healon®; Healon® GV; Healon® Yellow

Therapeutic Category Ophthalmic Agent, Viscoeleastic

Synonyms Hyaluronic Acid

Use Surgical aid in cataract extraction, intraocular implantation, corneal transplant, glaucoma filtration, and retinal attachment surgery

Usual Dosage Depends upon procedure (slowly introduce a sufficient quantity into eye)

Mechanism of Action Functions as a tissue lubricant and is thought to play an important role in modulating the interactions between adjacent tissues. Sodium hyaluronate is a polysaccharide which is distributed widely in the extracellular matrix of connective tissue in man. (Vitreous and aqueous humor of the eye, synovial fluid, skin, and umbilical cord.) Sodium hyaluronate forms a viscoelastic solution in water (at physiological pH and ionic strength) which makes it suitable for aqueous and vitreous humor in ophthalmic surgery.

Local Anesthetic/Vasoconstrictor Precautions No information available to require special precautions

Effects on Dental Treatment No effects or complications reported

(Continued)

Sodium Hyaluronate *(Continued)*

Other Adverse Effects 1% to 10%: Ocular: Corneal edema, corneal decompensation, transient postoperative increase in IOP, postoperative inflammatory reactions (iritis, hypopyon)

Drug Uptake
Absorption: Following intravitreous injection, diffusion occurs slowly

Pregnancy Risk Factor C

Comments Bring drug to room temperature before instillation into eye

Sodium Hyaluronate-Chrondroitin Sulfate *see* Chondroitin Sulfate-Sodium Hyaluronate *on page 203*

Sodium P.A.S. *see* Aminosalicylate Sodium *on page 47*

Sodium-PCA and Lactic Acid *see* Lactic Acid and Sodium-PCA *on page 487*

Sodium Phosphates *(sow' dee um fos' fates)*

Brand Names Fleet® Enema [OTC]; Fleet® Phospho®-Soda [OTC]

Therapeutic Category Electrolyte Supplement, Parenteral; Laxative, Saline; Phosphate Salt; Sodium Salt

Use Source of phosphate in large volume I.V. fluids; short-term treatment of constipation (oral/rectal) and to evacuate the colon for rectal and bowel exams; treatment and prevention of hypophosphatemia

Usual Dosage
Normal requirements elemental phosphorus: Oral:
0-6 months: 240 mg
6-12 months: 360 mg
1-10 years: 800 mg
>10 years: 1200 mg
Pregnancy lactation: Additional 400 mg/day
Adults RDA: 800 mg

I.V. doses should be incorporated into the patient's maintenance I.V. fluids whenever possible; intermittent I.V. infusion should be reserved for severe depletion situations and requires continuous EKG monitoring. It is difficult to determine total body phosphorus deficit due to redistribution into intracellular compartment or bone tissue; (it is recommended that repletion of severe hypophosphatemia (<1 mg/dL in adults) be done via I.V. route since large dose of oral phosphate may cause diarrhea and intestinal absorption may be unreliable). The following dosages are empiric guidelines. **Note:** Doses listed as mmol of phosphate.

Severe hypophosphatemia: I.V.:
Children:
Low dose: 0.08 mmol/kg over 6 hours; use if recent losses and uncomplicated
Intermediate dose: 0.16-0.24 mmol/kg over 4-6 hours; use if phosphorus level 0.5-1 mg/dL
High dose: 0.36 mmol/kg over 6 hours; use if serum phosphorus <0.5 mg/dL
Adults: 0.15-0.3 mmol/kg/dose over 12 hours, may repeat as needed to achieve desired serum level
Maintenance:
Children: 0.5-1.5 mmol/kg/24 hours I.V. or 2-3 mmol/kg/24 hours orally in divided doses
Adults: 50-70 mmol/24 hours I.V. or 50-150 mmol/24 hours orally in divided doses **or**

Children <4 years: Oral: 1 capsule (250 mg/8 mmol phosphorus) 4 times/day; dilute as instructed
Children >4 years and Adults: Oral: 1-2 capsules (250-500 mg/8-16 mmol phosphorus) 4 times/day; dilute as instructed
Phosphate maintenance electrolyte requirement in parenteral nutrition: 2 mmol/kg/24 hours or 35 mmol/kcal/24 hours; maximum: 15-30 mmol/24 hours

Laxative (Fleet®): Rectal:
Children 2-12 years: Contents of one 2.25 oz pediatric enema, may repeat
Children ≥12 years and Adults: Contents of one 4.5 oz enema as a single dose, may repeat

Laxative (Fleet® Phospho®-Soda): Oral:
Children 5-9 years: 5 mL as a single dose
Children 10-12 years: 10 mL as a single dose
Children ≥12 years and Adults: 20-30 mL as a single dose

Mechanism of Action As a laxative, exerts osmotic effect in the small intestine by drawing water into the lumen of the gut, producing distention and promoting peristalsis and evacuation of the bowel; phosphorous participates in bone deposition, calcium metabolism, utilization of B complex vitamins, and as a buffer in acid-base equilibrium

Local Anesthetic/Vasoconstrictor Precautions No information available to require special precautions

Effects on Dental Treatment No effects or complications reported

Other Adverse Effects 1% to 10%:
Cardiovascular: Edema, hypotension
Endocrine & metabolic: Hypocalcemia, hypernatremia, hyperphosphatemia, calcium phosphate precipitation
Gastrointestinal: Nausea, vomiting, diarrhea
Renal: Acute renal failure

Drug Uptake
Onset of action:
Cathartic: 3-6 hours
Rectal: 2-5 minutes
Absorption: Oral: ~1% to 20%

Pregnancy Risk Factor C

Comments Sodium content of 1 mmol PO_4 in injection: 1.3 mEq

Sodium Salicylate (sow' dee um sa lis' i late)

Brand Names Uracel®

Therapeutic Category Analgesic, Non-narcotic

Use Treatment of minor pain or fever; arthritis

Local Anesthetic/Vasoconstrictor Precautions No information available to require special precautions

Effects on Dental Treatment No effects or complications reported

Other Adverse Effects 1% to 10%:
Dermatologic: Rash, urticaria
Gastrointestinal: Nausea, vomiting, GI distress, GI ulcers, GI bleeding
Hematologic: Platelet inhibition
Hepatic: Hepatotoxicity
Respiratory: Bronchospasm/wheezing

Comments Sodium content of 1 g: 6.25 mEq; less effective than an equal dose of aspirin in reducing pain or fever; patients hypersensitive to aspirin may be able to tolerate

Sodium Sulamyd® see Sodium Sulfacetamide on this page

Sodium Sulfacetamide (sow' dee um sul fa see' ta mide)

Brand Names AK-Sulf®; Bleph®-10; Cetamide®; Ophthacet®; Sebizon®; Sodium Sulamyd®; Sulf-10®; Sulfair®; Sulten-10®

Therapeutic Category Antibiotic, Ophthalmic

Use Treatment and prophylaxis of conjunctivitis due to susceptible organisms; corneal ulcers; adjunctive treatment with systemic sulfonamides for therapy of trachoma; topical application in scaling dermatosis (seborrheic); bacterial infections of the skin

Usual Dosage
Children >2 months and Adults: Ophthalmic:
Ointment: Apply to lower conjunctival sac 1-4 times/day and at bedtime
Solution: Instill 1-3 drops several times daily up to every 2-3 hours in lower conjunctival sac during waking hours and less frequently at night
Children >12 years and Adults: Topical:
Seborrheic dermatitis: Apply at bedtime and allow to remain overnight; in severe cases, may apply twice daily
Secondary cutaneous bacterial infections: Apply 2-4 times/day until infection clears

Mechanism of Action Interferes with bacterial growth by inhibiting bacterial folic acid synthesis through competitive antagonism of PABA

Local Anesthetic/Vasoconstrictor Precautions No information available to require special precautions

Effects on Dental Treatment No effects or complications reported

Other Adverse Effects
1% to 10%: Local: Irritation, stinging, burning
<1%:
Central nervous system: Headache
Dermatologic: Stevens-Johnson syndrome, exfoliative dermatitis, toxic epidermal necrolysis
Ocular: Blurred vision, browache
(Continued)

Sodium Sulfacetamide *(Continued)*

Sensitivity reactions: Hypersensitivity reactions

Drug Interactions Decreased effect: Silver, gentamicin (antagonism)

Drug Uptake

Serum half-life: 7-13 hours

Pregnancy Risk Factor C

Sodium Sulfacetamide and Fluorometholone

(sow' dee um sul fa see' ta mide & flure oh meth' oh lone)

Brand Names FML-S® Ophthalmic Suspension

Therapeutic Category Antibiotic, Ophthalmic; Anti-inflammatory Agent, Ophthalmic

Use Steroid-responsive inflammatory ocular conditions where infection is present or there is a risk of infection

Local Anesthetic/Vasoconstrictor Precautions No information available to require special precautions

Effects on Dental Treatment No effects or complications reported

Sodium Sulfacetamide and Phenylephrine

(sow' dee um sul fa see' ta mide & fen il ef' rin)

Brand Names Vasosulf® Ophthalmic

Therapeutic Category Antibiotic, Ophthalmic; Ophthalmic Agent, Vasoconstrictor

Local Anesthetic/Vasoconstrictor Precautions No information available to require special precautions

Effects on Dental Treatment No effects or complications reported

Sodium Sulfacetamide and Prednisolone Acetate

(sow' dee um sul fa see' ta mide & pred niss' oh lone as' e tate)

Brand Names Blephamide®; Cetapred®; Metimyd®; Vasocidin®

Therapeutic Category Antibiotic, Ophthalmic; Corticosteroid, Ophthalmic

Use Steroid-responsive inflammatory ocular conditions where infection is present or there is a risk of infection; ophthalmic suspension may be used as an otic preparation

Usual Dosage Children >2 months and Adults: Ophthalmic:

Ointment: Apply to lower conjunctival sac 1-4 times/day

Solution: Instill 1-3 drops every 2-3 hours while awake

Mechanism of Action Interferes with bacterial growth by inhibiting bacterial folic acid synthesis through competitive antagonism of PABA; decreases inflammation by suppression of migration of polymorphonuclear leukocytes and reversal of increased capillary permeability; suppresses the immune system by reducing activity and volume of the lymphatic system

Local Anesthetic/Vasoconstrictor Precautions No information available to require special precautions

Effects on Dental Treatment No effects or complications reported

Other Adverse Effects

1% to 10%: Local: Burning, stinging

<1%:

Central nervous system: Vertigo, seizures, psychoses, pseudotumor cerebri, headache

Dermatologic: Stevens-Johnson syndrome, skin atrophy

Endocrine & metabolic: Cushing's syndrome, pituitary-adrenal axis suppression, growth suppression

Gastrointestinal: Peptic ulcer, nausea, vomiting

Neuromuscular & skeletal: Muscle weakness, osteoporosis, fractures

Ocular: Cataracts, glaucoma

Drug Interactions Decreased effect: Silver, gentamicin, vaccines, toxoids

Pregnancy Risk Factor C

Sodium Sulfacetamide and Sulfur *see* Sulfur and Sodium Sulfacetamide *on page 813*

Sodium Tetradecyl Sulfate (sow' dee um tetra dek' il sul' fate)

Brand Names Sotradecol® Injection

Therapeutic Category Sclerosing Agent

Use Treatment of small, uncomplicated varicose veins of the lower extremities; endoscopic sclerotherapy in the management of bleeding esophageal varices

Usual Dosage I.V.: Test dose: 0.5 mL given several hours prior to administration of larger dose; 0.5-2 mL in each vein, maximum: 10 mL per treatment session; 3% solution reserved for large varices

Mechanism of Action Acts by irritation of the vein intimal endothelium
Local Anesthetic/Vasoconstrictor Precautions No information available to require special precautions
Effects on Dental Treatment No effects or complications reported
Other Adverse Effects
1% to 10%:
Central nervous system: Headache
Dermatologic: Urticaria
Gastrointestinal: Mucosal lesions, nausea, vomiting
Local: Discoloration at the site of injection, pain, ulceration at the site, sloughing and tissue necrosis following extravasation
Respiratory: Pulmonary edema
<1%:
Dermatologic: Hives
Gastrointestinal: Esophageal perforation
Respiratory: Asthma
Pregnancy Risk Factor C

Sodium Thiosulfate (sow' dee um thye oh sul' fate)
Brand Names Tinver® Lotion
Therapeutic Category Antidote, Cyanide; Antifungal Agent, Topical
Use
Parenteral: Used alone or with sodium nitrite or amyl nitrite in cyanide poisoning or arsenic poisoning; reduce the risk of nephrotoxicity associated with cisplatin therapy; local infiltration (in diluted form) of selected chemotherapy extravasation
Topical: Treatment of tinea versicolor
Usual Dosage
Cyanide and nitroprusside antidote: I.V.:
Children <25 kg: 50 mg/kg after receiving 4.5-10 mg/kg sodium nitrite; a half dose of each may be repeated if necessary
Children >25 kg and Adults: 12.5 g after 300 mg of sodium nitrite; a half dose of each may be repeated if necessary

Cyanide poisoning: I.V.: Dose should be based on determination as with nitrite, at rate of 2.5-5 mL/minute to maximum of 50 mL. See table.

Variation of Sodium Nitrite and Sodium Thiosulfate Dose With Hemoglobin Concentration*

Hemoglobin (g/dL)	Initial Dose Sodium Nitrite (mg/kg)	Initial Dose Sodium Nitrite 33% (mL/kg)	Initial Dose Sodium Thiosulfate 25% (mL/kg)
7	5.8	0.19	0.95
8	6.6	0.22	1.10
9	7.5	0.25	1.25
10	8.3	0.27	1.35
11	9.1	0.30	1.50
12	10.0	0.33	1.65
13	10.8	0.36	1.80
14	11.6	0.39	1.95

*Adapted from Berlin DM Jr, "The Treatment of Cyanide Poisoning in Children," *Pediatrics*, 1970, 46:793.

Cisplatin rescue should be given before or during cisplatin administration: I.V. infusion (in sterile water): 12 g/m^2 over 6 hours or 9 g/m^2 I.V. push followed by 1.2 g/m^2 continuous infusion for 6 hours

Arsenic poisoning: I.V.: 1 mL first day, 2 mL second day, 3 mL third day, 4 mL fourth day, 5 mL on alternate days thereafter

Children and Adults: Topical: 20% to 25% solution: Apply a thin layer to affected areas twice daily
Mechanism of Action
Cyanide toxicity: Increases the rate of detoxification of cyanide by the enzyme rhodanese by providing an extra sulfur
Cisplatin toxicity: Complexes with cisplatin to form a compound that is nontoxic to either normal or cancerous cells
Local Anesthetic/Vasoconstrictor Precautions No information available to require special precautions
(Continued)

Sodium Thiosulfate *(Continued)*

Effects on Dental Treatment No effects or complications reported
Other Adverse Effects 1% to 10%:
Cardiovascular: Hypotension
Central nervous system: Coma, CNS depression secondary to thiocyanate intoxication, psychosis, confusion
Dermatologic: Contact dermatitis
Local: Irritation
Neuromuscular & skeletal: Weakness
Otic: Tinnitus
Drug Uptake
Serum half-life: 0.65 hour
Pregnancy Risk Factor C
Comments White, odorless crystals or powder with a salty taste; normal body burden: 1.5 mg/kg

Sodol® *see* Carisoprodol *on page 157*
Sofarin® *see* Warfarin Sodium *on page 903*
Solaquin® **[OTC]** *see* Hydroquinone *on page 439*
Solaquin Forte® *see* Hydroquinone *on page 439*
Solatene® *see* Beta-Carotene *on page 109*
Solfoton® *see* Phenobarbital *on page 680*
Solganal® *see* Aurothioglucose *on page 87*
Solu-Cortef® *see* Hydrocortisone *on page 436*
Solu-Medrol® *see* Methylprednisolone *on page 569*
Solurex L.A.® *see* Dexamethasone *on page 260*
Soma® *see* Carisoprodol *on page 157*
Soma® **Compound** *see* Carisoprodol *on page 157*
Somnos® *see* Chloral Hydrate *on page 180*
Soothe® **[OTC]** *see* Tetrahydrozoline Hydrochloride *on page 831*
Soprodol® *see* Carisoprodol *on page 157*
Sorbitrate® *see* Isosorbide Dinitrate *on page 474*
Soridol® *see* Carisoprodol *on page 157*

Sotalol Hydrochloride *(soe' ta lole hye droe klor' ide)*

Related Information
Cardiovascular Diseases *on page 912*
Brand Names Betapace®
Canadian/Mexican Brand Names Sotacor® (Canada)
Therapeutic Category Antianginal Agent; Antiarrhythmic Agent, Class II; Antiarrhythmic Agent, Class III; Antiarrhythmic Agent (Supraventricular & Ventricular); Beta-Adrenergic Blocker, Cardioselective
Use Treatment of documented ventricular arrhythmias, such as sustained ventricular tachycardia, that in the judgment of the physician are life-threatening

Unlabeled use: Supraventricular arrhythmias
Usual Dosage Sotalol should be initiated and doses increased in a hospital with facilities for cardiac rhythm monitoring and assessment. Proarrhythmic events can occur after initiation of therapy and with each upward dosage adjustment.

Children (oral): The safety and efficacy of sotalol in children have not been established
Supraventricular arrhythmias: 2-4 mg/kg/24 hours was given in 2 equal doses every 12 hours in 18 infants (≤2 months of age). All infants, except one with chaotic atrial tachycardia, were successful controlled with sotalol. Ten infants discontinued therapy between the ages of 7-18 months when it was no longer necessary. Median duration of treatment was 12.8 months.

Adults (oral):
Initial: 80 mg twice daily
Dose may be increased (gradually allowing 2-3 days between dosing increments in order to attain steady-state plasma concentrations and to allow monitoring of Q-T intervals) to 240-320 mg/day
Most patients respond to a total daily dose of 160-320 mg/day in 2-3 divided doses
Some patients, with life-threatening refractory ventricular arrhythmias, may require doses as high as 480-640 mg/day; however, these doses should only be prescribed when the potential benefit outweighs the increased of adverse events

Elderly patients: Age does not significantly alter the pharmacokinetics of sotalol, but impaired renal function in elderly patients can increase the terminal half-life, resulting in increased drug accumulation

Mechanism of Action

Beta-blocker which contains both beta-adrenoreceptor-blocking (Vaughan Williams Class II) and cardiac action potential duration prolongation (Vaughan Williams Class III) properties

Class II effects: Increased sinus cycle length, slowed heart rate, decreased A-V nodal conduction, and increased A-V nodal refractoriness

Class III effects: Prolongation of the atrial and ventricular monophasic action potentials, and effective refractory prolongation of atrial muscle, ventricular muscle, and atrioventricular accessory pathways in both the antegrade and retrograde directions

Sotalol is a racemic mixture of *d-* and *L*-sotalol; both isomers have similar Class III antiarrhythmic effects while the *L*-isomer is responsible for virtually all of the beta-blocking activity

Sotalol has both beta$_1$- and beta$_2$-receptor blocking activity

The beta-blocking effect of sotalol is a non-cardioselective [half maximal at about 80 mg/day and maximal at doses of 320-640 mg/day]. Significant beta blockade occurs at oral doses as low as 25 mg/day.

The Class III effects are seen only at oral doses of ≥160 mg/day

Local Anesthetic/Vasoconstrictor Precautions Use with caution; epinephrine has interacted with nonselective beta-blockers to result in initial hypertensive episode followed by bradycardia

Effects on Dental Treatment Non-cardioselective beta-blockers (ie, propranolol, nadolol) enhance the pressor response to epinephrine, resulting in hypertension and bradycardia. Many nonsteroidal anti-inflammatory drugs such as ibuprofen and indomethacin can reduce the hypotensive effect of beta-blockers after 3 or more weeks of therapy with the NSAID. Short-term NSAID use (ie, 3 days) requires no special precautions in patients taking beta-blockers.

Other Adverse Effects

>10%:

Cardiovascular: Bradycardia

Central nervous system: Mental depression

Endocrine & metabolic: Decreased sexual ability

1% to 10%:

Cardiovascular: Congestive heart failure

Central nervous system: Mental confusion, hallucinations, reduced peripheral circulation, anxiety, dizziness, drowsiness, nightmares, insomnia, weakness, tiredness

Dermatologic: Itching

Gastrointestinal: Constipation, diarrhea, nausea, vomiting, stomach discomfort

Respiratory: Breathing difficulties

<1%:

Cardiovascular: Chest pain, hypotension (especially with higher doses), Raynaud's phenomena

Dermatologic: Skin rash; red, crusted skin, skin necrosis after extravasation

Hematologic: Leukopenia

Local: Phlebitis

Miscellaneous: Diaphoresis, cold extremities

Drug Interactions Class Ia antiarrhythmics, such as quinidine, have the potential to prolong refractoriness of sotalol; sotalol should be administered with caution with calcium-blocking drugs because of possible additional effects on A-V conduction

Drug Uptake

Onset of action: Rapid, 1-2 hours

Peak effect: 2.5-4 hours

Absorption: Decreased 20% to 30% by meals compared to fasting

Serum half-life: 12 hours

Pregnancy Risk Factor B

Sotradecol® Injection *see* Sodium Tetradecyl Sulfate *on page 794*

Spancap® No. 1 *see* Dextroamphetamine Sulfate *on page 265*

Span-FF® [OTC] *see* Ferrous Fumarate *on page 359*

Sparine® *see* Promazine Hydrochloride *on page 732*

Spaslin® *see* Hyoscyamine, Atropine, Scopolamine, and Phenobarbital *on page 444*

Spasmoject® *see* Dicyclomine Hydrochloride *on page 273*

Spasmolin® *see* Hyoscyamine, Atropine, Scopolamine, and Phenobarbital *on page 444*

Spasmophen® *see* Hyoscyamine, Atropine, Scopolamine, and Phenobarbital *on page 444*

Spasquid® *see* Hyoscyamine, Atropine, Scopolamine, and Phenobarbital *on page 444*

Spec-T® **[OTC]** *see* Benzocaine *on page 102*

Spectam® *see* Spectinomycin Hydrochloride *on this page*

Spectazole™ *see* Econazole Nitrate *on page 306*

Spectinomycin Hydrochloride
(spek ti noe mye' sin hye droe klor' ide)
Related Information
Nonviral Infectious Diseases *on page 932*
Brand Names Spectam®; Trobicin®
Therapeutic Category Antibiotic, Miscellaneous
Use Treatment of uncomplicated gonorrhea (ineffective against syphilis)
Usual Dosage I.M.:
Children:
<45 kg: 40 mg/kg/dose 1 time
≥45 kg: See adult dose
Children >8 years who are allergic to PCNS/cephalosporins may be treated with oral tetracycline
Adults:
Uncomplicated urethral endocervical or rectal gonorrhea: 2 g deep I.M. or 4 g where antibiotic resistance is prevalent 1 time; 4 g (10 mL) dose should be given as two 5 mL injections, followed by doxycycline 100 mg twice daily for 7 days
Disseminated gonococcal infection: 2 g every 12 hours
Hemodialysis effects: 50% removed by hemodialysis
Mechanism of Action A bacteriostatic antibiotic that selectively binds to the 30s subunits of ribosomes, and thereby inhibiting bacterial protein synthesis
Local Anesthetic/Vasoconstrictor Precautions No information available to require special precautions
Effects on Dental Treatment No effects or complications reported
Other Adverse Effects <1%:
Central nervous system: Dizziness, headache, chills
Dermatologic: Urticaria, rash, pruritus
Gastrointestinal: Nausea, vomiting
Local: Pain at injection site
Drug Interactions No data reported
Drug Uptake
Duration of action: Up to 8 hours
Serum half-life: 1.7 hours
Time to peak serum concentration: Within 1 hour
Pregnancy Risk Factor B

Spectrobid® *see* Bacampicillin Hydrochloride *on page 92*

Spirapril (spye' ra pril)
Related Information
Cardiovascular Diseases *on page 912*
Brand Names Renormax®
Therapeutic Category Angiotensin-Converting Enzyme (ACE) Inhibitors
Use Management of mild to severe hypertension
Local Anesthetic/Vasoconstrictor Precautions No information available to require special precautions
Effects on Dental Treatment No effects or complications reported

Spironazide® *see* Hydrochlorothiazide and Spironolactone *on page 431*

Spironolactone (speer on oh lak' tone)
Related Information
Cardiovascular Diseases *on page 912*
Brand Names Aldactone®
Canadian/Mexican Brand Names Novo-Spiroton® (Canada)
Therapeutic Category Diuretic, Potassium Sparing
Use Management of edema associated with excessive aldosterone excretion; hypertension; primary hyperaldosteronism; hypokalemia; treatment of hirsutism; cirrhosis of liver accompanied by edema or ascites

Usual Dosage Administration with food increases absorption. To reduce delay in onset of effect, a loading dose of 2 or 3 times the daily dose may be administered on the first day of therapy. Oral:

Children:

Diuretic, hypertension: 1.5-3.5 mg/kg/day in divided doses every 6-24 hours

Diagnosis of primary aldosteronism: 125-375 mg/m²/day in divided doses

Vaso-occlusive disease: 7.5 mg/kg/day in divided doses twice daily (not FDA approved)

Adults:

Edema, hypertension, hypokalemia: 25-200 mg/day in 1-2 divided doses

Diagnosis of primary aldosteronism: 100-400 mg/day in 1-2 divided doses

Elderly: Initial: 25-50 mg/day in 1-2 divided doses, increasing by 25-50 mg every 5 days as needed

Mechanism of Action Competes with aldosterone for receptor sites in the distal renal tubules, increasing sodium chloride and water excretion while conserving potassium and hydrogen ions; may block the effect of aldosterone on arteriolar smooth muscle as well

Local Anesthetic/Vasoconstrictor Precautions No information available to require special precautions

Effects on Dental Treatment No effects or complications reported

Other Adverse Effects

1% to 10%:

Cardiovascular: Hypotension, edema, bradycardia, congestive heart failure

Central nervous system: Constipation, dizziness, fatigue, headache

Dermatologic: Rash

Gastrointestinal: Nausea

Respiratory: Dyspnea

<1%:

Cardiovascular: Flushing

Endocrine & metabolic: Hyperkalemia, dehydration, hyponatremia, gyneco-mastia, hyperchloremia, metabolic acidosis, postmenopausal bleeding

Genitourinary: Inability to achieve or maintain an erection

Drug Interactions Spironolactone potentiates the effects of other diuretics and antihypertensives; spironolactone has been shown to increase the half-life of digoxin; this may result in increased serum digoxin levels and digoxin toxicity

Drug Uptake

Serum half-life: 78-84 minutes

Time to peak serum concentration: Within 1-3 hours (primarily as the active metabolite)

Pregnancy Risk Factor D

Spironolactone and Hydrochlorothiazide see Hydrochlorothiazide and Spirono-lactone on page 431

Spirozide® see Hydrochlorothiazide and Spironolactone on page 431

Sporanox® see Itraconazole on page 477

Sportscreme® [OTC] see Triethanolamine Salicylate on page 868

S-P-T see Thyroid on page 844

SRC® Expectorant see Hydrocodone, Pseudoephedrine, and Guaifenesin on page 435

SSD™ see Silver Sulfadiazine on page 788

SSD-AF™ see Silver Sulfadiazine on page 788

SSKI® see Potassium Iodide on page 711

Stadol® see Butorphanol Tartrate on page 135

Stadol® NS see Butorphanol Tartrate on page 135

Stagesic® [5/500] see Hydrocodone and Acetaminophen on page 431

Stannous Fluoride see Fluoride on page 374

Stanozolol (stan oh′ zoe lole)

Brand Names Winstrol®

Therapeutic Category Anabolic Steroid

Use Prophylactic use against hereditary angioedema

Usual Dosage

Children: Acute attacks:

<6 years: 1 mg/day

6-12 years: 2 mg/day

Adults: Oral: Initial: 2 mg 3 times/day, may then reduce to a maintenance dose of 2 mg/day or 2 mg every other day after 1-3 months

Mechanism of Action Synthetic testosterone derivative with similar andro-genic and anabolic actions

(Continued)

Stanozolol *(Continued)*

Local Anesthetic/Vasoconstrictor Precautions No information available to require special precautions

Effects on Dental Treatment No effects or complications reported

Other Adverse Effects

Male:

Postpubertal:

>10%:

Dermatologic: Acne

Endocrine & metabolic: Bladder irritability, priapism, gynecomastia

1% to 10%:

Central nervous system: Insomnia

Endocrine & metabolic: Decreased libido, hepatic dysfunction, chills, prostatic hypertrophy (elderly)

Gastrointestinal: Nausea, diarrhea

Hematologic: Iron deficiency anemia, suppression of clotting factors

<1%: Hepatic: Hepatic necrosis, hepatocellular carcinoma

Prepubertal:

>10%:

Dermatologic: Acne

Endocrine & metabolic: Virilism

1% to 10%:

Central nervous system: Chills, insomnia, factors

Dermatologic: Hyperpigmentation

Gastrointestinal: Diarrhea, nausea

Hematologic: Iron deficiency anemia, suppression of clotting

<1%: Hepatic: Hepatic necrosis, hepatocellular carcinoma

Female:

>10%: Endocrine & metabolic: Virilism

1% to 10%:

Central nervous system: Chills, insomnia

Endocrine & metabolic: Hypercalcemia

Gastrointestinal: Nausea, diarrhea

Hematologic: Iron deficiency anemia, suppression of clotting factors

Hepatic: Hepatic dysfunction

<1%: Hepatic: Hepatic necrosis, hepatocellular carcinoma

Drug Interactions Stanozolol enhances the hypoprothrombinemic effects of oral anticoagulants; enhances the hypoglycemic effects of insulin and sulfonylureas (oral hypoglycemics)

Pregnancy Risk Factor X

Staphcillin® *see* Methicillin Sodium *on page 556*

Staticin® Topical *see* Erythromycin, Topical *on page 324*

Statrol® *see* Neomycin and Polymyxin B *on page 609*

Stavudine *(stav′ yoo deen)*

Related Information

Systemic Viral Diseases *on page 934*

Brand Names Zerit®

Therapeutic Category Antiviral Agent, Oral; Antiviral Agent, Parenteral

Use For the treatment of adults with advanced HIV infection who are intolerant to approved therapies with proven clinical benefit or who have experienced significant clinical or immunologic deterioration while receiving these therapies, or for whom such therapies are contraindicated

Usual Dosage

Adults: Oral:

≥60 kg: 40 mg every 12 hours

<60 kg: 30 mg every 12 hours

Dose may be cut in half if symptoms of peripheral neuropathy occur

Mechanism of Action Inhibits reverse transcriptase of the human immunodeficiency virus (HIV)

Local Anesthetic/Vasoconstrictor Precautions No information available to require special precautions

Effects on Dental Treatment No effects or complications reported

Other Adverse Effects

>10%: Neuromuscular & skeletal: Peripheral neuropathy

1% to 10%:

Central nervous system: Headache, chills/fever abdominal or back pain, malaise, asthenia, insomnia, anxiety, depression

Gastrointestinal: Nausea, vomiting, diarrhea, pancreatitis

Neuromuscular & skeletal: Myalgia
Drug Interactions No data reported
Drug Uptake
Peak serum level: 1 hour after administration
Serum half-life: 1-1.6 hours
Pregnancy Risk Factor C

Stay Trim® Diet Gum [OTC] *see* Phenylpropanolamine Hydrochloride *on page 687*

Stelazine® *see* Trifluoperazine Hydrochloride *on page 869*

Stemex® *see* Paramethasone Acetate *on page 659*

Sterapred® *see* Prednisone *on page 719*

Stilphostrol® *see* Diethylstilbestrol *on page 277*

Stimate™ *see* Desmopressin Acetate *on page 258*

St. Joseph® Cough Suppressant [OTC] *see* Dextromethorphan *on page 266*

St. Joseph® Measured Dose Nasal Solution [OTC] *see* Phenylephrine Hydrochloride *on page 685*

Stop® [OTC] *see* Fluoride *on page 374*

Streptase® *see* Streptokinase *on this page*

Streptokinase (strep toe kye' nase)
Related Information
Cardiovascular Diseases *on page 912*
Brand Names Kabikinase®; Streptase®
Therapeutic Category Thrombolytic Agent
Use Thrombolytic agent used in treatment of recent severe or massive deep vein thrombosis, pulmonary emboli, myocardial infarction, and occluded arteriovenous cannulas
Usual Dosage I.V.:
Children: Safety and efficacy not established; limited studies have used 3500-4000 units/kg over 30 minutes followed by 1000-1500 units/kg/hour
Clotted catheter: 25,000 units, clamp for 2 hours then aspirate contents and flush with normal saline
Adults: Antibodies to streptokinase remain for at least 3-6 months after initial dose: Administration requires the use of an infusion pump
An intradermal skin test of 100 units has been suggested to predict allergic response to streptokinase. If a positive reaction is not seen after 15-20 minutes, a therapeutic dose may be administered.
Guidelines for acute myocardial infarction (AMI): 1.5 million units over 60 minutes
Administration:
Dilute two 750,000 unit vials of streptokinase with 5 mL dextrose 5% in water (D$_5$W) each, gently swirl to dissolve
Add this dose of the 1.5 million units to 150 mL D$_5$W
This should be infused over 60 minutes; an in-line filter ≥0.45 micron should be used
Monitor for the first few hours for signs of anaphylaxis or allergic reaction. **Infusion should be slowed if lowering of 25 mm Hg in blood pressure or terminated if asthmatic symptoms appear.**
Begin heparin 5000-10,000 unit bolus followed by 1000 units/hour approximately 3-4 hours after completion of streptokinase infusion or when PTT is <100 seconds
Guidelines for acute pulmonary embolism (APE): 3 million unit dose over 24 hours
Administration:
Dilute four 750,000 unit vials of streptokinase with 5 mL dextrose 5% in water (D$_5$W) each, gently swirl to dissolve
Add this dose of 3 million units to 250 mL D$_5$W, an in-line filter ≥0.45 micron should be used
Administer 250,000 units (23 mL) over 30 minutes followed by 100,000 units/hour (9 mL/hour) for 24 hours
Monitor for the first few hours for signs of anaphylaxis or allergic reaction. **Infusion should be slowed if blood pressure is lowered by 25 mm Hg or if asthmatic symptoms appear.**
Begin heparin 1000 units/hour about 3-4 hours after completion of streptokinase infusion or when PTT is <100 seconds
Monitor PT, PTT, and fibrinogen levels during therapy
Thromboses: 250,000 units to start, then 100,000 units/hour for 24-72 hours depending on location
(Continued)

Streptokinase (Continued)

Cannula occlusion: 250,000 units into cannula, clamp for 2 hours, then aspirate contents and flush with normal saline

Mechanism of Action Activates the conversion of plasminogen to plasmin by forming a complex, exposing plasminogen-activating site, and cleaving a peptide bond that converts plasminogen to plasmin; plasmin degrades fibrin, fibrinogen and other procoagulant proteins into soluble fragments; effective both outside and within the formed thrombus/embolus

Local Anesthetic/Vasoconstrictor Precautions No information available to require special precautions

Effects on Dental Treatment No effects or complications reported

Other Adverse Effects

>10%:

Cardiovascular: Hypotension, arrhythmias, trauma arrhythmias

Dermatologic: Angioneurotic edema

Hematologic: Surface bleeding, internal bleeding, cerebral hemorrhage

Respiratory: Bronchospasm

Miscellaneous: Periorbital swelling, anaphylaxis

<1%:

Cardiovascular: Flushing

Central nervous system: Headache, chills, sweating, fever

Dermatologic: Rash, itching

Gastrointestinal: Nausea, vomiting

Hematologic: Anemia, eye hemorrhage

Neuromuscular & skeletal: Musculoskeletal pain

Respiratory: Bronchospasm

Miscellaneous: Epistaxis

Drug Interactions

Antifibrinolytic agents (aminocaproic acid) cause decreased effectiveness of streptokinase

Anticoagulants, antiplatelet agents cause increased risk of bleeding of streptokinase

Drug Uptake

Onset of action: Activation of plasminogen occurs almost immediately

Duration: Fibrinolytic effects last only a few hours, while anticoagulant effects can persist for 12-24 hours

Serum half-life: 83 minutes

Pregnancy Risk Factor C

Streptomycin Sulfate (strep toe mye' sin sul' fate)

Related Information

Nonviral Infectious Diseases on page 932

Therapeutic Category Antibiotic, Aminoglycoside; Antitubercular Agent

Use Combination therapy of active tuberculosis; used in combination with other agents for treatment of streptococcal or enterococcal endocarditis, mycobacterial infections, plague, tularemia, and brucellosis. Streptomycin is indicated for persons from endemic areas of drug-resistant *Mycobacterium tuberculosis* or who are HIV infected.

Usual Dosage Intramuscular (may also be given intravenous piggyback):

Tuberculosis therapy: **Note:** A four-drug regimen (isoniazid, rifampin, pyrazinamide and either streptomycin or ethambutol) is preferred for the initial, empiric treatment of TB. When the drug susceptibility results are available, the regimen should be altered as appropriate.

Patients with TB and without HIV infection:

OPTION 1:

Isoniazid resistance rate <4%: Administer daily isoniazid, rifampin, and pyrazinamide for 8 weeks followed by isoniazid and rifampin daily or directly observed therapy (DOT) 2-3 times/week for 16 weeks

If isoniazid resistance rate is not documented, ethambutol or streptomycin should also be administered until susceptibility to isoniazid or rifampin is demonstrated. Continue treatment for at least 6 months or 3 months beyond culture conversion.

OPTION 2: Administer daily isoniazid, rifampin, pyrazinamide, and either streptomycin or ethambutol for 2 weeks followed by DOT 2 times/week administration of the same drugs for 6 weeks, and subsequently, with isoniazid and rifampin DOT 2 times/week administration for 16 weeks

OPTION 3: Administer isoniazid, rifampin, pyrazinamide, and either ethambutol or streptomycin by DOT 3 times/week for 6 months

Patients with TB and with HIV infection: Administer any of the above OPTIONS 1, 2 or 3, however, treatment should be continued for a total of 9 months and at least 6 months beyond culture conversion

Note: Some experts recommend that the duration of therapy should be extended to 9 months for patients with disseminated disease, miliary disease, disease involving the bones or joints, or tuberculosis lymphadenitis

Children:
  Daily therapy: 20-30 mg/kg/day (maximum: 1 g/day)
  Directly observed therapy (DOT): Twice weekly: 25-30 mg/kg (maximum: 1.5 g)
  DOT: 3 times/week: 25-30 mg/kg (maximum: 1 g)
Adults:
  Daily therapy: 15 mg/kg/day (maximum: 1 g)
  Directly observed therapy (DOT): Twice weekly: 25-30 mg/kg (maximum: 1.5 g)
  DOT: 3 times/week: 25-30 mg/kg (maximum: 1 g)
  Enterococcal endocarditis: 1 g every 12 hours for 2 weeks, 500 mg every 12 hours for 4 weeks in combination with penicillin
  Streptococcal endocarditis: 1 g every 12 hours for 1 week, 500 mg every 12 hours for 1 week
  Tularemia: 1-2 g/day in divided doses for 7-10 days or until patient is afebrile for 5-7 days
  Plague: 2-4 g/day in divided doses until the patient is afebrile for at least 3 days
Elderly: 10 mg/kg/day, not to exceed 750 mg/day; dosing interval should be adjusted for renal function; some authors suggest not to give more than 5 days/week or give as 20-25 mg/kg/dose twice weekly

Mechanism of Action Inhibits bacterial protein synthesis by binding directly to the 30S ribosomal subunits causing faulty peptide sequence to form in the protein chain

Local Anesthetic/Vasoconstrictor Precautions No information available to require special precautions

Effects on Dental Treatment No effects or complications reported

Other Adverse Effects
1% to 10%:
  Neuromuscular & skeletal: Neuromuscular blockade
  Otic: Ototoxicity (auditory), ototoxicity (vestibular)
  Renal: Nephrotoxicity
<1%:
  Cardiovascular: Hypotension
  Central nervous system: Drug fever, headache, drowsiness, weakness
  Dermatologic: Skin rash
  Gastrointestinal: Nausea, vomiting
  Hematologic: Eosinophilia, anemia
  Neuromuscular & skeletal: Paresthesia, tremor, arthralgia
  Respiratory: Difficulty in breathing

Drug Interactions
Concurrent use of amphotericin, loop diuretics may increase nephrotoxicity of streptomycin

Drug Uptake
Absorption: Oral: Absorbed poorly; usually given parenterally
Time to peak serum concentration: Within 1 hour
Serum half-life:
  Adults: 2-4.7 hours, prolonged with renal impairment

Pregnancy Risk Factor D

Streptozocin (strep toe zoe' sin)

Brand Names Zanosar®

Therapeutic Category Antineoplastic Agent, Alkylating Agent (Nitrosourea)

Use Treat metastatic islet cell carcinoma of the pancreas, carcinoid tumor and syndrome, Hodgkin's disease, palliative treatment of colorectal cancer

Usual Dosage I.V. (refer to individual protocols): Children and Adults: 500 mg/m^2 for 5 days every 4-6 weeks until optimal benefit or toxicity occurs or may be given in single dose 1000 mg/m^2 at weekly intervals for 2 doses, then increased to 1500 mg/m^2; usual course of therapy: 4-6 weeks

Mechanism of Action Interferes with the normal function of DNA by alkylation and cross-linking the strands of DNA, and by possible protein modification

Local Anesthetic/Vasoconstrictor Precautions No information available to require special precautions

Effects on Dental Treatment No effects or complications reported
(Continued)

Streptozocin *(Continued)*

Other Adverse Effects

>10%:

Gastrointestinal: Nausea and vomiting in all patients usually 1-4 hours after infusion; diarrhea in 10% of patients; increased LFTs and hypoalbuminemia

Emetic potential: High (>90%)

Renal: Renal dysfunction occurs in 65% of patients; proteinuria, decreased Cl_{cr}, increased BUN, hypophosphatemia, and renal tubular acidosis; be careful with patients on other nephrotoxic agents; nephrotoxicity (25% to 75% of patients)

1% to 10%:

Gastrointestinal: Diarrhea

Hypoglycemia: Seen in 6% of patients; may be prevented with the administration of nicotinamide

Local: Pain at injection site

<1%:

Central nervous system: Confusion, lethargy, depression

Hematologic: Leukopenia, thrombocytopenia

Hepatic: Liver dysfunction

Myelosuppressive:

WBC: Mild

Platelets: Mild

Onset (days): 7

Nadir (days): 14

Recovery (days): 21

Secondary malignancy

Drug Interactions

Phenytoin results in negation of streptozocin cytotoxicity

Doxorubicin prolongs half-life of streptozocin and thus prolongs leukopenia and thrombocytopenia

Drug Uptake

Serum half-life: 35-40 minutes

Pregnancy Risk Factor C

Stresstabs® 600 Advanced Formula Tablets [OTC] *see* Vitamins, Multiple *on page 901*

Stuartnatal® 1 + 1 *see* Vitamins, Multiple *on page 901*

Stuart Prenatal® [OTC] *see* Vitamins, Multiple *on page 901*

Sublimaze® *see* Fentanyl *on page 357*

Sucralfate *(soo kral' fate)*

Related Information

Patients Undergoing Cancer Therapy *on page 967*

Brand Names Carafate®

Canadian/Mexican Brand Names Novo-Sucralate® (Canada); Sulcrate® (Canada); Sulcrate® Suspension Plus (Canada); Antepsin® (Mexico)

Therapeutic Category Gastrointestinal Agent, Miscellaneous

Synonyms Sucralfato (Mexico)

Use Short-term management of duodenal ulcers

Unlabeled uses: Gastric ulcers; maintenance of duodenal ulcers; suspension may be used topically for treatment of stomatitis due to cancer chemotherapy and other causes of esophageal and gastric erosions; GERD, esophagitis, treatment of NSAID mucosal damage, prevention of stress ulcers, post-schlerotherapy for esophageal variceal bleeding.

Usual Dosage Oral:

Children: Dose not established, doses of 40-80 mg/kg/day divided every 6 hours have been used

Stomatitis: 2.5-5 mL (1 g/15 mL suspension), swish and spit or swish and swallow 4 times/day

Adults:

Stress ulcer prophylaxis: 1 g 4 times/day

Stress ulcer treatment: 1 g every 4 hours

Duodenal ulcer:

Treatment: 1 g 4 times/day, 1 hour before meals or food and at bedtime for 4-8 weeks, or alternatively 2 g twice daily; treatment is recommended for 4-8 weeks in adults, the elderly will require 12 weeks

Maintenance: Prophylaxis: 1 g twice daily

Stomatitis: 1 g/15 mL suspension, swish and spit or swish and swallow 4 times/day

Mechanism of Action Forms a complex by binding with positively charged proteins in exudates, forming a viscous paste-like, adhesive substance, when combined with gastric acid adheres to the damaged mucosal area. This selectively forms a protective coating that protects the lining against peptic acid, pepsin, and bile salts.

Local Anesthetic/Vasoconstrictor Precautions No information available to require special precautions

Effects on Dental Treatment No effects or complications reported

Other Adverse Effects
1% to 10%: Gastrointestinal: Constipation
<1%:
Central nervous system: Dizziness, sleepiness, vertigo
Dermatologic: Rash, pruritus
Gastrointestinal: Diarrhea, nausea, gastric discomfort, indigestion, dry mouth
Neuromuscular & skeletal: Back pain

Drug Interactions Decreased effect:
Digoxin, phenytoin, theophylline, ciprofloxacin, itraconazole; because of the potential for sucralfate to alter the absorption of some drugs, separate administration (2 hours before or after) should be considered when alterations in bioavailability are believed to be critical
Antacids/cimetidine/ranitidine: Do not administer concomitantly with sucralfate; these types of drugs reduce acidity; sucralfate requires gastric acid for it's mechanism of action (ie, to form a gel in the stomach as a protective barrier)

Drug Uptake
Onset of action: Paste formation and ulcer adhesion occur within 1-2 hours
Duration: Up to 6 hours
Absorption: Oral: <5%

Pregnancy Risk Factor B

Sucralfato (Mexico) *see* Sucralfate *on previous page*

Sucrets® Cough Calmers [OTC] *see* Dextromethorphan *on page 266*

Sudafed® [OTC] *see* Pseudoephedrine *on page 749*

Sudafed® 12 Hour [OTC] *see* Pseudoephedrine *on page 749*

Sudafed® Plus Liquid [OTC] *see* Chlorpheniramine and Pseudoephedrine *on page 191*

Sudafed® Plus Tablet [OTC] *see* Chlorpheniramine and Pseudoephedrine *on page 191*

Sudex® *see* Guaifenesin and Pseudoephedrine *on page 409*

Sufedrin® [OTC] *see* Pseudoephedrine *on page 749*

Sufenta® *see* Sufentanil Citrate *on this page*

Sufentanil Citrate (soo fen' ta nil sit' rate)
Related Information
Narcotic Agonist Charts *on page 1019*
Brand Names Sufenta®
Therapeutic Category Analgesic, Narcotic
Use Analgesic supplement in maintenance of balanced general anesthesia
Usual Dosage
Children <12 years: 10-25 mcg/kg with 100% O_2, maintenance: 25-50 mcg as needed

Adults: Dose should be based on body weight. **Note:** In obese patients (ie, >20% above ideal body weight), use lean body weight to determine dosage.
1-2 mcg/kg with NO_2/O_2 for endotracheal intubation; maintenance: 10-25 mcg as needed
2-8 mcg/kg with NO_2/O_2 more complicated major surgical procedures; maintenance: 10-50 mcg as needed
8-30 mcg/kg with 100% O_2 and muscle relaxant produces sleep; at doses ≥8 mcg/kg maintains a deep level of anesthesia; maintenance: 10-50 mcg as needed

Mechanism of Action Binds with stereospecific receptors at many sites within the CNS, increases pain threshold, alters pain reception, inhibits ascending pain pathways; ultra short-acting narcotic

Local Anesthetic/Vasoconstrictor Precautions No information available to require special precautions

Effects on Dental Treatment No effects or complications reported

Other Adverse Effects
>10%:
Cardiovascular: Bradycardia, hypotension
Central nervous system: Drowsiness
Gastrointestinal: Nausea, vomiting
(Continued)

Sufentanil Citrate *(Continued)*
Respiratory: Respiratory depression
1% to 10%:
Cardiovascular: Cardiac arrhythmias, orthostatic hypotension
Central nervous system: Confusion, CNS depression
Gastrointestinal: Biliary spasm
Ocular: Blurred vision
<1%:
Cardiovascular: Bronchospasm, circulatory depression
Central nervous system: Convulsions, dysesthesia, paradoxical CNS excitation or delirium; mental depression, dizziness
Dermatologic: Skin rash, hives, itching
Respiratory: Laryngospasm
Miscellaneous: Cold, clammy skin; biliary or urinary tract spasm, physical and psychological dependence with prolonged use
Drug Interactions Increased effect/toxicity with CNS depressants, beta-blockers
Drug Uptake
Onset of action: 1-3 minutes
Duration: Dose dependent
Pregnancy Risk Factor C

Sugar-Free Liquid Pharmaceuticals *see page 1070*
Sular™ *see Nisoldipine on page 622*

Sulconazole Nitrate *(sul kon' a zole nye' trate)*
Brand Names Exelderm®
Therapeutic Category Antifungal Agent, Topical
Synonyms Sulconazol, Nitrato De (Mexico)
Use Treatment of superficial fungal infections of the skin, including tinea cruris (jock itch), tinea corporis (ringworm), tinea versicolor, and possibly tinea pedis (athlete's foot - cream only)
Usual Dosage Adults: Topical: Apply a small amount to the affected area and gently massage once or twice daily for 3 weeks (tinea cruris, tinea corporis, tinea versicolor) to 4 weeks (tinea pedis).
Mechanism of Action Substituted imidazole derivative which inhibits metabolic reactions necessary for the synthesis of ergosterol, an essential membrane component. The end result is usually fungistatic; however, sulconazole may act as a fungicide in *Candida albicans* and parapsilosis during certain growth phases.
Local Anesthetic/Vasoconstrictor Precautions No information available to require special precautions
Effects on Dental Treatment No effects or complications reported
Other Adverse Effects 1% to 10%: Local: Itching, burning, stinging, redness
Drug Interactions No data reported
Drug Uptake
Absorption: Topical: About 8.7% absorbed percutaneously
Pregnancy Risk Factor C

Sulconazol, Nitrato De (Mexico) *see Sulconazole Nitrate on this page*
Sulf-10® *see Sodium Sulfacetamide on page 793*

Sulfabenzamide, Sulfacetamide, and Sulfathiazole
(sul fa benz' a mide, sul fa see' ta mide, sul fa thye' a zol)
Brand Names Gyne-Sulf®; Sultrin™; Trysul®; Vagilia®; V.V.S.®
Therapeutic Category Antibiotic, Vaginal
Use Treatment of *Haemophilus vaginalis* vaginitis
Usual Dosage Adults:
Cream: Insert one applicatorful in vagina twice daily for 4-6 days; dosage may then be decreased to ½ to ¼ of an applicatorful twice daily
Tablet: Insert one intravaginally twice daily for 10 days
Mechanism of Action Interferes with microbial folic acid synthesis and growth via inhibition of para-aminobenzoic acid metabolism
Local Anesthetic/Vasoconstrictor Precautions No information available to require special precautions
Effects on Dental Treatment No effects or complications reported
Other Adverse Effects
>10%: Dermatologic: Local irritation, pruritus, urticaria
<1%: Dermatologic: Allergic reactions, Stevens-Johnson syndrome
Drug Interactions No data reported

Drug Uptake
Absorption: Absorption from the vagina is variable and unreliable
Pregnancy Risk Factor C

Sulfacet-R® Topical *see* Sulfur and Sodium Sulfacetamide *on page 813*

Sulfacytine (sul fa sye′ teen)
Brand Names Renoquid®
Therapeutic Category Antibiotic, Sulfonamide Derivative
Use Treatment of urinary tract infections
Local Anesthetic/Vasoconstrictor Precautions No information available to require special precautions
Effects on Dental Treatment No effects or complications reported
Other Adverse Effects
>10%:
Central nervous system: Fever, dizziness, headache
Dermatologic: Itching, skin rash, photosensitivity
Gastrointestinal: Anorexia, nausea, vomiting, diarrhea
1% to 10%:
Dermatologic: Stevens-Johnson syndrome
Hematologic: Granulocytopenia, leukopenia, thrombocytopenia, aplastic anemia, hemolytic anemia
Hepatic: Hepatitis
Miscellaneous: Lyell's syndrome
<1%:
Dermatologic: Photosensitivity
Endocrine & metabolic: Thyroid function disturbance
Genitourinary: Crystalluria
Hepatic: Jaundice
Renal: Hematuria, interstitial nephritis, acute nephropathy
Miscellaneous: Serum sickness-like reactions

Sulfadiazine (sul fa dye′ a zeen)
Brand Names Microsulfon®
Canadian/Mexican Brand Names Coptin® (Canada)
Therapeutic Category Antibiotic, Sulfonamide Derivative
Use Treatment of urinary tract infections and nocardiosis, rheumatic fever prophylaxis; adjunctive treatment in toxoplasmosis; uncomplicated attack of malaria
Usual Dosage Oral:
Congenital toxoplasmosis:
Newborns and Children <2 months: 100 mg/kg/day divided every 6 hours in conjunction with pyrimethamine 1 mg/kg/day once daily and supplemental folinic acid 5 mg every 3 days for 6 months
Children >2 months: 25-50 mg/kg/dose 4 times/day

Toxoplasmosis:
Children: 120-150 mg/kg/day, maximum dose: 6 g/day; divided every 6 hours in conjunction with pyrimethamine 2 mg/kg/day divided every 12 hours for 3 days followed by 1 mg/kg/day once daily (maximum: 25 mg/day) with supplemental folinic acid
Adults: 2-8 g/day divided every 6 hours in conjunction with pyrimethamine 25 mg/day and with supplemental folinic acid
Mechanism of Action Interferes with bacterial growth by inhibiting bacterial folic acid synthesis through competitive antagonism of PABA
Local Anesthetic/Vasoconstrictor Precautions No information available to require special precautions
Effects on Dental Treatment No effects or complications reported
Other Adverse Effects
>10%:
Central nervous system: Fever, dizziness, headache
Dermatologic: Itching, skin rash, photosensitivity
Gastrointestinal: Anorexia, nausea, vomiting, diarrhea
1% to 10%:
Dermatologic: Lyell's syndrome, Stevens-Johnson syndrome
Hematologic: Granulocytopenia, leukopenia, thrombocytopenia, aplastic anemia, hemolytic anemia
Hepatic: Hepatitis
<1%:
Endocrine & metabolic: Thyroid function disturbance
Hepatic: Jaundice
Renal: Interstitial nephritis, acute nephropathy, crystalluria, hematuria
(Continued)

Sulfadiazine *(Continued)*

Miscellaneous: Serum sickness-like reactions

Drug Interactions Decreased effect with PABA or PABA metabolites of drugs (eg, procaine, proparacaine, tetracaine, sunscreens); decreased effect of oral anticoagulants and oral hypoglycemic agents

Drug Uptake
Absorption: Oral: Well absorbed
Serum half-life: 10 hours
Time to peak serum concentration: Within 3-6 hours

Pregnancy Risk Factor B (D at term)

Sulfadiazine, Sulfamethazine, and Sulfamerazine

(sul fa dye′ a zeen sul fa meth′ a zeen & sul fa mer′ a zeen)

Therapeutic Category Antibiotic, Sulfonamide Derivative; Antibiotic, Vaginal

Synonyms Multiple Sulfonamides; Trisulfapyrimidines

Use Treatment of toxoplasmosis

Local Anesthetic/Vasoconstrictor Precautions No information available to require special precautions

Effects on Dental Treatment No effects or complications reported

Sulfadoxine and Pyrimethamine

(sul fa dox′ een & peer i meth′ a meen)

Brand Names Fansidar®

Therapeutic Category Antimalarial Agent

Use Treatment of *Plasmodium falciparum* malaria in patients in whom chloroquine resistance is suspected; malaria prophylaxis for travelers to areas where chloroquine-resistant malaria is endemic

Usual Dosage Children and Adults: Oral:
Treatment of acute attack of malaria: A single dose of the following number of Fansidar® tablets is used in sequence with quinine or alone:
2-11 months: $1/4$ tablet
1-3 years: $1/2$ tablet
4-8 years: 1 tablet
9-14 years: 2 tablets
>14 years: 2-3 tablets

Malaria prophylaxis:
The first dose of Fansidar® should be taken 1-2 days before departure to an endemic area (CDC recommends that therapy be initiated 1-2 days before such travel), administration should be continued during the stay and for 4-6 weeks after return. Dose = pyrimethamine 0.5 mg/kg/dose and sulfadoxine 10 mg/kg/dose up to a maximum of 25 mg pyrimethamine and 500 mg sulfadoxine/dose weekly.
2-11 months: $1/8$ tablet weekly **or** $1/4$ tablet once every 2 weeks
1-3 years: $1/4$ tablet once weekly **or** $1/2$ tablet once every 2 weeks
4-8 years: $1/2$ tablet once weekly **or** 1 tablet once every 2 weeks
9-14 years: $3/4$ tablet once weekly **or** $11/2$ tablets once every 2 weeks
>14 years: 1 tablet once weekly **or** 2 tablets once every 2 weeks

Mechanism of Action Sulfadoxine interferes with bacterial folic acid synthesis and growth via competitive inhibition of para-aminobenzoic acid; pyrimethamine inhibits microbial dihydrofolate reductase, resulting in inhibition of tetrahydrofolic acid synthesis

Local Anesthetic/Vasoconstrictor Precautions No information available to require special precautions

Effects on Dental Treatment No effects or complications reported

Other Adverse Effects
>10%:
Central nervous system: Ataxia, seizures, headache
Dermatologic: Photosensitivity
Gastrointestinal: Atrophic glossitis, vomiting, gastritis
Hematologic: Megaloblastic anemia, leukopenia, thrombocytopenia, pancytopenia
Neuromuscular & skeletal: Tremors
Miscellaneous: Hypersensitivity
1% to 10%:
Dermatologic: Stevens-Johnson syndrome
Hepatic: Hepatitis
<1%:
Dermatologic: Erythema multiforme, toxic epidermal necrolysis, rash
Endocrine & metabolic: Thyroid function dysfunction
Gastrointestinal: Anorexia, glossitis

Hepatic: Hepatic necrosis
Renal: Crystalluria
Respiratory: Respiratory failure
Drug Interactions
Decreased effect with PABA or PABA metabolites of local anesthetics
Increased toxicity with methotrexate, other sulfonamides, co-trimoxazole
Drug Uptake
Absorption: Oral: Well absorbed
Serum half-life:
Pyrimethamine: 80-95 hours
Sulfadoxine: 5-8 days
Time to peak serum concentration: Within 2-8 hours
Pregnancy Risk Factor C

Sulfair® see Sodium Sulfacetamide on page 793
Sulfalax® [OTC] see Docusate on page 295
Sulfamethoprim® see Trimethoprim and Sulfamethoxazole on page 874

Sulfamethoxazole (sul fa meth ox' a zole)
Brand Names Gantanol®; Urobak®
Canadian/Mexican Brand Names Apo-Sulfamethoxazole® (Canada)
Therapeutic Category Antibiotic, Sulfonamide Derivative
Synonyms Sulfametoxazol (Mexico)
Use Treatment of urinary tract infections, nocardiosis, toxoplasmosis, acute otitis media, and acute exacerbations of chronic bronchitis due to susceptible organisms
Usual Dosage Oral:
Children >2 months: 50-60 mg/kg as single dose followed by 50-60 mg/kg/day divided every 12 hours; maximum: 3 g/24 hours or 75 mg/kg/day
Adults: 2 g stat, 1 g 2-3 times/day; maximum: 3 g/24 hours
Mechanism of Action Interferes with bacterial growth by inhibiting bacterial folic acid synthesis through competitive antagonism of PABA
Local Anesthetic/Vasoconstrictor Precautions No information available to require special precautions
Effects on Dental Treatment No effects or complications reported
Other Adverse Effects
>10%:
Central nervous system: Fever, dizziness, headache
Dermatologic: Itching, skin rash, photosensitivity
Gastrointestinal: Anorexia, nausea, vomiting, diarrhea
1% to 10%:
Dermatologic: Lyell's syndrome, Stevens-Johnson syndrome
Hematologic: Granulocytopenia, leukopenia, thrombocytopenia, aplastic anemia, hemolytic anemia
Hepatic: Hepatitis
<1%:
Cardiovascular: Vasculitis
Endocrine & metabolic: Thyroid function disturbance
Hepatic: Jaundice
Renal: Crystalluria, hematuria, acute nephropathy, interstitial nephritis
Miscellaneous: Serum sickness-like reactions
Drug Interactions
Decreased effect with PABA or PABA metabolites of drugs (ie, procaine, proparacaine, tetracaine)
Increased effect of oral anticoagulants, oral hypoglycemic agents, and methotrexate
Drug Uptake
Absorption: Oral: 90%
Serum half-life: 9-12 hours, prolonged with renal impairment
Time to peak serum concentration: Within 3-4 hours
Pregnancy Risk Factor B (D at term)

Sulfamethoxazole and Phenazopyridine
(sul fa meth ox' a zole & fen az oh peer' i deen)
Brand Names Azo Gantanol®
Therapeutic Category Antibiotic, Sulfonamide Derivative
Use Treatment of urinary tract infections complicated with pain
Local Anesthetic/Vasoconstrictor Precautions No information available to require special precautions
Effects on Dental Treatment No effects or complications reported

Sulfamethoxazole and Trimethoprim *see* Trimethoprim and Sulfamethoxazole *on page 874*

Sulfametoxazol (Mexico) *see* Sulfamethoxazole *on previous page*

Sulfamylon® *see* Mafenide Acetate *on page 520*

Sulfanilamide (sul fa nil′ a mide)

Brand Names AVC™ Cream; AVC™ Suppository; Vagitrol®

Therapeutic Category Antifungal Agent, Vaginal

Use Treatment of vulvovaginitis caused by *Candida albicans*

Usual Dosage Adults: Female: Insert one applicatorful intravaginally once or twice daily continued through 1 complete menstrual cycle or insert one suppository intravaginally once or twice daily for 30 days

Mechanism of Action Interferes with microbial folic acid synthesis and growth via inhibition of para-aminiobenzoic acid metabolism

Local Anesthetic/Vasoconstrictor Precautions No information available to require special precautions

Effects on Dental Treatment No effects or complications reported

Other Adverse Effects

1% to 10%:

Dermatologic: Itching, skin rash, burning, irritation, exfoliative dermatitis, Stevens-Johnson syndrome

Gastrointestinal: Nausea, vomiting

Hematologic: Agranulocytosis, hemolytic anemia in patients with severe G-6-PD deficiency

Hepatic: Kernicterus, hepatic toxicity

Renal: Crystalluria

<1%: Irritation of penis of sexual partner

Drug Interactions No data reported

Pregnancy Risk Factor B (D at term)

Sulfasalazine (sul fa sal′ a zeen)

Brand Names Azulfidine®; Azulfidine® EN-tabs®

Canadian/Mexican Brand Names Apo-Sulfasalazine® (Canada); PMS-Sulfasalazine® (Canada); Salazopyrin® (Canada); Salazopyrin EN-Tabs® (Canada); S.A.S® (Canada)

Therapeutic Category 5-Aminosalicylic Acid Derivative; Anti-inflammatory Agent

Use Management of ulcerative colitis

Usual Dosage Oral:

Children >2 years: 40-60 mg/kg/day in 3-6 divided doses, not to exceed 6 g/day; maintenance dose: 20-30 mg/kg/day in 4 divided doses; not to exceed 2 g/day

Adults: 1 g 3-4 times/day, 2 g/day maintenance in divided doses; not to exceed 6 g/day

Mechanism of Action Acts locally in the colon to decrease the inflammatory response and systemically interferes with secretion by inhibiting prostaglandin synthesis

Local Anesthetic/Vasoconstrictor Precautions No information available to require special precautions

Effects on Dental Treatment No effects or complications reported

Other Adverse Effects

>10%:

Central nervous system: Fever, dizziness, headache

Dermatologic: Itching, skin rash, photosensitivity

Gastrointestinal: Anorexia, nausea, vomiting, diarrhea

Genitourinary: Reversible oligospermia

1% to 10%:

Dermatologic: Lyell's syndrome, Stevens-Johnson syndrome

Hematologic: Granulocytopenia, leukopenia, thrombocytopenia, aplastic anemia, hemolytic anemia

Hepatic: Hepatitis

<1%:

Endocrine & metabolic: Thyroid function disturbance

Hepatic: Jaundice

Renal: Interstitial nephritis, acute nephropathy, crystalluria, hematuria

Miscellaneous: Serum sickness-like reactions

Drug Interactions

Decreased effect with iron, digoxin and PABA or PABA metabolites of drugs (ie, procaine, proparacaine, tetracaine)

Decreased effect of oral anticoagulants, methotrexate, and oral hypoglycemic agents
Drug Uptake
Absorption: 10% to 15% of dose is absorbed as unchanged drug from the small intestine
Serum half-life: 5.7-10 hours
Pregnancy Risk Factor B (D at term)

Sulfatrim® *see* Trimethoprim and Sulfamethoxazole *on page 874*

Sulfatrim® DS *see* Trimethoprim and Sulfamethoxazole *on page 874*

Sulfinpyrazone (sul fin peer' a zone)
Brand Names Anturane®
Canadian/Mexican Brand Names Antazone® (Canada); Anturan® (Canada); Apo-Sulfinpyrazone® (Canada); Novo-Pyrazone® (Canada); Nu-Sulfinpyrazone® (Canada)
Therapeutic Category Uric Acid Lowering Agent
Use Treatment of chronic gouty arthritis and intermittent gouty arthritis

Unlabeled use: To decrease the incidence of sudden death postmyocardial infarction
Usual Dosage Adults: Oral: 100-200 mg twice daily; maximum daily dose: 800 mg
Mechanism of Action Acts by increasing the urinary excretion of uric acid, thereby decreasing blood urate levels; this effect is therapeutically useful in treating patients with acute intermittent gout, chronic tophaceous gout, and acts to promote resorption of tophi; also has antithrombic and platelet inhibitory effects
Local Anesthetic/Vasoconstrictor Precautions No information available to require special precautions
Effects on Dental Treatment No effects or complications reported
Other Adverse Effects
>10%: Gastrointestinal: Nausea, vomiting, stomach pain
1% to 10%: Dermatologic: Dermatitis, skin rash
<1%:
Cardiovascular: Flushing
Central nervous system: Dizziness, headache
Dermatologic: Rash
Hematologic: Anemia, leukopenia, increased bleeding time (decreased platelet aggregation)
Hepatic: Hepatic necrosis
Genitourinary: Urinary frequency, uric acid stones
Renal: Nephrotic syndrome
Drug Interactions
Decreased effect/levels of theophylline, verapamil; decreased uricosuric activity with salicylates, niacins
Increased effect of oral hypoglycemics and anticoagulants
Risk of acetaminophen hepatotoxicity is increased, but therapeutic effects may be reduced
Drug Uptake
Absorption: Complete and rapid
Serum half-life, elimination: 2.7-6 hours
Time to peak serum concentration: 1.6 hours
Pregnancy Risk Factor C

Sulfisoxasol (Mexico) *see* Sulfisoxazole *on this page*

Sulfisoxazole (sul fi sox' a zole)
Brand Names Gantrisin®
Canadian/Mexican Brand Names Novo-Soxazole® (Canada); Sulfizole® (Canada)
Therapeutic Category Antibiotic, Sulfonamide Derivative
Synonyms Sulfisoxasol (Mexico)
Use Treatment of urinary tract infections, otitis media, *Chlamydia*; nocardiosis; treatment of acute pelvic inflammatory disease in prepubertal children; often used in combination with trimethoprim
Usual Dosage
Oral (not for use in patients <2 months of age):
Children >2 months: 75 mg/kg stat, followed by 120-150 mg/kg/day in divided doses every 4-6 hours; not to exceed 6 g/day
Pelvic inflammatory disease: 100 mg/kg/day in divided doses every 6 hours; used in combination with ceftriaxone
(Continued)

Sulfisoxazole *(Continued)*

    Chlamydia trachomatis: 100 mg/kg/day in divided doses every 6 hours
   Adults: 2-4 g stat, 4-8 g/day in divided doses every 4-6 hours
    Pelvic inflammatory disease: 500 mg every 6 hours for 21 days; used in combination with ceftriaxone
    Chlamydia trachomatis: 500 mg every 6 hours for 10 days
   Elderly: 2 g stat, then 2-8 g/day in divided doses every 6 hours
   Ophthalmic: Children and Adults:
    Solution: Instill 1-2 drops to affected eye every 2-3 hours
    Ointment: Apply small amount to affected eye 1-3 times/day and at bedtime

Mechanism of Action Interferes with bacterial growth by inhibiting bacterial folic acid synthesis through competitive antagonism of PABA

Local Anesthetic/Vasoconstrictor Precautions No information available to require special precautions

Effects on Dental Treatment No effects or complications reported

Other Adverse Effects
  >10%:
    Central nervous system: Fever, dizziness, headache
    Dermatologic: Itching, skin rash, photosensitivity
    Gastrointestinal: Anorexia, nausea, vomiting, diarrhea
  1% to 10%:
    Dermatologic: Lyell's syndrome, Stevens-Johnson syndrome
    Hematologic: Granulocytopenia, leukopenia, thrombocytopenia, aplastic anemia, hemolytic anemia
    Hepatic: Hepatitis
  <1%:
    Endocrine & metabolic: Thyroid function disturbance
    Hepatic: Jaundice
    Renal: Interstitial nephritis, acute nephropathy, crystalluria, hematuria
    Miscellaneous: Serum sickness-like reactions

Drug Interactions
  Decreased effect with PABA or PABA metabolites of drugs (ie, procaine, proparacaine, tetracaine), thiopental
  Increased effect of oral anticoagulants, methotrexate and oral hypoglycemic agents

Drug Uptake
  Absorption: Sulfisoxazole acetyl is hydrolyzed in the GI tract to sulfisoxazole which is readily absorbed
  Serum half-life: 4-7 hours, prolonged with renal impairment
  Time to peak serum concentration: Within 2-3 hours

Pregnancy Risk Factor B (D at term)

Sulfisoxazole and Phenazopyridine

(sul fi sox' zole & fen az oh peer' i deen)

Brand Names Azo Gantrisin®

Therapeutic Category Antibiotic, Sulfonamide Derivative; Local Anesthetic, Urinary

Use Treatment of urinary tract infections and nocardiosis

Usual Dosage Adults: Oral: 4-6 tablets to start, then 2 tablets 4 times/day for 2 days, then continue with sulfisoxazole only

Mechanism of Action Interferes with bacterial growth by inhibiting bacterial folic acid synthesis through competitive antagonism of PABA; phenazopyridine exerts local anesthetic or analgesic action on urinary tract mucosa through an unknown mechanism

Local Anesthetic/Vasoconstrictor Precautions No information available to require special precautions

Effects on Dental Treatment No effects or complications reported

Other Adverse Effects
  >10%:
    Central nervous system: Fever, dizziness, headache
    Dermatologic: Itching, skin rash, photosensitivity
    Gastrointestinal: Anorexia, nausea, vomiting, diarrhea
  1% to 10%:
    Dermatologic: Lyell's syndrome, Stevens-Johnson syndrome
    Hematologic: Granulocytopenia, leukopenia, thrombocytopenia, aplastic anemia, hemolytic anemia
    Hepatic: Hepatitis
  <1%:
    Endocrine & metabolic: Thyroid function disturbance
    Hepatic: Jaundice

Renal: Crystalluria, hematuria, acute nephropathy, interstitial nephritis
Miscellaneous: Serum sickness-like reactions

Drug Interactions
Decreased effect with PABA or PABA metabolites of drugs (ie, procaine, proparacaine, tetracaine), thiopental
Increased effect of oral anticoagulants, methotrexate and oral hypoglycemic agents

Drug Uptake
Absorption: Sulfisoxazole acetyl is hydrolyzed in the GI tract to sulfisoxazole which is readily absorbed
Serum half-life: 4-7 hours, prolonged with renal impairment
Time to peak serum concentration: Within 2-3 hours

Pregnancy Risk Factor B (D at term)

Sulfoxaprim® *see* Trimethoprim and Sulfamethoxazole *on page 874*

Sulfoxaprim® DS *see* Trimethoprim and Sulfamethoxazole *on page 874*

Sulfur and Salicylic Acid (sul' fur & sal i sil' ik as' id)

Brand Names Aveeno® Cleansing Bar [OTC]; Fostex® [OTC]; Pernox® [OTC]; Sastid® Plain Therapeutic Shampoo and Acne Wash [OTC]; Sebulex® [OTC]

Therapeutic Category Antiseborrheic Agent, Topical

Synonyms Salicylic Acid and Sulfur

Use Therapeutic shampoo for dandruff and seborrheal dermatitis; acne skin cleanser

Local Anesthetic/Vasoconstrictor Precautions No information available to require special precautions

Effects on Dental Treatment No effects or complications reported

Other Adverse Effects Local: Topical preparations containing 2% to 5% sulfur generally are well tolerated, local irritation may occur, concentration >15% is very irritating to the skin, higher concentration (eg, 10% or higher) may cause systemic toxicity (eg, headache, vomiting, muscle cramps, dizziness, collapse)

Comments For external use only

Sulfur and Sodium Sulfacetamide
(sul' fur & sow' dee um sul fa see' ta mide)

Brand Names Novacet® Topical; Sulfacet-R® Topical

Therapeutic Category Acne Products

Synonyms Sodium Sulfacetamide and Sulfur

Use Aid in the treatment of acne vulgaris, acne rosacea and seborrheic dermatitis

Local Anesthetic/Vasoconstrictor Precautions No information available to require special precautions

Effects on Dental Treatment No effects or complications reported

Sulindac (sul in' dak)

Related Information
Nonsteroidal Anti-Inflammatory Agents, Comparative Dosages, and Pharmacokinetics *on page 1021*
Rheumatoid Arthritis, Osteoarthritis, and Joint Prostheses *on page 930*
Temporomandibular Dysfunction (TMD) *on page 963*

Brand Names Clinoril®

Canadian/Mexican Brand Names Apo-Sulin® (Canada); Novo-Sundac® (Canada)

Therapeutic Category Analgesic, Non-narcotic; Anti-inflammatory Agent; Nonsteroidal Anti-inflammatory Agent (NSAID), Oral

Use Management of inflammatory disease, rheumatoid disorders; acute gouty arthritis; structurally similar to indomethacin but acts like aspirin; safest NSAID for use in mild renal impairment

Usual Dosage Maximum therapeutic response may not be realized for up to 3 weeks. Oral:

Children: Dose not established
Adults: 150-200 mg twice daily or 300-400 mg once daily; not to exceed 400 mg/day

Mechanism of Action Inhibits prostaglandin synthesis by decreasing the activity of the enzyme, cyclo-oxygenase, which results in decreased formation of prostaglandin precursors

Local Anesthetic/Vasoconstrictor Precautions No information available to require special precautions

Effects on Dental Treatment No effects or complications reported
(Continued)

Sulindac (Continued)

Other Adverse Effects

>10%:

Central nervous system: Dizziness

Dermatologic: Skin rash

Gastrointestinal: Abdominal cramps, heartburn, indigestion, nausea

1% to 10%:

Cardiovascular: Fluid retention

Central nervous system: Headache, nervousness

Dermatologic: Itching

Gastrointestinal: Vomiting

Otic: Ringing in ears

<1%:

Cardiovascular: Congestive heart failure, hypertension, arrhythmias, hot flushes, tachycardia

Central nervous system: Epistaxis, confusion, hallucinations, aseptic meningitis, mental depression, drowsiness, insomnia

Dermatologic: Hives, erythema multiforme, toxic epidermal necrolysis, Stevens-Johnson syndrome, angioedema

Endocrine & metabolic: Polydipsia

Gastrointestinal: Gastritis, GI ulceration

Genitourinary: Cystitis

Hematologic: Agranulocytosis, anemia, hemolytic anemia, bone marrow depression, leukopenia, thrombocytopenia

Hepatic: Hepatitis

Neuromuscular & skeletal: Peripheral neuropathy

Ocular: Toxic amblyopia, blurred vision, conjunctivitis, dry eyes

Otic: Decreased hearing

Renal: Polyuria, acute renal failure

Respiratory: Allergic rhinitis, shortness of breath

Drug Interactions

Decreased effect: Aspirin may decrease sulindac serum concentrations

Increased toxicity: Sulindac may increase digoxin, methotrexate, and lithium serum concentrations; other nonsteroidal anti-inflammatories may increase adverse gastrointestinal effects of sulindac

Drug Uptake

Absorption: 90%

Serum half-life:

Parent drug: 7 hours

Active metabolite: 18 hours

Pregnancy Risk Factor B (D at term)

Sulten-10® see Sodium Sulfacetamide on page 793

Sultrin™ see Sulfabenzamide, Sulfacetamide, and Sulfathiazole on page 806

Sumacal® [OTC] see Glucose Polymers on page 400

Sumatriptan Succinate (soo′ ma trip tan suk′ si nate)

Brand Names Imitrex®

Canadian/Mexican Brand Names Imigran® (Mexico)

Therapeutic Category Antimigraine Agent

Use Acute treatment of migraine with or without aura

Unlabeled use: Cluster headaches

Usual Dosage Adults:

Oral: 25 mg (taken with fluids); maximum recommended dose is 100 mg. If a satisfactory response has not been obtained at 2 hours, a second dose of up to 100 mg may be given. Efficacy of this second dose has not been examined. If a headache returns, additional doses may be taken at intervals of at least 2 hours up to a daily maximum of 300 mg. There is no evidence that an initial dose of 100 mg provides substantially greater relief than 25 mg.

S.C.: 6 mg; a second injection may be administered at least 1 hour after the initial dose, but not more than 2 injections in a 24-hour period

Mechanism of Action Selective agonist for serotonin (5HT-$_{1-D}$ receptor) in cranial arteries to cause vasoconstriction and reduces sterile inflammation associated with antidromic neuronal transmission correlating with relief of migraine

Local Anesthetic/Vasoconstrictor Precautions No information available to require special precautions

Effects on Dental Treatment No effects or complications reported

Other Adverse Effects

>10%:

Central nervous system: Tingling, hot flushes, dizziness

Local: Injection site reaction
1% to 10%:
  Cardiovascular: Tightness in chest
  Central nervous system: Weakness, burning sensation, drowsiness, headache, numbness, neck pain
  Gastrointestinal: Abdominal discomfort, sweating
  Neuromuscular & skeletal: Myalgia
  Miscellaneous: Mouth discomfort, jaw discomfort
<1%:
  Dermatologic: Skin rashes
  Endocrine & metabolic: Polydipsia, dehydration, dysmenorrhea
  Renal: Dysuria, renal calculus
  Respiratory: Dyspnea
  Miscellaneous: Thirst, hiccups
Drug Interactions Increased toxicity: Ergot-containing drugs
Drug Uptake After S.C. administration:
  Serum half-life:
  Time to peak serum concentration: 5-20 minutes
Pregnancy Risk Factor C

Sumycin® see Tetracycline on page 829

Sunscreen, PABA-Free see Methoxycinnamate and Oxybenzone on page 564

SuperChar® [OTC] see Charcoal on page 179

Suplical® [OTC] see Calcium Carbonate on page 140

Supprelin™ see Histrelin on page 425

Suppress® [OTC] see Dextromethorphan on page 266

Suprax® see Cefixime on page 165

Suprofen (soo proe′ fen)
Brand Names Profenal®
Therapeutic Category Nonsteroidal Anti-Inflammatory Agent (NSAID), Ophthalmic
Use Inhibition of intraoperative miosis
Usual Dosage Adults: On day of surgery, instill 2 drops in conjunctival sac at 3, 2, and 1 hour prior to surgery; or 2 drops in sac every 4 hours, while awake, the day preceding surgery
Mechanism of Action Inhibits prostaglandin synthesis, acts on the hypothalamus heat-regulating center to reduce fever, blocks prostaglandin synthetase action which prevents formation of the platelet-aggregating substance thromboxane A_2; decreases pain receptor sensitivity.
Local Anesthetic/Vasoconstrictor Precautions No information available to require special precautions
Effects on Dental Treatment No effects or complications reported
Other Adverse Effects
1% to 10%: Topical: Transient burning or stinging, redness, iritis
<1%:
  Systemic: Chemosis, photophobia
  Topical: Discomfort, pain, punctate epithelial staining
Drug Interactions Decreased effect: When used concurrently with suprofen, acetylcholine chloride and carbachol may be ineffective
Drug Uptake
  Serum half-life, elimination: 2-4 hours
  Time to peak serum concentration: ~1 hour
Pregnancy Risk Factor C

Surbex® [OTC] see Vitamin B Complex on page 899

Surbex-T® **Filmtabs**® [OTC] see Vitamin B Complex With Vitamin C on page 900

Surbex® **with C Filmtabs**® [OTC] see Vitamin B Complex With Vitamin C on page 900

Surfak® [OTC] see Docusate on page 295

Surgicel® see Cellulose, Oxidized on page 174

Surgicel® **Absorbable Hemostat** see Cellulose, Oxidized Regenerated on page 175

Surmontil® see Trimipramine Maleate on page 876

Survanta® see Beractant on page 108

Susano® see Hyoscyamine, Atropine, Scopolamine, and Phenobarbital on page 444

Sus-Phrine® see Epinephrine (Dental) on page 313

Sustaire® see Theophylline/Aminophylline on page 832

Sutilains (soo' ti lains)
Brand Names Travase®

Therapeutic Category Enzyme, Topical Debridement

Use Promote debridement of necrotic debris, as an adjunct in the treatment of second and third degree burns, decubitus ulcers

Usual Dosage Children and Adults: Topical: Thoroughly cleanse and irrigate wound then apply ointment in a thin layer extending ¼" to ½" beyond the tissue being debrided; apply loose moist dressing; repeat 3-4 times/day

Mechanism of Action Enzymatically converts denatured proteins (necrotic soft tissue, hemoglobin and purulent exudate) to peptides and amino acids

Local Anesthetic/Vasoconstrictor Precautions No information available to require special precautions

Effects on Dental Treatment No effects or complications reported

Other Adverse Effects 1% to 10%:
Central nervous system: Pain
Dermatologic: Transient dermatitis
Hematologic: Bleeding
Neuromuscular & skeletal: Paresthesia

Drug Interactions Benzalkonium chloride, hexachlorophene, iodine, thimerosal, and silver nitrate decrease the actions of sutilains

Drug Uptake
Onset of action: Within 1 hour
Duration: 8-12 hours
Peak effect: May take 7 days for maximal effect to be achieved for burns or wounds and up to 14 days in decubital and peripheral vascular ulcers

Pregnancy Risk Factor B

Sween® Cream [OTC] *see* Methylbenzethonium Chloride *on page 566*

Swim-Ear® Otic [OTC] *see* Boric Acid *on page 118*

Syllact® [OTC] *see* Psyllium *on page 750*

Symadine® *see* Amantadine Hydrochloride *on page 41*

Symmetrel® *see* Amantadine Hydrochloride *on page 41*

Synalar® *see* Fluocinolone Acetonide *on page 372*

Synalar-HP® *see* Fluocinolone Acetonide *on page 372*

Synalgos® [OTC] *see* Aspirin *on page 78*

Synalgos®-DC *see* Dihydrocodeine, Acetaminophen, and Aspirin *on page 281*

Synarel® *see* Nafarelin Acetate *on page 598*

Synemol® *see* Fluocinolone Acetonide *on page 372*

Synthetic Lung Surfactant *see* Colfosceril Palmitate *on page 230*

Synthroid® *see* Levothyroxine Sodium *on page 498*

Syntocinon® *see* Oxytocin *on page 654*

Syracol-CF® [OTC] *see* Guaifenesin and Dextromethorphan *on page 408*

Systemic Considerations Related to Natural Products for Weight Loss *see page 979*

Systemic Viral Diseases *see page 934*

Sytobex® *see* Cyanocobalamin *on page 237*

Tac™-3 *see* Triamcinolone *on page 862*

TACE® *see* Chlorotrianisene *on page 189*

Tacrine Hydrochloride (tak' reen hye droe klor' ide)
Brand Names Cognex®

Therapeutic Category Cholinergic Agent

Use Treatment of mild to moderate dementia of the Alzheimer's type

Dose Adjustment Based Upon Transaminase Elevations

ALT	Regimen
≤3 x ULN*	Continue titration
>3 to ≤5 x ULN	Decrease dose by 40 mg/day, resume when ALT returns to normal
>5 x ULN	Stop treatment, may rechallenge upon return of ALT to normal

*ULN = upper limit of normal.

Usual Dosage Adults: Initial: 10 mg 4 times/day; may increase by 40 mg/day adjusted every 6 weeks; maximum: 160 mg/day; best administered separate from meal times; see table.

Patients with clinical jaundice confirmed by elevated total bilirubin (>3 mg/dL) should not be rechallenged with tacrine

Mechanism of Action A deficiency of cortical acetylcholine is believed to account for some of the clinical manifestations of mild to moderate dementia. Tacrine probably acts by elevating acetylcholine concentrations in the cortical areas by slowing the degradation of acetylcholine released by still intact cholinergic neurons.

Local Anesthetic/Vasoconstrictor Precautions No information available to require special precautions

Effects on Dental Treatment No effects or complications reported

Other Adverse Effects 1% to 10%:
Central nervous system: Sweating
Gastrointestinal: Diarrhea, nausea, abdominal discomfort
Genitourinary: Increased urination

Drug Interactions Increased effect of theophylline, cimetidine, succinylcholine, cholinesterase inhibitors, or cholinergic agonists

Pregnancy Risk Factor C

Tacrolimus (ta kroe' li mus)

Brand Names Prograf®

Therapeutic Category Immunosuppressant Agent

Use Potent immunosuppressive drug used in liver, kidney, heart, lung, or small bowel transplant recipients

Usual Dosage
Children:
I.V. continuous infusion: 0.1 mg/kg/day
Oral: 0.3 mg/kg/day
Adults:
I.V. continuous infusion: Initial (at least 6 hours after transplantation): 0.05-0.1 mg/kg/day
Oral (within 2-3 days): 0.15-0.3 mg/kg/day in divided doses every 12 hours; give 8-12 hours after discontinuation of the I.V. infusion; may gradually adjust (decrease) maintenance dose via pharmacokinetic monitoring

Mechanism of Action Suppressed humoral immunity (inhibits T-lymphocyte activation); produced by the fungus streptomyces tsukubaensis

Local Anesthetic/Vasoconstrictor Precautions No information available to require special precautions

Effects on Dental Treatment No effects or complications reported

Other Adverse Effects
>10%:
Cardiovascular: Hypertension
Central nervous system: Headache, insomnia, abdominal/back pain, fever, asthenia
Dermatologic: Pruritus
Endocrine & metabolic: Hypo-/hyperkalemia, hyperglycemia, hypomagnesemia
Gastrointestinal: Diarrhea, nausea, anorexia, vomiting
Hematologic: Anemia, leukocytosis
Hepatic: LFT abnormalities, ascites
Neuromuscular & skeletal: Tremors, paresthesias
Renal: Nephrotoxicity, elevated creatinine and BUN
Respiratory: Peripheral edema, pleural effusion, atelectasis, dyspnea
1% to 10%:
Dermatologic: Rash
Gastrointestinal: Constipation
Genitourinary: Urinary tract infection
Hematologic: Thrombocytopenia
Renal: Oliguria

Drug Interactions

Antacids: Tacrolimus absorption impaired (separate administration by at least 2 hours)

Nephrotoxic antibiotics potentially increase tacrolimus associated nephrotoxicity; amphotericin B potentially increases tacrolimus associated nephrotoxicity

Agents which may increase tacrolimus plasma concentrations and consequently effect and toxicity include erythromycin, clarithromycin, clotrimazole, fluconazole, itraconazole, ketoconazole, diltiazem, nicardipine, verapamil, (Continued)

Tacrolimus *(Continued)*

bromocriptine, cimetidine, danazol, metoclopramide, methylprednisolone, cyclosporine (synergistic immunosuppression)

Agents which may decrease tacrolimus plasma concentrations and consequently effect include rifampin, rifabutin, phenytoin, phenobarbital, and carbamazepine

Drug Uptake

Absorption: Better in small bowel patients with a closed stoma; unlike cyclosporine, clamping of the T-tube in liver transplant patients does not alter trough concentrations or AUC; food within 15 minutes of administration decreases absorption (27%); T_{max}: 0.5-4 hours

Serum half-life, elimination: 12 hours (range: 4-40 hours, twice as fast in children)

Pregnancy Risk Factor C

Tagamet® *see Cimetidine on page 207*

Talacen® *see Pentazocine Compound on page 672*

Talwin® *see Pentazocine on page 671*

Talwin® Compound *see Pentazocine Compound on page 672*

Talwin® NX *see Pentazocine on page 671*

Tambocor™ *see Flecainide Acetate on page 365*

Tamine® [OTC] *see Brompheniramine and Phenylpropanolamine on page 123*

Tamoxifen Citrate *(ta mox' i fen sit' rate)*

Brand Names Nolvadex®

Canadian/Mexican Brand Names Alpha-Tamoxifen® (Canada); Apo-Tamox® (Canada); Novo-Tamoxifen® (Canada); Tamofen® (Canada); Tamone® (Canada); Bilem® (Mexico); Cryoxifeno® (Mexico); Tamoxan® (Mexico); Taxus® (Mexico)

Therapeutic Category Antineoplastic Agent, Hormone (Antiestrogen)

Synonyms Tamoxifeno (Mexico)

Use Palliative or adjunctive treatment of advanced breast cancer

Unlabeled use: Treatment of mastalgia, gynecomastia, male breast cancer, and pancreatic carcinoma. Studies have shown tamoxifen to be effective in the treatment of primary breast cancer in elderly women. Comparative studies with other antineoplastic agents in elderly women with breast cancer had more favorable survival rates with tamoxifen. Initiation of hormone therapy rather than chemotherapy is justified for elderly patients with metastatic breast cancer who are responsive.

Usual Dosage Oral (refer to individual protocols):

Adults: 10-20 mg twice daily in the morning and evening

High-dose therapy is under investigation

Mechanism of Action Competitively binds to estrogen receptors on tumors and other tissue targets, producing a nuclear complex that decreases DNA synthesis and inhibits estrogen effects; nonsteroidal agent with potent antiestrogenic properties which compete with estrogen for binding sites in breast and other tissues; cells accumulate in the G_0 and G_1 phases; therefore, tamoxifen is cytostatic rather than cytocidal.

Local Anesthetic/Vasoconstrictor Precautions No information available to require special precautions

Effects on Dental Treatment No effects or complications reported

Other Adverse Effects

>10%:

Gastrointestinal: Little to mild nausea (10%), vomiting, weight gain

General: Flushing, increased bone and tumor pain and local disease flare shortly after starting therapy; this will subside rapidly, but patients should be aware of this since many may discontinue the drug due to the side effects; skin rash, hepatotoxicity

Myelosuppressive: Transient thrombocytopenia occurs in 24% of patients receiving 10-20 mg/day; platelet counts return to normal within several weeks in spite of continued administration; leukopenia has also been reported and does resolve during continued therapy; anemia has also been reported

1% to 10%:

Central nervous system: Lightheadedness, depression, dizziness, headache, lassitude, mental confusion, weakness

Dermatologic: Rash

Endocrine & metabolic: Hypercalcemia may occur in patients with bone metastases; galactorrhea and vitamin deficiency, menstrual irregularities

Genitourinary: Vaginal bleeding or discharge, endometriosis, priapism, possible endometrial cancer

Ocular: Ophthalmologic effects (visual acuity changes, cataracts, or retinopathy), corneal opacities

Thromboembolism: Tamoxifen has been associated with the occurrence of venous thrombosis and pulmonary embolism; arterial thrombosis has also been described in a few case reports

Drug Interactions
Increased toxicity:
Allopurinol results in exacerbation of allopurinol-induced hepatotoxicity
Cyclosporine may result in increased cyclosporine serum levels
Warfarin results in significant enhancement of the anticoagulant effects of warfarin; has been speculated that a decrease in antitumor effect of tamoxifen may also occur due to alterations in the percentage of active tamoxifen metabolites

Drug Uptake
Absorption: Well absorbed from GI tract
Time to peak serum concentration: Oral: Within 4-7 hours
Serum half-life: 7 days

Pregnancy Risk Factor D

Tamoxifeno (Mexico) *see* Tamoxifen Citrate *on previous page*

Tanoral® Tablet *see* Chlorpheniramine, Pyrilamine, and Phenylephrine *on page 195*

Tao® *see* Troleandomycin *on page 880*

Tapazole® *see* Methimazole *on page 556*

Taractan® *see* Chlorprothixene *on page 198*

Tavist® *see* Clemastine Fumarate *on page 214*

Tavist-D® *see* Clemastine and Phenylpropanolamine *on page 213*

Taxol® *see* Paclitaxel *on page 655*

Taxotere® *see* Docetaxel *on page 294*

Tazicef® *see* Ceftazidime *on page 171*

Tazidime® *see* Ceftazidime *on page 171*

3TC *see* Lamivudine *on page 489*

Tear Drop® Solution [OTC] *see* Artificial Tears *on page 75*

TearGard® Ophthalmic Solution [OTC] *see* Artificial Tears *on page 75*

Teargen® Ophthalmic Solution [OTC] *see* Artificial Tears *on page 75*

Tearisol® Solution [OTC] *see* Artificial Tears *on page 75*

Tears Naturale® Free Solution [OTC] *see* Artificial Tears *on page 75*

Tears Naturale® II Solution [OTC] *see* Artificial Tears *on page 75*

Tears Naturale® Solution [OTC] *see* Artificial Tears *on page 75*

Tears Plus® Solution [OTC] *see* Artificial Tears *on page 75*

Tears Renewed® Solution [OTC] *see* Artificial Tears *on page 75*

Tebamide® *see* Trimethobenzamide Hydrochloride *on page 873*

Tedral® *see* Theophylline, Ephedrine, and Phenobarbital *on page 836*

Tega-Cert® [OTC] *see* Dimenhydrinate *on page 286*

Tegison® *see* Etretinate *on page 349*

Tegopen® *see* Cloxacillin Sodium *on page 224*

Tegretol® *see* Carbamazepine *on page 151*

Tegretol-XR® *see* Carbamazepine *on page 151*

T.E.H.® *see* Theophylline, Ephedrine, and Hydroxyzine *on page 836*

Telachlor® *see* Chlorpheniramine Maleate *on page 191*

Teladar® *see* Betamethasone *on page 109*

Teldrin® [OTC] *see* Chlorpheniramine Maleate *on page 191*

Temaril® *see* Trimeprazine Tartrate *on page 871*

Temazepam (te maz' e pam)
Brand Names Restoril®
Therapeutic Category Benzodiazepine; Hypnotic; Sedative
Use Treatment of anxiety and as an adjunct in the treatment of depression; also may be used in the management of panic attacks; transient insomnia and sleep latency
Usual Dosage Adults: Oral: 15-30 mg at bedtime; 15 mg in elderly or debilitated patients
Mechanism of Action Benzodiazepine anxiolytic sedative that produces CNS depression at the subcortical level, except at high doses, whereby it works at the cortical level; causes minimal change in REM sleep patterns
(Continued)

Temazepam *(Continued)*

Local Anesthetic/Vasoconstrictor Precautions No information available to require special precautions

Effects on Dental Treatment Over 10% of patients will exhibit significant dry mouth; normal salivary flow returns with cessation of drug therapy

Other Adverse Effects

>10%:

Cardiovascular: Tachycardia, chest pain

Central nervous system: Drowsiness, fatigue, impaired coordination, light-headedness, memory impairment, insomnia, anxiety, depression, headache

Dermatologic: Rash

Endocrine & metabolic: Decreased libido

Gastrointestinal: Dry mouth, constipation, diarrhea, decreased salivation, nausea, vomiting, increased or decreased appetite

Neuromuscular & skeletal: Dysarthria

Ocular: Blurred vision

Miscellaneous: Sweating

1% to 10%:

Cardiovascular: Syncope, hypotension

Central nervous system: Confusion, nervousness, dizziness, akathisia

Dermatologic: Dermatitis

Gastrointestinal: Increased salivation

Neuromuscular & skeletal: Rigidity, tremor, muscle cramps

Otic: Tinnitus

Respiratory: Nasal congestion, hyperventilation weight gain or loss

<1%:

Central nervous system: Reflex slowing

Endocrine & metabolic: Menstrual irregularities

Hematologic: Blood dyscrasias

Miscellaneous: Drug dependence

Drug Interactions Increased effect of CNS depressants; contraindicated with alcohol

Drug Uptake

Serum half-life: 9.5-12.4 hours

Time to peak serum concentration: Within 2-3 hours

Pregnancy Risk Factor X

Temazin® Cold Syrup [OTC] *see* Chlorpheniramine and Phenylpropanolamine *on page 190*

Temovate® *see* Clobetasol Propionate *on page 216*

Temporomandibular Dysfunction (TMD) *see page 963*

Tempra® [OTC] *see* Acetaminophen *on page 14*

Tenex® *see* Guanfacine Hydrochloride *on page 413*

Teniposide *(ten i poe' side)*

Brand Names Vumon Injection

Therapeutic Category Antineoplastic Agent, Miscellaneous

Synonyms EPT; VM-26

Use Treatment of Hodgkin's and non-Hodgkin's lymphomas, acute lymphocytic leukemia, bladder carcinoma and neuroblastoma

Usual Dosage I.V.:

Children: 130 mg/m^2/week, increasing to 150 mg/m^2 after 3 weeks and up to 180 mg/m^2 after 6 weeks

Adults: 50-180 mg/m^2 once or twice weekly for 4-6 weeks or 20-60 mg/m^2/day for 5 days

Acute lymphoblastic leukemia (ALL): 165 mg/m^2 twice weekly for 8-9 doses **or** 250 mg/m^2 weekly for 4-8 weeks

Small cell lung cancer: 80-90 mg/m^2/day for 5 days

Mechanism of Action Inhibits mitotic activity; inhibits cells from entering mitosis

Local Anesthetic/Vasoconstrictor Precautions No information available to require special precautions

Effects on Dental Treatment No effects or complications reported

Other Adverse Effects

>10%:

Gastrointestinal: Mucositis, nausea, vomiting, diarrhea

Hematologic: Myelosuppression, leukopenia, neutropenia, thrombocytopenia

Miscellaneous: Infection

1% to 10%:
  Cardiovascular: Hypotension
  Central nervous system: Fever
  Dermatologic: Alopecia, rash
  Hematologic: Hemorrhage
  Miscellaneous: Hypersensitivity
<1%:
  Central nervous system: Peripheral neurotoxicity
  Endocrine & metabolic: Metabolic abnormalities
  Hepatic: Hepatic dysfunction
  Renal: Renal dysfunction
Drug Uptake
  Serum half-life: 5 hours
Pregnancy Risk Factor D

Tenoretic® *see* Atenolol and Chlorthalidone *on page 84*

Tenormin® *see* Atenolol *on page 83*

Tenuate® *see* Diethylpropion Hydrochloride *on page 276*

Tenuate® Dospan® *see* Diethylpropion Hydrochloride *on page 276*

Tepanil® *see* Diethylpropion Hydrochloride *on page 276*

Terak® Ophthalmic Ointment *see* Oxytetracycline and Polymyxin B *on page 653*

Terazol® *see* Terconazole *on page 823*

Terazosin (ter ay' zoe sin)
Related Information
  Cardiovascular Diseases *on page 912*
Brand Names Hytrin®
Therapeutic Category Alpha-Adrenergic Blockers - Peripheral-Acting (Alpha$_1$-Blockers)
Synonyms Terazosina (Mexico)
Use Management of mild to moderate hypertension; considered a step 2 drug in stepped approach to hypertension; benign prostate hypertrophy
Usual Dosage Adults: Oral:
  Hypertension: Initial: 1 mg at bedtime; slowly increase dose to achieve desired blood pressure, up to 20 mg/day; usual dose: 1-5 mg/day
  Dosage reduction may be needed when adding a diuretic or other antihypertensive agent; if drug is discontinued for greater than several days, consider beginning with initial dose and retitrate as needed; dosage may be given on a twice daily regimen if response is diminished at 24 hours and hypotensive is observed at 2-4 hours following a dose
  Benign prostatic hypertrophy: Initial: 1 mg at bedtime, increasing as needed; most patients require 10 mg day; if no response after 4-6 weeks of 10 mg/day, may increase to 20 mg/day
Mechanism of Action Alpha$_1$-specific blocking agent with minimal alpha$_2$ effects; this allows peripheral postsynaptic blockade, with the resultant decrease in arterial tone, while preserving the negative feedback loop which is mediated by the peripheral presynaptic alpha$_2$-receptors; terazosin relaxes the smooth muscle of the bladder neck, thus reducing bladder outlet obstruction
Local Anesthetic/Vasoconstrictor Precautions No information available to require special precautions
Effects on Dental Treatment No effects or complications reported
Other Adverse Effects
  >10%:
    Cardiovascular: Orthostatic hypotension
    Central nervous system: Dizziness, lightheadedness, drowsiness, headache, malaise
  1% to 10%:
    Cardiovascular: Edema, palpitations
    Central nervous system: Fatigue, nervousness
    Gastrointestinal: Dry mouth
    Genitourinary: Urinary incontinence
  <1%:
    Cardiovascular: Angina
    Central nervous system: Nightmares, drowsiness, hypothermia
    Dermatologic: Rash
    Endocrine & metabolic: Sexual dysfunction
    Gastrointestinal: Nausea, urinary frequency
    Genitourinary: Priapism
    Respiratory: Dyspnea, nasal congestion
(Continued)

Terazosin *(Continued)*

Drug Interactions Increased hypotensive effect with diuretics and antihypertensive medications (especially beta-blockers)

Drug Uptake
Absorption: Oral: Rapid
Serum half-life: 9.2-12 hours
Time to peak serum concentration: Within 1 hour

Pregnancy Risk Factor C

Terazosina (Mexico) *see* Terazosin *on previous page*

Terbenafina Clorhidrato De (Mexico) *see* Terbinafine *on this page*

Terbinafine (ter' bin a feen)

Brand Names Lamisil®

Therapeutic Category Antifungal Agent, Topical

Synonyms Terbenafina Clorhidrato De (Mexico)

Use Topical antifungal for the treatment of tinea pedis (athlete's foot), tinea cruris (jock itch), and tinea corporis (ring worm)

Unlabeled use: Cutaneous candidiasis and pityriasis versicolor

Usual Dosage Adults: Topical:
Athlete's foot: Apply to affected area twice daily for at least 1 week, not to exceed 4 weeks
Ringworm and jock itch: Apply to affected area once or twice daily for at least 1 week, not to exceed 4 weeks

Mechanism of Action Synthetic alkylamine derivative which inhibits squalene epoxidases which is a key enzyme in sterol biosynthesis in fungi to result in a deficiency in ergosterol within fungal cell wall and result in fungal cell death

Local Anesthetic/Vasoconstrictor Precautions No information available to require special precautions

Effects on Dental Treatment No effects or complications reported

Other Adverse Effects 1% to 10%: Local: Pruritus, contact dermatitis, irritation, stinging

Drug Interactions No data reported

Drug Uptake
Absorption: Topical: Limited

Pregnancy Risk Factor B

Terbutalina, Sulfato De (Mexico) *see* Terbutaline Sulfate *on this page*

Terbutaline Sulfate (ter byoo' ta leen sul' fate)

Related Information
Respiratory Diseases *on page 924*

Brand Names Brethaire®; Brethine®; Bricanyl®

Therapeutic Category Adrenergic Agonist Agent; Antiasthmatic; Beta-2-Adrenergic Agonist Agent; Bronchodilator

Synonyms Terbutalina, Sulfato De (Mexico)

Use Bronchodilator in reversible airway obstruction and bronchial asthma

Usual Dosage
Children <12 years:
Oral: Initial: 0.05 mg/kg/dose 3 times/day, increased gradually as required; maximum: 0.15 mg/kg/dose 3-4 times/day or a total of 5 mg/24 hours
S.C.: 0.005-0.01 mg/kg/dose to a maximum of 0.3 mg/dose every 15-20 minutes for 3 doses
Nebulization: 0.1-0.3 mg/kg/dose up to a maximum of 10 mg/dose every 4-6 hours
Inhalation: 1-2 inhalations every 4-6 hours

Children >12 years and Adults:
Oral:
12-15 years: 2.5 mg every 6 hours 3 times/day; not to exceed 7.5 mg in 24 hours
>15 years: 5 mg/dose every 6 hours 3 times/day; if side effects occur, reduce dose to 2.5 mg every 6 hours; not to exceed 15 mg in 24 hours
S.C.: 0.25 mg/dose repeated in 15-30 minutes for one time only; a total dose of 0.5 mg should not be exceeded within a 4-hour period
Nebulization: 0.1-0.3 mg/kg/dose every 4-6 hours
Inhalation: 2 inhalations every 4-6 hours; wait 1 minute between inhalations

Mechanism of Action Relaxes bronchial smooth muscle by action on beta$_2$-receptors with less effect on heart rate

Local Anesthetic/Vasoconstrictor Precautions No information available to require special precautions

Effects on Dental Treatment No effects or complications reported
Other Adverse Effects
>10%: Central nervous system: Nervousness, restlessness, trembling
1% to 10%:
Cardiovascular: Tachycardia, hypertension
Central nervous system: Dizziness, drowsiness, headache, weakness, insomnia
Gastrointestinal: Dry mouth, nausea, vomiting, bad taste in mouth
Neuromuscular & skeletal: Muscle cramps
Miscellaneous: Diaphoresis
<1%:
Cardiovascular: Chest pain, arrhythmias
Respiratory: Paradoxical bronchospasm
Drug Interactions
Decreased effect with beta-blockers
Increased toxicity with MAO inhibitors, TCAs
Drug Uptake
Onset of action:
Oral: 30-45 minutes
S.C.: Within 6-15 minutes
Serum half-life: 11-16 hours
Pregnancy Risk Factor B

Terconazole (ter kone' a zole)
Brand Names Terazol®
Canadian/Mexican Brand Names Fungistat® (Mexico); Fungistat® Dual (Mexico)
Therapeutic Category Antifungal Agent, Vaginal
Use Local treatment of vulvovaginal candidiasis
Usual Dosage Adults: Female: Insert 1 applicatorful intravaginally at bedtime for 7 consecutive days
Mechanism of Action Triazole ketal antifungal agent; involves inhibition of fungal cytochrome P-450. Specifically, terconazole inhibits cytochrome P-450-dependent 14-alpha-demethylase which results in accumulation of membrane disturbing 14-alpha-demethylsterols and ergosterol depletion.
Local Anesthetic/Vasoconstrictor Precautions No information available to require special precautions
Effects on Dental Treatment No effects or complications reported
Other Adverse Effects 1% to 10%: Genitourinary: Vulvar/vaginal burning
Drug Interactions No data reported
Drug Uptake Absorption: Extent of systemic absorption after vaginal administration may be dependent on the presence of a uterus; 5% to 8% in women who had a hysterectomy versus 12% to 16% in nonhysterectomy women
Pregnancy Risk Factor C
Dosage Forms
Cream, vaginal: 0.4% (45 g); 0.8% (20 g)
Suppository, vaginal: 80 mg (3s)
Generic Available No

Terfenadina (Mexico) see Terfenadine on this page

Terfenadine (ter fen' a deen)
Related Information
Dental Drug Interactions: Update on Drug Combinations Requiring Special Considerations on page 1022
Brand Names Seldane®
Canadian/Mexican Brand Names Apo-Terfenadine® (Canada); Novo-Terfenadine® (Canada); Keneter® (Mexico); Teldane® (Mexico)
Therapeutic Category Antihistamine
Synonyms Terfenadina (Mexico)
Use Perennial and seasonal allergic rhinitis and other allergic symptoms including urticaria; has drying effect in patients with asthma
Usual Dosage Oral:
Children:
3-6 years: 15 mg twice daily
6-12 years: 30 mg twice daily
Children >12 years and Adults: 60 mg twice daily
Mechanism of Action Competes with histamine for H_1-receptor sites on effector cells in the gastrointestinal tract, blood vessels, and respiratory tract; binds to lung receptors significantly greater than it binds to cerebellar receptors, resulting in a reduced sedative potential
(Continued)

Terfenadine *(Continued)*

Local Anesthetic/Vasoconstrictor Precautions No information available to require special precautions

Effects on Dental Treatment Up to 10% of patients taking terfenadine may have significant dry mouth which will disappear with cessation of drug therapy; no erythromycin products or antifungals (ketoconazole, itraconazole) should be given since cardiotoxicities could occur (See respective monographs in dental section)

Other Adverse Effects
1% to 10%:
Central nervous system: Headache, fatigue, nervousness, dizziness
Gastrointestinal: Appetite increase, weight increase, nausea, diarrhea, abdominal pain, dry mouth
Neuromuscular & skeletal: Arthralgia
Respiratory: Pharyngitis
<1%:
Cardiovascular: Edema, palpitations, hypotension, torsade de pointes
Central nervous system: Depression, epistaxis, slight drowsiness, sedation, dizziness, paradoxical excitement, insomnia
Dermatologic: Angioedema, photosensitivity, rash
Genitourinary: Urinary retention
Hepatic: Hepatitis
Neuromuscular & skeletal: Myalgia, paresthesia, tremor
Ocular: Blurred vision
Respiratory: Bronchospasm, thickening of bronchial secretions

Drug Interactions Serious cardiac events have occurred with elevated terfenadine levels
Increased effect with pseudoephedrine
Increased toxicity with ketoconazole, itraconazole, fluconazole, metronidazole, miconazole, erythromycin, troleandomycin, azithromycin, clarithromycin, cimetidine, bepridil, psychotropics, probucol, astemizole, carbamazepine

Drug Uptake
Duration of antihistaminic effect: Up to 12 hours
Serum half-life: 16-22 hours
Time to peak serum concentration: Within 1-2 hours

Pregnancy Risk Factor C
Dosage Forms Tablet: 60 mg
Dietary Considerations May be taken with food
Generic Available No

Terfenadine and Pseudoephedrine
(ter fen′ a deen & soo doe e fed′ rin)

Brand Names Seldane-D®
Therapeutic Category Antihistamine/Decongestant Combination
Use Perennial and seasonal allergic rhinitis and other allergic symptoms including urticaria; has drying effect in patients with asthma

Local Anesthetic/Vasoconstrictor Precautions
Pseudoephedrine: Use with caution since pseudoephedrine is a sympathomimetic amine which could interact with epinephrine to cause a pressor response
Terfenadine: No information available to require special precautions

Effects on Dental Treatment
Pseudoephedrine: Up to 10% of patients could also experience tachycardia & palpitations; use vasoconstrictor with caution
Terfenadine: Up to 10% of patients taking terfenadine may have significant dry mouth which will disappear with cessation of drug therapy; no erythromycin products or antifungals (ketoconazole, itraconazole) should be given since cardiotoxicities could occur (See respective monographs in dental section)

Other Adverse Effects
1% to 10%:
Central nervous system: Headache, fatigue, nervousness, dizziness
Gastrointestinal: Appetite (increased), weight increase, nausea, diarrhea, abdominal pain, dry mouth
Neuromuscular & skeletal: Arthralgia
Respiratory: Pharyngitis
<1%:
Cardiovascular: Edema, palpitations, hypotension, torsade de pointes
Central nervous system: Depression, sedation, dizziness, paradoxical excitement, insomnia, slight drowsiness
Dermatologic: Angioedema, photosensitivity, rash

    Genitourinary: Urinary retention
    Hepatic: Hepatitis
    Neuromuscular & skeletal: Myalgia, paresthesia, tremor
    Ocular: Blurred vision
    Respiratory: Epistaxis, thickening of bronchial secretions, bronchospasm

Terpin Hydrate (ter' pin hye' drate)
Therapeutic Category Expectorant
Use Symptomatic relief of cough
Local Anesthetic/Vasoconstrictor Precautions No information available to require special precautions
Effects on Dental Treatment No effects or complications reported

Terpin Hydrate and Codeine (ter' pin hye' drate & koe' deen)
Therapeutic Category Cough Preparation; Expectorant
Synonyms ETH and C
Use Symptomatic relief of cough
Local Anesthetic/Vasoconstrictor Precautions No information available to require special precautions
Effects on Dental Treatment No effects or complications reported

Terra-Cortril® Ophthalmic Suspension *see* Oxytetracycline and Hydrocortisone *on page 653*

Terramycin® IV *see* Oxytetracycline Hydrochloride *on page 653*

Terramycin® Ophthalmic Ointment *see* Oxytetracycline and Polymyxin B *on page 653*

Terramycin® w/Polymyxin B Ophthalmic Ointment *see* Oxytetracycline and Polymyxin B *on page 653*

Tesanone® *see* Testosterone *on this page*

Teslac® *see* Testolactone *on this page*

TESPA *see* Thiotepa *on page 841*

Tessalon® Perles *see* Benzonatate *on page 104*

Testex® *see* Testosterone *on this page*

Testoderm® *see* Testosterone *on this page*

Testolactone (tess toe lak' tone)
Brand Names Teslac®
Therapeutic Category Androgen
Use Palliative treatment of advanced disseminated breast carcinoma
Usual Dosage Adults: Female: Oral: 250 mg 4 times/day for at least 3 months; desired response may take as long as 3 months
Mechanism of Action Testolactone is a synthetic testosterone derivative without significant androgen activity. The drug inhibits steroid aromatase activity, thereby blocking the production of estradiol and estrone from androgen precursors such as testosterone and androstenedione. Unfortunately, the enzymatic block provided by testolactone is transient and is usually limited to a period of 3 months.
Local Anesthetic/Vasoconstrictor Precautions No information available to require special precautions
Effects on Dental Treatment No effects or complications reported
Other Adverse Effects 1% to 10%:
    Cardiovascular: Edema
    Dermatologic: Maculopapular rash
    Endocrine & metabolic: Hypercalcemia
    Gastrointestinal: Anorexia, diarrhea, nausea, swelling of tongue
    Neuromuscular & skeletal: Paresthesias, peripheral neuropathies
Drug Interactions No data reported
Drug Uptake
    Absorption: Oral: Absorbed well
Pregnancy Risk Factor C

Testosterona (Mexico) *see* Testosterone *on this page*

Testosterone (tess toss' ter one)
Brand Names Andro®; Andro-Cyp®; Andro-L.A.®; Andronate®; Andropository®; Andryl®; Delatest®; Delatestryl®; Depotest®; Depo®-Testosterone; Duratest®; Durathate®; Everone®; Histerone®; Tesanone®; Testex®; Testoderm®; Testrin® P.A.
Therapeutic Category Androgen
Synonyms Testosterona (Mexico)
(Continued)

Testosterone *(Continued)*

Use Androgen replacement therapy in the treatment of delayed male puberty; postpartum breast pain and engorgement; inoperable breast cancer; male hypogonadism

Usual Dosage

Delayed puberty: Males: Children: I.M.: 40-50 mg/m^2/dose (cypionate or enanthate) monthly for 6 months

Male hypogonadism: I.M.: 50-400 mg every 2-4 weeks

Initiation of pubertal growth: 40-50 mg/m^2/dose (cypionate or enanthate) monthly until the growth rate falls to prepubertal levels (~5 cm/year)

During terminal growth phase: 100 mg/m^2/dose (cypionate or enanthate) monthly until growth ceases

Maintenance virilizing dose: 100 mg/m^2/dose (cypionate or enanthate) twice monthly or 50-400 mg/dose every 2-4 weeks

Inoperable breast cancer: Adults: I.M.: 200-400 mg every 2-4 weeks

Hypogonadism: Males: Adults:

I.M.:

Testosterone or testosterone propionate: 10-25 mg 2-3 times/week

Testosterone cypionate or enanthate: 50-400 mg every 2-4 weeks

Postpubertal cryptorchism: Testosterone or testosterone propionate: 10-25 mg 2-3 times/week

Topical: Initial: 6 mg/day system applied daily applied on scrotal skin. If scrotal area is inadequate, start with a 4 mg/day system. Transdermal system should be worn for 22-24 hours. Determine total serum testosterone after 3-4 weeks of daily application. If patients have not achieved desired results after 6-8 weeks of therapy, another form of testosterone replacement therapy should be considered.

Mechanism of Action Principal endogenous androgen responsible for promoting the growth and development of the male sex organs and maintaining secondary sex characteristics in androgen-deficient males

Local Anesthetic/Vasoconstrictor Precautions No information available to require special precautions

Effects on Dental Treatment No effects or complications reported

Other Adverse Effects

\>10%:

Dermatologic: Acne

Endocrine & metabolic: Menstrual problems (amenorrhea), virilism, breast soreness

Genitourinary: Epididymitis, priapism, bladder irritability

1% to 10%:

Cardiovascular: Flushing, edema

Central nervous system: Excitation, aggressive behavior, sleeplessness, anxiety, mental depression, headache

Endocrine & metabolic: Prostatic hypertrophy, prostatic carcinoma, hirsutism (increase in pubic hair growth), impotence, testicular atrophy

Gastrointestinal: Nausea, vomiting, GI irritation

Hepatic: Hepatic dysfunction

<1%:

Endocrine & metabolic: Gynecomastia, hypercalcemia, leukopenia, suppression of clotting factors, polycythemia, hypoglycemia

Hepatic: Cholestatic hepatitis, hepatic necrosis

Miscellaneous: Hypersensitivity reactions

Drug Interactions Increased toxicity: Effects of oral anticoagulants may be enhanced

Drug Uptake

Duration of effect: Based upon the route of administration and which testosterone ester is used; the cypionate and enanthate esters have the longest duration, up to 2-4 weeks after I.M. administration

Serum half-life: 10-100 minutes

Pregnancy Risk Factor X

Testosterone and Estradiol *see* Estradiol and Testosterone *on page 326*

Testred® *see* Methyltestosterone *on page 570*

Testrin® **P.A.** *see* Testosterone *on previous page*

Tetanus Immune Globulin, Human

(tet' a nus i myun' glob' yoo lin hyu' min)

Related Information

Animal and Human Bites Guidelines *on page 976*

Brand Names Hyper-Tet®

Canadian/Mexican Brand Names Hyper-Tet® (Mexico); Tetanogamma® P (Mexico); Probi-Tet (Mexico)
Therapeutic Category Immune Globulin
Synonyms TIG
Use Passive immunization against tetanus; tetanus immune globulin is preferred over tetanus antitoxin for treatment of active tetanus; part of the management of an unclean, nonminor wound in a person whose history of previous receipt of tetanus toxoid is unknown or who has received less than three doses of tetanus toxoid
Usual Dosage I.M.:
Prophylaxis of tetanus:
Children: 4 units/kg; some recommend administering 250 units to small children
Adults: 250 units

Treatment of tetanus:
Children: 500-3000 units; some should infiltrate locally around the wound
Adults: 3000-6000 units

Tetanus Prophylaxis in Wound Management

Number of Prior Tetanus Toxoid Doses	Clean, Minor Wounds		All Other Wounds	
	Td*	TIG†	Td*	TIG†
Unknown or <3	Yes	No	Yes	Yes
≥3‡	No#	No	No¶	No

Adapted from Report of the Committee on Infectious Diseases, American Academy of Pediatrics, Elk Grove Village, IL: American Academy of Pediatrics, 1986.

*Adult tetanus and diphtheria toxoids; use pediatric preparations (DT or DTP) if the patient is <7 years old.

†Tetanus immune globulin.

‡If only three doses of fluid tetanus toxoid have been received, a fourth dose of toxoid, preferably an adsorbed toxoid, should be given.

#Yes, if >10 years since last dose.

¶Yes, if >5 years since last dose.

Mechanism of Action Passive immunity toward tetanus
Local Anesthetic/Vasoconstrictor Precautions No information available to require special precautions
Effects on Dental Treatment No effects or complications reported
Other Adverse Effects
>10%: Local: Pain, tenderness, erythema at injection site
1% to 10%:
Central nervous system: Fever (mild),
Dermatologic: Hives, angioedema
Neuromuscular & skeletal: Muscle stiffness
Miscellaneous: Anaphylaxis reaction
<1%: Local: Sensitization to repeated injections
Drug Uptake Absorption: Well absorbed
Pregnancy Risk Factor C
Comments Tetanus immune globulin is preferred over tetanus antitoxin for treatment of active tetanus

Tetanus Toxoid, Adsorbed (tet′ a nus toks′ oyd, ad sorbed′)
Canadian/Mexican Brand Names Tetanol® (Mexico)
Therapeutic Category Toxoid
Use Active immunization against tetanus
Usual Dosage Adults: I.M.:
Primary immunization: 0.5 mL; repeat 0.5 mL at 4-8 weeks after first dose and at 6-12 months after second dose
Routine booster doses are recommended only every 5-10 years
Mechanism of Action Tetanus toxoid preparations contain the toxin produced by virulent tetanus bacilli (detoxified growth products of *Clostridium tetani*). The toxin has been modified by treatment with formaldehyde so that is has lost toxicity but still retains ability to act as antigen and produce active immunity.
Local Anesthetic/Vasoconstrictor Precautions No information available to require special precautions
Effects on Dental Treatment No effects or complications reported
Other Adverse Effects
>10%: Local: Induration/redness at injection site
1% to 10%:
Central nervous system: Chills, fever
(Continued)

Tetanus Toxoid, Adsorbed *(Continued)*

Local: Sterile abscess at injection site
Miscellaneous: Allergic reaction
<1%:
Central nervous system: Fever >103°F, malaise, neurological disturbances
Local: Blistering at injection site
Miscellaneous: Arthus-type hypersensitivity reactions have occurred rarely in patients >25 years of age and who have received multiple booster doses

Drug Uptake Duration of immunization following primary immunization: ~10 years

Pregnancy Risk Factor C

Comments Routine booster doses are recommended only every 10 years

Tetanus Toxoid, Fluid (tet' a nus toks' oyd floo' id)

Canadian/Mexican Brand Names Tetinox® (Mexico); Toxoide Tetanico Myn® (Mexico)

Therapeutic Category Toxoid

Synonyms Tetanus Toxoid Plain

Use Active immunization against tetanus in adults and children

Usual Dosage

Anergy testing: Intradermal: 0.1 mL
Primary immunization (**Note:** Td, TD, DTaP/DTwP are recommended): Adults: Inject 3 doses of 0.5 mL I.M. or S.C. at 4- to 8-week intervals; give fourth dose 6-12 months after third dose
Booster doses: I.M., S.C.: 0.5 mL every 10 years

Mechanism of Action Tetanus toxoid preparations contain the toxin produced by virulent tetanus bacilli (detoxified growth products of *Clostridium tetani*). The toxin has been modified by treatment with formaldehyde so that is has lost toxicity but still retains ability to act as antigen and produce active immunity.

Local Anesthetic/Vasoconstrictor Precautions No information available to require special precautions

Effects on Dental Treatment No effects or complications reported

Other Adverse Effects

>10%: Local: Induration/redness at injection site
1% to 10%:
Central nervous system: Chills, fever
Local: Sterile abscess at injection site
Miscellaneous: Allergic reaction
<1%:
Central nervous system: Fever >103°F, malaise, neurological disturbances
Local: Blistering at injection site
Miscellaneous: Arthus-type hypersensitivity reactions

Pregnancy Risk Factor C

Comments Tetanus Toxoid, Adsorbed is preferred for all basic immunizing and recall reactions because of more persistent antitoxin titer induction

Tetanus Toxoid Plain *see* Tetanus Toxoid, Fluid *on this page*

Tetracaine Hydrochloride (tet' ra kane hye droe klor' ide)

Related Information

Mouth Pain, Cold Sore, Canker Sore Products *on page 1063*
Oral Nonviral Soft Tissue Ulcerations or Erosions *on page 955*
Oral Pain *on page 940*

Brand Names Pontocaine®; Viractin® [OTC]

Therapeutic Category Dental/Local Anesthetics; Local Anesthetic, Injectable; Local Anesthetic, Oral; Local Anesthetic, Topical

Use

Dental: Ester-type local anesthetic topically applied to nose and throat for various diagnostic procedures
Medical: Spinal anesthesia; local anesthesia in the eye for various diagnostic and examination purposes

Usual Dosage Children and Adults: Topical: Applied as a 1% cream to affected areas 3-4 times/day as needed

Mechanism of Action Local anesthetics bind selectively to the intracellular surface of sodium channels to block influx of sodium into the axon. As a result, depolarization necessary for action potential propagation and subsequent nerve function is prevented. The block at the sodium channel is reversible. When drug diffuses away from the axon, sodium channel function is restored and nerve propagation returns.

Local Anesthetic/Vasoconstrictor Precautions No information available to require special precautions

Effects on Dental Treatment No effects or complications reported

Other Adverse Effects 1% to 10%: Dermatologic: Contact dermatitis, burning, stinging, angioedema

Oral manifestations: No data reported

Contraindications Hypersensitivity to tetracaine or any component; ophthalmic secondary bacterial infection, patients with liver disease, CNS disease, meningitis (if used for epidural or spinal anesthesia), myasthenia gravis

Warnings/Precautions No pediatric dosage recommendations

Drug Interactions No data reported

Drug Uptake
Onset: Rapid
Duration of action: Topical: 1.5-3 hours

Pregnancy Risk Factor C

Breast-feeding Considerations No data reported

Dosage Forms
Cream: 1%
Cream (Viractin®): 2% (4 g)
Gel (Viractin®): 2% (4 g)

Dietary Considerations No data reported

Generic Available Yes

Tetracaine Hydrochloride, Benzocaine Butyl Aminobenzoate and Benzalkonium Chloride see Benzocaine, Butyl Aminobenzoate, Tetracaine, and Benzalkonium Chloride on page 103

Tetracaine With Dextrose (tet' ra kane with deks' trose)
Related Information
Oral Pain on page 940
Brand Names Pontocaine® With Dextrose Injection
Therapeutic Category Dental/Local Anesthetics; Local Anesthetic, Injectable
Use Spinal anesthesia (saddle block)
Local Anesthetic/Vasoconstrictor Precautions No information available to require special precautions
Effects on Dental Treatment No effects or complications reported

Tetraclear® [OTC] see Tetrahydrozoline Hydrochloride on page 831

Tetracycline (tet ra sye' kleen)
Related Information
Dental Drug Interactions: Update on Drug Combinations Requiring Special Considerations on page 1022
Oral Bacterial Infections on page 945
Oral Nonviral Soft Tissue Ulcerations or Erosions on page 955
Brand Names Achromycin®; Achromycin® V; Sumycin®; Tetracyn®
Canadian/Mexican Brand Names Apo-Tetra® (Canada); Novo-Tetra® (Canada); Nu-Tetra® (Canada); Acromicina® (Mexico); Ambotetra® (Mexico); Quimocyclar® (Mexico); Tetra-Atlantis® (Mexico); Zorbenal-G® (Mexico)
Therapeutic Category Acne Products; Antibiotic, Ophthalmic; Antibiotic, Tetracycline Derivative; Antibiotic, Topical
Use
Dental: Treatment of periodontitis associated with presence of *Actinobacillus actinomycetemcomitans* (AA). As adjunctive therapy in recurrent aphthous ulcers
Medical: In medicine for treatment of susceptible bacterial infections of both gram-positive and gram-negative organisms; also some unusual organisms including *Mycoplasma*, *Chlamydia*, and *Rickettsia*; may also be used for acne, exacerbations of chronic bronchitis, and treatment of gonorrhea and syphilis in patients that are allergic to penicillin
Usual Dosage Adults: 250 mg every 6 hours until improvement (usually 10 days or more)
Mechanism of Action Inhibits bacterial protein synthesis by binding with the 30S and possibly the 50S ribosomal subunit(s) of susceptible bacteria; may also cause alterations in the cytoplasmic membrane
Local Anesthetic/Vasoconstrictor Precautions No information available to require special precautions
Effects on Dental Treatment Tetracycline's are not recommended for use during pregnancy or in children ≤8 years of age since they have been reported to cause enamel hypoplasia and permanent teeth discoloration. The use of
(Continued)

Tetracycline *(Continued)*

tetracycline's should only be used in these patients if other agents are contra-indicated or alternative antimicrobials will not eradicate the organism. Long-term use associated with oral candidiasis.

Other Adverse Effects
>10%: Miscellaneous: Discoloration of teeth and enamel hypoplasia (infants)
1% to 10%:
  Dermatologic: Photosensitivity
  Gastrointestinal: Nausea, diarrhea

Oral manifestations: Opportunistic "superinfection" with *Candida albicans*

Contraindications Hypersensitivity to tetracycline or any component; do not administer to children ≤8 years of age

Warnings/Precautions Use of tetracyclines during tooth development may cause permanent discoloration of the teeth and enamel, hypoplasia and retar-dation of skeletal development and bone growth with risk being the greatest for children <4 years of age and those receiving high doses; use with caution in patients with renal or hepatic impairment and in pregnancy; dosage modifica-tion required in patients with renal impairment; pseudotumor cerebri has been reported with tetracycline use; outdated drug can cause nephropathy.

Drug Interactions Dairy products; calcium, magnesium or aluminum-containing antacids, iron, zinc, cimetidine causes decreased tetracycline absorption; methoxyflurane anesthesia when concurrent with tetracycline may cause fatal nephrotoxicity; warfarin with tetracyclines leads to increased anticoagulation; penicillin-tetracycline combination counteracts antibiotic effects of each; decreased effect of oral contraceptives

Drug Uptake
Absorption: Oral: 75%
Time to peak serum concentration: Oral: Within 2-4 hours
Serum half-life: Normal renal function: 8-11 hours
Influence of food: Decreases absorption

Pregnancy Risk Factor D; B (topical)

Breast-feeding Considerations May be taken while breast-feeding

Dosage Forms
Capsule: 100 mg, 250 mg, 500 mg
Suspension, oral: 125 mg/5 mL (60 mL, 480 mL)
Tablet: 250 mg, 500 mg

Dietary Considerations Should be taken 1 hour before or 2 hours after meals with adequate amounts of fluid; avoid taking antacids, iron, dairy products, or milk formulas within 3 hours of tetracyclines; decrease absorption of magne-sium, zinc, calcium, iron, and amino acids

Generic Available Yes

Comments *Helicobacter pylori:* Clinically effective treatment regimens include triple therapy with amoxicillin or tetracycline, metronidazole, and bismuth subsalicylate; amoxicillin, metronidazole, and H_2 receptor antagonist; or double therapy with amoxicillin and omeprazole. Adult dose of tetracycline against *H. pylori:* 250 mg 3 times/day to 500 mg 4 times/day

Selected Readings
Rams TE and Slots J, "Antibiotics in Periodontal Therapy: An Update," *Compendium*, 1992, 13(12):1130, 1132, 1134.

Tetracycline Periodontal Fibers
(tet ra sye' kleen per ee oh don' tal fye' bers)

Related Information
Dental Drug Interactions: Update on Drug Combinations Requiring Special Considerations *on page 1022*

Brand Names Actisite®

Therapeutic Category Antibacterial, Dental

Use
Dental: Treatment of adult periodontitis; as an adjunct to scaling and root planing for the reduction of pocket depth and bleeding on probing in selected patients with adult periodontitis
Medical: No data reported

Usual Dosage
Children: Has not been established
Adults: Insert fiber to fill the periodontal pocket; each fiber contains 12.7 mg of tetracycline in 23 cm (9 inches) and provides continuous release of drug for 10 days; fibers are to be secured in pocket with cyanoacrylate adhesive and left in place for 10 days

Mechanism of Action Tetracycline is an antibiotic which inhibits growth of susceptible microorganisms. Tetracycline binds primarily to the 30S subunits of bacterial ribosomes, and appears to prevent access of aminoacyl tRNA to the acceptor site on the mRNA-ribosome complex. The fiber releases tetracycline into the periodontal site at a rate of 2 mcg/cm/hour.

Local Anesthetic/Vasoconstrictor Precautions No information available to require special precautions

Effects on Dental Treatment No effects or complications reported

Other Adverse Effects 1% to 10%:
Dermatologic: Local erythema following removal
Miscellaneous: Discomfort from fiber placement

Oral manifestations: Gingival inflammation; pain in mouth; glossitis; candidiasis; staining of tongue

Contraindications Known hypersensitivity to tetracyclines

Warnings/Precautions Use of tetracyclines is not recommended during pregnancy because of interference with fetal bone and dental development

Drug Interactions No data reported

Drug Uptake
The fiber releases tetracycline at a rate of 2 mcg/cm/hour
Tissue fluid concentrations:
Gingival fluid: ~1590 mcg/mL of tetracycline per site over 10 days
Plasma: During fiber treatment of up to 11 teeth, the tetracycline plasma concentration was below any detectable levels (<0.1 mcg/mL)
Oral: 500 mg of tetracycline produces a peak plasma level of 3-4 mcg/mL
Saliva: ~50.7 mcg/mL of tetracycline immediately after fiber treatment of 9 teeth

Pregnancy Risk Factor C

Breast-feeding Considerations It is not known whether tetracycline from periodontal fibers is distributed into human breast milk

Dosage Forms Fibers 23 cm (9") in length; 12.7 mg of tetracycline hydrochloride per fiber

Dietary Considerations No data reported

Generic Available No

Comments A number of different facultative and obligate anaerobic bacteria have been found to be causative factors in periodontal disease. These include *Actinobacillus actinomycetemcomitans* (AA), *Fusobacterium nucleatum*, and *Porphyromonas gingivalis*. These bacteria are sensitive to tetracyclines at similar concentrations as those released from the tetracycline-impregnated fibers. Placement of tetracycline periodontal fibers into gingival pockets decreases inflammation, edema, pocket depth, and bleeding upon probing.

Tetracyn® *see* Tetracycline *on page 829*

Tetrahydrozoline Hydrochloride
(tet ra hye drozz′ a leen hye droe klor′ ide)

Brand Names Collyrium Fresh® [OTC]; Eye-Zine® [OTC]; Murine® Plus [OTC]; Ocu-Drop® [OTC]; Optigene® [OTC]; Soothe® [OTC]; Tetraclear® [OTC]; Tetra-Ide® [OTC]; Tyzine®; Visine® [OTC]; Visine A.C.® [OTC]

Therapeutic Category Adrenergic Agonist Agent; Adrenergic Agonist Agent, Ophthalmic; Nasal Agent, Vasoconstrictor; Ophthalmic Agent, Vasoconstrictor

Use Symptomatic relief of nasal congestion and conjunctival congestion

Usual Dosage
Nasal congestion: Intranasal:
Children 2-6 years: Instill 2-3 drops of 0.05% solution every 4-6 hours as needed, no more frequent than every 3 hours
Children >6 years and Adults: Instill 2-4 drops or 3-4 sprays of 0.1% solution every 3-4 hours as needed, no more frequent than every 3 hours

Conjunctival congestion: Ophthalmic: Adults: Instill 1-2 drops in each eye 2-4 times/day

Mechanism of Action Stimulates alpha-adrenergic receptors in the arterioles of the conjunctiva and the nasal mucosa to produce vasoconstriction

Local Anesthetic/Vasoconstrictor Precautions No information available to require special precautions

Effects on Dental Treatment No effects or complications reported

Other Adverse Effects
>10%: Local: Transient stinging, sneezing
1% to 10%:
Cardiovascular: Tachycardia, palpitations, increased blood pressure, heart rate
Central nervous system: Headache
Neuromuscular & skeletal: Tremor
(Continued)

Tetrahydrozoline Hydrochloride *(Continued)*

    Ocular: Blurred vision

Drug Interactions Increased toxicity: MAO inhibitors can cause an exaggerated adrenergic response if taken concurrently or within 21 days of discontinuing MAO inhibitor; beta-blockers can cause hypertensive episodes and increased risk of intracranial hemorrhage; anesthetics

Drug Uptake
    Onset of decongestant effect: Intranasal: Within 4-8 hours
    Duration: Ophthalmic vasoconstriction: 2-3 hours

Pregnancy Risk Factor C

Tetra-Ide® [OTC] *see* Tetrahydrozoline Hydrochloride *on previous page*

TG *see* Thioguanine *on page 838*

6-TG *see* Thioguanine *on page 838*

T/Gel® [OTC] *see* Coal Tar *on page 225*

T-Gen® *see* Trimethobenzamide Hydrochloride *on page 873*

T-Gesic® [5/500] *see* Hydrocodone and Acetaminophen *on page 431*

Thalitone® *see* Chlorthalidone *on page 199*

THAM-E® Injection *see* Tromethamine *on page 880*

THAM® Injection *see* Tromethamine *on page 880*

Theelin® *see* Estrone *on page 329*

Theo-24® *see* Theophylline/Aminophylline *on this page*

Theobid® *see* Theophylline/Aminophylline *on this page*

Theochron® *see* Theophylline/Aminophylline *on this page*

Theoclear® L.A. *see* Theophylline/Aminophylline *on this page*

Theo-Dur® *see* Theophylline/Aminophylline *on this page*

Theodur-Sprinkle® *see* Theophylline/Aminophylline *on this page*

Theo-G® *see* Theophylline and Guaifenesin *on page 836*

Theolair™ *see* Theophylline/Aminophylline *on this page*

Theolate® *see* Theophylline and Guaifenesin *on page 836*

Theon® *see* Theophylline/Aminophylline *on this page*

Theophylline/Aminophylline *(thee off' i lin)/(am in off' i lin)*

Related Information
    Dental Drug Interactions: Update on Drug Combinations Requiring Special Considerations *on page 1022*
    Respiratory Diseases *on page 924*

Brand Names Aerolate®; Aerolate III®; Aerolate JR®; Aerolate SR® S; Aminophyllin™; Aquaphyllin®; Asmalix®; Bronkodyl®; Constant-T®; Duraphyl™; Elixophyllin®; Elixophyllin® SR; LaBID®; Phyllocontin®; Quibron®-T; Quibron®-T/SR; Respbid®; Slo-bid™; Slo-Phyllin®; Sustaire®; Theo-24®; Theobid®; Theochron®; Theoclear® L.A.; Theo-Dur®; Theodur-Sprinkle®; Theolair™; Theon®; Theospan®-SR; Theovent®; Truphylline®

Canadian/Mexican Brand Names Apo-Theo® LA (Canada); Pulmophylline® (Canada); Phyllocontin® (Canada)

Therapeutic Category Antiasthmatic; Bronchodilator; Theophylline Derivative

Use Bronchodilator in reversible airway obstruction due to asthma, chronic bronchitis, and emphysema; for neonatal apnea/bradycardia

Usual Dosage Use ideal body weight for obese patients
    I.V.: Initial: Maintenance infusion rates:
        Children:
            6 weeks to 6 months: 0.5 mg/kg/hour
            6 months to 1 year: 0.6-0.7 mg/kg/hour

        Children >1 year and Adults:
            Treatment of acute bronchospasm: I.V.: Loading dose (in patients not currently receiving aminophylline or theophylline): 6 mg/kg (based on aminophylline) given I.V. over 20-30 minutes; administration rate should not exceed 25 mg/minute (aminophylline). See table.

Approximate I.V. Theophylline Dosage for Treatment of Acute Bronchospasm

Group	Dosage for next 12 h*	Dosage after 12 h*
Infants 6 wk to 6 mo	0.5 mg/kg/h	
Children 6 mo to 1 y	0.6-0.7 mg/kg/h	
Children 1-9 y	0.95 mg/kg/h (1.2 mg/kg/h)	0.79 mg/kg/h (1 mg/kg/h)
Children 9-16 y and young adult smokers	0.79 mg/kg/h (1 mg/kg/h)	0.63 mg/kg/h (0.8 mg/kg/h)
Healthy, nonsmoking adults	0.55 mg/kg/h (0.7 mg/kg/h)	0.39 mg/kg/h (0.5 mg/kg/h)
Older patients and patients with cor pulmonale	0.47 mg/kg/h (0.6 mg/kg/h)	0.24 mg/kg/h (0.3 mg/kg/h)
Patients with congestive heart failure or liver failure	0.39 mg/kg/h (0.5 mg/kg/h)	0.08-0.16 mg/kg/h (0.1-0.2 mg/kg/h)

*Equivalent hydrous aminophylline dosage indicated in parentheses.

Approximate I.V. maintenance dosages are based upon continuous infusions; bolus dosing (often used in children <6 months of age) may be determined by multiplying the hourly infusion rate by 24 hours and dividing by the desired number of doses/day; see table.

Maintenance Dose for Acute Symptoms

Population Group	Oral Theophylline (mg/kg/day)	I.V. Aminophylline
Premature infant or newborn - 6 wk (for apnea/bradycardia)	4	5 mg/kg/day
6 wk - 6 mo	10	12 mg/kg/day or continuous I.V. infusion*
Infants 6 mo-1 y	12-18	15 mg/kg/day or continuous I.V. infusion*
Children 1-9 y	20-24	1 mg/kg/hour
Children 9-12 y, and adolescent daily smokers of cigarettes or marijuana, and otherwise healthy adult smokers <50 y	16	0.9 mg/kg/hour
Adolescents 12-16 y (nonsmokers)	13	0.7 mg/kg/hour
Otherwise healthy nonsmoking adults (including elderly patients)	10 (not to exceed 900 mg/day)	0.5 mg/kg/hour
Cardiac decompensation, cor pulmonale and/or liver dysfunction	5 (not to exceed 400 mg/day)	0.25 mg/kg/hour

*For continuous I.V. infusion divide total daily dose by 24 = mg/kg/hour.

Dosage should be adjusted according to serum level measurements during the first 12- to 24-hour period; see table on following page

Oral theophylline: Initial dosage recommendation: Loading dose (to achieve a serum level of about 10 mcg/mL; loading doses should be given using a rapidly absorbed oral product **not** a sustained release product):

If no theophylline has been administered in the previous 24 hours: 4-6 mg/kg theophylline

If theophylline has been administered in the previous 24 hours: administer ½ loading dose or 2-3 mg/kg theophylline can be given in emergencies when serum levels are not available

On the average, for every 1 mg/kg theophylline given, blood levels will rise 2 mcg/mL

(Continued)

Theophylline/Aminophylline *(Continued)*

Dosage Adjustment After Serum Theophylline Measurement

Serum Theophylline		Guidelines
Within normal limits	10-20 mcg/mL	Maintain dosage if tolerated. Recheck serum theophylline concentration at 6- to 12-month intervals.*
Too high	20-25 mcg/mL	Decrease doses by about 10%. Recheck serum theophylline concentration after 3 days and then at 6- to 12-month intervals.*
	25-30 mcg/mL	Skip next dose and decrease subsequent doses by about 25%. Recheck serum theophylline.
	>30 mcg/mL	Skip next 2 doses and decrease subsequent doses by 50%. Recheck serum theophylline.
Too low	7.5-10 mcg/mL	Increase dose by about 25%.† Recheck serum theophylline concentration after 3 days and then at 6- to 12-month intervals.*
	5-7.5 mcg/mL	Increase dose by about 25% to the nearest dose increment† and recheck serum theophylline for guidance in further dosage adjustment (another increase will probably be needed, but this provides a safety check).

From Weinberger M and Hendeles L,"Practical Guide to Using Theophylline," *J Resp Dis*, 1981, 2:12-27.

*Finer adjustments in dosage may be needed for some patients.

†Dividing the daily dose into 3 doses administered at 8-hour intervals may be indicated if symptoms occur repeatedly at the end of a dosing interval.

Ideally, defer the loading dose if a serum theophylline concentration can be obtained rapidly. However, if this is not possible, exercise clinical judgment. If the patient is not experiencing theophylline toxicity, this is unlikely to result in dangerous adverse effects.

See table.

Oral Theophylline Dosage for Bronchial Asthma*

Age	Initial 3 Days	Second 3 Days	Steady-State Maintenance
<1 y	0.2 x (age in weeks) + 5		0.3 x (age in weeks) + 8
1-9 y	16 up to a maximum of 400 mg/24 h	20	22
9-12 y	16 up to a maximum of 400 mg/24 h	16 up to a maximum of 600 mg/24 h	20 up to a maximum of 800 mg/24 h
12-16 y	16 up to a maximum of 400 mg/24 h	16 up to a maximum of 600 mg/24 h	18 up to a maximum of 900 mg/24 h
Adults	400 mg/24 h	600 mg/24 h	900 mg/24 h

*Dose in mg/kg/24 hours of theophylline.

Increasing dose: The dosage may be increased in approximately 25% increments at 2- to 3-day intervals so long as the drug is tolerated or until the maximum dose is reached

Maintenance dose: In children and healthy adults, a slow-release product can be used; the total daily dose can be divided every 8-12 hours

Mechanism of Action Causes bronchodilatation, diuresis, CNS and cardiac stimulation, and gastric acid secretion by blocking phosphodiesterase which increases tissue concentrations of cyclic adenine monophosphate (cAMP) which in turn promotes catecholamine stimulation of lipolysis, glycogenolysis, and gluconeogenesis and induces release of epinephrine from adrenal medulla cells

Local Anesthetic/Vasoconstrictor Precautions No information available to require special precautions

Effects on Dental Treatment Do not prescribe any erythromycin product to patients taking theophylline products. Erythromycin will delay the normal metabolic inactivation of theophyllines leading to increased blood levels; this has resulted in nausea, vomiting and CNS restlessness

Other Adverse Effects See table.

Theophylline Serum Levels (mcg/mL)*	Adverse Reactions
15-25	GI upset, diarrhea, N/V, abdominal pain, nervousness, headache, insomnia, agitation, dizziness, muscle cramp, tremor
25-35	Tachycardia, occasional PVC
>35	Ventricular tachycardia, frequent PVC, seizure

*Adverse effects do not necessarily occur according to serum levels. Arrhythmia and seizure can occur without seeing the other adverse effects.

Uncommon at serum theophylline concentrations ≤20 mcg/mL

1% to 10%:

Cardiovascular: Tachycardia

Central nervous system: Nervousness, restlessness

Gastrointestinal: Nausea, vomiting

<1%: Allergic reactions:

Central nervous system: Insomnia, irritability, seizures

Dermatologic: Skin rash

Gastrointestinal: Gastric irritation

Neuromuscular & skeletal: Tremor

Drug Interactions Decreased effect/increased toxicity: Changes in diet may affect the elimination of theophylline; charcoal-broiled foods may increase elimination, reducing half-life by 50%; see table for factors affecting serum levels.

Factors Reported to Affect Theophylline Serum Levels

Decreased Theophylline Level	Increased Theophylline Level
Smoking (cigarettes, marijuana)	Hepatic cirrhosis
High protein/low carbohydrate diet	Cor pulmonale
Charcoal	CHF
Phenytoin	Fever/viral illness
Phenobarbital	Propranolol
Carbamazepine	Allopurinol (>600 mg/d)
Rifampin	Erythromycin
I.V. isoproterenol	Cimetidine
Aminoglutethimide	Troleandomycin
Barbiturates	Ciprofloxacin
Hydantoins	Oral contraceptives
Ketoconazole	Beta blockers
Sulfinpyrazone	Calcium channel blockers
Isoniazid	Corticosteroids
Loop diuretics	Disulfiram
Sympathomimetics	Ephedrine
	Influenza virus vaccine
	Interferon
	Macrolides
	Mexiletine
	Quinolones
	Thiabendazole
	Thyroid hormones
	Carbamazepine
	Isoniazid
	Loop diuretics

Pregnancy Risk Factor C

Theophylline and Guaifenesin (thee off' i lin & gwye fen' e sin)
Brand Names Bronchial®; Glycerol-T®; Lanophyllin-GG®; Quibron®; Slo-Phyllin® GG; Theo-G®; Theolate®
Therapeutic Category Antiasthmatic; Bronchodilator; Expectorant; Theophylline Derivative
Use Symptomatic treatment of bronchospasm associated with bronchial asthma, chronic bronchitis and pulmonary emphysema
Local Anesthetic/Vasoconstrictor Precautions No information available to require special precautions
Effects on Dental Treatment Do not prescribe any erythromycin product to patients taking theophylline products. Erythromycin will delay the normal metabolic inactivation of theophyllines leading to increased blood levels; this has resulted in nausea, vomiting and CNS restlessness

Theophylline, Ephedrine, and Hydroxyzine
(thee off' i lin, e fed' rin, & hye drox' i zeen)
Brand Names Hydrophen®; Marax®; T.E.H.®
Therapeutic Category Antiasthmatic; Bronchodilator; Theophylline Derivative
Use Possibly effective for controlling bronchospastic disorders
Local Anesthetic/Vasoconstrictor Precautions Use vasoconstrictors with caution since ephedrine may enhance cardiostimulation and vasopressor effects of sympathomimetics
Effects on Dental Treatment Do not prescribe any erythromycin product to patients taking theophylline products. Erythromycin will delay the normal metabolic inactivation of theophyllines leading to increased blood levels; this has resulted in nausea, vomiting and CNS restlessness

Theophylline, Ephedrine, and Phenobarbital
(thee off' i lin, e fed' rin, & fee noe bar' bi tal)
Brand Names Tedral®
Therapeutic Category Antiasthmatic; Bronchodilator; Theophylline Derivative
Synonyms Ephedrine, Theophylline and Phenobarbital
Use Prevention and symptomatic treatment of bronchial asthma; relief of asthmatic bronchitis and other bronchospastic disorders
Local Anesthetic/Vasoconstrictor Precautions Use vasoconstrictors with caution since ephedrine may enhance cardiostimulation and vasopressor effects of sympathomimetics
Effects on Dental Treatment Do not prescribe any erythromycin product to patients taking theophylline products. Erythromycin will delay the normal metabolic inactivation of theophyllines leading to increased blood levels; this has resulted in nausea, vomiting and CNS restlessness

Theospan®-SR *see* Theophylline/Aminophylline *on page 832*

Theovent® *see* Theophylline/Aminophylline *on page 832*

Therabid® [OTC] *see* Vitamins, Multiple on *page 901*

Thera-Combex® H-P Kapseals® [OTC] *see* Vitamin B Complex With Vitamin C *on page 900*

TheraCys™ *see* Bacillus Calmette-Guérin (BCG) Live *on page 93*

Thera-Flur® *see* Fluoride *on page 374*

Thera-Flur-N® *see* Fluoride *on page 374*

Theragran® [OTC] *see* Vitamins, Multiple *on page 901*

Theragran® Hematinic® *see* Vitamins, Multiple *on page 901*

Theragran® Liquid [OTC] *see* Vitamins, Multiple *on page 901*

Theragran-M® [OTC] *see* Vitamins, Multiple *on page 901*

Thera-Hist® Syrup [OTC] *see* Chlorpheniramine and Phenylpropanolamine *on page 190*

Theralax® [OTC] *see* Bisacodyl *on page 113*

Theramin® Expectorant [OTC] *see* Guaifenesin and Phenylpropanolamine *on page 409*

Theraplex Z® [OTC] *see* Pyrithione Zinc *on page 755*

Thermazene™ *see* Silver Sulfadiazine *on page 788*

Thiabendazole (thye a ben' da zole)
Brand Names Mintezol®
Therapeutic Category Anthelmintic
Use Treatment of strongyloidiasis, cutaneous larva migrans, visceral larva migrans, dracunculiasis, trichinosis, and mixed helminthic infections

Usual Dosage Purgation is not required prior to use; drinking of fruit juice aids in expulsion of worms by removing the mucous to which the intestinal tapeworms attach themselves.

Children and Adults: Oral: 50 mg/kg/day divided every 12 hours; maximum dose: 3 g/day
Strongyloidiasis: For 2 consecutive days
Cutaneous larva migrans: For 2-5 consecutive days
Visceral larva migrans: For 5-7 consecutive days
Trichinosis: For 2-4 consecutive days
Dracunculosis: 50-75 mg/kg/day divided every 12 hours for 3 days

Mechanism of Action Inhibits helminth-specific mitochondrial fumarate reductase

Local Anesthetic/Vasoconstrictor Precautions No information available to require special precautions

Effects on Dental Treatment No effects or complications reported

Other Adverse Effects
>10%:
Central nervous system: Numbness, seizures, hallucinations, delirium, dizziness, drowsiness, headache
Gastrointestinal: Anorexia, diarrhea, nausea, vomiting
Otic: Tinnitus
Miscellaneous: Drying of mucous membranes
1% to 10%: Dermatologic: Skin rash, Stevens-Johnson syndrome
<1%:
Central nervous system: Chills
Genitourinary: Malodor of urine
Hematologic: Leukopenia
Hepatic: Hepatotoxicity
Ocular: Blurred or yellow vision
Renal: Nephrotoxicity
Miscellaneous: Lymphadenopathy, hypersensitivity reactions

Drug Interactions Increased levels of theophylline and other xanthines

Drug Uptake
Absorption: Rapid and nearly complete
Time to peak serum concentration: Within 1-2 hours

Pregnancy Risk Factor C

Thiamine Hydrochloride (thye' a min hye droe klor' ide)
Brand Names Betalin®S; Biamine®
Canadian/Mexican Brand Names Betaxin® (Canada); Bewon® (Canada)
Therapeutic Category Vitamin, Water Soluble
Use Treatment of thiamine deficiency including beriberi, Wernicke's encephalopathy syndrome, and peripheral neuritis associated with pellagra, alcoholic patients with altered sensorium; various genetic metabolic disorders

Usual Dosage
Recommended daily allowance:
<6 months: 0.3 mg
6 months to 1 year: 0.4 mg
1-3 years: 0.7 mg
4-6 years: 0.9 mg
7-10 years: 1 mg
11-14 years: 1.1-1.3 mg
>14 years: 1-1.5 mg
Thiamine deficiency (beriberi):
Children: 10-25 mg/dose I.M. or I.V. daily (if critically ill), or 10-50 mg/dose orally every day for 2 weeks, then 5-10 mg/dose orally daily for 1 month
Adults: 5-30 mg/dose I.M. or I.V. 3 times/day (if critically ill); then orally 5-30 mg/day in single or divided doses 3 times/day for 1 month
Wenicke's encephalopathy: Adults: Initial: 100 mg I.V., then 50-100 mg/day I.M. or I.V. until consuming a regular, balanced diet
Dietary supplement (depends on caloric or carbohydrate content of the diet):
Children: 0.5-1 mg/day
Adults: 1-2 mg/day
Note: The above doses can be found in multivitamin preparations
Metabolic disorders: Oral: Adults: 10-20 mg/day (dosages up to 4 g/day in divided doses have been used)

Mechanism of Action An essential coenzyme in carbohydrate metabolism by combining with adenosine triphosphate to form thiamine pyrophosphate

Local Anesthetic/Vasoconstrictor Precautions No information available to require special precautions
(Continued)

Thiamine Hydrochloride *(Continued)*

Effects on Dental Treatment No effects or complications reported
Other Adverse Effects <1%:
Cardiovascular: Cardiovascular collapse and death
Central nervous system: Warmth, tingling
Dermatologic: Rash, angioedema
Drug Interactions No data reported
Drug Uptake
Absorption:
Oral: Adequate
I.M.: Rapid and complete
Pregnancy Risk Factor A (C if dose exceeds RDA recommendation)

Thiethylperazine Maleate *(thye eth il per' a zeen mal' ee ate)*

Brand Names Torecan®
Therapeutic Category Antiemetic
Use Relief of nausea and vomiting
Unlabeled use: Treatment of vertigo
Usual Dosage Children >12 years and Adults:
Oral, I.M., rectal: 10 mg 1-3 times/day as needed
I.V. and S.C. routes of administration are not recommended

Not dialyzable (0% to 5%)
Dosing comments in hepatic impairment: Use with caution
Mechanism of Action Blocks postsynaptic mesolimbic dopaminergic receptors in the brain; exhibits a strong alpha-adrenergic blocking effect and depresses the release of hypothalamic and hypophyseal hormones; acts directly on chemoreceptor trigger zone and vomiting center
Local Anesthetic/Vasoconstrictor Precautions No information available to require special precautions
Effects on Dental Treatment No effects or complications reported
Other Adverse Effects
>10%:
Central nervous system: Drowsiness, dizziness
Gastrointestinal: Dry mouth
Respiratory: Dry nose
1% to 10%:
Cardiovascular: Tachycardia, orthostatic hypotension
Central nervous system: Confusion, convulsions, extrapyramidal effects, tardive dyskinesia, fever, headache
Hematologic: Agranulocytosis
Hepatic: Cholestatic jaundice
Otic: Tinnitus
Drug Interactions Increased effect/toxicity with CNS depressants (eg, anesthetics, opiates, tranquilizers, alcohol), lithium, atropine, epinephrine, MAO inhibitors, TCAs
Drug Uptake
Onset of antiemetic effect: Within 30 minutes
Duration of action: ~4 hours
Pregnancy Risk Factor X

Thimerosal *(thye mer' oh sal)*

Brand Names Aeroaid® [OTC]; Mersol® [OTC]; Merthiolate® [OTC]
Therapeutic Category Antibacterial, Topical
Use Organomercurial antiseptic with sustained bacteriostatic and fungistatic activity
Local Anesthetic/Vasoconstrictor Precautions No information available to require special precautions
Effects on Dental Treatment No effects or complications reported

Thioguanine *(thye oh gwah' neen)*

Therapeutic Category Antineoplastic Agent, Antimetabolite
Synonyms 2-Amino-6-Mercaptopurine; TG; 6-TG; 6-Thioguanine; Tioguanine
Use Remission induction in acute myelogenous (nonlymphocytic) leukemia; treatment of chronic myelogenous leukemia and acute lymphocytic leukemia
Usual Dosage Total daily dose can be given at one time; offers little advantage over mercaptopurine; is sometimes ordered as 6-thioguanine, with 6 being part of the drug name and not some kind of unit or strength

Oral (refer to individual protocols):
  Children <3 years: Combination drug therapy for acute nonlymphocytic leukemia: 3.3 mg/kg/day in divided doses twice daily for 4 days
  Children and Adults: 2-3 mg/kg/day calculated to nearest 20 mg or 75-200 mg/m^2/day in 1-2 divided doses for 5-7 days or until remission is attained
Dosing comments in renal or hepatic impairment: Reduce dose
Mechanism of Action Purine analog that is incorporated into DNA and RNA resulting in the blockage of synthesis and metabolism of purine nucleotides
Local Anesthetic/Vasoconstrictor Precautions No information available to require special precautions
Effects on Dental Treatment No effects or complications reported
Other Adverse Effects
1% to 10%:
  Dermatologic: Skin rash
  Endocrine & metabolic: Hyperuricemia
  Gastrointestinal: Mild nausea or vomiting, anorexia, stomatitis, diarrhea
    Emetic potential: Low (<10%)
  Neuromuscular: Unsteady gait
<1%:
  Central nervous system: Neurotoxicity
  Dermatologic: Photosensitivity, skin rash
  Endocrine & metabolic: Hyperuricemia
  Hepatic: Hepatitis, jaundice, veno-occlusive hepatic disease
Drug Uptake
  Absorption: Oral: 30%
  Serum half-life, terminal: 11 hours
  Time to peak serum concentration: Within 8 hours
Pregnancy Risk Factor D

6-Thioguanine see Thioguanine *on previous page*
Thiola™ see Tiopronin *on page 849*

Thiopental Sodium (thye oh pen' tal sow' dee um)
Brand Names Pentothal® Sodium
Therapeutic Category Barbiturate; General Anesthetic, Intravenous; Sedative
Synonyms Tiopental Sodico (Mexico)
Use Induction of anesthesia; adjunct for intubation in head injury patients; control of convulsive states; treatment of elevated intracranial pressure
Usual Dosage I.V.:
Induction anesthesia:
  Children 1-12 years: 5-6 mg/kg
  Adults: 3-5 mg/kg

Maintenance anesthesia:
  Children: 1 mg/kg as needed
  Adults: 25-100 mg as needed

Increased intracranial pressure: Children and Adults: 1.5-5 mg/kg/dose; repeat as needed to control intracranial pressure

Seizures:
  Children: 2-3 mg/kg/dose, repeat as needed
  Adults: 75-250 mg/dose, repeat as needed

Rectal administration: (Patient should be NPO for no less than 3 hours prior to administration)
  Suggested initial doses of thiopental rectal suspension are:
    <3 months: 15 mg/kg/dose
    >3 months: 25 mg/kg/dose
  Note: The age of a premature infant should be adjusted to reflect the age that the infant would have been if full-term (eg, an infant, now age 4 months, who was 2 months premature should be considered to be a 2-month old infant).
  Doses should be rounded downward to the nearest 50 mg increment to allow for accurate measurement of the dose
  Inactive or debilitated patients and patients recently medicated with other sedatives, (eg, chloral hydrate, meperidine, chlorpromazine, and promethazine), may require smaller doses than usual

If the patient is not sedated within 15-20 minutes, a single repeat dose of thiopental can be given. The single repeat doses are:
  <3 months: <7.5 mg/kg/dose
  >3 months: 15 mg/kg/dose
(Continued)

Thiopental Sodium *(Continued)*

Adults weighing >90 kg should not receive >3 g as a total dose (initial plus repeat doses)

Children weighing >34 kg should not receive >1 g as a total dose (initial plus repeat doses)

Neither adults nor children should receive more than one course of thiopental rectal suspension (initial dose plus repeat dose) per 24-hour period

Mechanism of Action Interferes with transmission of impulses from the thalamus to the cortex of the brain resulting in an imbalance in central inhibitory and facilitatory mechanisms

Local Anesthetic/Vasoconstrictor Precautions No information available to require special precautions

Effects on Dental Treatment No effects or complications reported

Other Adverse Effects

>10%: Local: Pain on I.M. injection

1% to 10%: Gastrointestinal: Cramping, diarrhea, rectal bleeding

<1%:

Cardiovascular: Hypotension, peripheral vascular collapse, myocardial depression, cardiac arrhythmias

Central nervous system: Radial nerve palsy, seizures, headache, emergence delirium, prolonged somnolence and recovery, anxiety

Dermatologic: Erythema, pruritus, urticaria

Gastrointestinal: Nausea, vomiting, emesis

Hematologic: Hemolytic anemia

Local: Thrombophlebitis

Neuromuscular & skeletal: Tremor, involuntary muscle movement, twitching, rigidity

Respiratory: Respiratory depression, coughing, circulatory depression, rhinitis, apnea, laryngospasm, bronchospasm, sneezing, dyspnea

Miscellaneous: Hiccups, anaphylactic reactions

Drug Interactions Increased toxicity with CNS depressants (especially narcotic analgesics and phenothiazines), salicylates, sulfisoxazole

Drug Uptake

Onset of action: I.V.: Anesthesia occurs in 30-60 seconds

Duration: 5-30 minutes

Serum half-life: 3-11.5 hours, decreased in children vs adults

Pregnancy Risk Factor C

Thiophosphoramide *see* Thiotepa *on next page*

Thioridazine *(thye oh rid′ a zeen)*

Brand Names Mellaril®; Mellaril-S®

Canadian/Mexican Brand Names Apo-Thioridazine® (Canada); Novo-Ridazine® (Canada); PMS-Thioridazine® (Canada)

Therapeutic Category Antipsychotic Agent; Phenothiazine Derivative

Synonyms Tioridacina (Mexico)

Use Management of manifestations of psychotic disorders; depressive neurosis; alcohol withdrawal; dementia in elderly; behavioral problems in children

Usual Dosage Oral:

Children >2 years: Range: 0.5-3 mg/kg/day in 2-3 divided doses; usual: 1 mg/kg/day; maximum: 3 mg/kg/day

Behavior problems: Initial: 10 mg 2-3 times/day, increase gradually

Severe psychoses: Initial: 25 mg 2-3 times/day, increase gradually

Adults:

Psychoses: Initial: 50-100 mg 3 times/day with gradual increments as needed and tolerated; maximum: 800 mg/day in 2-4 divided doses; if >65 years, initial dose: 10 mg 3 times/day

Depressive disorders, dementia: Initial: 25 mg 3 times/day; maintenance dose: 20-200 mg/day

Not dialyzable (0% to 5%)

Mechanism of Action Blocks postsynaptic mesolimbic dopaminergic receptors in the brain; exhibits a strong alpha-adrenergic blocking effect and depresses the release of hypothalamic and hypophyseal hormones

Local Anesthetic/Vasoconstrictor Precautions No information available to require special precautions

Effects on Dental Treatment Significant hypotension may occur, especially when the drug is administered parenterally; orthostatic hypotension is due to alpha-receptor blockade, the elderly are at greater risk for orthostatic hypotension

Tardive dyskinesia; Prevalence rate may be 40% in elderly; development of the syndrome and the irreversible nature are proportional to duration and total cumulative dose over time

Extrapyramidal reactions are more common in elderly with up to 50% developing these reactions after 60 years of age; drug-induced **Parkinson's syndrome** occurs often; **Akathisia** is the most common extrapyramidal reaction in elderly

Increased confusion, memory loss, psychotic behavior, and agitation frequently occur as a consequence of anticholinergic effects

Antipsychotic associated sedation in nonpsychotic patients is extremely unpleasant due to feelings of depersonalization, derealization, and dysphoria

Other Adverse Effects

>10%:

Central nervous system: Pseudoparkinsonism, akathisia, dystonias, tardive dyskinesia (persistent), dizziness
Cardiovascular: Hypotension, orthostatic hypotension
Gastrointestinal: Constipation
Ocular: Pigmentary retinopathy
Respiratory: Basal congestion
Miscellaneous: Decreased sweating

1% to 10%:

Dermatologic: Increased sensitivity to sun, skin rash
Endocrine & metabolic: Changes in menstrual cycle, changes in libido, pain in breasts
Gastrointestinal: Weight gain, nausea, vomiting, stomach pain
Genitourinary: Difficulty in urination, ejaculatory disturbances
Neuromuscular & skeletal: Trembling of fingers

<1%:

Central nervous system: Neuroleptic malignant syndrome (NMS),
Dermatologic: Discoloration of skin (blue-gray)
Endocrine & metabolic: Galactorrhea
Genitourinary: Priapism
Hematologic: Agranulocytosis, leukopenia
Hepatic: Cholestatic jaundice, hepatotoxicity
Ocular: Cornea and lens changes, pigmentary retinopathy
Miscellaneous: Impairment of temperature regulation, lowering of seizures threshold

Drug Interactions

Decreased effect with anticholinergics
Decreased effect of guanethidine
Increased toxicity with CNS depressants, lithium (rare), tricyclic antidepressants (cardiotoxicity), propranolol, pindolol

Drug Uptake

Duration of action: 4-5 days
Serum half-life: 21-25 hours
Time to peak serum concentration: Within 1 hour

Pregnancy Risk Factor C

Thiotepa (thye oh tep′ a)

Therapeutic Category Antineoplastic Agent, Alkylating Agent

Synonyms TESPA; Thiophosphoramide; Triethylenethiophosphoramide; TSPA

Use Treatment of superficial tumors of the bladder; palliative treatment of adenocarcinoma of breast or ovary; lymphomas and sarcomas; meningeal neoplasms; control pleural, pericardial or peritoneal effusions caused by metastatic tumors; high-dose regimens with autologous bone marrow transplantation

Usual Dosage Refer to individual protocols. Dosing must be based on the clinical and hematologic response of the patient.

Children: Sarcomas: I.V.: 25-65 mg/m² as a single dose every 21 days
Adults:

I.M., I.V., S.C.: 30-60 mg/m² once per week
I.V. doses of 0.3-0.4 mg/kg by rapid I.V. administration every 1-4 weeks, or 0.2 mg/kg or 6-8 mg/m²/day for 4-5 days every 2-4 weeks
High-dose therapy for bone marrow transplant: I.V.: 500 mg/m²; up to 900 mg/m²
I.M. doses of 15-30 mg in various schedules have been given
Intracavitary: 0.6-0.8 mg/kg
Intrapericardial dose: Usually 15-30 mg

Mechanism of Action Alkylating agent that reacts with DNA phosphate groups to produce cross-linking of DNA strands leading to inhibition of DNA, (Continued)

Thiotepa (Continued)

RNA, and protein synthesis; mechanism of action has not been explored as thoroughly as the other alkylating agents, it is presumed that the azridine rings open and react as nitrogen mustard; reactivity is enhanced at a lower pH

Local Anesthetic/Vasoconstrictor Precautions No information available to require special precautions

Effects on Dental Treatment No effects or complications reported

Other Adverse Effects

Carcinogenesis: Like other alkylating agents, this drug is carcinogenic

>10%: Local: Pain at injection site

Hematopoietic: Dose-limiting toxicity which is dose-related and cumulative; moderate to severe leukopenia and severe thrombocytopenia have occurred. Anemia and pancytopenia may become fatal, so careful hematologic monitoring is required; intravesical administration may cause bone marrow suppression as well.

Myelosuppressive:
WBC: Moderate
Platelets: Severe
Onset (days): 7-10
Nadir (days): 14
Recovery (days): 28

1% to 10%:
Central nervous system: Dizziness, fever, headache
Dermatologic: Alopecia, rash, pruritus
Endocrine & metabolic: Hyperuricemia
Gastrointestinal: Stomatitis
Emetic potential: Low (<10%); nausea and vomiting rarely occur
Renal: Hematuria

<1%:
Central nervous system: Dizziness, fever
Dermatologic: Alopecia, rash
Gastrointestinal: Tightness of the throat, anorexia
Genitourinary: Hemorrhagic cystitis
Miscellaneous: Allergic reactions

Drug Uptake

Absorption: Following intracavitary instillation, the drug is unreliably absorbed (10% to 100%) through the bladder mucosa; variable I.M. absorption

Serum half-life, terminal: 109 minutes with dose-dependent clearance

Pregnancy Risk Factor D

Thiothixene (thye oh thix' een)

Brand Names Navane®

Therapeutic Category Antipsychotic Agent; Phenothiazine Derivative

Use Management of psychotic disorders

Usual Dosage

Children <12 years: Oral: 0.25 mg/kg/24 hours in divided doses (dose not well established)

Children >12 years and Adults: Mild to moderate psychosis:
Oral: 2 mg 3 times/day, up to 20-30 mg/day; more severe psychosis: Initial: 5 mg 2 times/day, may increase gradually, if necessary; maximum: 60 mg/day
I.M.: 4 mg 2-4 times/day, increase dose gradually; usual: 16-20 mg/day; maximum: 30 mg/day; change to oral dose as soon as able

Not dialyzable (0% to 5%)

Mechanism of Action Elicits antipsychotic activity by postsynaptic blockade of CNS dopamine receptors resulting in inhibition of dopamine-mediated effects; also has alpha-adrenergic blocking activity

Local Anesthetic/Vasoconstrictor Precautions No information available to require special precautions

Effects on Dental Treatment Significant hypotension may occur, especially when the drug is administered parenterally; orthostatic hypotension is due to alpha-receptor blockade, the elderly are at greater risk for orthostatic hypotension

Tardive dyskinesia: Prevalence rate may be 40% in elderly; development of the syndrome and the irreversible nature are proportional to duration and total cumulative dose over time

Extrapyramidal reactions are more common in elderly with up to 50% developing these reactions after 60 years of age; drug-induced **Parkinson's**

syndrome occurs often; **Akathisia** is the most common extrapyramidal reaction in elderly

Increased confusion, memory loss, psychotic behavior, and agitation frequently occur as a consequence of anticholinergic effects

Antipsychotic associated sedation in nonpsychotic patients is extremely unpleasant due to feelings of depersonalization, derealization, and dysphoria

Other Adverse Effects
>10%:
  Cardiovascular: Hypotension, orthostatic hypotension
  Central nervous system: Pseudoparkinsonism, akathisia, dystonias, tardive dyskinesia (persistent), dizziness
  Gastrointestinal: Constipation
  Ocular: Pigmentary retinopathy
  Respiratory: Nasal congestion
  Miscellaneous: Decreased sweating
1% to 10%:
  Dermatologic: Increased sensitivity to sun, skin rash
  Endocrine & metabolic: Changes in menstrual cycle, changes in libido, pain in breasts
  Gastrointestinal: Weight gain, nausea, vomiting, stomach pain
  Genitourinary: Difficulty in urination, ejaculatory disturbances
  Neuromuscular & skeletal: Trembling of fingers
<1%:
  Central nervous system: Neuroleptic malignant syndrome (NMS)
  Endocrine & metabolic: Galactorrhea
  Dermatologic: Discoloration of skin (blue-gray)
  Genitourinary: Priapism
  Hematologic: Agranulocytosis, leukopenia
  Hepatic: Cholestatic jaundice, hepatotoxicity
  Ocular: Fornea and lens changes, pigmentary retinopathy
  Miscellaneous: Impairment of temperature regulation, lowering of seizures threshold

Drug Interactions
  Decreased effect of guanethidine; decreased effect with anticholinergics
  Increased toxicity with CNS depressants, anticholinergics, alcohol
Drug Uptake
  Serum half-life: >24 hours with chronic use
Pregnancy Risk Factor C

Thorazine® see Chlorpromazine Hydrochloride on page 195
Thrombate III™ see Antithrombin III on page 71
Thrombinar® see Thrombin, Topical on this page

Thrombin, Topical (throm' bin, top' i kal)
Brand Names Thrombinar®; Thrombogen®; Thrombostat®
Therapeutic Category Hemostatic Agent
Use
  Dental & Medical: Hemostasis whenever minor bleeding from capillaries and small venules is accessible
Usual Dosage Use 1000-2000 units/mL of solution where bleeding is profuse; apply powder directly to the site of bleeding or on oozing surfaces; use 100 units/mL for bleeding from skin or mucosal surfaces
Mechanism of Action Catalyzes the conversion of fibrinogen to fibrin
Local Anesthetic/Vasoconstrictor Precautions No information available to require special precautions
Effects on Dental Treatment No effects or complications reported
Other Adverse Effects 1% to 10%:
  Central nervous system: Fever
  Miscellaneous: Allergic type reaction

  Oral manifestations: No data reported
Contraindications Hypersensitivity to thrombin or any component
Warnings/Precautions Do not inject, for topical use only
Drug Interactions No data reported
Pregnancy Risk Factor C
Breast-feeding Considerations No data reported
Dosage Forms Powder: 1000 units, 5000 units, 10,000 units, 20,000 units, 50,000 units
Dietary Considerations No data reported
Generic Available No
  (Continued)

Thrombin, Topical *(Continued)*

Comments Topical thrombin is not to be used in conjunction with oxidized cellulose

Thrombogen® *see* Thrombin, Topical *on previous page*

Thrombostat® *see* Thrombin, Topical *on previous page*

Thypinone® Injection *see* Protirelin *on page 747*

Thyrar® *see* Thyroid *on this page*

Thyro-Block® *see* Potassium Iodide *on page 711*

Thyroid *(thye' roid)*

Related Information
Endocrine Disorders & Pregnancy *on page 927*

Brand Names Armour® Thyroid; S-P-T; Thyrar®; Thyroid Strong®

Therapeutic Category Thyroid Product

Use Replacement or supplemental therapy in hypothyroidism; pituitary TSH suppressants (thyroid nodules, thyroiditis, multinodular goiter, thyroid cancer), thyrotoxicosis, diagnostic suppression tests

Usual Dosage Oral:
Children: See table.

Recommended Pediatric Dosage for Congenital Hypothyroidism

Age	Daily Dose (mg)	Daily Dose/kg (mg)
0-6 mo	15-30	4.8-6
6-12 mo	30-45	3.6-4.8
1-5 y	45-60	3-3.6
6-12 y	60-90	2.4-3
>12 y	>90	1.2-1.8

Adults: Initial: 15-30 mg; increase with 15 mg increments every 2-4 weeks; use 15 mg in patients with cardiovascular disease or myxedema. Maintenance dose: Usually 60-120 mg/day; monitor TSH and clinical symptoms.
Thyroid cancer: Requires larger amounts than replacement therapy

Mechanism of Action The primary active compound is T_3 (triiodothyronine), which may be converted from T_4 (thyroxine) and then circulates throughout the body to influence growth and maturation of various tissues; exact mechanism of action is unknown; however, it is believed the thyroid hormone exerts its many metabolic effects through control of DNA transcription and protein synthesis; involved in normal metabolism, growth, and development; promotes gluconeogenesis, increases utilization and mobilization of glycogen stores and stimulates protein synthesis, increases basal metabolic rate

Local Anesthetic/Vasoconstrictor Precautions No precautions with vasoconstrictor are necessary if patient is well controlled with thyroid preparations

Effects on Dental Treatment No effects or complications reported

Other Adverse Effects <1%:
Cardiovascular: Palpitations, tachycardia, cardiac arrhythmias, chest pain
Central nervous system: Nervousness, headache, insomnia, fever, clumsiness
Dermatologic: Hair loss
Endocrine & metabolic: Changes in menstrual cycle, shortness of breath
Gastrointestinal: Weight loss, increased appetite, diarrhea, abdominal cramps, vomiting, constipation
Neuromuscular & skeletal: Excessive bone loss with overtreatment (excess thyroid replacement), tremor, hand tremors, muscle aches
Miscellaneous: Heat intolerance, sweating

Drug Interactions
Decreased effect:
Thyroid hormones increase the therapeutic need for oral hypoglycemics or insulin
Cholestyramine can bind thyroid and reduce its absorption
Increased toxicity: Thyroid may potentiate the hypoprothrombinemic effect of oral anticoagulants

Drug Uptake
Absorption: T_4 is 48% to 79% absorbed; T_3 is 95% absorbed; desiccated thyroid contains thyroxine, liothyronine, and iodine (primarily bound); following absorption thyroxine is largely converted to liothyronine
Serum half-life:
Liothyronine: 1-2 days

Thyroxine: 6-7 days
Pregnancy Risk Factor A

Thyroid Strong® *see* Thyroid *on previous page*
Thyrolar® *see* Liotrix *on page 505*

Thyrotropin (thye roe troe' pin)
Brand Names Thytropar®
Therapeutic Category Diagnostic Agent, Hypothyroidism; Diagnostic Agent, Thyroid Function
Use Diagnostic aid to differentiate thyroid failure; diagnosis of decreased thyroid reserve, to differentiate between primary and secondary hypothyroidism and between primary hypothyroidism and euthyroidism in patients receiving thyroid replacement
Usual Dosage Adults: I.M., S.C.: 10 units/day for 1-3 days; follow by a radioiodine study 24 hours past last injection, no response in thyroid failure, substantial response in pituitary failure
Mechanism of Action Stimulates formation and secretion of thyroid hormone, increases uptake of iodine by thyroid gland
Local Anesthetic/Vasoconstrictor Precautions No information available to require special precautions
Effects on Dental Treatment No effects or complications reported
Other Adverse Effects <1%:
Cardiovascular: Tachycardia
Central nervous system: Fever, headache
Endocrine & metabolic: Menstrual irregularities
Gastrointestinal: Nausea, vomiting, increased bowel motility
Sensitivity reactions: Anaphylaxis with repeated administration
Drug Interactions No data reported
Drug Uptake
Serum half-life: 35 minutes, dependent upon thyroid state
Pregnancy Risk Factor C

Thyrotropin Releasing Hormone *see* Protirelin *on page 747*
Thytropar® *see* Thyrotropin *on this page*
Ticar® *see* Ticarcillin Disodium *on next page*
Ticarcilina Disodica (Mexico) *see* Ticarcillin Disodium *on next page*

Ticarcillin and Clavulanic Acid
(tye kar sil' in & klav yoo lan' ick as' id)
Brand Names Timentin®
Therapeutic Category Antibiotic, Penicillin
Use Treatment of infections of lower respiratory tract, urinary tract, skin and skin structures, bone and joint, and septicemia caused by susceptible organisms. Clavulanate expands activity of ticarcillin to include beta-lactamase producing strains of *S. aureus*, *H. influenzae*, *Enterobacteriaceae*, *Klebsiella*, *Citrobacter*, and *Serratia*
Usual Dosage I.V.:
Children: 200-300 mg of ticarcillin component/kg/day in divided doses every 4-6 hours
Adults: 3.1 g (ticarcillin 3 g plus clavulanic acid 0.1 g) every 4-6 hours; maximum: 18-24 g/day
Urinary tract infections: 3.1 g every 6-8 hours
Mechanism of Action Ticarcillin interferes with bacterial cell wall synthesis during active multiplication, causing cell wall death and resultant bactericidal activity against susceptible bacteria; clavulanic acid prevents degradation of ticarcillin by binding to the active site on beta-lactamase
Local Anesthetic/Vasoconstrictor Precautions No information available to require special precautions
Effects on Dental Treatment Prolonged use of penicillins may lead to development of oral candidiasis
Other Adverse Effects <1%:
Central nervous system: Convulsions, confusion, drowsiness, fever, Jarisch-Herxheimer reaction
Dermatologic: Rash
Endocrine & metabolic: Electrolyte imbalance
Hematologic: Hemolytic anemia, positive Coombs' reaction
Local: Thrombophlebitis
Neuromuscular & skeletal: Myoclonus
Renal: Acute interstitial nephritis
Miscellaneous: Hypersensitivity reactions, anaphylaxis
(Continued)

Ticarcillin and Clavulanic Acid *(Continued)*

Drug Interactions
Decreased effect: Tetracyclines cause decreased penicillin effectiveness; aminoglycosides cause physical inactivation of aminoglycosides in the presence of high concentrations of ticarcillin and potential toxicity in patients with mild-moderate renal dysfunction

Increased effect:
Probenecid causes increased penicillin levels
Neuromuscular blockers causes increased duration of blockade
Aminoglycosides cause synergistic efficacy

Drug Uptake
Serum half-life:
Clavulanate: 66-90 minutes
Ticarcillin: 66-72 minutes in patients with normal renal function; clavulanic acid does not affect the clearance of ticarcillin

Pregnancy Risk Factor B

Ticarcillin Disodium *(tye kar sil' in dye sow' dee um)*

Brand Names Ticar®
Therapeutic Category Antibiotic, Penicillin
Synonyms Ticarcilina Disodica (Mexico)
Use Treatment of susceptible infections such as septicemia, acute and chronic respiratory tract infections, skin and soft tissue infections, and urinary tract infections due to susceptible strains of *Pseudomonas*, *Proteus*, and *Escherichia coli* and *Enterobacter*; normally used with other antibiotics (ie, aminoglycosides)

Usual Dosage Ticarcillin is generally given I.M. only for the treatment of uncomplicated urinary tract infections
Children: I.V.: Serious Infections:200-300 mg/kg/day in divided doses every 4-6 hours; doses as high as 400 mg/kg/day divided every 4 hours have been used in acute pulmonary exacerbations of cystic fibrosis
Maximum dose: 24 g/day
Urinary tract infections: I.M., I.V.: 50-100 mg/kg/day in divided doses every 6-8 hours
Adults: I.V.: 1-4 g every 4-6 hours

Mechanism of Action Interferes with bacterial cell wall synthesis during active multiplication, causing cell wall death and resultant bactericidal activity against susceptible bacteria

Local Anesthetic/Vasoconstrictor Precautions No information available to require special precautions

Effects on Dental Treatment Prolonged use of penicillins may lead to development of oral candidiasis

Other Adverse Effects <1%:
Central nervous system: Convulsions, confusion, drowsiness, fever, Jarisch-Herxheimer reaction
Dermatologic: Rash
Endocrine & metabolic: Electrolyte imbalance
Hematologic: Hemolytic anemia, positive Coombs' reaction
Local: Thrombophlebitis
Neuromuscular & skeletal: Myoclonus
Renal: Acute interstitial nephritis
Miscellaneous: Hypersensitivity reactions, anaphylaxis

Drug Interactions
Decreased effect: Tetracyclines cause decreased ticarcillin effectiveness
Increased effect:
Probenecid causes increased ticarcillin levels
Neuromuscular blockers cause increased duration of blockade
Aminoglycosides cause synergistic efficacy

Drug Uptake
Absorption: I.M.: 86%
Serum half-life, adults: 1-1.3 hours, prolonged with renal impairment and/or hepatic impairment
Peak serum levels: I.M.: Within 30-75 minutes

Pregnancy Risk Factor B

TICE® BCG *see* Bacillus Calmette-Guérin (BCG) Live *on page 93*
Ticlid® *see* Ticlopidine Hydrochloride *on next page*
Ticlopidina (Mexico) *see* Ticlopidine Hydrochloride *on next page*

Ticlopidine Hydrochloride (tye kloe' pi deen hye droe klor' ide)
Brand Names Ticlid®
Therapeutic Category Antiplatelet Agent
Synonyms Ticlopidina (Mexico)
Use Platelet aggregation inhibitor that reduces the risk of thrombotic stroke in patients who have had a stroke or stroke precursors

> **Unlabeled use:** Protection of aortocoronary bypass grafts, diabetic microangiopathy, ischemic heart disease, prevention of postoperative DVT, reduction of graft loss following renal transplant

Usual Dosage Adults: Oral: 1 tablet twice daily with food

Mechanism of Action Ticlopidine is an inhibitor of platelet function with a mechanism which is different from other antiplatelet drugs. The drug significantly increases bleeding time. This effect may not be solely related to ticlopidine's effect on platelets. The prolongation of the bleeding time caused by ticlopidine is further increased by the addition of aspirin in *ex vivo* experiments. Although many metabolites of ticlopidine have been found, none have been shown to account for *in vivo* activity.

Local Anesthetic/Vasoconstrictor Precautions No information available to require special precautions

Effects on Dental Treatment No effects or complications reported

Other Adverse Effects
1% to 10%: Dermatologic: Skin rash
<1%:
Central nervous system: Epistaxis
Dermatologic: Ecchymosis
Gastrointestinal: Diarrhea, nausea, vomiting, GI pain
Hematologic: Neutropenia, thrombocytopenia
Hepatic: Increased liver function tests
Otic: Tinnitus
Renal: Hematuria

Drug Interactions
Decreased effect with antacids (decreased absorption), corticosteroids; decreased effect of digoxin, cyclosporine
Increased effect/toxicity of aspirin, anticoagulants, antipyrine, theophylline, cimetidine (increased levels), NSAIDs

Drug Uptake
Onset of action: Within 6 hours
Serum half-life, elimination: 24 hours

Pregnancy Risk Factor B

Ticon® *see* Trimethobenzamide Hydrochloride *on page 873*

TIG *see* Tetanus Immune Globulin, Human *on page 826*

Tigan® *see* Trimethobenzamide Hydrochloride *on page 873*

Tiject® *see* Trimethobenzamide Hydrochloride *on page 873*

Tilade® Inhalation Aerosol *see* Nedocromil Sodium *on page 607*

Timentin® *see* Ticarcillin and Clavulanic Acid *on page 845*

Timolol Maleate (tye' moe lole mal' ee ate)
Related Information
Cardiovascular Diseases *on page 912*
Brand Names Betimol® Ophthalmic; Blocadren® Oral; Timoptic® Ophthalmic; Timoptic-XE® Ophthalmic
Canadian/Mexican Brand Names Apo-Timol® (Canada); Apo-Timop® (Canada); Gen-Timolol® (Canada); Novo-Timol® (Canada); Nu-Timolol® (Canada); Imot® Ofteno (Mexico); Timoptol® (Mexico); Timoptol® XE (Mexico)
Therapeutic Category Antianginal Agent; Antiglaucoma Agent; Beta-Adrenergic Blocker, Noncardioselective; Beta-Adrenergic Blocker, Ophthalmic
Synonyms Timolol, Maleato De (Mexico)
Use Ophthalmic dosage form used to treat elevated intraocular pressure such as glaucoma or ocular hypertension; orally for treatment of hypertension and angina and reduce mortality following myocardial infarction and prophylaxis of migraine
Usual Dosage
Children and Adults: Ophthalmic: Initial: 0.25% solution, instill 1 drop twice daily; increase to 0.5% solution if response not adequate; decrease to 1 drop/day if controlled; do not exceed 1 drop twice daily of 0.5% solution

Adults: Oral:
Hypertension: Initial: 10 mg twice daily, increase gradually every 7 days, usual dosage: 20-40 mg/day in 2 divided doses; maximum: 60 mg/day
(Continued)

Timolol Maleate *(Continued)*

Prevention of myocardial infarction: 10 mg twice daily initiated within 1-4 weeks after infarction

Migraine headache: Initial: 10 mg twice daily, increase to maximum of 30 mg/day

Mechanism of Action Blocks both beta$_1$- and beta$_2$-adrenergic receptors, reduces intraocular pressure by reducing aqueous humor production or possibly outflow; reduces blood pressure by blocking adrenergic receptors and decreasing sympathetic outflow, produces a negative chronotropic and inotropic activity through an unknown mechanism

Local Anesthetic/Vasoconstrictor Precautions No information available to require special precautions

Effects on Dental Treatment No effects or complications reported

Other Adverse Effects

Ophthalmic:

1% to 10%:

Dermatologic: Alopecia

Ocular: Burning, stinging of eyes

<1%:

Dermatologic: Skin rash

Ocular: Blepharitis, conjunctivitis, keratitis, vision disturbances

Oral:

>10%: Endocrine & metabolic: Decreased sexual ability

1% to 10%:

Cardiovascular: Bradycardia, breathing difficulty, irregular heartbeat, reduced peripheral circulation

Central nervous system: Dizziness, itching, tiredness, weakness

<1%:

Cardiovascular: Chest pain, congestive heart failure

Central nervous system: Hallucinations, mental depression, anxiety, nightmares

Dermatologic: Skin rashes

Gastrointestinal: Diarrhea, nausea, vomiting, stomach discomfort

Neuromuscular & skeletal: Numbness in toes and fingers

Ocular: Dry sore eyes

Drug Interactions No data reported with ophthalmic preparation

Drug Uptake

Onset of hypotensive effect: Oral: Within 15-45 minutes

Peak effect: Within 0.5-2.5 hours

Duration of action: ~4 hours; intraocular effects persist for 24 hours after ophthalmic instillation

Serum half-life: 2-2.7 hours; prolonged with reduced renal function

Pregnancy Risk Factor C

Timolol, Maleato De (Mexico) *see* Timolol Maleate *on previous page*

Timoptic® Ophthalmic *see* Timolol Maleate *on previous page*

Timoptic-XE® Ophthalmic *see* Timolol Maleate *on previous page*

Tinactin® [OTC] *see* Tolnaftate *on page 855*

TinBen® [OTC] *see* Benzoin *on page 104*

TinCoBen® [OTC] *see* Benzoin *on page 104*

Tindal® *see* Acetophenazine Maleate *on page 20*

Tine Test *see* Tuberculin Purified Protein Derivative *on page 882*

Tinver® Lotion *see* Sodium Thiosulfate *on page 795*

Tioconazole *(tye oh kone' a zole)*

Brand Names Vagistat®

Therapeutic Category Antifungal Agent, Vaginal

Synonyms Tioconazol (Mexico)

Use Local treatment of vulvovaginal candidiasis

Usual Dosage Adults: Vaginal: Insert 1 applicatorful in vagina, just prior to bedtime, as a single dose

Mechanism of Action A 1-substituted imidazole derivative with a broad antifungal spectrum against a wide variety of dermatophytes and yeasts, usually at a concentration of ≤6.25 mg/L; has been demonstrated to be at least as active *in vitro* as other imidazole antifungals. *In vitro*, tioconazole has been demonstrated 2-8 times as potent as miconazole against common dermal pathogens including *Trichophyton mentagrophytes*, *T. rubrum*, *T. erinacei*, *T. tonsurans*, *Microsporum canis*, *Microsporum gypseum*, and *Candida albicans*. Both agents appear to be similarly effective against *Epidermophyton floccosum*.

Local Anesthetic/Vasoconstrictor Precautions No information available to require special precautions
Effects on Dental Treatment No effects or complications reported
Other Adverse Effects
1% to 10%: Genitourinary: Vulvar/vaginal burning
<1%: Genitourinary: Vulvar itching, soreness, swelling, or discharge; urinary frequency
Drug Interactions No data reported
Drug Uptake
Absorption: Intravaginal: Following application small amounts of drug are absorbed systemically (25%) within 2-8 hours
Serum half-life: 21-24 hours
Pregnancy Risk Factor C

Tioconazol (Mexico) see Tioconazole on previous page
Tioguanine see Thioguanine on page 838
Tiopental Sodico (Mexico) see Thiopental Sodium on page 839

Tiopronin (tye oh proe' nin)
Brand Names Thiola™
Therapeutic Category Urinary Tract Product
Use Prevention of kidney stone (cystine) formation in patients with severe homozygous cystinuric who have urinary cystine >500 mg/day who are resistant to treatment with high fluid intake, alkali, and diet modification, or who have had adverse reactions to penicillamine
Local Anesthetic/Vasoconstrictor Precautions No information available to require special precautions
Effects on Dental Treatment No effects or complications reported

Tioridacina (Mexico) see Thioridazine on page 840
Ti-Screen® [OTC] see Methoxycinnamate and Oxybenzone on page 564
Tisit® [OTC] see Pyrethrins on page 753
Titralac® [OTC] see Calcium Carbonate on page 140
Titralac® Plus Liquid [OTC] see Calcium Carbonate and Simethicone on page 141
TMP-SMZ see Trimethoprim and Sulfamethoxazole on page 874
TobraDex® see Tobramycin and Dexamethasone on next page
Tobramicina Sulfato De (Mexico) see Tobramycin on this page

Tobramycin (toe bra mye' sin)
Related Information
Antimicrobial Prophylaxis in Surgical Patients on page 1042
Brand Names Nebcin®; Tobrex®
Canadian/Mexican Brand Names Tobra® (Mexico); Trazil® Often y Trazil® Ungena (Mexico)
Therapeutic Category Antibiotic, Aminoglycoside; Antibiotic, Ophthalmic
Synonyms Tobramicina Sulfato De (Mexico)
Use Treatment of documented or suspected *Pseudomonas aeruginosa* infection; infection with a nonpseudomonal enteric bacillus which is more sensitive to tobramycin than gentamicin based on susceptibility tests; empiric therapy in cystic fibrosis and immunocompromised patients; topically used to treat superficial ophthalmic infections caused by susceptible bacteria
Usual Dosage Individualization is critical because of the low therapeutic index
Use of ideal body weight (IBW) for determining the mg/kg/dose appears to be more accurate than dosing on the basis of total body weight (TBW)
In morbid obesity, dosage requirement may best be estimated using a dosing weight of IBW + 0.4 (TBW - IBW)
Initial and periodic peak and trough plasma drug levels should be determined, particularly in critically ill patients with serious infections or in disease states known to significantly alter aminoglycoside pharmacokinetics (eg, cystic fibrosis, burns, or major surgery); 2-3 serum level measurements should be obtained after the initial dose to measure the half-life in order to determine the frequency of subsequent doses

Once daily dosing: Higher peak serum drug concentration to MIC ratios, demonstrated aminoglycoside postantibiotic effect, decreased renal cortex drug uptake, and improved cost-time efficiency are supportive reasons for the use of once daily dosing regimens for aminoglycosides. Current research indicates these regimens to be as effective for nonlife-threatening infections, with no higher incidence of nephrotoxicity, than those requiring multiple daily doses. Doses are determined by calculating the entire day's dose via usual
(Continued)

Tobramycin (Continued)

multiple dose calculation techniques and administering this quantity as a single dose. Doses are then adjusted to maintain mean serum concentrations above the MIC(s) of the causative organism(s). (Example: 2.5-5 mg/kg as a single dose; expected Cp_{max}: 10-20 mcg/mL and Cp_{min}: <1 mcg/mL). Further research is needed for universal recommendation in all patient populations and gram-negative disease; exceptions may include those with known high clearance (eg, children, patients with cystic fibrosis, or burns who may require shorter dosage intervals) and patients with renal function impairment for whom longer than conventional dosage intervals are usually required.

Children <5 years: I.M., I.V.: 2.5 mg/kg/dose every 8 hours

Children >5 years: 1.5-2.5 mg/kg/dose every 8 hours

Note: Some patients may require larger or more frequent doses if serum levels document the need (ie, cystic fibrosis or febrile granulocytopenic patients).

Adults: I.M., I.V.:

Severe life-threatening infections: 2-2.5 mg/kg/dose

Urinary tract infection: 1.5 mg/kg/dose

Synergy (for gram-positive infections): 1 mg/kg/dose

Children and Adults: Ophthalmic: Instill 1-2 drops of solution every 4 hours; apply ointment 2-3 times/day; for severe infections apply ointment every 3-4 hours, or solution 2 drops every 30-60 minutes initially, then reduce to less frequent intervals

Mechanism of Action Interferes with bacterial protein synthesis by binding to 30S and 50S ribosomal subunits resulting in a defective bacterial cell membrane

Local Anesthetic/Vasoconstrictor Precautions No information available to require special precautions

Effects on Dental Treatment No effects or complications reported

Other Adverse Effects

1% to 10%:

Renal: Nephrotoxicity

Neuromuscular & skeletal: Neurotoxicity (neuromuscular blockade)

Otic: Ototoxicity (auditory), ototoxicity (vestibular)

<1%:

Cardiovascular: Hypotension

Central nervous system: Drug fever, headache, drowsiness, weakness

Dermatologic: Skin rash

Gastrointestinal: Nausea, vomiting

Hematologic: Eosinophilia anemia

Neuromuscular & skeletal: Paresthesia, tremor, arthralgia

Ocular: Lacrimation, itching, edema of the eyelid, keratitis

Respiratory: Difficulty in breathing

Drug Interactions

Increased effect: Extended spectrum penicillins (synergistic)

Increased toxicity:

Neuromuscular blockers increase neuromuscular blockade

Amphotericin B, cephalosporins, loop diuretics cause increased risk of nephrotoxicity

Drug Uptake

Absorption: I.M.: Rapid and complete

Time to peak serum concentration:

I.M.: Within 30-60 minutes

I.V.: Within 30 minutes

Serum half-life:

Adults: 2-3 hours, directly dependent upon glomerular filtration rate

Adults with impaired renal function: 5-70 hours

Pregnancy Risk Factor C

Tobramycin and Dexamethasone

(toe bra mye' sin & dex a meth' a sone)

Brand Names TobraDex®

Therapeutic Category Antibiotic, Ophthalmic; Corticosteroid, Ophthalmic

Use Treatment of external ocular infection caused by susceptible gram-negative bacteria and steroid responsive inflammatory conditions of the palpebral and bulbar conjunctiva, lid, cornea, and anterior segment of the globe

Usual Dosage Children and Adults: Ophthalmic: Instill 1-2 drops of solution every 4 hours; apply ointment 2-3 times/day; for severe infections apply ointment every 3-4 hours, or solution 2 drops every 30-60 minutes initially, then reduce to less frequent intervals

Mechanism of Action Refer to individual monographs for Dexamethasone and Tobramycin

Local Anesthetic/Vasoconstrictor Precautions No information available to require special precautions

Effects on Dental Treatment No effects or complications reported

Other Adverse Effects 1% to 10%: Ocular: Allergic contact dermatitis, delayed wound healing, lacrimation, itching, edema of eyelid, keratitis, increased intraocular pressure, glaucoma, cataract formation

Drug Interactions Refer to individual monographs for Tobramycin and Dexamethasone

Drug Uptake
Absorption: Absorbed into the aqueous humor
Time to peak serum concentration: 1-2 hours after instillation in the cornea and aqueous humor

Pregnancy Risk Factor B

Tobrex® see Tobramycin on page 849

Tocainide Hydrochloride (toe kay' nide hye droe klor' ide)

Related Information
Cardiovascular Diseases on page 912

Brand Names Tonocard®

Therapeutic Category Antiarrhythmic Agent, Class I-B; Antiarrhythmic Agent (Supraventricular & Ventricular)

Use Suppress and prevent symptomatic life-threatening ventricular arrhythmias

Unlabeled use: Trigeminal neuralgia

Usual Dosage Adults: Oral: 1200-1800 mg/day in 3 divided doses, up to 2400 mg/day

Mechanism of Action Class 1B antiarrhythmic agent; suppresses automaticity of conduction tissue, by increasing electrical stimulation threshold of ventricle, HIS-Purkinje system, and spontaneous depolarization of the ventricles during diastole by a direct action on the tissues; blocks both the initiation and conduction of nerve impulses by decreasing the neuronal membrane's permeability to sodium ions, which results in inhibition of depolarization with resultant blockade of conduction

Local Anesthetic/Vasoconstrictor Precautions No information available to require special precautions

Effects on Dental Treatment No effects or complications reported

Other Adverse Effects
>10%:
Gastrointestinal: Nausea, dizziness, anorexia
Neuromuscular & skeletal: Tremor
Central nervous system: Nervousness, confusion, ataxia
1% to 10%:
Cardiovascular: Hypotension, tachycardia
Central nervous system: Ataxia
Dermatologic: Skin rash
Gastrointestinal: Vomiting, diarrhea
Neuromuscular & skeletal: Arthralgia, myalgia, paresthesia
Ocular: Blurred vision
<1%:
Cardiovascular: Bradycardia, palpitations
Hematologic: Agranulocytosis, anemia, leukopenia, neutropenia
Respiratory: Respiratory arrest
Miscellaneous: Sweating

Drug Interactions
Decreased plasma levels: Phenobarbital, phenytoin, rifampin, and other hepatic enzyme inducers, cimetidine and drugs which make the urine acidic
Increased effect of tocainide, allopurinol
Increased toxicity/levels of caffeine and theophylline

Drug Uptake
Absorption: Oral: Extensive, 99% to 100%
Serum half-life: 11-14 hours, prolonged with renal and hepatic impairment with half-life increased to 23-27 hours
Time to peak: Peak serum levels occur within 30-160 minutes

Pregnancy Risk Factor C

Tocophersolan (toe kof er soe' lan)
Brand Names Liqui-E®
Therapeutic Category Vitamin, Fat Soluble
Synonyms TPGS
Use Treatment of vitamin E deficiency resulting from malabsorption due to prolonged cholestatic hepatobiliary disease
Local Anesthetic/Vasoconstrictor Precautions No information available to require special precautions
Effects on Dental Treatment No effects or complications reported
Comments Studies indicate that TPGS is absorbed better than fat soluble forms of vitamin E in patients with impaired digestion and absorption and when coadministered with cyclosporin to transplant recipients it improves cyclosporin absorption. Due to these findings, this product has a valuable role in the liver transplant patient population.

Tofranil® *see* Imipramine *on page 451*
Tofranil-PM® *see* Imipramine *on page 451*

Tolazamide (tole az' a mide)
Related Information
Endocrine Disorders & Pregnancy *on page 927*
Brand Names Tolinase®
Therapeutic Category Antidiabetic Agent; Hypoglycemic Agent, Oral; Sulfonylurea Agent
Use Adjunct to diet for the management of mild to moderately severe, stable, noninsulin-dependent (type II) diabetes mellitus
Usual Dosage Oral (doses >1000 mg/day normally do not improve diabetic control):
Adults: Initial: 100 mg/day, increase at 2- to 4-week intervals; maximum dose: 1000 mg; give as a single or twice daily dose
Conversion from insulin → tolazamide
10 units day = 100 mg/day
20-40 units/day = 250 mg/day
>40 units/day = 250 mg/day and 50% of insulin dose
Doses >500 mg/day should be given in 2 divided doses
Mechanism of Action Stimulates insulin release from the pancreatic beta cells; reduces glucose output from the liver; insulin sensitivity is increased at peripheral target sites
Local Anesthetic/Vasoconstrictor Precautions No information available to require special precautions
Effects on Dental Treatment Use salicylates with caution in patients taking tolazamide because of potential increased hypoglycemia; NSAIDs such as ibuprofen and naproxen may be safely used. Tolazamide-dependent diabetics (noninsulin dependent, Type II) should be appointed for dental treatment in morning in order to minimize chance of stress-induced hypoglycemia.
Other Adverse Effects
>10%:
Central nervous system: Headache, dizziness
Gastrointestinal: Anorexia, nausea, vomiting, diarrhea, constipation, heartburn, epigastric fullness
1% to 10%: Dermatologic: Rash, urticaria, hives, photosensitivity
<1%:
Endocrine & metabolic: Hypoglycemia
Hematologic: Aplastic anemia, hemolytic anemia, bone marrow depression, thrombocytopenia, agranulocytosis
Hepatic: Cholestatic jaundice
Renal: Diuretic effect
Drug Interactions Increased toxicity: Monitor patient closely; large number of drugs interact with sulfonylureas including salicylates, anticoagulants, H_2 antagonists, TCA, MAO inhibitors, beta-blockers, thiazides
Drug Uptake
Onset of action: Oral: Within 4-6 hours
Duration: 10-24 hours
Serum half-life: 7 hours
Pregnancy Risk Factor D

Tolazoline Hydrochloride (tole az' oh leen hye droe klor' ide)
Brand Names Priscoline®
Therapeutic Category Alpha-Adrenergic Blocking Agent, Parenteral; Vasodilator, Coronary

Use Treatment of persistent pulmonary vasoconstriction and hypertension of the newborn (persistent fetal circulation), peripheral vasospastic disorders

Usual Dosage

Neonates: Initial: I.V.: 1-2 mg/kg over 10-15 minutes via scalp vein or upper extremity; maintenance: 1-2 mg/kg/hour; use lower maintenance doses in patients with decreased renal function. Also used in neonates for acute vasospasm "cath toes" at 0.25 mg/kg/hour (no load); maximum dose: 6-8 mg/kg/hour

Mechanism of Action Competitively blocks alpha-adrenergic receptors to produce brief antagonism of circulating epinephrine and norepinephrine; reduces hypertension caused by catecholamines and causes vascular smooth muscle relaxation (direct action); results in peripheral vasodilation and decreased peripheral resistance

Local Anesthetic/Vasoconstrictor Precautions No information available to require special precautions

Effects on Dental Treatment No effects or complications reported

Other Adverse Effects

>10%:

Cardiovascular: Hypotension,

Endocrine & metabolic: Hypochloremic alkalosis

Gastrointestinal: GI bleeding, abdominal pain

Hematologic: Thrombocytopenia

Local: Burning at injection site

Renal: Acute renal failure, oliguria

1% to 10%:

Cardiovascular: Peripheral vasodilation, tachycardia

Gastrointestinal: Nausea, diarrhea

Neuromuscular & skeletal: Increased pilomotor activity

<1%:

Cardiovascular: Hypertension, tachycardia, arrhythmias

Hematologic: Increased agranulocytosis, pancytopenia

Ocular: Mydriasis

Respiratory: Pulmonary hemorrhage

Miscellaneous: Increased secretions

Drug Interactions

Increased toxicity: Disulfiram reaction may possibly be seen with concomitant ethanol use

Drug Uptake

Time to peak serum concentration: Within 30 minutes

Pregnancy Risk Factor C

Tolbutamida (Mexico) *see* Tolbutamide *on this page*

Tolbutamide (tole byoo' ta mide)

Related Information

Endocrine Disorders & Pregnancy *on page 927*

Brand Names Orinase®

Canadian/Mexican Brand Names Apo-Tolbutamide® (Canada); Mobenol® (Canada); Novo-Butamide® (Canada); Artosin® (Mexico); Diaval® (Mexico); Rastinon® (Mexico)

Therapeutic Category Antidiabetic Agent; Hypoglycemic Agent, Oral; Sulfonylurea Agent

Synonyms Tolbutamida (Mexico)

Use Adjunct to diet for the management of mild to moderately severe, stable, noninsulin-dependent (type II) diabetes mellitus

Usual Dosage Divided doses may increase gastrointestinal side effects

Adults:

Oral: Initial: 500-1000 mg 1-3 times/day; usual dose should not be more than 2 g/day

I.V. bolus: 1 g over 2-3 minutes

Elderly: Oral: Initial: 250 mg 1-3 times/day; usual: 500-2000 mg; maximum: 3 g/day

Mechanism of Action A sulfonylurea hypoglycemic agent; its ability to lower elevated blood glucose levels in patients with functional pancreatic beta cells is similar to the other sulfonylurea agents; stimulates synthesis and release of endogenous insulin from pancreatic islet tissue. The hypoglycemic effect is attributed to an increased sensitivity of insulin receptors and improved peripheral utilization of insulin. Suppression of glucagon secretion may also contribute to the hypoglycemic effects of tolbutamide.

Local Anesthetic/Vasoconstrictor Precautions No information available to require special precautions

(Continued)

Tolbutamide *(Continued)*

Effects on Dental Treatment Use salicylates with caution in patients taking tolazamide because of potential increased hypoglycemia; NSAIDs such as ibuprofen and naproxen may be safely used. Tolbutamide-dependent diabetics (noninsulin dependent, Type II) should be appointed for dental treatment in morning in order to minimize chance of stress-induced hypoglycemia

Other Adverse Effects

>10%:

Central nervous system: Headache, dizziness

Gastrointestinal: Constipation, diarrhea, heartburn, anorexia, epigastric fullness

1% to 10%: Dermatologic: Skin rash, hives, photosensitivity

<1%:

Endocrine & metabolic: SIADH

Hematologic: Thrombocytopenia, agranulocytosis, hypoglycemia, leukopenia, aplastic anemia, hemolytic anemia, bone marrow depression

Hepatic: Cholestatic jaundice

Local: Thrombophlebitis

Otic: Tinnitus

Miscellaneous: Venospasm, disulfiram-type reactions, hypersensitivity reaction

Drug Interactions Increased toxicity: Monitor patient closely; large number of drugs interact with sulfonylureas including salicylates, anticoagulants, H_2 antagonists, TCA, MAO inhibitors, beta-blockers, thiazides

Drug Uptake

Peak hypoglycemic action:

Oral: 1-3 hours

I.V.: 30 minutes

Duration:

Oral: 6-24 hours

I.V.: 3 hours

Time to peak serum concentration: 3-5 hours

Absorption: Oral: Rapid

Serum half-life: Plasma: 4-25 hours

Pregnancy Risk Factor D

Tolectin® *see* Tolmetin Sodium *on this page*

Tolinase® *see* Tolazamide *on page 852*

Tolmetin Sodium *(tole′ met in sow′ dee um)*

Related Information

Nonsteroidal Anti-Inflammatory Agents, Comparative Dosages, and Pharmacokinetics *on page 1021*

Rheumatoid Arthritis, Osteoarthritis, and Joint Prostheses *on page 930*

Brand Names Tolectin®

Canadian/Mexican Brand Names Novo-Tolmetin® (Canada)

Therapeutic Category Analgesic, Non-narcotic; Nonsteroidal Anti-inflammatory Agent (NSAID), Oral

Use Treatment of rheumatoid arthritis and osteoarthritis, juvenile rheumatoid arthritis

Usual Dosage Oral:

Children ≥2 years:

Anti-inflammatory: Initial: 20 mg/kg/day in 3 divided doses, then 15-30 mg/kg/day in 3 divided doses

Analgesic: 5-7 mg/kg/dose every 6-8 hours

Adults: 400 mg 3 times/day; usual dose: 600 mg to 1.8 g/day; maximum: 2 g/day

Mechanism of Action Inhibits prostaglandin synthesis by decreasing the activity of the enzyme, cyclo-oxygenase, which results in decreased formation of prostaglandin precursors

Local Anesthetic/Vasoconstrictor Precautions No information available to require special precautions

Effects on Dental Treatment No effects or complications reported

Other Adverse Effects

>10%:

Dermatologic: Skin rash, dizziness

Gastrointestinal: Abdominal cramps, heartburn, indigestion, nausea

1% to 10%:

Cardiovascular: Fluid retention

Central nervous system: Headache, nervousness

Dermatologic: Itching
Gastrointestinal: Vomiting
Otic: Ringing in ears
<1%:
Cardiovascular: Congestive heart failure, hypertension, arrhythmias, tachycardia, hot flushes
Central nervous system: Epistaxis, confusion, hallucinations, aseptic meningitis, mental depression, drowsiness, insomnia
Dermatologic: Hives, erythema multiforme, toxic epidermal necrolysis, Stevens-Johnson syndrome, angioedema
Endocrine & metabolism: Polydipsia
Gastrointestinal: Gastritis, GI ulceration
Genitourinary: Cystitis
Hematologic: Agranulocytosis, anemia, hemolytic anemia, bone marrow depression, leukopenia, thrombocytopenia
Hepatic: Hepatitis
Neuromuscular & skeletal: Peripheral neuropathy
Ocular: Toxic amblyopia, blurred vision, conjunctivitis, dry eyes
Otic: Decreased hearing
Renal: Polyuria, acute renal failure
Respiratory: Allergic rhinitis, shortness of breath
Drug Interactions
Decreased effect with aspirin; decreased effect of thiazides, furosemide
Increased toxicity of digoxin, methotrexate, cyclosporine, lithium, insulin, sulfonylureas, potassium-sparing diuretics, aspirin
Drug Uptake
Absorption: Oral: Well absorbed
Time to peak serum concentration: Within 30-60 minutes
Pregnancy Risk Factor C (D at term)

Tolnaftate (tole naf' tate)
Brand Names Aftate® [OTC]; Footwork® [OTC]; Fungatin® [OTC]; Genaspor® [OTC]; NP-27® [OTC]; Tinactin® [OTC]; Zeasorb-AF® [OTC]
Canadian/Mexican Brand Names Pitrex® (Canada); Tinaderm® (Mexico)
Therapeutic Category Antifungal Agent, Topical
Synonyms Tolnaftato (Mexico)
Use Treatment of tinea pedis, tinea cruris, tinea corporis, tinea manuum, tinea versicolor infections
Usual Dosage Children and Adults: Topical: Wash and dry affected area; apply 1-3 drops of solution or a small amount of cream or powder and rub into the affected areas 2-3 times/day for 2-4 weeks
Mechanism of Action Distorts the hyphae and stunts mycelial growth in susceptible fungi
Local Anesthetic/Vasoconstrictor Precautions No information available to require special precautions
Effects on Dental Treatment No effects or complications reported
Other Adverse Effects 1% to 10%: Dermatologic: Pruritus, contact dermatitis, irritation, stinging
Drug Interactions No data reported
Drug Uptake Onset of action: Response may be seen 24-72 hours after initiation of therapy
Pregnancy Risk Factor C

Tolnaftato (Mexico) see Tolnaftate on this page
Tolu-Sed® DM [OTC] see Guaifenesin and Dextromethorphan on page 408
Tonocard® see Tocainide Hydrochloride on page 851
Topicort® see Desoximetasone on page 259
Topicort®-LP see Desoximetasone on page 259
TOPO see Topotecan Hydrochloride on this page

Topotecan Hydrochloride (toe poe tee' kan hye droe klor' ide)
Brand Names Hycamtin®
Therapeutic Category Antineoplastic Agent, Antibiotic
Synonyms Hycamptamine; SK and F 104864; SKF 104864; SKF 104864-A; TOPO; TPT
Use Treatment of ovarian cancer after failure of first-line chemotherapy
Usual Dosage
Children: A phase I study in pediatric patients by CCSG determined the recommended phase II dose to be 5.5 mg/mm² as a 24-hour continuous infusion
(Continued)

Topotecan Hydrochloride *(Continued)*

Adults: Most phase II studies currently utilize topotecan at 1.5-2.0 mg/mm^2/day for 5 days, repeated every 21-28 days. Alternative dosing regimens evaluated in phase I studies have included 21-day continuous infusion (recommended phase II dose: 0.53-0.7 mg/mm^2/day) and weekly 24-hour infusions (recommended phase II dose: 1.5 mg/mm^2/week).

Dose modifications: Dosage modification may be required for toxicity

Mechanism of Action Topotecan (TPT), like other camptothecin (CPT) analogues, is a potent inhibitor of topoisomerase I. Structure-activity studies have revealed a direct relationship between the ability of CPT analogues to inhibit topoisomerase I catalytic activity and their potency as cytotoxic agents.

Local Anesthetic/Vasoconstrictor Precautions No information available to require special precautions

Effects on Dental Treatment No effects or complications reported

Other Adverse Effects

>10%:
Central nervous system: Headache
Dermatologic: Alopecia
Gastrointestinal: Nausea, vomiting, diarrhea
Hematologic: Neutropenia
Respiratory: Dyspnea

1% to 10%:
Central nervous system: Paresthesia, fatigue
Gastrointestinal: Constipation, abdominal pain
Hepatic: AST and ALT elevations, bilirubin elevation

<1%:
Central nervous system: Arthralgia, myalgia
Gastrointestinal: Stomatitis

Drug Interactions Concurrent administration of TPT and G-CSF in clinical trials results in severe myelosuppression. Concurrent *in vitro* exposure to TPT and the topoisomerase II inhibitor etoposide results in no altered effect; sequential exposure results in potentiation. Concurrent exposure to TPT and 5-azacytidine results in potentiation both *in vitro* and *in vivo*.

Drug Uptake

Serum half-life: 3 hours

Generic Available No

Comments Constituted vial: When constituted with 2 mL of sterile water for injection, USP, each mL contains topotecan 2.5 mg and mannitol 50 mg with a pH of approximately 3.5. Final infusion preparation: Topotecan constituted solution should be further diluted in 5% dextrose injection, USP, preferably to the concentrations listed below. Topotecan should NOT be diluted in buffered solutions.

Toprol XL® [Succinate] *see* Metoprolol *on page 574*

TOPV *see* Poliovirus Vaccine, Live, Trivalent, Oral *on page 702*

Toradol® *see* Ketorolac Tromethamine *on page 484*

Torecan® *see* Thiethylperazine Maleate *on page 838*

Tornalate® *see* Bitolterol Mesylate *on page 116*

Torsemide *(tore' se mide)*

Related Information

Cardiovascular Diseases *on page 912*

Brand Names Demadex®

Therapeutic Category Diuretic, Loop

Use Management of edema associated with congestive heart failure and hepatic or renal disease; used alone or in combination with antihypertensives in treatment of hypertension; I.V. form is indicated when rapid onset is desired

Usual Dosage Adults: Oral, I.V.:

Congestive heart failure: 10-20 mg once daily; may increase gradually for chronic treatment by doubling dose until the diuretic response is apparent (for acute treatment, I.V. dose may be repeated every 2 hours with double the dose as needed)

Chronic renal failure: 20 mg once daily; increase as described above

Hepatic cirrhosis: 5-10 mg once daily with an aldosterone antagonist or a potassium-sparing diuretic; increase as described above

Hypertension: 5 mg once daily; increase to 10 mg after 4-6 weeks if an adequate hypotensive response is not apparent; if still not effective, an additional antihypertensive agent may be added

Mechanism of Action Inhibits reabsorption of sodium and chloride in the ascending loop of Henle and distal renal tubule, interfering with the chloride-binding cotransport system, thus causing increased excretion of water, sodium, chloride, magnesium, and calcium; does not alter GFR, renal plasma flow, or acid-base balance

Local Anesthetic/Vasoconstrictor Precautions No information available to require special precautions

Effects on Dental Treatment No effects or complications reported

Other Adverse Effects
>10%: Cardiovascular: Orthostatic hypotension
1% to 10%:
Central nervous system: Headache, dizziness, vertigo
Dermatologic: Photosensitivity, urticaria
Endocrine & metabolic: Electrolyte imbalance, dehydration, hyperuricemia
Gastrointestinal: Diarrhea, loss of appetite, stomach cramps or pain, pancreatitis
Ocular: Blurred vision
<1%:
Dermatologic: Skin rash
Endocrine & metabolic: Gout
Gastrointestinal: Pancreatitis, nausea
Hepatic: Hepatic dysfunction
Hematologic: Agranulocytosis, leukopenia, anemia, thrombocytopenia
Local: Redness at injection site
Otic: Ototoxicity
Renal: Nephrocalcinosis, prerenal azotemia, interstitial nephritis

Drug Interactions
Aminoglycosides: Ototoxicity may be increased; anticoagulant activity is enhanced
Beta-blockers: Plasma concentrations of beta-blockers may be increased
Cisplatin: Ototoxicity may be increased
Digitalis: Arrhythmias may occur with diuretic-induced electrolyte disturbances
Lithium: Plasma concentrations of lithium may be increased
NSAIDs: Torsemide efficacy may be decreased
Probenecid: Torsemide action may be reduced
Salicylates: Diuretic action may be impaired in patients with cirrhosis and ascites
Sulfonylureas: Glucose tolerance may be decreased
Thiazides: Synergistic effects may result

Drug Uptake
Onset of diuresis: 30-60 minutes
Peak effect: 1-4 hours
Duration: ~6 hours
Absorption: Oral: Rapid
Serum half-life: 2-4; 7-8 hours in cirrhosis (dose modification appears unnecessary)

Pregnancy Risk Factor B

Totacillin® *see* Ampicillin *on page 62*
Touro LA® *see* Guaifenesin and Pseudoephedrine *on page 409*
TPGS *see* Tocophersolan *on page 852*
TPT *see* Topotecan Hydrochloride *on page 855*
Trace-4® *see* Trace Metals *on this page*

Trace Metals (trace met' als)
Brand Names Chroma-Pak®; Iodopen®; Molypen®; M.T.E.-4®; M.T.E.-5®; M.T.E.-6®; Multe-Pak-4®; Neotrace-4®; Pedte-Pak-5®; Pedtrace-4®; P.T.E.-4®; P.T.E.-5®; Sele-Pak®; Selepen®; Trace-4®; Zinca-Pak®
Therapeutic Category Trace Element, Parenteral
Synonyms Chromium; Copper; Iodine; Manganese; Molybdenum; Neonatal Trace Metals; Selenium; Zinc
Use Prevent and correct trace metal deficiencies
Local Anesthetic/Vasoconstrictor Precautions No information available to require special precautions
Effects on Dental Treatment No effects or complications reported
Comments Persistent diarrhea or excessive gastrointestinal fluid losses from ostomy sites may grossly increase zinc losses

Tramadol Hydrochloride (tra' ma dole hye droe klor' ide)
Brand Names Ultram®
Canadian/Mexican Brand Names Tradol® (Mexico)
Therapeutic Category Analgesic, Non-narcotic
(Continued)

Tramadol Hydrochloride *(Continued)*

Use

Dental: Relief of moderate to moderately severe dental pain

Medical: Relief of moderate to moderately severe medical pain

Usual Dosage Adults: Oral: 50-100 mg every 4-6 hours, not to exceed 400 mg/ day

Mechanism of Action Binds to µ-opiate receptors in the CNS causing inhibition of ascending pain pathways, altering the perception of and response to pain; also inhibits the reuptake of norepinephrine and serotonin, which also modifies the ascending pain pathway

Local Anesthetic/Vasoconstrictor Precautions No information available to require special precautions

Effects on Dental Treatment No effects or complications reported

Other Adverse Effects >1%:

Central nervous system: Dizziness, drowsiness, restlessness

Gastrointestinal: Nausea, constipation

Miscellaneous: Sweating

Oral manifestations: No data reported

Contraindications Previous hypersensitivity to tramadol or any components; should not be administered in cases of acute intoxication with alcohol, hypnotics, centrally acting analgesics, opioids, or psychotropic drugs

Warnings/Precautions Elderly patients and patients with chronic respiratory disorders may be at greater risk of adverse events; liver disease; patients with myxedema, hypothyroidism, or hypoadrenalism should use tramadol with caution and at reduced dosages; not recommended during pregnancy or in nursing mothers

Drug Interactions Carbamazepine decreases half-life by 33% to 50%; increased toxicity with monoamine oxidase inhibitors (seizures); quinidine inhibits cytochrome P450IID6, thereby increasing tramadol serum concentrations; cimetidine increases tramadol half-life by 20% to 25%

Drug Uptake

Absorption: Oral: ~75%

Onset of action: ~1 hour

Time to peak serum concentration: 2 hours

Serum half-life, elimination: 6 hours

Influence of food: No effect on rate or extent of absorption

Pregnancy Risk Factor C

Breast-feeding Considerations No data reported

Dosage Forms Tablet: 50 mg

Dietary Considerations No data reported

Generic Available No

Comments Literature reports suggest that the efficacy of tramadol in oral surgery pain is equivalent to the combination of aspirin and codeine. One study (Olson et al 1990) showed acetaminophen and dextropropoxyphene combination to be superior to tramadol and another study (Mehlisch et al, 1990) showed tramadol to be superior to acetaminophen and dextropropoxyphene combination. Tramadol appears to be at least equal to if not better than codeine alone.

Selected Readings

Mehlisch DR, Minn F, and Brown P, "Tramadol Hydrochloride: Efficacy Compared to Codeine Sulfate, Acetaminophen With Dextropropoxyphene and Placebo in Dental Extraction Pain," *Clin Pharmacol Ther*, 1992.

Olson NZ, Sunshine A, O'Neill, et al, "Tramadol Hydrochloride: Oral Efficacy in Postoperative Pain," Presented at the American Pain Society 9th Annual Scientific Meeting, St Louis, MO, October, 1990.

Sunshine A, Olson NZ, Zighelboim I, et al, "Analgesic Oral Efficacy of Tramadol Hydrochloride in Postoperative Pain," *Clin Pharmacol Ther*,

Voorhees F, Leibold DG, Stumpf, et al, "Tramadol Hydrochloride: Efficacy Compared to Codeine Sulfate, Aspirin With Codeine Phosphate, and Placebo in Dental Extraction Pain," *Clin Pharmacol Ther*, 1992, 51:122.

Trandate® *see* Labetalol Hydrochloride *on page 486*

Trandolapril *(tran doe' la pril)*

Brand Names Mavik®

Therapeutic Category Angiotensin-Converting Enzyme (ACE) Inhibitors

Use Management of hypertension alone or in combination with other antihypertensive agents

Usual Dosage Adults:

Non-Black patients: 0.5-1 mg for those not receiving diuretics; increase dose at 0.5-1 mg increments at 1- to 2-week intervals; maximum dose: 4 mg/day

Black patients: Initiate doses of 1-2 mg; maximum dose: 4 mg/day

Dosing adjustment in renal impairment: Cl$_{cr}$ ≤30 mL/minute: Administer lowest doses

Mechanism of Action Trandolapril is an angiotensin-converting enzyme (ACE) inhibitor which prevents the formation of angiotensin II from angiotensin I. Trandolapril must undergo enzymatic hydrolysis, mainly in liver, to its biologically active metabolite, trandolaprilat. A CNS mechanism may also be involved in the hypotensive effect as angiotensin II increases adrenergic outflow from the CNS. Vasoactive kallikrein's may be decreased in conversion to active hormones by ACE inhibitors, thus, reducing blood pressure.

Local Anesthetic/Vasoconstrictor Precautions No information available to require special precautions

Effects on Dental Treatment No effects or complications reported

Other Adverse Effects

Cardiovascular: Tachycardia, chest pain, palpitations, orthostatic blood pressure changes, syncope, heart failure, hypotension, angioedema, cardiogenic shock

Central nervous system: Headache, fatigue, dizziness, malaise, vertigo, somnolence, ataxia, nervousness, insomnia, fever

Dermatologic: Rash, pruritus, alopecia, exfoliative dermatitis, urticaria, photosensitivity

Endocrine & metabolic: Hyperkalemia

Gastrointestinal: Dysgeusia, abdominal pain, nausea, vomiting, diarrhea, anorexia, constipation, dry mouth, loss of taste perception, glossitis

Genitourinary: Oliguria, impotence, decreased libido

Hematologic: Neutropenia, agranulocytosis

Hepatic: Hepatitis

Neuromuscular & skeletal: Arthritis, arthralgia, myalgia, paresthesias

Ocular: Blurred vision

Otic: Tinnitus

Renal: Oliguria, increase in BUN, increased serum creatinine, proteinuria, worsening renal failure

Respiratory: Chest pain, chronic cough (nonproductive, persistent - more frequent in women)

Miscellaneous: Sweating

Warnings/Precautions Neutropenia, agranulocytosis, angioedema, decreased renal function (hypertension, renal artery stenosis, CHF), hepatic dysfunction (elimination, activation), proteinuria, first-dose hypotension (hypovolemia, CHF, dehydrated patients at risk, eg, diuretic use, elderly), elderly (due to renal function changes); use with caution and modify dosage in patients with renal impairment; use with caution in patients with collagen vascular disease, CHF, hypovolemia, valvular stenosis, hyperkalemia (>5.7 mEq/L), anesthesia

Drug Interactions

ACE inhibitors (trandolapril) and potassium-sparing diuretics → additive hyperkalemic effect

ACE inhibitors (trandolapril) and indomethacin or nonsteroidal anti-inflammatory agents → reduced antihypertensive response to ACE inhibitors (trandolapril)

Allopurinol and trandolapril → neutropenia

Antacids and ACE inhibitors → ↓ absorption of ACE inhibitors

Phenothiazines and ACE inhibitors → ↑ ACE inhibitor effect

Probenecid and ACE inhibitors (trandolapril) → ↑ ACE inhibitors (trandolapril) levels

Rifampin and ACE inhibitors (trandolapril) → ↓ ACE inhibitor effect

Digoxin and ACE inhibitors → ↑ serum digoxin levels

Lithium and ACE inhibitors → ↑ lithium serum levels

Tetracycline and ACE inhibitors (trandolapril) → ↓ tetracycline absorption (up to 37%)

Food decreases trandolapril absorption; rate, but not extent, of ramipril and fosinopril is reduced by concomitant administration with food; food does not reduce absorption of enalapril, lisinopril, or benazepril; trandolapril has a decreased rate and extent (25% to 30%) of absorption when taken with a high fat meal

Drug Uptake

Absorption: Rapid

Half-life: 24 hours

Pregnancy Risk Factor C (first trimester); D (second & third trimester)

Generic Available No

Comments Patients taking diuretics are at risk for developing hypotension on initial dosing; to prevent this, discontinue diuretics 2-3 days prior to initiating

(Continued)

Trandolapril *(Continued)*

trandolapril; may restart diuretics if blood pressure is not controlled by trandolapril alone

Selected Readings

Bevan EG, McInnes GT, Aldigier JC, et al, "Effect of Renal Function on the Pharmacokinetics and Pharmacodynamics of Trandolapril," *Br J Clin Pharmacol*, 1993, 35(2):128-35.

Caren H and Brunner HR, "Pharmacologic Profile of Trandolapril, A New Angiotensin-Converting Enzyme Inhibitor," *Am J Heart*, 1993, 125(5 Part 2):1524-31.

Zannad F, "Trandolapril: How Does It Differ From Other Angiotensin-Converting Enzyme Inhibitors?" *Drugs*, 1993, 46(Suppl 2):172-81.

Tranexamic Acid *(tran ex am' ik as' id)*

Brand Names Cyklokapron® Injection; Cyklokapron® Oral

Therapeutic Category Antihemophilic Agent

Use Short-term use (2-8 days) in hemophilia patients during and following tooth extraction to reduce or prevent hemorrhage

Usual Dosage Children and Adults: I.V.: 10 mg/kg immediately before surgery, then 25 mg/kg/dose orally 3-4 times/day for 2-8 days

Alternatively:

Oral: 25 mg/kg 3-4 times/day beginning 1 day prior to surgery

I.V.: 10 mg/kg 3-4 times/day in patients who are unable to take oral

Mechanism of Action Forms a reversible complex that displaces plasminogen from fibrin resulting in inhibition of fibrinolysis; it also inhibits the proteolytic activity of plasmin

Local Anesthetic/Vasoconstrictor Precautions No information available to require special precautions

Effects on Dental Treatment No effects or complications reported

Other Adverse Effects

>10%: Gastrointestinal: Nausea, diarrhea, vomiting

1% to 10%:

Cardiovascular: Hypotension, thrombosis

Ocular: Blurred vision

<1%: Endocrine & metabolic: Unusual menstrual discomfort

Drug Uptake

Serum half-life: 2-10 hours

Pregnancy Risk Factor B

Transdermal-NTG® *see* Nitroglycerin *on page 623*

Transderm-Nitro® *see* Nitroglycerin *on page 623*

Transderm Scop® *see* Scopolamine *on page 781*

Trans-Ver-Sal® *see* Salicylic Acid *on page 777*

Tranxene® *see* Clorazepate Dipotassium *on page 222*

Tranylcypromine Sulfate *(tran il sip' roe meen sul' fate)*

Brand Names Parnate®

Therapeutic Category Antidepressant, Monoamine Oxidase Inhibitor

Use Symptomatic treatment of depressed patients refractory to or intolerant to tricyclic antidepressants or electroconvulsive therapy; has a more rapid onset of therapeutic effect than other MAO inhibitors, but causes more severe hypertensive reactions

Usual Dosage Adults: Oral: 10 mg twice daily, increase by 10 mg increments at 1- to 3-week intervals; maximum: 60 mg/day

Mechanism of Action Inhibits the enzymes monoamine oxidase A and B which are responsible for the intraneuronal metabolism of norepinephrine and serotonin and increasing their availability to postsynaptic neurons; decreased firing rate of the locus ceruleus, reducing norepinephrine concentration in the brain; agonist effects of serotonin

Local Anesthetic/Vasoconstrictor Precautions Attempts should be made to avoid use of vasoconstrictor due to possibility of hypertensive episodes with monoamine oxidase inhibitors

Effects on Dental Treatment Orthostatic hypotension in >10% of patients; meperidine should be avoided as an analgesic due to toxic reactions with MAO inhibitors

Other Adverse Effects

1% to 10%: Cardiovascular: Orthostatic hypotension

<1%:

Cardiovascular: Edema, hypertensive crises

Central nervous system: Drowsiness, hyperexcitability, headache

Dermatologic: Skin rash, photosensitivity

Gastrointestinal: Dry mouth, constipation

Genitourinary: Urinary retention

Hepatic: Hepatitis
Ocular: Blurred vision
Drug Interactions
Decreased effect of antihypertensives
Increased toxicity with disulfiram (seizures), fluoxetine and other serotonin-active agents (eg, paroxetine, sertraline), TCAs (cardiovascular instability), meperidine (cardiovascular instability), phenothiazine (hypertensive crisis), sympathomimetics (hypertensive crisis), sumatriptan (hypothetical), CNS depressants, levodopa (hypertensive crisis), tyramine-containing foods (eg, aged foods), dextroamphetamine (psychosis)
Drug Uptake
Onset of action: 2-3 weeks are required of continued dosing to obtain full therapeutic effect
Serum half-life: 90-190 minutes
Time to peak serum concentration: Within 2 hours
Pregnancy Risk Factor C

Trasylol® *see* Aprotinin *on page 72*
Travase® *see* Sutilains *on page 816*

Trazodone (traz' oh done)
Related Information
Vasoconstrictor Interactions With Antidepressants *on page 1108*
Brand Names Desyrel®
Therapeutic Category Antidepressant, Miscellaneous
Use Treatment of depression
Usual Dosage Oral: Therapeutic effects may take up to 4 weeks to occur; therapy is normally maintained for several months after optimum response is reached to prevent recurrence of depression

Children 6-18 years: Initial: 1.5-2 mg/kg/day in divided doses; increase gradually every 3-4 days as needed; maximum: 6 mg/kg/day in 3 divided doses
Adolescents: Initial: 25-50 mg/day; increase to 100-150 mg/day in divided doses
Adults: Initial: 150 mg/day in 3 divided doses (may increase by 50 mg/day every 3-7 days); maximum: 600 mg/day
Elderly: 25-50 mg at bedtime with 25-50 mg/day dose increase every 3 days for inpatients and weekly for outpatients, if tolerated; usual dose: 75-150 mg/day

Mechanism of Action Inhibits reuptake of serotonin and norepinephrine by the presynaptic neuronal membrane and desensitization of adenyl cyclase, down regulation of beta-adrenergic receptors, and down regulation of serotonin receptors

Local Anesthetic/Vasoconstrictor Precautions No information available to require special precautions

Effects on Dental Treatment Trazodone elicits anticholinergic effects, but occur much less frequently than with tricyclic antidepressants; more than 10% of patients will have significant dry mouth especially in the elderly which could contribute to periodontal diseases and oral discomfort

Other Adverse Effects
>10%:
Central nervous system: Dizziness, headache, confusion
Gastrointestinal: Nausea, bad taste in mouth, dry mouth
Neuromuscular & skeletal: Muscle tremors
1% to 10%:
Central nervous system: Weakness
Gastrointestinal: Diarrhea, constipation
Ocular: Blurred vision
<1%:
Cardiovascular: Hypotension, tachycardia, bradycardia
Central nervous system: Agitation, seizures, extrapyramidal reactions
Dermatologic: Skin rash
Genitourinary: Prolonged priapism, urinary retention
Hepatic: Hepatitis

Drug Interactions
Decreased effect: Clonidine, methyldopa, anticoagulants
Increased toxicity: Fluoxetine; increased effect/toxicity of phenytoin, CNS depressants, MAO inhibitors; digoxin serum levels increase

Drug Uptake
Onset of effect: Therapeutic effects take 1-3 weeks to appear
Serum half-life: 4-7.5 hours, 2 compartment kinetics
(Continued)

Trazodone *(Continued)*

Time to peak serum concentration: Within 30-100 minutes, prolonged in the presence of food (up to 2.5 hours)
Pregnancy Risk Factor C

Trecator®-SC *see* Ethionamide *on page 342*
Trendar® [OTC] *see* Ibuprofen *on page 447*
Trental® *see* Pentoxifylline *on page 675*

Tretinoin *(tret' i noyn)*

Brand Names Retin-A™
Canadian/Mexican Brand Names Retisol-A® (Canada); Stieva-A® (Canada); Stieva-A Forte® (Canada); Stieva-A® (Mexico); Stieva-A® 0.025% (Mexico)
Therapeutic Category Acne Products; Retinoic Acid Derivative; Vitamin, Topical
Synonyms Tretinoina (Mexico)
Use Treatment of acne vulgaris, photodamaged skin, and some skin cancers
Usual Dosage Children >12 years and Adults: Topical: Apply once daily before retiring; if stinging or irritation develops, decrease frequency of application. Relapses normally occur within 3-6 weeks after stopping medication.
Mechanism of Action Keratinocytes in the sebaceous follicle become less adherent which allows for easy removal; decreases microcomedone formation
Local Anesthetic/Vasoconstrictor Precautions No information available to require special precautions
Effects on Dental Treatment No effects or complications reported
Other Adverse Effects 1% to 10%:
Cardiovascular: Edema
Dermatologic: Excessive dryness, erythema, scaling of the skin, hyperpigmentation or hypopigmentation, photosensitivity, initial acne flare-up
Local: Stinging, blistering
Drug Interactions Increased toxicity: Sulfur, benzoyl peroxide, salicylic acid, resorcinol (potentiates adverse reactions seen with tretinoin)
Drug Uptake
Absorption: Topical: Minimum absorption occurs
Pregnancy Risk Factor C

Tretinoina (Mexico) *see* Tretinoin *on this page*
Trexan™ *see* Naltrexone Hydrochloride *on page 603*
TRH *see* Protirelin *on page 747*

Triacetin *(trye a see' tin)*

Brand Names Fungoid®; Ony-Clear® Nail
Therapeutic Category Antifungal Agent, Topical
Synonyms Glycerol Triacetate
Use Fungistat for athlete's foot and other superficial fungal infections
Local Anesthetic/Vasoconstrictor Precautions No information available to require special precautions
Effects on Dental Treatment No effects or complications reported

Triacin-C® *see* Triprolidine, Pseudoephedrine, and Codeine *on page 879*
Triam-A® *see* Triamcinolone *on this page*

Triamcinolone *(trye am sin' oh lone)*

Related Information
Corticosteroid Equivalencies Comparison *on page 1017*
Corticosteroids, Topical Comparison *on page 1018*
Oral Nonviral Soft Tissue Ulcerations or Erosions *on page 955*
Respiratory Diseases *on page 924*
Brand Names Amcort®; Aristocort® Forte; Aristocort® Intralesional Suspension; Aristocort® Tablet; Aristospan®; Azmacort™; Delta-Tritex®; Kenacort® Syrup; Kenacort® Tablet; Kenalog® Injection; Kenonel®; Nasacort®; Tac™-3; Triam-A®; Triamolone®; Tri-Kort®; Trilog®; Trilone®; Trisoject®
Canadian/Mexican Brand Names Zamacort® (Mexico); Ledercort® (Mexico); Kenacort® (Mexico)
Therapeutic Category Anti-inflammatory Agent; Corticosteroid, Inhalant; Corticosteroid, Systemic; Corticosteroid, Topical (Medium Potency)
Synonyms Triamcinolone Acetonide, Aerosol; Triamcinolone Acetonide, Parenteral; Triamcinolone Diacetate, Oral; Triamcinolone Diacetate, Parenteral; Triamcinolone Hexacetonide; Triamcinolone, Oral
Use Severe swelling or immunosuppression; nasal spray for symptoms of seasonal and perennial allergic rhinitis

Usual Dosage In general, single I.M. dose of 4-7 times oral dose will control patient from 4-7 days up to 3-4 weeks.

Children 6-12 years:
Oral inhalation: 1-2 inhalations 3-4 times/day, not to exceed 12 inhalations/day
I.M. (acetonide or hexacetonide): 0.03-0.2 mg/kg at 1- to 7-day intervals
Intra-articular, intrabursal, or tendon-sheath injection: 2.5-15 mg, repeated as needed

Children >12 years and Adults:
Intranasal: 2 sprays in each nostril once daily; may increase after 4-7 days up to 4 sprays once daily or 1 spray 4 times/day in each nostril
Topical: Apply a thin film 2-3 times/day
Oral: 4-48 mg/day
I.M.: Acetonide or hexacetonide: 60 mg (of 40 mg/mL), additional 20-100 mg doses (usual: 40-80 mg) may be given when signs and symptoms recur, best at 6-week intervals to minimize HPA suppression
Oral inhalation: 2 inhalations 3-4 times/day, not to exceed 16 inhalations/day
Intra-articular (hexacetonide): 2-20 mg every 3-4 weeks as hexacetonide salt
Intralesional (use 10 mg/mL) (diacetate or acetonide): 1 mg/injection site, may be repeated one or more times/week depending upon patients response; maximum; 30 mg at any one time; may use multiple injections if they are more than 1 cm apart
Intra-articular, intrasynovial, and soft-tissue injection (use 10 mg/mL or 40 mg/mL) (diacetate or acetonide): 2.5-40 mg depending upon location, size of joints, and degree of inflammation; repeat when signs and symptoms recur
Sublesional (as acetonide): Up to 1 mg per injection site and may be repeated one or more times weekly; multiple sites may be injected if they are 1 cm or more apart, not to exceed 30 mg
See table.

Triamcinolone Dosing

	Acetonide	Diacetate	Hexacetonide
Intrasynovial	2.5-40 mg	5-40 mg	
Intralesional	2.5-40 mg	5-48 mg	Up to 0.5 mg/sq inch affected area
Sublesional	1-30 mg	
Systemic I.M.	2.5-60 mg/d	~40 mg/wk	20-100 mg
Intra-articular		5-40 mg	2-20 average
large joints	5-15 mg		10-20 mg
small joints	2.5-5 mg		2-6 mg
Tendon sheaths	10-40 mg		
Intradermal	1 mg/site		

Mechanism of Action Decreases inflammation by suppression of migration of polymorphonuclear leukocytes and reversal of increased capillary permeability; suppresses the immune system by reducing activity and volume of the lymphatic system; suppresses adrenal function at high doses

Local Anesthetic/Vasoconstrictor Precautions No information available to require special precautions

Effects on Dental Treatment No effects or complications reported

Other Adverse Effects
>10%:
Gastrointestinal: Increased appetite, indigestion
Central nervous system: Insomnia, nervousness
1% to 10%:
Dermatologic: Hirsutism
Endocrine & metabolic: Diabetes mellitus
Neuromuscular & skeletal: Joint pain
Ocular: Cataracts
Respiratory: Epistaxis
<1%:
Central nervous system: Seizures, mood swings, headache, delirium, hallucinations, euphoria
Dermatologic: Skin atrophy, bruising, hyperpigmentation, acne
Endocrine & metabolic: Amenorrhea, sodium and water retention, Cushing's syndrome, hyperglycemia
Gastrointestinal: Abdominal distention, ulcerative esophagitis, pancreatitis
(Continued)

Triamcinolone *(Continued)*

Hematologic: Bone growth suppression
Neuromuscular & skeletal: Muscle wasting
Miscellaneous: Hypersensitivity reactions

Drug Uptake
Duration of action: Oral: 8-12 hours
Absorption: Topical: Systemic absorption may occur
Time to peak: I.M.: Within 8-10 hours
Serum half-life, biologic: 18-36 hours

Pregnancy Risk Factor C

Comments Triamcinolone 16 mg is equivalent to cortisone 100 mg (no mineral-ocorticoid activity)

Triamcinolone Acetonide, Aerosol *see* Triamcinolone *on page 862*

Triamcinolone Acetonide Dental Paste

(trye am sin' oh lone a see' toe nide den' tal paste)

Brand Names Kenalog® in Orabase®
Canadian/Mexican Brand Names Oracort® (Canada)
Therapeutic Category Anti-inflammatory Agent

Use
Dental: For adjunctive treatment and for the temporary relief of symptoms associated with oral inflammatory lesions and ulcerative lesions resulting from trauma
Medical: Localized inflammation responsive to steroids

Usual Dosage Press a small dab (about ¼ inch) to the lesion until a thin film develops. A larger quantity may be required for coverage of some lesions. For optimal results use only enough to coat the lesion with a thin film.

Mechanism of Action Decreases inflammation by suppression of migration of polymorphonuclear leukocytes and reversal of increased capillary permeability; suppresses the immune system by reducing activity and volume of the lymphatic system; suppresses adrenal function at high doses

Local Anesthetic/Vasoconstrictor Precautions No information available to require special precautions

Effects on Dental Treatment No effects or complications reported

Other Adverse Effects No data reported

Oral manifestations: No data reported

Contraindications Known hypersensitivity to triamcinolone; contraindicated in the presence of fungal, viral, or bacterial infections of the mouth or throat

Warnings/Precautions Patients with tuberculosis, peptic ulcer or diabetes mellitus should not be treated with any corticosteroid preparation without the advice of the patient's physician. Normal immune responses of the oral tissues are depressed in patients receiving topical corticosteroid therapy. Virulent strains of oral microorganisms may multiply without producing the usual warning symptoms of oral infections. The small amount of steroid released from the topical preparation makes systemic effects very unlikely. If local irritation or sensitization should develop, the preparation should be discontinued. If significant regeneration or repair of oral tissues has not occurred in seven days, re-evaluation of the etiology of the oral lesion is advised.

Drug Interactions No data reported

Drug Uptake
Absorption: Topical: Systemic absorption may occur
Serum half-life: Biological: 18-36 hours

Pregnancy Risk Factor C

Breast-feeding Considerations No data reported

Dosage Forms Tubes: 5 g; each g provides 1 mg (0.1%) triamcinolone in emollient dental paste containing gelatin, pectin, and carboxymethylcellulose sodium in a polyethylene and mineral oil gel base

Dietary Considerations No data reported

Generic Available Yes

Comments When applying to tissues, attempts to spread this preparation may result in a granular, gritty sensation and cause it to crumble. This preparation should be applied at bedtime to permit steroid contact with the lesion throughout the night.

Triamcinolone Acetonide, Parenteral *see* Triamcinolone *on page 862*
Triamcinolone Diacetate, Oral *see* Triamcinolone *on page 862*
Triamcinolone Diacetate, Parenteral *see* Triamcinolone *on page 862*
Triamcinolone Hexacetonide *see* Triamcinolone *on page 862*
Triamcinolone, Oral *see* Triamcinolone *on page 862*

Triaminic® Allergy Tablet [OTC] *see* Chlorpheniramine and Phenylpropanolamine *on page 190*

Triaminic® Cold Tablet [OTC] *see* Chlorpheniramine and Phenylpropanolamine *on page 190*

Triaminic® Expectorant [OTC] *see* Guaifenesin and Phenylpropanolamine *on page 409*

Triaminicol® Multi-Symptom Cold Syrup [OTC] *see* Chlorpheniramine, Phenylpropanolamine, and Dextromethorphan *on page 194*

Triaminic® Oral Infant Drops *see* Pheniramine, Phenylpropanolamine, and Pyrilamine *on page 680*

Triaminic® Syrup [OTC] *see* Chlorpheniramine and Phenylpropanolamine *on page 190*

Triamolone® *see* Triamcinolone *on page 862*

Triamterene (trye am' ter een)
Related Information
 Cardiovascular Diseases *on page 912*
Brand Names Dyrenium®
Therapeutic Category Diuretic, Potassium Sparing
Synonyms Triamtereno (Mexico)
Use Alone or in combination with other diuretics to treat edema and hypertension; decreases potassium excretion caused by kaliuretic diuretics
Usual Dosage Oral:
 Children: 2-4 mg/kg/day in 1-2 divided doses; maximum: 300 mg/day
 Adults: 100-300 mg/day in 1-2 divided doses; maximum dose: 300 mg/day
Mechanism of Action Competes with aldosterone for receptor sites in the distal renal tubules, increasing sodium, chloride, and water excretion while conserving potassium and hydrogen ions; may block the effect of aldosterone on arteriolar smooth muscle as well
Local Anesthetic/Vasoconstrictor Precautions No information available to require special precautions
Effects on Dental Treatment No effects or complications reported
Other Adverse Effects
 1% to 10%:
  Cardiovascular: Hypotension, edema, congestive heart failure, bradycardia
  Central nervous system: Dizziness, headache, fatigue
  Dermatologic: Rash
  Gastrointestinal: Constipation, nausea
  Respiratory: Dyspnea
 <1%:
  Cardiovascular: Flushing
  Endocrine & metabolic: Hyperkalemia, dehydration, hyponatremia, gynecomastia, hyperchloremic, metabolic acidosis, postmenopausal bleeding
  Genitourinary: Inability to achieve or maintain an erection
Drug Interactions
 Increased risk of hyperkalemia if given together with amiloride, spironolactone, angiotensin-converting enzyme (ACE) inhibitors
 Increased toxicity of amantadine (possibly by decreasing its renal excretion)
Drug Uptake
 Onset of action: Diuresis occurs within 2-4 hours
 Duration: 7-9 hours
 Absorption: Oral: Unreliable
Pregnancy Risk Factor D

Triamterene and Hydrochlorothiazide
(trye am' ter een & hye droe klor oh thye' a zide)
Related Information
 Cardiovascular Diseases *on page 912*
Brand Names Dyazide®; Maxzide®
Canadian/Mexican Brand Names Apo-Triazide® (Canada); Novo-Triamzide® (Canada); Nu-Triazide® (Canada)
Therapeutic Category Diuretic, Combination
Synonyms Triamtereno Hidroclorotiacida (Mexico)
Use Management of mild to moderate hypertension; treatment of edema in congestive heart failure and nephrotic syndrome
Usual Dosage Oral:
 Adults: 1-2 capsules twice daily after meals
 Elderly: Initial: 1 capsule/day or every other day
Mechanism of Action Competes with aldosterone for receptor sites in the distal renal tubules, increasing sodium, chloride, and water excretion while
(Continued)

Triamterene and Hydrochlorothiazide *(Continued)*

conserving potassium and hydrogen ions; may block the effect of aldosterone on arteriolar smooth muscle as well

Inhibits sodium reabsorption in the distal tubules causing increased excretion of sodium and water as well as potassium and hydrogen ions

Local Anesthetic/Vasoconstrictor Precautions No information available to require special precautions

Effects on Dental Treatment No effects or complications reported

Other Adverse Effects

1% to 10%: Gastrointestinal: Loss of appetite, nausea, vomiting, stomach cramps, diarrhea, upset stomach

<1%:
Central nervous system: Dizziness, fatigue
Dermatologic: Purpura
Endocrine & metabolic: Electrolyte disturbances
Hematologic: Aplastic anemia, agranulocytosis, hemolytic anemia, leukopenia, thrombocytopenia, megaloblastic anemia
Neuromuscular & skeletal: Muscle cramps
Ocular: Xanthopsia, transient blurred vision
Respiratory: Allergic pneumonitis, pulmonary edema, respiratory distress
Miscellaneous: Bright orange tongue, burning of tongue, cracked corners of mouth

Drug Interactions

Hydrochlorothiazide:
Decreased effect of oral hypoglycemics; decreased absorption with cholestyramine and colestipol
Increased effect with furosemide and other loop diuretics
Increased toxicity/levels of lithium

Triamterene:
Increased risk of hyperkalemia if given together with amiloride, spironolactone, angiotensin-converting enzyme (ACE) inhibitors
Increased toxicity of amantadine (possibly by decreasing its renal excretion)

Pregnancy Risk Factor C

Triamtereno Hidroclorotiacida (Mexico) *see* Triamterene and Hydrochlorothiazide *on previous page*

Triamtereno (Mexico) *see* Triamterene *on previous page*

Triapin® *see* Butalbital Compound *on page 133*

Triavil® *see* Amitriptyline and Perphenazine *on page 50*

Triazolam *(trye ay' zoe lam)*

Related Information

Dental Drug Interactions: Update on Drug Combinations Requiring Special Considerations *on page 1022*
Patients Requiring Sedation *on page 965*

Brand Names Halcion®

Canadian/Mexican Brand Names Apo-Triazo® (Canada); Gen-Triazolam® (Canada); Novo-Triolam® (Canada); Nu-Triazo® (Canada)

Therapeutic Category Benzodiazepine; Hypnotic; Sedative

Use

Dental: Oral premedication before dental procedures
Medical: Short-term treatment of insomnia

Usual Dosage Oral:

Children <18 years: Dosage not established
Adults: 0.25 mg taken the evening before oral surgery; or 0.25 mg 1 hour before procedure

Mechanism of Action Depresses all levels of the CNS, including the limbic and reticular formation, probably through the increased action of gamma-aminobutyric acid (GABA), which is a major inhibitory neurotransmitter in the brain

Local Anesthetic/Vasoconstrictor Precautions No information available to require special precautions

Effects on Dental Treatment No effects or complications reported

Other Adverse Effects >10%: Central nervous system: Drowsiness, fatigue, impaired coordination, lightheadedness, memory impairment, insomnia, anxiety, depression, headache

Oral manifestations: >10%: Dry mouth, decreased salivation

Contraindications Hypersensitivity to triazolam, or any component, cross-sensitivity with other benzodiazepines may occur; severe uncontrolled pain;

pre-existing CNS depression; narrow-angle glaucoma; not to be used in pregnancy or lactation

Warnings/Precautions May cause drug dependency; avoid abrupt discontinuance in patients with prolonged therapy or seizure disorders; not considered a drug of choice in the elderly

Drug Interactions Decreased effect with phenytoin, phenobarbital; increased effect/toxicity with CNS depressants, cimetidine, erythromycin

Drug Uptake
Onset of hypnotic effect: Within 15-30 minutes
Time to peak serum concentration: Oral: ~2 hours
Duration: 6-7 hours
Serum half-life: 1.7-5 hours

Pregnancy Risk Factor X

Breast-feeding Considerations No data reported

Dosage Forms Tablet: 0.125 mg, 0.25 mg

Dietary Considerations No data reported

Generic Available No

Selected Readings
Berthold CW, Schneider A, and Dionne RA, "Using Triazolam to Reduce Dental Anxiety," *J Am Dent Assoc*, 1993, 124(11):58-64.
Lieblich SE and Horswell B, "Attenuation of Anxiety in Ambulatory Oral Surgery Patients With Oral Triazolam," *J Oral Maxillofac Surg*, 1991, 49(8):792-7.

Triban® *see* Trimethobenzamide Hydrochloride *on page 873*

Tribavirin *see* Ribavirin *on page 767*

Tri-Chlor® *see* Trichloroacetic Acid *on this page*

Trichlormethiazide (trye klor meth eye' a zide)

Related Information
Cardiovascular Diseases *on page 912*

Brand Names Metahydrin®; Naqua®

Therapeutic Category Diuretic, Thiazide Type

Use Management of mild to moderate hypertension; treatment of edema in congestive heart failure and nephrotic syndrome

Usual Dosage Oral:
Children >6 months: 0.07 mg/kg/24 hours or 2 mg/m²/24 hours
Adults: 1-4 mg/day

Mechanism of Action The diuretic mechanism of action of the thiazides is primarily inhibition of sodium, chloride, and water reabsorption in the renal distal tubules, thereby producing diuresis with a resultant reduction in plasma volume. The antihypertensive mechanism of action of the thiazides is unknown. It is known that doses of thiazides produce greater reduction in blood pressure than equivalent diuretic doses of loop diuretics. There has been speculation that the thiazides may have some influence on vascular tone mediated through sodium depletion, but this remains to be proven.

Local Anesthetic/Vasoconstrictor Precautions No information available to require special precautions

Effects on Dental Treatment No effects or complications reported

Other Adverse Effects
1% to 10%: Endocrine & metabolic: Hypokalemia
<1%:
Cardiovascular: Hypotension
Dermatologic: photosensitivity
Endocrine & metabolic: Fluid and electrolyte imbalances (hypocalcemia, hypomagnesemia, hyponatremia); hyperglycemia
Hematologic: Rarely blood dyscrasias
Renal: Prerenal azotemia

Drug Interactions
Decreased effect of oral hypoglycemics; decreased absorption with cholestyramine and colestipol
Increased effect with furosemide and other loop diuretics
Increased toxicity/levels of lithium

Drug Uptake
Onset of of diuretic effect: Within 2 hours
Peak: 4 hours
Duration: 12-24 hours

Pregnancy Risk Factor D

Trichloroacetic Acid (trye klor oh a see' tik as' id)

Brand Names Tri-Chlor®

Therapeutic Category Keratolytic Agent

(Continued)

Trichloroacetic Acid *(Continued)*

Use Debride callous tissue

Local Anesthetic/Vasoconstrictor Precautions No information available to require special precautions

Effects on Dental Treatment No effects or complications reported

Tri-Clear® Expectorant [OTC] *see* Guaifenesin and Phenylpropanolamine *on page 409*

Tridesilon® *see* Desonide *on page 259*

Tridihexethyl Chloride *(trye dye hex e' thil klor' ide)*

Brand Names Pathilon®

Therapeutic Category Anticholinergic Agent; Antispasmodic Agent, Gastrointestinal

Use Adjunctive therapy in peptic ulcer treatment

Local Anesthetic/Vasoconstrictor Precautions No information available to require special precautions

Effects on Dental Treatment 1% to 10% dry mouth

Other Adverse Effects

>10%:
    Dermatologic: Dry skin
    Gastrointestinal: Constipation, dry mouth and throat
    Respiratory: Dry nose
    Miscellaneous: Decreased sweating
1% to 10%: Gastrointestinal: Difficulty in swallowing
<1%:
    Dermatologic: Rash
    Cardiovascular: Tachycardia
    Central nervous system: Confusion, headache, loss of memory, nausea, tiredness, drowsiness, nervousness, insomnia
    Gastrointestinal: Bloated feeling, vomiting
    Genitourinary: Urinary retention
    Ocular: Intraocular pressure (increased), blurred vision
    Neuromuscular & skeletal: Weakness

Tridil® *see* Nitroglycerin *on page 623*

Tridione® *see* Trimethadione *on page 872*

Triethanolamine Polypeptide Oleate-Condensate

(trye eth a nole' a meen pol ee pep' tide oh' lee ate-kon' den sate)

Brand Names Cerumenex®

Therapeutic Category Otic Agent, Cerumenolytic

Use Removal of ear wax (cerumen)

Usual Dosage Children and Adults: Otic: Fill ear canal, insert cotton plug; allow to remain 15-30 minutes; flush ear with lukewarm water as a single treatment; if a second application is needed for unusually hard impactions, repeat the procedure

Mechanism of Action Emulsifies and disperses accumulated cerumen

Local Anesthetic/Vasoconstrictor Precautions No information available to require special precautions

Effects on Dental Treatment No effects or complications reported

Other Adverse Effects <1%: Dermatologic: Mild erythema and pruritus, severe eczematoid reactions, localized dermatitis

Drug Interactions No data reported

Drug Uptake Onset of effect: Produces slight disintegration of very hard ear wax by 24 hours

Pregnancy Risk Factor C

Triethanolamine Salicylate *(trye eth a nole' a meen sa lis' i late)*

Brand Names Myoflex® [OTC]; Sportscreme® [OTC]

Therapeutic Category Analgesic, Topical

Use Relief of pain of muscular aches, rheumatism, neuralgia, sprains, arthritis on intact skin

Local Anesthetic/Vasoconstrictor Precautions No information available to require special precautions

Effects on Dental Treatment No effects or complications reported

Other Adverse Effects 1% to 10%:
    Central nervous system: Confusion, drowsiness
    Gastrointestinal: Nausea, vomiting, diarrhea
    Respiratory: Hyperventilation

Triethylenethiophosphoramide *see* Thiotepa *on page 841*
Trifed® [OTC] *see* Triprolidine and Pseudoephedrine *on page 878*
Trifed-C® *see* Triprolidine, Pseudoephedrine, and Codeine *on page 879*
Trifluoperacina, Clorhidrato De (Mexico) *see* Trifluoperazine Hydrochloride *on this page*

Trifluoperazine Hydrochloride
(trye floo oh per' a zeen hye droe klor' ide)
Brand Names Stelazine®
Canadian/Mexican Brand Names Flupazine® (Mexico)
Therapeutic Category Antipsychotic Agent; Phenothiazine Derivative
Synonyms Trifluoperacina, Clorhidrato De (Mexico)
Use Treatment of psychoses and management of nonpsychotic anxiety
Usual Dosage
Children 6-12 years: Psychoses:
Oral: Hospitalized or well supervised patients: Initial: 1 mg 1-2 times/day, gradually increase until symptoms are controlled or adverse effects become troublesome; maximum: 15 mg/day
I.M.: 1 mg twice daily
Adults:
Psychoses:
Outpatients: Oral: 1-2 mg twice daily
Hospitalized or well supervised patients: Initial: 2-5 mg twice daily with optimum response in the 15-20 mg/day range; do not exceed 40 mg/day
I.M.: 1-2 mg every 4-6 hours as needed up to 10 mg/24 hours maximum
Nonpsychotic anxiety: Oral: 1-2 mg twice daily; maximum: 6 mg/day; therapy for anxiety should not exceed 12 weeks; do not exceed 6 mg/day for longer than 12 weeks when treating anxiety; agitation, jitteriness, or insomnia may be confused with original neurotic or psychotic symptoms
Not dialyzable (0% to 5%)
Mechanism of Action Blocks postsynaptic mesolimbic dopaminergic receptors in the brain; exhibits a strong alpha-adrenergic blocking effect and depresses the release of hypothalamic and hypophyseal hormones
Local Anesthetic/Vasoconstrictor Precautions No information available to require special precautions
Effects on Dental Treatment Significant hypotension may occur, especially when the drug is administered parenterally; orthostatic hypotension is due to alpha-receptor blockade, the elderly are at greater risk for orthostatic hypotension

Tardive dyskinesia: Prevalence rate may be 40% in elderly; development of the syndrome and the irreversible nature are proportional to duration and total cumulative dose over time

Extrapyramidal reactions are more common in elderly with up to 50% developing these reactions after 60 years of age; drug-induced **Parkinson's syndrome** occurs often; **Akathisia** is the most common extrapyramidal reaction in elderly

Increased confusion, memory loss, psychotic behavior, and agitation frequently occur as a consequence of anticholinergic effects

Antipsychotic associated sedation in nonpsychotic patients is extremely unpleasant due to feelings of depersonalization, derealization, and dysphoria
Other Adverse Effects
>10%:
Cardiovascular: Hypotension, orthostatic hypotension
Central nervous system: Pseudoparkinsonism, akathisia, dystonias, tardive dyskinesia (persistent), dizziness
Gastrointestinal: Constipation
Ocular: Pigmentary retinopathy
Respiratory: Nasal congestion
Miscellaneous: Decreased sweating
1% to 10%:
Central nervous system: Dizziness
Genitourinary: Difficulty in urination, ejaculatory disturbances
Dermatologic: Increased sensitivity to sun, skin rash
Endocrine & metabolic: Changes in menstrual cycle, changes in libido, pain in breasts
Gastrointestinal: Weight gain, nausea, vomiting, stomach pain
Neuromuscular & skeletal: Trembling of fingers
<1%:
Central nervous system: Neuroleptic malignant syndrome (NMS)
(Continued)

Trifluoperazine Hydrochloride (Continued)

Dermatologic: Discoloration of skin (blue-gray)
Endocrine & metabolic: Galactorrhea
Genitourinary: Priapism
Hematologic: Agranulocytosis, leukopenia
Hepatic: Cholestatic jaundice, hepatotoxicity
Ocular: Cornea and lens changes, pigmentary retinopathy
Miscellaneous: Impairment of temperature regulation, lowering of seizures threshold

Drug Interactions

Decreased effect of anticonvulsants (increases requirements), guanethidine, anticoagulants; decreased effect with anticholinergics

Increased effect/toxicity with CNS depressants, metrizamide (increased seizures), propranolol, lithium (rare encephalopathy)

Drug Uptake

Serum half-life: >24 hours with chronic use

Pregnancy Risk Factor C

Triflupromazine Hydrochloride

(trye floo proe' ma zeen hye droe klor' ide)

Brand Names Vesprin®

Therapeutic Category Phenothiazine Derivative

Use Treatment of psychoses, nausea, vomiting, and intractable hiccups

Local Anesthetic/Vasoconstrictor Precautions No information available to require special precautions

Effects on Dental Treatment Significant hypotension may occur, especially when the drug is administered parenterally; orthostatic hypotension is due to alpha-receptor blockade, the elderly are at greater risk for orthostatic hypotension

Tardive dyskinesia: Prevalence rate may be 40% in elderly; development of the syndrome and the irreversible nature are proportional to duration and total cumulative dose over time

Extrapyramidal reactions are more common in elderly with up to 50% developing these reactions after 60 years of age; drug-induced **Parkinson's syndrome** occurs often; **Akathisia** is the most common extrapyramidal reaction in elderly

Increased confusion, memory loss, psychotic behavior, and agitation frequently occur as a consequence of anticholinergic effects

Antipsychotic associated sedation in nonpsychotic patients is extremely unpleasant due to feelings of depersonalization, derealization, and dysphoria

Trifluridine (trye flure' i deen)

Related Information

Systemic Viral Diseases *on page 934*

Brand Names Viroptic®

Therapeutic Category Antiviral Agent, Ophthalmic

Use Treatment of primary keratoconjunctivitis and recurrent epithelial keratitis caused by herpes simplex virus types I and II

Usual Dosage Adults: Instill 1 drop into affected eye every 2 hours while awake, to a maximum of 9 drops/day, until re-epithelialization of corneal ulcer occurs; then use 1 drop every 4 hours for another 7 days; do **not** exceed 21 days of treatment; if improvement has not taken place in 7-14 days, consider another form of therapy

Mechanism of Action Interferes with viral replication by incorporating into viral DNA in place of thymidine, inhibiting thymidylate synthetase resulting in the formation of defective proteins

Local Anesthetic/Vasoconstrictor Precautions No information available to require special precautions

Effects on Dental Treatment No effects or complications reported

Other Adverse Effects

1% to 10%: Ocular: Burning, stinging
<1%: Ocular: Palpebral edema, epithelial keratopathy, keratitis, stromal edema, increased intraocular pressure, hyperemia, hypersensitivity reactions

Drug Interactions No data reported

Drug Uptake Absorption: Ophthalmic instillation: Systemic absorption is negligible, while corneal penetration is adequate

Pregnancy Risk Factor C

Triglycerides, Medium Chain see Medium Chain Triglycerides on page 532
Trihexifenidico (Mexico) see Trihexyphenidyl Hydrochloride on this page
Trihexy® see Trihexyphenidyl Hydrochloride on this page

Trihexyphenidyl Hydrochloride
(trye hex ee fen' i dil hye droe klor' ide)

Brand Names Artane®; Trihexy®

Canadian/Mexican Brand Names Apo-Trihex® (Canada); PMS-Trihexyphenidyl® (Canada); Trihexyphen® (Canada); Novo-Hexidyl® (Canada); Hipokinon® (Mexico)

Therapeutic Category Anticholinergic Agent; Anti-Parkinson's Agent

Synonyms Trihexifenidico (Mexico)

Use Adjunctive treatment of Parkinson's disease; also used in treatment of drug-induced extrapyramidal effects and acute dystonic reactions

Usual Dosage Adults: Oral: Initial: 1-2 mg/day, increase by 2 mg increments at intervals of 3-5 days; usual dose: 5-15 mg/day in 3-4 divided doses

Mechanism of Action Thought to act by blocking excess acetylcholine at cerebral synapses; many of its effects are due to its pharmacologic similarities with atropine

Local Anesthetic/Vasoconstrictor Precautions No information available to require special precautions

Effects on Dental Treatment Over 10% of patients will experience significant dry mouth. Normal salivary flow will resume with cessation of drug therapy. Prolonged xerostomia may contribute to development of caries, periodontal disease, oral candidiasis and discomfort

Other Adverse Effects

>10%:

Gastrointestinal: Constipation, dry mouth
Miscellaneous: Decreased sweating; dry nose, throat, or skin

1% to 10%:

Endocrine & metabolic: Decreased flow of breast milk
Gastrointestinal: Difficulty in swallowing
Ocular: Increased sensitivity to light

<1%:

Cardiovascular: Orthostatic hypotension, ventricular fibrillation, tachycardia, palpitations
Central nervous system: Confusion, drowsiness, headache, loss of memory, weakness, tiredness, ataxia
Dermatologic: Skin rash
Gastrointestinal: Bloated feeling, nausea, vomiting
Genitourinary: Difficult urination
Ocular: Increased intraocular pain, blurred vision

Drug Interactions

Decreased effect of levodopa
Increased toxicity with narcotic analgesics, phenothiazines, TCAs, quinidine, levodopa, anticholinergics

Drug Uptake

Peak effect: Within 1 hour
Serum half-life: 3.3-4.1 hours
Time to peak serum concentration: Within 1-1.5 hours

Pregnancy Risk Factor C

Tri-Hydroserpine® see Hydralazine, Hydrochlorothiazide, and Reserpine on page 429

Tri-K® see Potassium Acetate, Potassium Bicarbonate, and Potassium Citrate on page 706

Trikates® see Potassium Acetate, Potassium Bicarbonate, and Potassium Citrate on page 706

Tri-Kort® see Triamcinolone on page 862

Trilafon® see Perphenazine on page 677

Tri-Levlen® see Ethinyl Estradiol and Levonorgestrel on page 337

Trilisate® see Choline Magnesium Salicylate on page 202

Trilog® see Triamcinolone on page 862

Trilone® see Triamcinolone on page 862

Trimazide® see Trimethobenzamide Hydrochloride on page 873

Trimeprazine Tartrate (trye mep' ra zeen tar' trate)

Brand Names Temaril®

Therapeutic Category Antihistamine; Phenothiazine Derivative
(Continued)

Trimeprazine Tartrate *(Continued)*

Use Perennial and seasonal allergic rhinitis and other allergic symptoms including urticaria

Usual Dosage Oral:

Children:

6 months to 3 years: 1.25 mg at bedtime or 3 times/day if needed

>3 years: 2.5 mg at bedtime or 3 times/day if needed

>6 years: Sustained release: 5 mg/day

Adults: 2.5 mg 4 times/day (5 mg every 12-hour sustained release)

Not dialyzable (0% to 5%)

Mechanism of Action Blocks postsynaptic mesolimbic dopaminergic receptors in the brain, exhibits a strong alpha-adrenergic blocking effect and depresses the release of hypothalamic and hypophyseal hormones; competes with histamine for the H_1-receptor; reduces stimuli to the brainstem reticular system

Local Anesthetic/Vasoconstrictor Precautions No information available to require special precautions

Effects on Dental Treatment Chronic use of antihistamines will inhibit salivary flow, particularly in elderly patients; this may contribute to periodontal disease and oral discomfort

Other Adverse Effects

>10%:

Central nervous system: Slight to moderate drowsiness

Respiratory: Thickening of bronchial secretions

1% to 10%:

Central nervous system: Headache, fatigue, nervousness, dizziness

Gastrointestinal: Appetite increase, weight increase nausea, diarrhea, abdominal pain, dry mouth

Neuromuscular & skeletal: Arthralgia

Respiratory: Pharyngitis

<1%:

Cardiovascular: Edema, hypotension, palpitations

Central nervous system: Depression, epistaxis, sedation, dizziness, paradoxical excitement, insomnia

Dermatologic: Angioedema, photosensitivity, rash

Genitourinary: Urinary retention

Hepatic: Hepatitis

Neuromuscular & skeletal: Myalgia, paresthesia, tremor

Ocular: Blurred vision

Respiratory: Bronchospasm

Drug Interactions Increased effect/toxicity with CNS depressants, alcohol, MAO inhibitors (avoid concomitant use), oral contraceptives, progesterone, reserpine, nylidrin

Drug Uptake

Absorption: Well absorbed

Serum half-life, elimination: 4.78 hours mean

Time to peak serum concentration:

Syrup: 3.5 hours

Tablet: 4.5 hours

Pregnancy Risk Factor C

Trimethadione *(trye meth a dye' one)*

Brand Names Tridione®

Therapeutic Category Anticonvulsant, Oxazolidinedione

Synonyms Troxidone

Use Control absence (petit mal) seizures refractory to other drugs

Local Anesthetic/Vasoconstrictor Precautions No information available to require special precautions

Effects on Dental Treatment No effects or complications reported

Other Adverse Effects

>10%:

Central nervous system: Dizziness, drowsiness, sedation, headache

Ocular: Double vision, photophobia

1% to 10%:

Central nervous system: Insomnia

Dermatologic: Alopecia

Gastrointestinal: Anorexia, stomach upset

Miscellaneous: Hiccups

<1%:
    Dermatologic: Exfoliative dermatitis
    Neuromuscular & skeletal: Myasthenia gravis syndrome
    Hematologic: Aplastic anemia, agranulocytosis, thrombocytopenia, exacerbation of porphyria
    Hepatic: Hepatitis
    Miscellaneous: Systemic lupus erythematosus (SLE), nephrosis

Trimethaphan Camsylate (trye meth' a fan kam' sil late)
Brand Names Arfonad®
Therapeutic Category Adrenergic Blocking Agent; Anticholinergic Agent; Ganglionic Blocking Agent
Use Immediate and temporary reduction of blood pressure in patients with hypertensive emergencies; controlled hypotension during surgery
Mechanism of Action Blocks transmission in both adrenergic and cholinergic ganglia by blocking stimulation from presynaptic receptors to postsynaptic receptors mediated by acetylcholine; possesses direct peripheral vasodilatory activity and is a weak histamine releaser
Local Anesthetic/Vasoconstrictor Precautions No information available to require special precautions
Effects on Dental Treatment No effects or complications reported
Other Adverse Effects 1% to 10%:
    Cardiovascular: Hypotension (especially orthostatic), tachycardia
    Central nervous system: Restlessness, weakness
    Dermatologic: Itching, urticaria
    Gastrointestinal: Anorexia, nausea, vomiting, dry mouth, adynamic ileus
    Genitourinary: Urinary retention
    Ocular: Mydriasis, cycloplegia
    Respiratory: Apnea, respiratory arrest
    Miscellaneous: Sodium and water retention
Drug Interactions
    Increased effect:
        Anesthetics, procainamide, diuretics, and other hypotensive agents may increase hypotensive effects of trimethaphan
        Effects of tubocurarine and succinylcholine may be prolonged by trimethaphan
Pregnancy Risk Factor C

Trimethobenzamide Hydrochloride
(trye meth oh ben' za mide hye droe klor' ide)
Brand Names Arrestin®; Tebamide®; T-Gen®; Ticon®; Tigan®; Tiject®; Triban®; Trimazide®
Therapeutic Category Antiemetic
Use Control of nausea and vomiting (especially for long-term antiemetic therapy); less effective than phenothiazines but may be associated with fewer side effects
Usual Dosage Rectal use is contraindicated in neonates and premature infants
    Children:
        Rectal: <14 kg: 100 mg 3-4 times/day
        Oral, rectal: 14-40 kg: 100-200 mg 3-4 times/day
    Adults:
        Oral: 250 mg 3-4 times/day
        I.M., rectal: 200 mg 3-4 times/day
Mechanism of Action Acts centrally to inhibit the medullary chemoreceptor trigger zone
Local Anesthetic/Vasoconstrictor Precautions No information available to require special precautions
Effects on Dental Treatment No effects or complications reported
Other Adverse Effects
    >10%: Central nervous system: Drowsiness
    1% to 10%:
        Cardiovascular: Hypotension
        Central nervous system: Dizziness, headache
        Gastrointestinal: Diarrhea
        Neuromuscular & skeletal: muscle cramps
    <1%:
        Central nervous system: Mental depression, convulsions, opisthotonus
        Dermatologic: Hypersensitivity skin reactions
        Hematologic: Blood dyscrasias
        Hepatic: Hepatic impairment
Drug Interactions Antagonism of oral anticoagulants may occur
(Continued)

Trimethobenzamide Hydrochloride *(Continued)*

Drug Uptake
Onset of antiemetic effect:
Oral: Within 10-40 minutes
I.M.: Within 15-35 minutes
Duration: 3-4 hours
Absorption: Rectal: ~60%
Pregnancy Risk Factor C

Trimethoprim *(trye meth' oh prim)*

Brand Names Proloprim®; Trimpex®
Therapeutic Category Antibiotic, Miscellaneous
Synonyms Trimetoprima (Mexico)
Use Treatment of urinary tract infections; acute otitis media in children; acute exacerbations of chronic bronchitis in adults; in combination with other agents for treatment of toxoplasmosis, *Pneumocystis carinii*
Usual Dosage Oral:
Children: 4 mg/kg/day in divided doses every 12 hours
Adults: 100 mg every 12 hours or 200 mg every 24 hours
Mechanism of Action Inhibits folic acid reduction to tetrahydrofolate, and thereby inhibits microbial growth
Local Anesthetic/Vasoconstrictor Precautions No information available to require special precautions
Effects on Dental Treatment No effects or complications reported
Other Adverse Effects
>10%: Dermatologic: Rash, pruritus
1% to 10%: Hematologic: Megaloblastic anemia
<1%:
Central nervous system: Fever
Dermatologic: Exfoliative dermatitis
Gastrointestinal: Nausea, vomiting, epigastric distress
Hepatic: Cholestatic jaundice
Hematologic: Thrombocytopenia, neutropenia, leukopenia
Miscellaneous: Increased LFTS, BUN, and serum creatinine
Drug Interactions Increased effect/toxicity/levels of phenytoin
Drug Uptake
Absorption: Oral: Readily and extensive
Serum half-life: 8-14 hours, prolonged with renal impairment
Time to peak serum concentration: Within 1-4 hours
Pregnancy Risk Factor C

Trimethoprim and Polymyxin B
(trye meth' oh prim & pol i mix' in bee)
Brand Names Polytrim® Ophthalmic
Therapeutic Category Antibiotic, Ophthalmic
Synonyms Polymyxin B and Trimethoprim
Use Treatment of surface ocular bacterial conjunctivitis and blepharoconjunctivitis
Local Anesthetic/Vasoconstrictor Precautions No information available to require special precautions
Effects on Dental Treatment No effects or complications reported
Other Adverse Effects 1% to 10%: Local: Burning, stinging, itching, increased redness

Trimethoprim and Sulfamethoxazole *(koe trye mox' a zole)*
Related Information
Animal and Human Bites Guidelines *on page 976*
Brand Names Bactrim™; Bactrim™ DS; Cotrim®; Cotrim® DS; Septra®; Septra® DS; Sulfamethoprim®; Sulfatrim®; Sulfatrim® DS; Sulfoxaprim®; Sulfoxaprim® DS; Trisulfam®; Uroplus® DS; Uroplus® SS
Canadian/Mexican Brand Names Apo-Sulfatrim® (Canada); Novo-Trimel® (Canada); Nu-Cotrimox® (Canada); Pro-Trin® (Canada); Roubac® (Canada); Trisulfa® (Canada); Trisulfa-S® (Canada); Anitrim® (Mexico); Bactelan® (Mexico); Batrizol® (Mexico); Ectaprim® (Mexico); Ectaprim-F® (Mexico); Enter-obacticel® (Mexico); Esteprim® (Mexico); Isobac® (Mexico); Kelfiprim® (Mexico); Metoxiprim® (Mexico); Syraprim® (Mexico); Trimesuxol® (Mexico); Trimetoger® (Mexico); Trimetox® (Mexico); Trimzol® (Mexico)
Therapeutic Category Antibiotic, Sulfonamide Derivative
Synonyms Co-trimoxazole; SMZ-TMP; Sulfamethoxazole and Trimethoprim; TMP-SMZ

Use

Oral treatment of urinary tract infections; acute otitis media in children; acute exacerbations of chronic bronchitis in adults; prophylaxis of *Pneumocystis carinii* pneumonitis (PCP)

I.V. treatment of documented PCP, empiric treatment of PCP in immune compromised patients; treatment of documented or suspected shigellosis, typhoid fever, *Nocardia asteroides* infection, or other infections caused by susceptible bacterial

Usual Dosage Dosage recommendations are based on the trimethoprim component

Children >2 months:

Mild to moderate infections: Oral, I.V.: 8 mg TMP/kg/day in divided doses every 12 hours

Serious infection/*Pneumocystis*: I.V.: 20 mg TMP/kg/day in divided doses every 6 hours

Urinary tract infection prophylaxis: Oral: 2 mg TMP/kg/dose daily

Prophylaxis of *Pneumocystis*: Oral, I.V.: 10 mg TMP/kg/day or 150 mg TMP/m^2/day in divided doses every 12 hours for 3 days/week; dose should not exceed 320 mg trimethoprim and 1600 mg sulfamethoxazole 3 days/week

Adults:

Urinary tract infection/chronic bronchitis: Oral: 1 double strength tablet every 12 hours for 10-14 days

Sepsis: I.V.: 20 TMP/kg/day divided every 6 hours

Pneumocystis carinii:

Prophylaxis: Oral, I.V.: 10 mg TMP/kg/day divided every 12 hours for 3 days/week

Treatment: I.V.: 20 mg TMP/kg/day divided every 6 hours

Mechanism of Action Sulfamethoxazole interferes with bacterial folic acid synthesis and growth via inhibition of dihydrofolic acid formation from para-aminobenzoic acid; trimethoprim inhibits dihydrofolic acid reduction to tetrahydrofolate resulting in sequential inhibition of enzymes of the folic acid pathway

Local Anesthetic/Vasoconstrictor Precautions No information available to require special precautions

Effects on Dental Treatment No effects or complications reported

Other Adverse Effects

>10%:

Dermatologic: Allergic skin reactions including rashes and urticaria, photosensitivity

Gastrointestinal: Nausea, vomiting, anorexia

1% to 10%:

Dermatologic: Stevens-Johnson syndrome, toxic epidermal necrolysis

Hematologic: Blood dyscrasias

Hepatic: Hepatitis

<1%:

Central nervous system: Confusion, depression, hallucinations, seizures, fever, ataxia

Dermatologic: Erythema multiforme

Gastrointestinal: Stomatitis, diarrhea, pseudomembranous colitis

Hematologic: Thrombocytopenia, megaloblastic anemia, granulocytopenia, aplastic anemia, hemolysis (with G-6-PD deficiency)

Hepatic: Hepatitis, kernicterus in neonates

Renal: Interstitial nephritis

Miscellaneous: Serum sickness

Drug Interactions Co-trimoxazole causes:

Decreased effect: Cyclosporines

Increased effect: Sulfonylureas and oral anticoagulants

Increased toxicity: Phenytoin, cyclosporines (nephrotoxicity), methotrexate (displaced from binding sites)

Drug Uptake

Absorption: Oral: 90% to 100%

Serum half-life:

SMX: 9 hours

TMP: 6-17 hours, both are prolonged in renal failure

Time to peak serum concentration: Within 1-4 hours

Pregnancy Risk Factor C

Trimetoprima (Mexico) see Trimethoprim *on previous page*

Trimetrexate Glucuronate (tri me trex' ate gloo ku ron' ate)

Brand Names Neutrexin™

Therapeutic Category Antibiotic, Miscellaneous

(Continued)

Trimetrexate Glucuronate *(Continued)*

Use Alternative therapy for the treatment of moderate-to-severe *Pneumocystis carinii* pneumonia (PCP) in immunocompromised patients, including patients with acquired immunodeficiency syndrome (AIDS), who are intolerant of, or are refractory to, co-trimoxazole therapy or for whom co-trimoxazole and pentamidine are contraindicated (concurrent folinic acid (leucovorin) must always be administered)

Usual Dosage Adults: I.V.: 45 mg/m^2 once daily over 60 minutes for 21 days; it is necessary to reduce the dose in patients with liver dysfunction, although no specific recommendations exist

Mechanism of Action Exerts an antimicrobial effect through potent inhibition of the enzyme dihydrofolate reductase (DHFR)

Local Anesthetic/Vasoconstrictor Precautions No information available to require special precautions

Effects on Dental Treatment No effects or complications reported

Other Adverse Effects 1% to 10%:
Central nervous system: Seizures, fever
Dermatologic: Rash
Gastrointestinal: Stomatitis, nausea, vomiting
Hematologic: Neutropenia, thrombocytopenia, anemia
Hepatic: Elevated liver function tests
Neuromuscular & skeletal: Peripheral neuropathy
Miscellaneous: Increased serum creatinine, flu-like illness, hypersensitivity reactions

Drug Interactions
Decreased effect of pneumococcal vaccine
Increased toxicity (infection rates) of yellow fever vaccine

Drug Uptake
Serum half-life: 15-17 hours

Pregnancy Risk Factor D

Trimipramine Maleate *(trye mi' pra meen mal' ee ate)*

Brand Names Surmontil®

Canadian/Mexican Brand Names Apo-Trimip® (Canada); Novo-Tripramine® (Canada); Nu-Trimipramine® (Canada); Rhotrimine® (Canada)

Therapeutic Category Antidepressant, Tricyclic

Use Treatment of various forms of depression, often in conjunction with psychotherapy

Usual Dosage Adults: Oral: 50-150 mg/day as a single bedtime dose up to a maximum of 200 mg/day outpatient and 300 mg/day inpatient

Mechanism of Action Increases the synaptic concentration of serotonin and/or norepinephrine in the central nervous system by inhibition of their reuptake by the presynaptic neuronal membrane

Local Anesthetic/Vasoconstrictor Precautions Use with caution; epinephrine, norepinephrine and levonordefrin have been shown to have an increased pressor response in combination with TCAs

Effects on Dental Treatment Long-term treatment with TCAs such as amoxapine increases the risk of caries by reducing salivation and salivary buffer capacity

Other Adverse Effects
>10%:
Central nervous system: Dizziness, drowsiness, headache,
Gastrointestinal: Dry mouth, constipation, increased appetite, nausea, weakness, unpleasant taste, weight gain
1% to 10%:
Cardiovascular: Arrhythmias, hypotension
Central nervous system: Confusion, delirium, hallucinations, nervousness, restlessness, parkinsonian syndrome, insomnia
Endocrine & metabolic: Sexual function impairment
Gastrointestinal: Diarrhea, heartburn
Genitourinary: Difficult urination
Neuromuscular & skeletal: Fine muscle tremors
Ocular: Blurred vision, eye pain
Miscellaneous: Excessive sweating
<1%:
Central nervous system: Anxiety, seizures
Dermatologic: Alopecia, allergic reactions, photosensitivity
Endocrine & metabolic: Breast enlargement, galactorrhea, SIADH
Genitourinary: Testicular swelling
Hematologic: Agranulocytosis, leukopenia, eosinophilia

Hepatic: Cholestatic jaundice, increased liver enzymes
Ocular: Increased intraocular pressure
Otic: Tinnitus
Miscellaneous: Trouble with gums, decreased lower esophageal sphincter tone may cause GE reflux

Drug Interactions

Decreased effect of guanethidine, clonidine; decreased effect with barbiturates, carbamazepine, phenytoin

Increased effect/toxicity with MAO inhibitors (hyperpyretic crises), CNS depressants, alcohol (CNS depression), methylphenidate (increased levels), cimetidine (decreased clearance), anticholinergics

Drug Uptake

Therapeutic plasma levels: Oral: Occurs within 6 hours
Serum half-life: 20-26 hours

Pregnancy Risk Factor C

Trimox® *see* Amoxicillin Trihydrate *on page 58*

Trimpex® *see* Trimethoprim *on page 874*

Trinalin® *see* Azatadine and Pseudoephedrine *on page 89*

Tri-Nefrin® Extra Strength Tablet [OTC] *see* Chlorpheniramine and Phenylpropanolamine *on page 190*

Tri-Norinyl® *see* Ethinyl Estradiol and Norethindrone *on page 339*

Triofed® [OTC] *see* Triprolidine and Pseudoephedrine *on next page*

Triostat™ *see* Liothyronine Sodium *on page 504*

Triotann® Tablet *see* Chlorpheniramine, Pyrilamine, and Phenylephrine *on page 195*

Trioxsalen (trye ox′ sa len)

Brand Names Trisoralen®

Therapeutic Category Psoralen

Use In conjunction with controlled exposure to ultraviolet light or sunlight for repigmentation of idiopathic vitiligo; increasing tolerance to sunlight with albinism; enhance pigmentation

Usual Dosage Children >12 years and Adults: Oral: 10 mg/day as a single dose, 2-4 hours before controlled exposure to UVA (for 15-35 minutes) or sunlight; do not continue for longer than 14 days

Mechanism of Action Psoralens are thought to form covalent bonds with pyrimidine bases in DNA which inhibit the synthesis of DNA. This reaction involves excitation of the trioxsalen molecule by radiation in the long-wave ultraviolet light (UVA) resulting in transference of energy to the trioxsalen molecule producing an excited state. Binding of trioxsalen to DNA occurs only in the presence of ultraviolet light. The increase in skin pigmentation produced by trioxsalen and UVA radiation involves multiple changes in melanocytes and interaction between melanocytes and keratinocytes. In general, melanogenesis is stimulated but the size and distribution of melanocytes is unchanged.

Local Anesthetic/Vasoconstrictor Precautions No information available to require special precautions

Effects on Dental Treatment No effects or complications reported

Other Adverse Effects

>10%:
Dermatologic: Itching
Gastrointestinal: Nausea

1% to 10%:
Central nervous system: Dizziness, headache, mental depression, insomnia, nervousness
Dermatologic: Severe burns from excessive sunlight or ultraviolet exposure
Gastrointestinal: Gastric discomfort

Drug Interactions No data reported

Drug Uptake

Peak photosensitivity: 2 hours
Duration: Skin sensitivity to light remains for 8-12 hours
Absorption: Rapid
Serum half-life, elimination: ~2 hours

Pregnancy Risk Factor C

Tripelennamine (tri pel enn′ a meen)

Brand Names PBZ®; PBZ-SR®

Therapeutic Category Antihistamine

Use Perennial and seasonal allergic rhinitis and other allergic symptoms including urticaria

(Continued)

Tripelennamine (Continued)

Usual Dosage Oral:
Children: 5 mg/kg/day in 4-6 divided doses, up to 300 mg/day maximum
Adults: 25-50 mg every 4-6 hours, extended release tablets 100 mg morning and evening up to 100 mg every 8 hours

Mechanism of Action Competes with histamine for H_1-receptor sites on effector cells in the gastrointestinal tract, blood vessels, and respiratory tract

Local Anesthetic/Vasoconstrictor Precautions No information available to require special precautions

Effects on Dental Treatment Chronic use of antihistamines will inhibit salivary flow, particularly in elderly patients; this may contribute to periodontal disease and oral discomfort

Other Adverse Effects
>10%:
Central nervous system: Slight to moderate drowsiness
Respiratory: Thickening of bronchial secretions
1% to 10%:
Central nervous system: Headache, fatigue, nervousness, dizziness
Gastrointestinal: Appetite increase, weight increase, nausea, diarrhea, abdominal pain, dry mouth
Neuromuscular & skeletal: Arthralgia
Respiratory: Pharyngitis
<1%:
Cardiovascular: Edema, palpitations, hypotension
Central nervous system: Depression, epistaxis, sedation, paradoxical excitement, insomnia
Dermatologic: Angioedema, photosensitivity, rash
Genitourinary: Urinary retention
Hepatic: Hepatitis
Neuromuscular & skeletal: Myalgia, paresthesia, tremor
Ocular: Blurred vision
Respiratory: Bronchospasm

Drug Interactions Increased effect/toxicity with alcohol, CNS depressants, MAO inhibitors

Drug Uptake
Onset of antihistaminic effect: Within 15-30 minutes
Duration: 4-6 hours (up to 8 hours with PBZ-SR®)

Pregnancy Risk Factor B

Triphasil® see Ethinyl Estradiol and Levonorgestrel *on page 337*

Tri-Phen-Chlor® see Chlorpheniramine, Phenyltoloxamine, Phenylpropanolamine, and Phenylephrine *on page 194*

Triphenyl® Expectorant [OTC] see Guaifenesin and Phenylpropanolamine *on page 409*

Triphenyl® Syrup [OTC] see Chlorpheniramine and Phenylpropanolamine *on page 190*

Triple Antibiotic® see Bacitracin, Neomycin, and Polymyxin B *on page 94*

Triposed® [OTC] see Triprolidine and Pseudoephedrine *on this page*

Triprolidina y Pseudoefedrina (Mexico) see Triprolidine and Pseudoephedrine *on this page*

Triprolidine and Pseudoephedrine
(trye proe′ li deen & soo doe e fed′ rin)

Brand Names Actagen® [OTC]; Actifed® [OTC]; Allerfrin® [OTC]; Allerphed® [OTC]; Aprodine® [OTC]; Cenafed® Plus [OTC]; Genac® [OTC]; Trifed® [OTC]; Triofed® [OTC]; Triposed® [OTC]

Therapeutic Category Antihistamine/Decongestant Combination

Synonyms Triprolidina y Pseudoefedrina (Mexico)

Use Temporary relief of nasal congestion, decongest sinus openings, running nose, sneezing, itching of nose or throat and itchy, watery eyes due to common cold, hay fever, or other upper respiratory allergies

Usual Dosage Oral:
Children:
Syrup:
4 months to 2 years: 1.25 mL 3-4 times/day
2-4 years: 2.5 mL 3-4 times/day
4-6 years: 3.75 mL 3-4 times/day
6-12 years: 5 mL every 4-6 hours; do not exceed 4 doses in 24 hours
Tablet: 1/2 every 4-6 hours; do not exceed 4 doses in 24 hours

Children >12 years and Adults:
Syrup: 10 mL every 4-6 hours; do not exceed 4 doses in 24 hours
Tablet: 1 every 4-6 hours; do not exceed 4 doses in 24 hours

Mechanism of Action Refer to Pseudoephedrine monograph

Triprolidine is a member of the propylamine (alkylamine) chemical class of H_1-antagonist antihistamines. As such, it is considered to be relatively less sedating than traditional antihistamines of the ethanolamine, phenothiazine, and ethylenediamine classes of antihistamines. Triprolidine has a shorter half-life and duration of action than most of the other alkylamine antihistamines. Like all H_1-antagonist antihistamines, the mechanism of action of triprolidine is believed to involve competitive blockade of H_1-receptor sites resulting in the inability of histamine to combine with its receptor sites and exert its usual effects on target cells. Antihistamines do not interrupt any effects of histamine which have already occurred. Therefore, these agents are used more successfully in the prevention rather than the treatment of histamine-induced reactions.

Local Anesthetic/Vasoconstrictor Precautions Use with caution since pseudoephedrine is a sympathomimetic amine which could interact with epinephrine to cause a pressor response

Effects on Dental Treatment Chronic use of antihistamines will inhibit salivary flow, particularly in elderly patients; this may contribute to periodontal disease and oral discomfort

Other Adverse Effects

>10%:
Cardiovascular: Tachycardia
Central nervous system: Slight to moderate drowsiness, nervousness, insomnia, transient stimulation
Respiratory: Thickening of bronchial secretions

1% to 10%:
Central nervous system: Headache, fatigue, weakness, dizziness
Gastrointestinal: Appetite increase, weight increase, nausea, diarrhea, abdominal pain, dry mouth
Genitourinary: Difficult urination
Neuromuscular & skeletal: Arthralgia
Renal: Dysuria
Respiratory: Pharyngitis
Miscellaneous: Diaphoresis

<1%:
Central nervous system: Depression, epistaxis, hallucinations, convulsions, paradoxical excitement, sedation
Cardiovascular: Edema, palpitations, hypotension
Dermatologic: Angioedema, rash, photosensitivity
Genitourinary: Urinary retention
Hepatic: Hepatitis
Neuromuscular & skeletal: Myalgia, paresthesia, tremor
Ocular: Blurred vision
Respiratory: Bronchospasm, shortness of breath, troubled breathing

Drug Interactions
Decreased effect of guanethidine, reserpine, methyldopa
Increased toxicity with MAO inhibitors (hypertensive crisis), sympathomimetics, CNS depressants, alcohol (sedation)

Pregnancy Risk Factor C

Triprolidine, Pseudoephedrine, and Codeine
(trye proe' li deen, soo doe e fed' rin, & koe' deen)

Brand Names Actagen-C®; Actifed® With Codeine; Allerfrin® w/Codeine; Aprodine® w/C; Triacin-C®; Trifed-C®

Therapeutic Category Antihistamine/Decongestant Combination; Cough Preparation

Use Symptomatic relief of cough

Local Anesthetic/Vasoconstrictor Precautions Use with caution since pseudoephedrine is a sympathomimetic amine which could interact with epinephrine to cause a pressor response

Effects on Dental Treatment Up to 10% of patients could experience tachycardia, palpitations, and dry mouth; use vasoconstrictor with caution

TripTone® Caplets® [OTC] see Dimenhydrinate on page 286

Tris Buffer see Tromethamine on next page

Tris(hydroxymethyl)aminomethane see Tromethamine on next page

Trisoject® see Triamcinolone on page 862

Trisoralen® see Trioxsalen on page 877

Tri-Statin® II *see* Nystatin and Triamcinolone *on page 632*

Trisulfam® *see* Trimethoprim and Sulfamethoxazole *on page 874*

Trisulfapyrimidines *see* Sulfadiazine, Sulfamethazine, and Sulfamerazine *on page 808*

Tri-Tannate® Plus *see* Chlorpheniramine, Ephedrine, Phenylephrine, and Carbetapentane *on page 191*

Tri-Tannate® Tablet *see* Chlorpheniramine, Pyrilamine, and Phenylephrine *on page 195*

Tritann® Pediatric *see* Chlorpheniramine, Pyrilamine, and Phenylephrine *on page 195*

Tritan® Tablet *see* Chlorpheniramine, Pyrilamine, and Phenylephrine *on page 195*

Tritec® *see* Ranitidine Bismuth Citrate *on page 763*

Tri-Vi-Flor® *see* Vitamins, Multiple *on page 901*

Trobicin® *see* Spectinomycin Hydrochloride *on page 798*

Trocal® [OTC] *see* Dextromethorphan *on page 266*

Troleandomycin (troe lee an doe mye' sin)
Brand Names Tao®
Therapeutic Category Antibiotic, Macrolide
Use Adjunct in the treatment of corticosteroid-dependent asthma due to its steroid-sparing properties; antibiotic with spectrum of activity similar to erythromycin
Usual Dosage Oral:
Children 7-13 years: 25-40 mg/kg/day divided every 6 hours (125-250 mg every 6 hours)
Adjunct in corticosteroid-dependent asthma: 14 mg/kg/day in divided doses every 6-12 hours not to exceed 250 mg every 6 hours; dose is tapered to once daily then alternate day dosing
Children >13 years and adults: 250-500 mg 4 times/day
Mechanism of Action Decreases methylprednisolone clearance from a linear first order decline to a nonlinear decline in plasma concentration. Tao® also has an undefined action independent of its effects on steroid elimination. Inhibits RNA-dependent protein synthesis at the chain elongation step; binds to the 50S ribosomal subunit resulting in blockage of transpeptidation.
Local Anesthetic/Vasoconstrictor Precautions No information available to require special precautions
Effects on Dental Treatment No effects or complications reported
Other Adverse Effects
>10%: Gastrointestinal: Abdominal cramping and discomfort
1% to 10%:
Dermatologic: Urticaria, skin rashes
Gastrointestinal: Nausea, vomiting, diarrhea
<1%:
Dermatologic: Rectal burning
Hepatic: Cholestatic jaundice
Drug Interactions Increased effect/toxicity/levels of astemizole, carbamazepine, ergot alkaloids, methylprednisolone, terfenadine, theophylline, and triazolam
Drug Uptake
Time to peak serum concentration: Within 2 hours
Pregnancy Risk Factor C

Tromethamine (troe meth' a meen)
Brand Names THAM-E® Injection; THAM® Injection
Therapeutic Category Alkalinizing Agent, Parenteral
Synonyms Tris Buffer; Tris(hydroxymethyl)aminomethane
Use Correction of metabolic acidosis associated with cardiac bypass surgery or cardiac arrest; to correct excess acidity of stored blood that is preserved with acid citrate dextrose (ACD); to prime the pump-oxygenator during cardiac bypass surgery; indicated in severe metabolic acidosis in patients in whom sodium or carbon dioxide elimination is restricted [eg, infants needing alkalinization after receiving maximum sodium bicarbonate (8-10 mEq/kg/24 hours)]
Usual Dosage Dose depends on buffer base deficit; when deficit is known: tromethamine (mL of 0.3 M solution) = body weight (kg) x base deficit (mEq/L); when base deficit is not known: 3-6 mL/kg/dose I.V. (1-2 mEq/kg/dose)

Metabolic acidosis with cardiac arrest:
I.V.: 3.5-6 mL/kg (1-2 mEq/kg/dose) into large peripheral vein; 500-1000 mL if needed in adults
I.V. continuous drip: Infuse slowly by syringe pump over 3-6 hours

Excess acidity of acid citrate dextrose priming blood: 14-70 mL of 0.3 molar solution added to each 500 mL of blood

Mechanism of Action Acts as a proton acceptor, which combines with hydrogen ions to form bicarbonate buffer, to correct acidosis

Local Anesthetic/Vasoconstrictor Precautions No information available to require special precautions

Effects on Dental Treatment No effects or complications reported

Other Adverse Effects
1% to 10%:
Cardiovascular: Venospasm
Local: Tissue irritation, necrosis with extravasation
<1%:
Endocrine & metabolic: Hyperkalemia, hypoglycemia
Hematologic: Increased blood coagulation time
Hepatic: Liver cell destruction from direct contact with THAM®
Respiratory: Apnea, respiratory depression
Miscellaneous: Hyperosmolality of serum

Drug Uptake
Absorption: 30% of dose is not ionized

Pregnancy Risk Factor C

Comments 1 mM = 120 mg = 3.3 mL = 1 mEq of THAM®

Tronolane® [OTC] *see* Pramoxine Hydrochloride *on page 714*

Tronothane® [OTC] *see* Pramoxine Hydrochloride *on page 714*

Tropicacyl® Ophthalmic *see* Tropicamide *on this page*

Tropicamide (troe pik′ a mide)

Brand Names I-Picamide® Ophthalmic; Mydriacyl® Ophthalmic; Tropicacyl® Ophthalmic

Therapeutic Category Ophthalmic Agent, Mydriatic

Synonyms Bistropamide

Use Short-acting mydriatic used in diagnostic procedures; as well as preoperatively and postoperatively; treatment of some cases of acute iritis, iridocyclitis, and keratitis

Usual Dosage Children and Adults (individuals with heavily pigmented eyes may require larger doses):
Cycloplegia: Instill 1-2 drops (1%); may repeat in 5 minutes
Exam must be performed within 30 minutes after the repeat dose; if the patient is not examined within 20-30 minutes, instill an additional drop Mydriasis: Instill 1-2 drops (0.5%) 15-20 minutes before exam; may repeat every 30 minutes as needed

Mechanism of Action Prevents the sphincter muscle of the iris and the muscle of the ciliary body from responding to cholinergic stimulation

Local Anesthetic/Vasoconstrictor Precautions No information available to require special precautions

Effects on Dental Treatment No effects or complications reported

Other Adverse Effects 1% to 10%:
Cardiovascular: Tachycardia, vascular congestion, edema, parasympathetic stimulations
Central nervous system: Drowsiness, headache
Dermatologic: Eczematoid dermatitis
Gastrointestinal: Dryness of the mouth
Local: Transient stinging
Ocular: Blurred vision, photophobia with or without corneal staining, increased intraocular pressure, follicular conjunctivitis

Drug Uptake
Onset of mydriasis: ~20-40 minutes
Duration: ~6-7 hours
Onset of cycloplegia: Within 30 minutes
Duration: <6 hours

Pregnancy Risk Factor C

Troxidone *see* Trimethadione *on page 872*

Truphylline® *see* Theophylline/Aminophylline *on page 832*

Trusopt® *see* Dorzolamide Hydrochloride *on page 296*

Trypsin, Balsam Peru, and Castor Oil
(trip′ sin, bal′ sam pe rue′, & kas′ tor oyl)

Brand Names Granulex

Therapeutic Category Enzyme, Topical Debridement; Protectant, Topical; Topical Skin Product
(Continued)

Trypsin, Balsam Peru, and Castor Oil *(Continued)*

Use Treatment of decubitus ulcers, varicose ulcers, debridement of eschar, dehiscent wounds and sunburn

Local Anesthetic/Vasoconstrictor Precautions No information available to require special precautions

Effects on Dental Treatment No effects or complications reported

Trysul® *see* Sulfabenzamide, Sulfacetamide, and Sulfathiazole *on page 806*

TSPA *see* Thiotepa *on page 841*

TST *see* Tuberculin Purified Protein Derivative *on this page*

T-Stat® Topical *see* Erythromycin, Topical *on page 324*

Tuberculin Purified Protein Derivative

(too ber' kyoo lin pure' eh fide pro' teen dah riv' ah tiv)

Brand Names Aplisol®; Tubersol®

Therapeutic Category Diagnostic Agent, Skin Test

Synonyms Mantoux; PPD; Tine Test; TST; Tuberculin Skin Test

Use Skin test in diagnosis of tuberculosis, to aid in assessment of cell-mediated immunity; routine tuberculin testing is recommended at 12 months of age and at every 1-2 years thereafter, before the measles vaccination

Usual Dosage Children and Adults: Intradermal: 0.1 mL about 4" below elbow; use $\frac{1}{4}$" to $\frac{1}{2}$" or 26- or 27-gauge needle; significant reactions are ≥5 mm in diameter

Interpretation of induration of tuberculin skin test injections: Positive: ≥10 mm; inconclusive: 5-9 mm; negative: <5 mm

Interpretation of induration of Tine test injections: Positive: >2 mm and vesiculation present; inconclusive: <2 mm (give patient Mantoux test of 5 TU/0.1 mL - base decisions on results of Mantoux test); negative: <2 mm or erythema of any size (no need for retesting unless person is a contact of a patient with tuberculosis or there is clinical evidence suggestive of the disease)

Mechanism of Action Tuberculosis results in individuals becoming sensitized to certain antigenic components of the *M. tuberculosis* organism. Culture extracts called tuberculins are contained in tuberculin skin test preparations. Upon intracutaneous injection of these culture extracts, a classic delayed (cellular) hypersensitivity reaction occurs. This reaction is characteristic of a delayed course (peak occurs >24 hours after injection, induration of the skin secondary to cell infiltration, and occasional vesiculation and necrosis). Delayed hypersensitivity reactions to tuberculin may indicate infection with a variety of nontuberculosis mycobacteria, or vaccination with the live attenuated mycobacterial strain of *M. bovis* vaccine, BCG, in addition to previous natural infection with *M. tuberculosis*.

Local Anesthetic/Vasoconstrictor Precautions No information available to require special precautions

Effects on Dental Treatment No effects or complications reported

Other Adverse Effects 1% to 10%:
Gastrointestinal: Ulceration
Dermatologic: Vesiculation
Neuromuscular & skeletal: Pain
Miscellaneous: Necrosis

Drug Uptake
Onset of action: Delayed hypersensitivity reactions to tuberculin usually occur within 5-6 hours following injection
Peak effect: Become maximal at 48-72 hours
Duration: Reactions subside over a few days

Pregnancy Risk Factor C

Comments Test dose: 0.1 mL intracutaneously; examine site at 48-72 hours after administration; whenever tuberculin is administered, a record should be made of the administration technique (Mantoux method, disposable multiple-puncture device), tuberculin used (OT or PPD), manufacturer and lot number of tuberculin used, date of administration, date of test reading, and the size of the reaction in millimeters (mm).

Tuberculin Skin Test *see* Tuberculin Purified Protein Derivative *on this page*

Tubersol® *see* Tuberculin Purified Protein Derivative *on this page*

Tuinal® *see* Amobarbital and Secobarbital *on page 55*

Tums® [OTC] *see* Calcium Carbonate *on page 140*

Tussafed® Drops *see* Carbinoxamine, Pseudoephedrine, and Dextromethorphan *on page 155*

Tussafin® Expectorant *see* Hydrocodone, Pseudoephedrine, and Guaifenesin *on page 435*

Tuss-Allergine® Modified T.D. Capsule see Caramiphen and Phenylpropanolamine on page 150

Tussar® SF Syrup see Guaifenesin, Pseudoephedrine, and Codeine on page 410

Tuss-DM® [OTC] see Guaifenesin and Dextromethorphan on page 408

Tuss-Genade® Modified Capsule see Caramiphen and Phenylpropanolamine on page 150

Tussigon® see Hydrocodone and Homatropine on page 434

Tussionex® see Hydrocodone and Chlorpheniramine on page 434

Tuss-LA® see Guaifenesin and Pseudoephedrine on page 409

Tussogest® Extended Release Capsule see Caramiphen and Phenylpropanolamine on page 150

Tuss-Ornade® Liquid see Caramiphen and Phenylpropanolamine on page 150

Tuss-Ornade® Spansule® see Caramiphen and Phenylpropanolamine on page 150

Tusstat® see Diphenhydramine Hydrochloride on page 288

Twin-K® see Potassium Citrate and Potassium Gluconate on page 710

Two-Dyne® see Butalbital Compound on page 133

Tylenol® [OTC] see Acetaminophen on page 14

Tylenol® Cold Effervescent Medication Tablet [OTC] see Chlorpheniramine, Phenylpropanolamine, and Acetaminophen on page 194

Tylenol® With Codeine see Acetaminophen and Codeine on page 15

Tylox® see Oxycodone and Acetaminophen on page 646

Typhoid Vaccine (tye´ foid vak seen´)

Brand Names Vivotif Berna™ Oral

Therapeutic Category Vaccine, Inactivated Bacteria

Synonyms Typhoid Vaccine Live Oral Ty21a

Use Promotes active immunity to typhoid fever for patients exposed to typhoid carrier or foreign travel to typhoid fever endemic area

Usual Dosage
S.C.:
Children 6 months to 10 years: 0.25 mL; repeat in ≥4 weeks (total immunization is 2 doses)
Children >10 years and Adults: 0.5 mL; repeat dose in ≥4 weeks (total immunization is 2 doses)
Booster: 0.25 mL every 3 years for children 6 months to 10 years and 0.5 mL every 3 years for children >10 years and adults
Oral: Adults:
Primary immunization: 1 capsule on alternate days (day 1, 3, 5, and 7)
Booster immunization: Repeat full course of primary immunization every 5 years

Mechanism of Action Virulent strains of *Salmonella typhi* cause disease by penetrating the intestinal mucosa and entering the systemic circulation via the lymphatic vasculature. One possible mechanism of conferring immunity may be the provocation of a local immune response in the intestinal tract induced by oral ingesting of a live strain with subsequent aborted infection. The ability of *Salmonella typhi* to produce clinical disease (and to elicit an immune response) is dependent on the bacteria having a complete lipopolysaccharide. The live attenuate Ty21a strain lacks the enzyme UDP-4-galactose epimerase so that lipopolysaccharide is only synthesized under conditions that induce bacterial autolysis. Thus, the strain remains avirulent despite the production of sufficient lipopolysaccharide to evoke a protective immune response. Despite low levels of lipopolysaccharide synthesis, cells lyse before gaining a virulent phenotype due to the intracellular accumulation of metabolic intermediates.

Local Anesthetic/Vasoconstrictor Precautions No information available to require special precautions

Effects on Dental Treatment No effects or complications reported

Other Adverse Effects
Oral:
1% to 10%:
Dermatologic: Skin rash
Gastrointestinal: Abdominal discomfort, stomach cramps, diarrhea, nausea, vomiting
<1%: Miscellaneous: Anaphylactic reaction
Injection: >10%: Local: Tenderness, erythema, induration, myalgia

Drug Uptake
Oral:
Onset of immunity to *Salmonella typhi*: Within about 1 week
Duration: ~5 years
(Continued)

Typhoid Vaccine *(Continued)*

Parenteral: Duration of immunity: ~3 years

Pregnancy Risk Factor C

Comments Inactivated bacteria vaccine; federal law requires that the date of administration, the vaccine manufacturer, lot number of vaccine, and the administering person's name, title and address be entered into the patient's permanent medical record

Typhoid Vaccine Live Oral Ty21a *see* Typhoid Vaccine *on previous page*

Tyzine® *see* Tetrahydrozoline Hydrochloride *on page 831*

UAD® Topical *see* Clioquinol and Hydrocortisone *on page 216*

UCB-P071 *see* Cetirizine Hydrochloride *on page 179*

ULR® *see* Guaifenesin, Phenylpropanolamine, and Phenylephrine *on page 410*

ULR-LA® *see* Guaifenesin and Phenylpropanolamine *on page 409*

Ultiva® *see* Remifentanil *on page 765*

Ultracef® *see* Cefadroxil Monohydrate *on page 162*

Ultram® *see* Tramadol Hydrochloride *on page 857*

Ultra Mide® *see* Urea *on this page*

Ultrase® MT12 *see* Pancrelipase *on page 657*

Ultrase® MT20 *see* Pancrelipase *on page 657*

Ultrase® MT24 *see* Pancrelipase *on page 657*

Ultra Tears® Solution [OTC] *see* Artificial Tears *on page 75*

Ultravate™ *see* Halobetasol Propionate *on page 416*

Unasyn® *see* Ampicillin Sodium and Sulbactam Sodium *on page 64*

Undecylenic Acid and Derivatives

(un de sil en' ik as' id & dah riv' ah tivs)

Brand Names Caldesene® Topical [OTC]; Cruex® Topical [OTC]; Fungoid® Topical Solution; Merlenate® Topical [OTC]; Pedi-Dri Topical; Pedi-Pro Topical [OTC]; Quinsana® Plus Topical [OTC]; Undoguent® Topical [OTC]

Therapeutic Category Antifungal Agent, Topical

Synonyms Zinc Undecylenate

Use Treatment of athlete's foot (tinea pedis), ringworm (except nails and scalp), prickly heat, jock itch (tinea cruris), diaper rash and other minor skin irritations due to superficial dermatophytes

Local Anesthetic/Vasoconstrictor Precautions No information available to require special precautions

Effects on Dental Treatment No effects or complications reported

Other Adverse Effects 1% to 10%: Dermatologic: Skin irritation, sensitization

Comments Ointment should be applied at night, powder may be applied during the day or used alone when a drying effect is needed

Undoguent® Topical [OTC] *see* Undecylenic Acid and Derivatives *on this page*

Unicap® [OTC] *see* Vitamins, Multiple *on page 901*

Uni-Decon® *see* Chlorpheniramine, Phenyltoloxamine, Phenylpropanolamine, and Phenylephrine *on page 194*

Unilax® [OTC] *see* Docusate and Phenolphthalein *on page 295*

Unipen® *see* Nafcillin Sodium *on page 599*

Unipres® *see* Hydralazine, Hydrochlorothiazide, and Reserpine *on page 429*

Uni-Pro® [OTC] *see* Ibuprofen *on page 447*

Uni-Tussin® [OTC] *see* Guaifenesin *on page 407*

Uni-tussin® DM [OTC] *see* Guaifenesin and Dextromethorphan *on page 408*

Univasc® *see* Moexipril Hydrochloride *on page 587*

Unna's Boot *See* Zinc Gelatin *on page 908*

Unna's Paste *see* Zinc Gelatin *on page 908*

Urabeth® *see* Bethanechol Chloride *on page 112*

Uracel® *see* Sodium Salicylate *on page 793*

Urea *(yoor ee' a)*

Brand Names Amino-Cerv™ Vaginal Cream; Aquacare® [OTC]; Carmol® [OTC]; Nutraplus® [OTC]; Rea-Lo® [OTC]; Ultra Mide®; Ureacin®-20 [OTC]; Ureacin®-40; Ureaphil®

Canadian/Mexican Brand Names Onyvul® (Canada); Uremol® (Canada); Urisec® (Canada); Velvelan® (Canada)

Therapeutic Category Diuretic, Osmotic; Topical Skin Product

Use Reduces intracranial pressure and intraocular pressure; topically promotes hydration and removal of excess keratin in hyperkeratotic conditions and dry skin; mild cervicitis

Usual Dosage

Children: I.V. slow infusion:
<2 years: 0.1-0.5 g/kg
>2 years: 0.5-1.5 g/kg

Adults:
I.V. infusion: 1-1.5 g/kg by slow infusion (1-2$\frac{1}{2}$ hours); maximum: 120 g/24 hours
Topical: Apply 1-3 times/day
Vaginal: Insert 1 applicatorful in vagina at bedtime for 2-4 weeks

Mechanism of Action Elevates plasma osmolality by inhibiting tubular reabsorption of water, thus enhancing the flow of water into extracellular fluid

Local Anesthetic/Vasoconstrictor Precautions No information available to require special precautions

Effects on Dental Treatment No effects or complications reported

Other Adverse Effects

>10%: Gastrointestinal: Nausea, vomiting

1% to 10%:
Central nervous system: Headache
Local: Transient stinging, local irritation, tissue necrosis from extravasation of I.V. preparation

<1%: Endocrine & metabolic: Electrolyte imbalance

Drug Interactions Decreased effect/toxicity/levels of lithium

Drug Uptake

Onset of therapeutic effect: I.V.: Maximum effects within 1-2 hours
Duration: 3-6 hours (diuresis can continue for up to 10 hours)
Serum half-life: 1 hour

Pregnancy Risk Factor C

Urea and Hydrocortisone (yoor ee' a & hye droe kor' ti sone)

Brand Names Carmol-HC® Topical

Therapeutic Category Corticosteroid, Topical (Low Potency); Topical Skin Product

Synonyms Hydrocortisone and Urea

Use Inflammation of corticosteroid-responsive dermatoses

Local Anesthetic/Vasoconstrictor Precautions No information available to require special precautions

Effects on Dental Treatment No effects or complications reported

Ureacin®-20 [OTC] see Urea on previous page
Ureacin®-40 see Urea on previous page
Ureaphil® see Urea on previous page
Urecholine® see Bethanechol Chloride on page 112
Urex® see Methenamine on page 555
Urised® see Methenamine on page 555
Urispas® see Flavoxate on page 364
Uri-Tet® see Oxytetracycline Hydrochloride on page 653
Urobak® see Sulfamethoxazole on page 809
Urocit®-K see Potassium Citrate on page 710
Urodine® see Phenazopyridine Hydrochloride on page 679
Urofolitropina (Mexico) see Urofollitropin on this page

Urofollitropin (yoor oh fol li troe' pin)

Brand Names Metrodin®

Canadian/Mexican Brand Names Fertinorm® H.P. (Mexico)

Therapeutic Category Ovulation Stimulator

Synonyms Urofolitropina (Mexico)

Use Induction of ovulation in patients with polycystic ovarian disease and to stimulate the development of multiple oocytes

Usual Dosage Adults: Female: I.M.: 75 units/day for 7-12 days, used with hCG may repeat course of treatment 2 more times

Mechanism of Action Preparation of follicle-stimulating hormone 75 IU with <1 IU of luteinizing hormone (LH) which is isolated from the urine of postmenopausal women. Follicle-stimulating hormone plays a role in the development of follicles. Elevated FSH levels early in the normal menstrual cycle are thought to play a significant role in recruiting a cohort of follicles for maturation. A single follicle is enriched with FSH receptors and becomes dominant over the rest of (Continued)

Urofollitropin *(Continued)*

the recruited follicles. The increased number of FSH receptors allows it to grow despite declining FSH levels. This dominant follicle secretes low levels of estrogen and inhibin which further reduces pituitary FSH output. The ovarian stroma, under the influence of luteinizing hormone, produces androgens which the dominant follicle uses as precursors for estrogens.

Local Anesthetic/Vasoconstrictor Precautions No information available to require special precautions

Effects on Dental Treatment No effects or complications reported

Other Adverse Effects

>10%:

Endocrine & metabolic: Ovarian enlargement

Local: Swelling at injection site, pain

1% to 10%:

Cardiovascular: Arterial thromboembolism

Central nervous system: Fever, chills

Dermatologic: Rash

Gastrointestinal: Nausea, vomiting, abdominal pain, diarrhea

Miscellaneous: Hyperstimulation syndrome

Drug Interactions No data reported

Drug Uptake

Serum half-life, elimination: 3.9 hours and 70.4 hours (FSH has two half-lives)

Pregnancy Risk Factor X

Urogesic® *see* Phenazopyridine Hydrochloride *on page 679*

Urokinase *(yoor oh kin' ase)*

Related Information

Cardiovascular Diseases *on page 912*

Brand Names Abbokinase®

Canadian/Mexican Brand Names Ukidan® (Mexico)

Therapeutic Category Thrombolytic Agent

Synonyms Uroquinasa (Mexico)

Use Thrombolytic agent used in treatment of recent severe or massive deep vein thrombosis, pulmonary emboli, myocardial infarction, and occluded arteriovenous cannulas; more expensive than streptokinase; not useful on thrombi over 1 week old

Usual Dosage

Children and Adults: Deep vein thrombosis: I.V.: Loading: 4400 units/kg over 10 minutes, then 4400 units/kg/hour for 12 hours

Adults:

Myocardial infarction: Intracoronary: 750,000 units over 2 hours (6000 units/minute over up to 2 hours)

Occluded I.V. catheters:

5000 units (use only Abbokinase® Open Cath) in each lumen over 1-2 minutes, leave in lumen for 1-4 hours, then aspirate; may repeat with 10,000 units in each lumen if 5000 units fails to clear the catheter; **do not infuse into the patient**; volume to instill into catheter is equal to the volume of the catheter

I.V. infusion: 200 units/kg/hour in each lumen for 12-48 hours at a rate of at least 20 mL/hour

Dialysis patients: 5000 units is administered in each lumen over 1-2 minutes; leave urokinase in lumen for 1-2 days, then aspirate

Clot lysis (large vessel thrombi): Loading: I.V.: 4400 units/kg over 10 minutes, increase to 6000 units/kg/hour; maintenance: 4400-6000 units/kg/hour adjusted to achieve clot lysis or patency of affected vessel; doses up to 50,000 units/kg/hour have been used. **Note:** Therapy should be initiated as soon as possible after diagnosis of thrombi and continued until clot is dissolved (usually 24-72 hours).

Acute pulmonary embolism: Three treatment alternatives: 3 million unit dosage

Alternative 1: 12-hour infusion: 4400 units/kg (2000 units/lb) bolus over 10 minutes followed by 4400 units/kg/hour (2000 units/lb); begin heparin 1000 units/hour approximately 3-4 hours after completion of urokinase infusion or when PTT is <100 seconds

Alternative 2: 2-hour infusion: 1 million unit bolus over 10 minutes followed by 2 million units over 110 minutes; begin heparin 1000 units/hour approximately 3-4 hours after completion of urokinase infusion or when PTT is <100 seconds

Alternative 3: Bolus dose only: 15,000 units/kg over 10 minutes; begin heparin 1000 units/hour approximately 3-4 hours after completion of urokinase infusion or when PTT is <100 seconds

Mechanism of Action Promotes thrombolysis by directly activating plasminogen to plasmin, which degrades fibrin, fibrinogen, and other procoagulant plasma proteins

Local Anesthetic/Vasoconstrictor Precautions No information available to require special precautions

Effects on Dental Treatment No effects or complications reported

Other Adverse Effects

>10%:

Cardiovascular: Hypotension, arrhythmias

Central nervous system: Angioneurotic edema

Endocrine & metabolic: Periorbital swelling

Hematologic: Bleeding at sites of percutaneous trauma

Respiratory: Bronchospasm

Miscellaneous: Anaphylaxis

<1%:

Central nervous system: Epistaxis, headache, chills

Dermatologic: Rash

Gastrointestinal: Nausea, vomiting

Hematologic: Anemia

Ocular: Eye hemorrhage

Miscellaneous: Sweating

Drug Interactions Increased toxicity (increased bleeding) with anticoagulants, antiplatelet drugs, aspirin, indomethacin, dextran

Drug Uptake

Onset of action: I.V.: Fibrinolysis occurs rapidly

Duration: 4 or more hours

Serum half-life: 10-20 minutes

Pregnancy Risk Factor B

Uro-KP-Neutral® see Potassium Phosphate and Sodium Phosphate on page 713

Uroplus® DS see Trimethoprim and Sulfamethoxazole on page 874

Uroplus® SS see Trimethoprim and Sulfamethoxazole on page 874

Uroquinasa (Mexico) see Urokinase on previous page

Ursodeoxycholic Acid see Ursodiol on this page

Ursodiol (er' soe dye ole)

Brand Names Actigall™

Canadian/Mexican Brand Names Ursofalk (Mexico)

Therapeutic Category Gallstone Dissolution Agent

Synonyms Ursodeoxycholic Acid

Use Gallbladder stone dissolution

Usual Dosage Adults: Oral: 8-10 mg/kg/day in 2-3 divided doses; use beyond 24 months is not established; obtain ultrasound images at 6-month intervals for the first year of therapy; 30% of patients have stone recurrence after dissolution

Mechanism of Action Decreases the cholesterol content of bile and bile stones by reducing the secretion of cholesterol from the liver and the fractional reabsorption of cholesterol by the intestines

Local Anesthetic/Vasoconstrictor Precautions No information available to require special precautions

Effects on Dental Treatment No effects or complications reported

Other Adverse Effects

1% to 10%: Gastrointestinal: Diarrhea

<1%:

Central nervous system: Fatigue, headache, pruritus

Dermatologic: Rash

Gastrointestinal: Nausea, vomiting, dyspepsia, metallic taste, abdominal pain, biliary pain, and constipation

Drug Uptake

Serum half-life: 100 hours

Pregnancy Risk Factor B

Comments Use beyond 24 months is not established; obtain ultrasound images at 6-month intervals for the first year of therapy; 30% of patients have stone recurrence after dissolution

Urticort® see Betamethasone on page 109

Utimox® *see* Amoxicillin Trihydrate *on page 58*
Vagilia® *see* Sulfabenzamide, Sulfacetamide, and Sulfathiazole *on page 806*
Vagistat® *see* Tioconazole *on page 848*
Vagitrol® *see* Sulfanilamide *on page 810*

Valacyclovir (val ay sye′ kloe veer)
Related Information
Systemic Viral Diseases *on page 934*
Brand Names Valtrex®
Therapeutic Category Antiviral Agent, Oral
Use Treatment of herpes zoster (shingles) in immunocompetent patients
Usual Dosage Oral: Adults: 1 g 3 times/day for 7 days
Dosing interval in renal impairment:
Cl_{cr}: 30-49 mL/minute: 1 g every 12 hours
Cl_{cr} 10-29 mL/minute: 1 g every 24 hours
Cl_{cr} <10 mL/minute: 500 mg every 24 hours

Hemodialysis effects: 33% removed during 4-hour session

Peritoneal dialysis effects: Limited information available; supplemental doses not required

Local Anesthetic/Vasoconstrictor Precautions No information available to require special precautions
Effects on Dental Treatment No effects or complications reported
Drug Uptake
Absorption: Rapid and converted to acyclovir and L-valine by first-pass/hepatic metabolism
Serum half-life:
Normal renal function: 2.5-3.3 hours

Valadol® [OTC] *see* Acetaminophen *on page 14*
Valergen® *see* Estradiol *on page 325*
Valertest No.1® Injection *see* Estradiol and Testosterone *on page 326*
Valisone® *see* Betamethasone *on page 109*
Valium® *see* Diazepam *on page 268*
Valpin® 50 *see* Anisotropine Methylbromide *on page 67*

Valproic Acid and Derivatives
(val proe′ ik as′ id & dah riv′ ah tives)
Brand Names Depakene®; Depakote®
Canadian/Mexican Brand Names Atemperator-S® (Mexico); Cryoval® (Mexico); Epival® (Mexico); Leptilan® (Mexico); Valprosid® (Mexico)
Therapeutic Category Anticonvulsant, Miscellaneous
Synonyms Valproico Acido (Mexico)
Use Management of simple and complex absence seizures; mixed seizure types; myoclonic and generalized tonic-clonic (grand mal) seizures; may be effective in partial seizures and infantile spasms
Usual Dosage Children and Adults:
Oral: Initial: 10-15 mg/kg/day in 1-3 divided doses; increase by 5-10 mg/kg/day at weekly intervals until therapeutic levels are achieved; maintenance: 30-60 mg/kg/day in 2-3 divided doses
Children receiving more than 1 anticonvulsant (ie, polytherapy) may require doses up to 100 mg/kg/day in 3-4 divided doses
Rectal: Dilute syrup 1:1 with water for use as a retention enema; loading dose: 17-20 mg/kg one time; maintenance: 10-15 mg/kg/dose every 8 hours

Not dialyzable (0% to 5%)
Dosing adjustment/comments in hepatic impairment: Reduce dose
Mechanism of Action Causes increased availability of gamma-aminobutyric acid (GABA), an inhibitory neurotransmitter, to brain neurons or may enhance the action of GABA or mimic its action at postsynaptic receptor sites
Local Anesthetic/Vasoconstrictor Precautions No information available to require special precautions
Effects on Dental Treatment No effects or complications reported
Other Adverse Effects
1% to 10%:
Gastrointestinal: Abdominal cramps, anorexia, diarrhea, nausea, vomiting, weight gain
Endocrine & metabolic: Change in menstrual cycle
<1%:
Central nervous system: Drowsiness, ataxia, irritability, confusion, restlessness, hyperactivity, headache

Dermatologic: Alopecia, erythema multiforme
Endocrine & metabolic: Hyperammonemia
Gastrointestinal: Pancreatitis
Hematologic: Thrombocytopenia, prolongation of bleeding time
Hepatic: Transient increased liver enzymes, liver failure
Neuromuscular & skeletal: Tremor, malaise
Ocular: Nystagmus, spots before eyes

Drug Interactions
Decreased effect of phenytoin, clonazepam, diazepam; decreased effect with phenobarbital, primidone, phenytoin, carbamazepine
Increased effect/toxicity with CNS depressants, alcohol, aspirin (bleeding), warfarin (bleeding)

Drug Uptake
Serum half-life:
Adults: 8-17 hours
Time to peak serum concentration: Within 1-4 hours; 3-5 hours after divalproex (enteric coated)

Pregnancy Risk Factor D

Valproico Acido (Mexico) *see* Valproic Acid and Derivatives *on previous page*

Valrelease® *see* Diazepam *on page 268*

Valtrex® *see* Valacyclovir *on previous page*

Vamate® *see* Hydroxyzine *on page 443*

Vancenase® *see* Beclomethasone Dipropionate *on page 97*

Vancenase® AQ *see* Beclomethasone Dipropionate *on page 97*

Vanceril® *see* Beclomethasone Dipropionate *on page 97*

Vancocin® *see* Vancomycin Hydrochloride *on this page*

Vancoled® *see* Vancomycin Hydrochloride *on this page*

Vancomycin Hydrochloride (van koe mye' sin hye droe klor' ide)
Related Information
Antimicrobial Prophylaxis in Surgical Patients *on page 1042*
Cardiovascular Diseases *on page 912*

Brand Names Lyphocin®; Vancocin®; Vancoled®

Canadian/Mexican Brand Names Vancocin® CP (Canada); Balcoran® (Mexico); Vanmicina® (Mexico)

Therapeutic Category Antibiotic, Miscellaneous

Use
Dental: Alternate antibiotic for the prevention of bacterial endocarditis in patients undergoing dental procedures. It is to be used in those patients considered high risk and not candidates for the standard regimen of prevention of bacterial endocarditis and who are allergic to ampicillin, amoxicillin, and penicillin.
Medical: Treatment of patients with the following infections or conditions:
Infections due to documented or suspected methicillin-resistant *S. aureus* or beta-lactam resistant coagulase negative *Staphylococcus*
Serious or life-threatening infections (ie, endocarditis, meningitis) due to documented or suspected staphylococcal or streptococcal infections in patients who are allergic to penicillins and/or cephalosporins
Empiric therapy of infections associated with gram-positive organisms; used orally for staphylococcal enterocolitis or for antibiotic-associated pseudomembranous colitis produced by *C. difficile*

Usual Dosage I.V.:
Children: 20 mg/kg; total pediatric dose should not exceed total adult dose
Adults: 1 g over 1 hour, starting 1 hour before procedure, no repeat dose necessary

Mechanism of Action Inhibits bacterial cell wall synthesis by blocking glycopeptide polymerization through binding tightly to D-alanyl-D-alanine portion of cell wall precursor

Local Anesthetic/Vasoconstrictor Precautions No information available to require special precautions

Effects on Dental Treatment No effects or complications reported

Other Adverse Effects
>10%: Cardiovascular: Hypotension accompanied by flushing and erythematous rash on face and upper body (red neck or red man syndrome)
1% to 10%:
Central nervous system: Chills, drug fever
Hematologic: Eosinophilia

Oral manifestations: No data reported
(Continued)

Vancomycin Hydrochloride (Continued)

Contraindications Hypersensitivity to vancomycin or any component; avoid in patients with previous severe hearing loss

Warnings/Precautions Use with caution in patients with renal impairment or those receiving other nephrotoxic or ototoxic drugs; dosage modification required in patients with impaired renal function (especially elderly)

Drug Interactions Increased toxicity with general anesthetic agents

Drug Uptake
Time to peak serum concentration: I.V.: Within 45-65 minutes
Serum half-life (biphasic):
Children >3 years: 2.2-3 hours
Adults: 5-11 hours, prolonged significantly with reduced renal function

Pregnancy Risk Factor C

Breast-feeding Considerations No data reported

Dosage Forms Powder for injection: 500 mg, 1 g, 2 g, 5 g, 10 g

Generic Available Yes

Selected Readings
Council on Dental Therapeutics, American Heart Association, "Preventing Bacterial Endocarditis," *J Am Dent Assoc*, 1991, 122(2):87-92.
Dajani AS, Bisno AL, Chung KJ, et al, "Prevention of Bacterial Endocarditis. Recommendations by the American Heart Association," *JAMA*, 1990, 264(22):2919-22.

Vanex-LA® *see* Guaifenesin and Phenylpropanolamine *on page 409*

Vanoxide® [OTC] *see* Benzoyl Peroxide *on page 104*

Vanoxide-HC® *see* Benzoyl Peroxide and Hydrocortisone *on page 105*

Van R Gingibraid® *see* Epinephrine, Racemic and Aluminum Potassium Sulfate *on page 314*

Vansil™ *see* Oxamniquine *on page 642*

Vantin® *see* Cefpodoxime Proxetil *on page 169*

Vapo-Iso® *see* Isoproterenol *on page 472*

Vaponefrin® *see* Epinephrine, Racemic *on page 314*

Varicella-Zoster Immune Globulin (Human)

(var i sel' a- zos' ter i myun' glob' yoo lin hyu' min)

Therapeutic Category Immune Globulin

Synonyms VZIG

Use Passive immunization of susceptible immunodeficient patients after exposure to varicella; most effective if begun within 96 hours of exposure

VZIG supplies are limited, restrict administration to those meeting the following criteria:

One of the following underlying illnesses or conditions:
Neoplastic disease (eg, leukemia or lymphoma)
Congenital or acquired immunodeficiency
Immunosuppressive therapy with steroids, antimetabolites or other immunosuppressive treatment regimens
Newborn of mother who had onset of chickenpox within 5 days before delivery or within 48 hours after delivery
Premature (≥28 weeks gestation) whose mother has no history of chickenpox
Premature (<28 weeks gestation or ≤1000 g VZIG) regardless of maternal history

One of the following types of exposure to chickenpox or zoster patient(s):
Continuous household contact
Playmate contact (>1 hour play indoors)
Hospital contact (in same 2-4 bedroom or adjacent beds in a large ward or prolonged face-to-face contact with an infectious staff member or patient)
Susceptible to varicella-zoster
Age of <15 years; administer to immunocompromised adolescents and adults and to other older patients on an individual basis

An acceptable alternative to VZIG prophylaxis is to treat varicella, if it occurs, with high-dose I.V. acyclovir

Usual Dosage High risk susceptible patients who are exposed again more than 3 weeks after a prior dose of VZIG should receive another full dose; there is no evidence VZIG modifies established varicella-zoster infections.

I.M.: Administer by deep injection in the gluteal muscle or in another large muscle mass. Inject 125 units/10 kg (22 lb); maximum dose: 625 units (5 vials); minimum dose: 125 units; do not give fractional doses. Do not inject I.V. See table.

VZIG Dose Based on Weight

Weight of Patient		Dose	
kg	lb	Units	No. of Vials
0-10	0-22	125	1
10.1-20	22.1-44	250	2
20.1-30	44.1-66	375	3
30.1-40	66.1-88	500	4
>40	>88	625	5

Mechanism of Action The exact mechanism has not been clarified but the antibodies in varicella-zoster immune globulin most likely neutralize the varicella-zoster virus and prevent its pathological actions

Local Anesthetic/Vasoconstrictor Precautions No information available to require special precautions

Effects on Dental Treatment No effects or complications reported

Other Adverse Effects

1% to 10%: Local: Discomfort at the site of injection (pain, redness, swelling)

<1%:

Central nervous system: Headache

Dermatologic: Rash, angioedema

Gastrointestinal: GI symptoms, malaise

Respiratory: Respiratory symptoms

Miscellaneous: Anaphylactic shock

Pregnancy Risk Factor C

Comments Should be administered within 96 hours of exposure

Vascor® see Bepridil Hydrochloride on page 108

Vaseretic® 5-12.5 see Enalapril and Hydrochlorothiazide on page 309

Vaseretic® 10-25 see Enalapril and Hydrochlorothiazide on page 309

Vasocidin® see Sodium Sulfacetamide and Prednisolone Acetate on page 794

VasoClear® [OTC] see Naphazoline Hydrochloride on page 605

Vasocon-A® [OTC] Ophthalmic see Naphazoline and Antazoline on page 604

Vasocon Regular® see Naphazoline Hydrochloride on page 605

Vasoconstrictor Interactions With Antidepressants see page 1108

Vasodilan® see Isoxsuprine Hydrochloride on page 476

Vasopressin (vay soe press' in)

Brand Names Pitressin®

Canadian/Mexican Brand Names Pressyn® (Canada)

Therapeutic Category Antidiuretic Hormone Analog; Hormone, Posterior Pituitary

Use Treatment of diabetes insipidus; prevention and treatment of postoperative abdominal distention; differential diagnosis of diabetes insipidus

Unlabeled use: Adjunct in the treatment of GI hemorrhage and esophageal varices

Usual Dosage

Diabetes insipidus (highly variable dosage; titrated based on serum and urine sodium and osmolality in addition to fluid balance and urine output):

Children: I.M., S.C.: 2.5-10 units 2-4 times/day as needed

Adults:

I.M., S.C.: 5-10 units 2-4 times/day as needed (dosage range 5-60 units/day)

Intranasal: Administer on cotton pledget or nasal spray

Abdominal distention: Adults: I.M.: 5 mg stat, 10 mg every 3-4 hours

GI hemorrhage: Children and Adults: Continuous I.V. infusion: 0.5 milliunit/kg/hour (0.0005 unit/kg/hour); double dosage as needed every 30 minutes to a maximum of 10 milliunits/kg/hour

Children: 0.01 units/kg/minute; continue at same dosage (if bleeding stops) for 12 hours, then taper off over 24-48 hours

Adults: I.V.: Initial: 0.2-0.4 unit/minute, then titrate dose as needed; if bleeding stops, continue at same dose for 12 hours, taper off over 24-48 hours

Mechanism of Action Increases cyclic adenosine monophosphate (cAMP) which increases water permeability at the renal tubule resulting in decreased urine volume and increased osmolality; causes peristalsis by directly stimulating the smooth muscle in the GI tract

(Continued)

891

Vasopressin *(Continued)*

Local Anesthetic/Vasoconstrictor Precautions No information available to require special precautions

Effects on Dental Treatment No effects or complications reported

Other Adverse Effects

1% to 10%:
Cardiovascular: Increased blood pressure, bradycardia, arrhythmias, venous thrombosis, vasoconstriction with higher doses, angina
Central nervous system: Pounding in the head, fever
Dermatologic: Urticaria
Gastrointestinal: Vertigo, flatulence, abdominal cramps, nausea, vomiting
Neuromuscular & skeletal: Tremor
Miscellaneous: Sweating, circumoral pallor

<1%:
Cardiovascular: Myocardial infarction
Miscellaneous: Allergic reaction, water intoxication

Drug Interactions

Decreased effect: Lithium, epinephrine, demeclocycline, heparin, and alcohol block antidiuretic activity to varying degrees
Increased effect: Chlorpropamide, phenformin, urea and fludrocortisone potentiate antidiuretic response

Drug Uptake

Nasal:
Onset of action: 1 hour
Duration: 3-8 hours
Parenteral: Duration of action: I.M., S.C.: 2-8 hours
Absorption: Destroyed by trypsin in GI tract, must be administered parenterally or intranasally

Nasal:
Serum half-life: 15 minutes

Pregnancy Risk Factor B

Vasosulf® Ophthalmic *see* Sodium Sulfacetamide and Phenylephrine *on page 794*

Vasotec® *see* Enalapril *on page 307*

V-Cillin K® *see* Penicillin V Potassium *on page 668*

VCR *see* Vincristine Sulfate *on page 896*

V-Dec-M® *see* Guaifenesin and Pseudoephedrine *on page 409*

Veetids® *see* Penicillin V Potassium *on page 668*

Velban® *see* Vinblastine Sulfate *on page 895*

Velosef® *see* Cephradine *on page 178*

Velosulin® Human *see* Insulin Preparations *on page 459*

Veltane® *see* Brompheniramine Maleate *on page 124*

Venlafaxine *(ven' la fax een)*

Related Information

Vasoconstrictor Interactions With Antidepressants *on page 1108*

Brand Names Effexor®

Therapeutic Category Antidepressant, Miscellaneous

Use Treatment of depression in adults; has demonstrated effectiveness for obsessive-compulsive disorder, although it has not been approved for this indication

Usual Dosage Adults: Oral: 75 mg/day, administered in 2 or 3 divided doses, taken with food; dose may be increased in 75 mg/day increments at intervals of at least 4 days, up to 225-375 mg/day

Mechanism of Action Venlafaxine and its active metabolite o-desmethylvenlafaxine (ODV) are potent inhibitors of neuronal serotonin and norepinephrine reuptake and weak inhibitors of dopamine reuptake; causes beta-receptor down regulation and reduces adenylcyclase coupled beta-adrenergic systems in the brain

Local Anesthetic/Vasoconstrictor Precautions No information available to require special precautions

Effects on Dental Treatment Over 10% of patients will experience significant dry mouth which may contribute to oral discomfort, especially in older patients

Other Adverse Effects

≥10%:
Central nervous system: Headache, somnolence, dizziness, insomnia, nervousness
Gastrointestinal: Nausea, dry mouth, constipation

Genitourinary: Abnormal ejaculation
Neuromuscular & skeletal: Weakness, neck pain
Miscellaneous: Sweating
1% to 10%:
Cardiovascular: Palpitations, hypertension, sinus tachycardia
Central nervous system: Anxiety, asthenia
Gastrointestinal: Weight loss, anorexia, vomiting, diarrhea, dysphagia
Genitourinary: Impotence
Neuromuscular & skeletal: Tremor
Ocular: Blurred vision
<1%: Central nervous system: Ear pain, seizures

Drug Interactions Increased toxicity: Cimetidine, MAO inhibitors (hyperpyrexic crisis); TCAs, fluoxetine, sertraline, phenothiazine, class 1C antiarrhythmics, warfarin; venlafaxine is a weak inhibitor of cytochrome P-450-2D6, which is responsible for metabolizing antipsychotics, antiarrhythmics, TCAs, and beta-blockers. Therefore, interactions with these agents are possible, however, less likely than with more potent enzyme inhibitors.

Drug Uptake
Absorption: Oral: 92% to 100%
Serum half-life: 3-7 hours (venlafaxine) and 11-13 hours (ODV)

Pregnancy Risk Factor C

Venoglobulin®-I *see* Immune Globulin, Intravenous *on page 454*
Venoglobulin®-S *see* Immune Globulin, Intravenous *on page 454*
Ventolin® *see* Albuterol *on page 27*
VePesid® *see* Etoposide *on page 348*

Verapamil Hydrochloride (ver ap' a mil hye droe klor' ide)

Related Information
Calcium Channel Blockers & Gingival Hyperplasia *on page 1010*
Cardiovascular Diseases *on page 912*

Brand Names Calan®; Calan® SR; Covera-HS®; Isoptin®; Isoptin® SR; Verelan®

Canadian/Mexican Brand Names Apo-Verap® (Canada); Novo-Veramil® (Canada); Nu-Verap® (Canada); Dilacoran® (Mexico); Dilacoran-HTA® (Mexico); Dilacoran-Retard® (Mexico); Veraken® (Mexico); Verdilac® (Mexico)

Therapeutic Category Antianginal Agent; Antiarrhythmic Agent, Class IV; Antiarrhythmic Agent (Supraventricular & Ventricular); Calcium Channel Blocker

Use Orally used for treatment of angina pectoris (vasospastic, chronic stable, unstable) and hypertension; I.V. for supraventricular tachyarrhythmias (PSVT, atrial fibrillation, atrial flutter)

Usual Dosage
Children: SVT:
I.V.:
<1 year: 0.1-0.2 mg/kg over 2 minutes; repeat every 30 minutes as needed
1-16 years: 0.1-0.3 mg/kg over 2 minutes; maximum: 5 mg/dose, may repeat dose in 15 minutes if adequate response not achieved; maximum for second dose: 10 mg/dose
Oral (dose not well established):
1-5 years: 4-8 mg/kg/day in 3 divided doses **or** 40-80 mg every 8 hours
>5 years: 80 mg every 6-8 hours
Adults:
SVT: I.V.: 5-10 mg (approximately 0.075-0.15 mg/kg), second dose of 10 mg (~0.15 mg/kg) may be given 15-30 minutes after the initial dose if patient tolerates, but does not respond to initial dose
Angina: Oral: Initial dose: 80-120 mg twice daily (elderly or small stature: 40 mg twice daily); range: 240-480 mg/day in 3-4 divided doses
Hypertension: Usual dose is 80 mg 3 times/day or 240 mg/day (sustained release); range 240-480 mg/day (no evidence of additional benefit in doses >360 mg/day)

Mechanism of Action Inhibits calcium ion from entering the "slow channels" or select voltage-sensitive areas of vascular smooth muscle and myocardium during depolarization; produces a relaxation of coronary vascular smooth muscle and coronary vasodilation; increases myocardial oxygen delivery in patients with vasospastic angina; slows automaticity and conduction of A-V node.

Local Anesthetic/Vasoconstrictor Precautions No information available to require special precautions

Effects on Dental Treatment Calcium channel blockers (CCB) have been reported to cause gingival hyperplasia (GH). Verapamil induced GH has (Continued)

Verapamil Hydrochloride *(Continued)*

appeared 11 months or more after subjects took daily doses of 240-360 mg. The severity of hyperplastic syndrome does not seem to be dose-dependent. Gingivectomy is only successful if CCB therapy is discontinued. GH regresses markedly one week after CCB discontinuance with all symptoms resolving in 2 months. If a patient must continue CCB therapy, begin a program of professional cleaning and patient plaque control to minimize severity and growth rate of gingival tissue.

Other Adverse Effects

1% to 10%:

Cardiovascular: Bradycardia; first, second, or third degree A-V block; congestive heart failure, hypotension, peripheral edema

Central nervous system: Dizziness, lightheadedness, nausea, tiredness, weakness

Dermatologic: Skin rash

Gastrointestinal: Constipation

<1%:

Cardiovascular: Chest pain, hypotension (excessive), tachycardia, flushing

Endocrine & metabolic: Galactorrhea

Gastrointestinal: Gingival hyperplasia

Drug Interactions

Increased toxicity/effect/levels:

H_2-blockers cause increased bioavailability of verapamil

Beta-blockers cause increased cardiac depressant effects on A-V conduction in combination with verapamil

Verapamil may cause increases in blood levels of the following drugs: Carbamazepine, cyclosporin, digitalis, quinidine, and theophylline; toxicities to all the above drugs could result

Drug Uptake

Oral (nonsustained tablets):

Peak effect: 2 hours

Duration: 6-8 hours

I.V.:

Peak effect: 1-5 minutes

Duration: 10-20 minutes

Serum half-life:

Infants: 4.4-6.9 hours

Adults: Single dose: 2-8 hours, increased up to 12 hours with multiple dosing; increased half-life with hepatic cirrhosis

Pregnancy Risk Factor C

Selected Readings

Wynn RL, "Update on Calcium Channel Blocker Induced Gingival Hyperplasia," *Pharmacol Today*, 1995, 43:218-22.

Verazinc® [OTC] *see* Zinc Supplements *on page 909*

Vercyte® *see* Pipobroman *on page 698*

Verelan® *see* Verapamil Hydrochloride *on previous page*

Vergon® [OTC] *see* Meclizine Hydrochloride *on page 530*

Vermizine® *see* Piperazine Citrate *on page 697*

Vermox® *see* Mebendazole *on page 529*

Verr-Canth™ *see* Cantharidin *on page 146*

Verrex-C&M® *see* Podophyllin and Salicylic Acid *on page 701*

Versacaps® *see* Guaifenesin and Pseudoephedrine *on page 409*

Versed® *see* Midazolam Hydrochloride *on page 580*

Vesprin® *see* Triflupromazine Hydrochloride *on page 870*

Vexol® Ophthalmic Suspension *see* Rimexolone *on page 772*

V-Gan® *see* Promethazine Hydrochloride *on page 733*

Vibazine® *see* Buclizine Hydrochloride *on page 125*

Vibramycin® *see* Doxycycline *on page 301*

Vibra-Tabs® *see* Doxycycline *on page 301*

Vicks® 44D Cough & Head Congestion *see* Pseudoephedrine and Dextromethorphan *on page 750*

Vicks® 44 Non-Drowsy Cold & Cough Liqui-Caps [OTC] *see* Pseudoephedrine and Dextromethorphan *on page 750*

Vicks Children's Chloraseptic® [OTC] *see* Benzocaine *on page 102*

Vicks Chloraseptic® Sore Throat [OTC] *see* Benzocaine *on page 102*

Vicks® DayQuil® Allergy Relief 4 Hour Tablet [OTC] *see* Brompheniramine and Phenylpropanolamine *on page 123*

Vicks® DayQuil® Sinus Pressure & Congestion Relief [OTC] *see* Guaifenesin and Phenylpropanolamine *on page 409*

Vicks Formula 44® [OTC] *see* Dextromethorphan *on page 266*

Vicks Formula 44® Pediatric Formula [OTC] *see* Dextromethorphan *on page 266*

Vicks® Sinex® Long-Acting Nasal Solution [OTC] *see* Oxymetazoline Hydrochloride *on page 649*

Vicks® Sinex® Nasal Solution [OTC] *see* Phenylephrine Hydrochloride *on page 685*

Vicks Vatronol® *see* Ephedrine Sulfate *on page 310*

Vicodin® [5/500] *see* Hydrocodone and Acetaminophen *on page 431*

Vicodin® ES [7.5/750] *see* Hydrocodone and Acetaminophen *on page 431*

Vicon-C® [OTC] *see* Vitamin B Complex With Vitamin C *on page 900*

Vicon Forte® *see* Vitamins, Multiple *on page 901*

Vicon® Plus [OTC] *see* Vitamins, Multiple *on page 901*

Vidarabina (Mexico) *see* Vidarabine *on this page*

Vidarabine (vye dare' a been)

Related Information
Oral Viral Infections *on page 951*
Systemic Viral Diseases *on page 934*

Brand Names Vira-A®

Canadian/Mexican Brand Names Adena® a Ungena (Mexico)

Therapeutic Category Antiviral Agent, Ophthalmic

Synonyms Vidarabina (Mexico)

Use Treatment of acute keratoconjunctivitis and epithelial keratitis due to herpes simplex virus; herpes simplex conjunctivitis

Usual Dosage
Children and Adults: Ophthalmic: Keratoconjunctivitis: Instill $1/2$" of ointment in lower conjunctival sac 5 times/day every 3 hours while awake until complete re-epithelialization has occurred, then twice daily for an additional 7 days

Mechanism of Action Inhibits viral DNA synthesis by blocking DNA polymerase

Local Anesthetic/Vasoconstrictor Precautions No information available to require special precautions

Effects on Dental Treatment No effects or complications reported

Other Adverse Effects Ocular: Burning, lacrimation, keratitis, photophobia, foreign body sensation, uveitis

Drug Interactions No data reported

Pregnancy Risk Factor C

Vi-Daylin® [OTC] *see* Vitamins, Multiple *on page 901*

Vi-Daylin/F® *see* Vitamins, Multiple *on page 901*

Videx® *see* Didanosine *on page 274*

Vinblastine Sulfate (vin blas' teen sul' fate)

Brand Names Alkaban-AQ®; Velban®

Canadian/Mexican Brand Names Lemblastine (Mexico)

Therapeutic Category Antineoplastic Agent, Mitotic Inhibitor

Synonyms Vincaleukoblastine; VLB

Use Palliative treatment of Hodgkin's disease; advanced testicular germinal-cell cancers; non-Hodgkin's lymphoma, histiocytosis, and choriocarcinoma

Usual Dosage Refer to individual protocols. Varies depending upon clinical and hematological response. Give at intervals of at least 7 days and only after leukocyte count has returned to at least 4000/mm³; maintenance therapy should be titrated according to leukocyte count. Dosage should be reduced in patients with recent exposure to radiation therapy or chemotherapy; single doses in these patients should not exceed 5.5 mg/m².

Children and Adults: I.V.: 4-20 mg/m² (0.1-0.5 mg/kg) every 7-10 days **or** 5-day continuous infusion of 1.4-1.8 mg/m²/day **or** 0.1-0.5 mg/kg/week

Hemodialysis effects: Not removed by hemodialysis

Mechanism of Action VLB binds to tubulin and inhibits microtubule formation, therefore, arresting the cell at metaphase by disrupting the formation of the mitotic spindle; it is specific for the M and S phases; binds to microtubular protein of the mitotic spindle causing metaphase arrest

Local Anesthetic/Vasoconstrictor Precautions No information available to require special precautions

Effects on Dental Treatment No effects or complications reported
(Continued)

895

Vinblastine Sulfate *(Continued)*

Other Adverse Effects

>10%: Alopecia

    Hematologic: May cause severe bone marrow depression and is the dose-limiting toxicity of vinblastine (unlike vincristine); severe granulocytopenia and thrombocytopenia may occur following the administration of vinblastine and nadir 7-10 days after treatment

1% to 10%:

    Cardiovascular: Tachycardia, orthostatic hypotension

    Central nervous system: Depression, malaise, seizures, headache

    Dermatologic: Rash, photosensitivity

    Endocrine & metabolic: Hyperuricemia

    Gastrointestinal: Paralytic ileus, stomatitis, nausea and vomiting are most common and are easily controlled with standard antiemetics; constipation, diarrhea, abdominal cramps, anorexia, metallic taste

        Emetic potential: Moderate (30% to 60%)

    Genitourinary: Urinary retention

    Hematologic: Bone marrow depression

    Neuromuscular & skeletal: Jaw pain, muscle pain

    Extravasation: vinblastine is a vesicant and can cause tissue irritation and necrosis if infiltrated; if extravasation occurs, follow institutional policy, which may include hyaluronidase and hot compresses

    Neurologic: Vinblastine rarely produces neurotoxicity at clinical doses; however, neurotoxicity may be seen, especially at high doses; if it occurs, symptoms are similar to vincristine toxicity: peripheral neuropathy, loss of deep tendon reflexes, weakness, and GI symptoms

<1%:

    Central nervous system: Neurotoxicity

    Dermatologic: Alopecia, dermatitis, photosensitivity

    Endocrine & metabolic: Hyperuricemia

    Gastrointestinal: Hemorrhagic colitis

    Respiratory: Bronchospasm

    Neuromuscular & skeletal: Paresthesias, pain, muscle pain

Drug Uptake

Absorption: Not reliably absorbed from the GI tract and must be given I.V.

Serum half-life (biphasic):

    Initial 0.164 hours

    Terminal: 25 hours

Pregnancy Risk Factor D

Vincaleukoblastine *see* Vinblastine Sulfate *on previous page*

Vincasar® PFS™ Injection *see* Vincristine Sulfate *on this page*

Vincristine Sulfate *(vin kris' teen sul' fate)*

Brand Names Oncovin® Injection; Vincasar® PFS™ Injection

Canadian/Mexican Brand Names Citomid (Mexico)

Therapeutic Category Antineoplastic Agent, Mitotic Inhibitor

Synonyms LCR; Leurocristine; VCR

Use Treatment of leukemias, Hodgkin's disease, neuroblastoma, malignant lymphomas, Wilms' tumor, and rhabdomyosarcoma

Usual Dosage Refer to individual protocols as dosages vary with protocol used. Adjustments are made depending upon clinical and hematological response and upon adverse reactions

Children: I.V. (maximum single dose: 2 mg):

    ≤10 kg or BSA <1 m^2: 0.05 mg/kg once weekly

    2 mg/m^2; may repeat every week

Adults: I.V.: 0.4-1.4 mg/m^2 (up to 2 mg maximum); may repeat every week

Mechanism of Action Binds to microtubular protein of the mitotic spindle causing metaphase arrest; cell-cycle phase specific in the M and S phases

Local Anesthetic/Vasoconstrictor Precautions No information available to require special precautions

Effects on Dental Treatment No effects or complications reported

Other Adverse Effects

>10%:

    Dermatologic: Alopecia: Occurs in 20% to 70% of patients

    Extravasation: Vincristine is a vesicant and can cause tissue irritation and necrosis if infiltrated; if extravasation occurs, follow institutional policy, which may include hyaluronidase and hot compresses

1% to 10%:

    Dermatologic: Skin rash

Gastrointestinal: Weight loss, paralytic ileus, constipation and possible paralytic ileus secondary to neurologic toxicity; oral ulceration, nausea, diarrhea, vomiting, bloating, abdominal cramps, anorexia, metallic taste

Cardiovascular: Hypotension (orthostatic)

Local: Phlebitis

Central nervous system: Neurotoxicity, seizures, CNS depression, cranial nerve paralysis

Neuromuscular & skeletal: Numbness, weakness, motor difficulties, jaw pain, leg pain, myalgias, cramping

Endocrine & metabolic: Hyperuricemia, SIADH

Myelosuppressive: Occasionally mild leukopenia and thrombocytopenia may occur

<1%: Gastrointestinal: Stomatitis

Neurologic: Alterations in mental status such as depression, confusion, or insomnia. Constipation, paralytic ileus, and urinary tract disturbances may occur. All patients should be on a prophylactic bowel management regimen. Cranial nerve palsies, headaches, jaw pain, optic atrophy with blindness have been reported. Intrathecal administration of vincristine has uniformly caused death, vincristine should **never** be administered by this route. Neurologic effects of vincristine may be additive with those of other neurotoxic agents and spinal cord irradiation.

Peripheral neuropathy: Frequently the dose-limiting toxicity of vincristine. Most frequent in patients >40 years of age; occurs usually after an average of 3 weekly doses, but may occur after just one dose. Manifested as loss of the deep tendon reflexes in the lower extremities, numbness, tingling, pain, paresthesias of the fingers and toes (stocking glove sensation), and "foot drop" or "wrist drop"

SIADH: Rarely occurs, but may be related to the neurologic toxicity; may cause symptomatic hyponatremia with seizures; the increase in serum ADH concentration usually subsides within 2-3 days after onset

Miscellaneous: Rash, photophobia, headache, weight loss, fever, hypertension, hypotension

Drug Uptake

Absorption: Oral: Poor

Serum half-life: Terminal: 24 hours

Pregnancy Risk Factor D

Vinorelbine Tartrate (vi nor' el been tar' trate)

Brand Names Navelbine®

Therapeutic Category Antineoplastic Agent, Mitotic Inhibitor

Use Treatment of nonsmall cell lung cancer (as a single agent or in combination with cisplatin)

Unlabeled use: Breast cancer, ovarian carcinoma (cisplatin-resistant), Hodgkin's disease

Usual Dosage Varies depending upon clinical and hematological response (refer to individual protocols)

Adults: I.V.: 30 mg/m^2 every 7 days

Mechanism of Action Semisynthetic *Vinca* alkaloid which binds to tubulin and inhibits microtubule formation, therefore, arresting the cell at metaphase by disrupting the formation of the mitotic spindle; it is specific for the M and S phases; binds to microtubular protein of the mitotic spindle causing metaphase arrest

Local Anesthetic/Vasoconstrictor Precautions No information available to require special precautions

Effects on Dental Treatment No effects or complications reported

Other Adverse Effects

1% to 10%:

Cardiovascular: Chest pain

Central nervous system: Fatigue

Endocrine & metabolic: SIADH

Gastrointestinal: Nausea, vomiting, constipation

Genitourinary: Hemorrhagic cystitis

Hematologic: Neutropenia, leukopenia (nadir 7-8 days with recovery by days 15-17), anemia

Hepatic: Transient elevation in liver enzymes

Local: Phlebitis at sight of infusion, vesicant with extravasation

Neuromuscular & skeletal: Decreased deep tendon reflexes, tumor pain, jaw pain, parasthesia

Respiratory: Acute reversible dyspnea, hypoxemia, interstitial pulmonary infiltrates

(Continued)

Vinorelbine Tartrate *(Continued)*

<1%:
Cardiovascular: Myocardial infarction
Dermatologic: Alopecia
Hematologic: Thrombocytopenia

Drug Uptake
Absorption: Not reliably absorbed from the GI tract and must be given I.V.
Serum half-life (triphasic):
Terminal: 27.7-43.6 hours

Pregnancy Risk Factor D

Vioform® **[OTC]** *see* Iodochlorhydroxyquin *on page 466*

Viokase® *see* Pancrelipase *on page 657*

Vira-A® *see* Vidarabine *on page 895*

Viractin® **[OTC]** *see* Tetracaine Hydrochloride *on page 828*

Viramune® *see* Nevirapine *on page 614*

Virazole® Aerosol *see* Ribavirin *on page 767*

Virilon® *see* Methyltestosterone *on page 570*

Viroptic® *see* Trifluridine *on page 870*

Viscoat® *see* Chondroitin Sulfate-Sodium Hyaluronate *on page 203*

Visine® [OTC] *see* Tetrahydrozoline Hydrochloride *on page 831*

Visine A.C.® [OTC] *see* Tetrahydrozoline Hydrochloride *on page 831*

Visken® *see* Pindolol *on page 694*

Vistacon-50® *see* Hydroxyzine *on page 443*

Vistaject-25® *see* Hydroxyzine *on page 443*

Vistaject-50® *see* Hydroxyzine *on page 443*

Vistaquel® *see* Hydroxyzine *on page 443*

Vistaril® *see* Hydroxyzine *on page 443*

Vistazine® *see* Hydroxyzine *on page 443*

Vistide® *see* Cidofovir *on page 205*

Vita-C® [OTC] *see* Ascorbic Acid *on page 76*

Vitacarn® Oral *see* Levocarnitine *on page 494*

Vitamin A *(vye' ta min aye)*

Brand Names Aquasol A® [OTC]
Canadian/Mexican Brand Names Arovit® (Mexico); A-Vicon® (Mexico); A-Vitex® (Mexico)
Therapeutic Category Vitamin, Fat Soluble
Synonyms Vitamina A (Mexico)
Use Dental and Medical: Treatment and prevention of vitamin A deficiency
Usual Dosage
RDA:
<1 year: 375 mcg
1-3 years: 400 mcg
4-6 years: 500 mcg•
7-10 years: 700 mcg•
>10 years: 800-1000 mcg•
Male: 1000 mcg
Female: 800 mcg
•mcg retinol equivalent (0.3 mcg retinol = 1 unit vitamin A)
Vitamin A supplementation in measles (recommendation of the World Health Organization): Children: Oral: Give as a single dose; repeat the next day and at 4 weeks for children with ophthalmologic evidence of vitamin A deficiency:
6 months to 1 year: 100,000 units
>1 year: 200,000 units
Note: Use of vitamin A in measles is recommended only for patients 6 months to 2 years of age hospitalized with measles and its complications **or** patients >6 months of age who have any of the following risk factors and who are not already receiving vitamin A: immunodeficiency, ophthalmologic evidence of vitamin A deficiency including night blindness, Bitot's spots or evidence of xerophthalmia, impaired intestinal absorption, moderate to severe malnutrition including that associated with eating disorders, or recent immigration from areas where high mortality rates from measles have been observed
Note: Monitor patients closely; dosages >25,000 units/kg have been associated with toxicity

Severe deficiency with xerophthalmia: Oral:
Children 1-8 years: 5000-10,000 units/kg/day for 5 days or until recovery occurs

Children >8 years and Adults: 500,000 units/day for 3 days, then 50,000 units/day for 14 days, then 10,000-20,000 units/day for 2 months
Deficiency (without corneal changes): Oral:
Children 1-8 years: 200,000 units every 4-6 months
Children >8 years and Adults: 100,000 units/day for 3 days then 50,000 units/day for 14 days
Malabsorption syndrome (prophylaxis): Children >8 years and Adults: Oral: 10,000-50,000 units/day of water miscible product
Dietary supplement: Oral:
Children:
6 months to 3 years: 1500-2000 units/day
4-6 years: 2500 units/day
7-10 years: 3300-3500 units/day
Children >10 years and Adults: 4000-5000 units/day

Mechanism of Action Needed for bone development, growth, visual adaptation to darkness, testicular and ovarian function, and as a cofactor in many biochemical processes

Local Anesthetic/Vasoconstrictor Precautions No information available to require special precautions

Effects on Dental Treatment No effects or complications reported

Other Adverse Effects 1% to 10%:
Central nervous system: Irritability, vertigo, lethargy, malaise, fever, headache
Dermatologic: Drying or cracking of skin
Endocrine & metabolic: Hypercalcemia
Gastrointestinal: Weight loss
Ocular: Visual changes
Miscellaneous: Hypervitaminosis A

Contraindications Hypervitaminosis A, hypersensitivity to vitamin A or any component

Warnings/Precautions Evaluate other sources of vitamin A while receiving this product; patients receiving >25,000 units/day should be closely monitored for toxicity

Drug Interactions
Decreased effect: Cholestyramine decreases absorption of vitamin A; neomycin and mineral oil may also interfere with vitamin A absorption
Increased toxicity: Retinoids may have additive adverse effects

Drug Uptake
Absorption: Vitamin A in dosages **not** exceeding physiologic replacement is well absorbed after oral administration; water miscible preparations are absorbed more rapidly than oil preparations; large oral doses, conditions of fat malabsorption, low protein intake, or hepatic or pancreatic disease reduces oral absorption

Pregnancy Risk Factor A (X if dose exceeds RDA recommendation)

Dosage Forms
Capsule: 10,000 units, 25,000 units, 50,000 units
Drops, oral (water miscible): 5000 units/0.1 mL (30 mL)
Injection: 50,000 units/mL (2 mL)

Generic Available Yes

Vitamina A (Mexico) *see* Vitamin A *on previous page*

Vitamin A and Vitamin D (vye′ ta min aye & vye′ ta min dee)
Brand Names A and D™ Ointment [OTC]
Therapeutic Category Protectant, Topical; Topical Skin Product
Use Temporary relief of discomfort due to chapped skin, diaper rash, minor burns, abrasions, as well as irritations associated with ostomy skin care
Local Anesthetic/Vasoconstrictor Precautions No information available to require special precautions
Effects on Dental Treatment No effects or complications reported
Other Adverse Effects Irritation

Vitamin B₅ *see* Pantothenic Acid *on page 658*

Vitamin B Complex (vye′ ta min bee kom′ pleks)
Brand Names Apatate® [OTC]; Gevrabon® [OTC]; Lederplex® [OTC]; Lipovite® [OTC]; Mega-B® [OTC]; Megaton™ [OTC]; Mucoplex® [OTC]; NeoVadrin® B Complex [OTC]; Orexin® [OTC]; Surbex® [OTC]
Therapeutic Category Vitamin, Water Soluble
Local Anesthetic/Vasoconstrictor Precautions No information available to require special precautions
Effects on Dental Treatment No effects or complications reported

Vitamin B Complex With Vitamin C
(vye′ ta min bee kom′ pleks with vye′ ta min see)

Brand Names Allbee® With C [OTC]; Surbex-T® Filmtabs® [OTC]; Surbex® with C Filmtabs® [OTC]; Thera-Combex® H-P Kapseals® [OTC]; Vicon-C® [OTC]

Therapeutic Category Vitamin, Water Soluble

Use Supportive nutritional supplementation in conditions in which water-soluble vitamins are required like GI disorders, chronic alcoholism, pregnancy, severe burns, and recovery from surgery

Local Anesthetic/Vasoconstrictor Precautions No information available to require special precautions

Effects on Dental Treatment No effects or complications reported

Vitamin B Complex With Vitamin C and Folic Acid
(vye′ ta min bee kom′ pleks with vye′ ta min see & foe′ lik as′ id)

Brand Names Berocca®; Folbesyn®; Nephrocaps® [OTC]

Therapeutic Category Vitamin, Water Soluble

Use Supportive nutritional supplementation in conditions in which water-soluble vitamins are required like GI disorders, chronic alcoholism, pregnancy, severe burns, and recovery from surgery

Local Anesthetic/Vasoconstrictor Precautions No information available to require special precautions

Effects on Dental Treatment No effects or complications reported

Vitamin E (vye′ ta min ee)

Brand Names Amino-Opti-E® [OTC]; Aquasol E® [OTC]; E-Complex-600® [OTC]; E-Vitamin® [OTC]; Vita-Plus® E Softgels® [OTC]; Vitec® [OTC]; Vite E® Creme [OTC]

Therapeutic Category Vitamin, Fat Soluble

Use Dental and Medical: Prevention and treatment hemolytic anemia secondary to vitamin E deficiency, dietary supplement

Usual Dosage One unit of vitamin E = 1 mg dl-alpha-tocopherol acetate. Oral:
Vitamin E deficiency:
Children (with malabsorption syndrome): 1 unit/kg/day of water miscible vitamin E (to raise plasma tocopherol concentrations to the normal range within 2 months and to maintain normal plasma concentrations)
Adults: 60-75 units/day
Prevention of vitamin E deficiency:
Adults: 30 units/day
Prevention of retinopathy of prematurity or BPD secondary to O_2 therapy: (American Academy of Pediatrics considers this use investigational and routine use is not recommended):
Retinopathy prophylaxis: 15-30 units/kg/day to maintain plasma levels between 1.5-2 µg/mL (may need as high as 100 units/kg/day)
Cystic fibrosis, beta-thalassemia, sickle cell anemia may require higher daily maintenance doses:
Cystic fibrosis: 100-400 units/day
Beta-thalassemia: 750 units/day
Sickle cell: 450 units/day
Recommended daily allowance:
Children:
1-3 years: 6 mg (9 units)
4-10 years: 7 mg (10.5 units)
Children >11 years and Adults:
Male: 10 mg (15 units)
Female: 8 mg (12 units)
Topical: Apply a thin layer over affected area

Mechanism of Action Prevents oxidation of vitamin A and C; protects poly-unsaturated fatty acids in membranes from attack by free radicals and protects red blood cells against hemolysis

Local Anesthetic/Vasoconstrictor Precautions No information available to require special precautions

Effects on Dental Treatment No effects or complications reported

Other Adverse Effects <1%:
Central nervous system: Weakness, headache
Dermatologic: Contact dermatitis with topical preparation
Gastrointestinal: Nausea, diarrhea, intestinal cramps
Ocular: Blurred vision
Miscellaneous: Gonadal dysfunction

Contraindications Hypersensitivity to drug or any components

Warnings/Precautions May induce vitamin K deficiency; necrotizing enterocolitis has been associated with oral administration of large dosages (eg, >200 units/day) of a hyperosmolar vitamin E preparation in low birth weight infants

Drug Interactions
Decreased absorption with mineral oil
Delayed absorption of iron
Increased effect of oral anticoagulants

Drug Uptake
Absorption: Oral: Depends upon the presence of bile; absorption is reduced in conditions of malabsorption, in low birth weight premature infants, and as dosage increases; water miscible preparations are better absorbed than oil preparations

Pregnancy Risk Factor A (C if dose exceeds RDA recommendation)

Dosage Forms
Capsule: 100 units, 200 units, 330 mg, 400 units, 500 units, 600 units, 1000 units
Capsule, water miscible: 73.5 mg, 147 mg, 165 mg, 330 mg, 400 units
Cream: 50 mg/g (15 g, 30 g, 60 g, 75 g, 120 g, 454 g)
Drops, oral: 50 mg/mL (12 mL, 30 mL)
Liquid, topical: 10 mL, 15 mL, 30 mL, 60 mL
Lotion: 120 mL
Oil: 15 mL, 30 mL, 60 mL
Ointment, topical: 30 mg/g (45 g, 60 g)
Tablet: 200 units, 400 units

Generic Available Yes

Vitamins, Multiple (vye′ ta mins mul′ ti pul)

Brand Names Adeflor®; Allbee® With C; Becotin® Pulvules®; Cefol® Filmtab®; Chromagen® OB [OTC]; Eldercaps® [OTC]; Filibon® [OTC]; Florvite®; LKV-Drops® [OTC]; Multi Vit® Drops [OTC]; M.V.I.®; M.V.I.®-12; M.V.I.® Concentrate; M.V.I.® Pediatric; Natabec® [OTC]; Natabec® FA [OTC]; Natabec® Rx; Natalins® [OTC]; Natalins® Rx; NeoVadrin® [OTC]; Niferex®-PN; Poly-Vi-Flor®; Poly-Vi-Sol® [OTC]; Pramet® FA; Pramilet® FA; Prenavite® [OTC]; Secran®; Stresstabs® 600 Advanced Formula Tablets [OTC]; Stuartnatal® 1 + 1; Stuart Prenatal® [OTC]; Therabid® [OTC]; Theragran® [OTC]; Theragran® Hematinic®; Theragran® Liquid [OTC]; Theragran-M® [OTC]; Tri-Vi-Flor®; Unicap® [OTC]; Vicon Forte®; Vicon® Plus [OTC]; Vi-Daylin® [OTC]; Vi-Daylin/F®

Canadian/Mexican Brand Names Clanda® (Mexico); Complan® (Mexico); Suplena® (Mexico); Vi-Syneral® (Mexico)

Therapeutic Category Vitamin

Use Dental and Medical: Dietary supplement

Usual Dosage Oral:

Children:
>2 years: Chew 1 tablet/day
≥4 years: 5 mL/day liquid

Adults: 1 tablet/day or 5 mL/day liquid

Local Anesthetic/Vasoconstrictor Precautions No information available to require special precautions

Effects on Dental Treatment No effects or complications reported

Other Adverse Effects 1% to 10%: Miscellaneous: Hypervitaminosis; refer to individual vitamin entries for individual reactions

Contraindications Hypersensitivity to product components

Warnings/Precautions RDA values are not requirements, but are recommended daily intakes of certain essential nutrients; periodic dental exams should be performed to check for dental fluorosis; use with caution in patients with severe renal or liver failure

Drug Interactions No data reported

Pregnancy Risk Factor A (C if used in doses above RDA recommendation)

Dosage Forms See table on following page

Vita-Plus® E Softgels® [OTC] *see* Vitamin E *on previous page*

Vitec® [OTC] *see* Vitamin E *on previous page*

Vite E® Creme [OTC] *see* Vitamin E *on previous page*

Vivactil® *see* Protriptyline Hydrochloride *on page 748*

Viva-Drops® Solution [OTC] *see* Artificial Tears *on page 75*

Vivotif Berna™ Oral *see* Typhoid Vaccine *on page 883*

V-Lax® [OTC] *see* Psyllium *on page 750*

VLB *see* Vinblastine Sulfate *on page 895*

VM-26 *see* Teniposide *on page 820*

Multivitamin Products Available

Product	Content Given Per	A IU	D IU	E IU	C mg	FA mg	B$_1$ mg	B$_2$ mg	B$_3$ mg	B$_6$ mg	B$_{12}$ mcg	Other
Drops/Liquid												
Theragran®	5 mL liquid	10,000	400		200		10	10	100	4.1	5	B$_5$ 21.4 mg
Vi-Daylin®	1 mL drops	1500	400	4.1	35		0.5	0.6	8	0.4	1.5	Alcohol <0.5%
Vi-Daylin® Iron	1 mL	1500	400	4.1	35		0.5	0.6	8	0.4		Fe 10 mg
Capsules/Tablets												
Allbee® with C	Tablet				300		15	10.2		5		Niacinamide 50 mg, pantothenic acid 10 mg
Vitamin B Complex	Tablet					400 mcg	1.5	1.7		2	6	Niacinamide 20 mg
Hexavitamin	Cap/Tab	5000	400		75	0.8	2	3	20			
Iberet®-Folic-500	Tablet				500	1	6	6	30	5	25	B$_5$ 10, Fe 105 mg
Stuartnatal 1+1	Tablet	4000	400	11	120	1	1.5	3	20	10	12	Cu, Zn 25 mg, Fe 65 mg, Ca 200 mg
Theragran® M	Tablet	5000	400	30	90	0.4	3	3.4	30	3	9	Cl, Cr, I, K, B$_5$ 10, Mg, Mn, Mo, P, Se, Zn 15 mg, Fe 27 mg, biotin 35 mcg, beta-carotene 1250 IU
Vi-Daylin®	Tablet	2500	400	15	60	0.3	1.05	1.2	13.5	1.05	4.5	
Injectables												
M.V.I.-12 injection	5 mL	3300	200	10	100	0.4	3	3.6	40	4	5	B$_5$ 15 mg, biotin 60 mcg
M.V.I.-12 unit vial	20 mL											
M.V.I. pediatric powder	5 mL	2300	400	7	80	0.14	1.2	1.4	17	1	1	B$_5$ 5 mg, biotin 20 mcg, vitamin K 200 mcg

Volmax® *see Albuterol on page 27*

Voltaren® *see Diclofenac on page 271*

Vontrol® *see Diphenidol Hydrochloride on page 289*

VōSol® HC Otic *see Acetic Acid, Propanediol Diacetate, and Hydrocortisone on page 19*

Vumon Injection *see Teniposide on page 820*

V.V.S.® *see Sulfabenzamide, Sulfacetamide, and Sulfathiazole on page 806*

Vytone® Topical *see Iodoquinol and Hydrocortisone on page 467*

VZIG *see Varicella-Zoster Immune Globulin (Human) on page 890*

Warfarin Sodium (war' far in sow' dee um)

Related Information
Cardiovascular Diseases *on page 912*

Dental Drug Interactions: Update on Drug Combinations Requiring Special Considerations *on page 1022*

Brand Names Coumadin®; Sofarin®

Canadian/Mexican Brand Names Warfilone® (Canada)

Therapeutic Category Anticoagulant

Use Prophylaxis and treatment of venous thrombosis, pulmonary embolism and thromboembolic disorders; atrial fibrillation with risk of embolism and as an adjunct in the prophylaxis of systemic embolism after myocardial infarction

Unlabeled use: Prevention of recurrent transient ischemic attacks and to reduce risk of recurrent myocardial infarction

Usual Dosage
Oral:

Children: 0.05-0.34 mg/kg/day; children <12 months of age may require doses at or near the high end of this range; consistent anticoagulation may be difficult to maintain in children <5 years of age

Adults: 5-15 mg/day for 2-5 days, then adjust dose according to results of prothrombin time; usual maintenance dose ranges from 2-10 mg/day

I.V. (administer as a slow bolus injection): 2-5 mg/day

Mechanism of Action Interferes with hepatic synthesis of vitamin K-dependent coagulation factors (II, VII, IX, X)

Local Anesthetic/Vasoconstrictor Precautions No information available to require special precautions

Effects on Dental Treatment Signs of warfarin overdose may first appear as bleeding from gingival tissue; consultation with prescribing physician is advisable prior to surgery to determine temporary dose reduction or withdrawal of medication

Other Adverse Effects
1% to 10%:

Dermatologic: Skin lesions, alopecia, skin necrosis

Gastrointestinal: Anorexia, nausea, vomiting, stomach cramps, diarrhea

Hematologic: Hemorrhage; leukopenia, unrecognized bleeding sites (eg, colon cancer) may be uncovered by anticoagulation

Respiratory: Hemoptysis

<1%:

Dermatologic: Skin rash

Gastrointestinal: Anorexia

Hematologic: Agranulocytosis

Hepatic: Hepatotoxicity

Renal: Renal damage

Miscellaneous: Mouth ulcers, fever, discolored toes (blue or purple)

Drug Interactions See tables.

Decreased Anticoagulant Effects

Induction of Enzymes		Increased Procoagulant Factors	Decreased Drug Absorption	Other
Barbiturates Carbamazepine Glutethimide Griseofulvin	Nafcillin Phenytoin Rifampin	Estrogens Oral contraceptives Vitamin K (including nutritional supplements)	Aluminum hydroxide Cholestyramine* Colestipol*	Ethchlorvynol Griseofulvin Spironolactone† Sucralfate

Decreased anticoagulant effect may occur when these drugs are administered with oral anticoagulants.

*Cholestyramine and colestipol may increase the anticoagulant effect by binding vitamin K in the gut; yet, the decreased drug absorption appears to be of more concern.

†Diuretic-induced hemoconcentration with subsequent concentration of clotting factors has been reported to decrease the effects of oral anticoagulants.

(Continued)

Warfarin Sodium *(Continued)*

Increased Bleeding Tendency

Inhibit Platelet Aggregation	Inhibit Procoagulant Factors	Ulcerogenic Drugs
Cephalosporins Dipyridamole Indomethacin Oxyphenbutazone Penicillin, parenteral Phenylbutazone Salicylates Sulfinpyrazone	Antimetabolites Quinidine Quinine Salicylates	Adrenal corticosteroids Indomethacin Oxyphenbutazone Phenylbutazone Potassium products Salicylates

Use of these agents with oral anticoagulants may increase the chances of hemorrhage.

Enhanced Anticoagulant Effects

Decrease Vitamin K	Displace Anticoagulant	Inhibit Metabolism	Other
Oral antibiotics Can ↑ or ↓ an INR Check an INR 3 days after a patient begins antibiotics to see the INR value and adjust the warfarin dose accordingly	Chloral hydrate Clofibrate Diazoxide Ethacrynic acid Miconazole Nalidixic acid Phenylbutazone Salicylates Sulfonamides Sulfonylureas Triclofos	Alcohol (acute ingestion)* Allopurinol Amiodarone Chloramphenicol Chlorpropamide Cimetidine Co-trimoxazole Disulfiram Metronidazole Phenylbutazone Phenytoin Propoxyphene Sulfinpyrazone Sulfonamides Tolbutamide	Acetaminophen Anabolic steroids Clofibrate Danazol Erythromycin Gemfibrozil Glucagon Influenza vaccine Ketoconazole Propranolol Ranitidine Sulindac Thyroid drugs

* The hypoprothrombinemic effect of oral anticoagulants has been reported to be both increased and decreased during chronic and excessive alcohol ingestion. Data are insufficient to predict the direction of this interaction in alcoholic patients.

Drug Uptake
Onset of anticoagulation effect: Oral: Within 36-72 hours
Absorption: Oral: Rapid
Serum half-life: 42 hours, highly variable among individuals
Pregnancy Risk Factor D

4-Way® Long Acting Nasal Solution [OTC] *see* Oxymetazoline Hydrochloride *on page 649*

Wehamine® *see* Dimenhydrinate *on page 286*

Wellbutrin® *see* Bupropion *on page 130*

Wellbutrin® SR *see* Bupropion *on page 130*

Wellcovorin® Injection *see* Leucovorin Calcium *on page 491*

Wellcovorin® Oral *see* Leucovorin Calcium *on page 491*

Westrim® LA [OTC] *see* Phenylpropanolamine Hydrochloride *on page 687*

Whitfield's Ointment [OTC] *see* Benzoic Acid and Salicylic Acid *on page 104*

Whole Root Rauwolfia *see* Rauwolfia Serpentina *on page 764*

Wigraine® *see* Ergotamine *on page 319*

Winstrol® *see* Stanozolol *on page 799*

Wolfina® *see* Rauwolfia Serpentina *on page 764*

Wyamycin® S *see* Erythromycin *on page 321*

Wycillin® *see* Penicillin G Procaine *on page 667*

Wydase® Injection *see* Hyaluronidase *on page 427*

Wygesic® *see* Propoxyphene and Acetaminophen *on page 741*

Wymox® *see* Amoxicillin Trihydrate *on page 58*

Wytensin® *see* Guanabenz Acetate *on page 411*

Xalatan® *see* Latanoprost *on page 490*

Xanax® *see* Alprazolam *on page 35*

Xero-Lube® [OTC] *see* Saliva Substitute *on page 778*

X-Prep® Liquid [OTC] *see* Senna *on page 785*

X-seb® T [OTC] *see* Coal Tar and Salicylic Acid *on page 226*

Xylocaine® *see* Lidocaine Hydrochloride *on page 502*

Xylocaine® With Epinephrine *see* Lidocaine and Epinephrine *on page 499*

Xylometazoline Hydrochloride
(zye loe met az' oh leen hye droe klor' ide)

Brand Names Otrivin® [OTC]

Therapeutic Category Adrenergic Agonist Agent; Nasal Agent, Vasoconstrictor

Use Symptomatic relief of nasal and nasopharyngeal mucosal congestion

Usual Dosage
Children 2-12 years: Instill 2-3 drops (0.05%) in each nostril every 8-10 hours
Children >12 years and Adults: Instill 2-3 drops or sprays (0.1%) in each nostril every 8-10 hours

Mechanism of Action Stimulates alpha-adrenergic receptors in the arterioles of the conjunctiva and the nasal mucosa to produce vasoconstriction

Local Anesthetic/Vasoconstrictor Precautions No information available to require special precautions

Effects on Dental Treatment No effects or complications reported

Other Adverse Effects 1% to 10%:
Cardiovascular: Palpitations
Central nervous system: Drowsiness, dizziness, seizures, headache
Ocular: Blurred vision, ocular irritation, photophobia
Miscellaneous: Sweating

Drug Interactions No data reported

Drug Uptake
Onset of action: Intranasal: Local vasoconstriction occurs within 5-10 minutes
Duration: 5-6 hours

Pregnancy Risk Factor C

Yellow Mercuric Oxide *see* Mercuric Oxide *on page 545*

Yocon® *see* Yohimbine Hydrochloride *on this page*

Yodoxin® *see* Iodoquinol *on page 466*

Yohimbine Hydrochloride (yo him' bine hye droe klor' ide)

Brand Names Aphrodyne™; Dayto Himbin®; Yocon®; Yohimex™

Therapeutic Category Impotency Agent

Use No FDA sanctioned indications

Local Anesthetic/Vasoconstrictor Precautions No information available to require special precautions

Effects on Dental Treatment No effects or complications reported

Yohimex™ *see* Yohimbine Hydrochloride *on this page*

Yutopar® *see* Ritodrine Hydrochloride *on page 773*

Zafirlukast (za fir' loo kast)

Brand Names Accolate®

Therapeutic Category Leukotriene Receptor Antagonist

Use Preventative and chronic treatment of asthma in adults and children 12 years and older

Usual Dosage Adults: Oral: 20 mg twice daily; take 1 hour before food or 2 hours after food

Mechanism of Action Leukotriene receptor antagonist; leukotriene selectively blocks a key mediator in early-phase and late-phase asthmatic response

Local Anesthetic/Vasoconstrictor Precautions No information available to require special precautions

Effects on Dental Treatment No effects or complications reported

Other Adverse Effects 1% to 10%:
Central nervous system: Headache, dizziness, fever, pain, asthenia
Gastrointestinal: Nausea, diarrhea, abdominal pain, vomiting, dyspepsia
Hepatic: SGPT elevation
Neuromuscular & skeletal: Myalgia, back pain
Miscellaneous: Infection

Warnings/Precautions Not indicated for reversal of acute asthma attacks, including status asthmaticus; there appears to be an increased risk of infections in patients >55 years of age that occurred equally in both sexes

Drug Interactions
Zafirlukast enhances anticoagulation of S-warfarin
(Continued)

Zafirlukast *(Continued)*

Coadministration with erythromycin resulted in a 40% decrease in plasma levels of zafirlukast; coadministration with theophylline resulted in a 30% decreased mean plasma level; coadministration with aspirin resulted in mean increased plasma levels of zafirlukast by 45%

Pregnancy Risk Factor B

Zalcitabina (Mexico) *see* Zalcitabine *on this page*

Zalcitabine (zal site' a been)
Related Information
Systemic Viral Diseases *on page 934*

Brand Names Hivid®

Therapeutic Category Antiviral Agent, Oral

Synonyms Zalcitabina (Mexico)

Use The FDA has approved zalcitabine for use in the treatment of HIV infections only in combination with zidovudine in adult patients with advanced HIV disease demonstrating a significant clinical or immunological deterioration

Usual Dosage Safety and efficacy in children <13 years of age have not been established

Adults: Monotherapy: 0.75 mg every 8 hours (2.25 mg total daily dose)

Combination therapy: 0.75 mg every 8 hours, given together with 200 mg of zidovudine (ie, total daily dose: 2.25 mg of zalcitabine and 600 mg of zidovudine); if zalcitabine is permanently discontinued or interrupted due to toxicities, decrease zidovudine dose to 100 mg every 4 hours

Mechanism of Action
Purine nucleoside analogue, zalcitabine or 2',3'-dideoxycitidine (ddC) has been found to have *in vitro* activity and is reported to be successful against HIV in short term clinical trials

Intracellularly, ddc is converted to active metabolite ddCTP; lack the presence of the 3'-hydroxyl group necessary for phosphodiester linkages during DNA replication. As a result viral replication is prematurely terminated. ddCTP acts as a competitor for binding sites on the HIV-RNA dependent DNA polymerase (reverse transcriptase) to further contribute to inhibition of viral replication.

Local Anesthetic/Vasoconstrictor Precautions No information available to require special precautions

Effects on Dental Treatment No effects or complications reported

Other Adverse Effects
>10%: Oral ulcers

1% to 10%:

Cardiovascular: Chest pain

Central nervous system: Headache, dizziness, myalgia, foot pain, fatigue

Dermatologic: Rash, pruritus

Gastrointestinal: Nausea, dysphagia, anorexia, abdominal pain, vomiting, diarrhea, weight decrease

Respiratory: Pharyngitis

<1%:

Cardiovascular: Edema, hypertension, palpitations, syncope, atrial fibrillation, tachycardia, heart racing

Central nervous system: Night sweats, fever, pain, malaise, asthenia

Endocrine & metabolic: Hyperglycemia, hypocalcemia

Gastrointestinal: Constipation, pancreatitis

Hepatic: Jaundice, hepatitis

Neuromuscular & skeletal: Myositis, peripheral neuropathy

Miscellaneous: Epistaxis

Drug Interactions Increased toxicity:
Amphotericin, foscarnet, and aminoglycosides may potentiate the risk of developing peripheral neuropathy or other toxicities associated with zalcitabine by interfering with the renal elimination of zalcitabine

Other drugs associated with peripheral neuropathy include chloramphenicol, cisplatin, dapsone, disulfiram, ethionamide, glutethimide, gold hydralazine, iodoquinol, isoniazid, metronidazole, nitrofurantoin, phenytoin, ribavirin, and vincristine

Concomitant use of zalcitabine with didanosine is not recommended

Drug Uptake
Absorption: Food decreases absorption by 39%

Serum half-life: 2.9 hours

Pregnancy Risk Factor C

Zanosar® *see* Streptozocin *on page 803*

Zantac® *see* Ranitidine Hydrochloride *on page 763*
Zarontin® *see* Ethosuximide *on page 343*
Zaroxolyn® *see* Metolazone *on page 573*
Zeasorb-AF® [OTC] *see* Tolnaftate *on page 855*
Zebeta® *see* Bisoprolol Fumarate *on page 115*
Zebrax® *see* Clidinium and Chlordiazepoxide *on page 214*
Zefazone® *see* Cefmetazole Sodium *on page 165*
Zephiran® [OTC] *see* Benzalkonium Chloride *on page 102*
Zephrex® *see* Guaifenesin and Pseudoephedrine *on page 409*
Zephrex LA® *see* Guaifenesin and Pseudoephedrine *on page 409*
Zerit® *see* Stavudine *on page 800*
Zestoretic® *see* Lisinopril and Hydrochlorothiazide *on page 507*
Zestril® *see* Lisinopril *on page 506*
Zetar® [OTC] *see* Coal Tar *on page 225*
Zetran® Injection *see* Diazepam *on page 268*
Ziac™ *see* Bisoprolol and Hydrochlorothiazide *on page 115*
Zidovudina (Mexico) *see* Zidovudine *on this page*

Zidovudine (zye doe' vue deen)

Related Information
Systemic Viral Diseases *on page 934*

Brand Names Retrovir®

Canadian/Mexican Brand Names Apo-Zidovudine® (Canada); Novo-AZT® (Canada); Dipedyne® (Mexico); Kenamil® (Mexico); Retrovir-AZT® (Mexico)

Therapeutic Category Antiviral Agent, Oral; Antiviral Agent, Parenteral

Synonyms Zidovudina (Mexico)

Use Management of patients with HIV infections who have had at least one episode of *Pneumocystis carinii* pneumonia or who have CD4 cell counts of ≤500/mm³; patients who have HIV-related symptoms or who are asymptomatic with abnormal laboratory values indicating HIV-related immunosuppression; does not reduce risk of transmitting HIV infections

Usual Dosage
Prevention of maternal-fetal HIV transmission:
  Neonatal: Oral: 2 mg/kg/dose every 6 hours for 6 weeks beginning 8-12 hours after birth; infants unable to receive oral dosing may receive 1.5 mg/kg I.V. infused over 30 minutes every 6 hours
  Maternal (>14 weeks gestation): Oral: 100 mg 5 times/day until the start of labor; during labor and delivery, administer zidovudine I.V. at 2 mg/kg over 1 hour followed by a continuous I.V. infusion of 1 mg/kg/hour until the umbilical cord is clamped
Asymptomatic/symptomatic HIV infection:
  Children 3 months to 12 years:
    Oral: 90-180 mg/m²/dose every 6 hours; maximum: 200 mg every 6 hours
    I.V.: 1-2 mg/kg/dose (infused over 1 hour) administered every 4 hours around-the-clock (6 doses/day)

  Adults:
    Asymptomatic HIV infection: Oral: 100 mg every 4 hours while awake (500 mg/day)
    Symptomatic HIV infection
      Oral: Initial: 200 mg every 4 hours (1200 mg/day), then after 1 month, 100 mg every 4 hours (600 mg/day)
      I.V.: 1-2 mg/kg/dose (infused over 1 hour) administered every 4 hours around-the-clock (6 doses/day)
      Patients should receive I.V. therapy only until oral therapy can be administered
  Combination therapy with zalcitabine: Oral: 200 mg with zalcitabine 0.75 mg every 8 hours

Mechanism of Action Zidovudine is a thymidine analog which interferes with the HIV viral RNA dependent DNA polymerase resulting in inhibition of viral replication

Local Anesthetic/Vasoconstrictor Precautions No information available to require special precautions

Effects on Dental Treatment No effects or complications reported

Other Adverse Effects
>10%:
  Central nervous system: Severe headache, insomnia
  Gastrointestinal: Nausea
  Hematologic: Anemia, leukopenia, neutropenia
(Continued)

Zidovudine *(Continued)*

1% to 10%:
Dermatologic: Rash, hyperpigmentation of nails (bluish-brown)
Hematologic: Changes in platelet count
<1%:
Central nervous system: Weakness, neurotoxicity, confusion, mania, seizures
Gastrointestinal: Anorexia
Hematologic: Bone marrow depression, granulocytopenia, thrombocytopenia, pancytopenia
Hepatic: Hepatotoxicity, cholestatic jaundice
Local: Tenderness
Ocular: Myopathy

Drug Interactions Increased toxicity: Coadministration with drugs that are nephrotoxic (amphotericin B), cytotoxic (flucytosine, vincristine, vinblastine, doxorubicin, interferon), inhibit glucuronidation or excretion (acetaminophen, cimetidine, indomethacin, lorazepam, probenecid, aspirin), or interfere with RBC/WBC number or function (acyclovir, ganciclovir, pentamidine, dapsone)

Drug Uptake
Absorption: Oral: Well absorbed (66% to 70%)
Serum half-life: Terminal: 60 minutes
Time to peak serum concentration: Within 30-90 minutes

Pregnancy Risk Factor C

ZilaDent® [OTC] *see* Benzocaine *on page 102*

Zinacef® *see* Cefuroxime *on page 173*

Zinc *see* Trace Metals *on page 857*

Zinc Acetate *see* Zinc Supplements *on next page*

Zinca-Pak® *see* Trace Metals *on page 857*

Zincate® *see* Zinc Supplements *on next page*

Zinc Chloride *(zink klor' ide)*

Therapeutic Category Trace Element, Parenteral

Use Cofactor for replacement therapy to different enzymes helps maintain normal growth rates, normal skin hydration and senses of taste and smell

Local Anesthetic/Vasoconstrictor Precautions No information available to require special precautions

Effects on Dental Treatment No effects or complications reported

Other Adverse Effects <1%:
Cardiovascular: Hypotension
Gastrointestinal: Indigestion, nausea, vomiting
Hematologic: Neutropenia, leukopenia
Hepatic: Jaundice
Respiratory: Pulmonary edema

Comments Clinical response may not occur for up to 6-8 weeks

Zincfrin® Ophthalmic [OTC] *see* Phenylephrine and Zinc Sulfate *on page 685*

Zinc Gelatin *(zink jel' ah tin)*

Brand Names Gelucast®

Therapeutic Category Protectant, Topical

Synonyms Dome Paste Bandage; Unna's Boot; Unna's Paste; Zinc Gelatin Boot

Use Protectant and to support varicosities and similar lesions of the lower limbs

Usual Dosage Apply externally as an occlusive boot

Local Anesthetic/Vasoconstrictor Precautions No information available to require special precautions

Effects on Dental Treatment No effects or complications reported

Other Adverse Effects 1% to 10%: Local: Irritation

Zinc Gelatin Boot *see* Zinc Gelatin *on this page*

Zincon® Shampoo [OTC] *see* Pyrithione Zinc *on page 755*

Zinc Oxide *(zink ok' side)*

Therapeutic Category Topical Skin Product

Synonyms Base Ointment; Lassar's Zinc Paste

Use Protective coating for mild skin irritations and abrasions; soothing and protective ointment to promote healing of chapped skin, diaper rash

Usual Dosage Children and Adults: Topical: Apply as required for affected areas several times daily

Mechanism of Action Mild astringent with weak antiseptic properties

Local Anesthetic/Vasoconstrictor Precautions No information available to require special precautions
Effects on Dental Treatment No effects or complications reported
Other Adverse Effects 1% to 10%:
Dermatologic: Skin sensitivity
Local: Irritation

Zinc Oxide, Cod Liver Oil, and Talc
(zink ok' side kod liv' er oyl & talc)
Brand Names Desitin® Topical [OTC]
Therapeutic Category Protectant, Topical
Use Relief of diaper rash, superficial wounds and burns, and other minor skin irritations
Usual Dosage Topical: Apply thin layer as needed
Local Anesthetic/Vasoconstrictor Precautions No information available to require special precautions
Effects on Dental Treatment No effects or complications reported
Other Adverse Effects 1% to 10%:
Dermatologic: Skin sensitivity
Local: Irritation

Zinc Sulfate see Zinc Supplements on this page

Zinc Supplements (zink)
Brand Names Eye-Sed® [OTC]; Orazinc® [OTC]; Verazinc® [OTC]; Zincate®
Therapeutic Category Mineral, Oral; Mineral, Parenteral; Trace Elements
Synonyms Zinc Acetate; Zinc Sulfate
Use Cofactor for replacement therapy to different enzymes helps maintain normal growth rates, normal skin hydration and senses of taste and smell; zinc supplement (oral and parenteral); may improve wound healing in those who are deficient. May be useful to promote wound healing in patients with pressure sores.
Mechanism of Action Provides for normal growth and tissue repair, is a cofactor for more than 70 enzymes; ophthalmic astringent and weak antiseptic due to precipitation of protein and clearing mucus from outer surface of the eye
Local Anesthetic/Vasoconstrictor Precautions No information available to require special precautions
Effects on Dental Treatment No effects or complications reported
Other Adverse Effects <1%:
Cardiovascular: Hypotension
Gastrointestinal: Indigestion, nausea, vomiting
Hematologic: Neutropenia, leukopenia
Hepatic: Jaundice
Respiratory: Pulmonary edema
Drug Interactions Decreased effect: Decreased penicillamine, decreased tetracycline effect reduced, iron decreased uptake of zinc, bran products, dairy products reduce absorption of zinc
Pregnancy Risk Factor C

Zinc Undecylenate see Undecylenic Acid and Derivatives on page 884
Zinecard® see Dexrazoxane on page 263
Zithromax™ see Azithromycin on page 90
ZNP® Bar [OTC] see Pyrithione Zinc on page 755
Zocor™ see Simvastatin on page 789
Zofran® see Ondansetron on page 637
Zoladex® Implant see Goserelin Acetate on page 404
Zolicef® see Cefazolin Sodium on page 164
Zoloft™ see Sertraline Hydrochloride on page 786

Zolpidem Tartrate (zole pi' dem tar' trate)
Brand Names Ambien™
Therapeutic Category Hypnotic; Sedative
Use Short-term treatment of insomnia
Usual Dosage Duration of therapy should be limited to 7-10 days
Adults: Oral: 10 mg immediately before bedtime; maximum dose: 10 mg
Elderly: 5 mg immediately before bedtime

Not dialyzable
Dosing adjustment in hepatic impairment: Decrease dose to 5 mg
Mechanism of Action Structurally dissimilar to benzodiazepine, however, has much or all of its actions explained by its effects on benzodiazepine (BZD)
(Continued)

Zolpidem Tartrate *(Continued)*

receptors, especially the omega-1 receptor; retains hypnotic and much of the anxiolytic properties of the BZD, but has reduced effects on skeletal muscle and seizure threshold.

Local Anesthetic/Vasoconstrictor Precautions No information available to require special precautions

Effects on Dental Treatment No effects or complications reported

Other Adverse Effects

1% to 10%:
Central nervous system: Headache, drowsiness, dizziness
Gastrointestinal: Nausea, diarrhea
Neuromuscular & skeletal: Myalgia

<1%:
Central nervous system: Amnesia, confusion
Gastrointestinal: Vomiting
Neuromuscular & skeletal: Falls, tremor

Drug Interactions Increased effect/toxicity with alcohol, CNS depressants

Drug Uptake
Onset of action: 30 minutes
Duration: 6-8 hours
Absorption: Rapid
Serum half-life: 2-2.6 hours, in cirrhosis increased to 9.9 hours

Pregnancy Risk Factor B

Dosage Forms Tablet: 5 mg, 10 mg

Zone-A Forte® *see* Pramoxine and Hydrocortisone *on page 714*

ZORprin® *see* Aspirin *on page 78*

Zostrix® [OTC] *see* Capsaicin *on page 147*

Zostrix®-HP [OTC] *see* Capsaicin *on page 147*

Zosyn™ *see* Piperacillin Sodium and Tazobactam Sodium *on page 696*

Zovirax® *see* Acyclovir *on page 23*

Z-PAKS™ *see* Azithromycin *on page 90*

Zydone® [5/500] *see* Hydrocodone and Acetaminophen *on page 431*

Zyloprim® *see* Allopurinol *on page 33*

Zymase® *see* Pancrelipase *on page 657*

Zyprexa® *see* Olanzapine *on page 635*

Zyrtec™ *see* Cetirizine Hydrochloride *on page 179*

ORAL MEDICINE

TABLE OF CONTENTS

Part I. Dental Management and Therapeutic Considerations in Medically Compromised Patients

Cardiovascular Diseases 912
Respiratory Diseases 924
Endocrine Disorders & Pregnancy 927
Rheumatoid Arthritis, Osteoarthritis, and Joint Prostheses 930
Nonviral Infectious Diseases 932
Systemic Viral Diseases 934

Part II.

Dental Management and Therapeutic Considerations in Patients With Specific Oral Conditions

Oral Pain 940
Oral Bacterial Infections 945
Oral Fungal Infections 948
Oral Viral Infections 951
Oral Nonviral Soft Tissue Ulcerations or Erosions 955
Dentin Hypersensitivity; High Caries Index; Xerostomia 959
Temporomandibular Dysfunction (TMD) 963

Other Oral Medicine Topics

Patients Requiring Sedation 965
Patients Undergoing Cancer Therapy 967
Chemical Dependency and Dental Practice 971
Animal and Human Bites Guidelines 976
Systemic Considerations Related to Natural Products for
    Weight Loss 979
Dental Office Emergencies 984

Suggested Readings 991-1001

CARDIOVASCULAR DISEASES

Cardiovascular disease is the most prevalent human disease affecting over 60 million Americans and this group of diseases accounts for more than 50% of all deaths in the United States. Surgical and pharmacologic therapy have resulted in many cardiovascular patients living healthy and profitable lives. Consequently, patients presenting to the dental office may require treatment planning modifications related to the medical management of their cardiovascular disease. For the purposes of this text, we will cover infective endocarditis and associated conditions, ischemic heart disease including angina pectoris and myocardial infarction, cardiac arrhythmias, congestive heart failure, and hypertension.

INFECTIVE ENDOCARDITIS

Infective endocarditis is a severe cardiac infection which is usually preceded by some form of bacteremia or fungemia. Microbial organisms circulating in the blood lodge on fibrinous vegetations present on the endocardium. This process most often involves defective valves that have been injured by some previous process occurring at the endocardium. The organisms gain entry via a variety of routes including the oral cavity, the genital urinary tract, or the gastrointestinal system. Damaged heart valves can become infected in an acute or subacute fashion leading to the terms subacute bacterial endocarditis or acute bacterial endocarditis. Because of the fibrinous accumulations on the valve leaflets, turbulent flow of the blood allows the microbes sufficient time to colonize these vegetations. Oftentimes, these predisposing valvular defects are evident as a heart murmur.

Rheumatic heart disease or rheumatic globular disease is the most common underlying heart defect associated with infective endocarditis accounting for nearly 60% of all cases. Congenital heart defects account for 10% to 20% and the remaining cases often do not demonstrate a specific predisposition. Hence, we have the relationship between rheumatic fever which is an autoimmune sequela to beta-hemolytic streptococcal infection. During the rheumatic fever, pericarditis or inflammation of the pericardial tissue can lead to damaged heart valves. These damaged heart valves can predispose the patient to infective endocarditis. It should be noted that not all patients who develop rheumatic fever are left with a cardiac murmur and, therefore, they may not be at risk of infective endocarditis. However, a history of rheumatic fever should be a tip-off to investigate further with evaluation regarding the presence of fibrinous vegetation around the heart which may have left the patient with a heart murmur.

Other common conditions, such as mitral valve prolapse, can also result in a turbulence of blood flow that could lead to an elevated risk of infective endocarditis.

The most commonly prescribed drugs for prevention of infective endocarditis are:

Amoxicillin Trihydrate (A-Cillin®; Amoxil®; Larotid®; Polymox®; Trimox®; Utimox®; Wymox®) *on page 58*

Ampicillin (Amcill®; Amplin®; Omnipen®; Penamp®; Polycillin®; Principen®; Totacillin®) *on page 62*

Clindamycin (Cleocin®) *on page 214*

Erythromycin (E.E.S.®; E-Mycin®; Eryc®; EryPed®; Ery-Tab®; Erythrocin®; Ilosone®; PCE®; Wyamicin®) *on page 321*

Gentamicin Sulfate (Garamycin®) *on page 396*

Vancomycin Hydrochloride (Lyphocin®; Vancocin®; Vancoled®) *on page 889*

Table 1. ABSOLUTE AND RELATIVE RISK FOR ENDOCARDITIS AMONG VARIOUS CARDIAC LESIONS
(Incidence Rate, Cases per 100,000 Patient-Years)

Lesion	Absolute	Relative
Prosthetic valves	308-630	(63-129)*
Prior native valve endocarditis, non-IVDU	300-740	(61-151)
Rheumatic heart disease	380-440	(78-90)
Congenital heart disease	120	(25)
Coarctation of the aorta		
Tetralogy of Fallot		
Bicuspid aortic valve		
Transposition of the aorta		
Patent ductus arteriosus		
Ventricular septal defect		
Mitral valve prolapse with regurgitant murmur	52	(11)
Hypertrophic cardiomyopathy		
Other acquired valvular dysfunction (eg, degenerative heart disease)		
Marfan's syndrome		

Table 2. CARDIAC LESIONS THAT RARELY PREDISPOSE TO ENDOCARDITIS

Isolated secundum type of atrial septal defect
Syphilitic aortitis
Previous coronary artery bypass graft
Mitral valve prolapse without murmur
Previous rheumatic heart disease without valvular dysfunction
Permanent cardiac pacemakers and implanted defibrillators
Surgical repair, without residua, of secundum atrial septal defect, ventricular septal defect, patent ductus arteriosus after 6 months

Adapted from Dajani AS, Bisno AL, Chung KJ, et al, "Prevention of Bacterial Endocarditis. Recommendations by the American Heart Association," *JAMA*, 1990, 264:2919.

Most dentists are acutely aware of the necessity to obtain an adequate history regarding the presence of heart murmur, the presence of rheumatic heart disease, or, at the very least, the presence of a previous history of rheumatic fever. Usually, in addition to the history and routine consultation, the patient may need special studies, including the echocardiogram. A full cardiac work-up will determine whether the patient has an organic murmur or a functional murmur. This decision is based on the location, type, and extent of any murmur detected. Organic murmurs generally are of the type that leave the patient at an elevated risk for infective endocarditis.

Table 3. CIRCUMSTANCES LIKELY TO LEAD TO TRANSIENT BACTEREMIA THAT CAN PRECEDE ENDOCARDITIS

Dental and periodontal procedure known to induce mucosal bleeding

Tonsillectomy and adenoidectomy

Bronchoscopy with rigid scope

Surgical procedure on the respiratory or intestinal mucosa

Gallbladder surgery

Esophageal dilatation and scleropathy for esophageal varices

Prostatic surgery

Vaginal hysterectomy

Cystoscopy or urethral dilatation

In the presence of infection, urethral catheterization or urologic surgery

In presence of infection, vaginal delivery, dilatation and curettage, therapeutic abortion, insertion and removal of intrauterine devices, sterilization procedures

Incision and drainage of infected tissue

Adapted from Dajani AS, Bisno AL, Chung KJ, et al, "Prevention of Bacterial Endocarditis. Recommendations by the American Heart Association," *JAMA*, 1990, 264:2919.

Table 4. PREVENTION OF BACTERIAL ENDOCARDITIS

Recommendations by the American Heart Association
(*JAMA*, 1990, 264:2919-22)

CARDIAC CONDITIONS*

Endocarditis Prophylaxis Recommended
Prosthetic cardiac valves, including bioprosthetic and homograft valves
Previous bacterial endocarditis, even in the absence of heart disease
Most congenital cardiac malformations
Rheumatic and other acquired valvular dysfunction, even after valvular surgery
Hypertrophic cardiomyopathy
Mitral valve prolapse with valvular regurgitation

Endocarditis Prophylaxis Not Recommended‡
Isolated secundum atrial septal defect
Surgical repair without residua beyond 6 months of secundum atrial septal defect, ventricular septal defect, or patent ductus arteriosus
Previous coronary artery bypass graft surgery
Mitral valve prolapse without valvular regurgitation†
Physiologic, functional, or innocent heart murmurs
Previous Kawasaki disease without valvular dysfunction
Previous rheumatic fever without valvular dysfunction
Cardiac pacemakers and implanted defibrillators

*This table lists selected conditions but is not meant to be all-inclusive.

†Individuals who have a mitral valve prolapse associated with thickening and/or redundancy of the valve leaflets may be at increased risk for bacterial endocarditis, particularly men who are 45 years of age or older.

‡In patients who have prosthetic heart valves, a previous history of endocarditis, or surgically constructed systemic-pulmonary shunts or conduits, physicians may choose to administer prophylactic antibiotics even for low-risk procedures that involve the lower respiratory, genitourinary, or gastrointestinal tracts.

Table 5. DENTAL OR SURGICAL PROCEDURES*

Endocarditis Prophylaxis Recommended
Dental procedures known to induce gingival or mucosal bleeding, including professional cleaning
Tonsillectomy and/or adenoidectomy
Surgical operations that involve intestinal or respiratory mucosa
Bronchoscopy with a rigid bronchoscope
Sclerotherapy for esophageal varices
Esophageal dilatation
Gallbladder surgery
Cystoscopy
Urethral dilatation
Urethral catheterization if urinary tract infection is present†
Urinary tract surgery if urinary tract infection is present†
Prostatic surgery
Incision and drainage of infected tissue†
Vaginal hysterectomy
Vaginal delivery in the presence of infection†

Endocarditis Prophylaxis Not Recommended‡
Dental procedures not likely to induce gingival bleeding, such as simple adjustment of orthodontic appliances or fillings above the gum line
Injection of local intraoral anesthetic (except intraligamentary injections)
Shedding of primary teeth
Tympanostomy tube insertion
Endotracheal intubation
Bronchoscopy with a flexible bronchoscope, with or without biopsy
Cardiac catheterization
Endoscopy with or without gastrointestinal biopsy
Cesarean section
In the absence of infection (for urethral catheterization, dilatation and curettage, uncomplicated vaginal delivery, therapeutic abortion, sterilization procedures, or insertion or removal of intrauterine devices

*This table lists selected conditions but is not meant to be all-inclusive.

†In addition to prophylactic regimen for genitourinary procedures, antibiotic therapy should be directed against the most likely bacterial pathogen.

‡In patients who have prosthetic heart valves, a previous history of endocarditis, or surgically constructed systemic-pulmonary shunts or conduits, physicians may choose to administer prophylactic antibiotics even for low-risk procedures that involve the lower respiratory, genitourinary, or gastrointestinal tracts.

The American Medical Association and the American Heart Association have provided precise guidelines (see "Table 6. Prophylactic Regimens for Bacterial Endocarditis") for antibiotic coverage prior to invasive procedures which may lead to a bacteremia and a subsequent elevated risk for infective endocarditis in these patients. These recommended regimens are currently under review. It is expected that new recommendations, likely affecting the requirements for follow-up dosing, will be forthcoming in the next year. Practitioners are advised to check the journals of the American Medical and Dental Associations for any recommendation changes. In any case, inappropriate use of antibiotics can be avoided by not only an adequate history but appropriate medical consultation or complete work-up prior to decisions regarding regular coverage for a potential murmur.

Table 6. PROPHYLACTIC REGIMENS FOR BACTERIAL ENDOCARDITIS

Genitourinary/gastrointestinal procedures*

Standard Regimen

Ampicillin, gentamicin, and amoxicillin	I.V. or I.M. administration of ampicillin, 2 g plus gentamicin, 1.5 mg/kg (not to exceed 80 mg) 30 minutes before procedure; followed by amoxicillin, 1.5 g orally 6 hours after initial dose; alternatively, the parenteral regimen may be repeated once 8 hours after initial dose.

Ampicillin/amoxicillin/penicillin-allergic patients

Vancomycin and gentamicin	I.V. administration of vancomycin 1 g over 1 hour, plus I.V. or I.M. administration of gentamicin, 1.5 mg/kg (not to exceed 80 mg) 1 hour before procedure; may be repeated once 8 hours after initial dose.

Alternate low-risk patients

Amoxicillin	3 g orally 1 hour before procedure; then 1.5 g 6 hours after initial dose

Dental, oral, or upper respiratory tract procedures in patients who are at risk*

Standard regimen

Amoxicillin	3 g orally 1 hour before procedure; then 1.5 g 6 hours after initial dose

Amoxicillin/penicillin-allergic patients

Erythromycin	Erythromycin ethylsuccinate, 800 mg, or erythromycin stearate, 1 g, orally 2 hours before procedure, then half the dose 6 hours after initial dose
or Clindamycin	300 mg orally 1 hour before procedure and 150 mg 6 hours after initial dose

Patients unable to take oral medications

Ampicillin	I.V. or I.M. administration of ampicillin, 2 g, 30 minutes before procedure; then I.V. or I.M. administration of ampicillin, 1 g or oral administration of amoxicillin, 1.5 g 6 hours after initial dose

Ampicillin/amoxicillin/penicillin-allergic patients unable to take oral medications

Clindamycin	I.V. administration of 300 mg 30 minutes before procedure and I.V. or oral administration of 150 mg 6 hours after initial dose

Patients considered high risk and not candidates for standard regimen†

Ampicillin, gentamicin, and amoxicillin	I.V. or I.M. administration of ampicillin, 2 g, plus gentamicin, 1.5 mg/kg (not to exceed 80 mg), 30 minutes before procedure; followed by amoxicillin, 1.5 g, orally 6 hours after initial dose; alternatively, the parenteral regimen may be repeated 8 hours after initial dose

Ampicillin/amoxicillin/penicillin-allergic patients considered high risk†

Vancomycin	I.V. administration of 1 g over 1 hour, starting 1 hour before procedure; no repeat dose necessary

*Initial pediatric doses are as follows: Ampicillin or amoxicillin: 50 mg/kg; erythromycin ethylsuccinate or erythromycin stearate: 20 mg/kg; clindamycin: 10 mg/kg; gentamicin: 2 mg/kg; and vancomycin: 20 mg/kg. Follow-up doses should be one half the initial dose. Total pediatric dose should not exceed total adult dose. The following weight ranges may also be used for the initial pediatric dose of amoxicillin: <15 kg: 750 mg; 15-30 kg: 1500 mg; and >30 kg: 3000 mg (full adult dose). Follow-up amoxicillin dose: 25 mg/kg.

†Includes those with prosthetic heart valves and other high-risk patients.

Adapted from Dajani AS, Bisno, AL, Chung KJ, et al, "Prevention of Bacterial Endocarditis. Recommendations by the American Heart Association," *JAMA*, 1990, 264:2919.

The penicillin drugs have long been used to prevent the occurrence of infective endocarditis. It should be noted, however, that even appropriate use of antibiotics may not preclude the development of endocarditis. Please see Table 6 for the complete regimens for coverage for chemoprophylaxis in the prevention of infective endocarditis.

ISCHEMIC HEART DISEASE

Any long-term decrease in the delivery of oxygen to the heart muscle can lead to the condition ischemic heart disease. Often arteriosclerosis and atherosclerosis result in a narrowing of the coronary vessels' lumina and are the most common causes of vascular ischemic heart disease. Other causes such as previous infarct, mitral valve regurgitation, and ruptured septa may also lead to ischemia in the heart muscle. The two most common major conditions that result from ischemic heart disease are angina pectoris and myocardial infarction. Sudden death, a third category, can likewise result from ischemia.

To the physician, the most common presenting sign or symptom of ischemic heart disease is chest pain. This chest pain can be of a transient nature as in angina pectoris or the result of a myocardial infarction. It is now believed that sudden death represents a separate occurrence that essentially involves the development of a lethal cardiac arrhythmia or coronary artery spasm leading to an acute shutdown of the heart muscle blood supply. Risk factors in patients for coronary atherosclerosis include cigarette smoking, elevated blood lipids, hypertension, as well as diabetes mellitus, age, and gender (male).

Lipid-lowering drugs include cholestyramine, colestipol, fluvastatin, gemfibrozil, lovastatin, nicotinic acid, pravastatin, probucol, and simvastatin (seen in the following list) have become standard treatments for patients with developing atherosclerosis in an attempt to lower blood cholesterol and thereby, indirectly reduce the risk of ischemia heart disease.

Lipid-Lowering Drugs

Cholestyramine Resin (Cholybar®; Questran®) *on page 201*

Clofibrate (Atromid-S®) *on page 217*

Colestipol Hydrochloride (Colestid®) *on page 229*

Dextrothyroxine Sodium (Choloxin®) *on page 266*

Fenofibrate (Lipidil®) *on page 356*

Fluvastatin (Lescol®) *on page 383*

Gemfibrozil (Lopid®) *on page 395*

Lovastatin (Mevacor®) *on page 516*

Niacin (Nicotinic Acid) *on page 614*

Pravastatin Sodium (Pravachol®) *on page 715*

Probucol (Lorelco®) *on page 725*

Simvastatin (Zocor™) *on page 789*

ANGINA PECTORIS

Angina pectoris is a symptomatic manifestation of ischemic heart disease characterized by thoracic pain resulting from oxygen deprivation to the heart muscle. Often metabolites build up in the vessels and the muscle tissue leading to the pain. Occasionally, the pain can radiate to the left arm or to the jaw. The pain is often midsternal and usually described as an extreme pressure sensation, not unlike an elephant sitting on one's chest (which we have all undoubtedly experienced). Three forms of angina pectoris are usually recognized. Stable angina includes chest pain that predictably is precipitated by overexertion, cold, or overactivity. Unstable angina pectoris usually is defined as a recent change in pattern of occurrence, usually a decreased threshold of stimulus and an unpredictable response to the major drug of choice, nitroglycerin. Prinzmetal's angina or variant angina often occurs due to spasm in a single large coronary artery and may have a cardiac dysrhythmia associated with it. Regardless of the type of angina pectoris, treatment includes control of risk factors, reducing oxygen demand to the myocardium, and increasing coronary blood flow.

The most common antianginal drugs fall into three categories. Nitrates are first-line drugs in the management of angina and include oral nitrate tablets or capsules. Nitrates can also be available as transcutaneous patches and are available in solution for I.V. administration. Beta-adrenergic blockers, the second category, are often used when a patient's angina responds poorly to nitrates.

Calcium channel blockers are also indicated for angina related to coronary vessel spasm with or without atherosclerosis. These drugs inhibit calcium ion passage through the slow channels of cell membranes. They tend to be used alone or in combination with nitrates and beta-blockers.

Selected antianginal drugs include:

Nitrates

Erythrityl Tetranitrate (Cardilate®) *on page 320*
Isosorbide Dinitrate (Dilitrate®; Iso-Bid®; Isonate®; Isordil®; Isotrate®; Sorbitrate®) *on page 474*
Isosorbide Mononitrate (Imdur®; Ismo™; Monoket®) *on page 474*
Nitroglycerin (various products) *on page 623*
Pentaerythritol Tetranitrate (Duotrate®; Peritrate®) *on page 669*

Beta-Adrenergic Blockers

Atenolol (Tenormin®) *on page 83*
Betaxolol Hydrochloride (Kerlone®) *on page 111*
Bisoprolol Fumarate (Zebeta®) *on page 115*
Carteolol Hydrochloride (Cartrol®; Ocupress®) *on page 158*
Nadolol (Corgard®) *on page 597*
Propranolol Hydrochloride (Betachron E-R®; Inderal®) *on page 743*
Sotalol (Betapace®) *on page 796*
Timolol Maleate (Blocadren®) *on page 847*

Calcium Channel Blockers

Amlodipine (Norvasc®) *on page 53*
Bepridil Hydrochloride (Vascor®) *on page 108*
Diltiazem (Cardizem®; Dilacor™ XR) *on page 284*
Nicardipine Hydrochloride (Cardene®) *on page 616*
Nifedipine (Adalat®; Procardia®) *on page 619*
Verapamil Hydrochloride (Calan®; Covera-HS®; Isoptin®; Verelan®) *on page 893*

The dental management of the patient with angina pectoris may include: sedation techniques for complicated procedures (see "Sedation" in Part II of this Oral Medicine section), to limit the extent of procedures, and to limit the use of local anesthesia containing 1:100,000 epinephrine to two carpules. Anesthesia without vasoconstrictor might also be selected. The appropriate use of vasoconstrictor in anesthesia, however, should be weighed against the necessity to maximize anesthesia. Please see Management of Office Emergencies in the Oral Medicine section. Complete history and appropriate referral and consultation with the patient's physician for those patients who are known to be at risk for angina pectoris is recommended.

MYOCARDIAL INFARCTION

Myocardial infarction is the leading cause of death in the United States. It is an acute irreversible ischemic event that produces an area of myocardial necrosis in the heart tissue. If a patient has a previous history of myocardial infarction, he/she may be taking a variety of drugs (ie, antihypertensives, lipid lowering drugs, ACE inhibitors, and antianginal medications) to not only prevent a second infarct, but to treat the long-term associated ischemic heart disease. Postmyocardial infarction patients are often taking anticoagulants such as warfarin and antiplatelet agents such as aspirin. Consultation with the prescribing physician by the dentist is necessary prior to invasive procedures. Temporary dose reduction may allow the dentist to proceed with most procedures.

Aspirin (various products) *on page 78*
Warfarin Sodium (Coumadin®) *on page 903*

Thrombolytic drugs, that might dissolve hemostatic plugs, may also be given on a short-term basis immediately following an infarct and include:

Alteplase (Activase®) *on page 37*
Anistreplase (Eminase®) *on page 67*
Streptokinase (Kabikinase®; Streptase®) *on page 801*
Urokinase (Abbokinase®) *on page 886*

Alteplase is also currently in use for acute myocardial infarction. Following myocardial infarction and rehabilitation, outpatients may be placed on anticoagulants (such as coumadin), diuretics, beta-adrenergic blockers, ACE inhibitors to reduce blood pressure, and calcium-channel blockers. Depending on the presence or absence of continued angina pectoris, patients may also be taking nitrates, beta-blockers, or calcium-channel blockers as indicated for treatment of angina.

BETA-ADRENERGIC BLOCKING AGENTS CATEGORIZED ACCORDING TO SPECIFIC PROPERTIES

Alpha-Adrenergic Blocking Activity

Labetalol Hydrochloride (Normodyne®, Trandate®) *on page 486*

Intrinsic Sympathomimetic Activity

Acebutolol Hydrochloride (Sectral®) *on page 12*

Pindolol (Visken®) *on page 694*

Long Duration of Action and Fewer CNS Effects

Acebutolol Hydrochloride (Sectral®) *on page 12*

Atenolol (Tenormin®) *on page 83*

Betaxolol Hydrochloride (Kerlone®) *on page 111*

Nadolol (Corgard®) *on page 597*

Beta₁-Receptor Selectivity

Acebutolol Hydrochloride (Sectral®) *on page 12*

Atenolol (Tenormin®) *on page 83*

Metoprolol (Lopressor®, Toprol XL®) *on page 574*

Non-Selective (blocks both beta₁ and beta₂ receptors)

Betaxolol Hydrochloride (Kerlone®) *on page 111*

Labetalol Hydrochloride (Normodyne®, Trandate®) *on page 486*

Nadolol (Corgard®) *on page 597*

Pindolol (Visken®) *on page 694*

Propranolol Hydrochloride (Inderal®) *on page 743*

Timolol Maleate (Blocadren®) *on page 847*

ARRHYTHMIAS

Abnormal cardiac rhythm can develop spontaneously and survivors of a myocardial infarction are often left with an arrhythmia. An arrhythmia is any alteration or disturbance in the normal rate, rhythm, or conduction through the cardiac tissue. This is known as a cardiac arrhythmia. Abnormalities in rhythm can occur in either the atria or the ventricles. Various valvular deformities, drug effects, and chemical derangements can initiate arrhythmias. These arrhythmias can be a slowing of the heart rate (<60 beats/minute) as defined in bradycardia or tachycardia resulting in a rapid heart beat (usually >150 beats/minute). The dentist will encounter a variety of treatments for management of arrhythmias. Usually, underlying causes such as reduced cardiac output, hypertension, and irregular ventricular beats will require treatment. Pacemaker therapy is also sometimes used. Indwelling pacemakers may require supplementation with antibiotics, and consultation with the physician is certainly appropriate. Sinus tachycardia is often treated with drugs such as:

Propranolol Hydrochloride (Betachron ER®; Inderal®) *on page 743*

Quinidine (Cardioquin®; Quinaglute®; Quinalan®; Quinidex®; Quinora®) *on page 759*

Beta-blockers are often used to slow cardiac rate and diazepam may be helpful when anxiety is a contributing factor in arrhythmia. When atrial flutter and atrial fibrillation are diagnosed, digitalis preparations such as digitoxin and digoxin are the drugs of choice.

Digitoxin (Crystodigin®) *on page 279*

Digoxin (Lanoxin®) *on page 280*

Patients with atrial fibrillation are also frequently placed on anticoagulants such as Coumadin®. (See Myocardial Infarction Section on previous page.)

Warfarin Sodium (Coumadin®) *on page 903*

The basis for anticoagulation therapy is that mitral stenosis may be the result of the long-term arrhythmia and there is concern over the possibility of stroke. Ventricular dysrhythmias are often treated with drugs such as quinidine, procainamide, lidocaine, beta-adrenergic agents, and calcium channel blockers. Quinidine is used for selected arrhythmias. Lidocaine is often used when there are ventricular dysrhythmias. Procainamide (Pronestyl®) or flecainide (Tambocor®) are alternative agents.

CLASSIFICATION OF ANTIARRHYTHMIC DRUGS

Supraventricular

Digitoxin (digitalis) (Crystodigin®) *on page 279*
Digoxin (Lanoxin®) *on page 280*

Supraventricular and Ventricular

Acebutolol Hydrochloride (Sectral®) *on page 12*
Adenosine (Adenocard®) *on page 25*
Amiodarone Hydrochloride (Cordarone®) *on page 48*
Atenolol (Tenormin®) *on page 83*
Bepridil Hydrochloride (Vascor®) *on page 108*
Bisoprolol Fumarate (Zebeta®) *on page 115*
Bretylium Tosylate (Bretylol®) *on page 119*
Diltiazem (Cardizem®; Dilacor™ XR) *on page 284*
Disopyramide Phosphate (Norpace®) *on page 292*
Encainide (Enkaid®) *on page 309*
Flecainide Acetate (Tambocor®) *on page 365*
Lidocaine Hydrochloride (Xylocaine®) *on page 502*
Mexiletine (Mexitil®) *on page 577*
Moricizine Hydrochloride (Ethmozine®) *on page 589*
Nicardipine Hydrochloride (Cardene®) *on page 616*
Phenytoin (Dilantin®) *on page 688*
Procainamide Hydrochloride (Pronestyl®) *on page 725*
Propafenone Hydrochloride (Rythmol®) *on page 735*
Propranolol Hydrochloride (Inderal®) *on page 743*
Quinidine (Cardioquin®; Quinaglute®; Quinalan®; Quinidex®; Quinora®) *on page 759*
Sotalol (Betapace®) *on page 796*
Tocainide Hydrochloride (Tonocard®) *on page 851*
Verapamil Hydrochloride (Calan®, Isoptin®) *on page 893*

Treatment of arrhythmias often can result in oral manifestations including oral ulcerations with drugs such as procainamide, lupus-like lesions, as well as xerostomia.

CONGESTIVE HEART FAILURE

Congestive heart failure is a clinical disease that occurs when the heart muscle gradually fails to deliver adequate oxygenated blood to the tissues. The chronically failing heart will attempt to compensate by three physiologic mechanisms: enlargement, increased heart rate, or dilitation. As the congestive heart failure becomes more profound, myocardial contractility diminishes and sodium and water retention increase leading to edema in the peripheral extremities. Edema is commonly seen in the patient with congestive heart failure. The failure of the heart may be right sided, left sided, or both. The treatment of congestive heart failure is usually rest with increased oxygenation.

The long-term treatment is to attempt to increase the strength and efficiency of the heart contractions, to avoid arrhythmias, and to reduce retention of water and sodium. Digitalis is one of the primary drugs used in treatment of congestive heart failure. It is usually prescribed in small doses and is coupled with diuretics and/or angiotensin-converting enzyme (ACE) inhibitors to decrease water retention. Nitrates and hydralazine are often given to patients with acute heart failure. The dentist may find that the patient is well compensated; however, treatment of CHF represents a complicated pharmacologic pattern necessary to be analyzed. Consultation with the managing physician regarding the patient's stability is recommended. Clinical signs of congestive heart failure might include distended neck veins, peripheral edema, and a ruddy complexion.

Digitoxin (Crystodigin®) *on page 279*
Digoxin (Lanoxin®) *on page 280*

Angiotensin-Converting Enzyme Inhibitors

Captopril (Capoten®) *on page 148*
Enalapril (Vasotec®) *on page 307*
Fosinopril (Monopril®) *on page 387*
Lisinopril (Prinivil®) *on page 506*
Quinapril Hydrochloride (Accupril®) *on page 756*
Ramipril (Altace™) *on page 762*
Trandolapril (Mavik®) *on page 858*

Direct-Acting Vasodilators

Hydralazine Hydrochloride (Apresoline®) *on page 428*

Nitrates

Erythrityl Tetranitrate (Cardilate®) *on page 320*
Isosorbide Dinitrate (Dilitrate®; Iso-Bid®; Isonate®; Isordil®;
    Isotrate®; Sorbitrate®) *on page 474*
Isosorbide Mononitrate (Imdur®; Ismo™; Monoket®) *on page 474*
Nitroglycerin (various products) *on page 623*
Pentaerythritol Tetranitrate (Duotrate®; Peritrate®) *on page 669*

HYPERTENSION

Adult blood pressure is usually measured in millimeters of mercury and represents systolic pressure that is exerted as the blood flows through the artery during a beat of the heart and the diastolic pressure when the blood is at rest between heart beats. Pulse pressure is a term commonly used and refers to the pressure difference between systolic and diastolic. Hypertension is a sustained elevated systolic or diastolic blood pressure (SBP and DBP). The definitions of elevated blood pressure and a referral scheme can be found in the following tables.

CLASSIFICATION OF BLOOD PRESSURE FOR ADULTS ≥18 YEARS OF AGE

Average DBP mm Hg	Average SBP mm Hg			
	<120	120-129	130-139	≥140
<80	Optimal*	Normal	High Normal	High
80-84	Normal	Normal	High Normal	High
85-89	High Normal	High Normal	High Normal	High
≥90	High	High	High	High

*Optimal blood pressure, with regard to cardiovascular risk, is SBP <120 mm Hg and DBP <80 mm Hg. However, unusually low readings should be evaluated for clinical significance.

Adapted from the *Joint National Committee Report*, October, 1992.

Category	Systolic (mm Hg)	Diastolic (mm Hg)	Category
Isolated systolic hypertension	>160	>120	Severe hypertension
Borderline systolic hypertension	140-159	105-120	Moderate hypertension
		90-104	Mild hypertension
Normal	<140	<90	Normal

Diastolic		
<85	Recheck at recall (within 2 years)	No restriction
85-89	Recheck at recall (within 1 year)	No restrictions
90-99	Recheck within 2 months; if still elevated, refer to physician promptly	No restrictions
100-109	Refer promptly to physician (within 1 month)	Limited elective care or emergency care
110-119	Refer promptly to physician (within 1 week)	Limited elective care or emergency care
≥120	Immediate referral to physician	Emergency care only
Systolic		
<140	Recheck at recall (within 2 years)	No restrictions
140-199	Recheck within 2 months; if still elevated, refer to physician promptly (within 2 months)	No restrictions
≥200	Refer promptly to physician	Limited elective care or emergency care

Generally, peripheral vascular resistance, intravascular fluid volume, and cardiac output determine the blood pressure of a patient. Selection of therapies for patients being treated for prolonged elevated blood pressure is generally dependent upon the severity of the condition, age, and the pharmacological stability related to other cardiac diseases. Nonpharmacologic management of the patient with elevated sustained blood pressure begins with diet restriction, avoidance of fatty foods, an exercise program, reduction in sodium intake, and cessation of smoking. If there is an inadequate response, pharmacologic management usually begins with a diuretic or a beta-adrenergic receptor blocker.

ACE inhibitors, calcium channel blockers, alpha-adrenergic blockers are currently gaining popularity as early treatment modalities, however, data on these agents reducing long-term morbidity and mortality are only now being published. If there is an inadequate response to these drugs, practitioners often increase drug dosage, substitute another drug, or add a second agent from a different class. If there is still inadequate response, a second or third agent can be added, along with a diuretic if one has not already been utilized. Different combinations of drugs are often used in treating African-American patients.

When given in combination, these drugs can create not only side effects including xerostomia and oral ulcerations, but profound reduction in blood pressure. The new drug classification Angiotensin Receptor Antagonists with the drug Losartan® representative is showing promise as an alternative therapy. The 1992 Report of the Joint National Commission on Detection, Evaluation, and Treatment of High Blood Pressure is being re-evaluated and it is hopeful that new guidelines will be released in a 1997 or early 1998 Commission Report.

CLASSIFICATION OF ANTIHYPERTENSIVES

DIURETICS

Thiazide-Type

Bendroflumethiazide (Naturetin®) *on page 101*
Benzthiazide (Exna®) *on page 105*
Chlorothiazide (Diurigen®, Diuril®) *on page 188*
Chlorthalidone (Hygroton®) *on page 199*
Hydrochlorothiazide (Esidrix®) *on page 430*
Hydroflumethiazide (Diucardin®; Saluron®) *on page 437*
Indapamide (Lozol®) *on page 455*
Metolazone (Mykrox®, Zaroxolyn®) *on page 573*
Methyclothiazide (Aquatensen®, Enduron®) *on page 565*
Polythiazide (Renese®) *on page 705*
Quinethazone (Hydromox®) *on page 758*
Trichlormethiazide (Metahydrin®; Naqua®) *on page 867*

Loop

Bumetanide (Bumenex®) *on page 126*
Ethacrynic Acid (Edecrin®) *on page 331*
Furosemide (Lasix®) *on page 391*
Torsemide (Demadex®) *on page 856*

Potassium-Sparing

Amiloride Hydrochloride (Midamor®) *on page 45*
Spironolactone (Aldactone®) *on page 798*
Triamterene (Dyrenium®) *on page 865*

Potassium-Sparing Combinations

Hydrochlorothiazide and Spironolactone (Aldactazide®; Alazide®; Spironazide®; Spirozide®) *on page 431*
Triamterene and Hydrochlorothiazide (Dyazide®; Maxide®) *on page 865*

ADRENERGIC INHIBITORS

Noncardioselective Beta-Adrenergic Blockers

Carteolol Hydrochloride (Cartrol®, Ocupress®) *on page 158*
Carvedilol (Coreg®) *on page 159*
Nadolol (Corgard®) *on page 597*
Penbutolol (Levatol®) *on page 664*
Pindolol (Visken®) *on page 694*
Propranolol Hydrochloride (Inderal®) *on page 743*
Timolol Maleate (Blocadren®) *on page 847*

Cardioselective Beta-Adrenergic Blockers

Acebutolol Hydrochloride (Sectral®) *on page 12*
Atenolol (Tenormin®) *on page 83*
Betaxolol Hydrochloride (Betoptic®, Kerlone®) *on page 111*
Bisoprolol (Zebeta™) *on page 115*

Metoprolol (Lopressor®, Toprol XL®) *on page 574*
Sotalol (Betapace®) *on page 796*

Combined Alpha- and Beta-Adrenergic Blockers
Labetalol Hydrochloride (Normodyne®, Trandate®) *on page 486*

Alpha-Adrenergic Blockers - Peripheral-Acting (Alpha₁-Blockers)
Doxazosin (Cardura®) *on page 298*
Guanadrel Sulfate (Hylorel®) *on page 411*
Guanethidine Sulfate (Ismelin®) *on page 412*
Prazosin Hydrochloride (Minipress®) *on page 717*
Reserpine (Serpasil®) *on page 765*
Terazosin (Hytrin®) *on page 821*

Alpha-Adrenergic Blockers - Central-Acting (Alpha₂-Agonists)
Clonidine (Catapres®) *on page 221*
Guanabenz Acetate (Wytensin®) *on page 411*
Guanfacine Hydrochloride (Tenex®) *on page 413*
Methyldopa (Aldomet®) *on page 566*

VASODILATORS
Direct-Acting
Hydralazine Hydrochloride (Apresoline®) *on page 428*
Minoxidil (Loniten®) *on page 583*

Angiotensin-Converting Enzyme Inhibitors
Benazepril Hydrochloride (Lotensin®) *on page 99*
Captopril (Capoten®) *on page 148*
Enalapril (Vasotec®) *on page 307*
Fosinopril (Monopril®) *on page 387*
Lisinopril (Prinivil®) *on page 506*
Moexipril Hydrochloride (Univasc®) *on page 587*
Quinapril Hydrochloride (Accupril®) *on page 756*
Ramipril (Altace™) *on page 762*
Spirapril (Renormax®) *on page 798*
Trandolapril (Mavik®) *on page 798*

Angiotensin-Converting Enzyme Inhibitors Combinations
Captopril and Hydrochlorothiazide (Capozide®) *on page 149*
Enalapril and Hydrochlorothiazide (Vasoretic®) *on page 309*
Lisinopril and Hydrochlorothiazide (Prinzide®; Zestoretic®) *on page 507*

Calcium Channel Blockers
Amlodipine (Norvasc®) *on page 53*
Bepridil Hydrochloride (Vascor®) *on page 108*
Diltiazem (Cardizem®, Dilacor™ XR) *on page 284*
Felodipine (Plendil®) *on page 354*
Isradipine (DynaCirc®) *on page 476*
Nicardipine Hydrochloride (Cardene®) *on page 616*
Nifedipine (Adalat®, Procardia®) *on page 619*
Nisoldipine (Sular™) *on page 622*
Verapamil Hydrochloride (Calan®, Isoptin®) *on page 893*

Angiotensin Receptor Antagonists
Losartan Potassium (Cozaar®) *on page 515*

The most common oral side effects of the management of the hypertensive patient are related to the antihypertensive drug therapy. A dry sore mouth can be caused by diuretics and central-acting adrenergic inhibitors. Occasionally, lichenoid reactions can occur in patients taking quinidine and methyldopa. The thiazides are occasionally also implicated. Lupus-like face rashes can be seen in patients taking calcium channel blockers as well as documented gingival hyperplasia in Appendix; see listing below.

Calcium Channel Blockers & Gingival Hyperplasia *on page 1010*

RESPIRATORY DISEASES

Diseases of the respiratory system put dental patients at increased risk in the dental office because of their decreased pulmonary reserve, the medications they may be taking, drug interactions between these medications, medications the dentist may prescribe, and in some patients with infectious respiratory diseases, a risk of disease transmission.

The respiratory system consists of the nasal cavity, the nasopharynx, the trachea, and the components of the lung including, of course, the bronchi, the bronchioles, and the alveoli. The diseases that affect the lungs and the respiratory system can be separated by location of affected tissue. Diseases that affect the lower respiratory tract are often chronic, although infections can also occur. Three major diseases that affect the lower respiratory tract are often encountered in the medical history for dental patients. These include chronic bronchitis, emphysema, and asthma. Diseases that affect the upper respiratory tract are usually of the infectious nature and include sinusitis and the common cold. The upper respiratory tract infections may also include a wide variety of nonspecific infections, most of which are also caused by viruses. Influenza produces upper respiratory type symptoms and is often caused by orthomyxoviruses. Herpangina is caused by the Coxsackie type viruses and results in upper respiratory infections in addition to pharyngitis or sore throat. One serious condition, known as croup, has been associated with *Haemophilus influenzae* infections. Other more serious infections might include respiratory syncytial virus, adenoviruses, and parainfluenza viruses.

The respiratory symptoms that are often encountered in both upper respiratory and lower respiratory disorders include cough, dyspnea (difficulty in breathing), the production of sputum, hemoptysis (coughing up blood), a wheeze, and occasionally chest pain. One additional symptom, orthopnea (difficulty in breathing when lying down) is often used by the dentist to assist in evaluating the patient with the condition, pulmonary edema. This condition results from either respiratory disease or congestive heart failure.

No effective drug treatments are available for the management of many of the upper respiratory tract viral infections. However, amantadine (sold under the brand name Symmetrel®) is a synthetic drug given orally (200 mg/day) and has been found to be effective against some strains of influenza. Treatment other than for influenza includes supportive care products available over the counter. These might include antihistamines for symptomatic relief of the upper respiratory congestion, antibiotics to combat secondary bacterial infections, and in severe cases, fluids when patients have become dehydrated during the illness (see Therapeutic Category Index for selection). The treatment of herpangina may include management of the painful ulcerations of the oropharynx. The dentist may become involved in managing these lesions in a similar way to those seen in other acute viral infections (see Viral Infection section).

SINUSITIS

Sinusitis also represents an upper respiratory infection that often comes under the purview of the practicing dentist. Acute sinusitis characterized by nasal obstruction, fever, chills, and midface head pain may be encountered by the dentist and discovered as part of a differential work-up for other facial or dental pain. Chronic sinusitis may likewise produce similar dental symptoms. Dental drugs of choice may include ephedrine or nasal drops, antihistamines, and analgesics. These drugs sometimes require supplementation with antibiotics. Most commonly, broad spectrum antibiotics, such as ampicillin, are prescribed. These are often combined with antral lavage to re-establish drainage from the sinus area. Surgical intervention such as a Caldwell-Luc procedure opening into the sinus is rarely necessary and many of the second generation antibiotics such as cephalosporins are used successfully in treating the acute and chronic sinusitis patient (see Bacterial Infection section).

LOWER RESPIRATORY DISEASES

Lower respiratory tract diseases, including asthma, chronic bronchitis, and emphysema are often identified in dental patients. Asthma is an intermittent respiratory disorder that produces recurrent bronchial smooth muscle spasm, inflammation, swelling of the bronchial mucosa, and hypersecretion of mucus. The incidence of childhood asthma appears to be increasing and may be related to the presence of pollutants such as sulfur dioxide and indoor cigarette smoke. The end result is widespread narrowing of the airways and decreased ventilation with increased airway resistance, especially to expiration. Asthmatic patients often suffer from asthmatic attacks when stimulated by respiratory tract infections, exercise, and cold air. Medications such as aspirin and some nonsteroidal anti-inflammatory agents as well as cholinergic and beta-adrenergic blocking drugs, can also trigger asthmatic attacks in addition to chemicals, smoke, and emotional anxiety.

The classical chronic obstructive pulmonary diseases (COPD) of chronic bronchitis and emphysema are both characterized by chronic airflow obstructions during normal ventilatory efforts. They often occur in combination in the same patient and their treatment is similar. One common finding is that the patient is often a smoker. The dentist can play a role in reinforcement of smoking cessation in patients with chronic respiratory diseases.

Treatments include a variety of drugs depending on the severity of the symptoms and the respiratory compromise upon full respiratory evaluation. Patients who are having acute and chronic obstructive pulmonary attacks may be susceptible to infection and antibiotics such as penicillin, ampicillin, tetracycline, or trimethoprim-sulfamethoxazole are often used to eradicate susceptible infective organisms. Corticosteroids, as well as a wide variety of respiratory stimulants, are available in inhalant and/or oral forms. In patients using inhalant medication, oral candidiasis is occasionally encountered.

Amantadine Hydrochloride (Symadine®; Symmetrel®) *on page 41*

Analgesics *on page 1113*
Antibiotics *on page 1117*
Antihistamines *on page 1123*
Decongestants *on page 1133*
Epinephrine (Dental) (Sus-Phrine®) *on page 313*

SPECIFIC DRUGS USED IN THE TREATMENT OF CHRONIC RESPIRATORY CONDITIONS

SYMPATHOMIMETIC AMINES

Beta$_2$-Selective

Albuterol (Proventil®,Ventolin®) *on page 27*
Bitolterol Mesylate (Tornalate®) *on page 116*
Isoetharine (Bronkosol®, Bronkometer®) *on page 470*
Metaproterenol Sulfate (Alupent®) *on page 550*
Pirbuterol Acetate (Maxair™) *on page 698*
Salmeterol Xinafoate (Serevent®) *on page 778*
Terbutaline Sulfate (Brethine®, Brethaire®) *on page 822*

Methylxanthines

Oxytriphylline (Choledyl®)
Theophylline/Aminophylline (Theo-Dur®,Slo-Bid®, Somophyllin®) *on page 832*

Mast Cell Stabilizer

Cromolyn Sodium (Intal®) *on page 235*
Nedocromil Sodium (Tilade®) *on page 607*

Corticosteroids

Beclomethasone Dipropionate (Beclovent®, Vanceril®) *on page 97*
Dexamethasone (Decadron® phosphate Respihaler®) *on page 260*
Flunisolide (Aerobid®) *on page 372*
Prednisone (Deltasone®; Liquid Pred®; Meticorten®; Prednicen-M®; Sterapred®) *on page 719*
Triamcinolone (Azmacort™) *on page 862*

Anticholinergics

Ipratropium Bromide (Atrovent®) *on page 467*

Other respiratory diseases include tuberculosis and sarcoidosis which are considered to be restrictive granulomatous respiratory diseases. Tuberculosis will be covered in "Nonviral Infectious Diseases." Sarcoidosis is a condition that at one time was thought to be similar to tuberculosis, however, it is a multisystem disorder of unknown origin which has as a characteristic lymphocytic and mononuclear phagocytic accumulation in epithelioid granulomas within the lung. It occurs worldwide but shows a slight increased prevalence in temperate climates. The treatment of sarcoidosis is usually one that corresponds to its usually benign course, however, many patients are placed on corticosteroids at the level of 40-60 mg of prednisone daily. This treatment is continued for a protracted period of time. As in any disease requiring steroid therapy, consideration of adrenal suppression is necessary. Alteration of steroid dosage prior to stressful dental procedures may be necessary, usually increasing the steroid dosage prior to and during the stressful procedures and then gradually returning the patient to the original dosage over several days. Even in the absence of evidence of adrenal suppression, consultation with the prescribing physician for appropriate dosing and timing of procedures is advisable.

Prednisone *on page 719*

RELATIVE POTENCY OF ENDOGENOUS AND SYNTHETIC CORTICOSTEROIDS

Agent	Equivalent Dose (mg)
Short-Acting (8-12 h)	
Cortisol	20
Cortisone	25
Intermediate-Acting (18-36 h)	
Prednisolone	5
Prednisone	5
Methylprednisolone	4
Triamcinolone	4
Long-Acting (36-54 h)	
Betamethasone	0.75
Dexamethasone	0.75

Potential drug interactions for the respiratory disease patient exist. An acute sensitivity to aspirin-containing drugs and some of the nonsteroidal anti-inflammatory drugs is a threat for the asthmatic patient. Barbiturates and narcotics may occasionally precipitate asthmatic attacks as well. Erythromycin, clarithromycin, and ketoconazole are contraindicated in patients who are taking theophylline due to potential enhancement of theophylline toxicity. Patients that are taking steroid preparations as part of their respiratory therapy may require alteration in dosing prior to stressful dental procedures. The physician should be consulted.

Barbiturates *on page 1129*
Clarithromycin *on page 212*
Erythromycin *on page 321*
Ketoconazole *on page 481*

ENDOCRINE DISORDERS & PREGNANCY

The human endocrine system manages metabolism and homeostasis. Numerous glandular tissues produce hormones that act in broad reactions with tissues throughout the body. Cells in various organ systems may be sensitive to the hormone, or they release, in reaction to the hormone, a second hormone that acts directly on another organ. Diseases of the endocrine system may have importance in dentistry. For the purposes of this section, we will limit our discussion to diseases of the thyroid tissues, diabetes mellitus, and conditions requiring the administration of synthetic hormones, and pregnancy.

THYROID

Thyroid diseases can be classified into conditions that cause the thyroid to be overactive (hyperthyroidism) and those that cause the thyroid to be underactive (hypothyroidism). Clinical signs and symptoms associated with hyperthyroidism may include goiter, heat intolerance, tremor, weight loss, diarrhea, and hyperactivity. Thyroid hormone production can be tested by TSH levels and additional screens may include radioactive iodine uptake or a pre-T_4 (tetraiodothyronine, thyroxine) assay or iodine index or total serum T_3 (triiodothyronine). The results of thyroid function tests may be altered by ingestion of antithyroid drugs such as propylthiouracil, estrogen-containing drugs, and organic and inorganic iodides. When a diagnosis of hyperthyroidism has been made, treatment usually begins with antithyroid drugs which may include propranolol coupled with radioactive iodides as well as surgical procedures to reduce thyroid tissue. Generally, the beta-blockers are used to control cardiovascular effects of excessive T_4. Propylthiouracil or methimazole are the most common antithyroid drugs used. The dentist should be aware that epinephrine is definitely contraindicated in patients with uncontrolled hyperthyroidism.

Diseases and conditions associated with hypothyroidism may include bradycardia, drowsiness, cold intolerance, thick dry skin, and constipation. Treatment of hypothyroidism is generally with replacement thyroid hormone until a euthyroid state is achieved. Various preparations are available, the most common is levothyroxine, commonly known as Synthroid® or Levothroid® and is generally the drug of choice for thyroid replacement therapy.

Drugs to Treat Hypothyroidism

> Levothyroxine Sodium (Levothroid®; Synthroid®) *on page 498*
> Liothyronine Sodium (Cytomel®; Tristat™) *on page 504*
> Liotrix (Euthroid®; Thyrolar®) *on page 505*
> Thyroid (Armour® Thyroid; S-P-T; Thyrar®; Thyroid Strong®) *on page 844*

Drugs to Treat Hyperthyroidism

> Methimazole (Tapazole®) *on page 556*
> Potassium Iodide (Iosat®; Pima®; Potassium Iodide Enseals®; SSKI®; Thyro-Block®) *on page 711*
> Propranolol Hydrochloride (Betachron E-R®; Inderal®) *on page 743*
> Propylthiouracil *on page 746*

DIABETES

Diabetes mellitus refers to a condition of prolonged hyperglycemia associated with either abnormal production or lack of production of insulin. Commonly known as Type 1 diabetes, insulin-dependent diabetes (IDDM) is a condition where there are absent or deficient levels of circulating insulin therefore triggering tissue reactions associated with prolonged hyperglycemia. The kidney's attempt to excrete the excess glucose and the organs that do not receive adequate glucose essentially are damaged. Small vessels and arterial vessels in the eye, kidney, and brain are usually at the greatest risk. Generally, blood sugar levels between 70-120 mg/dL are considered to be normal. Inadequate insulin levels allow glucose to rise to greater than the renal threshold which is 180 mg/dL, and such elevations prolonged lead to organ damage.

The goals of treatment of the diabetic are to maintain metabolic control of the blood glucose levels and to reduce the morbid effects of periodic hyperglycemia. Insulin therapy is the primary mechanism to attain management of consistent insulin levels. Insulin preparations are categorized according to their duration of action. Generally, NPH or intermediate-acting insulin and long-acting insulin can be used in combination with short-acting or regular insulin to maintain levels consistent throughout the day.

In Type 2 or noninsulin-dependent diabetes (NIDDM), the receptor for insulin in the tissues is generally down regulated and the glucose, therefore, is not utilized at an appropriate rate. There is perhaps a stronger genetic basis for noninsulin-dependent diabetes than for Type 1. Treatment of the diabetes Type 2 patient is generally directed toward early nonpharmacologic intervention, mainly weight reduction, moderate exercise, and lower plasma-glucose concentrations. Oral hypoglycemic agents as seen in the list below are often used to maintain blood sugar levels. Often 30% of Type 2 diabetics require insulin as well as oral hypoglycemics in order to manage their diabetes. Generally, the two classes of oral hypoglycemics are the sulfonylureas and the biguanides. The sulfonylureas are prescribed more frequently and they stimulate beta cell production of insulin, increased glucose utilization, and tend to normalize glucose metabolism in the liver. The uncontrolled diabetic may represent a challenge to the dental practitioner.

TYPES OF INSULIN

Type	Action	Duration (h)
Regular	Rapid	5-7
Semilente	Rapid	10-14
Lispro	Rapid	3.5 h
NPH	Intermediate	18-24
Lente	Intermediate	14-20
Ultralente	Prolonged	>36

ORAL HYPOGLYCEMIC DRUGS

Generic Name	Trade Name
First-Generation Sulfonylureas	
Acetohexamide	Dymelor®
Chlorpropamide	Diabinese®
Tolazamide	Tolinase®
Tolbutamide	Orinase®
Second-Generation Sulfonylureas	
Glimepiride	Amaryl®
Glipizide	Glucotrol®, Glucotrol XL®
Glyburide	Diaβeta®, Micronase®, Glynase™ PresTab™
Biguanides	
Metformin	Glucophage®

Oral Hypoglycemic Agents

Acarbose (Precose®) *on page 12*
Acetohexamide (Dymelor®) *on page 19*
Chlorpropamide (Diabinese®) *on page 197*
Glimepiride (Amaryl®) *on page 398*
Glipizide (Glucotrol®) *on page 399*
Glyburide (Diaβeta; Glynase™; PresTab™; Micronase®) *on page 401*
Insulin Preparations (various products) *on page 459*
Metformin Hydrochloride (Glucophage®) *on page 551*
Tolazamide (Tolinase®) *on page 852*
Tolbutamide (Orinase®) *on page 853*

Adjunct Therapy

Cisapride (Propulsid®) *on page 209*
Metoclopramide (Clopra®; Maxolon®; Octamide®; Reglan®) *on page 572*

Oral manifestations of uncontrolled diabetes might include abnormal neutrophil function resulting in a poor response to periodontal pathogens. Increased risk of gingivitis and periodontitis in these patients is common. Candidiasis is a frequent occurrence. Denture sore mouth may be more prominent and poor wound healing following extractions may be one of the complications encountered.

HORMONAL THERAPY

Two uses of hormonal supplementation include oral contraceptives and estrogen replacement therapy. Drugs used for contraception interfere with fertility by inhibiting release of follicle stimulating hormone, luteinizing hormone, and by preventing ovulation. There are few oral side effects; however, moderate gingivitis, similar to that seen during pregnancy, has been reported. The dentist should be aware that decreased effect of oral contraceptives has been reported with most antibiotics. See individual monographs for specific details. Drugs commonly encountered include:

Estradiol (various products) *on page 325*
Ethinyl Estradiol and Ethynodiol Diacetate (Demulen®) *on page 335*
Ethinyl Estradiol and Levonorgestrel (Levlen®, Nordette®, Tri-Level®, Triphasil™) *on page 337*
Ethinyl Estradiol and Norethindrone (Ortho-Novum™, Ortho-Novum™ 1/35) *on page 339*
Levonorgestrel (Norplant®) *on page 497*
Medroxyprogesterone Acetate (Amen®; Curretab®; Cycrin®; Depo-Provera®; Provera®) *on page 533*
Mestranol and Norethindrone (Ortho-Novum™ 1/50) *on page 547*
Mestranol and Norethynodrel (Enovid®) *on page 549*
Norethindrone (Aygestin®; Micronor®; Norlutate®; Norlutin®; Nor-Q.D.®) *on page 627*
Norgestrel (Ovrette®) *on page 629*

Estrogens or derivatives are usually prescribed as replacement therapy following menopause or cyclic irregularities and to inhibit osteoporosis. The following list of drugs may interact with antidepressants and barbiturates.

Chlorotrianisene (TACE®) *on page 189*
Estrogens, Conjugated (Premarin®) *on page 327*
Estrogens, Esterified (Estratab®; Menest®) *on page 328*
Estrogens and Medroxyprogesterone (Prempro®) *on page 327*
Estrogens With Methyltestosterone (Estratest®; Premarin®) *on page 329*
Estrone (Estronol®; Kestrone®; Theelin®) *on page 329*
Estropipate (Ogen®; Ortho-Est®) *on page 330*
Ethinyl Estradiol (Estinyl®) *on page 334*
Quinestrol (Estrovis®) *on page 757*

PREGNANCY

Normal endocrine and physiologic functions are altered during pregnancy. Endogenous estrogens and progesterone increase and placental hormones are secreted. Thyroid stimulating hormone and growth hormone also increase. Cardiovascular changes can result and increased blood volume can lead to blood pressure elevations and transient heart murmurs. Generally, in a normal pregnancy, oral gingival changes will be limited to gingivitis. Alteration of treatment plans might include limiting administration of all drugs to emergency procedures only during the first and third trimesters and medical consultation regarding the patients' status for all elective procedures. Limiting dental care throughout pregnancy to preventive procedures is not unreasonable.

RHEUMATOID ARTHRITIS, OSTEOARTHRITIS, AND JOINT PROSTHESES

Arthritis and its variations represent the most common chronic musculoskeletal disorders of man. The conditions can essentially be divided into rheumatoid, osteoarthritic, and polyarthritic presentations. Differences in age of onset and joint involvement exist and it is now currently believed that the diagnosis of each may be less clear than previously thought. These autoinflammatory diseases have now been shown to affect young and old alike. Criteria for a diagnosis of rheumatoid arthritis include a positive serologic test for rheumatoid factor, subcutaneous nodules, affected joints on opposite sides of the body, and clear radiographic changes. The hematologic picture includes moderate normocytic hypochromic anemia, mild leukocytosis, and mild thrombocytopenia. During acute inflammatory periods, C-reactive protein is elevated and IgG and IgM (rheumatoid factors) can be detected. Osteoarthritis lacks these diagnostic features.

Other systemic conditions, such as systemic lupus erythematosus and Sjögren's syndrome, are often found simultaneously with some of the arthritic conditions. The treatment of arthritis includes the use of slow-acting and rapid-acting anti-inflammatory agents ranging from the gold salts to aspirin (see following listings). Long-term usage of these drugs can lead to numerous adverse effects including bone marrow suppression, platelet suppression, and oral ulcerations. The dentist should be aware that steroids (usually prednisone) are often prescribed along with the listed drugs and are often used in dosages sufficient to induce adrenal suppression. Adjustment of dosing prior to invasive dental procedures may be indicated along with consultation with the managing physician. Alteration of steroid dosage prior to stressful dental procedures may be necessary, usually increasing the steroid dosage prior to and during the stressful procedures and then gradually returning the patient to the original dosage over several days. Even in the absence of evidence of adrenal suppression, consultation with the prescribing physician for appropriate dosing and timing of procedures is advisable.

Gold Salts

Auranofin (Ridaura®) *on page 87*
Aurothioglucose (Myochrysine®) *on page 87*

Metabolic Inhibitor

Methotrexate *on page 559*

Nonsteroidal Anti-inflammatory Agents

Diclofenac (Cataflam®, Voltaren®) *on page 271*
Diflunisal (Dolobid®) *on page 278*
Etodolac (Lodine®) *on page 347*
Fenoprofen Calcium (Nalfon®) *on page 356*
Flurbiprofen Sodium (Ansaid®) *on page 381*

Ibuprofen (Motrin®) *on page 447*
Indomethacin (Indocin®) *on page 457*
Ketoprofen (Orudis®) *on page 483*
Ketorolac (Toradol®) *on page 484*
Meclofenamate Sodium (Meclomen®) *on page 531*
Nabumetone (Relafen®) *on page 596*
Naproxen (Naprosyn®) *on page 606*
Oxaprozin (Daypro™) *on page 643*
Piroxicam (Feldene®) *on page 699*
Sulindac (Clinoril®) *on page 813*
Tolmetin Sodium (Tolectin®) *on page 854*

Salicylates

Aspirin *on page 78*
Choline Magnesium Salicylate (Trilisate®) *on page 202*
Salsalate (Argesic®-SA, Artha-G®, Disalcid®, Mono-Gesic®, Salflex®, Salgesic®, Salsitab®) *on page 779*

Other

Hydroxychloroquine Sulfate (Plaquenil®) *on page 440*
Prednisone *on page 719*

ANTI-INFLAMMATORY AGENTS USED IN THE TREATMENT OF RHEUMATOID ARTHRITIS, OSTEOARTHRITIS, AND JOINT PROSTHESES

Drug	Adverse Effects
SLOW-ACTING	
GOLD SALTS	
Aurothioglucose I.M. parenteral injection (Myochrysine®); Auranofin (Ridaura®)	GI intolerance, diarrhea; leukopenia, thrombocytopenia, and/or anemia; skin and oral eruptions; possible nephrotoxicity and hepatotoxicity
METABOLIC INHIBITOR	
Methotrexate	Oral ulcerations, leukopenia
OTHER	
Hydroxychloroquine (Plaquenil®)	Usually mild and reversible; ophthalmic complications
Prednisone	Insomnia, nervousness, indigestion, increased appetite
RAPID-ACTING	
SALICYLATES	
Aspirin	Inhibition of platelet aggregation; gastrointestinal (GI) irritation, ulceration, and bleeding; tinnitus; teratogenicity
Choline magnesium salicylate (Trilisate®)	GI irritation and ulceration, weakness, skin rash, hemolytic anemia, troubled breathing
Salsalate	
OTHER NONSTEROIDAL ANTI-INFLAMMATORY DRUGS	
Diclofenac (Cataflam®, Voltaren®); Diflunisal (Dolobid®); Etodolac (Lodine®); Fenoprofen calcium (Nalfon®); Flurbiprofen sodium (Ansaid®); Ibuprofen (Motrin®); Indomethacin (Indocin®); Ketoprofen (Orudis®); Ketorolac tromethamine (Toradol®); Meclofenamate (Meclomen®); Nabumetone (Relafen®); Naproxen (Naprosyn®); Oxaprozin (Daypro™); Phenylbutazone; Piroxicam (Feldene®); Salsalate (Argesic®-SA, Artha-G®, Disalcid®, Mono-Gesic®, Salflex®, Salgesic®, Salsitab®); Sulindac (Clinoril®); Tolmetin (Tolectin®)	GI irritation, ulceration, and bleeding; inhibition of platelet aggregation; displacement of protein-bound drugs (eg, oral anticoagulants, sulfonamides, and sulfonylureas); headache; vertigo; mucocutaneous rash or ulceration; parotid enlargement

JOINT PROSTHESES

A controversial subject in appropriate therapeutics involves concern over bacteremia in patients with orthopedic joint prostheses. The concern is that infection surrounding an artificial joint may lead to rejection of the prosthesis; when encountered, bacteremia is the common cause. The controversy arises since such infections are rarely caused by bacteria of oral origin. When the orthopedist is concerned, a penicillin-related drug is usually recommended; however, there is seldom consensus on the dosage and appropriate regimen. Consultation with the orthopedic surgeon is advisable and consideration must be given to the risk of overprescribing antibiotics.

NONVIRAL INFECTIOUS DISEASES

Nonviral infectious diseases are numerous. For the purposes of this text, discussion will be limited to tuberculosis, gonorrhea, and syphilis.

TUBERCULOSIS

Tuberculosis is caused by the organism *Mycobacterium tuberculosis* as well as a variety of other mycobacteria including *M. bovis*, *M. avium-intracellulare*, and *M. kansasii*. Diagnosis of tuberculosis can be made from a skin test and a positive chest x-ray as well as acid-fast smears of cultures from respiratory secretions. Nucleic acid probes and polymerase chain reaction (PCR) to identify nucleic acid of *M. tuberculosis* have recently become useful.

The treatment of tuberculosis is based on the general principle that multiple drugs should reduce infectivity within 2 weeks and that failures in therapy may be due to noncompliance with the long-term regimens necessary. General treatment regimens last 6-12 months.

Isoniazid-resistant and multidrug-resistant mycobacterial infections have become an increasingly significant problem in recent years. TB as an opportunistic disease in HIV-positive patients has also risen. Combination drug therapy has always been popular in TB management and the advent of new antibiotics has not diminished this need.

ANTITUBERCULOSIS DRUGS

Bactericidal Agents

Capreomycin Sulfate (Capastat®) *on page 147*
*Isoniazid (INH™; Laniazid®; Nydrazid®) *on page 471*
Kanamycin Sulfate (Kantrex®) *on page 479*
*Pyrazinamide *on page 752*
Rifabutin (Mycobutin®) *on page 769*
*Rifampin (Rifadin®; Rimactane®) *on page 769*
*Streptomycin Sulfate *on page 802*

Bacteriostatic Agents

Cycloserine (Seromycin® Pulvules®) *on page 242*
*Ethambutol Hydrochloride (Myambutol®) *on page 332*
Ethionamide (Trecaton® SC) *on page 342*
Para-Aminosalicylate Sodium *on page 658*

*Drugs of Choice

SEXUALLY TRANSMITTED DISEASES

Sexually transmitted diseases (STDs) represent a group of infectious diseases that include bacterial, fungal, and viral etiologies. Several related infections are covered elsewhere. Gonorrhea and syphilis will be covered here.

The management of a patient with a STD begins with identification. Paramount to the correct management of patients with a history of gonorrhea or syphilis is when the condition was diagnosed, how and with what agent it was treated, did the condition recur, and are there any residual signs and symptoms potentially indicating active disease. With universal precautions, the patient with *Neisseria gonorrhoea* or *Treponema pallidum* infection pose little threat to the dentist; however, diagnosis of oral lesions may be problematic. Gonococcal pharyngitis, primary syphilitic lesions (chancre), secondary syphilitic lesions (mucous patch), and tertiary lesions (gumma) may be identified by the dentist.

Drugs used in treatment of gonorrhea/syphilis include:

Cefixime (Suprax®) *on page 165*
Ceftriaxone Sodium (Rocephin®) *on page 172*
Ciprofloxacin Hydrochloride (Cipro™) *on page 208*
Doxycycline (alternate) (Doryx®; Doxy®; Doxychel®; Vibramycin®; Vibra-Tabs®) *on page 301*
Ofloxacin (Floxin®; Ocuflox™) *on page 634*
Penicillin G Benzathine, Parenteral (Bicillin® L-A; Permapen®) *on page 665*
Penicillin G, Parenteral, Aqueous (Pfizerpen®) *on page 666*
Spectinomycin Hydrochloride (alternate) (Spectam®; Trobicin®) *on page 798*

The drugs listed above are often used alone or in stepped regimens, particularly when there is concomitant *Chlamydia* infection or when there is evidence of disseminated disease. The proper treatment for syphilis depends on the state of the disease.

Current treatment regimens for syphilis include:

1°, 2°, early latent (<1 y)	Benzathine penicillin G I.M.: 2-4 million units x 1 (alternate doxycycline)
Latent (>1 y), gumma, or cardiovascular	As above but once weekly for 3 weeks
Neurosyphilis	Aqueous penicillin G I.V.: 12-24 million units/day for 14 days

SYSTEMIC VIRAL DISEASES

HEPATITIS

The hepatitis viruses are a group of DNA and RNA viruses that produce symptoms associated with inflammation of the liver. Currently, hepatitis A through G have been identified by immunological testing; however, hepatitis A through E have received most attention in terms of disease identification. Hepatitis A virus is an enteric virus that is a member of the Picornavirus family along with Coxsackie viruses and poliovirus. Previously known as infectious hepatitis, hepatitis A has been detected in humans for centuries. It causes acute hepatitis, often transmitted by oral-fecal contamination and having an incubation period of approximately 30 days. Typically, constitutional symptoms are present and jaundice may occur.

Drug therapy that the dentist may encounter in a patient being treated for hepatitis A would primarily include immunoglobulin. Hepatitis B virus is previously known as serum hepatitis and has particular trophism for liver cells. Hepatitis B virus causes both acute and chronic disease in susceptible patients. The incubation period is often long and the diagnosis might be made by serologic markers even in the absence of symptoms. No drug therapy for acute hepatitis B is known; however, chronic hepatitis has recently been successfully treated with alfa-interferon. There are vaccines available for hepatitis A and B. Hepatitis C virus was described in 1988 and has been formerly classified as non-A/non-B. It is clear that hepatitis C represents a high percentage of the transfusion-associated hepatitis that is seen. Treatment of acute hepatitis C infection is generally supportive. Interferon Alfa-2a therapy has been used with some success recently and interferon-alfa may be beneficial with hepatitis C related chronic hepatitis. Hepatitis D is previously known as the delta agent and is a virus that is incomplete in that it requires previous infection with hepatitis B in order to be manifested. Currently, no antiviral therapy is effective against hepatitis D. Hepatitis E virus is an RNA virus that represents a proportion of the previously classified as non-A/non-B diagnoses. There is currently no antiviral therapy against hepatitis E.

PRE-EXPOSURE PROPHYLAXIS FOR HEPATITIS B

Health care workers*

Special patient groups (eg. adolescents, infants born to HB_sAg–positive mothers, military personnel, etc)

  Hemodialysis patients†

  Recipients of certain blood products‡

Lifestyle factors

  Homosexual and bisexual men

  Intravenous drug abusers

  Heterosexually active persons with multiple sexual partners or recently acquired sexually transmitted diseases

Environmental factors

  Household and sexual contacts of HBV carriers

  Prison inmates

  Clients and staff of institutions for the mentally handicapped

  Residents, immigrants and refugees from areas with endemic HBV infection

  International travelers at increased risk of acquiring HBV infection

*The risk of hepatitis B virus (HBV) infection for health care workers varies both between hospitals and within hospitals. Hepatitis B vaccination is recommended for all health care workers with blood exposure.

†Hemodialysis patients often respond poorly to hepatitis B vaccination; higher vaccine doses or increased number of doses are required. A special formulation of one vaccine is now available for such persons (Recombivax HB®, 40 mcg/mL). The anti-HB_s (antibody to hepatitis B surface antigen) response of such persons should be tested after they are vaccinated, and those who have not responded should be revaccinated with 1-3 additional doses.

Patients with chronic renal disease should be vaccinated as early as possible, ideally before they require hemodialysis. In addition, their anti- HB_s levels should be monitored at 6- to 12-month intervals to assess the need for revaccination.

‡Patients with hemophilia should be immunized subcutaneously, not intramuscularly.

POSTEXPOSURE PROPHYLAXIS FOR HEPATITIS B*

Exposure	Hepatitis B Immune Globulin	Hepatitis B Vaccine
Perinatal	0.5 mL I.M. within 12 h of birth	0.5 mL† I.M. within 12 h of birth (no later than 7 d), and at 1 and 6 mo‡; test for HB$_s$Ag and anti-HB$_s$ at 12-15 mo
Sexual	0.06 mL/kg I.M. within 14 d of sexual contact; a second dose should be given if the index patient remains HB$_s$Ag-positive after 3 mo and hepatitis B vaccine was not given initially	1 mL I.M. at 0, 1, and 6 mo for homosexual and bisexual men and regular sexual contacts of persons with acute and chronic hepatitis B
Percutaneous; exposed person unvaccinated		
Source known HB$_s$Ag-positive	0.06 mL/kg I.M. within 24 h	1 mL I.M. within 7 d, and at 1 and 6 mo§
Source known, HB$_s$Ag status not known	Test source for HB$_s$Ag; if source is positive, give exposed person 0.06 mL/kg I.M. once within 7 d	1 mL I.M. within 7 d, and at 1 and 6 mo§
Source not tested or unknown	Nothing required	1 mL I.M. within 7 d, and at 1 and 6 mo
Percutaneous; exposed person vaccinated		
Source known HB$_s$Ag-positive	Test exposed person for anti-HB$_s$¶. If titer is protective, nothing is required; if titer is not protective, give 0.06 mL/kg within 24 h.	Review vaccination status#
Source known, HB$_s$Ag status not known	Test source for HB$_s$Ag and exposed person for anti-HB$_s$. If source is HB$_s$Ag-negative, or if source is HB$_s$Ag-positive but anti-HB$_s$ titer is protective, nothing is required. If source is HB$_s$Ag-positive and anti-HB$_s$ titer is not protective or if exposed person is a known nonresponder, give 0.06 mL/kg I.M. within 24 h. A second dose of hepatitis B immune globulin can be given 1 mo later if a booster dose of hepatitis B vaccine is not given.	Review vaccination status#
Source not tested or unknown	Test exposed person for anti-HB$_s$. If anti-HB$_s$ titer is protective, nothing is required. If anti-HB$_s$ titer is not protective, 0.06 mL/kg may be given along with a booster dose of hepatitis B vaccine.	Review vaccination status#

*HB$_s$Ag = hepatitis B surface antigen; anti-HB$_s$ = antibody to hepatitis B surface antigen; I.M. = intramuscularly; SRU = standard ratio units.

†Each 0.5 mL dose of plasma-derived hepatitis B vaccine contains 10 µg of HB$_s$Ag; each 0.5 mL dose of recombinant hepatitis B vaccine contains 5 µg (Merck Sharp & Dohme) or 10 µg (SmithKline Beecham) of HB$_s$Ag.

‡If hepatitis B immune globulin and hepatitis B vaccine are given simultaneously, they should be given at separate sites.

§If hepatitis B vaccine is not given, a second dose of hepatitis B immune globulin should be given 1 month later.

¶Anti-HB$_s$ titers <10 SRU by radioimmunoassay or negative by enzyme immunoassay indicate lack of protection. Testing the exposed person for anti-HB$_s$ is not necessary if a protective level of antibody has been shown within the previous 24 months.

#If the exposed person has not completed a three-dose series of hepatitis B vaccine, the series should be completed. Test the exposed person for anti-HB$_s$. If the antibody level is protective, nothing is required. If an adequate antibody response in the past is shown on retesting to have declined to an inadequate level, a booster dose (1 mL) of hepatitis B vaccine should be given. If the exposed person has inadequate antibody or is a known nonresponder to vaccination, a booster dose can be given along with one dose of hepatitis B immune globulin.

TYPES OF HEPATITIS VIRUS

Features	A	B	C	D	E
Incubation Period	2-6 wks	8-24 wks	2-52 wks	3-13 wks	3-6 wks
Onset	Abrupt	Insidious	Insidious	Abrupt	Abrupt
Symptoms					
Jaundice	Adults: 70% to 80%; Children: 10%	25%	25%	Varies	Unknown
Asymptomatic Patients	Adults: 50%; Children: Most	~75%	~75%	Rare	Rare
Routes of Transmission					
Fecal/Oral	Yes	No	No	No	Yes
Parenteral	Rare	Yes	Yes	Yes	No
Sexual	No	Yes	Possible	Yes	No
Perinatal	No	Yes	Possible	Possible	No
Water/Food	Yes	No	No	No	Yes
Sequelae (% of patients)					
Chronic state	No	Adults: 6% to 10%; Children: 25% to 50%; Infants: 70% to 90%	>75%	10% to 15%	No
Case-Fatality Rate	0.6%	1.4%	1% to 2%	30%	1% to 2%; Pregnant women: 20%

Hepatitis A Vaccine (Havrix®) *on page 421*

Hepatitis B Immune Globulin (H-BIG®, Hep-B-Gammagee®, HyperHep®) *on page 422*

Hepatitis B Vaccine (Engerix-B®, Recombivax HB®) *on page 422*

Immune Globulin, Intramuscular (Gamastan®, Gammar®) *on page 453*

Immune Globulin, Intravenous (Gamimune N®, Gammagard®, Gammagard® S/D, Polygam®, Polygam® S/D, Sandoglobulin®, Venoglobulin®-I, Venoglobulin®-S) *on page 454*

Interferon Alfa-2a (Roferon-A®) *on page 461*

HERPES

The herpes viruses not only represent a topic of specific interest to the dentist due to oral manifestations, but are widespread as systemic infections. Herpes simplex virus is also of interest because of its central nervous system infections and its relationship as one of the viral infections commonly found in AIDS patients. Oral herpes infections will be covered elsewhere. Treatment of herpes simplex primary infection includes acyclovir. Ganciclovir is an alternative drug and foscarnet is also occasionally used. Epstein-Barr virus is a member of the herpesvirus family and produces syndromes important in dentistry, including infectious mononucleosis with the commonly found oral pharyngitis and petechial hemorrhages, as well as being the causative agent of Burkitt's lymphoma. The relationship between Epstein-Barr virus to oral hairy leukoplakia in AIDS patients has not been shown to be one of cause and effect; however, the presence of Epstein-Barr in these lesions is consistent. Currently, there is no accepted treatment for Epstein-Barr virus, although acyclovir has been shown in *in vitro* studies to have some efficacy. Varicella-zoster virus is another member of the herpesvirus family and is the causative agent of two clinical entities, chickenpox and shingles or herpes zoster. Oral manifestations of both chickenpox and herpes zoster include vesicular eruptions often leading to confluent mucosal ulcerations. Acyclovir is the drug of choice for treatment of herpes zoster infections.

HIV

Human immunodeficiency virus represents a systemic infection that is of interest, not only because of the elevated infectious disease risk in dentistry, but because of oral manifestations and the incidence of oral complications in these patients.

NATURAL HISTORY OF HIV INFECTION/ORAL MANIFESTATIONS

Time From Transmission (Average)	Observation	CD4 Cell Count
0	Viral transmissions	Normal: 1000 ($\pm$500/mm^3)
2-4 weeks	Self limited infectious mononucleosis-like illness with fever, rash, leukopenia	Transient decrease
6-12 weeks	Seroconversion (rarely requires $\geq$3 months for seroconversion)	Normal
0-8 years	Healthy/asymptomatic HIV infection; peripheral generalized lymphadenopathy; HPV, thrush, OHL; RAU, periodontal diseases, salivary gland diseases; dermatitis	$\geq$500/mm^3 gradual reduction with average decrease of 50-80/mm^3/year
4-8 years	AIDS-related complex or early symptomatic HIV infection: Thrush, oral hairy leukoplakia, salivary gland diseases, ITP, xerostomia, dermatitis, shingles; RAU, herpes simplex, HPV, bacterial infection, periodontal diseases, molluscum contagiosum, other physical symptoms: fever, weight loss, fatigue	$\geq$300-500/mm^3
6-10 years	AIDS: Wasting syndrome, *Candida* esophagitis, Kaposi sarcoma, HIV-associated dementia, disseminated *M. avium*, lymphoma, herpes simplex >30 days; PCP; cryptococcal meningitis	<200/mm^3

Natural history indicates course of HIV infection in absence of antiretroviral treatment. Adapted from Bartlett JG, "A Guide to HIV Care from the AIDS Care Program of the Johns Hopkins Medical Institutions," 2nd ed.

CD4+ LYMPHOCYTE COUNT AND PERCENTAGE AS RELATED TO THE RISK OF OPPORTUNISTIC INFECTION

CD4+ Cells/mm^3	CD4+ Percentage*	Risk of Opportunistic Infection
>600	32-60	No increased risk
400-500	<29	Initial immune suppression
200-400	14-28	Appearance of opportunistic infections, some may be major
<200	<14	Severe immune suppression. AIDS diagnosis. Major opportunistic infections. Although variable, prognosis for surviving more than 3 years is poor.
<50	–	Although variable, prognosis for surviving more than 1 year is poor

*Several studies have suggested that the CD4+ percentage demonstrates less variability between measurements, as compared to the absolute CD4+ cell count. CD4+ percentages may therefore give a clearer impression of the course of disease.

HIV infection can result in increased risk of candidiasis, herpes simplex reactivation, Kaposi's sarcoma, aphthous ulcerations, and numerous other oral conditions that are discussed elsewhere in this text. Drug therapy for human immunodeficiency virus includes zidovudine, didanosine, and zalcitabine, commonly known as AZT, ddI, and ddC. Other drugs are used in combination such as protease inhibitors, lamivudine (3TC) (Epivir®) and saquinavir mesylate (Invirase®). In recent clinical trials, combination therapy has shown the greatest efficacy. Common oral complications include fungal overgrowth and antifungal therapy may be necessary. See "Management of Oral Fungal Infections" in this section.

ANTIVIRALS

ANTIVIRAL AGENTS OF ESTABLISHED THERAPEUTIC EFFECTIVENESS

Viral Infection	Drug
Cytomegalovirus	
Retinitis	Ganciclovir
	Foscarnet
Pneumonia	Ganciclovir
Hepatitis viruses	
Chronic hepatitis C	Interferon Alfa-2b
Chronic hepatitis B	Interferon Alfa-2b
Herpes simplex virus	
Oro-facial herpes	
First episode	Acyclovir
Recurrence	Acyclovir
	Penciclovir
Genital herpes	
First episode	Acyclovir
Recurrence	Acyclovir
Suppression	Acyclovir
Encephalitis	Acyclovir
Mucocutaneous disease in immunocompromised	Acyclovir
Neonatal	Acyclovir
Keratoconjunctivitis	Trifluridine
	Vidarabine
Human immunodeficiency virus-1	
AIDS, advanced ARC	Ritonavir
	Lamivudine
	Saquinavir Mesylate
	Zidovudine
	Didanosine
	Zalcitabine
Asymptomatic, CD4 <500	Zidovudine
Influenza A virus	Amantadine
	Rimantadine
Papillomavirus	
Condyloma acuminatum	Interferon Alfa-2b
Respiratory syncytial virus	Ribavirin
Varicella-zoster virus	
Varicella in normal children	Acyclovir
Varicella in immunocompromised	Acyclovir
Herpes zoster in immunocompromised	Acyclovir
Herpes zoster in normal hosts	Acyclovir
	Famciclovir

Acyclovir (Zovirax®) *on page 23*
Amantadine Hydrochloride (Symadine®; Symmetrel®) *on page 41*
Atovaquone (Mepron™) *on page 84*
Didanosine (ddl) (Videx®) *on page 274*
Famciclovir (Famvir™) *on page 352*
Foscarnet (Foscavir®) *on page 386*
Ganciclovir (Cytovene®) *on page 393*
Hepatitis B Immune Globulin *on page 422*
Immune Globulin, Intramuscular *on page 453*
Indinavir (Crixivan®) *on page 456*
Interferon Alfa-2a (Roferon-A®) *on page 461*
Interferon Alfa-2b (Intron® A) *on page 462*
Interferon Alfa-N3 (Alferon® N) *on page 463*
Lamivudine (Epivir®) *on page 489*
Penciclovir (Denavir®) (Approved, to be released)
Rifabutin (Mycobutin®) *on page 769*
Rimantadine Hydrochloride (Flumadine®) *on page 771*
Ritonavir (Norvir®) *on page 773*
Saquinavir Mesylate (Invirase®) *on page 780*
Stavudine (Zerit®) *on page 800*
Trifluridine (Viroptic®) *on page 870*
Valacyclovir (Valtrex®) *on page 888*
Vidarabine (Vira-A®) *on page 895*
Zalcitabine (ddC) (Hivid®) *on page 906*
Zidovudine (AZT) (Retrovir®) *on page 907*

PART II.

Dental Management and Therapeutic Considerations in Patients With Specific Oral Conditions and Other Oral Medicine Topics

This second part of the text focuses on therapies the dentist may choose to prescribe for patients suffering from oral disease or are in need of special care. Some overlap between these sections has resulted from systemic conditions that have oral manifestations and vice-versa. Cross-references to the descriptions and the monographs for individual drugs described elsewhere in this handbook allow for easy retrieval of information. Example prescriptions of selected drug therapies for each condition are presented so that the clinician can evaluate alternate approaches to treatment. Seldom is there a single drug of choice.

Those drug prescriptions listed represent prototype drugs and popular prescriptions and are examples only. The therapeutic index is available for cross-referencing if alternatives and additional drugs are sought.

ORAL PAIN

PAIN PREVENTION

For the dental patient, the prevention of pain aids in relieving anxiety and reduces the probability of stress during dental care. For the practitioner, dental procedures can be accomplished more efficiently in a "painless" situation. Appropriate selection and use of local anesthetics is one of the foundations for success in this arena. Local anesthetics listed below include drugs for the most commonly confronted dental procedures. Ester anesthetics have a higher incidence of allergic manifestations due to the formation of the metabolic by-product, para-aminobenzoic acid. The amides have an almost negligible allergic rate, however, at least one well documented case of amide allergy was reported be Seng, et al, in January of this year.

Bupivacaine Hydrochloride (Marcaine®; Sensorcaine®) *on page 127*

Bupivacaine With Epinephrine (Marcaine® With Epinephrine; Sensorcaine®) *on page 128*

Chloroprocaine Hydrochloride (Nescaine®) *on page 185*

Etidocaine Hydrochloride (With Epinephrine) (Duranest® Injection) *on page 345*

Lidocaine and Epinephrine (Octocaine® 50; Octocaine® 100; Xylocaine® With Epinephrine) *on page 499*

Lidocaine Hydrochloride (Dilocaine®; Nervocaine®; Xylocaine® Octocaine®) *on page 502*

Lidocaine Transoral (Dentipatch®) *on page 502*

Mepivacaine Dental Anesthetic (Carbocaine® 3%; Isocaine® 3%; Polocaine® 3%) *on page 541*

Mepivacaine With Levonordefrin (Carbocaine® 2% with Neo-Cobefrin®; Isocaine® 2%; Polocaine® 2%) *on page 542*

Prilocaine (Citanest® Plain 4%) *on page 721*

Prilocaine With Epinephrine (Citanest Forte® With Epinephrine) *on page 721*

Procaine Hydrochloride (Novocain®) *on page 727*

Propoxycaine and Procaine (Ravocaine® and Novocain® with Levophed®; Ravocaine® and Novocain® with Neo-Cobefrin®) *on page 739*

Ropivacaine Hydrochloride (Naropin®) *on page 775*

Tetracaine Hydrochloride (Pontocaine®; Viractin®) *on page 828*

Tetracaine With Dextrose (Pontocaine® with Dextrose Injection) *on page 829*

The selection of a vasoconstrictor with the local anesthetic must be based on the length of the procedure to be performed, the patient's medical status (epinephrine is contraindicated in patients with uncontrolled hyperthyroidism), and the need for hemorrhage control. The following table lists some of the common drugs with their duration of action. Transoral patches with lidocaine are now available (Dentipatch®) and the new long-acting amide injectable, Ropivacaine (Naropin®) may be useful for postoperative pain management.

DENTAL ANESTHETICS
(Average Duration by Route)

Product	Infiltration	Inferior Alveolar Block
Marcaine® HCl 0.5% with epinephrine 1:200,000 (bupivacaine and epinephrine)	60 minutes	5-7 hours
Carbocaine® HCl 3% (mepivacaine)	20 minutes	40 minutes
Carbocaine® HCl 2% with Neo-Cobefrin® 1:20,000 (mepivacaine HCl and levonordefrin)	50 minutes	60-75 minutes
Duranest® Injection (etidocaine)	5-10 hours	5-10 hours
Citanest® Plain 4% (prilocaine)	20 minutes	2.5 hours
Citanest Forte® With Epinephrine (prilocaine with epinephrine)	2.25 hours	3 hours
Lidocaine HCl 2% and epinephrine 1:100,000 (lidocaine and epinephrine)	60 minutes	90 minutes
Ravocaine® HCl 0.4% and Novocain® 2% with Levophed® 1:30,000 (propoxycaine and procaine with norepinephrine bitartrate)	30-40 minutes	60 minutes

The use of preinjection topical anesthetics can assist in pain prevention (see also Management of Oral Mucosal Ulcers of Viral and Nonviral Origin).

Benzocaine (Hurricane®; Numzident®; various other products) *on page 102*

Lidocaine Hydrochloride (Dilocaine®; Nervocaine®; Xylocaine® Octocaine®) *on page 502*

Tetracaine Hydrochloride (Pontocaine®; Viractin®) *on page 828*

PAIN MANAGEMENT

The patient with existing acute or chronic oral pain requires appropriate treatment and sensitivity on the part of the dentist, all for the purpose of achieving relief from the oral source of pain. Pain can be divided into mild, moderate, and severe levels and requires a subjective assessment by the dentist based on knowledge of the dental procedures to be performed, the presenting signs and symptoms of the patient, and the realization that most dental procedures are invasive often leading to pain once the patient has left the dental office. The practitioner must be aware that the treatment of the source of the pain is usually the best management. If infection is present, treatment of the infection will directly alleviate the patient's discomfort. However, a patient who is not in pain tends to heal better and it is wise to adequately cover the patient for any residual or recurrent discomfort suffered. Likewise, many of the procedures that the dentist performs have pain associated with them. Much of this pain occurs after leaving the dentist office due to an inflammatory process or a healing process that has been initiated. It is difficult to assign specific pain levels (mild, moderate, or severe) for specific procedures; however, the dentist should use his or her prescribing capacity judiciously so that overmedication is avoided.

The following categories of drugs and appropriate example prescriptions for each follow. These include management of mild pain with aspirin products, acetaminophen, and some of the nonsteroidal noninflammatory agents. Management of moderate pain includes codeine, Vicodin®, Vicodin ES®, Lorcet® 10/650; and Motrin® in the 800 mg dosage. Severe pain may require treatment with Percodan®, Percocet®, or Demerol®. All prescription pain preparations should be closely monitored for efficacy and discontinued if the pain persists or requires a higher level formulation.

The chronic pain patient represents a particular challenge for the practitioner. Some additional drugs that may be useful in managing the patient with chronic pain are covered in the temporomandibular dysfunction section of this text. It is always incumbent on the practitioner to reevaluate the diagnosis, source of pain, and treatment, whenever prolonged use of analgesics (narcotic or non-narcotic) is contemplated. Drugs such as Dilaudid® are not recommended for management of dental pain in most states.

Narcotic analgesics can be used on a short-term basis or intermittently in combination with non-narcotic therapy in the chronic pain patient. Judicious prescribing, monitoring, and maintenance by the practitioner is imperative, particularly whenever considering the use of a narcotic analgesic due to the abuse and addiction liabilities.

MILD PAIN

Acetaminophen (various products) *on page 14*

Aspirin (various products) *on page 78*

Diflunisal (Dolobid®) *on page 278*

Ibuprofen (various products) *on page 447*

Ketoprofen (Orudis®; Orudis KT®; Oruvail®) *on page 483*

Naproxen (Aleve®; Anaprox®; Naprosyn®) *on page 606*

OVER-THE-COUNTER PRESCRIPTION EXAMPLES

Rx

Aspirin 325 mg

Disp

Sig: Take 2-3 tablets every 4 hours

Rx

Ibuprofen 200 mg

Disp

Sig: Take 2-3 tablets every 4 hours, up to 3200 mg (16 tablets)/
day

Note: Ibuprofen is available over-the-counter as Motrin IB®, Advil®, Nuprin®, and many other brands in 200 mg tablets.

Note: NSAIDs should never be taken together, nor should they be combined with aspirin. NSAIDs have anti-inflammatory effects as well as analgesics. An allergy to aspirin constitutes a contradiction to all the new NSAIDs. Aspirin and the NSAIDs may increase post-treatment bleeding.

Rx

Acetaminophen 325 mg

Disp

Sig: Take 2-3 tablets every 4 hours

Products include: Tylenol®, Datril®, Anacin® 3, and many others

---

Note: Acetaminophen can be given if patient has allergy, bleeding problems, or stomach upset secondary to aspirin or NSAIDs.

Rx

Aleve® 220 mg

Disp

Sig: 1-2 tablets every 8 hours

Ingredient: Naproxen

Rx

Orudis KT® 12.5 mg

Disp

Sig: 1-2 tablets every 8 hours

Ingredient: Ketoprofen

PRESCRIPTION ONLY EXAMPLES

Rx

Ketoprofen 25 mg

Disp

Sig: 1-2 tablets every 8 hours

Rx

Dolobid® 500 mg

Disp 16 tablets

Sig: Take 2 tablets initially, then 1 tablet every 8-12 hours for pain

Ingredient: Diflunisal

MODERATE/MODERATELY SEVERE PAIN

Aspirin and Codeine (Empirin® With Codeine) *on page 80*

Dihydrocodeine, Acetaminophen, and Aspirin (Synalgos® DC) *on page 281*

Hydrocodone and Acetaminophen (Lortab®, Vicodin®) *on page 431*

Ibuprofen (various products) *on page 447*

The following is a guideline to use when prescribing codeine with either aspirin or acetaminophen (Tylenol®):

Codeine No. 2 = codeine 15 mg

Codeine No. 3 = codeine 30 mg

Codeine No. 4 = codeine 60 mg

Example: ASA No. 3 = aspirin 325 mg + codeine 30 mg

PRESCRIPTION EXAMPLES

Rx

Motrin® 800 mg*

Disp 16 tablets

Sig: Take 1 tablet 3 times/day

Ingredient: Ibuprofen

Note: For more severe pain, Motrin® (800 mg) can be given up to 4 times/day.

*Note: Also available as 600 mg

Rx

Tylenol® No. 3*

Disp 16 (sixteen) tablets

Sig: Take 1 tablet every 4 hours as needed for pain

Ingredients: Acetaminophen and codeine

*Note: Also available as #2 and #4

Rx

Synalgos® DC

Disp 16 (sixteen) capsules

Sig: Take 1 capsule every 4 hours as needed for pain

Ingredients: Dihydrocodeine 16 mg, aspirin 356.4 mg, and caffeine 30 mg

---

Rx

Vicodin®

Disp 16 (sixteen) tablets

Sig: Take 1 tablet every 4 hours for pain

Ingredients: Hydrocodone 5 mg and acetaminophen 500 mg

Note: Available as Vicodin ES® for use 1 tablet every 8-12 hours

---

Rx

Lortab® 5 mg*

Disp 16 (sixteen) tablets

Sig: Take 1 or 2 tablets every 4 hours for pain (do not exceed 8 tablets in 24 hours)

Ingredients: Hydrocodone 5 mg and acetaminophen 500 mg

Note: Available under other brand names with varying dosages and strengths

SEVERE PAIN

Meperidine Hydrochloride (Demerol®) *on page 539*

Oxycodone and Acetaminophen (Percocet®, Tylox®) *on page 646*

Oxycodone and Aspirin (Percodan®) *on page 647*

PRESCRIPTION EXAMPLES

Rx

Demerol® 50 mg*

Disp 16 (sixteen) tablets

Sig: Take 1 tablet every 4 hours for pain   No Refills

Ingredients: Meperidine

*Triplicate prescription required in some states

Rx

Percodan®*

Disp 16 (sixteen) tablets

Sig: Take 1 tablet every 4 hours for pain   No Refills

Ingredients: Oxycodone 4.88 mg and aspirin 325 mg

*Triplicate prescription required in some states

Rx

Percocet® tablets or Tylox® capsules*

Disp 16 (sixteen) tablets or capsules

Sig: Take 1 tablet every 4 hours for pain   No Refills

Ingredients: Oxycodone 5 mg and acetaminophen 325 mg
(Tylox® contains acetaminophen 500 mg)

*Triplicate prescription required in some states

ORAL BACTERIAL INFECTIONS

Dental infection can occur for any number of reasons, primarily involving pulpal and periodontal infections. Secondary infections of the soft tissues as well as sinus infections pose special treatment challenges. The drugs of choice in treating most oral infections have been selected because of their efficacy in providing adequate blood levels for delivery to the oral tissues and their proven usefulness in managing dental infections. Penicillin and erythromycin remain the two primary drugs for treatment of dental infections of pulpal origin. The management of soft tissue infections may require the use of additional drugs.

SINUS INFECTION TREATMENT

Sinus infections represent a common condition which may present with confounding dental complaints. Treatment is sometimes instituted by the dentist, but due to the often chronic and recurrent nature of sinus infections, early involvement of an otolaryngologist is advised. These infections may require antibiotics of varying spectrum as well as requiring the management of sinus congestion. Although amoxicillin is usually adequate, many otolaryngologists go directly to Augmentin®. Second generation cephalosporins and clarithromycin are sometimes used depending on the chronicity of the problem.

Amoxicillin and Clavulanic Acid (Augmentin®) *on page 57*
Amoxicillin Trihydrate *on page 58*
Chlorpheniramine Maleate (Chlor-Trimeton®) *on page 191*
Clarithromycin (Biaxin™ Filmtabs®) *on page 212*
Loratadine and Pseudoephedrine (Claritin-D®) *on page 513*
Oxymetazoline Hydrochloride (Afrin®) *on page 649*
Pseudoephedrine (Sudafed®) *on page 749*

PRESCRIPTION EXAMPLES

Rx

Amoxicillin 500 mg
Disp 21 capsules
Sig: Take 1 capsule 3 times/day

Rx

Augmentin® 500
Disp 30 tablets
Sig: Take 1 tablet 3 times/day

Ingredients: Amoxicillin 500 mg and clavulanate potassium 125 mg

The selected antibiotic should be used with a nasal decongestant and possibly an antihistamine.

Rx

Afrin® Nasal Spray (OTC)
Disp 15 mL
Sig: Spray 1 time in each nostril every 6-8 hours for no more than 3 days

Ingredient: Oxymetazoline

OR

Rx

Sudafed® 60 mg tablets (OTC)
Disp 30 tablets
Sig: Take 1 tablet every 4-6 hours as needed for congestion

Ingredient: Pseudoephedrine

Rx

> Chlor-Trimeton® 4 mg (OTC)
>
> Disp 14 tablets
>
> Sig: Take 1 tablet 2 times/day

Ingredient: Chlorpheniramine

PULPAL AND PERIODONTAL INFECTIONS

Regardless of the condition to be treated, consideration should always be given to managing and monitoring the course of the infection with observations at 24 and 72 hours to ensure efficacy of the drug selected. Due to the usual multiorganism etiology of most pulpal and periodontal dental infections, culture and sensitivity studies may not be pertinent. Penicillin, clindamycin, and erythromycin are first-line drugs of choice for most dental infections. Some periodontal infections respond well to tetracyclines and metronidazole. Although culturing oral infections is not always necessary, a complete listing of the spectrum of antibiotics available can be found in the Appendix. Oral antimicrobial rinses may be useful in periodontal infections.

Common Oral-Facial Infections and Antibiotics for Treatment *on page 1077*

Amoxicillin and Clavulanic Acid (Augmentin®) *on page 57*
Amoxicillin Trihydrate *on page 58*
Cephalexin Monohydrate (Cefanex®; C-Lexin®; Entacef®; Keflet®; Keflex®; Keftab®) *on page 176*
Chlorhexidine Gluconate (Peridex®; PerioGard®) *on page 184*
Clindamycin (Cleocin®) *on page 214*
Dicloxacillin (Dycill®; Dynapen®; Pathocil®) *on page 273*
Erythromycin (various products) *on page 321*
Metronidazole (Flagyl®; MetroGel®; Protostat®) *on page 576*
Mouthwash, Antiseptic (Listerine®) *on page 592*
Penicillin V Potassium (various products) *on page 668*
Tetracycline (Achromycin®; Sumycin®; Tetracyn®) *on page 829*

Note: Often penicillins are prescribed with a double or triple loading dose initially, then followed by the course described below.

PRESCRIPTION EXAMPLES

Rx

> Penicillin V potassium 500 mg
>
> Disp 28 tablets
>
> Sig: Take 1 tablet 4 times/day

Rx

> Augmentin® 500 mg
>
> Disp 28 tablets
>
> Sig: Take 1 tablet 4 times/day

Rx

> Erythromycin base 250 mg
>
> Disp 28 (enteric coated) tablets
>
> Sig: Take 1 tablet 4 times/day

Rx

Cephalexin 250 mg

Disp 28 capsules

Sig: Take 1 capsule 4 times/day

Rx

Dicloxacillin 250 mg

Disp 28 capsules

Sig: Take 2 capsules once every 6 hours

Rx

Clindamycin 300 mg (Cleocin®)

Disp 14 capsules

Sig: Take 1 capsule every 6 hours

Rx

Metronidazole 250 mg (Flagyl®)

Disp 40 tablets

Sig: Take 1 tablet 4 times/day

Rx

Chlorhexidine Gluconate .12% (Peridex® and PerioGard®)

Disp 1 bottle

Sig: 20 mL for 30 seconds 3 times/day

Rx

Listerine® (OTC)

Disp 1 bottle

Sig: 20 mL for 30 seconds twice daily

ORAL FUNGAL INFECTIONS

Oral fungal infections can result from alteration in oral flora, immunosuppression, and underlying systemic diseases that may allow the overgrowth of these opportunistic organisms. These systemic conditions might include diabetes, long-term xerostomia, adrenal suppression, anemia, and chemotherapy-induced myelosuppression for the management of cancer. Drugs of choice in treating fungal infections are amphotericin B, ciclopirox olamine, clotrimazole, itraconazole, ketoconazole, fluconazole, naftifine hydrochloride, nystatin, and oxiconazole. Patients being treated for fungal skin infections may also be using topical antifungal preparations coupled with a steroid such as triamcinolone. Clinical presentation might include pseudomembranous, atrophic, and hyperkeratotic forms. Fungus has also been implicated in denture stomatitis and symptomatic geographic tongue.

Nystatin (Mycostatin®) is effective topically in the treatment of candidal infections of the skin and mucous membrane. The drug is extremely well tolerated and appears to be nonsensitizing. In persons with denture stomatitis in which monilial organisms play at least a contributory role, it is important to soak the prosthesis overnight in a nystatin suspension. Nystatin ointment can be placed in the denture during the daytime much like a denture adhesive. Medication should be continued for at least 48 hours after disappearance of clinical signs in order to prevent relapse. Patients must be re-evaluated after 14 days of therapy. Predisposing systemic factors must be reconsidered if the oral fungal infection persists. Topical applications rely on contact of the drug with the lesions. Therefore, 4-5 times daily with a dissolving troche or pastille is appropriate. Concern over the presence of sugar in the troches and pastilles has led practitioners to sometimes prescribe the vaginal suppository formulation.

Amphotericin B (Fungizone®) on page 60
Clotrimazole (Mycelex®) troches on page 223
Fluconazole (Diflucan®) on page 367
Itraconazole (Sporanox®) on page 477
Ketoconazole (Nizoral®) on page 481
Nystatin (Mycostatin®) ointment or cream on page 632
Nystatin (Mycostatin®) oral suspension on page 632
Nystatin (Mycostatin®) pastilles on page 632
Nystatin (Mycostatin®) powder on page 632
Nystatin and Triamcinolone (Mycolog®) cream on page 632

Note: Consider Peridex® oral rinse, or Listerine® antiseptic oral rinse for long-term control in immunosuppressed patients.

PRESCRIPTION EXAMPLES

Rx

Mycostatin® pastilles

Disp 70 pastilles

Sig: Dissolve 1 tablet in mouth until gone, 4-5 times/day for 14 days

---

Ingredients: 200,000 units of nystatin per tablet

Special indications: Pastille is more effective than oral suspension due to prolonged contact

---

Rx

Mycostatin® oral suspension

Disp 60 mL (4 oz)

Sig: Use 1 teaspoonful 4-5 times/day; rinse and hold in mouth as long as possible before swallowing or spitting out (2 minutes); do not eat or drink for 30 minutes following application

---

Ingredients: Nystatin 100,000 units/mL; vehicle contains 50% sucrose and not more than 1% alcohol

Rx

Mycostatin® ointment or cream

Disp 15 g or 30 g tube

Sig: Apply liberally to affected areas 4-5 times/day; do not eat or drink for 30 minutes after application

Note: Denture wearers should apply to dentures prior to each insertion; for edentulous patients, we can also prescribe Mycostatin® powder (15 g) to be sprinkled on denture

Ingredients:

Cream: 100,000 units nystatin per g, aqueous vanishing cream base
Ointment: 100,000 units nystatin per g, polyethylene and mineral oil gel base

OR

Rx

Mycelex® troche 10 mg

Disp 70 tablets

Sig: Dissolve 1 tablet in mouth 5 times/day

Ingredients: Clotrimazole

Note: Tablets contain sucrose, risk of caries with prolonged use (>3 months); care must be exercised in diabetic patients

Rx

Fungizone® oral suspension

Disp 50 mL

Sig: 1 mL, swish and swallow 4 times/day between meals

MANAGEMENT OF FUNGAL INFECTIONS REQUIRING SYSTEMIC MEDICATION

If the patient is refractory to topical treatment, consideration of a systemic route might include Diflucan or Nizoral®. Also, when the patient cannot tolerate topical therapy, ketoconazole (Nizoral®) is an effective, well tolerated, systematic drug for mucocutaneous candidiasis. Concern over liver function and possible drug interactions must be considered.

PRESCRIPTION EXAMPLES

Rx

Nizoral® 200 mg

Disp 10 or 28 tablets

Sig: Take 1 tablet daily for 10-14 days

Ingredients: Ketoconazole

Note: To be used if *Candida* infection does not respond to mycostatin; potential for liver toxicity; liver function should be monitored with long-term use (>3 weeks)

Rx

Diflucan® 100 mg

Disp 15 tablets

Sig: Take 2 tablets the first day and 1 tablet a day for 10-14 days

Ingredients: Fluconazole

MANAGEMENT OF ANGULAR CHEILITIS

Angular cheilitis may represent the clinical manifestation of a multitude of etiologic factors. Cheilitis-like lesions may result from local habits, from a decrease in the intermaxillary space, or from nutritional deficiency. More commonly, angular cheilitis represents a mixed infection coupled with an inflammatory response involving *Candida albicans* and other organisms. The drug of choice is now formulated to contain nystatin and triamcinolone and the effect is excellent.

PRESCRIPTION EXAMPLE

Rx

Mycolog® (Squibb) cream

Disp 15 g tube

Sig: Apply to affected area after each meal and before bedtime

ORAL VIRAL INFECTIONS

Oral viral infections are most commonly caused by herpes simplex viruses and Coxsackie viruses. Oral pharyngeal infections and upper respiratory infections are commonly caused by the Coxsackie group A viruses. Soft tissue viral infections, on the other hand, are most often caused by the herpes simplex viruses. Herpes zoster or varicella-zoster virus, which is one of the herpes family of viruses, can likewise cause similar viral eruptions involving the mucosa.

The diagnosis of an acute viral infection is one that begins by ruling out bacterial etiology and having an awareness of the presenting signs and symptoms associated with viral infection. Acute onset and vesicular eruption on the soft tissues generally favors a diagnosis of viral infection. Unfortunately, vesicles do not remain for a great length of time in the oral cavity; therefore, the short-lived vesicles rupture leaving ulcerated bases as the only indication of their presence. These ulcers, however, are generally small in size and only when left unmanaged do they coalesce to form larger, irregular ulcerations. Distinction should be made between the commonly occurring intraoral ulcers (aphthous ulcerations) which do not have a viral etiology and the lesions associated with intraoral herpes. The management of an oral viral infection may be palliative for the most part; however, with the advent of acyclovir we now have a drug that can assist us in managing primary and secondary infection.

It should be noted that herpes can present as, a primary infection (gingivostomatitis), recurrent lip lesions (herpes labialis), and intraoral ulcers (recurrent intraoral herpes), three primary forms involving the oral and perioral tissues. Primary infection is one that is generally a systemic infection that leads to acute gingivostomatitis involving multiple tissues of the buccal mucosa, lips, tongue, floor of the mouth, and the gingiva. Treatment of primary infections utilizes acyclovir in combination with supportive care. Dyclonine 0.5%, a topical anesthetic used in combination with Benadryl® 0.5% in a saline vehicle, are found to be effective oral rinses in the symptomatic treatment of primary herpetic gingivostomatitis. Other agents available for symptomatic and supportive treatment include commercially available elixir of Benadryl®, Xylocaine® viscous, Ora-Jel® (OTC), Camphophenique® (OTC), and antibiotics to prevent secondary infections. Systemic supportive therapy should include forced fluids, high concentration protein, vitamin and mineral food supplements, and rest.

ANTIVIRALS

Acyclovir (Zovirax®) *on page 23*
Penciclovir (Denavir®) *on page 664*
Vidarabine (Vira-A®) *on page 895*

SUPPORTIVE THERAPY

Dyclonine Hydrochloride *on page 304*
Diphenhydramine Hydrochloride (Benadryl®) *on page 288*
Lidocaine Hydrochloride (Xylocaine®) *on page 502*

ANTIBIOTICS FOR PREVENTION OF SECONDARY BACTERIAL INFECTION

Erythromycin *on page 321*
Penicillin V Potassium *on page 668*

PRIMARY INFECTION

PRESCRIPTION EXAMPLE

Rx

Zovirax® 200 mg

Disp 70 capsules

Sig: Take 1 capsule every 4 hours (maximum: 5/day) for 2 weeks

---

Ingredient: Acyclovir

SUPPORTIVE CARE FOR PAIN AND PREVENTION OF SECONDARY INFECTION

Primary infections often become secondarily infected with bacteria, requiring antibiotics. Dietary supplement may be necessary. Options are presented due to variability in patient compliance and response.

PRESCRIPTION EXAMPLE

Rx

    Benadryl® powder 0.5% with dyclonine 0.5% in saline

    Disp 8 oz

    Sig: Rinse with 1 teaspoonful every 2 hours

Ingredient: Diphenhydramine and dyclonine

Rx

    Benadryl® elixir 12.5 mg/5 mL

    Disp 4 oz bottle

    Sig: Rinse with 1 teaspoonful for 2 minutes before each meal

Ingredient: Diphenhydramine

Rx

    Benadryl® elixir 12.5 mg/5 mL with Kaopectate®, 50% mixture by volume

    Disp 8 oz

    Sig: Rinse with 1 teaspoonful every 2 hours

Ingredients: Diphenhydramine and attapulgite

Rx

    Xylocaine® viscous 2%

    Disp 450 mL bottle

    Sig: Swish with 1 tablespoon 4 times/day and spit out

Ingredient: Lidocaine

Rx

    Penicillin V 250 mg tablets

    Disp 40 tablets

    Sig: 1 tablet 4 times/day

Rx

    Erythromycin 250 mg tablets

    Disp 40 tablets

    Sig: 1 tablet 4 times/day

Rx

    Meritene®

    Disp 1 lb can (plain, chocolate, eggnog flavors)

    Sig: Take 3 servings daily; prepare as indicated on can

Ingredients: (Doyle Pharmaceutical) Protein-vitamin-mineral food supplement

RECURRENT HERPETIC INFECTIONS

Following this primary infection, the herpesvirus remains latent until such time as it has the opportunity to recur. The etiology of this latent period and the degree of viral shedding present during latency is currently under study; however, it is thought that some trigger in the mucosa or the skin causes the virus to begin to replicate. This process may involve Langerhans cells which are immunocompetent antigen-presenting cells resident in all epidermal surfaces. The virus replication then leads to eruptions in tissues surrounding the mouth. The most common form of recurrence is the lip lesion or herpes labialis, however, intraoral recurrent herpes also occurs with some frequency. Prevention of recurrences has been attempted with drugs such as Lysine® (500-1000 mg/day). Response has been variable. Pain management during intraoral recurrences can be utilized as in primary infections.

Water-soluble bioflavonoid-ascorbic acid complex, now available as Peridin-C®, may be helpful in reducing the signs and symptoms associated with recurrent herpes simplex virus infections. As with all agents used, the therapy is more effective when instituted in the early prodromal stage of the disease process.

PRESCRIPTION EXAMPLE

Rx

        Citrus bioflavonoids and ascorbic acid tablets 400 mg (Peridin-C® from Beutlich Pharmaceutical)

        Disp 10 tablets

        Sig: Take 2 tablets at once, then 1 tablet tid for 3 days

---

PREVENTION

Where a recurrence is usually precipitated by exposure to sunlight, the lesion may be prevented by the application to the area of a sunscreen, with a high skin protection factor (SPF) in the range of 10-15.

PRESCRIPTION EXAMPLE

Rx

        PreSun® (OTC) 15 sunscreen lotion

        Disp 4 fluid oz

        Sig: Apply to susceptible area 1 hour before sun exposure

---

TREATMENT

Vidarabine (Vira-A®) possesses antiviral activity against herpes simplex types 1 and 2. The ophthalmic ointment may be used topically to treat recurrent mucosal and skin lesions. In the 3% strength, it does not penetrate well on the skin lesions thereby providing questionable relief of symptoms. If recommended, its use should be closely monitored. Penciclovir, an active metabolite of famciclovir, has been recently approved in a cream for treatment of recurrent herpes lesions. The drug is to be released in the near future; prescribing information will be available at that time.

PRESCRIPTION EXAMPLES

Rx

        Vira-A® ophthalmic ointment 3%

        Disp 3.5 g tube

        Sig: Apply to affected area 4 times/day

    Ingredient: Vidarabine

Rx

Zovirax® ointment 5% (3%)

Disp 15 g

Sig: Apply thin layer to lesions 6 times/day for 7 days

Ingredient: Acyclovir

Rx

Zovirax® 200 mg

Disp 70 capsules

Sig: Take 1 capsule every 4 hours (maximum: 5/day) for 2 weeks

Ingredient: Acyclovir

ORAL NONVIRAL SOFT TISSUE ULCERATIONS OR EROSIONS

RECURRENT APHTHOUS STOMATITIS

Kenalog® in Orabase is indicated for the temporary relief of symptoms associated with infrequent recurrences of minor aphthous lesions and ulcerative lesions resulting from trauma. More severe forms of recurrent aphthous stomatitis may be treated with an oral suspension of tetracycline. The agent appears to reduce the duration of symptoms and decrease the rate of recurrence by reducing secondary bacterial infection. Its use is contraindicated during the last half of pregnancy, infancy, and childhood to the age of 8 years. *Lactobacillus acidophilus* preparations (Bacid®, Lactinex®) are occasionally effective for reducing the frequency and severity of the lesions. Patients with long-standing history of recurrent aphthous stomatitis should be evaluated for iron, folic acid, and vitamin B$_{12}$ deficiencies. Regular use of Listerine® antiseptic has been shown in clinical trials to reduce the severity, duration, and frequency of aphthous stomatitis. Chlorhexidine oral rinses 20 mL x 30 sec bid or tid have also demonstrated efficacy in reducing the duration of aphthae. With both of these products, however, patient intolerance of the burning from the alcohol content is of concern. Viractin® has recently been approved for symptomatic relief.

Amlexanox (Aphthasol®) *on page 52*
Attapulgite (Kaopectate®) *on page 86*
Chlorhexidine Gluconate (Peridex®; PerioGard®) *on page 184*
Clobetasol Propionate (Temovate®) *on page 216*
Dexamethasone (Decadron®) *on page 260*
Diphenhydramine Hydrochloride (Benadryl®) *on page 288*
Fluocinonide (Lidex®) ointment with Orabase *on page 373*
Lactobacillus acidophilus and *Lactobacillus bulgaricus* (Bacid®; Lactinex®) *on page 488*
Metronidazole (Flagyl®) *on page 576*
Mouthwash, Antiseptic (Listerine®) *on page 592*
Prednisone *on page 719*
Tetracaine Hydrochloride (Pontocaine®; Viractin®) *on page 828*
Tetracycline liquid *on page 829*
Triamcinolone (Kenalog®) Acetonide Dental Paste *on page 862*

PRESCRIPTION EXAMPLES

Rx

Listerine® antiseptic (OTC)

20 mL x 30 sec bid

Rx

Peridex® oral rinse

Disp 1 bottle

Sig: 20 mL x 30 sec tid

Rx

PerioGard® oral rinse

Disp 1 bottle

Sig: 20 mL x 30 sec tid

Rx

Tetracycline capsules 250 mg

Disp 40 capsules

Sig: Suspend contents of 1 capsule in a teaspoonful of water; rinse for 2 minutes 4 times/day and swallow

Note: This comes as liquid 125 mg/5 mL which is convenient to use

Sig: Swish 5 mL for 2 minutes 4 times/day

Rx

Kenalog® in Orabase (Squibb) 0.1%

Disp 5 g tube

Sig: Coat the lesion with a film after each meal and at bedtime

BURNING TONGUE SYNDROME, GEOGRAPHIC TONGUE, MILD FORMS OF ORAL LICHEN PLANUS

Elixir of Benadryl®, a potent antihistamine, is used in the oral cavity primarily as a mild topical anesthetic agent for the symptomatic relief of certain allergic deficiencies which should be ruled out as possible etiologies for the oral condition under treatment. It is often used alone as well as in solutions with agents such as Kaopectate® or Maalox® to assist in coating the oral mucosa. Benadryl® can also be used in capsule form.

PRESCRIPTION EXAMPLE

Rx

Benadryl® elixir 12.5 mg/5 mL

Disp 4 oz bottle

Sig: Rinse with 1 teaspoonful for 2 minutes before each meal and swallow

Ingredient: Diphenhydramine

EROSIVE LICHEN PLANUS AND MAJOR APHTHAE

Elixir of dexamethasone (Decadron®), a potent anti-inflammatory agent, is used topically in the management of acute episodes of erosive lichen planus and major aphthae. Continued supervision of the patient during treatment is essential.

PRESCRIPTION EXAMPLE

Rx

Decadron® (Merck, Sharpe, & Dohme) elixir 0.5 mg/5 mL

Disp 100 mL bottle

Sig: Rinse with 1 teaspoonful for 2 minutes 4 times/day; do not swallow

Ingredient: Dexamethasone

For severe cases and when the oropharynx is involved, some practitioners have the patient swallow after a 2-minute rinse.

Allergy	Benadryl®
Aphthous	Benadryl®/Maalox® (compounded prescription)
	Benadryl®/Kaopectate® (compounded prescription)
	Lidex® in Orabase (compounded prescription)
	Kenalog® in Orabase
	Tetracycline mouth rinse
Oral inflammatory disease	Lidex® in Orabase (compounded prescription)
	Kenalog® in Orabase
	Prednisone
	Temovate® cream

The use of long-term steroids is always of concern due to possible adrenal suppression. If systemic steroids are contemplated for a protracted time, medical consultation is advisable.

PRESCRIPTION EXAMPLES

Rx

Benadryl® 50 mg

Disp 16 capsules

Sig: 3-4 times/day

Ingredient: Diphenhydramine hydrochloride

Special considerations: Use 3-4 times/day for 4 days depending on the duration of the allergic reaction; may cause drowsiness

---

Rx

Benadryl® syrup (mix 50/50) with Kaopectate®*

Disp 8 oz total

Sig: Use 2 teaspoons as rinse as needed to relieve pain or burning (use after meals)

---

*Note: Benadryl can be mixed with Maalox® if constipation is a problem

---

Rx

Kenalog® in Orabase®

Disp 5 mg

Sig: Apply thin layer to affected area 3 times/day

Rx

Lidex® ointment mixed 50/50 with Orabase®

Disp 30 g total

Sig: Apply thin layer to oral lesions 4-6 times/day

Ingredient: Fluocinonide 0.05%

Note: To be used for oral inflammatory lesions that do not respond to Kenalog® in Orabase®

Ingredient: Triamcinolone acetonide

Systemic steroids may be considered:

Rx

Prednisone 5 mg

Disp 60 tablets

Sig: Take 4 tablets in morning and 4 tablets at noon for 4 days; then decrease the total number of tablets by 1 each day until down to zero

Caution: Take medication with food

For a high potency corticosteroid:

Rx

Temovate® cream 0.05%

Disp 15 g tube

Sig: Apply locally 4-6 times/day

And for secondary infections:

Rx

Tetracycline liquid 125 mg/5 mL

Disp 100 mL

Sig: Rinse 1 tablespoonful in mouth 4 times/day then spit out; do not eat or drink for 30 minutes after using

Note: Tetracycline rinse is effective in approximately 33% of the patients with aphthous ulcers

NECROTIZING ULCERATING PERIODONTITIS (HIV Periodontal Disease)

Initial Treatment (In-Office)
Betadine rinse *on page 713*
Ensure patient has no iodine allergies
Gentle debridement

At-Home
Listerine® rinses
Peridex® rinse *on page 184*
Metronidazole (Flagyl®) 7-10 days *on page 576*

Follow-Up Therapy
Proper dental cleaning including scaling and root planing (repeat as needed)
Continue Peridex® rinse (indefinite) *on page 184*
Listerine® antiseptic rinse (20 mL for 30 seconds twice daily)

DENTIN HYPERSENSITIVITY; HIGH CARIES INDEX; XEROSTOMIA

DENTIN HYPERSENSITIVITY

Suggested steps in resolving dentin hypersensitivity (a thorough exam had ruled any other source for the problem).

Treatment Steps
- Home treatment with a desensitizing toothpaste containing potassium nitrate (used to brush teeth as well as a thin layer applied, each night for 2 weeks)
- If needed, in office potassium oxalate (Protect® by Butler) and/or in office fluoride iontophoresis
- If sensitivity is still not tolerable to the patient, consider pumice then dentin adhesive and unfilled resin or composite restoration overlaying a glass ionomer base

Home Products: All contain nitrate as active ingredient

Promise®
Denquel®
Sensodyne®

Dentifrice Products *on page 1051*

ANTICARIES AGENTS

Fluoride gel 0.4%, rinse 0.05% *on page 374*

FLUORIDE GELS

Oral Rinse Products *on page 1067*

Used for the prevention of demineralization of the tooth structure secondary to xerostomia. For patients with long-term or permanent xerostomia, daily application is accomplished using custom gel applicator trays. Patients with porcelain crowns should use a neutral pH fluoride.

1.1% neutral pH sodium fluoride
Thera-Flur-N® or Prevident® (Colgate Hoyt)
0.4% stannous fluoride
Gel-Kam® unflavored (Colgate Hoyt)

REMINERALIZING GEL

In addition to fluoride gel to remineralize enamel breakdown in severely xerostomic patients, applicator trays may be used.

Revive® (Dental Resources, Inc. Delano, MN)

Note: Many preparations are available over-the-counter so prescriptions sometimes are not required. If caries is severe, use fluoride gel in custom tray once daily as long as needed (years).

ANTIPLAQUE AGENTS

PRESCRIPTION EXAMPLES

Rx
Listerine® antiseptic (OTC) 20 mL for 30 seconds twice daily

Rx
Peridex® oral rinse 0.12% Disp 3 times 16 oz Sig: ½ oz, swish for 30 seconds 2-3 times/day

Rx

PerioGard® oral rinse

Disp 3 times 16 oz

Sig: ½ oz, swish for 30 seconds 2-3 times/day

Ingredient: Chlorhexidine

Peridex may:

- Stain teeth yellow to brown (can be removed with dental cleaning)
- Alter taste (temporary)
- Increase the deposition of calculus (reversible)

Chlorhexidine Gluconate (Peridex®) *on page 184*

XEROSTOMIA

Dry mouth associated with radiation therapy, drug therapy, aging, and Sjögren's disease may be managed by rinsing with a solution of sodium carboxymethylcellulose. It is a nonirritating agent that moistens and lubricates the oral tissues and may be used for prolonged periods of time without adverse effects. For dentulous patients, fluoride and electrolytes have been added to this solution to reduce caries susceptibility (Xero-Lube®). Consideration of alternative medical drug regimens in consult with the physician may assist in management. Numerous patients being treated for anxiety or depression are often susceptible to chronic xerostomia due to medications selected; see table on following page.

Pilocarpine (Dental) (Salagen®) *on page 693*

Saliva Substitute (Moi-Stir®; MouthKote®; Optimoist®; Salivart®; Xero-Lube®) *on page 693*

OTHER DRUGS IMPLICATED IN XEROSTOMIA

>10%	1% to 10%
Alprazolam	Acrivastine and Pseudoephedrine
Amitriptyline hydrochloride	Albuterol
Amoxapine	Amantadine hydrochloride
Anisotropine methylbromide	Amphetamine sulfate
Atropine sulfate	Astemizole
Belladonna and Opium	Azatadine maleate
Benztropine mesylate	Beclomethasone dipropionate
Bupropion	Bepridil hydrochloride
Chlordiazepoxide	Bitolterol mesylate
Clomipramine hydrochloride	Brompheniramine maleate
Clonazepam	Carbinoxamine and Pseudoephedrine
Clonidine	Chlorpheniramine maleate
Clorazepate dipotassium	Clemastine fumarate
Cyclobenzaprine	Clozapine
Desipramine hydrochloride	Cromolyn sodium
Diazepam	Cyproheptadine hydrochloride
Dicyclomine hydrochloride	Dexchlorpheniramine maleate
Diphenoxylate and Atropine	Dextroamphetamine sulfate
Doxepin hydrochloride	Dimenhydrinate
Ergotamine	Diphenhydramine hydrochloride
Estazolam	Disopyramide phosphate
Flavoxate	Doxazosin
Flurazepam hydrochloride	Dronabinol
Glycopyrrolate	Ephedrine sulfate
Guanabenz acetate	Flumazenil
Guanfacine hydrochloride	Fluvoxamine
Hyoscyamine sulfate	Gabapentin
Interferon Alfa-2a	Guaifenesin and Codeine
Interferon Alfa-2b	Guanadrel sulfate
Interferon Alfa-N3	Guanethidine sulfate
Ipratropium bromide	Hydroxyzine
Isoproterenol	Hyoscyamine, Atropine, Scopolamine, and Phenobarbital
Isotretinoin	Imipramine
Loratadine	Isoetharine
Lorazepam	Levocabastine hydrochloride
Loxapine	Levodopa
Maprotiline hydrochloride	Levodopa and Carbidopa
Methscopolamine bromide	Levorphanol tartrate
Molindone hydrochloride	Meclizine hydrochloride
Nabilone	Meperidine hydrochloride
Nefazodone	Methadone hydrochloride
Oxybutynin chloride	Methamphetamine hydrochloride
Oxazepam	Methyldopa
Paroxetine	Metoclopramide
Phenelzine sulfate	Morphine sulfate
Prochlorperazine	Nortriptyline hydrochloride
Propafenone hydrochloride	Ondansetron
Protriptyline hydrochloride	Oxycodone and Acetaminophen
Quazepam	Oxycodone and Aspirin
Reserpine	Pentazocine
Selegiline hydrochloride	Phenylpropanolamine hydrochloride
Temazepam	Prazosin hydrochloride
Thiethylperazine maleate	Promethazine hydrochloride
Trihexyphenidyl hydrochloride	Propoxyphene
Trimipramine maleate	Pseudoephedrine
Venlafaxine	Risperidone
	Sertraline hydrochloride
	Terazosin
	Terbutaline sulfate
	Terfenadine

PRESCRIPTION EXAMPLES

Rx

Sodium carboxymethylcellulose (Baker) 0.5% aqueous solution

Disp 8 oz

Sig: Use as a rinse frequently as needed to relieve symptoms of
dry mouth

Rx

Xero-Lube®*

Disp 1 bottle

Sig: Apply several drops or sprays to mouth as necessary for
dryness

Note: Consider topical treatment in custom trays for those patients
with severe xerostomia

*Note: Alternatives: Moi-Stir®; MouthKote®; Optimoist®; Salivart®

Systemic stimulation of saliva has been achieved in some patients using pilocarpine.

Rx

Salagen® 5 mg

Disp 120 tablets

Sig: 1 tablet 3-4 times/day, not top exceed 30 mg/day

Note: Patients should be treated for a minimum of 90 days
to achieve clinical effects.

TEMPOROMANDIBULAR DYSFUNCTION (TMD)

Temporomandibular dysfunction comprises a broad spectrum of signs and symptoms. Although TMD presents in patterns, diagnosis is often difficult. Evaluation and treatment is time-intensive and no single therapy or drug regimen has been shown to be universally beneficial. The Oral Medicine specialist in TMD management, the physical therapist interested in head and neck pain, and the Oral and Maxillofacial surgeon will all work together with the referring general dentist to accomplish successful patient treatment. Table 1 lists the wide variety of treatment alternatives available to the team. Depending on the diagnosis, one or more of the therapies might be selected. For organic diseases of the joint not responding to nonsurgical approaches, a wide variety of surgical techniques are available (Table 2).

ACUTE TMD

Acute TMD oftentimes presents alone or as an episode during a chronic pattern of signs and symptoms. Trauma such as a blow to the chin or the side of the face can result in acute TMD. Occasionally, similar symptoms will follow a lengthy wide open mouth dental procedure.

The condition usually presents as continuous deep pain in the TMJ. If edema is present in the joint, the condyle sometimes can be displaced which will cause abnormal occlusion of the posterior teeth on the affected side. The diagnosis is usually based on the history and clinical presentation. Management of the patient includes:

1. Restriction of all mandibular movement to function in a pain-free range of motion
2. Soft diet
3. NSAIDs (eg, Anaprox® DS 1 tablet every 12 hours for 7-10 days)
4. Moist heat applications to the affected area for 15-20 minutes, 4-6 times/day

Additional therapies could include referral to a physical therapist for ultrasound therapy 2-4 times/week and a single injection of steroid in the joint space. A team approach with an oral maxillofacial surgeon for this procedure may be helpful. Spray and stretch with Fluori-methane® is often helpful for rapid relief of trismus.

Dichlorodifluoromethane and Trichloromonofluoromethane (Fluori-methane®) *on page 270*

Nonsteroidal Anti-inflammatory Agent (NSAID), Oral *on page 1140*

CHRONIC TMD

Following diagnosis which is often problematic, the most common therapeutic modalities include:

- Explaining the problem to the patient
- Recommending a soft diet:
  - avoid chewing gum, salads, biting into large sandwiches, biting into hard fruit
  - diet should consist of soft foods such as eggs, yogurt, casseroles, soup, ground meat
- Reducing stress; moist heat application 4-6 times daily for 15-20 minutes coupled with a monitored exercise program will be beneficial. Usually, working with a physical therapist is ideal.
- Medications include analgesics, anti-inflammatories, tranquilizers, and muscle relaxants

MEDICATION OPTIONS

Most commonly used medication (NSAIDs):

Ibuprofen (Motrin®) *on page 447*
Naproxen (Anaprox®) *on page 606*
Flurbiprofen Sodium (Ansaid®) *on page 381*
Sulindac (Clinoril®) *on page 813*

Tranquilizers and muscle relaxants when used appropriately can provide excellent adjunctive therapy. These drugs should be primarily used for a short period of time to manage acute pain.

Common minor tranquilizers include:

Alprazolam (Xanax®) *on page 35*

Diazepam (Valium®) *on page 268*

Lorazepam (Ativan®) *on page 513*

Common muscle relaxants include:

Chlorzoxazone (Parafon® Forte DSC) *on page 200*

Methocarbamol (Robaxin®) *on page 557*

Orphenadrine Citrate (Norgesic® Forte) *on page 640*

Cyclobenzaprine Hydrochloride (Flexeril®) *on page 239*

Muscle relaxants and tranquilizers should generally be prescribed with an analgesic or NSAID to relieve pain as well

Narcotic analgesics can be used on a short-term basis or intermittently in combination with non-narcotic therapy in the chronic pain patient. Judicious prescribing, monitoring, and maintenance by the practitioner is imperative whenever considering the use of narcotic analgesics due to the abuse and addiction liabilities.

Table 1. TMD - NONSURGICAL THERAPIES

1. Moist heat and cold spray
2. Injections in muscle trigger areas (procaine)
3. Exercises (passive, active)
4. Medications
    a. Muscle relaxants
    b. Minerals
    c. Multiple vitamins (Ca, B_6, B_{12})
5. Orthopedic craniomandibular respositioning appliance (splints)
6. Biofeedback, acupuncture
7. Physiotherapy: TMJ muscle therapy
8. Myofunctional therapy
9. TENS (transcutaneous electrical neural stimulation), Myo-Monitor
10. Dental therapy
    a. Equilibration (coronoplasty)
    b. Restoring occlusion to proper vertical dimension of maxilla to mandible by orthodontics, dental restorative procedures, orthognathic surgery, permanent splint, or any combination of these

Table 2. TMD - SURGICAL THERAPIES

1. Cortisone injection into joint (with local anesthetic)
2. Bony and/or fibrous ankylosis: requires surgery (osteoarthrotomy with prosthetic appliance)
3. Chronic subluxation: requires surgery, depending on problem (possibly eminectomy and/or prosthetic implant)
4. Osteoarthritis: requires surgery, depending on problem
    a. Arthroplasty with implant
    b. Meniscectomy with implant
    c. Arthroplasty with repair of disc and/or implant
    d. Implant with Silastic insert
5. Rheumatoid arthritis
    a. Arthroplasty with implant with Silastic insert
    b. "Total" TMJ replacement
6. Tumors: require osteoarthrotomy — removal of tumor and restoring of joint when possible
7. Chronic disc displacement: requires repair of disc and possible removal of bone from condyle

PATIENTS REQUIRING SEDATION

Anxiety constitutes the most frequently found psychiatric problem in the general population. Anxiety can range from simple phobias to severe debilitating anxiety disorders. Functional results of this anxiety can, therefore, range from simple avoidance of dental procedures to panic attacks when confronting stressful situations such as seen in some patients regarding dental visits. Many patients claim to be anxious over dental care when in reality they simply have not been managed with modern techniques of local anesthesia, the availability of sedation, or the caring dental practitioner.

The dentist may detect anxiety in patients during the treatment planning evaluation phase of the care. The anxious person may appear overly alert, may lean forward in the dental chair during conversation or may appear concerned over time, possibly using this as a guise to require that they cut short their dental visit. Anxious persons may also show signs of being nervous by demonstrating sweating, tension in their muscles including their temporomandibular musculature, or they may complain of being tired due to an inability to obtain an adequate night's sleep.

The management of such patients requires a methodical approach to relaxing the patient, discussing their dental needs, and then planning, along with the patient the best way to accomplish dental treatment in the presence of their fears, both real or imagined. Consideration may be given to sedation to assist with managing the patient. This sedation can be oral or parenteral, or inhalation in the case of nitrous oxide. The dentist must be adequately trained in administering the sedative of choice, as well as in monitoring the patient during the sedated procedures. Numerous medications are available to achieve the level of sedation usually necessary in the dental office: Valium®, Ativan®, Xanax®, Vistaril®, Serax®, and Buspar® represent a few. Buspar® is soon to be available as a transdermal patch. These oral sedatives can be given prior to dental visits as outlined in the following prescriptions. They have the advantage of allowing the patient a good night's sleep prior to the day of the procedures and providing on the spot sedation during the procedures. Nitrous oxide represents an in the office administered sedative that is relatively safe, but requires additional training and carefully planned monitoring protocols of any auxiliary personnel during the inhalation procedures. Both the oral and the inhalation techniques can, however, be applied in a very useful manner to manage the anxious patient in the dental office.

Alprazolam (Xanax®) *on page 35*
Buspirone Hydrochloride (Buspar®) *on page 131*
Diazepam (Valium®) *on page 268*
Hydroxyzine (Vistaril®) *on page 443*
Lorazepam (Ativan®) *on page 513*
Nitrous Oxide *on page 625*
Oxazepam (Serax®) *on page 644*
Triazolam (Halcion®) *on page 866*

PRESCRIPTION EXAMPLES

Rx

Valium® 5 mg*

Disp 6 (six) tablets

Sig: Take 1 tablet in evening before going to bed and 1 tablet 1 hour before your appointment

---

Ingredient: Diazepam

*Note: Also available as 2 mg and 10 mg

Rx

Ativan® 1 mg*

Disp 4 (four) tablets

Sig: Take 2 tablets in evening before going to bed and take 2 tablets 1 hour before your appointment

---

Ingredient: Lorazepam

*Note: Also available as 0.5 mg and 2 mg

Rx

Xanax® 0.5 mg

Disp 4 (four) tablets

Sig: Take 1 tablet in evening before going to bed and 1 tablet 1 hour before your appointment

Ingredient: Alprazolam

Rx

Vistaril® 25 mg

Disp 16 capsules

Sig: Take 2 capsules in evening before going to bed and 2 capsules 1 hour before your appointment

Ingredient: Hydroxyzine

Rx

Halcion® 0.25 mg

Disp 4 (four) tablets

Sig: Take 1 tablet in evening before going to bed and 1 tablet 1 hour before your appointment

Ingredient: Triazolam

Rx

Serax® 10 mg

Disp 2 (two) tablets

Sig: Take 1 tablet before bed and 1 tablet 30 minutes before your appointment.

Ingredient: Oxazepam

PATIENTS UNDERGOING CANCER THERAPY

The dental management recommendations for patients undergoing chemotherapy, bone marrow transplantation, and/or radiation therapy for the treatment of cancer are based primarily on clinical observations. The following protocols will provide a conservative, consistent approach to the dental management of patients undergoing chemotherapy or bone marrow transplantation. Many of the cancer chemotherapy drugs produce oral side effects including mucositis, oral ulceration, dry mouth, acute infections, and taste aberrations. Cancer drugs include antibiotics, alkylating agents, antimetabolites, DNA inhibitors, hormones, and cytokines (see listing of Cancer Chemotherapy Regimens in Appendix).

Cancer Chemotherapy Regimens *on page 1011*

DENTAL PROTOCOL

All patients undergoing chemotherapy or bone marrow transplantation for malignant disease should have the following baseline:

A.   Panoramic radiograph

B.   Dental consultation and examination

C.   Dental prophylaxis and cleaning (if the neutrophil count is >1500/mm³ and the platelet count is >50,000/mm³

- Prophylaxis and cleaning will be deferred if the patient's neutrophil count is <1500 and the platelet count is <50,000. Oral hygiene recommendations will be made.

D.   Oral Hygiene. Patients should be encouraged to follow normal hygiene procedures. Addition of a chlorhexidine mouth rinse such as Peridex® or PerioGard® is usually helpful. If patient develops oral mucositis, tolerance of such alcohol-based products may be limited.

E.   If the patient develops mucositis, bacterial, viral, and fungal cultures should be obtained. Sucralfate suspension in either a pharmacy prepared form or Carafate® suspension as well as Benadryl® or Xylocaine® viscous can assist in helping the patient to tolerate food. Patients may also require systemic analgesics for pain relief depending on the presence of mucositis. Positive fungal cultures may require a nystatin swish and swallow prescription.

F.   The determination of performing dental procedures must be based on the goal of preventing infection during periods of neutropenia. Timing of procedures must be coordinated with the patient's hematologic status.

G.   If oral surgery is required, at least 7-10 days of healing should be allowed before the anticipated date of bone marrow suppression (eg, ANC of <1000/mm³ and/or platelet count of 50,000/mm³).

H.   Daily use of topical fluorides is recommended for those who have received radiation therapy to the head-neck region involving salivary glands. Any patients with prolonged xerostomia subsequent to graft versus host disease and/or chemotherapy can also be considered for fluoride supplement. Use the fluoride-containing mouthwashes (Act®, Fluorigard®, etc) each night before going to sleep; swish, hold 1-2 minutes, spit out or use prescription fluorides (gels or rinses); apply them daily for 3-4 minutes as directed; if the mouth is sore (mucositis), use flavorless/colorless gels (Thera-Flur®, Gel-Kam®). Improvement in salivary flow following radiation therapy to the head and neck has been noted with Salagen®. See "Oral Rinse Products" in Appendix.

Benzonatate (Tessalon Perles®) *on page 104*

Chlorhexidine Gluconate (Peridex®; PerioGard®) *on page 184*

Diphenhydramine Hydrochloride (Benadryl® elixir) *on page 288*

Lidocaine Hydrochloride (Xylocaine®) *on page 502*

Oral Rinse Products *on page 1067*

Pilocarpine (Dental) (Salagen®) *on page 693*

Povidone-Iodine (Betadine®) *on page 713*

Sucralfate (Carafate®) *on page 804*

PRESCRIPTION EXAMPLES

Rx

Peridex® or PerioGard® oral rinse

Disp 3 bottles

Sig: 20 mL x 30 sec tid; swish and expectorate

Ingredient: Chlorhexidine

Rx

Xylocaine® viscous 2%

Disp 450 mL bottles

Sig: Swish with 1 tablespoonful 4 times/day

Ingredient: Lidocaine

Rx

Betadine® mouthwash 0.8%

Disp 6 oz bottle

Sig: Rinse with 1 tablespoonful 4 times/day; do not swallow

Ingredient: Povidone-Iodine

Rx

Mycostatin® oral suspension 100,000 units/mL

Disp 60 mL bottle

Sig: 2 mL 4 times/day; hold in mouth for 2 minutes and swallow

---

Ingredient: Nystatin

When the oral mucous membranes are especially sensitive, nystatin "popsicles" can be made by adding 2 mL of nystatin oral suspension to the water in ice cube trays. Tessalon Perles® have been used ad lib to provide relief in painful mucositis.

Rx

Tessalon Perles®

Disp 50

Sig: Squeeze contents of capsule and apply to lesion

Ingredient: Benzonatate

ORAL CARE PRODUCTS

BACTERIAL PLAQUE CONTROL

Patients should use an extra soft bristle toothbrush and dental floss for removal of plaque. Sponge/foam sticks and lemon-glycerine swabs do not adequately remove bacterial plaque.

PRESCRIPTION EXAMPLE

Rx

Ultra Suave® toothbrush (Periodontal Health Brush Inc)

Biotene Supersoft® toothbrush (Laclede Products)

Chlorhexidine 0.12% (Peridex®, Procter & Gamble, or other preparations available in Canada and Europe) may be used to assist with bacterial plaque control.

SALIVA SUBSTITUTES

Carboxymethylcellulose or mucopolysaccharide*-based sprays for temporary relief from xerostomia include:

Glandosane®(Tsumura Medical) *on page 778*
Moi-Stir® (Kingswood Labs) *on page 778*
*Mouth-Kote® (Parnell Pharmaceuticals) *on page 778*
Optimoist® (Colgate Oral Pharmaceuticals) *on page 778*
Salivart® (Gebauer) *on page 778*
Xerolube® (Colgate Hoyt) *on page 778*

FLUORIDE GELS

Oral Rinse Products *on page 1067*

Used for the prevention of demineralization of the tooth structure secondary to xerostomia. For patients with long-term or permanent xerostomia, daily application is accomplished using custom gel applicator trays. Patients with porcelain crowns should use a neutral pH fluoride.

1.1% neutral pH sodium fluoride
Thera-Flur-N® or Prevident® (Colgate Hoyt) *on page 374*
0.4% stannous fluoride
Gel-Kam® unflavored (Colgate Hoyt) *on page 374*

REMINERALIZING GEL

In addition to fluoride gel to remineralize enamel breakdown in severely xerostomic patients, applicator trays may be used.

Revive® (Dental Resources, Inc. Delano, MN)

ORAL AND LIP MOISTURIZERS/LUBRICANTS

Mouth Pain, Cold Sore, Canker Sore Products *on page 1063*

Water-based gels should first be used to provide moisture to dry oral tissues.

Surgi-Lube® (Fougera)
K-Y Jelly® (Johnson & Johnson)
Oral Balance® (Laclede Products)
Mouth Moisturizer® (Sage Medical)

PALLIATION OF PAIN

Mouth Pain, Cold Sore, Canker Sore Products *on page 1063*

Palliative pain preparations should be monitored for efficacy.

* For relief of pain associated with isolated ulcerations, topical anesthetic and protective preparations may be used.

Orabase-B® with 20% benzocaine (Colgate-Hoyt) *on page 102*
Oratect Gel® with 15% benzocaine and protective film (MGI Pharma) *on page 102*
Ziladent® with 6% benzocaine and protective film (Zila Pharm) *on page 102*

* For generalized oral pain:

Chloraseptic Spray® (OTC) anesthetic spray without alcohol (Richardson Vicks) *on page 102*
Ulcer-Ease® anesthetic/analgesic mouthrinse (Med-Derm Pharmaceuticals)
Xylocaine® 2% viscous *on page 502*
May anesthetize swallowing mechanism and cause aspiration of food; caution patient against using too close to eating; lack of sensation may also allow patient to damage intact mucosa
Tantum Mouthrinse® (benzydamine hydrochloride); available only in Canada and Europe; may be diluted as required

PATIENT PREPARED PALLIATIVE MIXTURES

Coating agents:

Maalox® (Ciba Self-Medication) *on page 40*

Mylanta® (Merck) *on page 41*

Gelucil® (Parke-Davis) *on page 41*

Kaopectate® (Upjohn) *on page 86*

These products can be mixed with Benadryl® elixir 50:50

Diphenhydramine Hydrochloride (Benadryl®) *on page 288*

Mouth Pain, Cold Sore, Canker Sore Products *on page 1063*

Topical anesthetics (diphenhydramine chloride)

Benadryl® elixir or Benylin® cough syrup (Parke Davis) *on page 288*

Choose product with lowest alcohol and sucrose contents; ask pharmacist for assistance

PHARMACY PREPARATIONS

A Pharmacist may also prepare the following solutions for relief of generalized oral pain:

Benadryl-Lidocaine Solution

Diphenhydramine injectable 1.5 mL (50 mg/mL) *on page 288*

Xylocaine viscous 2% (45 mL) *on page 502*

Magnesium aluminum hydroxide solution (45 mL)

Swish and hold 1 teaspoonful in mouth for 30 seconds

Do not use too close to eating

Rx

Carafate suspension 1 g/10 mL

Disp 420 mL

Sig: Swish and hold 1 teaspoonful in mouth for 30 seconds

CHEMICAL DEPENDENCY AND DENTAL PRACTICE

INTRODUCTION

As long as history has been recorded, every society has used drugs that alter mood, thought, and feeling. In addition, pharmacological advances sometimes have been paralleled by physical as well as unfortunate behavioral dependence on agents initially consumed for therapeutic purposes.

In 1986, the American Dental Association passed a policy statement recognizing chemical dependency as a disease. In recognizing this disease, the Association mandated that dentists have a responsibility to include questions relating to a history of chemical dependency or more broadly substance abused in their health history questionnaire. A positive response may require the dentist to alter the treatment plan for the patient's dental care. This includes patients who are actively abusing alcohol, drugs, or patients who are in recovery. The use and abuse of drugs is not a topic that is usually found in the dental curriculum. Information about substance abuse is usually gleaned from newspapers, magazines, or just hearsay.

This chapter reviews street drugs, where they come from, signs and symptoms of the drug abuser, and some of the dental implications of treating patients actively using or in recovery from these substances. There are many books devoted to this topic that provide greater detail. The intent is to provide an overview of some of the most prevalent drugs, how patients abusing these drugs may influence dental treatment, and how to recognize some signs and symptoms of use and withdrawal.

Street drugs, like other drugs, can come from various sources. They may be derived from natural sources (ie, morphine and codeine). They may be semisynthetic, that is a natural product is chemically modified to produce another molecule (ie, morphine conversion to heroin). Street drugs may also be synthetic with no natural origin.

ALCOHOL

The chronic use of alcohol as well as that of other sedatives is associated with the development of depression. The risk of suicide among alcoholics is one of the highest of any diagnostic category. Cognitive deficits have been reported in alcoholics tested while sober. These deficits usually improve after weeks to months of abstinence. More severe recent memory impairment is associated with specific brain damage caused by nutritional deficiencies common in alcoholics.

Alcohol is toxic to many organ systems. As a result, the medical complications of alcohol abuse and dependence include liver disease, cardiovascular disease, endocrine and gastrointestinal effects, and malnutrition, in addition to CNS dysfunctions. Ethanol readily crosses the placental barrier, producing the *fetal alcohol syndrome*, a major cause of mental retardation.

Alcohol Withdrawal Syndrome Signs and Symptoms
Alcohol craving
Tremor, irritability
Nausea
Sleep disturbance
Tachycardia
Hypertension
Sweating
Perceptual distortion
Seizures (12-48 hours after last drink)
Delirium tremens (rare in uncomplicated withdrawal):
Severe agitation
Confusion
Visual hallucinations
Fever, profuse sweating
Tachycardia
Nausea, diarrhea
Dilated pupils

NICOTINE

Cigarette (nicotine) addiction is influenced by multiple variables. Nicotine itself produces reinforcement; users compare nicotine to stimulants such as cocaine or amphetamine, although its effects are of lower magnitude.

Nicotine is absorbed readily through the skin, mucous membranes, and of course, through the lungs. The pulmonary route produces discernible central nervous system effects in as little as 7 seconds. Thus, each puff produces some discrete reinforcement. With 10 puffs per cigarette, the 1 pack per day smoker reinforces the habit 200 times daily. The timing, setting, situation, and preparation all become associated repetitively with the effects of nicotine.

Nicotine has both stimulant and depressant actions. The smoker feels alert, yet there is some muscle relaxation. Nicotine activates the nucleus accumbens reward system in the brain. Increased extracellular dopamine has been found in this region after nicotine injections in rats. Nicotine affects other systems as well, including the release of endogenous opioids and glucocorticoids.

Nicotine Withdrawal Syndrome Signs and Symptoms
Irritability, impatience, hostility
Anxiety
Dysphoric or depressed mood
Difficulty concentrating
Restlessness
Decreased heart rate
Increased appetite or weight gain

Medications to assist users in breaking a nicotine habit are available.

Nicotine (Habitrol®, Nicoderm®, Nicorette® (OTC), Nicotrol® (OTC), ProStep®) *on page 617*

OPIATES

The opiates are most often called narcotics. The most common opiate found on the street is heroin. Heroin is the diacetyl derivative of morphine which is extracted from opium. Although commercial production of morphine involves extraction from the dried opium plant which grows in many parts of the world, some areas still harvest opium by making slits in the unripened seed pod. The pod secretes a white, viscous material which upon contact with the air turns a blackish-brown color. It is this off-white material that is called opium. The opium is then dried and smoked or processed to yield morphine and codeine. Actually, the raw opium contains several chemicals that are used medicinally or commercially. Much (it has been estimated that 50%) of the morphine is converted chemically into heroin which finds its way into the United States and then on the street. Heroin is a Schedule I drug and as such has no acceptable use in the United States today. In fact, possession is a violation of the Controlled Substances Act of 1970. The majority of the heroin found on the streets is from Southeast Asia and can be as concentrated as 100%.

The heroin user goes through many phases once the drug has been administered. When administered intravenously, the user initially feels a "rush" often described as an "orgasmic rush". This initial feeling is most likely due to the release of histamine resulting in cutaneous vasodilation, itching, and a flushed appearance. Shortly after this "rush" the user becomes euphoric. This euphoric stage often called "stoned" or being "high" lasts approximately 3-4 hours. During this stage, the user is lethargic, slow to react to stimuli, speech is slurred, pain reaction threshold is elevated, exhibits xerostomia, slowed heart rate, and the pupils may be constricted. Following the "high", the abuser is "straight" for about 2 hours, with no tell-tale signs of abuse. Approximately 6-8 hours following the last injection of heroin, the user begins to experience a runny nose, lacrimation, and abdominal muscle cramps as they begin the withdrawal from the drug. During this stage and the one that follows, the person may become agitated as they develop anxiety about where they are going to get their next "hit". The withdrawal signs and symptoms become more intense. For the next 3 days, the abuser begins to sweat profusely in combination with cutaneous vasoconstriction. The skin becomes cold and clammy, hence the term "cold turkey". Tachycardia, pupillary dilation, diarrhea, and salivation occur for the 3 days following the last injection. Withdrawal signs and symptoms may last longer than the average of 3 days or they may be more abrupt.

Opioid Withdrawal Signs and Symptoms

Symptoms	Signs
Regular Withdrawal	
Craving for opioids	Pupillary dilation
Restlessness, irritability	Sweating
Increased sensitivity to pain	Piloerection ("gooseflesh")
Nausea, cramps	Tachycardia
Muscle aches	Vomiting, diarrhea
Dysphoric mood	Increased blood pressure
Insomnia, anxiety	Yawning
	Fever
Protracted Withdrawal	
Anxiety	Cyclic changes in weight, pupil size, respiratory center sensitivity
Insomnia	
Drug craving	

Many of these patients who have been abusing opiates for any length of time will exhibit multiple carious lesions, particularly class V lesions. This increased caries rate is probably a result of the heroin-induced xerostomia, high intake of sweets, and lack of daily oral hygiene. Patients who are recovering from heroin or any opiate addiction should not be given any kind of opiate analgesic, whether it be for sedation or as a postoperative analgesic because of the increased chance of relapse. The nonsteroidal anti-inflammatory drugs (NSAIDs) should be used to control any postoperative discomfort. Patients who admit to a past history of intravenous heroin use or any intravenous drug for that matter, are at higher risk for subacute bacterial endocarditis (SBE), HIV disease, and hepatitis but with the exception of postoperative analgesia should present no special problem for dental care.

MARIJUANA

The number one most abused illegal drug by high school students today is marijuana. Marijuana is a plant that grows throughout the world, but is particularly suited for a warm, humid environment. There are three species of plant but the two most frequently cited are *Cannabis sativa* and *Cannabis indica*. All species possess a female and male plant. Although approximately 450 chemicals have been isolated from the plant, the major psychoactive ingredient is delta-9-tetrahydrocannabinol (THC). Of these 450 chemicals, there are about 23 psychoactive chemicals, THC being the most abundant. The highest concentration of THC is found in the bud of the female plant. The concentration of THC varies according to growing conditions and location on the plant but has increased from about 2% to 3% in marijuana sold in the 50s to about 30% sold on the streets today. Marijuana can be smoked in cigarettes (joints), pipes, water pipes (bongs), or baked in brownies, cakes, etc, and then ingested. However, smoking marijuana is more efficient and the "high" has a quicker onset. Marijuana is a Schedule I drug but has been promoted as a medicinal for the treatment of glaucoma, for increasing appetite in patients who have HIV disease, and to prevent the nausea associated with cancer chemotherapy. In response to this request, the FDA approved dronabinol (Marinol®), a synthetic THC and placed this drug in Schedule II to be prescribed by physicians for the indicated medical conditions.

Dronabinol (Marinol®) *on page 302*

An individual under the influence of marijuana may exhibit no signs or symptoms of intoxication. The pharmacologic effects are dose-dependent and depend to a large extent on the set and setting of the intoxicated individual. As the dose of THC increases, the person experiences euphoria or a state of well-being, often referred to as "mellowing out". Everything becomes comical, problems disappear, and their appetite for snack foods increases. This is called the "munchies". The marijuana produces time and spatial distortion, which contribute, as the dose increases, to a dysphoria characterized by paranoia and fear. Although there has never been a death reported from marijuana overdose, certainly the higher doses may produce such bizarre circumstances as to increase the chances of accidental death. THC is fat soluble. Daily consumption of marijuana will result in THC being stored in body fat which will result in detectable amounts of THC being found in the urine for as long as 60 days in some cases.

Marijuana Withdrawal Syndrome Signs and Symptoms
Restlessness
Irritability
Mild agitation
Insomnia
Restlessness
Sleep EEG disturbance
Nausea, cramping

Because of anxiety associated with dental visits, marijuana would be the most likely drug, after alcohol, to be used when coming to the dental office. But, unlike alcohol, marijuana may not produce any detectable odor on the breath nor any signs of intoxication. Fortunately, local anesthetics, analgesics, and antibiotics used by the general dentist do not interact with marijuana. The major concern with the marijuana intoxicated patient is a failure to follow directions while in the chair, and the inability to follow postoperative instructions.

COCAINE

Cocaine, referred to on the street as "snow", "nose candy", "girl", and many other euphemisms, has created an epidemic. This drug is like no other local anesthetic. Known for about the last two thousand years, cocaine has been used and abused by politicians, scientists, farmers, warriors, and of course, on the street. Cocaine is derived from the leaves of a plant called *Erythroxylon coca* which grows in South America. Ninety percent of the world's supply of cocaine originates in Peru, Bolivia, and Colombia. At last estimate, the United States consumes 75% of the world's supply. The plant grows to a height of approximately four feet and produces a red berry. Farmers go through the fields stripping the leaves from the plant three times a year. During the working day the farmers chew the coca leaves to suppress appetite and fight the fatigue of working the fields. The leaves are transported to a laboratory site where the cocaine is extracted by a process called maceration. It takes approximately 7-8 pounds of leaves to produce one ounce of cocaine.

On the streets of the United States, cocaine can be found in two forms. One form is as the hydrochloride salt. In this form, the cocaine can be "snorted" or it can be dissolved in water and injected intravenously. The other form of cocaine is as the free base. The free base form can be smoked. The free base form is sometimes referred to as "crack", "rock", or "free base". It is called crack because it cracks or pops when large pieces are smoked. It is called rock because it is so hard and difficult to break into smaller pieces. The most popular method of administration of cocaine is "snorting." In this method, small amounts of cocaine hydrochloride are divided into segments or "lines". The person uses any straw-like device to inhale one or more lines of the cocaine into their nose. Although the cocaine does not reach the lungs, enough cocaine is absorbed through the nasal mucosa to provide a "high" within 3-5 minutes. Rock or crack on the other hand is heated and inhaled from any device available. This form of cocaine does reach the lungs and provides a much faster onset of action as well as a more intense stimulation. There are dangers to the user with any form of cocaine. Undoubtedly the most dangerous form, though, is the intravenous route.

Cocaine Withdrawal Signs and Symptoms
Dysphoria, depression
Sleepiness, fatigue
Cocaine craving
Bradycardia

The cocaine user, regardless of how the cocaine was administered, presents the potential of a life-threatening situation in the dental operatory. The patient under the influence of cocaine could be compared to a car going 100 miles per hour. Blood pressure is elevated and heart rate is likely increased. The use of a local anesthetic with epinephrine in such a patient may result in a medical emergency. Such patients can be identified by their jitteriness, irritability, talkativeness, tremors, and short abrupt speech patterns. These same signs and symptoms may also be seen in a normal dental patient with preoperative dental anxiety; therefore, the dentist must be particularly alert in order to identify the potential cocaine abuser. If a patient is suspected, they should never be given a local anesthetic with vasoconstrictor for fear of exacerbating the cocaine-induced sympathetic response. Life-threatening episodes of cardiac arrhythmias and hypertensive crises have been reported when local anesthetic with vasoconstrictor was administered to a patient under the influence of cocaine. No local anesthetic used by any dentist can interfere with, nor test positive for cocaine in any urine testing screen. Therefore, the dentist needn't be concerned with any false drug use accusations associated with dental anesthesia.

PSYCHEDELIC AGENTS

Perceptual distortions that include hallucinations, illusions, and disorders of thinking such as paranoia can be produced by toxic doses of many drugs. These phenomena also may be seen during toxic withdrawal from sedatives such as alcohol. There are, however, certain drugs that have as their primary effect the production of perception, thought, or mood disturbances at low doses with minimal effects on memory and orientation. These are commonly called *hallucinogenic drugs*, but their use does not always result in frank hallucinations.

LSD: LSD is the most potent hallucinogenic drug and produces significant psyche-delic effects with a total dose of as little as 25-50 mcg. This drug is over 3000 times more potent than mescaline. LSD is sold on the illicit market in a variety of forms. A popular contemporary system involves postage stamp-sized papers impregnated with varying doses of LSD (50-300 mcg or more). A majority of street samples sold as LSD actually contain LSD. In contrast, the samples of mushrooms and other botanicals sold as sources of psilocybin and other psychedelics have a low proba-bility of containing the advertised hallucinogenics.

Phencyclidine (PCP): PCP deserves special mention because of its widespread availability and because its pharmacological effects are different from LSD. PCP was originally developed as an anesthetic in the 1950s and later abandoned because of a high frequency of postoperative delirium with hallucinations. It was classed as a dissociative anesthetic because, in the anesthetized state, the patient remains conscious with staring gaze, flat facies, and rigid muscles. It was discov-ered as a drug of abuse in the 1970s, first in an oral form and then in a smoked version enabling a better control over the dose.

INHALANTS

Anesthetic gases such as nitrous oxide or halothane are sometimes used as intoxicants by medical personnel. Nitrous oxide also is abused by food service employees because it is supplied for use as a propellant in disposable aluminum minitanks for whipping cream canisters. Nitrous oxide produces euphoria and analgesia and then loss of consciousness. Compulsive use and chronic toxicity rarely are reported, but there are obvious risks of overdose associated with the abuse of this anesthetic. Chronic use has been reported to cause peripheral neuropathy.

The dental team should be alert to the signs and symptoms of drug abuse and withdrawal. Further reading is recommended.

ANIMAL AND HUMAN BITES GUIDELINES

The dentist is often confronted with early management of animal and human bites. The following protocols may assist in appropriate care and referral.

WOUND MANAGEMENT

Irrigation: Critically important; irrigate all penetration wounds using 20 mL syringe, 19-gauge needle and >250 mL 1% povidone iodine solution. This method will reduce wound infection by a factor of 20. When there is high risk of rabies, use viricidal 1% benzalkonium chloride in addition to the 1% povidone iodine. Irrigate wound with normal saline after antiseptic irrigation.

Debridement: Remove all crushed or devitalized tissue remaining after irrigation; minimize removal on face and over thin skin areas or anywhere you would create a worse situation than the bite itself already has; do not extend puncture wounds surgically — rather, manage them with irrigation and antibiotics.

Suturing: Close most dog bites if <8 hours (<12 hours on face); do not routinely close puncture wounds, or deep or severe bites on the hands or feet, as these are at highest risk for infection. Cat and human bites should not be sutured unless cosmetically important. Wound edge freshening, where feasible, reduces infection; minimize sutures in the wound and use monofilament on the surface.

Immobilization: Critical in all hand wounds; important for infected extremities.

Hospitalization/I.V. Antibiotics: Admit for I.V. antibiotics all significant human bites to the hand, especially closed fist injuries, and bites involving penetration of the bone or joint (a high index of suspicion is needed). Consider I.V. antibiotics for significant established wound infections with cellulitis or lymphangitis, any infected bite on the hand, any infected cat bite, and any infection in an immunocompromised or asplenic patient. Outpatient treatment with I.V. antibiotics may be possible in selected cases by consulting with infectious disease.

LABORATORY ASSESSMENT

Gram's Stain: Not useful prior to onset of clinically apparent infection; examination of purulent material may show a predominant organism in established infection, aiding antibiotic selection; not warranted unless results will change your treatment.

Culture: Not useful or cost-effective prior to onset of clinically apparent infection.

X-ray: Whenever you suspect bony involvement, especially in craniofacial dog bites in very small children or severe bite/crush in an extremity; cat bites with their long needle like teeth may cause osteomyelitis or a septic joint, especially in the hand or wrist.

IMMUNIZATIONS

Tetanus: All bite wounds are contaminated. If not immunized in last 5 years, or if not current in a child, give DPT, DT, Td, or TT as indicated. For absent or incomplete primary immunization, give 250 units tetanus immune globulin (TIG) in addition.

Rabies: In the U.S. 30,000 persons are treated each year in an attempt to prevent 1-5 cases. Domestic animals should be quarantined for 10 days to prove need for prophylaxis. High risk animal bites (85% of cases = bat, skunk, raccoon) usually receive treatment consisting of:
- human rabies immune globulin (HRIG): 20 units/kg I.M. (unless previously immunized with HDCV)
- human diploid cell vaccine (HDCV): 1 mL I.M. on days 0, 3, 7, 14, and 28 (unless previously immunized with HDCV - then give only first 2 doses)

Tetanus Immune Globulin, Human *on page 826*
Rabies Immune Globulin, Human *on page 761*
Rabies Virus Vaccine *on page 761*

BITE WOUNDS AND PROPHYLACTIC ANTIBIOTICS

Parenteral vs Oral: If warranted, consider an initial I.V. dose to rapidly establish effective serum levels, especially if high risk, delayed treatment, or if patient reliability is poor.

Dog Bite:

1. Rarely get infected (~5%)

2. Infecting organisms: Staph coag negative, staph coag positive, alpha strep, diphtheroids, beta strep, *Pseudomonas aeruginosa*, gamma strep, *Pasteurella multocida*

3. Prophylactic antibiotics are seldom indicated. Consider for high risk wounds such as distal extremity puncture wounds, severe crush injury, bites occurring in cosmetically sensitive areas (eg, face), or in immunocompromised or asplenic patients.

Cat Bite:

1. Often get infected (~25% to 50%)

2. Infecting organisms: *Pasteurella multocida* (first 24 hours), coag positive staph, anaerobic cocci (after first 24 hours)

3. Prophylactic antibiotics are indicated in all cases.

Human Bite:

1. Intermediate infection rate (~15% to 20%)

2. Infecting organisms: Coag positive staph α, β, γ strep, *Haemophilus*, *Eikenella corrodens*, anaerobic streptococci, *Fusobacterium*, *Veillonella*, bacteroides.

3. Prophylactic antibiotics are indicated in almost all cases except superficial injuries.

   Amoxicillin Trihydrate (various products) *on page 58*
   Amoxicillin and Clavulanic Acid (Augmentin®) *on page 57*
   Cefazolin Sodium (Ancef®; Kefxol®; Zolicef®) *on page 164*
   Cefotetan Disodium (Cefotan®) *on page 168*
   Ceftriaxone Sodium (Rocephin®) *on page 172*
   Clindamycin (Cleocin®) *on page 214*
   Trimethoprim and Sulfamethoxazole (various products) *on page 874*
   Doxycycline (various products) *on page 301*
   Imipenem/Cilastatin (Primaxin®) *on page 451*

BITE WOUND ANTIBIOTIC REGIMENS

	Dog Bite	Cat Bite	Human Bite
Prophylactic Antibiotics			
Prophylaxis	No routine prophylaxis, consider if involves face or hand, or immunosuppressed or asplenic patients	Routine prophylaxis	Routine prophylaxis
Prophylactic antibiotic	Amoxicillin	Amoxicillin	Amoxicillin
Penicillin allergy	Doxycycline if >10 y or co-trimoxazole	Doxycycline if >10 y or co-trimoxazole	Doxycycline if >10 y or erythromycin and cephalexin*
Outpatient Oral Antibiotic Treatment (mild to moderate infection)			
Established infection	Amoxicillin and clavulanic acid	Amoxicillin and clavulanic acid	Amoxicillin and clavulanic acid
Penicillin allergy (mild infection only)	Doxycycline if >10 y	Doxycycline if >10 y	Cephalexin* or clindamycin
Outpatient Parenteral Antibiotic Treatment (moderate infections — single drug regimens)			
	Ceftriaxone	Ceftriaxone	Cefotetan
Inpatient Parenteral Antibiotic Treatment			
Established infection	Ampicillin + cefazolin	Ampicillin + cefazolin	Ampicillin + clindamycin
Penicillin allergy	Cefazolin*	Ceftriaxone*	Cefotetan* or imipenem
Duration of Prophylactic and Treatment Regimens			
Prophylaxis: 5 days			
Treatment: 10-14 days			

*Contraindicated if history of immediate hypersensitivity reaction (anaphylaxis) to penicillin.

SYSTEMIC CONSIDERATIONS RELATED TO NATURAL PRODUCTS FOR WEIGHT LOSS

Weight loss has become increasingly popular. Many people purchase "natural products" which contain various herbal and nutritional supplements to aid in weight loss. Natural products are often labeled by the public as completely safe for use in every situation and by all people. Many plant derivatives and nutritional supplements can positively or negatively influence pre-existing medical conditions or have the propensity to interact with a patient's current medications.

This chapter calls special attention to some of the individual ingredients in selected natural products for weight loss. This chapter is divided by body system with accompanying charts detailing some of the most commonly available natural weight loss products.

It is important to remember natural products, vitamin supplements, and some over-the-counter medications are not regulated by the Food and Drug Administration (FDA) resulting in variability among products and little control on claims of medicinal benefit.

CENTRAL NERVOUS SYSTEM

(Aconite, Ginseng, Xanthine derivatives)

Aconite and hawthorn have potentially sedating effects, and aconite also contains various alkaloids and traces of ephedrine. Some documented central nervous system (CNS) effects of aconite include sedation, vertigo, and incoordination. Hawthorn has been reported to exert a depressive effect on the CNS leading to sedation.

Ginseng, ma-huang, and xanthine derivatives can exert a stimulant effect on the central nervous system. Some of the CNS effects of ginseng include nervousness, insomnia, and euphoria. The action of ma-huang is due to the presence of ephedrine and pseudoephedrine. Ma-huang exerts a stimulant action on the CNS similar to decongestant/weight loss products (Dexatrim®, etc) thus causing nervousness, insomnia, and anxiety. Kola nut, green tea, guarana, and yerba mate contain varying amounts of caffeine, a xanthine derivative. Stimulant properties exerted by these herbs are expected to be comparable to those of caffeine, including insomnia, nervousness, and anxiety.

Products containing aconite and hawthorn should be used with caution in patients with known history of depression, vertigo, or syncope. Ginseng or xanthine derivatives should be avoided in patients with history of insomnia or anxiety. Use of natural products with these components may contribute to a worsening of a patient's pre-existing medical condition. Patients taking CNS-active medications should avoid or use extreme caution when using preparations containing any of the above components. These components may interact directly or indirectly with CNS-active medications causing an increase or decrease in overall effect.

CARDIOVASCULAR SYSTEM

CONGESTIVE HEART FAILURE

(Diuretics, Xanthine derivatives, Licorice, Ginseng, Aconite)

Alisma plantago, bearberry (*Arctostaphylos uva-ursi*), buchu (*Barosma betulina*), couch grass, dandelion, horsetail rush, juniper, licorice, and xanthine derivatives exert varying degrees of diuretic action. Many patients with congestive heart failure (CHF) are already taking a diuretic medication. By taking products containing one or more of these components, patients already on diuretic medications may increase their risk for dehydration.

Ginseng and licorice can potentially worsen congestive heart failure and edema by causing fluid retention. Aconite has varying effects on the heart that itself could lead to heart failure. Patients with CHF should be advised to consult with their healthcare provider before using products containing any of these components.

HYPERTENSION/HYPOTENSION

(Diuretics, Ginkgo biloba, Ginseng, Hawthorn, Ma-huang, Xanthine derivatives)

The stimulant properties of ginseng and ma-huang could worsen pre-existing hypertension. Elevated blood pressure has been reported as a side effect of ginseng. Although ma-huang contains ephedrine, a known vasoconstrictor, ma-huang's effect on blood pressure varies between individuals. Ma-huang can cause hypotension or hypertension. Due to its unpredictable effects, patients with pre-existing hypertension should use caution when using natural products containing ma-huang. Providers should caution patients with labile hypertension against the use of ginseng.

The diuretic effect of xanthine derivatives and other diuretic components could increase the effects of antihypertensive medications, increasing the risk for hypotension. Hawthorn and ginkgo biloba can cause vasodilation increasing the hypotensive effects of antihypertensive medication. Patients susceptible to hypotension or patients taking antihypertensive medication should use caution when taking products containing xanthine derivatives or diuretics. Patients with pre-existing hypertension or hypotension who wish to use products containing these components should be closely monitored by a healthcare professional for changes in blood pressure control.

ARRHYTHMIAS

(Ginseng)

It has been reported that ginseng may increase the risk of arrhythmias, although it is unclear whether this effect is due to the actual ingredient (ginseng) or other possible impurities. Patients at risk for arrhythmias should be cautioned against the use of products containing ginseng without first consulting with their healthcare provider.

GASTROINTESTINAL SYSTEM

PEPTIC ULCER DISEASE

(Betaine Hydrochloride, White Willow)

Betaine hydrochloride is a source of hydrochloric acid. The acid released from betaine hydrochloride could aggravate an existing ulcer. White willow, like aspirin, contains salicylates.

Aspirin has been known to induce gastric damage by direct irritation on the gastric mucosa and by an indirect systemic effect. As a result, patients with a history of peptic ulcer disease or gastritis are informed to avoid use of aspirin and other salicylate derivatives. These precautions should also apply to white willow. Patients with a history of peptic ulcer disease or gastritis should not use products containing white willow or betaine hydrochloride as either could exacerbate ulcers.

INFLAMMATORY BOWEL DISEASE

(Cascara Sagrada, Senna, Dandelion)

Cascara sagrada and senna are stimulant laxatives. Their laxative effect is exerted by stimulation of peristalsis in the colon and by inhibition of water and electrolyte secretion. The laxative effect produced by these herbs could induce an exacerbation of inflammatory bowel disease. Patients with a history of inflammatory bowel disease should avoid using products containing cascara sagrada or senna, and use caution when taking products containing dandelion which may also have a laxative effect.

OBSTRUCTION/ILEUS

(Glucomannan, Kelp, Psyllium)

Glucomannan, kelp, and psyllium act as bulk laxatives. In the presence of water, bulk laxatives swell or form a viscous solution adding extra bulk in the gastrointestinal tract. The resulting mass is thought to stimulate peristalsis. In the presence of an ileus, these laxatives could cause an obstruction.

If sufficient water is not consumed when taking a bulk laxative, a semisolid mass can form resulting in an obstruction. Any patient who wishes to take a natural product containing kelp, psyllium, or glucomannan should drink sufficient water to decrease the risk of obstruction. This may be of concern in particular disease states such as CHF or other cases where excess fluid intake may influence the existing disease presentation. Patients with a suspected obstruction or ileus should avoid using products containing kelp, psyllium, or glucomannan without consent of their primary healthcare provider.

HEMATOLOGIC SYSTEM

ANTICOAGULATION THERAPY & COAGULATION DISORDERS

(Horsetail Rush, Ginseng, Ginkgo Biloba, Guarana, White Willow)

Horsetail rush, ginseng, ginkgo biloba, guarana, and white willow can potentially affect platelet aggregation and bleeding time. Ginkgo biloba, ginseng, guarana, and white willow inhibit platelet aggregation resulting in an increase in bleeding time. Horsetail rush, on the other hand, may decrease bleeding time. Patients with coagulation disorders or patients on anticoagulation therapy may be sensitive to the effects on coagulation by these components and should, therefore, avoid use of products containing any of these components.

ENDOCRINE SYSTEM

DIABETES MELLITUS

(Chromium, Glucomannan, Ginseng, Hawthorn, Ma-huang, Periploca, Spirulina)

Ma-huang and spirulina both may increase glucose levels. This could cause a decrease in glucose control, thereby, increasing a patient's risk for hyperglycemia. Patients with diabetes or glucose intolerance should avoid using ma-huang and spirulina containing products.

Chromium, ginseng, glucomannan, periploca (*gymneme sylvestre*), and hawthorn should be used with caution in patients being treated for diabetes. These ingredients may reduce glucose levels increasing the risk for hypoglycemia in patients who are already taking a hypoglycemic agent. Patients with diabetes who wish to use products containing these ingredients should be closely monitored for fluctuations in blood glucose levels.

OTHER

PHENYLKETONURIA

(Aspartame, Spirulina)

Patients with phenylketonuria should not use products containing aspartame or spirulina. Aspartame, a common artificial sweetener, is metabolized to phenylalanine, while spirulina contains phenylalanine.

GOUT

(Diuretics, White Willow)

Patients with a history of gout should avoid using natural products containing components with diuretic action or white willow. By increasing urine output, ingredients with diuretic action may concentrate uric acid in the blood increasing the risk of gout in these patients. White willow, like aspirin, may inhibit excretion of urate resulting in an increase in uric acid concentration. The increase in urate levels could cause precipitation of uric acid resulting in an exacerbation of gout.

CONCLUSION

Due to the possible actions of the various natural products or weight loss products, patients should use precaution when starting any regimen that includes these supplements. Before taking any natural weight loss supplement, other concomitant diseases and medications should be evaluated for possible interactions.

NATURAL PRODUCTS SOLD FOR WEIGHT LOSS

Product (Distributor)	Other Ingredients
24 hour Diet Herbal Tea® (GNC)	Papaya (carcia papaya), moon daisy (leucanthemum vulgare), parsley (petroselinum hortense), citrus peel (citrus aurantium), spices, natural flavor, althaea
24 hour Diet Shake® (GNC)	Soy protein isolate, sodium/calcium caseinate, whey, corn syrup solids, fiber blend, Dutch cocoa, herbal blend (dahlulin, chickweed, schizandra, L-selenomethionate, inosine, CoQ10), sunflower oil, calcium blend
24 hour Diet Shake	Potassium chloride, natural/artificial flavors, magnesium oxide, soy lecithin, vitamin C, vitamin E, d-alpha tocopherol, vitamin A palmitate, niacinamide, zinc oxide, iron, copper gluconate, d-calcium panthenate
24 hour Diet Shake	Vitamin D_3, pyridoxine hydrochloride, riboflavin, thiamine mononitrate, cyanocobalamin, folate, biotin, potassium iodide
24 hour Dietgel: Energy for Dieters® (GNC)	Cayenne powder, cranberry concentrate, gotu kola
Chroma Plus Slim® (Richardson Labs)	L-carnitine USP, choline bitartrate, inositol, DL-methionine, potassium chloride, pantothenic acid, vitamin B_6, peppermint, bromelain
Chroma Slim for Men® (Richardson Labs)	L-carnitine USP, choline bitartrate, inositol, DL-methionine, pantothenic acid, vitamin B_6, peppermint, saw palmetto berries, cayenne, mustard seed powder, cinnamon, ginger root extract
Chroma Slim Plus Complete® (Richardson Labs)	Hydroxycitric acid, vanadyl sulfate, CoQ10, inositol, folate, potassium chloride, magnesium oxide, B_5 (cal d-pantothenate), niacin, whole food blend, mustard seed, cayenne
Citralean® (Advanced Research)	Hydroxycitric acid, vanadyl sulfate
Diet Fuel: Thermogenic Formula® (Twin Lab)	Hydroxycitric acid, L-carnitine, potassium phosphate, magnesium phosphate, citrus, bioflavonoids, ginger root powder, cayenne powder
Diet Max: Fat Control® (Kal, Inc)	Lotus leaf, cinnamon bark, stephania, rhaponticum, L-carnitine tartrate, niacin, choline bitartrate, pantothenic acid, vitamin B_6, capsicum powder, mustard powder, magnesium oxide/citrate, potassium citrate
Diet Max: Sweet Balance® (Kal, Inc)	Bittermelon, bay leaf powder, cinnamon powder, niacin, magnesium citrate/oxide, medium chain triglycerides, lecithin, oleic acid, natural mixed tocopherols
Excel: Fat Burner Formula® (Human Energy Co)	Garcinia cambogia, (hydroxycitric acid), cayenne
Fat Burners® (Action Labs, Inc)	Choline, inositol, methionine, vitamin B_6, bromelain (pineapple), potassium citrate, calcium ascorbate, L-carnitine, pantothine, corn silk, alfalfa
Fat Fighters® (Only Natural, Inc)	Oat bran, rice brain, apple pectin, carrot fiber, beef fiber, L-acidophilus, lecithin, choline bitartrate, inositol, L-carnitine, aloe vera, bromelain, CoQ10, calcium carbonate, magnesium hydroxide, potassium citrate
Ginseng Trim Maxx® (Body Breakthrough)	Locust plant (cassia augustifolia), gynostermma (pentaphyllum), lycii berry leaf
Metabo Lift Thermogenic Formula® (Twin Lab)	Cayenne
Slim Max® (USA Sports Labs)	Potassium, L-carnitine complex, vitamin B_6, bromelain
Super Diet Max With Chromium® (Natural Max Co)	Mustard seed powder, garcinia cambogia, schizandra extract

(continued)

Product (Distributor)	Other Ingredients
Super Dieters Tea® (Laci Le Beau)	Citrus reticulate (orange peel), carcia papaya, lonicera japonica (honeysuckle), chrysanthemum officinalis (German chamomile), spice, natural flavor, althaea officinalis
Thermachrome 5000	L-carnitine, ginger, boron proteinate, gotu kola, saw palmetto
Ultra Lean Herbal® (Schiff)	Garcinia cambogia extract, cayenne, iodine, potassium (glycerophosphate), magnesium (glycinate), cellulose, vegetable stearates
Ultra Lean Tablet® (Schiff)	Cayenne, iodine, potassium (glycerophosphate), magnesium (glycinate), vanadyl sulfate, cellulose, vegetable stearates, brindall berry extract (garcinia cambogia)

Adapted from Mistry MG and Mays DA, "Precautions Against Global Use of Natural Products for Weight Loss: A Review of Active Ingredients and Issues Concerning Concomitant Disease States," *Therapeutic Perspectives*, 1996, 10(1):2.

DENTAL OFFICE EMERGENCIES

Protocols should be established for most Office Emergencies. Recognition and rapid diagnosis lead to appropriate management. Major drugs discussed under the various headings are listed below.

Ammonia Spirit, Aromatic *on page 54*
Atropine Sulfate *on page 85*
Dexamethasone (Decadron®) *on page 260*
Diazepam (Valium®) *on page 268*
Diphenhydramine Hydrochloride (Benadryl®) *on page 288*
Epinephrine *on page 313*
Hydrocortisone *on page 436*
Isoproterenol *on page 472*
Naloxone Hydrochloride (Narcan®) *on page 602*
Meperidine Hydrochloride (Demerol®) *on page 539*
Methohexital Sodium (Brevital®) *on page 559*
Morphine Sulfate *on page 590*
Theophylline/Aminophylline *on page 832*

SYNCOPE (Fainting)

Cause: Decreased circulation of blood to the brain

Symptoms:

- Pallor
- Anxiety
- Nausea
- Diaphoresis
- Rapid pulse (tachycardia)
- Loss of consciousness
- Decreased blood pressure
- Dilatation of pupils

Treatment:

- Place patient in supine position, with feet slightly elevated
- Maintain airway
- Monitor vital signs
- Administer oxygen
- Place crushed ammonia carpule under nose
- Apply cold compress to face and neck
- Reassure and comfort patient

POSTURAL HYPOTENSION - ORTHOSTATIC HYPOTENSION (Syncope in Moving From the Supine to Upright Position)

Treatment:

- Place patient in supine position
- Maintain airway; check breathing
- Oxygen (as needed)
- Monitor vital signs
- Reposition patient slowly, after stable

AIRWAY OBSTRUCTION

Cause: Foreign body in larynx and pharynx

Symptoms:

- Choking
- Gagging
- Violent expiratory effort
- Substernal notch retraction
- Cyanosis
- Labored breathing
- Rapid pulse initially, then decreased pulse
- Cardiac arrest

Treatment:

- Place patient in supine position
- Tilt head backward
- Clear airway manually of debris (suction oral cavity)
- Check for respiratory sounds; ventilate if necessary
- Administer oxygen
- Perform Heimlich maneuver, if needed
- Place oropharyngeal or nasopharyngeal airway, if obstruction is visible, try to dislodge
- Perform cricothyrotomy, if unable to clear airway
- If foreign body passes, refer immediately for radiographic examination
- Child: Small child may be held upside down and four sharp blows delivered between shoulder blades

HYPERVENTILATION SYNDROME

Cause: Excessive loss of carbon dioxide, producing respiratory alkalosis

Symptoms:

- Rapid, shallow breathing
- Confusion
- Vertigo (dizziness)
- Paresthesia (numbness or tingling of extremities)
- Carpo-pedal spasm

Treatment:

- Position patient semi-reclining
- Calm and reassure patient vocally
- Instruct patient to breathe carbon dioxide enriched air through rebreathing bag
- Do **not** administer oxygen
- Administer medication to calm patient, if needed

BRONCHIAL ASTHMA

Cause: Spasm and constriction of the bronchi

Symptoms:

- Labored breathing
- Wheezing
- Anxiety
- Cyanosis

Treatment:

- Position patient semi-reclining
- Administer bronchodilator-mistometer
- Administer oxygen
- Administer parenteral medications:
    - Adult: I.M. epinephrine 1:1000 0.3 mL, repeat if necessary
    - Children: I.M. epinephrine 1:1000 0.1 mL, repeat if necessary
- I.V. medication optional:
    - Aminophylline: 250 mg (slowly)
    - Hydrocortisone sodium succinate: 100 mg

DRUG OVERDOSE
LOCAL ANESTHETIC

Cause: Drug overdose

> **Symptoms:** Excitement of central nervous system followed by depression
> - Apprehension
> - Anxiety
> - Restlessness
> - Confusion
> - Tremors
> - Rapid breathing
> - Rapid heart rate
>
> **Treatment:**
>   Mild Reaction:
> - Administer oxygen, if needed
> - Monitor vital signs
> - Administer anticonvulsant drug, if needed (ie, Valium® - I.V.)
> - Medical consult, if necessary
>   Severe Reaction:
> - Place patient in supine position
> - Suction mouth and throat
> - Manage seizures
> - Provide basic life support
> - Monitor vital signs
> - Administer anticonvulsant drug, if needed
> - Manage postseizure depression

EPINEPHRINE OVERDOSE

> **Treatment:**
> - Position patient semi-reclining
> - Monitor vital signs
> - Administer oxygen, if necessary (except during hyperventilation syndrome)
> - Reassure patient

SEDATIVE-HYPNOTIC OVERDOSE

> **Treatment:**
> - Place patient in supine position
> - Maintain airway
> - Monitor vital signs
> - Administer oxygen and artificially ventilate, if necessary
> - Administer Vasoxyl®, 20 mg I.V., for low blood pressure

NARCOTIC-ANALGESIC OVERDOSE

> **Treatment:**
> - Place patient in supine position
> - Maintain airway
> - Check ventilation
> - Artificial ventilation and oxygen, as needed
> - Administer Narcan® (naloxone) 0.4 mg I.M. or I.V.

DRUG REACTIONS - ALLERGY
URTICARIA OR PRURITUS

Cause: Allergy

> **Symptoms:**
> - Urticaria: Red eruption of face, neck, hands, and arms
> - Pruritus: Itching of above areas
>
> **Treatment:**
>   Immediate:
> - Administer epinephrine 0.3 mL of 1:1000 I.M. or I.V.
> - Administer antihistamine
> - Prescribe for oral antihistamine
> - Withdraw drug in question
>   Delayed:
> - Administer Benadryl® (diphenhydramine hydrochloride) 50 mg orally or I.M. every 6-8 hours
> - If severe, administer Benadryl® 10-50 mg I.V. initially
> - Withdraw drug in question

ANGIONEUROTIC EDEMA

Cause: Allergic reaction

> **Symptoms:**
> - Single localized sealing of lips, eyelids, cheeks, pharynx, and larynx

- Pruritus, urticaria, hoarseness, stridor, cyanosis

Treatment:

- Administer Benadryl® 10-50 mg I.M. or I.V.
- Administer epinephrine 0.2-0.5 mL, 1:1000 I.M. or S.C.
- Inject Solu-Cortef® 100 mg I.M. or Decadron® 4 mg I.V.
- Administer oxygen
- Give aminophylline 250 mg I.V., slowly
- Withdraw drug in question

ANAPHYLACTIC SHOCK

Cause: Allergic reaction

Symptoms:

- Progressive respiratory and circulatory failure
- Itching of nose and hands
- Flushed face
- Feeling of substernal depression
- Labored breathing, stridor
- Coughing
- Sudden hypotension
- Cyanosis
- Loss of consciousness
- Incontinence

Treatment:

- Place patient in supine position
- Clear airway
- Monitor vital signs
- Administer oxygen and ventilate manually, if necessary
- Administer aqueous epinephrine 1:1000, 0.2-0.5 mL I.M. or S.C. (Children: 0.125-0.25 mL I.V.)
- Give Decadron® 4 mg I.V., if necessary
- Start I.V. fluids (1000 mL or 500 mL of D_5W or Ringer's lactate)
- Give aminophylline 250 mg I.V. very slowly
- Apply tourniquet to injection site (if injection is in extremity)
- Transfer patient to hospital

SEIZURE DISORDERS

Cause:

- Intermittent disorder of nervous system caused by sudden discharge of cerebral neurons
- Idiosyncracy to drug

Symptoms:

- Excitement, tremor, followed by clonic-tonic convulsions
- Trance-like state

Treatment:

- Place patient on floor
- Loosen clothing and ensure safety of patient
- Maintain airway
- Administer Valium® 5-20 mg I.V. or Brevital® I.V. (Children: 5 mg I.V.) until cessation of seizure
- Be prepared for postseizure depression; support respiration

CEREBRAL VASCULAR ACCIDENTS

Cause: Obstruction of blood vessel of brain

Symptoms:

- Weakness
- Confusion
- Headache
- Dizziness
- Dysphagia
- Vital signs usually satisfactory
- Aphasia
- Nausea
- Paralysis
- Loss of consciousness

Treatment:

Transient Ischemic Attack

- Monitor vital signs
- Obtain medical consult with physician

CVA (Conscious Patient)

- Position patient semi-reclining
- Monitor vital signs
- Seek medical assistance

CVA (Unconscious Patient)

- Place patient in supine position
- Record vital signs
- Provide basic life support
- Transfer to hospital

RESPIRATORY ARREST

Cause:

- Respiratory obstruction
- Drug overdose
- Allergic reaction
- Cessation of breathing

Symptoms:

- Change in pattern of breathing to possible cessation of respirations
- Patient unable to breathe
- Cyanosis

Treatment:

- Place patient in supine position with firm back support
- Maintain airway
- Give oxygen and artificially ventilate
- Administer Narcan® 1 mL if due to narcotic depression
- Give CPR, if necessary
- Transfer to hospital

ANGINA PECTORIS

Cause:

- Insufficient blood supply to cardiac muscle
- May be precipitated by stress and anxiety

Symptoms:

- Pain in chest
- Vital signs satisfactory
- Patient history of angina; pain persists 3-5 minutes

Treatment:

- Position patient semi-reclining
- Administer oxygen
- Administer nitroglycerine 1/150 gr sublingually (may be repeated in 5 minutes)
- Reassure patient
- If history of angina or pain does not subside, suspect myocardial infarction

MYOCARDIAL INFARCTION

Cause: Occlusion of coronary vessels

Symptoms:
- Severe pain in chest which may radiate to neck, shoulder, and jaws
- Palpitations, tachycardia
- Dyspnea
- Cyanosis
- Diaphoresis
- Weakness
- Feeling of impending doom
- Pulse thready

Treatment:
- Position patient semi-reclining with firm back support
- Administer oxygen
- Reassure patient
- Inject morphine sulfate 10-15 mg I.M. or Demerol® 75-100 mg for pain
- Start I.V. fluids 1000 D_5W or Ringer's lactate
- Transfer to hospital

Management of Special Complications
- Arrhythmias: Do not administer drugs unless EKG is on site
- Sudden death: Administer CPR
- Transfer to hospital; accompany patient in ambulance

CARDIAC ARREST

A sudden emergency due to either actual standstill (asystole) or ventricular fibrillation with ineffective contractions; respiratory arrest may follow

Signs & symptoms:
- Collapse of blood pressure
- Dilated pupils
- Ashen skin
- No peripheral pulse
- Possible loss of respiration
- No heart sounds

Treatment: CPR
- Slap anterior left chest briskly, only if you witness the arrest
- Place patient in supine position with firm back support
- Make sure airway is open; suction mouth and pharynx; intubate, if necessary
- Closed chest cardiac massage 60/minute (CPR - adult)
- Give oxygen under positive pressure with AMBU resuscitator up to 8 L/minute
- If no AMBU or tracheal tube available, give 4 breaths (mouth to mouth); then start closed chest cardiac compression (60/minute)
- Start I.V. sodium bicarbonate I.V. 44.6 mEq (children: half the dose)
- Monitor EKG
- If in ventricular fibrillation: Defibrillate 200-400 watt/second (start at 200, if no result, move up to higher voltage)
- Keep patient warm
- Epinephrine 0.5 mL I.V. 1:1000 in 10 mL of saline
- Repeat sodium bicarbonate unless blood is pH normal
- May need other drugs (ie, $CaCl_2$, atropine, etc)

Transvenous pacemaker may be needed to reinitiate heartbeat
Possible open chest massage (very few indications and may not be any more effective than closed massage)

INSULIN SHOCK

Cause: Hypoglycemia or hyperinsulinism

Symptoms:
- Nervousness
- Confusion
- Profuse sweating
- Sudden onset
- Drooling from mouth
- Full and bounding pulse
- Convulsions
- Moist, pale skin
- Coma

Treatment:
- Administer oral sugar with orange juice

- If unconscious, administer 50% dextrose I.V.

DIABETIC ACIDOSIS

Cause: Hyperglycemia, insufficient insulin in the body to metabolize carbohydrates and fats, acidosis

Symptoms:
- Gradual onset
- Dry, flushed skin
- Dry mouth, intense thirst
- Exaggerated respirations (Kussmaul)
- Confusion
- Disoriented
- Stuporous
- Sweet breath
- Coma

Treatment:
- Call for medical assistance
- Position patient semi-reclining
- Maintain airway, administer oxygen
- Start I.V. and administer lactated Ringer's
- Keep warm
- Administer basic life support
- Transfer to hospital

ADRENAL INSUFFICIENCY

Cause: Insufficient corticosteroid output during a stimulus such as a stressful dental situation or infection

Symptoms:
- Weakness
- Pallor
- Cardiovascular attack
- Perspiration
- Thready, rapid pulse

Treatment:
- Administer oxygen
- Send for medical assistance
- Administer Decadron® 4 mg I.V. to adults, 1-4 mg I.V. to children

SUGGESTED READINGS

CANCER

American Cancer Society, *Cancer Facts and Figures* 1995, Atlanta, GA.

American Cancer Society, *Cancer Manual,* 8th ed, American Cancer Society, Boston, MA Division, 1990.

Barasch A, Gofa A, Krutchkoff DJ, et al, "Squamous Cell Carcinoma of the Gingiva. A Case Series Analysis," *Oral Surg, Oral Med, Oral Path*, 1995, 80(2):183-7.

Carl W, "Oral Complications of Local and Systemic Cancer Treatment," *Curr Opinions in Oncol,* 1995, 7(4):320-4.

Chambers MS, Toth BB, Martin W, et al, "Oral and Dental Management of the Cancer Patient: Prevention and Treatment of Complications," *Support Care Cancer,* 1995, 3(3):168-75.

Hobson RS and Clark JD, "Management of the Orthodontic Patient 'At Risk' From Infective Endocarditis," *Br Dent J,* 1995, 178(8):289-95.

Jullien JA, Downer MC, Zakrzewska JM, et al, "Evaluation of a Screening Test for the Early Detection of Oral Cancer and Precancer," *Comm Dental Health,* 1995, 12(1):3-7.

Messer NC, Yant WR, and Archer RD, "Developing Provider Partnerships in the Detection of Oral Cancer and the Prevention of Smokeless Tobacco Use," *Maryland Med J,* 1995, 44(10):788-91.

National Institutes of Health, Consensus Development Conference on Oral Complications of Cancer Therapies: Diagnosis, Prevention, and Treatment. NCI Monograph No. 9 U.S. Public Health Service, Washington, DC: U.S. Government Printing Office, 1990.

National Institutes of Health, Consensus Development Conference on Oral Complications of Cancer Therapies: Diagnosis, Prevention, and Treatment. (Final Conference Statement and Recommendations), *J Am Dent Assoc,* 1989, 119(1):179-83.

Partridge M and Langdon JD, "Oral Cancer: A Serious and Growing Problem," *Ann R Coll Surg Engl,* 1995, 77(5):321-2.

Peterson DE and Sonis ST, eds, *Oral Complications of Cancer Chemotherapy,* Boston, MA: Martinus and Nijhoff, 1983.

Peterson DE, Elias EG, and Sonis ST, eds, *Head and Neck Management of the Cancer Patient,* Boston, MA: Martinus and Nijhoff Publishers, 1986.

Sandmann BJ, Sokol SA, and Buck GW, "Formulation and Stability of an Oral Mouthwash to Treat Symptoms of Mucositis," *Int Pharm Abstracts,* 1996, 33(1).

Shaffer J and Wesler LF, "Reducing Low-Density Lipoprotein Cholesterol Levels in an Ambulatory Care System," *Arch Int Med,* 1995, 155:2330-5.

Silverman S, *Oral Cancer,* 3rd ed, Atlanta, GA: American Cancer Society, 1990.

Takinami S, Yahata H, Kanoshima A, et al, "Hepatocellular Carcinoma Metastatic to the Mandible," *Oral Surg, Oral Med, Oral Path,* 1995, 79(5):649-54.

Vigneswaran N, Tilashalski K, Rodu B, et al, "Tobacco Use and Cancer. A Reappraisal," *Oral Surg, Oral Med, Oral Path, Oral Rad Endod,* 1995, 80(2):178-82.

CARDIOVASCULAR

American Dental Association: *ADA Oral Health Care Guidelines: Patients With Cardiovascular Disease,* Chicago, IL: American Dental Association, 1989.

American Heart Association, *Textbook of Advanced Cardiac Life Support,* 2nd ed, American Heart Association, Dallas, TX, 1990.

Assael LA, "Acute Cardiac Care in Dental Practice," *Dent Clin N Am,* 1995, 39(3):555-65.

Dajani AS, Bisno AL, Chung KJ, et al, "Prevention of Bacterial Endocarditis. Recommendations by the American Heart Association," *J Am Med Assoc,* 1990, 244:2019.

Giuliani ER, Gersh BJ, McGoon, MD et al, , *Mayo Clinic Practice of Cardiology,* 3rd ed, St Louis, MO: Mosby-Year Book, Inc, 1996, 1698-814.

Gorgia H, et al, "Prevention of Tolerance to Hemodynamic Effects of Nitrates With Concomitant Use of Hydralazine in Patients With Chronic Heart Failure," *J Am Coll Cardiol,* 1995, 26(1):1575-80.

Grey AB, et al, "The Effect of Anti-Estrogen Tamoxifen on Cardiovascular Risk Factors in Normal Postmenopausal Women," *J Clin Endocrin Metab,* 1995, 80:3191-5.

Henning RJ and Grenvik A, *Critical Care Cardiology,* New York, NY: Churchill Livingston, 1989, 233.

Kerpen SJ, Kerpen HO, and Sachs SA, "Mitral Valve Prolapse: A Significant Cardiac Defect in the Development of Infective Endocarditis," *Spec Care Dentist,* 1984, 4(4):158-9.

McDonald CC, et al, "Cardiac and Vascular Morbidity in Women Receiving Adjuvant Tamoxifen for Breast Cancer in Randomized Trial," *Br Med J,* 1995, 311:977-80.

Murgatroyd FD and Camm AJ, "Atrial Arrhythmias," *Lancet,* 1993, 341(8856):1317-22.

Naegell B, et al, "Intermittent Pacemaker Dysfunction Caused by Digital Mobile Telephones," *J Am Coll Cardiol,* 1996, 27:1471-7.

Pabor M, et al , "Risk of Gastrointestinal Haemorrhage With Calcium Antagonists in Hypertensive Persons Over 67 Years Old," *Lancet,* 1996, 347(20):1061-5.

Pieper SJ and Stanton MS, "Narrow QRS Complex Tachycardias," *Mayo Clin Proc,* 1995, 70(4):371-5.

Pritchett EL, "Management of Atrial Fibrillation," *N Engl J Med,* 1992, 326(19):1264-71.

Textbook of Advanced Cardiac Life Support, 2nd ed, Dallas, TX: American Heart Association, 1990.

The Fifth Report of the Joint National Committee on Detection, Evaluation, and Treatment of High Blood Pressure (JNC V), *Arch Intern Med,* 1993, 153(2):154-83.

Tierney LM, McPhee SJ, Papadakis MA, et al, *Current Medical Diagnosis and Treatment,* East Norwalk, CT: Appleton & Lange, 1993.

Williams GH, "Hypertensive Vascular Disease," *Harrison's Principles in Internal Medicine,* 13th ed, Isselbacher KJ, et al, eds, New York, NY: McGraw-Hill, 1994, 1116-31.

CHEMICAL DEPENDENCY

American Psychiatric Association: *Diagnosis and Statistical Manual of Mental Disorders,* 4th (DSM IV) ed, Washington, DC: American Psychiatric Association, 1994.

Alterman AI, Droba M, Antelo RE, et al, "Amantadine May Facilitate Detoxification of Cocaine Addicts," *Drug and Alcohol Dependency,* 1992, 31(1):19-29.

Benowitz NL, Porchet H, Sheiner L, et al, "Nicotine Absorption and Cardiovascular Effects With Smokeless Tobacco Use: Comparison With Cigarettes and Nicotine Gum," *Clin Pharmacol Ther,* 1988, 44(1):23-8.

Gariti P, Auriacombe M, Incmikoski R, et al, "A Randomized Double-Blind Study of Neuroelectric Therapy in Opiate and Cocaine Detoxification," *J Substance Abuse,* 1992, 4(1):299-308.

Henningfield JE, "Nicotine Medications for Smoking Cessation," *N Engl J Med,* 1995, 333(18):196-1203.

Herkenham MA, "Localization of Cannabinoid Receptors in Brain: Relationship to Motor and Reward Systems," *Biological Basis of Substance Abuse,* Korenman SG and Barchas JD, eds, New York, NY: Oxford University Press, 1993, 187-200.

Higgins ST, Budney AJ, Bickel WK, et al, Presented at the Problems of Drug Dependence Symposium, College. 1994.

Kreek MJ, "Rationale for Maintenance Pharmacotherapy of Opiate Dependence," O'Brien CP and Barchas JD, eds, *Addictive States,* New York, NY: Raven Press, 1992, 205-30.

Leshner AI, "Molecular Mechanisms of Cocaine Addictions," *N Engl J Med,* 1996, 335(2):128-9.

Mendelson JH and Mello NK, "Management of Cocaine Abuse and Dependence," *Drug Therapy,* 1996, 334(15):965-72.

O'Brien CP, "Drug Addiction and Drug Abuse," *The Pharmacological Basis of Therapeutics,* 9th ed, Molinoff PB and Ruddon R, eds, New York, NY: McGraw-Hill, 1996, 557-77.

O'Brien CP, "Treatment of Alcoholism as a Chronic Disorder," *Toward a Molecular Basis of Alcohol Use and Abuse,* Jansson B, Jornvall H, Rydberg U, et al, eds, Basel, Switzerland: Birkhauser Verlag, 1994, Vol 71, EXS, 349-59.

Self DW, Barnhart WJ, Lehman DA, et al, "Opposite Modulation of Cocaine-Seeking Behavior," *Science,* 1996, 271(1):1586-9.

DIAGNOSIS AND MANAGEMENT OF PAIN

Beckett D, "Topical Guanethidine Relieves Dental Hypersensitivity and Pain," *J Royal Soc Med,* 1995, 88(1):60.

Berthold CW, Schneider A, and Dionne RA, "Using Triazolam to Reduce Dental Anxiety," *J Am Dent Assoc,* 1993, 124(1):58-64.

Brown RS, Hinderstein B, Reynolds DC, et al, "Using Anesthetic Localization to Diagnose Oral and Dental Pain: Review of Clinical and Experimental Evidence," *Pain,* 1995, 126(5):633-4, 637-41.

Coderre TJ, Katz J, Vaccarino AL, et al, "Contribution of Central Neuroplasticity to Pathological Pain: Review of Clinical and Experimental Evidence," *Pain,* 1993, 52:259.

Delcanho RE and Graff-Radford SB, "Chronic Paroxysmal Hemicrania Presenting as Toothache," *J Orofacial Pain,* 1993, 7:300.

Denson DD and Katz JA, "Nonsteroidal Anti-inflammatory Agents," *Practical Management of Pain,* 2nd ed, PP Raj, ed, St Louis, MO: Mosby Year Book, 1992.

Forbes JA, Butterworth GA, Burchfield WH, et al, "Evaluation of Ketorolac, Aspirin, and an Acetaminophen-Codeine Combination in Postoperative Oral Surgery Pain," *Pharmacotherapy,* 1990, 10(6 Pt 2):77S-93S.

Graff-Radford SB, "Headache Problems That Can Present as Toothache," *Dent Clin North Am,* 1991, 35(1):155-70.

Harvey M and Elliott M, "Transcutaneous Electrical Nerve Stimulation (TENS) for Pain Management During Cavity Preparations in Pediatric Patients," *ASDC J Dentistry Child,* 1995, 62(1):49-51.

Henry G, et al, "Postoperative Pain Experience With Flurbiprofen and Acetaminophen With Codeine," *J Dent Res,* 1992, 71:952.

Jaffe JH and Martin WR, "Opioid Analgesic and Antagonists," *The Pharmacological Basis of Therapeutics,* 8th ed, Gilman AG, Rall TW, Nies AD, et al, eds, New York, NY: Maxwell Pergamon MacMillan Publishing, 1990.

Kalso E and Vainio A, "Morphine and Oxycodone Hydrochloride in the Management of Cancer Pain," *Clin Pharmacol Ther,* 1990, 47(5):639-46.

Lee AG, "A Case Report. Jaw Claudication: A Sign of Giant Cell Arteritis," *J Am Dent Assoc,* 1995, 126(7):1028-9.

McQuay H, Carroll D, Jadad AR, et al, "Anticonvulsant Drugs for Management of Pain: A Systemic Review," *Br Med J,* 1995, 311(7012):1047-52.

Olin BR, Hebel SK, Connell SI, et al, *Drug Facts and Comparisons,* 1993, St Louis, MO: Facts and Comparisons, Inc.

Pendeville PE, van Boven MJ, Contreras V, et al, "Ketorolac Tromethamine for Postoperative Analgesia in Oral Surgery," *Acta Anaesth Belgium* 1995, 46(1):25-30.

Robertson S, Goodell H, and Wolff HG, "The Teeth as a Source of Headache and Other Pain," *Arch Neurol Psychiatry,* 1947, 57:277.

Sandler NA, Ziccardi AV, and Ochs M, "Differential Diagnosis of Jaw Pain in the Elderly," *J Am Dent Assoc* 1995, 126(9):1263-72.

Scully C, Eveson JW, and Porter SR, "Munchausen's Syndrome: Oral Presentations," *Br Dent J,* 1995, 178(2):65-7.

Seng GF, Kraus K, Cartwright G, et al, "Confirmed Allergic Reactions to Amide Local Anesthetics," *Gen Dent,* 1996, 44(1):52-4.

Ship JA, Grushka M, Lipton JA, et al, "Burning Mouth Syndrome: An Update" *J Am Dent Assoc,* 1995, 126(7):842-53.

Wright EF and Schiffman EL, "Treatment Alternatives for Patients With Masticatory Myofascial Pain," *J Am Dent Assoc,* 1995, 126(7):1030-9.

NATURAL PRODUCTS AND HERBALS

1995 Martindale - The Extra Pharmacopoeia, Vol 86, Roy Pharm Soc, GB, 1996.

Castleman M, "The Healing Herbs: The Ultimate Guide to the Curative Power of Nature's Medicines," Rodale Press, Emmaus, 1991.

Lust J, *The Herb Book,* New York, NY: Benedict Lust Publications, 1974.

Mistry MG and Mays DA, "Precautions Against Global Use of Natural Products for Weight Loss: A Review of Active Ingredients and Issues Concerning Concomitant Disease States," *Therapeutic Perspectives,* 1996, 10(1):2.

Murray M and Pizzorno J, *Encyclopedia of Natural Medicine,* 1991, Prima Publishing, Rockin.

Olin BR, Hebel SK, Connell SI, et al, *Drug Facts and Comparisons,* 1993, St Louis, MO: Facts and Comparisons, Inc.

Polunin M and Robbins C, *The Natural Pharmacy,* 1992, New York, NY: MacMillan Publishing.

Tyler VF, *The Honest Herbal: A Sensible Guide to the Use of Herbs and Related Remedies,* 1993, Birmingham, AL: The Hawthorn Press, Inc.

ORAL INFECTIONS

Baron EJ and Finegold SM, eds, "Gram-Negative Cocci (*Neisseria* and *Branhamella*)," Bailey and Scott's Diagnostic Microbiology, St Louis, MO: Mosby Year Book, 1990.

Borssen E and Sundquist G, "Actinomycosis of Infected Dental Root Canals," *Oral Surg, Oral Med, Oral Path,* 1981, 51(1):643-7.

1993 Sexually Transmitted Diseases Treatment Guidelines, Centers for Disease Control and Prevention, *MMWR Morb Mortal Wkly Rep,* 1993, 42(RR-14):1-102.

Chow AW, "Infections of the Oral Cavity, Neck, and Head," *Principles and Practice of Infectious Diseases,* 4th ed, Mandell GL, Benne** JE, Dolin R, eds, New York, NY: Churchill Livingstone, 1995, 593-605.

Crockett DN, O'Grady JF, and Reade PC, "*Candida* Species and *Candida albicans* Morphotypes in Erythematous Candidiasis, "*Oral Surg, Oral Med, Oral Path* 1992, 73(5):559-63.

Dajani A, Taubert K, Ferrieri P, et al, "Treatment of Acute Streptococcal Pharyngitis and Prevention of Rheumatic Fever: A Statement for Health Professionals," *Pediatrics*, 1995, 96(4):758-64.

Diz Dios P, Hermida AO, Alvarez CM, et al, "Fluconazole-Resistant Oral Candidiasis in HIV-Infected Patients," *AIDS*, 1995, 9(7):809-10.

Dobson RL, "Antimicrobial Therapy for Cutaneous Infections," *J Am Acad Dermatol*, 1990, 22(5):871-3.

Ferris DG, et al, "Treatment of Bacterial Vaginosis: A Comparison of Oral Metronidazole, Metronidazole Vaginal Gel, and Clindamycin Vaginal Cream," *J Fam Pract*, 1995, 41(Nov):443-9.

Fox RI, Luppi M, Kang HI, et al, "Reactivation of Epstein-Barr Virus in Sjögren's Syndrome," *Springer Seminar in Immunopathology*, 1991, 13(2):217-31.

Giunta JL and Fiumara NJ, "Facts About Gonorrhea and Dentistry," *Oral Surg, Oral Med, Oral Path*, 1986, 62(5):529-31.

Goldberg MH and Topazian R, "Odontogenic Infections and Deep Facial Space Infections of Dental Origin," *Oral and Maxillofacial Infections*, 3rd ed, Philadelphia, PA: WB Saunders, 1994, 232-6.

Goulden V and Goodfield MJ, "Treatment of Childhood Dermatophyte Infections With Oral Terbinafine," *Ped Dermatol*, 1995, 12(1):53-4.

Hanna J, "Cefadroxil in the Management of Facial Cellulitis of Odontogenic Origin," *Oral Med Oral Path* 1991, 71(4):496-8.

Hook I and Marra CM, "Acquired Syphilis in Adults," *N Engl J Med*, 1992, 326(16):1060-9.

Larsen PE, "Alveolar Osteitis After Surgical Removal of Impacted Mandibular Third Molars," *Oral Surg, Oral Med, Oral Path*, 1992, 73(4):393-7.

Lewis MA, Parkhurst CL, Douglas CW, et al, "Prevalence of Penicillin Resistant Bacteria in Acute Suppurative Oral Infection," *J Antimicro Chemo*, 1995, 35(6):785-91.

Musher DM, Hamill RJ, and Baughn RE, "Effect of Human Immunodeficiency Virus (HIV) Infection on the Course of Syphilis and on the Response to Treatment," *Ann Int Med*, 1990, 113(11):872-81.

Muzyka BC and Glick M, "A Review of Oral Fungal Infections and Appropriate Therapy," *J Am Dent Assoc*, 1995, 126(1):63-72.

Namavar F, Roosendaal R, Kuipers EJ, et al, "Presence of *Helicobacter pylori* in the Oral Cavity, Oesophagus, Stomach and Faeces of Patients With Gastritis," *Eur J Clin Micro Inf Dis* 1995, 14(3):234-7.

Nguyen AM, el-Zaatari FA, and Graham DY, "*Helicobacter pylori* in the Oral Cavity. A Critical Review of the Literature," *Oral Surg, Oral Med, Oral Path, Oral Radiol Endod*, 1995, 79(6):705-9.

Pogrel MA, "Complications of Third Molar Surgery," *Oral Maxillofacial Surg Clin N Am*, 1990, 2(1):441-8.

Schiodt M, "HIV-Associated Salivary Gland Disease: A Review," *Oral Surg, Oral Med, Oral Path*, 1992, 73(2):164-7.

Sjögren UD, Figdor L, Sprangberg, et al, "The Antimicrobial Effect of Calcium Hydroxide as a Short-Term Intracanal Dressing," *J Internat Endodon*, 1991, 24(3):119-24.

Talal N, Dauphinee MJ, Dang H, et al, "Detection of Serum Antibodies to Retroviral Proteins in Patients With Primary Sjögren's Syndrome (Auto-immune Exocrinopathy)," *Arthritis and Rheumatism*, 1990, 33(1):774-81.

Torabinejad M, Kettering JD, Megraw JC, et al, "Factors Associated With Endodontic Interappointment Emergencies of Teeth With Necrotic Pulps," *J Endodont,* 1988, 14:261.

Walton RE and Fouad A, "Endodontic Interappointment Flare-Ups. A Prospective Study of Incidence and Related Factors," *J Endodont,* 1992, 18:172.

Wheeler TT, Alberts MA, Dolan TA, et al, "Dental, Visual, Auditory and Olfactory Complications in Paget's Disease of Bone," *J Am Geriatr Soc,* 1995, 43(12):1384-91.

Williams JW, et al, "Randomized Controlled Trial of 3 vs 10 Days of Trimethoprim/Sulfamethoxazole for Acute Maxillary Sinusitis," *JAMA,* 1995, 273(Apr):1015-21.

Wormser GP, "Lyme Disease: Insights Into the Use of Antimicrobials for Prevention and Treatment in the Context of Experience With Other Spirochetal Infections," *Mt Sinai J Med,* 1995, 62(3):188-95.

ORAL LEUKOPLAKIA

Barker JN, Mitra RS, et al, "Keratinocytes as Initiators of Inflammation," *Lancet,* 1991, 337(8735):211-4.

Belton CM and Evesole LR, "Oral Hairy Leukoplakia: Ultrastructural Studies," *J Oral Pathol,* 1986, 15(1):493-9.

Boehncke WH, Kellner I, Konter U, et al, "Different Expression of Adhesion Molecules on Infiltrating Cells in Inflammatory Dermatoses," *J Am Acad Dermatol,* 1992, 26(6):907-13.

Chou MJ and Daniels TE, "Langerhans Cells Expressing HLA-DQ, HLA-DR, and T6 Antigens in Normal Oral Mucosa and Lichen Planus," *J Oral Pathol Med,* 1989, 18(10):573-6.

Corso B, Eversole LR, and Hutt-Fletcher L, "Hairy Leukoplakia: Epstein-Barr Virus Receptors on Oral Keratinocyte Plasma Membranes," *Oral Surg, Oral Med, Oral Path* 1989, 67(4):416-21.

Eisen D, Ellis CN, Duell EA, et al, "Effect of Topical Cyclosporine Rinse on Oral Lichen Planus," *N Engl J Med,* 1990, 323(5):290-4.

Greenspan D, Greenspan JS, Overby G, et al, "Risk Factors for Rapid Progression From Hairy Leukoplakia to AIDS: A Nested Case-Control Study, *J Acquired Imm Deficiency Syndrome* 1991, 4(7):652-8.

Regezi JA, Stewart JC, Lloyd RV, et al, "Immunohistochemical Staining of Langerhans Cells and Macrophages in Oral Lichen Planus," *Oral Surg, Oral Med, Oral Path,* 1985, 60(4):396-402.

Sciubba JJ, "Oral Leukoplakia," *Oral Biology and Medicine,* 1995, 6(2):147-60.

ORAL SOFT TISSUE DISEASES

Anhalt GJ, "Pemphigoid: Bullous and Cicatricial," *Dermatol Clin,* 1990, 8(4):701-16.

Berk MA and Lorincz AL, "The Treatment of Bullous Pemphigoid With Tetracycline and Niacinamide; A Preliminary Report," *Arch Dermatol,* 1986, 122(6):670-4.

den Besten P and Giambro N, "Treatment of Fluorosed and White-Spot Human Enamel With Calcium Sucrose Phosphate *in vitro,*" *Pediatr Dentistry* 1995, 17(5):340-5.

Firth NA and Reade PC, "Angiotensin-Converting Enzyme Inhibitors Implicated in Oral Mucosal Lichenoid Reactions," *Oral Surg, Oral Med, Oral Path,* 1989, 67(1):41-4.

Fritz K and Weston W, "Topical Glucocorticoids," *Ann Allergy* 1983, 50(1):68-76.

Gallant C and Kenny P, "Oral Glucocorticoids and Their Complications," *J Am Acad Dermatol,* 1986, 14(2):161-77.

Goupil MT, "Occupational Health and Safety Emergencies," *Dent Clin N Am,* 1995, 39(3):637-47.

Grady D, Ernster VL, Stillman L, et al, "Smokeless Tobacco Use Prevents Aphthous Stomatitis," *Oral Surg Oral Med Oral Pathol,* 1992, 74(4):463-5.

Hamuryudan V, Yurdakul S, Serdaroglu S, et al, "Topical Alpha Interferon in the Treatment of Oral Ulcers in Behcet's Syndrome: A Preliminary Report," *Clin Exper Rheumatol,* 1990, 8(1):51-4.

Hoover CA, Olson JA, and Greenspan JS, "Humoral Responses and Cross-Reactivity to Viridans Streptococci in Recurrent Aphthous Ulceration," *J Dent Research,* 1986, 65(8):1101-4.

Jungell P, "Oral Lichen Planus: A Review," *Int J Oral Maxilofac Surg,* 1991, 20(3):129-35.

Lindermann RA, Riviere GR, and Sapp JP, "Oral Mucosal Antigen Reactivity During Exacerbation and Remission Phases or Recurrent Aphthous Ulceration," *Oral Surg, Oral Med, Oral Pathol,* 1985, 60(3):281-4.

MacPhail LA, Greenspan D, Feigal DW, et al, "Recurrent Aphthous Ulcers in Association With HIV Infection," *Oral Surg, Oral Med, Oral Path,* 1991, 71(6):678-83.

Meiller TF, Kutcher MJ, Overholser CD, et al, "Effect of an Antimicrobial Mouthrinse on Recurrent Aphthous Ulcerations," *Oral Surg, Oral Med, Oral Pathol,* 1991, 72(4):425-9.

Moncarz V, Ulmansky M, and Lustmann J, "Lichen Planus: Exploring Its Malignant Potential," *J Am Dent Assoc,* 1993, 124:102.

Pederson A, Klausen B, Hougen H, et al, "T-Lymphocyte Subsets in Recurrent Aphthous Ulceration," *J Oral Pathol,* 1989, 18(1):59-60.

Porter SR, Scully C, and Flint S, "Hematological Status in Recurrent Aphthous Stomatitis Compared With Other Oral Disease," *Oral Surg, Oral Med, Oral Path,* 1988, 66(1):41-4.

Porter SR, Scully C, and Midda M, "Adult Linear Immunoglobulin, A Disease Manifesting as Desquamative Gingivitis," *Oral Surg, Oral Med, Oral Pathol,* 1990, 70(4):450-3.

Rodu B and Mattingly G, "Oral Mucosal Ulcers: Diagnosis and Management," *J Am Dent Assoc,* 1992, 123(10):83-6.

Rothman KJ, "Teratogenicity of High Vitamin A Intake," *N Engl J Med,* 1995, 333(Nov):1369-73.

Savage NW, "Oral Ulceration: Assessment of Treatment of Commonly Encountered Oral Ulcerative Disease," *Aust Fam Physician,* 1988, 17(4):247-50.

Schiodt M, Holmstrup P, Dabelsteen E, et al, "Deposits of Immunoglobulins, Complement, and Fibrinogen in Oral Lupus Erythematosus, Lichen Planus, and Leukoplakia," *Oral Surg, Oral Med, Oral Path,* 1981, 51(1):603-8.

Scully C and Porter S, "Recurrent Aphthous Stomatitis: Current Concepts of Etiology, Pathogenesis, and Management," *J Oral Pathol,* 1989, 18(1):21-7.

Shilhara T, Moriya N, Mochizuki T, et al, "Lichenoid Tissue Reaction Induced by Local Transfer of Ia-Reactive T-cell Clones: LTR by Epidermal Invasion of Cytotoxic Lymphokine Producing Autoreactive T Cells," *J Invest Dermatol,* 1987, 89(1):8-14.

Shohat-Zabarski R, Kalderon S, Klein T, et al, "Close Association of HLA-B51 in Persons With Recurrent Aphthous Stomatitis," *Oral Surg, Oral Med, Oral Pathol,* 1992, 74(4):455-8.

Van Dis ML and Vincent SD, "Diagnosis and Management of Autoimmune and Idiopathic Mucosal Diseases," *Dent Clin North Am,* 1992, 36(4):897-917.

Vincent SD and Lilly GE, "Clinical, Historic, and Therapeutic Features of Aphthous Stomatitis," *Oral Surg, Oral Med, Oral Pathol,* 1992, 74(1):79-86.

ORAL VIRAL DISEASES

Ades AE, Peckham CS, Dale GE, et al, "Prevalence of Antibodies to Herpes Simplex Virus Types 1 and 2 in Pregnant Women, and Estimated Rates of Infection," *J Epidemiol Comm Health,* 1989, 43(1):53-60.

Amsterdam JD, Maislin G, and Rybakowski J, "A Possible Antiviral Action of Lithium Carbonate in Herpes Simplex Virus Infections," *Biol Psychiatry,* 1990, 27(4):447-53.

Balfour J, Rotbart HA, Feldman S, et al, "Acyclovir Treatment of Varicella in Otherwise Healthy Adolescents. The Collaborative Acyclovir Varicella Study Group," *J Pediatr,* 1992, 120(4):627.

Carey WD and Patel G, "Viral Hepatitis in the 1990s, Part III, Hepatitis C, Hepatitis E, and Other Viruses," *Cleve Clin J Med,* 1992, 59(6):595-601.

Chang Y, et al, "Identification of Herpesvirus-Like DNA Sequences in AIDS-Associated Kaposi's Sarcoma," *Science,* 1994, 266(Dec 16):1865-9.

Corey L and Spear P, "Infections With Herpes Simplex Viruses," *N Engl J Med,* 1986, 314(11):686-91, 749-57.

Dolin R, "Antiviral Chemotherapy and Chemoprophylaxis," *Science,* 1985, 227(4692):1296-1303.

Ficarra G and Shillitoe EJ, "HIV-Related Infections of the Oral Cavity," *Oral Biol Med,* 1992, 3(3):297-31.

Fiddian A and Ivanyi L, "Topical Acyclovir in the Management of Recurrent *Herpes labialis,*" *Br J Dermatol* 1983, 3(3):297-31.

Gupta S, Govindarajan S, Cassidy WM, et al, "Acute Delta Hepatitis: Sero-logical Diagnosis With Particular Reference to Hepatitis Delta Virus RNA," *Am J Gastroenterol,* 1991, 86(9):1227-31.

Huff JC, Balfour J, et al, "Therapy of Herpes Zoster With Oral Acyclovir ," *Am J Med,* 1988, 85(2A):84-9.

Johnson RJ, Gretch DR, and Yamabe H, "Membranoproliferative Glomerulo-nephritis Associated With Hepatitis C Virus Infection," *N Engl J Med,* 1993, 327(7):465-70.

Markowitz M, et al, "A Preliminary Study of Ritonavir, an Inhibitor of HIV-1 Protease, to Treat HIV-1 Infection," *N Engl J Med,* 1995, 333(1):1534-9.

McCreary C, Bergin C, Pilkington R, et al, "Clinical Parameters Associated With Recalcitrant Oral Candidiasis in HIV Infection: A Preliminary Study," *Int J STD AIDS,* 1995, 6(3):204-7.

Robinson WS, "Hepatitis B Virus and Hepatitis D Virus," *Principles and Practice of Infectious Disease,* 4th ed, 1995, New York, NY: Churchill Living-stone. 1995.

Roizman B and Sears AE, "An Inquiry Into Mechanisms of Herpes Simplex Virus Latency," *Ann Reviews in Microbiol,* 1987, 41(1):543-71.

Rooney JF, Bryson Y, Mannix ML, et al, "Prevention of Ultraviolet Light-Induced *Herpes labialis* by Sunscreen," *Lancet* 1991, 338(8780):1419-22.

Snijders PJ, Schulten EA, Mulink H, et al, "Detection of Human Papillomavirus and Epstein-Barr Virus DNA Sequences in Oral Mucosa of HIV-Infected Patients by the Polymerase Chain Reaction," *Am J Pathol,* 1990, 137(3):659-66.

Spruance SL, Steward JC, Rowe NH, et al, "Treatment of Recurrent Herpes Simplex labialis With Oral Acyclovir," *J Infect Dis* 1990, 161(2):185-90.

Whitley RJ, Soong SF, Polin R, et al, "Early Vidarabine Therapy to Control the Complications of Herpes Zoster in Immunocompromised Patients," *N Engl J Med,* 1982, 307(1):971.

PERIODONTOLOGY

Barak S, Engelberg IS, and Hiss J, "Gingival Hyperplasia Caused by Nifedipine. Histopathologic Findings," *J Periodontol,* 1987, 58(9):639-42.

Carson HG and Rainone AD, "Occult Periodontal Disease With Heat Sensitivity: A Different Diagnostic Problem," *General Dentistry,* 1992, 23(3):191-5.

Checchi L, Trombelli L, and Nonato M, "Postoperative Infections and Tetracycline Prophylaxis in Periodontal Surgery: A Retrospective Study," *Quintessence Int,* 1992, 23(3):191-5.

Creath CJ, Steinmetz S, and Roebuck R, "A Case Report. Gingival Swelling Due to a Fingernail-Biting Habit," *J Am Dent Assoc,* 1995, 126(7):1019-21.

Crow HC and Ship JA, "Are Gingival and Periodontal Conditions Related to Salivary Gland Flow Rates in Healthy Individuals?" *J Am Dent Assoc,* 1995, 126(11):1154-20.

Dens F, Boute P, Otten J, et al, "Dental Caries, Gingival Health, and Oral Hygiene of Long-Term Survivors of Paediatric Malignant Diseases," *Arch Dis Child,* 1995, 72(2):129-32.

Harel-Raviv M, Ekler M, Lalani K, et al, "Nifedipine-Induced Gingival Hyperplasia. A Comprehensive Review and Analysis," *Oral Surg, Oral Med, Oral Path* 1995, 79(6):715-22.

Holt RD, Wilson M, and Musa S, "Mycoplasmas in Plaque and Saliva of Children and Their Relationship to Gingivitis," *J Periodontol,* 1995, 66(2):97-101.

Lareau D, Herzberg MC, and Nelson RD, "Human Neutrophil Migration Under Agarose to Bacteria Associated With the Development of Gingivitis," *J Periodontol,* 1984, 55(9):540-9.

Listgarten MA, "Pathogenesis of Periodontitis," *J Clin Periodontol,* 1986, 13(5):418-30.

Listgarten M, Lindhe J, and Heliden L, "Effect of Tetracycline and/or Scaling on Human Periodontal Disease," *J Clin Periodontol,* 1978, 5(1):246-71.

Loesche WJ, Syed SA, Laughton BE, et al, "The Bacteriology of Acute Necrotizing Ulcerative Gingivitis," *J Periodontol,* 1982, 53(1):223.

McLoughlin P, Newman L, and Brown A, "Oral Squamous Cell Carcinoma Arising in Phenytoin-Induced Hyperplasia," *Br Dent J,* 1995, 178(5):183-4.

Moghadam BK and Gier RE, "Common and Less Common Gingival Overgrowth Conditions," *Cutis* 1995, 56(1):46-8.

Mombelli A, Buser D, Lang NP, et al, "Suspected Periodontopathogens in Erupting Third Molar Sites of Periodontally Health Individuals," *J Clin Periodontol,* 1990, 17(1):48-54.

Moore L, Moore W, Cato E, et al, "Bacteriology of Human Gingivitis," *J Dental Research,* 1987, 66(1):989-95.

Navazesh M and Mulligan R, "Systemic Dissemination as a Result of Oral Infection in Individuals 50 Years of Age and Older," *Special Care Dentist,* 1995, 15(1):11-9.

Nery EB, Edson RG, Lee KK, et al, "Prevalence of Nifedipine-Induced Gingival Hyperplasia," *J Periodontol,* 1995, 66(7):572-8.

Nickoloff BJ, Griffiths CE, and Barker JN, "The Role of Adhesion Molecules, Chempotactic Factors, and Cytokinesin Inflammatory and Neoplastic Skin Diseases," *J Investigative Dermatol,* 1990, 94(Suppl 6):151S-7S.

Pinson M, Hoffman WH, Garnick JJ, et al, "Periodontal Disease and Type I Diabetes Mellitus in Children and Adolescents," *J Clin Periodontol,* 1995, 22(2):118-23.

Preber H and Bergstrom J, "Effect of Cigarette Smoking on Periodontal Healing Following Surgical Therapy," *J Clin Periodontol,* 1990, 17(5):324-8.

Ramfjord SP and Ash MM, "Periodontology and Periodontics: Modern Theory and Practice," St Louis, MO: Ishryalar Euro-America, 1989.

Ramsdale DR, Morris JL, and Hardy P,"Gingival Hyperplasia With Nifedipine," *Br Heart J,* 1995, 73(2):115.

Ransier A, Epstein JB, Lunn R, et al, "A Combined Analysis of a Toothbrush, Foam Brush, and a Chlorhexidine-Soaked Foam Brush in Maintaining Oral Hygiene," *Cancer Nurse,* 1995, 18(5):393-6.

Robertson PB and Greenspan JS, *Perspectives on Oral Manifestations of AIDS: Diagnosis and Management of HIV-Associated Infection,* Littleton, MA: PSG Publishing Co, 1988.

Wahlstrom E, Zamora JU, and Teichman S, "Improvement in Cyclosporine-Associated Gingival Hyperplasia With Azithromycin Therapy," *N Engl J Med,* 1995, 332(11):753-4.

RESPIRATORY DISEASES

"Asthma Mortality and Hospitalization Among Children and Young Adults - United States, 1980-1993," *Morb Mortal Wkly Rep,* 1996, 45:350-3.

Barnes PF and Barrows SA, "Tuberculosis in the 1990s," *Ann Intern Med,* 1993, 119(5):400-10.

Bass J, Farer LS, Hopewell PC, et al, "A New Tuberculosis," *N Engl J Med,* 1992, 326(10):703-5.

Cohen C, Krutchkoff DJ, and Eisenberg E, "Systemic Sarvoidosis: Report of Two Cases With Oral Lesions," *J Oral Surg,* 1981, 39(1):613-8.

DeLuke DM and Scuibba JJ, "Oral Manifestations of Sarvoidosis: Report of a Case Masquerading as a Neoplasm," *Oral Surg, Oral Med, Oral Path,* 1985, 59(2):184-8.

Drosos AA, Constantopoulos SH, Psychose D, et al, "The Forgotten Cause of Sicca Complex: Sarcoidosis," *J Rheumatol,* 1989, 16(12):1548-57.

Egman DH and Christiani DC, *Respiratory Disorders in Occupational Health: Recognizing and Preventing Work-Related Disease,* 2nd ed, Levy BS and Wegman DH, eds, Boston, MA: Little-Brown, 1988, 319-44.

Frieden TR, Sterling T, Paablos-Mendex A, et al, "The Emergence of Drug Resistant Tuberculosis in New York City," *N Engl J Med,* 1993, 328(8):521-6.

Murciano D, Auclair MH, Pariente R, et al, "A Randomized Controlled Trial of Theophylline in Patients With Severe Chronic Obstructive Pulmonary Disease," *N Engl J Med,* 1989, 320(23):1521-5.

Snider J, and Roper WL, "Treatment of Tuberculosis and Tuberculosis Infection in Adults and Children, American Thoracic Society and the Centers for Disease Control and Prevention," *Am J Respir Crit Care Med,* 1994, 149(5):1359-74.

TEMPOROMANDIBULAR DYSFUNCTION

Becker IM, "Occlusion as a Causative Factor in TMD. Scientific Basis to Occlusal Therapy, *NY State Dent J,* 1995, 61(9):54-7.

Bell WE, et al, *Temporomandibular Disorders: Classification Diagnosis, Management,* 3rd ed, Chicago, IL: Year Book Medical Publishers, 1990.

Bloch M, Riba H, Redensky D, et al, "Cranio-Mandibular Disorder in Children," *NY State Dent J,*1995, 61(3):48-50.

Canavan D and Gratt BM, "Electronic Thermography for the Assessment of Mild and Moderate Temporomandibular Joint Dysfunction," *Oral Surg, Oral Med, Oral Path,* 1996, 79(6):778-86.

SUGGESTED READINGS

Carlson CR, Okeson JP, Falace DA, et al, "Comparison of Psychologic and Physiological Functioning Between Patients With Masticatory Muscle Pain and Matched Controls," *J Orofacial Pain,* 1993, 7(1):15-22.

Clark GT and Takeuchi H, "Temporomandibular Dysfunction, Chromic Orofacial Pain and Oral Motor Disorders in the 21st Century," *J Calif Dent Assoc,* 1995, 23(4):44-6, 48-50.

Clayton JA, "Occlusion and Prosthodontics," *Dent Clin N Am,* 1995, 39(2):313-33.

CTD, "Temporomandibular Disorder Prosthodontics: Treatment and Management Goals. Report of the Committee on Temporomandibular Disorders of the American College of Prosthodontics," *J Prosthodontology,* 1995, 4(1):58-64.

dos Santos JJ, "Supportive Conservative Therapies for Temporomandibular Disorders," *Dent Clin N Am,* 1995, 39(2):459-77.

Kai S, Kai H, Nakayama E, et al, "Clinical Symptoms of Open Lock Position of the Condyle: Relation to Anterior Dislocation of the Temporomandibular Joint," *Oral Surg, Oral Med, Oral Pathol,* 1992, 74(2):143-8.

Lund JP, Donga R, Widmer CG, et al, "The Pain-Adaptation Model: a Discussion of the Relationship Between Chronic Musculoskeletal Pain and Motor Activity," *Can J Physiol Pharmacol,* 1991, 69(5):683-94.

Okeson JP, "Occlusion and Functional Disorders of the Masticatory System," *Dent Clin N Am,* 1995, 39(2):285-300.

Okeson JP, *The Management of Temporomandibular Disorders and Occlusion,* 3rd ed, St Louis, MO: Mosby Year Book, 1993.

Quinn JH, "Mandibular Exercises to Control Bruxism and Deviation Problems," *Cranio,* 1995, 13(1):30-4.

Schiffman E, Haley D, Baker C, et al, "Diagnostic Criteria for Screening Headache Patients for Temporomandibular Disorders," *Headache,* 1995, 35(3):121-4.

Widmark G, Kahnberg KE, Haraldson T, et al, "Evaluation of TMJ Surgery in Cases Not Responding to Conservative Treatment," *Cranio,* 1995, 13(1):44-9.

APPENDIX TABLE OF CONTENTS

Abbreviations and Measurements
Common Symbols & Abbreviations 1004
Apothecary / Metric Conversions 1006
Pounds - Kilograms Conversion 1007
Temperature Conversion.................................... 1007
Body Surface Area of Adults and Children.................. 1008
Average Weights and Surface Areas 1009

Calcium Channel Blockers & Gingival Hyperplasia
Some General Observations of CCB-Induced GH 1010

Cancer Chemotherapy
Cancer Chemotherapy Regimens - Adults 1011

Comparative Drug Charts
Corticosteroid Equivalencies Comparison................... 1017
Corticosteroids, Topical Comparison 1018
Narcotic Agonist Charts 1019
Nonsteroidal Anti-Inflammatory Agents, Comparative Dosages,
and Pharmacokinetics 1021

Dental Drug Interactions
Dental Drug Interactions: Update on Drug Combinations Requiring
Special Considerations 1022

Infectious Disease Information
Occupational Exposure to Bloodborne Pathogens (Universal
Precautions) 1030

Infectious Disease - Antimicrobial Activity Against Selected Organisms
Penicillins, Penicillin-Related Antibiotics & Other Antibiotics 1034
Cephalosporins, Aminoglycosides, Macrolides, & Quinolones 1038

Infectious Disease - Prophylaxis
Antimicrobial Prophylaxis in Surgical Patients 1042
Organisms Isolated in Head & Neck Infections 1044
Predominant Cultivable Microorganisms of the Oral Cavity 1045

Laboratory Values
Reference Values for Adults 1046

Over-the-Counter Dental Products
Artificial Saliva Products 1050
Dentifrice Products 1051
Denture Adhesive Products 1060
Denture Cleanser Products 1062
Mouth Pain, Cold Sore, Canker Sore Products 1063
Oral Rinse Products 1067

Sugar-Free Liquid Pharmaceuticals
Sugar-Free Liquid Pharmaceuticals Listing 1070

Miscellaneous
Allergic Skin Reactions to Drugs 1076
Common Oral-Facial Infections and Antibiotics for Treatment 1077
Controlled Substances 1078
Drugs Associated With Adverse Hematologic Effects 1079
Herbal Medicines 1081
Poison Information Centers................................ 1086
Prescription Writing 1100
Safe Writing Practices 1103
Top 200 Prescribed Drugs in 1995......................... 1104
Vasoconstrictor Interactions With Antidepressants 1108
What's New 1109

COMMON SYMBOLS & ABBREVIATIONS

µg	microgram
°C	degrees Celsius (Centigrade)
<	less than
>	greater than
≤	less than or equal to
≥	greater than or equal to
ABG	arterial blood gas
ACE	angiotensin-converting enzyme
ACLS	adult cardiac life support
ADH	antidiuretic hormone
AED	antiepileptic drug
ALL	acute lymphoblastic leukemia
ALT	alanine aminotransferase (was SGPT)
AML	acute myeloblastic leukemia
ANA	antinuclear antibodies
ANC	absolute neutrophil count
ANL	acute nonlymphoblastic leukemia
APTT	activated partial thromboplastin time
ASA (class I-IV)	classification of surgical patients according to their baseline health (eg, healthy ASA I and II or increased severity of illness ASA III or IV)
AST	aspartate aminotransferase (was SGOT)
A-V	atrial-ventricular
BMT	bone marrow transplant
BUN	blood urea nitrogen
cAMP	cyclic adenosine monophosphate
CBC	complete blood count
CHF	congestive heart failure
CI	cardiac index
Cl_{cr}	creatinine clearance
CNS	central nervous system
COPD	chronic obstructive pulmonary disease
CSF	cerebral spinal fluid
CT	computed tomography
CVA	cerebral vascular accident
CVP	central venous pressure
d	day
D_5W	dextrose 5% in water
$D_5/_{0.45}$ NaCl	dextrose 5% in sodium chloride 0.45%
$D_{10}W$	dextrose 10% in water
DIC	disseminated intravascular coagulation
DNA	deoxyribonucleic acid
DVT	deep vein thrombosis
EEG	electroencephalogram
EKG	electrocardiogram
ESR	erythrocyte sedimentation rate
E.T.	endotracheal
FEV_1	forced expiratory volume
FVC	forced vital capacity
g	gram
G-6-PD	glucose-6-phosphate dehydrogenase
GA	gestational age
GABA	gamma-aminobutyric acid
GE	gastroesophageal
GI	gastrointestinal
GU	genitourinary
h	hour
HIV	human immunodeficiency virus
HPLC	high performance liquid chromatography
IBW	ideal body weight
ICP	intracranial pressure
IgG	immune globulin G
I.M.	intramuscular
INR	international normalized ratio
I.O.	intraosseous

(continued)

I.V.	intravenous
IVH	intraventricular hemorrhage
IVP	intravenous push
I & O	input and output
IOP	intraocular pressure
I.T.	intrathecal
JRA	juvenile rheumatoid arthritis
kg	kilogram
L	liter
LDH	lactate dehydrogenase
LE	lupus erythematosus
LP	lumbar puncture
MAO	monoamine oxidase
MAP	mean arterial pressure
mcg	microgram
mg	milligram
MI	myocardial infarction
μmol	micromole
min	minute
mL	milliliter
mo	month
mOsm	milliosmoles
MRI	magnetic resonance image
ND	nasoduodenal
ng	nanogram
NG	nasogastric
NMDA	n-methyl-d-aspartate
nmol	nanomole
NPO	nothing per os (nothing by mouth)
NSAID	nonsteroidal anti-inflammatory drug
O.R.	operating room
OTC	over-the-counter (nonprescription)
PALS	pediatric advanced life support
PCA	postconceptional age
PCP	*Pneumocystis carinii* pneumonia
PCWP	pulmonary capillary wedge pressure
PDA	patent ductus arteriosus
PNA	postnatal age
PSVT	paroxysmal supraventricular tachycardia
PT	prothrombin time
PTT	partial thromboplastin time
PUD	peptic ulcer disease
PVC	premature ventricular contraction
qsad	add an amount sufficient to equal
RAP	right atrial pressure
RIA	radioimmunoassay
RNA	ribonucleic acid
S-A	sino-atrial
S.C.	subcutaneous
S_{cr}	serum creatinine
SIADH	syndrome of inappropriate antidiuretic hormone
S.L.	sublingual
SLE	systemic lupus erythematosus
SVR	systemic vascular resistance
SVT	supraventricular tachycardia
SWI	sterile water for injection
TT	thrombin time
UTI	urinary tract infection
V_d	volume of distribution
V_{dss}	volume of distribution at steady-state
y	year

*Other than drug synonyms

APOTHECARY/METRIC CONVERSIONS

Liquid Measures

Basic equivalent: 1 fluid ounce = 30 mL

Examples:

1 gallon	3800 mL	15 minims	1 mL
1 quart	960 mL	10 minims	0.6 mL
1 pint	480 mL	1 gallon	128 fluid ounces
8 fluid ounces	240 mL	1 quart	32 fluid ounces
4 fluid ounces	120 mL	1 pint	16 fluid ounces

Approximate Household Equivalents

1 teaspoonful	5 mL	1 tablespoonful	15 mL

Weights

Basic equivalents:

1 ounce = 30 g   15 grains = 1 g

Examples:

4 ounces	120 g	1/100 grain	600µg
2 ounces	60 g	1/150 grain	400µg
10 grains	600 mg	1/200 grain	300µg
7 1/2 grains	500 mg		
1 grain	60 mg	16 ounces	1 pound

Metric Conversions

Basic equivalents:

1 g	1000 mg	1 mg	1000 mcg

Examples:

5 g	5000 mg	5 mg	5000 mcg
0.5 g	500 mg	0.5 mg	500 mcg
0.05 g	50 mg	0.05 mg	50 mcg

Exact Equivalents

1 gram (g)	15.43 grains	0.1 mg	1/600 gr
1 milliliter (mL)	16.23 minims	0.12 mg	1/500 gr
1 minim ( )	0.06 milliliter	0.15 mg	1/400 gr
1 grain (gr)	64.8 milligrams	0.2 mg	1/300 gr
1 ounce (oz)	31.1 grams	0.5 mg	1/120 gr
1 ounce (oz)	28.35	0.8 mg	1/80 gr
1 pound (lb)	453.6 grams	1 mg	1/65 gr
1 kilogram (kg)	2.2 pounds		

Solids*

1/4 grain	15 mg	5 grains	300 mg
1/2 grain	30 mg	10 grains	600 mg
1 1/2 grain	100 mg		

*Use exact equivalents for compounding and calculations requiring a high degree of accuracy.

POUNDS-KILOGRAMS CONVERSION

1 pound = 0.45359 kilograms
1 kilogram = 2.2 pounds

lb	=	kg	lb	=	kg	lb	=	kg
1		0.45	70		31.75	140		63.50
5		2.27	75		34.02	145		65.77
10		4.54	80		36.29	150		68.04
15		6.80	85		38.56	155		70.31
20		9.07	90		40.82	160		72.58
25		11.34	95		43.09	165		74.84
30		13.61	100		45.36	170		77.11
35		15.88	105		47.63	175		79.38
40		18.14	110		49.90	180		81.65
45		20.41	115		52.16	185		83.92
50		22.68	120		54.43	190		86.18
55		24.95	125		56.70	195		88.45
60		27.22	130		58.91	200		90.72
65		29.48	135		61.24			

TEMPERATURE CONVERSION

Celsius to Fahrenheit = (°C x 9/5) + 32 = °F
Fahrenheit to Celsius = (°F - 32) x 5/9 = °C

°C	=	°F	°C	=	°F	°C	=	°F
100.0		212.0	39.0		102.2	36.8		98.2
50.0		122.0	38.8		101.8	36.6		97.9
41.0		105.8	38.6		101.5	36.4		97.5
40.8		105.4	38.4		101.1	36.2		97.2
40.6		105.1	38.2		100.8	36.0		96.8
40.4		104.7	38.0		100.4	35.8		96.4
40.2		104.4	37.8		100.1	35.6		96.1
40.0		104.0	37.6		99.7	35.4		95.7
39.8		103.6	37.4		99.3	35.2		95.4
39.6		103.3	37.2		99.0	35.0		95.0
39.4		102.9	37.0		98.6	0		32.0
39.2		102.6						

BODY SURFACE AREA OF ADULTS AND CHILDREN

Calculating Body Surface Area in Children
In a child of average size, find weight and corresponding surface area on the boxed scale to the left; or, use the nomogram to the right. Lay a straightedge on the correct height and weight points for the child, then read the intersecting point on the surface area scale.

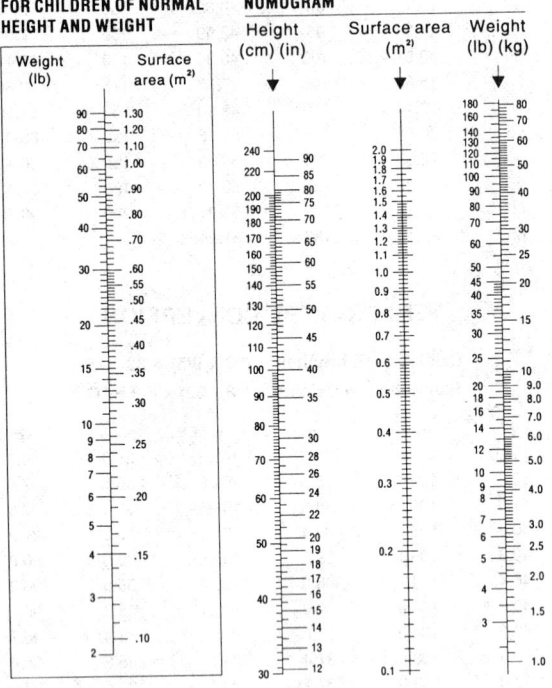

FOR CHILDREN OF NORMAL HEIGHT AND WEIGHT

Weight (lb)	Surface area (m²)

NOMOGRAM

Height (cm) (in)	Surface area (m²)	Weight (lb) (kg)

BODY SURFACE AREA FORMULA
(Adult and Pediatric)

$$BSA\ (m^2) = \sqrt{\frac{Ht\ (in)\ x\ Wt\ (lb)}{3131}} \quad \text{or, in metric: } BSA\ (m^2) = \sqrt{\frac{Ht\ (cm)\ x\ Wt\ (kg)}{3600}}$$

References
Lam TK, Leung DT, *N Engl J Med*, 1988, 318:1130, (Letter).
Mosteller RD, "Simplified Calculation of Body Surface Area", *N Engl J Med*, 1987, 317:1098.

AVERAGE WEIGHTS AND SURFACE AREAS

Average Weight and Surface Area of Preterm Infants, Term Infants, and Children

Age	Average Weight (kg)*	Approximate Surface Area (m²)
Weeks Gestation		
26	0.9-1	0.1
30	1.3-1.5	0.12
32	1.6-2	0.15
38	2.9-3	0.2
40 (term infant at birth)	3.1-4	0.25
Months		
3	5	0.29
6	7	0.38
9	8	0.42
Year		
1	10	0.49
2	12	0.55
3	15	0.64
4	17	0.74
5	18	0.76
6	20	0.82
7	23	0.90
8	25	0.95
9	28	1.06
10	33	1.18
11	35	1.23
12	40	1.34
Adult	70	1.73

*Weights from age 3 months and older are rounded off to the nearest kilogram.

CALCIUM CHANNEL BLOCKERS & GINGIVAL HYPERPLASIA

Generic Preparation	FDA Approval	Cases Cited in Literature	Common Name	Manufacturer
Amlodipine	1992	0	Norvasc®	Pfizer
Bepridil	1993	0	Vascor®	McNeil
Diltiazem	1982	>20	Cardizem®; Dilacor®	Marion Merrell Dow; Rorer
Felodipine	1992	1	Plendil®	Merck Sharpe Dome
Isradipine	1991	0	DynaCirc®	Sandoz
Nicardipine	1989	0	Cardene®	Syntex
Nifedipine	1982	>120	Adalat®; Procardia®	Miles; Pfizer
Nimodipine	1989	0	Nimotop®	Miles
Nitrendipine*		1	Baypress®	Miles
Verapamil	1982	7	Calan®; Isoptin®; Verelan®	GD Searle; Knoll; Lederle; Wyeth-Ayerst

*Not yet approved for use in the United States.

SOME GENERAL OBSERVATIONS OF CCB-INDUCED GH

Most of the reported cases listed in the Calcium Channel Blockers and Gingival Hyperplasia table have involved patients >50 years of age taking CCBs chronically for postmyocardial infarction syndrome, angina pain, essential hypertension, and Raynaud's syndrome. Nifedipine-induced GH has appeared between 1 and 9 months after a daily dose of 30-100 mg, verapamil-induced GH has appeared at 11 months or more after a daily dose of 240-360 mg, and diltiazem-induced GH has appeared between 1 and 24 months after a daily dose of 60-135 mg. As with phenytoin, there does not seem to be a dose-dependent effect of CCBs on the severity of the hyperplastic syndrome. Discontinuance of the CCB usually results in complete disappearance or marked regression of symptoms, with symptoms reappearing upon remedication. The time required after drug discontinuance for marked regression of GH has been one week. Complete disappearance of all symptoms usually takes two months. If gingivectomy is performed and the drug retained or resumed, the hyperplasia will usually recur. Only when the medication is discontinued or a switch to a non-CCB occurs will the gingivectomy usually be successful. One study of Nishikawa[1], et al, showed that if nifedipine could not be discontinued, hyperplasia did not recur after gingivectomy when extensive plaque control was carried out. If the CCB is changed to another class of cardiovascular agent, the gingival hyperplasia will probably regress and disappear. A switch to another CCB, however, will probably result in continued hyperplasia. For example, Giustiniani[2], et al, reported disappearance of symptoms within 15 days after discontinuance of verapamil, with the reoccurrence of symptoms after resumption with diltiazem. The reader is referred to the review of 1991[3] for descriptive clinical and histological findings of CCB-induced GH.

1. Nishikawa SI, Tada H, Hamasaki A, et al, "Nifedipine-Induced Gingival Hyperplasia: A Clinical and In Vitro Study," *J Periodontol*, 1991, 62(1):30-5.
2. Giustiniani S, Robestelli della Cuna F, and Marienei M, "Hyperplastic Gingivitis During Diltiazem Therapy," *Int J Cardiol*, 1987, 15(2):247-9.
3. Wynn RL, "Calcium Channel Blockers and Gingival Hyperplasia," *Gen Dent*, 1991, 240-3.

CANCER CHEMOTHERAPY REGIMENS

ADULT REGIMENS

Breast Cancer

AC

Doxorubicin (Adriamycin®, I.V., 45 mg/m², day 1
Cyclophosphamide, I.V., 500 mg/m², day 1

Repeat cycle every 21 days

ACe

Doxorubicin (Adriamycin®, I.V., 40 mg/m², day 1
Cyclophosphamide, P.O., 200 mg/m²/d, days 1-3 or 3-6

Repeat cycle every 21-28 days

CAF

Cyclophosphamide, P.O., 100 mg/m², days 1-14
Doxorubicin (Adriamycin®, I.V., 30 mg/m², days 1 & 8
Fluorouracil, I.V., 400-500 mg/m², days 1 & 8

Repeat cycle every 28 days

or

Cyclophosphamide, I.V., 500 mg/m², day 1
Doxorubicin (Adriamycin®, I.V., 50 mg/m², day 1
Fluorouracil, I.V., 500 mg/m², day 1

Repeat cycle every 21 days

or Dose Intensification of CAF*

Cyclophosphamide, I.V., 600 mg/m², day 1
Doxorubicin (Adriamycin®, I.V., 60 mg/m², day 1
Fluorouracil, I.V., 600 mg/m², day 1
G-CSF, I.V./S.C., 5 mcg/kg/dose

Repeat cycle every 21 days

*Preliminary data presented at ASCO (March, 1992) suggests better response with dose intensification.

CFM

Cyclophosphamide, I.V., 500 mg/m², day 1
Fluorouracil, I.V., 500 mg/m², day 1
Mitoxantrone, I.V., 10 mg/m², day 1

Repeat cycle every 21 days

CFPT

Cyclophosphamide, I.V., 150 mg/m², days 1-5
Fluorouracil, I.V., 300 mg/m², days 1-5
Prednisone, P.O., 10 mg tid, days 1-7
Tamoxifen, P.O., 10 mg bid, days 1-42

Repeat cycle every 42 days

CMF

Cyclophosphamide, P.O., 100 mg/m², days 1-14
Methotrexate, I.V., 40-60 mg/m², days 1 & 8
Fluorouracil, I.V., 400-600 mg/m², days 1 & 8

Repeat cycle every 28 days

or

Cyclophosphamide, I.V., 600 mg/m², days 1 & 8
Methotrexate, I.V., 40-60 mg/m², days 1 & 8
Fluorouracil, I.V., 400-600 mg/m², days 1 & 8

Repeat cycle every 28 days

CMFP

Cyclophosphamide, P.O., 100 mg/m², days 1-14
Methotrexate, I.V., 40-60 mg/m², days 1 & 8
Fluorouracil, I.V., 600-700 mg/m², days 1 & 8
Prednisone, P.O., 40 mg (first 3 cycles only), days 1-14

Repeat cycle every 28 days

CMFVP (Cooper's)

Cyclophosphamide, P.O., 2-2.5 mg/kg/d for 9 months
Methotrexate, I.V., 0.7 mg/kg/wk for 8 weeks then every other week for 7 months
Fluorouracil, I.V., 12 mg/kg/wk for 8 weeks then every other week for 7 months

Vincristine, I.V., 0.035 mg/kg (max 2 mg/wk) for 5 weeks then once
  monthly
Prednisone, P.O., 0.75 mg/kg/d, taper over next 40 days, discontinue,
  days 1-10

or

Cyclophosphamide, I.V., 400 mg/m^2, day 1
Methotrexate, I.V., 30 mg/m^2, days 1 & 8
Fluorouracil, I.V., 400 mg/m^2, days 1 & 8
Vincristine, I.V., 1 mg, days 1 & 8
Prednisone, P.O., 20 mg qid, days 1-7

Repeat cycle every 28 days

FAC

Fluorouracil, I.V., 500 mg/m^2, days 1 & 8
Doxorubicin (Adriamycin®), I.V., 50 mg/m^2, day 1
Cyclophosphamide, I.V., 500 mg/m^2, day 1

Repeat cycle every 21 days

IMF

Ifosfamide, I.V., 1.5 g/m^2, days 1 & 8
Mesna, I.V., 20% of ifosfamide dose, give immediately before and 4 and
  8 hours after ifosfamide infusion, days 1 & 8
Methotrexate, I.V., 40 mg/m^2, days 1 & 8
Fluorouracil, I.V., 600 mg/m^2, days 1 & 8

Repeat cycle every 28 days

NFL

Mitoxantrone (Novantrone®), I.V., 12 mg/m^2, day 1
Fluorouracil, I.V., 350 mg/m^2, days 1-3, given after leucovorin calcium
Leucovorin calcium, I.V., 300 mg/m^2, days 1-3

or

Mitoxantrone (Novantrone®), I.V., 10 mg/m^2, day 1
Fluorouracil, I.V., 1000 mg/m^2 continuous infusion, given after
leucovorin calcium, days 1-3
Leucovorin calcium, I.V., 100 mg/m^2, days 1-3

Repeat cycle every 21 days

VATH

Vinblastine, I.V., 4.5 mg/m^2, day 1
Doxorubicin (Adriamycin®), I.V., 45 mg/m^2, day 1
Thiotepa, I.V., 12 mg/m^2, day 1
Fluoxymesterone (Halotestin®), P.O., 30 mg qd, days 1-21

Repeat cycle every 21 days

Single-Agent Regimens

Doxorubicin, I.V., 60 mg/m^2, every 3 weeks
or
Doxorubicin, I.V., 20 mg/m^2, every week
or
Doxorubicin, I.V., 20 mg/m^2 continuous infusion, days 1-3, every 3 weeks

Mitomycin C, I.V., 8-10 mg/m^2, every 6-8 weeks

Paclitaxel, I.V., 175 mg/m^2 over 3-24 h, every 21 d
  Patient must be premedicated with:
  Dexamethasone 20 mg P.O., 12 and 6 h prior
  Diphenhydramine 50 mg I.V., 30 min prior
  Cimetidine 300 mg I.V., or ranitidine 50 mg I.V., 30 min prior

Vinblastine, I.V., 12 mg/m^2, every 3-4 weeks

Colon Cancer

F-CL

Fluorouracil, I.V., 375 mg/m^2, days 1-5
Calcium leucovorin, I.V., 200 mg/m^2, days 1-5

Repeat cycle every 28 days

or

Fluorouracil, I.V., 500 mg/m^2 weekly 1 h after initiating the calcium
  leucovorin infusion for 6 weeks
Calcium leucovorin, I.V., 500 mg/m^2, over 2 h, weekly for 6 weeks

Two-week break, then repeat cycle

FLe

Fluorouracil, I.V., 450 mg/m^{2}for 5 days, then, after a pause of 4 weeks, 450 mg/m^2, weekly for 48 weeks
Levamisole, P.O., 50 mg tid for 3 days, repeated every 2 weeks for 1 year

FMV

Fluorouracil, I.V., 10 mg/kg/d, days 1-5
Methyl-CCNU, P.O., 175 mg/m^2, day 1
Vincristine, I.V., 1 mg/m^2(max 2 mg), day 1

Repeat cycle every 35 days

FU/LV

Fluorouracil, I.V., 370-400 mg/m^2/d, days 1-5
Leucovorin calcium, I.V., 200 mg/m^2/d, commence infusion 15 min prior to fluorouracil infusion, days 1-5

Repeat cycle every 21 days

or

Fluorouracil, I.V., 1000 mg/m^2/d by continuous infusion, days 1-4
Leucovorin calcium, I.V., 200 mg/m^2/d, days 1-4

Repeat cycle every 28 days

Weekly 5FU/LV

Fluorouracil, I.V., 600 mg/m^{2}over 1 h given after leucovorin, repeat weekly x 6 then 2-week rest period = 1 cycle, days 1, 8, 15, 22, 29, 36
Leucovorin calcium, I.V., 500 mg/m^{2}over 2 h, days 1, 8, 15, 22, 29, 36

Repeat cycle every 56 days

5FU/LDLF

Fluorouracil, I.V., 370 mg/m^2/d, days 1-5
Leucovorin calcium, I.V., 20-25 mg/m^2/d, days 1-5

Repeat cycle every 28 days

Gastric Cancer

EAP

Etoposide, I.V., 120 mg/m^2, days 4, 5, 6
Doxorubicin (Adriamycin®), I.V., 20 mg/m^2, days 1, 7
Cisplatin (Platinol®), I.V., 40 mg/m^2, days 2, 8

Repeat cycle every 21 days

ELF

Etoposide, I.V., 120 mg/m^2, days 1-3
Leucovorin calcium, I.V., 300 mg/m^2, days 1-3
Fluorouracil, I.V., 500 mg/m^2, days 1-3

Repeat cycle every 21-28 days

FAM

Fluorouracil, I.V., 600 mg/m^2, days 1, 8, 29, & 36
Doxorubicin (Adriamycin®), I.V., 30 mg/m^2, days 1 & 29
Mitomycin C, I.V., 10 mg/m^2, day 1

Repeat cycle every 56 days

FAME

Fluorouracil, I.V., 350 mg/m^2, days 1-5, 36-40
Doxorubicin (Adriamycin®), I.V., 40 mg/m^2, days 1 & 36
Methyl-CCNU, P.O., 150 mg/m^2, day 1

Repeat cycle every 70 days

FAMTX

Methotrexate, IVPB, 1500 mg/m^2, day 1
Fluorouracil, IVPB, 1500 mg/m^{2}1 h after methotrexate, day 1
Leucovorin calcium, P.O., 15 mg/m^{2}q6h x 48 h 24 h after methotrexate, day 2
Doxorubicin (Adriamycin®), IVPB, 30 mg/m^2, day 15

Repeat cycle every 28 days

FCE

Fluorouracil, I.V., 900 mg/m^2/d continuous infusion, days 1-5
Cisplatin, I.V., 20 mg/m^2, days 1-5
Etoposide, I.V., 90 mg/m^2, days 1, 3, & 5

Repeat cycle every 21 days

PFL

Cisplatin (Platinol®), I.V., 25 mg/m^{2}continuous infusion, days 1-5
Fluorouracil, I.V., 800 mg/m^{2}continuous infusion, days 2-5
Leucovorin calcium, I.V., 500 mg/m^{2}continuous infusion, days 1-5
Repeat cycle every 28 days

Genitourinary Cancer

Bladder

CAP

Cyclophosphamide, I.V., 400 mg/m^2, day 1
Doxorubicin (Adriamycin®), I.V., 40 mg/m^2, day 1
Cisplatin (Platinol®), I.V., 60 mg/m^2, day 1
Repeat cycle every 21 days

CISCA

Cisplatin, I.V., 70-100 mg/m^2, day 2
Cyclophosphamide, I.V., 650 mg/m^2, day 1
Doxorubicin (Adriamycin®), I.V., 50 mg/m^2, day 1
Repeat cycle every 21-28 days

CMV

Cisplatin, I.V., 100 mg/m^{2}over 4 h start 12 h after MTX, day 2
Methotrexate, I.V., 30 mg/m^2, days 1 & 8
Vinblastine, I.V., 4 mg/m^2, days 1 & 8
Repeat cycle every 21 days

m-PFL

Methotrexate, I.V., 60 mg/m^2, day 1
Cisplatin (Platinol®), I.V., 25 mg/m^{2}continuous infusion, days 2-6
Fluorouracil, I.V., 800 mg/m^{2}continuous infusion, days 2-6
Leucovorin calcium, I.V., 500 mg/m^{2}continuous infusion, days 2-6
Repeat cycle every 28 days for 4 cycles

MVAC

Methotrexate, I.V., 30 mg/m^2, days 1, 15, 22
Vinblastine, I.V., 3 mg/m^2, days 2, 15, 22
Doxorubicin (Adriamycin®), I.V., 30 mg/m^2, day 2
Cisplatin, I.V., 70 mg/m^2, day 2
Repeat cycle every 28 days

Prostate

FL

Flutamide, P.O., 250 mg tid, days 1-28
Leuprolide acetate, S.C., 1 mg qd, days 1-28
Repeat cycle every 28 days

or

Flutamide, P.O., 250 mg tid, days 1-28
Leuprolide acetate depot, I.M., 7.5 mg, day 1
Repeat cycle every 28 days

FZ

Flutamide, P.O., 250 mg tid
Goserelin acetate (Zoladex®), S.C., 3.6 mg implant, every 28 days

L-VAM

Leuprolide acetate, S.C., 1 mg qd, days 1-28
Vinblastine, I.V., 1.5 mg/m^2/d continuous infusion, days 2-7
Doxorubicin (Adriamycin®), I.V., 50 mg/m^2 continuous infusion, day 1
Mitomycin C, I.V., 10 mg/m^2, day 2
Repeat cycle every 28 days

Testicular, Induction, Good Risk

BEP

Bleomycin, I.V., 30 units, days 2, 9, 16
Etoposide, I.V., 100 mg/m^2, days 1-5
Cisplatin (Platinol®), I.V., 20 mg/m^2, days 1-5
Repeat cycle every 21 days

PE

Cisplatin (Platinol®), I.V., 20 mg/m^2, days 1-5
Etoposide, I.V., 100 mg/m^2, days 1-5
Repeat cycle every 21 days

PVB

Cisplatin (Platinol®), I.V., 20 mg/m², days 1-5
Vinblastine, I.V., 6 mg/m², days 1, 2
Bleomycin, I.V., 30 units, weekly

Repeat cycle every 21-28 days

Testicular, Induction, Poor Risk

VIP

Etoposide (VePesid®), I.V., 75 mg/m², days 1-5
Ifosfamide, I.V., 1.2 g/m², days 1-5
Cisplatin (Platinol®), I.V., 20 mg/m², days 1-5
Mesna, I.V., 120 mg/m² then 1200 mg/m²/d continuous infusion, days 1-5

Repeat cycle every 21 days

VIP (Einhorn)

Vinblastine, I.V., 0.11 mg/kg, days 1-2
Ifosfamide, I.V., 1200 mg/m², days 1-5
Cisplatin (Platinol®), I.V., 20 mg/m², days 1-5
Mesna, I.V., 120 mg/m², then 1200 mg/m²/d continuous infusion, days 1-5

Repeat cycle every 21 days

Testicular, Induction, Salvage

VAB VI

Vinblastine, I.V., 4 mg/m², day 1
Dactinomycin (Actinomycin D), I.V., 1 mg/m², day 1
Bleomycin, I.V., 30 units push day 1, then 20 units/m²/d continuous infusion, days 1-3
Cisplatin, I.V., 120 mg/m², day 4
Cyclophosphamide, I.V., 600 mg/m², day 1

Repeat cycle every 21 days

VBP (PVB)

Vinblastine, I.V., 6 mg/m², days 1 & 2
Bleomycin, I.V., 30 units, days 1, 8, 15, (22)
Cisplatin (Platinol®), I.V., 20 mg/m², days 1-5

Repeat cycle every 21-28 days

Gestational Trophoblastic Cancer

DMC

Dactinomycin, I.V., 0.37 mg/m², days 1-5
Methotrexate, I.V., 11 mg/m², days 1-5
Cyclophosphamide, I.V., 110 mg/m², days 1-5

Repeat cycle every 21 days

Head and Neck Cancer

CAP

Cyclophosphamide, I.V., 500 mg/m², day 1
Doxorubicin (Adriamycin®), I.V., 50 mg/m², day 1
Cisplatin (Platinol®), I.V., 50 mg/m², day 1

Repeat cycle every 28 days

CF

Cisplatin, I.V., 100 mg/m², day 1
Fluorouracil, I.V., 1000 mg/m²/d continuous infusion, days 1-5

Repeat cycle every 21-28 days

CF

Carboplatin, I.V., 400 mg/m², day 1
Fluorouracil, I.V., 1000 mg/m²/d continuous infusion, days 1-5

Repeat cycle every 21-28 days

COB

Cisplatin, I.V., 100 mg/m², day 1
Vincristine (Oncovin®), I.V., 1 mg/m², days 2 & 5
Bleomycin, I.V., 30 units/d continuous infusion, days 2-5

Repeat cycle every 21 days

5-FU HURT

Hydroxyurea, P.O., 1000 mg q12h x 11 doses; start PM of admission, give 2 hours prior to radiation therapy, days 0-5

Fluorouracil, I.V., 800 mg/m^2/d continuous infusion, start AM after admission, days 1-5

Paclitaxel, I.V., 5-25 mg/m^2/d continuous infusion, start AM after admission; dose escalation study — refer to protocol, days 1-5

G-CSF, S.C., 5 mcg/kg/d, days 6-12, start ≥12 hours after completion of 5-FU infusion

5-7 cycles may be administered

MAP

Mitomycin C, I.V., 8 mg/m^2, day 1
Doxorubicin (Adriamycin®), I.V., 40 mg/m^2, day 1
Cisplatin (Platinol®), I.V., 60 mg/m^2, day 1

Repeat cycle every 28 days

MBC (MBD)

Methotrexate, I.M./I.V., 40 mg/m^2, days 1 & 15
Bleomycin, I.M./I.V., 10 units, days 1, 8, 15
Cisplatin, I.V., 50 mg/m^2, day 4

Repeat cycle every 21 days

MF

Methotrexate, I.V., 125-250 mg/m^2, day 1
Fluorouracil, I.V., 600 mg/m^2 beginning 1 h after methotrexate, day 1
Leucovorin calcium, I.V./P.O., 10 mg/m^2 q6h x 5 doses beginning 24 h after methotrexate

Repeat cycle every 7 days

PFL

Cisplatin (Platinol®), I.V., 100 mg/m^2, day 1
Fluorouracil, I.V., 600-800 mg/m^2/d continuous infusion, days 1-5
Leucovorin calcium, I.V., 200-300 mg/m^2/d, days 1-5

Repeat cycle every 21 days

PFL+IFN

Cisplatin (Platinol®), I.V., 100 mg/m^2, day 1
Fluorouracil, I.V., 640 mg/m^2/d continuous infusion, days 1-5
Leucovorin calcium, P.O., 100 mg q4h, days 1-5

CORTICOSTEROID EQUIVALENCIES COMPARISON

Glucocorticoid	Approximate Equivalent Dose (mg)	Routes of Administration	Relative Anti-inflammatory Potency	Relative Mineralocorticoid Potency	Half-life Plasma (min)	Half-life Biologic (h)
Short-Acting						
Cortisone	25	P.O., I.M.	0.8	2	30	8-12
Hydrocortisone	20	I.M., I.V.	1	2	80-118	
Intermediate-Acting						
Prednisone	5	P.O.	4	1	60	18-36
Prednisolone	5	P.O., I.M., I.V., intra-articular, intradermal, soft tissue injection	4	1	115-212	
Triamcinolone	4	P.O., I.M., intra-articular, intradermal, intrasynovial, soft tissue injection	5	0	200+	
Methylprednisolone	4	P.O., I.M., I.V.	5	0	78-188	
Long-Acting						
Dexamethasone	0.75	P.O., I.M., I.V., intra-articular, intradermal, soft tissue injection	25-30	0	110-210	36-54
Betamethasone	0.6-0.75	P.O., I.M., intra-articular, intradermal, intrasynovial, soft tissue injection	25	0	300+	

CORTICOSTEROIDS, TOPICAL COMPARISON

Steroid		Vehicle
Lowest Potency (may be ineffective for some indications)		
0.1%	Betamethasone	Cream
0.2%	Betamethasone (Celestone®)	Cream
0.05%	Desonide	Cream
0.04%	Dexamethasone (Hexadrol®)*	Cream
0.1%	Dexamethasone (Decadron® Phosphate, Decaderm®)*	Cream, gel
1%	Hydrocortisone	Cream, ointment, lotion
2.5%	Hydrocortisone	Cream, ointment
0.25%	Methylprednisolone acetate (Medrol®)	Ointment
1%	Methylprednisolone acetate (Medrol®)	Ointment
0.5%	Prednisolone (Meti-Derm®)	Cream
Low Potency		
0.01%	Betamethasone valerate (Valisone®, reduced strength)	Cream
0.1%	Clocortolone (Cloderm®)	Cream
0.03%	Flumethasone pivalate (Locorten®)	Cream
0.01%	Fluocinolone acetonide (Synalar®)*	Cream, solution
0.025%	Fluorometholone (Oxylone®)	Cream
0.025%	Flurandrenolide (Cordran®, Cordran® SP)*	Cream, ointment
0.2%	Hydrocortisone valerate (Westcort®)	Cream
0.025%	Triamcinolone acetonide (Kenalog®)*	Cream, ointment
Intermediate Potency		
0.025%	Betamethasone benzoate	Cream, gel, lotion
0.1%	Betamethasone valerate (Valisone®)*	Cream, ointment, lotion
0.05%	Desonide (Tridesilon®)	Cream, ointment
0.05%	Desoximetasone (Topicort® LP)	Cream
0.025%	Fluocinolone acetonide*	Cream, ointment
0.05%	Flurandrenolide (Cordran®, Cordran® SP)*	Cream, ointment, lotion
0.025%	Halcinonide (Halog®)	Cream, ointment
0.1%	Triamcinolone acetonide (Kenalog®)*	Cream, ointment
High Potency		
0.1%	Amcinonide (Cyclocort®)	Cream, ointment
0.05%	Betamethasone dipropionate (Diprosone®)	Cream, ointment, lotion
0.05%	Clobetasol dipropionate	Cream, ointment
0.25%	Desoximetasone (Topicort®)	Cream
0.05%	Diflorasone diacetate (Florone®, Maxiflor®)	Cream, ointment
0.2%	Fluocinolone (Synalar-HP®)	Cream
0.05%	Fluocinonide (Lidex®)*	Cream, ointment
0.1%	Halcinonide (Halog®)	Cream, ointment, solution
0.5%	Triamcinolone acetonide*	Cream, ointment

*Fluorinated.

NARCOTIC AGONIST CHARTS

Comparative Pharmacokinetics

Drug	Onset (min)	Peak (h)	Duration (h)	t ½ (h)	Average Dosing Interval (h)		Equianalgesic Doses* (mg)	
							I.M.	P.O.
Alfentanil	Immediate	ND	ND	1-2	—	—	ND	NA
Buprenorphine	15	1	4-8	2-3			0.4	—
Butorphanol	I.M.: 30-60 I.V.: 4-5	0.5-1	3-5	2.5-3.5	3	(3-6)	2	—
Codeine	P.O.: 30-60 I.M.: 10-30	0.5-1	4-6	3-4	3	(3-6)	120	200
Fentanyl	I.M.: 7-15 I.V.: Immediate	ND	1-2	1.5-6	1	(0.5-2)	0.1	NA
Hydrocodone	ND	ND	4-8	3.3-4.4	6	(4-8)	ND	ND
Hydromorphone	P.O.: 15-30	0.5-1	4-6	2-4	4	(3-6)	1.5	7.5
Levorphanol	P.O.: 10-60	0.5-1	4-8	12-16	6	(6-24)	2	4
Meperidine	P.O./I.M./ S.C.: 10-15 I.V.: ≤5	0.5-1	2-4	3-4	3	(2-4)	75	300
Methadone	P.O.: 30-60 I.V.: 10-20	0.5-1	4-6 (acute) >8 (chronic)	15-30	8	(6-12)	10	20
Morphine	P.O.: 15-60 I.V.: ≤5	P.O./I.M./ S.C.: 0.5-1 I.V.: 0.3	3-6	2-4	4	(3-6)	10	60# (acute) 30 (chronic)
Nalbuphine	I.M.: 30 I.V.: 1-3	1	3-6	5		—	10	—
Naloxone†	2-5	0.5-2	0.5-1	0.5-1.5	—	—	—	—
Oxycodone	P.O.: 10-15	0.5-1	4-6	3-4	4	(3-6)	NA	30
Oxymorphone	5-15	0.5-1	3-6				1	10‡
Pentazocine	15-20	0.25-1	3-4	2-3	3	(3-6)		
Propoxyphene	P.O.: 30-60	2-2.5	4-6	3.5-15	6	(4-8)	ND	130§-200¶
Sufentanil	1.3-3	ND	ND	2.5-3	—	—	0.02	NA

ND = no data available. NA = not applicable.

*Based on acute, short-term use. Chronic administration may alter pharmacokinetics and decrease the oral parenteral dose ratio. The morphine oral-parenteral ratio decreases to ~ 1.5-2.5:1 upon chronic dosing.

#Extensive survey data suggest that the relative potency of I.M.:P.O. morphine of 1:6 changes to 1:2-3 with chronic dosing.

†Narcotic antagonist.

‡Rectal.

§HCl salt.

¶Napsylate salt.

Comparative Pharmacology

Drug	Analgesic	Antitussive	Constipation	Respiratory Depression	Sedation	Nausea/Vomiting
Phenanthrenes						
Codeine	+	+++	+	+	+	+
Hydrocodone	+	+++		+		
Hydromorphone	++	+++	+	++	+	+
Levorphanol	++	++	++	++	++	+
Morphine	++	+++	++	++	++	++
Oxycodone	++	+++	++	++	++	++
Oxymorphone	++	+	++	+++		+++
Phenylpiperidines						
Alfentanil	++					
Fentanyl	++			+		+
Meperidine	++	+	+	++	+	
Sufentanil	+++					
Diphenylheptanes						
Methadone	++	++	++	++	+	+
Propoxyphene	+			+	+	+
Agonist/Antagonist						
Buprenorphine	++	N/A	+++	+++	++	++
Butorphanol	++	N/A	+++	+++	++	+
Dezocine	++		+	++	+	++
Nalbuphine	++	N/A	+++	+++	++	++
Pentazocine	++	N/A	+	++	++ or stimulation	++

NONSTEROIDAL ANTI-INFLAMMATORY AGENTS, COMPARATIVE DOSAGES, AND PHARMACOKINETICS

Drug	Maximum Recommended Daily Dose (mg)	Time to Peak Levels (h)†	Half-life (h)
Propionic Acids			
Fenoprofen (Nalfon®)	3200	1-2	2-3
Flurbiprofen (Ansaid®)	300	1.5	5.7
Ibuprofen	3200	1-2	1.8-2.5
Ketoprofen (Orudis®)	300	0.5-2	2-4
Naproxen (Naprosyn®)	1500	2-4	12-15
Naproxen sodium (Anaprox®)	1375	1-2	12-13
Acetic Acids			
Diclofenac sodium delayed release (Voltaren®)	225	2-3	1-2
Diclofenac potassium immediate release (Cataflam®)	200	1	1-2
Etodolac (Lodine®)	1200	1-2	7.3
Indomethacin (Indocin®)	200	1-2	4.5
Indomethacin SR	150	2-4	4.5-6
Ketorolac (Toradol®)	I.M.: 120‡ P.O.: 40	0.5-1	3.8-8.6
Sulindac (Clinoril®)	400	2-4	7.8 (16.4)§
Tolmetin (Tolectin®)	2000	0.5-1	1-1.5
Fenamates (Anthranilic Acids)			
Meclofenamate (Meclomen®)	400	0.5-1	2 (3.3)¶
Mefenamic acid (Ponstel®)	1000	2-4	2-4
Nonacidic Agent			
Nabumetone (Relafen®)	2000	3-6	24
Oxicam			
Piroxicam (Feldene®)	20	3-5	30-86

Dosage is based on 70 kg adult with normal hepatic and renal function.

†Food decreases the rate of absorption and may delay the time to peak levels.

‡150 mg on the first day.

§Half-life of active sulfide metabolite.

¶Half-life with multiple doses.

DENTAL DRUG INTERACTIONS: UPDATE ON DRUG COMBINATIONS REQUIRING SPECIAL CONSIDERATIONS

This update discussion includes 16 drug interaction monographs describing clinically important drug combinations requiring special considerations in dental practice. The actions which have resulted from these combinations range from life-threatening adverse effects to attenuation of the therapeutic effects of the interacting drug. The monographs are organized according to the four major groups of drugs used in dentistry: antibiotics, nonsteroidal anti-inflammatory drugs (including aspirin), epinephrine (vasoconstrictors), and narcotic analgesics. An additional monograph on Valium® and alcohol is included.

ANTIBIOTICS - ORAL CONTRACEPTIVES

Description of the Interaction

Case reports suggest that antibiotics used in dentistry can reduce the effectiveness of oral contraceptives resulting in breakthrough ovulation and unplanned pregnancies.

Mechanism

Estrogens, which are components of oral contraceptives, are activated in the intestine by bacteria and reabsorbed into the blood stream as active compounds to inhibit ovulation. Antibiotics reduce the bacteria population in the intestine, which may result in less activated estrogen available to inhibit ovulation.

Background Reports

Tetracyclines: One report described a woman on an estrogen-type oral contraceptive who became pregnant after a 5-day course of tetracycline[1]. Also, several cases of unintended pregnancy and menstrual irregularities have been reported following concurrent use of tetracyclines and oral contraceptives[2,3].

Penicillins: Ampicillin has been shown to reduce estrogen levels in women not taking oral contraceptives and there are reports of unplanned pregnancies in women taking ampicillin with oral contraceptives[4,5]. Concomitant use of penicillin with estrogen-containing oral contraceptives decreased the efficacy of the contraceptive and increased the incidence of breakthrough bleeding[6,7]. Since amoxicillin is closely related to other penicillins, it may also interact with oral contraceptives.

Cephalosporins: Cephalexin (Keflex®) has been reported to interact with oral contraceptives resulting in an unplanned pregnancy[8].

Erythromycins: Unlike ampicillin and tetracyclines, erythromycins have been implicated in only a few cases of oral contraceptive failure over the last 15 years and it is questionable whether erythromycin was the cause of those reported failures[9].

Management

If antibiotics are prescribed to oral contraceptive users, it is suggested that the patients be advised to use additional methods of birth control during both 7 to 10 day dosing, and the two-dose prophylaxis regimens. Any additional method of birth control should be continued through the remaining oral contraceptive cycle.

1. Bacon JF, et al, "Pregnancy Attributable to Interaction Between Tetracycline and Oral Contraceptives," *Br Med J*, 1980, 280-93.

2. Orme MLE, "The Clinical Pharmacology of Oral Contraceptive Steroids," *Br J Clin Pharmacol*, 1982, 14:31.

3. Back DJ, Grimmer SF, Orme ML, et al, "Evaluation of Committee on Safety of Medicines Yellow Card Reports on Oral Contraceptive-Drug Interactions With Anticonvulsants and Antibiotics," *Br J Clin Pharmacol*, 1988, 25(5):527-32.

4. Trybuchowski H, "Effect of Ampicillin on the Urinary Output of Steroidal Hormones in Pregnant and Nonpregnant Women," *Clin Chim Acta*, 1973, 45:9.

5. Aldercreutz H, et al, "Effect of Ampicillin Administration on Plasma Conjugated and Unconjugated Estrogen and Progesterone Levels in Pregnancy," *Am J Obstet Gynecol*, 1977, 128:266.

6. Proudfit CW, "Concurrent Oral Contraceptive and Antibiotic Therapy," *JAMA*, 1981, 246:2076.

7. True RJ, "Interaction Between Antibiotics and Oral Contraceptives," *JAMA*, 1982, 247:1408.

8. Bainton R, "Interaction Between Antibiotic Therapy and Contraceptive Medication," *Oral Surg Oral Med Oral Pathol*, 1986, 61(5):453-5.

9. Bainton R, "Interaction Between Antibiotic Therapy and Contraceptive Medication," *Oral Surg Oral Med Oral Pathol*, 1986, 61(5):453.

TETRACYCLINES - ANTACIDS (Containing Divalent or Trivalent Ions)

Description of the Interaction

Concomitant therapy with a tetracycline and an antacid containing aluminum, calcium, or magnesium products can reduce serum concentration and the efficacy of the tetracycline.

Mechanism

Aluminum, calcium, and magnesium ions can combine with the tetracycline molecule in the gastrointestinal tract to form a larger ionized molecule unable to be absorbed into the blood stream.

Background

The interaction between tetracyclines and antacids containing aluminum, calcium, and magnesium is well documented. Foods and dairy products containing calcium will also impair the absorption of tetracyclines. Some reports suggest that doxycycline and minocycline are minimally affected by antacids and dairy products[1,2].

Management

Tetracyclines should be given as far apart as possible from antacids and dairy products.

1. Welling PG, et al, "Bioavailability of Tetracycline and Doxycycline in Fasted and Nonfasted Subjects," *Antimicrob Agents Chemother*, 1977, 11:462.
2. *Anti-infective Drug Interactions. In Drug Interactions and Updates*, Hansten PD and Horn JR, eds, Malvern, PA: Lea and Febiger.

TETRACYCLINE - PENICILLIN

Description of the Interaction

Simultaneous tetracycline-penicillin therapy may impair the efficacy of penicillin.

Mechanism

Penicillin kills bacteria by inhibiting cell wall synthesis. Tetracycline inhibits protein synthesis in bacteria and this action has been shown to antagonize the cell wall inhibiting effect of penicillin.

Background

Most of the manufacturers product information contains warnings against using tetracyclines and penicillins together.

Management

Tetracycline-penicillin combination should never be used to treat oral infections. For penicillin two-dose prophylaxis, it would be prudent not to give to patients taking tetracycline. Reappoint if possible.

ERYTHROMYCIN - PENICILLIN

Description of the Interaction

Simultaneous erythromycin-penicillin therapy may impair the efficacy of penicillin.

Mechanism

Penicillin kills bacteria by inhibiting cell wall synthesis. Erythromycin inhibits protein synthesis in bacteria and this action may antagonize the cell wall inhibiting effect of penicillin.

Background

This interaction has not been sufficiently documented in clinical studies.

Management

Erythromycin-penicillin combination should not be used to treat oral infections. For penicillin two-dose prophylaxis, it would be prudent not to give to patients taking erythromycin. Reappoint if possible.

ERYTHROMYCIN - THEOPHYLLINE

Description of the Interaction

Erythromycins interact with theophylline, a bronchodilator, to result in symptoms suggestive of a relative overdose of theophylline. Resulting symptoms were nausea, vomiting, and seizures.

Mechanism

A recent study showed that erythromycin forms complexes with a specific enzyme that metabolizes theophylline and that this complex may explain the impairment of theophylline metabolic inactivation resulting in symptoms of theophylline overdose[1].

Background

An erythromycin regimen of 5 to 20 day daily dosing in theophylline patients caused increased blood levels, a longer half-life and decreased urinary clearance of the theophylline[2]. A more recent review indicated that many patients did not experience any interactions between the two drugs with 8 out of 22 studies reporting no change in theophylline kinetics after erythromycin dosing[3]. The interactions which have occurred have included all formulations of erythromycin. There have been no reported interactions between erythromycin and theophylline when using the prophylaxis dosing schedule.

Management

Patients taking theophylline and who may be at increased risk for theophylline toxicity should be given erythromycin with caution and only if there is absolutely no alternative to erythromycin. These patients should be monitored closely.

1. Delaforge M and Sartori E, "In Vivo Effects of Erythromycin, Oleandomycin, and Erythralosamine Derivatives on Hepatic Cytochrome P-450," *Biochem Pharmacol*, 1990, 40(2):223-8.
2. Cummins LH, et al, "Erythromycin's Effect on Theophylline Blood Levels. Correspondence," *Pediatrics*, 1977, 59:144-5.
3. Ludden TM, "Pharmacokinetic Interactions of the Macrolide Antibiotics," *Clin Pharmacokinet*, 1985, 10(1):63-79.

ERYTHROMYCIN - CARBAMAZEPINE (Tegretol®)

Description of the Interaction

Erythromycin has interacted with carbamazepine (Tegretol®), an antiepileptic, to cause increased blood levels resulting in carbamazepine toxicity[1]. Symptoms were drowsiness, dizziness, nausea, headache, and blurred vision.

Mechanism

This interaction is suggestive of an inhibition of the hepatic metabolizing enzymes by erythromycin which normally convert carbamazepine to inactive products.

Background

The increased blood levels of carbamazepine has occurred within one day of concomitant erythromycin therapy[1]. This effect has not been reported with the two-dose erythromycin, prophylaxis regimen.

Management

Patients taking carbamazepine and who may be at increased risk for carbamazepine toxicity should be given erythromycin with caution and only if there is absolutely no alternative to erythromycin. These patients should be monitored closely.

1. Ludden TM, "Pharmacokinetic Interactions of the Macrolide Antibiotics," *Clin Pharmacokinet*, 1985, 10(1):63.

ERYTHROMYCIN - TRIAZOLAM (Halcion®)

Description of the Interaction

Erythromycin has interacted with triazolam (Halcion®), a hypnotic type antianxiety agent, to cause increased blood levels resulting in triazolam toxicity. Resulting effects were psychomotor impairment and memory dysfunction.

Mechanism

This interaction is suggestive of an inhibition of the hepatic metabolizing enzymes by erythromycin which normally convert triazolam to inactive products.

Background

Erythromycin has caused significant increases in triazolam blood concentrations within 3 days after 333 mg erythromycin base 3 times/day and triazolam 0.5 mg daily[1].

Management

Patients taking triazolam should be given erythromycin with caution and only if there is absolutely no alternative to erythromycin. These patients should be closely monitored.

1. Phillips JP, "A Pharmacokinetic Drug Interaction Between Erythromycin and Triazolam," *J Clin Psychopharmacol*, 1986, 6(5):297-9.

ERYTHROMYCIN OR KETOCONAZOLE (Nizoral®) - TERFENADINE (Seldane®)

Description of the Interaction

Erythromycin and ketoconazole when administered to patients taking terfenadine (Seldane®), a drug for hayfever, may cause cardiotoxicities.

Mechanism

After oral administration and absorption from the stomach into the liver, 99% of terfenadine is metabolized to other products. Both erythromycin and ketoconazole have been shown to block this metabolism of terfenadine[1]. The resulting nonmetabolized terfenadine is excitatory to the heart and has caused ventricular arrhythmias.

Background

Ventricular arrhythmias from terfenadine and its interaction with ketoconazole were first reported by Monahan, et al[2]. They described the syndrome as torsade de pointes or "twisting of the points". This is a form of ventricular tachycardia associated with prolongation of the QT interval, with the name referring to the morphological features of the QRS complex that appear to twist around the axis of the complex. Terfenadine has also been shown to cause cardiotoxicities as the sole drug in overdose[3]. Another report has shown that erythromycin changes the pharmacokinetics and electrocardiographic pharmacodynamics of terfenadine in humans[4]. Nine subjects were given the recommended dose of terfenadine (60 mg every 12 hours) for 7 days then given erythromycin 500 mg every 8 hours in addition to terfenadine for a second week. Three of the subjects had detectable unmetabolized terfenadine levels after erythromycin and EKG data revealed changes in the normal sinus rhythm resembling cardiotoxicity.

Management

The concurrent use of erythromycin or ketoconazole in patients medicated with terfenadine is not recommended. The dentist should be aware that other drugs that are metabolic inhibitors may also precipitate this interaction with terfenadine. Patients at increased risk for this interaction are those with pre-existing myocardial conduction defects taking terfenadine.

1. Wynn RL, "Erythromycin and Ketoconazole (Nizoral®) are Associated With Terfenadine (Seldane®)-induced Ventricular Arrhythmias," *Gen Dent*, 1993, 41:27.
2. Monahan BP, Ferguson CL, Killeavy ES, et al, "Torsade de Pointes Occurring in Association With Terfenadine Use," *JAMA*, 1990, 264(21):2788-90.
3. Davies AJ, Harindra V, McEwan A, et al, "Cardiotoxic Effect With Convulsions in Terfenadine Overdose," *Br Med J*, 1989, 298(6669):325
4. Honig PK, Woosley RL, Zamani K, et al, "Erythromycin Changes Terfenadine Pharmacokinetics and Electrocardiographic Pharmacodynamics," *Clin Pharmacol Ther*, 1992, 51:156 (abstract).

IBUPROFEN (Motrin®, Advil®, Nuprin®) - ORAL ANTICOAGULANTS (Coumarins)

Description of the Interaction

Bleeding may occur when ibuprofen is administered to patients taking coumarin type anticoagulants.

Mechanism

Inhibition of prostaglandins by ibuprofen results in decreased platelet aggregation and interference with blood clotting, resulting in an enhancement of the anticoagulant effect of coumarins.

DENTAL DRUG INTERACTIONS

Background

Product information on ibuprofen in the 1995 edition of the *Physicians' Desk Reference* (PDR) states that Motrin® inhibits platelet aggregation, but the effect is quantitatively less and of shorter duration than aspirin. It goes on to state that bleeding has been reported when Motrin® had been administered to patients on coumarin-type anticoagulants and the clinician should use caution in these circumstances. Additional product information on naproxen, diflunisal, and flurbiprofen is listed in the same edition of the PDR. It advises caution when using naproxen with coumarins since interactions have been seen with other NSAIDs of this class; it states that diflunisal, when given with warfarin, resulted in prolongation of prothrombin time; and it states that serious clinical bleeding has been reported in patients taking flurbiprofen together with coumarins. Product information for warfarin (Coumadin®) in the 1995 PDR states that ibuprofen, naproxen, and diflunisal may be responsible for increased prothrombin time response of the warfarin. Flurbiprofen was not mentioned.

Management

It is suggested that ibuprofen (Motrin®, Advil®, Nuprin®) and other dental NSAIDs such as naproxen (Naprosyn®), naproxen sodium (Anaprox®, Aleve®), diflunisal (Dolobid®), flurbiprofen (ANSAID®), and ketorolac (Toradol® Oral), be used with caution (if at all) in patients taking coumarin-type anticoagulants. Use of other analgesics is preferred.

IBUPROFEN (Motrin®, Advil®, Nuprin®) - LITHIUM

Description of the Interaction

Concurrent administration of ibuprofen with lithium produces symptoms of lithium toxicity including nausea, vomiting, slurred speech, and mental confusion.

Mechanism

Prostaglandins stimulate renal lithium tubular secretion. NSAIDs inhibit prostaglandin-induced renal secretion of lithium, which increases lithium plasma levels and produces symptoms of lithium toxicity.

Background

Lithium is used for the treatment of acute mania and to prevent recurrent episodes of bipolar (manic-depressive) illness. The therapeutic lithium plasma concentration is extremely narrow (0.8-1.2 mEq/L) and drugs that cause lithium plasma levels to go outside this narrow therapeutic range will result in lithium toxicity. Of the four NSAIDs used in dentistry (ibuprofen, naproxen, diflunisal, and flurbiprofen) the former two have been well documented to interact with lithium. In 1980, Ragheb, et al, reported that a patient taking 2400 mg ibuprofen daily experienced nausea and drowsiness while stabilized on lithium[1]. The lithium plasma level increased from 0.8 to 1.0 mEq/L. Subsequently, in a study of 11 healthy volunteers, Kristoff, et al, observed that 400 mg of ibuprofen 4 times/day combined with 450 mg of lithium carbonate every 12 hours, increased lithium plasma levels within several days[2]. Decreased ability to concentrate, lightheadedness, and fatigue resulted from this interaction.

Ragheb reported that concomitant administration of lithium and ibuprofen (1.8 g/day) in nine patients with bipolar- or schizoid-type disorders resulted in significant increases (average 34%) in lithium plasma concentrations as well as decreases in lithium clearance[3]. Individual variations were observed, with increases in lithium levels ranging from 12% to 66% within 6 days of concomitant administration of ibuprofen. In this study, tremors occurred in three patients as a result of this interaction. Ragheb reported that patients older than 50 years were more susceptible to lithium toxicity. The 1993 edition of the *Physician's Desk Reference* (PDR) (in the monograph for Motrin®) warns that concomitant use of ibuprofen and lithium citrate or carbonate may elevate lithium plasma levels and reduce renal lithium clearance.

In a 1986 study by Ragheb and Powell, concomitant administration of naproxen and lithium has resulted in individual variations in plasma lithium levels (from increases of 0% to 42%[4]. In that study, lithium renal clearance decreased in patients who were taking daily doses of lithium (900 mg) and naproxen (750 mg) for 6 days. The monograph for Naprosyn® in the 1993 PDR cautions that concomitant use of naproxen and lithium could increase lithium plasma concentrations.

Interactions between diflunisal (Dolobid®) and lithium, and flurbiprofen (Ansaid®) and lithium have not been reported. Nor is any potential interaction between these two NSAIDs and lithium mentioned in the PDR. Interestingly, aspirin has been shown to affect plasma lithium levels in healthy subjects[5]. Lack of documentation about diflunisal and flurbiprofen does not mean these agents are safe to use in conjunction with lithium. NSAIDs should be used with caution by dental patients who are taking lithium. Substitution of NSAIDs with acetaminophen preparations may be warranted.

Management

Extreme caution is necessary in administering NSAIDs to lithium patients; use of analgesics other than NSAIDs is preferred.

1. Ragheb M, et al, "Interaction of Indomethacin and Ibuprofen With Lithium in Manic Patients Under a Steady-State Lithium Level," *J Clin Psychiatry*, 1980, 41:397.
2. Kristoff CA, Hayes PE, Barr WH, et al, "Effect of Ibuprofen on Lithium Plasma and Red Blood Cell Concentrations," *Clin Pharm*, 1986, 5(1):51-5.
3. Ragheb M, "Ibuprofen Can Increase Serum Lithium Level in Lithium Treated Patients," *J Clin Psychiatry*, 1987, 48(4):161-3.
4. Ragheb M and Powell AL, "Lithium Interaction With Sulindac and Naproxen," *J Clin Psychopharmacol*, 1986, 6(3):150-4.
5. Reimann IW, et al, "Indomethacin But Not Aspirin Increases Plasma Lithium Ion Levels," *Arch Gen Psychiatry*, 1983, 40:283.

ASPIRIN - ORAL ANTICOAGULANTS (Coumarins)

Description of the Interaction

Aspirin increases the risk of bleeding in patients taking oral anticoagulants.

Mechanism

Small doses of aspirin inhibit platelet function. Larger doses (>3 g/day) elicit a hypoprothrombinemic effect. Aspirin may also displace oral anticoagulants from plasma protein-binding sites. These actions of aspirin all contribute to increase the risk of bleeding in patients taking oral anticoagulants.

Background

There is much documentation in the literature confirming this interaction. One study using over 500 patients showed that excessive bleeding was about 3 times more common with warfarin (Coumadin®) plus aspirin (500 mg/day) than with warfarin alone[1]. Another study showed enhanced hypoprothrombinemia in warfarin patients during the first few days of aspirin therapy (1 g/day)[2]. There are other reports describing bleeding episodes due to concurrent therapy with aspirin and oral anticoagulants[3,4].

Management

Patients receiving oral anticoagulants should avoid aspirin and aspirin-containing products.

1. Chesebro JH, et al, "Trial of Combined Warfarin Therapy Plus dipyridamole or ASA Therapy in Prosthetic Heart Valve Replacement: Danger of ASA Compared With Dipyridamole," *Am J Cardiol*, 1983, 51:1537.
2. Donaldson DR, et al, "Assessment of the Interaction of Warfarin With Aspirin and Dipyridamole," *Thromb Haemost*, 1982, 47:77.
3. Starr KJ, et al, "Drug Interactions in Patients on Long-Term Oral Anticoagulant and Antihypertensive Adrenergic Neuron-Blocking Drugs," *Br Med J*, 1972, 4:133.
4. Udall JA, "Drug Interference With Warfarin Therapy," *Clin Med*, 1970, 77:20.

ASPIRIN - PROBENECID (Benemid®)

Description of the Interaction

Aspirin inhibits the uricosuric action of probenecid.

Mechanism

Unknown

Background

The inhibition of probenecid-induced uricosuria by aspirin is dose-dependent. Doses of aspirin of 1 g or less do not appear to affect probenecid uricosuria. Larger doses however, appear to considerably inhibit uricosuria. Conversely, probenecid appears to inhibit uricosuria following large doses of aspirin. Aspirin does not interfere with the actions of probenecid to inhibit the renal elimination of penicillins.

Management

It appears prudent to use a nonsalicylate-type analgesic (ie, acetaminophen or NSAID) in patients receiving probenecid as a uricosuric agent (treatment of gouty arthritis).

EPINEPHRINE (Vasoconstrictor) - TRICYCLIC ANTIDEPRESSANTS

Description of the Interaction

Use of epinephrine as vasoconstrictor in local anesthetic injections may cause a hypertensive interaction in patients taking tricyclic antidepressants.

Mechanism

Tricyclic antidepressants cause increases of norepinephrine in synaptic areas in the central nervous system and periphery. Epinephrine may add to the effects of norepinephrine resulting in vasoconstriction and transient hypertension.

Background

There is adequate information in the literature to confirm a hypertensive interaction between epinephrine, norepinephrine, and levonordefrin with TCAs. An I.V. infusion of epinephrine to healthy subjects receiving imipramine resulted in two- to four-fold increases in the pressor response to epinephrine[1,2]. Also, cardiac dysrhythmias were reported. Although these effects were seen with I.V. infusions, these reports suggested that caution should certainly be exercised if epinephrine is administered by other routes. I.V. infusions of norepinephrine to healthy subjects receiving imipramine resulted in a four- to eight-fold increase in the pressor response to norepinephrine[1,2] and a later study showed a two-fold increase in pressor response to norepinephrine[3]. Other tricyclics were associated with a three-fold increase in pressor response to norepinephrine[4]. This increased pressor response was probably due to tricyclic antidepressant-induced inhibition of norepinephrine reuptake. Similar effects have been reported with levonordefrin[5].

Management

The use of epinephrine in patients taking tricyclic type antidepressants is potentially dangerous. Use minimum amounts of vasoconstrictor with caution in patients on tricyclic antidepressants.

1. Boakes AJ, et al, "Interactions Between Sympathomimetic Amines and Antidepressant Agents in Man," Br Med J, 1973, 1:311.
2. Svedmyr N, "The Influence of a Tricyclic Antidepressive Agent (Protriptyline) on Some of the Circulatory Effects of Noradrenaline and Adrenalin in Man," Life Sci, 1968, 7:77.
3. Larochelle P, et al, "Responses to Tyramine and Norepinephrine After Imipramine and Trazodone," Clin Pharmacol Ther, 1979, 26:24.
4. Mitchell JR, "Guanethidine and Related Agents. III. Antagonism by Drugs Which Inhibit the Norepinephrine Pump in Man,"J Clin Invest, 1970, 49:1596.
5. Jastak JT and Yagiela JA, "Vasoconstrictors and Local Anesthesia: A Review and Rationale for Use," JADA, 1983, 107:623.

EPINEPHRINE (Vasoconstrictor) - MONOAMINE OXIDASE INHIBITORS

Description of Interaction

Use of epinephrine as vasoconstrictor in local anesthetic injections may cause a hypertensive interaction in patients taking monoamine oxides inhibitors.

Mechanism

Drugs which inhibit monoamine oxidase cause increases in the concentration of endogenous norepinephrine, serotonin, and dopamine in storage sites throughout the central nervous system. Epinephrine may add to the effects of norepinephrine resulting in vasoconstriction and transient hypertension.

Background

One study reported on four health subjects taking MAOIs and given I.V. epinephrine. There was no significant effect on heart rate or blood pressure[1]. This same study also showed a lack of interaction with norepinephrine and MAOI. Nevertheless, it is advisable that vasoconstrictors be used with caution in these patients. Hansten and Horn[2] report that MAOIs may slightly increase the pressor response to norepinephrine and epinephrine, an action which appeared to be due to receptor sensitivity by the MAOI.

Management

There is a potential for unexpected increases in blood pressure when using epinephrine vasoconstrictor in patients taking monoamine oxidase inhibitors. Use vasoconstrictor with caution in these patients.

1. Boakes AJ, et al, "Interactions Between Sympathomimetic Amines and Antidepressant Agents in Man," Br Med J, 1973, 1:311.

2. Hansten PD and Horn JR, eds, "Monoamine Oxidase Inhibitor Interactions," *Drug Interactions and Updates*, Malvern, PA: Lea and Febiger, 1990, 387-8.

NARCOTIC ANALGESICS - CIMETIDINE (Tagamet®)

Description of the Interaction

Cimetidine may increase the adverse effects of narcotic analgesics.

Mechanism

The hepatic metabolism of narcotic analgesics to inactive products may be inhibited by cimetidine. The central nervous system effects of narcotic analgesics and cimetidine may be additive.

Background

One study reported that cimetidine, when given to patients taking meperidine (Demerol®), reduced the rate of renal excretion of the narcotic, resulting in increased sedation, and an increase in respiratory depression[1]. Additional studies showed that cimetidine may inhibit the liver metabolism of meperidine and fentanyl, another narcotic analgesic thus exacerbating the sedative effects of both of these narcotics[2,3].

Management

Although the side effects of cimetidine on codeine, hydrocodone, and oxycodone are unknown, it is advised to use caution in prescribing these narcotic analgesics in dental patients taking cimetidine. Ranitidine (Zantac®) is probably less likely to interact with narcotic analgesics.

1. Guay DR, Meatherall RC, Chalmers JL, et al, "Cimetidine Alters Pethidine Disposition in Man," *Br J Clin Pharmacol*, 1984, 18(6):907-14.
2. Knodell RG, et al, "Drug Metabolism by Rat and Human Hepatic Microsomes in Response to Interaction With H₂-Receptor Antagonists," *Gastroenterol*, 1982, 82:84.
3. Lee HR, et al, "Effect of Histamine H2-Receptors on Fentanyl Metabolism," *Pharmacologist*, 1982, 24:145.

BENZODIAZEPINES - Diazepam (Valium®) - ALCOHOL

Description of the Interaction

Alcohol may enhance the adverse psychomotor effects of benzodiazepines such as Valium®. Combined use may result in dangerous inebriation, ataxia, and respiratory depression.

Mechanism

Alcohol and benzodiazepines have additive central nervous system depressant activity. Also, alcohol may increase the gastrointestinal absorption of diazepam[1,2] leading to symptoms of diazepam overdose.

Background

There is much documentation in the literature to confirm the serious interaction between alcohol and benzodiazepines. Many controlled studies have shown that benzodiazepines such as diazepam enhance the detrimental effects of alcohol on simulated driving, reaction times, and other psychomotor skills[3-6].

Management

Patients receiving benzodiazepines such as diazepam (Valium®) should be warned against taking any alcohol until the benzodiazepine is cleared from the body. This is usually 48-72 hours after the last dose. This interaction has been unpredictable and significant CNS depression and ataxia has occurred with only a single dose of diazepam (5 mg) along with a moderate amount of alcohol.

1. Hayes SL, et al, "Ethanol and Oral Diazepam Absorption," *N Engl J Med*, 1977, 296:186.
2. MacLeod SM, et al, "Diazepam Actions and Plasma Concentrations Following Ethanol Ingestion," *Eur J Clin Pharmacol*, 1977, 11:345.
3. Linnoila M, et al, "Effects of Diazepam and Codeine, Alone and in Combination With Alcohol, on Simulated Driving," *Clin Pharmacol Ther*, 1974, 15:368.
4. Linnoila M, "Effects of Diazepam, Chlordiazepoxide, Thioridazine, Haloperidol, Flupenthixole, and Alcohol on Psychomotor Skills Related to Driving," *Ann Med Exp Biol Fenn*, 1973, 51:125.
5. Linnoila M, et al, "Drug Interaction on Psychomotor Skills Related to Driving: Diazepam and Alcohol," *Eur J Clin Pharmacol*, 1973, 5:186.
6. Morland J, et al, " Combined Effects of Diazepam and Ethanol on Psychomotor Functions," *Acta Pharmacol Toxicol*, 1975, 34:5.

OCCUPATIONAL EXPOSURE TO BLOODBORNE PATHOGENS (UNIVERSAL PRECAUTIONS)

OVERVIEW AND REGULATORY CONSIDERATIONS

Every healthcare employee, from nurse to housekeeper, has some (albeit small) risk of exposure to HIV and other viral agents such as hepatitis B and Jakob-Creutzfeldt agent. The incidence of HIV-1 transmission associated with a percutaneous exposure to blood from an HIV-1 infected patient is approximately 0.3% per exposure.[1]In 1989, it was estimated that 12,000 United States healthcare workers acquired hepatitis B annually.[2] An understanding of the appropriate procedures, responsibilities, and risks inherent in the collection and handling of patient specimens is necessary for safe practice and is required by Occupational Safety and Health Administration (OSHA) regulations.

The Occupational Safety and Health Administration published its "Final Rule on Occupational Exposure to Bloodborne Pathogens" in the Federal Register on December 6, 1991. OSHA has chosen to follow the Center for Disease Control (CDC) definition of universal precautions. The Final Rule provides full legal force to universal precautions and requires employers and employees to treat blood and certain body fluids as if they were infectious. The Final Rule mandates that healthcare workers must avoid parenteral contact and must avoid splattering blood or other potentially infectious material on their skin, hair, eyes, mouth, mucous membranes, or on their personal clothing. Hazard abatement strategies must be used to protect the workers. Such plans typically include, but are not limited to, the following:

- safe handling of sharp items ("sharps") and disposal of such into puncture resistant containers
- gloves required for employees handling items soiled with blood or equipment contaminated by blood or other body fluids
- provisions of protective clothing when more extensive contact with blood or body fluids may be anticipated (eg, surgery, autopsy, or deliveries)
- resuscitation equipment to reduce necessity for mouth to mouth resuscitation
- restriction of HIV- or hepatitis B-exposed employees to noninvasive procedures

OSHA has specifically defined the following terms: **Occupational exposure** means reasonably anticipated skin, eye mucous membrane, or parenteral contact with blood or other potentially infectious materials that may result from the performance of an employee's duties. **Other potentially infectious materials** are human body fluids including semen, vaginal secretions, cerebrospinal fluid, synovial fluid, pleural fluid, pericardial fluid, peritoneal fluid, amniotic fluid, saliva in dental procedures, and body fluids that are visibly contaminated with blood, and all body fluids in situations where it is difficult or impossible to differentiate between body fluids; any unfixed tissue or organ (other than intact skin) from a human (living or dead); and HIV-containing cell or tissue cultures, organ cultures, and HIV- or HBV-containing culture medium or other solutions, and blood, organs, or other tissues from experimental animals infected with HIV or HBV. An **exposure incident** involves specific eye, mouth, other mucous membrane, nonintact skin, or parenteral contact with blood or other potentially infectious materials that results from the performance of an employee's duties.[3] It is important to understand that some exposures may go unrecognized despite the strictest precautions.

A written Exposure Control Plan is required. Employers must provide copies of the plan to employees and to OSHA upon request. Compliance with OSHA rules may be accomplished by the following methods.

- **Universal precautions (UPs)** means that all human blood and certain body fluids are treated as if known to be infectious for HIV, HBV, and other bloodborne pathogens. UPs do not apply to feces, nasal secretions, saliva, sputum, sweat, tears, urine, or vomitus unless they contain visible blood.
- **Engineering controls (ECs)** are physical devices which reduce or remove hazards from the workplace by eliminating or minimizing hazards or by isolating the worker from exposure. Engineering control devices include sharps disposal containers, self-resheathing syringes, etc.
- **Work practice controls (WPCs)** are practices and procedures that reduce the likelihood of exposure to hazards by altering the way in which a task is performed. Specific examples are the prohibition of two-handed recapping of needles, prohibition of storing food alongside potentially contaminated material, discouragement of pipetting fluids by mouth, encouraging handwashing after removal of gloves, safe handling of contaminated sharps, and appropriate use of sharps containers.

- **Personal protective equipment (PPE)** is specialized clothing or equipment worn to provide protection from occupational exposure. PPE includes gloves, gowns, laboratory coats (the type and characteristics will depend upon the task and degree of exposure anticipated), face shields or masks, and eye protection. Surgical caps or hoods and/or shoe covers or boots are required in instances in which gross contamination can reasonably be anticipated (eg, autopsies, orthopedic surgery). If PPE is penetrated by blood or any contaminated material, the item must be removed immediately or as soon as feasible. **The employer must provide and launder or dispose of all PPE at no cost to the employee.** Gloves must be worn when there is a reasonable anticipation of hand contact with potentially infectious material, including a patient's mucous membranes or nonintact skin. Disposable gloves must be changed as soon as possible after they become torn or punctured. Hands must be washed after gloves are removed. OSHA has revised the PPE standards, effective July 5, 1994, to include the requirement that the employer certify in writing that it has conducted a hazard assessment of the workplace to determine whether hazards are present that will necessitate the use of PPE. Also, verification that the employee has received and understood the PPE training is required.[4]

Housekeeping protocols: OSHA requires that all bins, cans, and similar receptacles, intended for reuse which have a reasonable likelihood for becoming contaminated, be inspected and decontaminated immediately or as soon as feasible upon visible contamination and on a regularly scheduled basis. Broken glass that may be contaminated must not be picked up directly with the hands. Mechanical means (eg, brush, dust pan, tongs, or forceps) must be used. Broken glass must be placed in a proper sharps container.

Employers are responsible for teaching appropriate clean-up procedures for the work area and personal protective equipment. A 1:10 dilution of household bleach is a popular and effective disinfectant. It is prudent for employers to maintain signatures or initials of employees who have been properly educated. If one does not have written proof of education of universal precautions teaching, then by OSHA standards, such education never happened.

Pre-exposure and postexposure protocols: OSHA's Final Rule includes the provision that employees, who are exposed to contamination, be offered the hepatitis B vaccine at no cost to the employee. Employees may decline; however, a declination form must be signed. The employee must be offered free vaccine if he/she changes his/her mind. Vaccination to prevent the transmission of hepatitis B in the healthcare setting is widely regarded as sound practice.[5] In the event of exposure, a confidential medical evaluation and follow-up must be offered at no cost to the employee. Follow-up must include collection and testing of blood from the source individual for HBV and HIV if permitted by state law if a blood sample is available. If a postexposure specimen must be specially drawn, the individual's consent is usually required. Some states may not require consent for testing of patient blood after accidental exposure. One must refer to state and/or local guidelines for proper guidance.

The employee follow-up must also include appropriate postexposure prophylaxis, counseling, and evaluation of reported illnesses. The employee has the right to decline baseline blood collection and/or testing. If the employee gives consent for the collection but not the testing, the sample must be preserved for 90 days in the event that the employee changes his/her mind within that time. Confidentiality related to blood testing must be ensured. **The employer does not have the right to know the results** of the testing of either the source individual or the exposed employee.

The Management of Occupational Exposure to HIV in the Workplace[6]

1. Likelihood of transmission of HIV-1 from occupational exposure is 0.2% per parenteral exposure (eg, needlestick) to blood from HIV infected patients.
2. Factors that increase risk for occupational transmission include advanced stages of HIV in source patient, hollow bore needle puncture, a poor state of health or inexperience of healthcare worker (HCW).
3. Immediate actions an exposed healthcare worker should take include aggressive first aid at the puncture site (eg, scrubbing site with povidone-iodine solution for 10 minutes) or at mucus membrane site (eg, saline irrigation of eye for 15 minutes). Then immediate reporting to the hospital's occupational medical service. The authors indicate that there is no direct evidence for the efficacy of their recommendations. Other institutions suggest rigorous scrubbing with soap.

4. After first aid is initiated, the healthcare worker should report exposure to a supervisor and to the institution's occupational medical service for evaluation.

5. Occupational medicine should perform a thorough investigation including identifying the HIV and hepatitis B status of the source, type of exposure, volume of inoculum, timing of exposure, extent of injury, appropriateness of first aid, as well as psychological status of the healthcare worker. HIV serologies should be performed on the healthcare worker. HIV risk counselling should begin at this point.

6. All parenteral exposures should be treated equally until they can be evaluated by the occupational medicine service, who will then determine the actual risk of exposure. Follow-up counselling sessions may be necessary.

7. Although the data are not clear, antiviral prophylaxis may be offered to healthcare workers who are parenterally or mucous membrane exposed. If used, antiretroviral prophylaxis should be initiated within 1-2 hours after exposure.

8. Counselling regarding risk of exposure, antiviral prophylaxis, plans for follow up, exposure prevention, sexual activity, and providing emotional support and response to concerns are necessary to support the exposed healthcare worker. Follow-up should consist of periodic serologic evaluation and blood chemistries and counts if antiretroviral prophylaxis is initiated. Additional information should be provided to healthcare workers who are pregnant or planning to become pregnant.

HAZARDOUS COMMUNICATION

Communication regarding the dangers of bloodborne infections through the use of labels, signs, information, and education is required. Storage locations (eg, refrigerators and freezers, waste containers) that are used to store, dispose of, transport, or ship blood or other potentially infectious materials require labels. The label background must be red or bright orange with the biohazard design and the word biohazard in a contrasting color. The label must be part of the container or affixed to the container by permanent means.

Education provided by a qualified and knowledgeable instructor is mandated. The sessions for employees must include:

- accessible copies of the regulation
- general epidemiology of bloodborne diseases
- modes of bloodborne pathogen transmission
- an explanation of the exposure control plan and a means to obtain copies of the written plan
- an explanation of the tasks and activities that may involve exposure
- the use of exposure prevention methods and their limitations (eg, engineering controls, work practices, personal protective equipment)
- information on the types, proper use, location, removal, handling, decontamination, and disposal of personal protective equipment)
- an explanation of the basis for selection of personal protective equipment
- information on the HBV vaccine, including information on its efficacy, safety, and method of administration and the benefits of being vaccinated (ie, the employee must understand that the vaccine and vaccination will be offered free of charge)
- information on the appropriate actions to take and persons to contact in an emergency involving exposure to blood or other potentially infectious materials
- an explanation of the procedure to follow if an exposure incident occurs, including the method of reporting the incident
- information on the postexposure evaluation and follow-up that the employer is required to provide for the employee following an exposure incident
- an explanation of the signs, labels, and color coding
- an interactive question-and-answer period

RECORD KEEPING

The OSHA Final Rule requires that the employer maintain both education and medical records. The medical records must be kept confidential and be maintained for the duration of employment plus 30 years. They must contain a copy of the employee's HBV vaccination status and postexposure incident information. Education records must be maintained for 3 years from the date the program was given.

OSHA has the authority to conduct inspections without notice. Penalties for cited violation may be assessed as follows.

Serious violations. In this situation, there is a substantial probability of death or serious physical harm, and the employer knew, or should have known, of the hazard. A violation of this type carries a mandatory penalty of up to $7000 for each violation.

Other-than-serious violations. The violation is unlikely to result in death or serious physical harm. This type of violation carries a discretionary penalty of up to $7000 for each violation.

Willful violations. These are violations committed knowingly or intentionally by the employer and have penalties of up to $70,000 per violation with a minimum of $5000 per violation. If an employee dies as a result of a willful violation, the responsible party, if convicted, may receive a personal fine of up to $250,000 and/or a 6-month jail term. A corporation may be fined $500,000.

Large fines frequently follow visits to laboratories, physicians' offices, and healthcare facilities by OSHA Compliance Safety and Health Offices (CSHOS). Regulations are vigorously enforced. A working knowledge of the final rule and implementation of appropriate policies and practices is imperative for all those involved in the collection and analysis of medical specimens.

Effectiveness of universal precautions in averting exposure to potentially infectious materials has been documented.[7] Compliance with appropriate rules, procedures, and policies, including reporting exposure incidents, is a matter of personal professionalism and prudent self-preservation.

References

Buehler JW and Ward JW, "A New Definition for AIDS Surveillance," *Ann Intern Med*, 1993, 118(5):390-2.
Brown JW and Blackwell H, "Complying With the New OSHA Regs, Part 1: Teaching Your Staff About Biosafety," *MLO*, 1992, 24(4)24-8. Part 2: "Safety Protocols No Lab Can Ignore," 1992, 24(5):27-9. Part 3: "Compiling Employee Safety Records That Will Satisfy OSHA," 1992, 24(6):45-8.
Department of Labor, Occupational Safety and Health Administration, "Occupational Exposure to Bloodborne Pathogens; Final Rule (29 CFR Part 1910.1030), "*Federal Register*, December 6, 1991, 64004-182.
Gold JW, "HIV-1 Infection: Diagnosis and Management," *Med Clin North Am*, 1992, 76(1):1-18.
"Hepatitis B Virus: A Comprehensive Strategy for Eliminating Transmission in the United States Through Universal Childhood Vaccination," Recommendations of the Immunization Practices Advisory Committee (ACIP), *MMWR Morb Mortal Wkly Rep*, 1991, 40(RR-13):1-25.
"Mortality Attributable to HIV Infection/AIDS — United States", *MMWR Morb Mortal Wkly Rep*, 1991, 40(3):41-4.
National Committee for Clinical Laboratory Standards, "Protection of Laboratory Workers From Infectious Disease Transmitted by Blood, Body Fluids, and Tissue," NCCLS Document M29-T, Villanova, PA: NCCLS, 1989, 9(1).
"Nosocomial Transmission of Hepatitis B Virus Associated With a Spring-Loaded Fingerstick Device — California," *MMWR Morb Mortal Wkly Rep*, 1990, 39(35):610-3.
Polish LB, Shapiro CN, Bauer F, et al, "Nosocomial Transmission of Hepatitis B Virus Associated With the Use of a Spring-Loaded Fingerstick Device," *N Engl J Med*, 1992, 326(11):721-5.
"Recommendations for Preventing Transmission of Human Immunodeficiency Virus and Hepatitis B Virus to Patients During Exposure-Prone Invasive Procedures," *MMWR Morb Mortal Wkly Rep*, 1991, 40(RR-8):1-9.
"Update: Acquired Immunodeficiency Syndrome — United States," *MMWR Morb Mortal Wkly Rep*, 1992, 41(26):463-8.
"Update: Transmission of HIV Infection During an Invasive Dental Procedure — Florida," *MMWR Morb Mortal Wkly Rep*, 1991, 40(2):21-7, 33.
"Update: Universal Precautions for Prevention of Transmission of Human Immunodeficiency Virus, Hepatitis B Virus, and Other Bloodborne Pathogens in Healthcare Settings," *MMWR Morb Mortal Wkly Rep*, 1988, 37(24):377-82, 387-8.

Footnotes

1. Henderson DK, Fahey BJ, Willy M, et al, "Risk for Occupational Transmission of Human Immunodeficiency Virus Type 1 (HIV-1) Associated With Clinical Exposures. A Prospective Evaluation," *Ann Intern Med*, 1990, 113(10):740-6.
2. Niu MT and Margolis HS, "Moving Into a New Era of Government Regulation: Provisions for Hepatitis B Vaccine in the Workplace, *Clin Lab Manage Rev*, 1989, 3:336-40.
3. Bruning LM, "The Bloodborne Pathogens Final Rule — Understanding the Regulation," *AORN Journal*, 1993, 57(2):439-40.
4. "Rules and Regulations," *Federal Register*, 1994, 59(66):16360-3.
5. Schaffner W, Gardner P, and Gross PA, "Hepatitis B Immunization Strategies: Expanding the Target," *Ann Intern Med*, 1993, 118(4):308-9.
6. Fahey BJ, Beekmann SE, Schmitt JM, et al, "Managing Occupational Exposures to HIV-1 in the Healthcare Workplace," *Infect Control Hosp Epidemiol*, 1993, 14(7):405-12.
7. Wong ES, Stotka JL, Chinchilli VM, et al, "Are Universal Precautions Effective in Reducing the Number of Occupational Exposures Among Healthcare Workers?" *JAMA*, 1991, 265(9):1123-8.

Penicillins, Penicillin-Related Antibiotics & Other Antibiotics

KEY TO TABLE

- **A** Recommended drug therapy
- **B** Alternate drug therapy
- **C** Organism is usually or always sensitive to this agent
- **D** Organism portrays variable sensitivity to this agent
- (Blank) This drug should not be used for this organism or insufficient data is available

GRAM-POSITIVE AEROBES — Bacilli (first 3 organism columns) and Cocci (remaining columns)

Staphylococcus columns: S. epidermidis (Methicillin-Resistant / Methicillin-Susceptible); S. aureus (Methicillin-Resistant / Methicillin-Susceptible)

Class	Antibiotic	Listeria monocytogenes	Corynebacterium jeikeium	Corynebacterium sp.	Streptococcus, Viridans Group	Streptococcus pneumoniae	Enterococcus sp. (Group D)	Streptococcus bovis (Group D)	Streptococcus agalactiae (Group B)	Streptococcus pyogenes (Group A)	S. epidermidis: Methicillin-Resistant	S. epidermidis: Methicillin-Susceptible	S. aureus: Methicillin-Resistant	S. aureus: Methicillin-Susceptible
Penicillins	Amoxicillin				C	C	C		C	C				
Penicillins	Ampicillin	A			C	C	C	A	C	C				
Penicillins	Penicillin G	A	B	B	A	A	A	A	A	A				A
Penicillins	Penicillin V				C	C	C	C	C	C				C
Penicillins	Azlocillin													
Penicillins	Mezlocillin				D	C	D	D	C	C				
Penicillins	Piperacillin				D	C	D	C	C	C				
Penicillins	Ticarcillin				D	C	D		C	C				
Penicillins	Cloxacillin				D							A		A
Penicillins	Dicloxacillin				D							A		A
Penicillins	Methicillin				D							A		A
Penicillins	Nafcillin				D							A		A
Penicillins	Oxacillin				D							A		A
Penicillin-Related Antibiotics	Amoxicillin/Clavulanate	C			C	C	C	C	C	C		C		C
Penicillin-Related Antibiotics	Ampicillin/Sulbactam	C			C	C	C	C	C	C		C		C
Penicillin-Related Antibiotics	Ticarcillin/Clavulanate				C	C	C	D	C	C		C		C
Penicillin-Related Antibiotics	Aztreonam													
Penicillin-Related Antibiotics	Imipenem/Cilastatin				C	C	C	D	C	C		C		C
Penicillin-Related Antibiotics	Piperacillin/Tazobactam				C	C	C	C	C	C		C		C
Other Antibiotics	Chloramphenicol	C				B		D						
Other Antibiotics	Clindamycin			D	D	C	D		C	C		B		B
Other Antibiotics	Co-trimoxazole	B				C					B	C	B	C
Other Antibiotics	Metronidazole													
Other Antibiotics	Rifampin			D							A	C	A	C
Other Antibiotics	Sulfonamides													
Other Antibiotics	Tetracyclines	C			C	C			C				A	D
Other Antibiotics	Vancomycin	D	A		B	B	B	B	B	B	A	B	A	B
UTI Agents	Indanyl Carbenicillin						D							
UTI Agents	Nitrofurantoin						D							

Penicillins, Penicillin-Related Antibiotics & Other Antibiotics

KEY TO TABLE

- **A** Recommended drug therapy
- **B** Alternate drug therapy
- **C** Organism is usually or always sensitive to this agent
- **D** Organism portrays variable sensitivity to this agent
- (Blank) This drug should not be used for this organism or insufficient data is available

GRAM-NEGATIVE AEROBES

Class	Drug	Yersinia enterocolitica	Shigella sp.	Serratia sp.	Salmonella sp.	Providencia sp.	Proteus sp.	Proteus mirabilis	Klebsiella pneumoniae	Escherichia coli	Enterobacter sp.[1]	Citrobacter sp.[1]	Neisseria meningitidis	Neisseria gonorrhoeae	Moraxella (Branhamella) catarrhalis
Penicillin	Amoxicillin				B			A		C			C	D	
	Ampicillin		A		B			A		A			C	D	
	Penicillin G												A	D	
	Penicillin V													D	
	Azlocillin														
	Mezlocillin			A		B	B	C	B	C	A	A		D	
	Piperacillin			A		B	B	C	B	C	A	A		D	
	Ticarcillin			A		B	B	C	D	C	A	A		D	
	Cloxacillin														
	Dicloxacillin														
	Methicillin														
	Nafcillin														
	Oxacillin														
Penicillin-Related Antibiotics	Amoxicillin/Clavulanate				C			C	C	C			C	C	A
	Ampicillin/Sulbactam		C		C			C	C	C			C	C	C
	Ticarcillin/Clavulanate	C	A	C	B	C	B	C	B	C	A	A	C	C	C
	Aztreonam	C	B	C	C	C	C	C	B	C	A	C		C	C
	Imipenem/Cilastatin	B	B	C	B	B	C	B	C	B	B	D		C	C
	Piperacillin/Tazobactam	C	A	C	B	C	B	C	B	C	A	A	C	C	C
Other Antibiotics	Chloramphenicol	C			B						C		B		
	Clindamycin														
	Co-trimoxazole	C	A	C	B	A	C	B	C	A	C	C			A
	Metronidazole														
	Rifampin												D		
	Sulfonamides			C		C			C	C	C		D		
	Tetracyclines	C	C				C	C		D			C	B	C
	Vancomycin														
UTI Agents	Indanyl Carbenicillin			C		C	C	C	C	C	C	C			
	Nitrofurantoin								C	C	C	C			

[1] *Citrobacter freundii, Citrobacter diversus, Enterobacter cloacae* and *Enterobacter aerogenes* often have significantly different antibiotic sensitivity patterns. Speciation and susceptibility testing are particularly important

Penicillins, Penicillin-Related Antibiotics & Other Antibiotics

KEY TO TABLE

- **A** Recommended drug therapy
- **B** Alternate drug therapy
- **C** Organism is usually or always sensitive to this agent
- **D** Organism portrays variable sensitivity to this agent
- (Blank) This drug should not be used for this organism or insufficient data is available

GRAM-NEGATIVE AEROBES — Other bacilli

Class	Drug	Vibrio cholerae	Xanthomonas maltophilia	Pseudomonas aeruginosa	Pasteurella multocida	Legionella pneumophila	Haemophilus influenzae	Haemophilus ducreyi	Gardnerella vaginalis	Francisella tularensis	Campylobacter jejuni	Brucella sp.	Bordetella pertussis	Alcaligenes	Acinetobacter sp.
Penicillin	Amoxicillin				C		B		C						
Penicillin	Ampicillin				C		B		B		D				
Penicillin	Penicillin G				A										
Penicillin	Penicillin V				C										
Penicillin	Azlocillin														
Penicillin	Mezlocillin			A	C		D								A
Penicillin	Piperacillin			A	C		D								A
Penicillin	Ticarcillin			A	C		D								A
Penicillin	Cloxacillin														
Penicillin	Dicloxacillin														
Penicillin	Methicillin														
Penicillin	Nafcillin														
Penicillin	Oxacillin														
Penicillin-Related Antibiotics	Amoxicillin/Clavulanate				B		B	B	C						C
Penicillin-Related Antibiotics	Ampicillin/Sulbactam				B		C	C	C						C
Penicillin-Related Antibiotics	Ticarcillin/Clavulanate		B	A	C		C								A
Penicillin-Related Antibiotics	Aztreonam			C			C								B
Penicillin-Related Antibiotics	Imipenem/Cilastatin			A			C								B
Penicillin-Related Antibiotics	Piperacillin/Tazobactam			A	C		C								A
Other Antibiotics	Chloramphenicol		C		C		B				A	C	C		
Other Antibiotics	Clindamycin								C		C				
Other Antibiotics	Co-trimoxazole	A	A				A	B					B	A	
Other Antibiotics	Metronidazole								A						
Other Antibiotics	Rifampin					A	D					D	A		
Other Antibiotics	Sulfonamides				C			C				C			
Other Antibiotics	Tetracyclines	A			C		C	C				B	A	C	
Other Antibiotics	Vancomycin														
UTI Agents	Indanyl Carbenicillin			D											C
UTI Agents	Nitrofurantoin														

Penicillins, Penicillin-Related Antibiotics & Other Antibiotics

KEY TO TABLE

A — Recommended drug therapy

B — Alternate drug therapy

C — Organism is usually or always sensitive to this agent

D — Organism portrays variable sensitivity to this agent

(Blank) This drug should not be used for this organism or insufficient data is available

		OTHERS									ANAEROBES			
											Gram -		Gram +	
	Drug	Treponema pallidum	Leptospira sp.	Borrelia burgdorferi (Lyme disease)	Rickettsia sp.	Ureaplasma urealyticum	Mycoplasma pneumoniae	Chlamydia trachomatis	Chlamydia pneumoniae (TWAR)	Chlamydia psittaci	Bacteroides sp.	Streptococcus, anaerobic	Clostridium perfringens	Clostridium difficile [2]
Penicillin	Amoxicillin			B							D	C	D	
	Ampicillin			B							C	C	D	
	Penicillin G	A	A	B							C	A	A	
	Penicillin V	C	C	B							C	C	C	
	Azlocillin													
	Mezlocillin										C	C	C	
	Piperacillin										C	C	C	
	Ticarcillin										C	C	C	
	Cloxacillin													
	Dicloxacillin													
	Methicillin													
	Nafcillin													
	Oxacillin													
Penicillin-Related Antibiotics	Amoxicillin/Clavulanate										C	C	C	
	Ampicillin/Sulbactam										C	C	C	
	Ticarcillin/Clavulanate										C	C	C	
	Aztreonam													
	Imipenem/Cilastatin										C	C	B	
	Piperacillin/Tazobactam										C	C	C	
Other Antibiotics	Chloramphenicol				A						C	C	C	D
	Clindamycin										A	B	B	
	Co-trimoxazole													
	Metronidazole										A	D	A	A
	Rifampin													
	Sulfonamides							D						
	Tetracyclines	B	B	A	A	A	A	A	B	B	D	C	C	
	Vancomycin											B		B
UTI Agents	Indanyl Carbenicillin													
	Nitrofurantoin													

[2] Vancomycin is effective orally only.

Cephalosporins, Aminoglycosides, Macrolides & Quinolones

KEY TO TABLE

- **A** Recommended drug therapy
- **B** Alternate drug therapy
- **C** Organism is usually or always sensitive to this agent
- **D** Organism portrays variable sensitivity to this agent
- (Blank) This drug should not be used for this organism or insufficient data is available

GRAM-POSITIVE AEROBES

Generation	Drug	Listeria monocytogenes	Corynebacterium jeikeium	Corynebacterium sp.	Streptococcus, Viridans Group	Streptococcus pneumoniae	Streptococcus bovis (Group D)	Enterococcus sp. (Group D)	Streptococcus agalactiae (Group B)	Streptococcus pyogenes (Group A)	Staphylococcus epidermidis: Methicillin-Susceptible	Staphylococcus epidermidis: Methicillin-Resistant	Staphylococcus aureus: Methicillin-Susceptible	Staphylococcus aureus: Methicillin-Resistant
1st Generation	Cefadroxil				B	B	C		B	B	B		B	
1st Generation	Cefazolin				B	B	C		B	B	B		B	
1st Generation	Cephalexin				B	B	C		B	B	B		B	
1st Generation	Cephalothin				B	B	C		B	B	B		B	
1st Generation	Cephapirin				B	B	C		B	B	B		B	
1st Generation	Cephradine				B	B	C		B	B	B		B	
2nd Generation and others	Cefaclor				C	C	C		C	C	D		D	
2nd Generation and others	Cefamandole				C	C	C		C	C	C		C	
2nd Generation and others	Cefmetazole				C	C	C		C	C	D		D	
2nd Generation and others	Cefonicid				C	C	C		C	C	D		D	
2nd Generation and others	Cefotetan				C	C	C		C	C	D		D	
2nd Generation and others	Cefoxitin				C	C	C		C	C	D		D	
2nd Generation and others	Cefpodoxime Proxetil				C	C	C		C	C	D		D	
2nd Generation and others	Cefprozil				C	C	D		C	C			D	
2nd Generation and others	Cefuroxime				C	C	C		C	C	D		D	
2nd Generation and others	Cefuroxime Axetil				C	C			C	C	C		C	
2nd Generation and others	Loracarbef				C	C	D		C	C	C		C	
3rd Generation	Cefixime				D	D			C	C				
3rd Generation	Cefoperazone				D	D	C		C	C	D		D	
3rd Generation	Cefotaxime				D	D	C		C	C	D		D	
3rd Generation	Ceftazidime				D				D		D		D	
3rd Generation	Ceftizoxime				D	D	C		C	C	D		D	
3rd Generation	Ceftriaxone				C	C	C		C	C	D		D	
Aminoglycosides	Amikacin	C	C					D	D					
Aminoglycosides	Gentamicin	A	B		A			D	A		A	D	A	D
Aminoglycosides	Netilmicin	C	C					C						
Aminoglycosides	Streptomycin							D	C					
Aminoglycosides	Tobramycin	C	C					D						D
Macrolides	Azithromycin	C			C	C			C	C				C
Macrolides	Clarithromycin	C			C	C			C	C				C
Macrolides	Erythromycin	C	C	A	C	B			B	B				C
Quinolones	Lomefloxacin		D		D	D	D	D	D	D	D	D	D	D
Quinolones	Ciprofloxacin		D		D	D	D	D	D	D	D	D	D	D
Quinolones	Norfloxacin							D	D					
Quinolones	Ofloxacin		D		D	D	D	D	D	D	D	D	D	D

Cephalosporins, Aminoglycosides, Macrolides & Quinolones

KEY TO TABLE

- **A** Recommended drug therapy
- **B** Alternate drug therapy
- **C** Organism is usually or always sensitive to this agent
- **D** Organism portrays variable sensitivity to this agent
- (Blank) This drug should not be used for this organism or insufficient data is available

GRAM-NEGATIVE AEROBES — Enteric bacilli and Cocci

Class	Drug	Yersinia enterocolitica	Shigella sp.	Serratia sp.	Salmonella sp.	Providencia sp.	Proteus mirabilis	Klebsiella pneumoniae	Escherichia coli	Enterobacter sp.[1]	Citrobacter sp.[1]	Neisseria meningitidis	Neisseria gonorrhoeae	Moraxella (Branhamella) catarrhalis
1st Generation	Cefadroxil						A	A	B					D
1st Generation	Cefazolin						A	A	B					D
1st Generation	Cephalexin						A	A	B					D
1st Generation	Cephalothin						A	A	B					D
1st Generation	Cephapirin						A	A	B					D
1st Generation	Cephradine						A	A	B					D
2nd Generation and others	Cefaclor						C	A	B				C	B
2nd Generation and others	Cefamandole					D	C	A	B				C	B
2nd Generation and others	Cefmetazole	D	C	C	C	D	C	A	B				C	B
2nd Generation and others	Cefonicid						C	A	B				C	B
2nd Generation and others	Cefotetan	C	C	C	C	D	C	A	B				C	B
2nd Generation and others	Cefoxitin			D	C	D	C	A	B				C	B
2nd Generation and others	Cefpodoxime Proxetil						C	A	B				C	B
2nd Generation and others	Cefprozil		C				C	D	B				C	B
2nd Generation and others	Ceftibuten													
2nd Generation and others	Cefuroxime	C	C			D	C	A	B				C	B
2nd Generation and others	Cefuroxime Axetil						C	A	B			C	C	B
2nd Generation and others	Loracarbef						C	C	B				C	B
3rd Generation	Cefepime					A								
3rd Generation	Cefixime		C	C			C	C	A	A			C	B
3rd Generation	Cefoperazone		B	A	A	A	A	C	A	A	A			B
3rd Generation	Cefotaxime	A	B	A	A	A	A	C	A	A	A	B	C	B
3rd Generation	Ceftazidime		B	A		A	A	C	A	A	A			B
3rd Generation	Ceftizoxime	A	B	A	A	A	A	C	A	A	A	B	C	B
3rd Generation	Ceftriaxone	A	B	A	A	A	A	C	A	A	A	B	A	B
Aminoglycosides	Amikacin	A		C		C	C	C	C	C	C			
Aminoglycosides	Gentamicin	A	D	C	D	D	C	C	C	C	C			
Aminoglycosides	Netilmicin	A	D	C	D	D	C	C	C	C	C			
Aminoglycosides	Streptomycin				D									
Aminoglycosides	Tobramycin	A		C	D	D	C	C	C	C	C			
Macrolides	Azithromycin											C	C	
Macrolides	Clarithromycin											C	C	
Macrolides	Dirithromycin													
Macrolides	Erythromycin												D	C
Quinolones	Lomefloxacin	C	C	C	C	C	C	C	C	C	D	C	C	C
Quinolones	Ciprofloxacin	C	B	C	B	C	C	C	C	C	C	C	A	C
Quinolones	Norfloxacin	C	C	C	C	C	C	C	C	C	C		C	
Quinolones	Ofloxacin	C	C	C	C	C	C	C	C	C	C	C	A	C

[1] *Citrobacter freundii, Citrobacter diversus, Enterobacter cloacae* and *Enterobacter aerogenes* often have significantly different antibiotic sensitivity patterns. Speciation and susceptibility testing are particularly important

INFECTIOUS DISEASE - ANTIMICROBIAL ACTIVITY AGAINST SELECTED ORGANISMS

Cephalosporins, Aminoglycosides, Macrolides & Quinolones

KEY TO TABLE

A — Recommended drug therapy

B — Alternate drug therapy

C — Organism is usually or always sensitive to this agent

D — Organism portrays variable sensitivity to this agent

(Blank) This drug should not be used for this organism or insufficient data is available

	GRAM-NEGATIVE AEROBES — Other bacilli											
	Vibrio cholerae	Xanthomonas maltophilia	Pseudomonas aeruginosa	Pasteurella multocida	Legionella pneumophila	Haemophilus ducreyi	Haemophilus influenzae	Campylobacter jejuni	Gardnerella vaginalis	Brucella sp.	Bordetella pertussis	Acinetobacter sp.
1st Generation												
Cefadroxil							D					
Cefazolin							D					
Cephalexin							D					
Cephalothin							D					
Cephapirin							D					
Cephradine							D					
2nd Generation and others												
Cefaclor							B					
Cefamandole			C				B					
Cefmetazole				D			C					
Cefonicid							C					
Cefotetan				D			C					
Cefoxitin				D			C					
Cefpodoxime Proxetil							B					
Cefprozil							B					
Cefuroxime							B					
Cefuroxime Axetil				D			B					
Loracarbef							B					
3rd Generation												
Cefixime							A					D
Cefoperazone		D	D	C			A	C				D
Cefotaxime		D	C				C					A
Ceftazidime		D	A				C					A
Ceftizoxime		D	C				C					A
Ceftriaxone		D	C				A					A
Aminoglycosides												
Amikacin		C	A				C		C			C
Gentamicin		C	A				C		C	C		C
Netilmicin		C	A				C		C			C
Streptomycin										C		
Tobramycin		C	A				C		C			C
Macrolides												
Azithromycin				D	B	C	C		C		C	
Clarithromycin				D	B	C			C		C	
Erythromycin				D	A			C	A		A	
Quinolones												
Lomefloxacin	C	C	D	C		C	C	D	B	C		D
Ciprofloxacin	C	B	A	C	B	C	B	C	B	C		C
Norfloxacin			C						B			D
Ofloxacin	C	B	D	C	C	C	C	C	B	C		C

Cephalosporins, Aminoglycosides, Macrolides & Quinolones

KEY TO TABLE

A Recommended drug therapy

B Alternate drug therapy

C Organism is usually or always sensitive to this agent

D Organism portrays variable sensitivity to this agent

(Blank) This drug should not be used for this organism or insufficient data is available

		OTHERS									ANAEROBES			
											Gram -	Gram +		
		Treponema pallidum	Leptospira sp.	Borrelia burgdorferi (Lyme disease)	Rickettsia sp.	Ureaplasma urealyticum	Mycoplasma pneumoniae	Chlamydia trachomatis	Chlamydia pneumoniae (TWAR)	Chlamydia psittaci	Bacteroides sp.	Streptococcus, anaerobic	Clostridium difficile [2]	Clostridium perfringens
1st Generation	Cefadroxil											B		
	Cefazolin											B		
	Cephalexin											B		
	Cephalothin											B		
	Cephapirin											B		
	Cephradine											B		
2nd Generation and others	Cefaclor													
	Cefamandole													
	Cefmetazole										C	C		C
	Cefonicid													
	Cefotetan										B	C		C
	Cefoxitin										B	C		C
	Cefpodoxime Proxetil													
	Cefprozil													
	Cefuroxime											C		C
	Cefuroxime Axetil													
	Loracarbef													
3rd Generation	Cefixime													
	Cefoperazone													D
	Cefotaxime			C							D	C		C
	Ceftazidime													D
	Ceftizoxime			C							D	C		C
	Ceftriaxone	C		A								C		
Aminoglycosides	Amikacin													
	Gentamicin													
	Netilmicin													
	Streptomycin													
	Tobramycin													
Macrolides	Azithromycin	D		C			B	C	C	C		D		D
	Clarithromycin	D		D			B	C	C	C		D		D
	Erythromycin	D		C			A	A	A	A		D		D
Quinolones	Lomefloxacin					D	D	D						
	Ciprofloxacin				D	D	D	D						
	Norfloxacin													
	Ofloxacin					D	D	D	C					

[2] Vancomycin is effective orally only.

ANTIMICROBIAL PROPHYLAXIS IN SURGICAL PATIENTS

Nature of Operation	Likely Pathogens	Recommended Drugs	Adult Dosage Before Surgery*
CLEAN			
Cardiac			
Prosthetic valve and other open-heart surgery	S. epidermidis, S. aureus, Corynebacterium, enteric gram-negative bacilli	Cefazolin **or** vancomycin‡	1 g I.V.
Vascular			
Arterial surgery involving the abdominal aorta, a prosthesis, or a groin incision	S. aureus, S. epidermidis, enteric gram-negative bacilli	Cefazolin **or** vancomycin‡	1 g I.V.
Lower extremity amputation for ischemia	S. aureus, S. epidermidis, enteric gram-negative bacilli, clostridia	Cefazolin **or** vancomycin‡	1 g I.V.
Neurosurgery			
Craniotomy	S. aureus, S. epidermidis	Cefazolin **or** vancomycin‡	1 g I.V.
Orthopedic			
Total joint replacement, internal fixation of fractures	S. aureus, S. epidermidis	Cefazolin **or** vancomycin‡	1 g I.V.
Ocular§	S. aureus, S. epidermidis, streptococci, enteric gram-negative bacilli, Pseudomonas	Gentamicin **or** tobramycin **or** combination of neomycin, gramicidin, and polymyxin B,	Multiple drops topically over 2-24 h
		cefazolin	100 mg subconjunctivally at end of procedure
CLEAN-CONTAMINATED			
Head and neck			
Entering oral cavity or pharynx	S. aureus, streptococci, oral anaerobes	Cefazolin **or**	2 g I.V.¶
		clindamycin	600 mg I.V.
Gastroduodenal			
High risk, gastric bypass, or percutaneous endoscopic gastrostomy only	Enteric gram-negative bacilli, gram-positive cocci	Cefazolin	1 g I.V.
Biliary tract			
High risk only	Enteric gram-negative bacilli, enterococci, clostridia	Cefazolin	1 g I.V.
Colorectal	Enteric gram-negative bacilli, anaerobes	Oral:	
		Neomycin plus erythromycin base	1 g of each at 1 PM, 2 PM, and 11 PM the day before the operation#
		Parenteral: Cefoxitin **or**	1 g I.V.¶
		cefotetan	1 g I.V.
Appendectomy	Enteric gram-negative bacilli, anaerobes	Cefoxitin **or**	1 g I.V.¶
		cefotetan	1 g I.V.
Vaginal or abdominal hysterectomy	Enteric gram-negative bacilli, anaerobes, group B streptococci, enterococci	Cefazolin **or** Cefoxitin **or**	1 g I.V.¶
		cefotetan	1 g I.V.
Cesarean section	Same as for hysterectomy	High risk only: Cefazolin	1 g I.V. after cord clamping
Abortion	Same as for hysterectomy	First trimester in patients with previous pelvic inflammatory disease:	

(continued)

Nature of Operation	Likely Pathogens	Recommended Drugs	Adult Dosage Before Surgery*
		Aqueous penicillin G **or**	1 million units I.V.
		doxycycline	100 mg P.O. 1 hour before abortion, then 200 mg P.O. 30 minutes after abortion
		Second trimester: Cefazolin	1 g I.V.
DIRTY			
Ruptured viscus	Enteric gram-negative bacilli, anaerobes, enterococci	Cefoxitin **or** clindamycin plus gentamicin	1 g I.V.
		cefotetan with or without gentamicin **or**	1 g I.V. 1.5 mg/kg q8h I.V.
		clindamycin plus gentamicin	600 mg I.V. q6h 1.5 mg/kg q8h I.V.
Traumatic wound•	*S. aureus*, group A streptococci, clostridia	Cefazolin	1 g q8h I.V.

*Parenteral prophylactic antimicrobials for clean and clean-contaminated surgery can be given as a single intravenous dose just before the operation. Cefazolin can also be given intramuscularly. For prolonged operations, additional intraoperative doses should be given every 4-8 hours for the duration of the procedure. For "dirty" surgery, therapy should usually be continued for 5-10 days.

‡For hospitals in which methicillin-resistant *S. aureus* and *S. epidermidis* frequently cause wound infection, or for patients allergic to penicillins or cephalosporin.

§In addition, at the end of the operation many ophthalmologists give a subconjunctival injection of an aminoglycoside such as gentamicin (10-20 mg), with or without a cephalosporin such as cefazolin (100 mg).

¶In controlled studies, 2 g were effective, while 0.5 g was not (JT Johnson and VL Yu, *Ann Surg*, 1988, 207:108).

#After appropriate diet and catharsis.

•For bite wounds, in which likely pathogens may also include oral anaerobes, *Eikenella corrodens* (humans), and *Pasteurella multocida* (dog and cat), some *Medical Letter* consultants recommend use of amoxicillin-clavulanic acid (Augmentin®) or ampicillin/sulbactam (Unasyn®).

ORGANISMS ISOLATED IN HEAD & NECK INFECTIONS

Organisms	Percentage Infections
Alpha hemolytic streptococci	41
Staphylococci aureas	27
Staphylococci epidermidis	23
Bacteroides sp	17
Streptococcus intermedius	7
Klebsiella pneumoniae	7
Beta hemolytic streptococci	7
Non A, Non B, Non D	7
Group A	7
Group B	5
Peptostreptococcus sp	6
Fungi	6
Mycobacteria tuberculosis	6
Actinobacter	5
Other anaerobic gram-negative rods	5
Proteus	3
Enterobacter	3
Anaerobic gram-negative cocci	3
Neisseria	3
Bacillus sp	3
Actinomyces	3
Other *Klebsiella* sp	3
Streptococcus pneumoniae	3
Bifidobacterium	3
Microaerophilic streptococci	3
Propionibacterium sp	3
Pseudomonas	1
Escherichia coli	1

PREDOMINANT CULTIVABLE MICROORGANISMS OF THE ORAL CAVITY

Type	Predominant Genus or Family
Aerobic or Facultative	
Gram-positive cocci	*Streptococcus* sp
	S. mutans
	S. sanguis
	S. mitior
	S. salivarius
Gram-positive rods	*Lactobacillus* sp
	Corynebacterium sp
Gram-negative cocci	*Moraxella* sp
Gram-negative rods	*Enterobacteriaceae* sp
Anaerobic	
Gram-positive cocci	*Peptostreptococcus* sp
Gram-positive rods	*Actinomyces* sp
	Eubacterium sp
	Lactobacillus sp
	Leptotrichia sp
Gram-negative cocci	*Veillonella* sp
Gram-negative rods	*Actinobacillus* sp
	Fusobacterium sp
	Prevotella sp
	Porphyromonas sp
	Bacteroides sp
	Campylobacter sp
Spirochetes	*Treponema* sp
Fungi	*Candida* sp

REFERENCE VALUES FOR ADULTS
Automated Chemistry (CHEMISTRY A)

Test	Values	Remarks
SERUM PLASMA		
Acetone	Negative	
Albumin	3.2-5 g/dL	
Alcohol, ethyl	Negative	
Aldolase	1.2-7.6 IU/L	
Ammonia	20-70 mcg/dL	Specimen to be placed on ice as soon as collected
Amylase	30-110 units/L	
Bilirubin, direct	0-0.3 mg/dL	
Bilirubin, total	0.1-1.2 mg/dL	
Calcium	8.6-10.3 mg/dL	
Calcium, ionized	2.24-2.46 mEq/L	
Chloride	95-108 mEq/L	
Cholesterol, total	≤220 mg/dL	Fasted blood required – normal value affected by dietary habits. This reference range is for a general adult population
HDL cholesterol	40-60 mg/dL	Fasted blood required – normal value affected by dietary habits
LDL cholesterol	65-170 mg/dL	LDLC calculated by Friewald formula... which has certain inaccuracies and is invalid at trig levels >300 mg/dL
CO_2	23-30 mEq/L	
Creatine kinase (CK) isoenzymes		
CK-BB	0%	
CK-MB	0%-3.9%	
CK-MM	96%-100%	

CK-MB levels must be both ≥4% and 10 IU/L to meet diagnostic criteria for CK-MB positive result consistent with myocardial injury.

Test	Values	Remarks
Creatine phosphokinase (CPK)	8-150 IU/L	
Creatinine	0.5-1.4 mg/dL	
Ferritin	13-300 ng/mL	
Folate	3.6-20 ng/dL	
GGT (gamma-glutamyltranspeptidase)		
male	11-63 IU/L	
female	8-35 IU/L	
GLDH	To be determined	
Glucose (2-h postprandial)	Up to 140 mg/dL	
Glucose, fasting	60-110 mg/dL	
Glucose, nonfasting (2-h postprandial)	60-140 mg/dL	
Hemoglobin A_{1c}	8	
Hemoglobin, plasma free	<2.5 mg/100 mL	
Hemoglobin, total glycosolated (Hb A_1)	4%-8%	
Iron	65-150 mcg/dL	
Iron binding capacity, total (TIBC)	250-420 mcg/dL	
Lactic acid	0.7-2.1 mEq/L	Specimen to be kept on ice and sent to lab as soon as possible
Lactate dehydrogenase (LDH)	56-194 IU/L	
Lactate dehydrogenase (LDH) isoenzymes		
LD_1	20%-34%	
LD_2	29%-41%	
LD_3	15%-25%	
LD_4	1%-12%	

(continued)

Test	Values	Remarks
LD₅	1%-15%	

Flipped LD₁/LD₂ ratios (>1 may be consistent with myocardial injury) particularly when considered in combination with a recent CK-MB positive result

Test	Values	Remarks
Lipase	23-208 units/L	
Magnesium	1.6-2.5 mg/dL	Increased by slight hemolysis
Osmolality	289-308 mOsm/kg	
Phosphatase, alkaline		
adults 25-60 y	33-131 IU/L	
adults 61 y or older	51-153 IU/L	
infancy-adolescence	Values range up to 3-5 times higher than adults	
Phosphate, inorganic	2.8-4.2 mg/dL	
Potassium	3.5-5.2 mEq/L	Increased by slight hemolysis
Prealbumin	>15 mg/dL	
Protein, total	6.5-7.9 g/dL	
SGOT (AST)	<35 IU/L	
SGPT (ALT)	<35 IU/L	
Sodium	134-149 mEq/L	
Transferrin	>200 mg/dL	
Triglycerides	45-155 mg/dL	Fasted blood required
Urea nitrogen (BUN)	7-20 mg/dL	
Uric acid		
male	2.0-8.0 mg/dL	
female	2.0-7.5 mg/dL	

CEREBROSPINAL FLUID

Test	Values	Remarks
Glucose	50-70 mg/dL	
Protein		
adults and children	15-45 mg/dL	CSF obtained by lumbar puncture
newborn infants	60-90 mg/dL	

On CSF obtained by cisternal puncture: About 25 mg/dL
On CSF obtained by ventricular puncture: About 10 mg/dL
Note: Bloody specimen gives erroneously high value due to contamination with blood proteins

URINE
(24-hour specimen is required for all these tests unless specified)

Test	Values	Remarks
Amylase	32-641 units/L	The value is in units/L and **not** calculated for total volume
Amylase, fluid (random samples)		Interpretation of value left for physician, depends on the nature of fluid
Calcium	Depends upon dietary intake	
Creatine		
male	150 mg/24 h	Higher value on children and during pregnancy
female	250 mg/24 h	
Creatinine	1000-2000 mg/24 h	
Creatinine clearance (endogenous)		
male	85-125 mL/min	A blood sample must accompany urine specimen
female	75-115 mL/min	
Glucose	1 g/24 h	
5-hydroxyindoleacetic acid	2-8 mg/24 h	
Iron	0.15 mg/24 h	Acid washed container required
Magnesium	146-209 mg/24 h	
Osmolality	500-800 mOsm/kg	With normal fluid intake
Oxalate	10-40 mg/24 h	
Phosphate	400-1300 mg/24 h	

Test	Values	Remarks
Potassium	25-120 mEq/24 h	Varies with diet; the interpretation of urine electrolytes and osmolality should be left for the physician
Sodium	40-220 mEq/24 h	
Porphobilinogen, qualitative	Negative	
Porphyrins, qualitative	Negative	
Proteins	0.05-0.1 g/24 h	
Salicylate	Negative	
Urea clearance	60-95 mL/min	A blood sample must accompany specimen
Urea N	10-40 g/24 h	Dependent on protein intake
Uric acid	250-750 mg/24 h	Dependent on diet and therapy
Urobilinogen	0.5-3.5 mg/24 h	For qualitative determination on random urine, send sample to urinalysis section in Hematology Lab
Xylose absorption test		
children	16%-33% of ingested xylose	
adults	>4 g in 5 h	

FECES

Fat, 3-day collection	<5 g/d	Value depends on fat intake of 100 g/d for 3 days preceding and during collection

GASTRIC ACIDITY

Acidity, total, 12 h	10-60 mEq/L	Titrated at pH 7

BLOOD GASES

	Arterial	Capillary	Venous
pH	7.35-7.45	7.35-7.45	7.32-7.42
pCO_2 (mm Hg)	35-45	35-45	38-52
pO_2 (mm Hg)	70-100	60-80	24-48
HCO_3 (mEq/L)	19-25	19-25	19-25
TCO_2 (mEq/L)	19-29	19-29	23-33
O_2 saturation (%)	90-95	90-95	40-70
Base excess (mEq/L)	-5 to +5	-5 to +5	-5 to +5

Complete Blood Count

	Hgb (g/dL)	Hct (%)	MCV (fL)	MCH (pg)	MCHC (%)	RBC (x 10^6/mm^3)	RDW	Plts (x 10^3/mm^3)
0-3 d	15-20	45-61	95-115	31-37	29-37	4-5.9	<18	250-450
1-2 wk	12.5-18.5	39-57	86-110	28-36	28-38	3.6-5.5	<17	250-450
1-6 mo	10-13	29-42	74-96	25-35	30-36	3.1-4.3	<16.5	300-700
7 mo - 2 y	10.5-13	33-38	70-84	23-30	31-37	3.7-4.9	<16	250-600
2-5 y	11.5-13	34-39	75-87	24-30	31-37	3.9-5	<15	250-550
5-8 y	11.5-14.5	35-42	77-95	25-33	31-37	4-4.9	<15	250-550
13-18 y	12-15.2	36-47	78-96	25-35	31-37	4.5-5.1	<14.5	150-450
Adult male	13.5-16.5	41-50	80-100	26-34	31-37	4.5-5.5	<14.5	150-450
Adult female	12-15	36-44	80-100	26-34	31-37	4-4.9	<14.5	150-450

WBC and Diff

	WBC (x 10^3/mm^3)	Segmented Neutrophils	Band Neutrophils	Eosinophils	Basophils	Lymphocytes	Atypical Lymphs	Monocytes	# of NRBCs
0-3 d	9-35	32-62	10-18	0-2	0-1	19-29	0-8	5-7	0-2
1-2 wk	5-20	14-34	6-14	0-2	0-1	36-45	0-8	6-10	0
1-6 mo	6-17.5	13-33	4-12	0-3	0-1	41-71	0-8	4-7	0
7 mo - 2 y	6-17	15-35	5-11	0-3	0-1	45-76	0-8	3-6	0
2-5 y	5.5-15.5	23-45	5-11	0-3	0-1	45-76	0-8	3-6	0
5-8 y	5-14.5	32-54	5-11	0-3	0-1	28-48	0-8	3-6	0
13-18 y	4.5-13	34-64	5-11	0-3	0-1	25-45	0-8	3-6	0
Adults	4.5-11	35-66	5-11	0-3	0-1	24-44	0-8	3-6	0

Sedimentation Rate, Westergren
Children: 0-20 mm/hour
Adult male: 0-15 mm/hour
Adult female: 0-20 mm/hour

Sedimentation Rate, Wintrobe
Children: 0-13 mm/hour
Adult male: 0-10 mm/hour
Adult female: 0-15 mm/hour

Reticulocyte Count
Newborns: 2%-6%
1-6 mo: 0%-2.8%
Adults: 0.5%-1.5%

ARTIFICIAL SALIVA PRODUCTS

Product/(Manufacturer)	Dosage Form	Ingredients
Glandosane (Tsumura Medical)	Spray	Sodium carboxymethylcellulose, sorbitol, sodium chloride, potassium chloride, calcium chloride dihydrate, magnesium chloride hexahydrate, dipotassium hydrogen phosphate
Moi-Stir 10[a] (KLI Corp)	Pump spray	Sodium carboxymethylcellulose, potassium chloride, dibasic sodium phosphate, methylparaben, propylparaben
Moi-Stir Mouth Moistening (Kingswood Labs)	Pump spray	Carboxymethylcellulose
Moi-Stir Oral Swabsticks[a] (Kingswood Labs)	Swab	Carboxymethylcellulose
MouthKote (Parnell)	Spray	Water, xylitol, sorbitol, yerba santa, citric acid, flavor, ascorbic acid, sodium benzoate, sodium saccharin
Optimoist (Colgate Oral Pharmaceuticals)	Liquid	Citric acid, calcium phosphate, sodium monofluorophosphate, preservative, sweetener, xylitol, polysorbate 20, flavor, hydroxyethylcellulose, sodium hydroxide
Saliva Substitute[a] (Roxane Labs)	Spray	Sorbitol, sodium carboxymethylcellulose, methylparaben
Salivart Synthetic Saliva[a] (Gebauer)	Aerosol spray	Sorbitol 3%, sodium carboxymethylcellulose 1%, potassium chloride 0.12%, sodium chloride 0.084%, calcium chloride dihydrate, magnesium chloride hexahydrate, potassium phosphate dibasic, nitrogen (as propellant)

[a]Carries American Dental Association (ADA) seal indicating safety and efficacy.

Reprinted with permission from *Handbook of Nonprescription Drugs*, 10th ed, *Product Updates*, Washington, DC, American Pharmaceutical Association, 1995, 272.

DENTIFRICE PRODUCTS

Product/ (Manufacturer)	Abrasive Ingredient	Therapeutic Ingredient	Foaming Agent
Aim AntiTartar Gel Formula with Fluoride (Chesebrough-Pond's)	Hydrated silica	Sodium monofluorophosphate 0.79% (fluoride 0.15%)	Sodium lauryl sulfate
	Other Ingredients: Sorbitol and related polyols, water, glycerin, zinc citrate trihydrate, SD alcohol 38B, flavor, cellulose gum, sodium saccharin, sodium benzoate, blue #1, yellow #10		
Aim Baking Soda Gel with Fluoride (Chesebrough-Pond's)	Hydrated silica	Sodium monofluorophosphate 0.79% (fluoride 0.15%)	Sodium lauryl sulfate
	Other Ingredients: Sorbitol and related polyols, water, glycerin, SD alcohol 38B, flavor, sodium bicarbonate, cellulose gum, sodium saccharin, sodium benzoate, blue #1, yellow #10		
Aim Regular Strength Gel with Fluoride (Chesebrough-Pond's)	Hydrated silica	Sodium monofluorophosphate 0.79% (fluoride 0.15%)	Sodium lauryl sulfate
	Other Ingredients: Sorbitol and other related polyols, water, glycerin, SD alcohol 38B, flavor, cellulose gum, sodium saccharin, sodium benzoate, blue #1, yellow #10		
Aquafresh Baking Soda Toothpaste (SmithKline Beecham)	Calcium carbonate, hydrated silica	Sodium monofluorophosphate	Sodium lauryl sulfate
	Other Ingredients: Calcium carrageenan, cellulose gum, colors, flavor, glycerin, PEG-8, sodium benzoate, sodium bicarbonate, sodium saccharin, sorbitol, titanium dioxide, water		
Aquafresh Extra Fresh Toothpaste[a] (SmithKline Beecham)	Hydrated silica, calcium carbonate	Sodium monofluorophosphate	Sodium lauryl sulfate
	Other Ingredients: Sorbitol, water, glycerin, PEG-8, titanium dioxide, cellulose gum, flavor, sodium saccharin, sodium benzoate, calcium carrageenan, colors		
Aquafresh for Kids Toothpaste[a] (SmithKline Beecham)	Hydrated silica, calcium carbonate	Sodium monofluorophosphate	Sodium lauryl sulfate
	Other Ingredients: Sorbitol, water, glycerin, PEG-8, titanium dioxide, cellulose gum, flavor, sodium saccharin, calcium carrageenan, sodium benzoate, colors		
Aquafresh Sensitive Toothpaste (SmithKline Beecham)	Hydrated silica	Potassium nitrate, sodium fluoride	Sodium lauryl sulfate
	Other Ingredients: Colors, flavors, glycerin, sodium benzoate, sodium saccharin, sorbitol, titanium dioxide, water, xanthan gum		
Aquafresh Tartar Control Toothpaste[a] (SmithKline Beecham)	Hydrated silica	Sodium fluoride	Sodium lauryl sulfate
	Other Ingredients: Tetrapotassium, pyrophosphate, tetrasodium pyrophosphate, sorbitol, glycerin, PEG-8, flavor, xanthan gum, sodium saccharin, sodium benzoate, D&C red #30 lake, FD&C blue #1, D&C yellow #10, titanium dioxide, water		
Aquafresh Triple Protection Toothpaste[a] (SmithKline Beecham)	Hydrated silica, calcium carbonate	Sodium monofluorophosphate	Sodium lauryl sulfate

(continued)

Product/ (Manufacturer)	Abrasive Ingredient	Therapeutic Ingredient	Foaming Agent
	Other Ingredients: PEG-8, sorbitol, cellulose gum, sodium benzoate, titanium dioxide, calcium, carrageenan, flavor, sodium saccharin, colors, water		
Aquafresh Whitening Toothpaste (SmithKline Beecham)	Hydrated silica	Sodium fluoride	Sodium lauryl sulfate
	Other Ingredients: D&C yellow #10, FD&C blue #1, flavor, glycerin, PEG-8, sodium benzoate, sodium hydroxide, sodium saccharin, sodium tripolyphosphate, sorbitol, titanium dioxide, water, xanthan gum		
Arm & Hammer Dental Care Baking Soda Tartar Control Toothpaste (Church & Dwight)	Sodium bicarbonate	Sodium fluoride	Sodium lauryl sulfate
	Other Ingredients: Water, glycerin, sodium pyrophosphates, sodium saccharin, PEG-8, flavor blend, sodium phosphates, cellulose gum, sodium lauroyl sarcosinate		
Arm & Hammer Dental Care Baking Soda Gel (Church & Dwight)	Hydrated silica, sodium bicarbonate	Sodium fluoride	Sodium lauryl sulfate
	Other Ingredients: Sorbitol, water, glycerin, PEG-8, flavor blend, cellulose gum, sodium lauroyl sarcosinate, sodium saccharin, FD&C blue #1, D&C yellow #10		
Arm & Hammer Dental Care Baking Soda Tartar Control Gel (Church & Dwight)	Sodium bicarbonate, hydrated silica	Sodium fluoride	Sodium lauryl sulfate
	Other Ingredients: Water, sorbitol, glycerin, sodium pyrophosphates, PEG-8, flavor, cellulose gum, sodium saccharin, sodium lauroyl sarcosinate, FD&C blue #1, D&C yellow #10		
Arm & Hammer Dental Care Baking Soda Tooth Powder (Church & Dwight)	Sodium bicarbonate	Sodium fluoride	
	Other Ingredients: Mint flavor, sodium saccharin, trisodium saccharin, trisodium magnesium oxide, PEG-8		
Arm & Hammer Dental Care Baking Soda Toothpaste (Church & Dwight)	Sodium bicarbonate	Sodium fluoride	Sodium lauryl sulfate
	Other Ingredients: Water, glycerin, sodium saccharin, PEG-8, flavor blend, cellulose gum, sodium lauroyl sarcosinate		
Arm & Hammer PerioxiCare Toothpaste (Church & Dwight)	Sodium bicarbonate, silica	Sodium fluoride	Sodium carbonate peroxide, sodium lauryl sulfate
	Other Ingredients: PEG-8, poloxamer 338, flavor, water, sodium saccharin, sodium lauroyl sarconsinate		
Caffree Anti-Stain Fluoride Toothpaste[a] (Block Drug)		Sodium monofluorophosphate	Sodium lauryl sulfate
	Other Ingredients: Water, diatomaceous earth, glycerin, sorbitol, aluminum silicate, titanium dioxide, hydroxyethylcellulose, flavor, sodium saccharin, methylparaben, propylparaben		
Close-Up Anti-Plaque Gel (Chesebrough-Pond's)	Hydrated silica	Stannous fluoride 0.41%	Sodium lauryl sulfate

(continued)

Product/ (Manufacturer)	Abrasive Ingredient	Therapeutic Ingredient	Foaming Agent
	Other Ingredients: Sorbitol, water, PEG-32, SD alcohol 38B, flavor, zinc citrate trihydrate, cellulose gum, sodium saccharin, sodium benzoate, sodium hydroxide, blue #1		
Close-Up Crystal Clear Mint Gel (Chesebrough-Ponds)	Hydrated silica	Sodium monofluorophosphate 0.79% (fluoride 0.15%)	Sodium lauryl sulfate
	Other Ingredients: Sorbitol, water, glycerin, SD alcohol 38B, flavor, cellulose gum, sodium saccharin, polysorbate 20, sodium benzoate, sodium chloride, blue #1, mica, red #33, titanium dioxide		
Close-Up Original Gel (Chesebrough-Pond's)	Hydrated silica	Sodium monofluorophosphate 0.79% (fluoride 0.15%)	Sodium lauryl sulfate
	Other Ingredients: Sorbitol, water, glycerin, SD alcohol 38B, flavor, cellulose gum, sodium saccharin, sodium benzoate, sodium chloride, red #33, red #40		
Close-Up Tartar Control Gel (Chesebrough-Pond's)	Hydrated silica	Sodium monofluorophosphate 0.79% (fluoride 0.15%)	Sodium lauryl sulfate
	Other Ingredients: Sorbitol and related polyols, water, glycerin, zinc citrate trihydrate, SD alcohol 38B, flavor, cellulose gum, sodium saccharin, sodium benzoate, sodium chloride, red #33, red #40		
Close-Up with Baking Soda Toothpaste (Chesebrough-Pond's)	Hydrated silica	Sodium monofluorophosphate 0.79% (fluoride 0.15%)	Sodium lauryl sulfate
	Other Ingredients: Sorbitol and related polyols, water, glycerin, SD alcohol 38B, flavor, sodium bicarbonate, cellulose gum, sodium saccharin, sodium benzoate, red #33, red #40, titanium dioxide		
Colgate Baking Soda Gel[a] (Colgate Oral Pharmaceuticals)	Hydrated silica	Sodium fluoride 0.243%	Sodium lauryl sulfate
	Other Ingredients: Glycerin, PEG-12, cellulose gum, flavor, sodium saccharin, FD&C blue #1, D&C yellow #10		
Colgate Baking Soda Tartar Control Gel or Toothpaste (Colgate Oral Pharmaceuticals)	Hydrated silica, sodium bicarbonate	Sodium fluoride 0.243%	Sodium lauryl sulfate
	Other Ingredients: Glycerin, tetrasodium pyrophosphate, PVM/MA copolymer, cellulose gum, flavor, sodium saccharin, sodium hydroxide, titanium dioxide (paste), FD&C blue #1, D&C yellow #10 (gel)		
Colgate Baking Soda Toothpaste[a] (Colgate Oral Pharmaceuticals)	Hydrated silica, sodium bicarbonate	Sodium fluoride 0.243%	Sodium lauryl sulfate
	Other Ingredients: Glycerin, cellulose gum, flavor, sodium saccharin, titanium dioxide		
Colgate Junior Gel[a] (Colgate Oral Pharmaceuticals)	Hydrated silica	Sodium fluoride 0.243%	Sodium lauryl sulfate
	Other Ingredients: Sorbitol, PEG-12, flavor, tetrasodium pyrophosphate, cellulose gum, sodium saccharin, mica, titanium dioxide, FD&C blue #1, D&C yellow #10		
Colgate Micro Cleansing Tartar Control Gel or Toothpaste[a] (Colgate Oral Pharmaceuticals)	Synthetic amorphous silica 27%, hydrated amorphous silica 3%	Sodium fluoride 0.243%	Sodium lauryl sulfate

Product/ (Manufacturer)	Abrasive Ingredient	Therapeutic Ingredient	Foaming Agent
	Other Ingredients: Water, sorbitol, glycerin, PEG-12, tetrasodium pyrophosphate, PVM/MA copolymer, cellulose gum, flavor, sodium hydroxide, titanium dioxide (Paste), sodium saccharin, carrageenan, FD&C blue #1 (gel)		
Colgate Peak Toothpaste (Colgate Oral Pharmaceuticals)	Hydrated silica, sodium bicarbonate, precipitated calcium carbonate		Sodium lauryl sulfate
	Other Ingredients: Glycerin, cellulose gum, flavor, sodium saccharin, titanium dioxide, sodium benzoate		
Colgate Toothpaste[a] (Colgate Oral Pharmaceuticals)	Dicalcium phosphate dihydrate	Sodium monofluorophosphate 0.76%	Sodium lauryl sulfate
	Other Ingredients: Glycerin, cellulose gum, tetrasodium pyrophosphate, sodium saccharin, flavor		
Colgate Winterfresh Gel[a] (Colgate Oral Pharmaceuticals)	Hydrated silica	Sodium fluoride 0.243%	Sodium lauryl sulfate
	Other Ingredients: Sorbitol, glycerin, PEG-12, flavor, tetrasodium pyrophosphate, cellulose gum, sodium saccharin, FD&C blue #1		
Crest Baking Soda Gel or Toothpaste[a] (mint) (Procter & Gamble)	Hydrated silica	Sodium fluoride	Sodium lauryl sulfate
	Other Ingredients: Sorbitol, water, sodium bicarbonate, glycerin, sodium carbonate, flavor, cellulose gum, sodium saccharin, titanium dioxide (paste), FD&C blue #1 (gel)		
Crest Baking Soda Tartar Control Gel or Toothpaste[a] (mint) (Procter & Gamble)	Hydrated silica	Sodium fluoride	Sodium lauryl sulfate
	Other Ingredients: Water, sodium bicarbonate, glycerin, sorbitol, tetrasodium pyrophosphate, PEG-6, sodium carbonate, flavor, cellulose gum, sodium saccharin, titanium dioxide (paste), FD&C blue #1 (gel)		
Crest Cavity Fighting Gel[a] (cool mint) (Procter & Gamble)	Hydrated silica	Sodium fluoride	Sodium lauryl sulfate
	Other Ingredients: Sorbitol, water, trisodium phosphate, flavor, sodium phosphate, xanthan gum, sodium saccharin, carbomer 956, FD&C blue #1		
Crest Cavity Fighting Toothpaste[a] (icy mint or regular flavor) (Procter & Gamble)	Hydrated silica	Sodium fluoride	Sodium lauryl sulfate
	Other Ingredients: Sorbitol, water, glycerin, mint, trisodium phosphate, flavor, sodium phosphate, cellulose gum (mint), xanthan gum (regular), sodium saccharin, carbomer 956, titanium dioxide, FD&C blue #1		
Crest for Kids, Sparkle Fun Gel[a] (Procter & Gamble)	Hydrated silica	Sodium fluoride	Sodium lauryl sulfate
	Other Ingredients: Sorbitol, water, trisodium phosphate, sodium phosphate, xanthan gum, flavor, sodium saccharin, carbomer 956, mica, titanium dioxide, FD&C blue #1		
Crest Sensitivity Protection Toothpaste[a] (mild mint) (Procter & Gamble)	Hydrated silica	Potassium nitrate, sodium fluoride	Sodium lauryl sulfate

(continued)

Product/ (Manufacturer)	Abrasive Ingredient	Therapeutic Ingredient	Foaming Agent
	Other Ingredients: Water, glycerin, sorbitol, trisodium phosphate, cellulose gum, flavor, xanthan gum, sodium saccharin, titanium dioxide		
Crest Tartar Control Gel[a] (fresh mint or smooth mint) (Procter & Gamble)	Hydrated silica	Sodium fluoride	Sodium lauryl sulfate
	Other Ingredients: Water, sorbitol, glycerin, tetrapotassium pyrophosphate, PEG-6, disodium pyrophosphate, tetrasodium pyrophosphate, flavor, xanthan gum, sodium saccharin, carbomer 956, FD&C blue #1, (fresh mint & smooth mint), FD&C yellow #5 (smooth mint)		
Crest Tartar Control Toothpaste[a] (original flavor) (Procter & Gamble)	Hydrated silica	Sodium fluoride	Sodium lauryl sulfate
	Other Ingredients: Water, sorbitol, glycerin, tetrapotassium pyrophosphate, PEG-6, disodium pyrophosphate, tetrasodium pyrophosphate, flavor, xanthan gum, sodium saccharin, carbomer 956, titanium dioxide, FD&C blue #1		
Dentagard Toothpaste[a] (Colgate Oral Pharmaceuticals)	Hydrated silica	Sodium monofluorophosphate 0.76%	Sodium lauryl sulfate
	Other Ingredients: Sorbitol, glycerin, PEG-12, flavor, sodium benzoate, titanium dioxide, cellulose gum, sodium saccharin, FD&C red #40		
Gleem Toothpaste (Procter & Gamble)	Hydrated silica	Sodium fluoride	Sodium lauryl sulfate
	Other Ingredients: Sorbitol, water, trisodium phosphate, flavor, sodium phosphate, xanthan gum, sodium saccharin, carbomer 956, titanium dioxide		
Interplak Toothpaste with Fluoride (Bausch & Lomb)	Hydrated silica	Sodium fluoride	Sodium lauryl sulfate
	Other Ingredients: Purified water, poloxamer 407, sorbitol, glycerin, flavor, dibasic sodium phosphate, sodium saccharin, monobasic sodium phosphate, sodium benzoate, D&C yellow #10		
Mentadent Fluoride Toothpaste with Baking Soda & Peroxide[a] (Chesebrough-Pond's)	Hydrated silica, sodium bicarbonate	Sodium fluoride 0.24% (fluoride 0.15%)	Sodium lauryl sulfate, hydrogen peroxide
	Other Ingredients: Water, sorbitol, glycerin, poloxamer 407, PEG-32, SD alcohol 38B, flavor, cellulose gum, sodium saccharin, phosphoric acid, blue #1, titanium dioxide		
Oral-B Sensitive Toothpaste with Fluoride (Oral-B Labs)	Hydrated silica	Potassium nitrate 5%, sodium fluoride 0.225%	Sodium lauryl sulfate
	Other Ingredients: Water, glycerin, cellulose gum, PEG-8, sodium saccharin, methylparaben, propylparaben, flavor		
Oral-B Sesame Street Toothpaste, Bubblegum, or Fruity[a] (Oral-B Labs)	Hydrated silica	Sodium fluoride 0.248%	Sodium lauryl sulfate
	Other Ingredients: Water, sorbitol, glycerin, xanthan gum, acesulfame K, carbomer 980, sodium hydroxide, FD&C red #3, methylparaben, propylparaben		
Oral-B Tooth and Gum Care Toothpaste (Oral-B Labs)	Calcium pyrophosphate	Stannous fluoride 0.4%	

Product/ (Manufacturer)	Abrasive Ingredient	Therapeutic Ingredient	Foaming Agent
	Other Ingredients: Water, glycerin, sorbitol, PEG-8, sodium saccharin, methylparaben, propylparaben, zinc citrate, flavor, PVM/MA copolymer		
Pearl Drops Baking Soda Whitening Toothpaste Tartar Control (Carter Wallace)	Hydrated silica, sodium bicarbonate	Sodium fluoride	Sodium lauryl sulfate
	Other Ingredients: Sorbitol, glycerin, tetrapotassium pyrophosphate, tetrasodium pyrophosphate, PEG-12, titanium dioxide, flavor, sodium saccharin, cellulose gum		
Pearl Drops Extra Strength Whitening Toothpaste (Carter-Wallace)	Hydrated silica, calcium pyrophosphate, dicalcium phosphate	Sodium monofluorophosphate	Sodium lauryl sulfate
	Other Ingredients: Sorbitol, glycerin, PEG-12, flavor, titanium dioxide, cellulose gum, trisodium phosphate, sodium phosphate, sodium saccharin		
Pearl Drops Whitening Gel or Paste, Tartar Control w/Fluoride (Carter-Wallace)	Hydrated silica	Sodium fluoride	Sodium lauryl sulfate
	Other Ingredients: Sorbitol, glycerin, tetrapotassium pyrophosphate, tetrasodium pyrophosphate, PEG-12, flavor, titanium dioxide (paste), cellulose gum, sodium saccharin, FD&C blue #1 (gel), FD&C yellow #10 (gel)		
Pearl Drops Whitening Toothpolish Gel (Carter-Wallace)	Hydrated silica	Sodium monofluorophosphate	Sodium lauryl sulfate
	Other Ingredients: Sorbitol, glycerin, PEG-12, flavor, cellulose gum, trisodium phosphate, sodium phosphate, sodium saccharin, FD&C blue #1		
Pearl Drops Whitening Toothpolish (regular or spearmint) (Carter-Wallace)	Aluminum hydroxide, hydrated silica	Sodium monofluorophosphate	Sodium lauryl sulfate
	Other Ingredients: Sorbitol, glycerin, PEG-12, flavor, titanium dioxide, cellulose gum, trisodium phosphate, sodium phosphate, sodium saccharin		
Pepsodent Baking Soda Toothpaste (Chesebrough-Pond's)	Hydrated silica	Sodium fluoride 0.24%	Sodium lauryl sulfate
	Other Ingredients: Sorbitol, water, sodium bicarbonate, PEG-32, SD alcohol 38B, flavor, cellulose gum, sodium saccharin, titanium dioxide		
Pepsodent Original Fluoride Toothpaste (Chesebrough-Pond's)	Hydrated silica	Sodium monofluorophosphate 0.79% (fluoride 0.15%)	Sodium lauryl sulfate
	Other Ingredients: Sorbitol and related polyols, water, glycerin, SD alcohol 38B, flavor, cellulose gum, sodium saccharin, sodium benzoate, titanium dioxide		
PeriGel Toothpaste System (Zila)	Sodium bicarbonate 59%	Sodium fluoride	Hydrogen peroxide 3%
Platinum Whitening Toothpaste with Fluoride (Colgate Oral Pharmaceuticals)		Sodium monofluorophosphate 0.76%	
Promise Toothpaste (Block Drug)	Silica	Potassium nitrate, sodium monofluorophosphate	Sodium lauryl sulfate

(continued)

Product/ (Manufacturer)	Abrasive Ingredient	Therapeutic Ingredient	Foaming Agent
	Other Ingredients: Water, dicalcium phosphate, hydroxyethylcellulose, flavor, sodium saccharin, methylparaben, propylparaben, D&C yellow #10, FD&C blue #1		
Pycopay Tooth Powder (Block Drug)	Sodium bicarbonate, calcium carbonate, tricalcium phosphate, magnesium carbonate		
	Other Ingredients: Sodium chloride, eugenol, methyl salicylate		
Rembrandt Brushing Gel with Peroxide (Den-Mat)		Sodium monofluorophosphate	Carbamide peroxide, sodium lauryl sulfate
	Other Ingredients: Glycerin, sodium citrate, carbomer, titanium dioxide, flavor, triethanolamine		
Rembrandt Whitening Sensitive Toothpaste (Den-Mat)		Sodium monofluorophosphate 0.76%, potassium nitrate	Sodium lauryl sulfate
	Other Ingredients: Dicalcium phosphate dihydrate, glycerin, sorbitol, water, alumina, papain, sodium citrate, flavor, sodium carboxymethylcellulose, sodium saccharin, methylparaben, citric acid, FD&C red #40		
Rembrandt Whitening Toothpaste (mint or regular) (Den-Mat)		Sodium monofluorophosphate 0.76%	Sodium lauryl sulfate
	Other Ingredients: Dicalcium phosphate dihydrate, water, glycerin, sorbitol, alumina, papain, sodium citrate, flavor, sodium carrageenan, sodium saccharin, methylparaben, citric acid, FD&C blue #1		
Revelation Toothpowder (Alvin Last)	Calcium carbonate		Vegetable soap powder
	Other Ingredients: Methyl salicylate, menthol		
Sensodyne Baking Soda Toothpaste (Dentco)	Sodium bicarbonate, hydrated silica, silica	Potassium nitrate, sodium fluoride	Sodium lauryl sulfate
	Other Ingredients: Water, glycerin, sorbitol, flavor, hydroxyethylcellulose, titanium dioxide, sodium saccharin		
Sensodyne Gel (cool mint) (Dentco)	Hydrated silica, silica	Potassium nitrate, sodium fluoride	
	Other Ingredients: Water, sorbitol, glycerin, sodium carboxyethylcellulose, sodium methyl cocoyl taurate, flavor, guar gum, sodium saccharin, methylparaben, propylparaben, sodium hydroxide, FD&C blue #1		
Sensodyne Toothpaste[a] (fresh mint) (Dentco)	Silica	Potassium nitrate, sodium monofluorophosphate	Sodium lauryl sulfate
	Other Ingredients: Water, dicalcium phosphate dihydrate, glycerin, sorbitol, dicalcium phosphate, hydroxyethylcellulose, flavor, sodium saccharin, methylparaben, propylparaben, D&C yellow #10, FD&C blue #1		
Sensodyne-SC Toothpaste[a] (Dentco)	Calcium carbonate, silica	Strontium chloride hexahydrate 10%	
	Other Ingredients: Water, glycerin, sorbitol, hydroxyethylcellulose, sodium methyl cocoyl taurate, flavor, PEG-40, stearate, titanium dioxide, sodium saccharin, methylparaben, propylparaben, D&C red #28		

Product/ (Manufacturer)	Abrasive Ingredient	Therapeutic Ingredient	Foaming Agent
Thermodent Toothpaste (Mentholatum)	Diatomaceous earth, silica	Strontium chloride hexahydrate	Sodium methyl cocoyl taurate
Other Ingredients: Sorbitol, glycerin, titanium dioxide, hydroxyethylcellulose, flavor, preservative			
Tom's Natural Baking Soda Toothpaste with Fluoride (Tom's of Maine)	Calcium carbonate, sodium bicarbonate	Sodium monofluorophosphate	Sodium lauryl sulfate
Other Ingredients: Glycerin, carrageenan, xylitol, peppermint oil			
Tom's Natural Toothpaste for Children with Fluoride (Tom's of Maine)	Calcium carbonate, hydrated silica	Sodium monofluorophosphate	Sodium lauryl sulfate
Other Ingredients: Glycerin, fruit extracts, carrageenan			
Tom's Natural Toothpaste with Calcium and Fluoride (Tom's of Maine)	Calcium carbonate	Sodium monofluorophosphate	Sodium lauryl sulfate
Other Ingredients: Glycerin, carrageenan, xylitol, spearmint and peppermint oil			
Tom's Natural Toothpaste with Propolis and Myrrh (Tom's of Maine)	Calcium carbonate		Sodium lauryl sulfate
Other Ingredients: Glycerin, carrageenan, oil of spearmint, peppermint, cassia, or fennel, propolis, myrrh			
Toothpaste Booster (Dental Concepts)			Hydrogen peroxide, sodium lauryl sulfate
Other Ingredients: Deionized water, cornstarch, sorbitol, propylene glycol, carbomer 940, menthol, sodium benzoate, potassium sorbate			
Topol Gel[a] (spearmint) (Dep)	Hydrated silica	Sodium monofluorophosphate	Sodium lauryl sulfate
Other Ingredients: Sorbitol, deionized water, glycerin, PEG-6, flavor, xanthan gum, sodium saccharin, methylparaben, propylparaben, zirconium silicate, FD&C blue #1, FD&C yellow #5			
Topol Plus Baking Soda Whitening Gel or Toothpaste (Dep)	Hydrated silica	Sodium monofluorophosphate	Sodium lauryl sulfate
Other Ingredients: Water, sorbitol (gel), glycerin, calcium carbonate (gel), sorbitol, PEG-6, disodium phosphate, flavor, xanthan gum, sodium saccharin, titanium dioxide, methylparaben, propylparaben, FD&C blue #1 (gel)			
Topol Toothpaste[a] (peppermint) (Dep)	Hydrated silica, sodium bicarbonate	Sodium monofluorophosphate	Sodium lauryl sulfate
Other Ingredients: Sorbitol, deionized water, glycerin, PEG-6, flavor, xanthan gum, titanium dioxide, sodium saccharin, methylparaben, propylparaben, zirconium silicate			
Triplex Toothpaste (CCA Industries)	Hydrated silica, sodium bicarbonate	Sodium fluoride	Calcium peroxide, sodium lauryl sulfate
Other Ingredients: Glycerin, sorbitol, urea, flavor, titanium dioxide, carbomer, sodium saccharin, ethyl cellulose, sodium benzoate			
Ultra Brite Baking Soda Toothpaste (Colgate Oral Pharmaceuticals)	Hydrated silica, sodium bicarbonate, alumina	Sodium monofluorophosphate 0.76%	Sodium lauryl sulfate
Other Ingredients: Glycerin, tetrasodium pyrophosphate, cellulose gum, flavor, sodium saccharin, titanium dioxide			

(continued)

Product/ (Manufacturer)	Abrasive Ingredient	Therapeutic Ingredient	Foaming Agent
Ultra Brite Gel[a] (Colgate Oral Pharmaceuticals)	Hydrated silica	Sodium monofluorophosphate 0.76%	Sodium lauryl sulfate
Other Ingredients: Sorbitol, PEG-12, flavor, cellulose gum, sodium saccharin, glycerin, FD&C blue #1, D&C red #33			
Ultra Brite Toothpaste (Colgate Oral Pharmaceuticals)	Hydrated silica, alumina	Sodium monofluorophosphate 0.76%	Sodium lauryl sulfate
Other Ingredients: Glycerin, cellulose gum, carrageenan gum, sodium benzoate, titanium dioxide, sodium saccharin, flavor			
Viadent Fluoride Gel (Colgate Oral Pharmaceuticals)	Hydrated silica	Sodium monofluorophosphate 0.8%, sanguinaria extract 0.075%	Sodium lauryl sulfate
Other Ingredients: Sodium saccharin, zinc chloride, teaberry flavor, sodium carboxymethylcellulose, sorbitol			
Viadent Fluoride Toothpaste (Colgate Oral Pharmaceuticals)	Hydrated silica	Sodium monofluorophosphate 0.8%, sanguinaria extract 0.075%	Sodium lauryl sulfate
Other Ingredients: Sorbitol, titanium dioxide, carboxymethylcellulose, flavor, sodium saccharin, citric acid, zinc chloride			
Viadent Original Toothpaste (Colgate Oral Pharmaceuticals)	Dicalcium phosphate	Sanguinaria extract 0.075%	Sodium lauryl sulfate
Other Ingredients: Glycerin, sorbitol, titanium dioxide, zinc chloride, carrageenan, flavor, sodium saccharin, citric acid			

[a]Carries American Dental Association (ADA) seal indicating safety and efficacy.
[b]Topical fluoride rinse

Reprinted with permission from *Handbook of Nonprescription Drugs,* 10th ed, *Product Updates,* Washington, DC, American Pharmaceutical Association, 1995, 265-71.

DENTURE ADHESIVE PRODUCTS

Product/(Manufacturer)	Dosage Form	Ingredients
Confident (Block Drug)	Cream	Carboxymethylcellulose gum 32%, ethylene oxide polymer 13%, petrolatum, liquid petrolatum, propylparaben
Corega (Block Drug)	Powder	Karaya gum 94.6%, water-soluble ethylene oxide polymer 5%, flavor
Dentrol (Block Drug)	Liquid	Carboxymethylcellulose sodium, ethylene oxide polymer, mineral oil, polyethylene, flavor, propylparaben
Denturite (Brimms Labs)	Liquid, powder	Liquid: Butyl phthalyl butyl glycolate, vinyl acetate, SDA alcohol Powder: Polyethyl methacrylate polymer
Effergrip[a] (Warner-Wellcome)	Cream	Carboxymethylcellulose sodium 24.8%, calcium sodium mixed salt of methyl vinyl ether-maleic anhydride 29.8%, preservatives, red lake blend
Ezo Cushions (Medtech Labs)	Pad	Paraffin wax, cotton
Fasteeth (Procter & Gamble)	Powder	Calcium/zinc poly (vinyl methyl ether maleate), sodium carboxymethylcellulose, cornstarch, silicon dioxide, peppermint oil, rectified
Fasteeth Extra Hold (Procter & Gamble)	Powder	Calcium/zinc poly (vinyl methyl ether maleate), sodium carboxymethylcellulose, silicon dioxide, peppermint oil, rectified
Fixodent (Procter & Gamble)	Cream	Calcium/zinc poly (vinyl methyl ether maleate), sodium carboxymethylcellulose, mineral oil, petrolatum, silicon dioxide, color
Fixodent Fresh (Procter & Gamble)	Cream	Calcium/zinc poly (vinyl methyl ether maleate), sodium carboxymethylcellulose, mineral oil, petrolatum, silicon dioxide, color, peppermint flavor, methyl lactate, menthol
Orafix (SmithKline Beecham)	Cream	Karaya gum 51%, petrolatum 30%, mineral oil 13%, peppermint oil 0.08%
Orafix Special[a] (SmithKline Beecham)	Cream	Gantrez MS955, sodium carboxymethylcellulose type 7H4XF, povidone K-90, white petrolatum, mineral oil, heavy, isopropyl palmitate, isopropyl myristate, flavors, colors
Plasti-Liner (Brimms Labs)	Strip	Polyethyl metacrylate polymer, butyl phthalyl butyl glycolate, triacetin
Poli-Grip (Block Drug)	Cream	Karaya gum 51%, petrolatum 36.7%, liquid petrolatum, magnesium oxide, propylparaben, flavor
Poly-Grip Super (Block Drug)	Cream	Carboxymethylcellulose sodium, ethylene oxide polymer, petrolatum, mineral oil flavor, propylparaben
Poli-Grip Super (Block Drug)	Powder	Calcium sodium methyl vinyl ether-maleic copolymer, carboxymethylcellulose sodium, flavor
Polident Dentu-Grip (Block Drug)	Cream	Carboxymethylcellulose gum 49%, ethylene oxide polymer 21%, flavor

(continued)

Product/(Manufacturer)	Dosage Form	Ingredients
Quik-Fix (Brimms Labs)	Liquid, powder	Liquid: Methyl methacrylate monomer, hydroxyethyl metacyclate monomer, colorstable concentrate, triacetin; Powder: Polyethyl methacrylate polymer
Rigident (Carter-Wallace)	Powder	Acacia gum, karaya gum, sodium borate
Rigident[a] (Carter-Wallace)	Cream	Carboxymethylcellulose sodium, calcium sodium salts of methyl vinyl ether maleic anhydride copolymer, petrolatum, mineral oil, talc, flavor, propylparaben, D&C red #27 aluminum lake
Sea-Bond (Combe)	Pad	Ethylene oxide polymer, sodium alginate
Wernet's (Block Drug)	Cream	Carboxymethylcellulose gum 32%, petrolatum, mineral oil, ethylene oxide polymer 13%, propylparaben, flavor 0.5%
Wernet's (Block Drug)	Powder	Karaya gum 94.6%, water-soluble ethylene oxide polymer 5%, flavor 0.4%

[a]Carries American Dental Association (ADA) seal indicating safety and efficacy.

Reprinted with permission from *Handbook of Nonprescription Drugs*, 10th ed, *Product Updates*, Washington, DC, American Pharmaceutical Association, 1995, 277.

DENTURE CLEANSER PRODUCTS

Product/(Manufacturer)	Dosage Form	Ingredients
Ban-A-Stain** (Brimms Labs)	Liquid	Phosphoric acid 25%, deionized water, imidurea, methylparaben, xanthan gum, alkyl phenoxy polyethoxy ethanol, oil of cassis, FD&C red #40
Complete[a] (Procter & Gamble)	Paste	Calcium carbonate, water, glycerin, sorbitol, cellulose gum, sodium lauryl sulfate, silica, flavor, magnesium aluminum silicate, sodium saccharin, methylparaben, propylparaben
Dentu-Creme (Dentco)	Paste	Dicalcium phosphate dihydrate, propylene glycol, calcium carbonate, silica, sodium lauryl sulfate, glycerin, hydroxyethylcellulose, flavor, magnesium aluminum silicate, sodium saccharin, methylparaben, propylparaben
Efferdent Antibacterial[a] (Warner-Wellcome)	Tablet	Potassium monopersulfate, sodium perborate monohydrate, sodium carbonate, sodium lauryl sulfoacetate, sodium bicarbonate, citric acid, magnesium stearate, flavor
Efferdent, 2 Layer (Warner-Wellcome)	Tablet	Sodium bicarbonate, sodium carbonate, citric acid, potassium monopersulfate, sodium perborate monohydrate, sodium lauryl sulfoacetate, flavor
Polident (Block Drug)	Tablet, powder	Potassium monopersulfate, sodium perborate monohydrate, sodium carbonate, surfactant, chelating agents (tablet), proteolytic enzyme (tablet), sodium acid pyrophosphate (powder), sodium bicarbonate, citric acid (tablet), fragrance
Rembrandt Daily Denture Renewal (Den-Mat)	Gel	Citroxain
Smokers' Polident (Block Drug)	Tablet	Sodium carbonate, potassium monopersulfate, citric acid, sodium bicarbonate, sodium perborate monohydrate, surfactant, chelating agents, proteolytic enzyme, fragrance

[a]Carries American Dental Association (ADA) seal indicating safety and efficacy.

Reprinted with permission from *Handbook of Nonprescription Drugs*, 10th ed, *Product Updates*, Washington, DC, American Pharmaceutical Association, 1995, 276.

MOUTH PAIN, COLD SORE, CANKER SORE PRODUCTS

Product/(Manufacturer)	Anesthetic/ Analgesic	Other Ingredients
Amosan Powder (Oral B Labs)		Sodium peroxyborate monohydrate, sodium bitartrate, saccharin, peppermint, menthol, and vanilla flavors
Anbesol Baby Gel (grape or original) (Whitehall-Robins)	Benzocaine 7.5%	Benzoic acid (grape), carbomer 934P, D&C red #33, disodium EDTA, FD&C blue #1 (grape), flavor, glycerin, methylparaben (grape), PEG-8, propylparaben (grape), saccharin, water
Anbesol Gel (Whitehall-Robins)	Benzocaine 6.3%, phenol 0.5%, camphor	Alcohol 70%, carbomer 934P, D&C red #33, D&C yellow #10, FD&C blue #1, FD&C yellow #6, flavor, glycerin
Anbesol Liquid (Whitehall-Robins)	Benzocaine 6.3%, phenol 0.5%, camphor, menthol	Alcohol 70%, glycerin, potassium iodide, povidone iodine
Anbesol Maximum Strength Gel (Whitehall-Robins)	Benzocaine 20%	Alcohol 60%, carbomer 934P, D&C yellow #10, FD&C blue #1, FD&C red #40, flavor, PEG-12, saccharin
Anbesol Maximum Strength Liquid (Whitehall-Robins)	Benzocaine 20%	Alcohol 60%, D&C yellow #10, FD&C blue #1, FD&C red #40, flavor, PEG-8, saccharin
Babee Teething Lotion (SSS Company)	Benzocaine 2.5%, menthol, camphor	Alcohol 20%, witch hazel
Benzodent Denture Analgesic Ointment[a] (Chattem)	Benzocaine 20%, eugenol	8-hydroxyquinoline sulfate, petrolatum, sodium CMC, color
Betadine Mouthwash/ Gargle (Purdue Frederick)		Povidone-iodine 0.5%, alcohol 8.8%
Blistex Medicated Lip Ointment (Blistex)	Menthol 0.6%, camphor 0.5%, phenol 0.5%	Allantoin 1%
Blistex Lip Medex Ointment (Blistex)	Camphor 1%, menthol 1%, phenol 0.5%	Petrolatum, cocoa butter, flavor, lanolin, mixed waxes, oil of cloves
Campho-Phenique Antiseptic Gel (Sterling Health)	Camphor 10.8%, phenol 4.7%	Eucalyptus oil
Campho-Phenique Cold Sore Gel[b] (Sterling Health)	Camphor 10.8%, phenol 4.7%	Eucalyptus oil
Campho-Phenique Liquid (Sterling Health)	Camphor 10.8%, phenol 4.7%	Eucalyptus oil
Chap Stick Medicated Lip Balm (jar or squeeze tube) (Whitehall-Robins)	Camphor 1%, menthol 0.6%, phenol 0.5%	Petrolatum 60% (jar), petrolatum 67% (squeeze tube), microcrystalline wax, mineral oil, cocoa butter, lanolin, paraffin wax (jar)
Chap Stick Medicated Lip Balm Stick (Whitehall-Robins)	Camphor 1%, menthol 0.6%, phenol 0.5%	Petrolatum 41%, paraffin wax, mineral oil, cocoa butter, 2-octyl dodecanol, arachadyl propionate, polyphenylmethylsiloxane 556, white wax, isopropyl lanolate, carnauba wax, isopropyl myristate, lanolin, fragrance, methylparaben, propylparaben, oleyl alcohol, cetyl alcohol
Cold Sore Lotion[b] (SSS Company)	Camphor, menthol	Alcohol 85%, gum benzoin 7%, thymol, eucalyptol
Curasore Liquid (SSS Company)		Ethyl ether, ethyl alcohol

(continued)

Product/(Manufacturer)	Anesthetic/Analgesic	Other Ingredients
Dent's 3 in 1 Toothache Relief (gel, gum, drops) (CS Dent)	Benzocaine 20%	Alcohol 74% (drops), chlorobutanol anhydrous 0.09% (drops), eugenol
Dent's Double-Action Kit (tablets, drops) (CS Dent)	Benzocaine 20% (drops)	Denatured alcohol 74%, chlorobutanol 0.09%, acetaminophen 325 mg (tablet), eugenol
Dent's Extra Strength Toothache Gum (CS Dent)	Benzocaine 20%	Petrolatum, cotton and wax base, beeswax, FD&C red #40 aluminum lake, eugenol
Dent's Maxi-Strength Toothache Treatment Drops (CS Dent)	Benzocaine 20%	Alcohol 74%, chlorobutanol 0.09%, propylene glycol, FD&C red #40, eugenol
Dent-Zel-Ite Oral Mucosal Analgesic Liquid (Alvin Last)	Benzocaine 5%, camphor	Alcohol 81%, wintergreen, glycerin
Dent-Zel-Ite Temporary Dental Filling Liquid (Alvin Last)	Camphor	Alcohol 55%, sandarac gum, methyl salicylate
Dent-Zel-Ite Toothache Relief Drops (Alvin Last)	Eugenol 85%, camphor	Alcohol 13.5%, wintergreen
GargleAid Granular Effervescent (Tec Labs)	Dyclonine HCl 69 mg	Sucrose, salt, sodium bicarbonate, citric acid, natural lemon flavor, sodium ascorbate
HDA Toothache Gel (SSS Company)	Benzocaine 6.5%	Clove oil
Herpecin-L Stick[b] (Campbell Labs)		Allantoin, padimate O, titanium dioxide
Hurricaine Aerosol (wild cherry) (Beutlich)	Benzocaine	Polyethylene glycol, saccharin, flavoring
Hurricaine Gel (wild cherry, pina colada, or watermelon) (Beutlich)	Benzocaine	Polyethylene glycol, saccharin, flavoring
Hurricaine Liquid (wild cherry or pina colada) (Beutlich)	Benzocaine	Polyethylene glycol, saccharin, flavoring
Isodettes Spray (Goody's)	Phenol 1.4%	Propylene glycol 10%, artificial and sodium hydroxide 0.0047%, natural wild cherry flavor 0.5%, artificial and natural eucalyptus flavor, FD&C red #40, water
Kank-A-Professional Strength Liquid[a] (Blistex)	Benzocaine 20%, benzyl alcohol	Benzoin tincture compound 0.5%, cetylpyridinium chloride, ethylcellulose, SD alcohol, dimethyl isosorbide, castor oil, flavor, tannic acid, propylene glycol, saccharin
Lip Medex Ointment (Blistex)	Camphor 1.0%, menthol 0.5%, phenol 0.5%	Petrolatum 73.7%
Lotion-Jel (CS Dent)	Benzocaine	Distilled water, methylparaben, propylparaben, propylene glycol, carbopol 934-P, methyl salicylate, FD&C red #40, 2.2' iminodiethanol
Medadyne Liquid (Vetco)	Benzocaine 10%, menthol, camphor	Benzalkonium chloride, tannic acid, flavors, SD alcohol, benzyl alcohol, thymol
Mouth Kote-PR Ointment (Parnell)	Benzyl alcohol 3.5%, diphenhydramine 1.25%	PEG 8, cellulose gum, PEG 75, poloxamer 407, yerba santa, flavor
Mouth Kote-PR Solution (Parnell)	Diphenhydramine 1.25%, benzyl alcohol 1%	Water, cetylpyridinium chloride, disodium EDTA flavor, sodium benzoate, sodium hydroxide, sodium saccharin, yerba santa

(continued)

Product/(Manufacturer)	Anesthetic/ Analgesic	Other Ingredients
Mouth Kote-OR Solution (Parnell)	Benzyl alcohol 1%, menthol	Water, sorbitol, sodium chloride, yerba santa, flavor, poloxamer 407, sodium saccharin, cetylpyridinium chloride, disodium EDTA
Numzident (Adult Strength) Gel (Goody's)	Benzocaine 10%	PEG 400 47.86%, glycerin 30%, PEG 3350 10%, sodium saccharin 1%, purified water 0.75%, cherry vanilla flavor 0.4%
Numzit Teething Gel (Goody's)	Benzocaine 7.5%	PEG 400 66.2%, PEG 3350 26.1%, sodium saccharin 0.036%, clove oil 0.09%, peppermint oil 0.018%, purified water 0.056%
Numzit Teething Lotion (Goody's)	Benzocaine 0.2%	Alcohol 12.1%, glycerin 2%, kelgin MV 0.5%, sodium saccharin 0.02%, methylparaben 0.1%, FD&C red #40 0.1%, FD&C blue #1 0.009%
Orabase Baby Gel[a] (Colgate Oral Pharmaceuticals)	Benzocaine 7.5%	Glycerin, PEG, carbopol, preservative, sweetener, flavor
Orabase Gel (Colgate Oral Pharmaceuticals)	Benzocaine 15%	Ethanol, PEG, hydroxyethyl chloride, tannic acid, salicylic acid, flavor, sodium saccharin
Orabase Lip Cream (Colgate Oral Pharmaceuticals)	Benzocaine 5%, menthol 0.5%, camphor, phenol	Allantoin 1%, sodium carboxymethylcellulose, veegum, Tween 80, phenonip, PEG, biopure, talc, kaolin, lanolin, petrolatum, oil of clove, aerosil
Orabase Plain Paste[a] (Colgate Oral Pharmaceuticals)		Pectin, gelatin, carboxymethylcellulose sodium, polyethylene, mineral oil, flavors, preservative, guar, tragacanth
Orabase-B with Benzocaine Paste[a] (Colgate Oral Pharmaceuticals)	Benzocaine 20%	Plasticized hydrocarbon gel, guar, carboxymethylcellulose, tragacanth, pectin, preservatives, flavors
Orajel Baby Gel (Del Labs)	Benzocaine 7.5%	FD&C red #40, flavor, glycerin, polyethylene glycols, sodium saccharin, sorbic acid, sorbitol
Orajel Baby Nighttime Formula Gel (Del Labs)	Benzocaine 10%	FD&C red #40, flavor, glycerin, polyethylene glycols, sodium saccharin, sorbic acid, sorbitol
Orajel Denture Gel (Del Labs)	Benzocaine 10%, eugenol	Chlorothymol, FD&C red #40, flavor, polyethylene glycols, purified water, sodium saccharin, sorbic acid
Orajel Maximum Strength Gel (Del Labs)	Benzocaine 20%	Clove oil, flavor, polyethylene glycols, sodium saccharin, sorbic acid
Orajel Mouth-Aid Gel (Del Labs)	Benzocaine 20%	Zinc chloride 0.1%, benzalkonium chloride 0.02%. allantoin, carbomer, edetate disodium, peppermint oil, polyethylene glycol, polysorbate 60, propyl gallate, polysorbate 60, glycol, purified water, povidone sodium saccharin propylene, sorbic acid, stearyl alcohol
Orajel Mouth-Aid Liquid (Del Labs)	Benzocaine 20%	Cetylpyridinium chloride 0.1%, ethylcellulose
Orajel Regular Strength Gel (Del Labs)	Benzocaine 10%	Clove oil, flavor, polyethylene glycols, sodium saccharin, sorbic acid

Product/(Manufacturer)	Anesthetic/ Analgesic	Other Ingredients
Orasol Liquid (Goldline Labs)	Benzocaine 6.3%, phenol 0.5%	Alcohol 70%
Painalay Sore Throat Gargle & Spray (Meditech Labs)	Phenol 0.5%	
Probax Ointment[b] (Fischer)		Propolis 2%, petrolatum, mineral oil
Red Cross Toothache Medication Drops (Mentholatum)	Eugenol 85%	Sesame oil
SensoGARD Gel[b] (Dentco)	Benzocaine 20%	Methylparaben, polycarbophil, polyethylene glycol, propylparaben, sorbitan monooleate
Sore Throat Spray (cherry, menthol, or mint) (Pharmaceutical Assoc)	Phenol 1.4%	
Tanac Liquid (Del Labs)	Benzocaine 10%	Benzalkonium chloride 0.125%, saccharin
Tanac Medicated Gel (Del Labs)	Dyclonine HCl 1.0%	Allantoin 0.5%
Tanac Roll-On Lotion (Del Labs)	Benzocaine 5%	Benzalkonium chloride 0.12%, sodium saccharin, glycerin, polyethylene glycol, tannic acid
Tanac Stick (Del Labs)	Benzocaine 7.5%	Benzalkonium chloride 0.125%
Throtoceptic Pump Spray (SSS Company)	Phenol 1.4%	Alum 0.5%, flavor
Tisol Solution (Parnell)	Benzyl alcohol 1%	Water, sorbitol, sodium chloride, yerba santa, poloxamer 407, menthol, saccharin, cetylpyridinium chloride, disodium EDTA
Vaseline Lip Therapy Ointment (Chesebrough-Ponds)	Camphor 0.8%, menthol 0.8%, phenol 0.5%	White petrolatum 92.8%, allantoin 1%
Viractin	Tetracaine 2%	
Vicks Chloraseptic Advanced Formula Sore Throat Spray (Procter & Gamble)	Phenol 1.4%	Colors, flavors, glycerin, purified water, saccharin, sodium
Vicks Chloraseptic Sore Throat Spray, Childrens (Procter & Gamble)	Phenol 0.5%	FD&C blue #1, FD&C red #40, flavor, glycerin, purified water, saccharin sodium, sorbitol
Vicks Chloraseptic Sore Throat Gargle, Menthol (Procter & Gamble)	Phenol 1.4%	D&C green #5, D&C yellow #10, FD&C green #3, flavor, glycerin, water, saccharin sodium
Zilactin Medicated Gel (Zila)	Benzyl alcohol 10%	Tannic acid, hydroxypropyl cellulose filmformer
Zilactin-L Liquid (Zila)	Lidocaine 2.5%	

[a]Carries American Dental Association (ADA) seal indicating safety and efficacy.

[b]For cold sore treatment only.

Reprinted with permission from *Handbook of Nonprescription Drugs*, 10th ed, *Product Updates*, Washington, DC, American Pharmaceutical Association, 1995, 278-81.

ORAL RINSE PRODUCTS

Product/(Manufacturer)	Antiseptic	Other Ingredients
Act[b] (Johnson & Johnson Cons)	Cetylpyridinium chloride, menthol, methyl salicylate	Sodium fluoride 0.05%, edetate calcium disodium, FD&C green #3, FD&C yellow #5, flavor, glycerin, monobasic sodium phosphate, dibasic sodium phosphate, poloxamer 407, polysorbate-20, potassium sorbate, propylene glycol, sodium benzoate, sodium saccharin, water
Act for Kids[ab] (Johnson & Johnson Cons)	Cetylpyridinium chloride	Sodium fluoride 0.05%, D&C red #33, dibasic sodium phosphate, edetate calcium disodium, flavors, glycerin, monobasic sodium phosphate, poloxamer 407, polysorbate-80, propylene glycol, sodium benzoate, sodium saccharin, water
Astring-O-Sol (Mentholatum)	SD alcohol 38-B, 75.6%, methyl salicylate	Water, myrrh extract, zinc chloride, citric acid
Cankaid (EE Dickinson)	Carbamide peroxide 10%	Citric acid monohydrate, sodium citrate dihydrate, edetate disodium
Cepacol Mouthwash/Gargle (JB Williams)	Alcohol 14%, cetylpyridinium chloride 0.05%	Edetate disodium, colors, flavors, glycerin, polysorbate 80, saccharin, sodium B phosphate, sodium phosphate, water
Cepacol Mouthwash/Gargle, Mint (JB Williams)	Alcohol 14.5%, cetylpyridinium chloride 0.5%	Colors, flavors, glucono delta-lactone, glycerin, poloxamer-407, sodium saccharin, sodium gluconate, water
Clear Choice (Bausch & Lomb)	Cetylpyridinium chloride	Glycerin, sodium phosphate, poloxamer 338, flavor, sodium saccharin, domiphen bromide
Fluorigard Anti-Cavity Fluoride Rinse[ab] (Colgate Oral Pharmaceuticals)		Sodium fluoride 0.05%
Gly-Oxide[c] (SmithKline Beecham)	Carbamide peroxide 10%	Citric acid, flavor, glycerin, propylene glycol, sodium stannate, water
Lavoris (Dep)	SD Alcohol 38-B	Water, glycerin, citric acid, poloxamer 407, water, saccharin, clove oil, polysorbate 80, zinc chloride, zinc oxide, sodium hydroxide, flavors, colors
Lavoris Crystal Fresh (Dep)	SD Alcohol 38-B	Purified water, glycerin, poloxamer 407, citric acid, zinc oxide, sodium hydroxide, saccharin, polysorbate 80, flavors
Listerine (Warner-Wellcome)[a] Topical Fluoride Rinse	Alcohol 26.9%, menthol, methyl salicylate, eucalyptol, thymol	
Listerine, Coolmint (Warner-Wellcome)[a]	Alcohol 21.6%, menthol, methyl salicylate, eucalyptol, thymol	Anetmole

(continued)

Product/(Manufacturer)	Antiseptic	Other Ingredients
Listerine, Freshburst[a] (Warner-Wellcome)	Alcohol 21.6%, eucalyptol, menthol, methyl salicylate, thymol	Glycerin, benzoic acid, poloxamer 407, sodium saccharin, sodium citrate, FD&C green #3, D&C yellow #10
Listermint with Fluoride (Warner-Wellcome)	Alcohol 6.65%	Sodium fluoride 0.02%, zinc chloride, glycerin, poloxamer 407, sodium lauryl sulfate, sodium citrate, flavor, sodium saccharin, citric acid, D&C yellow #10, FD&C green #3
Mouth Wash Antiseptic (Goldline Labs)	Alcohol 26.9%, eucalyptol 0.09%, thymol 0.06%, methyl salicylate 0.06%, menthol 0.04%	
MouthKote-FR (Parnell)		Sodium fluoride 0.04%, benzyl alcohol, menthol, water, xylitol, sorbitol, sodium chloride, yerba santa, poloxamer 407, cetylpyridinium chloride, disodium EDTA
Orajel Perioseptic[c] (Del Labs)	Carbamide peroxide 15%	Citric acid, edetate disodium, propylene glycol, purified water, sodium chloride, sodium, flavor, methylparaben saccharin
Oral-B Anti-Cavity Rinse Alcohol Free[b] (Oral-B Labs)	Cetylpyridinium chloride monohydrate	Sodium fluoride 0.05%, water, glycerin, cremophor RH40, flavor, methylparaben, sodium saccharin, sodium benzoate, propylparaben, FD&C blue #1
Oral-B Anti-Cavity Rinse[ab] (Oral-B Labs)		Sodium fluoride 0.05%, water, sodium benzoate, potassium sorbate, sodium saccharin, glycerin, PEG-40, FD&C blue #1, phosphoric acid
Oral-B Anti-Plaque Rinse (Oral-B Labs)	Alcohol 8%, cetylpyridinium chloride	Water, glycerin, sodium saccharin, methylparaben, propylparaben, FD&C blue #1, D&C yellow #10, poloxamer 407
Oral-B Anti-Plaque Rinse Alcohol Free (Oral-B Labs)	Cetylpyridinium chloride 0.05%	Water, glycerin, flavor, polysorbate 20, methylparaben, sodium saccharin, propylparaben, sodium benzoate, FD&C blue #1, D&C yellow #10
Peroxyl Hygienic Dental Rinse[c] (Colgate Oral Pharmaceuticals)	Alcohol 5%, hydrogen peroxide 1.5%	Pluronic F108, sorbitol, sodium saccharin, dye, polysorbate 20, mint flavor
Peroxyl Oral Spot Treatment Gel[c] (Colgate Oral Pharmaceuticals)	Hydrogen Peroxide 1.5%	Mint flavor, ethyl alcohol 5%, pluronic F108, polysorbate 20, sorbitol, sodium saccharin, dye, pluronic F127
Plax Advanced Formula, Clear Peppermint (Pfizer Consumer)	Alcohol 8.5%	Water, glycerin, tetrasodium pyrophosphate, benzoic acid, sodium lauryl sulfate, sodium benzoate, polomer 407, flavor, xanthan gum

(continued)

Product/(Manufacturer)	Antiseptic	Other Ingredients
Plax Advanced Formula, Original Flavor (Pfizer Consumer)	Alcohol 8.5%	Sodium lauryl sulfate, water, glycerin, sodium benzoate, tetrasodium pyrophosphate, benzoic acid, poloxamer 407, saccharin, flavor, xanthan gum
Plax Advanced Formula, Softmint (Pfizer Consumer)	Alcohol 8.5%	Sodium lauryl sulfate, water, glycerin, sodium benzoate, tetrasodium pyrophosphate, benzoic acid, poloxamer 407, saccharin, flavor, xanthan gum, flavor enhancer, FD&C blue #1, FD&C yellow #5
Scope Baking Soda Clean Mint (Procter & Gamble)	SD alcohol 38-F 9.9%, cetylpyridinium chloride, domiphen bromide	Water, sorbitol, sodium bicarbonate, poloxamer 407, polysorbate 80, sodium saccharin, flavor
Scope Original, Mint (Procter & Gamble)	SD alcohol 38-F 18.9%, cetylpyridinium chloride, domiphen bromide	Purified water, glycerin, sodium saccharin, sodium benzoate, flavor, benzoic acid, FD&C blue #1, FD&C yellow #5
Scope, Peppermint (Procter & Gamble)	SD alcohol 38-F 14%, cetylpyridinium chloride, domiphen bromide	Purified water, glycerin, poloxamer 407, sodium saccharin, sodium benzoate, N-ethylmethylcarboxamide, benzoic acid, FD&C blue #1
Tech 2000 (Care-Tech Labs)	Cetylpyridinium chloride	Water, glycerin, poloxamer 407, flavor, FD&C blue #1, FD&C yellow #5, nutritive dextrose or sucrose and/or calcium saccharin
Tom's of Maine Mouthwash (Tom's of Maine)	Menthol	Water, glycerin, aloe vera juice, witch hazel, poloxamer 335, spearmint oil, ascorbic acid
Viadent Oral Rinse (Colgate Oral Pharmaceuticals)	Alcohol 10%	Sanguinaria extract, glycerin, polysorbate 80, flavor, sodium saccharin, poloxamer 237, citric acid, zinc chloride 0.2%

[a]Carries American Dental Association (ADA) seal indicating safety and efficacy.

[b]Topical fluoride rinse

[c]Oral debriding agent/wound cleanser

Reprinted with permission from *Handbook of Nonprescription Drugs*, 10th ed, *Product Updates*, Washington, DC, American Pharmaceutical Association, 1995, 273-5.

SUGAR-FREE LIQUID PHARMACEUTICALS

The following sugar-free liquid preparations are listed by therapeutic category and alphabetically within each category. Please note that product formulations are subject to change by the manufacturer. Some of these products may contain sorbitol, xylitol, or other sweeteners which may be partially metabolized to provide calories.

Analgesics
Acetaminophen Elixir (various)
APAP/APAP Plus
Aspirin/Buffered Aspirin (Medique®)
Bufferin® A/F Nite Time
Children's Anacin-3® Infants Drops
Children's Myapap® Elixir
Children's Panadol® Drops, Liquid, and Chewable Tablets
Children's Tylenol® Chewable Tablets
Conex® Liquid
Conex® With Codeine Liquid
Dolanex® Elixir
Extra Strength Tylenol® PM
Febrol® and Febrol® EX
I-Prin®
Methadone Hydrochloride Intensol
MS-Aid®
Myapap® Drops
No Drowsiness Tylenol®
Pain-Off®
Paregoric USP (Abbott)
Sep-A-Soothe® II
St Joseph® Aspirin-Free Liquid and Drops
Tempra® Chewable Tablets
Tylenol® Drops

Antacids/Antiflatulents
Alcalak®
Aldroxicon®
Almag® Suspension
Aludrox® Suspension
Aluminum Hydroxide Suspension
Calglycine® Tablets
Camalox® Suspension
Citrocarbonate® Granules
Creamalin® Suspension
Delcid®
Di-Gel® Liquid (mint, lemon & orange flavored)
Digestamic®
Dimacid®
Gaviscon® Liquid
Gelusil® II
Gelusil® Liquid
Gelusil® Liquid Flavor Pack
Gelusil-M® Liquid
Kolantyl® Gel
Maalox® Plus Suspension
Maalox® Suspension
Maalox® Therapeutic Concentrate
Magnatril® Suspension
Magnesia and Alumina Oral Suspension USP (Abbott, Phillips Roxane)
Mallamint® Chewable Tablets
Marblen® Suspension and Tablets
Medi-Seltzer®/Plus
Milk of Bismuth
Milk of Magnesia USP
Mylanta® Liquid
Mylanta®-II Liquid
Mylicon® Drops
Nephrox® Suspension
Nutrajel®
Nutramag®
Pepto-Bismol® Liquid and Tablets
Phosphaljel® Suspension
Riopan Plus®

Riopan® Suspension
Silain-Gel® Liquid
Trisogel®
Titralac® Liquid
Titralac® Plus Liquid
WinGel® Liquid and Tablets

Antiasthmatics
Aerolate® Liquid
Alupent® Syrup
Choledyl® Pediatric Syrup
Droxine®
Elixophyllin® Elixir
Elixophyllin®-GG Liquid
Lanophyllin® Elixir
Lixolin® Liquid
Lufyllin® Elixir
Metaprel® Syrup
Mucomyst®-10
Mucomyst®-20
Mudrane® GG Elixir
Neothylline® Elixir
Neothylline® G
Organidin® Solution
Slo-Phyllin® 80 Syrup
Somophyllin® Oral Liquid
Somophyllin®-DF Oral Liquid
Tedral® Elixir and Suspension
Theolair™ 80 Syrup
Theolixir®
Theon® Syrup
Theo-Organidin® Elixir
Theophylline Elixir (Phillips Roxane)

Antidepressants
Sinequan® Oral Concentrate

Antidiarrheals
Corrective Mixture With Paregoric
Diasorb® Liquid and Tablets
Di-Gon® II
Diotame®
Donnagel®
Infantol® Pink
Kalicon® Suspension
Kaolin Mixture With Pectin NF (Abbott)
Kaolin-Pectin Suspension (Phillips Roxane)
Konsyl® Powder
Lomanate®
Lomotil® Liquid
Paregoric USP (various)
Parepectolin® (various)
Pepto-Bismol®
St Joseph® Antidiarrheal

Antiepileptics
Mysoline® Suspension
Paradione® Solution

Antihistamine-Decongestants
Actifed® With Codeine
Actifed® Syrup
Actidil® Syrup
Bromphen® Elixir
Dimetane® Decongestant Elixir
Dimetapp® Elixir
Hay-Febrol® Liquid
Isoclor® Liquid and Capsules
Naldecon® Pediatric Drops and Syrup
Naldecon® Syrup
Novahistine® Elixir
Phenergan® Fortis Syrup
Phenergan® Syrup
Rondec® DM Drops
Ryna® Liquid
S-T® Forte® Liquid

SUGAR-FREE LIQUID PHARMACEUTICALS

Tavist® Syrup
Trind® Liquid
Veltap® Elixir
Vistaril® Oral Suspension

Anti-Infectives
Augmentin® Suspension
Furadantin® Oral Suspension
Furoxone® Suspension
Humatin®
Mandelamine® Suspension/Forte®
Minocin® Suspension
Mycifradin® Sulfate Oral Solution
NegGram® Suspension
Proklar® Suspension
Sulfamethoxazole and Trimethoprim Suspension (Biocraft, Beecham,
    Burroughs Wellcome)
Vibramycin® Syrup

Antiparkinsonism Agents
Artane® Elixir

Antispasmodics
Antrocol® Elixir
Spasmophen® Elixir

Corticosteroids
Decadron® Elixir
Dexamethasone Solution (Roxane)
Dexamethasone Intensol Solution
Pediapred® Oral Liquid

Cough Medicines
Anatuss® With Codeine Syrup
Anatuss® Syrup
Brown Mixture NF (Lannett)
CCP® Caffeine Free
CCP® Cough/Cold Tablets
Cerose-DM®
Chlorgest-HD®
Codagest® Expectorant
Codiclear® DH Syrup
Codimal® DM
Colrex® Compound Elixir
Colrex® Expectorant
Conar® Syrup
Conar® Expectorant Syrup
Conex® Liquid
Conex® With Codeine Syrup
Contac Jr® Liquid
Day-Night Comtrex®
Decoral® Forte®
Dexafed® Cough Syrup
Dimetane®-DC Cough Syrup
Dimetane®-DX Cough Syrup
Entuss® Expectorant Liquid
Fedahist® Expectorant Syrup and Pediatric Drops
Guaificon®-DMS
Histafed® Pediatric Liquid
Hycomine® Syrup and Pediatric Syrup
Lanatuss® Expectorant
Medicon® D
Medi-Synal®
Naldecon-DX® Pediatric Drops and Syrup
Naldecon-DX® Adult Liquid
Non-Drowsy Comtrex®
Noratuss®-II Expectorant and Liquid
Organidin® Solution
Potassium Iodide Solution (various)
Prunicodeine®
Queltuss® Tablets
Robitussin-CF® Liquid
Robitussin® Night Relief Liquid
Rondec®-DM Drops
Rondec®-DM Syrup
Ryna® Liquid

Ryna-C® Liquid
Ryna-CX® Liquid
Scot-Tussin® DM Syrup
Scot-Tussin® Expectorant
Scot-Tussin® DM Cough Chasers
Silexin® Cough Syrup
Sorbutuss®
S-T® Expectorant, SF/D-F
S-T® Forte®, Sugar-Free
Sudodrin®/Sudodrin® Forte®
Terpin® Hydrate With Codeine Elixir (various)
Toclonol® Expectorant
Toclonol® Expectorant With Codeine
Tolu-Sed® Cough Syrup
Tolu-Sed® DM
Tricodene® Liquid
Trind-DM® Liquid
Tuss-Ornade®
Tussar® SF
Tussionex® Extended Release Suspension
Tussi-Organidin® Liquid
Tussirex® Sugar-Free

Dental Preparations and Fluoride Preparations
Cepacol® Mouthwash
Cepastat® Mouthwash and Gargle
Chloraseptic® Mouthwash and Gargle
Fluorigard® Mouthrinse
Fluorinse®
Flura-Drops®
Flura-Loz®
Flura® Tablets
Gel-Kam®
Karigel®
Karigel® N
Luride® Drops
Luride® SF Lozi-Tabs
Luride® 0.25 and 0.5 Lozi-Tabs
Luride® Lozi-Tabs
Pediaflor® Drops
Phos-Flur® Rinse/Supplement
Point-Two® Mouthrinse
Prevident® Disclosing Drops
Thera-Flur® Gel and Drops

Diagnostic Agents
Gastrografin®

Dietary Substitutes
Co-Salt®

Iron Preparations/Blood Modifiers
Amicar® Syrup
Beminal® Stress Plus With Iron
Chel-Iron® Drops
Chel-Iron® Liquid
Geritol® Complete Tablets
Geritonic™ Liquid
Hemo-Vite® Liquid
Iberet® Liquid
Iberet®-500 Liquid
Incremin® With Iron Syrup
Kovitonic® Liquid
Niferex®
Nu-Iron® Elixir
Vita-Plus H® Half Strength, Sugar-Free
Vita-Plus H®, Sugar-Free

Laxatives
Agoral® (plain, marshmallow, and raspberry)
Aromatic Cascara Fluidextract USP
Castor Oil
Castor Oil (flavored)
Castor Oil USP
Colace®, Liquid
Cologel®

SUGAR-FREE LIQUID PHARMACEUTICALS

Disonate™ Liquid
Doxinate® Solution
Emulsoil®
Fiberall® Powder
Haley's MO®
Hydrocil® Instant Powder
Hypaque® Oral Powder
Kondremul®
Kondremul® With Cascara
Kondremul® With Phenolphthalein
Konsyl® Powder
Liqui-Doss®
Magnesium Citrate Solution NF
Metamucil® Instant Mix (lemon-lime or orange)
Metamucil® SF Powder
Milk of Magnesia
Milk of Magnesia/Cascara Suspension
Milk of Magnesia/Mineral Oil Emulsion (various)
Milkinol® Liquid
Mineral Oil (various)
Neoloid® Liquid
Nu-LYTELY®
Phospho-Soda®
Sodium Phosphate & Biphosphate Oral Solution USP (Phillips Roxane)
Zymenol® Emulsion

Potassium Products
Cena-K® Solution
EM-K®-10% Liquid
K-G® Elixir
Kaochlor-Eff® Tablets for Solution
Kaochlor® S-F Solution
Kaon® Elixir (grape and lemon-lime flavor)
Kaon-Cl® 20% Liquid
Kay Ciel® Elixir
Kay Ciel® Powder
Kaylixir®
Klor-Con®/25 Powder
Klor-Con® EF Tablets
Klor-Con® Liquid 20%
Klor-Con® Powder
Klorvess® Effervescent Tablets
Klorvess® Granules
Kolyum® Liquid and Powder
Potachlor® 10% and 20% Liquid
Potasalan® Elixir
Potassine® Liquid
Potassium Chloride Oral Solution USP 5%, 10%, and 20% (various)
Potassium Gluconate Elixir NF
Rum-K® Solution
Tri-K® Liquid
Trikates® Solution

Sedatives-Tranquilizers-Antipsychotics
Butabarbital Sodium Elixir
Butisol Sodium® Elixir
Haldol® Concentrate
Loxitane® C Drops
Mellaril® Concentrate
Serentil® Concentrate
Thorazine® Concentrate

Vitamin Preparations-Nutritionals
Aquasol A® Drops
BioCal® Tablets
Bugs Bunny™ Chewable Tablets
Bugs Bunny™ Plus Iron Chewable Tablets
Bugs Bunny™ With Extra C Chewable Tablets
Bugs Bunny™ Plus Minerals Chewable Tablets
Calciferol™ Drops
Caltrate® 600 Tablets
Ce-Vi-Sol® Drops
Cod Liver Oil (various)
Decagen® Tablets
DHT™ Intensol Solution (Roxane)

Drisdol® in Propylene Glycol
Flintstones™ Complete Chewable Tablets
Flintstones™ With Extra C Chewable Tablets
Flintstones™ Plus Iron Chewable Tablets
Incremin® With Iron Liquid
Kandium® Drops Tablets
Lanoplex® Elixir
Lycolan® Elixir
Oyst-Cal® 500 Tablets
Pediaflor®
PMS® Relief
Poly-Vi-Flor® Drops
Poly-Vi-Flor®/Iron Drops
Poly-Vi-Sol® Drops
Poly-Vi-Sol®/Iron Drops
Posture® Tablets
Spiderman™ Children's Chewable Vitamin Tablets
Spiderman™ Children's Plus Iron Tablets
Theragran® Jr Children's Chewable Tablets
Tri-Vi-Flor® Drops
Tri-Vi-Sol® Drops
Tri-Vi-Sol®/Iron Drops
Vi-Daylin® ADC Drops
Vi-Daylin® ADC/Fluoride Drops
Vi-Daylin® ADC Plus Iron Drops
Vi-Daylin® Drops
Vi-Daylin®/Fluoride Drops
Vi-Daylin® Plus Iron Drops
Vitalize®

Miscellaneous

Altace™ Capsules
Bicitra® Solution
Cibalith-S® Syrup
Colestid® Granules
Dayto® Himbin® Liquid
Digoxin® Elixir (Roxane)
Duvoid®
Glandosane®
Lipomul®
Lithium Citrate Syrup
Nicorette® Chewing Gum
Polycitra®-K Solution
Polycitra®-LC Solution
Tagamet® Liquid

References:

Hill EM, Flaitz CM, and Frost GR, "Sweetener Content of Common Pediatric Oral Liquid Medications," *Am J Hosp Pharm*, 1988, 45(1):135-42.
Kumar A, Rawlings RD, and Beaman DC, "The Mystery Ingredients: Sweeteners, Flavorings, Dyes, and Preservatives in Analgesic/Antipyretic, Antihistamine/Decongestant, Cough and Cold, Antidiarrheal, and Liquid Theophylline Preparations," *Pediatrics*, 1993, 91(5):927-33.
"Sugar Free Products," *Drug Topics Red Book*, 1992, 17-8.

ALLERGIC SKIN REACTIONS TO DRUGS

Skin eruptions are the most common clinically observed form of drug "allergy." Cutaneous manifestations of hypersensitivity may include pruritus, urticaria, and angioedema; maculopapular, morbilliform, or erythematous rashes; erythema multiforme; eczema; erythema nodosum; photosensitivity reactions; and fixed drug eruptions. The most severe drug-related reactions are exfoliative dermatitis and vesiculobullous eruptions such as the Stevens-Johnson syndrome and toxic epidermal necrolysis (Lyell's syndrome). This table lists the incidence of drugs associated with cutaneous manifestations reported in 22,227 consecutive medical inpatients in the Boston Collaborative Drug Surveillance Program.

Drug	Reaction per 1000 Recipients
Sulfamethoxazole and trimethoprim	59
Ampicillin	52
Semisynthetic penicillins	36
Blood, whole human	35
Corticotropin	28
Erythromycin	23
Sulfisoxazole	17
Penicillin G	16
Gentamicin sulfate	16
Practolol	16
Cephalosporins	13
Quinidine	13
Plasma protein fraction	12
Dipyrone	11
Mercurial diuretics	9.5
Nitrofurantoin	9.1
Packed RBCs	8.1
Heparin	7.7
Chloramphenicol	6.8
Trimethobenzamide	6.6
Phenazopyridine	6.5
Methenamine	6.4
Nitrazepam	6.3
Barbiturates	4.7
Glutethimide	4.5
Indomethacin	4.4
Chlordiazepoxide	4.2
Metoclopramide	4.0
Diazepam	3.8
Propoxyphene	3.4
Isoniazid	3.0
Guaifenesin and theophylline	2.9
Nystatin	2.9
Chlorothiazide	2.8
Furosemide	2.6
Isophane insulin suspension	1.3
Phenytoin	1.1
Phytonadione	0.9
Flurazepam	0.5
Chloral hydrate	0.2

Reference:

Patterson R and Anderson J, "Allergic Reactions to Drugs and Biologic Agents," *JAMA*, 1982, 248:2637-45.

COMMON ORAL-FACIAL INFECTIONS
AND ANTIBIOTICS FOR TREATMENT

Pathogens	Infections	Antibiotics
Aerobic gram-positive cocci	Cellulitis	Primary
	Periapical abscess	
	Periodontal abscess	Penicillin VK
and	Acute suppurative pulpitis	
	Oral-nasal fistulas	Alternates
Anaerobes	Pericorinitis	
	Osteitis	Erythromycin
	Osteomyelitis	
	Postsurgical and post-traumatic infection	Clindamycin

CONTROLLED SUBSTANCES

Schedule I = C-I

The drugs and other substances in this schedule have no legal medical uses except research. They have a **high** potential for abuse. They include selected opiates such as heroin, opium derivatives, and hallucinogens.

Schedule II = C-II

The drugs and other substances in this schedule have legal medical uses and a **high** abuse potential which may lead to severe dependence. They include former "Class A" narcotics, amphetamines, barbiturates, and other drugs.

Schedule III = C-III

The drugs and other substances in this schedule have legal medical uses and a **lesser** degree of abuse potential which may lead to **moderate** dependence. They include former "Class B" narcotics and other drugs.

Schedule IV = C-IV

The drugs and other substances in this schedule have legal medial uses and **low** abuse potential which may lead to **moderate** dependence. They include barbiturates, benzodiazepines, propoxyphenes, and other drugs.

Schedule V = C-V

The drugs and other substances in this schedule have legal medical uses and **low** abuse potential which may lead to **moderate** dependence. They include narcotic cough preparations, diarrhea preparations, and other drugs.

Note: These are federal classifications. Your individual state may place a substance into a more restricted category. When this occurs, the more restricted category applies. Consult your state law.

DRUGS ASSOCIATED WITH ADVERSE HEMATOLOGIC EFFECTS

Drug	Red Cell Aplasia	Thrombo-cytopenia	Neutro-penia	Pancyto-penia	Hemolysis
Acetazolamide		+	+	+	
Allopurinol			+		
Amiodarone	+				
Amphotericin B				+	
Amrinone		++			
Asparaginase		+++	+++	+++	++
Barbiturates		+		+	
Benzocaine					++
Captopril			++		+
Carbamazepine		++	+		
Cephalosporins			+		++
Chloramphenicol		+	++	+++	
Chlordiazepoxide			+	+	
Chloroquine		+			
Chlorothiazides		++			
Chlorpropamide	+	++	+	++	+
Chlortetracycline				+	
Chlorthalidone			+		
Cimetidine		+	++	+	
Codeine		+			
Colchicine				+	
Cyclophosphamide		+++	+++	+++	+
Dapsone					+++
Desipramine		++			
Digitalis		+			
Digitoxin		++			
Erythromycin		+			
Estrogen		+		+	
Ethacrynic acid			+		
Fluorouracil		+++	+++	+++	+
Furosemide		+	+		
Gold salts	+	+++	+++	+++	
Heparin		++		+	
Ibuprofen			+		+
Imipramine			++		
Indomethacin		+	++	+	
Isoniazid		+		+	
Isosorbide dinitrate					+
Levodopa					++
Meperidine		+			
Meprobamate		+	+	+	
Methimazole			++		
Methyldopa		++			+++
Methotrexate		+++	+++	+++	++
Methylene blue					+
Metronidazole			+		
Nalidixic acid					+
Naproxen				+	
Nitrofurantoin			++		+
Nitroglycerine		+			
Penicillamine		++	+		
Penicillins		+	++	+	+++
Phenazopyridine					+++
Phenothiazines		+	++	+++	+
Phenylbutazone		+	++	+++	+
Phenytoin		++	++	++	+
Potassium iodide		+			
Prednisone		+			
Primaquine					+++
Procainamide			+		
Procarbazine		+	++	++	+
Propylthiouracil		+	++	+	+
Quinidine		+++	+		
Quinine		+++	+		

MISCELLANEOUS

(continued)

Drug	Red Cell Aplasia	Thrombo- cytopenia	Neutro- penia	Pancyto- penia	Hemolysis
Reserpine		+			
Rifampicin		++	+		+++
Spironolactone			+		
Streptomycin		+		+	
Sulfamethoxazole with trimethoprim			+		
Sulfonamides	+	++	++	++	++
Sulindac	+	+	+	+	
Tetracyclines		+			+
Thioridazine			++		
Tolbutamide		++	+	++	
Triamterene					+
Valproate	+				
Vancomycin			+		

+ = rare or single reports.

++ = occasional reports.

+++ = substantial number of reports.

Adapted from D'Arcy PF and Griffin JP, eds, *Iatrogenic Diseases*, New York, NY: Oxford University Press, 1986, 128-30.

HERBAL MEDICINES

CHEMICAL ANALYSIS OF SELECTED PRODUCTS

Herb		Main Components	Pharmacological Claim
Latin Name	Chinese Name		
Ledebouriella seseloides	Fang feng	Essential oils, alcohol derivatives, organic acids	Dispels "wind", antipyretic, analgesic antibacterial
Potentilla chinensis	Wei ling cai	Vitamin C, tannin, proteins, Ca++ salts	Antibacterial (antituberculosis) muscle relaxant, removes toxic "heats"
Akebia clematidie	Chuan mu tong	Aristolochic acid, akebin saponin	Reduces "heat", diuretic, antibacterial myocardial stimulant
Rehmannia glutinosa	Sheng di huang	Sterol, campesterol, rehmannin, alkaloids	Cardiotonic, diuretic, aids blood coagulation, anti-inflammatory
Paeonia lactiflora	Chi shao	Glycosides (eg, paeoninflorin), essential oils	Increases leucocyte cell count, removes "heat", eliminates blood stasis
Lophatherum gracile	Dan zhu ye	Arundoin, cylindrin, frieldelin	Diuretic, removes "heat", reduces "wind", antipyretic, antibacterial
Dictamnus dasycarpus	Bai xian pi	Dictamnine, alkaloids, psoralen, essential oils	Removes "damp heat", dispels "wind", antifungal
Tribulus terrestris	Ci ji li	Harmane, harmine	Hypotensive, diuretic, suppresses hyperactivity of liver, promotes blood circulation
Glycyrrhiza uralensis	Gan cao	Glycyrrhizin	Strengthens spleen and stomach, removes "heat" and toxins
Schizonepeta tenuifolia	Jing jie sui	Essential oils, D-methone, Di-limonene	Expels "wind", induces diaphoresis, reduces bleeding time

HERBS AND COMMON NATURAL AGENTS

The authors have chosen to include this list of natural products and proposed medical claims. However, due to limited scientific investigation to support these claims, this list is not intended to imply that these claims have been scientifically proven.

PROPOSED MEDICINAL CLAIMS

Herb	Medicinal Claim
Agrimony	Digestive disorders
Alfalfa	Source of carotene (vitamin A); contains natural fluoride
Allspice	General health
Aloe	Healing agent
Angelica root	Diseases of the lungs and heart; distaste for alcoholic beverages
Anise seed	Prevent gas
Arthritis tea	Treat osteoarthritis
Astragalus	Enhance energy reserves; used with ginseng
Barberry bark	Treat halitosis
Basil leaf	Remedy to inhibit vomiting
Bayberry bark	Relieve and prevent varicose veins
Bay leaf	Relieves cramps
Bee pollen	Renewal of enzymes, hormones, vitamins, amino acids, and others
Bergamot herb	Calming effect
Bilberry leaf	Increases night vision, reduces eye fatigue
Birch bark	Treat urinary problems; used for rheumatism
Blackberry leaf	Treat diarrhea
Black cohosh	Relieves menstrual cramps; same effects as estrogen
Blessed thistle (Holy thistle)	Aids circulation to the brain
Blueberry leaf	General medicinal
Blue Cohosh	Regulate menstrual flow; emergency remedy for allergic reactions to bee stings
Blue flag	Useful in the treatment of skin diseases and constipation
Blue violet	Relieves severe headaches
Boldo leaf	Stimulates digestion; treatment of gallstones
Boneset	Treatment of colds and flu
Borage leaf	Reduces high fevers
Bromelain	Fat melting enzyme; stimulates the metabolism
Buchu leaf	Diuretic; treatment of acute and chronic bladder and kidney disorders
Buckthorn bark	Expels worms and will remove warts
Burdock leaf and root	Treatment of severe skin problems and cases of arthritis
Butternut bark	Works well for constipation
Calamus root	General medicinal
Calendula flower	Mending and healing of cuts or wounds
Capsicum (Cayenne)	Normalizes blood pressure; stops bleeding on contact
Caraway seed	Aids digestion
Cascara sagrada bark	Remedies for chronic constipation and gallstones
Catnip	Benefits gas or cramps
Celery leaf and seed	Incontinence of urine
Centaury	Stimulates the salivary gland
Chamomile flower	Excellent for a nervous stomach; relieves cramping associated with the menstrual cycle
Chervil	Stimulant, mild diuretic, lowers blood pressure
Chickweed	Rich in vitamin C and minerals (calcium, magnesium, and potassium)
Chicory root	Effective in disorders of the kidneys, liver, and urinary canal

Herb	Medicinal Claim
Cinnamon bark	Prevents infection and indigestion; helps break down fats during digestion
Cleavers	Treatment of kidney and bladder disorders; useful in obstructions of the urinary organ
Cloves	General medicinal
Colombo root	Colon trouble
Coltsfoot herb and flower	Useful for asthma, bronchitis, and spasmodic cough
Coriander seed	Stomach tonic
Cornsilk	Prostate gland
Cranberry	Bladder or kidney infection
Cubeb berry	Chronic bladder trouble; increases flow of urine
Damiana leaf	Sexual impotency
Dandelion leaf and root	Detoxify poisons in the liver; beneficial in lowering blood pressure
Dill weed	General medicinal
Dong Quai root	Female troubles
Echinacea root	Treat strep throat, lymph glands
Eucalyptus leaf	General medicinal
Elder	General medicinal
Elecampane root	General medicinal
Eyebright herb	General medicinal
Fennel seed	Remedies for gas and acid stomach
Fenugreek seed	Allergies, coughs, digestion, emphysema, headaches, migraines, intestinal inflammation, ulcers, lungs, mucous membranes, and sore throat
Feverfew herb	Migraines; helps reduce inflammation in arthritis joints
Garlic capsules	"Nature's antibiotic"
Gentian	Digestive organs and increase circulation
Ginger root	Remedy for sore throat
Ginkgo biloba	Improves blood circulation to the brain
Ginseng root, Siberian	Resistance against stress; slows the aging process
Goldenseal	Treatment of bladder infections, cankers, mouth sores, mucous membranes, and ulcers
Gota kola	"Memory herb"; nerve tonic
Gravelroot (Queen of the Meadow)	Remedy for stones in the kidney and bladder
Green barley	Excellent antioxidant
Hawthorn	Strengthens and regulates the heart; relieves insomnia
Henna	External use only
Hibiscus flower	Stimulant for the intestines and kidneys
Holy thistle (Blessed thistle)	Remedy for migraine headaches
Hops flower	Insomnia; used to decrease the desire for alcohol
Horehound	Acute or chronic sore throat and coughs
Horsetail (Shavegrass)	Rich in minerals, especially silica; used to develop strong fingernails and hair, good for split ends
Ho shou wu	Rejuvenator
Hydrangea root	Backaches
Hyssop	Asthma
Juniper berry	Kidney ailments
Kava kava root	Induce sleep and help calm nervousness
Kelp	High contents of natural plant iodine, for proper function of the thyroid; high levels of natural calcium, potassium, and magnesium
Lavender flower	Flavor moderator
Lecithin	Break up cholesterol; prevent arteriosclerosis
Licorice root	Mild laxative

(continued)

Herb	Medicinal Claim
Ma-huang	Cleanses respiratory system
Malva flower	Soothes inflammation in the mouth and throat; helpful for earaches
Marjoram	Beneficial for a sour stomach or loss of appetite
Marshmallow leaf	Inflammation
Milk thistle herb	Liver detoxifier
Motherwort	Chest cold, nervousness
Mugwort	Used for rheumatism and gout
Mullein leaf	High in iron, magnesium, and potassium; sinuses; relieves swollen joints
Mustard seed	General medicinal
Myrrh gum	Removes bad breath; sinus problems
Nettle leaf	In combination with seawrack, will bring splendid results in weight loss; remedy for dandruff
Nutmeg	Gas
Oregano leaf	Settles the stomach after meals; helps treat colds
Oregon grape root	Useful in rheumatism
Papaya leaf	Digestive stimulant; contains the enzyme papain
Paprika (sweet)	Stimulates the appetite and gastric secretions
Parsley leaf	High in iron
Passion flower	Mild sedative
Patchouli leaf	Excellent seasoning
Pau d'arco	Protects immune system
Pennyroyal	Relieves high fevers and brings on perspiration
Peppermint leaf	Excellent for headaches
Plantain leaf	Useful for infection, hemorrhoids, and inflammation
Pleurisy root	Break up a cold
Poppy seed blue	Excellent in the making of breads and desserts
Prickly ash bark	Increases circulation
Prince's pine	Diuretic; for rheumatism and chronic kidney problems
Psyllium seed	Lubricant to the intestinal tract
Red clover	Purify the blood
Red raspberry leaf	Eases menstrual cramps
Rhubarb root	Powerful laxative
Rose hips	High content of vitamin C
Safflower	Eliminates buildup of uric and lactic acid in the body, the leading cause of gout
Saffron	Natural digestive aid
Sanicle	Cleansing herb
Sarsaparilla root	Remedy for rheumatism and gout; acts as a diuretic; same effects on the body as the male hormone testosterone
Sassafras leaf and root	Stimulates the action of the liver to clear toxins from the body
Saw palmetto berry	Mucus in the head and nose
Scullcap	Nerve sedative; hangover remedy
Seawrack (Bladderwrack)	Combat obesity
Senna leaf	Splendid laxative
Shepherd's purse	Remedy for diarrhea
Sheep sorrel	Remedy for kidney trouble
Slippery elm bark	Normalize bowel movement; beneficial for hemorrhoids and constipation
Solomon's seal root	Poultice for bruises
Speedwell	Used as a gargle for mouth and throat sores
Spikenard	Skin ailments such as acne, pimples, blackheads, rashes, and general skin problems
Star anise	Promotes appetite and relieves flatulence

(continued)

Herb	Medicinal Claim
St John's wort	Correct irregular menstruation
Strawberry leaf	Prevents diarrhea
Sumac berry and bark	Sores and cankers in the mouth
Summer savory leaf	Treats diarrhea, upset stomach, and sore throat
Thyme leaf	Relief of migraine headaches
Uva-ursi leaf	Digestive stimulant
Valerian root	Promotes sleep
Vervain	Remedy for fevers
White oak bark	Strong astringent
White willow bark	Used for minor aches and pains in the body
Wild alum root	Powerful astringent; used as rinse for sores in mouth and bleeding gums
Wild cherry	Asthma
Wild Oregon grape root	Chronic skin disease
Wild yam root	Helps expel gas
Wintergreen leaf	Valuable for colic and gas in the bowels
Witch hazel bark and leaf	Restores circulation; for stiff joints
Wood betony	Relieves pain in the face and head
Woodruff	Insomnia and hysteria
Wormwood	Aids bruises and sprains
Yarrow root	Unsurpasses for flue and fevers
Yellow dock root	Good in all skin problems
Yerba santa	Bronchial congestion
Yohimbe	Natural aphrodisiac
Yucca root	Reduces inflammation of the joints

POISON INFORMATION CENTERS

Updated from "Poisoning Hotlines," *Emergency Medicine*, 1994, 26:96-102; and American Association of Poison Control Centers, *Vet Hum Toxicol*, 1994, 36:484-6.

*Denotes certified Regional Poison Control Centers by the American Association of Poison Control Centers (October, 1994)

Centers in each state are listed alphabetically by city.

ALABAMA

Regional Poison Control Center*
The Children's Hospital of Alabama
1600 7th Ave, S
Birmingham, AL 35233
(800) 292-6678 (Alabama only)
(205) 933-4050
(205) 939-9201
(205) 939-9202

The Alabama Poison Center*
408-A Paul Bryant Dr
Tuscaloosa, AL 35401
(800) 462-0800 (Alabama only)
(205) 345-0600

ALASKA

Anchorage Poison Control Center
Providence Hospital Pharmacy
3200 Providence Dr
PO Box 6604
Anchorage, AK 99502
(800) 478-3193 (Alaska only)
(907) 261-3193

Fairbanks Poison Control Center
1650 Cowles St
Fairbanks, AK 99701
(907) 456-7182

ARIZONA

Samaritan Regional Poison Center*
Good Samaritan Regional Medical Center
1111 E McDowell Rd
Phoenix, AZ 85006
(602) 253-3334

Arizona Poison and Drug Information Center*
University of Arizona
Arizona Health Sciences Center
1501 N Campbell Ave, Rm 1156
Tucson, AZ 85724
(800) 362-0101 (Arizona only)
(602) 626-6016

ARKANSAS

Arkansas Poison and Drug Information Center
University of Arkansas for Medical Sciences
College of Pharmacy
Slot 522 (internal mailing)
4301 W Markham St
Little Rock, AR 72205
(800) 376-4766 (MDs and hospitals; Arkansas only)
(501) 661-6161
(501) 666-5532 (MDs and hospitals)

CALIFORNIA

Central California Regional Poison Control Center*
Valley Children's Hospital
3151 N Milbrook
Fresno, CA 93703
(209) 445-1222
(800) 346-5922 (Central CA only)

Los Angeles County Regional Drug and Poison Information Center
1200 N State St, Rm 1107A and B
Los Angeles, CA 90033
(800) 777-6476 (Los Angeles, Santa Barbara, and Ventura counties only)
(213) 222-3212
(213) 222-8086 (MDs and hospitals)

Chevron Emergency Information Center
100 Chevron Way
Richmond, CA 94802
(800)231-0623
(510)231-0149

UC, Davis Medical Center Regional Poison Control Center*
2315 Stockton Blvd
Sacramento, CA 95817
(800) 342-9293 (Northern California only)
(916) 734-3692

San Diego Regional Poison Center*
UCSD Medical Center
200 West Arbor Dr
San Diego, CA 92103
(800) 876-4766 (in 619 area code only)
(619) 543-6000

San Francisco Bay Area Regional Poison Control Center*
San Francisco General Hospital
1001 Potrero Ave, Building 80, Rm 230
San Francisco, CA 94110
(800) 523-2222

Santa Clara Valley Regional Poison Center*
Valley Health Center
750 S Bascom Ave, Suite 310
San Jose, CA 95128
(800) 662-9886 (CA only)
(408) 885-6000

COLORADO

Rocky Mountain Poison and Drug Center*
8802 E 9th Ave
Denver, CO 80220
(303) 629-1123

Interstate Centers
The Poison Control Center
Omaha, NE
(800) 955-9119

CONNECTICUT

Connecticut Poison Control Center
University of Connecticut Health Center
263 Farmington Ave
Farmington, CT 06030
(800) 343-2822 (Connecticut only)
(203) 679-3473 (Administration)
(203) 679-4346 (TDD)

DELAWARE

Interstate Centers
The Poison Control Center
Philadelphia, PA
(800) 722-7112

DISTRICT OF COLUMBIA

National Capital Poison Center*
George Washington University Medical Center
3201 New Mexico Ave, NW, Suite 310
Washington, DC 20016
(202) 625-3333
(202) 362-8563 (TTY)

Interstate Centers
Blue Ridge Poison Center
Charlottesville, VA
(800) 451-1428

FLORIDA

Florida Poison Information Center-Jacksonville*
University Medical Center
University of Florida Health Science Center-Jacksonville
655 W 8th St
Jacksonville, FL 32209
(800) 282-3171 (Florida only)
(904) 549-4480 (Jacksonville)

Tallahassee Memorial Regional Medical Center
1300 Miccosukee Road
Tallahassee, FL 32308
(904)681-5411

Florida Poison Information Center and Toxicology Resource Center*
Tampa General Hospital
 PO Box 1289
Tampa, FL 33601
(800) 282-3171 (Florida only)
 (813) 253-4444 (Tampa)

GEORGIA

Georgia Poison Center*
Grady Memorial Hospital
80 Butler St, SE
Box 26066
Atlanta, GA 30335
(800) 282-5846 (Georgia only)
(404) 616-9000

Medical Center of Central Georgia Poison Control Center
777 Hemlock St
Macon, GA 31208
(912) 633-1427

Savannah Regional Poison Control Center
Memorial Medical Center, Inc
4700 Waters Avenue
(912)355-5228
(912)356-8390

HAWAII

Hawaii Poison Center
Kapiolani Women's and Children's Medical Center
1319 Punahou St
 Honolulu, HI 96826
(800) 362-3585 (outer islands of Hawaii only)
 (800) 362-3586
(808) 941-4411

IDAHO

Idaho Poison Center
1055 North Curtis Road
Boise, ID 83706
(800) 632-8000 (Idaho only)
(208) 378-2707
(208) 378-2750

ILLINOIS

Chicago & Northeastern Illinois Regional Poison Control Center
Rush-Presbyterian-St Luke's Medical Center
1653 W Congress Pkwy, Rm 432 Kellogg
Chicago, IL 60612
(800) 942-5969 (Northern Illinois only)
(312) 942-5969

Swedish American Hospital
Rockford, IL
(800) 543-2022

Interstate Centers
Cardinal Glennon Children's Hospital Regional Poison Center
St Louis, MO
(800) 366-8888 (Western Illinois only)

INDIANA

Indiana Poison Center*
Methodist Hospital of Indiana
1701 N Senate Blvd
PO Box 1367
Indianapolis, IN 46206
(800) 382-9097 (Indiana only)
(317) 929-2323

Interstate Centers
Kentucky Regional Poison Center of Kosair Children's Hospital*
Louisville, KY
(502) 589-8222 (Southern Indiana only)

IOWA

Mid-Iowa Club Poison and Drug Information Center
Iowa Methodist Medical Center
1200 Pleasant St
Des Moines, IA 50309
(800) 362-2327 (Iowa only)
(515) 241-6254

Poison Control Center
University of Iowa Hospitals and Clinics
200 Hawkins Dr
Iowa City, IA 52242
(800) 272-6477 (Iowa only)

St Luke's Poison Center
St Luke's Regional Medical Center
2720 Stone Park Blvd
Sioux City, IA 51104
(800) 352-2222 (Western Iowa, Northeastern Nebraska, and Southern South Dakota only)
(712) 277-2222

Interstate Centers
McKennan Hospital Poison Center
Sioux Falls, SD
(800) 843-0505

KANSAS

Mid-America Poison Control Center
University of Kansas Medical Center

3901 Rainbow, Rm B-400
Kansas City, KS 66160
(800) 332-6633 (Kansas only)
(913) 588-6633 (Kansas and Northern Missouri only)

Stormont-Vail Regional Medical Center Emergency Department
1500 West 10th St
Topeka, KS 66604
(913) 354-6106

HCA Wesley Poison Control Center Medical Center
550 N Hillside Ave
Wichita, KS 67214
(316) 688-2277

Interstate Centers
Cardinal Glennon Children's Hospital Regional Poison Control Center
St Louis, MO
(800) 366-8888 (Topeka only)

KENTUCKY

Northern Kentucky Poison Information Center
St Luke Hospital
85 North Grand Avenue
Fort Thomas, KY 41075
(513)872-5111

Kentucky Regional Poison Center of Kosair Children's Hospital*
Medical Towers South, Ste 572
PO Box 35070
Louisville, KY 40232
(800) 722-5725 (Kentucky only)
(502) 629-7275

LOUISIANA

Terrebonne General Medical Center Drug and Poison Information Center
936 East Main St
Houma, LA 70360
(504)873-4067
(504)873-4069

Louisiana Drug and Poison Information Center*
Northeast Louisiana University School of Pharmacy
Sugar Hall
Monroe, LA 71209
(800) 256-9822 (Louisiana only)
(318) 362-5393

MAINE

Maine Poison Control Center
Maine Medical Center
22 Bramhall St
Portland, ME 04102
 (800) 442-6305 (Maine only)
(207) 871-2381 (ER)

MARYLAND

Maryland Poison Center*
University of Maryland School of Pharmacy
20 N Pine St
Baltimore, MD 21201
(800) 492-2414 (Maryland only)
(410) 528-7701

Interstate Centers
National Capital Poison Center*
3201 New Mexico Ave, NW, Suite 310
Washington, DC 20016
(202) 625-3333 (DC suburbs only)
(202) 362-8563 (TTY)

MASSACHUSETTS

Massachusetts Poison Control System*
300 Longwood Ave
Boston, MA 02115
(800) 682-9211
(617) 355-6609 (Administration)
(617) 355-6607 (Massachusetts)
(617) 232-2120 (Boston)

MICHIGAN

Poison Control Center*
Children's Hospital of Michigan
4160 John R, Ste 425
Detroit, MI 48201
(313) 745-5711

Blodgett Regional Poison Center
Blodgett Memorial Medical Center
1840 Wealthy St, SE
Grand Rapids, MI 49506
(800) 632-2727 (616 area code only)
(800) 356-3232 (TTY)
(616) 774-7851 (Administration)

MINNESOTA

Hennepin Regional Poison Center*
Hennepin County Medical Center
701 Park Ave
Minneapolis, MN 55415
(612) 347-3141
(612) 337-7474 (TDD)
(612) 337-7387 (Petline)

Minnesota Regional Poison Center*
St Paul-Ramsey Medical Center
8100 34th Ave, S
Minneapolis, MN 55440-1309
(800) 222-1222 (Minnesota only)
(612) 221-2113

Interstate Centers
McKennan Hospital Poison Center
Sioux Falls, SD
(800) 843-0505

MISSISSIPPI

Forrest General Hospital Poison Center
400 S 28th Ave
PO Box 16389
Hattiesburg, MS 39401
(601) 288-4235

Mississippi Regional Poison Control Center
University Medical Center
2500 N State St
Jackson, MS 39216
(601) 354-7660

MISSOURI

Children's Mercy Hospital
2401 Gillham Rd
Kansas City, MO 64108
(816) 234-3430

Cardinal Glennon Children's Hospital Regional Poison Center*
1465 S Grand Blvd
St Louis, MO 63104
(800) 366-8888
(314) 772-5200

MONTANA

Interstate Centers
Rocky Mountain Poison and Drug Center*
8802 E 9th Ave
Denver, CO 80204
(303) 629-1123

NEBRASKA

The Poison Center*
Childrens Memorial Hospital
8301 Dodge St
Omaha, NE 68114
 (800) 955-9119 (Nebraska and Wyoming only)
(402) 390-5555 (Omaha)

Interstate Centers
McKennan Hospital Poison Center
Sioux Falls, SD
(800) 843-0505

St Luke's Medical Poison Center
2720 Stone Park Blvd
Sioux City, IA 51104
(800) 352-2222 (Northeastern Nebraska only)

NEVADA

Interstate Centers
Rocky Mountain Poison and Drug Center
645 Bannock St
Denver, CO 80204
(800) 446-6179 (Las Vegas only)

Poison Center
Humana Hospital Sunrise
3186 Maryland Pkwy
Las Vegas, NV 89109
(800) 446-6179

Poison Center
Washoe Medical Center
77 Pringle Way
Reno, NV 89520
(702) 328-4144
(702) 328-4100

NEW HAMPSHIRE

New Hampshire Poison Information Center
Dartmouth Hitchcock Memorial Hospital
1 Medical Center Dr
Lebanon, NH 03756
(800) 562-8236 (New Hampshire only)
(603) 650-5000 (New Hampshire and bordering towns in Maine, Massachusetts, and Vermont only)

NEW JERSEY

New Jersey Poison Information and Education System*
Newark Beth Israel Medical Center
201 Lyons Ave
Newark, NJ 07112
(800) 962-1253

Warren Hospital Poison Control Center
185 Roseberry St
Phillipsburg, NJ 08865
(800) 962-1253
(908) 859-6768

NEW MEXICO

New Mexico Poison and Drug Information Center*
University of New Mexico
Health Sciences Library, Rm 125
Albuquerque, NM 87131
(800) 432-6866 (New Mexico only)
(505) 843-2551

NEW YORK

Western New York Regional Poison Control Center
Children's Hospital of Buffalo
219 Bryant St
Buffalo, NY 14222
(800) 888-7655 (New York only)
(716) 878-7654
(716) 878-7655

Long Island Regional Poison Control Center*
Winthrop-University Hospital
259 First St
Mineola, NY 11501
(516) 542-2323
(516) 542-2324
(516) 542-2325
(516) 542-3813

New York City Poison Control Center*
New York City Department of Health
455 First Ave, Rm 123
New York, NY 10016
(212) 340-4494
(212) POISONS (764-7667)
(212) 689-9014 (TDD)

Hudson Valley Regional Poison Center*
Phelps Memorial Hospital Center
701 N Broadway
North Tarrytown, NY 10591
(800) 336-6997 (New York only)
(914) 366-3030

Finger Lakes Regional Poison Center/Life Line
University of Rochester Medical Center
Box 321
601 Elmwood Ave
Rochester, NY 14642
(800) 333-0542
(716) 275-5151
(716) 275-2700 (TTY)

Central New York Regional Poison Control Center
SUNY Health Science Center at University Hospital
750 E Adams St
Syracuse, NY 13210
(800) 252-5655 (New York only)
(315) 476-4766

NORTH CAROLINA

Western NC Poison Control Center
Memorial Mission Hospital
509 Biltmore Ave
Asheville, NC 28801
(800) 542-4225 (North Carolina only)
(704) 255-4490

Carolinas Poison Center*
1012 S Kings Drive, Ste 206
PO Box 32861
Charlotte, NC 28232

(800) 84-TOXIN (848-6946)
(704) 355-4000

Duke University Regional Poison Control Center
Duke University Medical Center
PO Box 3007
Durham, NC 27710
(800) 672-1697 (North Carolina only)
(919) 684-8111

Triad Poison Center at Moses H Cone Memorial Hospital
1200 N Elm St
Greensboro, NC 27401
(800) 953-4001 (Alamance, Forsyth, Guilford, Rockingham, and Randolph counties only)
(910) 574-8105

Catawba Memorial Hospital
Poison Control Center
810 Fairgrove Church Rd, SE
Hickory, NC 28602
(704) 322-6649

NORTH DAKOTA

North Dakota Poison Information Center
St Luke's Hospitals
720 Fourth St, N
Fargo, ND 58122
(800) 732-2200 (North Dakota, Minnesota only)
 (800) 592-1889 (Southeast North Dakota only)
(710) 234-5575 (local)

Interstate Centers
St Luke's Midland Regional Medical Center
Poison Control Center
Aberdeen, SD
(800) 592-1889

OHIO

Akron Regional Poison Center
1 Perkins Square
Akron, OH 44308
(800) 362-9922 (Ohio only)
(330) 379-8562
(330) 379-8446 (TTY)

Cincinnati Drug & Poison Information Center and Regional Poison Control System*
PO Box 670144
Cincinnati, OH 45267-0144
(800) 872-5111 (Ohio only)
(513) 558-5111

Greater Cleveland Poison Control Center
11100 Euclid Ave
Cleveland, OH 44106
 (216) 231-4455

Central Ohio Poison Center*
700 Children's Dr
Columbus, OH 43205-2696
(800) 762-0727 (Ohio only)
(614) 461-2012
(614) 228-1323
(614) 228-2272 (TTY)
(800) 682-7625

Firelands Community Hospital Poison Information Center
1101 Decatur St
Sandusky, OH 44870
(419) 626-7423

Poison and Drug Information Center of Northwest Ohio
Medical College of Ohio
3000 Arlington Ave
Toledo, OH 43614
(800) 589-3897 (Northwestern Ohio and Southeastern Michigan only)
(419) 381-3897

Bethesda Poison Control Center
2951 Maple Ave
Zanesville, OH 43701
(614) 454-4000
(800) 686-4221 (Ohio only)

Interstate Centers
Northwest Regional Poison Center
Erie, PA
(800) 822-3232 (Northeastern Ohio only)

OKLAHOMA

Oklahoma Poison Control Center
Children's Hospital of Oklahoma
940 NE 13 St
Oklahoma City, OK 73104
(800) 522-4611 (Oklahoma only)
(405) 271-5454

OREGON

Oregon Poison Center*
Oregon Health Sciences University
3181 SW Sam Jackson Park Rd, CB550
Portland, OR 97201
(800) 452-7165 (Oregon only)
(503) 494-8968

PENNSYLVANIA

Central Pennsylvania Poison Center*
Milton S Hershey Medical Center
University Dr, PO Box 850
Hershey, PA 17033
(800) 521-6110

St Joseph Hospital and Health Care Center
250 College Ave
PO Box 3509
Lancaster, PA 17604
(717) 299-4546
(717) 291-8314
(717) 291-8425

The Poison Control Center*
3600 Sciences Center, Ste 220
Philadelphia, PA 19104-2641
(215) 386-2100

Pittsburgh Poison Center*
Children's Hospital of Pittsburgh
1 Children's Pl
3705 Fifth Ave
Pittsburgh, PA 15213
(412) 681-6669

Williamsport Hospital Poison Control Center
Williamsport Hospital
777 Rural Avenue
Williamsport, PA 17701
(717) 321-2000

Interstate Centers
Mahoning Valley Poison Center
Youngstown, OH
(800) 426-2348 (Lawrence and Mercer counties only)

RHODE ISLAND

Rhode Island Poison Center*
Rhode Island Hospital
593 Eddy St
Providence, RI 02903
 (401) 277-5727

SOUTH CAROLINA

Palmetto Poison Center
University of South Carolina
College of Pharmacy
Columbia, SC 29208
(800) 922-1117 (South Carolina and central Savannah River area of Georgia only)
(803) 777-1117 (Columbia area only)

SOUTH DAKOTA

Poison Control Center
St Luke's Midland Regional Medical Center
305 S State St
Aberdeen, SD 57401
(800) 592-1889 (South Dakota, North Dakota, Minnesota, and Wyoming only)
(605) 622-5678

McKennan Poison Control Center
McKennon Hospital
800 E 21 St
PO Box 5045
Sioux Falls, SD 57117
(800) 952-0123 (South Dakota only)
(800) 843-0505 (Iowa, Minnesota, and Nebraska only)
(605) 336-3894

Interstate Centers
St Luke's Poison Center
Sioux City, IA
(800) 352-2222 (Southeastern South Dakota only)

TENNESSEE

Southern Poison Center, Inc
847 Monroe Ave, Suite 230
Memphis, TN 38163
(901) 528-6048
(901) 448-6800
(800) 288-9999 (S Tennessee)

Middle Tennessee Regional Poison Center*
The Center for Clinical Toxicology
1161 21st Ave S
501 Oxford House
Nashville, TN 37232-4632
(800) 288-9999
(615) 936-2034 (local)

TEXAS

North Texas Poison Center*
Parkland Hospital
5201 Harry Hines Blvd
PO Box 35926
Dallas, TX 75235
(800) 441-0040 (Northern Texas only)
(214) 590-5000

West Texas Poison Control Center
RE Thomason General Hospital
4815 Alameda Ave
El Paso, TX 79905
(915) 521-7661

Southeast Texas Poison Center*
University of Texas Medical Branch
301 University Ave
Galveston, TX 77550-2780
(409) 765-1420 (Galveston only)
(713) 654-1701 (Houston)

Central Texas Poison Center at Scott and White
2401 S 31st S
Temple, TX 76508
(817) 774-2005

UTAH

Poison Control Center
Humana Hospital Davis Hospital and Medical Center
1600 W Antelope Dr
Layton, UT 84041
(801) 825-4357

Utah Poison Control Center*
410 Chipeta Way, Ste 230
Salt Lake City, UT 84108
(800) 456-7707 (Utah only)
(801) 581-2151

VERMONT

Vermont Poison Center
Medical Center Hospital of Vermont
111 Colchester Ave
Burlington, VT 05401
(802) 658-3456 (Vermont and bordering New York towns only)

Interstate Centers
New Hampshire Poison Information Center
Lebanon, NH
(603) 650-5000

VIRGINIA

Blue Ridge Poison Center*
University of Virginia Health Sciences Center
Blue Ridge Hospital
 Box 67
Charlottesville, VA 22901
(800) 451-1428
(804) 924-5543

Virginia Poison Center
Virginia Commonwealth University
MCV Station, Box 522
Richmond, VA 23298
(800) 552-6337 (Virginia only)
(804) 828-9123 (local Richmond and TDD)

Interstate Centers
National Capital Poison Center* (Northern VA only)
3201 New Mexico Ave, NW, Ste 310
Washington, DC 20016
(202) 625-3333
(202) 362-8563 (TTY)

WASHINGTON

Washington Poison Center*
155 NE 100th St, Ste 400
Seattle, WA 98125
(800) 732-6985
(800) 572-0638 (TDD)
(206) 526-2121
(206) 517-2394

WEST VIRGINIA

West Virginia Poison Center*
West Virginia University
Robert C. Byrd Health Sciences Center/Charleston Division
3110 MacCorkle Ave, SE
Charleston, WV 25304
(800) 642-3625 (West Virginia only)
(304) 348-4211

Poison Center
St Joseph's Hospital Center
19th St and Murdoch Ave
Parkersburg, WV 26101
(304) 424-4222

WISCONSIN

Regional Poison Control Center
University of Wisconsin Hospital and Clinics
600 Highland Ave
Madison, WI 53792
(608) 262-3702 (also TDD)

Milwaukee Poison Center
Children's Hospital of Wisconsin
9000 W Wisconsin Ave
PO Box 1997
Milwaukee, WI 53201
(414) 266-2222

WYOMING

Interstate Centers
The Poison Center
8301 Dodge St
 Omaha, NE 68114
(800) 955-9119 (NE and NY)
(402) 390-5555 (Omaha)

FOREIGN

†Denotes American Association of Poison Control Centers:
Canadian Poison Center members.

CANADA

Alberta

PADIS (Poison and Drug Information Service)†
Foothills Provincial General Hospital
 1403 29th St, NW
Calgary, Alberta T2N 2T9
(403) 670-1414 670-1059

British Columbia

BC Drug and Poison Information Centre†
St Paul's Hospital
1081 Burrard St
Vancouver, BC V6Z 1Y6
(604) 682-5050
(604) 682-2344

Manitoba

Poison Control Centre†
Children's Hospital
685 Bannatyne Ave
Winnipeg, Manitoba R3E OW1
(204) 787-2444

Nova Scotia

Izaak Walton Killan Children's Hospital
PO Box 3070
Halifax, Nova Scotia B3J 3G9
(800) 565-8161 (Prince Edward Island)
(902) 428-8161 (Nova Scotia)

Ontario

Provincial Regional Poison Control Centre
Children's Hospital
Eastern Ontario
401 Smyth Rd
Ottawa, Ontario K1H 8L1
(800) 267-1373
(613) 737-1100

Ontario Regional Poison Centre†
Hospital for Sick Children
555 University Ave
Toronto, Ontario M5G 1X8
(800) 263-9017
(416) 813-5823
(416) 813-5900

Quebec

Quebec Poison Control Center†
Centre Hospitalier de l'Universite Laval
2705 Boulevard Laurier; J-782
Sainte-Foy Quebec
Canada GIV 4G2
(418) 656-8090
(418) 654-2731

COSTA RICA

Centro Nacional de Control de Intoxicaciones
Hospital Nacional de Ninos
"Dr Carlos Saenz Herrera"
Apartado 1654
San Jose, Costa Rica
(506) 23-10-28

MEXICO

Centro Panamerico de Ecologia Humana y
Salud — Toxicologia
Rancho Guadalupe
Metepec, Edo de Mexico
Apartado 37-473
06696 Mexico, DF
52-(91-721)
6-44-04
6-43-44

PUERTO RICO

University of Puerto Rico
College of Pharmacy
GPO Box 5067
San Juan, Puerto Rico
(809) 758-2525 ext 1516
(809) 763-0196

PRESCRIPTION WRITING

Doctor's Name
Address
Phone Number

Patient's Name/Date

Patient's Address/Age

Rx

    Drug Name/Dosage Size

    Disp: Number of tablets, capsules, ounces to be dispensed (roman numerals added as precaution for abused drugs)

    Sig: Direction on how drug is to be taken

Doctor's signature

State license number

DEA number (if required)

PRESCRIPTION REQUIREMENTS

1. Date

2. Full name and address of patient

3. Name and address of prescriber

4. Signature of prescriber

If Class II drug, Drug Enforcement Agency (DEA) number necessary.

If Class II and Class III narcotic, a triplicate prescription form (in the state of California) is necessary and it must be handwritten by the prescriber.

COMMON ABBREVIATIONS

i, ii, iii	one, two, three
q	every (as in 'every' 6 hours)
d	day
h	hour
prn	as needed
b	twice
t	three
q	four

Example: tid = 3 times/day; q8h = every 8 hours
Note: IF IN DOUBT, WRITE IT OUT!

PRESCRIPTIONS FOR THE PROPHYLACTIC ANTIBIOTIC COVERAGE FOR THE PREVENTION OF BACTERIAL ENDOCARDITIS

Current American Heart Association
Dec, 1990 Guidelines

Premedication requirements for patients with valvular heart disease or congenital cardiac defects; if in doubt have patient consult their physician to need.

STANDARD REGIMEN

Rx

Amoxicillin 500 mg

Disp: 9 capsules

Sig: Take 6 capsules (3 g) 1 hour before procedure; then 3 capsules (1.5 g) 6 hours after initial dose

STANDARD REGIMEN FOR PATIENTS ALLERGIC TO AMOXICILLIN/ PENICILLIN

Rx

Erythromycin ethylsuccinate 400 mg

Disp: 3 tablets

Sig: Take 2 tablets (800 mg) 2 hours before procedure; then 1 tablet (400 mg) 6 hours after initial dose

OR

Rx

Erythromycin stearate 500 mg

Disp: 3 tablets

Sig: Take 2 tablets (1 g) 2 hours before procedure; then 1 tablet (500 mg) 6 hours after initial dose

OR

Rx

Clindamycin 150 mg

Disp: 3 capsules

Sig: Take 2 capsules (300 mg) 1 hour before procedure; then 1 capsule (150 mg) 6 hours after initial dose

Patients Unable to Take Oral Medication

Ampicillin — 2 g I.V. or I.M. 30 minutes before procedure; then 1 g I.V. or I.M.

OR

1.5 g of amoxicillin oral, 6 hours after initial dose

Patients Allergic to Ampicillin, Amoxicillin, Penicillin

Clindamycin — 300 mg I.V. 30 minutes before procedure; then 150 mg I.V. or oral 6 hours after initial dose

Vancomycin — 1 g I.V. given over 1 hour starting 1 hour before procedure; no repeat dose necessary

Patients at High Risk and NOT Candidates for Standard Regimen

Ampicillin, Gentamicin, and Amoxicillin	I.M. or I.V. 2 g ampicillin and 1.5 mg/kg (maximum: 80 mg) gentamicin 30 minutes before procedure, and 1.5 g amoxicillin 6 hours after **OR** repeat parenteral dose 8 hours after

Patients Allergic to Ampicillin, Amoxicillin, Penicillin

Vancomycin	1 g I.V. given over 1 hour starting 1 hour before procedure; no repeat dose needed

SAFE WRITING PRACTICES

Health professionals and their support personnel frequently produce handwritten copies of information they see in print; therefore, such information is subjected to even greater possibilities for error or misinterpretation on the part of others. Thus, particular care must be given to how drug names and strengths are expressed when creating written healthcare documents.

The following are a few examples of safe writing rules suggested by the Institute for Safe Medication Practices, Inc.*

1. There should be a space between a number and its units as it is easier to read. There should be no periods after the abbreviations mg or mL.

Correct	Incorrect
10 mg	10mg
100 mg	100mg

2. Never place a decimal and a zero after a whole number (2 mg is correct and 2.0 mg is incorrect). If the decimal point is not seen because it falls on a line or because individuals are working from copies where the decimal point is not seen, this causes a tenfold overdose.

3. Just the opposite is true for numbers less than one. Always place a zero before a naked decimal (0.5 mL is correct, .5 mL is **in** correct).

4. Never abbreviate the word unit. The handwritten U or u, looks like a 0 (zero) and may cause a tenfold overdose error to be made.

5. Q.D. is not a safe abbreviation for once daily, as when the Q is followed by a sloppy dot, it looks like QID which means 4 times daily.

6. O.D. is not a safe abbreviation for once daily, as it is properly interpreted as meaning "right eye" and has caused liquid medications such as saturated solution of potassium iodide and Lugol's solution to be administered incorrectly. There is no safe abbreviation for once daily. It must be written out in full.

7. Do not use chemical names such as 6-mercaptopurine or 6-thioguanine, as sixfold overdoses have been given when these were not recognized as chemical names. The proper names of these drugs are mercaptopurine or thioguanine.

8. Do not abbreviate drug names (5FC, 6MP, 5-ASA, MTX, HCTZ CPZ, PBZ, etc) as they are misinterpreted and cause error.

9. Do not use the apothecary system or symbols.

10. Do not abbreviate microgram as μg; instead use mcg as there is less likelihood of misinterpretation.

11. When writing an outpatient prescription, write a complete prescription. A complete prescription can prevent the prescriber, the pharmacist, and/or the patient from making a mistake and can eliminate the need for further clarification.

    The legible prescriptions should contain:

    a. patient's full name
    b. for pediatric or geriatric patients: their age (or weight where applicable)
    c. drug name, dosage form and strength; if a drug is new or rarely prescribed, print this information
    d. number or amount to be dispensed
    e. complete instructions for the patient, including the purpose of the medication
    f. when there are recognized contraindications for a prescribed drug, indicate to the pharmacist that you are aware of this fact (ie, when prescribing a potassium salt for a patient receiving an ACE inhibitor, write "K serum leveling being monitored")

*From "Safe Writing" by Davis NM, PharmD and Cohen MR, MS, Lecturers and Consultants for Safe Medication Practices, 1143 Wright Drive, Huntingdon Valley, PA 19006. Phone: (215) 947-7566.

TOP 200 PRESCRIBED DRUGS IN 1995

Brand Name	Generic Name
1. Premarin Tabs	Conjugated estrogens
2. Trimox	Co-trimoxazole
3. Synthroid	Levothyroxine
4. Amoxil	Amoxicillin
5. Zantac	Ranitidine
6. Lanoxin	Digoxin
7. Procardia XL	Nifedipine
8. Vasotec	Enalapril
9. Prozac	Fluoxetine
10. Proventil (inhaler)	Albuterol
11. Cardizem CD	Diltiazem
12. Hydrocodone w/APAP	Hydrocodone w/APAP
13. Zoloft	Sertraline
14. Coumadin Tabs	Warfarin
15. Augmentin	Amoxicillin & Clavulanate acid
16. Amoxicillin	Amoxicillin (Biocraft)
17. Triamterene w/HCTZ	Triamterene/HCTZ
18. Zestril	Lisinopril
19. APAP w/Codeine	APAP w/Codeine
20. Cipro	Ciprofloxacin
21. Propoxyphene N w/APAP	Propoxyphene N w/APAP
22. Biaxin	Clarithromycin
23. Furosemide Oral	Furosemide
24. Veetids	Penicillin
25. Ventolin (inhaler)	Albuterol
26. Prilosec	Omeprazole
27. Norvasc	Amlodipine
28. Claritin	Loratadine
29. Mevacor	Lovastatin
30. Ortho-Novum 7/7/7	Ethinyl estradiol & Norethindrone
31. Capoten	Captopril
32. Provera	Medroxyprogesterone
33. Paxil	Paroxetine
34. IBU	Ibuprofen
35. Cephalexin	Cephalexin (Biocraft)
36. Humulin N	Human insulin
37. Hytrin	Terazosin
38. Alprazolam	Alprazolam
39. Dilantin Kapseals	Phenytoin
40. APAP w/Codeine	APAP w/Codeine
41. Pepcid	Famotidine
42. Triphasil	Ethinyl estradiol & Levonorgestrel
43. Seldane	Terfenadine
44. Relafen	Nabumetone
45. Zocor	Simvastatin
46. K-Dur 20	Potassium chloride
47. Amitriptyline	Amitriptyline
48. Klonopin	Clonazepam
49. Cefaclor	Cefaclor
50. Zovirax	Acyclovir
51. Zithromax	Azithromycin
52. Estrace Tabs	Estradiol
53. Vancenase AQ	Beclomethasone dipropionate
54. Prinivil	Lisinopril
55. Ceftin	Cefuroxime axetil

(continued)

Brand Name	Generic Name
56. Cephalexin	Cephalexin
57. Ery-Tab	Erythromycin
58. Pravachol	Pravastatin
59. Ortho-Cept	Ethinyl estradiol & Desogestrel
60. Trimethoprim/sulfamethoxazole	Trimethoprim/sulfamethoxazole (Biocraft)
61. Hydrocodone w/APAP	Hydrocodone w/APAP
62. Ambien	Zolpidem
63. Estraderm	Estradiol
64. Levoxyl	Levothyroxine
65. Axid	Nizatidine
66. Lodine	Etodolac
67. Atenolol	Atenolol
68. Cefzil	Cefprozil
69. Atrovent	Ipratropium bromide
70. Xanax	Alprazolam
71. Calan SR	Verapamil
72. Glyburide	Glyburide (Copley)
73. Deltasone	Prednisone
74. Roxicet	Oxycodone w/APAP
75. Nitrostat	Nitroglycerine
76. Dyazide	Triamterene/HCTZ
77. Propoxyphene N w/APAP	Propoxyphene N w/APAP
78. Lotensin	Benazepril
79. Lorazepam	Lorazepam
80. Voltaren	Diclofenac
81. Daypro	Oxaprozin
82. Duricef	Cefadroxil
83. Verapamil SR	Verapamil
84. Propulsid	Cisapride
85. Lotrisone	Betamethasone dipropionate & Clotrimazole
86. Desogen	Ethinyl estradiol and Desogestrel
87. Prednisone Oral	Prednisone
88. Lasix Oral	Furosemide
89. Cimetidine	Cimetidine
90. Insulin syringe	
91. Humulin 70/30	Human insulin
92. Azmacort	Triamcinolone
93. Accupril	Quinapril
94. Hydrochlorothiazide	Hydrochlorothiazide
95. Cycrin	Medroxyprogesterone
96. Buspar	Buspirone
97. Medroxyprogesterone tablet	Medroxyprogesterone
98. Claritin D	Loratadine
99. Trimethoprim/sulfamethoxazole	Trimethoprim/sulfamethoxazole (Mutual Ph)
100. Lorazepam	Lorazepam
101. Naproxen	Naproxen
102. Nizoral Topical	Ketoconazole
103. Beconase AQ	Beclomethasone dipropionate
104. Darvocet N 100	Propoxyphene Nap w/APAP
105. Lo/Ovral 28	Ethinyl estradiol & Norgestrel
106. Seldane-D	Terfenadine/Pseudoephedrine
107. Retin-A	Tretinoin
108. Methylphenidate	Methylphenidate
109. Lorabid	Loracarbef
110. Alprazolam	Alprazolam
111. Trental	Pentoxifylline

(continued)

Brand Name	Generic Name
112. Adalat CC	Nifedipine
113. Ultram	Tramadol
114. Neomycin/Polymyxin/Hydrocortisone	Neomycin/Polymyxin/Hydrocortisone
115. Klor-Con	Potassium chloride
116. Atenolol	Atenolol
117. Potassium Chloride	Potassium Chloride
118. Timoptic	Timolol
119. Tri-Levlen	Ethinyl Estradiol & Levonorgestrel
120. Diflucan	Fluconazole
121. Glucotrol XL	Glipizide
122. Glynase Prestab	Glyburide
123. Ortho-Novum 1/35	Ethinyl estradiol & Norethindrone
124. Suprax	Cefixime
125. Lescol	Fluvastatin
126. Cardura	Doxazosin
127. Tegretol	Carbamazepine
128. Glipizide	Glipizide
129. Depakote	Divalproex
130. Lopressor	Metoprolol
131. Gemfibrozil	Gemfibrozil
132. Macrobid	Macrodantin
133. Diazepam	Diazepam
134. Ceclor	Cefaclor
135. Children's Motrin	Ibuprofen
136. Cyclobenzaprine	Cyclobenzaprine (Mylan)
137. Diabeta	Glyburide
138. Nitro-Dur	Nitroglycerine
139. Toradol Oral	Ketorolac
140. Doxycycline	Doxycycline (Zenith)
141. Albuterol Oral Liquid	Albuterol
142. Tenormin	Atenolol
143. Micronase	Glyburide
144. Cephalexin	Cephalexin
145. Imitrex	Sumatriptan
146. Propacet 100	Propoxyphene Nap w/APAP
147. Lorcet-10	Hydrocodone and acetaminophen
148. Lozol	Indapamide
149. Temazepam	Temazepam
150. Phenergan Supp	Promethazine
151. Verelan	Verapamil
152. Metoprolol	Metoprolol (Mylan)
153. Metoprolol	Metoprolol (CibaGeneva)
154. Altace	Ramipril
155. Humulin R	Human insulin
156. Terazol 7	Terconazole
157. Theo-Dur	Theophylline
158. Albuterol (neb solution)	Albuterol
159. Methylprednisolone tablet	Methylprednisolone
160. Dilacor XR	Diltiazem
161. Bactroban	Mupirocin
162. Erythrocin stearate	Erythromycin
163. Nortriptyline	Nortriptyline
164. Ritalin	Methylphenidate
165. Atenolol	Atenolol
166. Floxin	Ofloxacin

(continued)

Brand Name	Generic Name
167. Glucotrol	Glipizide
168. Demulen 1/35	Ethinyl estradiol & Ethynodiol diacetate
169. Cyclobenzaprine	Cyclobenzaprine (Schein)
170. Serevent	Salmeterol
171. Vanceril	Betamethasone
172. Dicyclomine	Dicyclomine
173. Hismanal	Astemizole
174. Loestrin FE	Ethinyl estradiol & Norethindrone w/FE
175. Cotrim	Co-trimoxazole
176. Sumycin	Tetracycline
177. Children's Advil	Ibuprofen
178. Vicodin	Hydrocodone and Acetaminophen
179. Carafate	Sucralfate
180. Effexor	Venlafaxine
181. Guaifenesin and Phenylpropanolamine	Guaifenesin and Phenylpropanolamine
182. Amoxicillin	Amoxicillin (Warn-Chil)
183. Glyburide	Glyburide (Greenstone)
184. Promethazine/Codeine	Promethazine/Codeine
185. Penicillin VK	Penicillin VK
186. Doxycycline	Doxycycline (Mutual Ph)
187. Erythromycin base	Erythromycin base
188. Toprol XL	Metoprolol
189. Principen	Ampicillin
190. Carisoprodol	N-isopropyl meprobamate
191. Tylenol w/codeine	APAP w/Codeine
192. Cephalexin	Cephalexin (Barr)
193. One Touch Test Strip	
194. Elocon	Mometasone furoate
195. Nasacort	Triamcinolone
196. Lorcet Plus	Hydrocodone w/APAP
197. Fiorinal w/Codeine	Butalbital w/Codeine
198. Valium	Diazepam
199. Oruvail	Ketoprofen
200. PCE Dispertab	Erythromycin

VASOCONSTRICTOR INTERACTIONS WITH ANTIDEPRESSANTS

Antidepressant	Effects With Epinephrine, Norepinephrine, Levonordefrin	Contraindicated	Recommendation
Bupropion (Wellbutrin®)	No adverse interactions reported	No	No precautions appear to be necessary
Fluoxetine (Prozac®)	No adverse interactions reported	No	No precautions appear to be necessary
Maprotiline (Ludiomil®)	Potential for inc pressor response	No	Same precaution as TCAs since it has similar pharmacology
Paroxetine (Paxil®)	No adverse interactions reported	No	No precautions appear to be necessary
Sertraline (Zoloft®)	No adverse interactions reported	No	No precautions appear to be necessary
TCAs	epi = inc pressor response; cardiac dysrhythmias; ne = inc pressor response; levo = inc pressor response	No	Potentially dangerous; use minimal amounts with caution in local anesthetics
Trazodone (Desyrel®)	No adverse interactions reported	No	No precautions appear to be necessary
Venlafaxine (Effexor®)	No adverse interactions reported	No	No precautions appear to be necessary

Reference: Wynn RL, "Antidepressant Medications", *Gen Dent*, 1992, 40(3):192-7.

NEW DRUGS INTRODUCED OR APPROVED BY THE FDA IN 1996

Brand Name	Generic Name	Use
Allegra®	fexofenadine	Nonsedating antihistamine
Albenza®	albendazole (Orphan Drug)	Antilarval
Avonex®	interferon beta 1b	Multiple sclerosis
Buphenyl®	sodium phenylbutyrate (Orphan Drug)	Adjunctive therapy in patients with urea cycle disorders
Camptosar®	irinotecan hydrochloride	Colon carcinoma
Cerebyx®	fosphenytoin sodium	Epilepsy
Combivent®	ipratropium & albuterol	Chronic obstructive pulmonary disease (COPD)
Crixivan®	indinavir sulfate	Antiviral for HIV infections
DaunoXome®	daunorubicin citrate liposome	Kaposi's sarcoma (HIV associated)
Differin®	adapalene	Acne vulgaris
Gemzar®	gemcitabine	Pancreatic carcinoma
Humalog®	insulin lispro (rDNA origin)	Diabetes mellitus
Hycamtin®	topotecan	Ovarian carcinoma
Mavik®	trandolapril	Hypertension
Maxipime®	cefepime	Third generation cephalosporin
Merrem®	meropenem	Broad-spectrum antibiotic
Norvir®	ritonavir	Antiviral for HIV infections
Redux®	dexfenfluramine	Management of obesity
Remeron®	mirtazapine	Depression
Sular™	nisoldipine	Hypertension
Taxotere®	docetaxel	Breast carcinoma
Tritec®	ranitidine bismuth citrate	Duodenal ulcer
Ultiva®	remifentanil	Analgesic
Vesanoid®	tretinoin (oral)	Leukemias
Viramune®	nevirapine	Antiviral used in combination with other antivirals for HIV
Vistide®	cidofovir	CMV retinitis in AIDS patients
Xalatan®	latanoprost	Glaucoma
Zyprexa®	olanzapine	Psychosis
Zyrtec™	cetirizine hydrochloride	Antihistamine

PENDING DRUGS OR DRUGS IN CLINICAL TRIALS

Alredase®	tolrestat	Controlling late complications of diabetes
Arkin-Z®	vesnarinone	Congestive heart failure agent
Astelin®	azelastine hydrochloride	Inhalation antihistamine
Baypress®	nitrendipine	Calcium channel blocker for hypertension
Berotec®	fenoterol	Beta-2 agonist for asthma
Catatrol®	viloxazine	Bicyclic antidepressant
Cipralan®	cifeline succinate	Antiarrhythmic agent
Combivent®	albuterol & ipratropium	Bronchodilator for asthma
Decabid®	indecainide hydrochloride	Antiarrhythmic agent
Delaprem®	hexoprenaline sulfate	Tocolytic agent
Denavir®	penciclovir	Herpes labialis
Dirame®	propiram	Opioid analgesic
DurAct®	bromfenac sodium	Non-narcotic analgesic
Eldisine®	vindesine sulfate	Antineoplastic

Brand Name	Generic Name	Use
Elmiron®	pentosan polysulfate sodium	Relief of interstitial pain
Enable®	tenidap sodium	Arthritis
Fareston®	toremifene citrate	Antiestrogen for breast cancer
Freedox®	triliazad mesylate	Prevents progressive neuronal degeneration
Frisium®	clobazam	Benzodiazepine
Gastrozepine®	pirenzepine	Antiulcer drug
Inhibace®	cilazapril	ACE inhibitor
Isoprinosine®	inosiplex	Immunomodulating drug
Lacipil®	lacidipine	Hypertension
Maxicam®	isoxicam	NSAID
Mentane®	velnacrine	Alzheimer's disease agent
Mentax®	butenafine hydrochloride	Athlete's foot
Micturin®	terodiline hydrochloride	Agent for urinary incontinence
Mogadon®	nitrazepam	Benzodiazepine
Motilium®	domperidone	Antiemetic
Napa®	acecainide	Antiarrhythmic agent
Naropin®	ropivacaine hydrochloride	Local anesthesia
Nilandron®	nilutamide	Prostate cancer
Pindac®	pinacidil	Antihypertensive
ProAmatine®	midodrine	Orthostatic hypotension
Prothiaden®	dothiepin hydrochloride	Tricyclic antidepressant
Reactine®	cetirizine	Antihistamine
Rimadyl®	caprofen	NSAID
Roxiam®	remoxipride	Antipsychotic agent
Sabril®	vigabatrin	Anticonvulsant
Selecor®	celiprolol hydrochloride	Beta-adrenergic blocker
Soriatane®	acitretin	Recalcitrant psoriasis
Spexil®	trospectomycin	Antibiotic, a spectinomycin analog
Targocoid®	teicoplanin	Antibiotic, similar to vancomycin
Tarka®	trandolapril & verapamil	Hypertension
Teczem®	diltiazem & enalapril	Hypertension
Tiamate®	diltiazem	Hypertension
Topamax®	topiramate	Epilepsy
Unicard®	dilevalol	Beta-adrenergic blocker
Zaditen®	ketotifen	Antiasthmatic
Zanaflex®	tizanidine hydrochloride	Multiple sclerosis

THERAPEUTIC CATEGORY INDEX

ABORTIFACIENT
Carboprost Tromethamine 156

ACNE PRODUCTS
Adapalene 25
Benzoyl Peroxide. 104
Benzoyl Peroxide and Hydrocortisone. 105
Clindamycin 214
Erythromycin and Benzoyl Peroxide 323
Erythromycin, Topical 324
Isotretinoin 475
Sulfur and Sodium Sulfacetamide .813
Tetracycline 829
Tretinoin 862

ADJUVANT THERAPY, PENICILLIN LEVEL PROLONGATION
Probenecid 724

ADRENAL CORTICOSTEROID
Corticotropin 233
Cortisone Acetate 233
Cosyntropin 235
Methylprednisolone 569
Paramethasone Acetate 659
Prednisolone 718
Prednisone 719

ADRENERGIC AGONIST AGENT
Albuterol 27
Amrinone Lactate. 65
Dobutamine Hydrochloride 294
Ephedrine Sulfate 310
Epinephrine 311
Epinephrine (Dental) 313
Ethylnorepinephrine Hydrochloride 345
Fenfluramine Hydrochloride 355
Isoetharine 470
Isoproterenol 472
Isoproterenol and Phenylephrine .473
Metaproterenol Sulfate 550
Oxymetazoline Hydrochloride 649
Phenylephrine Hydrochloride 685
Phenylpropanolamine Hydrochloride 687
Pseudoephedrine. 749
Pseudoephedrine and Dextromethorphan 750
Pseudoephedrine and Ibuprofen .750
Ritodrine Hydrochloride 773
Salmeterol Xinafoate 778
Terbutaline Sulfate 822
Tetrahydrozoline Hydrochloride 831
Xylometazoline Hydrochloride 905

ADRENERGIC AGONIST AGENT, OPHTHALMIC
Dipivefrin 290
Epinephryl Borate 315
Naphazoline Hydrochloride 605
Phenylephrine Hydrochloride 685
Tetrahydrozoline Hydrochloride 831

ADRENERGIC BLOCKING AGENT
Ergotamine 319
Trimethaphan Camsylate 873

ALDEHYDE DEHYDROGENASE INHIBITOR AGENT
Disulfiram. 293

ALKALINIZING AGENT, ORAL
Potassium Citrate 710

ALKALINIZING AGENT, PARENTERAL
Tromethamine 880

ALPHA-ADRENERGIC BLOCKING AGENT, OPHTHALMIC
Dapiprazole Hydrochloride. 251

ALPHA-ADRENERGIC BLOCKING AGENT, ORAL
Phenoxybenzamine Hydrochloride. 682

ALPHA-ADRENERGIC BLOCKING AGENT, PARENTERAL
Phentolamine Mesylate 684
Tolazoline Hydrochloride 852

ALPHA-ADRENERGIC BLOCKERS - PERIPHERAL-ACTING (ALPHA₁-BLOCKERS)

Clonidine 221
Doxazosin 298
Guanabenz Acetate 411
Guanadrel Sulfate 411
Guanethidine Sulfate 412
Guanfacine Hydrochloride 413
Methyldopa 566
Prazosin Hydrochloride 717
Reserpine 765
Terazosin 821

ALPHA-ADRENERGIC INHIBITORS, CENTRAL

Phentolamine Mesylate 684

ALPHA-2-ADRENERGIC AGONIST AGENT, OPHTHALMIC

Apraclonidine Hydrochloride 72
Brimonidine Tartrate 121

ALPHA-/BETA- ADRENERGIC BLOCKER

Labetalol Hydrochloride 486

ALPHA-GLUCOSIDASE INHIBITOR

Acarbose 12

AMEBICIDE

Chloroquine Phosphate 187
Iodoquinol 466
Metronidazole 576
Paromomycin Sulfate 660

5-AMINOSALICYLIC ACID DERIVATIVE

Mesalamine 546
Olsalazine Sodium 635
Sulfasalazine 810

AMMONIUM DETOXICANT

Lactulose 488
Neomycin Sulfate 611

AMPHETAMINE

Amphetamine Sulfate 59
Dextroamphetamine Sulfate 265
Methamphetamine Hydrochloride 553

AMYOTROPHIC LATERAL SCLEROSIS (ALS) AGENT

Riluzole 771

ANABOLIC STEROID

Oxymetholone 650
Stanozolol 799

ANALGESIC, NARCOTIC

Acetaminophen and Codeine 15
Alfentanil Hydrochloride 31
Aspirin and Codeine 80
Belladonna and Opium 98
Buprenorphine Hydrochloride 129
Butalbital Compound and Codeine 134
Butorphanol Tartrate 135
Codeine 227
Dezocine 267
Dihydrocodeine, Acetaminophen, and Aspirin 281
Fentanyl 357
Hydrocodone and Acetaminophen 431
Hydrocodone and Aspirin 433
Hydromorphone Hydrochloride 438
Levomethadyl Acetate Hydrochloride 496
Levorphanol Tartrate 497
Meperidine and Promethazine 538
Meperidine Hydrochloride 539
Methadone Hydrochloride 552
Morphine Sulfate 590
Nalbuphine Hydrochloride 600
Opium Alkaloids 638
Opium Tincture 639
Oxycodone and Acetaminophen 646
Oxycodone and Aspirin 647
Oxymorphone Hydrochloride 651
Paregoric 659
Pentazocine 671
Pentazocine Compound 672

(Continued)

THERAPEUTIC CATEGORY INDEX

ANALGESIC, NARCOTIC *(Continued)*

Propoxyphene 740
Propoxyphene and Acetaminophen 741
Propoxyphene and Aspirin 742
Remifentanil 765
Sufentanil Citrate 805

ANALGESIC, NON-NARCOTIC

Acetaminophen 14
Acetaminophen and Dextromethorphan 16
Acetaminophen and Diphenhydramine 16
Acetaminophen and Isometheptene Mucate .16
Acetaminophen and Phenyltoloxamine 17
Acetaminophen, Aspirin, and Caffeine 17
Acetaminophen, Chlorpheniramine, and Pseudoephedrine 17
Aspirin 78
Butalbital Compound 133
Chlorpheniramine and Acetaminophen 190
Chlorpheniramine, Phenylpropanolamine, and Acetaminophen 194
Choline Magnesium Salicylate 202
Choline Salicylate 202
Diclofenac 271
Diflunisal 278
Etodolac 347
Fenoprofen Calcium 356
Flurbiprofen Sodium 381
Ibuprofen 447
Indomethacin 457
Ketoprofen 483
Ketorolac Tromethamine 484
Meclofenamate Sodium 531
Mefenamic Acid 534
Methotrimeprazine Hydrochloride 562
Naproxen 606
Orphenadrine, Aspirin, and Caffeine 640
Oxyphenbutazone 652
Para-Aminosalicylate Sodium 658
Phenyltoloxamine, Phenylpropanolamine, and Acetaminophen 688
Piroxicam 699
Pseudoephedrine and Ibuprofen 750
Salsalate 779
Sodium Salicylate 793
Sulindac 813
Tolmetin Sodium 854
Tramadol Hydrochloride 857

ANALGESIC, TOPICAL

Capsaicin 147
Lidocaine and Prilocaine 501
Triethanolamine Salicylate 868

ANALGESIC, URINARY

Pentosan Polysulfate Sodium 674
Phenazopyridine Hydrochloride 679

ANDROGEN

Bicalutamide 113
Danazol 249
Ethinyl Estradiol and Fluoxymesterone 337
Fluoxymesterone 378
Methyltestosterone 570
Nandrolone 604
Oxandrolone 642
Testolactone 825
Testosterone 825

ANESTHETICS *see* DENTAL/LOCAL ANESTHETICS

ANGIOTENSIN-CONVERTING ENZYME (ACE) INHIBITORS

Amlodipine and Benazepril 54
Benazepril Hydrochloride 99
Captopril 148
Enalapril 307
Fosinopril 387
Lisinopril 506
Moexipril Hydrochloride 587
Quinapril Hydrochloride 756
Ramipril 762
Spirapril 798
Trandolapril 858

ANGIOTENSIN II ANTAGONIST
Losartan and Hydrochlorothiazide 515
Losartan Potassium 515

ANOREXIANT
Benzphetamine Hydrochloride.................................105
Dexfenfluramine Hydrochloride 262
Dextroamphetamine Sulfate 265
Diethylpropion Hydrochloride.................................276
Fenfluramine Hydrochloride..................................355
Mazindol 527
Phentermine Hydrochloride 683
Phenylpropanolamine Hydrochloride 687

ANTACID
Aluminum Carbonate 39
Aluminum Hydroxide 39
Aluminum Hydroxide and Magnesium Carbonate 40
Aluminum Hydroxide and Magnesium Hydroxide 40
Aluminum Hydroxide and Magnesium Trisilicate 41
Aluminum Hydroxide, Magnesium Hydroxide, and Simethicone 41
Calcium Carbonate 140
Calcium Carbonate and Simethicone 141
Magaldrate..520
Magaldrate and Simethicone 521
Magnesium Hydroxide 522
Magnesium Oxide 523

ANTHELMINTIC
Albendazole 27
Mebendazole 529
Niclosamide 617
Oxamniquine 642
Piperazine Citrate 697
Praziquantel..716
Pyrantel Pamoate 751
Thiabendazole 836

ANTIADRENAL AGENT
Aminoglutethimide 46
Mitotane 585

ANTIALCOHOLIC AGENT
Disulfiram..293

ANTIANDROGEN
Finasteride 363
Flutamide 382

ANTIANGINAL AGENT
Amlodipine 53
Atenolol 83
Bepridil Hydrochloride 108
Bisoprolol Fumarate...115
Carteolol Hydrochloride 158
Diltiazem 284
Erythrityl Tetranitrate 320
Isosorbide Dinitrate 474
Isosorbide Mononitrate 474
Nadolol 597
Nicardipine Hydrochloride 616
Nifedipine..619
Nitroglycerin 623
Pentaerythritol Tetranitrate 669
Propranolol Hydrochloride 743
Sotalol Hydrochloride.......................................796
Timolol Maleate 847
Verapamil Hydrochloride 893

ANTIANXIETY AGENT *see also* SEDATIVE, BENZODIAZEPINE
Alprazolam..35
Buspirone Hydrochloride 131
Diazepam..268
Doxepin Hydrochloride.......................................298
Hydroxyzine 443
Lorazepam 513
Meprobamate 543
Prazepam 715
Propiomazine Hydrochloride 737

ANTIARRHYTHMIC AGENT, CLASS I
Moricizine Hydrochloride 589

ANTIARRHYTHMIC AGENT, CLASS I-A
Disopyramide Phosphate....................................292
Procainamide Hydrochloride 725
Quinidine..759

ANTIARRHYTHMIC AGENT, CLASS I-B
Mexiletine...577
Phenytoin..688
Propranolol Hydrochloride 743
Tocainide Hydrochloride 851

ANTIARRHYTHMIC AGENT, CLASS I-C
Encainide Hydrochloride 309
Flecainide Acetate 365
Propafenone Hydrochloride 735

ANTIARRHYTHMIC AGENT, CLASS II
Acebutolol Hydrochloride 12
Propranolol Hydrochloride 743
Sotalol Hydrochloride....................................796

ANTIARRHYTHMIC AGENT, CLASS III
Amiodarone Hydrochloride 48
Bretylium Tosylate 119
Sotalol Hydrochloride....................................796

ANTIARRHYTHMIC AGENT, CLASS IV
Verapamil Hydrochloride 893

ANTIARRHYTHMIC AGENT (SUPRAVENTRICULAR)
Adenosine 25
Digitoxin..279
Digoxin..280

ANTIARRHYTHMIC AGENT (SUPRAVENTRICULAR & VENTRICULAR)
Acebutolol Hydrochloride 12
Amiodarone Hydrochloride 48
Bretylium Tosylate 119
Disopyramide Phosphate.................................292
Encainide Hydrochloride 309
Flecainide Acetate 365
Lidocaine Hydrochloride 502
Mexiletine...577
Moricizine Hydrochloride 589
Phenytoin..688
Procainamide Hydrochloride 725
Propafenone Hydrochloride 735
Propranolol Hydrochloride 743
Quinidine..759
Sotalol Hydrochloride....................................796
Tocainide Hydrochloride 851
Verapamil Hydrochloride 893

ANTIARRHYTHMIC AGENT, MISCELLANEOUS
Adenosine 25
Digitoxin..279
Digoxin..280

ANTIASTHMATIC
Albuterol 27
Aminophylline, Amobarbital, and Ephedrine 47
Bitolterol Mesylate 116
Isoetharine 470
Metaproterenol Sulfate 550
Nedocromil Sodium 607
Oxtriphylline 645
Pirbuterol Acetate 698
Salmeterol Xinafoate 778
Terbutaline Sulfate......................................822
Theophylline/Aminophylline 832
Theophylline and Guaifenesin 836
Theophylline, Ephedrine, and Hydroxyzine 836
Theophylline, Ephedrine, and Phenobarbital 836

ANTIBACTERIAL, DENTAL
Tetracycline Periodontal Fibers 830

ANTIBACTERIAL, ORAL RINSE
Chlorhexidine Gluconate 184

ANTIBACTERIAL, OTIC
Polymyxin B and Hydrocortisone........................704

ANTIBACTERIAL, TOPICAL
Benzalkonium Chloride 102
Gentian Violet 397
Hexachlorophene 424
Mafenide Acetate 520
Nitrofurazone 623
Povidone-Iodine 713
Silver Sulfadiazine 788
Thimerosal 838

ANTIBIOTIC, AMINOGLYCOSIDE
Amikacin Sulfate 44
Gentamicin Sulfate 396
Kanamycin Sulfate 479
Neomycin Sulfate 611
Netilmicin Sulfate 613
Streptomycin Sulfate 802
Tobramycin 849

ANTIBIOTIC, ANAEROBIC
Clindamycin 214
Metronidazole 576

ANTIBIOTIC, CARBACEPHEM
Loracarbef 512
Meropenem 545

ANTIBIOTIC, CEPHALOSPORIN (FIRST GENERATION)
Cefadroxil Monohydrate 162
Cefazolin Sodium 164
Cephalexin Monohydrate 176
Cephalothin Sodium 177
Cephapirin Sodium 177
Cephradine 178

ANTIBIOTIC, CEPHALOSPORIN (SECOND GENERATION)
Cefaclor 161
Cefamandole Nafate 163
Cefmetazole Sodium 165
Cefonicid Sodium 166
Cefotetan Disodium 168
Cefoxitin Sodium 168
Cefpodoxime Proxetil 169
Cefprozil 170
Cefuroxime 173

ANTIBIOTIC, CEPHALOSPORIN (THIRD GENERATION)
Cefixime 165
Cefoperazone Sodium 167
Cefotaxime Sodium 167
Ceftazidime 171
Ceftizoxime 171
Ceftriaxone Sodium 172

ANTIBIOTIC, CEPHALOSPORIN (FOURTH GENRATION)
Cefepime 164

ANTIBIOTIC, MACROLIDE
Azithromycin 90
Clarithromycin 212
Dirithromycin 291
Erythromycin 321
Erythromycin and Sulfisoxazole 323
Lincomycin 503
Troleandomycin 880

ANTIBIOTIC, MISCELLANEOUS
Clindamycin 214
Vancomycin Hydrochloride 889

ANTIBIOTIC, OPHTHALMIC
Bacitracin 93
Bacitracin and Polymyxin B 94
Bacitracin, Neomycin, and Polymyxin B 94
Bacitracin, Neomycin, Polymyxin B, and Hydrocortisone 95
Chloramphenicol 182
Chloramphenicol and Prednisolone 183
Chloramphenicol, Polymyxin B, and Hydrocortisone 183
Chlortetracyline Hydrochloride 199
Ciprofloxacin Hydrochloride 208
Erythromycin 321
Gentamicin Sulfate 396
Mercuric Oxide 545
(Continued)

ANTIBIOTIC, OPHTHALMIC *(Continued)*

Neomycin and Dexamethasone 609
Neomycin, Polymyxin B, and Dexamethasone 610
Neomycin, Polymyxin B, and Gramicidin 610
Neomycin, Polymyxin B, and Hydrocortisone 610
Neomycin, Polymyxin B, and Prednisolone .611
Oxytetracycline and Hydrocortisone 653
Oxytetracycline and Polymyxin B 653
Polymyxin B Sulfate 704
Prednisolone and Gentamicin 719
Sodium Sulfacetamide 793
Sodium Sulfacetamide and Fluorometholone 794
Sodium Sulfacetamide and Phenylephrine .794
Sodium Sulfacetamide and Prednisolone Acetate 794
Tetracycline 829
Tobramycin 849
Tobramycin and Dexamethasone 850
Trimethoprim and Polymyxin B 874

ANTIBIOTIC, OTIC

Bacitracin, Neomycin, Polymyxin B, and Hydrocortisone 95
Chloramphenicol 182
Neomycin, Polymyxin B, and Hydrocortisone 610

ANTIBIOTIC, PENICILLIN

Amoxicillin and Clavulanic Acid 57
Amoxicillin Trihydrate 58
Ampicillin 62
Ampicillin and Probenecid 63
Ampicillin Sodium and Sulbactam Sodium 64
Bacampicillin Hydrochloride 92
Carbenicillin 153
Cloxacillin Sodium 224
Dicloxacillin Sodium 273
Methicillin Sodium 556
Mezlocillin Sodium 578
Nafcillin Sodium 599
Oxacillin Sodium 641
Penicillin G Benzathine and Procaine Combined 665
Penicillin G Benzathine, Parenteral 665
Penicillin G, Parenteral, Aqueous 666
Penicillin G Potassium, Oral 667
Penicillin G Procaine 667
Penicillin V Potassium 668
Piperacillin Sodium 696
Piperacillin Sodium and Tazobactam Sodium 696
Ticarcillin and Clavulanic Acid 845
Ticarcillin Disodium 846

ANTIBIOTIC, QUINOLONE

Cinoxacin 207
Ciprofloxacin Hydrochloride 208
Enoxacin 310
Lomefloxacin Hydrochloride 509
Nalidixic Acid 601
Norfloxacin 628
Ofloxacin 634

ANTIBIOTIC, SULFONAMIDE DERIVATIVE

Erythromycin and Sulfisoxazole 323
Sulfacytine 807
Sulfadiazine 807
Sulfadiazine, Sulfamethazine, and Sulfamerazine 808
Sulfamethoxazole 809
Sulfamethoxazole and Phenazopyridine 809
Sulfisoxazole 811
Sulfisoxazole and Phenazopyridine 812
Trimethoprim and Sulfamethoxazole 874

ANTIBIOTIC, SULFONE

Dapsone 251

ANTIBIOTIC, TETRACYCLINE DERIVATIVE

Chlortetracycline Hydrochloride 199
Demeclocycline Hydrochloride 255
Doxycycline 301
Minocycline Hydrochloride 582
Oxytetracycline Hydrochloride 653
Tetracycline 829

ANTIBIOTIC, TOPICAL
Bacitracin 93
Bacitracin and Polymyxin B 94
Bacitracin, Neomycin, and Polymyxin B 94
Bacitracin, Neomycin, Polymyxin B, and Hydrocortisone 95
Bacitracin, Neomycin, Polymyxin B, and Lidocaine 95
Chlorhexidine Gluconate 184
Erythromycin, Topical 324
Gentamicin Sulfate 396
Mafenide Acetate 520
Meclocycline Sulfosalicylate 531
Metronidazole 576
Mupirocin 593
Neomycin and Hydrocortisone 609
Neomycin and Polymyxin B 609
Neomycin, Polymyxin B, and Hydrocortisone 610
Neomycin Sulfate 611
Oxychlorosene Sodium 646
Polymyxin B Sulfate 704
Silver Protein, Mild 787
Tetracycline 829

ANTIBIOTIC, URINARY IRRIGATION
Neomycin and Polymyxin B 609

ANTIBIOTIC, VAGINAL
Sulfabenzamide, Sulfacetamide, and Sulfathiazole 806
Sulfadiazine, Sulfamethazine, and Sulfamerazine 808

ANTIBIOTIC, MISCELLANEOUS
Aztreonam 91
Bacitracin 93
Capreomycin Sulfate 147
Chloramphenicol 182
Clofazimine Palmitate 217
Colistimethate Sodium 230
Colistin, Neomycin, and Hydrocortisone 231
Colistin Sulfate 231
Cycloserine 242
Furazolidone 391
Imipenem/Cilastatin 451
Methenamine 555
Nitrofurantoin 622
Pentamidine Isethionate 670
Rifabutin 769
Rifampin 769
Rifampin and Isoniazid 771
Rifampin, Isoniazid, and Pyrazinamide 771
Spectinomycin Hydrochloride 798
Trimethoprim 874
Trimetrexate Glucuronate 875

ANTICHOLINERGIC AGENT
Anisotropine Methylbromide 67
Atropine Sulfate 85
Belladonna 98
Benztropine Mesylate 106
Glycopyrrolate 403
Hyoscyamine, Atropine, Scopolamine, and Phenobarbital ...444
Hyoscyamine Sulfate 445
Ipratropium Bromide 467
Mepenzolate Bromide 538
Methantheline Bromide 554
Methscopolamine Bromide 564
Oxyphencyclimine Hydrochloride 652
Procyclidine Hydrochloride 730
Propantheline Bromide 736
Scopolamine 781
Tridihexethyl Chloride 868
Trihexyphenidyl Hydrochloride 871
Trimethaphan Camsylate 873

ANTICHOLINERGIC AGENT, OPHTHALMIC
Atropine Sulfate 85
Cyclopentolate Hydrochloride 240
Homatropine Hydrobromide 426
Scopolamine 781

ANTICHOLINERGIC AGENT, TRANSDERMAL
Scopolamine 781

ANTICOAGULANT
Dalteparin 249
Heparin 419
Warfarin Sodium 903

ANTICONVULSANT, BARBITURATE
Mephobarbital 540
Phenobarbital 680
Phenytoin With Phenobarbital 689
Primidone 723

ANTICONVULSANT, BENZODIAZEPINE
Clonazepam 220
Clorazepate Dipotassium 222
Diazepam 268
Prazepam 715

ANTICONVULSANT, HYDANTOIN
Ethotoin 344
Fosphenytoin 389
Mephenytoin 540
Phenytoin 688
Phenytoin With Phenobarbital 689

ANTICONVULSANT, OXAZOLIDINEDIONE
Trimethadione 872

ANTICONVULSANT, SUCCINIMIDE
Ethosuximide 343
Methsuximide 564
Phensuximide 683

ANTICONVULSANT, MISCELLANEOUS
Acetazolamide 18
Carbamazepine 151
Felbamate 354
Gabapentin 392
Lamotrigine 489
Magnesium Sulfate 524
Valproic Acid and Derivatives 888

ANTIDEPRESSANT, MISCELLANEOUS
Bupropion 130
Nefazodone 608
Trazodone 861
Venlafaxine 892

ANTIDEPRESSANT, MONOAMINE OXIDASE INHIBITOR
Isocarboxazid 469
Phenelzine Sulfate 679
Tranylcypromine Sulfate 860

ANTIDEPRESSANT, SELECTIVE SEROTONIN REUPTAKE INHIBITOR
Fluoxetine Hydrochloride 377
Fluvoxamine 384
Paroxetine 660
Sertraline Hydrochloride 786

ANTIDEPRESSANT, TETRACYCLIC
Maprotiline Hydrochloride 525
Mirtazapine 583

ANTIDEPRESSANT, TRICYCLIC
Amitriptyline and Chlordiazepoxide 49
Amitriptyline and Perphenazine 50
Amitriptyline Hydrochloride 51
Amoxapine 56
Clomipramine Hydrochloride 219
Desipramine Hydrochloride 257
Doxepin Hydrochloride 298
Imipramine 451
Nortriptyline Hydrochloride 629
Protriptyline Hydrochloride 748
Trimipramine Maleate 876

ANTIDIABETIC AGENT
Acetohexamide 19
Chlorpropamide 197
Glimepiride 398
Glipizide 399
Glyburide 401
Insulin Preparations 459
Tolazamide 852

Tolbutamide 853

ANTIDIARRHEAL
Attapulgite 86
Bismuth 114
Calcium Polycarbophil 146
Charcoal 179
Colistin Sulfate 231
Difenoxin and Atropine 277
Diphenoxylate and Atropine 289
Furazolidone 391
Hyoscyamine, Atropine, Scopolamine, Kaolin, and Pectin 445
Hyoscyamine, Atropine, Scopolamine, Kaolin, Pectin, and Opium 445
Kaolin and Pectin 480
Kaolin and Pectin With Opium 480
Lactobacillus acidophilus and *Lactobacillus bulgaricus* 488
Loperamide Hydrochloride 511
Opium Tincture 639
Paregoric 659

ANTIDIURETIC HORMONE ANALOG
Lypressin 519
Vasopressin 891

ANTIDOTE, ACETAMINOPHEN
Acetylcysteine 21

ANTIDOTE, ADSORBENT
Charcoal 179

ANTIDOTE, ALUMINUM TOXICITY
Deferoxamine Mesylate 253

ANTIDOTE, ANTICHOLINERGIC AGENT
Physostigmine 690

ANTIDOTE, ARSENIC TOXICITY
Dimercaprol 287

ANTIDOTE, BENZODIAZEPINE
Flumazenil 370

ANTIDOTE, CYANIDE
Sodium Thiosulfate 795

ANTIDOTE, CYCLOSERINE TOXICITY
Pyridoxine Hydrochloride 753

ANTIDOTE, EMETIC
Ipecac Syrup 467

ANTIDOTE, EXTRAVASATION
Hyaluronidase 427
Phentolamine Mesylate 684

ANTIDOTE, GOLD TOXICITY
Dimercaprol 287

ANTIDOTE, HEPARIN
Protamine Sulfate 747

ANTIDOTE, HYDRALAZINE TOXICITY
Pyridoxine Hydrochloride 753

ANTIDOTE, HYPERCALCEMIA
Calcitonin 138
Etidronate Disodium 346
Pamidronate Disodium 655
Plicamycin 700

ANTIDOTE, HYPERPHOSPHATEMIA
Aluminum Hydroxide 39
Calcium Carbonate 140

ANTIDOTE, HYPERSENSITIVITY REACTIONS
Diphenhydramine Hydrochloride 288
Epinephrine 311
Epinephrine (Dental) 313

ANTIDOTE, INSECT STING
Insect Sting Kit 459

ANTIDOTE, IRON TOXICITY
Deferoxamine Mesylate 253

ANTIDOTE, ISONIAZID TOXICITY
Pyridoxine Hydrochloride 753

ANTIDOTE, LEAD TOXICITY
Dimercaprol 287

ANTIDOTE, MALIGNANT HYPERTHERMIA
Dantrolene Sodium 250

ANTIDOTE, MERCURY TOXICITY
Dimercaprol 287

ANTIDOTE, METHOTREXATE
Leucovorin Calcium 491

ANTIDOTE, NARCOTIC AGONIST
Nalmefene Hydrochloride 601

ANTIDOTE, ORGANOPHOSPHATE POISONING
Atropine Sulfate 85

ANTIEMETIC
Buclizine Hydrochloride 125
Chlorpromazine Hydrochloride 195
Cisapride 209
Cyclizine 238
Dexamethasone 260
Dimenhydrinate 286
Diphenidol Hydrochloride 289
Dronabinol 302
Droperidol 303
Granisetron 405
Hydroxyzine 443
Loxapine 517
Meclizine Hydrochloride 530
Metoclopramide 572
Nabilone 596
Ondansetron 637
Perphenazine 677
Phosphorated Carbohydrate Solution 690
Prochlorperazine 728
Promethazine Hydrochloride 733
Propiomazine Hydrochloride 737
Thiethylperazine Maleate 838
Trimethobenzamide Hydrochloride 873

ANTIFLATULENT
Aluminum Hydroxide, Magnesium Hydroxide, and Simethicone 41
Charcoal 179
Magaldrate and Simethicone 521
Simethicone 788

ANTIFUNGAL AGENT, OPHTHALMIC
Natamycin 607

ANTIFUNGAL AGENT, ORAL NONABSORBED
Amphotericin B 60
Clotrimazole 223
Nystatin 632

ANTIFUNGAL AGENT, SYSTEMIC
Amphotericin B 60
Amphotericin B Lipid Complex 61
Fluconazole 367
Flucytosine 368
Griseofulvin 406
Itraconazole 477
Ketoconazole 481

ANTIFUNGAL AGENT, TOPICAL
Amphotericin B 60
Benzoic Acid and Salicylic Acid 104
Betamethasone and Clotrimazole 111
Butenafine Hydrochloride 135
Carbol-Fuchsin Solution 155
Ciclopirox Olamine 205
Clioquinol and Hydrocortisone 216
Clotrimazole 223
Econazole Nitrate 306
Gentian Violet 397
Haloprogin 418
Iodochlorhydroxyquin 466
Iodoquinol and Hydrocortisone 467
Ketoconazole 481
Miconazole 578
Naftifine Hydrochloride 600

Nystatin 632
Nystatin and Triamcinolone 632
Oxiconazole Nitrate 644
Sodium Thiosulfate 795
Sulconazole Nitrate 806
Terbinafine 822
Tolnaftate 855
Triacetin 862
Undecylenic Acid and Derivatives 884

ANTIFUNGAL AGENT, VAGINAL

Butoconazole Nitrate 135
Clotrimazole 223
Miconazole 578
Nystatin 632
Sulfanilamide 810
Terconazole 823
Tioconazole 848

ANTIGLAUCOMA AGENT

Acetazolamide 18
Betaxolol Hydrochloride 111
Carbachol 150
Carteolol Hydrochloride 158
Clonidine 221
Demecarium Bromide 255
Dichlorphenamide 271
Dipivefrin 290
Dorzolamide Hydrochloride 296
Echothiophate Iodide 305
Epinephrine 311
Epinephryl Borate 315
Isoflurophate 470
Isosorbide 473
Levobunolol Hydrochloride 493
Methazolamide 554
Metipranolol Hydrochloride 572
Phenylephrine Hydrochloride 685
Physostigmine 690
Pilocarpine 691
Pilocarpine and Epinephrine 693
Timolol Maleate 847

ANTIHEMOPHILIC AGENT

Antihemophilic Factor (Human) 68
Antihemophilic Factor (Porcine) 69
Antihemophilic Factor (Recombinant) 70
Desmopressin Acetate 258
Factor IX Complex (Human) 350
Tranexamic Acid 860

ANTIHISTAMINE

Astemizole 82
Azatadine Maleate 89
Bromodiphenhydramine and Codeine 122
Brompheniramine Maleate 124
Buclizine Hydrochloride 125
Cetirizine Hydrochloride 179
Chlorpheniramine and Acetaminophen 190
Chlorpheniramine Maleate 191
Clemastine Fumarate 214
Cyclizine 238
Cyproheptadine Hydrochloride 244
Dexchlorpheniramine Maleate 261
Dimenhydrinate 286
Diphenhydramine Hydrochloride 288
Fexofenadine Hydrochloride 361
Hydroxyzine 443
Loratadine 512
Meclizine Hydrochloride 530
Promethazine and Codeine 733
Promethazine Hydrochloride 733
Terfenadine 823
Trimeprazine Tartrate 871
Tripelennamine 877

ANTIHISTAMINE, INHALATION

Nedocromil Sodium 607

ANTIHISTAMINE/DECONGESTANT COMBINATION

Acetaminophen, Chlorpheniramine, and Pseudoephedrine 17
(Continued)

ANTIHISTAMINE/DECONGESTANT COMBINATION *(Continued)*

Acrivastine and Pseudoephedrine 22
Azatadine and Pseudoephedrine 89
Brompheniramine and Phenylephrine 122
Brompheniramine and Phenylpropanolamine 123
Brompheniramine and Pseudoephedrine 123
Brompheniramine, Phenylpropanolamine, and Codeine 125
Caramiphen and Phenylpropanolamine 150
Carbinoxamine and Pseudoephedrine 154
Carbinoxamine, Pseudoephedrine, and Dextromethorphan 155
Chlorpheniramine and Phenylephrine 190
Chlorpheniramine and Phenylpropanolamine 190
Chlorpheniramine and Pseudoephedrine 191
Chlorpheniramine, Ephedrine, Phenylephrine, and Carbetapentane
. 191
Chlorpheniramine, Phenindamine, and Phenylpropanolamine 192
Chlorpheniramine, Phenylephrine, and Codeine .192
Chlorpheniramine, Phenylephrine, and Dextromethorphan 193
Chlorpheniramine, Phenylephrine, and Methscopolamine 193
Chlorpheniramine, Phenylephrine, and Phenylpropanolamine 193
Chlorpheniramine, Phenylephrine, and Phenyltoloxamine 193
Chlorpheniramine, Phenylpropanolamine, and Acetaminophen 194
Chlorpheniramine, Phenylpropanolamine, and Dextromethorphan 194
Chlorpheniramine, Phenyltoloxamine, Phenylpropanolamine, and
Phenylephrine 194
Chlorpheniramine, Pseudoephedrine, and Codeine 195
Chlorpheniramine, Pyrilamine, and Phenylephrine 195
Chlorpheniramine, Pyrilamine, Phenylephrine, and Phenylpropanolamine
. 195
Clemastine and Phenylpropanolamine 213
Dexbrompheniramine and Pseudoephedrine 261
Hydrocodone, Phenylephrine, Pyrilamine, Phenindamine,
Chlorpheniramine, and Ammonium Chloride 435
Loratadine and Pseudoephedrine 513
Pheniramine, Phenylpropanolamine, and Pyrilamine 680
Phenyltoloxamine, Phenylpropanolamine, and Acetaminophen 688
Promethazine and Phenylephrine 733
Promethazine, Phenylephrine, and Codeine 734
Terfenadine and Pseudoephedrine 824
Triprolidine and Pseudoephedrine 878
Triprolidine, Pseudoephedrine, and Codeine 879

ANTIHYPERTENSIVE

Diazoxide 269
Lisinopril and Hydrochlorothiazide 507
Perindopril Erbumine 676
Phenoxybenzamine Hydrochloride 682
Phentolamine Mesylate 684
Prazosin Hydrochloride 717
Rauwolfia Serpentina 764

ANTIHYPERTENSIVE AGENT, COMBINATION

Atenolol and Chlorthalidone 84
Bisoprolol and Hydrochlorothiazide 115
Captopril and Hydrochlorothiazide 149
Chlorothiazide and Methyldopa 188
Chlorothiazide and Reserpine 189
Clonidine and Chlorthalidone 222
Enalapril and Hydrochlorothiazide 309
Hydralazine and Hydrochlorothiazide 428
Hydralazine, Hydrochlorothiazide, and Reserpine 429
Hydrochlorothiazide and Reserpine 431
Hydrochlorothiazide and Spironolactone 431
Hydroflumethiazide and Reserpine 438
Methyclothiazide and Cryptenamine Tannates 566
Methyclothiazide and Deserpidine 566
Methyclothiazide and Pargyline 566
Methyldopa and Hydrochlorothiazide 567
Prazosin and Polythiazide 717
Propranolol and Hydrochlorothiazide 743

ANTIHYPOGLYCEMIC AGENT

Diazoxide 269
Glucagon 400
Glucose 400

ANTI-INFECTIVE AGENT, ORAL

Carbamide Peroxide 152

ANTI-INFLAMMATORY AGENT see also NONSTEROIDAL ANTI-INFLAMMATORY AGENT (NSAID) ORAL

Aspirin ... 78
Beclomethasone Dipropionate ... 97
Betamethasone ... 109
Budesonide ... 126
Choline Magnesium Salicylate ... 202
Choline Salicylate ... 202
Colchicine ... 228
Cortisone Acetate ... 233
Dexamethasone ... 260
Diclofenac ... 271
Fenoprofen Calcium ... 356
Flunisolide ... 372
Hydrocortisone ... 436
Ibuprofen ... 447
Indomethacin ... 457
Ketoprofen ... 483
Ketorolac Tromethamine ... 484
Meclofenamate Sodium ... 531
Methylprednisolone ... 569
Naproxen ... 606
Olsalazine Sodium ... 635
Piroxicam ... 699
Pramoxine and Hydrocortisone ... 714
Prednisolone ... 718
Prednisone ... 719
Salsalate ... 779
Sulfasalazine ... 810
Sulindac ... 813
Triamcinolone ... 862
Triamcinolone Acetonide Dental Paste ... 864

ANTI-INFLAMMATORY, LOCALLY APPLIED

Amlexanox ... 52

ANTI-INFLAMMATORY AGENT, OPHTHALMIC

Fluorometholone ... 375
Medrysone ... 533
Rimexolone ... 772
Sodium Sulfacetamide and Fluorometholone ... 794

ANTI-INFLAMMATORY AGENT, RECTAL

Mesalamine ... 546

ANTIMALARIAL AGENT

Chloroquine and Primaquine ... 186
Chloroquine Phosphate ... 187
Halofantrine ... 416
Hydroxychloroquine Sulfate ... 440
Mefloquine Hydrochloride ... 535
Primaquine Phosphate ... 723
Pyrimethamine ... 754
Quinine Sulfate ... 760
Sulfadoxine and Pyrimethamine ... 808

ANTIMANIC AGENT

Lithium ... 508

ANTIMIGRAINE AGENT

Acetaminophen and Isometheptene Mucate ... 16
Sumatriptan Succinate ... 814

ANTIMICROBIAL MOUTH RINSE

Chlorhexidine Gluconate ... 184
Mouthwash, Antiseptic ... 592

ANTINEOPLASTIC AGENT, ADJUVANT

Aminoglutethimide ... 46

ANTINEOPLASTIC AGENT, ALKYLATING AGENT

Altretamine ... 38
Busulfan ... 131
Carboplatin ... 155
Cisplatin ... 210
Ifosfamide ... 449
Pipobroman ... 698
Thiotepa ... 841

ANTINEOPLASTIC AGENT, ALKYLATING AGENT (NITROGEN MUSTARD)

Chlorambucil ... 181
(Continued)

ANTINEOPLASTIC AGENT, ALKYLATING AGENT (NITROGEN MUSTARD) *(Continued)*

Cyclophosphamide 240
Melphalan 536

ANTINEOPLASTIC AGENT, ALKYLATING AGENT (NITROSOUREA)

Carmustine 157
Lomustine 510
Streptozocin 803

ANTINEOPLASTIC AGENT, ANTHRACYCLINE

Mitoxantrone Hydrochloride 586

ANTINEOPLASTIC AGENT, ANTIBIOTIC

Bleomycin Sulfate 117
Dactinomycin 248
Daunorubicin Hydrochloride 252
Doxorubicin Hydrochloride 299
Idarubicin 448
Mitomycin 584
Mitoxantrone Hydrochloride 586
Plicamycin 700
Topotecan Hydrochloride 855

ANTINEOPLASTIC AGENT, ANTIMETABOLITE

Cladribine 211
Cytarabine Hydrochloride 246
Floxuridine 366
Fludarabine Phosphate 368
Fluorouracil 376
Mercaptopurine 544
Methotrexate 559
Pentostatin 674
Thioguanine 838

ANTINEOPLASTIC AGENT, ANTIMICROTUBULAR

Paclitaxel 655

ANTINEOPLASTIC AGENT, HORMONE

Bicalutamide 113
Megestrol Acetate 535

ANTINEOPLASTIC AGENT, HORMONE (ANTIESTROGEN)

Tamoxifen Citrate 818

ANTINEOPLASTIC AGENT, HORMONE (GONADOTROPIN HORMONE-RELEASING ANTIGEN)

Leuprolide Acetate 492

ANTINEOPLASTIC AGENT, HORMONE (ESTROGEN/NITROGEN MUSTARD)

Estramustine Phosphate Sodium 326

ANTINEOPLASTIC AGENT, MITOTIC INHIBITOR

Etoposide 348
Vinblastine Sulfate 895
Vincristine Sulfate 896
Vinorelbine Tartrate 897

ANTINEOPLASTIC AGENT, NONIRRITANT

Pentostatin 674

ANTINEOPLASTIC AGENT, PURINE

Mercaptopurine 544

ANTINEOPLASTIC AGENT, MISCELLANEOUS

Aldesleukin 29
Asparaginase 77
Azacitidine 88
Dacarbazine 247
Docetaxel 294
Hydroxyurea 442
Interferon Alfa-2a 461
Interferon Alfa-2b 462
Interferon Alfa-N3 463
Irinotecan 468
Mitotane 585
Nilutamide 621
Pegaspargase 662
Procarbazine Hydrochloride 727
Teniposide 820

ANTIPARASITIC AGENT, TOPICAL

Lindane 504

Permethrin 676
Pyrethrins 753

ANTI-PARKINSON'S AGENT
Amantadine Hydrochloride. 41
Benztropine Mesylate 106
Biperiden 113
Bromocriptine Mesylate 121
Carbidopa 153
Ethopropazine Hydrochloride. 343
Levodopa 495
Levodopa and Carbidopa 495
Pergolide Mesylate 675
Procyclidine Hydrochloride 730
Selegiline Hydrochloride 784
Trihexyphenidyl Hydrochloride. 871

ANTIPLAQUE AGENT
Chlorhexidine Gluconate 184
Mouthwash, Antiseptic 592

ANTIPLATELET AGENT
Aspirin 78
Dipyridamole 290
Ticlopidine Hydrochloride. 847

ANTIPROTOZOAL
Atovaquone 84
Furazolidone 391
Metronidazole 576

ANTIPRURITIC, TOPICAL
Crotamiton 236
Lidocaine and Prilocaine 501

ANTIPSORIATIC AGENT, SYSTEMIC
Etretinate 349

ANTIPSORIATIC AGENT, TOPICAL
Anthralin 68
Calcipotriene 138
Coal Tar 225
Coal Tar and Salicylic Acid 226
Coal Tar, Lanolin, and Mineral Oil. 226

ANTIPSYCHOTIC AGENT
Acetophenazine Maleate 20
Amitriptyline and Chlordiazepoxide 49
Chlorpromazine Hydrochloride. 195
Chlorprothixene 198
Clozapine. 225
Droperidol 303
Fluphenazine 379
Haloperidol. 417
Loxapine. 517
Mesoridazine Besylate. 547
Molindone Hydrochloride 588
Olanzapine. 635
Perphenazine. 677
Prochlorperazine 728
Promazine Hydrochloride 732
Risperidone 772
Thioridazine 840
Thiothixene 842
Trifluoperazine Hydrochloride 869

ANTIPYRETIC
Acetaminophen 14
Acetaminophen and Dextromethorphan 16
Aspirin 78
Salsalate 779

ANTISEBORRHEIC AGENT, TOPICAL
Chloroxine 189
Coal Tar. 225
Coal Tar and Salicylic Acid 226
Coal Tar, Lanolin, and Mineral Oil. 226
Parachlorometaxylenol. 659
Pyrithione Zinc 755
Sulfur and Salicylic Acid 813

ANTISECRETORY AGENT
Octreotide Acetate 633

ANTISPASMODIC AGENT, GASTROINTESTINAL
Anisotropine Methylbromide 67
Atropine Sulfate 85
Belladonna 98
Clidinium and Chlordiazepoxide 214
Dicyclomine Hydrochloride 273
Glycopyrrolate 403
Hyoscyamine, Atropine, Scopolamine, and Phenobarbital 444
Hyoscyamine Sulfate 445
Mepenzolate Bromide 538
Methantheline Bromide 554
Methscopolamine Bromide 564
Oxyphencyclimine Hydrochloride 652
Propantheline Bromide 736
Tridihexethyl Chloride 868

ANTISPASMODIC AGENT, URINARY
Flavoxate 364
Oxybutynin Chloride 645

ANTITHYROID AGENT
Methimazole 556
Potassium Iodide 711
Propylthiouracil 746

ANTITRYPSIN DEFICIENCY AGENT
Alpha$_1$-Proteinase Inhibitor, Human 34

ANTITUBERCULAR AGENT
Aminosalicylate Sodium 47
Capreomycin Sulfate 147
Cycloserine 242
Ethambutol Hydrochloride 332
Ethionamide 342
Isoniazid 471
Pyrazinamide 752
Rifabutin 769
Rifampin 769
Rifampin and Isoniazid 771
Rifampin, Isoniazid, and Pyrazinamide 771
Streptomycin Sulfate 802

ANTITUSSIVE
Acetaminophen and Dextromethorphan 16
Benzonatate 104
Codeine 227
Dextromethorphan 266
Guaifenesin and Codeine 408
Guaifenesin and Dextromethorphan 408
Hydrocodone and Chlorpheniramine 434
Hydrocodone and Guaifenesin 434
Hydrocodone and Homatropine 434
Hydrocodone, Chlorpheniramine, Phenylephrine, Acetaminophen and
    Caffeine 435
Hydromorphone Hydrochloride 438
Promethazine and Codeine 733
Promethazine, Phenylephrine, and Codeine 734
Promethazine With Dextromethorphan 735
Pseudoephedrine and Dextromethorphan 750

ANTIUROLITHIC
Cysteamine 245

ANTIVIRAL AGENT, INHALATION THERAPY
Ribavirin 767

ANTIVIRAL AGENT, OPHTHALMIC
Idoxuridine 449
Trifluridine 870
Vidarabine 895

ANTIVIRAL AGENT, ORAL
Acyclovir 23
Amantadine Hydrochloride 41
Didanosine 274
Famciclovir 352
Indinavir 456
Lamivudine 489
Rimantadine Hydrochloride 771
Ritonavir 773
Saquinavir Mesylate 780
Stavudine 800

Valacyclovir 888
Zalcitabine 906
Zidovudine 907

ANTIVIRAL AGENT, PARENTERAL

Acyclovir 23
Cidofovir 205
Foscarnet 386
Ganciclovir 393
Nevirapine 614
Stavudine 800
Zidovudine 907

ANTIVIRAL AGENT, TOPICAL

Acyclovir 23
Penciclovir 664

ANXIOLYTIC *see* ANTIANXIETY AGENT

ASTRINGENT

Aluminum Chloride 39
Epinephrine, Racemic and Aluminum Potassium Sulfate 314

BARBITURATE

Amobarbital 54
Amobarbital and Secobarbital 55
Butabarbital Sodium 132
Butalbital Compound 133
Butalbital Compound and Codeine 134
Methohexital Sodium 559
Pentobarbital 672
Phenobarbital 680
Secobarbital Sodium 783
Thiopental Sodium 839

BENZODIAZEPINE

Alprazolam 35
Chlordiazepoxide 183
Clorazepate Dipotassium 222
Estazolam 324
Flurazepam Hydrochloride 380
Halazepam 415
Lorazepam 513
Midazolam Hydrochloride 580
Oxazepam 644
Prazepam 715
Quazepam 755
Temazepam 819
Triazolam 866

BETA-ADRENERGIC BLOCKER, CARDIOSELECTIVE

Acebutolol Hydrochloride 12
Atenolol 83
Betaxolol Hydrochloride 111
Bisoprolol Fumarate 115
Metoprolol 574
Sotalol Hydrochloride 796

BETA-ADRENERGIC BLOCKER, NONCARDIOSELECTIVE

Carteolol Hydrochloride 158
Carvedilol 159
Nadolol 597
Penbutolol Sulfate 664
Pindolol 694
Propranolol Hydrochloride 743
Timolol Maleate 847

BETA-ADRENERGIC BLOCKER, OPHTHALMIC

Betaxolol Hydrochloride 111
Carteolol Hydrochloride 158
Levobunolol Hydrochloride 493
Metipranolol Hydrochloride 572
Timolol Maleate 847

BETA-2-ADRENERGIC AGONIST AGENT

Albuterol 27
Bitolterol Mesylate 116
Metaproterenol Sulfate 550
Pirbuterol Acetate 698
Ritodrine Hydrochloride 773
Salmeterol Xinafoate 778
Terbutaline Sulfate 822

BILE ACID
Dehydrocholic Acid 254

BIOLOGICAL RESPONSE MODULATOR
Aldesleukin 29
Bacillus Calmette-Guérin (BCG) Live 93
Interferon Alfa-2b 462
Interferon Gamma-1B 465

BIPHOSPHONATE DERIVATIVE
Alendronate Sodium 30
Etidronate Disodium 346
Pamidronate Disodium 655

BLOOD MODIFIERS
Hemin 419
Pentastarch 671

BLOOD PRODUCT DERIVATIVE
Antihemophilic Factor (Human) 68
Antithrombin III 71
Factor IX Complex (Human) 350

BLOOD VISCOSITY REDUCER AGENT
Pentoxifylline 675

BRONCHODILATOR
Albuterol 27
Aminophylline, Amobarbital, and Ephedrine 47
Atropine Sulfate 85
Bitolterol Mesylate 116
Dyphylline 305
Epinephrine 311
Epinephrine (Dental) 313
Ethylnorepinephrine Hydrochloride 345
Ipratropium Bromide 467
Isoetharine 470
Isoproterenol 472
Metaproterenol Sulfate 550
Oxtriphylline 645
Pirbuterol Acetate 698
Salmeterol Xinafoate 778
Terbutaline Sulfate 822
Theophylline/Aminophylline 832
Theophylline and Guaifenesin 836
Theophylline, Ephedrine, and Hydroxyzine 836
Theophylline, Ephedrine, and Phenobarbital 836

CALCIUM CHANNEL BLOCKER
Amlodipine 53
Amlodipine and Benazepril 54
Bepridil Hydrochloride 108
Diltiazem 284
Felodipine 354
Isradipine 476
Nicardipine Hydrochloride 616
Nifedipine 619
Nimodipine 621
Nisoldipine 622
Verapamil Hydrochloride 893

CALCIUM SALT
Calcium Acetate 139
Calcium Carbonate 140
Calcium Chloride 141
Calcium Citrate 142
Calcium Glubionate 142
Calcium Gluceptate 143
Calcium Gluconate 143
Calcium Lactate 145
Calcium Phosphate, Tribasic 145

CALORIC AGENT
Fat Emulsion 353

CARBONIC ANHYDRASE INHIBITOR
Acetazolamide 18
Dichlorphenamide 271
Dorzolamide Hydrochloride 296
Methazolamide 554

CARDIAC GLYCOSIDE
Digitoxin 279

Digoxin 280

CARDIOPROTECTIVE AGENT
Dexrazoxane 263

CARDIOVASCULAR AGENT, OTHER
Milrinone Lactate 581

CENTRAL NERVOUS SYSTEM STIMULANT, AMPHETAMINE
Amphetamine Sulfate 59
Dextroamphetamine Sulfate 265
Methamphetamine Hydrochloride 553

CENTRAL NERVOUS SYSTEM STIMULANT, NONAMPHETAMINE
Caffeine, Citrated 136
Doxapram Hydrochloride 297
Methylphenidate Hydrochloride 568
Pemoline 663

CENTRALLY ACTING SKELETAL MUSCLE RELAXANT
Chlorzoxazone 200

CHOLINERGIC AGENT
Ambenonium Chloride 43
Bethanechol Chloride 112
Cisapride 209
Physostigmine 690
Pilocarpine (Dental) 693
Tacrine Hydrochloride 816

CHOLINERGIC AGENT, OPHTHALMIC
Acetylcholine Chloride 21
Carbachol 150
Demecarium Bromide 255
Isoflurophate 470
Physostigmine 690
Pilocarpine 691

COLONY STIMULATING FACTOR
Filgrastim 362
Sargramostim 780

CONTRACEPTIVE, IMPLANT (PROGESTIN)
Levonorgestrel 497

CONTRACEPTIVE, LOW ESTROGEN/PROGESTIN
Mestranol and Norethindrone 547

CONTRACEPTIVE, MONOPHASIC
Mestranol and Norethindrone 547

CONTRACEPTIVE, ORAL
Ethinyl Estradiol and Desogestrel 335
Ethinyl Estradiol and Ethynodiol Diacetate 335
Ethinyl Estradiol and Levonorgestrel 337
Ethinyl Estradiol and Norethindrone 339
Ethinyl Estradiol and Norgestimate 340
Ethinyl Estradiol and Norgestrel 341
Mestranol and Norethindrone 547
Mestranol and Norethynodrel 549
Norethindrone 627
Norgestrel 629

CONTRACEPTIVE, PROGESTIN ONLY
Levonorgestrel 497
Medroxyprogesterone Acetate 533
Norethindrone 627

CORTICOSTEROID, INHALANT
Beclomethasone Dipropionate 97
Budesonide 126
Dexamethasone 260
Flunisolide 372
Triamcinolone 862

CORTICOSTEROID, OPHTHALMIC
Bacitracin, Neomycin, Polymyxin B, and Hydrocortisone 95
Chloramphenicol and Prednisolone 183
Dexamethasone 260
Fluorometholone 375
Medrysone 533
Neomycin and Dexamethasone 609
Neomycin, Polymyxin B, and Hydrocortisone 610
Neomycin, Polymyxin B, and Prednisolone 611
Prednisolone 718
Prednisolone and Gentamicin 719
(Continued)

CORTICOSTEROID, OPHTHALMIC *(Continued)*

Rimexolone 772
Sodium Sulfacetamide and Prednisolone Acetate .794
Tobramycin and Dexamethasone 850

CORTICOSTEROID, OTIC

Bacitracin, Neomycin, Polymyxin B, and Hydrocortisone 95
Colistin, Neomycin, and Hydrocortisone 231
Neomycin, Polymyxin B, and Hydrocortisone 610
Polymyxin B and Hydrocortisone 704

CORTICOSTEROID, SYSTEMIC

Betamethasone 109
Cortisone Acetate 233
Dexamethasone 260
Hydrocortisone 436
Methylprednisolone 569
Prednisolone 718
Prednisone 719
Triamcinolone 862

CORTICOSTEROID, TOPICAL (LOW POTENCY)

Alclometasone Dipropionate 28
Bacitracin, Neomycin, Polymyxin B, and Hydrocortisone 95
Benzoyl Peroxide and Hydrocortisone 105
Clioquinol and Hydrocortisone 216
Desonide 259
Dexamethasone 260
Dibucaine and Hydrocortisone 270
Hydrocortisone 436
Iodoquinol and Hydrocortisone 467
Lidocaine and Hydrocortisone 501
Methylprednisolone 569
Neomycin and Hydrocortisone 609
Neomycin, Polymyxin B, and Hydrocortisone 610
Pramoxine and Hydrocortisone 714
Urea and Hydrocortisone 885

CORTICOSTEROID, TOPICAL (MEDIUM POTENCY)

Clocortolone Pivalate 216
Fluocinolone Acetonide 372
Flurandrenolide 380
Fluticasone Propionate 383
Mometasone Furoate 589
Nystatin and Triamcinolone 632
Prednicarbate 718
Triamcinolone 862

CORTICOSTEROID, TOPICAL (MEDIUM/HIGH POTENCY)

Amcinonide 43
Betamethasone 109
Betamethasone and Clotrimazole 111

CORTICOSTEROID, TOPICAL (HIGH POTENCY)

Desoximetasone 259
Diflorasone Diacetate 278
Fluocinonide 373
Halcinonide 415

CORTICOSTEROID, TOPICAL (VERY HIGH POTENCY)

Clobetasol Propionate 216
Halobetasol Propionate 416

COUGH PREPARATION

Bromodiphenhydramine and Codeine 122
Brompheniramine, Phenylpropanolamine, and Codeine 125
Carbinoxamine, Pseudoephedrine, and Dextromethorphan 155
Chlorpheniramine, Phenylephrine, and Codeine 192
Chlorpheniramine, Phenylephrine, and Dextromethorphan 193
Chlorpheniramine, Phenylpropanolamine, and Dextromethorphan 194
Chlorpheniramine, Pseudoephedrine, and Codeine 195
Guaifenesin and Codeine 408
Guaifenesin and Dextromethorphan 408
Guaifenesin, Phenylpropanolamine, and Dextromethorphan 410
Guaifenesin, Pseudoephedrine, and Codeine 410
Hydrocodone and Chlorpheniramine 434
Hydrocodone and Guaifenesin 434
Hydrocodone and Homatropine 434
Hydrocodone and Phenylpropanolamine 435
Hydrocodone, Chlorpheniramine, Phenylephrine, Acetaminophen and
 Caffeine 435

Hydrocodone, Phenylephrine, Pyrilamine, Phenindamine,
  Chlorpheniramine, and Ammonium Chloride 435
Hydrocodone, Pseudoephedrine, and Guaifenesin 435
Promethazine and Codeine 733
Promethazine, Phenylephrine, and Codeine 734
Promethazine With Dextromethorphan 735
Terpin Hydrate and Codeine 825
Triprolidine, Pseudoephedrine, and Codeine 879

DECONGESTANT
Guaifenesin and Phenylpropanolamine 409
Guaifenesin and Pseudoephedrine 409
Guaifenesin, Phenylpropanolamine, and Dextromethorphan 410
Guaifenesin, Phenylpropanolamine, and Phenylephrine 410
Guaifenesin, Pseudoephedrine, and Codeine 410
Hydrocodone and Phenylpropanolamine 435
Hydrocodone, Pseudoephedrine, and Guaifenesin 435
Phenylpropanolamine Hydrochloride 687
Propylhexedrine 745
Pseudoephedrine 749
Pseudoephedrine and Dextromethorphan 750
Pseudoephedrine and Ibuprofen 750

DECONGESTANT, NASAL
Naphazoline Hydrochloride 605
Oxymetazoline Hydrochloride 649
Phenindamine Tartrate 680

DECONGESTANT, OPHTHALMIC
Nitrous Oxide 625
Oxygen 649

DENTAL/LOCAL ANESTHETICS
Bupivacaine Hydrochloride 127
Bupivacaine With Epinephrine 128
Chloroprocaine Hydrochloride 185
Etidocaine Hydrochloride (With Epinephrine) 345
Lidocaine and Epinephrine 499
Lidocaine Hydrochloride 502
Mepivacaine Dental Anesthetic 541
Mepivacaine With Levonordefrin 542
Prilocaine 721
Prilocaine With Epinephrine 721
Procaine Hydrochloride 727
Propoxycaine and Procaine 739
Tetracaine Hydrochloride 828
Tetracaine With Dextrose 829

DEPIGMENTING AGENT
Hydroquinone 439

DIAGNOSTIC AGENT, CARDIAC FUNCTION
Indocyanine Green 457

DIAGNOSTIC AGENT, GALLBLADDER FUNCTION
Sincalide 789

DIAGNOSTIC AGENT, GASTRIC ACID SECRETORY FUNCTION
Pentagastrin 670

DIAGNOSTIC AGENT, HYPOTHYROIDISM
Thyrotropin 845

DIAGNOSTIC AGENT, OPHTHALMIC DYE
Proparacaine and Fluorescein 736

DIAGNOSTIC AGENT, PANCREATIC EXOCRINE INSUFFICIENCY
Bentiromide 101
Secretin 784

DIAGNOSTIC AGENT, PENICILLIN ALLERGY SKIN TEST
Benzylpenicilloyl-polylysine 107

DIAGNOSTIC AGENT, PHEOCHROMOCYTOMA
Phentolamine Mesylate 684

DIAGNOSTIC AGENT, PITUITARY FUNCTION
Sermorelin Acetate 786

DIAGNOSTIC AGENT, SKIN TEST
Histoplasmin 425
Skin Test Antigens, Multiple 790
Tuberculin Purified Protein Derivative 882

DIAGNOSTIC AGENT, THYROID FUNCTION
Protirelin 747
(Continued)

DIAGNOSTIC AGENT, THYROID FUNCTION *(Continued)*
Thyrotropin 845

DIAGNOSTIC AGENT, ZOLLINGER-ELLISON SYNDROME AND PANCREATIC EXOCRINE DISEASE
Secretin 784

DIETARY SUPPLEMENT
Levocarnitine 494
L-Lysine Hydrochloride 509
Methionine 557

DIURETIC, CARBONIC ANHYDRASE INHIBITOR
Acetazolamide 18
Dichlorphenamide 271
Methazolamide 554

DIURETIC, COMBINATION
Amiloride and Hydrochlorothiazide 45
Hydrochlorothiazide and Spironolactone 431
Triamterene and Hydrochlorothiazide 865

DIURETIC, LOOP
Bumetanide 126
Ethacrynic Acid 331
Furosemide 391
Torsemide 856

DIURETIC, OSMOTIC
Isosorbide 473
Urea 884

DIURETIC, POTASSIUM SPARING
Amiloride Hydrochloride 45
Spironolactone 798
Triamterene 865

DIURETIC, THIAZIDE TYPE
Bendroflumethiazide 101
Benzthiazide 105
Bisoprolol and Hydrochlorothiazide 115
Chlorothiazide 188
Chlorthalidone 199
Hydrochlorothiazide 430
Hydroflumethiazide 437
Indapamide 455
Losartan and Hydrochlorothiazide 515
Methyclothiazide 565
Metolazone 573
Polythiazide 705
Quinethazone 758
Trichlormethiazide 867

DIURETIC, MISCELLANEOUS
Caffeine and Sodium Benzoate 136

ELECTROLYTE SUPPLEMENT, ORAL
Potassium Acetate, Potassium Bicarbonate, and Potassium Citrate
. . . . 706
Potassium Acid Phosphate 707
Potassium Bicarbonate 707
Potassium Bicarbonate and Potassium Chloride, Effervescent 707
Potassium Bicarbonate and Potassium Citrate, Effervescent 707
Potassium Bicarbonate, Potassium Chloride, and Potassium Citrate
. . . . 708
Potassium Chloride 708
Potassium Chloride and Potassium Gluconate 709
Potassium Citrate and Citric Acid 710
Potassium Citrate and Potassium Gluconate 710
Potassium Gluconate 710
Potassium Phosphate and Sodium Phosphate 713

ELECTROLYTE SUPPLEMENT, PARENTERAL
Calcium Chloride 141
Magnesium Sulfate 524
Potassium Acetate 706
Potassium Chloride 708
Potassium Phosphate 711
Sodium Phosphates 792

ENZYME
Dornase Alfa 296

ENZYME, GLUCOCEREBROSIDASE
Alglucerase 32
Imglucerase 450

ENZYME, INTRADISCAL
Chymopapain 204

ENZYME, PROTEOLYTIC
Chymopapain 204

ENZYME, REPLACEMENT THERAPY
Pegademase Bovine 662

ENZYME, TOPICAL DEBRIDEMENT
Collagenase 232
Fibrinolysin and Desoxyribonuclease 362
Sutilains 816
Trypsin, Balsam Peru, and Castor Oil 881

ERGOT ALKALOID AND DERIVATIVE
Belladonna, Phenobarbital, and Ergotamine Tartrate 99
Bromocriptine Mesylate 121
Dihydroergotamine Mesylate 283
Ergoloid Mesylates 318
Ergonovine Maleate 319
Ergotamine 319
Methylergonovine Maleate 567
Methysergide Maleate 571
Pergolide Mesylate 675

ESTROGEN AND ANDROGEN COMBINATION
Estradiol and Testosterone 326
Estrogens and Medroxyprogesterone 327
Estrogens With Methyltestosterone 329

ESTROGEN DERIVATIVE
Chlorotrianisene 189
Dienestrol 275
Diethylstilbestrol 277
Estradiol 325
Estrogens, Conjugated 327
Estrogens, Esterified 328
Estrone 329
Estropipate 330
Ethinyl Estradiol 334
Ethinyl Estradiol and Fluoxymesterone 337
Polyestradiol Phosphate 702
Quinestrol 757

IMPOTENCY AGENT
Yohimbine Hydrochloride 905

EXPECTORANT
Guaifenesin 407
Guaifenesin and Codeine 408
Guaifenesin and Dextromethorphan 408
Guaifenesin and Phenylpropanolamine 409
Guaifenesin and Pseudoephedrine 409
Guaifenesin, Phenylpropanolamine, and Dextromethorphan 410
Guaifenesin, Phenylpropanolamine, and Phenylephrine 410
Guaifenesin, Pseudoephedrine, and Codeine 410
Hydrocodone, Pseudoephedrine, and Guaifenesin ... 435
Iodinated Glycerol 465
Potassium Iodide 711
Terpin Hydrate 825
Terpin Hydrate and Codeine 825
Theophylline and Guaifenesin 836

FOLIC ACID DERIVATIVE
Leucovorin Calcium 491

FLUORIDE
Fluoride 374

GALLSTONE DISSOLUTION AGENT
Ursodiol 887

GANGLIONIC BLOCKING AGENT
Mecamylamine Hydrochloride 530
Trimethaphan Camsylate 873

GASTRIC ACID SECRETION INHIBITOR
Lansoprazole 490
Omeprazole 636

GASTROINTESTINAL AGENT, STIMULANT
Dexpanthenol...263

GASTROINTESTINAL AGENT, MISCELLANEOUS
Chlorophyll..185
Glutamic Acid...400
Saliva Substitute..778
Sucralfate...804

GENERAL ANESTHETIC, INTRAVENOUS
Alfentanil Hydrochloride......................................31
Fentanyl..357
Ketamine Hydrochloride.......................................481
Methohexital Sodium..559
Propofol..738
Remifentanil...765
Thiopental Sodium..839

GLUCOCORTICOID
Budesonide..126

GOLD COMPOUND
Auranofin..87
Aurothioglucose...87
Gold Sodium Thiomalate.......................................404

GONADOTROPIN
Chorionic Gonadotropin.......................................203
Menotropins..538

GONADOTROPIN RELEASING HORMONE ANALOG
Goserelin Acetate..404
Histrelin..425
Leuprolide Acetate...492

GROWTH HORMONE
Human Growth Hormone...426

HEMOPHILIC AGENT
Anti-Inhibitor Coagulant Complex..............................70

HEMOSTATIC AGENT
Aminocaproic Acid...46
Aprotinin...72
Cellulose, Oxidized..174
Cellulose, Oxidized Regenerated..............................175
Collagen, Absorbable...231
Desmopressin Acetate...258
Gelatin, Absorbable..394
Microfibrillar Collagen Hemostat.............................579
Thrombin, Topical..843

HISTAMINE-2 ANTAGONIST
Cimetidine...207
Famotidine...352
Nizatidine...626
Ranitidine Bismuth Citrate...................................763
Ranitidine Hydrochloride.....................................763

HMG-COA REDUCTASE INHIBITOR
Fluvastatin..383
Lovastatin...516
Pravastatin Sodium...715
Simvastatin..789

HORMONE, POSTERIOR PITUITARY
Nafarelin Acetate..598
Vasopressin..891

***H. PYLORI* AGENT**
Ranitidine Bismuth Citrate...................................763

HYPERTHERMIA, TREATMENT
Dantrolene Sodium..250

HYPNOTIC
Amobarbital...54
Amobarbital and Secobarbital..................................55
Butabarbital Sodium..132
Chloral Hydrate..180
Chlordiazepoxide...183
Estazolam..324
Ethchlorvynol..334
Flurazepam Hydrochloride.....................................380
Glutethimide...401

Lorazepam 513
Midazolam Hydrochloride 580
Phenobarbital 680
Quazepam 755
Secobarbital Sodium 783
Temazepam 819
Triazolam 866
Zolpidem Tartrate 909

HYPOGLYCEMIC AGENT, ORAL
Acarbose 12
Acetohexamide 19
Chlorpropamide 197
Glimepiride 398
Glipizide 399
Glyburide 401
Metformin Hydrochloride 551
Tolazamide 852
Tolbutamide 853

IMMUNE GLOBULIN
Hepatitis B Immune Globulin 422
Immune Globulin, Intramuscular 453
Immune Globulin, Intravenous 454
Rabies Immune Globulin, Human 761
Rh_o(D) Immune Globulin 767
Tetanus Immune Globulin, Human 826
Varicella-Zoster Immune Globulin (Human) 890

IMMUNE MODULATOR
Levamisole Hydrochloride 493

IMMUNOSUPPRESSANT AGENT
Azathioprine 89
Cyclosporine 243
Lymphocyte Immune Globulin, Anti-thymocyte Globulin (Equine) 518
Muromonab-CD3 594
Mycophenolate Mofetil 595
Tacrolimus 817

INHALATION, MISCELLANEOUS
Cromolyn Sodium 235

INTERFERON
Interferon Alfa-2a 461
Interferon Alfa-2b 462
Interferon Alfa-N3 463
Interferon Beta-1b 464
Interferon Gamma-1B 465

INTRAVENOUS NUTRITIONAL THERAPY
Fat Emulsion 353

IRON SALT
Ferrous Fumarate 359
Ferrous Gluconate 360
Ferrous Sulfate 360
Ferrous Sulfate and Ascorbic Acid 361
Ferrous Sulfate, Ascorbic Acid, and Vitamin B-Complex 361
Ferrous Sulfate, Ascorbic Acid, Vitamin B-Complex, and Folic Acid

. 361
Iron Dextran Complex 468
Polysaccharide-Iron Complex 705

IRRIGATING SOLUTION
Citric Acid Bladder Mixture 211

KERATOLYTIC AGENT
Anthralin 68
Cantharidin 146
Podofilox 701
Podophyllin and Salicylic Acid 701
Podophyllum Resin 701
Salicylic Acid 777
Salicylic Acid and Lactic Acid 778
Salicylic Acid and Propylene Glycol 778
Trichloroacetic Acid 867

LAXATIVE, BOWEL EVACUANT
Polyethylene Glycol-Electrolyte Solution 703

LAXATIVE, BULK-PRODUCING
Calcium Polycarbophil 146
Malt Soup Extract 525
(Continued)

LAXATIVE, BULK-PRODUCING *(Continued)*
Psyllium 750

LAXATIVE, HYDROCHOLERETIC
Dehydrocholic Acid 254

LAXATIVE, HYPEROSMOLAR
Glycerin 402

LAXATIVE, LUBRICANT
Magnesium Hydroxide and Mineral Oil Emulsion 523

LAXATIVE, SALINE
Magnesium Citrate 521
Magnesium Hydroxide 522
Magnesium Hydroxide and Mineral Oil Emulsion 523
Magnesium Sulfate 524
Sodium Phosphates 792

LAXATIVE, STIMULANT
Bisacodyl 113
Cascara Sagrada 160
Castor Oil 161
Docusate and Phenolphthalein 295
Phenolphthalein 682
Senna 785

LAXATIVE, SURFACTANT
Docusate 295
Docusate and Casanthranol 295
Docusate and Phenolphthalein 295

LAXATIVE, MISCELLANEOUS
Lactulose 488

LIPID LOWERING DRUGS
Cholestyramine Resin 201
Clofibrate 217
Colestipol Hydrochloride 229
Dextrothyroxine Sodium 266
Fenofibrate 356
Fluvastatin 383
Gemfibrozil 395
Lovastatin 516
Niacin 614
Pravastatin Sodium 715
Probucol 725
Simvastatin 789

LEUKOTRIENE RECEPTOR ANTAGONIST
Zafirlukast 905

LOCAL ANESTHETIC, INJECTABLE
Articaine Hydrochloride with Epinephrine 74
Bupivacaine Hydrochloride 127
Bupivacaine With Epinephrine 128
Chloroprocaine Hydrochloride 185
Etidocaine Hydrochloride (With Epinephrine) 345
Lidocaine and Epinephrine 499
Lidocaine Hydrochloride 502
Mepivacaine Dental Anesthetic 541
Mepivacaine With Levonordefrin 542
Prilocaine 721
Prilocaine With Epinephrine 721
Procaine Hydrochloride 727
Propoxycaine and Procaine 739
Ropivacaine Hydrochloride 775
Tetracaine Hydrochloride 828
Tetracaine With Dextrose 829

LOCAL ANESTHETIC, OPHTHALMIC
Proparacaine and Fluorescein 736
Proparacaine Hydrochloride 737

LOCAL ANESTHETIC, ORAL
Benzonatate 104
Cetylpyridinium Chloride and Benzocaine 179
Dyclonine Hydrochloride 304
Tetracaine Hydrochloride 828

LOCAL ANESTHETIC, TOPICAL
Benzocaine 102
Benzocaine, Butyl Aminobenzoate, Tetracaine, and Benzalkonium
    Chloride 103

Benzocaine, Gelatin, Pectin, and Sodium Carboxymethylcellulose 103
Cocaine Hydrochloride. 226
Dibucaine 270
Dibucaine and Hydrocortisone 270
Dichlorodifluoromethane and Trichloromonofluoromethane 270
Ethyl Chloride 344
Ethyl Chloride and Dichlorotetrafluoroethane 344
Lidocaine and Hydrocortisone 501
Lidocaine and Prilocaine 501
Pramoxine and Hydrocortisone 714
Pramoxine Hydrochloride. 714
Tetracaine Hydrochloride. 828

LOCAL ANESTHETIC, TRANSORAL
Lidocaine Transoral 502

LOCAL ANESTHETIC, URINARY
Phenazopyridine Hydrochloride 679
Sulfisoxazole and Phenazopyridine 812

LUNG SURFACTANT
Beractant 108
Colfosceril Palmitate 230

LUTEINIZING HORMONE-RELEASING HORMONE ANALOG
Nafarelin Acetate 598

MAGNESIUM SALT
Magnesium Chloride 521
Magnesium Gluconate 522
Magnesium Hydroxide 522
Magnesium Sulfate 524

METABOLIC ALKALOSIS AGENT
Ammonium Chloride 54
Arginine Hydrochloride. 73

MINERAL, ORAL
Fluoride 374
Zinc Supplements 909

MINERAL, ORAL TOPICAL
Fluoride 374

MINERAL, PARENTERAL
Zinc Supplements 909

MINERALOCORTICOID
Fludrocortisone Acetate 369

MOUTHWASH
Mouthwash, Antiseptic. 592

MUCOLYTIC AGENT
Acetylcysteine 21

MUSCLE RELAXANT
Baclofen. 95
Carisoprodol 157
Chlorphenesin Carbamate 190
Chlorzoxazone 200
Cyclobenzaprine Hydrochloride 239
Dantrolene Sodium 250
Diazepam. 268
Meprobamate 543
Metaxalone 551
Methocarbamol 557
Methocarbamol and Aspirin 558
Orphenadrine, Aspirin, and Caffeine 640
Orphenadrine Citrate 640
Quinine Sulfate 760

NARCOTIC ANTAGONIST
Naloxone Hydrochloride. 602
Naltrexone Hydrochloride 603

NASAL AGENT, VASOCONSTRICTOR
Naphazoline Hydrochloride 605
Oxymetazoline Hydrochloride 649
Phenylephrine Hydrochloride 685
Phenylpropanolamine Hydrochloride 687
Tetrahydrozoline Hydrochloride 831
Xylometazoline Hydrochloride 905

NEUROLEPTIC AGENT
Pimozide 694

NITRATE
Erythrityl Tetranitrate 320
Isosorbide Dinitrate 474
Nitroglycerin 623
Pentaerythritol Tetranitrate 669

NONSTEROIDAL ANTI-INFLAMMATORY AGENT (NSAID)
Diflunisal 278
Etodolac 347
Flurbiprofen Sodium 381
Ibuprofen 447
Ketorolac Tromethamine 484
Naproxen 606

NONSTEROIDAL ANTI-INFLAMMATORY AGENT (NSAID), OPHTHALMIC
Diclofenac 271
Suprofen 815

NONSTEROIDAL ANTI-INFLAMMATORY AGENT (NSAID) ORAL
Aminosalicylate Sodium 47
Choline Magnesium Salicylate 202
Choline Salicylate 202
Diclofenac 271
Fenoprofen Calcium 356
Indomethacin 457
Ketoprofen 483
Meclofenamate Sodium 531
Mefenamic Acid 534
Nabumetone 596
Oxaprozin 643
Oxyphenbutazone 652
Piroxicam 699
Salsalate 779
Sulindac 813
Tolmetin Sodium 854

NONSTEROIDAL ANTI-INFLAMMATORY AGENT (NSAID), PARENTERAL
Indomethacin 457

NUTRITIONAL SUPPLEMENT
Cysteine Hydrochloride 246
Glucose Polymers 400
Lactase 487
Medium Chain Triglycerides 532

OPHTHALMIC AGENT, MIOTIC
Acetylcholine Chloride 21
Carbachol 150
Demecarium Bromide 255
Echothiophate Iodide 305
Isoflurophate 470
Pilocarpine 691
Pilocarpine and Epinephrine 693

OPHTHALMIC AGENT, MISCELLANEOUS
Artificial Tears 75
Balanced Salt Solution 96
Carboxymethylcellulose Sodium 156
Hydroxypropyl Cellulose 441
Hydroxypropyl Methylcellulose 442
Latanoprost 490
Levocabastine Hydrochloride 494
Lodoxamide Tromethamine 509
Methylcellulose 566
Phenylephrine and Zinc Sulfate 685
Silver Nitrate 787

OPHTHALMIC AGENT, MYDRIATIC
Atropine Sulfate 85
Cyclopentolate Hydrochloride 240
Homatropine Hydrobromide 426
Hydroxyamphetamine and Tropicamide 440
Hydroxyamphetamine Hydrobromide 440
Phenylephrine and Scopolamine 685
Phenylephrine Hydrochloride 685
Scopolamine 781
Tropicamide 881

OPHTHALMIC AGENT, OSMOTIC
Isosorbide 473

OPHTHALMIC AGENT, TOXIN
Botulinum Toxin Type A 118

OPHTHALMIC AGENT, VASOCONSTRICTOR
Dipivefrin 290
Epinephryl Borate 315
Naphazoline and Antazoline 604
Naphazoline and Pheniramine 605
Naphazoline Hydrochloride 605
Sodium Sulfacetamide and Phenylephrine .794
Tetrahydrozoline Hydrochloride 831

OPHTHALMIC AGENT, VISCOELEASTIC
Chondroitin Sulfate-Sodium Hyaluronate 203
Sodium Hyaluronate 791

OTIC AGENT, ANALGESIC
Antipyrine and Benzocaine 70

OTIC AGENT, ANTI-INFECTIVE
Acetic Acid, Propanediol Diacetate, and Hydrocortisone 19
Aluminum Acetate and Acetic Acid 39
Colistin, Neomycin, and Hydrocortisone 231
m-Cresyl Acetate 527

OTIC AGENT, CERUMENOLYTIC
Antipyrine and Benzocaine 70
Carbamide Peroxide 152
Triethanolamine Polypeptide Oleate-Condensate 868

OVULATION STIMULATOR
Chorionic Gonadotropin 203
Clomiphene Citrate 218
Menotropins 538
Urofollitropin 885

OXYTOCIC AGENT
Oxytocin 654

PANCREATIC ENZYME
Pancreatin 656
Pancrelipase 657

PEDICULOCIDE
Lindane 504
Pyrethrins 753

PHARMACEUTICAL AID
Benzoin 104
Boric Acid 118
Phenol 682

PHENOTHIAZINE DERIVATIVE
Amitriptyline and Perphenazine 50
Chlorpromazine Hydrochloride 195
Fluphenazine 379
Loxapine 517
Mesoridazine Besylate 547
Methotrimeprazine Hydrochloride 562
Perphenazine 677
Prochlorperazine 728
Promazine Hydrochloride 732
Promethazine Hydrochloride 733
Propiomazine Hydrochloride 737
Thioridazine 840
Thiothixene 842
Trifluoperazine Hydrochloride 869
Triflupromazine Hydrochloride 870
Trimeprazine Tartrate 871

PHOSPHATE SALT
Potassium Phosphate 711
Potassium Phosphate and Sodium Phosphate 713
Sodium Phosphates 792

PLASMA VOLUME EXPANDER
Dextran 263
Dextran 1 264
Hetastarch 423

PLATELET AGGREGATION INHIBITOR
Abciximab 12

PLASMA VOLUME EXPANDER, COLLOIDAL
Epoprostenol Sodium 317

POTASSIUM SALT
Potassium Acetate 706
Potassium Acetate, Potassium Bicarbonate, and Potassium Citrate
. . . . 706
Potassium Acid Phosphate 707
Potassium Bicarbonate 707
Potassium Bicarbonate and Potassium Chloride, Effervescent . . . 707
Potassium Bicarbonate and Potassium Citrate, Effervescent 707
Potassium Bicarbonate, Potassium Chloride, and Potassium Citrate
. . . . 708
Potassium Chloride 708
Potassium Chloride and Potassium Gluconate 709
Potassium Citrate and Citric Acid 710
Potassium Citrate and Potassium Gluconate 710
Potassium Gluconate 710
Potassium Phosphate 711
Potassium Phosphate and Sodium Phosphate 713

PROGESTIN DERIVATIVE
Hydroxyprogesterone Caproate 441
Levonorgestrel 497
Medroxyprogesterone Acetate 533
Megestrol Acetate 535
Mestranol and Norethindrone 547
Norethindrone 627
Norgestrel 629
Progesterone 731

PROSTAGLANDIN
Alprostadil 35
Carboprost Tromethamine 156
Misoprostol 584

PROTEASE INHIBITOR
Indinavir 456
Ritonavir 773

PROTECTANT, TOPICAL
Benzoin 104
Gelatin, Pectin, and Methylcellulose 395
Trypsin, Balsam Peru, and Castor Oil 881
Vitamin A and Vitamin D 899
Zinc Gelatin 908
Zinc Oxide, Cod Liver Oil, and Talc 909

PSORALEN
Methoxsalen 563
Trioxsalen 877

RAUWOLFIA ALKALOID
Rauwolfia Serpentina 764

RECOMBINANT HUMAN ERYTHROPOIETIN
Epoetin Alfa 315

RESPIRATORY STIMULANT
Ammonia Spirit, Aromatic 54
Caffeine, Citrated 136
Doxapram Hydrochloride 297

RETINOIC ACID DERIVATIVE
Isotretinoin 475
Tretinoin 862

SALICYLATE
Choline Magnesium Salicylate 202
Choline Salicylate 202
Para-Aminosalicylate Sodium 658
Salsalate 779

SALIVA SUBSTITUTE
Saliva Substitute 778

SCABICIDAL AGENT
Crotamiton 236
Lindane 504
Permethrin 676

SCLEROSING AGENT
Ethanolamine Oleate 333
Morrhuate Sodium 592
Sodium Tetradecyl Sulfate 794

SEDATIVE
Amobarbital 54

Butabarbital Sodium 132
Chloral Hydrate 180
Chlordiazepoxide 183
Clorazepate Dipotassium 222
Diazepam 268
Diphenhydramine Hydrochloride 288
Estazolam 324
Ethchlorvynol 334
Flurazepam Hydrochloride 380
Glutethimide 401
Hydroxyzine 443
Lorazepam 513
Methohexital Sodium 559
Methotrimeprazine Hydrochloride 562
Midazolam Hydrochloride 580
Pentobarbital 672
Phenobarbital 680
Promethazine Hydrochloride 733
Propiomazine Hydrochloride 737
Quazepam 755
Secobarbital Sodium 783
Temazepam 819
Thiopental Sodium 839
Triazolam 866
Zolpidem Tartrate 909

SERUM
Antirabies Serum, Equine Origin 71

SHAMPOOS
Chloroxine 189
Lindane 504
Selenium Sulfide 785

SKELETAL MUSCLE RELAXANT
Baclofen 95
Carisoprodol 157
Chlorphenesin Carbamate 190
Chlorzoxazone 200
Cyclobenzaprine Hydrochloride 239
Dantrolene Sodium 250
Diazepam 268
Meprobamate 543
Metaxalone 551
Methocarbamol 557
Methocarbamol and Aspirin 558
Orphenadrine, Aspirin, and Caffeine .640
Orphenadrine Citrate 640
Quinine Sulfate 760

SKELETAL MUSCLE RELAXANT, LONG ACTING
Aspirin and Meprobamate 81

SMOKING DETERRENT
Nicotine 617

SOAP
Hexachlorophene 424

SODIUM SALT
Sodium Phosphates 792

SOMATOSTATIN ANALOG
Octreotide Acetate 633

SPERMICIDE
Nonoxynol 9 627

STEROIDS *see* ANTI-INFLAMMATORY AGENT

STOOL SOFTENER
Docusate 295
Docusate and Casanthranol 295
Docusate and Phenolphthalein 295

SULFONYLUREA AGENT
Acetohexamide 19
Chlorpropamide 197
Glimepiride 398
Glipizide 399
Glyburide 401
Tolazamide 852
Tolbutamide 853

SUNSCREEN
Methoxycinnamate and Oxybenzone 564

THEOPHYLLINE DERIVATIVE
Dyphylline 305
Oxtriphylline 645
Theophylline/Aminophylline 832
Theophylline and Guaifenesin 836
Theophylline, Ephedrine, and Hydroxyzine 836
Theophylline, Ephedrine, and Phenobarbital 836

THIOXANTHENE DERIVATIVE
Chlorprothixene 198

THROMBOLYTIC AGENT
Alteplase 37
Anistreplase 67
Streptokinase 801
Urokinase 886

THYROID PRODUCT
Levothyroxine Sodium 498
Liothyronine Sodium 504
Liotrix 505
Thyroid 844

TOPICAL SKIN PRODUCT
Aluminum Sulfate and Calcium Acetate 41
Benzoyl Peroxide 104
Benzoyl Peroxide and Hydrocortisone 105
Camphor and Phenol 146
Camphor, Menthol, and Phenol 146
Capsaicin 147
Chlorophyll 185
Dextranomer 264
Glycerin, Lanolin, and Peanut Oil 402
Iodine 465
Lactic Acid and Sodium-PCA 487
Lactic Acid With Ammonium Hydroxide 487
Lanolin, Cetyl Alcohol, Glycerin, and Petrolatum 490
Masoprocol 526
Merbromin 544
Methylbenzethonium Chloride 566
Monobenzone 589
Silver Nitrate 787
Trypsin, Balsam Peru, and Castor Oil 881
Urea 884
Urea and Hydrocortisone 885
Vitamin A and Vitamin D 899
Zinc Oxide 908

TOPICAL SKIN PRODUCT, ACNE
Azelaic Acid 90
Meclocycline Sulfosalicylate 531

TOXOID
Tetanus Toxoid, Adsorbed 827
Tetanus Toxoid, Fluid 828

TRACE ELEMENTS
Zinc Supplements 909

TRACE ELEMENT, PARENTERAL
Trace Metals 857
Zinc Chloride 908

TRANQUILIZER, MINOR
Alprazolam 35
Buspirone Hydrochloride 131
Diazepam 268
Doxepin Hydrochloride 298
Hydroxyzine 443
Lorazepam 513
Meprobamate 543
Prazepam 715
Propiomazine Hydrochloride 737

URIC ACID LOWERING AGENT
Allopurinol 33
Probenecid 724
Sulfinpyrazone 811

URICOSURIC AGENT
Allopurinol 33

Colchicine 228
Colchicine and Probenecid 229

URINARY ACIDIFYING AGENT
Ammonium Chloride 54
Ascorbic Acid 76
Potassium Acid Phosphate 707
Sodium Ascorbate 791

URINARY TRACT PRODUCT
Acetohydroxamic Acid 20
Cellulose Sodium Phosphate 175
Finasteride 363
Tiopronin 849

VACCINE, INACTIVATED BACTERIA
Cholera Vaccine 201
Haemophilus b Conjugate Vaccine 414
Typhoid Vaccine 883

VACCINE, INACTIVATED VIRUS
Hepatitis A Vaccine 421
Hepatitis B Vaccine 422
Influenza Virus Vaccine 458
Rabies Virus Vaccine 761

VACCINE, LIVE BACTERIA
Bacillus Calmette-Guérin (BCG) Live 93
Meningococcal Polysaccharide Vaccine, Groups A, C, Y, and W-135
. 537
Rocky Mountain Spotted Fever Vaccine 775

VACCINE, LIVE VIRUS
Japanese Encephalitis Virus Vaccine, Inactivated 478
Measles and Rubella Vaccines, Combined .527
Measles, Mumps, and Rubella Vaccines, Combined 528
Measles Virus Vaccine, Live 529
Mumps Virus Vaccine, Live, Attenuated 593
Poliovirus Vaccine, Live, Trivalent, Oral 702
Rubella and Mumps Vaccines, Combined .775
Rubella Virus Vaccine, Live 776

VACCINE, LIVE VIRUS AND INACTIVATED VIRUS
Poliovirus Vaccine, Inactivated 702

VASOCONSTRICTOR
Epinephrine, Racemic 314
Epinephrine, Racemic and Aluminum Potassium Sulfate 314

VASODILATOR
Ethaverine Hydrochloride 334
Hydralazine Hydrochloride 428
Isoxsuprine Hydrochloride 476
Minoxidil 583
Nitroprusside Sodium 625
Papaverine Hydrochloride 658

VASODILATOR, CORONARY
Amyl Nitrite 66
Erythrityl Tetranitrate 320
Isosorbide Dinitrate 474
Isosorbide Mononitrate 474
Nitroglycerin 623
Pentaerythritol Tetranitrate 669
Phenoxybenzamine Hydrochloride 682
Phentolamine Mesylate 684
Prazosin Hydrochloride 717
Tolazoline Hydrochloride 852

VASODILATOR, PERIPHERAL
Cyclandelate 238
Flosequinan 366
Nylidrin Hydrochloride 631

VASOPRESSIN ANALOG, SYNTHETIC
Desmopressin Acetate 258

VITAMIN
Ferrous Sulfate and Ascorbic Acid 361
Ferrous Sulfate, Ascorbic Acid, and Vitamin B-Complex 361
Ferrous Sulfate, Ascorbic Acid, Vitamin B-Complex, and Folic Acid
. 361
Vitamins, Multiple 901

THERAPEUTIC CATEGORY INDEX

VITAMIN A DERIVATIVE
Isotretinoin 475

VITAMIN D ANALOG
Calcifediol 137
Calcitriol 139
Cholecalciferol 200
Dihydrotachysterol 283
Ergocalciferol 317

VITAMIN, FAT SOLUBLE
Beta-Carotene 109
Phytonadione 690
Tocophersolan 852
Vitamin A 898
Vitamin E 900

VITAMIN, TOPICAL
Tretinoin 862

VITAMIN, WATER SOLUBLE
Ascorbic Acid 76
Cyanocobalamin 237
Folic Acid 385
Hydroxocobalamin 439
Niacin 614
Niacinamide 615
Pantothenic Acid 658
Pyridoxine Hydrochloride 753
Riboflavin 768
Sodium Ascorbate 791
Thiamine Hydrochloride 837
Vitamin B Complex 899
Vitamin B Complex With Vitamin C 900
Vitamin B Complex With Vitamin C and Folic Acid 900

ALPHABETICAL INDEX

A-200™ Pyrinate [OTC] see Pyrethrins 753
A and D™ Ointment [OTC] see Vitamin A and Vitamin D 899
Abbokinase® see Urokinase 886
Abciximab 12
Abelcet™ Injection see Amphotericin B Lipid Complex 61
Abitrate® (Canada) see Clofibrate 217
ABLC see Amphotericin B Lipid Complex 61
Acanol® (Mexico) see Loperamide Hydrochloride 511
Acarbose 12
Accolate® see Zafirlukast 905
Accupril® see Quinapril Hydrochloride 756
Accutane® see Isotretinoin 475
Acebutolol Hydrochloride 12
Aceon® see Perindopril Erbumine 676
Acephen® [OTC] see Acetaminophen 14
Aceta® [OTC] see Acetaminophen 14
Acetaminofen (Mexico) see Acetaminophen 14
Acetaminophen 14
Acetaminophen and Codeine 15
Acetaminophen and Dextromethorphan 16
Acetaminophen and Diphenhydramine 16
Acetaminophen and Isometheptene Mucate 16
Acetaminophen and Phenyltoloxamine 17
Acetaminophen, Aspirin, and Caffeine 17
Acetaminophen, Chlorpheniramine, and Pseudoephedrine 17
Acetasol® HC Otic see Acetic Acid, Propanediol Diacetate, and
    Hydrocortisone 19
Acetazolam® (Canada) see Acetazolamide 18
Acetazolamide 18
Acetic Acid and Aluminum Acetate Otic see Aluminum Acetate and Acetic
    Acid 39
Acetic Acid, Propanediol Diacetate, and Hydrocortisone 19
Acetohexamide 19
Acetohydroxamic Acid 20
Acetophenazine Maleate 20
Acetoxyl® (Canada) see Benzoyl Peroxide 104
Acetylcholine Chloride 21
Acetylcysteine 21
Aches-N-Pain® [OTC] see Ibuprofen 447
Achromycin® see Tetracycline 829
Achromycin® V see Tetracycline 829
Aciclovir (Mexico) see Acyclovir 23
Acidulated Phosphate Fluoride see Fluoride 374
Acifur® (Mexico) see Acyclovir 23
A-Cillin® see Amoxicillin Trihydrate 58
Acimox® (Mexico) see Amoxicillin Trihydrate 58
Acloral® (Mexico) see Ranitidine Hydrochloride 763
Aclovate® see Alclometasone Dipropionate 28
Acnex® (Canada) see Salicylic Acid 777
Acnomel® B.P.5 (Canada) see Benzoyl Peroxide 104
Acnomel® (Canada) see Salicylic Acid 777
Acrivastine and Pseudoephedrine 22
Acromicina® (Mexico) see Tetracycline 829
ACT see Dactinomycin 248
ACT® [OTC] see Fluoride 374
Actagen® [OTC] see Triprolidine and Pseudoephedrine 878
Actagen-C® see Triprolidine, Pseudoephedrine, and Codeine 879
ACTH® see Corticotropin 233
Acthar® see Corticotropin 233
Acti-B$_{12}$® (Canada) see Hydroxocobalamin 439
Actidose-Aqua® [OTC] see Charcoal 179
Actidose® With Sorbitol [OTC] see Charcoal 179
Actifed® [OTC] see Triprolidine and Pseudoephedrine 878
Actifed® With Codeine see Triprolidine, Pseudoephedrine, and Codeine
   879
Actigall™ see Ursodiol 887
Actimmune® see Interferon Gamma-1B 465
Actinex® see Masoprocol 526
Actinomycin D see Dactinomycin 248
Actiprofen® (Canada) see Ibuprofen 447
Actisite® see Tetracycline Periodontal Fibers 830
Activase® see Alteplase 37
Acupril® (Mexico) see Quinapril Hydrochloride 756
Acutrim® Precision Release® [OTC] see Phenylpropanolamine Hydrochloride
   687
Acyclovir 23
Adagen™ see Pegademase Bovine 662
Adalat® see Nifedipine 619

Adalat® CC see Nifedipine 619
Adalat® Oros (Mexico) see Nifedipine 619
Adalat PA® (Canada) see Nifedipine 619
Adalat® Retard (Mexico) see Nifedipine 619
Adapalene 25
Adapin® see Doxepin Hydrochloride 298
Adeflor® see Vitamins, Multiple 901
Adena® a Ungena (Mexico) see Vidarabine 895
Adenocard® see Adenosine 25
Adenoscan® see Adenosine 25
Adenosine 25
Adipex-P® see Phentermine Hydrochloride 683
Adistan® (Mexico) see Astemizole 82
Adlone® see Methylprednisolone 569
ADR see Doxorubicin Hydrochloride 299
Adrenalin® (Dental) see Epinephrine 313
Adriamycin® PFS see Doxorubicin Hydrochloride 299
Adriamycin® RDF see Doxorubicin Hydrochloride 299
Adrucil® Injection see Fluorouracil 376
Adsorbocarpine® see Pilocarpine 691
Adsorbotear® Ophthalmic Solution [OTC] see Artificial Tears 75
Advil® [OTC] see Ibuprofen 447
Advil® Cold & Sinus Caplets [OTC] see Pseudoephedrine and Ibuprofen
. . . . 750
Aeroaid® [OTC] see Thimerosal 838
Aerobec® (Mexico) see Beclomethasone Dipropionate 97
AeroBid® see Flunisolide 372
AeroBid-M® see Flunisolide 372
Aerolate® see Theophylline/Aminophylline 832
Aerolate III® see Theophylline/Aminophylline 832
Aerolate JR® see Theophylline/Aminophylline 832
Aerolate SR® S see Theophylline/Aminophylline 832
Aerosporin® see Polymyxin B Sulfate 704
AeroZoin® [OTC] see Benzoin 104
222 AF® (Canada) see Acetaminophen 14
Afrin® Nasal Solution [OTC] see Oxymetazoline Hydrochloride 649
Afrinol® [OTC] see Pseudoephedrine 749
Aftate® [OTC] see Tolnaftate 855
A.F. Valdecasas® (Mexico) see Folic Acid 385
AgNO$_3$ see Silver Nitrate 787
AHA see Acetohydroxamic Acid 20
AHF see Antihemophilic Factor (Human) 68
Akarpine® see Pilocarpine 691
AKBeta® see Levobunolol Hydrochloride 493
AK-Chlor® see Chloramphenicol 182
AK-Con® see Naphazoline Hydrochloride 605
AK-Dilate® Ophthalmic Solution see Phenylephrine Hydrochloride 685
AK-Homatropine® Ophthalmic see Homatropine Hydrobromide 426
Akineton® see Biperiden 113
AK-Nefrin® Ophthalmic Solution see Phenylephrine Hydrochloride 685
Akne-Mycin® Topical see Erythromycin, Topical 324
AK-Neo-Dex® Ophthalmic see Neomycin and Dexamethasone 609
Akorazol® (Mexico) see Ketoconazole 481
AK-Pentolate® see Cyclopentolate Hydrochloride 240
AK-Poly-Bac® see Bacitracin and Polymyxin B 94
AK-Pred® see Prednisolone 718
AK-Spore® see Bacitracin, Neomycin, and Polymyxin B 94
AK-Spore H.C.® Ophthalmic Ointment see Bacitracin, Neomycin, Polymyxin
    B, and Hydrocortisone 95
AK-Spore H.C.® Ophthalmic Suspension see Neomycin, Polymyxin B, and
    Hydrocortisone 610
AK-Spore H.C.® Otic see Neomycin, Polymyxin B, and Hydrocortisone
. . . . 610
AK-Spore® Ophthalmic Solution see Neomycin, Polymyxin B, and Gramicidin
. . . . 610
AK-Sulf® see Sodium Sulfacetamide 793
AK-Taine® see Proparacaine Hydrochloride 737
AK-Tracin® see Bacitracin 93
AK-Trol® see Neomycin, Polymyxin B, and Dexamethasone 610
Akwa Tears® Solution [OTC] see Artificial Tears 75
AK-Zol® see Acetazolamide 18
Ala-Quin® Topical see Clioquinol and Hydrocortisone 216
Alazide® see Hydrochlorothiazide and Spironolactone 431
Albalon-A® Ophthalmic see Naphazoline and Antazoline 604
Albalon® Liquifilm® see Naphazoline Hydrochloride 605
Albendazole 27
Albenza® see Albendazole 27
Albert Docusate® (Canada) see Docusate 295

Albert® Glyburide (Canada) *see* Glyburide 401
Albuterol. 27
Alcaine® *see* Proparacaine Hydrochloride 737
Alclometasona (Mexico) *see* Alclometasone Dipropionate 28
Alclometasone Dipropionate 28
Alconefrin® Nasal Solution [OTC] *see* Phenylephrine Hydrochloride 685
Aldactazide® *see* Hydrochlorothiazide and Spironolactone 431
Aldactone® *see* Spironolactone 798
Aldesleukin. 29
Aldoclor® *see* Chlorothiazide and Methyldopa. 188
Aldomet® *see* Methyldopa 566
Aldoril® *see* Methyldopa and Hydrochlorothiazide 567
Alendronate Sodium 30
Alepsal® (Mexico) *see* Phenobarbital 680
Alersule Forte® *see* Chlorpheniramine, Phenylephrine, and Methscopolamine
. 193
Aleve® (Naproxen Sodium) (OTC) *see* Naproxen 606
Alfenta® *see* Alfentanil Hydrochloride 31
Alfenta® (Canada) *see* Alfentanil Hydrochloride 31
Alfentanil Hydrochloride 31
Alferon® N *see* Interferon Alfa-N3 463
Alfotax® (Mexico) *see* Cefotaxime Sodium 167
Algitrin® (Mexico) *see* Acetaminophen 14
Alglucerase 32
Alin® Depot (Mexico) *see* Dexamethasone 260
Alin® (Mexico) *see* Dexamethasone 260
Alkaban-AQ® *see* Vinblastine Sulfate 895
Alka-Mints® [OTC] *see* Calcium Carbonate 140
Alka-Seltzer® Plus Cold Liqui-Gels Capsules [OTC] *see* Acetaminophen,
    Chlorpheniramine, and Pseudoephedrine 17
Alkeran® *see* Melphalan 536
Allbee® With C [OTC] *see* Vitamin B Complex With Vitamin C. 900
Allbee® With C *see* Vitamins, Multiple 901
Allegra® *see* Fexofenadine Hydrochloride 361
Aller-Chlor® [OTC] *see* Chlorpheniramine Maleate 191
Allerdryl® (Canada) *see* Diphenhydramine Hydrochloride 288
Allerest® 12 Hour Capsule [OTC] *see* Chlorpheniramine and
    Phenylpropanolamine 190
Allerest® 12 Hour Nasal Solution [OTC] *see* Oxymetazoline Hydrochloride
. 649
Allerest® Eye Drops [OTC] *see* Naphazoline Hydrochloride 605
Allerest® Maximum Strength [OTC] *see* Chlorpheniramine and
    Pseudoephedrine 191
Allerfrin® [OTC] *see* Triprolidine and Pseudoephedrine 878
Allerfrin® w/Codeine *see* Triprolidine, Pseudoephedrine, and Codeine . . .879
Allergan® Ear Drops *see* Antipyrine and Benzocaine 70
Allergic Skin Reactions to Drugs 1076
AllerMax® [OTC] *see* Diphenhydramine Hydrochloride 288
Allernix® (Canada) *see* Diphenhydramine Hydrochloride 288
Allerphed® [OTC] *see* Triprolidine and Pseudoephedrine 878
Allopurinol 33
Aloid® (Mexico) *see* Miconazole 578
Alomide® *see* Lodoxamide Tromethamine 509
Alophen Pills® [OTC] *see* Phenolphthalein 682
Alopurinol (Mexico) *see* Allopurinol 33
Alpha₁-PI *see* Alpha₁-Proteinase Inhibitor, Human 34
Alpha₁-Proteinase Inhibitor, Human 34
Alpha-Baclofen® (Canada) *see* Baclofen 95
Alpha-Dextrano"40" (Mexico) *see* Dextran 263
Alphagan® *see* Brimonidine Tartrate 121
Alphamin® *see* Hydroxocobalamin 439
Alphamul® [OTC] *see* Castor Oil 161
AlphaNine® *see* Factor IX Complex (Human) 350
Alpha-Tamoxifen® (Canada) *see* Tamoxifen Citrate 818
Alphatrex® *see* Betamethasone 109
Alpidine® *see* Apraclonidine Hydrochloride 72
Alprazolam 35
Alprostadil 35
AL-R® [OTC] *see* Chlorpheniramine Maleate 191
Altace™ *see* Ramipril 762
Alteplase 37
Alter-H₂® (Mexico) *see* Ranitidine Hydrochloride .763
ALternaGEL® [OTC] *see* Aluminum Hydroxide 39
Altretamine 38
Alu-Cap® [OTC] *see* Aluminum Hydroxide 39
Aludrox® [OTC] *see* Aluminum Hydroxide and Magnesium Hydroxide 40
Aluminio, Hidroxido De (Mexico) *see* Aluminum Hydroxide. 39
Aluminum Acetate and Acetic Acid 39

ALPHABETICAL INDEX

Aluminum Carbonate 39
Aluminum Chloride. 39
Aluminum Hydroxide 39
Aluminum Hydroxide and Magnesium Carbonate .40
Aluminum Hydroxide and Magnesium Hydroxide .40
Aluminum Hydroxide and Magnesium Trisilicate .41
Aluminum Hydroxide, Magnesium Hydroxide, and Simethicone 41
Aluminum Sulfate and Calcium Acetate 41
Alupent® see Metaproterenol Sulfate 550
Alu-Tab® [OTC] see Aluminum Hydroxide 39
Amantadina, Clorhidrato De (Mexico) see Amantadine Hydrochloride 41
Amantadine Hydrochloride. 41
Amaphen® see Butalbital Compound. 133
Amaryl® see Glimepiride 398
Ambenonium Chloride 43
Ambenyl® Cough Syrup see Bromodiphenhydramine and Codeine 122
Ambien™ see Zolpidem Tartrate 909
Ambotetra® (Mexico) see Tetracycline. 829
Amcill® see Ampicillin 62
Amcinonida (Mexico) see Amcinonide. 43
Amcinonide 43
Amcort® see Triamcinolone 862
Ameblin® (Mexico) see Metronidazole 576
Amen® see Medroxyprogesterone Acetate 533
Amesec® [OTC] see Aminophylline, Amobarbital, and Ephedrine 47
A-Methapred® see Methylprednisolone 569
Amfepramone (Canada) see Diethylpropion Hydrochloride 276
Amgenal® Cough Syrup see Bromodiphenhydramine and Codeine 122
Amicar® see Aminocaproic Acid 46
Amikacina, Sulfato De (Mexico) see Amikacin Sulfate 46
Amikacin Sulfate 44
Amikafur® (Mexico) see Amikacin Sulfate 44
Amikayect® (Mexico) see Amikacin Sulfate 44
Amikin® see Amikacin Sulfate 44
Amikin® (Canada) see Amikacin Sulfate 44
Amikin® (Mexico) see Amikacin Sulfate 44
Amilorida Clorhidrato De (Mexico) see Amiloride Hydrochloride 45
Amiloride and Hydrochlorothiazide 45
Amiloride Hydrochloride. 45
2-Amino-6-Mercaptopurine see Thioguanine 838
Aminocaproic Acid 46
Aminocaproico, Acido (Mexico) see Aminocaproic Acid 46
Amino-Cerv™ Vaginal Cream see Urea 884
Aminoglutethimide 46
Amino-Opti-E® [OTC] see Vitamin E 900
Aminophyllin™ see Theophylline/Aminophylline 832
Aminophylline, Amobarbital, and Ephedrine 47
Aminosalicilico, Acido see Aminosalicylate Sodium 47
Aminosalicylate Sodium 47
Amiodarona, Clorhidrato De (Mexico) see Amiodarone Hydrochloride 48
Amiodarone Hydrochloride. 48
Ami-Tex LA® see Guaifenesin and Phenylpropanolamine 409
Amitone® [OTC] see Calcium Carbonate 140
Amitriptilina Clorhidrato De (Mexico) see Amitriptyline Hydrochloride 51
Amitriptyline and Chlordiazepoxide 49
Amitriptyline and Perphenazine 50
Amitriptyline Hydrochloride 51
Amlexanox 52
Amlodipina, Besilato De (Mexico) see Amlodipine .53
Amlodipine 53
Amlodipine and Benazepril 54
Ammonia Spirit, Aromatic 54
Ammonium Chloride 54
Ammonium Lactate see Lactic Acid With Ammonium Hydroxide 487
Amobarbital 54
Amobarbital and Secobarbital 55
Amobarbital® (Canada) see Amobarbital. 54
Amonidrin® [OTC] see Guaifenesin 407
Amoxapina (Mexico) see Amoxapine 56
Amoxapine 56
Amoxicillin and Clavulanic Acid 57
Amoxicillin Trihydrate. 58
Amoxifur® (Mexico) see Amoxicillin Trihydrate 58
Amoxil® see Amoxicillin Trihydrate 58
Amoxisol® (Mexico) see Amoxicillin Trihydrate 58
Amoxivet® (Mexico) see Amoxicillin Trihydrate 58
Amphetamine Sulfate. 59
Amphojel® [OTC] see Aluminum Hydroxide 39

ALPHABETICAL INDEX

Amphotericin B ... 60
Amphotericin B Lipid Complex ... 61
Ampicillin ... 62
Ampicillin and Probenecid ... 63
Ampicillin Sodium and Sulbactam Sodium ... 64
Ampicin® [Sodium] (Canada) *see* Ampicillin ... 62
Amplin® *see* Ampicillin ... 62
Amrinona, Lactato De (Mexico) *see* Amrinone Lactate ... 65
Amrinone Lactate ... 65
Amvisc® *see* Sodium Hyaluronate ... 791
Amyl Nitrite ... 66
Amytal® *see* Amobarbital ... 54
Anacin® [OTC] *see* Aspirin ... 78
Anacin-3® [OTC] *see* Acetaminophen ... 14
Anadrol® *see* Oxymetholone ... 650
Anafranil® *see* Clomipramine Hydrochloride ... 219
Ana-Kit® *see* Insect Sting Kit ... 459
Analphen® (Mexico) *see* Acetaminophen ... 14
Anamine® Syrup [OTC] *see* Chlorpheniramine and Pseudoephedrine ... 191
Anandron® (Can) *see* Nilutamide ... 621
Anapenil® (Mexico) *see* Penicillin V Potassium ... 668
Anaplex® Liquid [OTC] *see* Chlorpheniramine and Pseudoephedrine ... 191
Anapolon® (Canada) *see* Oxymetholone ... 650
Anaprox® (Naproxen Sodium) *see* Naproxen ... 606
Anapsique® (Mexico) *see* Amitriptyline Hydrochloride ... 51
Anaspaz® *see* Hyoscyamine Sulfate ... 445
Anatuss® [OTC] *see* Guaifenesin, Phenylpropanolamine, and Dextromethorphan ... 410
Anbesol® Maximum Strength [OTC] *see* Benzocaine ... 102
Ancef® *see* Cefazolin Sodium ... 164
Ancobon® *see* Flucytosine ... 368
Ancotil® (Canada) *see* Flucytosine ... 368
Andro® *see* Testosterone ... 825
Andro-Cyp® *see* Testosterone ... 825
Andro®/Fem Injection *see* Estradiol and Testosterone ... 326
Android® *see* Methyltestosterone ... 570
Andro-L.A.® *see* Testosterone ... 825
Androlone® *see* Nandrolone ... 604
Androlone®-D *see* Nandrolone ... 604
Andronate® *see* Testosterone ... 825
Andropository® *see* Testosterone ... 825
Andryl® *see* Testosterone ... 825
Anergan® *see* Promethazine Hydrochloride ... 733
Anexate® (Canada) *see* Flumazenil ... 370
Anexsia® 5/500 *see* Hydrocodone and Acetaminophen ... 431
Anexsia® 7.5/650 *see* Hydrocodone and Acetaminophen ... 431
Anexsia® 10/660 *see* Hydrocodone and Acetaminophen ... 431
Angiotrofen A.P.® (Mexico) *see* Diltiazem ... 284
Angiotrofen® (Mexico) *see* Diltiazem ... 284
Angiotrofen® Retard (Mexico) *see* Diltiazem ... 284
Anglopen® (Mexico) *see* Ampicillin ... 62
Animal and Human Bites Guidelines ... 976
Anisotropine Methylbromide ... 67
Anistal® (Mexico) *see* Ranitidine Hydrochloride ... 763
Anistreplase ... 67
Anitrim® (Mexico) *see* Trimethoprim and Sulfamethoxazole ... 874
Anodynos-DHC® [5/500] *see* Hydrocodone and Acetaminophen ... 431
Anoquan® *see* Butalbital Compound ... 133
Ansaid® *see* Flurbiprofen Sodium ... 381
Antabuse® *see* Disulfiram ... 293
Antagon-1® (Mexico) *see* Astemizole ... 82
Antalgin® Dialicels (Mexico) *see* Indomethacin ... 457
Antazoline-V® Ophthalmic *see* Naphazoline and Antazoline ... 604
Antazone® (Canada) *see* Sulfinpyrazone ... 811
Antepsin® (Mexico) *see* Sucralfate ... 804
Anthra-Derm® *see* Anthralin ... 68
Anthraforte® (Canada) *see* Anthralin ... 68
Anthralin ... 68
Anthranol® (Canada) *see* Anthralin ... 68
Anthranol® (Mexico) *see* Anthralin ... 68
Anthrascalp® (Canada) *see* Anthralin ... 68
AntibiOtic® Otic *see* Neomycin, Polymyxin B, and Hydrocortisone ... 610
Antihemophilic Factor (Human) ... 68
Antihemophilic Factor (Porcine) ... 69
Antihemophilic Factor (Recombinant) ... 70
Anti-Inhibitor Coagulant Complex ... 70
Antilirium® *see* Physostigmine ... 690
Antimicrobial Prophylaxis in Surgical Patients ... 1042

Antiminth® [OTC] *see* Pyrantel Pamoate 751
Antipyrine and Benzocaine 70
Antirabies Serum, Equine Origin 71
Anti-Rho(D)® (Mexico) *see* Rh₀(D) Immune Globulin 767
Antispas® *see* Dicyclomine Hydrochloride 273
Antithrombin III 71
Antithymocyte Globulin (Equine) *see* Lymphocyte Immune Globulin, Anti-
  thymocyte Globulin (Equine) 518
Antithymocyte Immunoglobulin *see* Lymphocyte Immune Globulin, Anti-
  thymocyte Globulin (Equine) 518
Anti-Tuss® Expectorant [OTC] *see* Guaifenesin 407
Antivert® *see* Meclizine Hydrochloride 530
Antralina (Mexico) *see* Anthralin 68
Antrizine® *see* Meclizine Hydrochloride 530
Anturan® (Canada) *see* Sulfinpyrazone 811
Anturane® *see* Sulfinpyrazone 811
Anxanil® *see* Hydroxyzine 443
Apacet® [OTC] *see* Acetaminophen 14
Apatate® [OTC] *see* Vitamin B Complex 899
Aphrodyne™ *see* Yohimbine Hydrochloride 905
Aphthasol® *see* Amlexanox 52
A.P.L.® *see* Chorionic Gonadotropin 203
Aplisol® *see* Tuberculin Purified Protein Derivative 882
Aplonidine *see* Apraclonidine Hydrochloride 72
Apo-Acetazolamide® (Canada) *see* Acetazolamide 18
Apo-Allopurinol® (Canada) *see* Allopurinol 33
Apo-Alpraz® (Canada) *see* Alprazolam 35
Apo-Amitriptyline® (Canada) *see* Amitriptyline Hydrochloride 51
Apo-Amoxi® (Canada) *see* Amoxicillin Trihydrate 58
Apo-Ampi® [Trihydrate] (Canada) *see* Ampicillin 62
Apo-ASA® (Canada) *see* Aspirin 78
Apo-Atenol® (Canada) *see* Atenolol 83
Apo-Bisacodyl® (Canada) *see* Bisacodyl 113
Apo® Bromocriptine (Canada) *see* Bromocriptine Mesylate 121
Apo-Cal® (Canada) *see* Calcium Carbonate 140
Apo-Capto® (Canada) *see* Captopril 148
Apo-Carbamazepine® (Canada) *see* Carbamazepine 151
Apo-C® (Canada) *see* Ascorbic Acid 76
Apo-Cephalex® (Canada) *see* Cephalexin Monohydrate 176
Apo-Chlordiazepoxide® (Canada) *see* Chlordiazepoxide 183
Apo-Chlorpromazine® (Canada) *see* Chlorpromazine Hydrochloride 195
Apo-Chlorpropamide® (Canada) *see* Chlorpropamide 197
Apo-Chlorthalidone® (Canada) *see* Chlorthalidone 199
Apo-Cimetidine® (Canada) *see* Cimetidine 207
Apo-Clomipramine® (Canada) *see* Clomipramine Hydrochloride ... 219
Apo-Clonidine® (Canada) *see* Clonidine 221
Apo-Clorazepate® (Canada) *see* Clorazepate Dipotassium 222
Apo-Cloxi® (Canada) *see* Cloxacillin Sodium 224
Apo-Diazepam® (Canada) *see* Diazepam 268
Apo-Diclo® (Canada) *see* Diclofenac 271
Apo-Diflunisal® (Canada) *see* Diflunisal 278
Apo-Diltiaz® (Canada) *see* Diltiazem 284
Apo-Dimenhydrinate® (Canada) *see* Dimenhydrinate 286
Apo-Dipyridamole® FC (Canada) *see* Dipyridamole 290
Apo-Dipyridamole® SC (Canada) *see* Dipyridamole 290
Apo-Doxepin® (Canada) *see* Doxepin Hydrochloride 298
Apo-Doxy® (Canada) *see* Doxycycline 301
Apo-Doxy® Tabs (Canada) *see* Doxycycline 301
Apo-Enalapril® (Canada) *see* Enalapril 307
Apo-Erythro® E-C (Canada) *see* Erythromycin 321
Apo-Famotidine® (Canada) *see* Famotidine 352
Apo-Ferrous® Gluconate (Canada) *see* Ferrous Gluconate 360
Apo-Ferrous® Sulfate (Canada) *see* Ferrous Sulfate 360
Apo-Fluphenazine® [Hydrochloride] (Canada) *see* Fluphenazine . 379
Apo-Flurazepam® (Canada) *see* Flurazepam Hydrochloride 380
Apo-Folic® (Canada) *see* Folic Acid 385
Apo-Furosemide® (Canada) *see* Furosemide 391
Apo-Gain® (Canada) *see* Minoxidil 583
Apo-Gemfibrozil® (Canada) *see* Gemfibrozil 395
Apo-Glyburide® (Canada) *see* Glyburide 401
Apo-Guanethidine® (Canada) *see* Guanethidine Sulfate 412
Apo-Hydralazine® (Canada) *see* Hydralazine Hydrochloride 428
Apo-Hydro® (Canada) *see* Hydrochlorothiazide 430
Apo-Hydroxyzine® (Canada) *see* Hydroxyzine 443
Apo-Ibuprofen® (Canada) *see* Ibuprofen 447
Apo-Imipramine® (Canada) *see* Imipramine 451
Apo-Indomethacin® (Canada) *see* Indomethacin 457
Apo-ISDN® (Canada) *see* Isosorbide Dinitrate 474

Apo-Keto® (Canada) *see* Ketoprofen 483
Apo-Keto-E® (Canada) *see* Ketoprofen 483
Apo-Lorazepam® (Canada) *see* Lorazepam 513
Apo-Meprobamate® (Canada) *see* Meprobamate 543
Apo-Methyldopa® (Canada) *see* Methyldopa 566
Apo-Metoclop® (Canada) *see* Metoclopramide 572
Apo-Metoprolol® (Type L) (Canada) *see* Metoprolol 574
Apo-Metronidazole® (Canada) *see* Metronidazole 576
Apo-Minocycline® (Canada) *see* Minocycline Hydrochloride 582
Apo-Nadol® (Canada) *see* Nadolol 597
Apo-Naproxen® (Canada) *see* Naproxen 606
Apo-Nifed® (Canada) *see* Nifedipine 619
Apo-Nitrofurantoin® (Canada) *see* Nitrofurantoin 622
Apo-Oxazepam® (Canada) *see* Oxazepam 644
Apo-Pen® VK (Canada) *see* Penicillin V Potassium 668
Apo-Perphenazine® (Canada) *see* Perphenazine 677
Apo-Pindol® (Canada) *see* Pindolol 694
Apo-Piroxicam® (Canada) *see* Piroxicam 699
Apo-Prazo® (Canada) *see* Prazosin Hydrochloride 717
Apo-Prednisone® (Canada) *see* Prednisone 719
Apo-Primidone® (Canada) *see* Primidone 723
Apo-Procainamide® (Canada) *see* Procainamide Hydrochloride 725
Apo-Propranolol® (Canada) *see* Propranolol Hydrochloride 743
Apo-Ranitidine® (Canada) *see* Ranitidine Hydrochloride 763
Apo-Salvent® (Canada) *see* Albuterol 27
Apo-Sulfamethoxazole® (Canada) *see* Sulfamethoxazole 809
Apo-Sulfasalazine® (Canada) *see* Sulfasalazine 810
Apo-Sulfatrim® (Canada) *see* Trimethoprim and Sulfamethoxazole 874
Apo-Sulfinpyrazone® (Canada) *see* Sulfinpyrazone 811
Apo-Sulin® (Canada) *see* Sulindac 813
Apo-Tamox® (Canada) *see* Tamoxifen Citrate 818
Apo-Terfenadine® (Canada) *see* Terfenadine 823
Apo-Tetra® (Canada) *see* Tetracycline 829
Apo-Theo® LA (Canada) *see* Theophylline/Aminophylline 832
Apo-Thioridazine® (Canada) *see* Thioridazine 840
Apo-Timol® (Canada) *see* Timolol Maleate 847
Apo-Timop® (Canada) *see* Timolol Maleate 847
Apo-Tolbutamide® (Canada) *see* Tolbutamide 853
Apo-Triazide® (Canada) *see* Triamterene and Hydrochlorothiazide 865
Apo-Triazo® (Canada) *see* Triazolam 866
Apo-Trihex® (Canada) *see* Trihexyphenidyl Hydrochloride 871
Apo-Trimip® (Canada) *see* Trimipramine Maleate 876
Apo-Verap® (Canada) *see* Verapamil Hydrochloride 893
Apo-Zidovudine® (Canada) *see* Zidovudine 907
Apraclonidine Hydrochloride 72
Apresazide® *see* Hydralazine and Hydrochlorothiazide 428
Apresolina® (Mexico) *see* Hydralazine Hydrochloride 428
Apresoline® *see* Hydralazine Hydrochloride 428
Aprodine® [OTC] *see* Triprolidine and Pseudoephedrine 878
Aprodine® w/C *see* Triprolidine, Pseudoephedrine, and Codeine 879
Apro-Flurbiprofen® (Canada) *see* Flurbiprofen Sodium 381
Aprotinin 72
Aquacare® [OTC] *see* Urea 884
Aquachloral® Supprettes® *see* Chloral Hydrate 180
AquaMEPHYTON® *see* Phytonadione 690
Aquaphyllin® *see* Theophylline/Aminophylline 832
AquaSite® Ophthalmic Solution [OTC] *see* Artificial Tears 75
Aquasol A® [OTC] *see* Vitamin A 898
Aquasol E® [OTC] *see* Vitamin E 900
Aquatag® *see* Benzthiazide 105
AquaTar® [OTC] *see* Coal Tar 225
Aquatensen® *see* Methyclothiazide 565
Aralen® Phosphate *see* Chloroquine Phosphate 187
Aralen® Phosphate With Primaquine Phosphate *see* Chloroquine and
    Primaquine 186
Aredia™ *see* Pamidronate Disodium 655
Arfonad® *see* Trimethaphan Camsylate 873
Argesic®-SA *see* Salsalate 779
Arginine Hydrochloride 73
Argyrol® S.S. 20% *see* Silver Protein, Mild 787
Aristocort® Forte *see* Triamcinolone 862
Aristocort® Intralesional Suspension *see* Triamcinolone 862
Aristocort® Tablet *see* Triamcinolone 862
Aristospan® *see* Triamcinolone 862
Arlidin® *see* Nylidrin Hydrochloride 631
Arm-a-Med® Isoetharine *see* Isoetharine 470
Arm-a-Med® Isoproterenol *see* Isoproterenol 472
Arm-a-Med® Metaproterenol *see* Metaproterenol Sulfate 550

A.R.M.® Caplet [OTC] see Chlorpheniramine and Phenylpropanolamine
. 190
Armour® Thyroid see Thyroid 844
Aromatic Ammonia Aspirols® see Ammonia Spirit, Aromatic. 54
Arovit® (Mexico) see Vitamin A 898
Arrestin® see Trimethobenzamide Hydrochloride 873
ARS see Antirabies Serum, Equine Origin 71
Artane® see Trihexyphenidyl Hydrochloride. 871
Artha-G® see Salsalate 779
Arthritis Foundation® Nighttime [OTC] see Acetaminophen and
    Diphenhydramine 16
Arthropan® [OTC] see Choline Salicylate 202
Articaine Hydrochloride with Epinephrine 74
Articulose-50® see Prednisolone 718
Artificial Saliva Products 1050
Artificial Tears 75
Artosin® (Mexico) see Tolbutamide 853
Artrenac® (Mexico) see Diclofenac 271
Artyflam® (Mexico) see Piroxicam 699
A.S.A. [OTC] see Aspirin 78
ASA® (Canada) see Aspirin 78
Asacol® see Mesalamine 546
Asaphen® (Canada) see Aspirin 78
Ascorbic® 500 (Canada) see Ascorbic Acid 76
Ascorbic Acid 76
Ascorbic Acid and Ferrous Sulfate see Ferrous Sulfate and Ascorbic Acid
. 361
Ascorbicap® [OTC] see Ascorbic Acid 76
Ascorbico, Acido (Mexico) see Ascorbic Acid 76
Ascriptin® [OTC] see Aspirin 78
Asendin® see Amoxapine 56
Asmalix® see Theophylline/Aminophylline 832
Asparaginase 77
Aspergum® [OTC] see Aspirin 78
Aspirin 78
Aspirin and Codeine 80
Aspirin and Meprobamate 81
Aspirin-Free Bayer® Select® Allergy Sinus Caplets [OTC] see
    Acetaminophen, Chlorpheniramine, and Pseudoephedrine 17
Astemina® (Mexico) see Astemizole 82
Astemizole 82
AsthmaNefrin® see Epinephrine, Racemic. 314
Astramorph™ PF Injection see Morphine Sulfate 590
Atarax® see Hydroxyzine 443
Atasol® (Canada) see Acetaminophen 14
Atemperator-S® (Mexico) see Valproic Acid and Derivatives 888
Atenolol 83
Atenolol and Chlorthalidone 84
ATG see Lymphocyte Immune Globulin, Anti-thymocyte Globulin (Equine)
. 518
Atgam® see Lymphocyte Immune Globulin, Anti-thymocyte Globulin (Equine)
. 518
Atiflan® (Mexico) see Naproxen 606
ATIII see Antithrombin III 71
Atiquim® (Mexico) see Naproxen 606
Atisuril® (Mexico) see Allopurinol 33
Ativan® see Lorazepam 513
ATnativ® see Antithrombin III 71
Atovaquone 84
Atozine® see Hydroxyzine 443
Atrofen™ see Baclofen 95
Atromid-S® see Clofibrate 217
Atropine Sulfate 85
Atrovent® see Ipratropium Bromide 467
A/T/S® Topical see Erythromycin, Topical 324
Attapulgite 86
Attenuvax® see Measles Virus Vaccine, Live 529
Augmentin® see Amoxicillin and Clavulanic Acid 57
Auralate® see Gold Sodium Thiomalate 404
Auralgan® see Antipyrine and Benzocaine 70
Auranofin 87
Aureomicina® (Mexico) see Chlortetracycline Hydrochloride 199
Aureomycin® see Chlortetracycline Hydrochloride. 199
Auro® Ear Drops [OTC] see Carbamide Peroxide 152
Aurothioglucose 87
Auroto® see Antipyrine and Benzocaine 70
Autoplex® T see Anti-Inhibitor Coagulant Complex 70
AVC™ Cream see Sulfanilamide 810

AVC™ Suppository see Sulfanilamide 810
Aveeno® Cleansing Bar [OTC] see Sulfur and Salicylic Acid 813
Aventyl® Hydrochloride see Nortriptyline Hydrochloride 629
A-Vicon® (Mexico) see Vitamin A 898
Avirax® (Canada) see Acyclovir 23
Avitene® see Microfibrillar Collagen Hemostat 579
A-Vitex® (Mexico) see Vitamin A 898
Avlosulfon® see Dapsone 251
Axid® see Nizatidine 626
Axotal® see Butalbital Compound 133
Ayercillin® (Canada) see Penicillin G Procaine 667
Aygestin® see Norethindrone 627
Azacitidine 88
AZA-CR see Azacitidine 88
Azactam® see Aztreonam 91
5-Azacytidine see Azacitidine 88
Azantac® (Mexico) see Ranitidine Hydrochloride 763
Azatadina, Maleato De (Mexico) see Azatadine Maleate 89
Azatadine and Pseudoephedrine 89
Azatadine Maleate 89
Azathioprine 89
Azatioprina (Mexico) see Azathioprine 89
Azatrilem® (Mexico) see Azathioprine 89
5-AZC see Azacitidine 88
Azdone® see Hydrocodone and Aspirin........................433
Azelaic Acid 90
Azelex® see Azelaic Acid....................................90
Azithromycin 90
Azmacort™ see Triamcinolone 862
Azo Gantanol® see Sulfamethoxazole and Phenazopyridine 809
Azo Gantrisin® see Sulfisoxazole and Phenazopyridine 812
Azo-Standard® see Phenazopyridine Hydrochloride 679
Azo Wintomylon® (Mexico) see Phenazopyridine Hydrochloride 679
Aztreonam 91
Azulfidine® see Sulfasalazine 810
Azulfidine® EN-tabs® see Sulfasalazine 810
Babee® Teething [OTC] see Benzocaine 102
BAC see Benzalkonium Chloride 102
B-A-C® see Butalbital Compound 133
Bacampicillin Hydrochloride 92
Bacid® [OTC] see Lactobacillus acidophilus and Lactobacillus bulgaricus
....488
Baciguent® [OTC] see Bacitracin 93
Baci-IM® see Bacitracin 93
Bacillus Calmette-Guérin (BCG) Live 93
Bacitin® (Canada) see Bacitracin.............................93
Bacitracin 93
Bacitracin and Polymyxin B 94
Bacitracin, Neomycin, and Polymyxin B 94
Bacitracin, Neomycin, Polymyxin B, and Hydrocortisone 95
Bacitracin, Neomycin, Polymyxin B, and Lidocaine 95
Baclofen 95
Bactelan® (Mexico) see Trimethoprim and Sulfamethoxazole 874
Bacticort® Otic see Neomycin, Polymyxin B, and Hydrocortisone ...610
Bactocill® see Oxacillin Sodium 641
Bactocin® (Mexico) see Ofloxacin 634
Bactrim™ see Trimethoprim and Sulfamethoxazole...............874
Bactrim™ DS see Trimethoprim and Sulfamethoxazole 874
Bactroban® see Mupirocin 593
Baker's P&S Topical [OTC] see Phenol 682
Balanced Salt Solution 96
Balcoran® (Mexico) see Vancomycin Hydrochloride 889
BAL in Oil® see Dimercaprol 287
Balminil® Decongestant (Canada) see Pseudoephedrine 749
Balminil-DM® (Canada) see Dextromethorphan 266
Balminil® Expectorant (Canada) see Guaifenesin 407
Balnetar® [OTC] see Coal Tar, Lanolin, and Mineral Oil 226
Bancap® see Butalbital Compound 133
Bancap HC® [5/500] see Hydrocodone and Acetaminophen........431
Banesin® [OTC] see Acetaminophen..........................14
Banophen® [OTC] see Diphenhydramine Hydrochloride 288
Banthine® see Methantheline Bromide 554
Bapadin® (Canada) see Bepridil Hydrochloride 108
Barbidonna® see Hyoscyamine, Atropine, Scopolamine, and Phenobarbital
....444
Barbilixir® (Canada) see Phenobarbital 680
Barbita® see Phenobarbital 680
Barc™ [OTC] see Pyrethrins 753

Baridium® see Phenazopyridine Hydrochloride 679
Barophen® see Hyoscyamine, Atropine, Scopolamine, and Phenobarbital
....444
Basaljel® [OTC] see Aluminum Carbonate 39
Base Ointment see Zinc Oxide 908
Batrizol® (Mexico) see Trimethoprim and Sulfamethoxazole 874
Bayer® Aspirin [OTC] see Aspirin 78
Bayer® Select® Chest Cold Caplets [OTC] see Acetaminophen and
    Dextromethorphan 16
BCG see Bacillus Calmette-Guérin (BCG) Live.......................93
BCNU see Carmustine 157
B-D Glucose® [OTC] see Glucose 400
Because® [OTC] see Nonoxynol 9 627
Beclodisk® (Canada) see Beclomethasone Dipropionate 97
Becloforte® (Canada) see Beclomethasone Dipropionate 97
Beclometasona (Mexico) see Beclomethasone Dipropionate 97
Beclomethasone Dipropionate 97
Beclovent® see Beclomethasone Dipropionate 97
Beconase® see Beclomethasone Dipropionate 97
Beconase AQ® see Beclomethasone Dipropionate 97
Beconase® Aqua (Mexico) see Beclomethasone Dipropionate 97
Becotide® 100 (Mexico) see Beclomethasone Dipropionate 97
Becotide® 250 (Mexico) see Beclomethasone Dipropionate 97
Becotide® Aerosol (Mexico) see Beclomethasone Dipropionate 97
Becotin® Pulvules® see Vitamins, Multiple..........................901
Beepen-VK® see Penicillin V Potassium 668
Beesix® see Pyridoxine Hydrochloride.............................753
Beknol® (Mexico) see Benzonatate 104
Beldin® [OTC] see Diphenhydramine Hydrochloride 288
Belix® [OTC] see Diphenhydramine Hydrochloride 288
Belladonna 98
Belladonna and Opium 98
Belladonna, Phenobarbital, and Ergotamine Tartrate 99
Bellergal-S® see Belladonna, Phenobarbital, and Ergotamine Tartrate 99
Bel-Phen-Ergot S® see Belladonna, Phenobarbital, and Ergotamine Tartrate
....99
Bemote® see Dicyclomine Hydrochloride 273
Benadon® (Mexico) see Pyridoxine Hydrochloride 753
Benadryl® [OTC] see Diphenhydramine Hydrochloride 288
Benaxima® (Mexico) see Cefotaxime Sodium 167
Benaxona® (Mexico) see Ceftriaxone Sodium 172
Benazepril Clorhidrato De (Mexico) see Benazepril Hydrochloride 99
Benazepril Hydrochloride......................................99
Bendroflumethiazide 101
Bendroflumetiacida (Mexico) see Bendroflumethiazide 101
Benecid® Probenecida Valdecasas (Mexico) see Probenecid...........724
Benemid® see Probenecid.....................................724
Benoquin® see Monobenzone 589
Benoxyl® see Benzoyl Peroxide 104
Bentiromide 101
Bentyl® Hydrochloride see Dicyclomine Hydrochloride 273
Bentylol® (Canada) see Dicyclomine Hydrochloride 273
Benuryl® (Canada) see Probenecid...............................724
Benylin® Cough Syrup [OTC] see Diphenhydramine Hydrochloride 288
Benylin® DM [OTC] see Dextromethorphan 266
Benylin® Expectorant [OTC] see Guaifenesin and Dextromethorphan 408
Benza® [OTC] see Benzalkonium Chloride 102
Benzac AC Wash® see Benzoyl Peroxide.........................104
Benzac W Wash® see Benzoyl Peroxide 104
Benzalkonium Chloride 102
Benzamycin® see Erythromycin and Benzoyl Peroxide...............323
Benzanil® (Mexico) see Penicillin G, Parenteral, Aqueous 666
Benzedrex® [OTC] see Propylhexedrine 745
Benzetacil® (Mexico) see Penicillin G Benzathine, Parenteral 665
Benzilfan® (Mexico) see Penicillin G Benzathine, Parenteral 665
Benzmethyzin see Procarbazine Hydrochloride.....................727
Benzocaine 102
Benzocaine and Antipyrine see Antipyrine and Benzocaine 70
Benzocaine and Cetylpyridinium Chloride see Cetylpyridinium Chloride and
    Benzocaine 179
Benzocaine, Butyl Aminobenzoate, Tetracaine, and Benzalkonium Chloride
....103
Benzocaine, Gelatin, Pectin, and Sodium Carboxymethylcellulose 103
Benzocol® [OTC] see Benzocaine 102
Benzodent® [OTC] see Benzocaine 102
Benzoic Acid and Salicylic Acid.................................104
Benzoin 104
Benzonatate 104

1157

Benzonatato (Mexico) *see* Benzonatate 104
Benzoyl Peroxide 104
Benzoyl Peroxide® *see* Benzoyl Peroxide 104
Benzoyl Peroxide and Hydrocortisone 105
Benzphetamine Hydrochloride 105
Benzthiazide 106
Benztropine Mesylate 106
Benzylpenicilloyl-polylysine 107
Bepridil Hydrochloride 108
Beractant 108
Berocca® *see* Vitamin B Complex With Vitamin C and Folic Acid 900
Berubigen® *see* Cyanocobalamin 237
Beta-2® *see* Isoetharine 470
Beta-Carotene 109
Betachron E-R® *see* Propranolol Hydrochloride 743
Betadine® [OTC] *see* Povidone-Iodine 713
9-Beta-D-ribofuranosyladenine *see* Adenosine 25
Betagan® *see* Levobunolol Hydrochloride 493
Betalin®S *see* Thiamine Hydrochloride 837
Betaloc® (Canada) *see* Metoprolol 574
Betaloc Durules® (Canada) *see* Metoprolol 574
Betamethasone 109
Betamethasone and Clotrimazole 111
Betapace® *see* Sotalol Hydrochloride 796
Betapen®-VK *see* Penicillin V Potassium 668
Betaseron® *see* Interferon Beta-1b 464
Betatrex® *see* Betamethasone 109
Beta-Val® *see* Betamethasone 109
Betaxin® (Canada) *see* Thiamine Hydrochloride 837
Betaxolol Hydrochloride 111
Bethanechol Chloride 112
Betimol® Ophthalmic *see* Timolol Maleate 847
Betnesol® [Disodium Phosphate] (Canada) *see* Betamethasone 109
Betoptic® *see* Betaxolol Hydrochloride 111
Betoptic® S *see* Betaxolol Hydrochloride 111
Bewon® (Canada) *see* Thiamine Hydrochloride 837
Bexophene® *see* Propoxyphene and Aspirin 742
Biamine® *see* Thiamine Hydrochloride 837
Biavax® II *see* Rubella and Mumps Vaccines, Combined 775
Biaxin™ Filmtabs® *see* Clarithromycin 212
Bicalutamide 113
Bicillin® C-R 900/300 Injection *see* Penicillin G Benzathine and Procaine
   Combined 665
Bicillin® C-R Injection *see* Penicillin G Benzathine and Procaine Combined
   665
Bicillin® L-A *see* Penicillin G Benzathine, Parenteral 665
Biclin® (Mexico) *see* Amikacin Sulfate 44
BiCNU® *see* Carmustine 157
Bilem® (Mexico) *see* Tamoxifen Citrate 818
Biltricide® *see* Praziquantel 716
Binotal® (Mexico) *see* Ampicillin 62
Biocal® [OTC] *see* Calcium Carbonate 140
Bioclate® *see* Antihemophilic Factor (Recombinant) 70
Bioderm® (Canada) *see* Bacitracin and Polymyxin B 94
Bion® Tears Solution [OTC] *see* Artificial Tears 75
Biosint® (Mexico) *see* Cefotaxime Sodium 167
Biperiden 113
Bisac-Evac® [OTC] *see* Bisacodyl 113
Bisacodilo (Mexico) *see* Bisacodyl 113
Bisacodyl 113
Bisacodyl Uniserts® *see* Bisacodyl 113
Bisco-Lax® [OTC] *see* Bisacodyl 113
Bismatrol® (subsalicylate) [OTC] *see* Bismuth 114
Bismuth 114
Bismuth Subgallate *see* Bismuth 114
Bismuth Subsalicylate *see* Bismuth 114
Bisoprolol and Hydrochlorothiazide 115
Bisoprolol Fumarate 115
Bistropamide *see* Tropicamide 881
Bitolterol Mesylate 116
Black Draught® [OTC] *see* Senna 785
Blanex® *see* Chlorzoxazone 200
Blastocarb (Mexico) *see* Carboplatin 155
Blastolem (Mexico) *see* Cisplatin 210
BlemErase® [OTC] *see* Benzoyl Peroxide 104
Blenoxane® *see* Bleomycin Sulfate 117
Bleolem (Mexico) *see* Bleomycin Sulfate 117
Bleomycin Sulfate 117

Bleph®-10 see Sodium Sulfacetamide 793
Blephamide® see Sodium Sulfacetamide and Prednisolone Acetate 794
BLM see Bleomycin Sulfate 117
Blocadren® Oral see Timolol Maleate 847
Blocan® (Mexico) see Cimetidine 207
Bluboro® [OTC] see Aluminum Sulfate and Calcium Acetate 41
Blue® [OTC] see Pyrethrins 753
Bonine® [OTC] see Meclizine Hydrochloride 530
Boric Acid 118
Borofax® Topical [OTC] see Boric Acid 118
Boropak® [OTC] see Aluminum Sulfate and Calcium Acetate 41
B&O Suprettes® see Belladonna and Opium..............................98
Botox® see Botulinum Toxin Type A 118
Botulinum Toxin Type A 118
BQ® Tablet [OTC] see Chlorpheniramine, Phenylpropanolamine, and
    Acetaminophen 194
Braccopril® (Mexico) see Pyrazinamide 752
Braxan® (Mexico) see Amiodarone Hydrochloride........................48
Breonesin® [OTC] see Guaifenesin 407
Brethaire® see Terbutaline Sulfate 822
Brethine® see Terbutaline Sulfate 822
Bretylate® (Canada) see Bretylium Tosylate 119
Bretylium Tosylate 119
Bretylol® see Bretylium Tosylate 119
Brevicon® see Ethinyl Estradiol and Norethindrone 339
Brevital® Sodium see Methohexital Sodium 559
Bricanyl® see Terbutaline Sulfate 822
Brietal® Sodium (Canada) see Methohexital Sodium 559
Brimonidine Tartrate 121
Brispen® (Mexico) see Dicloxacillin Sodium 273
Brofed® Elixir [OTC] see Brompheniramine and Pseudoephedrine 123
Bromaline® Elixir [OTC] see Brompheniramine and Phenylpropanolamine
   123
Bromanate® DC see Brompheniramine, Phenylpropanolamine, and Codeine
   125
Bromanate® Elixir [OTC] see Brompheniramine and Phenylpropanolamine
   123
Bromanyl® Cough Syrup see Bromodiphenhydramine and Codeine 122
Bromarest® [OTC] see Brompheniramine Maleate 124
Bromatapp® [OTC] see Brompheniramine and Phenylpropanolamine.........123
Brombay® [OTC] see Brompheniramine Maleate 124
Bromfed® Syrup [OTC] see Brompheniramine and Pseudoephedrine 123
Bromfed® Tablet [OTC] see Brompheniramine and Pseudoephedrine 123
Bromocriptina (Mexico) see Bromocriptine Mesylate....................121
Bromocriptine Mesylate 121
Bromodiphenhydramine and Codeine 122
Bromofeniramina Maleato De (Mexico) see Brompheniramine Maleate 124
Bromotuss® w/Codeine Cough Syrup see Bromodiphenhydramine and
    Codeine 122
Bromphen® [OTC] see Brompheniramine Maleate 124
Bromphen® DC w/Codeine see Brompheniramine, Phenylpropanolamine, and
    Codeine 125
Brompheniramine and Phenylephrine 122
Brompheniramine and Phenylpropanolamine 123
Brompheniramine and Pseudoephedrine.................................123
Brompheniramine Maleate 124
Brompheniramine, Phenylpropanolamine, and Codeine 125
Bromphen® Tablet [OTC] see Brompheniramine and Phenylpropanolamine
   123
Bronalide® (Canada) see Flunisolide 372
Bronchial® see Theophylline and Guaifenesin 836
Bronkephrine® Injection see Ethylnorepinephrine Hydrochloride 345
Bronkodyl® see Theophylline/Aminophylline 832
Bronkometer® see Isoetharine 470
Bronkosol® see Isoetharine 470
Brotane® [OTC] see Brompheniramine Maleate 124
BSS® Ophthalmic see Balanced Salt Solution...........................96
BTPABA see Bentiromide 101
Bucladin®-S Softab® see Buclizine Hydrochloride 125
Buclizine Hydrochloride 125
Budesonide 126
Bufferin® [OTC] see Aspirin 78
Bumedyl® (Mexico) see Bumetanide 126
Bumetanida (Mexico) see Bumetanide 126
Bumetanide 126
Bumex® see Bumetanide...126
Bupivacaine Hydrochloride 127
Bupivacaine With Epinephrine 128

Buprenex® *see* Buprenorphine Hydrochloride 129
Buprenorfina (Mexico) *see* Buprenorphine Hydrochloride 129
Buprenorphine Hydrochloride 129
Bupropion 130
Burinex® (Canada) *see* Bumetanide 126
Burow's Otic *see* Aluminum Acetate and Acetic Acid 39
BuSpar® *see* Buspirone Hydrochloride 131
Buspirona, Clorhidrato De (Mexico) *see* Buspirone Hydrochloride 131
Buspirone Hydrochloride 131
Busulfan. 131
Busulfano (Mexico) *see* Busulfan 131
Butabarbital Sodium. 132
Butace® *see* Butalbital Compound. 133
Butacortelone® (Mexico) *see* Ibuprofen 447
Butalan® *see* Butabarbital Sodium. 132
Butalbital Compound 133
Butalbital Compound and Codeine 134
Butenafine Hydrochloride 135
Buticaps® *see* Butabarbital Sodium. 132
Butisol Sodium® *see* Butabarbital Sodium 132
Butoconazole Nitrate 135
Butoconazol (Mexico) *see* Butoconazole Nitrate 135
Butorfanol (Mexico) *see* Butorphanol Tartrate .135
Butorphanol Tartrate 135
Buvacaina® (Mexico) *see* Bupivacaine Hydrochloride 127
Buvacaina® (Mexico) *see* Bupivacaine With Epinephrine 128
Byclomine® *see* Dicyclomine Hydrochloride 273
C7E3 *see* Abciximab 12
C8-CCK *see* Sincalide 789
Cafatine® *see* Ergotamine 319
Cafergot® *see* Ergotamine 319
Cafetrate® *see* Ergotamine 319
Caffeine and Sodium Benzoate 136
Caffeine, Citrated 136
Calan® *see* Verapamil Hydrochloride 893
Calan® SR *see* Verapamil Hydrochloride 893
Calcibind® *see* Cellulose Sodium Phosphate 175
Calci-Chew™ *see* Calcium Carbonate 140
Calcifediol 137
Calciferol™ *see* Ergocalciferol 317
Calcijex™ *see* Calcitriol 139
Calcilac® [OTC] *see* Calcium Carbonate 140
Calcimar® *see* Calcitonin 138
Calci-Mix™ *see* Calcium Carbonate. 140
Calciparine® Injection *see* Heparin 419
Calcipotriene 138
Calcite-500® (Canada) *see* Calcium Carbonate 140
Calcitonin 138
Calcitriol 139
Calcium Acetate. 139
Calcium Carbonate 140
Calcium Carbonate and Simethicone 141
Calcium Channel Blockers & Gingival Hyperplasia 1010
Calcium Chloride 141
Calcium Citrate 142
Calcium Glubionate 142
Calcium Gluceptate 143
Calcium Gluconate 143
Calcium Lactate 145
Calcium Leucovorin *see* Leucovorin Calcium 491
Calcium Pantothenate *see* Pantothenic Acid 658
Calcium Phosphate, Tribasic 145
Calcium Polycarbophil 146
Calderol® *see* Calcifediol 137
Caldesene® Topical [OTC] *see* Undecylenic Acid and Derivatives 884
Calm-X® [OTC] *see* Dimenhydrinate 286
Calmylin® Expectorant (Canada) *see* Guaifenesin 407
Cal Plus® *see* Calcium Chloride 141
Calsan® (Canada) *see* Calcium Carbonate 140
CalSup® [OTC] *see* Calcium Carbonate 140
Caltine® (Canada) *see* Calcitonin 138
Caltrate® [OTC] *see* Calcium Carbonate 140
Cam-ap-es® *see* Hydralazine, Hydrochlorothiazide, and Reserpine 429
Campho-Phenique® [OTC] *see* Camphor and Phenol. 146
Camphor and Phenol. 146
Camphor, Menthol, and Phenol. 146
Camptosar® *see* Irinotecan 468
Cancer Chemotherapy Regimens 1011

ALPHABETICAL INDEX

Cankaid® [OTC] see Carbamide Peroxide 152
Cantharidin...146
Cantil® see Mepenzolate Bromide 538
Capastat® Sulfate see Capreomycin Sulfate 147
Capital® and Codeine see Acetaminophen and Codeine 15
Capital® (Mexico) see Captopril 148
Capitrol® see Chloroxine 189
Capoten® see Captopril 148
Capotena® (Mexico) see Captopril 148
Capozide® see Captopril and Hydrochlorothiazide 149
Capreomycin Sulfate 147
Capsaicin 147
Captopril 148
Captopril and Hydrochlorothiazide 149
Carafate® see Sucralfate 804
Caramiphen and Phenylpropanolamine 150
Carampicillin Hydrochloride see Bacampicillin Hydrochloride 92
Carbachol 150
Carbac® (Mexico) see Loracarbef 512
Carbamazepine 151
Carbamide Peroxide 152
Carbazep® (Mexico) see Carbamazepine 151
Carbazina® (Mexico) see Carbamazepine 151
Carbecin® Inyectable (Mexico) see Carbenicillin 153
Carbenicilina, Disodica (Mexico) see Carbenicillin 153
Carbenicillin 153
Carbidopa 153
Carbinoxamine and Pseudoephedrine 154
Carbinoxamine, Pseudoephedrine, and Dextromethorphan 155
Carbiset® Tablet see Carbinoxamine and Pseudoephedrine 154
Carbiset-TR® Tablet see Carbinoxamine and Pseudoephedrine 154
Carbocaine® 2% with Neo-Cobefrin® see Mepivacaine With Levonordefrin
542
Carbocaine® 3% see Mepivacaine Dental Anesthetic 541
Carbodec® DM see Carbinoxamine, Pseudoephedrine, and
  Dextromethorphan 155
Carbodec® Syrup see Carbinoxamine and Pseudoephedrine 154
Carbodec® Tablet see Carbinoxamine and Pseudoephedrine 154
Carbodec TR® Tablet see Carbinoxamine and Pseudoephedrine 154
Carbol-Fuchsin Solution 155
Carbolic Acid see Phenol 682
Carbolit® (Mexico) see Lithium 508
Carboplatin 155
Carboplat (Mexico) see Carboplatin 155
Carboprost Tromethamine 156
Carbose D see Carboxymethylcellulose Sodium 156
Carboxymethylcellulose Sodium 156
Cardec® DM see Carbinoxamine, Pseudoephedrine, and Dextromethorphan
155
Cardec-S® Syrup see Carbinoxamine and Pseudoephedrine 154
Cardene® see Nicardipine Hydrochloride 616
Cardene® SR see Nicardipine Hydrochloride 616
Cardilate® see Erythrityl Tetranitrate 320
Cardinit® (Mexico) see Nitroglycerin 623
Cardio-Green® see Indocyanine Green 457
Cardioquin® see Quinidine 759
Cardiorona® (Mexico) see Amiodarone Hydrochloride 48
Cardiovascular Diseases 912
Cardipril® (Mexico) see Captopril 148
Cardizem® CD see Diltiazem 284
Cardizem® Injectable see Diltiazem 284
Cardizem® SR see Diltiazem 284
Cardizem® Tablet see Diltiazem 284
Cardura® see Doxazosin 298
Carisoprodol 157
Carmol® [OTC] see Urea 884
Carmol-HC® Topical see Urea and Hydrocortisone 885
Carmustine 157
Carnitor® Injection see Levocarnitine 494
Carnitor® Oral see Levocarnitine 494
Carnotprim Primperan® (Mexico) see Metoclopramide 572
Carnotprim Primperan® Retard (Mexico) see Metoclopramide 572
Carteolol Hydrochloride 158
Carter's Little Pills® [OTC] see Bisacodyl 113
Cartrol® see Carteolol Hydrochloride 158
Carvedilol 159
Casanthranol and Docusate see Docusate and Casanthranol 295
Cascara Sagrada 160

Casodex® see Bicalutamide 113
Castellani Paint see Carbol-Fuchsin Solution 155
Castor Oil...161
Cataflam® see Diclofenac 271
Catapres® see Clonidine 221
Catapresan-100® (Mexico) see Clonidine 221
Catapres-TTS® see Clonidine 221
Cauteridol® (Mexico) see Ranitidine Hydrochloride 763
Caverject® Injection see Alprostadil 35
CBDCA see Carboplatin 155
CCNU see Lomustine 510
2-CdA see Cladribine 211
CDDP see Cisplatin 210
Ceclor® see Cefaclor 161
Ceclor® CD see Cefaclor 161
Cecon® [OTC] see Ascorbic Acid 76
Cedocard-SR® (Canada) see Isosorbide Dinitrate 474
Cee-1000® T.D. [OTC] see Ascorbic Acid 76
CeeNU® Oral see Lomustine 510
Cefaclor 161
Cefadroxil Monohydrate 162
Cefadyl® see Cephapirin Sodium 177
Cefalotina Sal Sodica De (Mexico) see Cephalothin Sodium 177
Cefamandole Nafate 163
Cefamezin® (Mexico) see Cefazolin Sodium 164
Cefamox® (Mexico) see Cefadroxil Monohydrate 162
Cefanex® see Cephalexin Monohydrate 176
Cefaxim® (Mexico) see Cefotaxime Sodium 167
Cefaxona® (Mexico) see Ceftriaxone Sodium 172
Cefazolina (Mexico) see Cefazolin Sodium 164
Cefazolin Sodium..164
Cefepime 164
Cefixima (Mexico) see Cefixime 165
Cefixime..165
Cefizox® see Ceftizoxime 171
Cefmetazole Sodium 165
Cefobid® see Cefoperazone Sodium 167
Cefoclin® (Mexico) see Cefotaxime Sodium 167
Cefol® Filmtab® see Vitamins, Multiple 901
Cefonicidid (Mexico) see Cefonicid Sodium 166
Cefonicid Sodium..166
Cefoperazona (Mexico) see Cefoperazone Sodium 167
Cefoperazone Sodium 167
Cefotan® see Cefotetan Disodium 168
Cefotaxima (Mexico) see Cefotaxime Sodium 167
Cefotaxime Sodium 167
Cefotetan Disodium 168
Cefoxitin Sodium 168
Cefpodoxime Proxetil 169
Cefprozil...170
Cefradina (Mexico) see Cephradine 178
Ceftazidima (Mexico) see Ceftazidime 171
Ceftazidime 171
Ceftazim® (Mexico) see Ceftazidime 171
Ceftin® see Cefuroxime 173
Ceftina® (Mexico) see Cephalothin Sodium 177
Ceftizoxima (Mexico) see Ceftizoxime 171
Ceftizoxime 171
Ceftriaxona (Mexico) see Ceftriaxone Sodium 172
Ceftriaxone Sodium 172
Cefuroxima (Mexico) see Cefuroxime 173
Cefuroxime..173
Cefzil® see Cefprozil 170
Celek® 20 (Mexico) see Potassium Chloride 708
Celestone® see Betamethasone 109
CellCept® see Mycophenolate Mofetil 595
Cellufresh® [OTC] see Carboxymethylcellulose Sodium 156
Cellulose, Oxidized 174
Cellulose, Oxidized Regenerated..175
Cellulose Sodium Phosphate...175
Celluvisc® [OTC] see Carboxymethylcellulose Sodium 156
Celontin® see Methsuximide 564
Celontin® (Canada) see Methsuximide 564
Cel-U-Jec® see Betamethasone 109
Cenafed® [OTC] see Pseudoephedrine 749
Cenafed® Plus [OTC] see Triprolidine and Pseudoephedrine 878
Cena-K® see Potassium Chloride 708
Cenolate® see Sodium Ascorbate 791

Centrax® *see* Prazepam 715
Cēpacol® Anesthetic Troches [OTC] *see* Cetylpyridinium Chloride and
    Benzocaine 179
Cēpastat® [OTC] *see* Phenol 682
Cephalexin Monohydrate 176
Cephalothin Sodium 177
Cephapirin Sodium 177
Cephradine 178
Cephulac® *see* Lactulose 488
Ceporacin® (Canada) *see* Cephalothin Sodium 177
Ceporex® (Mexico) *see* Cephalexin Monohydrate 176
Ceptaz™ (Canada) *see* Ceftazidime 171
Cerebyx® *see* Fosphenytoin 389
Ceredase® Injection *see* Alglucerase 32
Cerespan® *see* Papaverine Hydrochloride 658
Cerezyme® *see* Imglucerase 450
Cerose-DM® [OTC] *see* Chlorpheniramine, Phenylephrine, and
    Dextromethorphan 193
Cerubidine® *see* Daunorubicin Hydrochloride 252
Cerumenex® *see* Triethanolamine Polypeptide Oleate-Condensate 868
Cesamet® *see* Nabilone 596
C.E.S.® (Canada) *see* Estrogens, Conjugated 327
Cetacaine® *see* Benzocaine, Butyl Aminobenzoate, Tetracaine, and
    Benzalkonium Chloride 103
Cetamide® *see* Sodium Sulfacetamide 793
Cetane® [OTC] *see* Ascorbic Acid 76
Cetapred® *see* Sodium Sulfacetamide and Prednisolone Acetate 794
Cetina® (Mexico) *see* Chloramphenicol 182
Cetirizine Hydrochloride 179
Cetylpyridinium Chloride and Benzocaine 179
Cevalin® *see* Ascorbic Acid 76
Ce-Vi-Sol® [OTC] *see* Ascorbic Acid 76
Ce-Vi-Sol® (Mexico) *see* Ascorbic Acid 76
Cevita® [OTC] *see* Ascorbic Acid 76
Cevitamic Acid (Canada) *see* Ascorbic Acid 76
Charcoaid® [OTC] *see* Charcoal 179
Charcoal 179
Charcocaps® [OTC] *see* Charcoal 179
Chemical Dependency and Dental Practice 971
Cheracol® *see* Guaifenesin and Codeine 408
Cheracol D® [OTC] *see* Guaifenesin and Dextromethorphan 408
Chibroxin™ *see* Norfloxacin 628
Children's Hold® [OTC] *see* Dextromethorphan 266
Children's Kaopectate® [OTC] *see* Attapulgite 86
Chlo-Amine® [OTC] *see* Chlorpheniramine Maleate 191
Chlorafed® Liquid [OTC] *see* Chlorpheniramine and Pseudoephedrine ...191
Chloral Hydrate 180
Chlorambucil 181
Chloramphenicol 182
Chloramphenicol and Prednisolone 183
Chloramphenicol, Polymyxin B, and Hydrocortisone 183
Chloraseptic® Oral [OTC] *see* Phenol 682
Chlorate® [OTC] *see* Chlorpheniramine Maleate 191
Chlordiazepoxide 183
Chlordiazepoxide and Amitriptyline *see* Amitriptyline and Chlordiazepoxide
   49
Chlordiazepoxide and Clidinium *see* Clidinium and Chlordiazepoxide ...214
Chloresium® [OTC] *see* Chlorophyll 185
Chlorhexidine Gluconate 184
2-Chlorodeoxyadenosine *see* Cladribine 211
Chloroethane *see* Ethyl Chloride 344
Chlorofon-F® *see* Chlorzoxazone 200
Chloromycetin® *see* Chloramphenicol 182
Chlorophylin *see* Chlorophyll 185
Chlorophyll 185
Chloroprocaine Hydrochloride 185
Chloroptic® *see* Chloramphenicol 182
Chloroptic-P® Ophthalmic *see* Chloramphenicol and Prednisolone 183
Chloroquine and Primaquine 186
Chloroquine Phosphate 187
Chlorothiazide 188
Chlorothiazide and Methyldopa 188
Chlorothiazide and Reserpine 189
Chlorotrianisene 189
Chloroxine 189
Chlorphed® [OTC] *see* Brompheniramine Maleate 124
Chlorphed®-LA Nasal Solution [OTC] *see* Oxymetazoline Hydrochloride
   649

Chlorphenesin Carbamate 190
Chlorpheniramine and Acetaminophen 190
Chlorpheniramine and Phenylephrine 190
Chlorpheniramine and Phenylpropanolamine 190
Chlorpheniramine and Pseudoephedrine 191
Chlorpheniramine, Ephedrine, Phenylephrine, and Carbetapentane 191
Chlorpheniramine Maleate 191
Chlorpheniramine, Phenindamine, and Phenylpropanolamine 192
Chlorpheniramine, Phenylephrine, and Codeine 192
Chlorpheniramine, Phenylephrine, and Dextromethorphan 193
Chlorpheniramine, Phenylephrine, and Methscopolamine 193
Chlorpheniramine, Phenylephrine, and Phenylpropanolamine 193
Chlorpheniramine, Phenylephrine, and Phenyltoloxamine 193
Chlorpheniramine, Phenylpropanolamine, and Acetaminophen 194
Chlorpheniramine, Phenylpropanolamine, and Dextromethorphan 194
Chlorpheniramine, Phenyltoloxamine, Phenylpropanolamine, and
   Phenylephrine 194
Chlorpheniramine, Pseudoephedrine, and Codeine 195
Chlorpheniramine, Pyrilamine, and Phenylephrine 195
Chlorpheniramine, Pyrilamine, Phenylephrine, and Phenylpropanolamine
   195
Chlor-Pro® [OTC] see Chlorpheniramine Maleate 191
Chlorpromanyl® (Canada) see Chlorpromazine Hydrochloride 195
Chlorpromazine Hydrochloride 195
Chlorprom® (Canada) see Chlorpromazine Hydrochloride 195
Chlorpropamide 197
Chlorprothixene 198
Chlor-Rest® Tablet [OTC] see Chlorpheniramine and Phenylpropanolamine
   190
Chlortetracycline Hydrochloride 199
Chlorthalidone 199
Chlor-Trimeton® [OTC] see Chlorpheniramine Maleate 191
Chlor-Trimeton® 4 Hour Relief Tablet [OTC] see Chlorpheniramine and
   Pseudoephedrine 191
Chlor-Tripolon® (Canada) see Chlorpheniramine Maleate 191
Chlorzoxazone 200
Cholac® see Lactulose 488
Cholan-HMB® see Dehydrocholic Acid 254
Cholecalciferol 200
Choledyl® see Oxtriphylline 645
Cholera Vaccine 201
Cholestyramine Resin 201
Choline Magnesium Salicylate 202
Choline Salicylate 202
Choline Theophyllinate see Oxtriphylline 645
Choloxin® see Dextrothyroxine Sodium 266
Cholybar® see Cholestyramine Resin 201
Chondroitin Sulfate-Sodium Hyaluronate 203
Chooz® [OTC] see Calcium Carbonate 140
Chorex® see Chorionic Gonadotropin 203
Chorionic Gonadotropin 203
Choron® see Chorionic Gonadotropin 203
Chromagen® OB [OTC] see Vitamins, Multiple 901
Chroma-Pak® see Trace Metals 857
Chromium see Trace Metals 857
Chronulac® see Lactulose 488
Chymex® see Bentiromide 101
Chymodiactin® see Chymopapain 204
Chymopapain 204
Cianocobalamina (Mexico) see Cyanocobalamin 237
Cibacalcin® see Calcitonin 138
Cibalith-S® see Lithium 508
Ciclofosfamida (Mexico) see Cyclophosphamide 240
Ciclopirox Olamine 205
Ciclosporina (Mexico) see Cyclosporine 243
Cidofovir 205
Cilag® (Mexico) see Acetaminophen 14
Cimetase® (Mexico) see Cimetidine 207
Cimetidina (Mexico) see Cimetidine 207
Cimetidine 207
Cimetigal® (Mexico) see Cimetidine 207
Cimogal® (Mexico) see Ciprofloxacin Hydrochloride 208
Cinobac® Pulvules® see Cinoxacin 207
Cinoxacin 207
Cinoxacino (Mexico) see Cinoxacin 207
Cipro™ see Ciprofloxacin Hydrochloride 208
Ciprofloxacin Hydrochloride 208
Ciproflox® (Mexico) see Ciprofloxacin Hydrochloride 208

Ciproflur® (Mexico) *see* Ciprofloxacin Hydrochloride 208
Ciproxina® (Mexico) *see* Ciprofloxacin Hydrochloride 208
Cisaprida (Mexico) *see* Cisapride 209
Cisapride 209
Cisplatin 210
Cisticid® (Mexico) *see* Praziquantel......................................716
Citanest® Forte (Canada) *see* Prilocaine With Epinephrine 721
Citanest Forte® with Epinephrine *see* Prilocaine With Epinephrine 721
Citanest® Octapresin (Mexico) *see* Prilocaine With Epinephrine 721
Citanest Plain 4% Injection *see* Prilocaine 721
Citax (Mexico) *see* Immune Globulin, Intravenous 454
Citoken® (Mexico) *see* Piroxicam 699
Citomid (Mexico) *see* Vincristine Sulfate 896
Citracal® [OTC] *see* Calcium Citrate 142
Citrate of Magnesia *see* Magnesium Citrate 521
Citric Acid and d-gluconic Acid Irrigant *see* Citric Acid Bladder Mixture
....211
Citric Acid Bladder Mixture 211
Citrovorum Factor *see* Leucovorin Calcium 491
Citrucel® [OTC] *see* Methylcellulose 566
Cladribine 211
Claforan® *see* Cefotaxime Sodium 167
Clamurid® (Canada) *see* Carbamide Peroxide 152
Clanda® (Mexico) *see* Vitamins, Multiple.................................901
Claripex® (Canada) *see* Clofibrate.......................................217
Clarithromycin 212
Claritin® *see* Loratadine 512
Claritin-D® *see* Loratadine and Pseudoephedrine 513
Claritin-D 24-Hour® *see* Loratadine and Pseudoephedrine 513
Clarityne® (Mexico) *see* Loratadine 512
Clavulin® (Canada) *see* Amoxicillin and Clavulanic Acid 57
Clavulin® (Mexico) *see* Amoxicillin and Clavulanic Acid 57
Clearasil® [OTC] *see* Benzoyl Peroxide...................................104
ClearAway® *see* Salicylic Acid...777
Clear Eyes® [OTC] *see* Naphazoline Hydrochloride 605
Clemastina (Mexico) *see* Clemastine Fumarate 214
Clemastine and Phenylpropanolamine 213
Clemastine Fumarate 214
Cleocin HCl® *see* Clindamycin...214
Cleocin Pediatric® *see* Clindamycin.....................................214
Cleocin Phosphate® *see* Clindamycin.....................................214
C-Lexin® *see* Cephalexin Monohydrate 176
Clidinium and Chlordiazepoxide 214
Clindamycin 214
Clindex® *see* Clidinium and Chlordiazepoxide............................214
Clinoril® *see* Sulindac 813
Clinoxide® *see* Clidinium and Chlordiazepoxide 214
Clioquinol and Hydrocortisone 216
Clioquinol® (Canada) *see* Iodochlorhydroxyquin 466
Clipoxide® *see* Clidinium and Chlordiazepoxide 214
Clobetasol Propionate 216
Clobetasol, Propionato De (Mexico) *see* Clobetasol Propionate 216
Clocortolone Pivalate 216
Cloderm® *see* Clocortolone Pivalate.....................................216
Clofazimine Palmitate 217
Clofibrate 217
Clomid® *see* Clomiphene Citrate 218
Clomifeno, Citrato De (Mexico) *see* Clomiphene Citrate 218
Clomiphene Citrate 218
Clomipramine Hydrochloride 219
Clomycin® [OTC] *see* Bacitracin, Neomycin, Polymyxin B, and Lidocaine
....95
Clonacepam (Mexico) *see* Clonazepam 220
Clonazepam 220
Clonidina (Mexico) *see* Clonidine 221
Clonidine 221
Clonidine and Chlorthalidone...222
Clonodifen® (Mexico) *see* Diclofenac....................................271
Clopra® *see* Metoclopramide...572
Cloracepato Dipotasico (Mexico) *see* Clorazepate Dipotassium 222
Clorafen® (Mexico) *see* Chloramphenicol.................................182
Cloranfenicol (Mexico) *see* Chloramphenicol.............................182
Clorazepate Dipotassium 222
Clorfeniramina, Maleato De (Mexico) *see* Chlorpheniramine Maleate.......191
Clor-K-Zaf® (Mexico) *see* Potassium Chloride............................708
Clorodiacepoxido (Mexico) *see* Chlordiazepoxide 183
Cloroquina, Defosfato De (Mexico) *see* Chloroquine Phosphate...........187
Clorpactin® WCS-90 *see* Oxychlorosene Sodium 646

Clorpropamida (Mexico) *see* Chlorpropamide 197
Clortalidona (Mexico) *see* Chlorthalidone 199
Clortetraciclina (Mexico) *see* Chlortetracyline Hydrochloride 199
Cloruro® De Potasio (Mexico) *see* Potassium Chloride 708
Clotrimazole 223
Cloxacillin Sodium 224
Cloxapen® *see* Cloxacillin Sodium 224
Clozapina (Mexico) *see* Clozapine 225
Clozapine 225
Clozaril® *see* Clozapine 225
Clysodrast® *see* Bisacodyl 113
Coal Tar 225
Coal Tar and Salicylic Acid 226
Coal Tar, Lanolin, and Mineral Oil 226
Cobalamin (Canada) *see* Cyanocobalamin 237
Cobex® *see* Cyanocobalamin 237
Cocaine Hydrochloride 226
Codafed® Expectorant *see* Guaifenesin, Pseudoephedrine, and Codeine
. 410
Codamine® *see* Hydrocodone and Phenylpropanolamine 435
Codamine® Pediatric *see* Hydrocodone and Phenylpropanolamine 435
Codehist® DH *see* Chlorpheniramine, Pseudoephedrine, and Codeine 195
Codeine 227
Codeine and Bromodiphenhydramine *see* Bromodiphenhydramine and
Codeine 122
Codeine and Butalbital Compound *see* Butalbital Compound and Codeine
. 134
Codiclear® DH *see* Hydrocodone and Guaifenesin .434
Codimal-A® *see* Brompheniramine Maleate 124
Codoxy® *see* Oxycodone and Aspirin 647
Codroxomin® *see* Hydroxocobalamin 439
Cogentin® *see* Benztropine Mesylate 106
Co-Gesic® [5/500] *see* Hydrocodone and Acetaminophen 431
Cognex® *see* Tacrine Hydrochloride 816
Co-Hist® [OTC] *see* Acetaminophen, Chlorpheniramine, and
Pseudoephedrine 17
Colace® [OTC] *see* Docusate 295
Co-Lav® *see* Polyethylene Glycol-Electrolyte Solution 703
Colax® [OTC] *see* Docusate and Phenolphthalein 295
Colax-C® (Canada) *see* Docusate 295
ColBENEMID® *see* Colchicine and Probenecid 229
Colchicina (Mexico) *see* Colchicine 228
Colchicine 228
Colchicine and Probenecid 229
Colchiquim-30® (Mexico) *see* Colchicine 228
Colchiquim® (Mexico) *see* Colchicine 228
Cold & Allergy® Elixir [OTC] *see* Brompheniramine and Phenylpropanolamine
. 123
Coldlac-LA® *see* Guaifenesin and Phenylpropanolamine 409
Coldloc® *see* Guaifenesin, Phenylpropanolamine, and Phenylephrine 410
Colestid® *see* Colestipol Hydrochloride 229
Colestipol, Clorhidrato De (Mexico) *see* Colestipol Hydrochloride 229
Colestipol Hydrochloride 229
Colestiramina (Mexico) *see* Cholestyramine Resin .201
Colfosceril Palmitate 230
Colistimethate Sodium 230
Colistin, Neomycin, and Hydrocortisone 231
Colistin Sulfate 231
CollaCote® *see* Collagen, Absorbable 231
Collagen, Absorbable 231
Collagenase 232
CollaPlug® *see* Collagen, Absorbable 231
CollaTape® *see* Collagen, Absorbable 231
Collyrium Fresh® [OTC] *see* Tetrahydrozoline Hydrochloride 831
Colovage® *see* Polyethylene Glycol-Electrolyte Solution 703
Columina® (Mexico) *see* Cimetidine 207
Coly-Mycin® M Parenteral *see* Colistimethate Sodium 230
Coly-Mycin® S Oral *see* Colistin Sulfate 231
Coly-Mycin® S Otic Drops *see* Colistin, Neomycin, and Hydrocortisone
. 231
CoLyte® *see* Polyethylene Glycol-Electrolyte Solution 703
Combantrin® (Mexico) *see* Pyrantel Pamoate 751
Combipres® *see* Clonidine and Chlorthalidone 222
Comfort® [OTC] *see* Naphazoline Hydrochloride 605
Comfort® Tears Solution [OTC] *see* Artificial Tears 75
Comhist® *see* Chlorpheniramine, Phenylephrine, and Phenyltoloxamine
. 193

Comhist® LA see Chlorpheniramine, Phenylephrine, and Phenyltoloxamine
....193
Common Oral-Facial Infections and Antibiotics for Treatment 1077
Compazine® see Prochlorperazine 728
Complan® (Mexico) see Vitamins, Multiple 901
Compound W® [OTC] see Salicylic Acid 777
Compoz® [OTC] see Diphenhydramine Hydrochloride 288
Comprecin® (Mexico) see Enoxacin 310
Condylox® see Podofilox 701
Conex® [OTC] see Guaifenesin and Phenylpropanolamine................409
Congess® Jr see Guaifenesin and Pseudoephedrine 409
Congess® Sr see Guaifenesin and Pseudoephedrine 409
Congestac® see Guaifenesin and Pseudoephedrine 409
Congestant® D [OTC] see Chlorpheniramine, Phenylpropanolamine, and
  Acetaminophen 194
Congest® (Canada) see Estrogens, Conjugated 327
Constant-T® see Theophylline/Aminophylline 832
Constilac® see Lactulose 488
Constulose® see Lactulose 488
Consupren® (Mexico) see Cyclosporine 243
Contac® Cough Formula Liquid [OTC] see Guaifenesin and
  Dextromethorphan 408
Control® [OTC] see Phenylpropanolamine Hydrochloride 687
Controlip® (Mexico) see Fenofibrate 356
Control-L™ [OTC] see Pyrethrins 753
Controlled Substances 1078
Contuss® see Guaifenesin, Phenylpropanolamine, and Phenylephrine........410
Contuss® XT see Guaifenesin and Phenylpropanolamine 409
Cool Mint Listerine® Antiseptic [OTC] see Mouthwash, Antiseptic 592
Cophene-B® see Brompheniramine Maleate 124
Cophene XP® see Hydrocodone, Pseudoephedrine, and Guaifenesin 435
Copper see Trace Metals 857
Coptin® (Canada) see Sulfadiazine 807
Co-Pyronil® 2 Pulvules® [OTC] see Chlorpheniramine and Pseudoephedrine
....191
Coradur® (Canada) see Isosorbide Dinitrate 474
Corax® (Canada) see Chlordiazepoxide 183
Cordarone® see Amiodarone Hydrochloride 48
Cordran® see Flurandrenolide 380
Cordran® SP see Flurandrenolide 380
Coreg® see Carvedilol 159
Corgard® see Nadolol 597
Corgonject® see Chorionic Gonadotropin 203
Coricidin® [OTC] see Chlorpheniramine and Acetaminophen 190
Coricidin D® [OTC] see Chlorpheniramine, Phenylpropanolamine, and
  Acetaminophen 194
Corogal® (Mexico) see Nifedipine 619
Corotrend® (Mexico) see Nifedipine 619
Corotrend® Retard (Mexico) see Nifedipine................................619
Corque® Topical see Clioquinol and Hydrocortisone 216
Correctol® [OTC] see Docusate and Phenolphthalein 295
Cortatrigen® Otic see Neomycin, Polymyxin B, and Hydrocortisone 610
Cortef® see Hydrocortisone 436
Corticaine® Topical see Dibucaine and Hydrocortisone 270
Corticosteroid Equivalencies Comparison 1017
Corticosteroids, Topical Comparison 1018
Corticotropin..233
Cortin® Topical see Clioquinol and Hydrocortisone 216
Cortisone Acetate 233
Cortisporin® Ophthalmic Ointment see Bacitracin, Neomycin, Polymyxin B,
  and Hydrocortisone 95
Cortisporin® Ophthalmic Suspension see Neomycin, Polymyxin B, and
  Hydrocortisone 610
Cortisporin® Otic see Neomycin, Polymyxin B, and Hydrocortisone 610
Cortisporin® Topical Cream see Neomycin, Polymyxin B, and Hydrocortisone
....610
Cortisporin® Topical Ointment see Bacitracin, Neomycin, Polymyxin B, and
  Hydrocortisone 95
Cortone® Acetate see Cortisone Acetate...................................233
Cortrosyn® see Cosyntropin 235
Coryphen® Codeine (Canada) see Aspirin and Codeine 80
Cosmegen® see Dactinomycin 248
Cosyntropin 235
Cotazym® see Pancrelipase 657
Cotazym-S® see Pancrelipase 657
Cotrim® see Trimethoprim and Sulfamethoxazole 874
Cotrim® DS see Trimethoprim and Sulfamethoxazole 874
Co-trimoxazole see Trimethoprim and Sulfamethoxazole 874

Coumadin® see Warfarin Sodium 903
Covera-HS® see Verapamil Hydrochloride 893
Cozaar® see Losartan Potassium 515
Credaxol® (Mexico) see Ranitidine Hydrochloride 763
Crema Blanca Bustillos (Mexico) see Hydroquinone 439
Cremisona® (Mexico) see Fluocinolone Acetonide 372
Creon® see Pancreatin 656
Creon® 10 see Pancrelipase 657
Creon® 20 see Pancrelipase 657
Cresylate® see m-Cresyl Acetate 527
Crixivan® see Indinavir 456
Cromoglicato Disodico (Mexico) see Cromolyn Sodium 235
Cromolyn Sodium 235
Crotamiton 236
Crotamiton (Mexico) see Crotamiton 236
Crude Coal Tar see Coal Tar 225
Cruex® Topical [OTC] see Undecylenic Acid and Derivatives 884
Cryocriptina® (Mexico) see Bromocriptine Mesylate 121
Cryopril® (Mexico) see Captopril 148
Cryosolona® (Mexico) see Methylprednisolone 569
Cryoval® (Mexico) see Valproic Acid and Derivatives 888
Cryoxifeno® (Mexico) see Tamoxifen Citrate 818
Cryptenamine Tannates and Methyclothiazide see Methyclothiazide and
    Cryptenamine Tannates.......................................566
Crystamine® see Cyanocobalamin 237
Crysticillin® A.S. see Penicillin G Procaine 667
Crystodigin® see Digitoxin 279
CSP see Cellulose Sodium Phosphate 175
C-Span® [OTC] see Ascorbic Acid 76
Curretab® see Medroxyprogesterone Acetate 533
Cutivate™ see Fluticasone Propionate 383
Cyanocobalamin 237
Cyanoject® see Cyanocobalamin 237
Cyclan® see Cyclandelate 238
Cyclandelate 238
Cyclizine 238
Cyclobenzaprine Hydrochloride 239
Cyclocort® see Amcinonide 43
Cyclogyl® see Cyclopentolate Hydrochloride 240
Cyclomen® (Canada) see Danazol 249
Cyclopentolate Hydrochloride 240
Cyclophosphamide 240
Cycloserine 242
Cyclospasmol® see Cyclandelate 238
Cyclosporine 243
Cycoflex® see Cyclobenzaprine Hydrochloride 239
Cycrin® see Medroxyprogesterone Acetate 533
Cyklokapron® Injection see Tranexamic Acid 860
Cyklokapron® Oral see Tranexamic Acid..........................860
Cylert® see Pemoline 663
Cymevene® (Mexico) see Ganciclovir 393
Cyomin® see Cyanocobalamin 237
Cyproheptadine Hydrochloride 244
Cystagon® see Cysteamine 245
Cysteamine 245
Cysteine Hydrochloride 246
Cystospaz® see Hyoscyamine Sulfate 445
Cystospaz-M® see Hyoscyamine Sulfate 445
Cytadren® see Aminoglutethimide 46
Cytarabine Hydrochloride 246
Cytomel® see Liothyronine Sodium 504
Cytosar-U® see Cytarabine Hydrochloride 246
Cytotec® see Misoprostol 584
Cytovene® see Ganciclovir 393
Cytoxan® see Cyclophosphamide 240
D₃ see Cholecalciferol 200
Dacarbazine...247
Dacodyl® [OTC] see Bisacodyl 113
Dactinomycin 248
Dafloxen® (Mexico) see Naproxen 606
Dairy Ease® [OTC] see Lactase 487
Dakrina® Ophthalmic Solution [OTC] see Artificial Tears 75
Daktarin® (Mexico) see Miconazole 578
Dalacin® C [Hydrochloride] (Canada) see Clindamycin 214
Dalacin® C (Mexico) see Clindamycin 214
Dalalone L.A.® see Dexamethasone 260
Dalgan® see Dezocine 267
Dalisol® (Mexico) see Folic Acid 385

Dalisol (Mexico) *see* Leucovorin Calcium 491
Dallergy® *see* Chlorpheniramine, Phenylephrine, and Methscopolamine
.... 193
Dallergy-D® Syrup *see* Chlorpheniramine and Phenylephrine 190
Dalmane® *see* Flurazepam Hydrochloride 380
Dalteparin 249
Damason-P® *see* Hydrocodone and Aspirin 433
Danazol 249
Danocrine® *see* Danazol 249
Dantrium® *see* Dantrolene Sodium 250
Dantrolene Sodium 250
Daonil® (Mexico) *see* Glyburide 401
Dapa® [OTC] *see* Acetaminophen 14
Dapacin® Cold Capsule [OTC] *see* Chlorpheniramine, Phenylpropanolamine,
and Acetaminophen 194
Dapiprazole Hydrochloride 251
Dapsone 251
Daranide® *see* Dichlorphenamide 271
Daraprim® *see* Pyrimethamine 754
Daraprim® (Mexico) *see* Pyrimethamine 754
Daricon® *see* Oxyphencyclimine Hydrochloride 652
Darvocet-N® *see* Propoxyphene and Acetaminophen 741
Darvocet-N® 100 *see* Propoxyphene and Acetaminophen 741
Darvon® *see* Propoxyphene 740
Darvon® Compound-65 Pulvules® *see* Propoxyphene and Aspirin 742
Darvon-N® *see* Propoxyphene 740
Darvon-N® Compound (contains caffeine) (Canada) *see* Propoxyphene and
Aspirin 742
Darvon®-N With ASA *see* Propoxyphene and Aspirin 742
Darvon-N® with ASA (Canada) *see* Propoxyphene and Aspirin 742
Datril® [OTC] *see* Acetaminophen 14
Daunomycin *see* Daunorubicin Hydrochloride 252
Daunorubicin Hydrochloride 252
Daypro™ *see* Oxaprozin 643
Dayto Himbin® *see* Yohimbine Hydrochloride 905
DC 240® Softgels® [OTC] *see* Docusate 295
DCF *see* Pentostatin 674
DDAVP® *see* Desmopressin Acetate 258
Deavynfar® (Mexico) *see* Chlorpropamide 197
Debrisan® [OTC] *see* Dextranomer 264
Debrox® [OTC] *see* Carbamide Peroxide 152
Decadron® *see* Dexamethasone 260
Decadronal® (Mexico) *see* Dexamethasone 260
Decadron®-LA *see* Dexamethasone 260
Deca-Durabolin® *see* Nandrolone 604
Decaject-L.A.® *see* Dexamethasone 260
Decholin® *see* Dehydrocholic Acid 254
Declomycin® *see* Demeclocycline Hydrochloride 255
Decofed® Syrup [OTC] *see* Pseudoephedrine 749
Decohistine® DH *see* Chlorpheniramine, Pseudoephedrine, and Codeine
.... 195
Decohistine® Expectorant *see* Guaifenesin, Pseudoephedrine, and Codeine
.... 410
Deconamine® SR *see* Chlorpheniramine and Pseudoephedrine 191
Deconamine® Syrup [OTC] *see* Chlorpheniramine and Pseudoephedrine
.... 191
Deconamine® Tablet [OTC] *see* Chlorpheniramine and Pseudoephedrine
.... 191
Deconsal® II *see* Guaifenesin and Pseudoephedrine 409
Decorex® (Mexico) *see* Dexamethasone 260
Defen-LA® *see* Guaifenesin and Pseudoephedrine 409
Deferoxamine Mesylate 253
Deficol® [OTC] *see* Bisacodyl 113
Degest® 2 [OTC] *see* Naphazoline Hydrochloride 605
Dehist® *see* Brompheniramine Maleate 124
Dehydral® (Canada) *see* Methenamine 555
Dehydrobenzperidol® (Mexico) *see* Droperidol 303
Dehydrocholic Acid 254
Dekasol-L.A.® *see* Dexamethasone 260
Deladiol® *see* Estradiol 325
Deladumone® Injection *see* Estradiol and Testosterone 326
Delatest® *see* Testosterone 825
Delatestryl® *see* Testosterone 825
Delaxin® *see* Methocarbamol 557
Delestrogen® *see* Estradiol 325
Delfen® [OTC] *see* Nonoxynol 9 627
Del-Mycin® Topical *see* Erythromycin, Topical 324
Delsym® [OTC] *see* Dextromethorphan 266

Delta-Cortef® *see* Prednisolone 718
Delta-D® *see* Cholecalciferol 200
Deltasone® *see* Prednisone 719
Delta-Tritex® *see* Triamcinolone 862
Demadex® *see* Torsemide 856
Demazin® Syrup [OTC] *see* Chlorpheniramine and Phenylpropanolamine
. . . . 190
Demecarium Bromide 255
Demeclociclina (Mexico) *see* Demeclocycline Hydrochloride 255
Demeclocycline Hydrochloride 255
Demerol® *see* Meperidine Hydrochloride 539
4-demethoxydaunorubicin *see* Idarubicin 448
Demolox® (Mexico) *see* Amoxapine 56
Demulen® *see* Ethinyl Estradiol and Ethynodiol Diacetate 335
Denavir® *see* Penciclovir 664
Denorex® [OTC] *see* Coal Tar 225
Dental Drug Interactions: Update on Drug Combinations Requiring Special
    Considerations 1022
Dental Office Emergencies 984
Dentifrice Products 1051
Dentin Hypersensitivity; High Caries Index; Xerostomia 959
Dentipatch® *see* Lidocaine Transoral 502
Denture Adhesive Products 1060
Denture Cleanser Products 1062
Denvar® (Mexico) *see* Cefixime 165
Deoxycoformycin *see* Pentostatin 674
2′-deoxycoformycin *see* Pentostatin 674
Depakene® *see* Valproic Acid and Derivatives 888
Depakote® *see* Valproic Acid and Derivatives 888
depAndrogyn® Injection *see* Estradiol and Testosterone 326
depGynogen® *see* Estradiol 325
depMedalone® *see* Methylprednisolone 569
Depo®-Estradiol *see* Estradiol 325
Depogen® *see* Estradiol 325
Depoject® *see* Methylprednisolone 569
Depo-Medrol® *see* Methylprednisolone 569
Deponit® *see* Nitroglycerin 623
Depopred® *see* Methylprednisolone 569
Depo-Provera® *see* Medroxyprogesterone Acetate 533
Depotest® *see* Testosterone 825
Depo-Testadiol® Injection *see* Estradiol and Testosterone 326
Depotestogen® Injection *see* Estradiol and Testosterone 326
Depo®-Testosterone *see* Testosterone 825
Deproist® Expectorant with Codeine *see* Guaifenesin, Pseudoephedrine, and
    Codeine 410
Derifil® [OTC] *see* Chlorophyll 185
Dermacomb® *see* Nystatin and Triamcinolone 632
Dermalog® Simple (Mexico) *see* Halcinonide 415
Derma-Smoothe/FS® *see* Fluocinolone Acetonide 372
Dermasone® (Canada) *see* Clobetasol Propionate 216
Dermatop® *see* Prednicarbate 718
Dermatovate® (Mexico) *see* Clobetasol Propionate 216
Dermazin® (Canada) *see* Silver Sulfadiazine 788
Dermifun® (Mexico) *see* Miconazole 578
Dermovate® (Canada) *see* Clobetasol Propionate 216
Dermoxyl® [OTC] *see* Benzoyl Peroxide 104
Desferal® Mesylate *see* Deferoxamine Mesylate 253
Desipramina, Clorhidrato De (Mexico) *see* Desipramine Hydrochloride 257
Desipramine Hydrochloride 257
Desitin® Topical [OTC] *see* Zinc Oxide, Cod Liver Oil, and Talc 909
Desmopressin Acetate 258
Desocort® (Canada) *see* Desonide 259
Desogen® *see* Ethinyl Estradiol and Desogestrel 335
Desogestrel and Ethinyl Estradiol *see* Ethinyl Estradiol and Desogestrel
. . . . 335
Desonide 259
DesOwen® *see* Desonide 259
Desoximetasone 259
Desoxyn® *see* Methamphetamine Hydrochloride 553
Desoxyribonuclease and Fibrinolysin *see* Fibrinolysin and
    Desoxyribonuclease 362
Despec® Liquid *see* Guaifenesin, Phenylpropanolamine, and Phenylephrine
. . . . 410
Desquam-E® *see* Benzoyl Peroxide 104
Desquam-X® *see* Benzoyl Peroxide 104
Desyrel® *see* Trazodone 861
Detensol® (Canada) *see* Propranolol Hydrochloride 743

Detussin® Expectorant *see* Hydrocodone, Pseudoephedrine, and Guaifenesin
....435
Devrom® (subgallate) [OTC] *see* Bismuth 114
Dexacidin® *see* Neomycin, Polymyxin B, and Dexamethasone............610
Dex-A-Diet® [OTC] *see* Phenylpropanolamine Hydrochloride 687
Dexamethasone...260
Dexamethasone and Neomycin *see* Neomycin and Dexamethasone 609
Dexasone L.A.® *see* Dexamethasone 260
Dexasporin® *see* Neomycin, Polymyxin B, and Dexamethasone 610
Dexatrim® [OTC] *see* Phenylpropanolamine Hydrochloride.....................687
Dexbrompheniramine and Pseudoephedrine.....................................261
Dexchlor® *see* Dexchlorpheniramine Maleate..................................261
Dexchlorpheniramine Maleate 261
Dexedrine® *see* Dextroamphetamine Sulfate..................................265
Dexfenfluramine Hydrochloride..262
Dexone® *see* Dexamethasone..260
Dexone L.A.® *see* Dexamethasone 260
Dexpanthenol...263
Dexrazoxane 263
Dextran 263
Dextran 1..264
Dextran 40 *see* Dextran..263
Dextran 70 *see* Dextran..263
Dextran, High Molecular Weight *see* Dextran 263
Dextran, Low Molecular Weight *see* Dextran 263
Dextranomer 264
Dextroamphetamine Sulfate...265
Dextroclorofeniramina (Mexico) *see* Dexchlorpheniramine Maleate 261
Dextromethorphan...266
Dextrometorfano (Mexico) *see* Dextromethorphan 266
Dextrose, Levulose and Phosphoric Acid *see* Phosphorated Carbohydrate
Solution 690
Dextrothyroxine Sodium..266
Dey-Dose® Isoproterenol *see* Isoproterenol 472
Dey-Dose® Metaproterenol *see* Metaproterenol Sulfate 550
Dey-Lute® Isoetharine *see* Isoetharine 470
Dezocine 267
DHAD *see* Mitoxantrone Hydrochloride 586
DHC Plus® *see* Dihydrocodeine, Acetaminophen, and Aspirin 281
D.H.E. 45® *see* Dihydroergotamine Mesylate 283
DHS® Tar [OTC] *see* Coal Tar 225
DHS Zinc® [OTC] *see* Pyrithione Zinc..755
DHT™ *see* Dihydrotachysterol 283
Diaβeta® *see* Glyburide 401
Diabetic Tussin® DM [OTC] *see* Guaifenesin and Dextromethorphan........408
Diabinese® *see* Chlorpropamide...197
Dialose® [OTC] *see* Docusate..295
Dialose® Plus Capsule [OTC] *see* Docusate and Casanthranol 295
Dialose® Plus Tablet [OTC] *see* Docusate and Phenolphthalein..............295
Dialume® [OTC] *see* Aluminum Hydroxide 39
Diamine T.D.® [OTC] *see* Brompheniramine Maleate 124
Diamox® *see* Acetazolamide...18
Diamox® Sequels® *see* Acetazolamide..18
Diaparene® [OTC] *see* Methylbenzethonium Chloride.........................566
Diapid® *see* Lypressin 519
Diasorb® [OTC] *see* Attapulgite 86
Diaval® (Mexico) *see* Tolbutamide...853
Diazemuls® (Canada) *see* Diazepam 268
Diazepam...268
Diazoxide...269
Diazoxido (Mexico) *see* Diazoxide...269
Dibacilina® (Mexico) *see* Ampicillin...62
Dibasona® (Mexico) *see* Dexamethasone 260
Dibent® *see* Dicyclomine Hydrochloride.......................................273
Dibenzyline® *see* Phenoxybenzamine Hydrochloride 682
Dibucaine...270
Dibucaine and Hydrocortisone...270
Dibufen® (Mexico) *see* Ibuprofen..447
DIC *see* Dacarbazine...247
Dicarbosil® [OTC] *see* Calcium Carbonate 140
Dichlorodifluoromethane and Trichloromonofluoromethane...................270
Dichlorotetrafluoroethane and Ethyl Chloride *see* Ethyl Chloride and
Dichlorotetrafluoroethane 344
Dichlorphenamide 271
Diclofenac 271
Diclofenaco (Mexico) *see* Diclofenac..271
Diclofenamide *see* Dichlorphenamide 271
Diclotride® (Mexico) *see* Hydrochlorothiazide 430

Dicloxacillin Sodium 273
Dicyclomine Hydrochloride 273
Dicycloverine Hydrochloride see Dicyclomine Hydrochloride 273
Didanosina (Mexico) see Didanosine 274
Didanosine 274
Didrex® see Benzphetamine Hydrochloride 105
Didronel® see Etidronate Disodium 346
Dienestrol 275
Diethylpropion Hydrochloride 276
Diethylstilbestrol 277
Difenoxin and Atropine 277
Differin® see Adapalene 25
Diflorasone Diacetate 278
Diflucan® see Fluconazole 367
Diflunisal 278
Di-Gel® [OTC] see Aluminum Hydroxide, Magnesium Hydroxide, and
  Simethicone 41
Digepepsin® see Pancreatin 656
Digitaline® (Canada) see Digitoxin 279
Digitoxin 279
Digoxin 280
Digoxina (Mexico) see Digoxin 280
Dihidroergotamina (Mexico) see Dihydroergotamine Mesylate 283
Dihistine® DH see Chlorpheniramine, Pseudoephedrine, and Codeine 195
Dihistine® Expectorant see Guaifenesin, Pseudoephedrine, and Codeine
  410
Dihydrocodeine, Acetaminophen, and Aspirin 281
Dihydroergotamine Mesylate 283
Dihydrotachysterol 283
Dihydroxypropyl Theophylline see Dyphylline 305
Dilacoran-HTA® (Mexico) see Verapamil Hydrochloride 893
Dilacoran® (Mexico) see Verapamil Hydrochloride 893
Dilacoran-Retard® (Mexico) see Verapamil Hydrochloride 893
Dilacor™ XR see Diltiazem 284
Dilantin® see Phenytoin 688
Dilantin® With Phenobarbital see Phenytoin With Phenobarbital 689
Dilatrate®-SR see Isosorbide Dinitrate 474
Dilaudid® see Hydromorphone Hydrochloride 438
Dilaudid-HP® see Hydromorphone Hydrochloride 438
Dilocaine® see Lidocaine Hydrochloride 502
Dilor® see Dyphylline 305
Diltiazem 284
Diltiazem, Clorhidrato De (Mexico) see Diltiazem 284
Dimaphen® Elixir [OTC] see Brompheniramine and Phenylpropanolamine
  123
Dimaphen® Tablets [OTC] see Brompheniramine and Phenylpropanolamine
  123
Dimenhidrinato (Mexico) see Dimenhydrinate 286
Dimenhydrinate 286
Dimercaprol 287
Dimetabs® see Dimenhydrinate 286
Dimetane® [OTC] see Brompheniramine Maleate 124
Dimetane®-DC see Brompheniramine, Phenylpropanolamine, and Codeine
  125
Dimetane® Decongestant Elixir [OTC] see Brompheniramine and
  Phenylephrine 122
Dimetapp® 4-Hour Liqui-Gel Capsule [OTC] see Brompheniramine and
  Phenylpropanolamine 123
Dimetapp® Elixir [OTC] see Brompheniramine and Phenylpropanolamine
  123
Dimetapp® Extentabs® [OTC] see Brompheniramine and
  Phenylpropanolamine 123
Dimetapp® Sinus Caplets [OTC] see Pseudoephedrine and Ibuprofen 750
Dimetapp® Tablet [OTC] see Brompheniramine and Phenylpropanolamine
  123
Dimethyl Triazeno Imidazol Carboxamide see Dacarbazine 247
Diminex® (Mexico) see Phentermine Hydrochloride 683
Dimodan® (Mexico) see Disopyramide Phosphate 292
Dinate® see Dimenhydrinate 286
Diochloram® (Canada) see Chloramphenicol 182
Diocto® [OTC] see Docusate 295
Diocto C® [OTC] see Docusate and Casanthranol 295
Diocto-K® [OTC] see Docusate 295
Diocto-K Plus® [OTC] see Docusate and Casanthranol 295
Dioctolose Plus® [OTC] see Docusate and Casanthranol 295
Diodoquin® (Canada) see Iodoquinol 466
Dioeze® [OTC] see Docusate 295
Diomycin® (Canada) see Erythromycin 321

Dionephrine® (Canada) see Phenylephrine Hydrochloride 685
Dioval® see Estradiol 325
Dipalmitoylphosphatidylcholine see Colfosceril Palmitate 230
Dipedyne® (Mexico) see Zidovudine 907
Dipentum® see Olsalazine Sodium 635
Diphen® Cough [OTC] see Diphenhydramine Hydrochloride 288
Diphenhydramine Hydrochloride 288
Diphenidol Hydrochloride 289
Diphenoxylate and Atropine 289
Diphenylan Sodium® see Phenytoin 688
Diphtheria CRM₁₉₇ Protein Conjugate see Haemophilus b Conjugate Vaccine
. . . . 414
Diphtheria Toxoid Conjugate see Haemophilus b Conjugate Vaccine 414
Dipiridamol (Mexico) see Dipyridamole 290
Dipivefrin 290
Diprivan® Injection see Propofol 738
Diprolene® see Betamethasone 109
Diprolene® AF see Betamethasone 109
Diprolene® Glycol [Dipropionate] (Canada) see Betamethasone 109
Diprosone® see Betamethasone 109
Dipyridamole 290
Dirinol® (Mexico) see Dipyridamole 290
Dirithromycin 291
Disalcid® see Salsalate 779
Disanthrol® [OTC] see Docusate and Casanthranol 295
Discase® see Chymopapain 204
Disobrom® [OTC] see Dexbrompheniramine and Pseudoephedrine 261
Disolan® [OTC] see Docusate and Phenolphthalein 295
Disonate® [OTC] see Docusate 295
Disophrol® Chrontabs® [OTC] see Dexbrompheniramine and
    Pseudoephedrine 261
Disophrol® Tablet [OTC] see Dexbrompheniramine and Pseudoephedrine
. . . . 261
Disopiramida (Mexico) see Disopyramide Phosphate 292
Disopyramide Phosphate 292
Di-Spaz® see Dicyclomine Hydrochloride 273
Dispos-a-Med® Isoproterenol see Isoproterenol 472
Disulfiram 293
Ditropan® see Oxybutynin Chloride 645
Diucardin® see Hydroflumethiazide 437
Diuchlor® (Canada) see Hydrochlorothiazide 430
Diupres-250® see Chlorothiazide and Reserpine 189
Diupres-500® see Chlorothiazide and Reserpine 189
Diurigen® see Chlorothiazide 188
Diuril® see Chlorothiazide 188
Diutensin® see Methyclothiazide and Cryptenamine Tannates 566
Dixaparine® (Mexico) see Heparin 419
Dixarit® (Canada) see Clonidine 221
Dizmiss® [OTC] see Meclizine Hydrochloride 530
DNR see Daunorubicin Hydrochloride 252
Dobuject® (Mexico) see Dobutamine Hydrochloride 294
Dobutamina, Clorhidrato De (Mexico) see Dobutamine Hydrochloride 294
Dobutamine Hydrochloride 294
Dobutrex® see Dobutamine Hydrochloride 294
Docetaxel 294
Docucal-P® [OTC] see Docusate and Phenolphthalein 295
Docusate 295
Docusate and Casanthranol 295
Docusate and Phenolphthalein 295
DOK® [OTC] see Docusate 295
Doktors® Nasal Solution [OTC] see Phenylephrine Hydrochloride 685
Dolacet® [5/500] see Hydrocodone and Acetaminophen 431
Dolac® Inyectable (Mexico) see Ketorolac Tromethamine 484
Dolac® Oral (Mexico) see Ketorolac Tromethamine 484
Dolaren® (Carisoprodol with Diclofenac) (Mexico) see Carisoprodol 157
Dolene® see Propoxyphene 740
Dolobid® see Diflunisal 278
Dolo Pangavit D® (Mexico) see Diclofenac 271
Dolophine® see Methadone Hydrochloride 552
Domeboro® Topical [OTC] see Aluminum Sulfate and Calcium Acetate
. . . . 41
Dome Paste Bandage see Zinc Gelatin 908
Donnamor® see Hyoscyamine, Atropine, Scopolamine, and Phenobarbital
. . . . 444
Donnapectolin-PG® see Hyoscyamine, Atropine, Scopolamine, Kaolin, Pectin,
    and Opium 445
Donnapine® see Hyoscyamine, Atropine, Scopolamine, and Phenobarbital
. . . . 444

Donna-Sed® see Hyoscyamine, Atropine, Scopolamine, and Phenobarbital 444
Donnatal® see Hyoscyamine, Atropine, Scopolamine, and Phenobarbital 444
Donphen® see Hyoscyamine, Atropine, Scopolamine, and Phenobarbital 444
Dopamet® (Canada) see Methyldopa 566
Dopar® see Levodopa 495
Dopram® Injection see Doxapram Hydrochloride 297
Doral® see Quazepam 755
Dorcol® [OTC] see Acetaminophen 14
Dormicum® (Mexico) see Midazolam Hydrochloride 580
Dornase Alfa 296
Doryx® see Doxycycline 301
Dorzolamide Hydrochloride 296
DOS® Softgel® [OTC] see Docusate 295
Dovonex® see Calcipotriene 138
Doxapram Hydrochloride 297
Doxazosin 298
Doxepin Hydrochloride 298
Doxidan® [OTC] see Docusate and Phenolphthalein 295
Doxil® Injection see Doxorubicin Hydrochloride 299
Doxinate® [OTC] see Docusate 295
Doxolem (Mexico) see Doxorubicin Hydrochloride 299
Doxorubicin Hydrochloride 299
Doxy® see Doxycycline 301
Doxychel® see Doxycycline 301
Doxycin® (Canada) see Doxycycline 301
Doxycycline 301
Doxytec® (Canada) see Doxycycline 301
DPPC see Colfosceril Palmitate 230
Dramamine® [OTC] see Dimenhydrinate 286
Dramilin® see Dimenhydrinate 286
Drenison® (Canada) see Flurandrenolide 380
Dri-Ear® Otic [OTC] see Boric Acid 118
Driken® (Mexico) see Iron Dextran Complex 468
Drisdol® see Ergocalciferol 317
Dristan® Long Lasting Nasal Solution [OTC] see Oxymetazoline
    Hydrochloride 649
Dristan® Sinus Caplets [OTC] see Pseudoephedrine and Ibuprofen 750
Drithocreme® see Anthralin 68
Drithocreme® HP 1% see Anthralin 68
Dritho-Scalp® see Anthralin 68
Drixoral® [OTC] see Dexbrompheniramine and Pseudoephedrine 261
Drixoral® Cough & Congestion Liquid Caps [OTC] see Pseudoephedrine and
    Dextromethorphan 750
Drixoral® Cough & Sore Throat Liquid Caps [OTC] see Acetaminophen and
    Dextromethorphan 16
Drixoral® Nasal (Canada) see Oxymetazoline Hydrochloride 649
Drixoral® Non-Drowsy [OTC] see Pseudoephedrine 749
Drixoral® Syrup [OTC] see Brompheniramine and Pseudoephedrine 123
Dronabinol 302
Droperidol 303
Drotic® Otic see Neomycin, Polymyxin B, and Hydrocortisone ... 610
Drugs Associated With Adverse Hematologic Effects 1079
Dry Eyes® Solution [OTC] see Artificial Tears 75
Dry Eye® Therapy Solution [OTC] see Artificial Tears 75
Dryox® [OTC] see Benzoyl Peroxide 104
DSMC Plus® [OTC] see Docusate and Casanthranol 295
D-S-S® [OTC] see Docusate 295
D-S-S Plus® [OTC] see Docusate and Casanthranol 295
DSS With Casanthranol see Docusate and Casanthranol 295
DTIC see Dacarbazine 247
DTIC-Dome® see Dacarbazine 247
Duadacin® Capsule [OTC] see Chlorpheniramine, Phenylpropanolamine, and
    Acetaminophen 194
Dulcolan® (Mexico) see Bisacodyl 113
Dulcolax® [OTC] see Bisacodyl 113
DuoCet™ [5/500] see Hydrocodone and Acetaminophen 431
Duo-Cyp® Injection see Estradiol and Testosterone 326
Duofilm® Solution see Salicylic Acid and Lactic Acid 778
Duo-Medihaler® Aerosol see Isoproterenol and Phenylephrine .. 473
Duo-Trach® see Lidocaine Hydrochloride 502
Duotrate® see Pentaerythritol Tetranitrate 669
DuP 753 see Losartan Potassium 515
Duphalac® see Lactulose 488
Duplex® T [OTC] see Coal Tar 225

Durabolin® see Nandrolone 604
Duracef® (Mexico) see Cefadroxil Monohydrate 162
Duradoce® (Mexico) see Hydroxocobalamin 439
Duradyne DHC® [5/500] see Hydrocodone and Acetaminophen 431
Dura-Estrin® see Estradiol 325
Duragen® see Estradiol 325
Duragesic™ see Fentanyl 357
Dura-Gest® see Guaifenesin, Phenylpropanolamine, and Phenylephrine 410
Duralone® see Methylprednisolone 569
Duralutin® see Hydroxyprogesterone Caproate 441
Duramorph® Injection see Morphine Sulfate 590
Duranest® with Epinephrine see Etidocaine Hydrochloride (With Epinephrine) 345
Duraphyl™ see Theophylline/Aminophylline 832
Durater® (Mexico) see Famotidine 352
Duratest® see Testosterone 825
Duratestrin® Injection see Estradiol and Testosterone 326
Durathate® see Testosterone 825
Duration® Nasal Solution [OTC] see Oxymetazoline Hydrochloride 649
Dura-Vent® see Guaifenesin and Phenylpropanolamine 409
Duricef® see Cefadroxil Monohydrate 162
Durogesic® (Mexico) see Fentanyl 357
Durrax® see Hydroxyzine 443
Duvoid® see Bethanechol Chloride 112
DV® Cream see Dienestrol 275
Dwelle® Ophthalmic Solution [OTC] see Artificial Tears 75
Dyazide® see Triamterene and Hydrochlorothiazide 865
Dycill® see Dicloxacillin Sodium 273
Dyclone® see Dyclonine Hydrochloride 304
Dyclonine Hydrochloride 304
Dyflex® see Dyphylline 305
Dymelor® see Acetohexamide 19
Dynabac® see Dirithromycin 291
DynaCirc® see Isradipine 476
DynaCirc SRO® (Mexico) see Isradipine 476
Dyna-Hex® [OTC] see Chlorhexidine Gluconate 184
Dynapen® see Dicloxacillin Sodium 273
Dyphylline 305
Dyrenium® see Triamterene 865
7E3 see Abciximab 12
Easprin® see Aspirin 78
Ecapresan® (Mexico) see Captopril 148
Ecaten® (Mexico) see Captopril 148
Echothiophate Iodide 305
E-Complex-600® [OTC] see Vitamin E 900
Econazole Nitrate 306
Econopred® see Prednisolone 718
Econopred® Plus see Prednisolone 718
Ecostatin® (Canada) see Econazole Nitrate 306
Ecotrin® [OTC] see Aspirin 78
Ectaprim-F® (Mexico) see Trimethoprim and Sulfamethoxazole 874
Ectaprim® (Mexico) see Trimethoprim and Sulfamethoxazole 874
Ectasule® see Ephedrine Sulfate 310
Ed A-Hist® Liquid see Chlorpheniramine and Phenylephrine 190
Edecrin® see Ethacrynic Acid 331
Edenol® (Mexico) see Furosemide 391
E.E.S.® see Erythromycin 321
Efedrina (Mexico) see Ephedrine Sulfate 310
Efedron® see Ephedrine Sulfate 310
Effer-K™ see Potassium Bicarbonate and Potassium Citrate, Effervescent 707
Effer-Syllium® [OTC] see Psyllium 750
Effexor® see Venlafaxine 892
Efidac/24® [OTC] see Pseudoephedrine 749
Efodine® [OTC] see Povidone-Iodine 713
Efudex® Topical see Fluorouracil 376
Efudix® (Mexico) see Fluorouracil 376
Elantan® (Mexico) see Isosorbide Mononitrate 474
Elase-Chloromycetin® Topical see Fibrinolysin and Desoxyribonuclease 362
Elase® Topical see Fibrinolysin and Desoxyribonuclease 362
Elavil® see Amitriptyline Hydrochloride 51
Eldepryl® see Selegiline Hydrochloride 784
Eldercaps® [OTC] see Vitamins, Multiple 901
Eldopaque® [OTC] see Hydroquinone 439
Eldopaque Forte® see Hydroquinone 439
Eldoquin® [OTC] see Hydroquinone 439

Eldoquin Forte® *see* Hydroquinone 439
Electrolyte Lavage Solution *see* Polyethylene Glycol-Electrolyte Solution
.... 703
Elimite™ *see* Permethrin 676
Elixophyllin® *see* Theophylline/Aminophylline 832
Elixophyllin® SR *see* Theophylline/Aminophylline 832
Elmiron® *see* Pentosan Polysulfate Sodium 674
Elocom® (Canada) *see* Mometasone Furoate 589
Elocon® *see* Mometasone Furoate 589
Elomet® (Mexico) *see* Mometasone Furoate 589
E-Lor® *see* Propoxyphene and Acetaminophen 741
Elspar® *see* Asparaginase 77
Eltor® (Canada) *see* Pseudoephedrine 749
Eltroxin™ *see* Levothyroxine Sodium 498
Eltroxin® (Canada) *see* Levothyroxine Sodium 498
Emcyt® *see* Estramustine Phosphate Sodium 326
Emecheck® [OTC] *see* Phosphorated Carbohydrate Solution 690
Emetrol® [OTC] *see* Phosphorated Carbohydrate Solution 690
Emgel™ Topical *see* Erythromycin, Topical 324
Eminase® *see* Anistreplase 67
Emko® [OTC] *see* Nonoxynol 9 627
EMLA® *see* Lidocaine and Prilocaine 501
Empirin® [OTC] *see* Aspirin 78
Empirin® With Codeine *see* Aspirin and Codeine 80
Emulsan 20% (Mexico) *see* Fat Emulsion 353
Emulsoil® [OTC] *see* Castor Oil 161
E-Mycin® *see* Erythromycin 321
Enaladil® (Mexico) *see* Enalapril 307
Enalapril 307
Enalapril and Hydrochlorothiazide 309
Encainide Hydrochloride 309
Encare® [OTC] *see* Nonoxynol 9 627
Endantadine® (Canada) *see* Amantadine Hydrochloride 41
Endep® *see* Amitriptyline Hydrochloride 51
End Lice® [OTC] *see* Pyrethrins 753
Endocet® (Canada) *see* Oxycodone and Acetaminophen 646
Endocrine Disorders & Pregnancy 927
Endodan® (Canada) *see* Oxycodone and Aspirin 647
Endolor® *see* Butalbital Compound 133
Enduron® *see* Methyclothiazide 565
Enduronyl® *see* Methyclothiazide and Deserpidine 566
Enduronyl® Forte *see* Methyclothiazide and Deserpidine 566
Ener-B® [OTC] *see* Cyanocobalamin 237
Engerix-B® *see* Hepatitis B Vaccine 422
Enhanced-potency Inactivated Poliovirus Vaccine *see* Poliovirus Vaccine,
    Inactivated 702
Eni® (Mexico) *see* Ciprofloxacin Hydrochloride 208
Enisyl® [OTC] *see* L-Lysine Hydrochloride 509
Enkaid® *see* Encainide Hydrochloride 309
Enomine® *see* Guaifenesin, Phenylpropanolamine, and Phenylephrine 410
Enovid® *see* Mestranol and Norethynodrel 549
Enovil® *see* Amitriptyline Hydrochloride 51
Enoxacin 310
Enoxacina (Mexico) *see* Enoxacin 310
Entacef® *see* Cephalexin Monohydrate 176
Enterobacticel® (Mexico) *see* Trimethoprim and Sulfamethoxazole 874
Enteropride® (Mexico) *see* Cisapride 209
Entex® *see* Guaifenesin, Phenylpropanolamine, and Phenylephrine 410
Entex® LA *see* Guaifenesin and Phenylpropanolamine 409
Entex® PSE *see* Guaifenesin and Pseudoephedrine 409
Entocort® (Canada) *see* Budesonide 126
Entrophen® (Canada) *see* Aspirin 78
Enulose® *see* Lactulose 488
Enzone® *see* Pramoxine and Hydrocortisone 714
E Pam® (Canada) *see* Diazepam 268
Ephedrine Sulfate 310
Ephedrine, Theophylline and Phenobarbital *see* Theophylline, Ephedrine, and
    Phenobarbital 836
Ephedsol® *see* Ephedrine Sulfate 310
E-Pilo-x® Ophthalmic *see* Pilocarpine and Epinephrine 693
Epimorph® (Canada) *see* Morphine Sulfate 590
Epinal® *see* Epinephryl Borate 315
Epinephrine 311
Epinephrine (Dental) 313
Epinephrine, Racemic 314
Epinephrine, Racemic and Aluminum Potassium Sulfate 314
Epinephryl Borate 315
Epitol® *see* Carbamazepine 151

Epival® (Mexico) *see* Valproic Acid and Derivatives 888
Epivir® *see* Lamivudine 489
EPO *see* Epoetin Alfa 315
Epoetin Alfa 315
Epogen® *see* Epoetin Alfa 315
Epoprostenol Sodium... 317
Eprex® (Mexico) *see* Epoetin Alfa 315
Epsom Salts *see* Magnesium Sulfate 524
EPT *see* Teniposide 820
Equagesic® *see* Aspirin and Meprobamate 81
Equalactin® Chewable Tablet [OTC] *see* Calcium Polycarbophil ... 146
Equanil® *see* Meprobamate 543
Ercaf® *see* Ergotamine 319
Ergamisol® *see* Levamisole Hydrochloride 493
Ergocaf® (Mexico) *see* Ergotamine 319
Ergocalciferol 317
Ergocalciferol (Mexico) *see* Ergocalciferol 317
Ergoloid Mesylates.. 318
Ergomar® (Canada) *see* Ergotamine 319
Ergometrine Maleate (Canada) *see* Ergonovine Maleate 319
Ergonovina (Mexico) *see* Ergonovine Maleate 319
Ergonovine Maleate 319
Ergostat® *see* Ergotamine 319
Ergotamina Tartrato De (Mexico) *see* Ergotamine 319
Ergotamine... 319
Ergotrate® Maleate *see* Ergonovine Maleate.................... 319
Eridium® *see* Phenazopyridine Hydrochloride 679
Eritromicina y Sulfisoxasol (Mexico) *see* Erythromycin and Sulfisoxazole 323
Eritroquim® (Mexico) *see* Erythromycin 321
ERO Ear® [OTC] *see* Carbamide Peroxide 152
Ervevax (Mexico) *see* Measles Virus Vaccine, Live 529
Erybid® (Canada) *see* Erythromycin 321
Eryc® *see* Erythromycin 321
Erycette® Topical *see* Erythromycin, Topical................... 324
EryDerm® Topical *see* Erythromycin, Topical 324
Erygel® Topical *see* Erythromycin, Topical 324
Erymax® Topical *see* Erythromycin, Topical 324
EryPed® *see* Erythromycin 321
Ery-sol® Topical *see* Erythromycin, Topical 324
Ery-Tab® *see* Erythromycin 321
Erythrityl Tetranitrate 320
Erythro-Base® (Canada) *see* Erythromycin 321
Erythrocin® *see* Erythromycin 321
Erythromycin 321
Erythromycin and Benzoyl Peroxide 323
Erythromycin and Sulfisoxazole 323
Erythromycin, Topical 324
Erythropoietin *see* Epoetin Alfa 315
Eryzole® *see* Erythromycin and Sulfisoxazole 323
Esgic® *see* Butalbital Compound 133
Esidrix® *see* Hydrochlorothiazide 430
Eskalith® *see* Lithium 508
E-Solve-2® Topical *see* Erythromycin, Topical 324
Esoterica® Facial [OTC] *see* Hydroquinone.................... 439
Esoterica® Regular [OTC] *see* Hydroquinone 439
Esoterica® Sensitive Skin Formula [OTC] *see* Hydroquinone 439
Esoterica® Sunscreen [OTC] *see* Hydroquinone 439
Espotabs® [OTC] *see* Phenolphthalein 682
Estar® [OTC] *see* Coal Tar 225
Estazolam 324
Esteprim® (Mexico) *see* Trimethoprim and Sulfamethoxazole ... 874
Estinyl® *see* Ethinyl Estradiol............................... 334
Estivin® II [OTC] *see* Naphazoline Hydrochloride 605
Estrace® *see* Estradiol 325
Estra-D® *see* Estradiol 325
Estraderm® *see* Estradiol 325
Estradiol 325
Estradiol and Testosterone 326
Estradurin® *see* Polyestradiol Phosphate 702
Estra-L® *see* Estradiol 325
Estramustine Phosphate Sodium 326
Estratab® *see* Estrogens, Esterified.......................... 328
Estratest® H.S. Oral *see* Estrogens With Methyltestosterone ... 329
Estratest® Oral *see* Estrogens With Methyltestosterone 329
Estra-Testrin® Injection *see* Estradiol and Testosterone 326
Estro-Cyp® *see* Estradiol 325
Estrogenos Conjugados (Mexico) *see* Estrogens, Conjugated 327

Estrogens and Medroxyprogesterone 327
Estrogens, Conjugated 327
Estrogens, Esterified 328
Estrogens With Methyltestosterone 329
Estroject-L.A.® see Estradiol 325
Estrone 329
Estronol® see Estrone 329
Estropipate 330
Estrouis® (Canada) see Estropipate 330
Estrovis® see Quinestrol 757
Ethacrynic Acid 331
Ethambutol Hydrochloride 332
Ethamolin® see Ethanolamine Oleate 333
ETH and C see Terpin Hydrate and Codeine 825
Ethanolamine Oleate 333
Ethaquin® see Ethaverine Hydrochloride 334
Ethatab® see Ethaverine Hydrochloride 334
Ethaverine Hydrochloride 334
Ethavex-100® see Ethaverine Hydrochloride 334
Ethchlorvynol 334
Ethinyl Estradiol 334
Ethinyl Estradiol and Desogestrel 335
Ethinyl Estradiol and Ethynodiol Diacetate 335
Ethinyl Estradiol and Fluoxymesterone 337
Ethinyl Estradiol and Levonorgestrel 337
Ethinyl Estradiol and Norethindrone 339
Ethinyl Estradiol and Norgestimate 340
Ethinyl Estradiol and Norgestrel 341
Ethionamide 342
Ethmozine® see Moricizine Hydrochloride 589
Ethopropazine Hydrochloride 343
Ethosuximide 343
Ethotoin 344
Ethyl Chloride 344
Ethyl Chloride and Dichlorotetrafluoroethane 344
Ethylnorepinephrine Hydrochloride 345
Ethylphenylhydantoin see Ethotoin 344
Etibl® (Canada) see Ethambutol Hydrochloride 332
Etidocaine Hydrochloride (With Epinephrine) 345
Etidronate Disodium 346
Etinilestradiol and Noretindrona (Mexico) see Ethinyl Estradiol and
   Norethindrone 339
Etinilestradiol (Mexico) see Ethinyl Estradiol 334
Etodolac 347
Etoposide 348
Etopos® (Mexico) see Etoposide 348
Etrafon® see Amitriptyline and Perphenazine 50
Etretinate 349
ETS-2%® Topical see Erythromycin, Topical 324
Eudal-SR® see Guaifenesin and Pseudoephedrine 409
Euglucon® (Canada) see Glyburide 401
Euglucon® (Mexico) see Glyburide 401
Eulexin® see Flutamide 382
Eulexin® (Mexico) see Flutamide 382
Eurax® see Crotamiton 236
Euthroid® see Liotrix 505
Eutirox® (Mexico) see Levothyroxine Sodium 498
Eutron® see Methyclothiazide and Pargyline 566
Evac-Q-Mag® [OTC] see Magnesium Citrate 521
Evac-U-Gen® [OTC] see Phenolphthalein 682
Evac-U-Lax® [OTC] see Phenolphthalein 682
Evalose® see Lactulose 488
Everone® see Testosterone 825
E-Vista® see Hydroxyzine 443
E-Vitamin® [OTC] see Vitamin E 900
Excedrin®, Extra Strength [OTC] see Acetaminophen, Aspirin, and Caffeine
   17
Excedrin® IB [OTC] see Ibuprofen 447
Excedrin® P.M. [OTC] see Acetaminophen and Diphenhydramine 16
Exelderm® see Sulconazole Nitrate 806
Exidine® Scrub [OTC] see Chlorhexidine Gluconate 184
Ex-Lax® [OTC] see Phenolphthalein 682
Ex-Lax®, Extra Gentle Pills [OTC] see Docusate and Phenolphthalein 295
Exna® see Benzthiazide 105
Exosurf® Neonatal™ see Colfosceril Palmitate 230
Exsel® see Selenium Sulfide 785
Extendryl® SR see Chlorpheniramine, Phenylephrine, and Methscopolamine
   193

Extra Action Cough Syrup [OTC] see Guaifenesin and Dextromethorphan
....408
Eye-Lube-A® Solution [OTC] see Artificial Tears 75
Eye-Sed® [OTC] see Zinc Supplements 909
Eye-Zine® [OTC] see Tetrahydrozoline Hydrochloride 831
Ezide® see Hydrochlorothiazide 430
Facicam® (Mexico) see Piroxicam 699
Factor IX Complex (Human) 350
Factor VIII see Antihemophilic Factor (Human) 68
Factor VIII Recombinant see Antihemophilic Factor (Recombinant) 70
Famciclovir 352
Famotidina (Mexico) see Famotidine 352
Famotidine 352
Famoxal® (Mexico) see Famotidine 352
Famvir™ see Famciclovir 352
Fansidar® see Sulfadoxine and Pyrimethamine 808
Faraxen® (Mexico) see Naproxen 606
Farmotex® (Mexico) see Famotidine 352
Fastin® see Phentermine Hydrochloride 683
Fat Emulsion 353
Febrin® (Mexico) see Acetaminophen 14
Fedahist® Expectorant [OTC] see Guaifenesin and Pseudoephedrine 409
Fedahist® Tablet [OTC] see Chlorpheniramine and Pseudoephedrine 191
Feen-a-Mint® [OTC] see Phenolphthalein 682
Feen-a-Mint® Pills [OTC] see Docusate and Phenolphthalein 295
Feiba VH Immuno® see Anti-Inhibitor Coagulant Complex 70
Felbamate 354
Felbatol™ see Felbamate 354
Feldene® see Piroxicam 699
Felodipina (Mexico) see Felodipine 354
Felodipine 354
Femcet® see Butalbital Compound 133
Femilax® [OTC] see Docusate and Phenolphthalein 295
Femiron® [OTC] see Ferrous Fumarate 359
Femogen® (Canada) see Estrone 329
Femstal® (Mexico) see Butoconazole Nitrate 135
Femstat® see Butoconazole Nitrate 135
Fenazopiridina (Mexico) see Phenazopyridine Hydrochloride 679
Fenesin™ see Guaifenesin 407
Fenfluramine Hydrochloride 355
Fenilefrina (Mexico) see Phenylephrine Hydrochloride 685
Fenilpropanolamina (Mexico) see Phenylpropanolamine Hydrochloride 687
Fenobarbital (Mexico) see Phenobarbital 680
Fenofibrate 356
Fenofibrato (Mexico) see Fenofibrate 356
Fenoprofen Calcium 356
Fenoprofeno Calcico (Mexico) see Fenoprofen Calcium 356
Fentanest® (Mexico) see Fentanyl 357
Fentanyl 357
Fentanyl Oralet® see Fentanyl 357
Fentermina (Mexico) see Phentermine Hydrochloride 683
Feosol® [OTC] see Ferrous Sulfate 360
Feostat® [OTC] see Ferrous Fumarate 359
Ferancee® [OTC] see Ferrous Sulfate and Ascorbic Acid 361
Feratab® [OTC] see Ferrous Sulfate 360
Fergon® [OTC] see Ferrous Gluconate 360
Fer-In-Sol® [OTC] see Ferrous Sulfate 360
Fer-Iron® [OTC] see Ferrous Sulfate 360
Fermalac® (Canada) see Lactobacillus acidophilus and Lactobacillus
    bulgaricus 488
Ferndex see Dextroamphetamine Sulfate 265
Fero-Grad 500® [OTC] see Ferrous Sulfate and Ascorbic Acid 361
Fero-Gradumet® [OTC] see Ferrous Sulfate 360
Ferospace® [OTC] see Ferrous Sulfate 360
Ferralet® [OTC] see Ferrous Gluconate 360
Ferralyn® Lanacaps® [OTC] see Ferrous Sulfate 360
Ferra-TD® [OTC] see Ferrous Sulfate 360
Ferromar® [OTC] see Ferrous Sulfate and Ascorbic Acid 361
Ferro-Sequels® [OTC] see Ferrous Fumarate 359
Ferrous Fumarate 359
Ferrous Gluconate 360
Ferrous Sulfate 360
Ferrous Sulfate and Ascorbic Acid 361
Ferrous Sulfate, Ascorbic Acid, and Vitamin B-Complex 361
Ferrous Sulfate, Ascorbic Acid, Vitamin B-Complex, and Folic Acid ...361
Fertinorm® H.P. (Mexico) see Urofollitropin 885
Ferval® Ferroso (Mexico) see Ferrous Fumarate 359
Feverall™ [OTC] see Acetaminophen 14

Fexofenadine Hydrochloride 361
Fiberall® [OTC] see Psyllium 750
Fiberall® Chewable Tablet [OTC] see Calcium Polycarbophil 146
FiberCon® Tablet [OTC] see Calcium Polycarbophil 146
Fiber-Lax® Tablet [OTC] see Calcium Polycarbophil 146
Fibrepur® (Canada) see Psyllium 750
Fibrinolysin and Desoxyribonuclease 362
Filgrastim 362
Filibon® [OTC] see Vitamins, Multiple 901
Finasteride 363
Fiorgen PF® see Butalbital Compound 133
Fioricet® see Butalbital Compound 133
Fiorinal® see Butalbital Compound 133
Fiorinal® With Codeine see Butalbital Compound and Codeine 134
Fisopred® (Mexico) see Prednisolone 718
Flagenase® (Mexico) see Metronidazole 576
Flagyl® see Metronidazole 576
Flamazine® (Canada) see Silver Sulfadiazine 788
Flamicina® (Mexico) see Ampicillin 62
Flanax® (Mexico) see Naproxen 606
Flarex® see Fluorometholone 375
Flatulex® [OTC] see Simethicone 788
Flavorcee® [OTC] see Ascorbic Acid 76
Flavoxate 364
Flebocortid® [Sodium Succinate] (Mexico) see Hydrocortisone 436
Flecainida, Acetato De (Mexico) see Flecainide Acetate 365
Flecainide Acetate 365
Fleet® Babylax® Rectal [OTC] see Glycerin 402
Fleet® Enema [OTC] see Sodium Phosphates 792
Fleet® Flavored Castor Oil [OTC] see Castor Oil 161
Fleet® Laxative [OTC] see Bisacodyl 113
Fleet® Phospho®-Soda [OTC] see Sodium Phosphates 792
Flexaphen® see Chlorzoxazone 200
Flexen® (Mexico) see Naproxen 606
Flexeril® see Cyclobenzaprine Hydrochloride 239
Flodine® (Canada) see Folic Acid 385
Flogen® (Mexico) see Naproxen 606
Flogosan® (Mexico) see Piroxicam 699
Flolan® Injection see Epoprostenol Sodium 317
Flonase™ see Fluticasone Propionate 383
Florinef® Acetate see Fludrocortisone Acetate 369
Florone® see Diflorasone Diacetate 278
Florone® E see Diflorasone Diacetate 278
Floropryl® see Isoflurophate 470
Florvite® see Vitamins, Multiple 901
Flosequinan 366
Floxacin® (Mexico) see Norfloxacin 628
Floxil® (Mexico) see Ofloxacin 634
Floxin® see Ofloxacin 634
Floxstat® (Mexico) see Ofloxacin 634
Floxuridine 366
Fluconazole 367
Flucytosine 368
Fludara® see Fludarabine Phosphate 368
Fludarabine Phosphate 368
Fludrocortisone Acetate 369
Flufenacina (Mexico) see Fluphenazine 379
Flu-Imune® see Influenza Virus Vaccine 458
Fluken® (Mexico) see Flutamide 382
Flulem (Mexico) see Flutamide 382
Flumadine® see Rimantadine Hydrochloride 771
Flumazenil 370
Flunisolide 372
Fluocinolona, Acetonido De (Mexico) see Fluocinolone Acetonide 372
Fluocinolone Acetonide 372
Fluocinonide 373
Fluocinonido (Mexico) see Fluocinonide 373
Fluogen® see Influenza Virus Vaccine 458
Fluonex® see Fluocinonide 373
Fluonid® see Fluocinolone Acetonide 372
Fluoracaine® see Proparacaine and Fluorescein 736
Fluoride 374
Fluorigard® [OTC] see Fluoride 374
Fluori-Methane® see Dichlorodifluoromethane and
    Trichloromonofluoromethane 270
Fluorinse® see Fluoride 374
Fluoritab® see Fluoride 374
Fluorodeoxyuridine see Floxuridine 366

Fluorometholone 375
Fluor-Op® see Fluorometholone 375
Fluoroplex® Topical see Fluorouracil 376
Fluorouracil 376
5-Fluorouracil see Fluorouracil 376
Fluoro-uracil® (Mexico) see Fluorouracil 376
Fluoxac® (Mexico) see Fluoxetine Hydrochloride 377
Fluoxetina Clorhidrato De (Mexico) see Fluoxetine Hydrochloride 377
Fluoxetine Hydrochloride 377
Fluoximesterona (Mexico) see Fluoxymesterone 378
Fluoxymesterone 378
Fluoxymesterone and Estradiol see Ethinyl Estradiol and Fluoxymesterone
. 337
Flupazine® (Mexico) see Trifluoperazine Hydrochloride 869
Fluphenazine 379
Flura® see Fluoride 374
Flura-Drops® see Fluoride 374
Flura-Loz® see Fluoride 374
Flurandrenolide 380
Flurazepam Hydrochloride 380
Flurbiprofen Sodium 381
5-Flurocytosine see Flucytosine 368
Fluro-Ethyl® Aerosol see Ethyl Chloride and Dichlorotetrafluoroethane 344
Flurosyn® see Fluocinolone Acetonide 372
Flutamide 382
Fluticasone Propionate 383
Fluvastatin 383
Fluviral® (Canada) see Influenza Virus Vaccine 458
Fluvoxamine 384
Fluzone® see Influenza Virus Vaccine 458
FML® see Fluorometholone 375
FML® Forte see Fluorometholone 375
FML-S® Ophthalmic Suspension see Sodium Sulfacetamide and
Fluorometholone 794
Folbesyn® see Vitamin B Complex With Vitamin C and Folic Acid 900
Folex® see Methotrexate 559
Folic Acid 385
Folico Acido (Mexico) see Folic Acid 385
Folinic Acid see Leucovorin Calcium 491
Folitab® (Mexico) see Folic Acid 385
Follutein® see Chorionic Gonadotropin 203
Folvite® see Folic Acid 385
Footwork® [OTC] see Tolnaftate 855
Formula Q® [OTC] see Quinine Sulfate 760
5-Formyl Tetrahydrofolate see Leucovorin Calcium 491
Fortaz® see Ceftazidime 171
Fortum® (Mexico) see Ceftazidime 171
Fosamax® see Alendronate Sodium 30
Foscarnet 386
Foscavir® see Foscarnet 386
Fosinopril 387
Fosinopril Sodico (Mexico) see Fosinopril 387
Fosphenytoin 389
Fostex® [OTC] see Sulfur and Salicylic Acid 813
Fostex® BPO [OTC] see Benzoyl Peroxide 104
Fotexina® (Mexico) see Cefotaxime Sodium 167
Fototar® [OTC] see Coal Tar 225
Fragmin® see Dalteparin 249
Fraxiparine® (Mexico) see Heparin 419
Fresh Burst Listerine® Antiseptic [OTC] see Mouthwash, Antiseptic 592
Froben® (Canada) see Flurbiprofen Sodium 381
Froben-SR® (Canada) see Flurbiprofen Sodium 381
Froxal® (Mexico) see Cefuroxime 173
FS Shampoo® see Fluocinolone Acetonide 372
5-FU see Fluorouracil 376
FUDR® see Floxuridine 366
Fulvicin® P/G see Griseofulvin 406
Fulvicin-U/F® see Griseofulvin 406
Fulvina® P/G (Mexico) see Griseofulvin 406
Fumasorb® [OTC] see Ferrous Fumarate 359
Fumerin® [OTC] see Ferrous Fumarate 359
Fungatin® [OTC] see Tolnaftate 855
Fungiquim® (Mexico) see Miconazole 578
Fungistat® Dual (Mexico) see Terconazole 823
Fungistat® (Mexico) see Terconazole 823
Fungizone® see Amphotericin B 60
Fungoid® see Triacetin 862
Fungoid® Topical Solution see Undecylenic Acid and Derivatives 884

Furacin® *see* Nitrofurazone 623
Furadantin® *see* Nitrofurantoin 622
Furadantina® (Mexico) *see* Nitrofurantoin 622
Furalan® *see* Nitrofurantoin 622
Furan® *see* Nitrofurantoin 622
Furanite® *see* Nitrofurantoin 622
Furazolidona (Mexico) *see* Furazolidone 391
Furazolidone 391
Furosemida (Mexico) *see* Furosemide 391
Furosemide 391
Furoside® (Canada) *see* Furosemide 391
Furoxona® Gotas (Mexico) *see* Furazolidone 391
Furoxona® Tabletas (Mexico) *see* Furazolidone 391
Furoxone® *see* Furazolidone 391
Fursemide (Canada) *see* Furosemide 391
Fustaren® Retard (Mexico) *see* Diclofenac 271
Fuxen® (Mexico) *see* Naproxen 606
Fuxol® (Mexico) *see* Furazolidone 391
G-1® *see* Butalbital Compound 133
Gabapentin 392
Galecin® (Mexico) *see* Clindamycin 214
Galedol® (Mexico) *see* Diclofenac 271
Galidrin® (Mexico) *see* Ranitidine Hydrochloride 763
Gamastan® *see* Immune Globulin, Intramuscular 453
Gamikal® (Mexico) *see* Amikacin Sulfate 44
Gamimune® N *see* Immune Globulin, Intravenous 454
Gammabulin Immuno (Canada) *see* Immune Globulin, Intramuscular 453
Gammagard® *see* Immune Globulin, Intravenous 454
Gammagard® S/D *see* Immune Globulin, Intravenous 454
Gammar® *see* Immune Globulin, Intramuscular 453
Ganciclovir 393
Ganciclovir Sodico (Mexico) *see* Ganciclovir 393
Gantanol® *see* Sulfamethoxazole 809
Gantrisin® *see* Sulfisoxazole 811
Garalen® (Mexico) *see* Gentamicin Sulfate 396
Garamicina® (Mexico) *see* Gentamicin Sulfate 396
Garamycin® *see* Gentamicin Sulfate 396
Gas-Ban DS® [OTC] *see* Aluminum Hydroxide, Magnesium Hydroxide, and
    Simethicone 41
Gas Relief® [OTC] *see* Simethicone 788
Gastrec® (Mexico) *see* Ranitidine Hydrochloride 763
Gastrocrom® *see* Cromolyn Sodium 235
Gastrosed™ *see* Hyoscyamine Sulfate 445
Gas-X® [OTC] *see* Simethicone 788
Gaviscon®-2 Tablet [OTC] *see* Aluminum Hydroxide and Magnesium
    Trisilicate 41
Gaviscon® Liquid [OTC] *see* Aluminum Hydroxide and Magnesium Carbonate
   40
Gaviscon® Tablet [OTC] *see* Aluminum Hydroxide and Magnesium Trisilicate
   41
G-CSF *see* Filgrastim 362
Gee Gee® [OTC] *see* Guaifenesin 407
Gelafundin® (Mexico) *see* Gelatin, Absorbable 394
Gelatin, Absorbable 394
Gelatina Desdoblada Pulimerizado De (Mexico) *see* Gelatin, Absorbable
    394
Gelatin, Pectin, and Methylcellulose 395
Gelfoam® Topical *see* Gelatin, Absorbable 394
Gelisyn® (Mexico) *see* Fluocinonide 373
Gel Kam® *see* Fluoride 374
Gelpirin® [OTC] *see* Acetaminophen, Aspirin, and Caffeine 17
Gel-Tin® [OTC] *see* Fluoride 374
Gelucast® *see* Zinc Gelatin 908
Gelusil® [OTC] *see* Aluminum Hydroxide, Magnesium Hydroxide, and
    Simethicone 41
Gemfibrozil 395
Genabid® *see* Papaverine Hydrochloride 658
Genac® [OTC] *see* Triprolidine and Pseudoephedrine 878
Genagesic® *see* Propoxyphene and Acetaminophen 741
Genahist® *see* Diphenhydramine Hydrochloride 288
Genamin® Cold Syrup [OTC] *see* Chlorpheniramine and
    Phenylpropanolamine 190
Genamin® Expectorant [OTC] *see* Guaifenesin and Phenylpropanolamine
    409
Genapap® [OTC] *see* Acetaminophen 14
Genasoft® Plus [OTC] *see* Docusate and Casanthranol 295
Genaspor® [OTC] *see* Tolnaftate 855

Genatap® Elixir [OTC] see Brompheniramine and Phenylpropanolamine
.... 123
Genatuss® [OTC] see Guaifenesin 407
Genatuss DM® [OTC] see Guaifenesin and Dextromethorphan ... 408
Gen-Clobetasol® (Canada) see Clobetasol Propionate 216
Genenicina® (Mexico) see Gentamicin Sulfate 396
Gen-Glybe® (Canada) see Glyburide......................... 401
Gen-K® see Potassium Chloride 708
Genkova® (Mexico) see Gentamicin Sulfate 396
Gen-Minoxidil® (Canada) see Minoxidil 583
Gen-Nifedipine® (Canada) see Nifedipine 619
Genora® 0.5/35 see Ethinyl Estradiol and Norethindrone 339
Genora® 1/35 see Ethinyl Estradiol and Norethindrone......... 339
Genora® 1/50 see Mestranol and Norethindrone 547
Genoxal® (Mexico) see Cyclophosphamide 240
Gen-Pindolol® (Canada) see Pindolol 694
Genpril® [OTC] see Ibuprofen 447
Genrex® (Mexico) see Gentamicin Sulfate 396
Gentab-LA® see Guaifenesin and Phenylpropanolamine 409
Gentamicin and Prednisolone see Prednisolone and Gentamicin ... 719
Gentamicin Sulfate....................................... 396
Gentarim® (Mexico) see Gentamicin Sulfate 396
Gentian Violet 397
Gen-Timolol® (Canada) see Timolol Maleate 847
Gentran® see Dextran 263
Gen-Triazolam® (Canada) see Triazolam 866
Gen-XENE® see Clorazepate Dipotassium 222
Geocillin® see Carbenicillin 153
Geopen® (Canada) see Carbenicillin 153
Geref® Injection see Sermorelin Acetate 786
Geridium® see Phenazopyridine Hydrochloride 679
German Measles Vaccine see Rubella Virus Vaccine, Live 776
Germinal® see Ergoloid Mesylates 318
Gesterol® see Progesterone 731
Gesterol® L.A. see Hydroxyprogesterone Caproate 441
Gevrabon® [OTC] see Vitamin B Complex 899
GG-Cen® [OTC] see Guaifenesin 407
Gimalxina® (Mexico) see Amoxicillin Trihydrate 58
Ginedisc® (Mexico) see Estradiol 325
Gingi-Aid® Gingival Retraction Cord see Aluminum Chloride ... 39
Gingi-Aid® Solution see Aluminum Chloride 39
Glandosane® Spray [OTC] see Saliva Substitute 778
Glibenclamida (Mexico) see Glyburide 401
Glibenil® (Mexico) see Glyburide 401
Glimepiride... 398
Glioten® (Mexico) see Enalapril 307
Glipicida (Mexico) see Glipizide........................... 399
Glipizida (Mexico) see Glipizide 399
Glipizide 399
Glucagon 400
Glucal® (Mexico) see Glyburide 401
Glucocerebrosidase see Alglucerase 32
Glucophage® see Metformin Hydrochloride 551
Glucophage® Forte (Mexico) see Metformin Hydrochloride 551
Glucose 400
Glucose Polymers 400
Glucotrol® see Glipizide 399
Glucotrol® XL see Glipizide 399
Glukor® see Chorionic Gonadotropin 203
Glutamic Acid.. 400
Glutethimide 401
Glutose® [OTC] see Glucose 400
Glyate® [OTC] see Guaifenesin 407
Glyburide 401
Glycate® [OTC] see Calcium Carbonate 140
Glycerin 402
Glycerin, Lanolin, and Peanut Oil 402
Glycerol see Glycerin 402
Glycerol-T® see Theophylline and Guaifenesin 836
Glycerol Triacetate see Triacetin 862
Glycofed® see Guaifenesin and Pseudoephedrine 409
Glycopyrrolate 403
Glycotuss® [OTC] see Guaifenesin 407
Glycotuss-DM® [OTC] see Guaifenesin and Dextromethorphan ... 408
Glynase™ PresTab™ see Glyburide 401
Gly-Oxide® [OTC] see Carbamide Peroxide 152
Glytuss® [OTC] see Guaifenesin 407
GM-CSF see Sargramostim............................... 780

Go-Evac® see Polyethylene Glycol-Electrolyte Solution 703
Gold Sodium Thiomalate 404
GoLYTELY® see Polyethylene Glycol-Electrolyte Solution 703
Gonak™ [OTC] see Hydroxypropyl Methylcellulose 442
Gonic® see Chorionic Gonadotropin 203
Gonioscopic Ophthalmic Solution see Hydroxypropyl Methylcellulose 442
Goniosol® [OTC] see Hydroxypropyl Methylcellulose 442
Goody's® Headache Powders see Acetaminophen, Aspirin, and Caffeine
. . . . 17
Goserelin Acetate 404
Graneodin-B® (Mexico) see Benzocaine 102
Granisetron 405
Granulex see Trypsin, Balsam Peru, and Castor Oil 881
Granulocyte Colony Stimulating Factor see Filgrastim 362
Granulocyte-Macrophage Colony Stimulating Factor see Sargramostim
. . . . 780
Gravol® (Canada) see Dimenhydrinate 286
Grifulvin® V see Griseofulvin 406
Grisactin® see Griseofulvin 406
Grisactin® Ultra see Griseofulvin 406
Griseofulvin 406
Griseofulvina (Mexico) see Griseofulvin 406
Grisovin-FP® (Canada) see Griseofulvin 406
Grisovin-FP® (Mexico) see Griseofulvin 406
Gris-PEG® see Griseofulvin 406
Grunicina® (Mexico) see Amoxicillin Trihydrate 58
Guaifed® [OTC] see Guaifenesin and Pseudoephedrine 409
Guaifed-PD® see Guaifenesin and Pseudoephedrine 409
Guaifenesin 407
Guaifenesina Dextrometorfano (Mexico) see Guaifenesin and
    Dextromethorphan 408
Guaifenesina (Mexico) see Guaifenesin 407
Guaifenesin and Codeine 408
Guaifenesin and Dextromethorphan 408
Guaifenesin and Hydrocodone see Hydrocodone and Guaifenesin 434
Guaifenesin and Phenylpropanolamine 409
Guaifenesin and Pseudoephedrine 409
Guaifenesin, Phenylpropanolamine, and Dextromethorphan 410
Guaifenesin, Phenylpropanolamine, and Phenylephrine 410
Guaifenesin, Pseudoephedrine, and Codeine 410
Guaifenex® see Guaifenesin, Phenylpropanolamine, and Phenylephrine
. . . . 410
Guaifenex® PPA 75 see Guaifenesin and Phenylpropanolamine 409
Guaifenex PSE® see Guaifenesin and Pseudoephedrine 409
GuaiMax-D® see Guaifenesin and Pseudoephedrine 409
Guaipax® see Guaifenesin and Phenylpropanolamine 409
Guaitab® see Guaifenesin and Pseudoephedrine 409
Guaituss AC® see Guaifenesin and Codeine 408
Guai-Vent/PSE® see Guaifenesin and Pseudoephedrine 409
Guanabenz Acetate 411
Guanadrel Sulfate 411
Guanethidine Sulfate 412
Guanfacine Hydrochloride 413
Gugecin® (Mexico) see Cinoxacin 207
GuiaCough® [OTC] see Guaifenesin and Dextromethorphan 408
Guiatex® see Guaifenesin, Phenylpropanolamine, and Phenylephrine 410
Guiatuss® [OTC] see Guaifenesin 407
Guiatuss CF® [OTC] see Guaifenesin, Phenylpropanolamine, and
    Dextromethorphan 410
Guiatuss DAC® see Guaifenesin, Pseudoephedrine, and Codeine 410
Guiatuss DM® [OTC] see Guaifenesin and Dextromethorphan 408
Guiatussin® DAC see Guaifenesin, Pseudoephedrine, and Codeine 410
Guiatussin® with Codeine see Guaifenesin and Codeine 408
Guiatuss PE® [OTC] see Guaifenesin and Pseudoephedrine 409
Gum Benjamin see Benzoin 104
G-well® see Lindane 504
Gynergen® (Canada) see Ergotamine 319
Gyne-Sulf® see Sulfabenzamide, Sulfacetamide, and Sulfathiazole 806
Gyno-Daktarin® (Mexico) see Miconazole 578
Gyno-Daktarin® V (Mexico) see Miconazole 578
Gynogen L.A.® see Estradiol 325
Gynol II® [OTC] see Nonoxynol 9 627
H₂Oxyl® (Canada) see Benzoyl Peroxide 104
Habitrol™ see Nicotine 617
Haemaccel® (Mexico) see Gelatin, Absorbable 394
Haemophilus b Conjugate Vaccine 414
Haemophilus b Oligosaccharide Conjugate Vaccine see Haemophilus b
    Conjugate Vaccine 414

Haemophilus b Polysaccharide Vaccine *see Haemophilus* b Conjugate
  Vaccine 414
Halazepam 415
Halcinonida (Mexico) *see* Halcinonide 415
Halcinonide 415
Halcion® *see* Triazolam 866
Haldol® *see* Haloperidol 417
Haldol® Decanoate *see* Haloperidol 417
Haldrone® *see* Paramethasone Acetate 659
Halenol® [OTC] *see* Acetaminophen 14
Haley's M-O® [OTC] *see* Magnesium Hydroxide and Mineral Oil Emulsion
 523
Halfan® *see* Halofantrine 416
Halobetasol Propionate 416
Halofantrine 416
Halog® *see* Halcinonide 415
Halog®-E *see* Halcinonide 415
Haloperidol 417
Haloperil® (Mexico) *see* Haloperidol 417
Haloprogin 418
Halotestin® *see* Fluoxymesterone 378
Halotex® *see* Haloprogin 418
Halotussin® [OTC] *see* Guaifenesin 407
Halotussin® AC *see* Guaifenesin and Codeine 408
Halotussin® DAC *see* Guaifenesin, Pseudoephedrine, and Codeine 410
Halotussin® DM [OTC] *see* Guaifenesin and Dextromethorphan .408
Halotussin® PE [OTC] *see* Guaifenesin and Pseudoephedrine 409
Haltran® [OTC] *see* Ibuprofen 447
Havrix® *see* Hepatitis A Vaccine 421
Hayfebrol® Liquid [OTC] *see* Chlorpheniramine and Pseudoephedrine 191
HbCV *see Haemophilus* b Conjugate Vaccine 414
H-BIG® *see* Hepatitis B Immune Globulin 422
Head & Shoulders® [OTC] *see* Pyrithione Zinc 755
Healon® *see* Sodium Hyaluronate 791
Healon® GV *see* Sodium Hyaluronate 791
Healon® Yellow *see* Sodium Hyaluronate 791
Helberina (Mexico) *see* Heparin 419
Helidac® Combination *see* Metronidazole 576
Helminzole® (Mexico) *see* Mebendazole 529
Hemabate™ *see* Carboprost Tromethamine 156
Hemiacidrin *see* Citric Acid Bladder Mixture 211
Hemin 419
Hemobion® 200 (Mexico) *see* Ferrous Sulfate 360
Hemobion® 400 (Mexico) *see* Ferrous Sulfate 360
Hemocyte® [OTC] *see* Ferrous Fumarate 359
Hemodent® Gingival Retraction Cord *see* Aluminum Chloride 39
Hemofil® M *see* Antihemophilic Factor (Human) 68
Henexal® (Mexico) *see* Furosemide 391
Hepalac® *see* Lactulose 488
Heparin 419
Heparin Cofactor I *see* Antithrombin III 71
Heparin Lock Flush *see* Heparin 419
Heparin Sodium, Heparin Calcium *see* Heparin 419
Hepatitis A Vaccine 421
Hepatitis B Immune Globulin 422
Hepatitis B Vaccine 422
Hep-B-Gammagee® *see* Hepatitis B Immune Globulin 422
Hep-Lock® Injection *see* Heparin 419
Herbal Medicines 1081
Herklin® (Mexico) *see* Lindane 504
Herplex® *see* Idoxuridine 449
HES *see* Hetastarch 423
Hespan® *see* Hetastarch 423
Hetastarch 423
Hexachlorophene 424
Hexadrol® *see* Dexamethasone 260
Hexalen® *see* Altretamine 38
Hexit® (Canada) *see* Lindane 504
Hexlixate® *see* Antihemophilic Factor (Recombinant) 70
H.H.R.® *see* Hydralazine, Hydrochlorothiazide, and Reserpine 429
Hibiclens® [OTC] *see* Chlorhexidine Gluconate 184
Hibistat® [OTC] *see* Chlorhexidine Gluconate 184
Hib Polysaccharide Conjugate *see Haemophilus* b Conjugate Vaccine 414
HibTITER® *see Haemophilus* b Conjugate Vaccine 414
Hidralacina Clorhidrato De (Mexico) *see* Hydralazine Hydrochloride 428
Hidramox® (Mexico) *see* Amoxicillin Trihydrate 58
Hidroclorotiacida (Mexico) *see* Hydrochlorothiazide 430
Hidroquinona (Mexico) *see* Hydroquinone 439

Hidroxicloroquina Sulfato De (Mexico) see Hydroxychloroquine Sulfate
....440
Hidroxiprogesterona Caproato De (Mexico) see Hydroxyprogesterone
Caproate 441
Hidroxocobalamina (Mexico) see Hydroxocobalamin 439
Higroton® 50 (Mexico) see Chlorthalidone................................199
Hipokinon® (Mexico) see Trihexyphenidyl Hydrochloride...................871
Hiprex® see Methenamine..555
Hip-Rex® (Canada) see Methenamine.....................................555
Hismanal® see Astemizole...82
Histaject® see Brompheniramine Maleate................................124
Histalet Forte® Tablet see Chlorpheniramine, Pyrilamine, Phenylephrine, and
Phenylpropanolamine 195
Histalet® Syrup [OTC] see Chlorpheniramine and Pseudoephedrine 191
Histalet X® see Guaifenesin and Pseudoephedrine 409
Histatab® Plus Tablet [OTC] see Chlorpheniramine and Phenylephrine
....190
Hista-Vadrin® Tablet see Chlorpheniramine, Phenylephrine, and
Phenylpropanolamine 193
Histerone® see Testosterone 825
Histolyn-CYL® Injection see Histoplasmin................................425
Histoplasmin...425
Histoplasmosis Skin Test Antigen see Histoplasmin 425
Histor-D® Syrup see Chlorpheniramine and Phenylephrine.................190
Histor-D® Timecelles® see Chlorpheniramine, Phenylephrine, and
Methscopolamine 193
Histrelin...425
Histrodrix® [OTC] see Dexbrompheniramine and Pseudoephedrine 261
Hi-Vegi-Lip® see Pancreatin 656
Hivid® see Zalcitabine 906
HMS Liquifilm® Ophthalmic see Medrysone 533
Hold® DM [OTC] see Dextromethorphan...................................266
Homatropine and Hydrocodone see Hydrocodone and Homatropine 434
Homatropine Hydrobromide 426
Honvol® (Canada) see Diethylstilbestrol 277
Horse Anti-human Thymocyte Gamma Globulin see Lymphocyte Immune
Globulin, Anti-thymocyte Globulin (Equine) 518
H.P. Acthar® Gel see Corticotropin 233
Humalog® see Insulin Preparations 459
Human Growth Hormone..426
Humate-P® see Antihemophilic Factor (Human) 68
Humatin® see Paromomycin Sulfate 660
Humatrope® see Human Growth Hormone 426
Humibid® DM [OTC] see Guaifenesin and Dextromethorphan 408
Humibid® L.A. see Guaifenesin 407
Humibid® Sprinkle see Guaifenesin 407
Humorsol® see Demecarium Bromide 255
Humulin® 50/50 see Insulin Preparations 459
Humulin® 70/30 see Insulin Preparations 459
Humulin® L see Insulin Preparations 459
Humulin® N see Insulin Preparations 459
Humulin® R see Insulin Preparations 459
Humulin® U see Insulin Preparations 459
Hurricane® [OTC] see Benzocaine 102
Hyaluronic Acid see Sodium Hyaluronate 791
Hyaluronidase 427
Hyate®:C see Antihemophilic Factor (Porcine) 69
Hybalamin® see Hydroxocobalamin.......................................439
Hybolin™ Decanoate see Nandrolone 604
Hybolin™ Improved see Nandrolone 604
Hycamptamine see Topotecan Hydrochloride 855
Hycamtin® see Topotecan Hydrochloride 855
HycoClear Tuss® see Hydrocodone and Guaifenesin 434
Hycodan® see Hydrocodone and Homatropine 434
Hycomine® see Hydrocodone and Phenylpropanolamine 435
Hycomine® Compound see Hydrocodone, Chlorpheniramine, Phenylephrine,
Acetaminophen and Caffeine 435
Hycomine® Pediatric see Hydrocodone and Phenylpropanolamine..........435
Hycotuss® Expectorant Liquid see Hydrocodone and Guaifenesin 434
Hydeltrasol® see Prednisolone 718
Hydeltra-T.B.A.® see Prednisolone 718
Hydergine® see Ergoloid Mesylates 318
Hydergine® LC see Ergoloid Mesylates...................................318
Hydralazine and Hydrochlorothiazide 428
Hydralazine Hydrochloride 428
Hydralazine, Hydrochlorothiazide, and Reserpine 429
Hydrap-ES® see Hydralazine, Hydrochlorothiazide, and Reserpine 429
Hydrate® see Dimenhydrinate 286

Hydrazide® see Hydralazine and Hydrochlorothiazide................................428
Hydrea® see Hydroxyurea...442
Hydrex® see Benzthiazide..105
Hydrisalic™ see Salicylic Acid..777
Hydrobexan® see Hydroxocobalamin..439
Hydrocet® [5/500] see Hydrocodone and Acetaminophen...............................431
Hydrochlorothiazide...430
Hydrochlorothiazide and Amiloride see Amiloride and Hydrochlorothiazide
....45
Hydrochlorothiazide and Hydralazine see Hydralazine and
    Hydrochlorothiazide...428
Hydrochlorothiazide and Methyldopa see Methyldopa and Hydrochlorothiazide
....567
Hydrochlorothiazide and Reserpine...431
Hydrochlorothiazide and Spironolactone..431
Hydrocil® [OTC] see Psyllium..750
Hydro-Cobex® see Hydroxocobalamin...439
Hydrocodone and Acetaminophen...431
Hydrocodone and Aspirin...433
Hydrocodone and Chlorpheniramine..434
Hydrocodone and Guaifenesin...434
Hydrocodone and Homatropine...434
Hydrocodone and Phenylpropanolamine...435
Hydrocodone, Chlorpheniramine, Phenylephrine, Acetaminophen and
    Caffeine..435
Hydrocodone, Phenylephrine, Pyrilamine, Phenindamine, Chlorpheniramine,
    and Ammonium Chloride...435
Hydrocodone, Pseudoephedrine, and Guaifenesin.....................................435
Hydrocortisone..436
Hydrocortisone and Clioquinol see Clioquinol and Hydrocortisone...................216
Hydrocortisone and Dibucaine see Dibucaine and Hydrocortisone.....................270
Hydrocortisone and Iodochlorhydroxyquin see Clioquinol and Hydrocortisone
....216
Hydrocortisone and Pramoxine see Pramoxine and Hydrocortisone.....................714
Hydrocortisone and Urea see Urea and Hydrocortisone...............................885
Hydrocortone® Acetate see Hydrocortisone..436
Hydrocortone® Phosphate see Hydrocortisone..436
Hydro-Crysti-12® see Hydroxocobalamin...439
HydroDIURIL® see Hydrochlorothiazide..430
Hydro-Ergoloid® see Ergoloid Mesylates..318
Hydroflumethiazide..437
Hydroflumethiazide and Reserpine..438
Hydro-Fluserpine® see Hydroflumethiazide and Reserpine............................438
Hydrogesic® [5/500] see Hydrocodone and Acetaminophen.............................431
Hydromagnesium aluminate see Magaldrate...520
Hydromet® see Hydrocodone and Homatropine...434
Hydromorphone Hydrochloride...438
Hydromox® see Quinethazone..758
Hydropane® see Hydrocodone and Homatropine..434
Hydro-Par® see Hydrochlorothiazide..430
Hydrophen® see Theophylline, Ephedrine, and Hydroxyzine...........................836
Hydropres® see Hydrochlorothiazide and Reserpine..................................431
Hydroquinone..439
Hydro-Serp® see Hydrochlorothiazide and Reserpine.................................431
Hydroserpine® see Hydrochlorothiazide and Reserpine...............................431
Hydrotropine® see Hydrocodone and Homatropine.....................................434
Hydroxacen® see Hydroxyzine...443
Hydroxocobalamin..439
Hydroxyamphetamine and Tropicamide..440
Hydroxyamphetamine Hydrobromide...440
Hydroxycarbamide see Hydroxyurea..442
Hydroxychloroquine Sulfate..440
Hydroxydaunomycin Hydrochloride see Doxorubicin Hydrochloride.....................299
Hydroxyethylcellulose see Artificial Tears..75
Hydroxyethyl Starch see Hetastarch..423
Hydroxyprogesterone Caproate..441
Hydroxypropyl Cellulose...441
Hydroxypropyl Methylcellulose...442
Hydroxyurea...442
Hydroxyzine...443
Hy-Gestrone® see Hydroxyprogesterone Caproate.....................................441
Hygroton® see Chlorthalidone..199
Hylorel® see Guanadrel Sulfate..411
Hylutin® see Hydroxyprogesterone Caproate...441
Hyoscyamine, Atropine, Scopolamine, and Phenobarbital.............................444
Hyoscyamine, Atropine, Scopolamine, Kaolin, and Pectin............................445
Hyoscyamine, Atropine, Scopolamine, Kaolin, Pectin, and Opium.....................445
Hyoscyamine Sulfate...445

Hyosophen® *see* Hyoscyamine, Atropine, Scopolamine, and Phenobarbital 444
Hy-Pam® *see* Hydroxyzine 443
Hyperab® *see* Rabies Immune Globulin, Human 761
HyperHep® *see* Hepatitis B Immune Globulin 422
Hyperstat® I.V. *see* Diazoxide 269
Hyper-Tet® *see* Tetanus Immune Globulin, Human 826
Hyper-Tet® (Mexico) *see* Tetanus Immune Globulin, Human 826
Hy-Phen® [5/500] *see* Hydrocodone and Acetaminophen 431
HypoTears PF Solution [OTC] *see* Artificial Tears 75
HypoTears Solution [OTC] *see* Artificial Tears 75
HypRho®-D *see* Rh₀(D) Immune Globulin 767
HypRho®-D Mini-Dose *see* Rh₀(D) Immune Globulin 767
Hyprogest® *see* Hydroxyprogesterone Caproate 441
Hysone® Topical *see* Clioquinol and Hydrocortisone 216
Hytakerol® *see* Dihydrotachysterol 283
Hytinic® [OTC] *see* Polysaccharide-Iron Complex 705
Hytrin® *see* Terazosin 821
Hytuss® [OTC] *see* Guaifenesin 407
Hytuss-2X® [OTC] *see* Guaifenesin 407
Hyzaar® *see* Losartan and Hydrochlorothiazide 515
Hy-Zide® *see* Hydralazine and Hydrochlorothiazide 428
Hyzine-50® *see* Hydroxyzine 443
Iberet-Folic-500® *see* Ferrous Sulfate, Ascorbic Acid, Vitamin B-Complex, and Folic Acid 361
Iberet®-Liquid [OTC] *see* Ferrous Sulfate, Ascorbic Acid, and Vitamin B-Complex 361
Ibuprin® [OTC] *see* Ibuprofen 447
Ibuprofen 447
Ibuprohm® [OTC] *see* Ibuprofen 447
Ibu-Tab® *see* Ibuprofen 447
Idamycin® *see* Idarubicin 448
Idarubicin 448
Idoxuridina (Mexico) *see* Idoxuridine 449
Idoxuridine 449
IDR *see* Idarubicin 448
Idulamine® (Mexico) *see* Azatadine Maleate 89
Ifex® Injection *see* Ifosfamide 449
Ifosfamide 449
Ifoxan® (Mexico) *see* Ifosfamide 449
IL-2 *see* Aldesleukin 29
Ilopan® *see* Dexpanthenol 263
Ilopan-Choline® *see* Dexpanthenol 263
Ilosone® *see* Erythromycin 321
Ilotycin® Ophthalmic *see* Erythromycin, Topical 324
Ilozyme® *see* Pancrelipase 657
Imdur™ *see* Isosorbide Mononitrate 474
I-Methasone® *see* Dexamethasone 260
Imglucerase 450
Imidazole Carboxamide *see* Dacarbazine 247
Imigran® (Mexico) *see* Sumatriptan Succinate 814
Imipenem/Cilastatin 451
Imipramine 451
Imitrex® *see* Sumatriptan Succinate 814
Immune Globulin, Intramuscular 453
Immune Globulin, Intravenous 454
Imodium® *see* Loperamide Hydrochloride 511
Imodium® A-D [OTC] *see* Loperamide Hydrochloride 511
Imogam® *see* Rabies Immune Globulin, Human 761
Imot® Ofteno (Mexico) *see* Timolol Maleate 847
Imovax® Rabies I.D. Vaccine *see* Rabies Virus Vaccine 761
Imovax® Rabies Vaccine *see* Rabies Virus Vaccine 761
Imuran® *see* Azathioprine 89
I-Naphline® *see* Naphazoline Hydrochloride 605
Inapsine® *see* Droperidol 303
Indapamide 455
Inderal® *see* Propranolol Hydrochloride 743
Inderalici® (Mexico) *see* Propranolol Hydrochloride 743
Inderal® LA *see* Propranolol Hydrochloride 743
Inderide® *see* Propranolol and Hydrochlorothiazide 743
Indinavir 456
Indochron E-R® *see* Indomethacin 457
Indocid® (Canada) *see* Indomethacin 457
Indocid® (Mexico) *see* Indomethacin 457
Indocid-SR® (Canada) *see* Indomethacin 457
Indocin® *see* Indomethacin 457
Indocin® I.V. *see* Indomethacin 457
Indocin® SR *see* Indomethacin 457

Indocyanine Green 457
Indometacina (Mexico) see Indomethacin 457
Indomethacin 457
Infectious Disease - Antimicrobial Activity Against Selected Organisms
. . . . 1034
InFed™ Injection see Iron Dextran Complex 468
Inflamase® see Prednisolone 718
Inflamase® Mild see Prednisolone 718
Influenza Virus Vaccine 458
Infumorph™ Injection see Morphine Sulfate 590
INH™ see Isoniazid 471
Inhepar (Mexico) see Heparin 419
Inhibitron® (Mexico) see Omeprazole 636
Inocor® see Amrinone Lactate 65
Insect Sting Kit 459
Insogen® (Mexico) see Chlorpropamide 197
Insta-Char® [OTC] see Charcoal 179
Insta-Glucose® [OTC] see Glucose 400
Insulina Lenta® (Mexico) see Insulin Preparations 459
Insulina (Mexico) see Insulin Preparations 459
Insulina NPH® (Mexico) see Insulin Preparations 459
Insulina Regular® (Mexico) see Insulin Preparations 459
Insulin Preparations 459
Intacglobin® (Mexico) see Immune Globulin, Intravenous 454
Intal® see Cromolyn Sodium 235
Intercept™ [OTC] see Nonoxynol 9 627
Interferon Alfa-2a 461
Interferon Alfa-2b 462
Interferon Alfa-N3 463
Interferon Beta-1b 464
Interferon Gamma-1B 465
Interleukin-2 see Aldesleukin 29
Intralipid® see Fat Emulsion 353
Intravenous Fat Emulsion see Fat Emulsion 353
Intron® A see Interferon Alfa-2b 462
Inversine® see Mecamylamine Hydrochloride 530
Invirase® see Saquinavir Mesylate 780
Iodex® Regular see Povidone-Iodine 713
Iodinated Glycerol 465
Iodine 465
Iodine see Trace Metals 857
Iodochlorhydroxyquin 466
Iodochlorhydroxyquin and Hydrocortisone see Clioquinol and Hydrocortisone
. . . . 216
Iodopen® see Trace Metals 857
Iodoquinol 466
Iodoquinol and Hydrocortisone 467
Ionamin® see Phentermine Hydrochloride 683
Ionil® [OTC] see Salicylic Acid 777
Iophen® see Iodinated Glycerol 465
Iophen DM® [OTC] see Guaifenesin and Dextromethorphan 408
Iopidine® see Apraclonidine Hydrochloride 72
Iosat® see Potassium Iodide 711
I-Paracaine® see Proparacaine Hydrochloride 737
I-Parescein® see Proparacaine and Fluorescein 736
Ipecac Syrup 467
I-Pentolate® see Cyclopentolate Hydrochloride 240
I-Phrine® Ophthalmic Solution see Phenylephrine Hydrochloride 685
I-Picamide® Ophthalmic see Tropicamide 881
IPOL™ see Poliovirus Vaccine, Inactivated 702
Ipratropium Bromide 467
IPV see Poliovirus Vaccine, Inactivated 702
Ircon® [OTC] see Ferrous Fumarate 359
Irinotecan 468
Iron Dextran Complex 468
Ismelin® see Guanethidine Sulfate 412
Ismo™ see Isosorbide Mononitrate 474
Ismotic® see Isosorbide 473
Isobac® (Mexico) see Trimethoprim and Sulfamethoxazole 874
Iso-Bid® see Isosorbide Dinitrate 474
Isocaine® HCl 2% see Mepivacaine With Levonordefrin 542
Isocaine® HCl 3% see Mepivacaine Dental Anesthetic 541
Isocarboxazid 469
Isoclor® Expectorant see Guaifenesin, Pseudoephedrine, and Codeine
. . . . 410
Isodine® [OTC] see Povidone-Iodine 713
Isoetharine 470
Isoflurophate 470

Isoket® (Mexico) *see* Isosorbide Dinitrate 474
Isollyl Improved® *see* Butalbital Compound 133
Isomeprobamate (Canada) *see* Carisoprodol 157
Isonate® *see* Isosorbide Dinitrate 474
Isoniazid...471
Isonipecaine (Canada) *see* Meperidine Hydrochloride 539
Isopro® *see* Isoproterenol 472
Isoproterenol 472
Isoproterenol and Phenylephrine 473
Isoptin® *see* Verapamil Hydrochloride 893
Isoptin® SR *see* Verapamil Hydrochloride 893
Isopto® Carbachol *see* Carbachol 150
Isopto® Carpine® *see* Pilocarpine 691
Isopto® Eserine® *see* Physostigmine 690
Isopto® Frin Ophthalmic Solution *see* Phenylephrine Hydrochloride ...685
Isopto® Homatropine Ophthalmic *see* Homatropine Hydrobromide 426
Isopto® Hyoscine *see* Scopolamine 781
Isopto® Plain Solution [OTC] *see* Artificial Tears 75
Isopto® Tears Solution [OTC] *see* Artificial Tears 75
Isorbid® (Mexico) *see* Isosorbide Dinitrate...............................474
Isordil® *see* Isosorbide Dinitrate..474
Isosorbide 473
Isosorbide Dinitrate 474
Isosorbide Mononitrate 474
Isotrate® *see* Isosorbide Dinitrate 474
Isotretinoin 475
Isotrex® (Canada) *see* Isotretinoin 475
Isovex® *see* Ethaverine Hydrochloride....................................334
Isox® (Mexico) *see* Itraconazole 477
Isoxsuprine Hydrochloride 476
Isradipine 476
Isuprel® *see* Isoproterenol 472
Italnik® (Mexico) *see* Ciprofloxacin Hydrochloride 208
Itch-X® [OTC] *see* Pramoxine Hydrochloride 714
Itraconazole 477
Itranax® (Mexico) *see* Itraconazole 477
Iveegam® (Canada) *see* Immune Globulin, Intramuscular 453
IVIG *see* Immune Globulin, Intravenous 454
Jaa Amp® [Trihydrate] (Canada) *see* Ampicillin...........................62
Jaa-Prednisone® (Canada) *see* Prednisone 719
Janimine® *see* Imipramine 451
Japanese Encephalitis Virus Vaccine, Inactivated 478
Jenest-28™ *see* Ethinyl Estradiol and Norethindrone 339
JE-VAX® *see* Japanese Encephalitis Virus Vaccine, Inactivated ...478
Just Tears® Solution [OTC] *see* Artificial Tears...........................75
K⁺8® *see* Potassium Chloride 708
Kabikinase® *see* Streptokinase 801
Kadian® Capsule *see* Morphine Sulfate...................................590
Kalcinate® *see* Calcium Gluconate 143
Kaliolite® (Mexico) *see* Potassium Chloride.............................708
Kanamycin Sulfate 479
Kantrex® *see* Kanamycin Sulfate...479
Kaochlor-Eff® *see* Potassium Bicarbonate, Potassium Chloride, and
    Potassium Citrate 708
Kaochlor® S-F *see* Potassium Chloride 708
Kaodene® [OTC] *see* Kaolin and Pectin 480
Kaolin and Pectin 480
Kaolin and Pectin With Opium 480
Kaon® *see* Potassium Gluconate...710
Kaon-CL® *see* Potassium Chloride 708
Kaopectate® Advanced Formula [OTC] *see* Attapulgite 86
Kaopectate® II [OTC] *see* Loperamide Hydrochloride 511
Kaopectate® Maximum Strength Caplets *see* Attapulgite 86
Kao-Spen® [OTC] *see* Kaolin and Pectin 480
Kapectolin® [OTC] *see* Kaolin and Pectin 480
Kapectolin PG® *see* Hyoscyamine, Atropine, Scopolamine, Kaolin, Pectin,
    and Opium 445
Karidium® *see* Fluoride 374
Karigel® *see* Fluoride 374
Karigel®-N *see* Fluoride 374
Kasof® [OTC] *see* Docusate 295
Kato® *see* Potassium Chloride...708
Kaybovite-1000® *see* Cyanocobalamin 237
Kaylixir® *see* Potassium Gluconate 710
K+ Care® Effervescent *see* Potassium Bicarbonate 707
K-Dur® *see* Potassium Chloride...708
Keduril® (Mexico) *see* Ketoprofen 483
Kedvil® (Mexico) *see* Ibuprofen 447

Keflet® *see* Cephalexin Monohydrate 176
Keflex® *see* Cephalexin Monohydrate 176
Keflin® *see* Cephalothin Sodium 177
Keftab® *see* Cephalexin Monohydrate 176
Kefurox® *see* Cefuroxime 173
Kefzol® *see* Cefazolin Sodium 164
K-Electrolyte® Effervescent *see* Potassium Bicarbonate 707
Kelfiprim® (Mexico) *see* Trimethoprim and Sulfamethoxazole 874
Kemadrin® *see* Procyclidine Hydrochloride 730
Kenacort® (Mexico) *see* Triamcinolone 862
Kenacort® Syrup *see* Triamcinolone 862
Kenacort® Tablet *see* Triamcinolone 862
Kenalog® Injection *see* Triamcinolone 862
Kenalog® in Orabase® *see* Triamcinolone Acetonide Dental Paste 864
Kenamil® (Mexico) *see* Zidovudine 907
Kenaprol® (Mexico) *see* Metoprolol 574
Keneter® (Mexico) *see* Terfenadine 823
Kenolan® (Mexico) *see* Captopril 148
Kenonel® *see* Triamcinolone 862
Kenzoflex® (Mexico) *see* Ciprofloxacin Hydrochloride 208
Keralyt® *see* Salicylic Acid 777
Keralyt® Gel *see* Salicylic Acid and Propylene Glycol 778
Kerlone® *see* Betaxolol Hydrochloride 111
Kestrone® *see* Estrone 329
Ketalar® *see* Ketamine Hydrochloride 481
Ketalin® (Mexico) *see* Ketamine Hydrochloride 481
Ketamine Hydrochloride 481
Ketoconazole 481
Ketoprofen 483
Ketoprofeno (Mexico) *see* Ketoprofen 483
Ketorolac Tromethamine 484
Key-Pred® *see* Prednisolone 718
Key-Pred-SP® *see* Prednisolone 718
K-G® Elixir *see* Potassium Gluconate 710
K-Gen® Effervescent *see* Potassium Bicarbonate 707
Kinesed® *see* Hyoscyamine, Atropine, Scopolamine, and Phenobarbital
.... 444
Kinestase® (Mexico) *see* Cisapride 209
Kinevac® *see* Sincalide 789
Klaricid® (Mexico) *see* Clarithromycin 212
Klerist-D® Tablet [OTC] *see* Chlorpheniramine and Pseudoephedrine 191
Klonopin™ *see* Clonazepam 220
K-Lor™ *see* Potassium Chloride 708
Klor-con® *see* Potassium Chloride 708
Klor-Con®/EF *see* Potassium Bicarbonate and Potassium Citrate,
Effervescent 707
Kloromin® [OTC] *see* Chlorpheniramine Maleate 191
Klorvess® *see* Potassium Chloride 708
Klorvess® Effervescent *see* Potassium Bicarbonate and Potassium Chloride,
Effervescent 707
Klotrix® *see* Potassium Chloride 708
Klyndaken® (Mexico) *see* Clindamycin 214
K-Lyte® *see* Potassium Bicarbonate and Potassium Citrate, Effervescent
.... 707
K-Lyte/CL® *see* Potassium Bicarbonate and Potassium Chloride, Effervescent
.... 707
K-Lyte® Effervescent *see* Potassium Bicarbonate 707
Kōate®-HP *see* Antihemophilic Factor (Human) 68
Kōate®-HS *see* Antihemophilic Factor (Human) 68
KoGENate® *see* Antihemophilic Factor (Human) 68
Kolephrin® GG/DM [OTC] *see* Guaifenesin and Dextromethorphan 408
Kolyum® *see* Potassium Chloride and Potassium Gluconate 709
Konakion® *see* Phytonadione 690
Konsyl® [OTC] *see* Psyllium 750
Konsyl-D® [OTC] *see* Psyllium 750
Konȳne® 80 *see* Factor IX Complex (Human) 350
Koromex® [OTC] *see* Nonoxynol 9 627
K-Phos® Neutral *see* Potassium Phosphate and Sodium Phosphate 713
K-Phos® Original *see* Potassium Acid Phosphate 707
K-Profen® (Mexico) *see* Ketoprofen 483
K-Tab® *see* Potassium Chloride 708
Ku-Zyme® HP *see* Pancrelipase 657
K-Vescent® *see* Potassium Bicarbonate and Potassium Citrate, Effervescent
.... 707
Kwelcof® *see* Hydrocodone and Guaifenesin 434
Kwell® *see* Lindane 504
Kwellada® (Canada) *see* Lindane 504
Kytril® *see* Granisetron 405

LA-12® see Hydroxocobalamin 439
Labetalol Hydrochloride 486
LaBID® see Theophylline/Aminophylline 832
Lac-Hydrin® see Lactic Acid With Ammonium Hydroxide 487
Lacril® Ophthalmic Solution [OTC] see Artificial Tears 75
Lacrisert® see Hydroxypropyl Cellulose 441
Lactaid® [OTC] see Lactase 487
Lactase 487
Lacteol® Fort (Mexico) see Lactobacillus acidophilus and Lactobacillus
    bulgaricus 488
Lactic Acid and Salicylic Acid see Salicylic Acid and Lactic Acid 778
Lactic Acid and Sodium-PCA 487
Lactic Acid With Ammonium Hydroxide 487
LactiCare® [OTC] see Lactic Acid and Sodium-PCA 487
Lactinex® [OTC] see Lactobacillus acidophilus and Lactobacillus bulgaricus
    488
Lactobacillus acidophilus and Lactobacillus bulgaricus 488
Lactrase® [OTC] see Lactase 487
Lactulose 488
Lactulose PSE® see Lactulose 488
Ladakamycin see Azacitidine 88
Ladogal® (Mexico) see Danazol 249
Lamictal® see Lamotrigine 489
Lamisil® see Terbinafine 822
Lamivudine 489
Lamotrigina (Mexico) see Lamotrigine 489
Lamotrigine 489
Lampicin® (Mexico) see Ampicillin 62
Lamprene® see Clofazimine Palmitate 217
Lanexat® (Mexico) see Flumazenil 370
Laniazid® see Isoniazid 471
Lanolin, Cetyl Alcohol, Glycerin, and Petrolatum 490
Lanophyllin-GG® see Theophylline and Guaifenesin 836
Lanorinal® see Butalbital Compound 133
Lanoxicaps® see Digoxin 280
Lanoxin® see Digoxin 280
Lansoprazole 490
Lanvisone® Topical see Clioquinol and Hydrocortisone 216
Largactil® (Canada) see Chlorpromazine Hydrochloride 195
Largon® Injection see Propiomazine Hydrochloride 737
Lariam® see Mefloquine Hydrochloride 535
Larodopa® see Levodopa 495
Larotid® see Amoxicillin Trihydrate 58
Lasan™ see Anthralin 68
Lasan HP-1™ see Anthralin 68
Lasix® see Furosemide 391
L-asparaginase see Asparaginase 77
Lassar's Zinc Paste see Zinc Oxide 908
Latanoprost 490
Latotryd® (Mexico) see Erythromycin 321
Lauricin® (Mexico) see Erythromycin 321
Lax-Pills® [OTC] see Phenolphthalein 682
LazerSporin-C® Otic see Neomycin, Polymyxin B, and Hydrocortisone . . . 610
L-Carnitine see Levocarnitine 494
LCD see Coal Tar 225
LCR see Vincristine Sulfate 896
Leche De Magnesia Normex (Mexico) see Magnesium Hydroxide 522
Ledercillin® VK see Penicillin V Potassium 668
Ledercort® (Mexico) see Triamcinolone 862
Ledermicina® (Mexico) see Demeclocycline Hydrochloride 255
Lederpax® (Mexico) see Erythromycin 321
Lederplex® [OTC] see Vitamin B Complex 899
Ledertrexate® (Mexico) see Methotrexate 559
Ledoxina® (Mexico) see Cyclophosphamide 240
Legatrin® [OTC] see Quinine Sulfate 760
Lemblastine (Mexico) see Vinblastine Sulfate 895
Lenoltec® With Codeine (Canada) see Acetaminophen and Codeine 15
Lenpryl® (Mexico) see Captopril 148
Lente® Iletin® I see Insulin Preparations 459
Lente® Iletin® II see Insulin Preparations 459
Lente® Insulin see Insulin Preparations 459
Lente® L see Insulin Preparations 459
Lentopenil® (Mexico) see Penicillin G, Parenteral, Aqueous 666
Leponex® (Mexico) see Clozapine 225
Leptilan® (Mexico) see Valproic Acid and Derivatives 888
Leptopsique® (Mexico) see Perphenazine 677
Lertamine® (Mexico) see Loratadine 512
Lescol® see Fluvastatin 383

Lesterol® (Mexico) see Probucol 725
Leucomax® (Mexico) see Sargramostim 780
Leucovorin Calcium 491
Leukeran® see Chlorambucil 181
Leukine™ see Sargramostim 780
Leunase® (Mexico) see Asparaginase 77
Leuprolide Acetate 492
Leuprorelin Acetate see Leuprolide Acetate 492
Leurocristine see Vincristine Sulfate 896
Leustatin™ see Cladribine 211
Levamisole Hydrochloride 493
Levate® (Canada) see Amitriptyline Hydrochloride 51
Levatol® see Penbutolol Sulfate 664
Levlen® see Ethinyl Estradiol and Levonorgestrel 337
Levobunolol Hydrochloride 493
Levocabastine Hydrochloride 494
Levocarnitine 494
Levodopa 495
Levodopa and Carbidopa 495
Levo-Dromoran® see Levorphanol Tartrate 497
Levomepromazine see Methotrimeprazine Hydrochloride 562
Levomethadyl Acetate Hydrochloride 496
Levonorgestrel 497
Levoprome® see Methotrimeprazine Hydrochloride 562
Levora® see Ethinyl Estradiol and Levonorgestrel 337
Levorphanol Tartrate 497
Levo-T™ see Levothyroxine Sodium 498
Levothroid® see Levothyroxine Sodium 498
Levothyroxine Sodium 498
Levotiroxina (Mexico) see Levothyroxine Sodium 498
Levoxyl™ see Levothyroxine Sodium 498
Levsin® see Hyoscyamine Sulfate 445
Levsinex® see Hyoscyamine Sulfate 445
Levulose, Dextrose and Phosphoric Acid see Phosphorated Carbohydrate
  Solution 690
Librax® see Clidinium and Chlordiazepoxide 214
Libritabs® see Chlordiazepoxide 183
Librium® see Chlordiazepoxide 183
Lice-Enz® (Canada) see Pyrethrins 753
Lida-Mantle HC® Topical see Lidocaine and Hydrocortisone 501
Lidemol® (Canada) see Fluocinolone Acetonide 372
Lidex® see Fluocinonide 373
Lidex-E® see Fluocinonide 373
Lidocaine and Epinephrine 499
Lidocaine and Hydrocortisone 501
Lidocaine and Prilocaine 501
Lidocaine Hydrochloride 502
Lidocaine Transoral 502
Lidox® see Clidinium and Chlordiazepoxide 214
Limbitrol® see Amitriptyline and Chlordiazepoxide 49
Lincocin® see Lincomycin 503
Lincomicina (Mexico) see Lincomycin 503
Lincomycin 503
Linctus Codeine Blac (Canada) see Codeine 227
Linctus With Codeine Phosphate (Canada) see Codeine 227
Lindane 504
Lindano (Mexico) see Lindane 504
Lioresal® see Baclofen 95
Liothyronine Sodium 504
Liotrix 505
Lipancreatin see Pancrelipase 657
Lipidil® see Fenofibrate 356
Lipocin (Mexico) see Fat Emulsion 353
Liposyn® see Fat Emulsion 353
Lipovite® [OTC] see Vitamin B Complex 899
Liquaemin® Injection see Heparin 419
Liqui-Char® [OTC] see Charcoal 179
Liquid Pred® see Prednisone 719
Liqui-E® see Tocophersolan 852
Liquifilm® Forte Solution [OTC] see Artificial Tears 75
Liquifilm® Tears Solution [OTC] see Artificial Tears 75
Liroken® (Mexico) see Diclofenac 271
Lisinopril 506
Lisinopril and Hydrochlorothiazide 507
Listerine® Antiseptic [OTC] see Mouthwash, Antiseptic 592
Listermint® with Fluoride [OTC] see Fluoride 374
Lithane® see Lithium 508
LithelIm® 300 (Mexico) see Lithium 508

Lithium 508
Lithobid® *see* Lithium 508
Lithonate® *see* Lithium 508
Lithostat® *see* Acetohydroxamic Acid 20
Lithotabs® *see* Lithium 508
Lito Carbonato De (Mexico) *see* Lithium 508
Livostin® *see* Levocabastine Hydrochloride 494
Livostin® Nasal (Mexico) *see* Levocabastine Hydrochloride 494
Livostin® Oftalmico (Mexico) *see* Levocabastine Hydrochloride . . . 494
LKV-Drops® [OTC] *see* Vitamins, Multiple 901
L-Lysine Hydrochloride 509
LMD® *see* Dextran 263
Lobac® *see* Chlorzoxazone 200
Lodimol® (Mexico) *see* Dipyridamole 290
Lodine® *see* Etodolac 347
Lodine® Retard (Mexico) *see* Etodolac 347
Lodine® XL *see* Etodolac 347
Lodosyn® *see* Carbidopa 153
Lodoxamide Tromethamine 509
Loestrin® *see* Ethinyl Estradiol and Norethindrone 339
Lofene® *see* Diphenoxylate and Atropine 289
Logen® *see* Diphenoxylate and Atropine 289
Logoderm® (Mexico) *see* Alclometasone Dipropionate 28
Lomanate® *see* Diphenoxylate and Atropine 289
Lomefloxacin Hydrochloride 509
Lomefloxacino Clorhidato De (Mexico) *see* Lomefloxacin Hydrochloride
. . . . 509
Lomodix® *see* Diphenoxylate and Atropine 289
Lomotil® *see* Diphenoxylate and Atropine 289
Lomustine 510
Loniten® *see* Minoxidil 583
Lonox® *see* Diphenoxylate and Atropine 289
Lo/Ovral® *see* Ethinyl Estradiol and Norgestrel 341
Loperamide Hydrochloride 511
Lopid® *see* Gemfibrozil 395
Lopremone *see* Protirelin 747
Lopresor® (Mexico) *see* Metoprolol 574
Lopressor® [Tartrate] *see* Metoprolol 574
Loprox® *see* Ciclopirox Olamine 205
Lorabid™ *see* Loracarbef 512
Loracarbef 512
Loracepam (Mexico) *see* Lorazepam 513
Loratadina (Mexico) *see* Loratadine 512
Loratadine 512
Loratadine and Pseudoephedrine 513
Lorazepam 513
Lorcet® [5/500] *see* Hydrocodone and Acetaminophen 431
Lorcet®-HD [5/500] *see* Hydrocodone and Acetaminophen 431
Lorcet® Plus [7.5/650] *see* Hydrocodone and Acetaminophen . . . 431
Lorelco® *see* Probucol 725
Loroxide® [OTC] *see* Benzoyl Peroxide 104
Lortab® 2.5/500 *see* Hydrocodone and Acetaminophen 431
Lortab® 5/500 *see* Hydrocodone and Acetaminophen 431
Lortab® 7.5/500 *see* Hydrocodone and Acetaminophen 431
Lortab® 10/500 *see* Hydrocodone and Acetaminophen 431
Lortab® 10/650 *see* Hydrocodone and Acetaminophen 431
Lortab® ASA *see* Hydrocodone and Aspirin 433
Lortab® Elixir *see* Hydrocodone and Acetaminophen 431
Lortab® Solution *see* Hydrocodone and Acetaminophen 431
Losartan and Hydrochlorothiazide 515
Losartan Potassium 515
Losec® (Canada) *see* Omeprazole 636
Lotensin® *see* Benazepril Hydrochloride 99
Lotrel™ *see* Amlodipine and Benazepril 54
Lotrisone® *see* Betamethasone and Clotrimazole 111
Lovastatin 516
Lovastatina (Mexico) *see* Lovastatin 516
Lowadina® (Mexico) *see* Loratadine 512
Low-Quel® *see* Diphenoxylate and Atropine 289
Loxapac® (Canada) *see* Loxapine 517
Loxapine 517
Loxitane® *see* Loxapine 517
Lozide® (Canada) *see* Indapamide 455
Lozol® *see* Indapamide 455
L-PAM *see* Melphalan 536
L-Sarcolysin *see* Melphalan 536
Lubriderm® [OTC] *see* Lanolin, Cetyl Alcohol, Glycerin, and Petrolatum
. . . . 490

LubriTears® Solution [OTC] *see* Artificial Tears 75
Lucrin Depot (Mexico) *see* Leuprolide Acetate 492
Lucrin (Mexico) *see* Leuprolide Acetate 492
Ludiomil® *see* Maprotiline Hydrochloride 525
Lufyllin® *see* Dyphylline 305
Luminal® *see* Phenobarbital 680
Lupron® *see* Leuprolide Acetate 492
Lupron® Depot *see* Leuprolide Acetate 492
Lupron® Depot-Ped *see* Leuprolide Acetate 492
Luride® *see* Fluoride 374
Luride® Lozi-Tab® *see* Fluoride 374
Luride®-SF Lozi-Tab® *see* Fluoride 374
Luritran® (Mexico) *see* Erythromycin 321
Luvox® *see* Fluvoxamine 384
Lycolan® Elixir [OTC] *see* L-Lysine Hydrochloride 509
Lyderm® (Canada) *see* Fluocinonide 373
Lymphocyte Immune Globulin, Anti-thymocyte Globulin (Equine) 518
Lyphocin® *see* Vancomycin Hydrochloride 889
Lyposyn (Mexico) *see* Fat Emulsion 353
Lypressin 519
Lysatec-rt-PA® (Canada) *see* Alteplase 37
Lysodren® *see* Mitotane 585
Maalox® [OTC] *see* Aluminum Hydroxide and Magnesium Hydroxide 40
Maalox® Plus [OTC] *see* Aluminum Hydroxide, Magnesium Hydroxide, and
  Simethicone 41
Maalox® Therapeutic Concentrate [OTC] *see* Aluminum Hydroxide and
  Magnesium Hydroxide 40
Macrobid® *see* Nitrofurantoin 622
Macrodantin® *see* Nitrofurantoin 622
Macrodantina® (Mexico) *see* Nitrofurantoin 622
Macrodex® *see* Dextran 263
Madel® (Mexico) *see* Phenazopyridine Hydrochloride 679
Mafenide Acetate 520
Magaldrate 520
Magaldrate and Simethicone 521
Magalox Plus® [OTC] *see* Aluminum Hydroxide, Magnesium Hydroxide, and
  Simethicone 41
Magnesio, Hidroxido De (Mexico) *see* Magnesium Hydroxide 522
Magnesio, Oxide De (Mexico) *see* Magnesium Oxide 523
Magnesium Chloride 521
Magnesium Citrate 521
Magnesium Gluconate 522
Magnesium Hydroxide 522
Magnesium Hydroxide and Aluminum Hydroxide *see* Aluminum Hydroxide
  and Magnesium Hydroxide 40
Magnesium Hydroxide and Mineral Oil Emulsion 523
Magnesium Oxide 523
Magnesium Sulfate 524
Magonate® [OTC] *see* Magnesium Gluconate 522
Maigret-50 *see* Phenylpropanolamine Hydrochloride 687
Malatal® *see* Hyoscyamine, Atropine, Scopolamine, and Phenobarbital
 444
Malival® y Malival® AP (Mexico) *see* Indomethacin 457
Mallergan-VC® With Codeine *see* Promethazine, Phenylephrine, and Codeine
 734
Malotuss® [OTC] *see* Guaifenesin 407
Malt Soup Extract 525
Maltsupex® [OTC] *see* Malt Soup Extract 525
Mandelamine® *see* Methenamine 555
Mandol® *see* Cefamandole Nafate 163
Manganese *see* Trace Metals 857
Manoplax® *see* Flosequinan 366
Mantoux *see* Tuberculin Purified Protein Derivative 882
Maolate® *see* Chlorphenesin Carbamate 190
Maox® *see* Magnesium Oxide 523
Mapluxin® (Mexico) *see* Digoxin 280
Maprotilina, Clorhidrato De (Mexico) *see* Maprotiline Hydrochloride 525
Maprotiline Hydrochloride 525
Marax® *see* Theophylline, Ephedrine, and Hydroxyzine 836
Marazide® *see* Benzthiazide 105
Marbaxin® *see* Methocarbamol 557
Marcaine® *see* Bupivacaine Hydrochloride 127
Marcaine® with Epinephrine *see* Bupivacaine With Epinephrine 128
Marezine® [OTC] *see* Cyclizine 238
Margesic® H [5/500] *see* Hydrocodone and Acetaminophen 431
Marinol® *see* Dronabinol 302
Marmine® [OTC] *see* Dimenhydrinate 286
Marnal® *see* Butalbital Compound 133

Marovilina® (Mexico) *see* Ampicillin 62
Marplan® *see* Isocarboxazid 469
Marpres® *see* Hydralazine, Hydrochlorothiazide, and Reserpine 429
Masoprocol 526
Massé® Breast Cream [OTC] *see* Glycerin, Lanolin, and Peanut Oil 402
Matulane® *see* Procarbazine Hydrochloride 727
Mavik® *see* Trandolapril 858
Maxair™ *see* Pirbuterol Acetate 698
Maxaquin® *see* Lomefloxacin Hydrochloride 509
Max-Caro® [OTC] *see* Beta-Carotene 109
Maxeran® (Canada) *see* Metoclopramide 572
Maxiflor® *see* Diflorasone Diacetate 278
Maximum Strength Anbesol® [OTC] *see* Benzocaine 102
Maximum Strength Orajel® [OTC] *see* Benzocaine 102
Maxipime® *see* Cefepime 164
Maxitrol® *see* Neomycin, Polymyxin B, and Dexamethasone 610
Maxivate® *see* Betamethasone 109
Maxolon® *see* Metoclopramide 572
Maxzide® *see* Triamterene and Hydrochlorothiazide 865
Mazanor® *see* Mazindol 527
Mazepine® (Canada) *see* Carbamazepine 151
Mazindol 527
m-Cresyl Acetate 527
MCT Oil® [OTC] *see* Medium Chain Triglycerides 532
Measles and Rubella Vaccines, Combined 527
Measles, Mumps, and Rubella Vaccines, Combined 528
Measles Virus Vaccine, Live 529
Measurin® [OTC] *see* Aspirin 78
Mebaral® *see* Mephobarbital 540
Mebendazole 529
Mebensole® (Mexico) *see* Mebendazole 529
Mecamylamine Hydrochloride 530
Meclan® *see* Meclocycline Sulfosalicylate 531
Meclizine Hydrochloride 530
Meclocycline Sulfosalicylate 531
Meclofenamate Sodium 531
Meclomen® *see* Meclofenamate Sodium 531
Meclomid® (Mexico) *see* Metoclopramide 572
Meclozina, Clorhidrato De (Mexico) *see* Meclizine Hydrochloride 530
Medasarvin (Mexico) *see* Leucovorin Calcium 491
Medigesic® *see* Butalbital Compound 133
Medihaler-Iso® *see* Isoproterenol 472
Medilax® [OTC] *see* Phenolphthalein 682
Medilium® (Canada) *see* Chlordiazepoxide 183
Medimet® (Canada) *see* Methyldopa 566
Medipren® [OTC] *see* Ibuprofen 447
Medi-Quick® *see* Bacitracin, Neomycin, and Polymyxin B 94
Meditran® (Canada) *see* Meprobamate 543
Medium Chain Triglycerides 532
Medralone® *see* Methylprednisolone 569
Medrol® *see* Methylprednisolone 569
Medroxyprogesterone Acetate 533
Medrysone 533
Medsaplatin (Mexico) *see* Cisplatin 210
Medsaposide® (Mexico) *see* Etoposide 348
Mefenamic Acid 534
Mefenamico, Acido (Mexico) *see* Mefenamic Acid 534
Mefloquine Hydrochloride 535
Mefoxin® *see* Cefoxitin Sodium 168
Mega-B® [OTC] *see* Vitamin B Complex 899
Megace® *see* Megestrol Acetate 535
Megacillin® Susp (Canada) *see* Penicillin G Benzathine, Parenteral 665
Megaton™ [OTC] *see* Vitamin B Complex 899
Megestrol Acetate 535
Melanex® *see* Hydroquinone 439
Mellaril® *see* Thioridazine 840
Mellaril-S® *see* Thioridazine 840
Melphalan 536
Menadol® [OTC] *see* Ibuprofen 447
Menest® *see* Estrogens, Esterified 328
Meni-D® *see* Meclizine Hydrochloride 530
Meningococcal Polysaccharide Vaccine, Groups A, C, Y, and W-135 537
Menomune®-A/C/Y/W-135 *see* Meningococcal Polysaccharide Vaccine,
    Groups A, C, Y, and W-135 537
Menotropins 538
Mentax® *see* Butenafine Hydrochloride 135
Mepenzolate Bromide 538
Mepergan® *see* Meperidine and Promethazine 538

Meperidine and Promethazine 538
Meperidine Hydrochloride 539
Mephenytoin 540
Mephobarbital 540
Mephyton® *see* Phytonadione 690
Mepivacaine Dental Anesthetic 541
Mepivacaine With Levonordefrin 542
Meprobamate 543
Meprobamate and Aspirin *see* Aspirin and Meprobamate 81
Mepron™ *see* Atovaquone 84
Meprospan® *see* Meprobamate 543
Merbromin 544
Mercaptopurine 544
6-Mercaptopurine *see* Mercaptopurine 544
Mercuric Oxide 545
Mercurochrome® *see* Merbromin 544
Merlenate® Topical [OTC] *see* Undecylenic Acid and Derivatives 884
Meronem® *see* Meropenem 545
Meropenem 545
Merrem® I.V. *see* Meropenem 545
Mersol® [OTC] *see* Thimerosal 838
Merthiolate® [OTC] *see* Thimerosal 838
Meruvax® II *see* Rubella Virus Vaccine, Live 776
Mesalamine 546
Mesantoin® *see* Mephenytoin 540
Mesoridazine Besylate 547
Mestatin® (Canada) *see* Nystatin 632
Mestranol and Norethindrone 547
Mestranol and Norethynodrel 549
Metahydrin® *see* Trichlormethiazide 867
Metamucil® [OTC] *see* Psyllium 750
Metamucil® Instant Mix [OTC] *see* Psyllium 750
Metandren® *see* Methyltestosterone 570
Metaprel® *see* Metaproterenol Sulfate 550
Metaproterenol Sulfate 550
Metasep® [OTC] *see* Parachlorometaxylenol 659
Metaxalone 551
Metforma (Mexico) *see* Metformin Hydrochloride 551
Metformin Hydrochloride 551
Methadone Hydrochloride 552
Methadose® (Canada) *see* Methadone Hydrochloride 552
Methamphetamine Hydrochloride 553
Methantheline Bromide 554
Methanthelinium Bromide *see* Methantheline Bromide 554
Methazolamide 554
Methenamine 555
Methergine® *see* Methylergonovine Maleate 567
Methicillin Sodium 556
Methimazole 556
Methionine 557
Methocarbamol 557
Methocarbamol and Aspirin 558
Methohexital Sodium 559
Methotrexate 559
Methotrimeprazine Hydrochloride 562
Methoxsalen 563
Methoxycinnamate and Oxybenzone 564
Methoxypsoralen *see* Methoxsalen 563
8-Methoxypsoralen *see* Methoxsalen 563
Methscopolamine Bromide 564
Methsuximide 564
Methyclothiazide 565
Methyclothiazide and Cryptenamine Tannates 566
Methyclothiazide and Deserpidine 566
Methyclothiazide and Pargyline 566
Methylbenzethonium Chloride 566
Methylcellulose 566
Methyldopa 566
Methyldopa and Chlorothiazide *see* Chlorothiazide and Methyldopa 188
Methyldopa and Hydrochlorothiazide 567
Methylergonovine Maleate 567
Methylmorphine (Canada) *see* Codeine 227
Methylone® *see* Methylprednisolone 569
Methylphenidate Hydrochloride 568
Methylprednisolone 569
Methyltestosterone 570
Methysergide Maleate 571
Meticorten® *see* Prednisone 719

Metifenidato, Clorhidrato De (Mexico) see Methylphenidate Hydrochloride
....568
Metildopa (Mexico) see Methyldopa 566
Metilergometrina, Maleato De (Mexico) see Methylergonovine Maleate
....567
Metimyd® see Sodium Sulfacetamide and Prednisolone Acetate 794
Metipranolol Hydrochloride 572
Metoclopramida (Mexico) see Metoclopramide 572
Metoclopramide 572
Metolazone 573
Metoprolol 574
Metotrexato (Mexico) see Methotrexate 559
Metoxiprim® (Mexico) see Trimethoprim and Sulfamethoxazole 874
Metreton® see Prednisolone 718
Metrodin® see Urofollitropin 885
MetroGel® see Metronidazole 576
Metro I.V.® see Metronidazole 576
Metronidazole 576
Mevacor® see Lovastatin 516
Meval® (Canada) see Diazepam 268
Mexiletina (Mexico) see Mexiletine 577
Mexiletine 577
Mexitil® see Mexiletine 577
Mezlin® see Mezlocillin Sodium 578
Mezlocillin Sodium 578
Miacalcin® see Calcitonin 138
Micatin® [OTC] see Miconazole 578
Miconazole 578
Micostatin® (Mexico) see Nystatin 632
Micostyl® (Mexico) see Econazole Nitrate 306
MICRhoGAM™ see Rh₀(D) Immune Globulin 767
Microfibrillar Collagen Hemostat 579
Microgynon® (Mexico) see Ethinyl Estradiol and Levonorgestrel 337
Micro-K® see Potassium Chloride 708
Microlut® (Mexico) see Levonorgestrel 497
Micronase® see Glyburide 401
microNefrin® see Epinephrine, Racemic 314
Micronor® see Norethindrone 627
Microrgan® (Mexico) see Ciprofloxacin Hydrochloride 208
Microsulfon® see Sulfadiazine 807
Microtid® (Mexico) see Ranitidine Hydrochloride 763
Midamor® see Amiloride Hydrochloride 45
Midazolam Hydrochloride 580
Midol® 200 [OTC] see Ibuprofen 447
Midol® PM [OTC] see Acetaminophen and Diphenhydramine 16
Midotens® (Mexico) see Labetalol Hydrochloride 486
Midrin® see Acetaminophen and Isometheptene Mucate 16
Miflex® see Chlorzoxazone 200
Milezzol® (Mexico) see Metronidazole 576
Milontin® see Phensuximide 683
Milrinone Lactate 581
Miltown® see Meprobamate 543
Mini-Gamulin® Rh see Rh₀(D) Immune Globulin 767
Minims® Pilocarpine (Canada) see Pilocarpine 691
Minipress® see Prazosin Hydrochloride 717
Minitran® see Nitroglycerin 623
Minizide® see Prazosin and Polythiazide 717
Minociclina (Mexico) see Minocycline Hydrochloride 582
Minocin® see Minocycline Hydrochloride 582
Minocin® IV see Minocycline Hydrochloride 582
Minocycline Hydrochloride 582
Minodiab® (Mexico) see Glipizide 399
Minodyl® see Minoxidil 583
Minofen® (Mexico) see Acetaminophen 14
Minoxidil 583
Mintezol® see Thiabendazole 836
Minute-Gel® see Fluoride 374
Miochol® see Acetylcholine Chloride 21
Miostat® see Carbachol 150
Miradon® (Canada) see Anisotropine Methylbromide 67
Mirtazapine 583
Misoprostol 584
Misostol (Mexico) see Mitoxantrone Hydrochloride 586
Mithracin® see Plicamycin 700
Mitomycin 584
Mitomycin-C see Mitomycin 584
Mitotane 585
Mitoxantrone Hydrochloride 586

Mitran® see Chlordiazepoxide 183
Mitroken® (Mexico) see Ciprofloxacin Hydrochloride 208
Mitrolan® Chewable Tablet [OTC] see Calcium Polycarbophil 146
MK594 see Losartan Potassium 515
M-KYA® [OTC] see Quinine Sulfate 760
MMR see Measles, Mumps, and Rubella Vaccines, Combined 528
M-M-R® II see Measles, Mumps, and Rubella Vaccines, Combined 528
Moban® see Molindone Hydrochloride 588
Mobenol® (Canada) see Tolbutamide 853
Modane® [OTC] see Phenolphthalein 682
Modane® Bulk [OTC] see Psyllium 750
Modane® Plus [OTC] see Docusate and Phenolphthalein 295
Modane® Soft [OTC] see Docusate 295
Modecate® [Fluphenazine Decanoate] (Canada) see Fluphenazine 379
Modecate® Enanthate [Fluphenazine Enanthate] (Canada) see Fluphenazine
. 379
Modicon™ see Ethinyl Estradiol and Norethindrone 339
Moditen® Hydrochloride (Canada) see Fluphenazine 379
Moducal® [OTC] see Glucose Polymers 400
Moduretic® see Amiloride and Hydrochlorothiazide 45
Moexipril Hydrochloride 587
Moi-Stir® [OTC] see Saliva Substitute 778
Moisture® Ophthalmic Drops [OTC] see Artificial Tears .75
Molindone Hydrochloride 588
Mol-Iron® [OTC] see Ferrous Sulfate 360
Molybdenum see Trace Metals 857
Molypen® see Trace Metals 857
Mometasona, Furoata De (Mexico) see Mometasone Furoate 589
Mometasone Furoate 589
MOM/Mineral Oil Emulsion see Magnesium Hydroxide and Mineral Oil
    Emulsion 523
Monistat™ see Miconazole 578
Monistat-Derm™ see Miconazole 578
Monistat i.v.™ see Miconazole 578
Monitan® (Canada) see Acebutolol Hydrochloride 12
Monobenzone 589
Monocid® see Cefonicid Sodium 166
Monocidur® (Mexico) see Cefonicid Sodium 166
Monoclate-P® see Antihemophilic Factor (Human) 68
Monoclonal Antibody see Muromonab-CD3 594
Monoethanolamine (Canada) see Ethanolamine Oleate 333
Mono-Gesic® see Salsalate 779
Monoket® see Isosorbide Mononitrate 474
Mono-Mack® (Mexico) see Isosorbide Mononitrate 474
Mononine® see Factor IX Complex (Human) 350
Monopril® see Fosinopril 387
8-MOP see Methoxsalen 563
More Attenuated Enders Strain see Measles Virus Vaccine, Live 529
More-Dophilus® [OTC] see Lactobacillus acidophilus and Lactobacillus
    bulgaricus 488
Morfina (Mexico) see Morphine Sulfate 590
Moricizine Hydrochloride 589
Morphine-HP® (Canada) see Morphine Sulfate 590
Morphine Sulfate 590
Morrhuate Sodium 592
Motofen® see Difenoxin and Atropine 277
Motrin® see Ibuprofen 447
Motrin® IB [OTC] see Ibuprofen 447
Motrin® IB Sinus [OTC] see Pseudoephedrine and Ibuprofen 750
MouthKote® [OTC] see Saliva Substitute 778
Mouth Pain, Cold Sore, Canker Sore Products 1063
Mouthwash, Antiseptic 592
6-MP see Mercaptopurine 544
M-R-VAX® II see Measles and Rubella Vaccines, Combined 527
MS Contin® Oral see Morphine Sulfate 590
MS-IR® (Canada) see Morphine Sulfate 590
MSIR® Oral see Morphine Sulfate 590
MS/L® see Morphine Sulfate 590
MS/S® see Morphine Sulfate 590
MST-Continus® (Mexico) see Morphine Sulfate 590
MTC see Mitomycin 584
M.T.E.-4® see Trace Metals 857
M.T.E.-5® see Trace Metals 857
M.T.E.-6® see Trace Metals 857
Mucomyst® see Acetylcysteine 21
Mucoplex® [OTC] see Vitamin B Complex 899
Mucosil™ see Acetylcysteine 21
Multe-Pak-4® see Trace Metals 857

Multipax® (Canada) see Hydroxyzine 443
Multiple Sulfonamides see Sulfadiazine, Sulfamethazine, and Sulfamerazine
.... 808
Multitest CMI® see Skin Test Antigens, Multiple 790
Multi Vit® Drops [OTC] see Vitamins, Multiple....................... 901
Mumps, Measles and Rubella Vaccines, Combined see Measles, Mumps,
    and Rubella Vaccines, Combined 528
Mumpsvax® see Mumps Virus Vaccine, Live, Attenuated 593
Mumps Virus Vaccine, Live, Attenuated 593
Munobal® (Mexico) see Felodipine 354
Mupiban® (Mexico) see Mupirocin 593
Mupirocin 593
Murine® Ear Drops [OTC] see Carbamide Peroxide 152
Murine® Plus [OTC] see Tetrahydrozoline Hydrochloride 831
Murine® Solution [OTC] see Artificial Tears 75
Murocel® Ophthalmic Solution [OTC] see Artificial Tears 75
Murocoll-2® Ophthalmic see Phenylephrine and Scopolamine 685
Muromonab-CD3 594
Muro's Opcon® see Naphazoline Hydrochloride 605
Mus-Lac® see Chlorzoxazone 200
Mutamycin® see Mitomycin 584
M.V.I.® see Vitamins, Multiple 901
M.V.I.®-12 see Vitamins, Multiple 901
M.V.I.® Concentrate see Vitamins, Multiple 901
M.V.I.® Pediatric see Vitamins, Multiple........................... 901
Myambutol® see Ethambutol Hydrochloride.......................... 332
Mycelex® Troche see Clotrimazole 223
Mycifradin® Sulfate see Neomycin Sulfate 611
Mycobutin® see Rifabutin 769
Mycogen® II see Nystatin and Triamcinolone 632
Mycolog®-II see Nystatin and Triamcinolone 632
Myconel® see Nystatin and Triamcinolone 632
Mycophenolate Mofetil 595
Mycostatin® see Nystatin 632
Myco-Triacet® II see Nystatin and Triamcinolone 632
Mydfrin® Ophthalmic Solution see Phenylephrine Hydrochloride....... 685
Mydriacyl® Ophthalmic see Tropicamide 881
Myfungar® (Mexico) see Oxiconazole Nitrate 644
Mykrox® see Metolazone 573
Mylanta® [OTC] see Aluminum Hydroxide, Magnesium Hydroxide, and
    Simethicone 41
Mylanta® Gas [OTC] see Simethicone............................... 788
Mylanta®-II [OTC] see Aluminum Hydroxide, Magnesium Hydroxide, and
    Simethicone 41
Myleran® see Busulfan 131
Mylicon® [OTC] see Simethicone.................................... 788
Mylosar® see Azacitidine 88
Myminic® Expectorant [OTC] see Guaifenesin and Phenylpropanolamine
.... 409
Myochrysine® see Gold Sodium Thiomalate 404
Myoflex® [OTC] see Triethanolamine Salicylate 868
Myotonachol™ see Bethanechol Chloride............................ 112
Myphetane DC® see Brompheniramine, Phenylpropanolamine, and Codeine
.... 125
Myphetapp® [OTC] see Brompheniramine and Phenylpropanolamine 123
Mysoline® see Primidone 723
Mytelase® Caplets® see Ambenonium Chloride 43
Mytrex® see Nystatin and Triamcinolone............................ 632
Mytussin® [OTC] see Guaifenesin 407
Mytussin® AC see Guaifenesin and Codeine 408
Mytussin® DAC see Guaifenesin, Pseudoephedrine, and Codeine 410
Mytussin® DM [OTC] see Guaifenesin and Dextromethorphan 408
Nabilone.. 596
Nabumetone 596
Nadolol 597
Nadopen-V® (Canada) see Penicillin V Potassium 668
Nadostine® (Canada) see Nystatin 632
Nafarelin Acetate 598
Nafazair® see Naphazoline Hydrochloride 605
Nafazolina, Clorhidrato De (Mexico) see Naphazoline Hydrochloride .. 605
Nafcil™ see Nafcillin Sodium 599
Nafcillin Sodium 599
Naftifine Hydrochloride 600
Naftin® see Naftifine Hydrochloride 600
Nalbufina, Clorhidrato De (Mexico) see Nalbuphine Hydrochloride 600
Nalbuphine Hydrochloride 600
Naldecon® see Chlorpheniramine, Phenyltoloxamine, Phenylpropanolamine,
    and Phenylephrine 194

Naldecon® DX Adult Liquid [OTC] *see* Guaifenesin, Phenylpropanolamine, and Dextromethorphan 410
Naldecon-EX® Children's Syrup [OTC] *see* Guaifenesin and Phenylpropanolamine 409
Naldecon® Senior DX [OTC] *see* Guaifenesin and Dextromethorphan 408
Naldecon® Senior EX [OTC] *see* Guaifenesin 407
Naldelate® *see* Chlorpheniramine, Phenyltoloxamine, Phenylpropanolamine, and Phenylephrine 194
Nalfon® *see* Fenoprofen Calcium 356
Nalgest® *see* Chlorpheniramine, Phenyltoloxamine, Phenylpropanolamine, and Phenylephrine 194
Nalidixic Acid 601
Nalidixio Acido (Mexico) *see* Nalidixic Acid 601
Nallpen® *see* Nafcillin Sodium 599
Nalmefene Hydrochloride 601
Naloxone Hydrochloride 602
Nalspan® *see* Chlorpheniramine, Phenyltoloxamine, Phenylpropanolamine, and Phenylephrine 194
Naltrexone Hydrochloride 603
Nandrolone 604
Naphazoline and Antazoline 604
Naphazoline and Pheniramine 605
Naphazoline Hydrochloride 605
Naphcon® [OTC] *see* Naphazoline Hydrochloride 605
Naphcon-A® Ophthalmic [OTC] *see* Naphazoline and Pheniramine 605
Naphcon Forte® *see* Naphazoline Hydrochloride 605
Naprodil® (Mexico) *see* Naproxen 606
Naprosyn® (Naproxen Base) *see* Naproxen 606
Naproxen 606
Naqua® *see* Trichlormethiazide 867
Narcan® *see* Naloxone Hydrochloride 602
Narcotic Agonist Charts 1019
Nardil® *see* Phenelzine Sulfate 679
Naropin® *see* Ropivacaine Hydrochloride 775
Nasabid™ *see* Guaifenesin and Pseudoephedrine 409
Nasacort® *see* Triamcinolone 862
Nasahist B® *see* Brompheniramine Maleate 124
Nasalcrom® *see* Cromolyn Sodium 235
Nasalide® *see* Flunisolide 372
Natabec® [OTC] *see* Vitamins, Multiple 901
Natabec® FA [OTC] *see* Vitamins, Multiple 901
Natabec® Rx *see* Vitamins, Multiple 901
Natacyn® *see* Natamycin 607
Natalins® [OTC] *see* Vitamins, Multiple 901
Natalins® Rx *see* Vitamins, Multiple 901
Natamycin 607
Natulan® (Mexico) *see* Procarbazine Hydrochloride 727
Nature's Tears® Solution [OTC] *see* Artificial Tears 75
Naturetin® *see* Bendroflumethiazide 101
Naus-A-Way® [OTC] *see* Phosphorated Carbohydrate Solution 690
Nausetrol® [OTC] *see* Phosphorated Carbohydrate Solution 690
Navane® *see* Thiothixene 842
Navelbine® *see* Vinorelbine Tartrate 897
Naxen® (Canada) *see* Naproxen 606
Naxen® (Mexico) *see* Naproxen 606
Naxil® (Mexico) *see* Naproxen 606
Naxodol® (Carisoprodol with Naproxen) (Mexico) *see* Carisoprodol 157
Nazil® Ofteno (Mexico) *see* Naphazoline Hydrochloride 605
N-B-P® Ointment *see* Bacitracin, Neomycin, and Polymyxin B 94
ND-Stat® *see* Brompheniramine Maleate 124
Nebcin® *see* Tobramycin 849
NebuPent™ *see* Pentamidine Isethionate 670
Nedocromil Sodium 607
N.E.E.® 1/35 *see* Ethinyl Estradiol and Norethindrone 339
Nefazodone 608
NegGram® *see* Nalidixic Acid 601
Nelova™ 0.5/35E *see* Ethinyl Estradiol and Norethindrone 339
Nelova™ 1/50M *see* Mestranol and Norethindrone 547
Nelova™ 10/11 *see* Ethinyl Estradiol and Norethindrone 339
Nembutal® *see* Pentobarbital 672
Neo-Calglucon® [OTC] *see* Calcium Glubionate 142
Neo-Codema® (Canada) *see* Hydrochlorothiazide 430
Neo-Cortef® Ophthalmic *see* Neomycin and Hydrocortisone 609
Neo-Cortef® Topical *see* Neomycin and Hydrocortisone 609
NeoDecadron® Ophthalmic *see* Neomycin and Dexamethasone 609
NeoDecadron® Topical *see* Neomycin and Dexamethasone 609
Neo-Dexameth® Ophthalmic *see* Neomycin and Dexamethasone 609
Neodol® (Mexico) *see* Acetaminophen 14

Neo-Durabolic see Nandrolone 604
Neo-Estrone® (Canada) see Estrogens, Esterified 328
Neo-Estrone® (Canada) see Estrone...329
Neofed® [OTC] see Pseudoephedrine..749
Neo-fradin® see Neomycin Sulfate...611
Neoloid® [OTC] see Castor Oil 161
Neomicol® (Mexico) see Miconazole...578
Neomixin® see Bacitracin, Neomycin, and Polymyxin B 94
Neomycin and Dexamethasone...609
Neomycin and Hydrocortisone..609
Neomycin and Polymyxin B...609
Neomycin, Polymyxin B, and Dexamethasone................................610
Neomycin, Polymyxin B, and Gramicidin......................................610
Neomycin, Polymyxin B, and Hydrocortisone.................................610
Neomycin, Polymyxin B, and Prednisolone....................................611
Neomycin Sulfate...611
Neonatal Trace Metals see Trace Metals.....................................857
Neopap® [OTC] see Acetaminophen...14
Neoquess® see Dicyclomine Hydrochloride....................................273
Neosar® see Cyclophosphamide..240
Neosporin® see Bacitracin, Neomycin, and Polymyxin B 94
Neosporin® Cream [OTC] see Neomycin and Polymyxin B 609
Neosporin® G.U. Irrigant see Neomycin and Polymyxin B 609
Neosporin® Oftalmico (Mexico) see Neomycin, Polymyxin B, and Gramicidin
....610
Neosporin® Ophthalmic Solution see Neomycin, Polymyxin B, and Gramicidin
....610
Neostrata® HQ (Canada) see Hydroquinone...................................439
Neo-Synephrine® 12 Hour Nasal Solution [OTC] see Oxymetazoline
   Hydrochloride...649
Neo-Synephrine® Nasal Solution [OTC] see Phenylephrine Hydrochloride
....685
Neo-Synephrine® Ophthalmic Solution see Phenylephrine Hydrochloride
....685
Neo-Tabs® see Neomycin Sulfate...611
Neothylline® see Dyphylline...305
Neotopic® (Canada) see Bacitracin, Neomycin, and Polymyxin B 94
Neotrace-4® see Trace Metals..857
Neotricin HC® Ophthalmic Ointment see Bacitracin, Neomycin, Polymyxin B,
   and Hydrocortisone...95
NeoVadrin® [OTC] see Vitamins, Multiple....................................901
NeoVadrin® B Complex [OTC] see Vitamin B Complex 899
Nephrocaps® [OTC] see Vitamin B Complex With Vitamin C and Folic Acid
....900
Nephro-Fer™ [OTC] see Ferrous Fumarate....................................359
Nephron® see Epinephrine, Racemic 314
Nephronex® (Canada) see Nitrofurantoin......................................622
Nephrox Suspension [OTC] see Aluminum Hydroxide.........................39
Neptazane® see Methazolamide..554
Nervocaine® see Lidocaine Hydrochloride.....................................502
Nesacaine® see Chloroprocaine Hydrochloride................................185
Nesacaine®-MPF see Chloroprocaine Hydrochloride 185
Nestrex® see Pyridoxine Hydrochloride.......................................753
Netilmicina Sulfato De (Mexico) see Netilmicin Sulfate......................613
Netilmicin Sulfate...613
Netromicina® (Mexico) see Netilmicin Sulfate................................613
Netromycin® see Netilmicin Sulfate...613
Neucalm® see Hydroxyzine..443
Neugal® (Mexico) see Ranitidine Hydrochloride 763
Neugeron® (Mexico) see Carbamazepine 151
Neupogen® Injection see Filgrastim...362
Neuramate® see Meprobamate..543
Neurontin® see Gabapentin..392
Neurosine® (Mexico) see Buspirone Hydrochloride..........................131
Neutra-Phos® see Potassium Phosphate and Sodium Phosphate.............713
Neutra-Phos®-K see Potassium Phosphate..................................711
Neutrexin™ see Trimetrexate Glucuronate...................................875
Neutrogena® [OTC] see Benzoyl Peroxide...................................104
Neutrogena® T/Derm see Coal Tar..225
Nevirapine 614
New Decongestant® see Chlorpheniramine, Phenyltoloxamine,
   Phenylpropanolamine, and Phenylephrine..................................194
N.G.T.® see Nystatin and Triamcinolone......................................632
Niac® [OTC] see Niacin..614
Niacels™ [OTC] see Niacin..614
Niacin...614
Niacinamide...615
Nicardipina (Mexico) see Nicardipine Hydrochloride.........................616

Nicardipine Hydrochloride 616
Niclocide® *see* Niclosamide 617
Niclosamide 617
Nicobid® [OTC] *see* Niacin 614
Nicoderm® *see* Nicotine 617
Nicolan® (Mexico) *see* Nicotine 617
Nicolar® [OTC] *see* Niacin 614
Nicorette® *see* Nicotine 617
Nicorette® Plus (Canada) *see* Nicotine 617
Nicotine 617
Nicotinell®-TTS (Mexico) *see* Nicotine 617
Nicotinex [OTC] *see* Niacin 614
Nicotrol® *see* Nicotine 617
Nidryl® [OTC] *see* Diphenhydramine Hydrochloride 288
Nifedipine 619
Nifedipino (Mexico) *see* Nifedipine 619
Nifedipres® (Mexico) *see* Nifedipine 619
Niferex® [OTC] *see* Polysaccharide-Iron Complex 705
Niferex®-PN *see* Vitamins, Multiple 901
Nilandron® *see* Nilutamide 621
Niloric® *see* Ergoloid Mesylates 318
Nilstat® *see* Nystatin 632
Nilutamide 621
NIM *see* Bleomycin Sulfate 117
Nimodipina (Mexico) *see* Nimodipine 621
Nimodipine 621
Nimotop® *see* Nimodipine 621
Nipent™ Injection *see* Pentostatin 674
Nipride® *see* Nitroprusside Sodium 625
Nisoldipine 622
Nistaquim® (Mexico) *see* Nystatin 632
Nitradisc® (Mexico) *see* Nitroglycerin 623
Nitro-Bid® *see* Nitroglycerin 623
Nitrocine® *see* Nitroglycerin 623
Nitroderm-TTS® (Mexico) *see* Nitroglycerin 623
Nitrodisc® *see* Nitroglycerin 623
Nitro-Dur® *see* Nitroglycerin 623
Nitrofurantoin 622
Nitrofurantoina (Mexico) *see* Nitrofurantoin 622
Nitrofurazona (Mexico) *see* Nitrofurazone 623
Nitrofurazone 623
Nitrogard® *see* Nitroglycerin 623
Nitroglicerina (Mexico) *see* Nitroglycerin 623
Nitroglycerin 623
Nitroglyn® *see* Nitroglycerin 623
Nitrol® *see* Nitroglycerin 623
Nitrolingual® *see* Nitroglycerin 623
Nitrong® *see* Nitroglycerin 623
Nitropress® *see* Nitroprusside Sodium 625
Nitroprusside Sodium 625
Nitrostat® *see* Nitroglycerin 623
Nitrous Oxide 625
Nivoflox® (Mexico) *see* Ciprofloxacin Hydrochloride 208
Nix™ [OTC] *see* Permethrin 676
Niyaplat (Mexico) *see* Cisplatin 210
Nizatidina (Mexico) *see* Nizatidine 626
Nizatidine 626
Nizoral® *see* Ketoconazole 481
N-Methylhydrazine *see* Procarbazine Hydrochloride 727
Nobesine® (Canada) *see* Diethylpropion Hydrochloride 276
Noctec® *see* Chloral Hydrate 180
Nolahist® [OTC] *see* Phenindamine Tartrate 680
Nolamine® *see* Chlorpheniramine, Phenindamine, and Phenylpropanolamine
. . . . 192
Nolex® LA *see* Guaifenesin and Phenylpropanolamine 409
Nolvadex® *see* Tamoxifen Citrate 818
Nonoxynol 9 627
Nonsteroidal Anti-Inflammatory Agents, Comparative Dosages, and
  Pharmacokinetics 1021
Nonviral Infectious Diseases 932
Norboral® (Mexico) *see* Glyburide 401
Norcet® [5/500] *see* Hydrocodone and Acetaminophen 431
Nordet® (Mexico) *see* Ethinyl Estradiol and Levonorgestrel 337
Nordette® *see* Ethinyl Estradiol and Levonorgestrel 337
Nordiol® (Mexico) *see* Ethinyl Estradiol and Levonorgestrel 337
Nordryl® *see* Diphenhydramine Hydrochloride 288
Norethin™ 1/35E *see* Ethinyl Estradiol and Norethindrone 339
Norethin™ 1/50M *see* Mestranol and Norethindrone 547

Norethindrone 627
Noretindrona (Mexico) *see* Norethindrone 627
Norfenon® (Mexico) *see* Propafenone Hydrochloride 735
Norflex™ *see* Orphenadrine Citrate 640
Norfloxacin 628
Norfloxacina (Mexico) *see* Norfloxacin 628
Norgesic® *see* Orphenadrine, Aspirin, and Caffeine 640
Norgesic® Forte *see* Orphenadrine, Aspirin, and Caffeine 640
Norgestimate and Ethinyl Estradiol *see* Ethinyl Estradiol and Norgestimate
....340
Norgestrel 629
Norinyl® 1+35 *see* Ethinyl Estradiol and Norethindrone 339
Norinyl® 1+50 *see* Mestranol and Norethindrone 547
Norisodrine® *see* Isoproterenol 472
Norlutate® *see* Norethindrone 627
Norlutin® *see* Norethindrone 627
Normodyne® *see* Labetalol Hydrochloride 486
Noroxin® *see* Norfloxacin 628
Norpace® *see* Disopyramide Phosphate 292
Norpanth® *see* Propantheline Bromide 736
Norplant® *see* Levonorgestrel 497
Norpramin® *see* Desipramine Hydrochloride 257
Nor-Q.D.® *see* Norethindrone 627
Nortriptilina Clorhidrato De (Mexico) *see* Nortriptyline Hydrochloride ...629
Nortriptyline Hydrochloride 629
Norvasc® *see* Amlodipine 53
Norvas® (Mexico) *see* Amlodipine 53
Norvir® *see* Ritonavir 773
Nositrol® [Sodium Succinate] (Mexico) *see* Hydrocortisone 436
Nöstrilla® *see* Oxymetazoline Hydrochloride 649
Nöstrilla® Long Acting Nasal Solution [OTC] *see* Oxymetazoline
  Hydrochloride 649
Nostril® Nasal Solution [OTC] *see* Phenylephrine Hydrochloride ..685
Novacef® (Mexico) *see* Cefixime 165
Novacet® Topical *see* Sulfur and Sodium Sulfacetamide 813
Novafed® *see* Pseudoephedrine 749
Novahistine® DH *see* Chlorpheniramine, Pseudoephedrine, and Codeine
....195
Novahistine® Elixir [OTC] *see* Chlorpheniramine and Phenylephrine ...190
Novahistine® Expectorant *see* Guaifenesin, Pseudoephedrine, and Codeine
....410
Novamoxin® (Canada) *see* Amoxicillin Trihydrate 58
Novantrone® *see* Mitoxantrone Hydrochloride 586
Novantrone® (Mexico) *see* Mitoxantrone Hydrochloride 586
Novasen® (Canada) *see* Aspirin 78
Noviken-N® (Mexico) *see* Nifedipine 619
Novo-Aloprazol® (Canada) *see* Alprazolam 35
Novo-Atenol® (Canada) *see* Atenolol 83
Novo-AZT® (Canada) *see* Zidovudine 907
Novo-Butamide® (Canada) *see* Tolbutamide 853
Novocain® *see* Procaine Hydrochloride 727
Novo-Captopril® (Canada) *see* Captopril 148
Novo-Carbamaz® (Canada) *see* Carbamazepine 151
Novo-Chlorhydrate® (Canada) *see* Chloral Hydrate 180
Novo-Chlorpromazine® (Canada) *see* Chlorpromazine Hydrochloride ..195
Novo-Cimetidine® (Canada) *see* Cimetidine 207
Novo-Clobetasol® (Canada) *see* Clobetasol Propionate 216
Novo-Clonidine® (Canada) *see* Clonidine 221
Novo-Clopate® (Canada) *see* Clorazepate Dipotassium 222
Novo-Cloxin® (Canada) *see* Cloxacillin Sodium 224
Novo-Cromolyn® (Canada) *see* Cromolyn Sodium 235
Novo-Cycloprine® (Canada) *see* Cyclobenzaprine Hydrochloride 239
Novo-Difenac® (Canada) *see* Diclofenac 271
Novo-Difenac-SR® (Canada) *see* Diclofenac 271
Novo-Diflunisal® (Canada) *see* Diflunisal 278
Novo-Digoxin® (Canada) *see* Digoxin 280
Novo-Diltazem® (Canada) *see* Diltiazem 284
Novo-Dipam® (Canada) *see* Diazepam 268
Novo-Dipiradol® (Canada) *see* Dipyridamole 290
Novo-Doxepin® (Canada) *see* Doxepin Hydrochloride 298
Novo-Doxylin® (Canada) *see* Doxycycline 301
Novo-Famotidine® (Canada) *see* Famotidine 352
Novo-Fibrate® (Canada) *see* Clofibrate 217
Novo-Flupam® (Canada) *see* Flurazepam Hydrochloride 380
Novo-Flurprofen® (Canada) *see* Flurbiprofen Sodium 381
Novo-Folacid® (Canada) *see* Folic Acid 385
Novo-Furan® (Canada) *see* Nitrofurantoin 622
Novo-Gesic-C8® (Canada) *see* Acetaminophen and Codeine 15

Novo-Gesic-C15® (Canada) see Acetaminophen and Codeine.............15
Novo-Gesic-C30® (Canada) see Acetaminophen and Codeine.............15
Novo-Glyburide® (Canada) see Glyburide.....................401
Novo-Hexidyl® (Canada) see Trihexyphenidyl Hydrochloride..............871
Novo-Hydrazide® (Canada) see Hydrochlorothiazide.............430
Novo-Hydroxyzine® (Canada) see Hydroxyzine 443
Novo-Hylazin® (Canada) see Hydralazine Hydrochloride 428
Novo-Keto-EC® (Canada) see Ketoprofen.....................483
Novo-Lexin® (Canada) see Cephalexin Monohydrate 176
Novolin® 70/30 see Insulin Preparations.....................459
Novolin® L see Insulin Preparations 459
Novolin® N see Insulin Preparations 459
Novolin® R see Insulin Preparations 459
Novo-Lorazepam® (Canada) see Lorazepam 513
Novo-Medopa® (Canada) see Methyldopa 566
Novo-Mepro® (Canada) see Meprobamate 543
Novo-Metformin® (Canada) see Metformin Hydrochloride.............551
Novo-Methacin® (Canada) see Indomethacin..................457
Novo-Metoprolol® (Canada) see Metoprolol 574
Novo-Mucilax® (Canada) see Psyllium 750
Novo-Naprox® (Canada) see Naproxen....................606
Novo-Nidazol® (Canada) see Metronidazole..................576
Novo-Nifedin® (Canada) see Nifedipine....................619
Novo-Oxazepam® (Canada) see Oxazepam 644
Novo-Pen-VK® (Canada) see Penicillin V Potassium 668
Novo-Pindol® (Canada) see Pindolol.....................694
Novo-Piroxicam® (Canada) see Piroxicam 699
Novo-Poxide® (Canada) see Chlordiazepoxide.................183
Novo-Pramine® (Canada) see Imipramine...................451
Novo-Prazin® (Canada) see Prazosin Hydrochloride..............717
Novo-Prednisolone® (Canada) see Prednisolone................718
Novo-Prednisone® (Canada) see Prednisone.................719
Novo-Profen® (Canada) see Ibuprofen 447
Novo-Propamide® (Canada) see Chlorpropamide...............197
Novo-Propoxyn® (Canada) see Propoxyphene.................740
Novo-Propoxyn Compound (contains caffeine) (Canada) see Propoxyphene
   and Aspirin..........................742
Novo-purol® (Canada) see Allopurinol....................33
Novo-Pyrazone® (Canada) see Sulfinpyrazone 811
Novo-Ranidine® (Canada) see Ranitidine Hydrochloride.............763
Novo-Reserpine® (Canada) see Reserpine 765
Novo-Ridazine® (Canada) see Thioridazine..................840
Novo-Rythro® Encap (Canada) see Erythromycin 321
Novo-Salmol® (Canada) see Albuterol....................27
Novo-Secobarb® (Canada) see Secobarbital Sodium..............783
Novo-Selegiline® (Canada) see Selegiline Hydrochloride............784
Novo-Semide® (Canada) see Furosemide...................391
Novo-Soxazole® (Canada) see Sulfisoxazole 811
Novo-Spiroton® (Canada) see Spironolactone.................798
Novo-Sucralate® (Canada) see Sucralfate...................804
Novo-Sundac® (Canada) see Sulindac....................813
Novo-Tamoxifen® (Canada) see Tamoxifen Citrate...............818
Novo-Terfenadine® (Canada) see Terfenadine 823
Novo-Tetra® (Canada) see Tetracycline 829
Novo-Thalidone® (Canada) see Chlorthalidone.................199
Novo-Timol® (Canada) see Timolol Maleate 847
Novo-Tolmetin® (Canada) see Tolmetin Sodium 854
Novo-Triamzide® (Canada) see Triamterene and Hydrochlorothiazide........865
Novo-Trimel® (Canada) see Trimethoprim and Sulfamethoxazole.........874
Novo-Triolam® (Canada) see Triazolam 866
Novo-Tripramine® (Canada) see Trimipramine Maleate.............876
Novo-Tryptin® (Canada) see Amitriptyline Hydrochloride.............51
Novo-Veramil® (Canada) see Verapamil Hydrochloride.............893
Novo-Zolamide® (Canada) see Acetazolamide..................18
Nozolon® (Mexico) see Gentamicin Sulfate..................396
NP-27® [OTC] see Tolnaftate 855
NPH Iletin® I see Insulin Preparations....................459
NPH Insulin see Insulin Preparations....................459
NPH-N see Insulin Preparations......................459
NSC-102816 see Azacitidine........................88
NTZ® Nasal Solution [OTC] see Oxymetazoline Hydrochloride..........649
Nu-Alprax® (Canada) see Alprazolam....................35
Nu-Amoxi® (Canada) see Amoxicillin Trihydrate 58
Nu-Ampi® [Trihydrate] (Canada) see Ampicillin 62
Nu-Atenol® (Canada) see Atenolol.....................83
Nubain® see Nalbuphine Hydrochloride...................600
Nu-Capto® (Canada) see Captopril.....................148
Nu-Carbamazepine® (Canada) see Carbamazepine 151

Nu-Cephalex® (Canada) *see* Cephalexin Monohydrate....................176
Nu-Cimet® (Canada) *see* Cimetidine........................207
Nu-Clonidine® (Canada) *see* Clonidine........................221
Nu-Cloxi® (Canada) *see* Cloxacillin Sodium....................224
Nucofed® *see* Guaifenesin, Pseudoephedrine, and Codeine............410
Nucofed® Pediatric Expectorant *see* Guaifenesin, Pseudoephedrine, and
   Codeine....................410
Nu-Cotrimox® (Canada) *see* Trimethoprim and Sulfamethoxazole..........874
Nucotuss® *see* Guaifenesin, Pseudoephedrine, and Codeine............410
Nu-Diclo® (Canada) *see* Diclofenac........................271
Nu-Diflunisal® (Canada) *see* Diflunisal......................278
Nu-Diltiaz® (Canada) *see* Diltiazem........................284
Nu-Doxycycline® (Canada) *see* Doxycycline....................301
Nu-Famotidine® (Canada) *see* Famotidine....................352
Nu-Flurprofen® (Canada) *see* Flurbiprofen Sodium................381
Nu-Gemfibrozil® (Canada) *see* Gemfibrozil....................395
Nu-Glyburide® (Canada) *see* Glyburide......................401
Nu-Hydral® (Canada) *see* Hydralazine Hydrochloride..............428
Nu-Ibuprofen® (Canada) *see* Ibuprofen......................447
Nu-Indo® (Canada) *see* Indomethacin........................457
Nu-Iron® [OTC] *see* Polysaccharide-Iron Complex................705
Nu-Ketoprofen® (Canada) *see* Ketoprofen....................483
Nu-Ketoprofen-E® (Canada) *see* Ketoprofen..................483
Nullo® [OTC] *see* Chlorophyll........................185
Nu-Loraz® (Canada) *see* Lorazepam........................513
NuLYTELY® *see* Polyethylene Glycol-Electrolyte Solution............703
Nu-Medopa® (Canada) *see* Methyldopa......................566
Nu-Metop® (Canada) *see* Metoprolol........................574
Numorphan® *see* Oxymorphone Hydrochloride..................651
Numzitdent® [OTC] *see* Benzocaine........................102
Numzit Teething® [OTC] *see* Benzocaine....................102
Nu-Naprox® (Canada) *see* Naproxen........................606
Nu-Nifedin® (Canada) *see* Nifedipine......................619
Nu-Pen-VK® (Canada) *see* Penicillin V Potassium................668
Nupercainal® [OTC] *see* Dibucaine........................270
Nu-Pindol® (Canada) *see* Pindolol........................694
Nu-Pirox® (Canada) *see* Piroxicam........................699
Nu-Prazo® (Canada) *see* Prazosin Hydrochloride................717
Nuprin® [OTC] *see* Ibuprofen........................447
Nu-Prochlor® (Canada) *see* Prochlorperazine..................728
Nu-Propranolol® (Canada) *see* Propranolol Hydrochloride............743
Nu-Ranit® (Canada) *see* Ranitidine Hydrochloride................763
Nu-Sulfinpyrazone® (Canada) *see* Sulfinpyrazone................811
Nu-Tears® II Solution [OTC] *see* Artificial Tears..................75
Nu-Tears® Solution [OTC] *see* Artificial Tears..................75
Nu-Tetra® (Canada) *see* Tetracycline........................829
Nu-Timolol® (Canada) *see* Timolol Maleate....................847
Nutraplus® [OTC] *see* Urea........................884
Nu-Triazide® (Canada) *see* Triamterene and Hydrochlorothiazide........865
Nu-Triazo® (Canada) *see* Triazolam........................866
Nu-Trimipramine® (Canada) *see* Trimipramine Maleate............876
Nutropin® *see* Human Growth Hormone....................426
Nu-Verap® (Canada) *see* Verapamil Hydrochloride................893
Nyaderm® PMS-Nystatin® (Canada) *see* Nystatin................632
Nydrazid® *see* Isoniazid........................471
Nylidrin Hydrochloride........................631
Nystatin........................632
Nystatin and Triamcinolone........................632
Nytol® [OTC] *see* Diphenhydramine Hydrochloride................288
Occlucort® (Canada) *see* Betamethasone....................109
Occucoat™ *see* Hydroxypropyl Methylcellulose..................442
Occupational Exposure to Bloodborne Pathogens (Universal Precautions)
........................1030
OCL® *see* Polyethylene Glycol-Electrolyte Solution................703
Octamide® *see* Metoclopramide........................572
Octicair® Otic *see* Neomycin, Polymyxin B, and Hydrocortisone........610
Octocaine® *see* Lidocaine Hydrochloride....................502
Octocaine® 50 *see* Lidocaine and Epinephrine..................499
Octocaine® 100 *see* Lidocaine and Epinephrine..................499
Octostim® (Canada) *see* Desmopressin Acetate..................258
Octreotide Acetate........................633
Ocu-Carpine® *see* Pilocarpine........................691
OcuCoat® Ophthalmic Solution [OTC] *see* Artificial Tears............75
OcuCoat® PF Ophthalmic Solution [OTC] *see* Artificial Tears..........75
Ocu-Drop® [OTC] *see* Tetrahydrozoline Hydrochloride..............831
Ocuflox™ *see* Ofloxacin........................634
Ocupress® *see* Carteolol Hydrochloride....................158
Ocusert® Pilo *see* Pilocarpine........................691

Ocusert Pilo-20® see Pilocarpine...691
Ocusert Pilo-40® see Pilocarpine...691
Ocutricin® see Bacitracin, Neomycin, and Polymyxin B........................94
Ocutricin® HC Otic see Neomycin, Polymyxin B, and Hydrocortisone.........610
Ocutricin® Ophthalmic Solution see Neomycin, Polymyxin B, and Gramicidin
....610
Oestrillin® (Canada) see Estrone...329
Oestrogel® (Mexico) see Estradiol..325
Ofloxacin..634
Ofloxacina (Mexico) see Ofloxacin..634
Ogen® see Estropipate..330
OKT3 see Muromonab-CD3...594
Olanzapine...635
Olsalazine Sodium..635
Omeprazole...636
Omeprazol (Mexico) see Omeprazole..636
Omifin® (Mexico) see Clomiphene Citrate......................................218
OmniHIB® see Haemophilus b Conjugate Vaccine.................................414
Omnipen® see Ampicillin...62
OMS® Oral see Morphine Sulfate...590
Oncaspar® see Pegaspargase...662
Oncovin® Injection see Vincristine Sulfate...................................896
Ondansetron..637
Ony-Clear® Nail see Triacetin..862
Onyvul® (Canada) see Urea..884
OP-CCK see Sincalide...789
Opcon® see Naphazoline Hydrochloride...605
o,p'-DDD see Mitotane..585
Ophthacet® see Sodium Sulfacetamide..793
Ophthaine® see Proparacaine Hydrochloride....................................737
Ophthalgan® Ophthalmic see Glycerin..402
Ophthetic® see Proparacaine Hydrochloride....................................737
Ophthochlor® see Chloramphenicol...182
Ophthocort® Ophthalmic see Chloramphenicol, Polymyxin B, and
    Hydrocortisone...183
Opium Alkaloids..638
Opium Tincture...639
Opticrom® (Canada) see Cromolyn Sodium.......................................235
Optigene® [OTC] see Tetrahydrozoline Hydrochloride...........................831
Optimine® see Azatadine Maleate...89
Optimoist® [OTC] see Saliva Substitute.......................................778
OptiPranolol® see Metipranolol Hydrochloride.................................572
Optised® Ophthalmic [OTC] see Phenylephrine and Zinc Sulfate.................685
OPV see Poliovirus Vaccine, Live, Trivalent, Oral............................702
Orabase®-B [OTC] see Benzocaine..102
Orabase® HCA see Hydrocortisone..436
Orabase®-O [OTC] see Benzocaine..102
Orabase® Plain [OTC] see Gelatin, Pectin, and Methylcellulose................395
Orabase® With Benzocaine [OTC] see Benzocaine, Gelatin, Pectin, and
    Sodium Carboxymethylcellulose..103
Oracort® (Canada) see Triamcinolone Acetonide Dental Paste...................864
Orafer® (Mexico) see Ferrous Sulfate...360
Orajel® Brace-Aid Oral Anesthetic [OTC] see Benzocaine......................102
Orajel® Brace-Aid Rinse [OTC] see Carbamide Peroxide........................152
Orajel® Maximum Strength [OTC] see Benzocaine...............................102
Orajel® Mouth-Aid [OTC] see Benzocaine......................................102
Oral Bacterial Infections..945
Oral Fungal Infections...948
Oral Nonviral Soft Tissue Ulcerations or Erosions............................955
Oral Pain..940
Oral Rinse Products...1067
Oral Viral Infections..951
Oraminic® II see Brompheniramine Maleate.....................................124
Oramorph SR™ Oral see Morphine Sulfate.......................................590
Oranor® (Mexico) see Norfloxacin...628
Orap™ see Pimozide...694
Orasept® [OTC] see Benzocaine..102
Orasol® [OTC] see Benzocaine...102
Orasone® see Prednisone..719
Oratect® [OTC] see Benzocaine..102
Orazinc® [OTC] see Zinc Supplements..909
Orbenin® (Canada) see Cloxacillin Sodium.....................................224
Ordrine AT® Extended Release Capsule see Caramiphen and
    Phenylpropanolamine..150
Oretic® see Hydrochlorothiazide..430
Oreton® Methyl see Methyltestosterone..570
Orexin® [OTC] see Vitamin B Complex..899
Orfenadrina (Mexico) see Orphenadrine Citrate................................640

Organidin® see Iodinated Glycerol 465
Orimune® see Poliovirus Vaccine, Live, Trivalent, Oral 702
Orinase® see Tolbutamide 853
ORLAAM® see Levomethadyl Acetate Hydrochloride 496
Ormazine see Chlorpromazine Hydrochloride 195
Ornade® Spansule® see Chlorpheniramine and Phenylpropanolamine 190
Orphenadrine, Aspirin, and Caffeine 640
Orphenadrine Citrate 640
Ortho®0.5/35 (Canada) see Ethinyl Estradiol and Norethindrone 339
Ortho-Cept® see Ethinyl Estradiol and Desogestrel 335
Orthoclone® OKT3 see Muromonab-CD3 594
Orthoclone® OKT3 (Mexico) see Muromonab-CD3 594
Ortho-Cyclen® see Ethinyl Estradiol and Norgestimate 340
Ortho® Dienestrol see Dienestrol 275
Ortho-Est® see Estropipate 330
Ortho-Novum™ 1/35 see Ethinyl Estradiol and Norethindrone 339
Ortho-Novum™ 1/50 see Mestranol and Norethindrone 547
Ortho-Novum™ 7/7/7 see Ethinyl Estradiol and Norethindrone 339
Ortho-Novum™ 10/11 see Ethinyl Estradiol and Norethindrone 339
Ortho Tri-Cyclen® see Ethinyl Estradiol and Norgestimate 340
Or-Tyl® see Dicyclomine Hydrochloride 273
Orudis® see Ketoprofen 483
Orudis KT® [OTC] see Ketoprofen 483
Oruvail® see Ketoprofen 483
Os-Cal® 250 [OTC] see Calcium Carbonate 140
Os-Cal® 500 [OTC] see Calcium Carbonate 140
Osmoglyn® Ophthalmic see Glycerin 402
Ostoforte®(Canada) see Ergocalciferol 317
Otic Domeboro® see Aluminum Acetate and Acetic Acid 39
Otobiotic® Otic see Polymyxin B and Hydrocortisone 704
Otocalm® Ear see Antipyrine and Benzocaine 70
Otocort® Otic see Neomycin, Polymyxin B, and Hydrocortisone 610
Otomycin-HPN® Otic see Neomycin, Polymyxin B, and Hydrocortisone
. . . . 610
Otosporin® Otic see Neomycin, Polymyxin B, and Hydrocortisone 610
Otrivin® [OTC] see Xylometazoline Hydrochloride 905
Otrozol® (Mexico) see Metronidazole 576
Ovcon® 35 see Ethinyl Estradiol and Norethindrone 339
Ovcon® 50 see Ethinyl Estradiol and Norethindrone 339
Ovol® (Canada) see Simethicone 788
Ovral® see Ethinyl Estradiol and Norgestrel 341
Ovrette® see Norgestrel 629
Oxacillin Sodium 641
Oxamniquine 642
Oxandrine® see Oxandrolone 642
Oxandrolone 642
Oxaprozin 643
Oxazepam 644
Oxcodan® (Canada) see Oxycodone and Aspirin 647
Oxicanol® (Mexico) see Piroxicam 699
Oxiconazole Nitrate 644
Oxiconazol, Nitrato De (Mexico) see Oxiconazole Nitrate 644
Oxifungol® (Mexico) see Fluconazole 367
Oxiken® (Mexico) see Dobutamine Hydrochloride 294
Oxistat® see Oxiconazole Nitrate 644
Oxitetraciclina (Mexico) see Oxytetracycline Hydrochloride 653
Oxitocina (Mexico) see Oxytocin 654
Oxitopisa® (Mexico) see Oxytocin 654
Oxitraklin® (Mexico) see Oxytetracycline Hydrochloride 653
Oxpam® (Canada) see Oxazepam 644
Oxsoralen® Topical see Methoxsalen 563
Oxsoralen-Ultra® Oral see Methoxsalen 563
Oxtriphylline 645
Oxy-5® [OTC] see Benzoyl Peroxide 104
Oxy-10® [OTC] see Benzoyl Peroxide 104
Oxybutynin Chloride 645
Oxycel® see Cellulose, Oxidized 174
Oxychlorosene Sodium 646
Oxycocet® (Canada) see Oxycodone and Acetaminophen 646
Oxycodone and Acetaminophen 646
Oxycodone and Aspirin 647
Oxyderm® (Canada) see Benzoyl Peroxide 104
Oxydess® II see Dextroamphetamine Sulfate 265
Oxygen 649
Oxymetazoline Hydrochloride 649
Oxymetholone 650
Oxymorphone Hydrochloride 651
Oxyphenbutazone 652

Oxyphencyclimine Hydrochloride 652
Oxytetracycline and Hydrocortisone 653
Oxytetracycline and Polymyxin B 653
Oxytetracycline Hydrochloride 653
Oxytocin 654
Ozoken® (Mexico) see Omeprazole 636
P-071 see Cetirizine Hydrochloride 179
Paclitaxel 655
Pactens® (Mexico) see Naproxen 606
Palafer® (Canada) see Ferrous Fumarate 359
PALS® [OTC] see Chlorophyll 185
Pamelor® see Nortriptyline Hydrochloride 629
Pamidronate Disodium 655
Pamine® see Methscopolamine Bromide 564
p-Aminoclonidine see Apraclonidine Hydrochloride 72
Pamprin IB® [OTC] see Ibuprofen 447
Panadol® [OTC] see Acetaminophen 14
Pancrease® see Pancrelipase 657
Pancrease® MT 4 see Pancrelipase 657
Pancrease® MT 10 see Pancrelipase 657
Pancrease® MT 16 see Pancrelipase 657
Pancreatin 656
Pancrelipase 657
Panhematin® see Hemin 419
PanOxyl® [OTC] see Benzoyl Peroxide 104
PanOxyl®-AQ see Benzoyl Peroxide 104
Panscol® see Salicylic Acid 777
Panthoderm® [OTC] see Dexpanthenol 263
Pantomicina® (Mexico) see Erythromycin 321
Pantopon® see Opium Alkaloids 638
Pantothenic Acid 658
Papaverine Hydrochloride 658
Para-Aminosalicylate Sodium 658
Paracetamol (Mexico) see Acetaminophen 14
Parachlorometaxylenol 659
Paraflex® see Chlorzoxazone 200
Parafon Forte™ DSC see Chlorzoxazone 200
Paramethasone Acetate 659
Paraplatin® see Carboplatin 155
Paraxin® (Mexico) see Chloramphenicol 182
Par Decon® see Chlorpheniramine, Phenyltoloxamine, Phenylpropanolamine,
   and Phenylephrine 194
Paredrine® see Hydroxyamphetamine Hydrobromide 440
Paregoric 659
Paremyd® Ophthalmic see Hydroxyamphetamine and Tropicamide 440
Parepectolin® see Kaolin and Pectin With Opium 480
Pargen Fortified® see Chlorzoxazone 200
Par Glycerol® see Iodinated Glycerol 465
Pargyline and Methyclothiazide see Methyclothiazide and Pargyline 566
Parhist SR® see Chlorpheniramine and Phenylpropanolamine 190
Parlodel® see Bromocriptine Mesylate 121
Parnate® see Tranylcypromine Sulfate 860
Paromomycin Sulfate 660
Paroxetina (Mexico) see Paroxetine 660
Paroxetine 660
Parsidol® see Ethopropazine Hydrochloride 343
Partuss® LA see Guaifenesin and Phenylpropanolamine 409
PAS see Para-Aminosalicylate Sodium 658
Pathilon® see Tridihexethyl Chloride 868
Pathocil® see Dicloxacillin Sodium 273
Patients Requiring Sedation 965
Patients Undergoing Cancer Therapy 967
Pavabid® see Papaverine Hydrochloride 658
Pavagen® see Papaverine Hydrochloride 658
Pavased® see Papaverine Hydrochloride 658
Pavaspan® see Papaverine Hydrochloride 658
Pavasull® see Papaverine Hydrochloride 658
Pavatab® see Papaverine Hydrochloride 658
Pavatine® see Papaverine Hydrochloride 658
Pavatym® see Papaverine Hydrochloride 658
Paveral Stanley Syrup With Codeine Phosphate (Canada) see Codeine
   227
Paverolan® see Papaverine Hydrochloride 658
Paxil™ see Paroxetine 660
Paxipam® see Halazepam 415
PBZ® see Tripelennamine 877
PBZ-SR® see Tripelennamine 877
PCE® see Erythromycin 321

PCMX *see* Parachlorometaxylenol 659
Pebegal® (Mexico) *see* Benzonatate 104
Pectin and Kaolin *see* Kaolin and Pectin........................... 480
Pedameth® *see* Methionine 557
PediaCare® Oral *see* Pseudoephedrine 749
Pediacof® *see* Chlorpheniramine, Phenylephrine, and Codeine 192
Pediaflor® *see* Fluoride 374
Pediapred® *see* Prednisolone 718
PediaProfen™ *see* Ibuprofen 447
Pediatrix® (Canada) *see* Acetaminophen 14
Pediazole® *see* Erythromycin and Sulfisoxazole 323
Pedi-Boro® [OTC] *see* Aluminum Sulfate and Calcium Acetate 41
Pedi-Cort V® Topical *see* Clioquinol and Hydrocortisone 216
Pedi-Dri Topical *see* Undecylenic Acid and Derivatives 884
PediOtic® Otic *see* Neomycin, Polymyxin B, and Hydrocortisone 610
Pedi-Pro Topical [OTC] *see* Undecylenic Acid and Derivatives 884
Pedituss® *see* Chlorpheniramine, Phenylephrine, and Codeine 192
Pedte-Pak-5® *see* Trace Metals 857
Pedtrace-4® *see* Trace Metals..................................... 857
PedvaxHIB™ *see* *Haemophilus* b Conjugate Vaccine 414
Pegademase Bovine 662
Peganone® *see* Ethotoin 344
Pegaspargase 662
PEG-L-asparaginase *see* Pegaspargase 662
Pemoline 663
Penamp® *see* Ampicillin 62
Penbutolol Sulfate 664
Penciclovir 664
Penetrex™ *see* Enoxacin... 310
Penicilina G Procainica (Mexico) *see* Penicillin G Procaine 667
Penicillin G Benzathine and Procaine Combined 665
Penicillin G Benzathine, Parenteral 665
Penicillin G, Parenteral, Aqueous 666
Penicillin G Potassium, Oral 667
Penicillin G Procaine 667
Penicillin G Procaine and Benzathine Combined *see* Penicillin G Benzathine
    and Procaine Combined 665
Penicillin V Potassium 668
Penicil® (Mexico) *see* Penicillin G Procaine 667
Penipot® (Mexico) *see* Penicillin G Procaine 667
Penprocilina® (Mexico) *see* Penicillin G Procaine 667
Pentacarinat® (Mexico) *see* Pentamidine Isethionate 670
Pentaerythritol Tetranitrate....................................... 669
Pentagastrin 670
Pentam-300® *see* Pentamidine Isethionate 670
Pentamidina (Mexico) *see* Pentamidine Isethionate 670
Pentamidine Isethionate 670
Pentamycetin® (Canada) *see* Chloramphenicol 182
Pentasa® *see* Mesalamine 546
Pentaspan® *see* Pentastarch...................................... 671
Pentastarch 671
Pentazocine 671
Pentazocine Compound... 672
Pentobarbital 672
Pentolair® *see* Cyclopentolate Hydrochloride 240
Pentosan Polysulfate Sodium 674
Pentostatin 674
Pentothal® Sodium *see* Thiopental Sodium 839
Pentoxifilina (Mexico) *see* Pentoxifylline 675
Pentoxifylline 675
Pentrax® [OTC] *see* Coal Tar 225
Pentrexyl® (Mexico) *see* Ampicillin 62
Pen.Vee® K *see* Penicillin V Potassium 668
Pen-Vi-K® (Mexico) *see* Penicillin V Potassium.................... 668
Pepcid® [OTC] *see* Famotidine 352
Pepcidine® (Mexico) *see* Famotidine 352
Peptavlon® *see* Pentagastrin 670
Pepto-Bismol® (subsalicylate) [OTC] *see* Bismuth 114
Pepto® Diarrhea Control [OTC *see* Loperamide Hydrochloride 511
Peptol® (Canada) *see* Cimetidine 207
Percocet® *see* Oxycodone and Acetaminophen 646
Percocet-Demi® (Canada) *see* Oxycodone and Acetaminophen 646
Percodan® *see* Oxycodone and Aspirin.............................. 647
Percodan®-Demi *see* Oxycodone and Aspirin 647
Percogesic® [OTC] *see* Acetaminophen and Phenyltoloxamine 17
Perdiem® Plain [OTC] *see* Psyllium................................ 750
Perfectoderm® [OTC] *see* Benzoyl Peroxide 104
Perfenacina (Mexico) *see* Perphenazine 677

Pergolida, Mesilato De (Mexico) see Pergolide Mesylate 675
Pergolide Mesylate 675
Pergonal® see Menotropins 538
Periactin® see Cyproheptadine Hydrochloride 244
Peri-Colace® [OTC] see Docusate and Casanthranol 295
Peridane® (Mexico) see Pentoxifylline 675
Peridex® see Chlorhexidine Gluconate 184
Perindopril Erbumine 676
PerioGard® see Chlorhexidine Gluconate 184
Peritrate® see Pentaerythritol Tetranitrate 669
Peritrate® SA see Pentaerythritol Tetranitrate 669
Permapen® see Penicillin G Benzathine, Parenteral 665
Permax® see Pergolide Mesylate 675
Permethrin 676
Permitil® see Fluphenazine 379
Pernox® [OTC] see Sulfur and Salicylic Acid 813
Perphenazine 677
Perphenazine and Amitriptyline see Amitriptyline and Perphenazine 50
Persa-Gel® see Benzoyl Peroxide 104
Persantine® see Dipyridamole 290
Pertofrane® see Desipramine Hydrochloride 257
Pertussin® CS [OTC] see Dextromethorphan 266
Pertussin® ES [OTC] see Dextromethorphan 266
Pethidine Hydrochloride (Canada) see Meperidine Hydrochloride 539
Pfizerpen® see Penicillin G, Parenteral, Aqueous 666
Pfizerpen®-AS see Penicillin G Procaine 667
PGE₁ see Alprostadil 35
Pharmacal® (Canada) see Calcium Carbonate 140
Pharmaflur® see Fluoride 374
Phazyme® [OTC] see Simethicone 788
Phenameth® DM see Promethazine With Dextromethorphan 735
Phenaphen® With Codeine see Acetaminophen and Codeine 15
Phenazine® see Promethazine Hydrochloride 733
Phenazo® (Canada) see Phenazopyridine Hydrochloride 679
Phenazodine® see Phenazopyridine Hydrochloride 679
Phenazopyridine Hydrochloride 679
Phencen® see Promethazine Hydrochloride 733
Phen DH® w/Codeine see Chlorpheniramine, Pseudoephedrine, and Codeine
. . . . 195
Phenelzine Sulfate 679
Phenerbel-S® see Belladonna, Phenobarbital, and Ergotamine Tartrate
. . . . 99
Phenergan® see Promethazine Hydrochloride 733
Phenergan® VC Syrup see Promethazine and Phenylephrine 733
Phenergan® VC With Codeine see Promethazine, Phenylephrine, and
Codeine 734
Phenergan® With Codeine see Promethazine and Codeine 733
Phenergan® With Dextromethorphan see Promethazine With
Dextromethorphan 735
Phenetron® see Chlorpheniramine Maleate 191
Phenhist® Expectorant see Guaifenesin, Pseudoephedrine, and Codeine
. . . . 410
Phenindamine Tartrate 680
Pheniramine and Naphazoline see Naphazoline and Pheniramine 605
Pheniramine, Phenylpropanolamine, and Pyrilamine 680
Phenobarbital 680
Phenol 682
Phenolax® [OTC] see Phenolphthalein 682
Phenolphthalein 682
Phenolphthalein, White see Phenolphthalein 682
Phenolphthalein, Yellow see Phenolphthalein 682
Phenoxybenzamine Hydrochloride 682
Phensuximide 683
Phentermine Hydrochloride 683
Phentolamine Mesylate 684
Phenylalanine Mustard see Melphalan 536
Phenylephrine and Chlorpheniramine see Chlorpheniramine and
Phenylephrine 190
Phenylephrine and Scopolamine 685
Phenylephrine and Zinc Sulfate 685
Phenylephrine Hydrochloride 685
Phenylfenesin® L.A. see Guaifenesin and Phenylpropanolamine 409
Phenylpropanolamine and Brompheniramine see Brompheniramine and
Phenylpropanolamine 123
Phenylpropanolamine and Caramiphen see Caramiphen and
Phenylpropanolamine 150
Phenylpropanolamine and Chlorpheniramine see Chlorpheniramine and
Phenylpropanolamine 190

Phenylpropanolamine and Guaifenesin *see* Guaifenesin and
    Phenylpropanolamine 409
Phenylpropanolamine and Hydrocodone *see* Hydrocodone and
    Phenylpropanolamine 435
Phenylpropanolamine Hydrochloride 687
Phenyltoloxamine, Phenylpropanolamine, and Acetaminophen 688
Phenylzin® Ophthalmic [OTC] *see* Phenylephrine and Zinc Sulfate 685
Phenytoin 688
Phenytoin With Phenobarbital 689
Pherazine® w/DM *see* Promethazine With Dextromethorphan 735
Pherazine® With Codeine *see* Promethazine and Codeine 733
Phicon® [OTC] *see* Pramoxine Hydrochloride 714
Phillips'® LaxCaps® [OTC] *see* Docusate and Phenolphthalein 295
Phillips'® Milk of Magnesia [OTC] *see* Magnesium Hydroxide 522
pHisoHex® *see* Hexachlorophene 424
pHiso® Scrub *see* Hexachlorophene 424
Phos-Ex® *see* Calcium Acetate 139
Phos-Flur® *see* Fluoride 374
PhosLo® *see* Calcium Acetate 139
Phospholine Iodide® *see* Echothiophate Iodide 305
Phosphorated Carbohydrate Solution 690
Phosphoric Acid, Levulose and Dextrose *see* Phosphorated Carbohydrate
    Solution 690
Phrenilin® *see* Butalbital Compound 133
Phrenilin® Forte® *see* Butalbital Compound 133
Phyllocontin® *see* Theophylline/Aminophylline 832
Phyllocontin® (Canada) *see* Theophylline/Aminophylline 832
Phylloquinone (Canada) *see* Phytonadione 690
Physostigmine 690
Phytomenadione (Canada) *see* Phytonadione 690
Phytonadione 690
Pilagan® *see* Pilocarpine 691
Pilocar® *see* Pilocarpine 691
Pilocarpine 691
Pilocarpine and Epinephrine 693
Pilocarpine (Dental) 693
Pilopine HS® *see* Pilocarpine 691
Piloptic® *see* Pilocarpine 691
Pilostat® *see* Pilocarpine 691
Pima® *see* Potassium Iodide 711
Pimozide 694
Pindolol 694
Pink Bismuth® (subsalicylate) [OTC] *see* Bismuth 114
Pin-Rid® [OTC] *see* Pyrantel Pamoate 751
Pin-X® [OTC] *see* Pyrantel Pamoate 751
Piperacilina (Mexico) *see* Piperacillin Sodium 696
Piperacillin Sodium 696
Piperacillin Sodium and Tazobactam Sodium 696
Piperazine Citrate 697
Pipobroman 698
Pipracil® *see* Piperacillin Sodium 696
Pirazinamida (Mexico) *see* Pyrazinamide 752
Pirbuterol Acetate 698
Piridoxina (Mexico) *see* Pyridoxine Hydrochloride 753
Pirimetamina (Mexico) *see* Pyrimethamine 754
Piroxan® (Mexico) *see* Piroxicam 699
Piroxen® (Mexico) *see* Piroxicam 699
Piroxicam 699
Pisacaina® (Mexico) *see* Lidocaine and Epinephrine 499
Pisacina® (Mexico) *see* Lidocaine Hydrochloride 502
Pitocin® *see* Oxytocin 654
Pitressin® *see* Vasopressin 891
Pitrex® (Canada) *see* Tolnaftate 855
Pix Carbonis *see* Coal Tar 225
Placidyl® *see* Ethchlorvynol 334
Plaquenil® *see* Hydroxychloroquine Sulfate 440
Plasil® (Mexico) *see* Metoclopramide 572
Platinol® *see* Cisplatin 210
Platinol®-AQ *see* Cisplatin 210
Plendil® *see* Felodipine 354
Plicamycin 700
PMS-Amantadine® (Canada) *see* Amantadine Hydrochloride 41
PMS-Baclofen® (Canada) *see* Baclofen 95
PMS-Benztropine® (Canada) *see* Benztropine Mesylate 106
PMS-Bethanechol® Chloride (Canada) *see* Bethanechol Chloride .. 112
PMS-Bisacodyl® (Canada) *see* Bisacodyl 113
PMS-Carbamazepine® (Canada) *see* Carbamazepine 151
PMS®-Chloral Hydrate (Canada) *see* Chloral Hydrate 180

PMS-Cholestyramine® (Canada) *see* Cholestyramine Resin 201
PMS-Clonazepam® (Canada) *see* Clonazepam 220
PMS-Cyproheptadine® (Canada) *see* Cyproheptadine Hydrochloride 244
PMS-Desipramine® (Canada) *see* Desipramine Hydrochloride 257
PMS®-Diazepam (Canada) *see* Diazepam 268
PMS-Dimenhydrinate® (Canada) *see* Dimenhydrinate 286
PMS-Docusate Calcium® (Canada) *see* Docusate 295
PMS®-Erythromycin (Canada) *see* Erythromycin 321
PMS-Ferrous® Sulfate (Canada) *see* Ferrous Sulfate 360
PMS-Flupam® (Canada) *see* Flurazepam Hydrochloride 380
PMS-Fluphenazine® [Hydrochloride] (Canada) *see* Fluphenazine 379
PMS-Hydromorphone® (Canada) *see* Hydromorphone Hydrochloride 438
PMS®-Hydroxyzine (Canada) *see* Hydroxyzine 443
PMS-Imipramine® (Canada) *see* Imipramine 451
PMS-Isoniazid® (Canada) *see* Isoniazid 471
PMS-Ketoprofen® (Canada) *see* Ketoprofen 483
PMS-Levothyroxine® Sodium (Canada) *see* Levothyroxine Sodium 498
PMS®-Lidocaine Viscous (Canada) *see* Lidocaine Hydrochloride 502
PMS-Lindane® (Canada) *see* Lindane 504
PMS-Loperamine® (Canada) *see* Loperamide Hydrochloride 511
PMS-Lorazepam® (Canada) *see* Lorazepam 513
PMS-Methylphenidate® (Canada) *see* Methylphenidate Hydrochloride 568
PMS-Nylidrin® (Canada) *see* Nylidrin Hydrochloride 631
PMS-Opium & Beladonna (Canada) *see* Belladonna and Opium 98
PMS-Oxazepam® (Canada) *see* Oxazepam 644
PMS-Perphenazine® (Canada) *see* Perphenazine 677
PMS-Prochlorperazine® (Canada) *see* Prochlorperazine 728
PMS-Procyclidine® (Canada) *see* Procyclidine Hydrochloride 730
PMS-Progesterone® (Canada) *see* Progesterone 731
PMS-Propranolol® (Mexico) *see* Propranolol Hydrochloride 743
PMS-Pseudoephedrine® (Canada) *see* Pseudoephedrine 749
PMS-Pyrazinamide® (Canada) *see* Pyrazinamide 752
PMS-Sodium Cromoglycate® (Canada) *see* Cromolyn Sodium 235
PMS-Sulfasalazine® (Canada) *see* Sulfasalazine 810
PMS-Thioridazine® (Canada) *see* Thioridazine 840
PMS-Trihexyphenidyl® (Canada) *see* Trihexyphenidyl Hydrochloride 871
Podocon-25® *see* Podophyllum Resin 701
Podofilm® (Canada) *see* Podophyllum Resin 701
Podofilox 701
Podofin® *see* Podophyllum Resin 701
Podophyllin and Salicylic Acid 701
Podophyllum Resin 701
Point-Two® *see* Fluoride 374
Poison Information Centers 1086
Poladex® *see* Dexchlorpheniramine Maleate 261
Polaramine® *see* Dexchlorpheniramine Maleate 261
Polargen® *see* Dexchlorpheniramine Maleate 261
Poliovirus Vaccine, Inactivated 702
Poliovirus Vaccine, Live, Trivalent, Oral 702
Polocaine® 2% *see* Mepivacaine With Levonordefrin 542
Polocaine® 3% *see* Mepivacaine Dental Anesthetic 541
Polocaine® and Levonordefrin (Canada) *see* Mepivacaine With Levonordefrin
. . . . 542
Polocaine® (Canada) *see* Mepivacaine Dental Anesthetic 541
Polycillin® *see* Ampicillin 62
Polycillin-PRB® *see* Ampicillin and Probenecid 63
Polycitra®-K *see* Potassium Citrate and Citric Acid 710
Polycose® [OTC] *see* Glucose Polymers 400
Polyestradiol Phosphate 702
Polyethylene Glycol-Electrolyte Solution 703
Polyflex® *see* Chlorzoxazone 200
Polygam® *see* Immune Globulin, Intravenous 454
Polygam® S/D *see* Immune Globulin, Intravenous 454
Poly-Histine CS® *see* Brompheniramine, Phenylpropanolamine, and Codeine
. . . . 125
Polymox® *see* Amoxicillin Trihydrate 58
Polymyxin B and Hydrocortisone 704
Polymyxin B and Oxytetracycline *see* Oxytetracycline and Polymyxin B
. . . . 653
Polymyxin B and Trimethoprim *see* Trimethoprim and Polymyxin B 874
Polymyxin B Sulfate 704
Polymyxin E *see* Colistin Sulfate 231
Poly-Pred® *see* Neomycin, Polymyxin B, and Prednisolone 611
Polysaccharide-Iron Complex 705
Polysporin® *see* Bacitracin and Polymyxin B 94
Polytar® [OTC] *see* Coal Tar 225
Polythiazide 705
Polytopic® (Canada) *see* Bacitracin and Polymyxin B 94

Polytrim® Ophthalmic see Trimethoprim and Polymyxin B 874
Poly-Vi-Flor® see Vitamins, Multiple 901
Polyvinyl Alcohol see Artificial Tears 75
Poly-Vi-Sol® [OTC] see Vitamins, Multiple..............................901
Ponderal® (Canada) see Fenfluramine Hydrochloride......................355
Pondimin® see Fenfluramine Hydrochloride 355
Ponstan-500® (Mexico) see Mefenamic Acid..............................534
Ponstan® (Canada) see Mefenamic Acid 534
Ponstel® see Mefenamic Acid 534
Pontocaine® see Tetracaine Hydrochloride 828
Pontocaine® With Dextrose Injection see Tetracaine With Dextrose 829
Porcelana® [OTC] see Hydroquinone 439
Pork NPH Iletin® II see Insulin Preparations 459
Pork Regular Iletin® II see Insulin Preparations 459
Posipen® (Mexico) see Dicloxacillin Sodium 273
Posture® [OTC] see Calcium Phosphate, Tribasic 145
Potasalan® see Potassium Chloride 708
Potassium Acetate...706
Potassium Acetate, Potassium Bicarbonate, and Potassium Citrate 706
Potassium Acid Phosphate 707
Potassium Bicarbonate 707
Potassium Bicarbonate and Potassium Chloride, Effervescent 707
Potassium Bicarbonate and Potassium Citrate, Effervescent 707
Potassium Bicarbonate, Potassium Chloride, and Potassium Citrate 708
Potassium Chloride 708
Potassium Chloride and Potassium Gluconate 709
Potassium Citrate 710
Potassium Citrate and Citric Acid 710
Potassium Citrate and Potassium Gluconate 710
Potassium Gluconate..710
Potassium Iodide 711
Potassium Iodide Enseals® see Potassium Iodide 711
Potassium Phosphate 711
Potassium Phosphate and Sodium Phosphate 713
Povidone-Iodine 713
PPD see Tuberculin Purified Protein Derivative 882
Pramet® FA see Vitamins, Multiple 901
Pramidal® (Mexico) see Loperamide Hydrochloride......................511
Pramilet® FA see Vitamins, Multiple 901
Pramosone® see Pramoxine and Hydrocortisone 714
Pramotil® (Mexico) see Metoclopramide 572
Pramoxine and Hydrocortisone 714
Pramoxine Hydrochloride 714
Pravachol® see Pravastatin Sodium 715
Pravastatin Sodium 715
Prax® [OTC] see Pramoxine Hydrochloride............................714
Prazepam 715
Prazidec® (Mexico) see Omeprazole 636
Praziquantel 716
Prazosin and Polythiazide 717
Prazosin Hydrochloride 717
Precaptil® (Mexico) see Captopril 148
Precose® see Acarbose...12
Predair® see Prednisolone 718
Predaject® see Prednisolone 718
Predalone T.B.A.® see Prednisolone 718
Predcor® see Prednisolone 718
Predcor-TBA® see Prednisolone 718
Pred Forte® see Prednisolone 718
Pred-G® Ophthalmic see Prednisolone and Gentamicin 719
Pred Mild® see Prednisolone 718
Prednicarbate..718
Prednicen-M® see Prednisone 719
Prednisolone 718
Prednisolone and Gentamicin 719
Prednisone..719
Predominant Cultivable Microorganisms From Various Sites of the Oral
    Cavity 1045
Prefrin™ Ophthalmic Solution see Phenylephrine Hydrochloride 685
Pregnyl® see Chorionic Gonadotropin 203
Prelone® see Prednisolone 718
Premarin® see Estrogens, Conjugated 327
Premarin® With Methyltestosterone Oral see Estrogens With
    Methyltestosterone 329
Premphase™ see Estrogens and Medroxyprogesterone 327
Prempro™ see Estrogens and Medroxyprogesterone 327
Prenavite® [OTC] see Vitamins, Multiple 901
Pre-Par® see Ritodrine Hydrochloride 773

Pre-Pen® *see* Benzylpenicilloyl-polylysine 107
Prepulsid® (Canada) *see* Cisapride 209
Prescription Writing 1100
Presoken® (Mexico) *see* Diltiazem 284
Presoquim® (Mexico) *see* Diltiazem 284
Pressyn® (Canada) *see* Vasopressin 891
PreSun® 29 [OTC] *see* Methoxycinnamate and Oxybenzone 564
Prevacid® *see* Lansoprazole 490
PreviDent® *see* Fluoride 374
Prilocaine 721
Prilocaine With Epinephrine 721
Prilosec™ *see* Omeprazole 636
Primacor® *see* Milrinone Lactate 581
Primaquine Phosphate 723
Primaxin® *see* Imipenem/Cilastatin 451
Primidone 723
Primolut® Depot (Mexico) *see* Hydroxyprogesterone Caproate 441
Principen® *see* Ampicillin 62
Princol® (Mexico) *see* Lincomycin 503
Prinivil® *see* Lisinopril 506
Prinzide® *see* Lisinopril and Hydrochlorothiazide 507
Priscoline® *see* Tolazoline Hydrochloride 852
Privine® *see* Naphazoline Hydrochloride 605
Pro-Amox® (Canada) *see* Amoxicillin Trihydrate 58
Proampacin® *see* Ampicillin and Probenecid 63
Pro-Ampi® [Trihydrate] (Canada) *see* Ampicillin 62
Proaqua® *see* Benzthiazide 105
proartinal® (Mexico) *see* Ibuprofen 447
Probalan® *see* Probenecid 724
Pro-Banthine® *see* Propantheline Bromide 736
Proben-C® *see* Colchicine and Probenecid 229
Probenecid 724
Probenecid and Colchicine *see* Colchicine and Probenecid 229
Probi-Rho(D) (Mexico) *see* Rh₀(D) Immune Globulin 767
Probi-Tet (Mexico) *see* Tetanus Immune Globulin, Human 826
Probucol 725
Procainamide Hydrochloride 725
Procaine Hydrochloride 727
Pro-Cal-Sof® [OTC] *see* Docusate 295
Procan® SR *see* Procainamide Hydrochloride 725
Procarbazine Hydrochloride 727
Procardia® *see* Nifedipine 619
Procardia XL® *see* Nifedipine 619
Prochlorperazine 728
Procrit® *see* Epoetin Alfa 315
Proctofoam® [OTC] *see* Pramoxine Hydrochloride 714
Proctofoam®-HC *see* Pramoxine and Hydrocortisone 714
Procyclid® (Canada) *see* Procyclidine Hydrochloride 730
Procyclidine Hydrochloride 730
Procytox® (Canada) *see* Cyclophosphamide 240
Prodiem® Plain (Canada) *see* Psyllium 750
Profasi® HP *see* Chorionic Gonadotropin 203
Profenal® *see* Suprofen 815
Profenid® 200 (Mexico) *see* Ketoprofen 483
Profenid-IM® (Mexico) *see* Ketoprofen 483
Pro-Fenid® (Mexico) *see* Ketoprofen 483
Profen II® *see* Guaifenesin and Phenylpropanolamine 409
Profen LA® *see* Guaifenesin and Phenylpropanolamine 409
Profilate® OSD *see* Antihemophilic Factor (Human) 68
Profilnine® Heat-Treated *see* Factor IX Complex (Human) 350
Progestaject® *see* Progesterone 731
Progesterona (Mexico) *see* Progesterone 731
Progesterone 731
Progesterone Oil (Canada) *see* Progesterone 731
Proglycem® *see* Diazoxide 269
Prograf® *see* Tacrolimus 817
ProHIBiT® *see* Haemophilus b Conjugate Vaccine 414
Pro-Indo® (Canada) *see* Indomethacin 457
Proken® M (Mexico) *see* Metoprolol 574
Prolaken® (Mexico) *see* Metoprolol 574
Prolamine® [OTC] *see* Phenylpropanolamine Hydrochloride 687
Prolastin® Injection *see* Alpha₁-Proteinase Inhibitor, Human 34
Proleukin® *see* Aldesleukin 29
Prolixin® *see* Fluphenazine 379
Prolixin Decanoate® *see* Fluphenazine 379
Prolixin Enanthate® *see* Fluphenazine 379
Proloprim® *see* Trimethoprim 874
Pro-Lorazepam® (Canada) *see* Lorazepam 513

Promazine Hydrochloride 732
Prometa® see Metaproterenol Sulfate 550
Prometh® see Promethazine Hydrochloride 733
Promethazine and Codeine 733
Promethazine and Phenylephrine 733
Promethazine Hydrochloride 733
Promethazine, Phenylephrine, and Codeine 734
Promethazine VC Plain Syrup see Promethazine and Phenylephrine 733
Promethazine VC Syrup see Promethazine and Phenylephrine 733
Promethazine With Dextromethorphan 735
Prometh VC Plain Liquid see Promethazine and Phenylephrine 733
Promine® see Procainamide Hydrochloride 725
Promit® see Dextran 1 264
Pronaxil® (Mexico) see Naproxen 606
Pronestyl® see Procainamide Hydrochloride 725
Propacet® see Propoxyphene and Acetaminophen 741
Propaderm® (Canada) see Beclomethasone Dipropionate 97
Propadrine see Phenylpropanolamine Hydrochloride 687
Propafenona, Clorhidrato De (Mexico) see Propafenone Hydrochloride
. . . . 735
Propafenone Hydrochloride 735
Propagest® [OTC] see Phenylpropanolamine Hydrochloride 687
Propantheline Bromide 736
Proparacaine and Fluorescein 736
Proparacaine Hydrochloride 737
Propine® see Dipivefrin 290
Propiomazine Hydrochloride 737
Pro-Piroxicam® (Canada) see Piroxicam 699
Proplex® T see Factor IX Complex (Human) 350
Propofol 738
Propoxycaine and Procaine 739
Propoxyphene 740
Propoxyphene and Acetaminophen 741
Propoxyphene and Aspirin 742
Propranolol and Hydrochlorothiazide 743
Propranolol Hydrochloride 743
Propulsid® see Cisapride 209
Propylene Glycol and Salicylic Acid see Salicylic Acid and Propylene Glycol
. . . . 778
Propylhexedrine 745
Propylthiouracil 746
Propyl-Thyracil® (Canada) see Propylthiouracil 746
Prorazin® (Canada) see Prochlorperazine 728
Prorex® see Promethazine Hydrochloride 733
Proscar® see Finasteride 363
Pro-Sof® [OTC] see Docusate 295
Pro-Sof® Plus [OTC] see Docusate and Casanthranol 295
ProSom™ see Estazolam 324
Prostaglandin E$_1$ see Alprostadil 35
Prostaphlin® see Oxacillin Sodium 641
ProStep® see Nicotine 617
Prostin VR Pediatric® Injection see Alprostadil 35
Protamine Sulfate 747
Prothazine-DC® see Promethazine and Codeine 733
Protilase® see Pancrelipase 657
Protirelin 747
Protostat® see Metronidazole 576
Pro-Trin® (Canada) see Trimethoprim and Sulfamethoxazole 874
Protriptyline Hydrochloride 748
Protropin® see Human Growth Hormone 426
Provatene® [OTC] see Beta-Carotene 109
Proventil® see Albuterol 27
Provera® see Medroxyprogesterone Acetate 533
Proxigel® [OTC] see Carbamide Peroxide 152
Prozac® see Fluoxetine Hydrochloride 377
Prozoladex® (Mexico) see Goserelin Acetate 404
PRP-D see Haemophilus b Conjugate Vaccine 414
Prulet® [OTC] see Phenolphthalein 682
P&S® [OTC] see Salicylic Acid 777
Pseudo-Car® DM see Carbinoxamine, Pseudoephedrine, and
Dextromethorphan 155
Pseudoefedrina (Mexico) see Pseudoephedrine 749
Pseudoephedrine 749
Pseudoephedrine and Azatadine see Azatadine and Pseudoephedrine
. . . . 89
Pseudoephedrine and Chlorpheniramine see Chlorpheniramine and
Pseudoephedrine 191

Pseudoephedrine and Dexbrompheniramine *see* Dexbrompheniramine and
   Pseudoephedrine 261
Pseudoephedrine and Dextromethorphan 750
Pseudoephedrine and Guaifenesin *see* Guaifenesin and Pseudoephedrine
  409
Pseudoephedrine and Ibuprofen 750
Pseudo-Gest Plus® Tablet [OTC] *see* Chlorpheniramine and
   Pseudoephedrine 191
Psorcon™ *see* Diflorasone Diacetate 278
psoriGel® [OTC] *see* Coal Tar 225
Psyllium 750
P.T.E.-4® *see* Trace Metals 857
P.T.E.-5® *see* Trace Metals 857
Pulmicort® (Canada) *see* Budesonide 126
Pulmophylline® (Canada) *see* Theophylline/Aminophylline 832
Pulmozyme® *see* Dornase Alfa 296
Puralube® Tears Solution [OTC] *see* Artificial Tears 75
Purge® [OTC] *see* Castor Oil 161
Puri-Clens™ [OTC] *see* Methylbenzethonium Chloride 566
Purinethol® *see* Mercaptopurine 544
Purinol® (Canada) *see* Allopurinol 33
PVF® K (Canada) *see* Penicillin V Potassium 668
P-V-Tussin® *see* Hydrocodone, Phenylephrine, Pyrilamine, Phenindamine,
   Chlorpheniramine, and Ammonium Chloride 435
P₂E𝑥® Ophthalmic *see* Pilocarpine and Epinephrine 693
Pyocidin-Otic® *see* Polymyxin B and Hydrocortisone .704
Pyonto® [OTC] *see* Pyrethrins 753
Pyrantel Pamoate 751
Pyrazinamide 752
Pyrethrins 753
Pyridiate® *see* Phenazopyridine Hydrochloride 679
Pyridium® *see* Phenazopyridine Hydrochloride 679
Pyridoxine Hydrochloride 753
Pyrimethamine 754
Pyrinyl II® [OTC] *see* Pyrethrins 753
Pyrithione Zinc 755
Pyronium® (Canada) *see* Phenazopyridine Hydrochloride 679
Quadra-Hist® *see* Chlorpheniramine, Phenyltoloxamine,
   Phenylpropanolamine, and Phenylephrine 194
Quadrax® (Mexico) *see* Ibuprofen 447
Quazepam 755
Quemicetina® (Mexico) *see* Chloramphenicol 182
Questran® *see* Cholestyramine Resin 201
Questran® Light *see* Cholestyramine Resin 201
Quibron® *see* Theophylline and Guaifenesin 836
Quibron®-T *see* Theophylline/Aminophylline 832
Quibron®-T/SR *see* Theophylline/Aminophylline 832
Quiess® *see* Hydroxyzine 443
Quilagen® (Mexico) *see* Gentamicin Sulfate 396
Quimocyclar® (Mexico) *see* Tetracycline 829
Quinaglute® Dura-Tabs® *see* Quinidine 759
Quinalan® *see* Quinidine 759
Quinamm® *see* Quinine Sulfate 760
Quinapril Hydrochloride 756
Quinaprilo, Clorhidrato De (Mexico) *see* Quinapril Hydrochloride 756
Quinestrol 757
Quinethazone 758
Quinidex® Extentabs® *see* Quinidine 759
Quinidina (Mexico) *see* Quinidine 759
Quinidine 759
Quini Durules® (Mexico) *see* Quinidine 759
Quinine Sulfate 760
Quinora® *see* Quinidine 759
Quinsana® Plus Topical [OTC] *see* Undecylenic Acid and Derivatives 884
Quiphile® *see* Quinine Sulfate 760
Q-vel® *see* Quinine Sulfate 760
Rabies Immune Globulin, Human 761
Rabies Virus Vaccine 761
Racet® Topical *see* Clioquinol and Hydrocortisone 216
Racovel® (Mexico) *see* Levodopa and Carbidopa 495
Radiostol® (Canada) *see* Ergocalciferol 317
Ramace® (Mexico) *see* Ramipril 762
Ramipril 762
Ramses® [OTC] *see* Nonoxynol 9 627
Randikan® (Mexico) *see* Kanamycin Sulfate 479
Ranifur® (Mexico) *see* Ranitidine Hydrochloride 763
Ranisen® (Mexico) *see* Ranitidine Hydrochloride 763
Ranitidina (Mexico) *see* Ranitidine Hydrochloride 763

Ranitidine Bismuth Citrate 763
Ranitidine Hydrochloride 763
Rapifen® (Mexico) see Alfentanil Hydrochloride 31
Rastinon® (Mexico) see Tolbutamide 853
Raudixin® see Rauwolfia Serpentina 764
Rauverid® see Rauwolfia Serpentina 764
Rauwolfia Serpentina 764
Ravocaine® and Novocain® with Levophed® see Propoxycaine and Procaine
. . . . 739
Ravocaine® and Novocain® with Neo-Cobefrin® see Propoxycaine and
Procaine 739
Raxedin® (Mexico) see Loperamide Hydrochloride 511
Rea-Lo® [OTC] see Urea 884
Recombinate® see Antihemophilic Factor (Recombinant) 70
Recombivax HB® see Hepatitis B Vaccine 422
Redisol® see Cyanocobalamin 237
Redoxon® (Canada) see Ascorbic Acid 76
Redoxon® Forte (Mexico) see Ascorbic Acid 76
Redux® see Dexfenfluramine Hydrochloride 262
Reese's® Pinworm Medicine [OTC] see Pyrantel Pamoate 751
Reference Values for Adults 1046
Refresh® Ophthalmic Solution [OTC] see Artificial Tears 75
Refresh® Plus Ophthalmic Solution [OTC] see Artificial Tears 75
Regaine® (Mexico) see Minoxidil 583
Regitine® see Phentolamine Mesylate 684
Reglan® see Metoclopramide 572
Regulace® [OTC] see Docusate and Casanthranol 295
Regular (Concentrated) Iletin® II U-500 see Insulin Preparations 459
Regular Iletin® I see Insulin Preparations 459
Regular Insulin see Insulin Preparations 459
Regular Purified Pork Insulin see Insulin Preparations 459
Regulax SS® [OTC] see Docusate 295
Reguloid® [OTC] see Psyllium 750
Regutol® [OTC] see Docusate 295
Rela® see Carisoprodol 157
Relafen® see Nabumetone 596
Relaxadon® see Hyoscyamine, Atropine, Scopolamine, and Phenobarbital
. . . . 444
Relefact® TRH Injection see Protirelin 747
Relief® Ophthalmic Solution see Phenylephrine Hydrochloride 685
Remeron® see Mirtazapine 583
Remifentanil 765
Renacidin® see Citric Acid Bladder Mixture 211
Renedil® (Canada) see Felodipine 354
Renese® see Polythiazide 705
Renitec® (Mexico) see Enalapril 307
Renoquid® see Sulfacytine 807
Renormax® see Spirapril 798
Rentamine® see Chlorpheniramine, Ephedrine, Phenylephrine, and
Carbetapentane 191
ReoPro™ see Abciximab 12
Repan® see Butalbital Compound 133
Reposans-10® see Chlordiazepoxide 183
Resaid® see Chlorpheniramine and Phenylpropanolamine 190
Rescaps-D® S.R. Capsule see Caramiphen and Phenylpropanolamine
. . . . 150
Rescon Liquid [OTC] see Chlorpheniramine and Phenylpropanolamine
. . . . 190
Reserpina (Mexico) see Reserpine 765
Reserpine 765
Reserpine and Chlorothiazide see Chlorothiazide and Reserpine 189
Reserpine and Hydrochlorothiazide see Hydrochlorothiazide and Reserpine
. . . . 431
Respa-1st® see Guaifenesin and Pseudoephedrine 409
Respaire®-60 SR see Guaifenesin and Pseudoephedrine 409
Respaire®-120 SR see Guaifenesin and Pseudoephedrine 409
Respbid® see Theophylline/Aminophylline 832
Respinol-G® see Guaifenesin, Phenylpropanolamine, and Phenylephrine
. . . . 410
Respiratory Diseases 924
Resporal® [OTC] see Dexbrompheniramine and Pseudoephedrine 261
Restoril® see Temazepam 819
Retin-A™ see Tretinoin 862
Retisol-A® (Canada) see Tretinoin 862
Retrovir® see Zidovudine 907
Retrovir-AZT® (Mexico) see Zidovudine 907
Revapol® (Mexico) see Mebendazole 529
Revex® see Nalmefene Hydrochloride 601

Rēv-Eyes™ *see* Dapiprazole Hydrochloride 251
Revitalose® C-1000® (Canada) *see* Ascorbic Acid .76
R-Gen® *see* Iodinated Glycerol 465
R-Gene® *see* Arginine Hydrochloride 73
rGM-CSF *see* Sargramostim 780
Rheaban® [OTC] *see* Attapulgite 86
Rheomacrodex® *see* Dextran 263
Rhesonativ® *see* Rh$_o$(D) Immune Globulin 767
Rheumatoid Arthritis, Osteoarthritis, and Joint Prostheses 930
Rheumatrex® *see* Methotrexate 559
Rhinalar® (Canada) *see* Flunisolide 372
Rhinall® Nasal Solution [OTC] *see* Phenylephrine Hydrochloride 685
Rhinaris-F® (Canada) *see* Flunisolide 372
Rhinatate® Tablet *see* Chlorpheniramine, Pyrilamine, and Phenylephrine
195
Rhindecon® *see* Phenylpropanolamine Hydrochloride 687
Rhinocort™ *see* Budesonide 126
Rhinosyn-DMX® [OTC] *see* Guaifenesin and Dextromethorphan 408
Rhinosyn® Liquid [OTC] *see* Chlorpheniramine and Pseudoephedrine 191
Rhinosyn-PD® Liquid [OTC] *see* Chlorpheniramine and Pseudoephedrine
191
Rh$_o$(D) Immune Globulin 767
Rhodis® (Canada) *see* Ketoprofen 483
Rhodis-EC® (Canada) *see* Ketoprofen 483
RhoGAM™ *see* Rh$_o$(D) Immune Globulin 767
Rhoprolene® (Canada) *see* Betamethasone 109
Rhoprosone® (Canada) *see* Betamethasone 109
Rhotral® (Canada) *see* Acebutolol Hydrochloride 12
Rhotrimine® (Canada) *see* Trimipramine Maleate 876
rHuEPO-α *see* Epoetin Alfa 315
Rhythmin® *see* Procainamide Hydrochloride 725
Ribavirin 767
Riboflavin 768
Riboflavina (Mexico) *see* Riboflavin 768
RID® [OTC] *see* Pyrethrins 753
Ridaura® *see* Auranofin 87
Ridene® (Mexico) *see* Nicardipine Hydrochloride 616
Rifabutin 769
Rifadin® *see* Rifampin 769
Rifadin® (Canada) *see* Rifampin 769
Rifamate® *see* Rifampin and Isoniazid 771
Rifampicina (Mexico) *see* Rifampin 769
Rifampin 769
Rifampin and Isoniazid 771
Rifampin, Isoniazid, and Pyrazinamide 771
Rifater® *see* Rifampin, Isoniazid, and Pyrazinamide 771
Rilutek® *see* Riluzole 771
Riluzole 771
Rimactane® *see* Rifampin 769
Rimactane® (Canada) *see* Rifampin 769
Rimantadine Hydrochloride 771
Rimevax (Mexico) *see* Rubella Virus Vaccine, Live .776
Rimexolone 772
Riobin® *see* Riboflavin 768
Riopan® [OTC] *see* Magaldrate 520
Riopan Plus® [OTC] *see* Magaldrate and Simethicone 521
Risperdal® *see* Risperidone 772
Risperidona (Mexico) *see* Risperidone 772
Risperidone 772
Ritalin® *see* Methylphenidate Hydrochloride 568
Ritalin-SR® *see* Methylphenidate Hydrochloride 568
Ritmolol® (Mexico) *see* Metoprolol 574
Ritodrine Hydrochloride 773
Ritonavir 773
Rivotril® (Canada) *see* Clonazepam 220
Rivotril® (Mexico) *see* Clonazepam 220
RMS® Rectal *see* Morphine Sulfate 590
Robafen AC *see* Guaifenesin and Codeine 408
Robafen® CF [OTC] *see* Guaifenesin, Phenylpropanolamine, and
 Dextromethorphan 410
Robafen DM® [OTC] *see* Guaifenesin and Dextromethorphan 408
Robaxin® *see* Methocarbamol 557
Robaxisal® *see* Methocarbamol and Aspirin 558
Robicillin® VK *see* Penicillin V Potassium 668
Robidrine® (Canada) *see* Pseudoephedrine 749
Robinul® *see* Glycopyrrolate 403
Robinul® Forte *see* Glycopyrrolate 403
Robitussin® [OTC] *see* Guaifenesin 407

Robitussin® A-C *see* Guaifenesin and Codeine 408
Robitussin-CF® [OTC] *see* Guaifenesin, Phenylpropanolamine, and
    Dextromethorphan 410
Robitussin® Cough Calmers [OTC] *see* Dextromethorphan 266
Robitussin®-DAC *see* Guaifenesin, Pseudoephedrine, and Codeine 410
Robitussin®-DM [OTC] *see* Guaifenesin and Dextromethorphan 408
Robitussin-PE® [OTC] *see* Guaifenesin and Pseudoephedrine 409
Robitussin® Pediatric [OTC] *see* Dextromethorphan .266
Robitussin® Severe Congestion Liqui-Gels [OTC] *see* Guaifenesin and
    Pseudoephedrine 409
Robomol® *see* Methocarbamol 557
Rocaltrol® *see* Calcitriol 139
Rocephin® *see* Ceftriaxone Sodium 172
Rocky Mountain Spotted Fever Vaccine 775
Rofact® (Canada) *see* Rifampin. 769
Roferon-A® *see* Interferon Alfa-2a 461
Rogaine® *see* Minoxidil 583
Rogal® (Mexico) *see* Piroxicam 699
Rogitine® (Canada) *see* Phentolamine Mesylate 684
Rolaids® Calcium Rich [OTC] *see* Calcium Carbonate 140
Rolatuss® Plain Liquid *see* Chlorpheniramine and Phenylephrine 190
Romazicon™ *see* Flumazenil 370
Rondamine®-DM Drops *see* Carbinoxamine, Pseudoephedrine, and
    Dextromethorphan 155
Rondec®-DM *see* Carbinoxamine, Pseudoephedrine, and Dextromethorphan
   155
Rondec® Drops *see* Carbinoxamine and Pseudoephedrine 154
Rondec® Filmtab® *see* Carbinoxamine and Pseudoephedrine 154
Rondec® Syrup *see* Carbinoxamine and Pseudoephedrine 154
Rondec-TR® *see* Carbinoxamine and Pseudoephedrine 154
Ropivacaine Hydrochloride 775
Roubac® (Canada) *see* Trimethoprim and Sulfamethoxazole 874
Rowasa® *see* Mesalamine 546
Roxanol™ Oral *see* Morphine Sulfate 590
Roxanol Rescudose® *see* Morphine Sulfate 590
Roxanol SR™ Oral *see* Morphine Sulfate 590
Roxicet® *see* Oxycodone and Acetaminophen 646
Roxiprin® *see* Oxycodone and Aspirin 647
R-Tannamine® Tablet *see* Chlorpheniramine, Pyrilamine, and Phenylephrine
   195
R-Tannate® Tablet *see* Chlorpheniramine, Pyrilamine, and Phenylephrine
   195
RTCA *see* Ribavirin 767
Rubella and Measles Vaccines, Combined *see* Measles and Rubella
    Vaccines, Combined 527
Rubella and Mumps Vaccines, Combined 775
Rubella, Measles and Mumps Vaccines, Combined *see* Measles, Mumps,
    and Rubella Vaccines, Combined 528
Rubella Virus Vaccine, Live 776
Rubeola Vaccine *see* Measles Virus Vaccine, Live. 529
Rubex® *see* Doxorubicin Hydrochloride 299
Rubidomycin Hydrochloride *see* Daunorubicin Hydrochloride 252
Rubilem (Mexico) *see* Daunorubicin Hydrochloride 252
Rubramin® (Canada) *see* Cyanocobalamin 237
Rubramin-PC® *see* Cyanocobalamin 237
Rufen® *see* Ibuprofen 447
Rum-K® *see* Potassium Chloride 708
Ru-Tuss® DE *see* Guaifenesin and Pseudoephedrine 409
Ru-Tuss® Liquid *see* Chlorpheniramine and Phenylephrine 190
Ru-Vert-M® *see* Meclizine Hydrochloride 530
Rymed® *see* Guaifenesin and Pseudoephedrine. 409
Rymed-TR® *see* Guaifenesin and Phenylpropanolamine 409
Ryna-C® Liquid *see* Chlorpheniramine, Pseudoephedrine, and Codeine
   195
Rynacrom® (Canada) *see* Cromolyn Sodium 235
Ryna-CX® *see* Guaifenesin, Pseudoephedrine, and Codeine 410
Ryna® Liquid [OTC] *see* Chlorpheniramine and Pseudoephedrine 191
Rynatan® Pediatric Suspension *see* Chlorpheniramine, Pyrilamine, and
    Phenylephrine 195
Rynatan® Tablet *see* Chlorpheniramine, Pyrilamine, and Phenylephrine
   195
Rynatuss® Pediatric Suspension *see* Chlorpheniramine, Ephedrine,
    Phenylephrine, and Carbetapentane 191
Rythmol® *see* Propafenone Hydrochloride. 735
S-2® *see* Epinephrine, Racemic 314
S5614 *see* Dexfenfluramine Hydrochloride 262
Sabin Vaccine *see* Poliovirus Vaccine, Live, Trivalent, Oral 702
Sabulin® (Canada) *see* Albuterol 27

Safe Tussin 30 Liquid® [OTC] see Guaifenesin and Dextromethorphan 408
Safe Writing Practices 1103
SalAc® [OTC] see Salicylic Acid 777
Salacid® see Salicylic Acid 777
Salagen® see Pilocarpine (Dental) 693
Salazopyrin® (Canada) see Sulfasalazine 810
Salazopyrin EN-Tabs® (Canada) see Sulfasalazine 810
Salbulin® (Mexico) see Albuterol 27
Salbutalan® (Mexico) see Albuterol 27
Salbutamol (Mexico) see Albuterol 27
Saleto-200® [OTC] see Ibuprofen 447
Saleto-400® see Ibuprofen 447
Salflex® see Salsalate 779
Salgesic® see Salsalate 779
Salicilico, Acido (Mexico) see Salicylic Acid 777
Salicylic Acid 777
Salicylic Acid and Benzoic Acid see Benzoic Acid and Salicylic Acid 104
Salicylic Acid and Lactic Acid 778
Salicylic Acid and Podophyllin see Podophyllin and Salicylic Acid 701
Salicylic Acid and Propylene Glycol 778
Salicylic Acid and Sulfur see Sulfur and Salicylic Acid 813
Saligel™ see Salicylic Acid 777
Salivart® [OTC] see Saliva Substitute 778
Saliva Substitute 778
Salk Vaccine see Poliovirus Vaccine, Inactivated 702
Salmeterol, Hidroxinaftoato De (Mexico) see Salmeterol Xinafoate 778
Salmeterol Xinafoate 778
Salofalk® (Mexico) see Aminosalicylate Sodium 47
Salsalate 779
Salsitab® see Salsalate 779
Sal-Tropine® see Atropine Sulfate 85
Saluron® see Hydroflumethiazide 437
Salutensin® see Hydroflumethiazide and Reserpine 438
Salutensin-Demi® see Hydroflumethiazide and Reserpine 438
Sandimmune® see Cyclosporine 243
Sandimmun® Neoral (Mexico) see Cyclosporine 243
Sandoglobulin® see Immune Globulin, Intravenous 454
Sandoglubolina® (Mexico) see Immune Globulin, Intravenous 454
Sandostatin® see Octreotide Acetate 633
Sandostatina® (Mexico) see Octreotide Acetate 633
Sani-Supp® Suppository [OTC] see Glycerin 402
Sanorex® see Mazindol 527
Sansert® see Methysergide Maleate 571
Santyl® see Collagenase 232
Saquinavir Mesylate 780
Sargramostim 780
Sarna [OTC] see Camphor, Menthol, and Phenol 146
S.A.S® (Canada) see Sulfasalazine 810
Sastid® Plain Therapeutic Shampoo and Acne Wash [OTC] see Sulfur and
   Salicylic Acid 813
Scabene® see Lindane 504
Scabisan® Shampoo (Mexico) see Lindane 504
Scleromate™ see Morrhuate Sodium 592
Scopolamine 781
Scopolamine and Phenylephrine see Phenylephrine and Scopolamine 685
Scot-Tussin® [OTC] see Guaifenesin 407
Scot-Tussin® DM Cough Chasers [OTC] see Dextromethorphan 266
Sebaquin® [OTC] see Iodoquinol 466
Sebizon® see Sodium Sulfacetamide 793
Sebulex® [OTC] see Sulfur and Salicylic Acid 813
Sebulon® [OTC] see Pyrithione Zinc 755
Secobarbital and Amobarbital see Amobarbital and Secobarbital 55
Secobarbital Sodium 783
Seconal™ see Secobarbital Sodium 783
Secran® see Vitamins, Multiple 901
Secretin 784
Secretin-Ferring Injection see Secretin 784
Sectral® see Acebutolol Hydrochloride 12
Sedapap-10® see Butalbital Compound 133
Sefulken® (Mexico) see Diazoxide 269
Seldane® see Terfenadine 823
Seldane-D® see Terfenadine and Pseudoephedrine 824
Selegiline Hydrochloride 784
Selenium see Trace Metals 857
Selenium Sulfide 785
Sele-Pak® see Trace Metals 857
Selepen® see Trace Metals 857

ALPHABETICAL INDEX

Selestoject® *see* Betamethasone 109
Selestoject® [Sodium Phosphate] (Canada) *see* Betamethasone 109
Seloken® (Mexico) *see* Metoprolol 574
Selopres® (Mexico) *see* Metoprolol 574
Selsun® *see* Selenium Sulfide 785
Selsun Blue® [OTC] *see* Selenium Sulfide 785
Selsun Gold® for Women [OTC] *see* Selenium Sulfide 785
Semicid® [OTC] *see* Nonoxynol 9 627
Semprex-D® *see* Acrivastine and Pseudoephedrine 22
Senna 785
Senna-Gen® [OTC] *see* Senna 785
Senokot® [OTC] *see* Senna 785
Senolax® [OTC] *see* Senna 785
Sensorcaine® *see* Bupivacaine Hydrochloride 127
Sensorcaine®-MPF *see* Bupivacaine Hydrochloride 127
Sensorcaine® With Epinephrine (Canada) *see* Bupivacaine With Epinephrine
.... 128
Septa® *see* Bacitracin, Neomycin, and Polymyxin B 94
Septisol® *see* Hexachlorophene 424
Septra® *see* Trimethoprim and Sulfamethoxazole 874
Septra® DS *see* Trimethoprim and Sulfamethoxazole 874
Ser-A-Gen® *see* Hydralazine, Hydrochlorothiazide, and Reserpine 429
Ser-Ap-Es® *see* Hydralazine, Hydrochlorothiazide, and Reserpine 429
Serathide® *see* Hydralazine, Hydrochlorothiazide, and Reserpine 429
Serax® *see* Oxazepam 644
Serentil® *see* Mesoridazine Besylate 547
Serevent® *see* Salmeterol Xinafoate 778
Sermorelin Acetate 786
Serocryptin® (Mexico) *see* Bromocriptine Mesylate 121
Seromycin® Pulvules® *see* Cycloserine 242
Serophene® *see* Clomiphene Citrate 218
Serozide® (Mexico) *see* Etoposide 348
Serpalan® *see* Reserpine 765
Serpasil® *see* Reserpine 765
Sertan® (Canada) *see* Primidone 723
Sertraline Hydrochloride 786
Serutan® [OTC] *see* Psyllium 750
Serzone® *see* Nefazodone 608
Shur-Seal® [OTC] *see* Nonoxynol 9 627
Siblin® [OTC] *see* Psyllium 750
Sigafam® (Mexico) *see* Famotidine 352
Silace-C® [OTC] *see* Docusate and Casanthranol 295
Silain® [OTC] *see* Simethicone 788
Silaminic® Cold Syrup [OTC] *see* Chlorpheniramine and
  Phenylpropanolamine 190
Silaminic® Expectorant [OTC] *see* Guaifenesin and Phenylpropanolamine
.... 409
Sildicon-E® [OTC] *see* Guaifenesin and Phenylpropanolamine 409
Siltussin-CF® [OTC] *see* Guaifenesin, Phenylpropanolamine, and
  Dextromethorphan 410
Silvadene® *see* Silver Sulfadiazine 788
Silver Nitrate 787
Silver Protein, Mild 787
Silver Sulfadiazine 788
Simethicone 788
Simethicone and Calcium Carbonate *see* Calcium Carbonate and
  Simethicone 141
Simethicone and Magaldrate *see* Magaldrate and Simethicone 521
Simron® [OTC] *see* Ferrous Gluconate 360
Simvastatin 789
Sinaplin® (Mexico) *see* Ampicillin 62
Sinarest® 12 Hour Nasal Solution *see* Oxymetazoline Hydrochloride 649
Sinarest® Nasal Solution [OTC] *see* Phenylephrine Hydrochloride 685
Sincalide 789
Sine-Aid® IB [OTC] *see* Pseudoephedrine and Ibuprofen 750
Sinedol® 500 (Mexico) *see* Acetaminophen 14
Sinedol® (Mexico) *see* Acetaminophen 14
Sinemet® *see* Levodopa and Carbidopa 495
Sinequan® *see* Doxepin Hydrochloride 298
Sinuberase® (Mexico) *see* Lactobacillus acidophilus and Lactobacillus
  bulgaricus 488
Sinubid® *see* Phenyltoloxamine, Phenylpropanolamine, and Acetaminophen
.... 688
Sinufed® Timecelles® *see* Guaifenesin and Pseudoephedrine 409
Sinumist®-SR Capsulets® *see* Guaifenesin 407
Sinusol-B® *see* Brompheniramine Maleate 124
Sinutab® Tablets [OTC] *see* Acetaminophen, Chlorpheniramine, and
  Pseudoephedrine 17

SK and F 104864 *see* Topotecan Hydrochloride........................855
Skelaxin® *see* Metaxalone.....................................551
Skelex® *see* Chlorzoxazone...................................200
SKF 104864 *see* Topotecan Hydrochloride........................855
SKF 104864-A *see* Topotecan Hydrochloride......................855
Skin Test Antigens, Multiple...................................790
Slo-bid™ *see* Theophylline/Aminophylline........................832
Slo-Niacin® [OTC] *see* Niacin..................................614
Slo-Phyllin® *see* Theophylline/Aminophylline.....................832
Slo-Phyllin® GG *see* Theophylline and Guaifenesin...............836
Slow FE® [OTC] *see* Ferrous Sulfate............................360
Slow-K® *see* Potassium Chloride...............................708
Slow-Mag® [OTC] *see* Magnesium Chloride......................521
SMZ-TMP *see* Trimethoprim and Sulfamethoxazole.................874
Snaplets-EX® [OTC] *see* Guaifenesin and Phenylpropanolamine.........409
Sodium Ascorbate..791
Sodium Benzoate and Caffeine *see* Caffeine and Sodium Benzoate.........136
Sodium Cellulose Phosphate *see* Cellulose Sodium Phosphate..........175
Sodium Cromoglycate (Canada) *see* Cromolyn Sodium...............235
Sodium Fluoride *see* Fluoride.................................374
Sodium Hyaluronate.......................................791
Sodium Hyaluronate-Chrondroitin Sulfate *see* Chondroitin Sulfate-Sodium
    Hyaluronate...203
Sodium P.A.S. *see* Aminosalicylate Sodium.......................47
Sodium-PCA and Lactic Acid *see* Lactic Acid and Sodium-PCA..........487
Sodium Phosphates..792
Sodium Salicylate...793
Sodium Sulamyd® *see* Sodium Sulfacetamide.....................793
Sodium Sulfacetamide.....................................793
Sodium Sulfacetamide and Fluorometholone......................794
Sodium Sulfacetamide and Phenylephrine........................794
Sodium Sulfacetamide and Prednisolone Acetate....................794
Sodium Sulfacetamide and Sulfur *see* Sulfur and Sodium Sulfacetamide
   813
Sodium Tetradecyl Sulfate..................................794
Sodium Thiosulfate..795
Sodol® *see* Carisoprodol..................................157
Sofarin® *see* Warfarin Sodium...............................903
Sofoton® *see* Phenobarbital................................680
Solaquin® [OTC] *see* Hydroquinone..........................439
Solaquin Forte® *see* Hydroquinone..........................439
Solatene® *see* Beta-Carotene..............................109
Solfoton® *see* Phenobarbital...............................680
Solganal® *see* Aurothioglucose.............................87
Solium® (Canada) *see* Chlordiazepoxide......................183
Soltric® (Mexico) *see* Mebendazole.........................529
Solu-Cortef® *see* Hydrocortisone...........................436
Solugel® (Canada) *see* Benzoyl Peroxide......................104
Solu-Medrol® *see* Methylprednisolone.......................569
Solurex L.A.® *see* Dexamethasone..........................260
Soma® *see* Carisoprodol..................................157
Soma® Compound *see* Carisoprodol.........................157
Somnol® (Canada) *see* Flurazepam Hydrochloride................380
Somnos® *see* Chloral Hydrate..............................180
Som Pam® (Canada) *see* Flurazepam Hydrochloride..............380
Soothe® [OTC] *see* Tetrahydrozoline Hydrochloride..............831
Sopamycetin® (Canada) *see* Chloramphenicol..................182
Sophipren® Ofteno (Mexico) *see* Prednisolone.................718
Sophixin® Ofteno (Mexico) *see* Ciprofloxacin Hydrochloride........208
Soprodol® *see* Carisoprodol..............................157
Sorbitrate® *see* Isosorbide Dinitrate..........................474
Soridol® *see* Carisoprodol................................157
Sotacor® (Canada) *see* Sotalol Hydrochloride..................796
Sotalol Hydrochloride......................................796
Sotradecol® Injection *see* Sodium Tetradecyl Sulfate.............794
Spancap® No. 1 *see* Dextroamphetamine Sulfate................265
Span-FF® [OTC] *see* Ferrous Fumarate.......................359
Sparine® *see* Promazine Hydrochloride.......................732
Spaslin® *see* Hyoscyamine, Atropine, Scopolamine, and Phenobarbital
   444
Spasmoject® *see* Dicyclomine Hydrochloride...................273
Spasmolin® *see* Hyoscyamine, Atropine, Scopolamine, and Phenobarbital
   444
Spasmophen® *see* Hyoscyamine, Atropine, Scopolamine, and Phenobarbital
   444
Spasquid® *see* Hyoscyamine, Atropine, Scopolamine, and Phenobarbital
   444
Spec-T® [OTC] *see* Benzocaine.............................102
Spectam® *see* Spectinomycin Hydrochloride...................798

Spectazole™ see Econazole Nitrate 306
Spectinomycin Hydrochloride. 798
Spectrobid® see Bacampicillin Hydrochloride 92
Spirapril 798
Spironazide® see Hydrochlorothiazide and Spironolactone 431
Spironolactone 798
Spironolactone and Hydrochlorothiazide see Hydrochlorothiazide and
    Spironolactone 431
Spirozide® see Hydrochlorothiazide and Spironolactone 431
Sporanox® see Itraconazole 477
Sportscreme® [OTC] see Triethanolamine Salicylate 868
S-P-T see Thyroid 844
SRC® Expectorant see Hydrocodone, Pseudoephedrine, and Guaifenesin
   435
SSD™ see Silver Sulfadiazine 788
SSD-AF™ see Silver Sulfadiazine 788
SSKI® see Potassium Iodide 711
Stadol® see Butorphanol Tartrate 135
Stadol® NS see Butorphanol Tartrate 135
Stagesic® [5/500] see Hydrocodone and Acetaminophen 431
Stannous Fluoride see Fluoride 374
Stanozolol 799
Staphcillin® see Methicillin Sodium 556
Statex® (Canada) see Morphine Sulfate 590
Staticin® Topical see Erythromycin, Topical 324
Statrol® see Neomycin and Polymyxin B 609
Stavudine 800
Stay Trim® Diet Gum [OTC] see Phenylpropanolamine Hydrochloride 687
Stelazine® see Trifluoperazine Hydrochloride 869
Stemex® see Paramethasone Acetate 659
Stenox® (Mexico) see Fluoxymesterone 378
Sterapred® see Prednisone 719
Stieva-A® 0.025% (Mexico) see Tretinoin 862
Stieva-A® (Canada) see Tretinoin 862
Stieva-A Forte® (Canada) see Tretinoin 862
Stieva-A® (Mexico) see Tretinoin 862
Stilphostrol® see Diethylstilbestrol 277
Stimate™ see Desmopressin Acetate 258
St. Joseph® Cough Suppressant [OTC] see Dextromethorphan 266
St. Joseph® Measured Dose Nasal Solution [OTC] see Phenylephrine
    Hydrochloride 685
Stop® [OTC] see Fluoride 374
Streptase® see Streptokinase 801
Streptokinase 801
Streptomycin Sulfate 802
Streptozocin 803
Stresstabs® 600 Advanced Formula Tablets [OTC] see Vitamins, Multiple
   901
Stuartnatal® 1 + 1 see Vitamins, Multiple 901
Stuart Prenatal® [OTC] see Vitamins, Multiple 901
Sublimaze® see Fentanyl 357
Sucralfate 804
Sucralfato (Mexico) see Sucralfate 804
Sucrets® Cough Calmers [OTC] see Dextromethorphan 266
Sudafed® [OTC] see Pseudoephedrine 749
Sudafed® 12 Hour [OTC] see Pseudoephedrine .749
Sudafed® Plus Liquid [OTC] see Chlorpheniramine and Pseudoephedrine
   191
Sudafed® Plus Tablet [OTC] see Chlorpheniramine and Pseudoephedrine
   191
Sudex® see Guaifenesin and Pseudoephedrine 409
Sufedrin® [OTC] see Pseudoephedrine 749
Sufenta® see Sufentanil Citrate 805
Sufentanil Citrate 805
Sugar-Free Liquid Pharmaceuticals 1070
Sular™ see Nisoldipine 622
Sulconazole Nitrate 806
Sulconazol, Nitrato De (Mexico) see Sulconazole Nitrate 806
Sulcrate® (Canada) see Sucralfate 804
Sulcrate® Suspension Plus (Canada) see Sucralfate 804
Sulf-10® see Sodium Sulfacetamide 793
Sulfabenzamide, Sulfacetamide, and Sulfathiazole 806
Sulfacet-R® Topical see Sulfur and Sodium Sulfacetamide 813
Sulfacytine 807
Sulfadiazine 807
Sulfadiazine, Sulfamethazine, and Sulfamerazine 808
Sulfadoxine and Pyrimethamine 808
Sulfair® see Sodium Sulfacetamide 793

Sulfalax® [OTC] *see* Docusate 295
Sulfamethoprim® *see* Trimethoprim and Sulfamethoxazole 874
Sulfamethoxazole 809
Sulfamethoxazole and Phenazopyridine 809
Sulfamethoxazole and Trimethoprim *see* Trimethoprim and Sulfamethoxazole
. 874
Sulfametoxazol (Mexico) *see* Sulfamethoxazole 809
Sulfamylon® *see* Mafenide Acetate 520
Sulfanilamide 810
Sulfasalazine 810
Sulfatrim® *see* Trimethoprim and Sulfamethoxazole .874
Sulfatrim® DS *see* Trimethoprim and Sulfamethoxazole 874
Sulfinpyrazone 811
Sulfisoxasol (Mexico) *see* Sulfisoxazole 811
Sulfisoxazole 811
Sulfisoxazole and Phenazopyridine 812
Sulfizole® (Canada) *see* Sulfisoxazole 811
Sulfoxaprim® *see* Trimethoprim and Sulfamethoxazole 874
Sulfoxaprim® DS *see* Trimethoprim and Sulfamethoxazole 874
Sulfur and Salicylic Acid 813
Sulfur and Sodium Sulfacetamide 813
Sulindac 813
Sulten-10® *see* Sodium Sulfacetamide 793
Sultrin™ *see* Sulfabenzamide, Sulfacetamide, and Sulfathiazole 806
Sumacal® [OTC] *see* Glucose Polymers 400
Sumatriptan Succinate 814
Sumycin® *see* Tetracycline 829
Sunscreen, PABA-Free *see* Methoxycinnamate and Oxybenzone 564
SuperChar® [OTC] *see* Charcoal 179
Suplena® (Mexico) *see* Vitamins, Multiple 901
Suplical® [OTC] *see* Calcium Carbonate 140
Supprelin™ *see* Histrelin 425
Suppress® [OTC] *see* Dextromethorphan 266
Supradol® (Mexico) *see* Naproxen 606
Suprax® *see* Cefixime 165
Suprofen 815
Surbex® [OTC] *see* Vitamin B Complex 899
Surbex-T® Filmtabs® [OTC] *see* Vitamin B Complex With Vitamin C 900
Surbex® with C Filmtabs® [OTC] *see* Vitamin B Complex With Vitamin C
. 900
Surfak® [OTC] *see* Docusate 295
Surgicel® *see* Cellulose, Oxidized 174
Surgicel® Absorbable Hemostat *see* Cellulose, Oxidized Regenerated 175
Surmontil® *see* Trimipramine Maleate 876
Survanta® *see* Beractant 108
Susano® *see* Hyoscyamine, Atropine, Scopolamine, and Phenobarbital
. 444
Sus-Phrine® *see* Epinephrine (Dental) 313
Sustaire® *see* Theophylline/Aminophylline 832
Sutilains 816
Sween® Cream [OTC] *see* Methylbenzethonium Chloride 566
Swim-Ear® Otic [OTC] *see* Boric Acid 118
Sydolil® (Mexico) *see* Ergotamine 319
Syllact® [OTC] *see* Psyllium 750
Symadine® *see* Amantadine Hydrochloride 41
Symmetrel® *see* Amantadine Hydrochloride 41
Synalar® *see* Fluocinolone Acetonide 372
Synalar-HP® *see* Fluocinolone Acetonide 372
Synalar® Simple (Mexico) *see* Fluocinolone Acetonide 372
Synalgos® [OTC] *see* Aspirin 78
Synalgos®-DC *see* Dihydrocodeine, Acetaminophen, and Aspirin 281
Synarel® *see* Nafarelin Acetate 598
Syn-Captopril® (Canada) *see* Captopril 148
Syn-Diltiazem® (Canada) *see* Diltiazem 284
Synemol® *see* Fluocinolone Acetonide 372
Syn-Flunisolide® (Canada) *see* Flunisolide 372
Syngestal® (Mexico) *see* Norethindrone 627
Syn-Minocycline® (Canada) *see* Minocycline Hydrochloride 582
Syn-Nadolol® (Canada) *see* Nadolol 597
Synphasic® (Canada) *see* Ethinyl Estradiol and Norethindrone 339
Syn-Pindol® (Canada) *see* Pindolol 694
Synthetic Lung Surfactant *see* Colfosceril Palmitate .230
Synthroid® *see* Levothyroxine Sodium 498
Syntocinon® *see* Oxytocin 654
Syntocinon® (Mexico) *see* Oxytocin 654
Syracol-CF® [OTC] *see* Guaifenesin and Dextromethorphan 408
Syraprim® (Mexico) *see* Trimethoprim and Sulfamethoxazole 874
Systemic Considerations Related to Natural Products for Weight Loss 979

ALPHABETICAL INDEX

Systemic Viral Diseases 934
Systen® (Mexico) *see* Estradiol 325
Sytobex® *see* Cyanocobalamin 237
Tabalon® (Mexico) *see* Ibuprofen 447
Tac™-3 *see* Triamcinolone 862
TACE® *see* Chlorotrianisene 189
Tacex® (Mexico) *see* Ceftriaxone Sodium 172
Tacrine Hydrochloride 816
Tacrolimus 817
Tafil® (Mexico) *see* Alprazolam 35
Tagal® (Mexico) *see* Ceftazidime 171
Tagamet® *see* Cimetidine 207
Talacen® *see* Pentazocine Compound 672
Taloken® (Mexico) *see* Ceftazidime 171
Talpramin® (Mexico) *see* Imipramine 451
Talwin® *see* Pentazocine 671
Talwin® Compound *see* Pentazocine Compound 672
Talwin® NX *see* Pentazocine 671
Tambocor™ *see* Flecainide Acetate 365
Tamine® [OTC] *see* Brompheniramine and Phenylpropanolamine 123
Tamofen® (Canada) *see* Tamoxifen Citrate 818
Tamone® (Canada) *see* Tamoxifen Citrate 818
Tamoxan® (Mexico) *see* Tamoxifen Citrate 818
Tamoxifen Citrate 818
Tamoxifeno (Mexico) *see* Tamoxifen Citrate .818
Tanoral® Tablet *see* Chlorpheniramine, Pyrilamine, and Phenylephrine
195
Tantaphen® (Canada) *see* Acetaminophen 14
Tao® *see* Troleandomycin 880
Tapazole® *see* Methimazole 556
Taporin® (Mexico) *see* Cefotaxime Sodium 167
Taractan® *see* Chlorprothixene 198
Taro-Ampicillin® [Trihydrate] (Canada) *see* Ampicillin 62
Taro-Atenol® (Canada) *see* Atenolol 83
Taro-Cloxacillin® (Canada) *see* Cloxacillin Sodium 224
Taro-Sone® (Canada) *see* Betamethasone 109
Tasedan® (Mexico) *see* Estazolam 324
Tavist® *see* Clemastine Fumarate 214
Tavist-D® *see* Clemastine and Phenylpropanolamine 213
Taxol® *see* Paclitaxel 655
Taxotere® *see* Docetaxel 294
Taxus® (Mexico) *see* Tamoxifen Citrate 818
Tazicef® *see* Ceftazidime 171
Tazidime® *see* Ceftazidime 171
3TC *see* Lamivudine 489
Tear Drop® Solution [OTC] *see* Artificial Tears .75
TearGard® Ophthalmic Solution [OTC] *see* Artificial Tears 75
Teargen® Ophthalmic Solution [OTC] *see* Artificial Tears 75
Tearisol® Solution [OTC] *see* Artificial Tears 75
Tears Naturale® Free Solution [OTC] *see* Artificial Tears 75
Tears Naturale® II Solution [OTC] *see* Artificial Tears 75
Tears Naturale® Solution [OTC] *see* Artificial Tears 75
Tears Plus® Solution [OTC] *see* Artificial Tears 75
Tears Renewed® Solution [OTC] *see* Artificial Tears 75
Tebamide® *see* Trimethobenzamide Hydrochloride 873
Tebrazid® (Canada) *see* Pyrazinamide 752
Tecnal® (Canada) *see* Butalbital Compound 133
Tecprazin (Mexico) *see* Praziquantel 716
Tedral® *see* Theophylline, Ephedrine, and Phenobarbital 836
Teejel® (Canada) *see* Choline Salicylate 202
Tega-Cert® [OTC] *see* Dimenhydrinate 286
Tegison® *see* Etretinate 349
Tegopen® *see* Cloxacillin Sodium 224
Tegretol® *see* Carbamazepine 151
Tegretol-XR® *see* Carbamazepine 151
T.E.H.® *see* Theophylline, Ephedrine, and Hydroxyzine 836
Telachlor® *see* Chlorpheniramine Maleate 191
Teladar® *see* Betamethasone 109
Teldane® (Mexico) *see* Terfenadine 823
Teldrin® [OTC] *see* Chlorpheniramine Maleate 191
Temaril® *see* Trimeprazine Tartrate 871
Temazepam 819
Temazin® Cold Syrup [OTC] *see* Chlorpheniramine and Phenylpropanolamine
190
Temgesic® (Mexico) *see* Buprenorphine Hydrochloride 129
Temovate® *see* Clobetasol Propionate 216
Temperal® (Mexico) *see* Acetaminophen 14
Temporomandibular Dysfunction (TMD) 963

Tempra® [OTC] *see* Acetaminophen 14
Tenex® *see* Guanfacine Hydrochloride 413
Teniposide 820
Tenoretic® *see* Atenolol and Chlorthalidone 84
Tenormin® *see* Atenolol 83
Tenuate® *see* Diethylpropion Hydrochloride 276
Tenuate® Dospan® *see* Diethylpropion Hydrochloride 276
Tepanil® *see* Diethylpropion Hydrochloride 276
Terak® Ophthalmic Ointment *see* Oxytetracycline and Polymyxin B 653
Terazol® *see* Terconazole 823
Terazosin 821
Terazosina (Mexico) *see* Terazosin 821
Terbenafina Clorhidrato De (Mexico) *see* Terbinafine 822
Terbinafine 822
Terbutalina, Sulfato De (Mexico) *see* Terbutaline Sulfate 822
Terbutaline Sulfate 822
Terconazole 823
Terfenadina (Mexico) *see* Terfenadine 823
Terfenadine 823
Terfenadine and Pseudoephedrine 824
Terpin Hydrate 825
Terpin Hydrate and Codeine 825
Terra-Cortril® Ophthalmic Suspension *see* Oxytetracycline and
  Hydrocortisone 653
Terramicina® (Mexico) *see* Oxytetracycline Hydrochloride 653
Terramycin® IV *see* Oxytetracycline Hydrochloride 653
Terramycin® Ophthalmic Ointment *see* Oxytetracycline and Polymyxin B
 653
Terramycin® w/Polymyxin B Ophthalmic Ointment *see* Oxytetracycline and
  Polymyxin B 653
Tesalon® (Mexico) *see* Benzonatate 104
Tesanone® *see* Testosterone 825
Teslac® *see* Testolactone 825
TESPA *see* Thiotepa 841
Tessalon® Perles *see* Benzonatate 104
Testex® *see* Testosterone 825
Testoderm® *see* Testosterone 825
Testolactone 825
Testosterona (Mexico) *see* Testosterone 825
Testosterone 825
Testosterone and Estradiol *see* Estradiol and Testosterone 326
Testred® *see* Methyltestosterone 570
Testrin® P.A. *see* Testosterone 825
Tetanogamma® P (Mexico) *see* Tetanus Immune Globulin, Human 826
Tetanol® (Mexico) *see* Tetanus Toxoid, Adsorbed 827
Tetanus Immune Globulin, Human 826
Tetanus Toxoid, Adsorbed 827
Tetanus Toxoid, Fluid 828
Tetanus Toxoid Plain *see* Tetanus Toxoid, Fluid 828
Tetinox® (Mexico) *see* Tetanus Toxoid, Fluid 828
Tetra-Atlantis® (Mexico) *see* Tetracycline 829
Tetracaine Hydrochloride 828
Tetracaine Hydrochloride, Benzocaine Butyl Aminobenzoate and
  Benzalkonium Chloride *see* Benzocaine, Butyl Aminobenzoate,
  Tetracaine, and Benzalkonium Chloride 103
Tetracaine With Dextrose 829
Tetraclear® [OTC] *see* Tetrahydrozoline Hydrochloride 831
Tetracycline 829
Tetracycline Periodontal Fibers 830
Tetracyn® *see* Tetracycline 829
Tetrahydrozoline Hydrochloride 831
Tetra-Ide® [OTC] *see* Tetrahydrozoline Hydrochloride 831
TG *see* Thioguanine 838
6-TG *see* Thioguanine 838
T/Gel® [OTC] *see* Coal Tar 225
T-Gen® *see* Trimethobenzamide Hydrochloride 873
T-Gesic® [5/500] *see* Hydrocodone and Acetaminophen 431
Thalitone® *see* Chlorthalidone 199
THAM-E® Injection *see* Tromethamine 880
THAM® Injection *see* Tromethamine 880
Theelin® *see* Estrone 329
Theo-24® *see* Theophylline/Aminophylline 832
Theobid® *see* Theophylline/Aminophylline 832
Theochron® *see* Theophylline/Aminophylline 832
Theoclear® L.A. *see* Theophylline/Aminophylline 832
Theo-Dur® *see* Theophylline/Aminophylline 832
Theodur-Sprinkle® *see* Theophylline/Aminophylline 832
Theo-G® *see* Theophylline and Guaifenesin 836

Theolair™ *see* Theophylline/Aminophylline 832
Theolate® *see* Theophylline and Guaifenesin 836
Theon® *see* Theophylline/Aminophylline 832
Theophylline/Aminophylline 832
Theophylline and Guaifenesin 836
Theophylline, Ephedrine, and Hydroxyzine 836
Theophylline, Ephedrine, and Phenobarbital 836
Theospan®-SR *see* Theophylline/Aminophylline 832
Theovent® *see* Theophylline/Aminophylline 832
Therabid® [OTC] *see* Vitamins, Multiple 901
Thera-Combex® H-P Kapseals® [OTC] *see* Vitamin B Complex With Vitamin
    C 900
TheraCys™ *see* Bacillus Calmette-Guérin (BCG) Live 93
Thera-Flur® *see* Fluoride 374
Thera-Flur-N® *see* Fluoride 374
Theragran® [OTC] *see* Vitamins, Multiple 901
Theragran® Hematinic® *see* Vitamins, Multiple 901
Theragran® Liquid [OTC] *see* Vitamins, Multiple 901
Theragran-M® [OTC] *see* Vitamins, Multiple 901
Thera-Hist® Syrup [OTC] *see* Chlorpheniramine and Phenylpropanolamine
    190
Theralax® [OTC] *see* Bisacodyl 113
Theramin® Expectorant [OTC] *see* Guaifenesin and Phenylpropanolamine
    409
Theraplex Z® [OTC] *see* Pyrithione Zinc 755
Thermazene™ *see* Silver Sulfadiazine 788
Thiabendazole 836
Thiamine Hydrochloride 837
Thiethylperazine Maleate 838
Thimerosal 838
Thioguanine 838
6-Thioguanine *see* Thioguanine 838
Thiola™ *see* Tiopronin 849
Thiopental Sodium 839
Thiophosphoramide *see* Thiotepa 841
Thioridazine 840
Thiotepa 841
Thiothixene 842
Thorazine® *see* Chlorpromazine Hydrochloride 195
Thrombate III™ *see* Antithrombin III 71
Thrombinar® *see* Thrombin, Topical 843
Thrombin, Topical 843
Thrombogen® *see* Thrombin, Topical 843
Thrombostat® *see* Thrombin, Topical 843
Thypinone® Injection *see* Protirelin 747
Thyrar® *see* Thyroid 844
Thyro-Block® *see* Potassium Iodide 711
Thyroid 844
Thyroid Strong® *see* Thyroid 844
Thyrolar® *see* Liotrix 505
Thyrotropin 845
Thyrotropin Releasing Hormone *see* Protirelin 747
Thytropar® *see* Thyrotropin 845
Ticar® *see* Ticarcillin Disodium 846
Ticarcilina Disodica (Mexico) *see* Ticarcillin Disodium 846
Ticarcillin and Clavulanic Acid 845
Ticarcillin Disodium 846
TICE® BCG *see* Bacillus Calmette-Guérin (BCG) Live 93
Ticlid® *see* Ticlopidine Hydrochloride 847
Ticlopidina (Mexico) *see* Ticlopidine Hydrochloride 847
Ticlopidine Hydrochloride 847
Ticon® *see* Trimethobenzamide Hydrochloride 873
Tienam® (Mexico) *see* Imipenem/Cilastatin 451
TIG *see* Tetanus Immune Globulin, Human 826
Tigan® *see* Trimethobenzamide Hydrochloride 873
Tiject® *see* Trimethobenzamide Hydrochloride 873
Tilade® Inhalation Aerosol *see* Nedocromil Sodium 607
Tilazem® (Mexico) *see* Diltiazem 284
Timentin® *see* Ticarcillin and Clavulanic Acid 845
Timolol Maleate 847
Timolol, Maleato De (Mexico) *see* Timolol Maleate 847
Timoptic® Ophthalmic *see* Timolol Maleate 847
Timoptic-XE® Ophthalmic *see* Timolol Maleate 847
Timoptol® (Mexico) *see* Timolol Maleate 847
Timoptol® XE (Mexico) *see* Timolol Maleate 847
Tinactin® [OTC] *see* Tolnaftate 855
Tinaderm® (Mexico) *see* Tolnaftate 855
TinBen® [OTC] *see* Benzoin 104

TinCoBen® [OTC] see Benzoin ... 104
Tindal® see Acetophenazine Maleate ... 20
Tine Test see Tuberculin Purified Protein Derivative ... 882
Tinver® Lotion see Sodium Thiosulfate ... 795
Tioconazole ... 848
Tioconazol (Mexico) see Tioconazole ... 848
Tioguanine see Thioguanine ... 838
Tiopental Sodico (Mexico) see Thiopental Sodium ... 839
Tiopronin ... 849
Tioridacina (Mexico) see Thioridazine ... 840
Tiroidine® (Mexico) see Levothyroxine Sodium ... 498
Ti-Screen® [OTC] see Methoxycinnamate and Oxybenzone ... 564
Tisit® [OTC] see Pyrethrins ... 753
Titralac® [OTC] see Calcium Carbonate ... 140
Titralac® Plus Liquid [OTC] see Calcium Carbonate and Simethicone ... 141
TMP-SMZ see Trimethoprim and Sulfamethoxazole ... 874
TobraDex® see Tobramycin and Dexamethasone ... 850
Tobra® (Mexico) see Tobramycin ... 849
Tobramicina Sulfato De (Mexico) see Tobramycin ... 849
Tobramycin ... 849
Tobramycin and Dexamethasone ... 850
Tobrex® see Tobramycin ... 849
Tocainide Hydrochloride ... 851
Tocophersolan ... 852
Toesen® (Canada) see Oxytocin ... 654
Tofranil® see Imipramine ... 451
Tofranil-PM® see Imipramine ... 451
Tolazamide ... 852
Tolazoline Hydrochloride ... 852
Tolbutamida (Mexico) see Tolbutamide ... 853
Tolbutamide ... 853
Tolectin® see Tolmetin Sodium ... 854
Tolinase® see Tolazamide ... 852
Tolmetin Sodium ... 854
Tolnaftate ... 855
Tolnaftato (Mexico) see Tolnaftate ... 855
Tolu-Sed® DM [OTC] see Guaifenesin and Dextromethorphan ... 408
Tonocard® see Tocainide Hydrochloride ... 851
Topactin® (Canada) see Fluocinonide ... 373
Topicort® see Desoximetasone ... 259
Topicort®-LP see Desoximetasone ... 259
Topilene® (Canada) see Betamethasone ... 109
Topisone® (Canada) see Betamethasone ... 109
TOPO see Topotecan Hydrochloride ... 855
Topotecan Hydrochloride ... 855
Toprol XL® [Succinate] see Metoprolol ... 574
Topsyn® (Canada) see Fluocinonide ... 373
TOPV see Poliovirus Vaccine, Live, Trivalent, Oral ... 702
Toradol® see Ketorolac Tromethamine ... 484
Torecan® see Thiethylperazine Maleate ... 838
Tornalate® see Bitolterol Mesylate ... 116
Torsemide ... 856
Totacillin® see Ampicillin ... 62
Touro LA® see Guaifenesin and Pseudoephedrine ... 409
Toxoide Tetanico Myn® (Mexico) see Tetanus Toxoid, Fluid ... 828
TPGS see Tocophersolan ... 852
TPT see Topotecan Hydrochloride ... 855
Trace-4® see Trace Metals ... 857
Trace Metals ... 857
Tradol® (Mexico) see Tramadol Hydrochloride ... 857
Tramadol Hydrochloride ... 857
Trandate® see Labetalol Hydrochloride ... 486
Trandolapril ... 858
Tranexamic Acid ... 860
Transdermal-NTG® see Nitroglycerin ... 623
Transderm-Nitro® see Nitroglycerin ... 623
Transderm Scop® see Scopolamine ... 781
Trans-Planta® (Canada) see Salicylic Acid ... 777
Trans-Ver-Sal® see Salicylic Acid ... 777
Trans-Ver-Sal® (Canada) see Salicylic Acid ... 777
Tranxene® see Clorazepate Dipotassium ... 222
Tranylcypromine Sulfate ... 860
Trasylol® see Aprotinin ... 72
Travase® see Sutilains ... 816
Travel Aid® (Canada) see Dimenhydrinate ... 286
Travel Tabs® (Canada) see Dimenhydrinate ... 286
Trazil® Often y Trazil® Ungena (Mexico) see Tobramycin ... 849
Trazodone ... 861

Trecator®-SC see Ethionamide 342
Tremytoine® (Canada) see Phenytoin 688
Trendar® [OTC] see Ibuprofen............................. 447
Trental® see Pentoxifylline 675
Tretinoin.. 862
Tretinoina (Mexico) see Tretinoin 862
Trexan™ see Naltrexone Hydrochloride.................. 603
TRH see Protirelin 747
Triacetin.. 862
Triacin-C® see Triprolidine, Pseudoephedrine, and Codeine............ 879
Triadapin® (Canada) see Doxepin Hydrochloride 298
Triaken® (Mexico) see Ceftriaxone Sodium 172
Triam-A® see Triamcinolone 862
Triamcinolone 862
Triamcinolone Acetonide, Aerosol see Triamcinolone 862
Triamcinolone Acetonide Dental Paste 864
Triamcinolone Acetonide, Parenteral see Triamcinolone 862
Triamcinolone Diacetate, Oral see Triamcinolone 862
Triamcinolone Diacetate, Parenteral see Triamcinolone 862
Triamcinolone Hexacetonide see Triamcinolone 862
Triamcinolone, Oral see Triamcinolone 862
Triaminic® Allergy Tablet [OTC] see Chlorpheniramine and
    Phenylpropanolamine 190
Triaminic® Cold Tablet [OTC] see Chlorpheniramine and
    Phenylpropanolamine 190
Triaminic® Expectorant [OTC] see Guaifenesin and Phenylpropanolamine
    409
Triaminicol® Multi-Symptom Cold Syrup [OTC] see Chlorpheniramine,
    Phenylpropanolamine, and Dextromethorphan 194
Triaminic® Oral Infant Drops see Pheniramine, Phenylpropanolamine, and
    Pyrilamine 680
Triaminic® Syrup [OTC] see Chlorpheniramine and Phenylpropanolamine
    190
Triamolone® see Triamcinolone............................ 862
Triamterene 865
Triamterene and Hydrochlorothiazide 865
Triamtereno Hidroclorotiacida (Mexico) see Triamterene and
    Hydrochlorothiazide..................................... 865
Triamtereno (Mexico) see Triamterene 865
Triapin® see Butalbital Compound 133
Triavil® see Amitriptyline and Perphenazine.............. 50
Triazolam 866
Triban® see Trimethobenzamide Hydrochloride 873
Tribavirin see Ribavirin 767
Tri-Chlor® see Trichloroacetic Acid 867
Trichlormethiazide 867
Trichloroacetic Acid 867
Tri-Clear® Expectorant [OTC] see Guaifenesin and Phenylpropanolamine
    409
Tridesilon® see Desonide 259
Tridihexethyl Chloride 868
Tridil® see Nitroglycerin 623
Tridione® see Trimethadione 872
Triethanolamine Polypeptide Oleate-Condensate 868
Triethanolamine Salicylate 868
Triethylenethiophosphoramide see Thiotepa 841
Trifed® [OTC] see Triprolidine and Pseudoephedrine.. 878
Trifed-C® see Triprolidine, Pseudoephedrine, and Codeine 879
Trifluoperacina, Clorhidrato De (Mexico) see Trifluoperazine Hydrochloride
    869
Trifluoperazine Hydrochloride 869
Triflupromazine Hydrochloride 870
Trifluridine 870
Triglycerides, Medium Chain see Medium Chain Triglycerides 532
Trihexifenidico (Mexico) see Trihexyphenidyl Hydrochloride 871
Trihexy® see Trihexyphenidyl Hydrochloride............ 871
Trihexyphen® (Canada) see Trihexyphenidyl Hydrochloride 871
Trihexyphenidyl Hydrochloride 871
Tri-Hydroserpine® see Hydralazine, Hydrochlorothiazide, and Reserpine
    429
Tri-K® see Potassium Acetate, Potassium Bicarbonate, and Potassium Citrate
    706
Trikates® see Potassium Acetate, Potassium Bicarbonate, and Potassium
    Citrate 706
Tri-Kort® see Triamcinolone................................ 862
Trilafon® see Perphenazine 677
Tri-Levlen® see Ethinyl Estradiol and Levonorgestrel .. 337
Trilisate® see Choline Magnesium Salicylate............ 202

Trilog® see Triamcinolone 862
Trilone® see Triamcinolone 862
Trimazide® see Trimethobenzamide Hydrochloride 873
Trimeprazine Tartrate 871
Trimesuxol® (Mexico) see Trimethoprim and Sulfamethoxazole 874
Trimethadione 872
Trimethaphan Camsylate 873
Trimethobenzamide Hydrochloride 873
Trimethoprim 874
Trimethoprim and Polymyxin B 874
Trimethoprim and Sulfamethoxazole 874
Trimetoger® (Mexico) see Trimethoprim and Sulfamethoxazole 874
Trimetoprima (Mexico) see Trimethoprim 874
Trimetox® (Mexico) see Trimethoprim and Sulfamethoxazole 874
Trimetrexate Glucuronate 875
Trimipramine Maleate 876
Trimox® see Amoxicillin Trihydrate 58
Trimpex® see Trimethoprim 874
Trimzol® (Mexico) see Trimethoprim and Sulfamethoxazole 874
Trinalin® see Azatadine and Pseudoephedrine 89
Tri-Nefrin® Extra Strength Tablet [OTC] see Chlorpheniramine and
      Phenylpropanolamine 190
Tri-Norinyl® see Ethinyl Estradiol and Norethindrone 339
Trinovum® (Mexico) see Ethinyl Estradiol and Norethindrone 339
Triofed® [OTC] see Triprolidine and Pseudoephedrine 878
Triostat™ see Liothyronine Sodium 504
Triotann® Tablet see Chlorpheniramine, Pyrilamine, and Phenylephrine
      195
Trioxsalen 877
Tripelennamine 877
Triphasil® see Ethinyl Estradiol and Levonorgestrel 337
Tri-Phen-Chlor® see Chlorpheniramine, Phenyltoloxamine,
      Phenylpropanolamine, and Phenylephrine 194
Triphenyl® Expectorant [OTC] see Guaifenesin and Phenylpropanolamine
      409
Triphenyl® Syrup [OTC] see Chlorpheniramine and Phenylpropanolamine
      190
Triple Antibiotic® see Bacitracin, Neomycin, and Polymyxin B 94
Triposed® [OTC] see Triprolidine and Pseudoephedrine 878
Triprolidina y Pseudoefedrina (Mexico) see Triprolidine and Pseudoephedrine
      878
Triprolidine and Pseudoephedrine 878
Triprolidine, Pseudoephedrine, and Codeine 879
Triptil® (Canada) see Protriptyline Hydrochloride 748
TripTone® Caplets® [OTC] see Dimenhydrinate 286
Tris Buffer see Tromethamine 880
Tris(hydroxymethyl)aminomethane see Tromethamine 880
Trisoject® see Triamcinolone 862
Trisoralen® see Trioxsalen 877
Tri-Statin® II see Nystatin and Triamcinolone 632
Trisulfa® (Canada) see Trimethoprim and Sulfamethoxazole 874
Trisulfam® see Trimethoprim and Sulfamethoxazole 874
Trisulfapyrimidines see Sulfadiazine, Sulfamethazine, and Sulfamerazine
      808
Trisulfa-S® (Canada) see Trimethoprim and Sulfamethoxazole....... 874
Tritace® (Mexico) see Ramipril 762
Tri-Tannate® Plus see Chlorpheniramine, Ephedrine, Phenylephrine, and
      Carbetapentane 191
Tri-Tannate® Tablet see Chlorpheniramine, Pyrilamine, and Phenylephrine
      195
Tritann® Pediatric see Chlorpheniramine, Pyrilamine, and Phenylephrine
      195
Tritan® Tablet see Chlorpheniramine, Pyrilamine, and Phenylephrine 195
Tritec® see Ranitidine Bismuth Citrate............................. 763
Tri-Vi-Flor® see Vitamins, Multiple 901
Trixilem (Mexico) see Daunorubicin Hydrochloride 252
Trobicin® see Spectinomycin Hydrochloride 798
Trocal® [OTC] see Dextromethorphan 266
Troleandomycin 880
Tromethamine 880
Tromigal® (Mexico) see Erythromycin 321
Trompersantin® (Mexico) see Dipyridamole........................... 290
Tronolane® [OTC] see Pramoxine Hydrochloride 714
Tronothane® [OTC] see Pramoxine Hydrochloride 714
Tropicacyl® Ophthalmic see Tropicamide 881
Tropicamide 881
Tropyn® Z (Mexico) see Atropine Sulfate 85
Troxidone see Trimethadione 872

Truphylline® see Theophylline/Aminophylline 832
Trusopt® see Dorzolamide Hydrochloride 296
Trypsin, Balsam Peru, and Castor Oil 881
Tryptanol® (Mexico) see Amitriptyline Hydrochloride 51
Trysul® see Sulfabenzamide, Sulfacetamide, and Sulfathiazole 806
TSPA see Thiotepa 841
TST see Tuberculin Purified Protein Derivative 882
T-Stat® Topical see Erythromycin, Topical 324
Tubasal® (Canada) see Aminosalicylate Sodium 47
Tuberculin Purified Protein Derivative 882
Tuberculin Skin Test see Tuberculin Purified Protein Derivative 882
Tubersol® see Tuberculin Purified Protein Derivative 882
Tuinal® see Amobarbital and Secobarbital 55
Tums® [OTC] see Calcium Carbonate 140
Tussafed® Drops see Carbinoxamine, Pseudoephedrine, and
    Dextromethorphan 155
Tussafin® Expectorant see Hydrocodone, Pseudoephedrine, and Guaifenesin
    435
Tuss-Allergine® Modified T.D. Capsule see Caramiphen and
    Phenylpropanolamine 150
Tussar® SF Syrup see Guaifenesin, Pseudoephedrine, and Codeine 410
Tuss-DM® [OTC] see Guaifenesin and Dextromethorphan 408
Tuss-Genade® Modified Capsule see Caramiphen and Phenylpropanolamine
    150
Tussigon® see Hydrocodone and Homatropine 434
Tussionex® see Hydrocodone and Chlorpheniramine 434
Tuss-LA® see Guaifenesin and Pseudoephedrine 409
Tussogest® Extended Release Capsule see Caramiphen and
    Phenylpropanolamine 150
Tuss-Ornade® Liquid see Caramiphen and Phenylpropanolamine 150
Tuss-Ornade® Spansule® see Caramiphen and Phenylpropanolamine 150
Tusstat® see Diphenhydramine Hydrochloride 288
Twin-K® see Potassium Citrate and Potassium Gluconate 710
Two-Dyne® see Butalbital Compound 133
Tylenol® [OTC] see Acetaminophen 14
Tylenol® Cold Effervescent Medication Tablet [OTC] see Chlorpheniramine,
    Phenylpropanolamine, and Acetaminophen 194
Tylenol® With Codeine see Acetaminophen and Codeine 15
Tylex® 750 (Mexico) see Acetaminophen 14
Tylex® CD (Mexico) see Acetaminophen and Codeine 15
Tylox® see Oxycodone and Acetaminophen 646
Typhoid Vaccine 883
Typhoid Vaccine Live Oral Ty21a see Typhoid Vaccine 883
Tyzine® see Tetrahydrozoline Hydrochloride 831
UAD® Topical see Clioquinol and Hydrocortisone 216
UCB-P071 see Cetirizine Hydrochloride 179
Ukidan® (Mexico) see Urokinase 886
Ulcedine® (Mexico) see Cimetidine 207
ULR® see Guaifenesin, Phenylpropanolamine, and Phenylephrine 410
ULR-LA® see Guaifenesin and Phenylpropanolamine 409
Ulsen® (Mexico) see Omeprazole 636
Ultiva® see Remifentanil 765
Ultracaine DS® (Canada) see Articaine Hydrochloride with Epinephrine
   74
Ultracaine DS Forte® (Canada) see Articaine Hydrochloride with Epinephrine
   74
Ultracef® see Cefadroxil Monohydrate 162
Ultracef® (Mexico) see Ceftizoxime 171
Ultram® see Tramadol Hydrochloride 857
Ultra Mide® see Urea 884
Ultraquin® (Canada) see Hydroquinone 439
Ultrase® MT12 see Pancrelipase 657
Ultrase® MT20 see Pancrelipase 657
Ultrase® MT24 see Pancrelipase 657
Ultra Tears® Solution [OTC] see Artificial Tears 75
Ultravate™ see Halobetasol Propionate 416
Unamol® (Mexico) see Cisapride 209
Unasyn® see Ampicillin Sodium and Sulbactam Sodium 64
Unasyna® (Mexico) see Ampicillin Sodium and Sulbactam Sodium 64
Unasyna® Oral (Mexico) see Ampicillin Sodium and Sulbactam Sodium
   64
Undecylenic Acid and Derivatives 884
Undoguent® Topical [OTC] see Undecylenic Acid and Derivatives 884
Unicap® [OTC] see Vitamins, Multiple 901
Uni-Decon® see Chlorpheniramine, Phenyltoloxamine, Phenylpropanolamine,
    and Phenylephrine 194
Unilax® [OTC] see Docusate and Phenolphthalein 295
Unipen® see Nafcillin Sodium 599

Unipres® see Hydralazine, Hydrochlorothiazide, and Reserpine 429
Uni-Pro® [OTC] see Ibuprofen 447
Uni-Tussin® [OTC] see Guaifenesin 407
Uni-tussin® DM [OTC] see Guaifenesin and Dextromethorphan 408
Univasc® see Moexipril Hydrochloride 587
Unizuric® 300 (Mexico) see Allopurinol 33
Unna's Boot see Zinc Gelatin 908
Unna's Paste see Zinc Gelatin 908
Urabeth® see Bethanechol Chloride 112
Uracel® see Sodium Salicylate 793
Urasal® (Canada) see Methenamine 555
Urea 884
Urea and Hydrocortisone 885
Ureacin®-20 [OTC] see Urea 884
Ureacin®-40 see Urea 884
Ureaphil® see Urea 884
Urecholine® see Bethanechol Chloride 112
Uremol® (Canada) see Urea 884
Urex® see Methenamine 555
Uridon® (Canada) see Chlorthalidone 199
Urisec® (Canada) see Urea 884
Urised® see Methenamine 555
Urispas® see Flavoxate 364
Uri-Tet® see Oxytetracycline Hydrochloride 653
Uritol® (Canada) see Furosemide 391
Urobak® see Sulfamethoxazole 809
Urocit®-K see Potassium Citrate 710
Urodine® see Phenazopyridine Hydrochloride 679
Urofolitropina (Mexico) see Urofollitropin 885
Urofollitropin 885
Urogesic® see Phenazopyridine Hydrochloride 679
Urokinase 886
Uro-KP-Neutral® see Potassium Phosphate and Sodium Phosphate 713
Uroplus® DS see Trimethoprim and Sulfamethoxazole 874
Uroplus® SS see Trimethoprim and Sulfamethoxazole 874
Uroquinasa (Mexico) see Urokinase 886
Urovalidin® (Mexico) see Phenazopyridine Hydrochloride 679
Urozide® (Canada) see Hydrochlorothiazide 430
Ursodeoxycholic Acid see Ursodiol 887
Ursodiol 887
Ursofalk (Mexico) see Ursodiol 887
Urticort® see Betamethasone 109
Utimox® see Amoxicillin Trihydrate 58
Utrogestan® (Mexico) see Progesterone 731
Uvega® (Mexico) see Lidocaine and Epinephrine 499
Vadosilan® 20 (Mexico) see Isoxsuprine Hydrochloride 476
Vadosilan® (Mexico) see Isoxsuprine Hydrochloride .476
Vagilia® see Sulfabenzamide, Sulfacetamide, and Sulfathiazole 806
Vagistat® see Tioconazole 848
Vagitrol® see Sulfanilamide 810
Valacyclovir 888
Valadol® [OTC] see Acetaminophen 14
Valergen® see Estradiol 325
Valertest No.1® Injection see Estradiol and Testosterone 326
Valisone® see Betamethasone 109
Valium® see Diazepam 268
Valpin® 50 see Anisotropine Methylbromide 67
Valproic Acid and Derivatives 888
Valproico Acido (Mexico) see Valproic Acid and Derivatives 888
Valprosid® (Mexico) see Valproic Acid and Derivatives 888
Valrelease® see Diazepam 268
Valtrex® see Valacyclovir 888
Vamate® see Hydroxyzine 443
Vancenase® see Beclomethasone Dipropionate 97
Vancenase® AQ see Beclomethasone Dipropionate 97
Vanceril® see Beclomethasone Dipropionate 97
Vancocin® see Vancomycin Hydrochloride 889
Vancocin® CP (Canada) see Vancomycin Hydrochloride 889
Vancoled® see Vancomycin Hydrochloride 889
Vancomycin Hydrochloride 889
Vanex-LA® see Guaifenesin and Phenylpropanolamine 409
Vanmicina® (Mexico) see Vancomycin Hydrochloride 889
Vanoxide® [OTC] see Benzoyl Peroxide 104
Vanoxide-HC® see Benzoyl Peroxide and Hydrocortisone 105
Van R Gingibraid® see Epinephrine, Racemic and Aluminum Potassium
    Sulfate 314
Vansil™ see Oxamniquine 642
Vantin® see Cefpodoxime Proxetil 169

Vapocet® (Canada) see Hydrocodone and Acetaminophen 431
Vapo-Iso® see Isoproterenol 472
Vaponefrin® see Epinephrine, Racemic................................314
Varicella-Zoster Immune Globulin (Human).......................890
Vascor® see Bepridil Hydrochloride 108
Vaseretic® 5-12.5 see Enalapril and Hydrochlorothiazide 309
Vaseretic® 10-25 see Enalapril and Hydrochlorothiazide 309
Vasocidin® see Sodium Sulfacetamide and Prednisolone Acetate 794
VasoClear® [OTC] see Naphazoline Hydrochloride 605
Vasocon-A® [OTC] Ophthalmic see Naphazoline and Antazoline 604
Vasocon Regular® see Naphazoline Hydrochloride 605
Vasoconstrictor Interactions With Antidepressants 1108
Vasodilan® see Isoxsuprine Hydrochloride 476
Vasopressin 891
Vasosulf® Ophthalmic see Sodium Sulfacetamide and Phenylephrine ..794
Vasotec® see Enalapril 307
Vatrix-S® (Mexico) see Metronidazole 576
V-Cillin K® see Penicillin V Potassium 668
VCR see Vincristine Sulfate 896
V-Dec-M® see Guaifenesin and Pseudoephedrine 409
Veetids® see Penicillin V Potassium 668
Velban® see Vinblastine Sulfate 895
Velosef® see Cephradine...178
Velosulin® Human see Insulin Preparations 459
Velsay® (Mexico) see Naproxen 606
Veltane® see Brompheniramine Maleate 124
Velvelan® (Canada) see Urea 884
Venlafaxine 892
Venoglobulin®-I see Immune Globulin, Intravenous................454
Venoglobulin®-S see Immune Globulin, Intravenous 454
Ventolin® see Albuterol 27
VePesid® see Etoposide 348
Veracef® (Mexico) see Cephradine 178
Veraken® (Mexico) see Verapamil Hydrochloride 893
Verapamil Hydrochloride 893
Verazinc® [OTC] see Zinc Supplements 909
Vercyte® see Pipobroman 698
Verdilac® (Mexico) see Verapamil Hydrochloride 893
Verelan® see Verapamil Hydrochloride 893
Vergon® [OTC] see Meclizine Hydrochloride 530
Vermicol® (Mexico) see Mebendazole 529
Vermizine® see Piperazine Citrate 697
Vermox® see Mebendazole 529
Verr-Canth™ see Cantharidin 146
Verrex-C&M® see Podophyllin and Salicylic Acid 701
Versacaps® see Guaifenesin and Pseudoephedrine 409
Versed® see Midazolam Hydrochloride 580
Versel® (Canada) see Selenium Sulfide 785
Vertisal® (Mexico) see Metronidazole 576
Vesprin® see Triflupromazine Hydrochloride 870
Vexol® Ophthalmic Suspension see Rimexolone 772
V-Gan® see Promethazine Hydrochloride 733
Vibazine® see Buclizine Hydrochloride 125
Vibramicina® (Mexico) see Doxycycline 301
Vibramycin® see Doxycycline 301
Vibra-Tabs® see Doxycycline.......................................301
Vicks® 44D Cough & Head Congestion see Pseudoephedrine and
   Dextromethorphan 750
Vicks® 44 Non-Drowsy Cold & Cough Liqui-Caps [OTC] see
   Pseudoephedrine and Dextromethorphan 750
Vicks Children's Chloraseptic® [OTC] see Benzocaine 102
Vicks Chloraseptic® Sore Throat [OTC] see Benzocaine 102
Vicks® DayQuil® Allergy Relief 4 Hour Tablet [OTC] see Brompheniramine
   and Phenylpropanolamine 123
Vicks® DayQuil® Sinus Pressure & Congestion Relief [OTC] see Guaifenesin
   and Phenylpropanolamine 409
Vicks Formula 44® [OTC] see Dextromethorphan 266
Vicks Formula 44® Pediatric Formula [OTC] see Dextromethorphan ...266
Vicks® Sinex® Long-Acting Nasal Solution [OTC] see Oxymetazoline
   Hydrochloride..649
Vicks® Sinex® Nasal Solution [OTC] see Phenylephrine Hydrochloride ...685
Vicks Vatronol® see Ephedrine Sulfate 310
Vicodin® [5/500] see Hydrocodone and Acetaminophen 431
Vicodin® ES [7.5/750] see Hydrocodone and Acetaminophen 431
Vicon-C® [OTC] see Vitamin B Complex With Vitamin C 900
Vicon Forte® see Vitamins, Multiple 901
Vicon® Plus [OTC] see Vitamins, Multiple 901
Vidarabina (Mexico) see Vidarabine 895

Vidarabine 895
Vi-Daylin® [OTC] *see* Vitamins, Multiple 901
Vi-Daylin/F® *see* Vitamins, Multiple 901
Videx® *see* Didanosine 274
Viken® (Mexico) *see* Cefotaxime Sodium 167
Vilona® (Mexico) *see* Ribavirin 767
Vilona Pediatrica® (Mexico) *see* Ribavirin 767
Vinblastine Sulfate 895
Vincaleukoblastine *see* Vinblastine Sulfate 895
Vincasar® PFS™ Injection *see* Vincristine Sulfate 896
Vincristine Sulfate 896
Vinorelbine Tartrate 897
Vioform® [OTC] *see* Iodochlorhydroxyquin 466
Viokase® *see* Pancrelipase 657
Vira-A® *see* Vidarabine 895
Viractin® [OTC] *see* Tetracaine Hydrochloride 828
Viramune® *see* Nevirapine 614
Virazide® (Mexico) *see* Ribavirin 767
Virazole® Aerosol *see* Ribavirin 767
Virilon® *see* Methyltestosterone 570
Viroptic® *see* Trifluridine 870
Viscoat® *see* Chondroitin Sulfate-Sodium Hyaluronate 203
Visderm® (Mexico) *see* Amcinonide 43
Visine® [OTC] *see* Tetrahydrozoline Hydrochloride 831
Visine A.C.® [OTC] *see* Tetrahydrozoline Hydrochloride 831
Visken® *see* Pindolol 694
Vistacon-50® *see* Hydroxyzine 443
Vistaject-25® *see* Hydroxyzine 443
Vistaject-50® *see* Hydroxyzine 443
Vistaquel® *see* Hydroxyzine 443
Vistaril® *see* Hydroxyzine 443
Vistazine® *see* Hydroxyzine 443
Vistide® *see* Cidofovir 205
Vi-Syneral® (Mexico) *see* Vitamins, Multiple 901
Vita-C® [OTC] *see* Ascorbic Acid 76
Vitacarn® Oral *see* Levocarnitine 494
Vitamin A 898
Vitamina A (Mexico) *see* Vitamin A 898
Vitamin A and Vitamin D 899
Vitamin B$_5$ *see* Pantothenic Acid 658
Vitamin B Complex 899
Vitamin B Complex With Vitamin C 900
Vitamin B Complex With Vitamin C and Folic Acid 900
Vitamin E 900
Vitamins, Multiple 901
Vita-Plus® E Softgels® [OTC] *see* Vitamin E 900
Vitec® [OTC] *see* Vitamin E 900
Vite E® Creme [OTC] *see* Vitamin E 900
Vito Reins® (Canada) *see* Phenazopyridine Hydrochloride 679
Vivactil® *see* Protriptyline Hydrochloride 748
Viva-Drops® Solution [OTC] *see* Artificial Tears 75
Vivol® (Canada) *see* Diazepam 268
Vivotif Berna™ Oral *see* Typhoid Vaccine 883
V-Lax® [OTC] *see* Psyllium 750
VLB *see* Vinblastine Sulfate 895
VM-26 *see* Teniposide 820
Volmax® *see* Albuterol 27
Volmax® (Canada) *see* Albuterol 27
Voltaren® *see* Diclofenac 271
Vomisen® (Mexico) *see* Dimenhydrinate 286
Vontrol® *see* Diphenidol Hydrochloride 289
VöSol® HC Otic *see* Acetic Acid, Propanediol Diacetate, and Hydrocortisone
. . . . 19
Vumon Injection *see* Teniposide 820
V.V.S.® *see* Sulfabenzamide, Sulfacetamide, and Sulfathiazole . . . 806
Vytone® Topical *see* Iodoquinol and Hydrocortisone 467
VZIG *see* Varicella-Zoster Immune Globulin (Human) 890
Warfarin Sodium 903
Warfilone® (Canada) *see* Warfarin Sodium 903
4-Way® Long Acting Nasal Solution [OTC] *see* Oxymetazoline Hydrochloride
. . . . 649
Waytrax® (Mexico) *see* Ceftazidime 171
Wehamine® *see* Dimenhydrinate 286
Wellbutrin® *see* Bupropion 130
Wellbutrin® SR *see* Bupropion 130
Wellcovorin® Injection *see* Leucovorin Calcium 491
Wellcovorin® Oral *see* Leucovorin Calcium 491
Westrim® LA [OTC] *see* Phenylpropanolamine Hydrochloride 687

Whitfield's Ointment [OTC] see Benzoic Acid and Salicylic Acid 104
Whole Root Rauwolfia see Rauwolfia Serpentina 764
Wigraine® see Ergotamine...319
Wimpred® (Canada) see Prednisone...719
Winasorb® (Mexico) see Acetaminophen 14
Winstrol® see Stanozolol 799
Wolfina® see Rauwolfia Serpentina 764
Wyamycin® S see Erythromycin 321
Wycillin® see Penicillin G Procaine 667
Wydase® Injection see Hyaluronidase 427
Wygesic® see Propoxyphene and Acetaminophen 741
Wymox® see Amoxicillin Trihydrate 58
Wytensin® see Guanabenz Acetate..411
Xalatan® see Latanoprost 490
Xanax® see Alprazolam 35
Xero-Lube® [OTC] see Saliva Substitute 778
Xitocin® (Mexico) see Oxytocin 654
X-Prep® Liquid [OTC] see Senna 785
X-seb® T [OTC] see Coal Tar and Salicylic Acid 226
Xylocaina® (Mexico) see Lidocaine and Epinephrine 499
Xylocaine® (Mexico) see Lidocaine Hydrochloride............................502
Xylocaine® see Lidocaine Hydrochloride 502
Xylocaine® With Epinephrine see Lidocaine and Epinephrine 499
Xylocard® (Canada) see Lidocaine Hydrochloride 502
Xylometazoline Hydrochloride 905
Yectamicina® (Mexico) see Gentamicin Sulfate 396
Yectamid® (Mexico) see Amikacin Sulfate 44
Yellow Mercuric Oxide see Mercuric Oxide 545
Yocon® see Yohimbine Hydrochloride 905
Yodoxin® see Iodoquinol 466
Yohimbine Hydrochloride 905
Yohimex™ see Yohimbine Hydrochloride 905
Yutopar® see Ritodrine Hydrochloride 773
Zafirlukast 905
Zalcitabina (Mexico) see Zalcitabine 906
Zalcitabine 906
Zamacort® (Mexico) see Triamcinolone 862
Zanosar® see Streptozocin 803
Zantac® see Ranitidine Hydrochloride 763
Zantirel® (Mexico) see Salmeterol Xinafoate 778
Zapex® (Canada) see Oxazepam 644
Zarontin® see Ethosuximide 343
Zaroxolyn® see Metolazone 573
Zeasorb-AF® [OTC] see Tolnaftate 855
Zebeta® see Bisoprolol Fumarate 115
Zebrax® see Clidinium and Chlordiazepoxide 214
Zefazone® see Cefmetazole Sodium 165
Zephiran® [OTC] see Benzalkonium Chloride 102
Zephrex® see Guaifenesin and Pseudoephedrine 409
Zephrex LA® see Guaifenesin and Pseudoephedrine 409
Zerit® see Stavudine 800
Zestoretic® see Lisinopril and Hydrochlorothiazide 507
Zestril® see Lisinopril 506
Zetar® [OTC] see Coal Tar 225
Zetran® Injection see Diazepam 268
Ziac™ see Bisoprolol and Hydrochlorothiazide 115
Zidovudina (Mexico) see Zidovudine 907
Zidovudine 907
ZilaDent® [OTC] see Benzocaine 102
Zinacef® see Cefuroxime 173
Zinc see Trace Metals 857
Zinc Acetate see Zinc Supplements 909
Zinca-Pak® see Trace Metals 857
Zincate® see Zinc Supplements...909
Zinc Chloride 908
Zincfrin® Ophthalmic [OTC] see Phenylephrine and Zinc Sulfate 685
Zinc Gelatin 908
Zinc Gelatin Boot see Zinc Gelatin 908
Zincon® Shampoo [OTC] see Pyrithione Zinc 755
Zinc Oxide 908
Zinc Oxide, Cod Liver Oil, and Talc 909
Zinc Sulfate see Zinc Supplements 909
Zinc Supplements 909
Zinc Undecylenate see Undecylenic Acid and Derivatives 884
Zinecard® see Dexrazoxane 263
Zinnat® (Mexico) see Cefuroxime 173
Zithromax™ see Azithromycin 90
ZNP® Bar [OTC] see Pyrithione Zinc.......................................755

Zocor™ *see* Simvastatin 789
Zofran® *see* Ondansetron 637
Zoladex® Implant *see* Goserelin Acetate 404
Zoldan-A® (Mexico) *see* Danazol 249
Zolicef® *see* Cefazolin Sodium 164
Zoloft™ *see* Sertraline Hydrochloride 786
Zolpidem Tartrate 909
Zonal® (Mexico) *see* Fluconazole 367
Zone-A Forte® *see* Pramoxine and Hydrocortisone 714
Zorbenal-G® (Mexico) *see* Tetracycline 829
ZORprin® *see* Aspirin 78
Zostrix® [OTC] *see* Capsaicin 147
Zostrix®-HP [OTC] *see* Capsaicin 147
Zosyn™ *see* Piperacillin Sodium and Tazobactam Sodium .. 696
Zovirax® *see* Acyclovir 23
Z-PAKS™ *see* Azithromycin 90
Zydone® [5/500] *see* Hydrocodone and Acetaminophen ... 431
Zyloprim® *see* Allopurinol 33
Zymase® *see* Pancrelipase 657
Zymerol® (Mexico) *see* Cimetidine 207
Zyprexa® *see* Olanzapine 635
Zyrtec™ *see* Cetirizine Hydrochloride 179

NOTES

NOTES

NOTES

NOTES

"Lexi-Comp's Clinical Reference Library™ (CRL) has established the new standard for quick reference information"

Lexi-Comp's information products are available in both print and electronic (CD-ROM) media. They can be acquired as specialized individual information sources (book and CD-ROM) or as a horizontally integrated comprehensive Clinical Reference Library™ (CRL). The Clinical Reference Library™, which includes 9 integrated reference handbooks, provides quick access to 20,000 pages of practical clinical knowledge for healthcare professionals, educators, and students.

Features & Available Modules

- Stedman's Medical Dictionary
- Calculations
- Symptoms Analysis Module*
- Drug Identification Module*
- MedCoach™*
- Patient Analysis*

---

*Not included in all packages.

DRUG INFORMATION HANDBOOK 4th Edition 96/97

by Charles Lacy, PharmD; Lora L. Armstrong, BSPharm; Naomi Ingrim, PharmD; and Leonard L. Lance, BSPharm

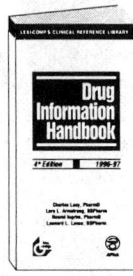

Specifically compiled and designed for the healthcare professional requiring quick access to concisely stated comprehensive data concerning clinical use of medications.

The Drug Information Handbook is an ideal portable drug information resource, containing 994 drug monographs. Each monograph typically provides the reader with up to 28 key points of data concerning clinical use and dosing of the medication. Material provided in the Appendix section is recognized by many users to be, by itself, well worth the purchase of the handbook.

PEDIATRIC DOSAGE HANDBOOK 4th Edition 97/98

by Carol K. Taketomo, PharmD; Jane Hurlburt Hodding, PharmD; and Donna M. Kraus, PharmD

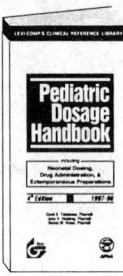

Special considerations must frequently be taken into account when dosing medications for the pediatric patient. This highly regarded quick reference handbook is a compilation of recommended pediatric doses based on current literature as well as the practical experience of the authors and their many colleagues who work every day in the pediatric clinical setting.

The Pediatric Dosage Handbook 4th Edition includes neonatal dosing, drug administration, and extemporaneous preparations for 592 medications used in pediatric medicine.

GERIATRIC DOSAGE HANDBOOK 3rd Edition 97/98

by Todd P. Semla, PharmD; Judith L. Beizer, PharmD; and Martin D. Higbee, PharmD

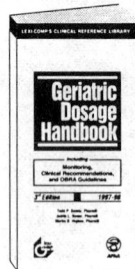

Many physiologic changes occur with aging, some of which affect the pharmacokinetics or pharmacodynamics of medications. Strong consideration should also be given to the effect of decreased renal or hepatic functions in the elderly as well as the probability of the geriatric patient being on multiple drug regimens.

Healthcare professionals working with nursing homes and assisted living facilities will find the 646 drug monographs contained in this handbook to be an invaluable source of helpful information.

DRUG INFORMATION HANDBOOK FOR THE ALLIED HEALTH PROFESSIONAL 4th Edition 97/98

by Leonard L. Lance, BSPharm; Charles Lacy, PharmD; and Morton P. Goldman, PharmD

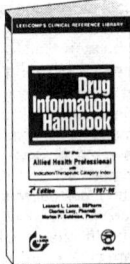

Working with clinical pharmacists, hospital pharmacy and therapeutics committees, and hospital drug information centers, the authors have assisted hundreds of hospitals in developing institution specific formulary reference documentation.

The most current basic drug and medication data from those clinical settings have been reviewed, coalesced, and cross-referenced to create this unique handbook. The handbook offers quick access to abbreviated monographs for over 1383 generic drugs.

This is a great tool for physician assistants, medical records personnel, medical transcriptionists and secretaries, pharmacy technicians, and other allied health professionals.

INFECTIOUS DISEASES HANDBOOK 2nd Edition 97/98

by Carlos M. Isada MD; Bernard L. Kasten Jr. MD; Morton P. Goldman PharmD; Larry D. Gray PhD; and Judith A. Aberg MD

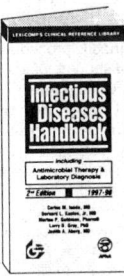

This four-in-one quick reference is concerned with the identification and treatment of infectious diseases. A unique feature of the handbook is that entries in each of the four sections of the book (164 disease syndromes, 143 organisms, 231 laboratory tests, and 222 antimicrobials) contain related information and cross-referencing to one or more of the other three sections.

The disease syndrome section provides straight-forward information on the clinical presentation, differential diagnosis, diagnostic tests, and drug therapy recommended for treatment of more common infectious diseases. The organism section presents discussion of the microbiology, epidemiology, diagnosis, and treatment of each organism. The laboratory diagnosis section describes performance of specific tests and procedures. The antimicrobial therapy section presents important facts and considerations regarding each drug product included.

POISONING & TOXICOLOGY HANDBOOK 2nd Edition 96/97

by Jerrold B. Leikin, MD and Frank P. Paloucek, PharmD

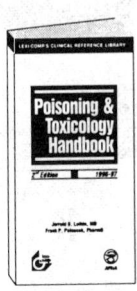

A six-in-one reference wherein each major entry contains information relative to one or more of the other sections. This handbook offers comprehensive concisely-stated monographs covering 539 medicinal agents, 210 nonmedicinal agents, 259 biological agents, 250 laboratory tests, 70 antidotes, and 180 pages of exceptionally useful appendix material.

A truly unique reference that presents signs and symptoms of acute overdose along with considerations for overdose treatment. Ideal reference for emergency situations.

ABORATORY TEST HANDBOOK - CONCISE (New!)

David S. Jacobs, MD, FACP, FCAP; Wayne R. DeMott, MD, FCAP; Harold J. Grady, PhD; becca T. Horvat, PhD; Douglas W. Huestis, MD; Bernard L. Kasten Jr., MD, FCAP

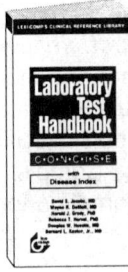

The authors of Lexi-Comp's highly regarded Laboratory Test Handbook have selected and extracted key information for presentation in this portable abridged version. It contains more than 800 test entries for quick reference and is ideal for residents, nurses, and medical students or technologists requiring information concerning patient preparation, specimen collection and handling, and test result interpretation.

LABORATORY TEST HANDBOOK 4th Edition 1996

by David S. Jacobs MD, FACP; Wayne R. DeMott, MD, FACP; Harold J. Grady, PhD; Rebecca T. Horvat, PhD; Douglas W. Huestis, MD; and Bernard L. Kasten Jr., MD, FACP

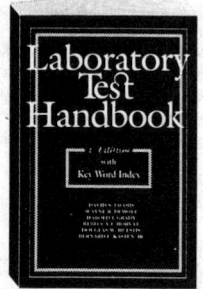

This is a single reference source that contains difficult to find general and interpretive information pertinent to the use of over 900 clinical laboratory tests.

Includes sections on Molecular Pathology and Trace Elements and each test entry in a section is complete in itself providing the user with the test name, synonyms, patient care recommendations, specimen requirements, reference ranges, methodology, footnotes, and references. Updated CPT and ICD-9 coding is also provided. This handbook delivers answers to many typical questions posed about laboratory tests. An extremely useful reference for practitioners and other healthcare professionals.

DIAGNOSTIC PROCEDURE HANDBOOK

by Joseph A. Golish, MD

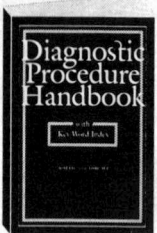

An ideal companion to the Laboratory Test Handbook this publication details 295 diagnostic procedures including: Allergy, Immunology/Rheumotology, Infectious Disease, Cardiology, Critical Care, Gastroenterology, Nephrology, Urology, Hematology, Neurology, Ophthalmology, Pulmonary Function, Pulmonary Medicine, Computed Tomography, Diagnostic Radiology, Invasive Radiology, Magnetic Resonance Imaging, Nuclear Medicine, and Ultrasound. A great reference handbook for healthcare professionals at any level of training and experience.

Enhance your practice management system!

with

Drug Information Handbook for Dentistry on CD-ROM

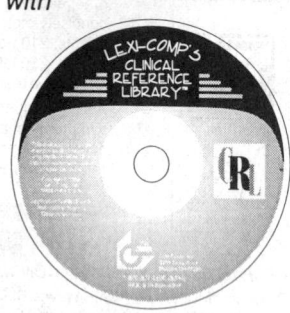

This product efficiently provides patient specific drug analysis reports which will *increase productivity* and *improve patient care* while saving you time and mone Any dental professional or administrative assistant can quickly produce a medication summary report specific t each individual patient with the help of Lexi-Comp's Support Modules included on the Drug Infomation for Dentistry CD-ROM.